Joslin's
DIABETES
MELLITUS

Editors

ALEXANDER MARBLE, M.D.

Physician, Joslin Clinic and New England Deaconess Hospital; President Emeritus, Joslin Diabetes Center; Clinical Professor of Medicine, Emeritus, Harvard Medical School

LEO P. KRALL, M.D., D. Sc. (Hon.)

Director, Education Division, Joslin Diabetes Center; Physician, Joslin Clinic and New England Deaconess Hospital; Lecturer on Medicine, Harvard Medical School; President, International Diabetes Federation

ROBERT F. BRADLEY, M.D.

President, Joslin Diabetes Center; Physician, Joslin Clinic and New England Deaconess Hospital; Physician, Brookline Hospital, Brookline, MA; Associate Clinical Professor of Medicine, Harvard Medical School; Senior Associate in Medicine, Brigham and Women's Hospital

A. RICHARD CHRISTLIEB, M.D.

Physician, Joslin Clinic and New England Deaconess Hospital; Associate in Medicine, Brigham and Women's Hospital; Associate Professor of Medicine, Harvard Medical School

J. STUART SOELDNER, M.D.

Senior Investigator, Elliott P. Joslin Research Laboratory; Associate Professor of Medicine, Brigham and Women's Hospital, Harvard Medical School; Associate Staff, New England Deaconess Hospital; Physician, Brigham and Women's Hospital

Joslin's
DIABETES MELLITUS

TWELFTH EDITION

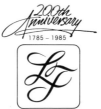

Lea & Febiger   *Philadelphia • 1985*

Lea & Febiger
600 South Washington Square
Philadelphia, PA 19106-4198
U.S.A.
(215) 922-1330

FIRST EDITION, 1916
SECOND EDITION, 1917
THIRD EDITION, 1923
FOURTH EDITION, 1928
FIFTH EDITION, 1935
SIXTH EDITION, 1937
SEVENTH EDITION, 1940
EIGHTH EDITION, 1946
NINTH EDITION, 1952
TENTH EDITION, 1959
ELEVENTH EDITION, 1971
   REPRINTED 1973
TWELFTH EDITION, 1985

Library of Congress Cataloging in Publication Data

Joslin, Elliott Proctor, 1869–1962.
  Joslin's Diabetes mellitus.

  Bibliography: p.
  Includes index.
  1. Diabetes. I. Title. II. Title: Diabetes mellitus.
[DNLM: 1. Diabetes mellitus. WK 810 J83t]
RC660.J6 1985   616.4'62   84-917
ISBN 0-8121-0763-2

PRINTED IN THE UNITED STATES OF AMERICA

Print Number: 3   2   1

Preface

The first edition of this book was written by Dr. Elliott P. Joslin and published in 1916, 5 years before the discovery of insulin. This Twelfth Edition comes more than 60 years after insulin became generally available. In these 6 decades, extraordinary advances have been made in knowledge regarding diabetes and its complications. In recent years, new developments have taken place at breathtaking speed. The most important of these is the wider acceptance by those interested in diabetes of the concept that careful control of the blood glucose provides the best insurance currently available for the prevention, amelioration, or postponement of the dread complications of angiopathy and neuropathy in their varied manifestations. This concept is eminently logical and is used in the treatment of other diseases with the aim of restoring bodily structure and function to or toward normal insofar as possible. A deterrent to greater acceptance of this principle in diabetes has been the lack of controlled, prospective, clinical studies indicating a positive relationship between the degree of metabolic control and the frequency and extent of late complications. Fortunately, enough information has become available during the past several years to convince most clinicians and investigators as to the benefits of control. Further longitudinal studies are needed, and fortunately under way, to determine the feasibility and effect of attempts to maintain excellent biochemical control over a prolonged period.

As in the past, this present edition is designed as a text book of diabetes containing to a reasonable degree currently available information regarding all phases of diabetes and its complications. With a few exceptions, the contributors are present or past members of the Joslin Diabetes Center and the New England Deaconess Hospital. An attempt has been made to maintain a logical flow of content from the opening chapter with its summary of current concepts to the final chapter with information and comments regarding everyday living with diabetes now and in the future. In the chapters devoted to treatment, procedures outlined include not only those used by authors, but also alternate methods when applicable. Duplication of material has been avoided by reference to other chapters.

For the most part, this edition represents a complete re-writing rather than a revision. New chapters include those regarding epidemiology, immunology, animal models, metabolic fuels, exercise, education, diabetes in the elderly, hypertension, and sexual disorders.

The first patient of the Joslin Clinic series was seen by Dr. Elliott P. Joslin in 1897. Today the number of patients seen exceeds 140,000, and the records of this diabetic population have often been called a "gold mine" of information regarding diabetes. Indeed, over the years much valuable information has been extracted, analyzed, and published in journals and in editions of this text. These data have been most useful in indicating the health problems confronting the diabetic patient and the effect of treatment, as well as in discovering at an early stage patient trends in mortality and causes of death. As shown in this volume, both past and present data have permitted epidemiologic studies of a longitudinal nature. It is our hope to maintain a registry of patients for whom basic information is obtained at first visit, so that at any time in the future data from any desired segment of this diabetic population may be extracted.

In the early planning stage of this edition, we had the cooperation of Drs. Kelly M. West and William B. Hadley. Each had his productive life cut short suddenly at too early an age. In his training period, Kelly was a Joslin Clinic Fellow and later became a pioneer in the field of epidemiology as applied to diabetes, leaving as a legacy his remarkable book on the subject. Bill, for more than 25 years an active member of the Joslin Clinic staff, was beloved and respected by patients and colleagues alike.

As is obvious from the number of contributors, the writing of the book has been a team effort as, indeed, must be the case in the present day for almost all treatises on science and medicine. There certainly has been no dearth of material and, in fact, one of the problems has been to keep up with rapidly advancing events, making necessary changes up until the last moment. We are deeply grateful to these contributors who, in addition to carrying on their regular work in the laboratory or clinic, have taken time, often from week-ends or vacation, to prepare chapters or sections of chapters regarding subjects in which they have had interest and personal experience. Their work has truly been a labor of love. We thank also others who have helped in the preparation of the monograph. These include the secretaries who have worked efficiently and loyally in typing, photocopying and other necessary activities. In special tribute, we express our deep gratitude to our associate, Mrs. Frances L. Wolf, who with much talent, hard work, and uncommon devotion has had such a large part in bringing this volume to completion.

We have greatly appreciated the patience, forbearance, and cooperation willingly given by Lea & Febiger, publishers of this text through 12 editions and almost 7 decades, who in 1985 celebrate their 200th anniversary.

Boston, Massachusetts

Alexander Marble
Leo P. Krall
Robert F. Bradley
A. Richard Christlieb
J. Stuart Soeldner

Contributors*

Nicolas N. Abourizk, M.D., Director, Diabetes Care Center, St. Francis Hospital and Medical Center; Assistant Professor of Medicine, University of Connecticut School of Medicine; both at Hartford, CT.

Lloyd M. Aiello, M.D., Director, William P. Beetham Eye Research and Treatment Unit, Joslin Clinic; Ophthalmologist, New England Deaconess Hospital and Massachusetts Eye and Ear Infirmary; Associate Clinical Professor of Ophthalmology, Harvard Medical School.

Thomas T. Aoki, M.D., Professor of Medicine and Chief of the Division of Endocrinology, University of California at Davis Medical Center, Davis, CA.

A. Cader Asmal, M.D., Ph.D., Physician, Joslin Clinic and New England Deaconess Hospital; Assistant Professor of Medicine, Harvard Medical School.

Donald M. Barnett, M.D., Physician, Joslin Clinic and New England Deaconess Hospital; Assistant Clinical Professor of Medicine, Harvard Medical School.

Peter Berchtold, M.D., Professor of Medicine, University of Düsseldorf, Düsseldorf, West Germany.

Michael Berger, M.D., Professor of Medicine, University of Düsseldorf, Düsseldorf, West Germany.

Murray M. Bern, M.D., Section Chief of Hematology, New England Deaconess Hospital; Assistant Professor of Medicine, Harvard Medical School.

William L. Black, M.D., Physician, Joslin Clinic and New England Deaconess Hospital; Clinical Instructor in Medicine, Harvard Medical School.

Michael J. Bradbury, M.D., Ophthalmologist, Retina Consultants and St. Vincent's Hospital; Associate in Ophthalmology, University of Massachusetts Medical School, all at Worcester, MA. Assistant in Ophthalmology, Massachusetts Eye and Ear Infirmary.

Stuart J. Brink, M.D., Clinical Instructor in Pediatrics, Harvard Medical School; Associate in Medicine, Children's Hospital Medical Center, Boston; Staff Pediatrician, New England Diabetes and Endocrinology Center, Chestnut Hill, MA.

Jose C. Briones, M.D., Staff Ophthalmologist, Glendora Community Hospital and Foot Hill Presbyterian Hospital, both in Glendora, CA, and at Queen of the Valley Hospital, West Covina, CA; Clinical Instructor of Ophthalmology, Jules Stein Eye Institute, University of California at Los Angeles.

Michael Brownlee, M.D., Assistant Professor, Laboratory of Medical Biochemistry, The Rockefeller University; Adjunct Assistant Professor of Medicine, Cornell University Medical College; Assistant Physician, The New York Hospital, New York, NY.

Edward J. Busick, Jr., M.D., Physician, Joslin Clinic and New England Deaconess Hospital; Clinical Instructor in Medicine, Harvard Medical School.

*All addresses are Boston, MA 02215 unless otherwise indicated.

CONTRIBUTORS

George F. Cahill, Jr., M.D., Director of Research, Howard Hughes Medical Institute; Professor of Medicine, Harvard Medical School; Physician, Brigham and Women's Hospital; Vice-President, Joslin Diabetes Center.

A. Richard Christlieb, M.D., Physician, Joslin Clinic and New England Deaconess Hospital; Associate in Medicine, Brigham and Women's Hospital; Associate Professor of Medicine, Harvard Medical School.

Ramachandiran Cooppan, M.B., Ch.B., F.R.C.P.(C), Physician, Joslin Clinic and New England Deaconess Hospital; Instructor in Medicine, Harvard Medical School.

Lee N. Cunningham, D.P.E., Associate Professor of Physical Education, Fitchburg State College, Fitchburg, MA; Research Associate, Elliott P. Joslin Research Laboratory.

John A. D'Elia, M.D., Director, Renal Unit, Joslin Clinic, and Chief, Renal Unit Section, New England Deaconess Hospital; Attending Physician, New England Baptist Hospital; Assistant Professor of Medicine, Harvard Medical School.

Robert E. Desautels, M.D., Urologist, New England Deaconness Hospital; Associate in Surgery, Brigham and Women's Hospital; Assistant Clinical Professor of Surgery, Harvard Medical School.

John C. Donovan, D.P.M., Staff Podiatrist, Our Lady of Lourdes Memorial Hospital and United Health Services Hospital, Binghamton, New York.

Thomas F. Drury, Ph.D., Chief, Health Status Measurement Branch, Office of Analysis and Epidemiology Program, National Center for Health Statistics, U.S. Department of Health and Human Services, Hyattsville, Maryland; Member of, and NCHS liaison to, the National Diabetes Data Group, National Institute of Arthritis, Diabetes, and Digestive and Kidney Diseases, National Institutes of Health, Bethesda, Maryland.

George S. Eisenbarth, M.D., Ph.D., Senior Investigator, Elliott P. Joslin Research Laboratory; Associate Professor of Medicine, Harvard Medical School.

Paul S. Entmacher, M.D., Vice-President and Chief Medical Director, Metropolitan Life Insurance Company, New York, New York.

Kenneth R. Falchuk, M.D., Director, Gastrointestinal Endoscopy Unit, New England Deaconess Hospital; Assistant Professor of Medicine, Harvard Medical School.

B. Dan Ferguson, M.D., Physician, Joslin Clinic and New England Deaconess Hospital; Clinical Instructor in Medicine, Harvard Medical School.

Thomas M. Flood, M.D., Medical Director, Atlanta Hospital and Regional Diabetes Center, Atlanta, Georgia.

Om P. Ganda, M.D., Physician, Joslin Clinic and New England Deaconess Hospital; Senior Investigator, Elliott P. Joslin Research Laboratory; Assistant Professor of Medicine, Brigham and Women's Hospital and Harvard Medical School.

Gisella Gaspar Garan, M.D., Physician, Joslin Clinic and New England Deaconess Hospital. Physician, Brookline Hospital, Brookline, MA.

Gary W. Gibbons, M.D., Surgeon and Co-Director of Vascular Laboratory, New England Deaconess Hospital; Assistant Clinical Professor of Surgery, Harvard Medical School.

Beverly N. Halford, R.D., M.P.H., Director, Nutrition Unit, Joslin Diabetes Center.

Sami J. Harawi, M.D., Associate Pathologist, Mallory Institute of Pathology; Assistant Professor of Pathology, Boston University Medical School.

John W. Hare, M.D., Physician, Joslin Clinic and New England Deaconess Hospital; Consultant in Medicine, Lying-in Unit, Brigham and Women's Hospital; Assistant Professor of Medicine, Harvard Medical School.

David M. Holmes, M.D., Consultant, Mental Health Unit, Joslin Diabetes Center; Chief of Clinical Psychiatry, Boston Veterans Administration Medical Center; Associate Clinical Professor of Psychiatry, Tufts University School of Medicine.

Allen P. Joslin, M.D., Physician Emeritus, Joslin Clinic; Honorary Physician, New England Deaconess Hospital.

C. Ronald Kahn, M.D., Professor of Medicine, Harvard Medical School; Director, Elliott P. Joslin Research Laboratory; Chief, Division of Diabetes and Metabolism, Brigham and Women's Hospital.

Antoine Kaldany, M.D., Physician, Joslin Clinic and New England Deaconess Hospital; Junior Associate in Medicine, Brigham and Women's Hospital; Assistant Professor of Medicine, Harvard Medical School.

George P. Kozak, M.D., Physician, Joslin Clinic and New England Deaconess Hospital; Junior Associate in Medicine, Brigham and Women's Hospital; Associate Clinical Professor of Medicine, Harvard Medical School.

Leo P. Krall, M.D., D.Sc. (Hon.), Director, Education Division, Joslin Diabetes Center; Physician, Joslin Clinic and New England Deaconess Hospital; Lecturer on Medicine, Harvard Medical School; President, International Diabetes Federation.

Stanley Kranczer, Manager, Statistical Bureau, Metropolitan Life Insurance Company, New York, New York.

Andrzej S. Królewski, M.D., Ph.D., Lecturer on Medicine, Harvard Medical School, Research Associate, Department of Epidemiology, Harvard School of Public Health and Elliott P. Joslin Research Laboratory, Joslin Diabetes Center.

Merle A. Legg, M.D., Chairman, Department of Pathology, New England Deaconess Hospital and New England Baptist Hospital; Associate Professor of Pathology at New England Deaconess Hospital, Harvard Medical School.

Joan B. Leibovich, A.C.S.W., L.I.C.S.W., Mental Health Unit, Joslin Diabetes Center.

O. Stevens Leland, Jr., M.D., Chief, Cardiology Section, New England Deaconess Hospital; Assistant Clinical Professor of Medicine, Harvard Medical School.

Simeon Locke, M.D., Chief, Neurology Section, New England Deaconess Hospital; Associate Clinical Professor of Neurology, Harvard Medical School

Paul B. Madden, M.Ed., Camp Administrator and Director; Youth Counselor; Joslin Diabetes Center.

Peter C. Maki, M.D., Staff Cardiologist, Arizona Heart Institute, St. Joseph's Hospital, and Good Samaritan Hospital, Phoenix, AZ.

Alexander Marble, M.D., Physician, Joslin Clinic and New England Deaconess Hospital; President Emeritus, Joslin Diabetes Center; Clinical Professor of Medicine, Emeritus, Harvard Medical School.

Donald G. Miller, M.D., Physician, Joslin Clinic; Assistant Director, Nutrition Support Service, New England Deaconess Hospital; Clinical Instructor in Medicine, Harvard Medical School.

John P. Mordes, M.D., Assistant Professor of Medicine, University of Massachusetts Medical School, Worcester, MA.

Stephen Podolsky, M.D., Chief, Endocrinology and Metabolism Section, Boston Veterans Administration Outpatient Clinic; Consultant in Diabetes, West Roxbury Veterans Administration Medical Center; Assistant Clinical Professor of Medicine, Harvard Medical School.

Lawrence I. Rand, M.D., Ophthalmologist, Joslin Clinic and New England Deaconess Hospital; Director of Research, William P. Beetham Eye Research and Treatment Unit, Joslin Clinic; Instructor in Ophthalmology, Harvard Medical School.

Aldo A. Rossini, M.D., Associate Professor of Medicine, Division of Metabolism, University of Massachusetts Medical School, Worcester, MA.

John L. Rowbotham, M.D., Surgeon, New England Deaconess Hospital; Senior Associate in Surgery, Brigham and Women's Hospital; Assistant Clinical Professor in Surgery, Harvard Medical School.

John G. Sebestyen, M.D., Ophthalmologist, New England Deaconess Hospital and Newton-Wellesley Hospital; Associate Surgeon, Massachusetts Eye and Ear Infirmary; Clinical Instructor in Ophthalmology, Harvard Medical School.

Robert J. Smith, M.D., Associate Investigator, Howard Hughes Medical Institute; Senior Investigator, Elliott P. Joslin Research Laboratory; Assistant Professor of Medicine, Harvard Medical School; Junior Associate in Medicine, Brigham and Women's Hospital.

John F. Sullivan, D.M.D., Staff Periodontist, New England Deaconess Hospital and New England Baptist Hospital; Clinical Instructor in Oral Medicine and Oral Pathology, Harvard School of Dental Medicine.

Daniel Tarsy, M.D., Physician, New England Deaconess Hospital; Associate Professor of Neurology, Boston University School of Medicine; Lecturer on Neurology, Harvard Medical School.

Charles Trey, M.D., Lecturer on Medicine, Harvard Medical School; Section Chief, Division of Gastroenterology, New England Deaconess Hospital; Senior Associate in Medicine, Brigham and Women's Hospital.

Louis Vignati, M.D., Physician, Joslin Clinic and New England Deaconess Hospital; Instructor in Medicine, Harvard Medical School; Junior Associate in Medicine, Brigham and Women's Hospital.

Mohammed Zafer Wafai, M.D., Ophthalmologist, King Khalid Eye Specialists' Hospital, Riyadh, Saudi Arabia.

James H. Warram, M.D., Lecturer on Epidemiology, Department on Epidemiology, Harvard School of Public Health; Consultant in Epidemiology, Elliott P. Joslin Research Laboratory, Joslin Diabetes Center.

Larry A. Weinrauch, M.D., Research Associate, Renal Unit, Joslin Clinic; Assistant in Medicine, New England Deaconess Hospital; Physician, Mount Auburn Hospital, Cambridge, MA; Clinical Instructor in Medicine, Harvard Medical School.

Jeffrey N. Weiss, M.D., Ophthalmologist and Associate Investigator, William P. Beetham Eye Research and Treatment Unit, Joslin Clinic; Surgeon, New England Deaconess Hospital; Instructor in Ophthalmology, Harvard Medical School.

Samuel M. Wentworth, M.D., Pediatrician, Hendricks County Hospital, Danville, IN, and Methodist Hospital, Indianapolis, IN.

Frank C. Wheelock, Jr., M.D., Section Chief of Vascular Surgery, New England Deaconess Hospital; Associate Clinical Professor of Surgery, Harvard Medical School.

Donna Younger, M.D., Director of Youth Division, Joslin Diabetes Center; Physician, Joslin Clinic and New England Deaconess Hospital; Consultant in Medicine, Brigham and Women's Hospital; Assistant Clinical Professor of Medicine, Harvard Medical School.

Walter S. Zawalich, Ph.D., Associate Professor, Schools of Nursing and Medicine, Yale University, New Haven, CT.

Contents

     KENNETH R. FALCHUK, CHARLES TREY, JOHN F. SULLIVAN,
     AND B. DAN FERGUSON

41. Lipoatrophic Diabetes 834
     ALDO A. ROSSINI

42. Diverse Abnormalities Associated with Diabetes 843
     STEPHEN PODOLSKY AND ALEXANDER MARBLE

43. Hypoglycemia 867
     ROBERT J. SMITH

44. Diabetes in its Psychosocial Context 882
     DAVID M. HOLMES

45. Life Cycle in Diabetes: Socioeconomic Aspects 907
     LEO P. KRALL, PAUL S. ENTMACHER, AND THOMAS F. DRURY

     Appendices 937

     Index 961

Joslin's
DIABETES
MELLITUS

1 Current Concepts of Diabetes

George F. Cahill, Jr.

HISTORICAL SURVEY

Knowledge of diabetes dates back to centuries before Christ. The Egyptian Papyrus Ebers (ca. 1500 B.C.) described an illness associated with the passage of much urine. Celsus (30 B.C. to 50 A.D.) recognized the disease but it was not until two centuries later that another Greek physician, the renowned Aretaeus of Cappadocia, gave the name diabetes (a siphon). He made the first complete clinical description, describing it as "a melting down of the flesh and limbs into urine."

In the 3rd to 6th centuries A.D., scholars in China, Japan and India wrote of a condition with polyuria in which the urine was sweet and sticky. However, although it had been known for centuries that diabetic urine tasted sweet, it remained for Willis in 1674 to add the observation "as if imbued with honey and sugar." The name diabetes mellitus (mellitus = honey) was thus established. A century after Willis, Dobson demonstrated that the sweetness was, indeed, due to sugar.

From the time of the earliest recorded history of diabetes, progress in the understanding of the disorder came slowly until the middle of the 19th century. However, over these centuries gradually the course and complications of the disease were recognized. Gangrene had been described by Avicenna, an Arab physician, in about 1000 A.D. Its hereditary tendency was described ("passed with the seed") as well as two general varieties, one with the classic acute symptoms noted above (Type I or IDDM in today's terminology) and the other with "torpor, indolence and corpulence" (Type II or NIDDM).

Within the past century an association was established with a disturbance in the beta cells, clustered as tiny islets of tissue in the exocrine pancreas. These islets were first noted in fish by Brockman early in the 19th century, but they bear the name of Langerhans who described them in mammals in 1869. Soon after, the German scientists, von Mering and Minkowski, found that surgical removal of the pancreas produced diabetes in the dog. At the turn of the century, an American, Opie, noted the beta cells in the islets to be damaged in humans dying of the disease.

The diabetes world was overwhelmed with joy in 1921 when a young surgeon, Frederick Banting, and his graduate student assistant, Charles Best, working in Toronto through the summer on an almost nonexistent budget in a laboratory loaned them temporarily by a vacationing professor, prepared active extracts of pancreas which lowered the elevated glucose levels of diabetic dogs. It is often said that their research protocol was so unsophisticated that an outright disapproval would be given today by any review group. Within months, children with diabetes who were slowly wasting away due to metabolic starvation as their flesh literally melted into sweet urine, regained strength promptly after starting treatment with insulin. Instead of death within weeks or months, life returned to almost normal, except for the need for insulin injections two or more times daily. Fortunately, there were no regulating agencies requiring years of testing in experimental animals prior to its release to the public!

ROLE OF INSULIN

Before tracing the most recent developments, further definition of diabetes and the physiologic role of insulin need to be discussed. In simplest

1

terms, insulin is the body's signal whose concentration controls both storage and mobilization of fuels. A high insulin level promotes storage in tissue, whereas a low level favors a movement of fuels back into the blood stream. Thus, after a meal, an increase in insulin release from the beta cells results in higher insulin levels in blood; this in turn signals liver, muscle, and fat to take up the extra fuel, especially glucose derived from the ingested carbohydrates. In the liver, the glucose is stored as glycogen or fat, and in muscle it is used to furnish immediate energy or stored. For example, after a carbohydrate-containing meal, the heart uses glucose as its sole fuel, provided that adequate insulin release has occurred from the beta cells.

In adipose tissue, insulin signals glucose uptake and synthesis of fat and removal from the blood of droplets of ingested and digested fat, the chylomicrons, as well as fat made in the liver and released into the blood as very low density lipoproteins (VLDL). Finally, the increase of insulin plays a role in the replenishment of muscle proteins from diet-derived amino acids.

From the above, it is obvious that a deficient release of insulin is an inadequate signal to tissues to remove various fuels, particularly glucose, from the blood. The level of blood glucose therefore rises higher and stays elevated for a longer period of time, i.e., a "diabetic" type of response or impaired glucose tolerance. This is clinically tested by giving a standard glucose load orally and determining glucose levels in the blood over several hours. A normal person has a whole blood glucose level after an overnight fast of approximately 70 to 100 mg/dl, and at 1 hour the rise is to less than 160 mg/dl and by 2 hours to less than 120 mg/dl (levels in plasma are approximately 15% higher). Values over these are suspect, except in older people in whom allowance may be made for age. This will be discussed in detail in Chapters 15 and 25.

In the fasting state the body must be supplied with fuel released from stores in liver, muscle and fat, and one of the signals for the mobilization is a low plasma insulin level. Thus after an overnight fast, the brain continues to require glucose at a rate of 100 to 150 g a day, ⅓ to ¼ of the total resting energy requirement, and this is met by glucose released from the liver into the blood stream. Other tissues, such as the heart, cease using glucose when insulin levels are too low, and instead use fatty acids released from fat stores; the signal for this release also is a low plasma insulin level. The critical factor is that the precise level of insulin plays the controlling role. Glucagon, released by the alpha cells in the islets of Langerhans, may also participate in liver glucose production; this will be discussed subsequently. Likewise, norepinephrine

released from sympathetic nerve endings in adipose tissue counters the effect of insulin and promotes the release of free fatty acids from adipose tissue.

In the normal meal-eating person, therefore, plasma insulin levels oscillate between a fed (high insulin) and fasted (low-insulin) state, requiring the beta cells to be able to release or not release insulin depending on the nutritional state and blood substrate levels, especially glucose.

Too Much or Too Little Insulin. With the above as background, situations in which there is too much or too little insulin can be described. Starting with too much insulin, the liver is signaled *not* to release glucose into the blood, and, if insulin levels are far too high, muscle and fat are signaled to remove glucose. The result is a rapidly falling glucose level which continues until the concentration is too low to provide the brain with fuel. At first there may be feelings of hunger, anxiety, and restlessness, together with sweating, tachycardia, and palpitation, as adrenalin is released as an emergency counterbalance. If the glucose falls still lower, the condition may progress to confusion and eventually unconsciousness or, very rarely, death. If the insulin production by the beta cells is minimally elevated, it may take a day or more of total starvation to unmask the slight but abnormal excess. This forms the basis for a test used frequently in the diagnosis of the rare tumors of the beta cells which produce excess insulin.

With slight deficits in insulin production, there still may be adequate insulin to control the situation in the fasted state. However, as described earlier, in the fed state, failure to increase insulin levels rapidly and sufficiently results in decreased glucose tolerance so that blood glucose levels rise higher and for a longer period of time. Thus in mild insulin deficiency, the fasting blood glucose may be normal, but tolerance be decreased, whether carbohydrate is ingested as glucose or as a part of an ordinary mixed meal. With more severe degrees of insulin deficiency, basal insulin needs may not be met, and as a result, the fasting or basal blood glucose level is elevated analogous to the inability of a warmer refrigerator to turn on a defective thermostat and activate the compressor. Fasting hyperglycemia indicates a moderate to marked insulin deficiency, and the higher the glucose, the more severe the deficit. In a person or animal with little if any insulin, the fasting glucose level rises to above the concentration at which the kidneys can retain glucose (over 180 ± mg/dl); glucose "spills" into the urine, followed by the production by the liver of more and more glucose at the expense of body protein. Thus, again, the "flesh melteth into sweet urine."

In milder or less severe insulin-deficient diabetes, glucose may appear in the urine only after meals and not in the fasted or basal state. In more severe insulin-deficient states, the few functioning beta cells, if any, release as much insulin as they can, and any excess glucose ingested elevates the blood glucose to a higher level, resulting in even greater loss of glucose in the urine, dehydration, hypovolemia, and shock.

Another significant factor is that when insulin production is low as in fasting, as glucose is produced by the liver, organic acids (ketones or ketoacids) derived from fats are also produced by the liver, even in nondiabetic persons. In markedly insulin-deficient states, these organic acids can be both overproduced and underutilized so that the problems associated with the high glucose level and its urinary ''spillage'' are compounded further by acidosis and loss in the urine, along with ketones, of body minerals such as the basic ions, sodium and potassium. The dehydration, acidosis, collapse of circulation and shock constitute diabetic ketoacidosis or coma which was almost uniformly fatal prior to the availability of insulin.

With this introduction concerning the role of insulin, and its excesses and deficiencies, it is easier to discuss the clinical problems as well as their emotional and social impacts and the various approaches to therapy and hoped-for cure.

DIABETES: A DEFINITION

What is diabetes mellitus? A single clear answer cannot be given, but a generalization is that it is a grouping of anatomic and chemical problems resulting from a number of factors in which an absolute or relative deficiency of insulin or its function usually is present. It tends to run in families; is associated with accelerated atherosclerosis, and predisposes to certain specific microvascular abnormalities including retinopathy, nephropathy and neuropathy. It doubles the risk for stroke, increases the risk for heart attacks 2- to 3-fold, and for peripheral vascular problems, particularly in the feet, 50-fold. It wipes out the relative protection that normal young females have against developing coronary artery disease as compared to their male counterparts, so that diabetic males and females are at equal risk, with the males two to three times the nondiabetic males, and the diabetic females 20 times the nondiabetic females. There are other problems, such as the lessening of resistance to infection shared by these subjects, especially if the diabetes is poorly controlled.

The clinician until recently spoke of two broad varieties of diabetes, although in reality they form a spectrum of insulin deficiency. The individual totally or almost totally lacking insulin is termed a ''juvenile-onset,'' or ''insulin-dependent'' or ''ketosis-prone'' type of diabetic, since without insulin, death may occur in ketoacidosis within a matter of days. As indicated by the term, those afflicted are usually children or adolescents and the mean age at onset of 12 to 13 years is synchronous with the adolescent growth spurt.

At the other end of the spectrum is the ''stable'' or ''maturity-onset'' or ''noninsulin-dependent'' individual in whom the diagnosis is most frequently made in the 5th or 6th decade. These persons show only a relative deficiency of insulin, and although many may need supplemental insulin by injection and therefore be insulin-requiring, ketoacidosis and death will usually not occur if exogenous insulin is withheld. In many there may even be an absolute increase in insulin levels when compared to normals, but this is usually related to their accompanying obesity and/or physical inactivity. Fajans in Ann Arbor has reported families in which the maturity-onset type of diabetes appears frequently in young people and, conversely, clinicians have long noted that typical juvenile-onset type of diabetes may occur even in quite elderly persons, so that the designations are not totally applicable. Most data do suggest, however, that the vast majority of children diagnosed as diabetic eventually depend on insulin therapy and the vast majority of adults (except those who developed the disease in childhood and have been on insulin therapy) have the milder form of insulin deficiency. This formed the basis for the terminologies as suggested by committees both in the United States and abroad of insulin-dependent diabetes mellitus (IDDM; Type I) for the juvenile-onset type and noninsulin-dependent diabetes mellitus (NIDDM: Type II) for maturity-onset type, although as noted above, some of these individuals may require insulin for appropriate control.

According to current concepts, the two broad groups can be subdivided into smaller subgroups which may or may not be variations of the two general types. In one broad group, ''IDDM'' or Type I, there is a correlation with certain inherited histocompatibility antigen types encoded on chromosome 6 and with various degrees of both serologic and cell-mediated autoimmunity. Viral inflammation at or near the time of onset has also been indicted in its pathogenesis. This type almost always ends in total insulin deficiency. The other broad group (NIDDM or Type II) does not have correlations with histocompatibility genes, viruses or autoimmunity, and usually has some remaining beta cell function, often requiring insulin but not dependent on insulin for life. See Chapters 3 and 15 for descriptions of the other categories and their subgroups.

EXTENT OF THE PROBLEM

Prevalence. The absolute numbers of diabetics in the United States can only be approximated because of the imperfect distinction between normal and diabetic, particularly in older people. Approximately 1.25 million take insulin, of whom 200,000 to 300,000 could be considered as truly having IDDM. Surveys in Michigan and Minnesota found approximately 1 in 600 children of school age to be diabetic. Of the milder variety of diabetes, approximately 1 to 1.5 million are on oral antidiabetic agents and another 2 to 3 million are on diet alone. But here again, the cut-off, as arbitrarily determined by glucose tolerance, is somewhat discretionary. An estimated 3 to 4 million more have glucose intolerance, so mild that in most it is asymptomatic and undiagnosed. Thus perhaps a total of 10,000,000 persons in the United States have the disease, but this is probably a high estimate unless the glucose intolerance of the aged be considered diabetes, in which case the number may be even higher.

The Economic Impact. This impact, however, is far greater. An estimated annual cost of $4 billion has been attributed to complications resulting directly from diabetes; treatment of a single gangrenous foot may cost over $10,000 in hospitalization alone. Of the several hundred thousand juveniles, 40 to 50% will die as a result of nephropathy, some 10 to 20% will become blind, and all will have premature atherosclerosis and shortening of life expectancy to two-thirds of that of the nondiabetic. Now that attempts at better control are being more broadly applied, one may hope that statistics in the future may reflect a much brighter outlook.

THERAPY: GENERAL COMMENTS

Returning to the historic aspects, the preparation of an active pancreatic extract (insulin) by Banting and Best in 1921 and its prompt use in the treatment of diabetes, particularly the juvenile-onset type (IDDM), were thought to have solved this problem. At least death from ketoacidosis was vastly reduced except for a few percent who were either undiagnosed or mismanaged. In 1936, the Dane, Hagedorn, by cocrystallization with protamine prepared insulins which were much longer acting, supposedly simplifying therapy by a single daily injection instead of multiple injections. However, in the 1940s and particularly in the 1950s, subjects now in their 4th and 5th decades who had been "saved" by insulin, were developing the so-called specific "complications." After 20 years of diabetes, 80% had retinopathy and of all of these subjects, one-half were destined to die of kidney failure within another 10 to 15 years. These complications had been noted infrequently prior to insulin, because in that era the juvenile-onset type diabetic usually died in ketoacidosis within two years of onset. The same complications, particularly neuropathy, were also noted in the maturity-onset type diabetic, but less frequently and usually to a less severe degree.

A serendipitous observation of a woman in Sweden who developed post-partum pituitary deficiency and experienced a reversal of the progress of the retinal complications of diabetes, led to a wave of pituitary gland removals in the 1960s. This was accomplished either by surgery or by external radiation or by more elegant procedures as freezing or insertion of radioactive materials directly into the gland, resulting in transient ameliorization of the retinopathy in many. But the morbidity of the procedure in addition to its only average slight benefit has now made it almost obsolete. Noteworthy is the fact that pituitary gland removal had little ameliorative effect on the progress of the kidney problems.

To discuss present and future therapy, the pathophysiology of the disease needs to be expanded further. When a normal person eats, signals are released from the intestinal wall which sensitize the beta cells to release more insulin into the blood as a response to a rise in glucose and amino acid concentrations. These signals, the intestinal factors, are by themselves excellent stimuli for insulin release; they have not as yet been completely characterized. Apparently they permit the body to gauge the size of the ingested load and prepare the beta cell accordingly. As a result, as the fuel (food) is digested and end-products are absorbed into the blood, the level of insulin signals the tissues to remove them at the same rate, and blood levels of fuels change relatively little. All this requires secretory accuracy on the part of the beta cells, as well as a rapid "on and off" response. As discussed previously, the average diabetic is apparently deficient in beta cell function or in the response of the tissues to insulin, and the intestinal or "gut" factors do not appear to be at fault.

INSULIN STRUCTURE AND PLASMA CONTENT

Insulin is a small protein made up in humans of 51 amino acids in two chains closely connected by molecules of sulfur (see Chapter 5). As shown by Steiner and colleagues in Chicago in 1968, it is made in the beta cells, first as a long single chain of over 80 amino acids and then the two ends are folded back on each other and are connected by sulfur bridges followed by splitting off of a segment of amino acids, the connecting or " C-peptide" fragment. The insulin molecules along with the connecting fragment are then stored in the beta cells, packed together into tiny crystalline granules. When the beta cell is stimulated, the granules are pulled to the surface and the insulin molecules are released into the blood as shown by the electron microscopic studies of Lacy in St. Louis and Orci in Geneva, Switzerland. The inactive C-peptide fragment is also released from the granule at the same time.

In the blood, insulin is carried to the various tissues where it reacts with specific "receptors" on the cell membranes, as a key fits into a lock. This in turn initiates as yet unidentified signals inside the cell which direct the cell to increase glucose transport; or various enzymatic activities to store fuel, such as protein or fat synthesis; or to initiate glucose metabolism; or many other processes. Insulin in blood is removed within minutes, in a more or less passive fashion dependent on its concentration, and thus the rate of release of insulin is the locus where the level of insulin is controlled.

So why diabetes? In the juvenile type diabetic or IDDM, if death occurs soon after development of the disease, the beta cells are found to be deficient in number and to be lacking in insulin and also to be surrounded in most cases by lymphocytic inflammatory cells. If death occurs years later, few, if any, beta cells can be found, and should there be any, they are grossly disarranged. In the maturity-onset type diabetic or NIDDM, the beta cells may be decreased in number and there may be some abnormalities of aging such as fibrosis or amyloid deposition, but often the cells may look relatively normal.

The second major advance in diabetes research and management, one almost as significant as that of Banting and Best, took place in 1959 when two workers at the Bronx Veterans Administration Hospital, the late Solomon Berson and his colleague, Rosalyn Yalow, developed an immunoassay technique for measuring the level of insulin in biologic fluids, using antibodies to insulin produced in a guinea pig injected with beef insulin. Dr. Yalow subsequently received the Nobel Prize for this and related contributions. The amino acid composition of insulin differs among animal species, and this difference (in addition to trace amounts of slightly altered insulin) is capable of initiating an immune response in an animal receiving insulin parenterally from another species. At times this difference may be a problem in humans, in which case insulin that is closer in chemical composition to human insulin must be used. Pork insulin, for example, differs from human insulin by a single amino acid in contrast to beef, which differs by four amino acids.

As shown by immunoassay, when insulin is pro-

duced in a normal person, fasting levels of 10 to 15 millionths of a unit per milliliter of serum are found (1 part in 1 billion parts water), and after a meal, these levels increase 5- to 10-fold. In the untreated juvenile diabetic, little or no insulin is found. Surprisingly, in the maturity-onset type, normal or even increased levels of insulin may be uncovered. This was originally a perplexing observation but is now explained, at least in part, by overnutrition, obesity, and inactivity—factors which create insulin resistance, thereby decreasing the capacity of insulin to be effective metabolically (see Chapter 3).

OBESITY

Kipnis and colleagues in St. Louis as well as Karam, Grodsky, and Forsham in San Francisco have shown that obese nondiabetics have two to three times higher insulin levels than normals, whereas fat diabetics have lower levels than fat nondiabetics (but frequently still higher than normals) signifying a relative insulin deficiency in the fat diabetic. Thus obesity, overnutrition, and inactivity cause a need for higher insulin levels to control metabolism. This explained the earlier paradoxical finding of normal or even increased levels of insulin in the maturity-onset diabetics by Yalow and Berson, since many of their subjects were obese. So, in summary, diabetes is due to an absolute or relative deficiency in insulin in almost all cases except for exquisitely rare situations where there may be truly an independent inability for insulin to work on tissues.

Excesses of certain other hormones have also been noted, such as glucagon, a hormone secreted by the alpha cells of the islets of Langerhans, and growth hormone, secreted by the pituitary gland. Unger of Dallas, Texas, has shown that for any given level of blood glucose, the diabetic has a higher glucagon level. Similar data have been shown for the growth hormone. However, the closer the diabetic state approaches normal by insulin injection, the closer to normal the levels of glucagon and growth hormone become, so a primary defect in these is not likely.

COMPLICATIONS OF DIABETES

Why are the beta cells deficient? Furthermore, does this deficiency lead directly to the complications and, finally, how can this progression be interrupted or reversed? And what research efforts are being made in these directions?

Macroangiopathy. The accelerated atherosclerosis in the diabetic is as complex, or even more so, than in the nondiabetic population. Its particular predilection for the vessels of the lower extremities, leading to vascular insufficiency, and in many to gangrene and amputation, is particularly note-worthy. Several explanations are given. The tendency of the diabetic to mishandle fuels, particularly fat, leads to higher circulating lipid levels, especially of low density lipoproteins (LDL) which may become incorporated into blood vessel walls. Another possibility is the ubiquitous alteration in the smallest blood vessels, the microangiopathy, which may lead to increased blood vessel wall leakage of proteins and fats and thereby to more severe atherosclerosis. The third, and currently the most interesting, is that the diabetic has a diffuse cellular abnormality leading to early senescence of certain cells, and this premature aging particularly hits the blood vessel cells and subsequently damages blood vessel walls. Other atherogenic factors include an increasing tendency of platelets to aggregate and decreased levels of high density lipoproteins (HDL) which are thought to be protective against atherosclerosis. The University Group Diabetes Program has indicated that minor alterations in the levels of blood glucose in diabetes by means of insulin or an oral antidiabetic agent, do not effectively alter the progress of atherosclerosis. However, carefully performed prospective studies to test the effect of meticulous glycemic control have not been carried out for sufficiently long periods. The current interest in attempts to maintain euglycemia as closely as possible (short of hypoglycemia) by means of multiple injections of insulin daily or the use of insulin "pumps" combined with self-monitoring of the blood glucose, are important though difficult steps in the right direction.

Microangiopathy. Retinopathy and nephropathy, the special scourges of the juvenile-onset diabetic, appear to be altered by reduction in glucose levels. Once insulin became available, certain physicians, particularly the late Elliott P. Joslin, urged the juvenile diabetic to balance food and insulin as precisely as possible by weighing food, testing the urine for glucose 4 times daily, and maintaining a strict insulin/meal/exercise/sleep schedule. Over the years, Joslin's colleagues continued this philosophy, whereas many others pointed out that even subjects attempting this rigid lifestyle became blind and died in renal failure, including many Joslin patients. Thus a "free" school developed on one hand and a "tight control" school on the other. Statistics, although relatively soft since they were collected retrospectively, suggested that the "tight control" subjects developed these microvascular complications less severely and at a later time. However, there was much overlap and many felt it better to enjoy a less restricting lifestyle since, as they reasoned, the complications would occur anyway. The problem, of course, is that it is almost impossible with injected insulin to mimic

the exquisitely accurate on-off feedback system that so closely regulates glucose concentration in the normal. The analogy can again be made to a refrigerator in which, instead of being regulated normally by a thermostat, the cooling unit is timed to run an arbitrarily selected 15 or 20 minutes each hour independent of whether the machine is too hot or too cold, resulting obviously in wild swings in one direction or the other.

The late pathologist, Kimmelstiel, discovered many decades ago that the blood vessel wall or basement membrane of the diabetic was thicker than that of the nondiabetic. In the past decade, Siperstein and Williamson independently have shown the increased thickness of the basement membrane to be ubiquitous throughout the body in the diabetic. Thus, electron microscopic examination of a piece of muscle of a diabetic, as from the thigh, shows a doubling in the anatomic thickness of capillary basement membranes. According to Williamson, the abnormal thickness is correlated with the duration and probably the severity of the diabetes. Workers in Aarhus, Denmark, have shown that within 2 to 3 years of developing diabetes, the capillaries in kidney glomeruli already show abnormalities. Later, these changes progress further to cause increased permeability and destruction of the glomeruli. In the eye, the thickened membrane also becomes more permeable and weaker, leading to the formation of capillary microaneurysms. Fragile capillaries rupture with release of blood into the retina. Cogan and Kuwabara, originally at the Howe Institute at the Massachusetts Eye and Ear Infirmary, noted that early in diabetic retinopathy, certain cells, the pericytes or mural cells, surrounding the capillaries, appeared to die prematurely supporting the early cell senescence hypothesis in diabetes.

The real argument is whether these small blood vessel lesions, which are anathema primarily to the juvenile diabetic, but also affect a large share of the maturity-onset group, are an independent expression of the hereditary disease process or are secondary to the abnormal metabolism resulting from the absolute or relative insulin deficiency. The importance of the question cannot be overemphasized, since in the first case, attempts to mimic the normal physiology with precise insulin injection and food ingestion would be a waste of time, and, in the second, it should be the basis of therapy. Anecdotally, as mentioned before, patients with closer control do appear to do better, but if one takes a random blood glucose determination of the average "well-controlled" diabetic, it is usually still almost double that of the normal. If one tries to achieve even better control, episodes of too much insulin may occur and hypoglycemic "reactions" then become not only distressing, but also potentially dangerous.

Engerman and Bloodworth in Madison, Wisconsin, and Mauer in Minneapolis, as well as others, working with animals with experimental diabetes, have shown clearly that accurate correction of the blood glucose elevation in dogs and rats tends to normalize the problems in the eye and kidney. In Paris, Tchobroutsky and his colleagues took two comparable groups of patients and in a prospective study showed that an intense effort to regulate glucose levels in one group by daily multiple injections and numerous testings of blood glucose levels did diminish the progress of the retinopathy as compared to the group treated by more conventional methods. Thus the almost religious teachings of Joslin, now over 60 years old, are being corroborated today by studies in humans and animals. Pirart of Brussels has also reported on results in an extensive series of patients again showing a beneficial effect of control.

In parallel to anatomic studies, Beisswenger and Spiro have isolated the blood vessel wall from normal and diabetic kidneys and have shown that the diabetic basement membrane differs in composition due to slight changes in amino acids and their attached sugar molecules. In rats, the enzymatic machinery attaching these sugars to basement membrane is increased when the rats are made diabetic, and it is corrected with insulin therapy. Although their work is extremely complicated, and some controversy exists, it strongly suggests that "tight control" when achievable, is warranted on biochemical as well as clinical evidence.

If the retinopathy, nephropathy and, probably, neuropathy result from insulin deficiency and hyperglycemia, three routes are available for correction of the lesion, and all are being actively pursued at the moment: pancreatic transplantation, a mechanical "pancreas" which determines glucose concentration and injects insulin accordingly and finally, prevention or possibly reversal of the initial process by immunologic mechanisms. Winegrad in Philadelphia and Gabbay and co-workers at the Children's Medical Center in Boston are studying the biochemistry of tissues as affected by high glucose levels and closely related products resulting from the elevated glucose to see if the processes can be inhibited by drugs or other agents at the tissue level. So far, using experimental neuropathy in diabetic rats as a model, alteration of the defect with these materials has been successful. As a result, clinical trials are being initiated.

Glycosylation: An Index of Control. For over a decade, a unique type of hemoglobin has been characterized, namely hemoglobin A_{1c}. About 5% of the hemoglobin in the red cells of a normal individual is of this special variety. In diabetics it may be 2 to 4 times higher, and the difference has been shown to be due to a glucose molecule chemically bound to hemoglobin. The higher the glucose concentration, the more hemoglobin A_{1c} is formed in the red cell. This results in a small but relatively insignificant alteration in the red cell's ability to carry oxygen to tissues. But the important point is that if hemoglobin becomes connected to glucose because there is too high a glucose concentration, what about other proteins? Perhaps this is why animals go to such physiologic extremes to keep glucose concentrations below certain critical levels. Could this be the reason why membranes such as those in small vessels in the eye and kidney get into trouble? This is currently under intense investigation in a number of laboratories and is a most exciting area for research since preliminary evidence suggests that this is the case. Glycosylation of a large number of proteins is now being demonstrated, including serum albumin, myelin, red cell membrane proteins and many others.

A recent major development in the treatment of one specific complication of diabetes, retinopathy, has been the use of photocoagulation. As mentioned earlier, the capillaries develop microaneurysms which burst, bleed, and then new blood vessels and scarring follow. Using either intense light or laser beams, the lesions can literally be coagulated to prevent their bursting or their further growth and scarring. In addition, if multiple small coagulation spots are scattered about, even in unaffected tissues, there appears to be a quieting down of the abnormal process elsewhere in the eye. The long term results of this procedure have been evaluated by a large scale multi-center study supported by the National Eye Institute, and its beneficial effects have been clearly established.

INSULIN-DEPENDENT DIABETES

The second approach is to the beta cell itself. Why does it fail in the juvenile diabetic and in a few years become almost totally nonfunctional insofar as insulin production is concerned? Why in the maturity-onset diabetic is its function impaired and unable to keep up with body needs, particularly if there is obesity?

Returning to the IDDM or juvenile diabetic, it has been known for years that the signs and symptoms of diabetes usually develop rapidly, within days to weeks. Typically, the child becomes listless, inattentive in school, thirsty (polydipsia), urinates frequently (polyuria), is hungry (polyphagia) yet loses weight, becomes weak and, unless diagnosed and treated, may die in ketoacidosis. If treated with insulin, there may be a "remission" lasting weeks or months during which little injected insulin or none at all is needed. This is followed by a type of diabetes not dissimilar to that in the maturity-onset patient, with a single injection of insulin daily frequently causing near normal or normal blood glucose levels. This "honeymoon" phase, as termed by Priscilla White, may last for a few weeks to a few years, and then the diabetes of the child, usually now about 14 to 18 years old, becomes labile or "brittle." Usually two daily insulin injections are then needed, and glucose levels are either too high with much glucose spilling in the urine, or too low with frequent insulin reactions, sometimes so severe as to cause unconsciousness.

Rubenstein and Steiner in Chicago have developed an immunoassay, using the Berson and Yalow principle, to measure C-peptide. This C-peptide is the connecting fragment that is stored with insulin in the beta cell and is released as insulin is released. Measuring insulin itself is of no value, since the subjects are injecting themselves with commercially prepared pork or beef insulin (free of C-peptide) which the immunoassay for insulin cannot distinguish from human insulin. By measuring the C-peptide, they have found that during the brief remission and "honeymoon" phase, endogenous insulin is still being produced. In other words, the juvenile diabetic still has some functioning beta cells during this phase of the disease, and this is probably why the diabetes is relatively easy to control during this period.

The Beta Cell. What about the life history of the beta cell itself? Nature could not have put it in a worse place for the researcher, unless perhaps, in the center of the brain! Being buried in the pancreas, the surgeon is loath to take a snip, let alone touch the pancreas. Besides, the gland is located deep in the posterior part of the abdomen, a place inaccessible for sampling except by major surgery. So we know little about the life history of the human beta cell except for one most important review by the Belgian pathologist, Gepts, who studied material from 22 autopsies of juvenile diabetics dying soon after developing the disease. In two-thirds, round inflammatory cells of lymphocyte type were found about the beta cells, associated with beta cell necrosis. But what about the beta cells even in the normal human? Nondiabetic fat people have more beta cells to meet the increased insulin levels needed by obesity. So beta cells can divide in experimental animals and humans (as first conclusively shown by the pathologist Arthur Like using electronmicroscopy).

Workers in Toronto, Geneva, Sweden (both Uppsala and Umea) and Boston have shown the beta cell to have poor replicating potential. To clarify this point, we must remind ourselves that the capacity of cells in the adult to divide is highly variable. By the time we finish childhood we have all the brain cells and muscle cells (particularly heart) that we will ever have—a depressing fact! Blood cells, skin cells and cells lining the gut are always dying and being replaced by new ones. Other cells, for example, liver, can divide if more cells are needed, as after removal of a part of the liver or after hepatitis. What about the beta cell? It can divide, but only with much stimulation, and as Logothetopoulous in Toronto and Chick in Boston have shown, only one or perhaps two divisions can occur. Thus again, could diabetes simply be due to too early senescence of certain cells and perhaps the beta cells are the first important ones to go? Does obesity cause a person to use up a limited life-long supply of beta cells or beta cell function?

This is highly plausible, particularly in the maturity-onset type diabetic, especially when we know that aging itself results in deficient beta cell function in the population at large. As mentioned before, most nonagenarians have a diabetic type glucose tolerance test as compared to subjects in early or mid-life. Goldstein in Hamilton, Ontario, in collaboration with Littlefield at Johns Hopkins and Soeldner of Boston have shown that skin fibroblasts, if taken from older diabetics and grown in tissue culture, age more rapidly than similar cells that are taken from nondiabetics and maintained identically in tissue culture. So the concept that there is an hereditary defect in cellular replication, and that the beta cells in the maturity-onset diabetic are involved in this premature aging, is most provocative.

How can one then explain the relatively sudden demise of the beta cells in the juvenile diabetic? For years anecdotal reports of diabetes following mumps, measles, or even colds, have been sporadically published. Thus a virus etiology was frequently suggested. In the mid 1960s, Gamble and Taylor collected data on newly diagnosed juvenile diabetics in England and found clusters of new cases appearing in relation to clusters of Coxsackie B virus endemics, strongly suggesting that this virus was playing an etiologic role. Similar clusters of diabetics were noted in the United States in Erie County, New York and St. Petersburg, Florida. John Craighead, a virologist and pathologist in Burlington, Vermont, at the same time had shown that a strain of encephalomyocarditis virus could cause acute diabetes in mice and even in certain subhuman primates, so no longer were the correlations between virus and juvenile diabetes in humans considered anecdotal. Another fact has appeared within the past few years: juvenile type diabetes appears more frequently in families in which there is thyroid or adrenal failure and also in which auto-antibodies against thyroid and adrenal tissues can be detected. Most recently, newly diagnosed juvenile diabetics have been found to have in their blood antibodies against human pancreas tissue as well as to contain lymphocytes which can attack beta cell components specifically; that is, they also possess cell-mediated autoimmunity.

Recent data independently collected by Irvine and Bottazzo in the United Kingdom and by Eisenbarth using Joslin Clinic material have shown that the islet-cell antibodies may precede the development of the diabetes by months or even years and this may be associated with progressive deterioration of glucose tolerance. Thus the classic "explosive" onset might merely reflect the demise of the remaining beta cells.

So today one hypothesis is that a virus may initiate damage to the beta cells in a juvenile diabetic and this may lead to some sort of destructive process which eventually causes death to all or nearly all the beta cells. Of most importance, further knowledge of this chain of events may provide clues as to how the process can be interrupted. If certain viruses can be associated with juvenile diabetes, prior immunization against the virus could be attempted. But, to be considered is the relative rarity of juvenile type diabetes with its incidence of 1:10,000 to 1:15,000 children annually. This represents only 2 to 4 new juvenile diabetics per year in a city of 100,000 people, so even if a specific virus be characterized, the cost-benefit of immunization may present a major problem. On the other hand, if one considers the life-long cost of treatment of the cumulative number of IDDM patients, such could be justified.

In studies in Erie County, New York, Sultz has found juvenile diabetes to be correlated with mumps occurring a year or more earlier than the onset of diabetes, suggesting that the mumps virus may reside for a long time as a "slow" virus in the beta cells and eventually cause their demise. The possible role of mumps vaccination in altering the incidence of juvenile diabetes is currently under study.

To compound the problem further, another paradox has distinguished diabetes from most other metabolic diseases, namely, its hereditability. The familial nature of the disease has been previously emphasized. The best tool of the geneticists, that of identical versus fraternal twins brought up in a similar environment, has been used in studying diabetes. Gottlieb and Root and subsequently Tattersall and Pyke, noted that in almost all NIDDM or maturity-onset type sets of identical twins, *both* had diabetes. The paradox is that in less than half

of IDDM or juvenile diabetics, the identical twin has the disease. Tattersall and Pyke noted that in the latter group, if the second of the twins did not develop diabetes within 2 to 3 years of the first, rarely did the disease develop at all. This suggests that heredity is more important in maturity-onset disease (could it again be an early β-cell senescence?), while environment (? virus) appears to be important in the juvenile-onset type. Nevertheless, in each there is a significant contribution of the other: environment in NIDDM and heredity in IDDM.

Three studies, those of Singhal in Canada, Cudworth in the United Kingdom, and Nerup in Copenhagen, have provided another breakthrough in our knowledge of juvenile diabetes. The surfaces of body cells contain specific factors, which distinguish each person from each other (unless the other is an identical twin). These inherited tissue antigens provide major problems in organ transplantation, but can be characterized by "tissue typing," analogous to typing of red blood cell antigens before transfusion. The three groups of workers noted that certain tissue transplant antigens, particularly HLA B8 and B15, and DW3 and DW4, were more prevalent in juvenile diabetics than in the general population. Maturity-onset type diabetics tested for these factors were indistinguishable from the general population. These and other transplant antigens can be correlated with certain other diseases involved in cellular immunity (allergies, multiple sclerosis, ankylosing spondylitis, etc.). Perhaps the specific surface properties on the beta cell make it more susceptible to virus invasion or else permit an autoimmune destructive process, genetically predetermined and linked to the HLA genes above, to be initiated once the virus has started things. The inflammatory cell invasion noted in human juvenile diabetics as described by Gepts would be in keeping with these thoughts.

Current research efforts in Boston, St. Louis, Minneapolis, London, etc. are heavily directed to clarifying the interrelationships between the viruses, beta cell involvement, the autoimmune process, beta cell replication and the tissue transplant antigens, with the hope that prevention or intervention could be feasible. Immunologic intervention has been successful in reversing diabetes in one animal model, the BB rat, and very early trials in man are being initiated.

On the other side, much research is involved in how insulin works on peripheral tissues. If the effect of insulin on cells could be amplified, the relative insulin deficiency of the maturity-onset type of diabetic (NIDDM) could be corrected. Thus, how insulin works on cells, particularly the initial reaction with the cell membrane, is under intense investigation, especially at the National Institutes of Health in Bethesda, Maryland, by Roth and colleagues. The other approach is to try to get more insulin out of the beta cells in the maturity-onset diabetic, and to this purpose, the oral hypoglycemic agents were developed and have been employed extensively although their use remains somewhat controversial. The effectiveness and safety of the sulfonylureas have been questioned by workers in the University Group Diabetes Program. On the other hand, many clinicians regard them as safe and, in carefully selected patients, effective for at least a few to several years. Another problem, of course, is why fat people need more insulin. This returns to the approach of trying to amplify the action of insulin.

Pancreas Transplants. If the complications of the person with insulin-dependent diabetes result from inability of conventional insulin treatment to bring about normalization of glucose and other fuels, therapy should logically be directed to a more physiologic insulin delivery system. As of Dec. 31, 1983, 397 transplantations of total or partial pancreas in diabetics had been done since 1966 (personal communication from Dr. D.E.W. Sutherland). Several grafts have functioned for over 2 years and a few, as long as 41–70 months. However, there are multiple problems. First, since the pancreas produces digestive juices, these must be drained somewhere or else the ducts must be occluded. This has been accomplished by a variety of methods but at the University of Minnesota, where most transplants have been done, the procedure currently being used is that of segmental grafts from living donors with occlusion of acinar ducts by synthetic polymers or other agents. Secondly, the operation has been mainly limited to subjects requiring immunosuppression therapy for a kidney transplant needed for already established kidney failure resulting from the long-standing diabetes. And, thirdly, fresh pancreases need to be found, either from patients who have just died or by use of a pancreatic segment from a living donor, preferably a close relative. The logistics pose a tremendous problem. For a more extensive discussion of pancreas transplantation, see Chapter 20.

Some workers including Najarian in Minneapolis, are trying to use injected human islet cell tissue in humans, following the experimental animal work of Lazarow, Lacy, Chick, Seltzer and others who have corrected diabetes in rats and mice with injections of large amounts of islet tissue or of beta cells grown in tissue culture. These animals, however, are pure inbred strains, and thus immunorejection is not a problem. Recently, Lacy has shown that islets can be accepted by nonrelated

mouse strains and even between rats and mice if resident lymphocytes are removed by one of several procedures. Equally as promising is the potential to rescue, possibly by immune intervention, the patient's own beta cells during the early stages of the disease, while there are still some present.

Newer Methods of Insulin Delivery. The other approach to a better insulin delivery system is the mechanical route. Now that cardiac pacemakers are a standard part of life, is an artificial beta cell possible? Albisser and colleagues in Toronto have connected a glucose analyzer to a catheter placed in a vein, and the analyzer to a computer regulating insulin injection back into the subject, a "closed loop" automatic device. This machine can control glucose levels even better than those achieved in a nondiabetic individual but, unfortunately, it requires continuous blood sampling from an indwelling catheter and the apparatus weighs 100 pounds. The problem in miniaturization is the capacity to detect glucose and only glucose. Soeldner in Boston and Bessman in Los Angeles have been trying to develop electrodes which can be implanted and which will either generate an electric current or can alter an electric current proportional to glucose concentration. Some of these experimental models have worked for several months in experimental animals, but the success has been limited and variable and much more bioengineering needs to be done. The project is, however, feasible and may reach practical development before the techniques for rejuvenating beta cells. Until closed-loop systems with feedback control become available, many are trying open loop continuous insulin delivery systems with "insulin pumps" to optimize control, with much success. Simply increasing glucose control by using home glucose monitoring and a heightened awareness by the patient of the entire problem has been shown by some studies to work as well as the insulin pump.

DIABETES RESEARCH AND EDUCATION

Finally, there is no question but that a disease which affects perhaps 10,000,000 Americans, which is the leading cause of new blindness, which kills annually several hundred thousands due to its effects on small blood vessels and its marked acceleration of atherosclerosis, formerly received only minimal publicity and emotional and financial support. In the early 1970s, less than $8 million of the National Institutes of Health (NIH) budget of $1.5 billion was directed to diabetes. Because of this, Congress passed Public Law 93-354, the National Diabetes Research and Education Act. This law set up a Commission which first met on March 10, 1975 and 9 months later reported to Congress its findings, urging that more support be given to diabetes research as well as provision for better education to the professionals and para-professionals who in turn educate the patients. This presumes that better glucose control by conventional means does decrease the specific complications, at least until investigators can develop biologic or mechanical systems that return the glucose control back to normal. In the late 1970s, over 100 million federal dollars were spent annually in diabetes research, not only for basic investigation dealing directly with the disease and its complications, but also for research into methods for teaching patients, for delivery of care to remote populations, and for many other efforts to improve the life of the diabetic in general. The National Institutes of Health, as part of their expanded diabetes program, initially set up 11 diabetes centers at major university-hospital medical centers, and these have markedly furthered diabetes research and education.

In summary, much has happened in the past decade since the last edition of this monograph appeared, and this update attempts to bring these new developments into a readable perspective. The rapid strides in knowledge and treatment that have taken place in recent years presage well for the future of the diabetic.

REFERENCES

In the foregoing summary of "Current Concepts," no attempt is made to document each item. However, the publications listed below furnish guides to further reading. In addition, articles in the journals DIABETES, DIABETOLOGIA, and DIABETES CARE as well as in many other publications attest to the continuing and extraordinary worldwide interest in diabetes and constitute "required reading" for anyone working in the field.

1. Allen, F.M., Stillman, E., Fitz, R.: Total Dietary Regulation in the Treatment of Diabetes. New York, Rockefeller Institute for Medical Research. Monograph No. 11, 1919, pp. 1–78.
2. Binder, C., Lauritzen, T., Faber, O., Pramming, S.: Insulin pharmacokinetics. Diabetes Care 7:188, 1984.
3. Bratusch-Marrain, P.R.: Insulin-counteracting hormones: their impact on glucose metabolism. Diabetologia 24:74, 1983.
4. Cahill, G.F., Jr., Etzwiler, D.D., Freinkel, N.: "Control" and diabetes. N. Engl. J. Med. 294:1004, 1976.
5. Cahill, G.F., Jr., McDevitt, H.O.: Insulin-dependent diabetes mellitus: the initial lesion. N. Engl. J. Med. 304:1454, 1981.
6. Craighead, J.E.: Current views on the etiology of insulin-dependent diabetes mellitus. N. Engl. J. Med. 299:1439, 1978.
7. Cryer, P.E., Gerich, J.E.: Relevance of glucose counter-regulatory systems to patients with diabetes: critical roles of glucagon and epinephrine. Diabetes Care 6:95, 1983.
8. Doniach, D., Bottazzo, G.F., Cudworth, A.G.: Etiology of Type I diabetes mellitus: heterogeneity and immunological events leading to clinical onset. Ann. Rev. Med. 34:13, 1983.
9. Ellenberg, M., Rifkin, H. (Eds.): Diabetes Mellitus. Theory and Practice. 3rd Ed. New Hyde Park, New York, Medical Examination Publishing Co., 1982.
10. Foster, D.W.: Diabetes mellitus. In: J.B. Stanbury, J.B. Wyngaarden, D.S. Fredrickson, et al. (Eds.): The Metabolic Basis of Inherited Disease, 5th Ed. New York, McGraw-Hill Book Co., 1983, pp. 99–117.
11. Gepts, W., LeCompte, P.M.: The pancreatic islets in diabetes. Am. J. Med. 70:105, 1981.
12. National Diabetes Data Group: Classification and diagnosis of diabetes mellitus and other categories of glucose intolerance. Diabetes 28:1039, 1979.
13. Orci, L.: Macro- and microdomains in the endocrine pancreas. Diabetes 31:538, 1982.
14. Skyler, J.S., Cahill, G.F., Jr.: Symposium on diabetes mellitus. Parts I–III. Am. J. Med. 70:101–214; 325–378; 579–630, 1981.

2 Epidemiology of Diabetes Mellitus

Andrzej S. Królewski and James H. Warram

INTRODUCTION

"Epidemiology is the study of the distribution and determinants of disease frequency in man."[1] While its predominant purpose is the understanding of disease etiology and the identification of preventive measures, knowledge of the distribution of disease is also useful in planning health services, and epidemiologic methods provide the most powerful tools available for evaluating the functioning of those services.

In the application of epidemiologic methods to diabetes, we can distinguish the following steps:

1. Determination of the frequency of diabetes and comparisons of its frequency in different populations or in different segments of the same population (*descriptive epidemiology*). The pattern of differences within and among populations is referred to as the distribution of diabetes.

2. Formulation of causal hypotheses to explain the distribution or the development of a model for the delivery of services.

3. Testing the etiologic hypothesis or health service model through experimental or observational studies of specific groups of individuals. These last two steps are called *analytic epidemiology*. Further discussion of epidemiologic methods can be found in Chapter 12, and the interested reader should consult a textbook on the subject.[1]

In this chapter the distribution of diabetes in man will be reviewed and, to emphasize its salient features, some hypotheses regarding the causes of diabetes will be examined in terms of their ability to explain or account for that distribution. First, however, it is necessary to define some of the indices used to measure disease frequency in populations.

Measures of Disease Frequency

In order to express disease frequency in a manner suitable for comparisons, the count or number of cases is divided by the total number of individuals in the population to obtain rates, typically expressed as the number of cases per 100, per 1000, or per 100,000 population. In determining these rates, it is important to distinguish between events (such as death or onset of diabetes) and states (such as having diabetes). Rates based on a count of events are *incidence rates* and require specification of the period of time during which the events occurred, typically a year. By convention, if it is not specified, one can assume it to be a year. Rates based on a count of the individuals having diabetes, i.e., being in a particular state, are *prevalence rates*. Unlike incidence rates, prevalence rates do not specify a period of time since the measurement is thought of as being taken at a moment in time. For a chronic disease such as diabetes, the prevalence rate greatly exceeds the incidence rate.

While both indices are valid measures of disease frequency in a population, the purposes for which each is useful are quite different. Incidence measures the probability of becoming diabetic and is useful for studying etiology and evaluating preventive measures. The prevalence rate indicates the probability of having diabetes and is useful in planning for health care facilities and manpower. The importance of distinguishing between these two measures, incidence and prevalence, must be emphasized in diabetes. The prevalence rate reflects not only the rate of appearance of diabetes in the population, but how long cases remain alive and, therefore, counted. For example, a marked increase in the prevalence of insulin-dependent diabetes followed the discovery of insulin. Increased prevalence in that instance reflected a favorable change. In contrast, an increase in incidence rate is always unfavorable and a decrease favorable.

Although historically the *mortality rate* due to diabetes has been the primary index of the occurrence of diabetes in populations,[2-4] it cannot now be considered an accurate measure of such. If a population has access to medical facilities, diabetes is not typically a fatal disease. When death occurs, it is usually many years after the onset of diabetes and is generally attributed to some other condition present at the time of death. Studies of death certificates of diabetic patients have indicated that approximately 50% contained no mention of diabetes. Furthermore, only 25% of those mentioning diabetes listed it as the underlying cause of death. Thus, only one-eighth of these deaths would have been included in national mortality statistics for this disease.[5,6]

When indices of disease frequency are calculated separately according to some characteristic, such as age, sex or race, they are referred to as *specific rates* as opposed to *crude rates*. Crude rates are simply the total number of new cases or existing cases divided by the total number of individuals in the population. In the case of diabetes, there are enormous differences among age-specific rates for incidence and prevalence. As a result, there can be large differences between crude rates for populations which are due to modest differences in their age distributions. Meaningful comparisons, therefore, must be based on age-specific rates.

Such comparisons between rates are commonly expressed as *relative risks*. Relative risk is the ratio of the rate of disease in one population to the rate of disease in another population. If the two populations have similar rates, the relative risk will be near unity; whereas if their rates differ, the relative risk will deviate from unity.

Distribution of Diabetes Mellitus

For the study of etiologic factors, the incidence rate is the most informative measure of the frequency of diabetes. The basic assumption here is that causal factors necessarily operate prior to the initiation of the disease. Of the measures discussed, the incidence rate is closest in time to causal factors and reflects the operation of those factors more directly than other measures. It also follows that incidence should be counted from the earliest possible stage of the disease. However, in the case of diabetes there is some difficulty in adhering to this principle. Insulin-dependent diabetes (IDDM) is easily recognized and virtually all cases are ascertained in a society with access to medical care. Recognition of new cases of non-insulin-dependent diabetes (NIDDM), however, has a variable likelihood which depends upon the severity of symptoms, diagnostic activity of the medical care system, and the pathophysiologic and therapeutic concepts about the disease that determine diagnostic criteria.

Data on the incidence rates of diabetes ascertained through medical care institutions in the population of Rochester, Minnesota, are shown in Figure 2–1. The medical records were reviewed to find all residents for whom a diagnosis of diabetes had been made and, after checking the records against criteria for a diagnosis of diabetes, the age-specific incidence rates were computed.[7-9] The graph shows that the risk of acquiring diabetes increased in each successive age group. However, instead of rising steadily throughout life, the risk leveled off between the 2nd and 3rd decade and again after age 70. This suggests that there might be two superimposed processes, one centered on the 2nd decade and the other on the 6th and 7th decades of life. There was almost a 100-fold difference between incidence rates for very young and very old persons. It is important to recognize that somewhat different results might have been obtained if the entire population of Rochester had been subjected to repeated screening with a diagnostic test for diabetes. New cases would have been detected near their time of onset, rather than after a variable period of unrecognized diabetes, which would have shifted some of the cases to younger age groups. Incidence rates based on repeated screening must then be distinguished from rates based on the ordinary diagnostic activity of medical care institutions.

An informative technique for summarizing such a set of age-specific rates is the *cumulative incidence rate*.[10,11] If a group or cohort of individuals are followed from birth to age 20, the cumulative incidence rate by age 20 would be the proportion of persons who had developed diabetes before that age. Note that if no one in the cohort had died by age 20, then the cumulative incidence rate at age 20 and the prevalence rate among 20 year olds would be identical. However, since there is usually some loss due to death, prevalence rates are less

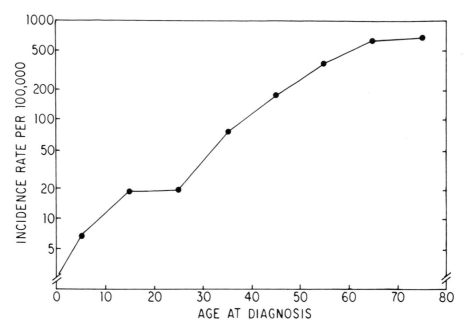

Fig. 2–1. Average annual incidence rates of diabetes mellitus according to age; Rochester, MN, 1960 to 1969. Rates are for diagnosis based on original study criteria (Adapted from ref. 9).

than cumulative incidence rates, particularly at older ages. By analogy with the cohort situation, the age-specific incidence rates for Rochester can be accumulated over age to obtain cumulative incidence rates for a hypothetical cohort exposed to these rates at appropriate ages. The age-specific rates from Rochester would yield the following cumulative incidence rates for a cohort of 1000 white newborns: two to three will have diabetes by the age of 20 years, 5 by age 30, 12 by age 40, 29 by age 50, 63 by age 60 and 123 by age 70.†️ As expected, these cumulative incidence estimates agree with age-specific prevalence rates in Rochester for young age groups but are higher than the prevalence rates for older age groups.[7]

Classification of Diabetes Mellitus

Basic to the calculation of a disease rate is the definition of affected individuals. Various sets of diagnostic criteria have been proposed for diabetes, and there is considerable literature regarding the lack of comparability between criteria (for reviews see refs. 12 and 13) and the loose or liberal inter-

pretation of these criteria in practice.[14] Recently, there has also been interest in the heterogeneity to be found within the diagnostic category of diabetes mellitus. To facilitate investigation of this heterogeneity, classification schemes for types of diabetes mellitus have been proposed by the National Diabetes Data Group[15] and World Health Organization[16] (See also Chapters 3 and 15).

In principle, there are two dimensions along which classification criteria can be developed: manifestations and causes. Manifestational criteria group patients according to the manner in which the illness appears, such as symptom pattern, age at diagnosis, type of therapy needed, proneness to ketosis, or insulin secretory capacity. Causal criteria group patients according to some prior experience judged to be an etiologic factor. In the case of diabetes this might be pancreatitis, Coxsackie B4 infection, or the presence of obesity. For purposes of prevention, it is necessary to think of types of diabetes in such terms. At present, however, our knowledge of the etiology of diabetes is sparse, so the new classifications are only alternative groupings of patients according to the dimension of manifestations. The hope is that a particular grouping will closely approach an etiologic classification. However, this goal may be futile since congruence between causes and manifestations may not exist. Once the etiology is known, it may be that persons whose illness has resulted from a particular cause may have different clinical presentations or even fail to develop diabetes. Con-

---

†️Ratios of cumulative incidence rates are used extensively in this text. Technically, these are *rate ratios* while relative measures of age-specific incidence rates are *risk ratios*. Risk ratios, usually estimated by the *odds ratio* in case-control studies (see Chapter 12 and ref. 1), reflect the situation at a particular age, whereas, rate ratios reflect the cumulative effect over a range of ages. In this text, relative risk will be used to refer to either of these measures.

versely, persons presenting similar symptoms may have different causes for those symptoms.

For purposes of classification, most of the literature that has accumulated so far regarding the epidemiology of diabetes has used one manifestational criterion, namely age at onset. While the proposed classifications[15] are more specific, they have little impact from the standpoint of population studies. Figure 2–2 presents data on the incidence rates of IDDM and NIDDM diagnosed in medical care facilities in Denmark[17,18] and Great Britain[19] according to age at onset. As can be seen, most cases of IDDM occur below age 25 while little NIDDM has occurred by that age.

The new criteria do contribute significantly to population based studies by distinguishing the asymptomatic category, impaired glucose tolerance (IGT), which was previously included in the category of diabetes. Since data on the distribution and determinants of IGT are sparse at present, this category has been omitted from this review. The following discussion is grouped, then, into insulin-dependent diabetes and non-insulin-dependent diabetes. The very sensitive and non-specific criteria used in diagnosing NIDDM in much of the existing literature resulted in this second section being to some extent about IGT as well.

EPIDEMIOLOGY OF INSULIN-DEPENDENT DIABETES (IDDM)

The studies reviewed in this section defined IDDM variously as diabetes with onset before the age of 15 years, before the age of 20 years, and in a few instances, as insulin-requiring diabetes regardless of age at onset. Incidence rates have been used as the measure of the frequency of occurrence insofar as possible. In some instances cumulative incidence rates to particular ages have been used as descriptive summaries of age-specific rates. Prevalence rates and mortality rates have been resorted to as indirect measures when incidence rates were not available.

Distribution According to Sex and Age

Insulin-dependent diabetes rarely occurs during the first 6 months of life. Gamble found only a few cases in a large registry of juvenile diabetics in Great Britain.[20] A sharp increase in incidence begins at about 9 months of age and continues to rise until the age group of 10 to 14 years. Table 2–1 shows the incidence rates according to sex and age in four countries. Within each population the lowest incidence was among children age 0 to 4 years and the highest in those 10 to 14 years, regardless of sex. After that peak, incidence rates decline. The relationship with age is clearly seen in Figure 2–2 in which the incidence rates of IDDM are presented according to age in Denmark for ages 0 to 29[18] and in England and Wales for ages 18 to 50.[19] Table 2–1 also shows cumulative incidence rates for the development of IDDM during the first 20 years of life. In every country except the German Democratic Republic, males had a slightly

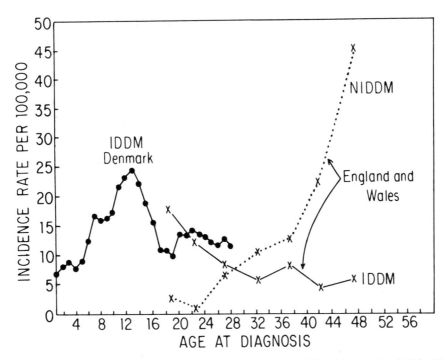

Fig. 2–2. Incidence rates of IDDM and NIDDM according to age in Denmark[18] and England and Wales.[19]

Table 2–1. Average Annual Incidence Rates per 100,000 of IDDM in Some White Populations According to Age and Sex

Age	German Democratic Republic, 1971–81[21]		Scotland 1968–76[22]		Pennsylvania, USA 1965–76[23]		Finland 1970–79[24]	
	M	F	M	F	M	F	M	F
0–4	} 4.7	} 5.4	7.3	6.8	6.8	6.2	17.2	14.4
5–9			12.0	10.8	19.6	17.4	28.7	28.7
10–14	} 9.5	} 9.3	20.0	20.1	20.8	24.1	39.5	35.1
15–19			19.6	15.3	14.7	8.9	29.3	18.9
Cumulative incidence rate by age 20	142	147	297	255	310	283	573	486

greater probability of developing diabetes than females.

Data regarding the incidence of IDDM with onset after the age of 30 years are scarce. In a population study in Copenhagen, the rate was 9.6/100,000 when stringent criteria for a diagnosis of IDDM were used to obtain a conservative estimate. If the criteria were relaxed to include all patients treated with insulin at the beginning of diabetes as IDDM, the incidence rate rose to over 50/100,000.[25] Using similar criteria, a study in Warsaw, Poland, found age-and-sex-specific incidence rates between 30 and 50/100,000 for ages 30 to 59.[26] In the German Democratic Republic, where diabetics throughout the country are registered, incidence rates for insulin-treated diabetes rose progressively from 10/100,000 for the age group 20 to 29 to 30/100,000 for age group 70 and over.[21] These rates are similar to those for insulin-treated diabetes in Rochester, Minnesota, between 1960–1969.[8] However, when the Rochester cases were reviewed and stringent criteria for a diagnosis of IDDM applied, only one-fifth of the insulin-treated cases could be classified as IDDM. The resulting age-specific incidence rates for IDDM varied between 4 and 8/100,000/year, which is similar to the rates shown in Figure 2–2. In all three of these studies of IDDM incidence after age 30, males had slightly higher incidence rates than females.

For health care planning as well as for genetic studies, it is important to know prevalence rates of IDDM according to age. To illustrate that age-specific prevalence rates can be estimated from age-specific incidence rates, data from two studies of the Danish population during the 1970s are summarized in Table 2–2. There is little difference between the prevalence rates obtained in one study[27] and cumulative incidence rates as computed from age-specific incidence rates obtained in the other.[17,25] Prevalence rates for IDDM increase from

0.5/1000 in the youngest age group to 6/1000 for ages 60 to 69 and were slightly lower among females than males.

Variation over Time

Variability in the occurrence of diabetes according to time can be an important etiologic clue arising from epidemiologic investigations. It allows one to look for factors which have a similar pattern of variability over time that can be considered as possible causes. First of all, long-term trends need to be assessed in order to determine whether the occurrence of diabetes in a population is epidemic or non-epidemic in character.

There are only a few sources of data that contribute to such an analysis. These are presented in Figure 2–3. The only data regarding the occurrence of diabetes at the beginning of the century are mortality rates in the population of Massachusetts.[28] For the age group 0–19 they varied from 3.5 to 4.3/100,000 per year during the first 25 years of the century and then declined with the introduction of insulin. Due to the usually short duration of survival before insulin was available, mortality rates could represent fairly accurately the incidence of juvenile onset IDDM but would underestimate it if persons died without a diagnosis of the disease. The next source of information about the occurrence of diabetes came from the National Health Survey carried out in 1935–1936 in a sample of the United States population.[29] The prevalence rates obtained in that survey can be used to estimate that the incidence rate in children under 15 years of age was 4/100,000/year, which was similar to the mortality rates for diabetes in Massachusetts at the beginning of the century. In the 1960s, an extensive retrospective study of the occurrence of several childhood diseases was conducted in Erie County, New York. Diabetes occurring between the ages of 1 and 15 years was one of the diseases studied. By reviewing medical records, it was pos-

Table 2–2. Age-specific Prevalence Rates of IDDM per 1000 Compared to Cumulative Incidence Rates at the Same Ages (Data from Denmark)

		Age groups						
		0–9	10–19	20–29	30–39	40–49	50–59	60–69
Prevalence Rate[27]	M	0.5	2.1	3.5	4.3	5.0	4.8	5.6
	F	0.4	1.9	2.3	3.5	3.3	4.1	6.0
Cumulative Incidence Rate*		0.4	2.1	3.4	4.5	5.4	6.4	7.4

*Computed for the midpoints of the age intervals (ages 5, 15, 25, 35, 45, 55 and 65) using incidence rates from Christy et al.[17] and Christau et al.[25]

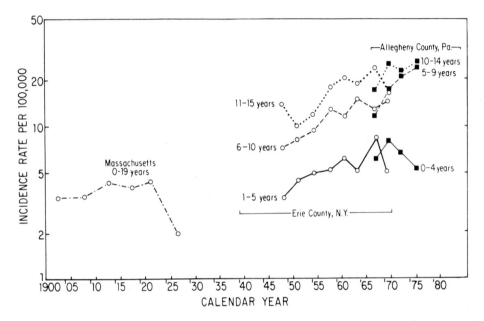

Fig. 2–3. Average annual incidence rates of IDDM in the United States, 1900 to 1976, according to age. Rates shown were based on mortality rates for diabetes in Massachusetts, 1900 to 1925,[28] and incidence rates for diagnoses of IDDM in the Erie County, NY, survey of childhood diseases, 1946 to 1972,[32] and the Allegheny County, PA, registry of IDDM, 1965 to 1976.[23]

sible to identify all the new cases of diabetes which had occurred in this population during the period 1946 to 1961[30,31] and later updated until 1972.[32] Incidence rates were calculated by using county population data for the same years. As can be seen in Figure 2–3, there was some increase in the occurrence of diabetes during the 25 years of observation. This was particularly evident among children aged 6 to 15 years. Another source of data is the Allegheny County study.[23] All new cases of IDDM in residents of the county in the age range 0 to 19 years were identified in a manner similar to that in the Erie County study. The period of observation was 1965–1976. Figure 2–3 shows close agreement between the data from Allegheny and Erie Counties as well as a continuing increase in the occurrence of IDDM, particularly in age group 5 to 9.

In *summary*, there has been some increase in the incidence of IDDM in the white, juvenile population of northeastern United States during the last 75 years. However, it is difficult to assess when the increase began as well as to estimate its magnitude because the evidence relies heavily on data from early in this century which may have been biased by incomplete ascertainment of cases.

Data from other countries regarding this issue are compatible with this interpretation. For example, there has been a small increase in the incidence rates in the German Democratic Republic (GDR) between 1964 and 1979.[21] In Finland, where the incidence of IDDM among children is several times higher than in the GDR, a similar small increase was found between 1970 and 1979.[24] The current incidence rate is much higher than that found in a study there in the 1950s.[33] However, the method of ascertainment used in the earlier study was less reliable than that in the more recent study. Also, in a large study in Scotland, a significant increase was observed during the period 1968–1976 in the incidence of IDDM as assessed by the frequency of first hospitalizations for newly diagnosed cases.[22] Contrary to these findings, there has been no increase in the occurrence of diabetes in the population 0 to 14 years of age in Denmark; incidence rates in 1970–1975 were exactly the same as in 1925.[17,18]

In addition to long-term trends over time, variability with time might be evidenced in year to year differences or seasonal differences within years. Seasonal variability has attracted much attention (see Chapter 24). The first data on this issue were presented in 1926.[34] A summary of most of the papers on this topic is presented in Table 2–3. Only two of 14 studies failed to find evidence of seasonality in the incidence of IDDM. All other studies found one peak in winter and another in the summer or early fall. It is interesting that in the United States population, seasonality was more pronounced among young children aged 0 to 6, whereas in Great Britain and Scandinavia it was more pronounced in the 5 to 14 age group. Seasonality has not been found after the age of 19 in studies in which it has been looked for. In the Joslin Clinic population seasonality was particularly pronounced among children 0 to 14 who did not have a family history of diabetes.[35] Most authors used the date of diagnosis as the initial date although studies have indicated that the onset of symptoms is typically 1 to 2 months earlier (see Chapter 12). Taking this into account, it would appear that one peak occurs in the late fall and early winter (except for two states in southern United States) and the second peak in summer. A study of seasonal incidence in Cuba, where there is little seasonal variation in climate, found a single peak which coincided with the return of children to school in the fall.[44] This could be due to exposure to infections which precipitate the appearance of symptoms in asymptomatic cases or a temporal cluster of cases resulting from closer observation of the children in a school setting.

The existing literature on variability from year to year shows a barely perceptible variation in the incidence rates.[18,21,22,24] Data from Great Britain suggest that variability within a year was greater than the year to year variability.[20]

Table 2–3. Summary of Findings in Studies of the Seasonal Occurrence of IDDM

Population and year(s) of observation	No. of patients	Age of patients (years)	Date used for onset of diabetes	Peak months	Ages with most pronounced seasonality
North America					
Mayo Clinic[34] (1926)	317	0–40	diagnosis	February	not considered
Joslin Clinic[35] (1964–1973)	1142	0–20	diagnosis	Jan.–Feb. July–August	0–9
Pittsburgh, PA[36] (1964–1974)	673	0–14	hospital admission	January	0–6
Montreal, Que[37] (1971–1977)	522	0–17	symptoms	no seasonality	not considered
Galveston, TX[36] (1972–1975)	741	0–14	symptoms	Feb.–March November	0–6
Gainesville, FL[36] (1962–1977)	976	0–14	symptoms	Jan.–May	0–6
Europe					
London[38] (1955–1968)	2816	0–39	diagnosis	January October	0–19
United Kingdom[39] (1973–1974)	2000	0–15	diagnosis	Dec.–March Sept.–Oct.	5–15
Edinburgh[40] (1964–1977)	502	10–69	symptoms	Nov.–Feb.	10–19
Sweden[41] (1970–1975)	359	0–14	insulin begun	January September	not considered
Denmark[18] (1970–1976)	792	0–29	diagnosis	January August	not considered
Southern Hemisphere					
Melbourne[36] (1920–1975)	851	0–14	symptoms	May–Aug.	6–14
New Zealand[42] (1968–1972)	578	0–20	hospital admission	no seasonality	not considered
Chile[43] (1935–1978)	525	0–30	symptoms	June January	0–19

Table 2–4. Incidence Rates of IDDM among Children Aged 0 to 14 in Various Countries

Country	Incidence rate per 100,000/year	Period of observation
Tokyo, Japan (age 5–16)[45]	0.6	1975–78
Santo Domingo, D.R.[46]	1.7	1971–80
Cuba[44]	2.3	1980
Slovenia, Yugoslavia[a]	2.7	1970–74
France[47]	3.7	1975
Venice, Italy[a]	4.7	1975
German Democratic Republic[b] [21]	7.4	1964–79
Montreal, Canada[37]	9.0	1970–75
Toronto, Canada[b] [48]	9.0	1976–78
New Zealand[42]	9.0	1968–72
Pennsylvania, USA (nonwhites)[23]	9.7	1965–76
Scotland[b] [22]	13.8	1968–76
Denmark[18]	13.7	1970–75
Norway[49]	17.6	1973–77
Pennsylvania, USA (whites)[23]	18.2	1965–76
Sweden[50]	22.6	1977–80
Finland[24]	29.0	1970–79

[a.] Quoted from ref. 47.
[b.] Age group 0 to 19.

Table 2–5. Prevalence Rates of IDDM among Children in Various Countries

Country	Prevalence rate per 1000	Year of observation	Age of population in years
Tokyo, Japan[45]	0.06	1977	0–18
Cuba[44]	0.15	1980	0–14
Israel[51,52]	0.16	1963	2–16
	0.24	1968	2–16
Slovenia, Yugoslavia[a]	0.22	1974	0–14
Venice, Italy[a]	0.26	1975	0–13
France[47]	0.24	1975	0–14
Poland[a]	0.42	1975	0–16
German Democratic Republic[21]	0.50	1979	0–19
U.S. Health Interview Survey, Non-Whites[b]	0.30	1964–66[c]	0–14
	1.03	1973,75[d]	0–14
Denmark[18]	0.83	1973	0–14
U.S. Health Interview Survey, Whites[b]	0.80	1964–66[c]	0–14
	1.17	1973,75[d]	0–14
Sweden[50]	1.48	1980	0–14
Finland[24]	1.90	1979	0–14

[a]Quoted from ref. 47.
[b]Computed from unpublished survey data supplied by Thomas F. Drury, Ph.D., National Center for Health Statistics (see refs. 53 and 54).
[c]Average prevalence from three surveys.
[d]Average prevalence from two surveys.

Geographic Distribution

Interest in the epidemiology of diabetes during the last decade has resulted in the publication of a number of papers on the incidence rates in various parts of the world. This permits international comparisons and the examination of geographic patterns in the occurrence of IDDM. In Table 2–4 are incidence rates for the population aged 0 to 14 in various parts of the world. The lowest rates are in Japan, the Caribbean and southern Europe, while the highest rates are in Scandinavia and the white population of Pennsylvania in the United States. The registries in northern Europe are well established and probably achieve good ascertainment of cases. Information regarding the completeness of registration in those countries with low rates is not available for assessing how much of the north-south difference might be due to incomplete ascertainment.

As confirmation of the results for incidence rates, data on prevalence rates from a similar set of countries are presented in Table 2–5. Although prevalence rates are a less direct measure of diabetes occurrence than incidence rates, in the population under age 20 they are a reasonably close measure since there is little removal of cases due to mortality which is low in that age group. Once again the lowest rates are in Japan, Cuba, Israel, and southern Europe, while the highest are in Finland, Sweden and the United States.

In addition to international differences, regional variation within countries has been examined. In Sweden the highest incidence and prevalence rates were observed in one northern area.[41,50,55] In Norway the lowest mean annual incidence (6.8/100,000/year) was found in the northern part of the country; whereas, an incidence of about 20/100,000 was found in southern Norway.[49] In Finland, incidence and prevalence rates were lower in the north (the region nearest Sweden) than in the rest of the country, and highest in the eastern region.[24] In part this parallels population density. An inverse relationship with population density was found in a large study in Scotland.[22] However, in Denmark the incidence of diabetes was similar in urban and rural areas, but there were substantial differences in incidence rates between the northern and southern parts of the city of Copenhagen.[17,18,56]

Distribution According to Race and Socio-economic Status

Data on the occurrence of diabetes among the non-white population of the United States were included in Tables 2–4 and 2–5. The incidence rate for non-whites was half that for whites. In the Erie County study,[30,31] for which the period of observation was from 1946–1961, the incidence among non-whites was less than half the rate for whites. In the Allegheny County study[23] between 1965 and 1976, i.e., after the Erie County study, the non-white incidence rate was higher than in Erie

County. The prevalence rates in Table 2–5 are from the National Health Surveys conducted between 1964 and 1976. Taken in time sequence, these data suggest that there has been an increase over time in the occurrence of IDDM in non-white children as well as in white children.

Although comparable data on black populations in Africa are not available, there have been reports which suggest that true IDDM occurs in African blacks.[57–60,63,64] Similarly, there have been reports of the occurrence of IDDM in Thailand,[61] in India,[62] and among Indians who migrated to South Africa.[63,64] Although IDDM is rare in China[65] and Japan,[45] some of its epidemiologic and clinical characteristics have been shown to be similar to those in Caucasians.[66,67]

In *summary,* the accumulated data suffice only to show (in a qualitative sense) that IDDM occurs in most racial and ethnic groups. While this is not evidence against the hypothesis that IDDM is primarily a Caucasian disease,[68,69] reliable assessment of the magnitude of racial differences in its rate of occurrence will require large studies. For example, in China only 2 cases were found in a study of 20,000 children and adolescents.[65] If large differences between races are confirmed, one must then consider to what extent they are due to environmental factors as opposed to genetic variation among races. The large variability among Caucasian populations in the incidence and prevalence rates of IDDM (Tables 2–4 and 2–5) can be interpreted as evidence that there are important environmental factors influencing the occurrence of IDDM in that race.

Surprisingly, there are scant data on the occurrence of IDDM according to socio-economic status. The earliest report on this issue was the Erie County Community Register of Childhood Diseases mentioned before. These authors used census data regarding average income to calculate prevalence rates according to residence in low, middle or high income census tracts.[31] They did not find any difference according to this measure of socioeconomic status. The same approach was used by authors who studied the incidence of IDDM in Montreal, Canada, during the years 1971–1977.[70] They divided Montreal census tracts into five strata according to average household income as reported in the census. The lowest incidence of IDDM was found among children from the lowest average income strata, and the highest among children in the two highest income strata. The difference between the lowest and highest was almost 2-fold, 6.4 and 11.9/100,000/year.

In a recently published analysis of the Allegheny County study, the incidence rates for IDDM did not vary according to average household income

of census tracts.[71] As noted earlier, a substantial difference in the occurrence of IDDM was found between the southern (20.0/100,000) and the northern parts (10.5/100,000) of Copenhagen.[56] In the southern part of the city, the age distribution of the population was younger, there was less property per family and more individuals per room, and higher percentages of unskilled workers and working women than in the northern part. One other study possibly points to socio-economic differences as a determinant of IDDM. An investigation conducted in Israel in the early 1960s computed prevalence rates of juvenile onset diabetes according to the country of birth of the patient's father.[51] They found the highest prevalence among children whose parents immigrated from Europe and America, and the lowest among children whose parents immigrated from Africa and Asia. These two populations of families differed in many other respects, including socio-economic status.

Occurrence Subsequent to Infections

Based on clinical observation, there have been persistent claims that diabetes can have an infectious etiology, and various agents have been suggested as possible etiologic factors (for reviews see references 20 and 72). Epidemiologic evidence relative to the involvement of infectious diseases in the etiology of IDDM can be examined by comparing the distribution of diabetes with the distribution of these infectious diseases in the same population. In Figure 2–4 are presented the number of

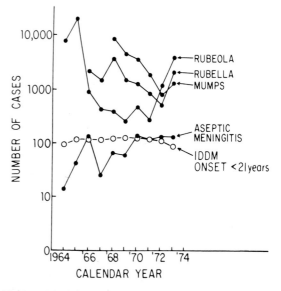

Fig. 2–4. Number of recently diagnosed IDDM registering at Joslin Clinic, 1964 to 1973, and number of cases of various viral infections reported to the Massachusetts Department of Public Health during the same period (Adapted from ref. 35).

patients with recently diagnosed IDDM presenting to Joslin Clinic during the years 1964–1973.[35] On the same figure for comparison, are the numbers of various reportable infectious diseases registered in Massachusetts during the same years. The number of new diabetics is remarkably constant from year to year, while pronounced variability from year to year characterizes these infectious diseases. Similarly, when the age distribution of IDDM is compared to that of infectious diseases, there is no disease which has a peak occurrence at age 10 to 14 years as diabetes has.

Another means of studying the possible infectious origin of diabetes is sero-epidemiology. If viruses play a direct role in the development of diabetes, significant elevation of antibody titers should be found in a greater proportion of recently diagnosed diabetics in comparison with similar persons without diabetes. In the first study of this question, slightly higher antibody titers to Coxsackie B4 virus were found in patients tested within 3 months of the onset of diabetes than in patients with longer duration and in nondiabetic patients.[73] Almost all of the 123 diabetic patients were over the age of 15, and some were over the age of 40 and not insulin-dependent. In another study in the United Kingdom, newly diagnosed IDDM and a control group matched for age and time of serum collection were tested for neutralizing antibody for Coxsackie B4.[74] Again evidence of past infection with Coxsackie B4 virus was more common in diabetics than in the controls in the age groups 10 to 19 and 20 + . However, among children aged 0 to 9, these antibodies were detected more frequently among nondiabetic controls than among diabetics. Similar results were obtained by Anderson in Copenhagen.[75]

In a study at the Joslin Clinic, 156 patients with IDDM were tested within 6 months of onset for antibodies to Coxsackie B1-6, mumps, and cytomegalovirus.[76] Three groups of age-matched controls (and sex-matched when possible) were tested; these consisted of siblings, playmates or friends, and individuals unknown to the proband but residing in the same community. In no instance was the proportion of positive titers ($>$ 1:20 for Coxsackie B1-6, and $>$ 1:8 for mumps and cytomegalovirus) significantly higher in the diabetics than in matched controls.

There are only two prospective studies where the development of diabetes subsequent to outbreaks of Coxsackie B virus has been examined. Hierholzer and Farris[77] investigated 126 children several years after an outbreak of Coxsackie B3 and B4, and Dippe and co-workers[78] examined 335 Aleuts in the Pribilof Islands 6 years after an outbreak of Coxsackie B4 infection in which 60% of the islanders experienced illness diagnosed clinically and confirmed serologically. In neither study did diabetes develop as a sequela to infection. However, these negative results do not exclude the possibility that IDDM is a sequela with an incidence too low to be detected in such small populations.

Thus while there have been a few case studies implicating infection with Coxsackie B virus in the development of IDDM,[79–81] population studies do not corroborate the association. A role of infectious agents in the etiology of IDDM cannot be ruled out, but any mechanism linking the two must be complex rather than simple. For example, what mechanism would explain the curious finding in several of these studies that IDDM patients with onset before age 10 had less frequent evidence of infection with Coxsackie B3 and B4 virus than controls?[74–76,82]

Familial Occurrence

Some diseases have a higher occurrence rate in relatives of affected individuals than in the general population but do not follow a pattern within family pedigrees which fits with any known genetic model for inheritance. Such diseases are commonly investigated not only by geneticists, but also by epidemiologists to find out to what extent the familial occurrence may be explained by environmental factors, which are shared by family members, as opposed to genetically determined susceptibility.[83] The goal for the following discussion is not to survey genetic hypotheses regarding the familial occurrence of IDDM (none of which has gained wide support), but to review the available empirical data on familial occurrence of IDDM and to examine whether their pattern and variability suggest a role for environmental factors in IDDM etiology. The approach[84,85] involves examination of the same indices of IDDM frequency, which have been discussed earlier, in relatives of IDDM probands and comparisons with available data on its frequency in the general population.

There are several published studies which allow the computation of age-specific incidence rates of diabetes for the siblings of IDDM probands in various populations and at different times. The results of three such studies are summarized in Table 2–6. For comparison purposes, incidence rates at the same ages in a general population are shown as reported in the Allegheny County study.[23] While the incidence rates are slightly higher in the London series,[86] the striking finding is their similarity to the Mayo series[87] and even the Pittsburgh series,[88,89] which was assembled 3 decades later. In all series of siblings, the pattern according to age was similar to that observed in the general popu-

Table 2–6.   Incidence Rate per 1000 per Year of Diabetes among Siblings of Juvenile Onset Diabetics in Several Populations According to Age

Age	London series (1950)[a] Index cases aged 0 to 14	Mayo Clinic series (1952)[b] Index cases aged 0 to 14	Pittsburgh offspring study (1981)[88] Index cases aged 0 to 17	White population of Allegheny County Pennsylvania[23] 1964–1976
0–4	0.65	0.82	0.49	0.06
5–9	2.90		1.24	0.18
10–14	3.37	2.69	3.83	0.22
15–19	3.11		1.18	0.12
Cumulative incidence rate by age 20	49.3	34.9	33.4	2.9

a. Computed from data published by Harris.[86]
b. Computed from data published by Steinberg et al.[87]

lation but 5 to 20 times higher. The relative risk was particularly high for siblings in the age group 10 to 14.

Cumulative incidence rates by age 20 were calculated to summarize each series and to show that the risk of developing diabetes among siblings in each series was about 11 to 17 times that of the general population. It is important to note that the Pittsburgh and Allegheny County studies determined the incidence rates of IDDM, specifically in the index cases and siblings, while the other two studies did not distinguish the type of diabetes in siblings. Non-insulin-dependent diabetes (NIDDM) represents a small fraction of cases of diabetes occurring by age 20, and presumably these rates were not affected appreciably by the absence of this distinction.

A shortcoming of the data in Table 2–6 is that the period of follow-up was short; ideally, the siblings should be followed through adult life. There are two such studies in which siblings were followed to age 60. One was conducted in Copenhagen[90] and the second at the Joslin Clinic.[91] In both studies, index cases were diagnosed primarily in the 1920s and 1930s and their siblings were followed until the late 1960s. In the Danish study the selection criterion for index cases was a diagnosis of diabetes before age 20, whereas in the Joslin Clinic study, insulin requirement was an added criterion. Cumulative incidence rates of diabetes, regardless of type, among siblings in each series were computed by life table methods and are presented in Table 2–7. The similarity between the rates for siblings observed in Copenhagen and Boston is remarkable. Since these tabulations do not distinguish the type of diabetes occurring in the siblings, they are not informative with regard to the incidence of IDDM in adult siblings. For the

Table 2–7.   Cumulative Incidence Rates per 1000 of Diabetes at Specified Ages for Siblings of Juvenile Onset Probands and the General Population of Denmark

Population studied	Age in years				
	10	20	30	40	50
Copenhagen series[90]	11	51	59	69	105
Joslin Clinic series*	12	31	53	83	104
General population**	1.2	3.0	4.0	5.0	6.0

*Reanalysis of data collected by Gottlieb.[91,92]
**Computed from incidence rates for Danish population.[17,25]

Joslin Clinic series, the type of treatment and history of ketosis among siblings were obtained. Preliminary analysis shows that almost all diabetes appearing among the siblings prior to age 40 required treatment with insulin.[92] Thus, by comparing the Joslin data with the cumulative incidence rates for IDDM in the Danish population (Table 2–2), one can estimate that the excess risk for siblings is 10-fold by age 10 and 17-fold by age 50.

The Joslin study also examined the occurrence of diabetes in siblings of diabetics diagnosed in the 1960s after age 25. The probands were divided into those treated with insulin from the first year of diabetes and those not requiring insulin. Cumulative incidence rates of IDDM were calculated by the use of life table techniques. Siblings of probands with IDDM diagnosed between ages 25 and 44 had cumulative incidence rates of IDDM almost identical to those shown in Table 2–7. On the other hand, siblings of probands with IDDM diagnosed after age 44 had a cumulative incidence rate for IDDM similar to the general population.[92]

With these results, no doubt remains that IDDM occurs in siblings of index cases far in excess of its occurrence in the general population, and that the excess rate of occurrence continues many years after the diagnosis of the first case in the family. This has important implications with regard to published studies of the time interval between primary and secondary cases in families. Affected pairs of siblings in the British Diabetic Association Register have been analyzed by Gamble[93] who reported an unusual clustering of sibling pairs which occurred within an interval of 6 months, suggesting an environmental agent, perhaps infectious in nature. In contrast to Gamble's results, the Pittsburgh investigators[88,89] found no excess risk for siblings during the first year or two after onset of the first case in the family. They found, instead, significant correlation between the ages at onset for affected sibling pairs. However, this similarity of ages at onset could have been coincidental since all siblings in a family tend to be of a somewhat similar age. In light of the results of the Joslin study, both the British and Pittsburgh studies were short-term and underestimated the number of long intervals between diagnoses in affected sibling pairs. Our analysis of the Danish and Joslin data showed closer clustering of ages at onset than dates of onset in families.[92]

Exposure to environmental factors can be sex-related and transmission of an agent within a family may be influenced by sex-specific patterns of contact between siblings. Both in the Pittsburgh[89] and the Joslin studies,[92] the occurrence of diabetes was identical among brothers and sisters of index cases. The same was true when the analysis was done separately for male and female probands, i.e., there was no evidence for greater transmission of a hypothetical agent from brother to brother, sister to sister, brother to sister or sister to brother. The same conclusion can be drawn from a Canadian study.[94]

Another opportunity to examine whether the familial occurrence of diabetes is of genetic or environmental etiology is the study of twins. The premise of this type of study is that monozygotic twins carry identical genotypes while dizygotic twins are no more similar genetically than non-twin siblings. More frequent concordance for diabetes among monozygotic twins than dizygotic twins is, therefore, evidence of a genetic etiology for diabetes. In Table 2–8 twin studies are summarized. Various definitions of IDDM and methods of ascertainment were used and most series are tiny. In the largest, the British study,[99] overall concordance was reported to be 54.4%; however, this figure includes twin pairs followed for short intervals

Table 2–8. Frequency of Concordant Occurrence of Diabetes among Monozygotic and Dizygotic Twins

	Monozygotic twins		Dizygotic twins	
Authors	No. of pairs	Concordant occurrence of diabetes	No. of pairs	Concordant occurrence of diabetes
Then Berg* 1934[95,96]	12	3(25%)†	17	—†
Harvald & Houge* 1964[97]	6	6(100%)	12	2
Gottlieb & Root* 1968[98]	19	3(16%)	26	—
Barnett et al.** 1981[99]	147	80(54%)	—	—

*Index cases had juvenile onset diabetes.
**Index cases had IDDM disregarding age of onset.
†Diabetes diagnosed on the basis of GTT in unaffected twins by authors was disregarded since it was not IDDM.

after the diagnosis in the index twin. To adjust for this, life table methods should be used. One can be approximated from the data as published and yields an estimate of 73% concordance within 15 years after the diagnosis in the first twin. This study did not include a group of dizygotic twins, but the few results from the other studies are consistent with the concordance rate observed in non-twin sibling pairs.

From these data, one can conclude that genetic determinants are important in the development of IDDM, but the relative magnitude of the genetic contribution cannot be estimated precisely. The British study was not population-based; rather, it depended upon voluntary registration of twins, and the authors stated, "...the method of ascertainment has almost certainly led to a bias towards discovery of concordant as against discordant twin pairs as they have a double chance of recognition."[99] Thus, this study sheds uncertain light on the concordance rate for IDDM in identical twins, not only because of inappropriate methods of analysis, but also because of selection bias. Unfortunately, none of the studies in Table 2–8 was designed to meet the basic requirements for drawing inferences regarding the concordance rate.[100,101]

Another issue in twin studies is the interpretation of the concordance rate. Its interpretation is relatively simple if there is justification for assuming a Mendelian mode of inheritance, but if more complicated models of inheritance must be considered, its interpretation is not obvious.[102–104] For example, if inheritance is multifactorial, then a concordance rate of 50% for a disease as rare as IDDM implies that heritability of liability is much greater than 50%.

Parent-offspring pairs are another relationship which can be examined for familial aggregation of

IDDM. This can be done retrospectively by searching for affected parents of index cases, or prospectively by following a cohort of offspring of a diabetic parent. Earlier in this century, this type of study was impossible since few cases of IDDM survived long enough to have children. The diabetes that could be found in parents of index cases was primarily NIDDM.[105] In Canada in the 1960s, Simpson studied the parents of juvenile onset index cases and found juvenile onset diabetes in 0.4% of the fathers and 0.16% of the mothers who were alive and under the age of 50.[94] Inclusion of parental diabetes diagnosed after age 20 increased the prevalence rates to 1.4% and 0.86% for fathers and mothers, respectively.

In the Pittsburgh study, which consisted of index cases diagnosed between 1964 and 1980, IDDM in parents was more frequent than in the previous study: 3.7% of fathers and 1.4% of mothers.[89] The highest prevalence of IDDM that has been found in parents was in a study conducted in the whole of Sweden in 1977–1980.[50] IDDM was found in 6.1% of the fathers and 2.9% of the mothers of newly diagnosed children with IDDM. Unfortunately, neither study compared the ages at onset in parent-child pairs or looked for clustering of their dates of onset.

In these studies, the prevalence rates of IDDM in the corresponding general populations are unknown, so calculation of relative risks of IDDM for children of insulin-dependent parents is impossible. However, if the Danish data in Table 2–2 are assumed to be applicable to Pittsburgh and Sweden and the prevalence rate in the 5th decade is taken as the reference point, relative risks for the last two studies can be estimated. These indicate that the risk for children of an insulin-dependent parent is 4 to 14 times the risk in the general population, and the risk is higher for children of diabetic fathers than diabetic mothers.

Prospective studies of the risk of IDDM in the offspring of insulin-dependent probands are few, and the duration of follow-up is short. Two of them are the Danish[90] and Joslin Clinic[91] studies cited above with regard to the occurrence of IDDM in siblings. In these studies, the offspring of the index cases were traced and the occurrence of IDDM ascertained. The authors found an excess of diabetes in offspring relative to the general population which was similar to that observed in siblings. A reanalysis of the affected parent-offspring pairs showed that IDDM appeared in the offspring at an age very close to the age of appearance in the parent. Also analysis of the risk in offspring according to the sex of the diabetic parent revealed a significant difference between offspring of diabetic fathers and diabetic mothers. Offspring of a diabetic father had a cumulative incidence of IDDM by age 20 which was 30 times that in the general population, while offspring of diabetic mothers had an incidence rate only 7 times that in the general population.[106] There were some differences between the Danish and Joslin series, but the overall pattern was the same. Simpson's large study of Canadian diabetics cited above[94] also found a higher prevalence rate of diabetes in the offspring of diabetic fathers than of diabetic mothers. These results agree with the observation in retrospective studies of the prevalence of IDDM in parents of index cases that the prevalence rates were higher for fathers than for mothers. Although one must consider that the lower prevalence of IDDM in mothers of index cases could be due to smaller family sizes when the mother is diabetic than when the father is diabetic, the agreement between retrospective and prospective findings suggest that IDDM is inherited more through the father than the mother. An alternative hypothesis is that the IDDM-susceptible fetuses were selectively lost during pregnancy.[106]

In *summary*, the evidence from family studies does not provide any leads to environmental factors as determinants of the familial aggregation of IDDM. Although no genetic model of inheritance has gained wide acceptance, the similarity in the magnitude of the excess risk in all first degree relatives of index cases, in various populations and at various times, supports a significant role for genetic factors. Moreover, the tendency for cases within a family to cluster around an age at onset rather than a time of onset also suggests a genetic etiology, although the mechanism must be complex. The need for an understanding of the mode of inheritance of IDDM is particularly important in the light of the improvement in survival of patients with IDDM (see Chapter 12) and the improved care of diabetic pregnancies. If the inheritance of IDDM is due to one or only a few loci, then the improved survival and fecundity of patients with IDDM would have increased the frequency of the diabetic gene(s) in the population, and one can suppose that some of the rise in the incidence of IDDM during the last 40 years (Fig. 2–3) could be attributed to that increase. If true, such a possibility would have important implications as far as prevention of IDDM in the population is concerned. On the other hand, if the genetic determinants of IDDM are polygenic, the issue is moot.

Distribution According to HLA Antigens

The HLA system was discovered in the search for tissue types that could be the basis for matching donors and recipients of transplanted organs. It was first identified as a series of antigenic specificities on peripheral white blood cells by using sera produced by fetal-maternal stimulation. Expression of these specificities is controlled by a set of genes on a segment of chromosome 6 which has been named the HLA region. The HLA region is now known to include a number of closely linked gene loci controlling cell surface determinants (HLA: A, B, C, DR), certain components of the complement system[107,108] and, according to Bodmer, enough DNA to control the amino acid sequence of at least 100 peptide products of the same approximate size as HLA A, B and C with unknown function and polymorphicity.[109]

In the early 1970s, certain HLA antigens were shown to be positively associated with IDDM but not with NIDDM.[110–112] The occurrence of IDDM in relation to HLA antigens has been studied by two different approaches: population studies (chiefly case-control studies) and family studies.

Population studies. The association between a particular HLA antigen and diabetes in population studies is usually expressed in terms of the odds ratio. This is an approximate measure of the relative risk for that antigen and can be interpreted as the ratio of the probability of IDDM developing in a carrier of the antigen to the probability of its developing in a non-carrier.[113,114] Although associations of IDDM with various HLA-B antigens[110–112] were first recognized, certain DR antigens have since been shown to be more strongly associated with the disease.[115] In all populations studied, IDDM has been confined largely to individuals who carry HLA-DR 3 and/or DR 4, regardless of the frequency of occurrence of IDDM in the population (Table 2–9). In Japan, where HLA-DR 3 is extremely rare, an analogous relationship was found with HLA-DR 8.[115] While the data presented at the Eighth International Histocompatibility Workshop appeared to suggest that HLA-DR 4 was particularly associated with very early onset IDDM and DR 3 was associated with onset in the second or later decades,[115] this has not been substantiated in subsequent studies.[119,120]

Another observation found in all populations was that individuals who carry both HLA-DR 3 and DR 4 were particularly susceptible to IDDM. Data on the relationship of IDDM risk to HLA-DR phenotype are summarized for various populations in Table 2–10. Individuals who were typable only as DR 3 or DR 4 had lower relative risks than DR 3/4 heterozygotes; therefore, they have been combined with those who had DR 3 or DR 4 in combination with some other DR antigen. Although the estimates of relative risk varied among the various studies and the differences between phenotypes were not always statistically significant, the pattern

Table 2–9. Proportion of Individuals with HLA DR3 and/or DR4 among Patients with IDDM and Healthy Controls in Several Countries

Country	IDDM with HLA DR 3 and/or 4		Controls with HLA DR 3 and/or 4	
	No.	(percent)	No.	(percent)
China[67]	31	74.2	105	29.5
Israel[116]				
Non-Ashkenazim	42	92.8	38	34.2
Ashkenazim	50	96.0	52	59.6
Basques[117]	50	96.1	50	38.0
France[118]	53	87.0	116	32.0
Germany[a]	74	86.5	53	58.5
United Kingdom[119]	122	97.5	110	59.1
Denmark[120]	93	91.4	260	57.4
U.S.A.				
Blacks[121][b]	55	80.0	56	35.7
Whites[122]	134	94.7	263	51.0

[a.] Computed from data presented in ref. 115.
[b.] Reanalysis of data in ref. 121 provided by Acton, R.T., Barger, B.O., Go, R.C.P., and Roseman, J.M.

was quite consistent, i.e., HLA-DR 3/4 had the highest relative risk.

These data suggest that populations could be screened for DR 3 and DR 4 antigens in order to identify children at high risk of developing IDDM. The results of such a screening program in a North American Caucasian population can be predicted from the frequencies of these antigens in patients with IDDM,[122] their frequencies in nondiabetics[122] and the cumulative incidence of IDDM by age 20 which can be estimated to be about 310/100,000 in the White U.S. population (see Table 2–1). Using these figures, one can estimate that the cumulative incidence of IDDM per 1000 by age 20 would be 15.1 for individuals carrying both DR 3 and DR 4 (Table 2–11), 4.7 for those carrying either DR 3 or DR 4 but not both, and 0.3 for those who have neither antigen. Therefore, while the risk of diabetes for individuals carrying both DR 3 and DR 4 would be quite high relative to individuals who carry neither (relative risk approximately 50), the absolute risk for those with a positive screening test for DR 3 and/or DR 4 would still be quite low. In other populations, particularly those with a lower frequency of IDDM, the probability of an individual with DR 3 and/or DR 4 developing IDDM might be even lower than we have estimated for North American Caucasians.

Despite the consistency of the data on the association between IDDM and HLA-DR antigens, it does not contribute to an understanding of the variability of the occurrence of IDDM in various populations. Examination of the phenotype frequencies presented in Table 2–9 reveals that they do not vary as much among populations as the

Table 2–10. Risk of IDDM in Individuals with HLA-DR3 and/or DR4 Relative to Individuals Without these Antigens as Reported for Various Populations [Relative Risk Expressed as the Odds Ratio (O.R.)[a]]

HLA-DR Phenotype	China[67]	Israel[116]	Basques[117]	England[119]	Denmark[120]	U.S.A. Blacks[d]	U.S.A. Whites[122]
3/4	27.0 (3/1)[b]	116.0 (37/3)	248.0 (16/1)	132.0 (62/7)	44.4 (32/10)	19.6 (6/1)	46.1 (35/14)
4/X[c]	3.2 (6/17)	12.8 (41/30)	6.6 (3/7)	16.5 (33/30)	6.6 (35/74)	14.2 (13/3)	18.2 (66/67)
3/X[c]	8.3 (14/15)	8.5 (9/10)	42.0 (30/11)	12.8 (24/28)	3.8 (18/65)	5.1 (25/16)	9.0 (26/53)
X/X	1.0 (8/72)	1.0 (5/47)	1.0 (2/31)	1.0 (3/45)	1.0 (8/111)	1.0 (11/36)	1.0 (7/129)
Total number	31/105	92/90	51/120	122/110	93/260	55/56	134/263

[a] The odds ratio is approximately equal to the relative risk (see ref. 1, page 273, for definition) for a particular phenotype in comparison to individuals without DR3 or DR4.

[b] In parentheses are the numbers of diabetics and controls, respectively, with the indicated phenotype.

[c] "X" indicates antigens DR1, 2, 5, 6, 7, 8 or blank with the following exception: Homozygous DR3/3 and DR4/4 had lower odds ratios than DR3/4 so they have been included with DR3/X and DR4/X, respectively.

[d] Reanalysis of data in ref. 121 provided by Acton, R.T., Barger, B.O., Go, R.C.P., and Roseman, J.M.

Table 2–11. Estimated Risk of IDDM by Age 20 According to the Presence of HLA Antigens, DR3 or DR4

IDDM status	DR3/4	DR3 or DR4 present	DR3 and DR4 absent	Total[b]
Present[a]	81	213	16	310
Absent[a]	5283	45559	48848	99690
Total	5364	45772	48864	100,000
Cumulative incidence by age 20 per 1000 individuals	15.1	4.7	0.3	3.1

[a] Expected numbers calculated from the phenotype distribution in U.S.A. whites shown in Table 2–10 (data from ref. 122).

[b] Based on cumulative incidence in white males in general population shown in column 5 of Table 2–1 (data from ref. 23). If cumulative incidence for white females had been used, all figures in bottom row would be slightly smaller.

occurrence of IDDM as summarized in Tables 2–5 and 2–6. However, a definitive analysis of this question must await more representative estimates of HLA phenotype frequencies in these populations.

Family studies. The subjects of this type of study are families with at least two diabetic children. Each child inherits one set of HLA-A, B, C and DR antigens, called a haplotype, from each parent, usually *en bloc*.[109] If IDDM were not in any way related to the HLA system, then among diabetic sib-pairs 25% would have identical HLA-haplotypes, each having received the same set from each parent. Further, 50% would share just one HLA-haplotype, and 25% of the pairs would not have any HLA-haplotypes in common. For the Eighth International Histocompatibility Workshop,[115] Svejgaard, Platz and Ryder summarized data for 263 affected IDDM sib-pairs and found a different distribution according to shared HLA-

haplotypes: 59% had both identical, 37% shared one, and only 5% shared no haplotype. The implication of these findings is that a sibling who has two HLA haplotypes identical to those in a diabetic sib has the highest probability of developing IDDM; while a sibling who has no HLA haplotype in common with a diabetic sib has the lowest risk.

Using the frequencies of shared haplotypes among affected sibling pairs[115] and data from the Pittsburgh Study on the occurrence of IDDM in a second sibling,[88] one can estimate the risk of IDDM in siblings according to the number of HLA-haplotypes shared with an affected sibling. If one assumes that 25% of all sibs of the diabetic probands have two identical to the proband, 50% have one in common with the proband, and 25% have neither in common with the proband, and further assumes that the secondary cases (there were 65 in that study) have the distribution of shared haplotypes previously described for affected sib-pairs, then one can calculate incidence rates in siblings according to haplotype similarity to the proband. The results are presented in Table 2–12. The lowest incidence rate would be among those with neither HLA-haplotype in common with their diabetic sib. Translated into cumulative incidence by age 20, this works out to 6/1000, which would be about twice the rate in the general population. Siblings with one HLA-haplotype in common with their diabetic sib would have a cumulative incidence of 24/1000 by age 20 which is 7.7 times the rate in the general population. Siblings with both HLA-haplotypes identical to their diabetic sib would have a cumulative incidence of 76/1000 by age 20, which is 25 times the risk in the general population.

Partial confirmation of this theoretical expectation was found in a study in Great Britain.[123] Perhaps due to some selection bias in their study sample and unjustified assumptions about the occurrence of diabetes in siblings, these authors estimated the cumulative incidence rate of IDDM in HLA identical siblings to be 300/1000 by age 30. This is far too high to be consistent with any empirical data on the occurrence of IDDM in siblings (see Table 2–6). Even if all secondary cases in these studies occurred among HLA identical siblings, the cumulative incidence by age 30 for them would be between 120 to 200/1000.

In another report from the same study, two of the previously reported secondary cases were HLA-A, B and C non-identical with the proband, but due to recombination, they were DR identical or DR haplo-identical.[119] If further substantiated, this unusual finding would suggest that HLA-DR identity is the important common factor rather than identity of the whole HLA haplotype and that DR 3 or DR 4 possibly play a direct role in the etiology of IDDM.

In *summary*, studies of HLA in relatives of patients wth IDDM, as well as in populations, concur in pointing to an association of this disease with two antigens, HLA-DR 3 and DR 4. Possibly, the antigens themselves may be directly involved in

the pathogenesis of IDDM. The fact that incidence rates for IDDM vary from country to country so much more than the frequencies of HLA-DR 3 and DR 4 phenotypes, suggests that the two DR antigens may play a permissive role rather than act alone. The other factor(s) responsible might be environmental in origin or another gene locus or loci. As far as the first possibility is concerned, support is found in two pieces of evidence; namely, large variability between countries and an increase in the occurrence of IDDM over time. Data on the familial occurrence of IDDM, on the other hand, favor the second possibility. Several genetic models have been proposed which allow for a second locus in addition to one associated with DR.[124-126] While these can fit or explain the available data on familial aggregation of IDDM, much more data (particularly in large pedigrees) will be required to choose a best model from among the alternatives. With regard to further research in this area, it is important to realize that the second locus is not necessarily linked to the HLA region.

EPIDEMIOLOGY OF NON-INSULIN-DEPENDENT DIABETES (NIDDM)

In this review, diabetes which occurs in adults will be considered as equivalent to NIDDM. This substitution of an age at diagnosis criterion for more specific classification criteria is a reasonable approximation since new cases of IDDM are rare, relative to NIDDM, in adult populations. According to a study of the population of Rochester, Minnesota, among new cases of diabetes occurring after the age of 30, less than 10% were treated with insulin and only half of these were diagnosed as IDDM.[8] Moreover, since the incidence of IDDM before age 30 is also low, prevalent cases of diabetes in age groups 30 years and older consist mainly of NIDDM. Insofar as possible, incidence data have been used, and prevalence rates resorted to only as confirmation of the incidence findings or as a substitute where incidence data were lacking.

Table 2–12. Estimated Risk of IDDM among Siblings of IDDM Probands According to the Number of HLA-haplotypes Shared with the Proband

Sibling's HLA-haplotype similarity to IDDM proband	Number of siblings[a]	Person-years of observation[a]	Number of siblings with IDDM[b]	Incidence rates per 1000 per year	Cumulative incidence rate by age 20 per 1000
Two identical	620	9976	38	3.81	76.2
One identical	1240	19952	24	1.20	24.0
Neither identical	620	9976	3	0.30	6.0
Total	2482[c]	39904[c]	65[c]	1.63	32.6

[a.] Expected distribution under assumption of random assortment of parental haplotypes in offspring.
[b.] Expected distribution for affected sib-pairs based on data in ref. 115.
[c.] Data from ref. 88.

Distribution According to Age, Sex, Method of Ascertainment and Diagnostic Criteria

Data are scarce on the incidence of NIDDM in the population below age 30. In the German Democratic Republic, where diabetes is a registered disease, the incidence rates of NIDDM in ages below 30 have been in the range of 5 to 30 per 100,000 per year.[21] Unfortunately, there is no procedure for verifying the diagnosis of reported cases. The new World Health Organization (WHO) criteria for a diagnosis of NIDDM were used in a study in Great Britain (Fig. 2–2) to determine the incidence rates for ages 18 to 35.[19] Rates much lower than in the GDR were found, ranging from 3 to 7/100,000 per year. These rates agree with the findings in Rochester, Minnesota.[8] The extent to which undiagnosed diabetes exists in this age group is unknown, as well as how long such cases would remain undiagnosed if they exist.

Table 2–13 summarizes data from several sources on the incidence of NIDDM in the adult white population of the U.S. according to age,

Table 2–13. Average Annual Incidence Rates of NIDDM per 100,000 in White Populations of the U.S. According to Age, Method of Ascertainment and Criteria for Diagnosis

Age group	Framingham, MA[a] 1954–1968	Health Interview Surveys[b] 1964, 1965, 1966	Rochester, MN[c] 1960–1969
20–29	—	73	19
30–39	—	112	74
40–49	230	248	173
50–59	465	454	348
60–69	604	570	640
70–79	939	572	673

Methods of Ascertainment and Criteria for Diagnosis

Framingham, MA
  The study population was screened every 2 years. Patients with a casual blood glucose ≥150 were referred to private physicians for confirmation of a diagnosis of diabetes. Physicians' diagnoses were accepted as final.
Health Interview Surveys
  All interviewees reporting that during the preceding 12 months a physician had given them a diagnosis of diabetes for the first time were considered new diagnoses of diabetes (incident cases)
Rochester, MN
  All diagnoses of diabetes during the study interval were identified in the medical records of the population of Rochester. Diagnoses in the records were considered valid only if they met specific criteria which resemble those of the NDDG.

  [a] Reanalysis of data in ref. 127 supplied by Peter W. Wilson, M.D.
  [b] Analysis of unpublished data in ref. 53 provided by Thomas F. Drury, Ph.D., National Center for Health Statistics.
  [c] Combined data for males and females in ref. 9.

method of ascertainment and criteria for the diagnosis of diabetes. The first set of rates came from 14 years of follow-up in the Framingham Study, a continuing prospective observation of about 5000 men and women. Individuals who fulfilled National Diabetes Data Group (NDDG) criteria for NIDDM or impaired glucose tolerance (IGT) were considered as incident cases of diabetes.[127] The rates increased from 230/100,000 per year at ages 40 to 49 to 939/100,000/year at ages 70 to 79 years. The second set of incidence rates came from the Health Interview Surveys, conducted by the National Center for Health Statistics in 1964, 1965 and 1966, of representative samples of the U.S. population.[53] Individuals who reported that during the preceding 12 months a physician had given them a diagnosis of diabetes for the first time were considered incident cases. As can be seen, the incidence rates based on the surveys were almost identical to those obtained in Framingham except for the oldest age group.

It is important to keep in mind that the diagnoses of cases identified in the surveys were not verified, and the Framingham cases were not analyzed separately for NIDDM and IGT. Indirect evidence of the relative contributions of IGT and NIDDM to these rates can be assessed by comparing these two sets of rates with the third set, which was obtained in a study of the residents of Rochester, Minnesota.[7,8] There, all new diagnoses of diabetes made by medical care providers were ascertained from medical records for the period 1945–1969, and the diagnoses were verified against criteria adopted for the study. Almost half of the cases in that community did not fulfill the requirements for a diagnosis by these criteria. The incidence rates shown in the table, based on the verified new cases which had occurred during the period 1960–1969,[8,9] were lower than the rates found in the other two studies. Subsequent examination of the Rochester data using NDDG criteria showed that 187 patients out of 1135 failed to meet these more stringent criteria.[9] If these cases are considered nondiabetics, then the differences between Rochester rates and the other two studies would be larger. These differences, which are largest below age 60, can be considered as an indirect measurement of the incidence of false positive diagnoses of diabetes and/or IGT in the white U.S. population.

Confirmation of this interpretation can be found in the results of the Rand Health Insurance Study.[128] Nearly 8000 people in 2750 families were enrolled in the study in six sites across the United States. The sites represent the four Census Regions of the country, and each was sampled to yield a mixture of urban and rural residents with over-sampling of low-income families. Each enrollee completed a

Medical History Questionnaire which (among other things) inquired about use of insulin or oral hypoglycemic agents and previous diagnosis of diabetes. A random sample of 3268 of the enrollees age 18 to 65 also underwent a screening examination with a glucose load. Some results of this study are summarized in Table 2–14. As can be seen, 1.26% of the group reported a prior diagnosis of diabetes and were taking some sort of treatment for it or, if not on treatment, had a high post-challenge blood glucose which was considered confirmation of the diagnosis. Age-specific prevalence rates of diabetes fulfilling these criteria ranged from 1.33 to 3.22% between ages 30 and 60. The rest of those who reported a diagnosis of diabetes (1.5% of the total group) did not have IGT, let alone diabetes, on the screening glucose challenge. On the other hand, 1.1% of the total group had evidence of undiagnosed impairment of glucose tolerance. The proportion of such patients increased with age from 0.61% in the age group 30 to 39 to 3.22% in the age group 50 to 59. Some of these individuals would have met NDDG criteria for NIDDM if the glucose challenge had been repeated.

In all the studies presented in Table 2–13, the incidence rates increased markedly with age, and if one takes the data for the Rochester population as the most reliable estimates of NIDDM incidence rates, then the increase between ages 25 and 75 is about 34-fold. The profound effect of age cannot be seen so clearly in analyzing prevalence data. Patients with an early age at diagnosis are selectively removed from the population by mortality after long durations of diabetes, so they do not contribute to the prevalence rates at older ages. The link between aging and the risk of NIDDM

Table 2–14. Prevalence of Diabetes Based on Medical History Questionnaire and Screening Examination[a]

Diabetic status	Number	Percent
Previous Diagnosis of Diabetes by Physician		
Confirmed	41	1.26
Unconfirmed[b]	49	1.50
Without previous diagnosis of diabetes		
Post Challenge Blood Glucose		
≥200 mg/dl	35	1.07
160–199 mg/dl	79	2.42
<160 mg/dl	3059	93.75
Total	3263	100.00

[a] Blood glucose determined in serum 2 hours post challenge with a dose of glucose based on estimated body surface area. Data from ref. 128.

[b] Among individuals not taking insulin or an oral agent, post challenge blood glucose <160 mg/dl.

should be taken into account in generating etiological hypotheses.

Another variable which is frequently discussed in the literature is the occurrence of diabetes according to sex. Although incidence rates for each sex separately were not shown in Table 2–13, age-specific rates for males in all three studies were higher than female rates until age 60. At older ages, female rates were similar or higher than males. Figure 2–5 shows age-specific prevalence rates of diagnosed diabetes as reported by a representative sample of the U.S. white population which was interviewed for the 1975 Health Interview Survey.[54] Prevalence rates for women and men were quite similar and showed the same pattern of increase with age. One must keep in mind the previous discussion which indicated that some part of the magnitude of these rates may represent IGT rather than NIDDM.

Variation over Time

The earliest population study of the occurrence of diabetes was conducted in Oxford, Massachusetts, in 1946.[129] A repeat survey conducted in 1963[130] showed no evidence of a change in the prevalence rate of diabetes for the middle-aged group. Individuals aged 34 to 55 at the second examination, who had been only 17 to 38 years old at the first examination 17 years earlier, had acquired a prevalence rate of diabetes by 1963 equal to that found in 1946 in individuals aged 34 to 55. In the study cited earlier from Rochester, Minnesota, of diabetes ascertained through medical care institutions, incidence rates for two time periods, 1945–1959 and 1960–1969, were compared in detail.[8] Incidence rates for the "severe" form of NIDDM were almost identical in the two time periods. There was, however, a significant increase of mild NIDDM and IGT in the later period.

The previously cited Health Interview Surveys conducted by the National Center for Health Statistics are another large data source which can be examined for changes in the incidence of diabetes. Incidence rates for diabetes were determined in representative samples of the U.S. population in 1964, 1965 and 1966[53] and again in similar samples in 1973 and 1975.[54] The results from these two periods, summarized in Table 2–15, show that diabetes was diagnosed almost twice as frequently in the 1970s as in the 1960s, regardless of age or race. This increase in the incidence of diabetes diagnoses resulted in a steady increase in the prevalence of diabetes in all age groups uniformly (Fig. 2–6).[131]

While this increased frequency of new diagnoses could reflect a real increase in the occurrence of diabetes, it could be partly or entirely an artifact.

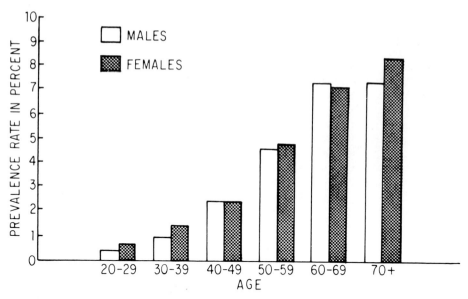

Fig. 2–5. Prevalence rates of diagnosed diabetes according to age as reported by a representative sample of the U.S. white population in the 1975 National Health Interview Survey. Rates were calculated from unpublished data provided by Thomas F. Drury, Ph.D., National Center for Health Statistics.[54]

Table 2–15. Incidence Rates per 100,000 of Diabetes Diagnosed in a 12-Month Interval as Reported in Interviews of Representative Samples of the U.S. Population in Two Time Periods According to Age and Race[a]

| | Whites
Health Interview Surveys | | Blacks
Health Interview Surveys | |
Age	1964–1966	1973, 1975	1964–1968	1973, 1975
20–29	73	114	89	210
30–39	112	240	190	387
40–49	248	312	347	760
50–59	454	580	697	852
60–69	570	818	693	724

[a] Computed from unpublished survey data supplied by Thomas F. Drury, Ph.D., National Center for Health Statistics (see refs. 53 and 54).

Increases in the frequency of diagnosis of diabetes could result from ascertainment of asymptomatic cases which had been overlooked previously or from a broadening of the criteria for the diagnosis to include lesser degrees of glucose intolerance. Before concluding that a real increase in the diabetes has occurred, one must exclude these other possibilities. During the 1960s, enthusiasm for screening and early diagnosis of asymptomatic diabetes on the basis of glucose tolerance tests was mounting.[132] This coincided with an increased use of batteries of laboratory tests due to the introduction of automated laboratory equipment, as well as increases in the utilization of medical facilities throughout the population. For example, in 1963–1964 about 64% of the middle-aged population visited a physician during a year,[133] while 10 years later 75% visited a physician at least once a year, and most made more than one visit.[134]

These factors could account for a substantial increase in the incidence of diagnoses of diabetes and, therefore, raise doubts about the conclusiveness of the evidence for an increase in the disease itself. These doubts are reinforced by the results of the two studies previously cited. In the Rand Study, half of the patients who reported a diagnosis of diabetes did not manifest glucose intolerance,[128] and in the Rochester study, insufficient evidence for a diagnosis of diabetes was found in the medical records of about half of the patients with that diagnosis.[7] Further evidence can be found in the Health Interview Surveys. For the diabetics identified by interview, tables showing their distribution according to age and type of hypoglycemic treatment were published for the 1965 survey[53] and again a decade later for the 1976 survey.[135] By combining this information with the age-specific prevalence rates for all diabetes, it was possible to calculate treatment-specific prevalence rates. The largest increase in the later survey was for diabetes treated with diet or by no treatment at all. The smallest increase was for diabetes treated by insulin.

In *summary*, there is evidence that the increase in the incidence and prevalence of NIDDM which has taken place over the last 20 years could be attributable to a broadening of diagnostic criteria and more complete ascertainment of cases. Evi-

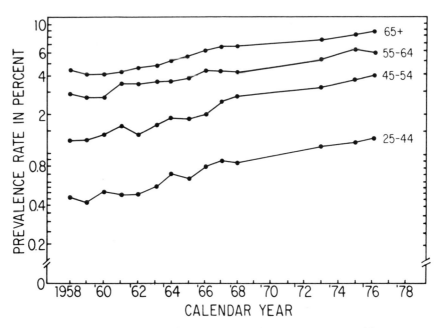

Fig. 2–6. Prevalence of diagnosed diabetes according to age and calendar year as reported by representative samples of the U.S. population, all races (Adapted from ref. 131).

dence for a real increase in the occurrence of NIDDM, then, remains in doubt.

The other studies[21,136] of variability in the occurrence of NIDDM over time have all suffered from the same drawbacks as the Health Interview Surveys which have already been discussed.

Ethnic and Geographic Distribution

Although the literature on geographic and ethnic differences in the occurrence of diabetes is enormous, much of it is unsuitable for examining the distribution of NIDDM. Earlier reports, particularly, were based on death certificate data rather than diagnoses, while other studies were based on non-random samples of the population or used glycosuria as a screening test. Also findings were often published only as crude rates rather than age-specific rates, so comparisons between countries with different age distributions cannot be made. During the last 2 decades, however, more accurate approaches have been used to determine the occurrence of diabetes in diverse populations around the world. While these provide a basis for comparative analysis, the findings must be interpreted cautiously due to the lack of a standardized definition of diabetes which can inflate or diminish true differences in disease frequency. Careful attention should be given to sample sizes, as well, since small samples give unreliable rates. In order to focus consideration on geographic and ethnic differences specifically, the following discussion concentrates on (but is not limited to) prevalence and

incidence rates for urban, middle-aged men because information is extensive for this particular category.

Incidence rates of NIDDM in the United States and various other countries are summarized in Table 2–16 according to the method of case ascertainment and the criteria used for a diagnosis of diabetes. In the upper half of the table are rates based on cases ascertained through diagnoses in medical records, while in the lower half the rates are based on systematic screening so that undiagnosed cases were ascertained as well. The incidence rate for cases diagnosed by physicians was several times higher in the United States than in two European countries. In the screened populations, the rates were higher but the difference between the United States and Scandinavian countries persisted. Higher rates were found in Israel, and extremely high rates in unusual populations such as the Pima Indians of Arizona and the Micronesians of Nauru. The relatively high incidence found in Israel perhaps resulted from the use of very sensitive but non-specific criteria for evaluating the glucose tolerance tests. While these results may not be comparable with those for U.S. men for this reason, they can be used for comparisons among groups in Israel.[141] The investigators found, for example, that men born in Asia had twice the incidence of diabetes as those born in Central and Eastern Europe. Those born in Southern Europe or Africa had rates in between.

Prevalence rates of NIDDM in the United States

Table 2–16. Incidence Rates per 1000 per year of NIDDM in Middle-aged Men as Obtained in Various Studies According to Diagnostic Criteria and Ascertainment Method

Population	Age group 40–49	Age group 50–59	Criteria for Diagnosis	Method of Ascertainment
Whites, U.S. National Health Survey, 1964–66[b]	2.9	4.4	physician's diagnosis	interview, no verification
Blacks, U.S. National Health Survey, 1964–66[b]	2.0	5.4	physician's diagnosis	interview, no verification
Rochester, Minn. 1960–69[9]	1.9	5.0	verified physician's diagnosis	medical records
Edinburgh, U.K. 1965–69[136]	0.8	1.6	physician's diagnosis	medical records
Oslo, Norway 1961–64[137]	0.3	0.7	physician's diagnosis	medical records
Periodic Health Exam. Pennsylvania, 1951–64[138]	4.9	8.5	fasting BG ≥130 mg/dl	periodic examination
Framingham, Mass. 1954–68[c]	3.0	5.7	casual BG ≥150 mg/dl then non-specific[a]	biennial screening
Goteborg, Sweden 1963–73[139]	—	2.8	—	occupational screening
Oslo, Norway 1960–69[140]	1.2		—	occupational screening
Israel 1963–68[141]	6.0	10.0	casual BG≥130 mg/dl then non-specific[a]	re-examination after 2.5 and 5 years
Nauru, Micronesia 1975–79[142]	15.1	40.5	2-h post glucose BG≥200 mg/dl	re-examination after 5 years
Pima Indians, Ariz. 1964–75[143]	57.0	49.9	2-h post glucose BG≥200 mg/dl	biennial examination

[a] "non-specific" refers to criteria which, according to NDDG criteria, includes some IGT.
[b] Analysis of unpublished data in ref. 53 provided by Thomas F. Drury, Ph.D., National Center for Health Statistics.
[c] Reanalysis of data in ref. 127 supplied by Peter W. Wilson, M.D.

and various other populations are summarized in Table 2–17. Those obtained in several studies in the United States during the 1970s were among the highest. In contrast, European rates were half or less than U.S. rates even though less specific diagnostic criteria were used in the European studies. This substantial variability in the occurrence of diabetes among Caucasians points to an environmental component in the development of diabetes in this race.

In Asia, Japanese men had a prevalence rate of diabetes similar to that of men on the Kamchatka Peninsula in the Soviet Union. Interestingly, studies of Japanese migrants to Hawaii have found much higher prevalence rates, approaching those in the U.S. population.[157,158] A very low prevalence of diabetes was observed in China.[65] This characteristic of the Chinese population can be seen in other countries where they have immigrated. In a large study conducted in Singapore, the Chinese population had the lowest prevalence of diabetes, while the Indian population had the highest.[159] Unfortunately, the results of that study cannot be compared directly with other studies of these ethnic groups. A high prevalence rate for Indians can be seen in Table 2–17. In a large study conducted in the western part of India, the prevalence rates obtained were the highest among Asian countries. The criteria for a diagnosis of diabetes in that study, however, were very sensitive and non-specific. Nonetheless, significant variablility within India

was found in a study using the same criteria.[160] Men in New Delhi had a prevalence only one-fifth that shown in the table, and intermediate values were found in four cities in other parts of the country. Indian immigrants in other countries are characterized by high prevalence rates of diabetes.[159,161,162] How these prevalence rates in Indian migrants compare with the region from which they emigrated is unknown.

Another ethnic group which appears to have high prevalence rates of diabetes are Arabs. Prevalence rates for diabetes in Saudi Arabia and Tunis are similar to U.S. rates even though relatively restrictive criteria were used for diagnosis. In a study conducted in Kuwait, where only diagnosed diabetes was ascertained, the prevalence rate for this age group was 6.6% for Kuwaiti and 6.8% for non-Kuwaiti.[165] In the latter group, Egyptians and Indians had particularly high prevalence rates.

Information is particularly scarce regarding the occurrence of NIDDM in Africa. The available data[166–168] are not sufficient to draw any conclusions about its occurrence in the black populations of Africa. Some data are available, however, on black populations in the Western Hemisphere. As was shown in Table 2–15, diabetes is significantly more frequent in U.S. blacks than in U.S. whites. It is worth noting that this difference exists despite the fact that blacks are less frequent users of medical care than whites in this country.[133,134] There have been no studies of screened populations of blacks

Table 2–17. Prevalence Rates (Percents) of Diabetes, Ascertained by Screening,[a] in Middle-aged Men as Obtained in Various Studies According to Diagnostic Criteria

Population	Age group 40–49	Age group 50–59	Date of Study	Verification of known cases	Criteria for detected cases
United States					
Oxford, MA*†[144]	3.9	4.4	1947	yes	intermediate
Sudbury, MA*†[144]	2.9	3.6	1964	yes	intermediate
Tecumseh, MI[146]	9.4	9.0	1971	—	non-specific[b]
Rancho Bernardo, CA[145]	8.6	14.1	1972–74	—	FBG > 140 mg/dl[b]
Rand, random sample of US†[128]	4.1	6.4	1974–75	yes	intermediate[b]
HANES II, a random sample of US*[147]	7.5	7.7	1976–80	—	specific[b]
Europe					
Reykjavik, Iceland[c]	1.3	3.5	1967–68	—	specific
Bergen, Norway[149,150]	0.9	2.4	1956	—	non-specific
Glostrup, Denmark[151,152]		2.6	1964	—	FBG ≥ 130 mg/dl[b]
Lodz, Poland†[153]		2.3	1973	—	non-specific
Dushambe, USSR†[154]	1.1	3.7	1970	—	non-specific
Asia					
Kamchatka, USSR[155]	1.8	4.3	1971–79	—	non-specific
Tokyo, Japan[156]	2.3	5.1	1973	—	non-specific
Shanghai, China[65]	1.3	2.5	1979	—	intermediate
Ahmedabad, India, urban area[160]	4.6	13.6	1975	—	non-specific
Middle East and North Africa					
Al-Kharj, Saudi Arabia*[163]		9.6	1980	—	specific
Tunisia, random sample[164]	4.9	9.0	1977	—	FBG > 150 mg/dl[b]
Black Populations in Africa and Elsewhere					
Cape Town, South Africa[166]		8.0	1969	yes	intermediate
Trinidad[162]	2.5	2.6	1961–62	—	GTT in glucosurics
Lawrence Tavern, Jamaica*[169]	14.5	10.6	1969	—	non-specific

*Age groups 45–54, 55–64.
†Males and females.
[a] In most studies, screening was performed in two stages; e.g., a casual blood glucose followed by a glucose tolerance test (GTT) for those with high values. The GTT criteria have been labeled "specific" if they resemble NDDG criteria, or "non-specific" if they resemble criteria which include IGT. Some studies used criteria which were "intermediate."
[b] Only first screening test used; no confirmatory test.
[c] Reanalysis of data in ref. 148 supplied by Gunnar Sigurdsson, M.D.

to assess precisely the magnitude of diabetes prevalence or its determinants.

There have been, however, many studies of the occurrence of NIDDM among American Indians (for a review see reference 170). These have shown enormous variability from very low rates in certain tribes[171,172] to those for the Pimas of Arizona, the highest rates known.[143]

In *summary*, large variability in the occurrence of NIDDM between countries and within racial or ethnic groups points to an important role for environmental factors as determinants of the development of NIDDM.

Distribution According to Obesity

Obesity is such a common condition that patients with diabetes may also be obese just by coincidence. As early as 1921, Dr. Elliott P. Joslin was the first to suggest that the association between diabetes and obesity was more than coincidence.[173] Unfortunately, his study suffered from certain

methodologic shortcomings, so he overestimated the excess occurrence of obesity in diabetics relative to nondiabetics. Summarized in Table 2–18 is a methodologically correct analysis which is similar to that proposed by Dr. Joslin. The data on diabetic patients were collected between 1957 and 1963[174] and, together with Framingham Heart Study data,[175] were analyzed for the purposes of this chapter. This case-control analysis shows that newly diagnosed diabetics had a higher prevalence of obesity than an age-matched comparison group of nondiabetics in Framingham. The relative risks shown in the table measure the excess risk of acquiring diabetes in the various categories of obesity relative to the risk in non-obese individuals. Thus, individuals with a Framingham relative weight of 120% or greater (corresponding to a relative weight of 140% or more of ideal body weight according to the 1959 Metropolitan Life Insurance Tables) had a risk of diabetes 2.3 times higher than individuals with Framingham relative weights of 90 to

Table 2–18.   Relative Risk[a] of Diabetes According to Degree of Obesity Estimated from the Distribution of Relative Weight[b] in Diabetics at Diagnosis[c] (Aged 45–59) and a Random Sample of the Population of Framingham[d] (Aged 45–59)

Framingham Relative Weight	Diabetics		Controls		Relative risk
	No.	%	No.	%	
<90	246	19.3	359	15.0	1.83
90–99	216	17.0	580	24.2	1.00
100–109	273	21.4	638	26.7	1.15
110–119	202	15.9	416	17.4	1.30
120+	337	26.5	400	16.7	2.26
Total	1274	100.0	2393	100.0	

[a] Relative risk for each weight category was calculated with the "90–99" category as the reference group using the odds ratio (see ref. 1, page 273, for definition).

[b] Framingham Relative Weight (see ref. 181 for derivation).

[c] Patients first seen at Joslin Clinic (1957–1963) within 1 year of diagnosis in ref. 174.

[d] Data from ref. 175.

99%. It has been well documented that many patients who develop diabetes have had some weight loss in the period before diagnosis. Taking this into account, the estimates of relative risk for obese individuals in Table 2–18 should be viewed as conservative. Presumably, such weight loss before diagnosis accounts for the observation of an excess number of diabetics among underweight individuals.

Evidence of this association has been found in many cross-sectional studies.[65,160,176] Figure 2–7 shows an example from the Health Interview Survey of a representative sample of the U.S. population in 1976. In addition to questions on the occurrence of diabetes, surveyed individuals were asked for their height and weight.[177] These were used to group individuals into three categories according to their body mass index, a measure of obesity. Prevalence rates of diagnosed diabetes were calculated for age-and-sex-specific categories. Among young adults, NIDDM was frequent only among the most obese. Prevalence rates increased with age, but in each age group, they also increased markedly with obesity. In each category blacks had higher prevalence rates than whites, but the pattern was the same for the two races. These prevalence rates are underestimates for obese individuals and overestimates for non-obese for the same reason discussed with regard to Table 2–18. Some proportion of these reported diagnoses represents IGT rather than NIDDM, but there is no way to assess how that proportion varies with age or sex.

A relationship between obesity and the devel-

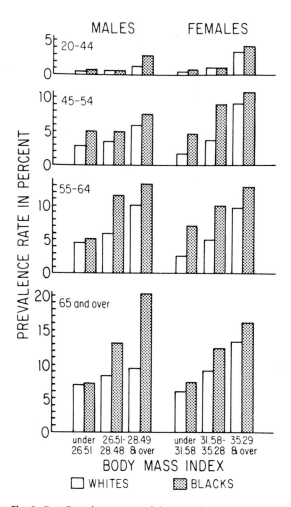

Fig. 2–7.   Prevalence rates of diagnosed diabetes according to age, sex, race and obesity as reported by representative sample of the U.S. population in the 1976 National Health Interview Survey (Adapted from ref. 177).

opment of NIDDM has also been found in prospective studies. The first was a follow-up of 13,148 middle-aged men participating in a periodic health examination program between 1950 and 171964.[178] Men with body weight 125% or more of ideal according to Metropolitan Life Insurance Standards had a risk of developing diabetes 1.5 times higher than those with weights less than 110% of ideal. Other prospective studies have yielded higher relative risks. For example, in a 10-year-follow-up of middle-aged men in Oslo, Norway, moderate obesity at the beginning of the study increased the risk of diabetes severalfold, while severe obesity increased the risk by a factor of twelve relative to non-obese individuals.[140] The number of cases in this study was small, however, so the estimates are imprecise. In the prospective studies of diabetes in Pima Indians, the incidence of NIDDM was strongly related to preceding obesity, increasing steadily from 10.9 cases/1000 person years for subjects with body mass index of 20–25 to 72.2 cases/1000 person years for those with a body mass index of 40 or more.[179] The relationship between relative weight and diabetes risk was investigated further in a population study in Tecumseh, Michigan.[180] In addition to finding a relationship between relative weight and risk of diabetes, the authors suggested that risk is related also to a centralized pattern of fat distribution, as indicated by subscapular skinfold thickness. It should be noted, however, that the relationship with skinfold measurements was stronger among men than women and stronger below age 55 than at older ages. These younger segments of the population were probably more muscular, so body mass index would not have been as good an indicator of obesity as a direct measure of skinfold thickness. Thus, these results could be interpreted as supporting nothing more than the superiority of skinfold thickness as a measure of obesity, particularly at younger ages. Furthermore, the Tecumseh data show a similar relationship with triceps skinfold thickness which does not support their hypothesis of a special role for central fatness.

No other prospective studies have elaborated further the nature of the relationship between obesity and the development of NIDDM. Specifically, it is not known whether the onset of obesity in childhood has the same impact as obesity which appears later in life. Is there an age at which excess weight gain is particularly dangerous? How long must it be present in order to have a significant effect?

The finding that obesity is an important risk factor for NIDDM suggests that some of the variation in the occurrence of NIDDM according to age, race, nationality and time might be due to variation in the occurrence of obesity. Prevalence rates of diagnosed diabetes increase with age, independently of obesity, as shown in Figure 2–7. However, the increase is less than that shown in Figure 2–5. The discrepancy results from the fact that the prevalence of obesity also increases with age as shown in Table 2–19. This table also shows that the prevalence of obesity in the United States did not increase between 1961 and 1973, so the huge increase in the incidence and prevalence of diagnosed diabetes during that interval cannot be attributed to increased obesity. Figure 2–7 also shows that blacks have higher prevalence rates of diabetes than whites, even after controlling for age and body mass index. West and Kalbfleisch showed that some of the international variation in diabetes prevalence rates could be explained by differences in obesity.[182] However, not all differences can be explained by variability in the prevalence of obesity.

Table 2–19. Prevalence of Obesity Defined as Weight Exceeding 120% of Desirable Weight[a] in Two Time Periods According to Age and Sex (Data from U.S. Health Examination Survey 1960–62 and Health and Nutrition Examination Survey 1971–74)[b]

	Men		Women	
Age	1960–62 %	1971–74 %	1960–62 %	1971–74 %
25–34	13.3	13.6	14.8	17.1
35–44	14.9	17.0	23.2	24.3
45–54	16.7	15.8	28.9	27.8
55–64	15.8	15.1	38.6	34.7
65–74	14.6	13.4	38.8	31.5

[a] Estimated from regression equation of weight on height for men and women ages 20–29 years, obtained from Health and Nutrition Examination Survey 1971–74.

[b] Data for this table were selected from Table 2 on page 5 of ref. 181.

For example, prevalence rates of diabetes in Poland are about one-third those in the United States, although the relative weight distributions for the two countries are similar.[183] The same can be found in a comparison between Denmark,[152] for example, and the United States.[184] Also the study of diabetes in Israel found that the differences in the incidence of diabetes between men born in Eastern Europe and men born in Asia persisted after adjustment for body mass index.[141]

Other Factors Related to the Distribution of NIDDM

In addition to the factors previously discussed, many studies have found lower prevalence rates of diabetes in rural populations than among urban dwellers. This difference has been seen regardless of the method of ascertaining cases or the criteria used for diagnosis.[160,185–192] Unfortunately, in most of these studies, the authors did not take into account differences between urban and rural populations in the prevalence of obesity. However, in two studies which compared urban and rural populations this difference persisted after controlling for sex, age, and obesity. In Polynesians of Western Samoa, marked differences in the prevalence of abnormal glucose tolerance were seen after age and weight standardization.[191] A study of diabetes in Puerto Rican men revealed prevalence rates in urban areas that were twice those in rural areas.[192] Comparisons within age-specific groups showed a higher prevalence of diabetes among lean urban dwellers than among lean rural dwellers, but among obese individuals, there was no urban-rural difference.

These findings suggest that some aspect of urban living, operating independently of obesity, contributes to a higher prevalence of diabetes. An effect of exercise might be responsible for the lower occurrence of diabetes in rural males. There are, however, scant population data on this issue. Diet is another factor which should be considered as a possible explanation for urban/rural differences, as well as international variation. This issue was reviewed by West[193] who considered the evidence inconclusive. Given the cross-sectional nature of the studies, the non-specificity of the diagnoses of diabetes and the crude data on nutrient intake used in the literature, one must conclude that the question has not been addressed adequately. Extensive population studies in India found that the rural population, which has a low prevalence of diabetes, also has a high intake of carbohydrates.[160] Moreover, studies of Japanese migrants to Hawaii are of interest as far as the role of diet is concerned. Diabetes prevalence in the Japanese of Hawaii is significantly higher than in the Japanese of Hiroshima after adjustment for age and body weight.[157,158] Dietary intake of animal protein, animal fat and simple carbohydrates was higher, and that of complex carbohydrates lower, in migrants than in Hiroshima subjects. Moreover, serum insulin levels were significantly higher in migrants (diabetic and nondiabetic) than in Hiroshima subjects. In migrants, serum insulin levels were unrelated to physical activity, strengthening the possibility that they might be due to dietary factors. It is not known what nutrient(s) in the diet were responsible for the higher insulin levels in the migrants. Possibly, over a long period of time, their diet composition may have caused an increased insulin resistance in peripheral tissues and subsequently a higher prevalence of diabetes.

Another characteristic of the migrants was that in the period after their migration they were poor and engaged in hard labor. After the end of World War II their standard of living improved rapidly, a history which has been noted in some other populations which have a high prevalence of NIDDM.[194]

It is worthwhile to consider whether the mechanisms underlying this phenomenon are also responsible for variability in the prevalence of NIDDM in the U.S. according to socio-economic status. Figure 2–8 shows prevalence rates of diagnosed diabetes (reported in interviews of a representative sample of the U.S. population for the 1976 Health Interview Survey) according to level of education, separately for whites and blacks. Prevalence rates are lower in people with higher education, regardless of sex or obesity, and the difference is more evident in whites than blacks. The same pattern was found among young as well as older individuals. Similar results were obtained

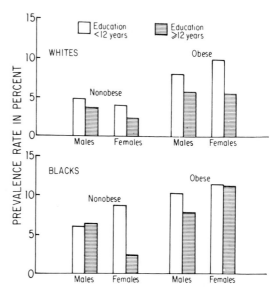

Fig. 2–8. Prevalence rates of diagnosed diabetes in the age group 45–64 according to sex, race, obesity and years of education as reported by a representative sample of the U.S. population in the 1976 National Health Interview Survey. Rates were calculated from unpublished data provided by Thomas F. Drury, Ph.D, National Center for Health Statistics.[54]

when the sample was stratified by income level instead of education. The true differences could be larger since the chance of a diagnosis being made might have been higher for the educated than the uneducated. A similar relationship with education was found in the incidence study in Israel[141] and in the population of Tecumseh, Michigan.[180] Also cross-sectional studies of Oklahoma Indians have found an inverse relationship between the prevalence of diabetes and years of schooling.[195] There is no obvious explanation for this association with level of education, but diabetes is not the only disease which is inversely related to education or income level. Low levels of education or income are associated with higher incidence and prevalence rates for hypertension as well.[196–200]

These observations point to some factors, independent of age and obesity, which increase the occurrence of NIDDM. They might be related to some nutrients or to unknown characteristics of a population in transition from one lifestyle to another. In the U.S. population they are associated with low educational level or low socio-economic status.

REFERENCES

1. MacMahon, B., Pugh, T.F.: Epidemiology, Principles and Methods. Boston, Little, Brown & Co., 1970, pp.1 and 241–282.
2. Joslin, E.P., Dublin, L.I., Marks, H.H.: Studies in diabetes mellitus. I. Characteristics and trends of diabetes

mortality throughout the world. Am. J. Med. Sci. *186*:753, 1933.

3. Joslin, E.P., Dublin, L.I., Marks, H.H.: Studies in diabetes mellitus. II. Its incidence and the factors underlying its variance. Am. J. Med. Sci. *187*:433, 1934.

4. West, K.M.: Epidemiology of Diabetes and its Vascular Lesions. New York, Elsevier North-Holland, Inc. 1978, p. 159–189.

5. Tokuhata, G.K., Miller, W., Digon, E., et al.: Diabetes mellitus: An underestimated health problem. J. Chron. Dis. *28*:23, 1975.

6. Fuller, J.H., Elford, J., Goldblatt, P., Adelstein, A.M.: Diabetes mortality: New light on an underestimated public health problem. Diabetologia *24*:336, 1983.

7. Palumbo, P.J., Labarthe, D.R.: The incidence of diabetes mellitus in Rochester, Minnesota, 1945–1969. In: R. Levine and R. Luft (eds.): Advances in Metabolic Disorders. Vol. 9. New York, Academic Press, 1978, pp. 13–28.

8. Melton, L.J., Palumbo, P.J., Chu, C.: Incidence of diabetes mellitus by clinical type. Diabetes Care *6*:75, 1983.

9. Melton, L.J., Palumbo, P.J., Dwyer, M.S., Chu, C.: Impact of recent changes in diagnostic criteria on the apparent natural history of diabetes mellitus. Am. J. Epidemiol. *117*:559, 1983.

10. Miettinen, O.: Estimability and estimation in case-referent studies. Am. J. Epidemiol. *103*:226, 1976.

11. Merrell, M., Shulman, L.E.: Determination of prognosis in chronic disease, illustrated by systemic lupus erythematosus. J. Chron. Dis. *1*:12, 1955.

12. West, K.M.: Epidemiology of Diabetes and its Vascular Lesions. New York, Elsevier North-Holland, Inc. 1978, p. 67–126.

13. Massari, V., Eschwege, E., Valleron, A.J.: Imprecision of new criteria for the oral glucose tolerance test. Diabetologia *24*:100, 1983.

14. West, K.M.: Substantial differences in the diagnostic criteria used by diabetes experts. Diabetes *24*:641, 1975.

15. National Diabetes Data Group: Classification and diagnosis of diabetes mellitus and other categories of glucose intolerance. Diabetes *28*:1039, 1979.

16. WHO Expert Committee on Diabetes Mellitus. Second Report. Geneva, World Health Organization, 1980, Technical Report Series 646.

17. Christy, M., Green, A., Christau, B., et al.: Epidemiologic studies of insulin-dependent diabetes mellitus. Diabetes Care *2*:127, 1979.

18. Christau, B., Kromann, H., Christy, M., et al.: Incidence of insulin-dependent diabetes mellitus (0–29 years at onset) in Denmark. Acta Med. Scand. Suppl. *62*:54, 1979.

19. Barker, D.J., Gardner, M.J., Power, C.: Incidence of diabetes amongst people aged 18–50 years in nine British towns: A collaborative study. Diabetologia *22*:421, 1982.

20. Gamble, D.R.: The epidemiology of insulin dependent diabetes, with particular reference to the relationship of virus infection to its etiology. Epidemiologic Reviews *2*:49, 1980.

21. Michaelis, D., Heinke, P., Albrecht, G., Jutzi, E.: Prevalence and incidence rates of type 1 diabetes in GDR during a period of 16 years. Abstract presented at 16th Annual Meeting of European Diabetes Epidemiology Study Group. 1981, Visegrad, Hungary. See also Diabetologia *19*:299, 1980. (And personal communication.)

22. Patterson, C.C., Thorogood, M., Smith, P.G., et al.: Epidemiology of type 1 (insulin dependent) diabetes in Scotland 1968–1976: Evidence of an increasing incidence. Diabetologia *24*:238, 1983.

23. LaPorte, R.E., Fishbein, H.A., Drash, A.L., et al.: The Pittsburgh insulin-dependent diabetes mellitus (IDDM)

registry. The incidence of insulin-dependent diabetes mellitus in Allegheny County, Pennsylvania (1965–1976). Diabetes *30*:279, 1981.

24. Reunanen, A., Akerblom, H.K., Kaar, M.L.: Prevalence and ten-year (1970–1979) incidence of insulin-dependent diabetes mellitus in children and adolescents in Finland. Acta Paediatr. Scand. *71*:893, 1982.

25. Christau, B., Molbak, A.G.: Incidence of insulin dependent diabetes mellitus in groups older than 30 years. Abstract presented at 16th Annual Meeting of European Diabetes Epidemiology Study Group, 1981, Visegrad, Hungary. See also Diabetologia *23*:160, 1982.

26. Krolewski, A.S.: Morbidity and mortality due to coronary heart disease among diabetics according to methods of hypoglycemic treatment. Doctoral thesis, Medical Academy, Warsaw, Poland, 1977.

27. Green, A., Hauge, M., Holm, N.V., Rasch, L.L.: Epidemiological studies of diabetes mellitus in Denmark. II. A prevalence study based on insulin prescriptions. Diabetologia *20*:468, 1981.

28. Hamblen, A.D., Joslin, E.P.: Deaths from diabetes in Massachusetts, 1900–1925. J.A.M.A. *88*:243, 1927.

29. Spiegelman, M., Marks, H.H.: Age and sex variations in the prevalence and onset of diabetes mellitus. Am. J. Pub. Health *36*:26, 1946.

30. Sultz, H.A., Schlesinger, E.R., Mosher, W.E.: The Erie County survey of long-term childhood illness: II. Incidence and prevalence. Am. J. Publ. Health *58*:491, 1968.

31. Sultz, H.A., Schlesinger, E.R., Mosher, W.E., Feldman, J.G.: Long-term childhood illness. Pittsburgh, University of Pittsburgh Press, 1972, pp. 223–248.

32. North, A.F., Jr., Gorwitz, K., Sultz, H.A.: A secular increase in the incidence of juvenile diabetes mellitus. J. Pediatr. *91*:706, 1977.

33. Somersalo, O.: Studies of childhood diabetes. I. Incidence in Finland. Ann. Paediatr. Fenn. *1*:239, 1955.

34. Adams, S.F.: The seasonal variation in the onset of acute diabetes. Arch. Intern. Med. *37*:861, 1926.

35. Gleason, R.E., Kahn, C.B., Funk, I.B., Craighead, J.E.: Seasonal incidence of insulin-dependent diabetes (IDDM) in Massachusetts, 1964–1973. Int. J. Epid. *11*:39, 1982.

36. Fleegler, F.M., Rogers, K.D., Drash, A., et al.: Age, sex, and season of onset of juvenile diabetes in different geographic areas. Pediatrics *63*:374, 1979.

37. West, R., Belmonte, M.M., Colle, E., et al.: Epidemiologic survey of juvenile-onset diabetes in Montreal. Diabetes *28*:690, 1979.

38. Gamble, D.R., Taylor, K.W.: Seasonal incidence of diabetes mellitus. Br. Med. J. *3*:631, 1969.

39. Bloom, A., Hayes, T.M., Gamble, D.R.: Register of newly diagnosed diabetic children. Br. Med. J. *3*:580, 1975.

40. Gray, R.S., Duncan, L.J.P., Clark, B.F.: Seasonal onset of insulin dependent diabetes in relation to sex and age at onset. Diabetologia *17*:29, 1979.

41. Sterky, G., Holmgren, G., Gustavson,, K.H., et al.: The incidence of diabetes mellitus in Swedish children 1970–1975. Acta Paediatr. Scand. *67*:139, 1978.

42. Crossley, J.R., Upsdell, M.: The incidence of juvenile diabetes mellitus in New Zealand. Diabetologia *18*:29, 1980.

43. Durruty, P., Ruiz, F., Garcia de los Rios, M.: Age at diagnosis and seasonal variation in the onset of insulin-dependent diabetes in Chile (Southern Hemisphere). Diabetologia *17*:357, 1979.

44. Diaz, O., Carvajal, F., Paz, M.P., et al.: Variaciones estacionales del debut de la diabetes mellitus an menores de 15 anos. Cuba 1980. Abstracts of the 1st National

Congress of Endocrinology, Havana, Cuba, December 9–12, 1981. (Also personal communication.)

45. Kitagawa, T., Owada, M., Mano, T., Fujita, H.: The epidemiology of childhood diabetes mellitus in the Tokyo metropolitan area. In: J.S. Melish, J. Hanna, S. Baba, (eds.): Genetic Environmental Interaction in Diabetes Mellitus. Proceedings of the Third Symposium on Diabetes Mellitus in Asia and Oceania, Honolulu, February 6–7, 1981. Amsterdam, Excerpta Medica, 1982, pp. 45–50.

46. Hazoury, B.J., Estrada, M.M., Nunez, M., et al.: Epidemiologia de la diabetes juvenil (Tipo 1) en Santo Domingo, R.D. Inden 6:33, 1981.

47. Lestradet, H., Besse, J.: Prevalence et incidence du diabete juvenile insulino-dependant en France. Diabete Metab. 3:229, 1977.

48. Ehrlich, R.M., Walsh, L.J., Falk, J.A., et al.: The incidence of type 1 (insulin-dependent) diabetes in Toronto. Diabetologia 22:289, 1982.

49. Joner, G., and Sovik, O.: Incidence, age at onset and seasonal variation of diabetes mellitus in Norwegian children 1973–1977. Acta Paediatr. Scand. 70:329, 1981.

50. Dahlquist, G., Gustavsson, K.H., Holmgren, G., et al.: The incidence of diabetes mellitus in Swedish children 0–14 years of age. A prospective study 1977–1980. Acta Paediatr. Scand. 71:7, 1982.

51. Cohen, T.: Juvenile diabetes in Israel. Israel J. Med. Sci. 7:1558, 1971.

52. Cohen, T.: Trends in frequency of juvenile diabetes mellitus in Israel. Israel J. Med. Sci. 8:844, 1972.

53. Characteristics of persons with diabetes, United States, July 1964–June 1965. U.S. Public Health Service, National Center for Health Statistics. PHS Publ. No. 1000 Ser. 10, No. 40, Washington, D.C., U.S. Government Printing Office, 1967 (Also unpublished data from surveys conducted between July 1965–June 1966 and between July 1966–June 1967).

54. Prevalence of chronic conditions of the genitourinary, nervous, endocrine, metabolic, and blood and blood forming systems and of other selected chronic conditions, United States, 1973. U.S. Public Health Service, National Center for Health Statistics. PHS Publ. No. (HRA)77–1536, Ser. 10, No. 109, Washington, D.C., U.S. Government Printing Office, 1977. (Also unpublished data from surveys conducted in 1975 and 1976).

55. Hagglof, B., Holmgren, G., Wall, S.: Incidence of insulin-dependent diabetes mellitus among children in a North-Swedish population 1938–1982. Hum. Hered. 32:408, 1982.

56. Christau, B., Kromann, A.H., Anderson, O., et al.: Incidence, seasonal and geographical patterns of juvenile onset insulin-dependent diabetes mellitus in Denmark. Diabetologia 13:281, 1977.

57. Lester, F.T.: Juvenile diabetes mellitus in Ethiopians. Trans. R. Soc. Trop. Med. Hyg. 73:663, 1978.

58. Lester, F.T.: The clinical pattern of diabetes mellitus in Ethiopians. Abstracts of the 11th Congress of the International Diabetes Federation, Nairobi, Kenya, 1982. Amsterdam, Excerpta Medica, 1982, p.76.

59. Gicheru, K., Gitau, W.: Control parameters in diabetes mellitus. East African Med. J. 56:631, 1979.

60. Thomas, S.E.: A review of diabetic hyperglycaemic comas—Kenyatta National Hospital 1978–1980, East African Med. J. 57:877, 1980.

61. Tandhanand, S., Inthuprapa, M.: Diabetic ketoacidosis in the tropics. In: W.K. Waldhausl (ed.): Diabetes 1979. Proceedings of the 10th Congress of the International Diabetes Federation. Amsterdam, Excerpta Medica, 1980, pp. 812–815.

62. Seshiah, V., Sundaram, A., Hariharan, R.S., et al.: Heterogeneity of diabetes mellitus in the young in Madras, South India. Abstracts of the 11th Congress of the International Diabetes Federation, Nairobi, Kenya, 1982. Amsterdam, Excerpta Medica, 1982, p. 79.

63. Asmal, A.C., Jialal, I., Leary, W.P., et al.: Insulin-dependent diabetes mellitus with early onset in Blacks and Indians. S. Afr. Med. J. 60:91, 1981.

64. Omar, M.A.K., Asmal, A.C.: Clinical pattern of diabetes mellitus in young Africans and Indians in Natal. Abstracts of the 11th Congress of the International Diabetes Federation, Nairobi, Kenya, 1982. Amsterdam, Excerpta Medica, 1982, p. 78.

65. Shanghai Diabetes Research Cooperative Group: Diabetes mellitus survey in Shanghai. Chinese Med. J. 93:663, 1980.

66. Miki, E., Maruyama, H.: Childhood diabetes mellitus in Japan. In: S. Tsuji, M. Wada (eds.): Diabetes Mellitus in Asia. Proceedings of a Symposium, Kobe, Japan, 1970. Amsterdam, Excerpta Medica International Congress Series No. 221, 1971, pp. 69–75.

67. Zhao Tong-mao, Chi Zhi-sheng, Wang Heng, et al.: HLA and diabetes mellitus in Chinese. Chinese Med. J.95:609, 1982.

68. MacDonald, M.J.: Hypothesis: the frequencies of juvenile diabetes in American blacks and caucasians are consistent with dominant inheritance. Diabetes 29:110, 1980.

69. Cudworth, A.G., Wolf, E.: The genetic susceptibility to type 1 (insulin-dependent) diabetes mellitus. Clin. Endocrinol. Metab. 11:389, 1982.

70. Colle, E., Siemiatycki, J., West, R., et al.: Incidence of juvenile onset diabetes in Montreal—demonstration of ethnic differences and socio-economic class differences. J. Chron. Dis. 34:611, 1981.

71. LaPorte, R.E., Orchard, T.J., Kuller, L.H., et al.: The Pittsburgh insulin dependent diabetes mellitus registry. The relationship of insulin dependent diabetes mellitus incidence to social class. Am. J. Epidemiol. 114:379, 1981.

72. Craighead, J.E.: Viral diabetes mellitus in man and experimental animals. Am. J. Med. 70:127, 1981.

73. Gamble, D.R., Kinsley, M.L., Fitzgerald, M.G., et al.: Viral antibodies in diabetes mellitus. Br. Med. J. 3:627,1969.

74. Gamble, D.R., Taylor, K.W., Cumming, H.: Coxsackie viruses and diabetes mellitus. Br. Med. J. 4:260, 1973.

75. Andersen, O.O., Christy, M., Arnung, K., et al.: Viruses and diabetes. In: J.S. Bajaj, (ed.): Diabetes. Proceedings of the 9th Congress of the International Diabetes Federation, New Delhi, 1976. Amsterdam, Excerpta Medica, 1977, pp. 294–298.

76. Craighead, J.E., Gleason, R.E., Funk, I.B., et al.: Prospective virological assessment of recent onset type 1 diabetics in Massachusetts. Unpublished data.

77. Hierholzer, J.C., Farris, W.A.: Follow-up of children infected in a Coxsackie virus B-3 and B-4 outbreak: No evidence of diabetes mellitus. J. Infect. Dis. 129:741, 1974.

78. Dippe, S.E., Bennett, P.H., Miller, M., et al.: Lack of causal association between Coxsackie B4 virus infection and diabetes. Lancet 1:1314, 1975.

79. Gibbs, P.: Three cases of acute ketotic diabetes mellitus with myocarditis: A common viral origin? Br. Med. J. 3:781, 1974.

80. Notkins, A.L.: Virus-induced diabetes mellitus. Arch. Virol. 54:1, 1977.

81. Yoon, J.W., Austin, M., Onodera, T., Notkins, A.L.: Virus induced diabetes. N. Engl. J. Med. 300:1173, 1979.

82. Palmer, J.P., Cooney, M.K., Ward, R.H., et al.: Reduced

Coxsackie antibody titers in type 1 (insulin-dependent) diabetic patients presenting during an outbreak of Coxsackie B3 and B4 infection. Diabetologia. 22:426, 1982.

83. MacMahon, B.: Epidemiologic approaches to family resemblance. In: N.E. Morton, Chin Ski Chung (eds.): Genetic Epidemiology. New York, Academic Press, 1978. p. 3–11.

84. Weiss, K.M., Chakraborty, R., Majumder, P.P., et al.: Problems in the assessment of relative risk of chronic disease among biological relatives of affected individuals. J. Chron. Dis. 35:539, 1982.

85. Green, A.: Empirical risk estimation for relatives of insulin-dependent diabetics: theoretical considerations and practical applications. In: J. Kobberling, R. Tattersall (eds.): The Genetics of Diabetes Mellitus. Proceedings of the Serono Symposia, Vol. 47. London, Academic Press, 1982, p. 21–26.

86. Harris, H.: The familial distribution of diabetes mellitus: a study of the relatives of 1241 diabetic propositi. Ann. Eugenics 15:95, 1950.

87. Steinberg, A.G., Wilder, R.M.: A study of the genetics of diabetes mellitus. Am. J. Hum. Genet. 4:113, 1952.

88. Wagener, D., Kuller, L., Orchard, T., et al.: Pittsburgh diabetes mellitus study. II. Secondary attack rates in families with insulin-dependent diabetes mellitus. Am. J. Epidemiol. 115:868, 1982.

89. Wagener, D.K., Sacks, J.M., LaPorte, R.E., MacGregor, J.M.: The Pittsburgh study of insulin-dependent diabetes mellitus. Risk for diabetes among relatives of IDDM. Diabetes 31:136, 1982.

90. Degnbol, B., Green, A.: Diabetes mellitus among first and second degree relatives of early onset diabetics. Ann. Hum. Genet. 42:25, 1978.

91. Gottlieb, M.S.: Diabetes in offspring and siblings of juvenile and maturity onset type diabetics. J. Chron. Dis. 33:331, 1980.

92. Warram, J.H., Krolewski, A.S., Gottlieb, M.S.: Clustering of ages of onset of IDD in affected siblings. Paper in preparation.

93. Gamble, D.R.: An epidemiological study of childhood diabetes affecting two or more siblings. Diabetologia 19:341, 1980.

94. Simpson, N.E.: Heritabilities of liability to diabetes when sex and age at onset are considered. Ann. Hum. Genet. 32:283, 1969.

95. Then Berg, H.: Zur Frage der psychischen und neurologischen Erscheinungen bei Diabeteskranken und deren Verwandten. Z. ges. Neurol. Psychiat. 165:278, 1939.

96. Then Berg, H.: Genetic aspects of diabetes mellitus. Foreign letters. J.A.M.A. 112:1091, 1939.

97. Harvald, B., Hauge, M.: Selection in diabetes in modern society. Acta Med. Scand. 173:459, 1963.

98. Gottlieb, M.S., Root, H.F.: Diabetes mellitus in twins. Diabetes 17:693, 1968.

99. Barnett, A.H., Eff, C., Leslie, R.D.G., Pyke, D.A.: Diabetes in identical twins. A study of 200 pairs. Diabetologia 20:87, 1981.

100. Allen, G., Harvald, B., Shields, J.: Measures of twin concordance. Acta Genet. (Basel). 17:475, 1967.

101. Allen, G., Hrubec, Z.: Twin concordance. A more general model. Acta Genet. Med. Gemellol. 28:3, 1979.

102. Smith, C.: Heritability of liability and concordance in monozygous twins. Ann. Hum. Genet. (Lond.) 34:85, 1970.

103. Smith, C.: Correlation in liability among relatives and concordance in twins. Further results. Hum. Hered. 22:97, 1972.

104. Smith, C.: Concordance in twins: methods and interpretation. Am. J. Hum. Genet. 26:454, 1974.

105. Joslin, E.P., Dublin, L.I., Marks, H.H.: Studies in diabetes mellitus. V. Heredity. Am. J. Med. Sci. 193:8, 1937.

106. Warram, J.H., Krolewski, A.S., Gottlieb, M.S., Kahn, C.R.: Differences in risk of insulin-dependent diabetes in offspring of diabetic mothers and diabetic fathers. N. Engl. J. Med. 311:149, 1984.

107. Bodmer, W.F.: HLA structure and function; a contemporary view. Tissue Antigens. 17:9, 1981.

108. Svejgaard, A., Jakobsen, B.K., Morling, N., et al.: Genetics of the HLA system. In: J. Kobberling, R. Tattersall (eds.): The Genetics of Diabetes Mellitus. Proceedings of the Serono Symposia, Vol. 47. London, Academic Press, 1982, p. 27–34.

109. Bodmer, W.F.: Gene clusters, genome organization, and complex phenotypes. When the sequence is known, what will it mean? Am. J. Hum. Genet. 33:664, 1981.

110. Singal, D.P., Blajchman, M.A.: Histocompatibility (HLA) antigens, lymphocytoxic antibodies and tissue antibodies in patients with diabetes mellitus. Diabetes 22:429, 1973.

111. Nerup, J., Platz, P., Anderson, O.O., et al.: HL-A antigens and diabetes mellitus. Lancet 2:864, 1974.

112. Cudworth, A.G., Woodrow, J.C.: HL-A system and diabetes mellitus. Diabetes 24:345, 1975.

113. Green, A.: The epidemiologic approach to studies of association between HLA and disease. I. The basic measures, concepts and estimation procedures. Tissue Antigens 19:245, 1982.

114. Green, A.: The epidemiologic approach to studies of association between HLA and disease. II. Estimation of absolute risks, etiologic and preventive fraction. Tissue Antigens 19:259, 1982.

115. Svejgaard, A., Platz, P., Ryder, L.P.: Insulin dependent diabetes mellitus; joint results of the 8th Workshop Study. In: P.I. Terasaki (ed.): Histocompatibility Testing 1980. Los Angeles, UCLA Press, 1980, pp. 638–651.

116. Brautbar, C., Karp, M., Amar, A., et al.: Genetics of insulin dependent diabetes mellitus in Israel: Population and family study. Hum. Immunol. 3:1, 1981.

117. Cambon-de Mouzon, A., Ohayon, E., Hauptmann, G., et al.: HLA-A, B, C, DR antigens, Bf, C4 and glyoxalase I (GLO) polymorphisms in French Basques with insulin-dependent diabetes mellitus (IDDM). Tissue Antigens 19:366, 1982.

118. Deschamps, I., Lestradet, H., Bonaiti, C., et al.: HLA genotype studies in juvenile insulin-dependent diabetes. Diabetologia 19:189, 1980.

119. Wolf, E., Spencer, K.M., Cudworth, A.G.: The genetic susceptibility to type 1 (insulin-dependent) diabetes: Analysis of the HLA-DR association. Diabetologia 24:224, 1983.

120. Platz, P., Jakobsen, B.K., Morling, N., et al.: HLA-D and -DR antigens in genetic analysis of insulin dependent diabetes mellitus. Diabetologia 21:108, 1981.

121. Reitnauer, P.J., Roseman, J.M., Barger, B.O., et al.: HLA associations with insulin-dependent diabetes mellitus in a sample of the American Black population. Tissue Antigens 17:286, 1981. (And personal communication).

122. Barbosa, J., Bach, F.H., Rich, S.S: Genetic heterogeneity of diabetes and HLA. Clin. Genet. 21:25, 1982.

123. Gorsuch, A.N., Spencer, K.M., Lister, J., et al.: Can future type 1 diabetes be predicted? A study in families of affected children. Diabetes 31:862, 1982.

124. Thomson, G.: A two locus model for juvenile diabetes. Ann. Hum. Genet. 43:383, 1980.

125. Clerget-Darpoux, F., Bonaiti-Pellie, C., Deschamps, I.,

et al.: Juvenile insulin-dependent diabetes: a possible susceptibility gene in interaction with HLA. Ann. Hum.
Genet. 45:199, 1981.

126. Morton, N.E., Green, A., Dunsworth, T., et al.: Heterozygous expression of insulin-dependent diabetes mellitus (IDDM) determinants in the HLA system. Am. J.
Hum. Genet. 35:201, 1983.

127. Wilson, P.W., McGee, D.L., Kannel, W.B.: Obesity,
very low density lipoproteins, and glucose intolerance
over fourteen years. The Framingham study. Am. J. Epidemiol. 114:697, 1981. (Also personal communication.)

128. Brook, R.H., Lohr, K.N., Berman, D.M., et al.: Con-
ceptualization and measurement of physiologic health for
adults. Vol.7 Diabetes mellitus. Santa Monica, The Rand
Corporation, 1981, R-2262/7-HHS. (Also personal communication.)

129. Wilkerson, H.L.C., Krall, L.P.: Diabetes in a New England Town. A study of 3516 persons in Oxford, Massachusetts. J.A.M.A. 135:209, 1947.

130. O'Sullivan, J.B.: Population retested for diabetes after 17
years: new prevalence study in Oxford, Massachusetts.
Diabetologia 5:211, 1969.

131. National Diabetes Data Group, NIH.: Prevalence and incidence of diabetes in the U.S. Unpublished data from
U.S. National Health Surveys, U.S. Public Health Service
and National Center for Health Statistics.

132. Conn, J.W., Fajan, S.S.: The prediabetic states. Am. J.
Med. 31:839, 1961.

133. Wilder, C.S.: Physician visits; interval of visits and children's routine checkup. United States, July, 1963–June,
1964. National Center for Health Statistics, Series 10,
No. 19, U.S. DHEW Publication. Washington, D.C.,
U.S. Government Printing Office, June 1965.

134. Gentile, A.: Physician visits, volume and interval since
last visit. United States–1975. National Center for Health
Statistics, Series 10, No. 128, U.S. DHEW Publication
No. (PHS) 79–1556. Hyattsville, Md. U.S. Government
Printing Office, April 1979.

135. Sayetta, R.B., Murphy, R.S.: Summary of current diabetes-related data from National Center for Health Statistics. Diabetes Care 2:105, 1979.

136. Falconer, D.S., Duncan, L.J.P., Smith, C.: A statistical
and genetical study of diabetes. I. Prevalence and morbidity. Ann. Hum. Genet.(Lond.) 34:347, 1971.

137. Ustvedt, H.J., Olsen, E.: Incidence of diabetes mellitus
in Oslo, Norway 1956–65. Br. J. Prev. Soc. Med.
31:251, 1977.

138. Ipsen, J., Clark, T.W., Elsom, K.O., Roberts, N.J.: Diabetes and heart disease: Periodic health examination programs. Am. J. Publ. Health 59:1595, 1969.

139. Larsson, B., Bjorntorp, P., Tibblin, G.: The health consequences of moderate obesity. Internat. J. Obes. 5:97,
1981.

140. Westlund, K., Nicholaysen, R.: Ten-year mortality and
morbidity related to serum cholesterol. Scand. J. Clin.
Lab. Invest. 30(Suppl.127):3, 1972.

141. Medalie, J.H., Herman, J.B., Goldbourt, U., Papier,
C.M.: Variations in incidence of diabetes among 10,000
adult Israeli males and the factors related to their development. In: R. Levine and R. Luft (eds.): Advances in
Metabolic Disorders. Vol. 9. New York, Academic Press,
1978, pp. 93–110.

142. Zimmet, P., Pinkstone, G., Whitehouse, S., Thoma, K.:
The high incidence of diabetes mellitus in the Micronesian
population of Nauru. Acta Diab. Lat. 19:75, 1982.

143. Knowler, W.C., Bennett, P.H., Hamman, R.F., et al.:
Diabetes incidence and prevalence in Pima Indians: A 19-
fold greater incidence than in Rochester, Minnesota. Am.
J. Epidemiol. 108:497, 1978.

144. O'Sullivan, J.B., Acheson, R.M.: Comparison of diabetes prevalence rates in Oxford (1946) and Sudbury
(1964). In: R. Levine and R. Luft (eds.): Advances in
Metabolic Disorders. Vol. 9. New York, Academic Press,
1978, pp. 1–11.

145. Barrett-Connor, E.: The prevalence of diabetes mellitus
in an adult community as determined by history of fasting
hyperglycemia. Am. J. Epidemiol. 111:705, 1980.

146. Ostrander, L.D., Lamphiear, D.E., Block, W.D.: Diabetes among men in general population. Prevalence and
associated physiological findings. Arch. Intern. Med.
136:415, 1976.

147. Bennett, P.H., Harris, M., Murphy, R.S.: Geographic
and ethnic differences in diabetes frequency in the Amer-
icas. In: E.N. Mngola (ed.): Diabetes 1982, Proceedings
of the 11th Congress of the International Diabetes Federation. Amsterdam, Excerpta Medica, 1983, pp.
131–136.

148. Sigurdsson, G., Gottskalksson, G., Thorsteinsson, T., et
al.: Community screening for glucose intolerance in middle-aged Icelandic men. Deterioration to diabetes over a
period of 7.5 years. Acta Med. Scand. 210:21, 1981.
(Also personal communication.)

149. Jorde, R.: The diabetes survey in Bergen, Norway, 1956.
An epidemiologic study and a study of blood sugar values
related to sex, age and weight. Bergen and Oslo, Norwegian Universities Press, 1962.

150. Aspevik, A., Jorde, R., Raeder, S.: The diabetes survey
in Bergen, Norway, 1956. A ten-year follow-up of an
epidemiologic study and a study of blood sugar values
related to sex, age and weight. Acta Med. Scand.
196:161, 1974.

151. Schroll, M., Hagerup, L.: Relationship of fasting blood
glucose to prevalence of ecg abnormalities and 10yr risk
of mortality from cardiovascular diseases in men born in
1914; from the Glostrup population studies. J. Chron. Dis.
32:699, 1979.

152. Hagerup, L., Eriksen, M., Schroll, M., et al.: The Glostrup population studies collection of epidemiologic tables.
Reference values for use in cardiovascular population
studies. Scand. J. Soc. Med. Suppl. 20, 1980.

153. Mroszczyk, M., Gdulewicz, T., Torzecka, W., et al.:
Cukrzyca w probie losowej trzech dzielnic Lodzi. Zdr.
Publ. 87:169, 1976. (See also Diabetologia 21:520,
1982.)

154. Samokhvalova, M.A., Dzhuraeva-Akhmedova, S.D.,
Zhukovsky, G.S., et al.: Study of diabetes mellitus incidence. Probl. Endocrynol. 22:27, 1976.

155. Burlak, S.I.: Prevalence and risk of diabetes mellitus in
the population of the Kamchatka region. Probl. Endocrynol. 28:17, 1982.

156. Toyota, T., Kudo, M., Goto, Y., et al.: Prevalence of
diabetes mellitus in rural and urban population in Japan.
In: S. Baba, I. Fukui, and Y. Goto (eds.): Diabetes Mellitus in Asia. Amsterdam, Excerpta Medica, 1976, pp.
35–40.

157. Kawate, R., Yamakido, M., Nishimoto, Y., et. al.: Diabetes mellitus and its vascular complications in Japanese
migrants on the island of Hawaii. Diabetes Care 2:161,
1979.

158. Kawate, R., Yamakido, M., Nishimoto, Y.: Migrant studies among the Japanese in Hiroshima and Hawaii. In:
W.K. Waldhausl (ed.): Diabetes 1979, Proceedings of the
10th Congress of the International Diabetes Federation.
Amsterdam, Excerpta Medica, 1980, pp. 526–531.

159. Cheah, J.S., Tan, B.Y.: Diabetes among different races
in a similar environment. In: W. Waldhausl, (ed.): Dia-

betes, 1979. Proceedings of the 10th Congress of the International Diabetes Federation. Amsterdam, Excerpta Medica, 1980, pp. 512–516.

160. Gupta, O.P., Joshi, M.H., Dave, S.K.: Prevalence of diabetes in India. In: R. Levine and R. Luft (eds.): Advances in Metabolic Disorders. Vol. 9. New York, Academic Press, 1978, pp. 147–165.

161. Jackson, W.P.U.: Epidemiology of diabetes in South Africa. In: R. Levine and R. Luft (eds.): Advances in Metabolic Disorders. Vol. 9. New York, Academic Press, 1978, pp. 112–146.

162. Poon-King, T., Henry, M.V., Rampersad, F.: Prevalence and natural history of diabetes in Trinidad. Lancet 1:155, 1968.

163. Bacchus, R.A., Bell, J.L., Madkour, M., Kilshaw, B.: The prevalence of diabetes mellitus in male Saudi Arabs. Diabetologia 23:330, 1982.

164. Henry-Amar, M., Papoz, L., Ben Khalifa, F., et al.: Prevalence du diabete dans le gouvernorat de Tunis a partir d'un echantillon representatif. Rev. Epidem et Sante Publ. 29:1, 1981.

165. Jayyab, A.K.A.: Preliminary survey of diabetes in Kuwait. Diab. Croat. 9(Suppl.1): 90, 1980.

166. Marine, N., Vinik, A.I., Edelstein, O., Jackson, W.P.U.: Diabetes hyperglycaemia and glycosuria among Indians, Malays and Africans (Bantu) in Cape Town, South Africa. Diabetes 18:840, 1969.

167. Wicks, A.C.B., Castle, W.M., Gelfand, M.: Effect of time on the prevalence of diabetes in the urban African of Rhodesia. Diabetes 22:733, 1973.

168. Imperato, P.J., Handelsman, M.B., Fofana, B., Sow, O.: The prevalence of diabetes mellitus in three population groups in the Republic of Mali. Trans. R. Soc. Trop. Med. Hyg. 70:155, 1976.

169. Florey, C. du V., McDonald, H., Miall, W.E.: The prevalence of diabetes in a rural population of Jamaican adults. Int. J. Epid. 1:157, 1972.

170. West, K.M.: Diabetes in American Indians. In: R. Levine and R. Luft (eds.): Advances in Metabolic Disorders. Vol. 9. New York, Academic Press, 1978, pp. 29–48.

171. Mouratoff, G.J., Carroll, N.V., Scott, E.M.: Diabetes mellitus in Eskimos. J.A.M.A. 199:961, 1967.

172. Mouratoff, G.J., Carroll, N.V., Scott, E.M.: Diabetes mellitus in Athabaskan Indians in Alaska. Diabetes 18:29, 1969.

173. Joslin, E.P.: The prevention of diabetes mellitus. J.A.M.A. 76:79, 1921.

174. Kanarek, P.H., Balodimos, M.C., Marble, A.: Survival and causes of death among diabetic patients treated with insulin, tolbutamide, or diet alone. Unpublished manuscript.

175. Population alive with specified events by sex, age and level of characteristic at exam. Section 9. In: W.B. Kannel and T. Gordon: The Framingham Study. An Epidemiological Investigation of Cardiovascular Disease. D.H.E.W. Publication (NIH). 1968.

176. Rimm, A.A., Werner, L.H., van Yserloo, B., Bernstein, R.A.: Relationship of obesity and disease in 73,532 weight-conscious women. Public Health Reports 90:44, 1975.

177. Bonham, G.S., Brock, D.B.: The relationship of diabetes with race, sex and obesity. Am. Stat. Assn., 1982 Proc. of the Social Statistic Section, pp. 397–402.

178. Dunn, J.P., Ipsen, J., Elsom, K.O., Ohtani, M.: Risk factors in coronary artery disease, hypertension and diabetes. Am. J. Med. Sci. 259:309, 1970.

179. Knowler, W.C., Pettitt, D.J., Savage, P.J., Bennett, P.H.: Diabetes incidence in Pima Indians: Contributions of obesity and parental diabetes. Am. J. Epidemiol. 113:144, 1981.

180. Butler, W.J., Ostrander, L.D., Carman, W.J., Lamphiear, D.E.: Diabetes mellitus in Tecumseh, Michigan. Prevalence, incidence, and associated conditions. Am. J. Epidemiol. 116:971, 1982.

181. Obesity in America: An overview. In: G.A. Bray (ed.): Obesity in America. U.S. Department of Health, Education, and Welfare. NIH Publication No. 79–359, 1979, pp. 1–19.

182. West, K.M., Kalbfleisch, J.M.: Influence of nutritional factors on prevalence of diabetes. Diabetes 20:99, 1971.

183. Kopczynski, J.: Height and weight of adults in Cracow. II. Weight for height. Epidemiol. Review 26:381, 1972.

184. Abraham, S., Carroll, M.D., Najjar, M.F., et al.: Obese and overweight adults in the United States. U.S. Public Health Service, National Center for Health Statistics, DHHS Publ. No. (PHS)83–1680 Ser. 11, No. 230, Hyattsville, MD, U.S. Government Printing Office, 1983.

185. Czyzyk, A., Kasperska, T.: O czestosci wystepowania cukrzycy w Polsce w swietle badan masowych. Pol. Arch. Med. Wewn. 33:1376, 1964.

186. Mincu, I., Dumitrescu, S., Campeanu, S., et al.: Epidemiological researches on diabetes mellitus in Roumanian urban and rural population. Diabetologia 8:12, 1972.

187. Christacopoulos, P.D., Karamanos, B.G., Tountas, C.D., et al.: The prevalence of diabetes mellitus (DM) and non-diabetic glycosuria (NDG) in a rural population of Greece. Diabetologia 11:335, 1975.

188. Katsilambros, N., Steryotis, J., Moiras, N., et al.: Prevalence of diabetes among glycosuric individuals in an urban area of Greece. Acta Diabet. Lat. 14:211, 1977.

189. Zhong Xue-li: Diabetes mellitus survey in China. Chinese Med. J. 95:423, 1982.

190. Zimmet, P., Faaiuso, J., Ainuu, J., et al.: The prevalence of diabetes in the rural and urban Polynesian population of Western Samoa. Diabetes 30:45, 1981.

191. Taylor, R., Zimmet, P.: Obesity and diabetes in Western Samoa. Int. J. Obesity 5:367, 1981.

192. Cruz-Vidal, M., Costas, R., Jr., Garcia-Palmieri, M.R., et al.: Factors related to diabetes mellitus in Puerto Rican men. Diabetes 28:300, 1979.

193. West, K.M.: Epidemiology of diabetes and its vascular lesions. New York, Elsevier North-Holland, Inc., 1978, pp. 248–274.

194. Zimmet, P.: Epidemiology of diabetes and its macrovascular manifestations in Pacific populations. The medical effects of social progress. Diabetes Care 2:144, 1979.

195. Lee, E.T., Anderson, P.S., Bryan, J., et al.: Diabetes, parental diabetes, obesity and education in Oklahoma Indians. Diabetes 31(Suppl.2):97A, 1982.

196. Harburg, E., Erfurt, J.C., Hauenstein, L.S., et al.: Socioecological stress, suppressed hostility, skin color and Black-White male blood pressure: Detroit. Psychosom. Med. 35:276, 1973.

197. Syme, S.L., Oakes, T.W., Friedman, G.D., et al.: Social class and racial differences in blood pressure. Am. J. Pub. Hlth. 64:619, 1974.

198. Blood pressure of persons 18–74, United States, 1971–1975. U.S. Public Health Service, National Center for Health Statistics. PHS Publ. No. 1000, Ser. 11, No. 150, Washington, D.C., U.S. Government Printing Office, 1975.

199. Dyer, A.R., Stamler, L., Shekelle, R.B., et al.: The relationship of education to blood pressure. Findings in 40,000 employed Chicagoans. Circulation 54:987, 1976.

200. Dischinger, P.C., Apostolides, A.Y., Entwisle, G., Hebel, J.R.: Hypertension incidence in an inner-city black population. J. Chron. Dis. 34:405, 1981.

3 Pathophysiology of Diabetes Mellitus: An Overview

C. Ronald Kahn

Diabetes mellitus is a complex syndrome (or syndromes) characterized by (1) hyperglycemia, secondary to deranged secretion and/or action of insulin; (2) specific microvascular complications, including thickening of capillary basement membranes, retinopathy and nephropathy; (3) macrovascular disease, i.e., accelerated atherosclerosis, and (4) a variety of other complications including neuropathy, complicated pregnancy, and increased tendency to infection. In addition, in the untreated state there is accelerated catabolism of both fat and protein. While none of these findings is absolutely specific for diabetes, it is clear that diabetes mellitus should not be considered simply as synonymous with hyperglycemia, since there are many conditions in which there is impaired glucose tolerance which are not generally associated with the same spectrum of complications.[1] These include acute stress (infection, surgery, trauma), hyperlipidemia, other endocrine disorders, pancreatic disease and a large number of complex genetic syndromes (Table 3–1; Chapters 9, 15, 42).

CLASSIFICATION AND PATHOGENESIS

Even eliminating these other causes of hyperglycemia, primary diabetes is still a heterogeneous disease. At the extremes are the two common types: Type I or insulin-dependent diabetes mellitus (IDDM), formerly called juvenile-onset diabetes, and Type II or non-insulin-dependent diabetes mellitus (NIDDM), formerly called maturity-onset diabetes. These differ both in clinical presentation and presumed etiology. While this simple binary classification is useful and provides a comfortable ''shorthand'' for describing these complex syndromes, the condition of many patients appears to lie between these two extremes and may be difficult

Table 3–1. Classification of Diabetes Mellitus and Other States of Glucose Intolerance*

I. Diabetes Mellitus
  A. Type I, or insulin-dependent diabetes (formerly juvenile-onset diabetes)
  B. Type II, or non-insulin-dependent diabetes (formerly maturity-onset diabetes)
  C. Other types**
II. Secondary Diabetes
  A. Pancreatic disease (chronic pancreatitis, hemochromatosis, pancreatectomy, etc.)
  B. Hormonal (Cushing's syndrome, acromegaly, pheochromocytoma)
  C. Drug or chemical induced (chlorothiazide, phenytoin, etc.)
  D. Insulin receptor abnormalities (acanthosis nigricans, lipodystrophy, etc.)
  E. Genetic syndromes (ataxia telangiectasia, progeria, Laurence-Moon-Biedl syndrome, myotonic dystrophy)
III. Impaired glucose tolerance (formerly chemical diabetes)
IV. Gestational diabetes

*Adapted from ref. 6.
**This was not included in original classification but almost certainly other or intermediate types exist.

to classify. A precise understanding of the pathogenesis of each of these types of diabetes is essential if we wish to develop an appropriate and optimal therapy.

An important point to keep in mind when considering the pathogenesis of diabetes is the lingering controversy concerning the relationship of the various complications to hyperglycemia.[2] The simplest notion would be that all of the complications are secondary to hyperglycemia (see Table 3–2A). Other possibilities exist, however, as described in Table 3–2B and 3–2C.

Whatever the exact order of events, the most striking early abnormality in diabetes mellitus is the development of hyperglycemia. Since insulin is the major humoral modulator of glucose homeostasis in all types of diabetes, hyperglycemia may be considered the result of a *deficiency of insulin action*. This deficiency may occur as a result of a relative or absolute lack of insulin itself, or as a result of *resistance to insulin action* at the

Table 3–2. Possibilities Regarding the Primary Defect in the Pathogenesis of Diabetes and Its Complications

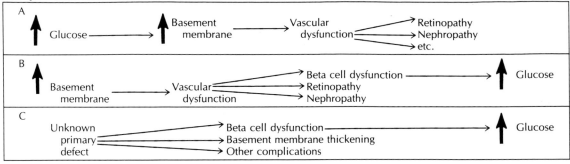

target cell level. Although the detailed pathogenesis of diabetes will be considered in other chapters of this text, the attempt here will be to provide a brief overview of some current concepts concerning the etiology of the disease and the relative importance of insulin deficiency and alterations in insulin action in the hyperglycemia of the two common forms of primary diabetes.

INSULIN-DEPENDENT DIABETES MELLITUS (IDDM)

Insulin-dependent (Type I) diabetes is clearly associated with an absolute deficiency of insulin secretion. The insulin deficiency is easily demonstrable when one measures circulating insulin levels in either the basal or stimulated state (Fig. 3–1). In the Type I diabetic, insulin deficiency is present at the time of onset of the disease and throughout the entire clinical course, although some residual beta cell function may be seen (as demonstrated by C-peptide measurements) and transient periods

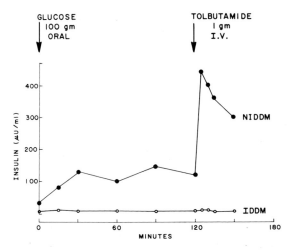

Fig. 3–1. Insulin secretion after a sequential oral glucose tolerance test and tolbutamide tolerance test as demonstrated in a patient with IDDM and a patient with NIDDM.

of remission can occur producing the so-called "honeymoon" phase of the disease.[3] This marked decrease in insulin secretory capacity is due to an actual loss of beta cell mass (Table 3–3), and extracts of pancreas reveal low or undetectable levels of insulin.[4,5]

Role of Autoimmunity

The loss of insulin secretion in IDDM appears to result from an autoimmune process which is directed at the insulin-producing beta cells of the pancreas and ultimately leads to their destruction and the development of the syndrome (Fig. 3–2). This autoimmune process itself is probably triggered by some environmental factor(s) in a genetically susceptible individual. Exactly what these factors are is unknown, but animal studies suggest viruses or toxins as likely candidates (Chapter 7). Although the autoimmune process is reviewed in detail in Chapter 4, we should briefly consider this hypothesis here.

The first clue that an immune mechanism may be involved in diabetes came from the association between IDDM and other endocrine deficiencies of autoimmune etiology, such as those of the adrenal or thyroid glands.[6] Patients with IDDM were also found to have a remarkable increase in the prevalence of other organ-specific autoantibodies in their sera.[6,7]

Direct evidence for cell-mediated autoimmunity directed against the endocrine pancreas, however, did not come until 1971 when it was found that the migration of leukocytes from patients with IDDM was inhibited by exposure to antigens prepared from the endocrine pancreas.[8] Lymphocytes from diabetic subjects have also been found to have adherence and cytotoxicity against cultured insulinoma cells.[9] These changes in lymphocyte function are accompanied by alterations in the circulating lymphocyte populations. Increases in certain T-lymphocyte populations have been seen in acute IDDM in both man[10] and the BB rat,[11] an animal

Table 3–3.   Features of Insulin-Dependent (IDDM) and Noninsulin-Dependent Diabetes Mellitus (NIDDM)

	IDDM	NIDDM
Clinical Features		
Age at onset	Usually <30	Usually >40
Onset	Often rapid	Insidious
Weight	Non-obese	Often obese
Ketosis	Common	Rare
Complications	Frequent	Frequent
Epidemiology		
Prevalence	0.5%	2%
Sex	Slight male predominance	Female predominance
Seasonal variation	Present	?
Genetics		
Concordance in identical twins	<50%	>90%
HLA association	Present	Absent
Pathology		
Islet mass	Severely reduced	Moderately reduced
Insulitis at onset	Present in 50 to 70%	?
Immunology		
Associated with other endocrinopathies	Frequent	Infrequent
Anti-islet cell immunity		
Humoral	60 to 80% at onset	5–20%
Cell-mediated	35 to 50% at onset	<5%

Modified from Christy, Deckert and Nerup.[6]

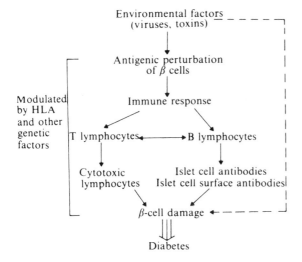

Fig. 3–2. Possible pathogenesis of insulin-dependent diabetes mellitus.

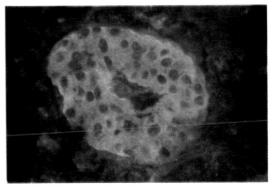

Fig. 3–3. Immunofluorescent staining of an islet of Langerhans by serum from a patient with IDDM which contains anti-islet cell antibodies.

model of IDDM. Passive transfer of diabetes from mouse to mouse and even man to mouse using lymphocytes from affected animals has also been reported,[12] but has been challenged as a number of groups have not been able to confirm the finding.

Despite the strong suspicion that autoantibodies might be important in IDDM, it was not until 1974 that autoantibodies against some component in the islet cell cytoplasm were detected in patients with diabetes and other autoimmune endocrinopathies[13] (Fig. 3–3). Similar autoantibodies were soon confirmed in other patients who did not have polyen-

docrine failure and have now been found in over 2,000 diabetic patients.[14] The exact prevalence of these autoantibodies depends on the duration of the disease. Within the first 1 to 2 weeks of onset, they are detectable in up to 85% of diabetic children. This percentage rapidly declines, reaching 25% by 2 to 5 years after diagnosis. The autoantibodies are present in 1 to 2% of normal controls, and their prevalence is increased in first-degree relatives of patients with IDDM and in patients with NIDDM. They are invariably of the IgG class, and, in most cases, react with the cytoplasm of all four major types of islet cells—the insulin-secreting beta cells, glucagon-secreting alpha cells, somatostatin-secreting delta cells and pancreatic polypeptide-secreting (PP) cells.

There is a serious question as to whether these autoantibodies are pathogenic in IDDM since antibodies are present to all cell types, but only beta cells are destroyed. Complement-fixing autoantibodies seem to correlate more closely with the disease.[15] Recent studies have suggested that these antibodies may be present in the non-diabetic siblings of affected children and serve as a predictive marker of impending development of IDDM.[16]

Islet cell antibodies have also been detected that react with the surface membranes of islet cells.[17,18] Like the islet cell cytoplasm autoantibodies, the membrane-directed autoantibodies are most prevalent in early-onset diabetes. In the presence of complement, these cell surface autoantibodies stimulate chromium release from radiolabeled islets and inhibit insulin release, suggesting direct cytotoxicity to islet cells.[19] Cell surface autoantibodies, however, are also found in the sera of some non-diabetic first-degree relatives of patients with IDDM.

The antigens at which the cytoplasmic and cell surface autoantibodies are directed remain to be identified. One recent study found that most of the sera which contain islet cell surface antibodies react with a protein of molecular weight 64,000 present in human islet cell lysates.[20] Hopefully, the determination of the nature of the antigen will provide a clue as to the earliest lesion in IDDM.

Circulating immune complexes have also been identified in patients with IDDM.[21] In contrast to the other immune markers, they are present not only in those patients with recent onset of IDDM, but also in later phases, and in patients with NIDDM. Some of these may be immune complexes involving anti-insulin antibodies, but the widespread nature of their occurrence suggests that other antigens must be involved also.

Exactly what initiates the autoimmune response remains unknown. Several animal studies suggest that in a genetically susceptible individual, a virus or toxin may be the triggering factor (see also Chapter 7). Diabetes-like syndromes can be produced in mice by infection with encephalomyocarditis virus or reovirus.[22-24] Reovirus also triggers production of autoantibodies that react with antigens on the surface of islet and pituitary cells, as well as antibodies that react with the hormones secreted by these cells. Insulitis and diabetes-like syndromes can also be produced by injection of low doses of beta cell toxins, such as streptozotocin.[22] In a series of elegant studies Notkins and coworkers have shown that the effect of these environmental factors may be additive, and clearly varies with the genetic background of the animal.[23,24]

In humans, the precise nature of the genetic influence in the pathogenesis of diabetes mellitus remains unclear as IDDM occurs concordantly in only about 50% of identical twin pairs.[25,26] Alleles of the major histocompatibility system (the HLA system) are clearly associated with the occurrence of IDDM.[6,14,27,28] Both HLA types DR3 and DR4 are associated with a 3- to 5-fold increase in risk for IDDM, and the risk of disease to the double heterozygote—the individual with DR3 and DR4—increases almost 10-fold, suggesting that the effect of these antigens involves independent mechanisms. Since HLA antigens B8 and B15 are in linkage disequilibrium with DR3 and DR4 they show similar associations. Interestingly, HLA B8/DR3 are also associated with a persistence of islet cell surface autoantibodies in patients with IDDM, whereas HLA B15/DR4 are associated with the development of high titer insulin antibodies.[6,14]

Based on all of these observations it is possible to derive a pathogenetic model for IDDM such as that shown in Figure 3–2. Any rational approach to therapy should be based on this model, although we must always realize that many parts remain unproven. Since IDDM once established is a disease of insulin deficiency and decreased beta cell mass, therapy of the disease must include hormone replacement. At present this may mean insulin therapy of conventional type or by an open-loop infusion pump. In the future, closed-loop insulin infusion devices (artificial beta cell), islet cell transplantation, and even genetic engineering may offer a more physiologic approach to replacement.

The recognition of a possibly important role for autoimmunity in the development of IDDM has led to attempts to suppress the immune response. In mouse and rat models of IDDM, immune suppression by irradiation, neonatal thymectomy, antilymphocyte serum or bone marrow transplant decreases the incidence of clinical disease.[29] At present it is too soon to know whether these techniques will alter the course of the human disease, but they certainly present hope for the prevention of diabetes and provide the first new approach to the therapy of IDDM since the introduction of insulin over 60 years ago.

NON-INSULIN-DEPENDENT DIABETES MELLITUS (NIDDM)

Non-insulin-dependent diabetes is by far the more common form of the disease, but its pathogenesis remains even less clear and more controversial than that of IDDM. NIDDM is not associated with any specific HLA alloantigens, but is clearly genetically influenced since it occurs in identical twins with almost total concordance.[25,26] NIDDM is associated with obesity in more than

80% of patients, suggesting the possibility that this type of diabetes may be due to a disordered mechanism of appetite regulation or energy expenditure. Finally, and most importantly, in contrast to the patients with IDDM, Type II diabetics have considerable preservation of the beta cell mass[4,5,30] and often secrete substantial quantities of insulin into the circulation (Fig. 3–1). This has led to the idea that in NIDDM there is resistance of the peripheral tissues to respond to insulin.[31,32] There is still considerable controversy as to which of these two factors (decreased insulin secretion and insulin resistance) is the major or primary one in the pathogenesis of Type II diabetes,[33] and it seems likely that in fact there is an interplay of both leading to the final disease manifestations (Fig. 3–4). It is, however, worthwhile to consider each of these briefly.

Insulin Secretion

Studies of islet cell morphology have suggested that in contrast to the pancreas of the patients with IDDM which has little beta cell mass, that of the patient with NIDDM has about 50% of the normal level.[4,5] This is consistent with the data on extractable insulin content and it is therefore not surprising that with the advent of radioimmunoassay, investigators found substantial amounts of immunoreactive insulin in the plasma of patients with NIDDM.[30,34] Virtually all studies have shown that in the basal state most individuals with NIDDM have normal or even elevated levels of plasma insulin, the latter often but not always related to the presence of obesity in this group.[35] Furthermore, this insulin appears to be normal, both in its relative proportion of proinsulin to insulin and its bioactivity.[36]

Although basal insulin levels in the Type II diabetic may be normal, several different varieties of abnormalities have been identified in insulin secretion after stimulation of the beta cell. In virtually all Type II diabetics, there is a loss of acute (first) phase insulin release to glucose given intravenously.[37] Second-phase responses to glucose and responses to other insulin secretagogues often remain normal suggesting a specific defect in glucorecognition.[38,39] Interestingly, many patients who do not respond to glucose intravenously will still secrete insulin during oral glucose tolerance testing. The insulin response to the oral glucose challenge may be similar to or even greater than that observed in normal individuals, but is usually somewhat reduced when compared to that in a group of obese, nondiabetic patients.[35]

One interesting observation in this population is that the lack of gluco-recognition is linked to the level of hyperglycemia.[40] With mild to moderate degrees of glucose intolerance, insulin secretion is elevated above normal, peaking when the plasma glucose value at 2 hours after the glucose load, reaches about 200 mg/dl. With more severe degrees of glucose intolerance, the secretion of insulin in response to the oral glucose load is reduced, generating a curve for beta cell function reminiscent of the "Starling curve" for cardiac function (Fig.

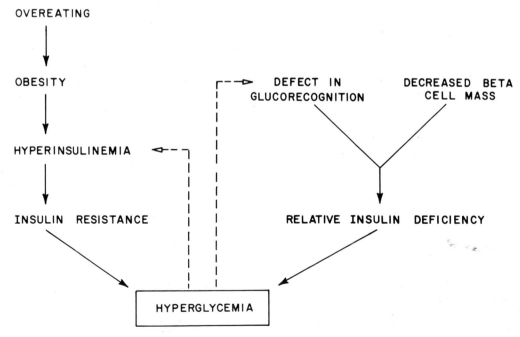

Fig. 3–4. Possible pathogenesis of non-insulin-dependent diabetes mellitus.

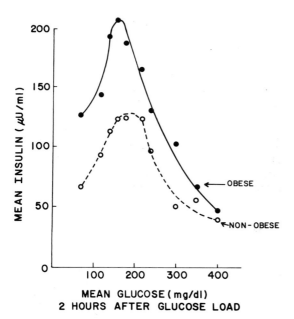

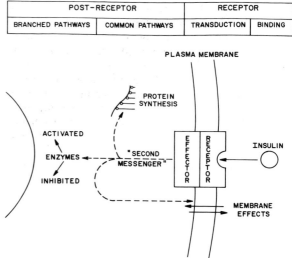

POST-RECEPTOR		RECEPTOR	
BRANCHED PATHWAYS	COMMON PATHWAYS	TRANSDUCTION	BINDING

Fig. 3–6. Cellular defects in insulin action in the patient with NIDDM.

Fig. 3–5. Insulin secretion as a function of hyperglycemia 2 hours after an oral glucose load in a population of Pima Indians with NIDDM. (Redrawn from ref. 40.)

3–5). This impairment of the beta cell function is reversible, at least in the early phases of the disease. Thus, if the blood glucose is lowered by treatment with a restricted diet, oral hypoglycemic agents, or insulin, beta cell function improves and insulin secretion is increased.[41]

Insulin Resistance

The finding of normal or elevated plasma levels of insulin in patients with Type II diabetes suggests the presence of some form of insulin resistance or reduced insulin sensitivity.[31,32] This has been confirmed by direct measurements of the effects of exogenous insulin in these patients. Whether one uses simple testing of tolerance to insulin given intravenously or more sophisticated procedures such as the "glucose-clamp" with graded insulin infusion, it is clear that NIDDM is associated with a decrease in response to exogenous, as well as endogenous, insulin. This is most marked in the patients with obesity, but also occurs in non-obese Type II diabetics and in some nondiabetic obese subjects as well.

The resistance to insulin present in the patient with NIDDM can occur as a result of defects at several levels in the action of insulin (Fig. 3–6) (see also references 42 and 43 and Chapter 6). The first step in insulin action is the binding of insulin to its receptor on the plasma membrane of the cell. This is a high molecular weight membrane glycoprotein (mol. wt. ~350,000) which binds insulin

and transmits some form of signal to initiate the changes in cellular metabolism associated with the effects of insulin.[44] Decreased numbers of insulin receptors were first found in the setting of obesity and NIDDM[45] (Fig. 3–7), but there are now a number of studies which demonstrate a similar decrease in insulin receptor number in the non-obese Type II diabetic also.[31,32,43,46] This defect is present on all cells except those of the brain, and appears to be due to a regulatory effect of insulin on its own receptor concentration.[47] Thus, the higher the basal insulin concentration, the lower the receptor concentration. Furthermore, any manipulation which lowers the insulin level (e.g., dietary restriction, streptozotocin, diazoxide) is associated with a return in receptor concentration toward normal.[31,42,43,45] Not surprisingly, when cells from a diabetic are placed in a long-term culture away from the endogenous hyperinsulinemia, insulin receptor content also returns to normal.[48]

While it is clear that there is a decrease in insulin binding in the Type II diabetic, it is not at all clear if this defect is of a sufficient degree to explain all of the insulin resistance. Thus a number of investigators have proposed that there must also be a defect (or defects) at some more distal step in the pathway of insulin action.[32,42,43] Most workers have termed this a "post-receptor" defect, implying some alteration at one of the *intracellular* steps in insulin action. However, the exact nature of the defect(s) remains unclear, and it is possible that the additional defect is still at the level of the receptor, but involves its signal transduction, rather than its binding capability.

Whatever the cause of the post-binding (post-

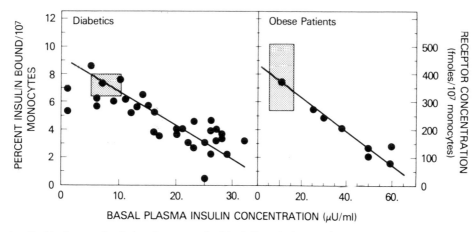

Fig. 3–7. Insulin binding to circulating monocytes in thin (left) and obese (right) patients with NIDDM. (Redrawn from refs. 31 and 43.)

receptor) defect, it appears to be related to the degree of metabolic abnormality. Treatment of the Type II diabetic with diet or insulin will substantially reverse this defect, even when the receptor abnormality persists.[49] Furthermore, a similar post-binding defect is observed in Type I diabetes.[50]

Identifying the Primary Defect

As is apparent from the foregoing discussion, patients with NIDDM have a variety of qualitative and quantitative abnormalities in both insulin secretion and insulin action. However, which if any of these constitutes the primary defect remains uncertain. We can summarize the findings discussed above as follows: (1) Although the number of pancreatic beta cells is reduced in the patient with Type II diabetes, the number is certainly adequate to maintain euglycemia assuming that function is normal. (2) Beta cells in Type II diabetes have impaired secretory ability, particularly in response to glucose, but this defect appears to be reversible (at least early in the disease) by lowering blood glucose. (3) There is peripheral resistance to insulin action both at the receptor and post-receptor levels. These defects in insulin action appear to be acquired and could probably be overcome if endogenous insulin secretion could be maximally increased.

It seems likely therefore that the pathogenesis of Type II diabetes is multifactorial (Fig. 3–4). In the obese patient, the primary lesion may be overeating which leads to an increased insulin secretion, insulin receptor down-regulation, insulin resistance, and ultimately glucose intolerance.[42] In non-obese patients, the primary lesion may well be at the target cell with some form of post-receptor defect in insulin action leading to hyperglycemia, hyperinsulinemia, and secondary changes in the insulin receptor.[43] In both cases, however, hyper-

glycemia would not occur if the pancreas could increase insulin secretion appropriately. Thus, there must be some lesion in the beta cell, as well, which limits insulin output and leads to clinical diabetes.[33]

With such a poor understanding of the pathophysiology, it is not surprising that therapy of the Type II diabetic is often more difficult than that of Type I patients. In the established Type II patients, attempts have been made both to increase insulin secretion by the remaining pancreas and to improve insulin responsiveness in peripheral tissues. The most effective therapy is at the process of overeating seen in the obese Type II patient, but whether or not this approaches the primary defect is as yet unknown.

REFERENCES

1. National Diabetes Data Group: Classification and diagnosis of diabetes mellitus and other categories of glucose intolerance. Diabetes 28:1039, 1979.
2. Flier, J.S., Roth, J.: Diabetes Mellitus. Introduction. In: K.L. Melmon, H.F. Morelli (Eds.): Clinical Pharmacology: Basic Principles in Therapeutics. 2nd Ed. New York, Macmillan Publishing Co., 1978, pp. 515–523.
3. Rubenstein, A.H., Kuzuya, H., Horowitz, D.L.: Clinical significance of circulating C-peptide in diabetes mellitus and hypoglycemic disorders. Arch. Intern. Med. 137:625, 1977.
4. Maclean, N., Ogilvie, R.F.: Quantitative estimation of the pancreatic islet tissue in diabetic subjects. Diabetes 4:367, 1955.
5. Westermark, P., Wilander, E.: The influence of amyloid deposits on the islet cell volume in maturity onset diabetes mellitus. Diabetologia 15:417, 1978.
6. Christy, M., Deckert, T., Nerup, J.: Immunity and autoimmunity in diabetes mellitus. Clin. Endocrinol. Metab. 6:305, 1977.
7. MacCuish, A.C., Irvine, W.J.: Autoimmunological aspects of diabetes mellitus. Clin. Endocrinol. Metab. 4:435, 1975.
8. Nerup, J., Anderson, O.O., Bendixen, C.T., et al.: Antipancreatic cellular hypersensitivity in diabetes mellitus. Diabetes 20:424, 1971.

9. Huang, S.W., MacLaren, N.I.: Insulin-dependent diabetes: a disease of autoaggression. Science 192:64, 1976.

10. Jackson, R., Morris, M.A., Haynes, B., Eisenbarth, G.S.: Increased circulating Ia-antigen bearing T cells in Type I diabetes mellitus. N. Engl. J. Med. 306:785, 1982.

11. Poussier, P., Nakhooda, A.F., Jalk, J.A., et al.: Lymphopenia and abnormal lymphocyte subsets in the "BB" rat: relationship to the diabetic syndrome. Endocrinology 110:1825, 1982.

12. Buschard, K., Madsbad, S., Rygaard, J.: Passive transfer of diabetes mellitus from man to mouse. Lancet 1:908, 1978.

13. Bottazzo, G.F., Florin-Christensen, A., Doniach, D.: Islet cell antibodies in diabetes mellitus with autoimmune polyendocrine deficiencies. Lancet 2:1279, 1974.

14. Kahn, C.R., Flier, J.S.: Immunologic aspects of endocrine disease. In: C.W. Parker (Ed.): Clinical Immunology, Vol. 2. Philadelphia, W.B. Saunders Co., 1980, pp. 815–866.

15. Bottazzo, G.F., Dean, B.M., Gorsuch, A.N., et al.: Complement-fixing islet cell antibodies in Type I diabetes: possible monitors of active beta-cell damage. Lancet 1:668, 1980.

16. Gorsuch, A.N., Lister, J., Dean, B.M., et al.: Evidence for a long prediabetic period in Type I (insulin-dependent) diabetes mellitus. Lancet 1:1363, 1981.

17. Maclaren, N.K., Huang, S.W., Fogh, J.: Antibody to cultured human insulinoma cells in insulin-dependent diabetes. Lancet 1:997, 1975.

18. Lernmark, A., Freedman, Z.R., Hofmann, C., et al.: Islet cell surface antibodies in juvenile diabetes mellitus. N. Engl. J. Med. 299:375, 1978.

19. Dobersen, M.J., Scharff, J.E., Ginsberg-Fellner, F., Notkins, A.L.: Cytotoxic autoantibodies to beta cells in the serum of patients with insulin-dependent diabetes mellitus. N. Engl. J. Med. 303:1493, 1980.

20. Baekkeskov, S., Neilsen, J.H., Marner, B., et al.: Autoantibodies in newly diagnosed diabetic children immunoprecipitate human pancreatic islet cell proteins. Nature 298:167, 1982.

21. DiMaria, U., Iavicoli, M., Andreani, D.: Circulating immune complexes in diabetes. Diabetologia 19:89, 1980.

22. Mordes, J.P., Rossini, A.A.: Animal models of diabetes. Am. J. Med. 70:353, 1981.

23. Toniolo, A., Onodera, T., Yoon, J.W., Notkins, A.L.: Induction of diabetes by cumulative environmental insults from viruses and chemicals. Nature 228:383, 1980.

24. Onodera, T., Ray, V.R., Melez, K.A., et al.: Virus-induced diabetes mellitus: autoimmunity and polyendocrine disease prevented by immunosuppression. Nature 297:66, 1982.

25. Barnett, A.H., Eff, C., Leslie, R.D.G., Pyke, D.A.: Diabetes in identical twins—a study of 200 pairs. Diabetologia 20:87, 1981.

26. Ganda, O.P., Soeldner, J.S., Gleason, R.E., et al.: Monozygotic triplets with discordance for diabetes mellitus and diabetic microangiopathy. Diabetes 26:469, 1977.

27. Nerup, J., Platz, P., Anderson, O.O., et al.: HLA antigens and diabetes mellitus. Lancet 2:864, 1974.

28. Cudworth, A.G., Woodrow, J.C.: Evidence for HLA linked genes in "juvenile" diabetes mellitus. Br. Med. J. 3:133, 1975.

29. Like, A.A., Rossini, A.A., Guberski, D.L., et al.: Spontaneous diabetes mellitus: reversal and prevention in the BB/W rat with antiserum to rat lymphocytes. Science 206:1421, 1979.

30. Holman, R.R., Turner, R.C.: Maintenance of basal plasma glucose and insulin concentrations in maturity-onset diabetes. Diabetes 28:227, 1979.

31. Bar, R.S., Harrison, L.C., Muggeo, M., et al.: Regulation of insulin receptors in normal and abnormal physiology in man. Adv. Intern. Med. 24:23, 1979.

32. Kolterman, O.G., Gray, R.S., Griffin, J., et al.: Receptor and post-receptor defects contribute to the insulin resistance in non-insulin-dependent diabetes mellitus. J. Clin. Invest. 68:957, 1981.

33. Weir, G.C.: Non-insulin-dependent diabetes mellitus: interplay between B-cell inadequacy and insulin resistance. Am. J. Med. 73:461, 1982.

34. Yalow, R.S., Berson, S.A.: Immunoassay of endogenous plasma insulin in man. J. Clin. Invest. 39:1157, 1960.

35. Perley, M., Kipnis, D.M.: Plasma insulin response to glucose and tolbutamide of normal weight and obese diabetic and nondiabetic subjects. Diabetes 15:867, 1966.

36. Gavin, J.R., III, Kahn, C.R., Gorden, P., et al.: Radioreceptor assay of insulin: comparison of plasma and pancreatic insulins and proinsulins. J. Clin. Endocrinol. Metab. 41:438, 1975.

37. Seltzer, H.S., Allen, E.W., Herron, A.L., Brennan, M.T.: Insulin secretion in response to glycemic stimulus: relations of delayed initial release to carbohydrate intolerance in mild diabetes mellitus. J. Clin. Invest. 46:323, 1967.

38. Deckert, T., Lauridsen, U.B., Madsen, S.N., Morgensen, P.: Insulin response to glucose, tolbutamide, secretin, and isoprenaline in maturity-onset diabetes mellitus. Dan. Med. Bull. 19:222, 1972.

39. Palmer, J.P., Benson, J.W., Walter, R.M., Ensinck, J.W.: Arginine stimulated acute phase of insulin and glucagon secretion in diabetic subjects. J. Clin. Invest. 58:565, 1976.

40. Savage, P.J., Dippe, S.E., Bennett, P.H., et al.: Hyperinsulinemia and hypoinsulinemia-insulin responses to oral carbohydrates over a wide spectrum of glucose tolerance. Diabetes 24:363, 1975.

41. Hidaka, H., Nagulesparan, M., Kimes, I., et al.: Improvement of insulin secretion but not insulin resistance after short-term control of plasma glucose in obese Type II diabetics. J. Clin. Endocrinol. Metab. 54:217, 1982.

42. Kahn, C.R.: The role of insulin receptors in insulin resistant states. Metabolism 29:455, 1980.

43. Olefsky, J.M., Reaven, G.M.: Insulin binding in diabetes, relationships with plasma insulin levels and insulin sensitivity. Diabetes 26:680, 1977.

44. Kahn, C.R., Baird, K.L., Flier, J.S., et al.: Insulin receptors, receptor antibodies, and the mechanism of insulin action. Rec. Prog. Horm. Res. 37:477, 1981.

45. Archer, J.A., Gorden, P., Roth, J.: Defect in insulin binding to receptors in obese man: amelioration with caloric restriction. J. Clin. Invest. 55:166, 1975.

46. DePirro, R., Fusco, A., Lauro, R.: Erythrocyte insulin receptors in non-insulin-dependent diabetes mellitus. Diabetes 29:96, 1980.

47. Gavin, J.R., III, Roth, J., Neville, D.M., Jr., et al.: Insulin-dependent regulation of insulin receptor concentrations: a direct demonstration in cell culture. Proc. Natl. Acad. Sci. USA 71:84, 1974.

48. Howard, M.J., Hidaka, H., Ishibashi, F., et al.: Type II diabetes and insulin resistance: evidence for lack of inherent cellular defects in insulin sensitivity. Diabetes 30:562, 1981.

49. Scarlett, J.A., Gray, R.S., Griffin, J., et al.: Insulin treatment reverses the insulin resistance of Type II diabetes mellitus. Diabetes Care 5:353, 1982.

50. Pedersen, O., Hjøllund, E.: Insulin receptor binding to fat and blood cells and insulin action in fat cells from insulin-dependent diabetics. Diabetes 31:706, 1982.

4 Diabetes Mellitus and the Immune System

Antoine Kaldany, Edward J. Busick, and
George S. Eisenbarth

Although knowledge of the immune system has recently been enriched by an unprecedented proliferation of discoveries in fundamental immunology, the understanding of the diseases associated with immunologic aberrations is just beginning to benefit from these fundamental advances. The concept of ''autoimmunity'' has changed markedly during the last few years, and appears to involve genetic, immunologic, and viral factors interacting through complicated mechanisms still poorly understood.

Ideally, in order to be considered an autoimmune phenomenon, a pathologic process should meet a series of criteria, delineated by Milgrom and Witebsky[1] in 1962: (a) the presence of either a circulating antibody or cell-mediated immune reaction against antigens of the target organs; (b) identification of a specific antigen within the involved organ which is the target of the immune response; (c) immunization of experimental animals with this specific antigen must elicit an immune response; (d) the disease must be produced in an experimental animal; and (e) the disease can be transferred from an immunized animal to a normal recipient by serum and/or immunologically competent cells. Hopefully, as knowledge progresses, an additional fundamental criterion will be added, namely that ''immunotherapy'' can prevent or cure the disease. Like many clinical disorders presumed to have an autoimmune etiology, diabetes fulfills some, but not all of the above criteria.

The predisposition to develop an autoimmune disease may be determined partially by genetic factors. Most autoimmune conditions occur more frequently in the families of affected individuals,[2] and in many instances, women are more frequently affected than men.[3] Also, in animal models of human diseases,[4] genetic factors clearly determine disease susceptibility.

The study of transplantation (or histocompatibility) antigens led to the definition of a major histocompatibility complex (MHC) in man and in several species of animals, including mice.[5] More recent work has demonstrated the importance of various MHC genes in immune responsiveness (Ir genes) and disease susceptibility and, in particular, susceptibility to insulin-dependent diabetes (IDDM). Neither the exact mechanisms by which Ir genes function nor the reasons for the association between specific MHC genes and certain diseases, are well understood. The current status of the MHC has recently been reviewed.[6-8]

AUTOIMMUNE ASPECTS OF DIABETES IN MAN

In the following discussion, we shall review and discuss the "autoimmune" aspects of diabetes mellitus in man, some important animal models of "autoimmune" insulitis and diabetes, and the immunogenicity of insulin as it may relate to the diabetic syndrome. A distinct form of "autoimmune" diabetes secondary to anti-insulin receptor antibodies is discussed in Chapter 3.

Immunopathogeneic Aspects of Diabetes

Insulitis. As early as 1940, von Meyenberg introduced the name "insulitis" to describe the inflammatory lesions present in the islets of Langerhans of some diabetics.[9] These lesions are characterized by inflammatory infiltration, predominantly lymphocytic, with or without cellular degeneration, and with or without fibrosis (which appears at a later stage). Such lymphocytic infiltration of the islets already had been described by Schmidt,[10] Weichselbaum,[11] and Heiberg[12] at the beginning of the century, well before the discovery of insulin. Their pioneering work was reviewed by Kraus in 1929.[13]

It was not until the studies of LeCompte in 1958,[14] however, that the presence of these inflammatory cells was considered significant in the genesis of the diabetic syndrome. In 1965, Gepts confirmed LeCompte's findings and reported insulitis in 15 of 22 patients with diabetes of recent onset. Insulitis was not seen in the pancreas of those diabetics who had survived for longer than 1 year.[15,16] Although additional studies noted lymphocytic infiltration in the islets of young persons with a short history of diabetes,[17-19] the exact frequency of insulitis is still controversial since others have found only a small proportion of cases affected.[20] In elderly diabetics, insulitis appears to be extremely rare, since only two case reports have been published to date.[21]

We were able recently to detect with emission computerized tomography scanning, active infiltration of indium[111]-labeled peripheral blood lymphocytes in an acutely diabetic 14-year-old patient (Fig. 4–1).[22]

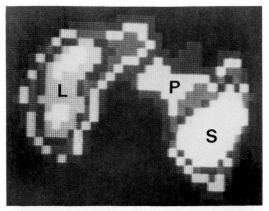
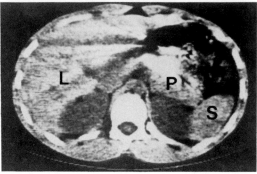

Fig. 4–1. Anatomic correlation between abdominal x-ray CT scan and emission CT scan of case #1. Single photon ECT body images of the indium oxine scan and liver-spleen sulfur colloid scan combined by computer processing on a Digital PDP-11 computer. (S = spleen; P = pancreas; L = liver.) (From Kaldany et al.[22] with permission of author and publishers.)

The primary problem, therefore, is to determine the significance of insulitis in the pathogenesis of diabetes mellitus. It may be the result of an environmental aggressor, e.g., a virus, acting either directly or by triggering an autoimmune reaction resulting in beta cell damage and death. Although not specific, the histologic characteristics of the lesions are compatible with either hypothesis. At this time there is uncertainty concerning the exact incidence of insulitis in newly diagnosed insulin-dependent diabetes (IDDM) and the role of insulitis as an integral part of the pathogenetic process of the disease is unproven.

Viruses and Diabetes. Since the initial report linking mumps and diabetes was published in 1899,[23] many such associations have been evoked with mumps,[24-26] rubella,[27-30] Coxsackie B4[31-34] and, to a much lesser extent, with infectious hepatitis,[35] influenza and mononucleosis.[36] For more exhaustive listing of references, see Craighead's review.[37] We shall review two lines of evidence, based on viral antibody titers and epidemiologic data.

Viral Antibody Titers. One would expect to find significant differences in viral antibody titers between patients with IDDM and healthy controls. In 1969, Gamble[32] found that levels of circulating antibodies to Coxsackie B4 virus were significantly higher in persons with IDDM of recent onset than in control subjects. In a later series, Gamble et al. confirmed the high prevalence of anti-Coxsackie B4 antibodies in those insulin-dependent diabetics with disease of short duration, especially in the 10–19-year age group.[34] Yet when cellular immunity to Coxsackie virus was investigated by the leukocyte migration inhibition test, no difference was found between juvenile insulin-dependent diabetics and age- and sex- matched controls.[38] Furthermore, Dippe et al. were unable to detect an increased incidence of diabetes in an isolated population of one of the Pribilof Islands in the Aleutian chain, five years after a severe epidemic of Coxsackie B4 virus.[39] Neither did Weaver et al. (quoted in Maugh's review[40]) in Belfast find a significant difference between diabetics and controls regarding antibody titers to Coxsackie B4.

Epidemiologic Data. The epidemiologic evidence linking diabetes and viruses has long been limited to the temporal association of viral diseases with the onset of diabetes. Diabetes occurs in a large percentage of patients with the congenital rubella syndrome.[27–30] A seasonal variation in the incidence of juvenile diabetes was reported first in 1926 by Adams.[41] In 1969, Gamble and Taylor in Great Britain reported a seasonal incidence of diabetes in patients below the age of 20 years.[31] In a more recent review, Gamble confirmed the seasonal pattern, eliciting one major peak at 11 to 12 years and secondary peaks at 5, and 8 to 9 years.[42] These peaks may be related to school entry at 4 to 5 years, transfer to elementary school at 7 to 8 years and to secondary school at 11 to 12 years.[42] Although these epidemiologic features could result from other influences, virus infection may provide a plausible explanation. Moreover, as discussed below, virus-induced diabetes in animals, and evidence for Coxsackie B4 virus antibodies in juvenile diabetics,[31–34] give circumstantial support to this hypothesis. Recent studies indicating that subclinical beta cell destruction may precede overt diabetes by some years[43] are a serious challenge, however, to the theory of acute viral-induced diabetes. If chronic progressive beta cell destruction is the rule, then the winter peaks may simply represent the development of overt hyperglycemia due to the stress of infection.

Yoon et al.[44] isolated Coxsackie B4 virus from the pancreas of a 10-year-old boy who died 7 days after the onset of acute IDDM following an influenza-like illness, providing the first evidence of virus-induced IDDM in humans. The child appears to have died from encephalitis and no data are provided concerning his prior metabolic status, but pathologic studies indicated chronic islet damage in this child. (W. Gepts: oral communication at IV International Workshop on Autoimmunity in Diabetes, April, 1983.) There have been no further reports concerning the isolated virus to assist in evaluating its pathogenic significance.

AUTOANTIBODIES AND DIABETES

Islet Cell Antibodies

The presence of islet cell antibodies (ICA) in diabetics has been the focus of widespread interest. Although originally discovered in those with IDDM and coexisting polyendocrine autoimmune disorders, circulating islet cell antibodies have been reported in uncomplicated IDDM as well as in a subgroup of patients with non-insulin-dependent diabetes (NIDDM).[45]

Insulin-Dependent Diabetes (IDDM). All available series show a high prevalence of ICA in recently diagnosed IDDM (Fig. 4–2). Nearly one-half of the recently diagnosed children with IDDM tested by Lendrum et al. had circulating ICA. In contrast, thyrogastric antibodies were detected in only 6% of the juveniles, and these were found only in older children.[46–48]

Three groups have recently completed extensive and representative screening of large populations.[49–51] Their combined results are shown in Table 4–1. The overall prevalence of ICA in IDDM was 20.2%. Whether or not circulating ICA are detected in IDDM depends largely on the duration of the disease. Lendrum et al. found ICA in 85% of patients with IDDM immediately after onset of the disease; they became less frequent as the duration of symptoms became longer.[50]

In most patients with IDDM, circulating ICA titers tend to decrease gradually and possibly disappear; however, in a sizeable percentage of cases, they remain stable for several years. Furthermore, ICA have been detected in nondiabetic patients: (a) the overall incidence of ICA in the general population has been reported to vary from 0.9 to 1.7%; (b) of 522 patients with documented autoimmune disorders, 31 (6%) were found to have circulating ICA; and (c) ICA have been detected in relatives of patients with IDDM, as well as in healthy playmates of children with newly diagnosed IDDM.[45] The measurement of cytoplasmic anti-ICA is still unfortunately an area with almost as much "art" as "science," depending on the availability of pancreases from human cadavers. The difficulties as-

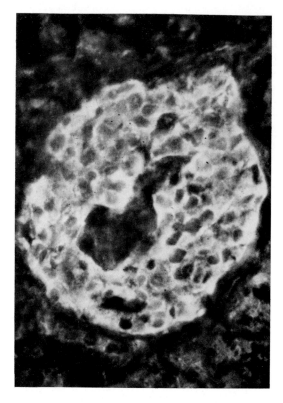

Fig. 4–2. Anti-"cytoplasmic" anti-islet antibody. Indirect immunofluorescence using serum from a patient with Type I diabetes and frozen normal human pancreas. This staining pattern is not typical but is the best staining one sees with human serum positive for anti-islet antibodies.

Table 4–1. Islet Cell Antibodies in Sera of Diabetic Patients and Nondiabetic Controls

Subjects Tested		Islet Cell Antibodies Present	
Status	Number	Number	Percent
Diabetic			
Insulin dependent	1848	540	29.2
Noninsulin dependent	851	54	6.3
Nondiabetic	1716	22	1.3

Numbers include the combined data of Irvine et al.,[49] Lendrum et al.,[50] and Del Prete et al.[51] Taken from Kaldany[45] with permission of author and publisher.

sociated with the assay almost certainly explain some of the divergent results in the literature.

Data are accumulating to indicate that anti-islet antibodies and progressive beta cell dysfunction in relatives (monozygotic twins and first degree relatives) precede by years the development of overt diabetes.[43,52] In particular, the Barts-Windsor study, by screening a population of first degree relatives of patients with Type I diabetes, found approximately 10% with anti-islet antibodies. All

patients who developed diabetes within a 3-year follow-up had anti-islet antibodies at the initial measurement.[53] Ganda and colleagues in an ongoing prospective study of insulin release in monozygotic twins have identified several twins who have developed Type I diabetes. In these individuals, anti-islet antibodies preceded the development of diabetes and, more importantly, were associated with slow progressive loss of first phase insulin release in response to glucose given intravenously.[52,54] The chronic loss of insulin secretory ability can precede hyperglycemia by years. Approximately 1 year prior to the onset of overt diabetes, there is often a complete loss of response to intravenous glucose, while response to intravenous glucagon, oral glucose, intravenous arginine and intravenous tolbutamide are relatively preserved (intravenous glucagon > intravenous arginine or oral glucose > intravenous tolbutamide > intravenous glucose).[54]

Non-Insulin-Dependent Diabetes (NIDDM).
The prevalence of islet cell antibodies (ICA) in NIDDM varies from 6 to 8%. Of the 851 patients with NIDDM reported to date, 54 or 6.3% had documented circulating islet cell antibodies (Table 4–1).

Irvine et al.[55] found circulating ICA in the sera of 20 patients with NIDDM treated with oral hypoglycemic agents. On long-term follow-up (4 years), only 2 patients (10%) remained stable while 13 patients (65%) required insulin and 5 patients (25%) required a combination of oral hypoglycemic agents at maximal dosage.[56] In contrast, only 14 of 150 (9.3%) patients lacking ICA required insulin over a mean period of 50 months. It appeared that NIDDM with circulating ICA represented an earlier stage of a disease process, culminating in IDDM. In fact, a greater prevalence of IDDM was found in family members of patients with NIDDM and circulating ICA.[55,56] In an extensive survey of patients with autoimmune disorders, Irvine et al. identified and followed 36 such patients with circulating ICA. Fourteen of these patients (38.9%) had an abnormal glucose tolerance test (GTT) and an additional 4 (11%) developed insulin-dependent diabetes.[56]

Although the above series of reports are relatively recent, and much may still be learned from longer follow-up, it appears that in some cases of NIDDM and latent diabetes, circulating ICA may serve as markers for future insulin dependence. One question that remains to be answered is: Do ICA cause future beta cell failure, or do they reflect ongoing cell damage? We suspect that the anti-ICA are only a small part of the immunologic process leading to beta cell destruction. In particular in the "BB" rat model of Type I diabetes, Koevary and colleagues have demonstrated that concanavalin-A-treated splenic cells can transfer diabetes, but no one has created diabetes in animals by transferring anti-islet cell antibodies.[57]

Islet Cell Antibodies and HLA Antigens. Several reports have confirmed an association between some HLA antigens and insulin-dependent diabetes. HLA-DW3,DR3, and more recently DW4,DR4 have been found to be increased in Caucasian diabetic populations. HLA-B8 and DW3,DR3 are increased also in auto-immune disorders such as Addison's disease, Graves' disease and hypogonadotrophic hypogonadism. As one would expect, there is an association between HLA-B8 and islet cell antibodies (Table 4–2). This correlation becomes stronger if ICA persist for more than 5 years after the onset of diabetes. No data are yet available for DW4 and ICA.[58]

Antibody to Cultured Human Insulinoma Cells. MacLaren et al. incubated sera from 39 patients with IDDM with a cultured human cell line initially considered an insulinoma.[59] These cells had been maintained in cell cultures since 1959. Positive immunofluorescence or cytoadherence and the presence of IgM and IgA were observed in the sera of 34 of 39 insulin-dependent diabetics. In contrast, only two of 15 non-insulin-dependent diabetics and one of 30 nondiabetic controls reacted with the cell cultures.

Autoantibodies to Glucagon and Somatostatin-Producing Cells. In 1976, Bottazzo and Lendrum reported the presence of autoantibodies which had reacted against either glucagon or somatostatin-producing cells with a specific granular intracellular fluorescence. Of 1,279 sera tested, 13 (1.0%) gave specific alpha cell fluorescence and 4 (0.31%) gave specific somatostatin cell fluorescence. This specificity was confirmed by double staining techniques, and the antibodies were of either IgG or IgM class. These autoantibodies are clearly distinct from the so-called islet cell antibodies: In some instances islet cell antibodies

were identified as IgG. Some A cell antibodies reacted as IgG and others as IgM. The absence of plasma membrane staining indicates that circulating antibodies fail to react with plasma membrane determinants.[60]

The exact significance of these antibodies is unclear, since they were found in diabetics as well as in normal controls. The reported cases are too few in number to permit speculation on their eventual role in the pathogenesis of any endocrine disorder.

Autoantibodies to Beta Cells. After pre-treating diabetic sera with peroxidase, Sorenson et al.[61] obtained indirect IgG fluorescence staining of beta cells only. Once again, the staining was "intracytoplasmic." The significance of such antibodies is uncertain because sera from 12 patients with cystic fibrosis and 19 nondiabetic controls gave similar fluorescence of beta cells only.

Complement-Fixing Islet Cell Antibodies. Bottazzo et al.[62] reported the presence of complement-fixing ICA in IDDM. In their study, these were more closely related to the onset of clinical disease than are the conventional islet-cell antibodies and they tend to disappear more rapidly. Indirect immunofluorescence produces an often diffuse and confluent cytoplasmic staining. Presence of complement fractions of C3, C1q and C4 suggest that complement may be activated by the classical pathway.

Islet Cell Surface Antibodies. Pre-incubation of cultures with viable ob/ob mouse islet cells in serum from patients with Type I diabetes revealed the presence of antibodies directed against islet cell plasma membranes.[63] Identical immunofluorescence patterns were obtained by utilizing serum from islet-immunized or virus-infected mice with glucose intolerance.

More recently, Lernmark et al.[64] detected circulating islet cell surface antibodies in 28 of 88 (32%) insulin-treated patients with juvenile diabetes by using cultured rat islet cells. Islet cell surface fluorescence was inhibited by pre-absorption of serum to islet cells, but not to other tissues. Unfortunately, whether or not these antibodies are specific for beta cells, remains to be proven.

Cytotoxic Anti-Islet Antibodies. Doberson and colleagues demonstrated cytotoxic anti-islet antibodies reacting with normal rat islet cells[65] and Eisenbarth and colleagues, such antibodies reacting with a rat insulinoma cell line (RINm5F).[66] These cytotoxic antibodies may be beta cell specific.

Despite the finding of anti-cell surface antibodies, their true significance is unknown. With such assays there are more false positives and more false negatives than with the standard immunofluorescent assays using frozen tissue sections. In partic-

Table 4–2. Association of Islet Cell Antibodies (ICA) and HLA-B8 in Diabetes

Subjects Tested	Number	HLA-B8 Frequency Percent
Normal population	300	28
Diabetic		
ICA negative	20	35
ICA positive	99	60
ICA positive ≤ 1 yr*	56	55
ICA positive >5 yr*	35	71

*After diagnosis of diabetes.

Taken from Kaldany[45] with permission of author and publisher.

ular in one series, thyroiditis patients appeared to have as high a prevalence of such antibodies as patients with diabetes.[64] Whereas evidence is accumulating that when properly measured, anti-"cytoplasmic" anti-islet antibodies predict disease development, there are little data available as to the predictability of anti-"surface" antibodies.

Other Auto-Antibodies in Diabetes Mellitus. Patients with polyendocrine autoimmune disorders often have circulating autoantibodies to thyroglobulin and cells of thyroid, adrenal, and gastric parietal origin. These antibodies are usually seen in conjunction with circulating islet cell antibodies, and occur more frequently in individuals possessing the HLA-A1, B8, DW3 haplotype. The peculiarities of this type of IDDM were discussed above.[67,68]

Hormone-producing tissues seem particularly vulnerable to assault by autoimmune disease mechanisms. Multiple gland failures coexist with diabetes and overt autoimmunity more often than can be expected by chance alone. Thyrogastric autoimmune diseases such as pernicious anemia,[69–71] thyrotoxicosis,[72] Hashimoto's thyroiditis,[73] and primary hypothyroidism[74] have all been reported to occur with increased frequency in diabetics as well as in their first degree relatives.[72] The most impressive example is idiopathic Addison's disease (autoimmune adrenalitis), in which the prevalence of overt diabetes is approximately 14%,[75] i.e., about 6 times higher than in the general population. Diabetes may coexist with multiple autoimmune disorders, notably the combination of adrenalitis and thyroiditis (Schmidt's syndrome) and frequently appears in familial endocrinopathies.[68,75] These clinical observations are complemented and largely confirmed by the discovery of circulating organ-specific autoantibodies. Most investigators record a 2-fold to 4-fold increase in the prevalence of thyrogastric cytoplasmic antibodies in diabetic sera.[71] Intrinsic factor antibody occurs with similar frequency, and adrenal antibody may be 30 times more common in diabetic than in nondiabetic populations.[71]

In a review including 972 diabetics, Irvine summarized data concerning circulating autoantibodies to thyroid, gastric mucosa, and adrenal cortex.[49] All three types of antibodies were found to be significantly increased in IDDM, with no correlation between age at onset or duration of diabetes and the incidence of antibodies. Conversely, antibodies to the intrinsic factor were found in both insulin-dependent and insulin-independent diabetics above the age of 40 years. In these patients, achlorhydria was found in 83% of those tested by gastric analysis. Yet, although the Schilling test may be depressed, vitamin B_{12} levels were normal in virtually

all patients, thus the term of "latent pernicious anemia" in older diabetics.[71]

In addition, a subset of patients with IDDM also have other HLA-DR3 associated autoimmune diseases such as celiac disease and myasthenia gravis. This is of particular clinical importance in patients evaluated for "diabetic enteropathy" to exclude celiac disease. In some families, Schmidt's syndrome (polyendocrine autoimmune syndrome Type II) is inherited in an autosomal dominant manner.[68]

Organ-Specific Cell-Mediated Autoimmunity in Diabetes Mellitus.

Cell-mediated autoimmunity in diabetes mellitus has been studied by many investigators. Lymphocytes obtained from insulin-dependent diabetics showed abnormal production of migration inhibitory factor when tested in vitro with pancreatic islet extracts.[76–80] Identical results were obtained when lymphocytes from patients with IDDM were incubated with insulin or B-chain, but not when incubated with A-chain preparations.[81] Similarly, these lymphocytes underwent active in vitro blastogenesis when cultured with insulin or B-chain.[82,83] Furthermore, Vel'Bri reported similar phenomena with lymphocytes from patients who were never treated with insulin.[84] More recently, Huang and Maclaren[85] found abnormal cytoadherence and direct cytotoxicity of lymphocytes from insulin-dependent patients against cultured insulinoma cells.

Monoclonal Antibody T Cell Typing

The development of techniques to enumerate T cell populations has progressed rapidly. These methods have been applied to study patients with Type I diabetes, using monoclonal antibodies to distinguish T cell subsets. These antibodies can be divided into two groups: (1) those marking apparently functionally distinct T cell subsets (T4, T8, 3A1) and (2) those reacting with activated T cells—Ia antigens (e.g., L243), the transferrin receptor (5E9) and a 120,000 dalton glycoprotein antigen (4F2). Our own studies using these monoclonals have revealed a marked abnormality among T cells expressing the L243 antigen (i.e., Ia positive cells) in patients with early Type I diabetes.[86,87] In a series of autoimmune disorders including Graves' disease, Ia positive T cells are elevated and thus are not specific for Type I diabetes.[88] We find approximately 70% of patients with Type I diabetes are positive for anti-islet antibodies and 70% for Ia positive T cells, and more than 90% of patients are positive for one or the other marker. Studies have not been carried out to define whether individuals who are negative for both markers have a different form of diabetes (e.g., Maturity Onset Diabetes of the Young—MODY).

THE MAJOR HISTOCOMPATIBILITY COMPLEX AND DIABETES MELLITUS

The HLA System

The term HLA represents the major histocompatibility complex (MHC) in man. As in other vertebrates, it controls three different sets of characters: (1) alloantigenicity; (2) some components of the complement system; and (3) some immune responses.[89]

The HLA system consists of two categories of closely linked genes on the short arm of the sixth chromosome:

(a) HLA-A, B, and C genes, controlling antigens present on all nucleated cell surfaces that are detectable by serologic techniques and linked to B2 microglobulin—a nonpolymorphic peptide coded for on chromosome 15;

(b) HLA-D and DR genes, controlling antigens present on only some cells (macrophages, B lymphocytes) and *not* associated with B2 microglobulin. HLA-D antigens are defined by cell culture techniques such as mixed lymphocyte culture (MLC) and primed lymphocyte typing (PLT), while HLA-DR antigens are recognized by serologic methods. Whether HLA-D/DR are products of the same locus or of closely linked loci remains to be determined.[90]

The HLA system is extremely polymorphic at each locus (except those controlling complement components). There is pronounced linkage disequilibrium between these various loci, i.e., some HLA antigens occur much more frequently in the same individual than would be expected from their individual frequencies (example: HLA-A1-B8-DR3). This phenomenon may be important for the understanding of HLA and disease associations.

HLA and Disease: Methods of Study

Two approaches are used in studying the association between HLA and disease:

Population Studies. These involve the typing of a number of unrelated patients and analysis of HLA antigen frequencies in comparison with a "normal" population of the *same ethnic origin* as the patients. The strength of association between a given HLA antigen and the disease is expressed as the relative risk (RR).

Family Studies. These require the testing of families in which more than one member is affected with diabetes. Such studies are often difficult to carry out because varying penetrance and age at onset have to be taken into account. Furthermore, families with accumulated cases represent biased samples, as it is possible they carry more disease susceptibility than families with only one patient. Nevertheless, family studies are essential for adequate analysis of haplotype inheritance and "longitudinal" transmission of disease.[90]

HLA and Insulin-Dependent Diabetes (IDDM)

Many studies found a strong association between specific HLA alleles and IDDM and, in particular between IDDM and HLA-B8 and B15.[91,92] In addition, a negative correlation between IDDM and HLA-B7 has been noted.[93] Workers have reported a degree of positive association between HLA-DR3 and HLA-DR4 and IDDM, higher than with other antigens studied.[94] Indeed, the specific allelic associations vary among ethnic groups. IDDM in the Japanese is strongly associated with factors in the HLA complex; the specific association is with BW54, a Japanese variant of BW22 and with HLA-DR4.[95,96]

Within families, disease correlates with inheritance of common sixth chromosome. Thus less than 2% of siblings who share neither sixth chromosome (identified by HLA typing) with a diabetic sibling, will develop IDDM[95,96] and some 30% of HLA identical siblings are expected to be diabetic by age 30 years.

The exact pathogenic role of the HLA molecules is not defined. Recently a family of HLA-DR(1a) molecules have been characterized and a direct role for such antigens in influencing the response to soluble antigens proved in mice. Although the great majority of patients with Type I diabetes are DR3 or DR4 positive, most individuals who are DR3 or DR4 positive are normal. This suggests that these molecules are "necessary" but not sufficient for the development of diabetes, and other genes (probably also on the sixth chromosome) influence disease susceptibility. To speculate, DR3 and DR4 probably are associated with a high immunologic response to islet cell antigens (DR3) and insulin (DR4, see later discussion) accounting for their association with Type I diabetes.

ANIMAL MODELS OF AUTOIMMUNE INSULITIS AND DIABETES

Spontaneous diabetes is observed in many animal species. In addition, animals can be rendered diabetic by means of surgery, viral infection, or the administration of various hormones and chemical agents. We shall limit our review to those animal models of IDDM pertinent to autoimmune insulitis. For a comprehensive review, the reader is referred to Chapter 7. The following is a review of various experimental models of "autoimmune" diabetes.

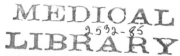

Passive Induction of Insulitis by Transfer of Antisera

In 1965, Lacy and Wright[97] injected guinea pig anti-bovine insulin antiserum into rats to neutralize their endogenous insulin and produce a diabetic state. However, none of the animals became diabetic and in only a few animals, did the authors find mononuclear and eosinophilic leukocytes within some of the islets. The main result observed was an interstitial inflammation of the exocrine part of the pancreas. Similarly, Logothetopoulos and Bell[98] observed transient islet inflammation in mice which were injected with guinea pig alloantiserum.

A more chronic model of this so-called "polymorphocellular immune complex" type of insulitis was later produced by Freytag in 1972;[99] the protocol involved repeated injections into mice of guinea pig anti-insulin (bovine) serum. This model was characterized by the presence of greater numbers of lymphocytes and fewer eosinophils in and around the islets. This polymorphocellular insulitis is comparable to an immune complex-type reaction, with a local Arthus phenomenon at the islet level. Diazoxide, which inhibits insulin secretion from the beta cells, also prevents the induction of polymorphocellular insulitis.[100] The finding of this polymorphocellular type of insulitis in mice is significant because similar infiltrates are frequently observed in the pancreas of the newborn of diabetic mothers.

Active Induction of Experimental Insulitis in Animals Immunized with Insulin

"Lymphoidcellular immune insulitis" was observed in the pancreas of some species following immunization with heterologous or homologous insulin in Freund's adjuvant. Lymphocytic infiltration of the pancreatic islets has been demonstrated only in cows, sheep, and rabbits. Twenty years ago, Renold et al.[101,102] reported the first observation in cattle immunized with bovine and porcine insulin in Freund's adjuvant. The lymphocytic infiltration of the islets was of variable degree, and few islets showed fibrosis. Despite widespread destruction of the beta cell mass, none of the animals became diabetic. Similar experiments in sheep produced severe pancreatic islet damage. The animals had high serum titers of anti-insulin antibodies and strongly positive skin tests for delayed hypersensitivity to insulin, but none became diabetic.[103]

Similar lymphoidcellular insulitis may also be produced in rabbits following immunization with bovine but not porcine insulin in Freund's adjuvant. Despite severe islet and beta cell damage and atrophy, and high titers of anti-insulin antibodies,

only a few animals developed transient glucose intolerance.[104–108]

In guinea pigs, immunization with insulin resulted in high titers of antibodies, but no insulitis.[109]

Experimental Virus-Induced Insulitis

Although the insulitis lesion may be the expression of an immunopathologic process, one should keep in mind that viral infections often produce similar mononuclear cell infiltrates. This question, though crucial, remains unresolved in man.

Since Gamble et al.[34] found antibodies against certain viruses more frequently in juveniles with IDDM than in control groups, we have to consider that virus infections may occur that result in IDDM without clinically overt pancreatitis. Craighead et al.[110–112] and From et al.[113] were able to induce insulitis with glucose intolerance by infecting mice with live M variant of the encephalomyocarditis (EMC) virus. The lesion was associated with macrophage and lymphocyte infiltration of the pancreas. Although the exact mechanism of islet cell damage is still undetermined, degranulation of beta cells is a hallmark of the disease process. More recently, a similar insulitis produced by cytomegalovirus (CMV) in mice has received considerable attention. Typical CMV viral inclusions are found in many pancreatic beta cells of infected mice.[114–117]

The host's genetic background plays a major role in the animal's susceptibility to viral infection and the development of insulitis. While 80% of DBA mice become diabetic, NMRI-mice always remain non-diabetic when injected with EMC virus.[118–120]

Streptozotocin-Induced Insulitis

Like and Rossini reported a unique model of insulitis and insulin-dependent diabetes in the mouse.[121] Multiple intraperitoneal or intravenous injections of small subdiabetogenic doses of streptozotocin in CD-1 male mice, produced a progressive increase in plasma glucose within 5 to 6 days after the injections, associated with pronounced insulitis and induction of Type C viruses within beta cells. The importance of cell-mediated immunity in the genesis of insulitis was demonstrated by the partial protective effect of rabbit anti-mouse lymphocyte serum prior to the administration of streptozotocin.[122]

The genetic background of the host is of paramount importance in the pathogenesis of this model: of eight strains of mice studied by Rossini et al.,[123] only C57BL/KsJ developed insulitis and hyperglycemia comparable to that observed in CD-1 mice. In two mouse strains (DBA/2J and BALB/cJ) having an H-2^d haplotype similar to the C57BL/KsJ, only mild insulitis and glucose intolerance were observed. These data suggest that although playing a role, the major histocompatibility complex genes, as presently defined, cannot be the only determinants of the severity of hypergylcemia and insulitis in this model.

Spontaneous IDDM Model in Wistar Rats ("BB" Rats)

Although laboratory animal models exist that are analogous to the juvenile-onset IDDM and maturity-onset NIDDM types of human disease, a new spontaneously diabetic syndrome in nonobese outbred Wistar rats of both sexes, deserves special mention here.[124–130] This model displays hyperglycemia, insulin deficiency, glucagon excess and ketosis, with dramatic inflammatory lesions of insulitis during active beta cell destruction. These "BB" rats develop IDDM between 60 and 120 days of age. The development of diabetes appears to be independent of any environmental influence. The prevalence of diabetes is unaltered when pups are raised in a germ-free environment. Most importantly, diabetes can now be routinely prevented by multiple forms of immunotherapy including neonatal thymectomy, anti-lymphocyte globulin, cyclosporin A, and bone marrow transplantation.[131–133] That both immunologic ablative and restorative therapies are successful, probably relate to the severe T cell immunodeficiency of these animals.[134] BB rats inherit in an autosomal recessive fashion a severe T-cell lymphopenia which is necessary but not sufficient for the development of diabetes. It is likely that in addition to this lymphopenia gene, one or more additional genes determine that beta cells are the target of the disordered immunity. Koevary and colleagues have demonstrated that diabetes can be transferred by activated BB spleen cells to immunodeficient but not normal rats.[57] The BB rats are an important model for disordered immunoregulation leading to diabetes, but do differ from man in the severity of their T-cell deficiency.

IMMUNOGENICITY OF INSULIN: ANTI-INSULIN ANTIBODIES AND THE DIABETIC SYNDROME

The dependence of IDDM patients on commercial insulin preparations makes discussion of the immunologic aspects of insulin therapy mandatory. These patients must take daily injections of a polypeptide extracted from pancreases of other species by acid alcohol and then purified and chemically treated to alter the duration of action after the injection. (At present, relatively few patients are taking the newly introduced "human insulin" prepared by recombinant DNA technique.)

In 1938, Glen and Eaton noted that serum from a patient requiring 1,000 units of insulin per day could protect mice from insulin-induced convulsions.[135] By 1950, sera from nine such patients were reported.[136] In 1956, Berson et al. first reported the presence of insulin-binding antibodies in the sera of diabetics treated with insulin.[137] However, albeit confirmation of these findings by others,[138,139] an accurate assessment of the immunogenicity of various insulin preparations was complicated by the presence of protein impurities.[140,141] Many of these impurities are now removed from insulin preparations by gel filtration and/or ion exchange chromatography.[140]

Antigenicity of Various Insulin Preparations

Although most investigators agree that virtually all available insulin preparations are immunogenic, it is clear that some preparations are much more antigenic than others. Comparing the antigenicity of various porcine and bovine lente insulins prepared from either conventional USP-grade insulin, or the more purified "single-peak" and "single-component" insulins, Chance et al. found that bovine preparations were the most immunogenic, while porcine "single-component" insulin was found to be the least immunogenic.[142] These findings are in agreement with earlier reports[143,144] that certain impurities play a role in insulin immunogenicity.[140,145,146] However, the data reported by Chance et al.[142] with porcine "single-peak" insulin indicated that although it was practically devoid of proinsulin (0.05%), this preparation was as immunogenic as conventional USP porcine insulin. Thus, some of the insulin-like molecules, such as desamino insulins and insulin ethyl ester(s) usually found in the "single-peak" preparation, may play an important role in insulin immunogenicity.[147] These are truly artifactual molecules created during large-scale insulin processing such as acid-alcohol extraction procedures. Immunogenicity studies with these insulin-like components are limited. Root et al.[140] found that only porcine A-component was immunogenic while bovine A and B components were equally immunogenic.

Since most authorities concur that lente (USP single-peak and single component) bovine preparations are significantly more immunogenic than USP porcine insulin, this becomes of practical concern, since most of the insulin preparations in the world consist wholly or partly of bovine insulin. Furthermore, Tantillo et al.[148] found that mixed bovine-porcine single-peak insulin was as immunogenic as mixed USP insulins.

The pharmaceutical form of insulin plays a major role as to its immunogenicity.[138] Thus, so-called regular preparations of bovine single-component insulin are much less immunogenic than the lente form which has poor solubility at neutral pH and may therefore act as an adjuvant. Conversely, long-acting forms of highly purified porcine insulin preparations maintain a low immunogenicity.[142,143]

Davidson and DeBra[149] used sulfated beef insulin (introduced in Canada in 1964 by Maloney and colleagues[150]) to treat patients with immunologic insulin resistance. Their results suggested that this form of insulin was much less antigenic than regular preparations, and produced a better clinical response than pork insulin.

Even human insulin when injected subcutaneously is now known to be antigenic and in all probability induces titers of antibodies similar to those of the purest porcine insulins.[151]

Anti-Insulin Antibodies: Characterization and Significance

An ideal method for measuring anti-insulin antibodies is not currently available. Some methods are influenced by the concentration of insulin in plasma.[151] With the most commonly used methods, insulin antibodies are characterized by the amount of labeled or unlabeled insulin bound to immunoglobulins. However, few comparisons of different methods are available, and the results of most published studies can be evaluated only against their own control material.

The major factors determining the antigenicity of insulin preparations are summarized below:

(a) The injection trauma and the sharp increase of local insulin concentration.

(b) The species of insulin: the antigenicity of bovine insulin preparations is more pronounced than the antigenicity of pure porcine insulin preparations in man (see above).

(c) Acidity and particle size: low pH increases the antigenicity of insulin preparations. Soluble insulin is less antigenic than regular (crystalline) insulin, and small crystals less than large.[139]

(d) Degree of purity (see above).

(e) Patient's age: young patients produce more antibodies than elderly patients.[152]

(f) Previous insulin treatment: if insulin therapy is interrupted and resumed, a secondary antibody response is to be expected.[138]

(g) Genetic factors: the highest titers of anti-insulin antibodies have been found in HLA-B15, HLA-DR4 individuals, while HLA-B7 diabetics have only minor antibody production.[92]

Clinically, insulin antigenicity may be responsible for a number of side effects. Severe allergic reactions caused by injection of insulin have been known since the early days of insulin treatment.[153,154] The introduction of more purified insulin preparations has significantly reduced the incidence of such reactions. Once a patient is

sensitized, administration of even highly purified insulin may induce allergic reactions.[153] If skin testing with a highly purified regular porcine insulin in a patient with a clinically important allergic reaction induces a positive result, desensitization should be considered (see Chapter 19).

Immunologically induced insulin resistance may or may not coexist with insulin allergy and is usually due to circulating IgG insulin antibodies. In spite of high doses of insulin, the effect on blood glucose levels may be minimal and ketoacidosis is not often observed. The insulin-binding capacity of the patient's serum is usually very high. Fortunately, life-threatening insulin resistance is extremely rare. Treatment should aim at lowering insulin requirements (caloric restriction), increasing insulin sensitivity (exercise), increasing endogenous insulin production (sulfonylureas), and replacing the insulin in use with a highly purified pork insulin preparation. During the acute phase, the patient should be maintained on a continuous intravenous infusion of insulin. For further discussion of the treatment of both immunogenic and nonimmunogenic insulin resistance, see Chapter 19.

Insulin antibodies may significantly shorten the length of the remission period when present.[144] Presumably, insulin antibodies are able to bind and "neutralize" or "eliminate" the patient's endogenous insulin.

It is uncertain whether circulating insulin-insulin antibody complexes play a role in the development of chronic diabetic complications. Andersen[155] reported a positive correlation between circulating insulin antibodies and the early development of proliferative retinopathy and/or nephropathy. Although it is generally agreed that insulin antibodies are not likely the cause of diabetic microangiopathy, they could well modify the course of the complications in at least two ways:

(a) By interfering with the metabolic action of insulin.

(b) By forming immune complexes which adhere

Table 4–3. Evidence that Insulin-Dependent Diabetes (IDDM) May Be an Autoimmune Disease in Humans

1. Overt diabetes is preceded by the development of
   a. Islet cell antibodies and
   b. Ia positive T cells.
2. These developments lead to progressive loss of beta cell function, as shown in serial glucose tolerance tests.
3. Transplantation of a pancreatic segment from the non-diabetic identical twin of a patient with IDDM may result in insulitis in the graft with specific beta cell destruction.*

*Sutherland et al.[159a]

to vascular walls, bind and activate complement, and elicit inflammation and destruction (intermediate size immune complexes are most pathogenic in this context). Fölling has shown that complement-binding intermediate size insulin-anti-insulin complexes may develop during immunization against insulin.[156] Wehner et al.[141,157] found changes in the basement membrane of glomerular capillaries in rabbits and mice treated with antigenic insulin preparations but not in animals treated with purified insulin preparations of low antigenicity. These findings, however, were not confirmed by Hägg[158] or by Westberg and Michael.[159]

Final Comment

There is increasing evidence that insulin-dependent diabetes (IDDM) in humans is an autoimmune disease (Table 4–3). In light of current long-term morbidity and mortality of "IDDM" and in view of the success of immunotherapy in preventing diabetes in the BB rat, a number of centers are developing immunotherapeutic protocols in an attempt to block beta-cell destruction in human patients.[160–164] To date no successful randomized trials have been reported, although the results of several pilot studies are encouraging.

It is apparent that there are significant risks associated with current forms of immunotherapy; therefore, it is crucial that the efficacy and side effects of such treatment be carefully evaluated in randomized trials prior to their introduction (if ever) into general practice. Without evaluation and monitoring, such therapy has the potential of doing more harm than good. At present, immunotherapy of IDDM should be attempted only with the overview of a Human Investigations Committee.

REFERENCES

1. Milgrom, F., Witebsky, E.: Autoantibodies and autoimmune diseases. J.A.M.A. 181:706, 1962.
2. Brown, D.L., Dacie, J.V., Worlledge, S. (revised by D.L. Brown): Autoallergic blood diseases. In: P.J. Lachmann, D.K. Peters (Eds.): Clinical Aspects of Immunology, 4th Ed. Oxford, Blackwell Scientific Publications, 1982, pp. 747–776.
3. Hooper, B.A., Whittingham, S., Mathews, J.D., et al.: Autoimmunity in a rural community. Clin. Exp. Immunol. 12:79, 1972.
4. Holmes, M.C, Burnet, F.M.: The characteristics of F₁ and backcross hybrids between "high leukaemia" (AKR) and "autoimmune" (NZB) mouse strains. Aust. J. Exp. Biol. Med. Sci. 44:235, 1966.
5. Klein, J.: The major histocompatibility complex of the mouse. Science 203:516, 1979.
6. H.O. McDevitt (Ed.): Ir Genes and Ia Antigens. Proceedings of the 3rd Ir Gene Workshop Held at Asilomar, Calif. Dec. 13–16, 1976. New York, Academic Press, 1978.
7. Carpenter, C.B.: Autoimmunity and HLA. J. Clin. Immunol. 2:157, 1982.
8. Schaller, J.G., Hansen, J.A.: HLA relationships to disease. Hosp. Pract. 16:41, 1981.
9. von Meyenberg, Von H.: Über 'Insulitis' bei Diabetes. Schweiz. Med. Wschr. 21:554, 1940.
10. Schmidt, M.B.: Über die Beziehung der Langerhans'schen Inseln des Pankreas zum Diabetes mellitus. Münch. Med. Wschr. 49:51, 1902.
11. Weichselbaum, A.: Über die Veränderungen des Pankreas bei Diabetes mellitus. Sitzungber. Kais. Akad. Wssnsch. Mat-Nat. Kl. 119:73, 1910.
12. Heiberg, K.A.: Über Diabetes bei Kindern. Arch. Kinderheilk. 56:403, 1911.
13. Kraus, E.J.: Die pathologisch-anatomischen Veränderungen des Pankreas beim Diabetes mellitus. In: F. Henke, O. Lubarsch (Eds.): Handbuch des speziellen pathologischen Anatomie und Histologie. Vol. 5. Part 2 Berlin, Springer, 1929, pp. 622–747.
14. LeCompte, P.M.: "Insulitis" in early juvenile diabetes. Arch. Pathol. 66:450, 1958.
15. Gepts, W.: Pathologic anatomy of the pancreas in juvenile diabetes mellitus. Diabetes 14:619, 1965.
16. Nagler, W., Taylor, H.: Diabetic coma with acute inflammation of islets of Langerhans. J.A.M.A. 184:723, 1963.
17. Crome, L., Erdohazi, M., Rivers, R.P.: Fulminating diabetes with lymphocytic thyroiditis. Arch. Dis. Childhood 42:677, 1967.
18. Steiner, M.: Insulitis beim perakuten Diabetes des Kindes. Klin. Wschr. 46:417, 1968.
19. Ogilvie, R.F.: The endocrine pancreas in human and experimental diabetes. In: M.P. Cameron, M. O'Connor (Eds.): Aetiology of Diabetes Mellitus and its Complications. Ciba Foundation Colloquia on Endocrinology. Vol. 15. Boston, Little, Brown and Company, 1964, pp. 49–74.
20. Doniach, I., Morgan, A.G.: Islets of Langerhans in juvenile diabetes mellitus. Clin. Endocrinol. (Oxf.) 2:233, 1973.
21. LeCompte, P.M., Legg, M.A.: Insulitis (lymphocytic infiltration of pancreatic islets) in late-onset diabetes. Diabetes 21:762, 1972.
22. Kaldany, A, Hill, T., Wentworth, S., et al.: Trapping of peripheral blood lymphocytes in the pancreas of patients with acute-onset insulin-dependent diabetes mellitus. Diabetes 31:463, 1982.
23. Harris, H.F.: A case of diabetes mellitus quickly following mumps. On the pathological alterations of the salivary glands, closely resembling those found in the pancreas, in a case of diabetes mellitus. Boston Med. Surg. J. 140:465, 1899.
24. Hinden, E.: Mumps followed by diabetes. Lancet 1:1381, 1962.
25. McCrae, W.M.: Diabetes mellitus following mumps. Lancet 1:1300, 1963.
26. Dacou-Voutetakis, C., Constantinidis, M., Moschos, A., et al.: Diabetes mellitus following mumps. Insulin reserve. Am. J. Dis. Child. 127:890, 1974.
27. Forrest. J.M., Menser, M.A., Harley, J.D.: Diabetes mellitus and congenital rubella. Pediatrics 44:445, 1969.
28. Forrest, I.M., Menser, M.A., Burgess, J.A.: High frequency of diabetes mellitus in young adults with congenital rubella. Lancet 2:332, 1971.
29. Menser, M.A., Reye, R.D.: The pathology of congenital rubella: a review written by request. Pathology 6:215, 1974.
30. Menser, M.A., Forrest, J.M., Honeyman, M.: Diabetes, HLA antigens, and congenital rubella. Lancet 2:1508, 1974.
31. Gamble, D.R., Taylor, K.W.: Seasonal incidence of diabetes mellitus. Br. Med. J. 3:631, 1969.

32. Gamble, D.R., Kinsley, M.L., FitzGerald, M.G.: Viral antibodies in diabetes mellitus. Br. Med. J. 3:627, 1969.

33. Craighead, J.E.: The role of viruses in the pathogenesis of pancreatic disease and diabetes mellitus. Progr. Med. Virol. 19:161, 1975.

34. Gamble, D.R., Taylor, K.W., Cumming, H.: Coxsackie viruses and diabetes mellitus. Br. Med. J. 4:260, 1973.

35. Adi, F.C.: Diabetes mellitus associated with epidemic of infectious hepatitis in Nigeria. Br. Med. J. 1:183, 1974.

36. Burgess, J.A., Kirkpatrick, K.L., Menser, M.A.: Fulminant onset of diabetes during an attack of infectious mononucleosis. Med. J. Aust. 2:706, 1974.

37. Craighead, J.E.: Current views on the etiology of insulin-dependent diabetes mellitus. N. Engl. J. Med. 299:1439, 1978.

38. Richens, E.R., Ancil, R.J., Hartog, M.: Autoimmunity and viral infection in diabetes mellitus. Clin. Exp. Immunol. 23:40, 1976.

39. Dippe, S.E., Bennett, P.H., Miller, M., et al.: Lack of causal association between Coxsackie B4 virus infection and diabetes. Lancet 1:1314, 1975.

40. Maugh, T.H., II: Diabetes: Epidemiology suggests a viral connection. Science 188:347, 1975.

41. Adams, S.F.: The seasonal variation in the onset of acute diabetes. The age and sex factors in 1000 diabetic patients. Arch. Intern. Med. 37:861, 1926.

42. Gamble, D.R.: Viral and epidemiological studies. Proc. R. Soc. Med. 68:256, 1975.

43. Srikanta, S., Ganda, O.P., Eisenbarth, G.S., Soeldner, J.S.: Islet cell antibodies and beta cell function in monozygotic triplets and twins initially discordant for Type I diabetes mellitus. N. Engl. J. Med. 308:322, 1983.

44. Yoon, J-W., Austin, M., Onodera, T., Notkins, A.L.: Virus induced diabetes mellitus: Isolation of a virus from the pancreas of a child with diabetic ketoacidosis. N. Engl. J. Med. 300:1173, 1979.

45. Kaldany, A.: Autoantibodies to islet cells in diabetes mellitus. Diabetes 28:102, 1979.

46. Lendrum, R., Walker, G.: Serum antibodies in human pancreatic disease. Gut 16:365, 1975.

47. Bottazzo, G.F., Florin-Christensen, A., Doniach D.: Islet-cell antibodies in diabetes mellitus with autoimmune polyendocrine deficiencies. Lancet 2:1279, 1974.

48. MacCuish, A.C., Barnes, E.W., Irvine, W.J., Duncan, L.J.P.: Antibodies to pancreatic islet cells in insulin-dependent diabetics with co-existent autoimmune disease. Lancet 2:1529, 1974.

49. Irvine, W.J., McCallum, C.J., Gray, R.S., et al.: Pancreatic islet-cell antibodies in diabetes mellitus correlated with duration and type of diabetes, coexistent autoimmune disease, and HLA type. Diabetes 26:138, 1977.

50. Lendrum, R., Walker, G., Cudworth, A.G., et al.: Islet-cell antibodies in diabetes mellitus. Lancet 2:1273, 1976.

51. DelPrete, G.F., Betterle, C., Padovan, D., et al.: Incidence and significance of islet cell autoantibodies in different types of diabetes mellitus. Diabetes 26:909, 1977.

52. Srikanta, S., Ganda, O.P., Jackson, R.A., et al.: Type I diabetes mellitus in monozygotic twins. Chronic progressive beta cell dysfunction. Ann. Intern. Med. 99:320, 1983.

53. Gorsuch, A.N., Spencer, K.M., Lister, J., et al.: Evidence for a long prediabetic period in Type I (insulin-dependent) diabetes mellitus. Lancet 2:1363, 1981.

54. Ganda, O.P., Srikanta, S., Brink, S.J., et al.: Differential sensitivity to β-cell secretagogues in "early" Type I diabetes mellitus. Diabetes 33:516, 1984.

55. Irvine, W.J., Gray, R.S., McCallum, C.J.: Pancreatic islet-cell antibody as a marker for asymptomatic and latent diabetes and prediabetes. Lancet 2:1097, 1976.

56. Irvine, W.J., McCallum, C.J., Gray, R.S., Duncan, L.P.J.: Clinical and pathogenic significance of pancreatic islet-cell antibodies in diabetics treated with oral hypoglycemic agents. Lancet 1:1025, 1977.

57. Koevary, S., Rossini, A.A., Stoller, W., Chick, W.: Passive transfer of diabetes in the BB/w rat. Science 220:727, 1983.

58. Bottazzo, G.F., Doniach, D.: Pancreatic autoimmunity and HLA antigens. Lancet 2:800, 1976.

59. Maclaren, N.K., Huang, S.W., Fogh, J.: Antibody to cultured human insulinoma cells in insulin-dependent diabetes. Lancet 1:997, 1975.

60. Bottazzo, G.F., Lendrum, R.: Separate autoantibodies to human pancreatic glucagon and somatostatin cells. Lancet 2:873, 1976.

61. Sorenson, R.L., Shank, R.D., Elde, R.P.: Immunoperoxidase demonstration of human serum globulin binding to islet tissue. Diabetes 24:230, 1975.

62. Bottazzo, G.F., Dean, B.M., Gorsuch, A.N., et al.: Complement-fixing islet-cell antibodies in Type I diabetes: possible monitors of active beta-cell damage. Lancet 1:668, 1980.

63. Kromann, H., Lernmark, A., Vestergaard, B.F., et al.: H-2 influence on experimental diabetes induced by heterologous and homologous immunization and by virus (Abstr.). Diabetologia 13:410, 1977.

64. Lernmark, A., Freedman, Z.R., Hofman, C., et al.: Islet-cell-surface antibodies in juvenile diabetes mellitus. N. Engl. J. Med. 299:375, 1978.

65. Doberson, M.J., Schraff, J.E., Ginsberg-Fellner, F., Notkins, A.L.: Cytotoxic autoantibodies to beta cells in the serum of patients with insulin-dependent diabetes mellitus. N. Engl. J. Med. 303:1493, 1980.

66. Eisenbarth, G.S., Morris, M.A., Scearce, R.M.: Cytotoxic antibodies to cloned rat islet cells in serum of patients with diabetes mellitus. J. Clin. Invest. 67:403, 1981.

67. Doberson, M.J.: Humoral autoimmunity in insulin-dependent (Type I) diabetes mellitus. Surv. Immunol. Res. 1:329, 1982.

68. Eisenbarth, G.S., Jackson, R.: Immunogenetics of polyglandular failure and related disease. In: N.R. Farid (Ed.): HLA in Endocrine and Metabolic Disorders. New York, Academic Press, 1981, pp. 235–264.

69. Ungar, B., Whittingham, S., Francis, C.M.: Intrinsic factor antibody, parietal cell antibody, and latent pernicious anaemia in diabetes mellitus. Lancet 2:415, 1968.

70. Wright, R.: Gastrointestinal disorders. In: W.J. Irvine (Ed.): Medical Immunology. New York, McGraw-Hill Book Co., 1979, p. 165.

71. Irvine, W.J., Clarke, B.F., Scarth, L., et al.: Thyroid and gastric autoimmunity in patients with diabetes mellitus. Lancet 2:163, 1970.

72. Perlman, L.V.: Familial incidence of diabetes in hyperthyroidism. Ann. Intern. Med. 55:796, 1961.

73. Masi, A.T., Hartmann, W.H., Hanan, B.H., et al.: Hashimoto's disease: a clinico-pathological study with matched controls. Lancet 1:123, 1965.

74. Ganz, K., Kozak, G.P.: Diabetes mellitus and primary hypothyroidism. Arch. Intern. Med. 134:430, 1974.

75. Irvine, W.J.: Immunological aspects of diabetes mellitus. In: J. Pierluissi (Ed.): Endocrine Pancreas and Diabetes. Amsterdam, Excerpta Medica, 1979, p. 281.

76. Nerup, J., Andersen, O.O., Bendixen, G., Egberg, J.: Pancreatic cellular hypersensitivity in diabetes mellitus. Diabetes 20:424, 1971.

77. Nerup, J., Andersen, O.O., Bendixen, G.: Antipancreatic cellular hypersensitivity in diabetes mellitus. II. Acta Allergol. 28:223, 1973.

78. Nerup, J., Andersen, O.O., Bendixen, G., Egberg, J.:

Antipancreatic cellular hypersensitivity in diabetes mellitus. III. Acta Allergol. *28*:231, 1973.

79. MacCuish, A.C., Jordan, J., Campbell, C.J.: Cell mediated immunity to human pancreas in diabetes mellitus. Diabetes *23*:693, 1974.

80. Nerup, J., Andersen, O.O., Bendixen, G., et al.: Cellular hypersensitivity to islet antigens in diabetes. In: P.A. Bastenie, W. Gepts (Eds.): Immunity and Autoimmunity in Diabetes Mellitus. Amsterdam, Excerpta Medica, 1974, p. 107.

81. Faulk, W.P., Girard, J.P., Welscher, H.D.: Cell-mediated immunity to insulin and its polypeptide chains in man. In: Ibid. p. 89.

82. MacCuish, A.C., Jordan, J., Campbell, C.J., et al.: Cell-mediated immunity in newly diagnosed diabetics. Diabetes *24*:36, 1974.

83. Faulk, W.P., Girard, J.D., Welscher, H.D.: Cell-mediated immunity to insulin and its polypeptide chains in insulin-treated diabetics. Int. Arch. Allergy Applied Immunol. *48*:364, 1975.

84. Vel'Bri, S.K.: Cellular immunological reactions to insulin and pancreatic tissue in diabetics not treated with insulin. Probl. Endokrinol. (Mosk.) *23*:15, 1977.

85. Huang, S.W., Maclaren, N.: Insulin dependent diabetes: a disease of autoaggression. Science *192*:64, 1976.

86. Jackson, R.A., Morris, M.A., Haynes, B.F., Eisenbarth, G.S.: Increased circulating Ia-antigen bearing T cells in Type I diabetes mellitus. N. Engl. J. Med. *306*:785, 1982.

87. Buse, J., Rowley, R.F., Eisenbarth, G.S.: Disordered cellular immunity in Type I diabetes of man and the BB rat. Surv. Immunol. Res. *1*:339, 1982.

88. Jackson, R., Bowring, M., Morris, M., et al.: Increased circulating Ia positive T cells in recent onset Graves' disease and insulin-dependent diabetes. 63rd Annual Meeting, The Endocrine Society, 1981. (Abstr. 450) p. 195.

89. Dausset, J., Svejgaard, A. (Eds.): HLA and Disease. Copenhagen, Munksgaard, 1977. pp. 1–316.

90. G. Möller (Ed.): Ir Genes and T Lymphocytes. Immunol. Rev. 38, 1978. pp. 3–162.

91. Nerup, J., Christy, M., Kromann, H., et al.: Genetic susceptibility and resistance to insulin-dependent diabetes mellitus. In: W.J. Irvine (Ed.): Immunology of Diabetes. Edinburgh, Teviot Scientific Publ., 1980, pp. 55–66.

92. Nerup, J., Cathelineau, C., Seignalet, J., Thomsen, M.: HLA and endocrine disease. In: J. Dausset, A. Svejgaard (Eds.): HLA and Disease. Copenhagen, Munksgaard, 1977, pp. 149–167.

93. Cudworth, A.G., Fentenstein, H.: HLA genetic heterogeneity in IDDM. Br. Med. Bull. *34*:285, 1978.

94. Platz, P., Thomsen, M., Svejgaard, A., et al.: More on the genetics of juvenile diabetes. (Letter to Editor). N. Engl. J. Med. *298*:1200, 1978.

95. Mimura, G.: Present status and future view of the genetic study of diabetes mellitus. In: G. Mimura, S. Baba, Y. Goto, K. Köbberling (Eds.): Clinico-Genetic Genesis of Diabetes Mellitus. Cong. Series 597. Amsterdam, Excerpta Medica, 1982, pp. viii–xxviii.

96. Gorsuch, A.N., Spencer, K.M., Lister, J., et al.: Can future Type I diabetes be predicted? A study in families of affected children. Diabetes *31*:862, 1982.

97. Lacy, P.E., Wright, P.H.: Allergic interstitial pancreatitis in rats injected with guinea pig anti-insulin serum. Diabetes *14*:634, 1965.

98. Logothetopoulos, J., Bell, E.G.: Histological and autoradiographic studies of the islets of mice injected with insulin antibody. Diabetes *15*:205, 1968.

99. Freytag, G.H.: Immunopathologie des Diabetes mellitus. Stuttgart, Gustav Fisher, 1972.

100. Klöppel, G.: "Insulin" induced insulitis. Acta Endocrinol. (Kbh.) *83*(Suppl.205):131, 1976.

101. Renold, A.E., Soeldner, J.S., Steinke, J.: Immunological studies with homologous and heterologous insulin in the cow. Ciba Found. Coll. Endocrinol. *15*:122, 1964.

102. Renold, A.E., Steinke, J., Soeldner, J.S., et al.: Immunological response to the prolonged administration of heterologous and homologous insulin in cattle. J. Clin. Invest. *45*:702, 1966.

103. Renold, A.E., Gonet, A., Crofford, O.B., Vecchio, D.: Metabolic regulation in heterogeneous systems: some new questions about diabetes mellitus. Fed. Proc. *25*:827, 1966.

104. Toreson, W.E., Feldman, R., Lee, J.C., Grodsky, G.M.: Pathology of diabetes mellitus produced in rabbits by means of immunization with beef insulin. Am. J. Clin. Pathol. *42*:531, 1964.

105. Toreson, W.E., Lee, J.C., Grodsky, G.M.: The histopathology of immune diabetes in the rabbit. Am. J. Pathol. *52*:1099, 1968.

106. Grodsky, G.M., Feldman, R., Toreson, W.E., Lee, J.C.: Diabetes mellitus in rabbits immunized with insulin. Diabetes *15*:579, 1966.

107. Lee, J.C., Grodsky, G.M., Caplan, C.J., Craw, L.: Experimental immune diabetes in the rabbit. Am. J. Pathol. *57*:597, 1969.

108. Klöppel, G., Altenähr, E., Freytag, G.: Studies on ultrastructure and immunology of the insulitis in rabbits immunized with insulin. Virchows Arch. Pathol. Anat. *356*:15, 1972.

109. Morse, J.H.: Rapid production and detection of insulin-binding antibodies in rabbits and guinea pigs. Proc. Soc. Exp. Biol. Med. *101*:722, 1959.

110. Craighead, J.E.: Pathogenicity of the M and E variants of the Encephalomyocarditis (EMC) virus. I. Myocardiotropic and neurotropic properties. Am. J. Pathol. *48*:333, 1966.

111. Craighead, J.E.: Pathogenicity of the M and E variants of the Encephalomyocarditis (EMC) virus: II. Lesions of the pancreas, parotid and lacrimal glands. Am. J. Pathol. *48*:375, 1966.

112. Craighead, J.E., McLane, M.F.: Diabetes mellitus: induction in mice by encephalomyocarditis virus. Science *162*:913, 1968.

113. From, G.L.A., Craighead, J.E., McLane, M.F., Steinke, J.: Virus-induced diabetes in mice. Metabolism *17*:1154, 1968.

114. Smith, M.G., Vellios, F.: Inclusion disease or generalized salivary gland virus infection. Arch. Pathol. *50*:862, 1926.

115. Wyatt, J.P., Saxton, J., Lee, R.S., Pinkerton, H.: Generalized cytomegalic inclusion disease. J. Pediatr. *36*:271, 1950.

116. Craighead, J.E.: Animal model of human disease. Am. J. Pathol. *78*:537, 1975.

117. Craighead, J.E.: Inflammatory lesions of the islets of Langerhans. In: R.O. Greep, E.B. Astwood, D.F. Steiner, N. Freinkel (Eds.): Handbook of Physiology. Sect. 7. Endocrinology, v. 1. Endocrine Pancreas. Washington, American Physiological Society, 1972, pp. 315, 321.

118. Münterfering, H.: Zur Pathologie des Diabetes mellitus der weissen Maus bei der EMC-Virusinfektion. Histologische, elektronenmikroskopische und quantitativ morphologische Befunde an den Langerhansschen Inseln. Virchows Arch. Pathol. Anat. *356*:207, 1972.

119. Münterfering, H., Schmidt, W.A.K., Körber, W.: Experimenteller Beitrag zur Virusgenese des Diabetes mellitus bei der weissen Maus. Verh. Dtsch. Ges. Pathol. *54*:669, 1970.

120. Münterfering, H., Schmidt, W.A.K., Körber, W.: Zur Virusgenese des Diabetes mellitus bei der weissen Maus. Dtsch. Med. Wschr. *96*:693, 1971.
121. Like, A.A., Rossini, A.A.:Streptozotocin-induced pancreatic insulitis: new model of diabetes mellitus. Science *193*:415, 1976.
122. Rossini, A.A., Like, A.A., Chick, W.L., et al.: Studies of streptozotocin-induced insulitis and diabetes. Proc. Natl. Acad. Sci. USA *74*:2485, 1977.
123. Rossini, A.A, Appel, M.C., Williams, R.M., Like, A.A.: Genetic influence of the streptozotocin-induced insulitis and hyperglycemia. Diabetes *26*:916, 1977.
124. Nakhooda, A.F., Like, A.A., Chappel, C.I., et al.: The spontaneously diabetic Wistar rat. Metabolic and morphologic studies. Diabetes *26*:100, 1977.
125. Nakhooda, A.F., Like, A.A., Chappel, C.I., et al.: The spontaneously diabetic Wistar rat (the "BB" rat). Studies prior to and during development of the overt syndrome. Diabetologia *14*:199, 1978.
126. Nakhooda, A.F., Poussier, P., Marliss, E.B.: Insulin and glucagon secretion in BB Wistar rats with impaired glucose tolerance. Diabetologia *24*:58, 1983.
127. Rossini, A.A., Williams, R.M., Mordes, J.F., et al.: Spontaneous diabetes in the gnotobiotic BB/W rat. Diabetes *28*:1031, 1979.
128. Like, A.A., Williams, R.M., Kislauskis, E., Rossini, A.A.: Neonatal thymectomy prevents spontaneous diabetes in biobreeding Worcester (BB/w) rat. (Abstr.) Clin. Res. *29*:542, 1981.
129. Rossini, A.A., Williams, R.M., Appel, M.C., Like, A.A.: Animal models of Type I diabetes. In: W.J. Irvine (Ed.): Immunology of Diabetes. Edinburgh, Teviot Scientific Publications, 1980, pp. 275–290.
130. Jackson, R., Rassi, N., Crump, T., et al.: The BB diabetic rat. Profound T-cell lymphocytopenia. Diabetes *30*:887, 1981.
131. Like, A.A., Anthony, M., Guberski, D.L., Rossini, A.A: Spontaneous diabetes mellitus in the BB/W rat. Effects of glucocorticoids, cyclosporin-A, and antiserum to rat lymphocytes. Diabetes *32*:326, 1983.
132. Naji, A., Silvers, W.K., Bellgrau, D., et al.: Prevention of diabetes in rats by bone marrow transplantation. Ann. Surg. *194*:328, 1981.
133. Like, A.A., Rossini, A.A., Guberski, D.L., et al.: Spontaneous diabetes mellitus: reversal and prevention in the BB/W rat with antiserum to rat lymphocytes. Science *206*:1421, 1979.
134. Jackson, R., Kadison, P., Buse, J., et al.: Lymphocyte abnormalities in the BB rat. Metabolism *32*(Suppl. 1):83, 1983.
135. Glen, A., Eaton, J.C.: Insulin antagonism. Q.J. Med. *7*:271, 1938.
136. Davidson, J.K., III, Eddleman, E.E., Jr.: Insulin resistance: review of the literature and report of a case associated with carcinoma of the pancreas. Arch. Intern. Med. *86*:727, 1950.
137. Berson, S.A., Yalow, R.S., Bauman, A., et al.: Insulin I[131] metabolism in humans. Circulating insulin-binding globulin in insulin-treated diabetics. J. Clin. Invest. *35*:170, 1956.
138. Deckert, T., Grundahl, E.: The antigenicity of pig insulin. Diabetologia *6*:15, 1970.
139. Andersen, O.O.: Insulin antibody formation. II. The influence of species difference and method of administration. Acta Endocrinol. (Kbh) *72*:33, 1973.
140. Root, M.A., Chance, R.E., Galloway, J.A.: Immunogenicity of insulin. Diabetes *21*:657, 1972.

141. Wehner, H., Huber, H., Kronenberg, K.H.: The glomerular basement membrane of the rabbit kidney on long-term treatment with heterologous insulin preparations of different purity. Diabetologia *9*:255, 1973.
142. Chance, R.E., Root, M.A., Galloway, J.A.: The immunogenicity of insulin preparations. Acta Endocrinol. (Kbh.) *83*(Suppl. 205):185, 1976.
143. Deckert, T., Andersen, O.O., Poulsen, J.E.: The clinical significance of highly purified pig insulin preparations. Diabetologia *10*:703, 1974.
144. Andersen, O.O.: The clinical importance of insulin-binding antibodies. Acta Endocrinol. *78*:723, 1975.
145. Deckert, T., Andersen, O.O., Grundahl, E., Kerp, L.: Isoimmunization of man by recrystallized human insulin. Diabetologia *8*:358, 1972.
146. Czyzyk, A., Lawecki, J., Rogala, H., et al.: Serum levels of insulin-binding antibodies in diabetic patients treated with monocomponent insulin. Diabetologia *10*:233, 1974.
147. Klöppel, G., Freytag, G.: Insulin antibodies and immune insulitis in rabbits immunized with bovine or porcine insulin components. Horm. Metabol. Res. *7*:25, 1975.
148. Tantillo, J.J., Karam, J.H., Burrill, K.C., et al.: Immunogenicity of "single peak" beef-pork insulin in diabetic subjects. Diabetes *23*:276, 1974.
149. Davidson, J.K., DeBra, D.W.: Immunologic insulin resistance. Diabetes *27*:307, 1978.
150. Maloney, P.J., Aprile, M.A., Wilson, S.: Sulfated insulin for treatment of insulin resistant diabetes. J. New Drugs *4*:258, 1964.
151. Skyler, J.: Human insulin of recombinant DNA origin: clinical potential. Diabetes Care *5*(Suppl. 2):181, 1982.
152. Andersen, O.O.: Insulin antibody formation. I. The influence of age, sex, infections, insulin dosage and regulation of diabetes. Acta Endocrinol. (Kbh) *71*:126, 1972.
153. Galloway, J.A., Root, M.A.: New forms of insulin. Diabetes *21*(Suppl.):637, 1972.
154. Kumar, D.: Antiinsulin IgE in diabetics. J. Clin. Endocrinol. Metab. *45*:1159, 1977.
155. Andersen, O.O.: Clinical significance of anti-insulin antibodies. Acta Endocrinol. (Kbh) (Suppl.)205:231, 1976.
156. Fölling, I.: Insulin-anti-insulin complexes. Acta Endocrinol. (Kbh) (Suppl.) *205*:199, 1976.
157. Wehner, H.: The influence of insulin and insulin antibodies on the glomerular structure. Acta Endocrinol. (Kbh) (Suppl.) *205*:241, 1976.
158. Hägg, E.: On the pathogenesis of glomerular lesions in the alloxan diabetic rat. Acta Med. Scand. (Suppl.) *558*:1, 1974.
159. Westberg, G.N., Michael, A.F.: Immunohistopathology of diabetic glomerulosclerosis. Diabetes *21*:163, 1972.
159a.Sutherland, D.E.R.: Personal communication.
160. Elliott, R.B., Crossley, J.R., Berryman, C.C., James, A.G.: Partial preservation of pancreatic beta cell function in children with diabetes. Lancet *2*:1, 1981.
161. Ludvigsson, J., Heding, L., Liedén, G., et al.: Plasmapheresis in the initial treatment of insulin-dependent diabetes mellitus in children. Br. Med. J. *286*:176, 1983.
162. Leslie, R.D.G., Pyke, D.A.: Immunosuppression of acute insulin-dependent diabetes. In: W.J. Irvine (Ed.): Immunology of Diabetes. Edinburgh, Teviot Scientific Publications, 1980, pp. 345–347.
163. Eisenbarth, G.S., Srikanta, S., Jackson, R., et al.: Immunotherapy of recent onset Type I diabetes mellitus. Clin. Res. *31*:500A, 1983.
164. Stiller, C.R., Lauparis, A., Dupre, J., et al.: Cyclosporine for treatment of early Type I diabetes: preliminary results (Letter to the Editor). N. Engl. J. Med. *308*:1226, 1983.

5 Insulin Biosynthesis, Structure, Storage, and Release

Walter S. Zawalich

Because glucose is an indispensable metabolic fuel, its levels in man are precisely regulated. Various homeostatic mechanisms have evolved to insure that the tissues of the body have prompt access to glucose, should the need arise. The liver, for example, a principal depot for glucose storage, is quite sensitive to the actions of the catecholamines and glucagon, releasing glucose into the blood stream in response to their stimulation.[1,2] Under normal conditions, however, the greatest excursions of blood glucose are usually produced by the ingestion of a carbohydrate-containing meal. Prompt and efficient uptake of the exogenous carbohydrate for subsequent utilization depends on an adequate delivery of insulin to insulin-sensitive targets, primarily liver, muscle and adipose tissue.[3] It has been suggested that a deficient or delayed insulin response to glucose levels in blood underlies in part the glucose intolerance which manifests itself as diabetes.[4] It is the primary function of the beta cell of the islets of Langerhans to analyze substrate levels and, if necessary, to release insulin. Cellular secretory activity may be tempered by hormonal and neuronal influences and several important metabolic fuels. Most available evidence suggests, however, that glucose is the principal physiologic regulator of the beta cell activity and hence, insulin levels.[5,6] Glucose has profound short and long-term effects on the capacity of the beta cells to secrete insulin. It is perhaps not coincidental that glucose also affects the processes which regulate insulin synthesis and storage, in addition to secretion.[7]

Rapid advances in our understanding of the beta cells have been made in the past decade. Most important, perhaps, is the realization that they possess the capacity to alter their responsiveness to various stimulants, depending on environmental conditions. For example, the prior dietary status of the organism (excessive food intake, starvation) may determine to a large extent the subsequent secretory activity of the beta cell. This chapter concerns itself with the factors which control the biosynthesis, storage and perhaps most importantly, the release of insulin from the pancreatic beta cell.

INSULIN BIOSYNTHESIS

For the purpose of discussion, the biosynthesis of insulin can be divided conveniently into several well-defined stages (Fig. 5–1). The genetic information which will initiate biosynthesis is, of course, present in the beta cell deoxyribonucleic acid (DNA). It is here that the amino acid sequence of the protein is encoded. In a process requiring ribonucleic acid (RNA) polymerase, a messenger (m) RNA is transcribed from the gene. Insulin mRNA has a half-life of approximately 2 hours.[8] With the development of systems for the cell-free translation of messenger RNA, particularly wheat germ ribosomal systems, the polypeptide products encoded in insulin mRNA have been examined.[9] The initial translation product has been termed preproinsulin.[10] In the rat, preproinsulin differs from proinsulin by an additional 23 amino acid residues attached to the N-terminal region of the nascent polypeptide. While the exact structure of human

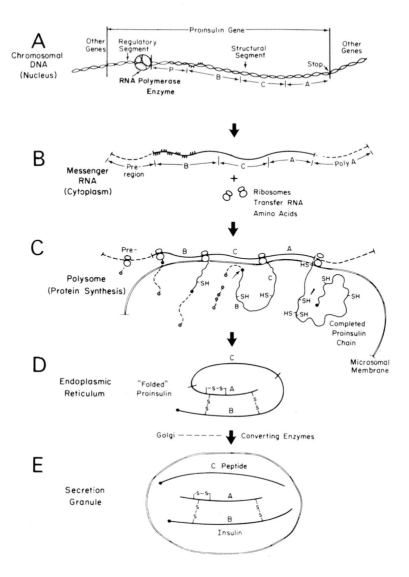

Fig. 5–1. Simplified scheme depicting the biochemical events involved in insulin formation. A. The DNA segment containing the insulin (or more correctly, the preproinsulin) gene is transcribed by a DNA-directed RNA polymerase, resulting in the synthesis of a preproinsulin messenger RNA. B. In the cytoplasm, the necessary machinery and components are assembled. C. The initial product of (m)RNA translation, the "pre" portion of the nascent insulin molecule, facilitates the association of the ribosomes with the endoplasmic reticulum. This "pre" portion appears to be cleaved from the developing peptide before synthesis of the entire molecule is completed. D. In the cisternal spaces of the endoplasmic reticulum, peptide chain folding and sulfhydryl oxidation occur. E. Biochemical changes in the secretory granules represent the final stages of the synthetic process. In the granule formed by the Golgi apparatus, conversion of proinsulin and C-peptide occurs. Although the process may be initiated in the Golgi apparatus, it appears to continue for several hours as the granules collect in the cytosol. (From Steiner and Tager,[154] with permission of the authors and publisher.)

proinsulin is known (Fig. 5–2), that of human preproinsulin has yet to be precisely determined. The "pre" portion of the molecule has a half-life of about 1 minute,[12] may be cleaved before the synthesis of the protein is completed, and probably serves to facilitate the association of ribosomal-bound messenger RNA with the membrane of the endoplasmic reticulum.[13]

The odyssey of the proinsulin molecule continues in the cisternal spaces of the endoplasmic reticulum which serve as a system of collecting channels where peptide chain folding and sulfhydryl oxidation occur.[14] This latter intramolecular event results in the union of the peptide fractions destined to become the A and B chains of insulin. An energy-requiring process assures transfer from the

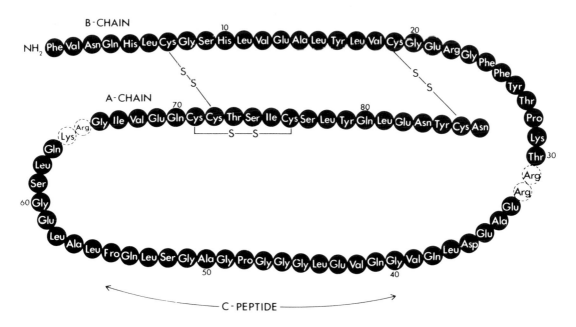

Fig. 5–2. Structure of human proinsulin. The circles in broken lines indicate the sites of cleavage, a process occurring in the secretory granule. (From Oyer et al.,[11] with permission of the authors and publisher.)

rough endoplasmic reticulum to the Golgi apparatus.[15] It is here that insulin granules are first recognizable, although these initially appear immature and less dense than the fully developed granules.[16] The Golgi apparatus is responsible for the synthesis of the membranous sac surrounding the developing granule.[17] By facilitating fusion with the cell membrane, this sac may play a vital role in the process of granule extrusion from the cell.[18] In the developing granules, several important cellular processes occur. First, the proinsulin is cleaved to insulin and connecting C-peptide, a process involving proteolytic cleavage by some as yet undefined enzyme system.[19,20] Second, zinc is taken up and together with insulin, forms what appear to be microcrystals of zinc insulin, the probable storage form of the hormone.[17] Because these conversion processes occur in the membranous sac of the developing granule, C-peptide and zinc are sequestered here to be released with insulin upon appropriate beta cell stimulation. Furthermore, because the proteolytic conversion process also appears to be imperfect, some proinsulin is also released along with insulin.[21]

Transport of Granules to Cell Surface. Since beta cell stimulation must obviously include an increase in the transport of the granules to the surface of the cell, several groups have attempted to characterize the systems involved. It was initially postulated that Brownian movement might be sufficiently rapid to account for stimulated secretion.[22] Lacy and coworkers, however, suggested the in-

volvement of a microtubular-microfilamentous system to account for granule movement.[23] In several reports,[24,25] using compounds known to disrupt or stabilize microtubules, they demonstrated that exposure to these agents blocked insulin secretion from the beta cell. Interestingly, cytochalasin B, a fungal metabolite known to interfere with microfilament organization, potentiated the insulin secretory response of the islets to glucose and tolbutamide.[26] Orci and co-workers[27] suggested that the cortical band of microfilaments noted in the beta cell may act as a type of sphincter or barrier for granule extrusion. Disruption of this band by cytochalasin B presumably removed this barrier and subsequently potentiated islet secretory responsiveness. As described by Lacy and Greider,[28] the microtubular-filamentous system can be considered a single functional unit whose primary objective upon appropriate stimulation, is the orderly translocation of beta cell granules to the cell's surface. While the involvement of calcium with this system appears unquestionable,[29] its site of action as well as the contractile proteins involved, remains a fertile area of research.

Emiocytosis. The final step in the release of insulin from the beta cell involves the fusion of the membranous sacs surrounding the granule with the plasma membrane. Obviously the continuity of both membranes must be breached, releasing insulin into the extracellular space for subsequent transport to distant tissues. Little is known about this final process termed emiocytosis (also called exocytosis in other systems), or the intracellular events which dominate the beta cell post-stimulation.[30] Whether the restructuring or recycling of the plasma membrane plays any role in the heightened secretory responsiveness noted after intense stimulation[31] remains to be determined.

The scenario depicted up to now does little justice to the dynamic nature of the beta cell. All the processes described are probably under some type of regulation, although through necessity and design, only several have been well studied. This does not imply that some processes are more important than others, but that some are more amenable to investigation. Serious deficiencies still exist in our understanding of the completed process from the initiation of transcription to emiocytosis. However, particularly well studied are the factors which stimulate insulin biosynthesis and a few words seem warranted about this aspect of cellular activity.

Factors Stimulating Insulin Biosynthesis. Insulin biosynthesis by the beta cell is remarkably sensitive to alterations of the ambient glucose concentration within the physiologic range.[7,8,32,33] Although the effect is dependent upon further catabolism of glucose[32] and is evidently related to both transcriptional (increase in messenger RNA) and post-transcriptional (perhaps a preferential translation of preformed insulin messenger RNA) events,[8] the underlying mediator or mediators have yet to be identified. In the case of glucose, the hexose does not have to actually stimulate secretion in order to stimulate insulin biosynthesis because the effect on the latter process[34] is still noted, even in the absence of extracellular calcium which totally abolishes secretion.[35] Based on studies gleaned from numerous reports, several generalities about insulin biosynthesis can be made. Compounds which are well metabolized by the beta cell are best able to augment biosynthesis. Consequently, glucose, mannose,[32] glyceraldehyde,[36] and N-acetylglucosamine,[37] compounds avidly utilized by the beta cell, promote this effect while poorly metabolized hexoses such as fructose are impotent.[38] Several metabolized non-sugars also augment biosynthesis. Thus, leucine,[39] alpha-ketoisocaproate[40,41] and several ribonucleosides[42] stimulate the synthetic process. The biosynthetic effect can easily be dissociated from secretion since several compounds, most notably sulfonylureas, stimulate the secretion but not the biosynthesis of insulin. In fact, sulfonylureas have been reported to suppress insulin biosynthesis.[43] Taken together, it does appear that a common metabolic intermediate or a co-factor generated during substrate catabolism, augments both the biosynthesis and release of the hormone (Fig. 5–3). While the

advantages of coupling both of these processes are obvious, the nature of the intracellular trigger generated during metabolism and how it interacts, directly or indirectly with either DNA, DNA-directed RNA polymerase, messenger RNA, or other cellular components, remains a matter for speculation.

Genetic Mutants of Insulin. Until the last few years, it was tacitly assumed by many workers that the myriad components, ranging from the gene to the synthetic machinery involved in insulin biosynthesis, displayed little heterogeneity. This concept reflected to a large extent the technical limitations in analyzing these processes. More recently, however, several variant insulins displaying decreased biological activity have been identified and their possible pathogenic involvement in diabetes suggested.[43a–43c]

Insertions of 1.5 to 3.4 kilobase pairs in the 5′-flanking region have been found in DNA obtained from some patients with non-insulin-dependent diabetes (NIDDM). It is not clear whether other alterations of the genetic component of the insulin gene (chromosome 11) might be present. While it does appear unlikely that insulins displaying abnormal structure and biological activity due to genetic mutations account for an appreciable number of persons with NIDDM, this area does remain most fertile for further research activity.

STIMULUS-SECRETION COUPLING IN THE PANCREATIC BETA CELL

The machinery for insulin biosynthesis functions to maintain insulin stores at appropriate levels. While some spontaneous discharge of the hormone occurs, granules are rapidly mobilized by various stimulants. Attempts to define the nature of the sensor system of the beta cell which allows for extreme flexibility in responding to chemically diverse stimulants, has occupied the efforts of numerous investigators. Rapid advances in this area have been made possible by both improved islet isolation techniques[44,45] and because of the application of radioisotopic tracers to assess metabolic fluxes.[46,47]

Quite simply, two major theories have evolved to explain the stimulant action of glucose on insulin secretion by the pancreatic beta cell and these will be discussed here in some detail. The first theory, the "substrate-site" theory, envisions a metabolite of glucose or a co-factor generated during its catabolism as being the actual stimulant for insulin secretion.[48–50] An alternative "glucose receptor" (glucoreceptor) theory has also been formulated, which suggests that the nonmetabolized intact glucose molecule is the actual stimulant for secretion.[51,52]

Reports in the early 1960s suggested that only

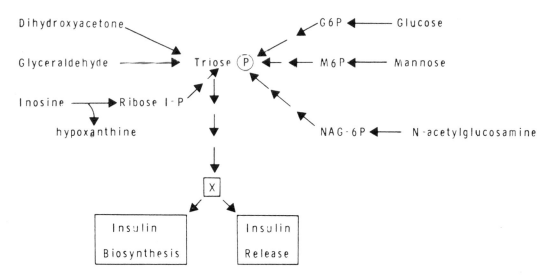

Fig. 5–3. Effects of several sugars and their derivatives on insulin biosynthesis and secretion. According to Ashcroft[60] these can be explained by their ability to generate a common metabolic intermediate—a triose phosphate. The precise nature of the intracellular trigger generated by this compound remains a matter for speculation, although reduced pyridine nucleotides and phosphoenolpyruvate have been implicated in the process (See text).

those sugars capable of being catabolized by islet cells were stimulants of secretion.[48,49] Thus, glucose and mannose, whose metabolism was inferred but not measured, stimulated secretion, while the nonmetabolized sugars, 3-0-methylglucose and 2-deoxyglucose or poorly metabolized fructose, were ineffective. Studies employing mannoheptulose, a 7-carbon sugar which blocks both glucose and mannose phosphorylation and further utilization, supported the concept that the metabolism of the hexose was a requirement for induced secretion.[49,53] The observation that both glyceraldehyde and dihydroxyacetone were metabolized by pancreatic beta cells and stimulated insulin secretion, gave added impetus to this theory.[36,54–56] Most importantly, neither the secretory nor metabolic functions of glyceraldehyde were affected by mannoheptulose.[54,57] Because the three-carbon compound pyruvate had little secretory activity,[48,49] it was suggested that the ultimate trigger for insulin secretion was probably generated at or below the level of the triose phosphates and prior to pyruvate formation (Fig. 5–3). Furthermore, results with metabolic inhibitors have generally been consistent with a key role of the catabolism of the molecule as regulating insulin secretion.[57] Probably the inhibitor of choice is mannoheptulose, which appears to affect only the metabolic and releasing functions of glucose and mannose and leaves largely intact the secretory responsiveness to various other stimulants including leucine,[54] glyceraldehyde,[54] and N-acetylglucosamine.[58] As a result of this latter situation, it has been suggested and later verified, that islets possess a distinct N-acetylglucosamine kinase re-

sponsible for the phosphorylation of this compound.[59]

INTRACELLULAR FATE OF GLUCOSE AND THE POSSIBLE NATURE OF THE INTRACELLULAR TRIGGER FOR STIMULATED SECRETION

The difficulties in delineating the role that glucose metabolism plays in coupling the ambient hexose level to the insulin secretory apparatus and in identifying the nature of the glucose sensor system involved, can be best appreciated if the factors controlling the uptake and metabolic fate of the sugar are briefly considered. Two distinct issues are involved—what factors regulate usage and what is the nature of the metabolic signal generated. In regard to the first point, and as suggested by Ashcroft,[60] the "glucose sensor system can perhaps be identified as the rate-limiting step for glucose utilization." In this context the enzymic apparatus, particularly those enzymes catalyzing rate-limiting reactions, assume primary importance. Without going into exhaustive detail, the glucose sensor system can be best identified with the high K_m glucose-phosphorylating enzyme, glucokinase, known to exist in the islet.[60–62] This enzyme possesses the necessary kinetic properties, K_m and V_{max}, to accurately couple glucose concentration and metabolic flux. It is competitively blocked by mannoheptulose and its activity is reduced by fasting, two conditions associated with impaired secretion.[62] That the activities of the low K_m hexokinase and high K_m glucokinase determine the pattern of glucose usage observed with the intact islets seems probable (Fig. 5–4).

After its phosphorylation in the beta cell, several pathways remain accessible to glucose-6-phosphate:[11] conversion to glycogen,[2] oxidation via the pentose cycle, and the glycolytic pathway.[3] However, little glucose is converted into glycogen[46] and only a few percent appears to traverse the pentose

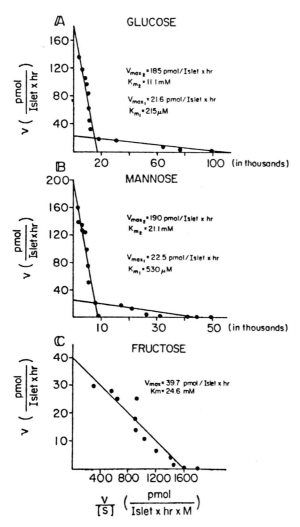

cycle.[46,63] Most glucose-6-phosphate appears to be glycolyzed.[64] Recently, however, Ammon and co-workers have emphasized the importance of the pentose cycle in the regulation of secretion.[65,66] Earlier published reports demonstrated that little glucose-6-phosphate was oxidized via this cycle and that its activity was even decreased with stimulated secretion.[46] Ammon has taken issue with these studies, arguing that the high levels of insulin which are allowed to accumulate under these static, batch-type incubations with isolated islets, have yielded results of questionable physiologic significance. He has further demonstrated quite convincingly an inhibitory effect of high insulin levels both on the fraction of glucose which traverses the pentose cycle,[65,66] an effect which may obscure its importance in regulating secretion under more physiologic conditions, and on NAD(P)H levels. Based on these studies, it was concluded that the reduced pyridine nucleotide NAD(P)H may function as the intracellular trigger for secretion.[67] If correct, these provocative results seem to imply that only a small fraction of the glucose utilized by the islet may be concerned with generating the ultimate triggering species for secretion. Although interesting, this theory needs further validation. In particular, the effects of glyceraldehyde, a potent stimulant of secretion which enters the glycolytic pathway at the triose phosphate step, on the levels of NAD(P)H, remain to be assessed. In a series of comprehensive investigations, Malaisse and co-workers[68–70] have proposed a preeminent role for the reduced pyridine nucleotide NADH as the intracellular regulator of induced secretion. Because its generation is coupled to the formation of reduced pyridine nucleotides, it might also be inferred from these as well as other studies[71] that the beta cell may in some manner be influenced by small and perhaps localized pH changes which occur as a result of an increase in metabolic flux. This notion has received support from studies demonstrating that intracellular pH influences secretory responsiveness;[71a] that glucose augments H^+ efflux from the islet;[68] and that alpha-ketoisocaproate, an insulin secretagogue at least as potent as glucose, produces a dose-related decrease in intracellular pH.[71b] Presumably, the protons generated during substrate catabolism influence calcium levels in the beta cell by either inhibiting its efflux from the cell or by making it available from intracellular (probably mitochondrial) stores.[71c]

A viable alternative to the role of NADH, NAD(P)H, or hydrogen ion, as the intracellular trigger for induced secretion has been forwarded by Ashcroft and co-workers.[72,73] Under a variety of conditions, they have noted that the level of phosphoenolpyruvate generated during glycolysis

Fig. 5–4. Glucose, mannose, and fructose usage by intact islets of Langerhans. These Eadie-Hofstee plots are based on a detailed analysis of glucose, mannose, and fructose utilization rates noted over a wide range of hexose concentrations (1 micromolar–100 millimolar). The composite nature of the systems regulating glucose and mannose usage are apparent while only one system regulates fructose metabolism. In these plots, hexose usage rate V in picomols/islet/hour is plotted against V/S where S is the substrate concentration. The intercept of each line with the ordinate determines the maximal rate of hexose usage (V_{max}) by the system while the K_m (the concentration resulting in the half-maximal usage rate) is determined by dividing the V_{max} by the intercept of the line on the abscissa. These values have been calculated and are given in the figure.

from 2-phosphoglycerate is correlated with stimulated secretion. As attractive as this hypothesis may appear, it has yet to be vigorously tested. Most importantly, the effect of leucine and alpha keto-isocaproate on the intracellular concentration of this high-energy phosphate compound remains to be reported. To briefly summarize, then, the state of the art: Reports in the literature suggest that pyridine nucleotide levels,[69,74] hydrogen ions,[71c] redox state,[69] phosphoenolpyruvate[72] or the phosphate potential[74] of the beta cell may play a crucial role in regulating secretion. Whatever the nature of the intracellular trigger, however, it must somehow affect calcium mobilization and handling by the islet cell and it is the increase in intracellular calcium that in some manner stimulates or is related to secretion.

THE ROLE OF CALCIUM IN STIMULUS-SECRETION COUPLING

If there is any consensus among the investigators studying stimulus-secretion coupling of pancreatic islets, it is that the sine qua non for release is the mobilization of calcium. Thus, insulin secretion provoked by a variety of chemically distinct stimulants, is markedly obtunded in the absence of this cation.[35,76,77] The beta cell has at its disposal at least several mechanisms to increase intracellular calcium. Most obviously, because of the decisive concentration gradient existing across the plasma membrane, a small change in calcium permeability might be expected to result in significant intracellular accumulation of calcium. This has been documented.[78] Early studies by Malaisse also demonstrated that calcium efflux from the cell was decreased by an increasing glucose concentration which, if all other processes remained constant, would elevate intracellular calcium.[79] Perhaps even more important is the mobilization of calcium from intracellular stores, primarily the endoplasmic reticulum[80] and mitochondria.[81] As suggested in several reports, the generation of metabolic intermediates or perhaps cyclic AMP (known to increase with glucose stimulation[82]) may result in the liberation of bound intracellular calcium. Hellmann has suggested that the mobilization of a plasma membrane-bound pool of calcium may play a crucial role, particularly during the first phase of release, in the stimulus-secretion coupling process.[83] In summary, then, while calcium remains essential for release, how it is precisely mobilized and from what specific compartment, remains enigmatic. Once elevated, calcium somehow results in an activation of the microtubular-microfilamentous system and an accelerated movement of secretory granules to the cell surface. In fact, such movement is dependent on calcium.[29]

THE PERMISSIVE EFFECT OF GLUCOSE

The role of glucose as the primary stimulant for induced secretion has often overshadowed its role in determining the secretory effectiveness of other molecules. Nowhere is this permissive effect more apparent than with studies on fructose. It has long been known that by itself even in exorbitant concentrations, fructose is incapable of inducing insulin secretion.[49,84] However, in the presence of a basal, non-stimulatory glucose concentration, the combination of these previously documented impotent molecules becomes an effective mixture to provoke secretion.[84,85] It was not until detailed studies on hexose usage by the islets were performed that this puzzling observation was settled.[85] It was found that glucose and mannose only stimulated secretion once their usage rates by the islet exceeded approximately 40 to 50 picomols/islet/hour. In other words, a substantial amount of the hexose, fully one-fourth the maximal metabolic capacity of the islets, could be metabolized before secretion occurred. Once this threshold was exceeded, however, release was dramatically accelerated. Moreover, a detailed analysis of glucose and mannose usage by intact islets revealed the involvement of two systems differing in K_m and V_{max}[87] (Fig. 5-4). The low K_m system contributes about 15% to total glucose/mannose usage and its kinetic characteristics hardly qualify it as a key component regulating usage at physiologic levels. Rather, it is the high K_m system, perhaps reflecting the activity of glucokinase (which, incidentally phosphorylates mannose as well), that appears particularly responsive to glucose concentrations found in vivo. That the activities of the low and high K_m hexokinases present in islets are responsible for these patterns of hexose usage, seems likely. Fructose usage, on the other hand, is regulated by one system, possessing a high K_m and limited maximal velocity (V_{max}). Its usage by this system, even at 50 millimolar, never approaches 40 to 50 picomols/islet/hour, a rate essential to stimulate release. Its ineffectiveness can then be easily explained by its inability to be utilized as well as glucose or mannose by the islets. Furthermore, it was found that fructose did not interfere with glucose usage and vice versa. Because of this, it was assumed that the usage rates of the hexoses might simply be additive and that it might be possible to predict insulin release in response to different glucose and fructose concentrations, based on data derived solely from glucose (Table 5-1). This has been demonstrated not only for glucose and fructose combinations, but also for N-acetylglucosamine and glucose mixtures.[58] In short, it would appear that the initial chemical structure of the stimulants,

Table 5–1. Metabolism and Insulin Release with Combinations of Glucose and Fructose

Stimulus Combination (mM)		Additive Metabolic Rate (pmol/islet/h)	Predicted Insulin Release (μU/min/100 islets)	Actual Insulin Release* (μU/min/100 islets)
Glucose	Fructose			
2.75	5.5	39.6	None	—†
2.75	10.0	43.7	None	—†
2.75	15.0	46.7	10	10 ± 4‡
2.75	27.5	63.7	86	77 ± 14
5.5	5.5	73.6	144	137 ± 4
5.5	10.0	77.7	170	181 ± 9
5.5	27.5	97.7	274	258 ± 13
8	5.5	93.6	259	268 ± 24
8	10.0	97.7	274	275 ± 4
8	27.5	117.7	321	322 ± 30

*Actual Insulin Release refers to the levels of hormone in the final 5-minute perifusate sample, corrected for basal release.

†The first two fructose concentrations tested with basal glucose caused a decrease in basal insulin release from 20 ± 2 to 13 ± 2 μU/min/100 islets.

‡Mean ± SE.

All islets were perifused for 30 min. without any added substrate and for an additional 20 min. in the presence of the hexose combinations indicated, which provided the actual insulin release data. Insulin release was predicted from the additive metabolic rates obtained with glucose and fructose combinations. A plot made of glucose usage versus glucose-induced insulin release provided the basis for the predicted values of insulin released by the various hexose combinations. (From Zawalich et al.[85] with permission of the authors and publisher.)

at least in the case for the hexoses and hexose derivatives, is not as important as once thought. Rather, the ability of the islets to utilize the substrates at rates sufficient to exceed a crucial threshold, is of primary importance. Consequently, in attempting to delineate and to identify the rate-limiting steps for both insulin secretion and glucose utilization by islet tissue, the enzymic composition of the beta cell assumes a preeminent position.

The physiologic and clinical correlates of the permissive or potentiating action of glucose merit closer scrutiny. Although only fructose has been studied in extensive detail, many compounds rely on glucose for their effectiveness. Circulating amino acids, particularly after a protein meal, can be expected to increase, and in the presence of glucose, become effective stimulants of insulin secretion.[88] The orally effective sulfonylureas, at least at therapeutic levels, are essentially ineffective in stimulating secretion without the concomitant presence of glucose.[89,90] In fact, even if the primary stimulant action of glucose is impaired in Type II diabetes, its ability to potentiate secretion due to other stimulants, appears to remain intact.[91,92] This has led Halter et al.[93] to speculate that the hyperglycemia in Type II diabetes may augment the stimulatory effectiveness of otherwise weak provocateurs such as arginine. Consequently, the heightened potentiating or permissive effect of glucose on these stimuli would tend to compensate for defective glucose-induced insulin release. A further corollary is that non-glucose stimulants such as amino acids may result in hyperinsulinemia even when the primary responsiveness of the beta cell to glucose is impaired.

ALTERNATIVE EXPLANATIONS FOR GLUCOSE-INDUCED INSULIN SECRETION. THE "GLUCORECEPTOR" HYPOTHESIS

Up to now, major emphasis has been placed on the notion that the metabolism of glucose is essential for triggering release of insulin. There is by no means unanimous agreement on this proposal, and it is perhaps at this point that the alternative concept, the glucoreceptor theory, should be discussed. The theory has received support from several observations: first, the ability of iodoacetate to dissociate the fuel and releasing function of glucose, provided pyruvate is present as an alternate fuel;[94] second, the inability to identify the metabolite or co-factor which might be important in stimulating insulin secretion;[95] and third, the observation that the alpha-anomer of glucose was more effective than the beta-anomer in stimulating insulin secretion from the beta cell.[96,97] These last studies were probably undertaken in response to the report by Rossini and co-workers that the alpha-anomer of glucose was more effective than the beta-anomer in preventing the diabetogenic action of alloxan.[98] In fact, since studies with alloxan and several other structurally related compounds have been used to bolster the "glucoreceptor" theory, the results obtained with these interesting compounds merit closer scrutiny.

It has been known for many years that alloxan is an extremely potent inducer of beta cell necrosis.[99,100] Studies by Tomita et al.[101] demonstrated that an initial effect of alloxan was a rapid inhibition of glucose-induced insulin secretion, an effect which could be blocked by simultaneous exposure of the beta cell to glucose, mannose or 3-0-methylglucose. This was in accordance with previous in vivo studies which showed that the diabetogenic action of alloxan was considerably attenuated by the same compounds.[100,102,103] Based on these and other studies,[104,105] it was suggested that alloxan was interacting with a glucoreceptor moiety, possibly membrane-bound, and that the interaction between alloxan and the receptor not only blocked insulin secretion, but was also related in some manner to the subsequently induced necrosis.[106,107] Furthermore, it has also been demonstrated that alloxan induces a transient release of insulin,[106,108] a result which would be consistent with its interaction at a "glucoreceptor" moiety. However, several objections were raised to this intriguing concept. First, alloxan blocks insulin secretion in response to many stimulants.[109,110] Second, 3-0-methylglucose has no effect on glucose-induced insulin secretion,[111] but completely blocks alloxan action. In addition, it has been demonstrated that alloxan, at least in lymphocytes, transiently stimulates the flow of glucose via the pentose cycle,[112,113] an effect which conceivably might account for its ability to transiently augment insulin secretion by the islet. (Incidentally if this observation is confirmed in islet tissue, this would add considerable support to the argument of Ammon and co-workers as to the importance of the pentose cycle in regulating insulin secretion.) Furthermore, at least in batch-incubation studies, alloxan depresses glucose utilization and glucose oxidation, effects which may take several minutes to develop.[109,114,115] Suffice it to say that results obtained with alloxan are amenable to various interpretations and that it is difficult at this time to ascribe its effects as being solely due to its binding to a putative glucoreceptor molecule.

STUDIES ON ALPHA- AND BETA-ANOMERS OF GLUCOSE AND MANNOSE

Studies utilizing the alpha- and beta-anomers of glucose as both stimulants of insulin secretion and metabolic fuels initially led to a state of uncertainty regarding the nature of the interaction between glucose and the beta cell.[116,117] While most available information up until that point appeared to support the substrate-site theory, the observation that the alpha anomer of glucose induced significantly more insulin release from the beta cell than did the beta anomer[96,97] and the further observation that there appeared to be indiscriminate metabolism of both hexose anomers by the islet, tended to argue against this theory.[116,117] Consequently, albeit indirectly, the "glucoreceptor" model received some support from these observations. Subsequently, however, Malaisse and co-workers[118] demonstrated in rat islets that there was a preferential capacity of the islet to utilize alpha glucose and that this effect could be ascribed to a preferential isomerization of alpha-glucose-6-phosphate by phosphoglucose isomerase. Unfortunately, there is as yet no means to reconcile the differences between the opposing reports concerning the metabolism of alpha- and beta-D-glucose. However, the controversy continues since Niki and co-workers have published results showing that the alpha anomer of mannose is a more potent secretagogue than is the beta anomer.[119] Furthermore, phosphomannose isomerase,

at least that isolated from yeast, is stereospecific for beta-mannose-6-phosphate.[120] Whether similar specificity is observed with phosphomannose isomerase isolated from islets is yet to be determined, as is the ability of islets to utilize alpha and beta mannose. However, Niki has used these observations to support the notion that a direct recognition of the glucose or mannose molecules by glucoreceptors is involved with stimulating insulin secretion.

In regard to the first two observations supporting the glucoreceptor theory and mentioned at the beginning of this section (that of studies with iodoacetate and metabolite and co-factor measurements made during the early phases of insulin secretion), it has since been shown that while iodoacetate does indeed block the fuel function of glucose, it also blocks the insulin releasing function of the hexose, an effect which cannot be overcome by the addition of pyruvate.[111,121] Furthermore, metabolite and co-factor measurements made not only on isolated islets, but also from the isolated perfused pancreas have shown rapid activation of islet cell metabolism, certainly rapid enough to account for stimulated secretion.[68,71,122] It has been suggested[71] that the metabolite and co-factor measurements made in previous studies[95] may have been obscured somewhat by the nutritional state of the animal since some of the measurements were made on animals that had been fasted overnight, a situation which can be expected to somewhat blunt islet metabolic and secretory capacity.[62,123] The discrepant results obtained with iodoacetate remain to be explained.

BIPHASIC HORMONE SECRETION FROM THE PANCREATIC BETA CELL

In the appropriate in vivo or in vitro system, an elevation of the ambient glucose level results in a biphasic release of insulin from the pancreatic beta cell.[6,25,124,125] Whether a similar sensor system is involved in the regulation of both phases has not been established, although the available evidence does suggest a single regulatory process.[126] If the metabolism of the substrate underlies this pattern of secretion, the secretory response noted may be due to oscillations of enzyme activity, metabolite and/or co-factor levels, or some combination of these factors. Grodsky[127] has suggested that the two phases may be reflections of the fact that two storage pools for insulin exist in the beta cell. One pool is labile and rapidly depleted. It represents a readily available storage form of the hormone and may be the principal contributor to the first phase of release. The second pool is large, slowly mobilized, and may be the main source of hormone for the second slowly rising phase of secretion

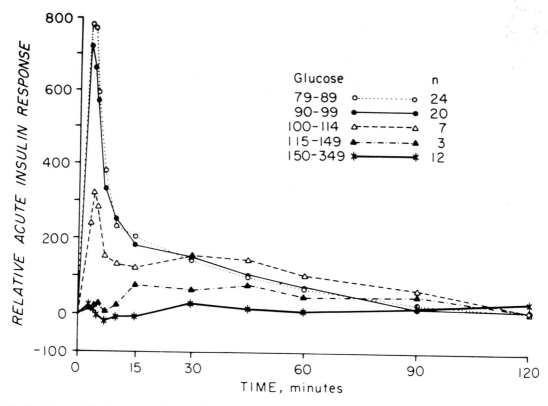

Fig. 5–5. Mean relative incremental insulin levels following intravenous glucose in arbitrarily divided subgroups of subjects based on fasting glucose levels. Note the presence of acute insulin response in subjects with fasting glucose levels below 115 mg/dl and the absence of the response above 115 mg/dl. (From Brunzell et al.[130] with permission of the authors and publisher.)

noted with prolonged stimulus presentation. Whether different storage pools exist for the hormone or whether a different sensor system regulates each phase, remain important topics for further experimentation. It does seem clear, however, that the ability of the beta cell to respond promptly to a glucose stimulus is of prime importance in regulating glucose disposal in man, implying a key physiologic role for the rapid first phase of hormone secretion.[128,129] Intravenous glucose tolerance tests have demonstrated a strongly positive correlation between the acute insulin response (defined as the area above the fasting insulin level from 3 to 5 minutes after glucose stimulation and probably corresponding to the first phase of release noted in other systems) and Kg, the glucose disappearance rate.[130] In individuals with carbohydrate intolerance, a reduction or complete obliteration of the AIR (acute insulin release), particularly when the fasting plasma glucose exceeds 115 mg/dl, is a characteristic finding (Fig. 5–5).[91,130] In markedly obese hyperglycemic individuals[131] or in Type II diabetics,[132–134] a reduction in fasting blood glucose brought about by caloric restriction restores to some extent β-cell responsiveness to glucose and

improves glucose tolerance. Whether sustained hyperglycemia elevates the threshold for glucose-induced insulin release or alters beta cell metabolism of the hexose, inducing some type of refractory state, remains undetermined. It is clear that hyperglycemia alters the chemosensitivity of the beta cell to glucose, its most important physiologic stimulant. The consequence of this state of affairs is an exacerbation of an already critical situation. The fact that a return toward euglycemia restores sensitivity further underscores the resilient nature and adaptive character of these cells.

EFFECTS OF ALTERED CALORIC INTAKE ON THE CHEMOSENSITIVITY OF THE PANCREATIC BETA CELL

Effect of Starvation. Caloric deprivation results in both decreased basal plasma insulin levels and an impaired secretory response to glucose.[135,136] In the rat, the effect is evident as early as 16 to 24 hours after food removal, provided only a moderate glucose concentration is employed to provoke the beta cell (Fig. 5–6).[123,137] Higher glucose levels result in an insulin response identical to that ob-

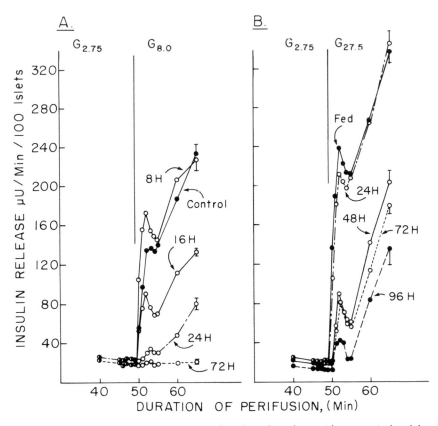

Fig. 5–6. Effect of total caloric deprivation on glucose-induced insulin release. Islets were isolated from rats fasted for various times given in the figure, perifused with 2.75 millimolar glucose for 30 minutes to establish basal secretory rates and then stimulated for 20 minutes with either 8 or 27.5 millimolar glucose. After 16 hours of caloric restriction, the response to moderate glucose stimulus (8 millimolar) is impaired while that to 27.5 millimolar glucose is unaffected. Further caloric restriction, however, obtunded even the response to this level of the hexose. (Used by permission of publisher[123]).

served in control animals.[138] These results suggest an altered K_m value for the overall secretory response without any change in the maximal secretory capacity. Furthermore, after 48 hours of starvation, the ability of islets to catabolize glucose is also impaired, and the levels of several metabolic intermediates are reduced.[123,137,138] Malaisse and co-workers[62] have attributed the blunted secretory response in the rat to a diminished activity of either glucokinase or phosphofructokinase, a result consistent with the impaired usage of the hexose. While there is little doubt that glucose metabolism is impaired in fasted animals, that this is the sole disturbance produced by caloric deprivation remains questionable. The fact that short-term fasting (24 hours or less) is associated with impaired secretion, yet normal glucose usage, supports this notion.[123,137]

Effect of Re-feeding. An area which has received little experimental interest concerns the factors responsible for the reinduction of islet cell chemosensitivity after re-feeding. In analogy to the situation noted for liver enzymes, particularly glu-

cokinase,[139,140] it has been suggested that an inducible receptor system exists in the pancreatic islet.[136] Studies by several groups have demonstrated that while a prompt return of glucose sensitivity can be demonstrated with re-feeding, adequate levels of carbohydrate must be included in the re-fed diet.[123,136,141] Thus, re-feeding rats a diet high in fat and protein but low in or devoid of carbohydrate has little effect on restoring islet cell responsiveness.[136,141] Further, injections of glucose, calorically negligible and insufficient to affect body weight, maintain beta cell responsiveness.[136] These observations support a key role of the hexose in the maintenance of certain enzyme systems responsible for glucose metabolism and, pari passu, insulin secretion.

Effects of Excessive Caloric Intake. There is little doubt that some degree of enzyme induction is responsible for the restoration of islet cell metabolic and secretory responsiveness noted by re-feeding previously fasted animals. Whether excessive caloric intake in some persons results in over-induction of the enzyme systems regulating

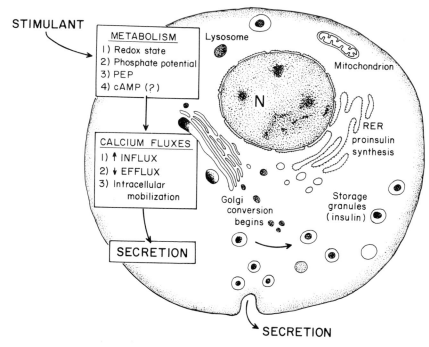

Fig. 5–7. Secretory cycle of the pancreatic beta cell. Schematically illustrated here are the organelles involved in insulin biosynthesis and the biochemical events which stimulate both this process and insulin secretion. From available evidence, it is proposed that stimulant metabolism changes several cell parameters. These include alterations in the levels of: (A) reduced pyridine nucleotides and hence redox state of the cell; (B) high-energy phosphate compounds and hence the phosphate potential; (C) phosphoenolpyruvate (PEP); and (D) cyclic adenosine 3-5-monophosphate (cAMP). Involving perhaps more than one mechanism, these metabolic changes increase the availability of free calcium within the cell and it is the combination of this cation with the microtubular-microfilamentous system that stimulates emiocytosis. Abbreviations: RER = rough endoplasmic reticulum. (Adapted and modified from Steiner et al.[34])

both these parameters remains an intriguing issue. In both normal individuals fed high-carbohydrate diets[142] and in moderately diabetic patients increasing their caloric intake,[143] heightened islet secretory responsiveness and a degree of hyperinsulinemia have been noted. Whether the hyperinsulinemia is simply a result of excessive beta cell stimulation, and the insulin resistance noted a type of adaptive response to prevent periodic hypoglycemia,[144] are matters of utmost importance. Perhaps the induction of obesity, produced by giving normal rats a highly palatable diet, will provide us with a useful model to study these issues.[145] In any event, the results of various studies, particularly those employing starvation to depress islet responsiveness and re-feeding to restore it, suggest that the beta cell is in some type of dynamic equilibrium with the circulating level of fuel substrates. The role played by other stimulants of secretion in maintaining and supporting this state of affairs, particularly amino acids, has not yet been thoroughly investigated.[146,147] However, and consistent with this line of reasoning, there exists a recent report showing that in obese individuals the protein con-

tent of the diet may contribute to the observed hyperinsulinemia.[148]

Effect of Exercise. Similar to fasting, physical training produces a hypoinsulinemic state.[149,150] The effect is evident from an analysis of both basal insulin levels and those observed after glucose tolerance testing. The hypoinsulinemia cannot be ascribed to changes in the circulating levels of catecholamines, known inhibitors of insulin secretion, since these levels are not elevated, at least in the basal state.[151] Using isolated islets obtained from exercising rats, a markedly diminished secretory response to glucose has been noted, identifying yet another condition altering beta cell chemosensitivity.[152] The changes responsible for reduced insulin secretion have not yet been examined. Because training is associated with increased peripheral tissue sensitivity to insulin, probably as a consequence of the hypoinsulinemic state, glucose disposal rates are normal.[150,153] The significance of these observations to man, particularly obese individuals or Type II diabetics, remains to be established.

The secretory cycle of the beta cell is schematically illustrated in Figure 5–7. Stimulant metabolism initiates a complex cascade of events aimed at activating the microtubular-microfilamentous system, culminating in emiocytosis and hormone release. Whether one, several or all the processes listed under metabolism contribute to cellular activation is not fully known. It does appear certain, however, that the metabolism of the substrate alters not only calcium fluxes within the beta cell but also promotes insulin biosynthesis, thus militating against hormone depletion. Not obvious from the figure, but hopefully apparent in the text, is the idea that these cellular processes and hence beta cell sensitivity to stimulation, are under the long-term control of dietary intake and physical activity and thus can be modulated to the benefit or detriment of the organism. The physiologic and clinical implications of this situation should be readily apparent even to the casual observer.

REFERENCES

1. Issekutz, B.I., Jr., Allen, M.: Effect of catecholamines and methylprednisolone on carbohydrate metabolism of dogs. Metabolism 21:48, 1972.
2. Kibler, R.F., Taylor, W.J., Myers, J.D.: The effect of glucagon on net splanchnic balances of glucose, amino acid, nitrogen, urea, ketones, and oxygen in man. J. Clin. Invest. 43:904, 1964.
3. Cahill, G.F.: Physiology of insulin in man. Diabetes 20:785, 1971.
4. Kipnis, D.M.: Insulin secretion in diabetes mellitus. Ann. Intern. Med. 69:891, 1968.
5. Goodner, C.J., Porte, D., Jr.: Determinants of basal islet secretion in man. In: D.F. Steiner, N. Freinkel (Eds.): Handbook of Physiology, Endocrinology, I. Baltimore, Williams & Wilkins, 1972, p. 597.
6. Cerasi, E.: Mechanisms of glucose stimulated insulin secretion in health and in diabetes: some re-evaluations and proposals. Diabetologia 11:1, 1975.
7. Morris, G.E., Korner, A.: The effect of glucose on insulin biosynthesis by isolated islets of Langerhans of the rat. Biochim. Biophys. Acta 208:404, 1970.
8. Permutt, M.A., Kipnis, D.M.: Insulin biosynthesis. I. On the mechanism of glucose stimulation. J. Biol. Chem. 247:1194, 1972.
9. Lomedico, P.T., Saunders, G.F.: Preparation of pancreatic mRNA: cell-free translation of an insulin-immunoreactive polypeptide. Nucleic Acids Res. 3:381, 1976.
10. Chan, S.J., Keim, P., Steiner, D.F.: Cell-free synthesis of rat preproinsulin: characterization and partial amino acid sequence determination. Proc. Natl. Acad. Sci. USA 73:1964, 1976.
11. Oyer, P.E., Cho, S., Peterson, J.D., Steiner, D.F.: Studies on human proinsulin. Isolation and amino acid sequence of the human pancreatic C-peptide. J. Biol. Chem. 246:1375, 1971.
12. Patzelt, C., Labrecque, A.D., Duguid, J.R., et al.: Detection and kinetic behavior of preproinsulin in pancreatic islets. Proc. Natl. Acad. Sci. (USA) 75:1260, 1978.
13. Blobel, G., Dobberstein, B.: Transfer of proteins across membranes. I. Presence of proteolytically processed and unprocessed nascent immunoglobulin light chains on membrane-bound ribosomes of murine myeloma. J. Cell. Biol. 67:835, 1975.
14. Palade, G.: Intracellular aspects of the process of protein synthesis. Science 189:347, 1975.
15. Howell, S.L.: Role of ATP in the intracellular translocation of proinsulin and insulin in the rat pancreatic beta cell. Nature (New Biol.) 235:85, 1972.
16. Munger, B.L.: A light and electron microscopic study of cellular differentiation in the pancreatic islets of the mouse. Am. J. Anat. 103:275, 1958.
17. Greider, M.H., Howell, S.L., Lacy, P.E.: Isolation and properties of secretory granules from rat islets of Langerhans. II. Ultrastructure of the beta granule. J. Cell. Biol. 41:162, 1969.
18. Blaschko, H., Firemark, H., Smith, A.D., Winkler, H.: Lipids of the adrenal medulla. Lysolecithin, a characteristic constituent of chromaffin granules. Biochem. J. 104:545, 1967.
19. Kemmler, W., Steiner, D.F.: Conversion of proinsulin to insulin in a subcellular fraction from rat islets. Biochem. Biophys. Res. Commun. 41:1223, 1970.
20. Grant, P.T., Combs, T.L.: Proinsulin, a biosynthetic precursor of insulin. Biochemistry 6:69, 1970.
21. Rubenstein, A.H., Melani, F., Pilkis, S., Steiner, D.F.: Proinsulin: Secretion, metabolism, immunological and biological properties. Postgrad. Med. J. 45(Suppl. I):476, 1969.
22. Matthews, E.K.: Electrical activity in islet cells and insulin secretions. Acta Diabetol. Lat. 7 Suppl. I.:3, 506, 1970.
23. Lacy, P.E., Howell, S.L., Young, D.A., Fink, C.J.: New hypothesis of insulin secretion. Nature 219:1177, 1968.
24. Malaisse, W.J., Malaisse-Lagae, F., Walker, M.O., Lacy, P.E.: The stimulus-secretion coupling of glucose-induced insulin release. V. The participation of a microtubular-microfilamentous system. Diabetes 20:257, 1971.
25. Lacy, P.E., Walker, M.M., Fink, C.J.: Perifusion of isolated rat islets in vitro: Participation of the microtubular system in the biphasic release of insulin. Diabetes 21:987, 1972.
26. Lacy, P.E., Klein, N.J., Fink, C.J.: Effect of cytochalasin B on the biphasic release of insulin in perifused rat islets. Endocrinology 92:1458, 1973.
27. Orci, L., Gabbay, K.H., Malaisse, W.J.: Pancreatic beta cell web. Its possible role in insulin secretion. Science 175:1128, 1972.
28. Lacy, P.E., Greider, M.H.: Anatomy and ultrastructural organization of pancreatic islets. In: L.J. DeGroot (Ed.): Endocrinology, Vol. 2, New York, Grune & Stratton, 1979, p. 907.
29. Lacy, P.E., Finke, E.H., Codilla, R.C.: Cinemicrographic studies on beta cell granule movement in monolayer culture of islet cells. Lab. Invest. 33:570, 1975.
30. Lacy, P.E.: Beta cell secretion—from the standpoint of a pathologist. Diabetes 19:895, 1970.
31. Grodsky, G.M., Landahl, H., Curry, D., Bennett, L.L.: In vitro studies suggesting a two compartment model for insulin secretion. In: S. Falkmer, B. Hellman, I-B Täljedal (Eds.): Structure and Metabolism of the Pancreatic Islets. Oxford, Pergamon, 1970, p. 409.
32. Lin, B.J., Haist, R.E.: Insulin biosynthesis: Effects of carbohydrates and related compounds. Can. J. Physiol. Pharmacol. 47:791, 1969.
33. Clark, J.L., Steiner, D.F.: Insulin biosynthesis: demonstration of two proinsulins. Proc. Natl. Acad. Sci. USA 62:278, 1969.
34. Steiner, D.F., Kemmler, W., Clark, J.L., et al.: The biosynthesis of insulin. In: D.F. Steiner, N. Freinkel (Eds.): Handbook of Physiology. Endocrinology I. Baltimore, Williams & Wilkins, 1972, p. 175.
35. Grodsky, G.M., Bennett, L.L.: Cation requirement for insulin secretion in the isolated perfused pancreas. Diabetes 15:910, 1966.

36. Jain, K., Logothetopoulos, J., Zucker, P.: The effects of D- and L-glyceraldehyde on glucose oxidation, insulin secretion and insulin biosynthesis of the rat. Biochim. Biophys. Acta *399*:384, 1975.

37. Ashcroft, S.J.H., Crossley, J.R., Crossley, P.C.: The effect of N-acetylglucosamines on the biosynthesis and secretion of insulin in rat. Biochem. J. *154*:701, 1976.

38. Lin, B.J., Haist, R.E.: Insulin biosynthesis: The monoaminergic mechanisms and the specificity of "glucoreceptor." Endocrinology *96*:1247, 1975.

39. Anderson, A.: Stimulation of insulin biosynthesis in isolated mouse islets by leucine, 2-aminonorbornane-2-carboxylic acid and alphaketoisocaproic acid. Biochim. Biophys. Acta *437*:345, 1976.

40. Hutton, J.C., Sener, A., Herchuelz, A., et al.:Similarities in the stimulus-secretion coupling mechanisms of glucose and 2-keto acid-induced insulin release. Endocrinology *106*:203, 1980.

41. Hutton, J.C., Sener, A., Malaisse, W.J.: The metabolism of 4-methyl-2-oxopentanoate in rat pancreatic islets. Biochem. J. *184*:291, 1979.

42. Jain, K., Logothetopoulos, J.: Metabolic signals produced by purine ribonucleosides stimulate proinsulin biosynthesis and insulin secretion. Biochem. J. *170*:461, 1978.

43. Schatz, H., Nierle, C., Pfeiffer, E.F.: (Pro-) insulin biosynthesis and the release of newly synthesized (pro-) insulin from isolated islets of rat pancreas in the presence of amino acids and sulphonylureas. Eur. J. Clin. Invest. *5*:477, 1975.

43a.Rotwein, P., Chyn, R., Chergwin, J., et al.: Polymorphism in the 5'-flanking region of the human insulin gene and its possible relation to Type II diabetes. Science *213*:1117, 1981.

43b.Owerbach, D., Nerup, J.: Restriction fragment length polymorphism of the insulin gene in diabetes mellitus. Diabetes *31*:275, 1982.

43c.Kwok, S.C.M., Steiner, D.F., Rubenstein, A.H., Tager, H.S.: Identification of a point mutation in the human insulin gene giving rise to a structurally abnormal insulin (Insulin Chicago). Diabetes *32*:872, 1983.

44. Moskalewski, S.: Isolation and culture of the islets of Langerhans of the guinea pig. Gen. Comp. Endocrinol. *5*:342, 1965.

45. Lacy, P.E., Kostianovsky, M.: Method for the isolation of intact islets of Langerhans from the rat pancreas. Diabetes *16*:35, 1967.

46. Ashcroft, S.J.H., Weerasinghe, L.C.C., Bassett, J.M., Randle, P.J.: The pentose cycle and insulin release in mouse pancreatic islets. Biochem. J. *126*:525, 1972.

47. Hellman, B., Idahl, L-Å., Lernmark, Å., et al.: The pancreatic β-cell recognition of insulin secretagogues. Effects of calcium and sodium on glucose metabolism and insulin release. Biochem. J. *138*:33, 1974.

48. Grodsky, G.M., Batts, A.A., Bennett, L.L., et al.: Effects of carbohydrates on secretion of insulin from the isolated rat pancreas. Am. J. Physiol. *205*:638, 1963.

49. Goore, H.G., Randle, P.J.: Regulation of insulin secretion studied with pieces of rabbit pancreas incubated *in vitro*. Biochem. J. *93*:66, 1964.

50. Ashcroft, S.J.H., Bassett, J.M., Randle, P.J.: Insulin secretion mechanisms and glucose metabolism in isolated islets. Diabetes *21*(Suppl. 2):538, 1972.

51. Cerasi, E., Luft, R.: Diabetes mellitus. A disorder of cellular transmission? Horm. Metab. Res. *2*:246, 1970.

52. Matschinsky, F.M., Ellerman, J.E., Krzanowski, J., et al.: The dual function of glucose in islets of Langerhans. J. Biol. Chem. *246*:1007, 1971.

53. Malaisse, W.J., Lea, M.A., Malaisse-Lagae, F.: The effect of mannoheptulose on the phosphorylation of glucose

and the secretion of insulin by islets of Langerhans. Metabolism *17*:126, 1968.

54. Ashcroft, S.J.H., Chatra, L., Weerasinghe, C., Randle, P.J.: Inter-relationship of islet metabolism, adenosine triphosphate content, and insulin release. Biochem. J. *132*:223, 1973.

55. Hellman, B., Idahl, L-Å., Lernmark, Å., et al.: The pancreatic β-cell recognition of insulin secretagogues. Comparisons of glucose with glyceraldehyde isomers and dihydroxyacetone. Arch. Biochem. Biophys. *162*:448, 1974.

56. Malaisse, W.J., Herchuelz, A., Levy, J., et al.: The stimulus-secretion coupling of glucose-induced insulin release. XIX. The insulinotropic effect of glyceraldehyde. Mol. Cell. Endocrinol. *4*:1, 1976.

57. Zawalich, W.S., Dye, E.S., Rognstad, R., Matschinsky, F.M.: On the biochemical nature of triose- and hexose-stimulated insulin secretions. Endocrinology *103*:2027, 1978.

58. Zawalich, W.S., Dye, E.S., Matschinsky, F.M.: Metabolism and insulin-releasing capabilities of glucosamine and N-acetylglucosamine in isolated rat islets. Biochem. J. *180*:145, 1979.

59. Ashcroft, S.J.H.: The control of insulin release by sugars. In: R. Porter and D.W. Fitzsimons (Eds.): Polypeptide Hormones: Molecular and Cellular Aspects. Ciba Fdn. Symposium *41* (New Series). Amsterdam, Elsevier/Excerpta Medica, 1975, p. 117.

60. Ashcroft, S.J.H.: Glucoreceptor mechanisms and the control of insulin release and biosynthesis. Diabetologia *18*:5, 1980.

61. Matschinsky, F.M., Ellerman, J.E.: Metabolism of glucose in the islets of Langerhans. J. Biol. Chem. *243*:2730, 1968.

62. Malaisse, W.J., Sener, A., Levy, J.: The stimulus-secretion coupling of glucose-induced insulin release. Fasting-induced adaptation of key glycolytic enzymes in isolated islets. J. Biol. Chem. *251*:1731, 1976.

63. Snyder, P.J., Kashket, S., O'Sullivan, J.B.: Pentose cycle in isolated islets during glucose-stimulated insulin release. Am. J. Physiol. *219*:876, 1970.

64. Malaisse, W.J., Sener, A., Levy, J., Herchuelz, A.: The stimulus-secretion coupling of glucose-induced insulin release. XXII. Qualitative and quantitative aspects of glycolysis in isolated islets. Acta Diabet. Lat. *13*:202, 1976.

65. Ammon, H.P.T., Verspohl, E.: Pyridine nucleotides in pancreatic islets during inhibition of insulin release by exogenous insulin. Endocrinology *99*:1469, 1976.

66. Verspohl, E.J., Händel, M., Ammon, H.P.T.: Pentose-phosphate shunt activity of rat pancreatic islets: its dependence on glucose concentration. Endocrinology *105*:1269, 1979.

67. Ammon, H.P.T., Verspohl, E.J.: Effect of methylene blue on pyridine nucleotides and insulin secretion of rat pancreatic islets. Diabetologia *17*:41, 1979.

68. Malaisse, W.J., Hutton, J.C., Kawazu, S., et al.: The stimulus-secretion coupling of glucose-induced insulin release. XXXV. The links between metabolic and cationic events. Diabetologia *16*:331, 1979.

69. Malaisse, W.J., Sener, A., Herchuelz, A., Hutton, J.C.: Insulin release: the fuel hypothesis. Metabolism *28*:373, 1979.

70. Malaisse, W.J., Hutton, J.C., Kawazu, S., Sener, A.: The stimulus-secretion coupling of glucose-induced insulin release. Metabolic effects of menadione in isolated islets. Eur. J. Biochem. *87*:121, 1978.

71. Trus, M.D., Hintz, C.S., Weinstein, J.B., et al.: A comparison of the effects of glucose and acetylcholine on

insulin release and intermediary metabolism in rat pancreatic islets. J. Biol. Chem. 254:3921, 1979.

71a. Smith, J.S., Pace, C.S.: Modification of glucose-induced insulin release by alterations of pH. Diabetes 32:61, 1983.

71b. Hutton, J.C., Sener, A., Malaisse, W.J.: The metabolism of 4-methyl-2-oxopentanoate in rat pancreatic islets. Biochem. J. 184:291, 1979.

71c. Malaisse, W.J., Herchuelz, A., Sener, A.: The possible significance of intracellular pH in insulin release. Life Sciences 26:1367, 1980.

72. Sugden, M.C., Ashcroft, S.J.H.: Phosphoenolpyruvate in rat pancreatic islets: A possible intracellular trigger of insulin release? Diabetologia 13:481, 1977.

73. Sugden, M.C., Ashcroft, S.J.H.: Effects of phosphoenolpyruvate, other glycolytic intermediates and methylxanthines on calcium uptake by a mitochondrial fraction from rat pancreatic islets. Diabetologia 15:173, 1978.

74. Watkins, D., Cooperstein, S.J., Lazarow, A.: Stimulation of insulin secretion by pyridine nucleotides. Endocrinology 88:1380, 1971.

75. Freinkel, N., Younsi, C.E., Bonnar, J., Dawson, R.M.C.: Rapid transient efflux of phosphate ions from pancreatic islets as an early action of insulin secretagogues. J. Clin. Invest. 54:1179, 1974.

76. Curry, D.L., Bennett, L.L., Grodsky, G.M.: Requirement for calcium ion in insulin secretion by the perfused rat pancreas. Am. J. Physiol. 214:174, 1968.

77. Milner, R.D.G., Hales, C.N.: The role of calcium and magnesium in insulin secretion from rabbit pancreas studied in vitro. Diabetologia 3:47, 1967.

78. Hellman, B., Sehlin, J., Täljedal, I-B.: Effects of glucose on $^{45}CA + +$ uptake by pancreatic islets as studied with the lanthanum method. J. Physiol. London 254:639, 1976.

79. Malaisse, W.J., Brisson, G.R., Baird, L.E.: Stimulus-secretion coupling of glucose-induced insulin release. X. Effect of glucose on ^{45}CA efflux from perifused islets. Am. J. Physiol. 224:389, 1973.

80. Sehlin, J.: Calcium uptake by subcellular fractions of pancreatic islets: Effects of nucleotides and theophylline. Biochem. J. 156:63, 1976.

81. Schäfer, H.J., Klöppel, G.: The significance of calcium in insulin secretion. Ultrastructural studies on identification and localization of calcium in activated and inactivated B-cells of mice. Virchows Arch. A. 362:231, 1974.

82. Charles, M.A., Fanska, R., Schmid, F.G., et al.: Adenosine 3',5'-monophosphate in pancreatic islets: Glucose-induced insulin release. Science 179:569, 1973.

83. Hellman, B., Sehlin, J., Täljedal, I-B.: Calcium and secretion: Distinction between two pools of glucose-sensitive calcium in pancreatic islets. Science 194:1421, 1976.

84. Curry, D.L., Curry, K.P., Gomez, M.: Fructose potentiation of insulin secretion. Endocrinology 91:1493, 1972.

85. Zawalich, W.S., Rognstad, R., Pagliara, A.S., Matschinsky, F.M.: A comparison of the utilization rates and hormone-releasing actions of glucose, mannose, and fructose in isolated pancreatic islets. J. Biol. Chem. 252:8519, 1977.

86. Curry, D.L.: Fructose potentiation of mannose-induced insulin secretion. Am. J. Physiol. 226;1073, 1975.

87. Zawalich, W.S, Weill, V.: Unpublished observations.

88. Pagliara, A.S., Stillings, S.N., Hover, B., et al.: Glucose modulation of amino acid-induced glucagon and insulin release in the isolated perfused pancreas. J. Clin. Invest. 54:819, 1974.

89. Grodsky, G.M., Lee, J.C., Fanska, R., Smith, D.: Insulin secretion from the in vitro perfused pancreas of the rat: Effect of Ro-6-4563 and other sulfonylureas. In: U.C.

Duback, A. Richert (Eds.): International Symposium on Recent Hypoglycemic Sulfonylureas: Mechanisms of Action and Clinical Indications. Bern, Huber, 1971, p. 83.

90. Cerasi, E., Chowers, I., Luft, R., Widström, A.: The significance of the blood glucose level for plasma insulin response to intravenously administered tolbutamide in healthy subjects. Diabetologia 5:343, 1969.

91. Palmer, J.P., Benson, J.W., Walter, R.M., Ensinck, J.W.: Arginine-stimulated acute phase of insulin and glucagon secretion in diabetic subjects. J. Clin. Invest. 58:565, 1976.

92. Halter, J.B., Porte, D., Jr.: Mechanism of impaired acute insulin release in adult onset diabetes: studies with isoproterenol and secretin. J. Clin. Endocrinol. Metab. 46:952, 1978.

93. Halter, J.B., Graf, R.J., Porte, D., Jr.: Potentiation of insulin secretory responses by plasma glucose levels in man: Evidence that hyperglycemia in diabetes compensates for impaired glucose potentiation. J. Clin. Endocrinol. Metab. 48:946, 1979.

94. Matschinsky, F.M., Ellerman, J.: Dissociation of the insulin releasing and the metabolic functions of hexoses in the islets of Langerhans. Biochem. Biophys. Res. Commun. 50:193, 1973.

95. Matschinsky, F.M., Landgraf, R., Ellerman, J., Kotler-Brajtburg, J.: Glucoreceptor mechanisms in islets of Langerhans. Diabetes 21(Suppl. 2):555, 1972.

96. Niki, A., Niki, H., Miwa, I., Okuda, J.: Insulin secretion by anomers of D-glucose. Science 186:150, 1974.

97. Grodsky, G.M., Fanska, R., West, L., Manning, M.: Anomeric specificity of glucose-stimulated insulin release: Evidence for a glucoreceptor? Science 186:536, 1974.

98. Rossini, A.A., Berger, M., Shadden, J., Cahill, G.F., Jr.: Beta cell protection to alloxan necrosis by anomers of D-glucose. Science 183:424, 1974.

99. Rerup, C.C.: Drugs producing diabetes through damage of the insulin secreting cells. Pharmacol. Rev. 22:485, 1970.

100. Scheynius, A., Täljedal, I-B.: On the mechanism of glucose protection against alloxan toxicity. Diabetologia 7:252, 1971.

101. Tomita, T., Lacy, P.E., Matschinsky, F.M., McDaniel, M.L.: Effect of alloxan on insulin secretion in isolated rat islets perifused in vitro. Diabetes 23:517, 1974.

102. Bhattacharya, G.: On the protection against alloxan diabetes by hexoses. Science 120:841, 1954.

103. Zawalich, W.S., Beidler, L.M.: Glucose and alloxan interactions in the pancreatic islets. Am. J. Physiol. 224:963, 1973.

104. McDaniel, M.L., Roth, C.E., Fink, C.J., Lacy, P.E.: Effect of anomers of D-glucose on alloxan inhibition of insulin release in isolated perifused pancreatic islets. Endocrinology 99:535, 1976.

105. Niki, A., Niki, H., Miwa, I., Lin, B.J.: Interaction of alloxan and anomers of D-glucose on glucose-induced insulin secretion and biosynthesis in vitro. Diabetes 25:574, 1976.

106. Weaver, D.C., McDaniel, M.L., Naber, S.P., et al.: Alloxan stimulation and inhibition of insulin release from isolated rat islets of Langerhans. Diabetes 27:1205, 1978.

107. Niki, A., Niki, H.: Hexose anomers, insulin release and diabetes mellitus. Biomed. Res. 1:189, 1980.

108. Pagliara, A.S., Stillings, S.N., Zawalich, W.S., et al.: Glucose and 3-0-methylglucose protection against alloxan poisoning of pancreatic alpha and beta cells. Diabetes 26:973, 1977.

109. Henquin, J.C., Malvaux, P., Lambert, A.E.: Alloxan-induced alteration of insulin release, rubidium efflux, and

glucose metabolism in rat islets stimulated by various secretagogues. Diabetologia *16*:253, 1979.

110. Tomita, T.: Effect of alloxan on arginine- and leucine-induced insulin secretion in isolated islets. FEBS Lett. *72*:79, 1976.

111. Zawalich, W.S., Pagliara, A.S., Matschinsky, F.M.: Effects of iodoacetate, mannoheptulose, and 3-0-methyl-glucose on the secretory function and metabolism of isolated pancreatic islets. Endocrinology *100*:1276, 1977.

112. Ishibashi, F., Hidaka, H., Fields, R.M., et al.: Alloxan action on glucose metabolism in cultured fibroblasts. I. Stimulation and inhibition of glucose utilization. Am. J. Physiol. *204*:E640, 1981.

113. Ishibashi, F., Bennett, P.H., Howard, B.V.: Alloxan action on glucose metabolism in cultured fibroblasts. II. Effects on pentose-monophosphate shunt and tricarboxylic acid pathways. Am. J. Physiol. *240*:E645, 1981.

114. Zawalich, W.S., Karl, R.C., Matschinsky, F.M.: Effects of alloxan on glucose-stimulated insulin secretion, glucose metabolism, and cyclic adenosine 3′,5′-monophosphate levels in rat isolated islets of Langerhans. Diabetologia *16*:115, 1979.

115. Borg, L.A.H., Eide, S.J., Andersson, A., Hellerström, C.: Effects *in vitro* of alloxan on the glucose metabolism of mouse pancreatic B-cells. Biochem. J. *182*:797, 1979.

116. Idahl, L-Å, Sehlin, J., Täljedal, I-B.: Metabolic and insulin-releasing activities of D-glucose anomers. Nature *254*:75, 1975.

117. Idahl, L-Å, Rahemtulla, F., Sehlin, J., Täljedal, I-B.: Further studies on the metabolism of D-glucose anomers in pancreatic islets. Diabetes *25*:450, 1976.

118. Malaisse, W.J., Sener, A., Koser, M., Herchuelz, A.: Stimulus-secretion coupling of glucose-induced insulin release. Metabolism of α- and β-D-glucose in isolated islets. J. Biol. Chem. *251*:5936, 1976.

119. Niki, A., Niki, H., Miwa, I.: Effect of anomers of D-mannose on insulin release from perfused rat pancreas. Endocrinology *105*:1051, 1979.

120. Rose, I.A., O'Connell, E.L., Schray, K.J.: Mannose 6-phosphate: Anomeric form used by phosphomannose isomerase and its l-epimerization by phosphoglucose isomerase. J. Biol. Chem. *248*:2232, 1973.

121. Sener, A., Pipeleers, D.G., Levy, J., Malaisse, W.J.: The stimulus-secretion coupling of glucose-induced insulin release. XXVI. Are the secretory and fuel functions of glucose dissociable by iodoacetate? Metabolism *27*:1505, 1978.

122. Idahl, L-Å.: Dynamics of pancreatic β-cell responses to glucose. Diabetologia *9*:403, 1973.

123. Zawalich, W.S., Dye, E.S., Pagliara, A.S., et al.: Starvation diabetes in the rat: Onset, recovery, and specificity of reduced responsiveness of pancreatic beta cells. Endocrinology *104*:1344, 1979.

124. Grodsky, G.M., Curry, D.L., Bennett, L.L., Rodrigo, J.J.: Factors influencing different rates of insulin release *in vitro*. In: R. Levine, E.E. Pfeiffer (Eds.): Mechanism and Regulation of Insulin Secretion. Acta Diabetol. Lat. *6*(Suppl. 1):140, 1968.

125. Grodsky, G.M., Curry, D., Landahl, H., Bennett, L.L.: Further studies on the dynamic aspects of insulin release *in vitro* with evidence for a two-compartmental storage system. Acta Diabetol. Lat. *6*(Suppl. 1):544, 1969.

126. Hedeskov, C.J.: Mechanism of glucose-induced insulin secretion. Physiol. Rev. *60*:442, 1980.

127. Grodsky, G.M.: A threshold distribution hypothesis for package storage of insulin and its mathematical modeling. J. Clin. Invest. *51*:2047, 1972.

128. Cerasi, E., Luft, R.: The plasma insulin response to glu-cose infusion in healthy subjects and in diabetes mellitus. Acta Endocrinol. (Kbh) *55*:278, 1967.

129. Seltzer, H.S., Allen, E.W., Herron, A.L., Jr., Brennan, M.T.: Insulin secretion in response to glycemic stimulus: relation of delayed initial release to carbohydrate intolerance in mild diabetes mellitus. J. Clin. Invest. *46*:323, 1967.

130. Brunzell, J.D., Robertson, R.P., Lerner, R.L., et al.: Relationships between fasting plasma glucose levels and insulin secretion during intravenous glucose tolerance tests. J. Clin. Endocrinol. Metab. *42*:222, 1976.

131. Stanik, S., Marcus, R.: Insulin secretion improves following dietary control of plasma glucose in severely hyperglycemic obese patients. Metabolism *29*:346, 1980.

132. Rudnick, P.A., Taylor, K.W.: Effect of prolonged carbohydrate restriction on serum insulin levels in mild diabetics. Br. Med. J. *1*:1125, 1965.

133. Doar, J.W.H., Thompson, M.E., Wilde, C.E., Sewell, P.F.J.: Influence of treatment with diet alone on oral glucose tolerance test and plasma sugar and insulin levels in patients with maturity-onset diabetes mellitus. Lancet. *1*:1263, 1975.

134. Savage, P.J., Bennion, L.J., Flock, E.V., et al.: Diet-induced improvement of abnormalities in insulin and glucagon secretion and in insulin receptor binding in diabetes mellitus. J. Clin. Endocrinol. Metab. *48*:999, 1979.

135. Cahill, G.F., Jr., Herrera, M.G., Morgan, A.P., et al.: Hormone-fuel interrelationships during fasting. J. Clin. Invest. *45*:1751, 1966.

136. Grey, N.J., Goldring, S., Kipnis, D.M.: The effect of fasting, diet and actinomycin D on insulin secretion in the rat. J. Clin. Invest. *49*:881, 1970.

137. Wolters, G.H.J., Konijnendijk, W., Bouman, P.R.: Effects of fasting on insulin secretion, islet glucose metabolism, and the cyclic adenosine 3′,5′-monophosphate content of rat pancreatic islets *in vitro*. Diabetes *26*:530, 1977.

138. Hedeskov, C.J., Capito, K.: The effect of starvation on insulin secretion and glucose metabolism in mouse pancreatic islets. Biochem. J. *140*:423, 1974.

139. DiPietro, D.L., Weinhouse, S.: Hepatic glucokinase in the fed, fasted, and alloxan-diabetic rat. J. Biol. Chem. *235*:2542, 1960.

140. Sharma, C., Manjeshwar, R., Weinhouse, S.: Effects of diet and insulin on glucose-adenosine triphosphate phosphotransferases of rat liver. J. Biol. Chem. *238*:3840, 1963.

141. Turner, D.S., Young, D.A.B.: The effect of fasting and selective re-feeding on insulin release in the rat. Acta Endocrinol. *72*:46, 1973.

142. Kolterman, O.G., Greenfield, M., Reaven, G.M., et al.: Effect of a high carbohydrate diet on insulin binding to adipocytes and on insulin action *in vivo* in man. Diabetes *28*:731, 1979.

143. Yingvorapant, N., Wendorff, H., Field, J.B.: Increased insulin secretion associated with increased caloric intake in mild noninsulin-dependent diabetics. J. Clin. Endocrinol. Metab. *50*:83, 1980.

144. Grey, N., Kipnis, D.M.: The effect of diet composition on the hyper-insulinemia of obesity. N. Engl. J. Med. *285*:827, 1971.

145. Sclafani, A., Springer, D.: Dietary obesity in adult rats: Similarities to hypothalamic and human obesity syndromes. Physiol. Behav. *17*:461, 1976.

146. Fajans, S.S., Floyd, J.C., Jr., Knopf, R.F., Conn. J.W.: Effect of amino acids and proteins on insulin secretion in man. Recent Prog. Hormone Res. *23*:617, 1967.

147. Felig, P., Marliss, E., Cahill, G.F.: Plasma amino acid

levels and insulin secretion in obesity. N. Engl. J. Med. *281*:811, 1969.

148. Schteingart, D.E., McKenzie, A.K., Victoria, R.S., Tsao, H.S.: Suppression of insulin secretion by protein deprivation in obesity. Metabolism *28*:943, 1979.

149. Lohmann, D., Liebold, F., Heilmann, W., et al.: Diminished insulin response in highly trained athletes. Metabolism *27*:521, 1978.

150. Berger, M., Kemmer, F.W., Becker, K., et al.: Effect of physical training on glucose tolerance and on glucose metabolism of skeletal muscle in anaesthetized normal rats. Diabetologia *16*:179, 1979.

151. Hartley, L.H., Mason, J.W., Hogan, R.P., et al.: Multiple hormonal responses to prolonged exercise in relation to physcial training. J. Appl. Physiol. *33*:607, 1972.

152. Zawalich, W.S., Maturo, S.A., Felig, P.: Physical training: decreased insulin secretion and liver glucokinase in the rat. Clin. Res. *29*:683A,1981 (Abstract).

153. Mondon, C.E., Dolkas, C.B., Reaven, G.M.: Site of enhanced insulin sensitivity in exercise-trained rats at rest. Am. J. Physiol. *239*:E169, 1980.

154. Steiner, D.F., Tager, H.S.: Biosynthesis of insulin and glucagon. In: L.J. DeGroot (Ed.): Endocrinology (Vol. 2). New York, Grune & Stratton, 1979, p. 921.

6 Insulin Transport and Action at Target Cells

Michael Berger and Peter Berchtold

The ability of insulin to fulfill its complex functions as a main hormonal regulator of metabolic processes depends not only on its adequate and appropriately regulated secretion rate, but also on its rapid transport to the target cells, its interaction with them, their responsiveness, and the subsequent degradation and excretion of the hormone. Circulating insulin levels are regulated both by changing rates of insulin secretion into the blood stream and the rapid degradation of the hormone in the liver and the kidney. The velocity of alteration of insulin secretion, balanced by the continuously rapid degradation, results in a half-life of circulating insulin of approximately 4 minutes. Thus, rapid oscillations of circulating insulin levels ensure the possibility of altering metabolic processes quickly. As described in Chapter 5, this extremely complex and capable regulatory system can be disturbed by deficiencies of insulin secretion.

On the other hand, disruption of the regulation of the serum insulin level and the efficacy of circulating insulin can also occur at various steps of its distribution, interaction with the target cell, and subsequent elimination. Such interferences include several forms of insulin resistance:

1. The transport of insulin in the blood stream can be delayed by insulin-binding antibodies or other non-specific circulating factors which interfere with the transport of insulin from the β-cell to its target organs. In this way, the kinetics of both the half-life of insulin disappearance in the blood and the biologic effects of insulin can be substantially altered.

2. The interaction of insulin with its target cell can be disturbed by diminution of receptor density or decrease of receptor affinity or by a direct inhibition of the binding process. These forms of insulin-resistant states include obesity, immobilization, hypercorticism, acromegaly, and the presence of insulin receptor antibodies. On the other hand, insulin receptor interactions can be facilitated by increased receptor numbers and/or receptor affinity such as in trained athletes, anorexia nervosa or other states of hyperinsulinemia, thereby resulting in increased insulin sensitivity.

3. The responsiveness of the target cell can be impaired by post-receptor defects, such as alterations of the transformation of the insulin receptor interaction to transmembrane or intracellular signals. Furthermore, the responsiveness of the cell can be inhibited by certain changes in the metabolic or hormonal milieu of the target cells.

4. Finally, the regulation of insulinemia and the metabolic effectiveness of insulin can be disturbed by decreased metabolic clearance rates of insulin, such as in advanced kidney and liver disease.

Most of these disorders of insulin transport, its various actions, and its subsequent degradation are associated with differing degrees of insulin resistance. In some cases a specific pathophysiologic defect can be identified as the cause for the diminished effectiveness of the hormone. In most of these disease states, a combination of various disorders is responsible for the insulin resistance. Nevertheless, recent developments in this area have deepened insight into the mechanisms and the various disturbances of insulin action which may lead to more specific and successful means of treatment.

This chapter will focus upon the various steps involved in insulin transport, interaction with target cells, effects on transmembrane transport, intracellular insulin effects, and various other actions of insulin. Wherever possible, abnormalities of these physiologic processes will be discussed in relation to pathologic disorders and disease states.

TRANSPORT OF INSULIN FROM THE BETA-CELL TO ITS TARGET ORGAN

Assessment of the steps involved in the transport of insulin from the islets of Langerhans to its target organs has long been hampered by the lack of appropriate methods to measure insulin in plasma. In fact, to date the nature of circulating insulin remains an enigma (Fig. 6–1). The fraction of insulin under particular scrutiny at present is the free immunoprecipitable insulin which can be identified by radioimmunoassay using specific insulin antibodies (IRI). In addition, many studies suggest that a substantial percentage of pancreatic insulin circulates in association with serum protein fractions, predominantly α- and β-globulins. The physiologic significance of these associations, however, remains controversial. Similarly, various hypothetical circulating insulin antagonists such as synalbumin[3] are, at present, not considered to be of particular relevance.

In any case, the predominant fraction of pancreatic insulin appears to circulate "freely," i.e. non-protein-associated. In addition to the immunoreactive insulin fraction, several other components exhibiting insulin-like biologic effects have been described; most notable are non-suppressible insulin-like activities (NSILA) (also termed Insulin-Like Growth Factors or IGF)[4-6] and the non-suppressible insulin-like protein.[7] The insulin-like polypeptides, some of which have already been chemically characterized, do not react with insulin

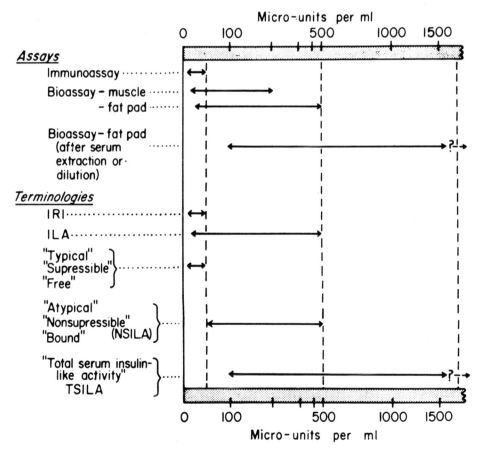

Fig. 6–1. Comparison of the magnitude of "insulin" moieties and their terminology of fasting serum. (Taken from Soeldner[1] with permission of the author.) It is of note that IRI includes a varying percentage of proinsulin-radioimmunoactivity. For further differentiation of NSILA, see Hall et al.[2]

antibodies, yet they do exhibit biologic effects assigned to insulin.

One component mentioned above, NSILA, has been particularly well described; it is closely related to somatomedins and tissue growth factors. The regulatory significance of these polypeptides for the main metabolic functions of insulin remains poorly understood. Some of those non-suppressible insulin-like activities have been mentioned in connection with the etiology of hypoglycemia induced by certain extra-pancreatic tumors, most notably fibrosarcomas.[8] In other work, it has been shown that in certain insulinopenic states there is a relative hypersecretion of proinsulin due presumably to the inability of the beta cell to store insulin normally[9] or to arrange proinsulin in secretory granules for adequate conversion to insulin. This proinsulin in the serum is less active biologically and may vary substantially in amount.[10]

Despite this apparent variety of insulin and insulin-like components in the circulation, most of the contemporary literature concentrates on the immunoreactive plasma insulin (IRI), the measurement of which has become a standard laboratory procedure ever since its first description by Yalow and Berson.[11] A particular problem arises in patients who have developed circulating insulin antibodies as a consequence of subcutaneous treatment with exogenous bovine or porcine insulin. Depending upon the antibody titer, a variable fraction of the intact IRI will be reversibly bound to the antibody fraction. Thus, the antibody might serve as a potentially useful reservoir of intact insulin or it might neutralize the effect of high doses of exogenous insulin, leading in certain cases to massive insulin resistance.

Various methods have been described to distinguish between free and antibody-bound insulin. They can, however, represent only an approximation since the steady state between free and antibody-bound insulin determined in vitro will not necessarily be identical with the status in vivo.

Consequently, most of the available data regarding the transport route of insulin and circulating levels of the hormone are based on studies in subjects not receiving exogenous insulin. Radioimmunoassay procedures have been used or the evidence deduced from experiments involving labeled insulin preparations. Most studies of insulin distribution have been carried out in rodents, using either iodinated insulin preparations[12] or, more recently, semisynthetic tritiated insulin.[13] It appears that the distribution of insulin in the body is rapid and that only 1 to 2% is excreted radioimmunologically intact in the urine. Insulin covers a distribution space of approximately 12%, the anatomic projection of which is not entirely clear.[14]

Even early distribution studies in rat organs, however, have suggested that part of the injected insulin penetrates across cell membrane barriers.[15]

Several attempts have been made to assess the half-life of disappearance, i.e., the metabolic clearance rate of exogenous insulin. Because of differences in the labeled hormones used, the results of those studies have varied considerably.[12,16] It appears that the distribution of intravenously injected insulin and its subsequent disappearance follows a multicompartmental, mathematical model. There is, however, little evidence at present as to what these hypothetical compartments actually represent in anatomic terms. Most recent studies in man report a half-life of serum insulin of 4 to 5 minutes. However, the clearance rate of endogenous insulin is probably even faster, since unlike the intravenous experiments on insulin pharmacokinetics, pancreatic insulin must first pass through the liver—a major site of degradation of insulin in the body.

Additional studies, preferably using semisynthetic ^{3}H-insulin and a chromatographic evaluation of the insulin degradation products,[13,17–19] are needed in order to define insulin distribution and clearance rates in normal man and in association with pathologic disorders. The predominant roles of the liver and kidney as insulin concentration, degradation and elimination sites, have been amply documented,[12] and the delay in disappearance curves for intravenously injected labeled insulin preparations has been documented in association with loss of hepatic and renal function.[20–22] Both chronic liver and renal disease may be associated with increased sensitivity to exogenous insulin. Recent studies by Halban et al.[13] have offered further insight into the various roles of the liver and the kidneys in removal of insulin from the circulation.

It is of note that so far no pathologic state of insulin resistance in association with increased insulin degradation has been found to interfere with the transport of the hormone from the β-cell to its target organ. In this context, Paulsen et al.[23] reported a rare disorder of severe resistance against subcutaneously injected insulin, possibly because of increased subcutaneous insulin degradation. This disorder might be treatable by inhibition of insulin degradation.[24,25]

In conclusion, the level of plasma insulin depends on the rates of its secretion and its degradation at a given point in time. It presently appears that acute oscillations of circulating insulin levels result from rapid alterations of insulin secretion in the presence of a consistently fast insulin degradation rate. Abnormalities of degradation can be instrumental in disturbing both insulin kinetics and effects. Thus, decreased degradation rates, such as in advanced liver and kidney disease, can increase the sensitivity to exogenous insulin and may induce hyperinsulinemia resulting in peripheral insulin resistance. Increased insulin degradation rates, such as reported in some cases of increased degradation of subcutaneously injected insulin, can result in massive insulin resistance. Pathologic states in association with increased degradation of endogenous insulin have not yet been reported.

INTERACTION OF INSULIN WITH THE TARGET CELL

The Insulin Receptor Concept

The interaction of insulin with its target cells has been the focus of attention ever since direct actions on metabolic processes have been described. What was first a hypothetical concept of hormone-binding to insulin-sensitive cells later evolved into the recognition of a specific hormone receptor interaction at the cell surface. Such an interaction between insulin and its membrane-based receptor is thought to be instrumental in the mechanism of any insulin action.[25a] The insulin receptor is a glycoprotein structure whose primary function is to identify the insulin molecule and to bind it. As with other hormone-receptor interactions,[26] the binding of insulin to its receptor is highly specific and reversible.

The association of insulin to its receptor, i.e., the formation of the hormone-receptor complex, represents the initial interaction of insulin with its target cell. The metabolic consequences depend on the effector system to which the receptor is coupled and the sequence of stimulus-response. Furthermore, the receptor does not appear to be a mere transmitter between the extracellular insulin molecule and the intracellular effector system; rather, regulatory processes and functions appear to be operational at the level of the insulin receptor interaction. Thus, the impact of the ambient extracellular insulin concentrations on intracellular metabolic events can be modulated by changes in the numbers of the receptors per cell and/or by alterations of the affinity of the receptor for insulin. These two mechanisms are believed to affect significantly the modulation of insulin action. Disturbances of the insulin receptor interactions are associated with and/or causally related to disease states,[26] especially those involving various forms of insulin resistance. In addition, it should be noted that other intracellular sites also exist for modulating insulin action.

Characterization of the Insulin Receptor

Many studies suggest that insulin exerts its action primarily at the cell membrane.[27–29] As early as 1950, Stadie et al.[30] reported that insulin induces an increase in glycogen synthesis in the isolated rat diaphragm, which persists even when insulin is removed. The hypothesis that insulin initiates its biologic effects through an interaction with the cell surface[31] was confirmed subsequently by findings in various studies among which were the following:

(a) Insulin action on various in vitro systems can be blocked rapidly by the addition of insulin antibodies to the incubation medium.

(b) Insulin cell-surface interaction is closely associated with the biologic effect of the hormone.[32]

(c) Insulin retains its biologic effects on isolated adipocytes even if it is firmly bound to sepharose beads[33] (although this observation was challenged by Butcher et al. on methodologic grounds[34]).

(d) The initial binding of labeled insulin is made visible by autoradiographic electron microscopic analysis.[35,36]

(e) Successful attempts to localize the receptor morphologically have been reported.[37–39]

Assessment of the insulin receptor and its interaction with the hormone depend on the availability of suitable insulin tracers. To this end, any labeled insulin preparation should be indistinguishable from active insulin in its binding characteristics, its degradation and its biologic activity when brought into contact with in vivo or in vitro systems. The iodinated insulin preparations initially in use in these studies were quite crude and suffered from various disadvantages. Later, it became possible to purify mono-iodinated insulins in such a way that the iodination and purification procedures would leave the insulin molecule undamaged; thus, the mono-iodinated ^{125}I-insulin as prepared by Freychet et al.[40,41] has been demonstrated both to stimulate glucose metabolism in adipocytes and to bind to adipocyte and various plasma membrane preparations. From a theoretical point of view, it would probably be advantageous to employ mono-tritiated semi-synthetic insulin preparations for any such studies.[13,42] However, the specific activity of presently available preparations of tritiated insulin is too low to render these insulin tracers useful for insulin receptor studies.

In order to study the interaction of insulin with its receptor, it appears preferable to employ both a homogeneous insulin and a homogeneous receptor preparation. Especially in earlier investigations, isolated cells (such as adipocytes and hepatocytes) and homogeneous plasma membrane preparations were used as sources of receptor.[43] However, some criticism has been directed to the fact that cell isolation procedures (especially if they involve a crude collagenase digestion of tissues) might damage the structures of the cell surface.

Currently, isolated cells are allowed to recover

in tissue culture before being used in receptor studies. Alternatively, various blood cells such as monocytes or erythrocytes and, to an increasing extent, cell membrane preparations and purified organelles, are employed as a source of homogeneous genuine receptor populations. Typically, insulin-binding studies are performed by incubating the receptor preparations with labeled insulin, such as ^{125}I-insulin, and varying concentrations of cold insulin. Subsequently, the bound hormone is separated from the free insulin tracer in the incubation medium at unphysiologically low temperatures. In order to accept such a simple competitive binding process as the insulin receptor interaction, several requirements must be fulfilled.

1. Most importantly, the association of labeled insulin to the (receptor carrying) preparation must be specific. The iodinated insulin can be replaced from its binding site only by an excessive amount of cold insulin. With a few exceptions (such as somatomedin, NSILA, IGF, etc.), the insulin receptor binds exclusively intact insulin. Depending on the source of the receptor population studied, a variable percentage of insulin tracer will be bound non-specifically. This basically unsaturable component represents binding of insulin to various structures other than its specific receptor, and this has to be corrected for.

2. Another source of error is the fact that, again depending on the source of the receptor bearing biologic material and the temperature of the incubation medium, a variable amount of insulin will be degraded during the incubation period. The degradation of insulin must be taken into account, preferably by direct measurement of labeled non-insulin material, using column chromatography techniques or other approaches. On the basis of a substantial amount of experience over several years, appropriate assay conditions for binding experiments have been described, such as the optimal temperature, pH and the ionic environment of the incubation system. As a result, it is now possible to characterize the kinetics of a specific binding process of insulin to its receptor in a variety of cell populations and fractions from the various species.[25a,46]

Assessment of the Insulin-Receptor Interaction. After correcting for non-specific binding and degradation of insulin, the kinetics of the binding process between insulin and its specific receptor can be assessed by varying the amount of labeled and cold insulin in the incubation medium and subsequent analysis of the ratio of bound to free labeled insulin. The two most important quantifications of the insulin receptor interaction kinetics in any given biologic material are:

(a) the total number of receptors and

(b) the insulin-receptor binding affinity.

Using the Scatchard plot analysis of the experimental data, these can be calculated: the abscissal intercept of the curve indicating the total number of receptors, and the slope of the line indicating binding affinity. For the insulin receptor, however, binding affinity does not appear to be a constant parameter over a wide range of insulin concentration. Rather, the Scatchard analysis of the insulin-binding data quite consistently is curvilinear, suggesting that binding affinity decreases with increasing insulin concentration in the incubation medium. This has been interpreted to indicate "negative cooperativity" between insulin receptor sites.[47] The relatively high affinity of unoccupied receptors gives way to a progressively decreasing affinity as neighboring receptors are forming insulin receptor complexes.

In addition to negative cooperativity, other reasons for the curvilinearity have been suggested, such as operational heterogeneity of insulin receptors[48] and several different binding components in biologic materials.[49,50] Further studies will be necessary to resolve these apparent discrepancies and to put these observations into pathophysiologic perspective. Thus, although the hypothesis of negative cooperativity has not remained unchallenged,[50,51] it has gained wide acceptance and proved to be a helpful guide in explaining clinical and pathophysiologic phenomena (see below).

In this context, it may not be possible in all instances to transfer information about the receptor number and the receptor affinity to insulin obtained from measurements in intact blood cells to the insulin-binding kinetics at the surface of fat, liver, or muscle cells. It should be noted that at least in humans, most receptor analyses have been performed in cells (monocytes and erythrocytes) which are unresponsive or only slightly responsive to the various metabolic actions of insulin; only in a limited number of studies in humans have isolated adipocytes been used for insulin-binding studies. The significance of specific insulin-binding in tissues or cells hitherto not considered as insulin targets, is at present poorly understood. Nevertheless, it is generally assumed that insulin-binding studies employing circulating cells at low temperatures in vitro reflect insulin binding by the main target cells of the hormone in vivo, i.e., hepatocytes, adipocytes, and muscle cells.[52]

The receptor concept has been solidly confirmed by extensive studies correlating the binding of insulin to target cells, such as adipocytes, and the biologic effect of insulin in these cells (Fig. 6–2). However, it has been found that a mere 10% receptor occupancy is required to elicit maximal biologic insulin effects. This surprising phenomenon

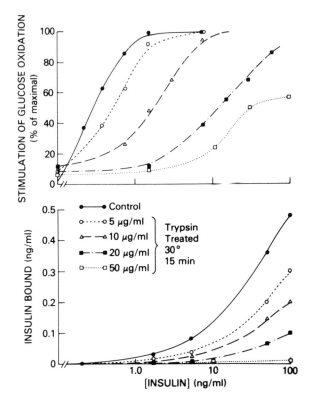

Fig. 6–2. Effect of a change in receptor concentration (R_o) on insulin binding and action in isolated adipocytes. Isolated rat adipocytes were treated with 0 to 50 μg/ml of trypsin for 15 minutes at 30°C. An equal amount of soybean trypsin inhibitor was added, and the cells were washed three times. Following this, glucose oxidation (upper figure) and insulin binding (lower figure) were assessed in the usual fashion. (Reprinted from Kahn[58] by permission of the author and publisher)

has led to the concept of "spare receptors" (Fig. 6–3).[53-57]

Physicochemical Characterization of the Insulin Receptor. Many attempts have been made to characterize the physicochemical structure of the insulin receptor. Initial findings, even before the receptor concept was formulated, suggested that the interaction of insulin with the target cell might depend on the integrity of sulfhydryl groups located at the cell surface and the disulfide bridges of the insulin molecule. Recent studies, however, suggest that this is not the case. Rather, the binding of insulin to its receptor appears to occur by a process dependent on interactions of hydrophobic processes and hydrogen bonds.[60] In other experiments, trypsin digestion was found to abolish the receptor capacity of intact cells and various cell membrane preparations. In culture the receptor reappeared, a process which was suppressible by protein synthesis blocking agents.[52,61] It was of note that at low

concentrations, trypsin had somewhat of an intrinsic insulin-like effect.

These and other experiments have confirmed that the insulin receptor is an integral part of the cell membrane and of protein structure. More direct attempts to characterize chemically the insulin receptor have dissociated the receptor from cell membranes by dissolving with various detergents;[44,58] such receptors have maintained at least some of the characteristics of receptors bound to membrane. Preliminary purification by means of various electrophoretic and chromatographic procedures, seems to indicate that the insulin receptor might be a glycoprotein consisting of 4 subunits of an estimated total molecular weight of approximately 200,000 to 1,000,000,[62,63] which in the presence of insulin, disintegrates into smaller components of as yet unidentified chemical and functional characteristics.[64] Only recently, Kasuga et al.[64a] were able to demonstrate in cultured human lymphocytes that 95,000-dalton (beta) subunits of the insulin receptor were selectively phosphorylated; this phosphorylation process was stimulated by insulin in a dose-dependent fashion.

Further analysis of the insulin receptor is necessary in order to understand its detailed physicochemical and molecular characteristics and thereby gain insight into the functional behavior of the receptor,[25a] its information transmitter function, possible receptor aggregation[65,66] or redistribution[67] and its subsequent internalization (Fig. 6–4).

Regulation of the Insulin Receptor. The binding kinetics of insulin-insulin receptor interactions are by no means a constant feature of any biologic system. By contrast, the insulin-receptor interaction is subjected to regulatory influences which appear to be important effectors of the biologic action of insulin.[25a] The insulin-binding kinetics can be regulated in two ways:

1. by alteration of the receptor affinity (indicated by an alteration of the slope of the Scatchard analysis of competitive binding experiments), and

2. by alteration of the receptor density, i.e., the number of receptors per cell surface.

The first possibility is generally believed to be involved in short-term regulation of the binding kinetics, whereas changes in the insulin receptor number seem to represent chronic adaptive responses. Cells seem able to regulate their capacity and kinetics to bind insulin specifically and thus to modulate their insulin sensitivity, i.e., their biologic response to changes in ambient insulin concentrations. This can be achieved by alteration of the receptor affinity to insulin (acute regulation) or of the total receptor number (chronic regulatory process) or by the simultaneous use of both of these possibilities. Studies by Pezzino et al.[68] have dem-

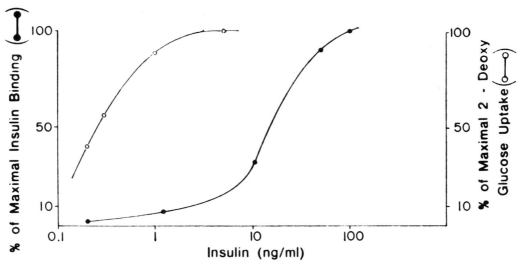

Fig. 6–3. Demonstration of "spare" insulin receptors in isolated rat fat cells. Open circles represent the percent of maximal insulin stimulated 2-deoxy glucose uptake as a function of insulin concentration. Closed circles represent the percent of maximal specific insulin binding. The maximal biological effect is reached at an insulin concentration of 5 μg/ml, at which point only about 10% of the available receptor sites are filled. (Reprinted from Olefsky[59] by permission of the author and publisher.)

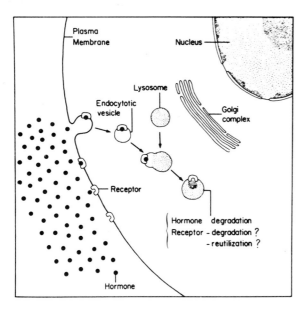

Fig. 6–4. Diagrammatic hypothesis of insulin's interaction with a target cell: according to this view, insulin initially binds to a specific cell surface receptor, and the insulin-receptor-complex may then be redistributed in the plane of the membrane. The ligand is then internalized by the cell by adsorptive pinocytosis into a membrane bound vesicle which fuses with lysosomes. Subsequently, insulin is degraded and the membrane vesicle containing the receptor is either degraded or reutilized. (Reprinted from Gorden et al.[67] by permission of the authors and publisher.)

onstrated, however, that insulin in vivo can reduce acutely the receptor number of rat hepatocytes.

Short-term fasting induces a *rapid increase in receptor affinity*,[69] presumably due to a decrease in the rate of dissociation of the insulin receptor complex. Similar accelerated receptor affinity has been reported following exercise. At present, the mechanisms for these acute augmentations of receptor affinity are unknown, but it is tempting to speculate that they are causally related to the abrupt fall in circulating insulin levels seen in both of these situations. In contrast, relatively sharp decrease of receptor affinity to insulin can be seen after glucocorticoid treatment, following the ingestion of carbohydrate[70] or food[71] and within 5 hours of the institution of hyperinsulinemia or hyperglycemia.[72] *Chronic regulation* of insulin binding by alteration of the receptor concentration at the cell surface is characteristically seen in all states of chronic hyperinsulinemia, most notably obesity (see below) and, in addition, in patients with insulinomas.[73] It appears that chronic exposure of the cell surface to high insulin concentration leads to a decrease in receptor numbers, i.e., to a "down regulation" of receptors. This concept has been confirmed by observations in vitro: the decrease in receptor density was proportional to both the magnitude of insulin levels and the time of exposure.[74,75] In addition, this hypothesis of the self-regulation of the insulin receptor number has been confirmed by the contrasting observation that various states of hypoinsulinemia, such as diabetes mellitus[76] and anorexia nervosa,[77] are associated with increased insulin receptor numbers. As in the hyperinsulinemic states, in some studies insulin receptor density could be normalized when serum insulin concentrations reverted to normal. Conversely, in obesity, caloric restriction is associated with an increase in receptor numbers, presumably because of the respective alterations in circulating insulin levels.[69] While the ambient insulin concentration is probably the most important modulator of the insulin receptor number and its affinity to insulin, additional possible regulators of the insulin-receptor action have been suggested, such as ketone bodies;[78] growth hormone;[79,80] glucocorticoids;[80] possibly drugs such as sulfonylureas[80a] or biguanides;[80b] and changes in the dietary intake of fat and carbohydrates.[81–83] In several studies, strenuous physical exercise and training were associated with increased insulin-receptor affinity.[84,85] Further recent studies on T-lymphocytes suggest that more complicated mechanisms, possibly genetic in nature, may be responsible for the decreased receptor density in obesity and adult-onset diabetes.[86]

Pathology of the Insulin Receptor in Insulin-Resistant States. Various alterations in insulin sensitivity have been related to changes of receptor density and/or affinity at the target cells. Since it became generally accepted that hormone action can be effectively modulated at the level of the insulin receptor (see above), several pathologic states of decreased insulin sensitivity have been investigated with particular attention to disturbances of the insulin binding process. In fact, in a variety of disease states, parallel changes in insulin binding and insulin action have been observed.[25a] These include conditions in which both binding and action of insulin are increased, e.g., anorexia nervosa, growth hormone deficiency and glucocorticoid deficiency. In other disease states, both insulin binding and action are decreased, as in growth hormone and glucocorticoid excess, uremia, obesity, NIDDM, severe insulin resistance and acanthosis nigricans. On the other hand, in some conditions insulin binding and insulin action are dissociated. Thus, in starvation, insulin binding is increased whereas insulin action is decreased; when a high carbohydrate diet is used, insulin binding is decreased and action increased.

Because of the nature of the insulin receptor interaction and the existence of overabundant "spare receptors", any decrease of receptor number and/or affinity causes the dose-response curve for insulin action to shift to the right,[87] a decrease in insulin action at submaximal insulin concentrations and a normal insulin effect at maximally effective concentrations of insulin. Therefore, the clinical state of insulin resistance can be explained only partially by an alteration of the insulin receptor

number and/or affinity leading to reduced insulin sensitivity. Decrease of the maximal biologic response to insulin seems to be due to postreceptor alterations. Both types of disturbance of insulin action have been described separately as well as in combination (Fig. 6–5).

Most extensive observations of the interrelation between alterations of insulin sensitivity and insulin receptor interactions have been made with respect to the insulin resistance associated with obesity. Both in animal models[58,88,89] and in man,[90] a consistent diminution of insulin receptor concentrations has been described.[60] In some models, the receptor affinity as well as certain characteristics of the insulin receptor interactions were unaltered; the disturbance at the receptor level was limited to a decrease in receptor number per cell surface area.[58,89]

In vivo studies in obese man, reporting a shift to the right of the dose-response curves for certain insulin actions, are compatible with these observations. These findings suggest that a decrease in receptor number may play an important role in the development of insulin insensitivity in obese man. In fact, a linear correlation between insulin binding and insulin sensitivity in vivo has been observed in such subjects.[90,91] Consistent with this hypothesis is the enhancement of both insulin sensitivity and insulin binding with hypocaloric diets and/or weight reduction programs.[69,92–94]

It must be added that in contrast, some studies

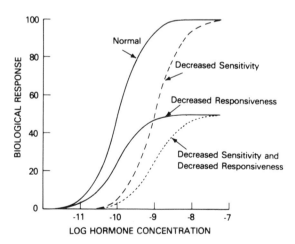

Fig. 6–5. Type of resistance to hormone action. The figure shows four dose-response curves for hormonal responses. In each case, the biologic response may be regarded as being defined by two separate terms: (a) the maximal response that can be achieved at any hormone concentration (in the ideal case this is a true plateau); and (b) the dose-response for the hormone that exists between no effect and the maximal response, i.e., the sensitivity of the response of the hormone. (Reprinted from Kahn[58] by permission of the author and publisher.)

have revealed no alteration of the insulin receptor binding in obese patients despite significant degrees of hyperinsulinemia.[95,96] These and other observations might indicate a certain heterogeneity of the obesity syndrome[55] and, more importantly, the involvement of metabolic abnormalities causing insulin resistance beyond the receptor level.

Clinically more important is the insulin resistance in NIDDM. As in nondiabetic obese patients, a parallel decrease of insulin sensitivity and insulin binding (due to a reduced number of receptors) has been described. While the majority of these patients are overweight, the decrease in insulin sensitivity cannot be satisfactorily explained by the accompanying obesity. In any case, insulin insensitivity does occur in nonobese patients with NIDDM and the degree of insulin resistance appears to be more pronounced in obese patients with NIDDM than in nondiabetic obese controls.[92]

It has been demonstrated repeatedly that monocytes, erythrocytes, and adipocytes from patients with NIDDM, obese or nonobese, with proven resistance to insulin, have a reduced number of insulin receptors. Those present, however, are functionally unaltered.[87,92,97–99] Close correlation between the receptor density and circulating insulin levels supports a down-regulation of receptor numbers by hyperinsulinemia as the mechanism of this decrease, as has been shown in nondiabetic subjects. However, factors other than hyperinsulinemia must be considered as possible causes of diminution of receptor number in NIDDM (see above).[92] Furthermore, it has been shown that apart from insulinemia, receptor numbers may be affected by an overall improvement of metabolic control or by the action of certain drugs.[100] Even more complicated is the relationship between insulin receptor binding and insulin resistance in NIDDM with severe fasting hyperglycemia. Although these patients are markedly resistant to insulin, the diminution of insulin binding is no greater than in patients with impaired glucose tolerance and mild insulin insensitivity.

Clearly, factors other than insulinemia can regulate the insulin receptor density, and factors other than insulin receptor numbers are operative in regulating insulin sensitivity in NIDDM. Insulin resistance due to glucocorticoid excess is associated with a decrease in receptor affinity;[52,80] and in acromegaly, a diminution of receptor density and an increase in a certain compartment of the receptor affinity have been noted.[79] In both cases of insulin resistance, however, postreceptor alterations appear to be the main reason for the relative ineffectiveness of endogenous and exogenous insulin. Furthermore, the glucose intolerance found in patients with uremia is not associated with a parallel decrease in insulin binding,[101] and the decrease in insulin receptors in Duchenne muscular dystrophy is not associated with impaired glucose metabolism.[101a]

In some instances of insulin resistance (in patients who are obese and in obese patients with NIDDM), the diminished response to insulin may be due to post-receptor defects as well as to receptor defects. These insulin-binding studies have offered a deeper insight into the pathophysiology of the diabetic state and allowed for some rationalization of therapeutic maneuvers. Thus, Beck-Nielsen et al.[102,103] have demonstrated in a group of obese NIDDM patients that treatment with a hypocaloric diet for 1 year normalized circulating glucose and insulin levels, as well as insulin sensitivity. These changes were associated with a parallel increase in insulin-binding to monocytes (Fig 6–6).

In a number of rare diseases and disorders, studies on the interrelationships between disturbances of insulin sensitivity and insulin binding allow a clarification of the underlying mechanisms.[104–107] Kahn et al.[89] describe two groups of patients with extreme insulin resistance associated with distinct disturbances of the insulin receptor interaction. One group consists of younger female patients with severe insulin resistance accompanied by hirsutism, mild virilism, polycystic ovaries and acanthosis nigricans. In these, a *primary* defect of insulin binding to monocytes due to a persistent diminution of receptor density has been found. In another group of somewhat older females with insulin resistance and additional symptoms of autoimmune disease, a circulating antibody against the insulin receptor has been reported. This anti-receptor antibody has been well characterized, and it is generally accepted that it interferes with the binding process of insulin to receptors, thus causing insulin resistance. So far, it has been difficult to prove the validity of therapeutic action (such as immunosuppressive therapy) in these patients since without treatment the severity of the syndrome may undergo dramatic change and even spontaneous remission.

Possible disturbance of insulin receptor interaction by hypothetical circulating interference factors or by a genuine diminution of receptor density as the cause for insulin resistance have been reported also in lipoatrophic diabetes[108] and ataxia telangiectasia.[108a] In other equally rare cases of insulin resistance, normal insulin-binding characteristics have been found, suggesting that the defects are postreceptor in nature.[58,107]

Post-Receptor Defects in Insulin Resistance. As outlined above (Fig. 6–5), any decrease in insulin responsiveness, i.e., a diminution of the V_{max} of a biologic effect of the hormone, can hardly be

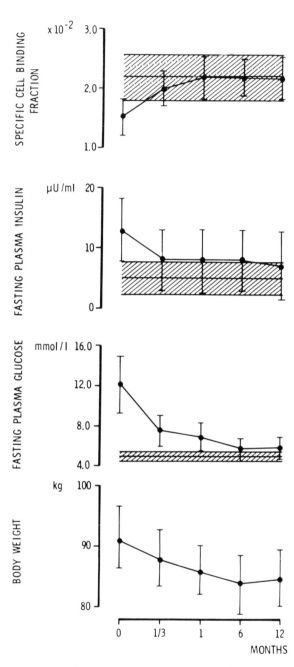

Fig. 6–6. Changes in specific binding of insulin to monocytes in ten obese nonketotic diabetics before and during treatment with a hypocaloric diet for 1 year. (Reprinted from Beck-Nielsen et al.[102] by permission of the authors and publisher.)

explained solely on the basis of a disturbed interaction between insulin and its receptor; rather, such a decrease points to a post-receptor disturbance of insulin action. In large adipocytes from obese rodents, the glucose *transport* process shows a decreased sensitivity to insulin, i.e., a rightward shift of the dose-response curve[54,109] without an alter-

ation of the K_m for insulin-stimulated glucose transport. This phenomenon can be explained by the associated decrease in receptor number. By contrast, even the maximally insulin-stimulated glucose oxidation rates are greatly diminished in these large fat cells,[54,109] indicating a decrease in V_{max} of the glucose oxidation stimulated by insulin (Figs. 6–7a and 6–7b), suggesting a postreceptor, intracellular defect of glucose metabolism. Likewise, studies by Kemmer et al.,[110] LeMarchand-Brustel,[111] and Crettaz et al.[112] confirm that intracellular defects of glucose metabolism are the major reason for the insulin resistance of skeletal muscle in obese rodents.

Various possible mechanisms for this intracellular metabolic lesion have been proposed,[44,112] several of which might be operative simultaneously. Crettaz and Jeanrenaud[113] have reviewed various abnormalities found in adipocytes from different species of obese rodents in a synopsis (Tables 6–1 and 6–2). Thus, in a variety of tissues of obese rodents, intracellular metabolic disturbances of glucose utilization appear to be more important in the etiology of insulin resistance than the concomitant alterations in receptor binding. In fact, at least in adipose tissue and skeletal muscle of rodents, insulin binding and the metabolic actions of insulin may vary in opposite directions, alterations of insulin binding being completely bypassed by changes in intracellular insulin effect.[113]

It has been suggested repeatedly that in man the impairment of insulin binding may play an important role in the pathophysiology of insulin resistance associated with obese or non-obese NIDDM. Whether the insulin resistance in obesity is due to reduced insulin sensitivity or to reduced insulin responsiveness or to both, is a question that so far has not been definitively resolved. In fact, this may well depend on the type of obesity and on the duration and degree of the hyperinsulinemia syndrome; also, it may vary from tissue to tissue. In addition, it appears plausible that one should assume a longitudinal view as to the progressive evolution of insulin resistance as a predominant feature in the "diabesity" syndrome. Such a dynamic view has offered substantial insight into the progression of the metabolic syndrome of insulin resistance in various animal models.[113,114] Similarly, in man various phases of what appears to be a hypothetic progression of a syndrome—obesity, hyperinsulinemia, impaired glucose tolerance, diabetes—can be observed. Whether there is, in fact, a longitudinal progression of these phases in a given obese subject is presently controversial; however, older studies, such as the one by Ogilvie[115] seem to support such a view.[116]

In a cross-sectional study of obese subjects with

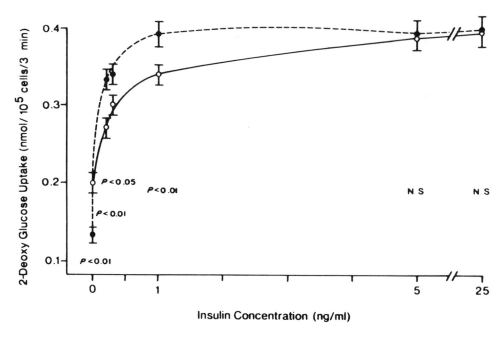

Fig. 6–7a. Insulin sensitivity of glucose transport and glucose oxidation of small (●) and large (○) adipocytes. (a) *Glucose transport* as measured by the uptake of *2-deoxy glucose uptake*. Cells were preincubated with or without insulin (at the indicated concentrations) for 45 minutes at 24°C. Uptake was measured at the end of a 3-minute incubation with 2-^{14}C-deoxy glucose (0.125mM). The maximal response is similar in both size cells but the dose-response curve of the large adipocyte is shifted to the right, which is the predicted functional consequence of a decrease in insulin binding. (Reprinted from Olefsky[54] by permission of the author and publisher.)

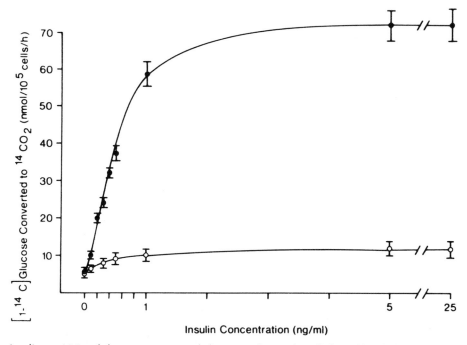

Fig. 6–7b. Insulin sensitivity of glucose transport and glucose oxidation of small (●) and large (○) adipocytes. (b) *Oxidation of 1-^{14}C-glucose*. Cells were preincubated with the indicated insulin concentrations at 37°C for 60 minutes. Rates of glucose oxidation are severely depressed in the large adipocytes even at the maximally effective insulin concentrations. (Reprinted from Olefsky[54] by permission of the author and publisher.)

Table 6–1. Main Abnormalities of Insulin-Resistant Large Adipocytes Observed in Different Types of Obesity Syndromes (Compared to Normal Small Adipocytes)*

Number of insulin receptors (per cell, per cell surface area)	Decreased
Basal glucose transport	Increased or normal
Insulin-stimulated glucose transport	Decreased sensitivity and decreased responsiveness
Coupling between IR and glucose transport system	Apparently normal
Overall basal glucose metabolism	Decreased
Overall insulin-stimulated glucose metabolism	Decreased sensitivity and decreased responsiveness
Basal intracellular abnormalities of glucose metabolism	Normal oxidation via Embden-Myerhof pathway and Krebs cycle
	Decreased oxidation via pentose shunt pathway
	Decreased total lipid synthesis from glucose, with very markedly decreased TGFA synthesis and relatively increased TGG
Insulin-sensitive intracellular pathways of glucose metabolism	Decreased sensitivity (relative) + decreased responsiveness (moderate-to-no response)
Basal intracellular abnormalities of lipid metabolism	Decreased acetyl-CoA carboxylase activity
	Increased lipolysis
	Increased intracellular FFA
	Increased esterification capacity of FA
Other basal abnormality of lipid metabolism	Increased LPL activity

IR = insulin-receptor complexes; TGFA = triglyceride fatty acids; TGG = triglyceride glycerol; FFA = free fatty acids; FA = fatty acids; LPL = lipoprotein lipase. "Basal" means non-insulin-stimulated.
*From Crettaz and Jeanrenaud[113] with permission of the authors and publisher.

Table 6–2. Main Abnormalities of Insulin-Resistant Muscles in Different Types of Obesities*

Number of insulin receptors	Decreased
Basal glucose transport and/or phosphorylation	Decreased
Insulin-stimulated glucose transport and/or phosphorylation	Decreased sensitivity and decreased responsiveness
Coupling between IR and glucose transport system	Apparently normal
Insulin-stimulated de novo glycogen synthesis	Decreased sensitivity and decreased responsiveness
Insulin-stimulated glycolysis	Decreased sensitivity and decreased responsiveness

IR = insulin-receptor complexes. "Basal" means non-insulin-stimulated.
*From Crettaz and Jeanrenaud[113] with permission of the authors and publisher.

varying degrees of glucose intolerance, Koltermann et al.[117] ascribed distinct metabolic abnormalities to some of these phases: all obese patients had both a decreased insulin sensitivity (right-shifted dose-response curves for insulin as assessed with the glucose clamp technique) and a decreased insulin receptor number per adipocyte surface. The maximal insulin-stimulated disposal rates of glucose were normal in some obese subjects with minor degrees of glucose intolerance, hyperinsulinemia, smaller adipocytes, and early onset of obesity. This indicates that no post-receptor defect of glucose metabolism was involved. In another subgroup of obese patients of comparable degree of adiposity, but with even higher serum insulin levels, larger fat cells, higher degree of glucose intolerance and later onset of obesity, maximal insulin-stimulated glucose disposal rates were markedly decreased, thus indicating, in addition, a post-receptor defect of glucose metabolism. These data suggest that there is a continuous spectrum of metabolic disturbances in obese man in which progressive degrees of hyperinsulinemia, insulin resist-

ance, and impairment of glucose tolerance are associated with decreased insulin responsiveness and post-receptor, intracellular lesions of glucose metabolism, in addition to the decreased insulin sensitivity associated with decreased insulin binding prevalent in obesity.

Earlier studies had suggested that impairment of insulin responsiveness in overt obese or nonobese NIDDM is also associated with postreceptor defects of insulin-stimulated glucose metabolism at the cellular level. Consequently, at least in cross-sectional studies, a continuum of metabolic disturbances exists in obese subjects, from glucose-tolerant persons to those overtly NIDDM. The phases of this interaction of insulin with its target cells progress from a mere impairment of the formation of insulin receptor complexes to defects of intracellular glucose utilization independent of the insulin receptor interaction. In a more recent study, Marshall and Olefsky[75] were able to confirm this concept by in vitro experiments involving the incubation of isolated adipocytes in the presence of high insulin levels. Short-term incubation was associated with a decrease in receptor numbers (i.e., insulin sensitivity), whereas more prolonged incubation induced an additional postreceptor defect in the glucose transport system.

Yet to be clarified are the possible consequences of this hypothetical concept with regard to other processes of insulin interaction with the cell, such as degradation and internalization of the hormone. At present, it remains unknown whether the intracellular lesions of insulin-stimulated glucose metabolism are:

(1) a direct result of hyperinsulinemia in these patients; or

(2) a long-term consequence of the disturbed insulin receptor interaction (reduced insulin binding due to a diminished number of receptors); or

(3) a defect of the second messenger system; or

(4) metabolic interference by inhibition of certain glycolytic pathways.

As long as no direct attempt to ameliorate intracellular inhibition of glucose metabolism is possible, any pathophysiologically based therapeutic approach in insulin-resistant NIDDM should be directed to improving the insulin receptor interaction by decreasing the hyperinsulinemia (via diet, fasting and drugs) and by facilitating the insulin receptor interaction (by physical activity and drugs).

THE SECOND MESSENGER CONCEPT OF INSULIN ACTION

The rapid initiation and/or modulation of various biologic processes within the cell following the interaction of insulin with its receptor structures at the plasma cell membrane has, for a long time, called for the hypothesis of a second messenger or a mediator system of some sort (Fig. 6–8). The function of such a pulse-transmitting system would be to initiate certain biologic responses within the cell following the formation of the insulin receptor complex at the cell surface. Initially, energy-rich phosphates were considered possible candidates for such a chemical mediator system; later, cation fluxes and other not yet purified mediators of peptide(-like) nature were suggested.

The observation that insulin stimulates the $(Na^+ K^+)$-ATPase in a variety of tissues[118] led to the hypothesis that the sodium pump might represent the transducer system of insulin action.[119,120] In sharp contrast to this hypothesis, in a variety of experiments using isolated adipocytes, a negative correlation was found between the activity of the sodium pump and insulin-like actions.[118] Thus, a mere acceleration of trans-membrane sodium influx now appears an unlikely candidate for the hypothetical second messenger system for insulin action. Similarly, earlier claims that Mg^{++} influx into the cell might trigger metabolic intracellular insulin

actions, have not been generally accepted. At present, like that of several other ions and substances, the role of Mg^{++} seems to be limited to a "permissive" action with respect to the metabolic actions of insulin.

Considerable attention has been paid to the possible importance of Ca^{++} ion fluxes in mediating insulin action as recently reviewed by Czech.[109,121,122] While alterations of Ca^{++} fluxes remain a hypothetical explanation of the transduction process between insulin binding and intracellular insulin effects,[123,124] the cited experimental evidence is highly controversial. In different tissues, both a fall and a rise of intracellular free calcium levels have been suggested.[118] These apparent contradictions may be related to species or organ-specific differences or to compartmentalization of intracellular calcium spaces.

As noted earlier, one line of evidence supports the hypothesis that the second messenger of insulin action involves the modulation of intracellular levels of energy-rich phosphates. In this context, the effect of insulin was initially thought to be mediated by a decrease in cellular cyclic-AMP levels[125–128] brought about by stimulation of phosphodiesterase activity,[129–134] possibly via the protein, calmodulin.[135,136] However, in a variety of studies, no such inverse correlation could be observed between cellular cAMP levels and insulin action.[76,120,137–141]

More recently, the effect of insulin on protein kinases and phosphatase has been investigated, especially since major metabolic actions of the hormone, such as the modulation of glycogen synthase, pyruvate dehydrogenase and pyruvate kinase, are dependent on insulin-sensitive phosphoenzymes. In some studies, insulin was shown to stimulate protein phosphorylase activities, such as the rat heart glycogen synthase D phosphatase,[142] and various investigators have demonstrated the inhibition of protein-kinase activities by insulin.[143] Presently unresolved is whether these effects of insulin on phosphatase protein-kinase cycles are mediated via an alteration of cyclic-AMP or cyclic-GMP levels.[118] Different chemical mediator systems for insulin action have been postulated by Larner and his associates[144] and Cheng et al.[145] These hypothetical messengers as extracted from skeletal muscle cells following exposure to insulin in vivo, have been shown to activate pyruvate dehydrogenase (PDH)[146] and glycogen-synthase-phosphatase[145] and to inhibit cyclic-AMP-dependent protein-kinase activities[145] in an insulin-like manner. This activity might represent the actual insulin mediator, at least for some processes. At present, the chemical characteristics of the peptide(-like) substance(s) and the location of their

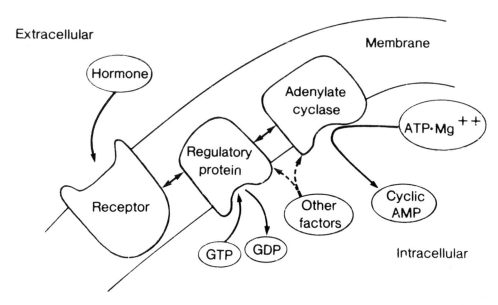

Fig. 6–8. Hypothetical model for a hormonal system in which adenylate cyclase is activated. The binding of hormone to receptor enhances the association of guanosine triphosphate (GTP) to a guanyl nucleotide regulatory protein. The GTP-regulatory complex then activates adenylate cyclase. Other factors (see text) can also activate adenylate cyclase; these factors may react directly with the enzyme or could affect the regulatory protein. After its activation, the enzyme converts adenosine triphosphate (ATP), in an ATP·Mg++ complex, to cyclic adenosine monophosphate (cAMP). (Reprinted from Baxter[26] with permission of the author and publisher).

origin within the cell or plasma membrane remain to be clarified. Nevertheless, this hypothetic chemical mediator is an attractive possibility for an insulin mediator or second messenger system to transfer information signals from the insulin receptor complex at the cell surface to intracellular structures.[144]

INSULIN INTERNALIZATION

Some investigators have questioned the absolute need for a second messenger or transmitter system in order to induce insulin action at intracellular locations. The internalization of insulin, as well as the existence of specific insulin-binding sites at various intracellular structures and organelles has been convincingly demonstrated.[67] In several different cell populations, some fractions of the labeled insulin at the cell surface can subsequently be taken up ("internalized") by the cell (Figs. 6–9 and 6–10).

It remains to be clarified as to what extent the internalized insulin molecules have been damaged or degraded. In addition, the mechanism of the penetration of insulin into the cell is still under investigation. Thus, it is not now known whether native insulin enters the cell by pinocytosis, or whether the insulin receptor complexes are internalized as such. The latter alternative appears to be possible in view of observations that high insulin levels in vivo can acutely reduce the number of specific insulin receptors on liver cell plasma membranes.[68] In fact, the down-regulation of receptor numbers in states of hyperinsulinemia might be caused by the increased formation of insulin receptor complexes and their subsequent internalization.[67] Furthermore, it is unclear how far the insulin molecule penetrates into the cell and with which intracellular structures it associates. A predominant association of the internalized insulin with lysosomes, as suggested in some studies[147,148] would favor the concept that the penetration of the hormone is part of the degradation process. In later studies, however, internalized tracer insulin was also found associated with rough endoplasmic reticulum and the cell nucleus,[52] suggesting additional physiologic significance of the internalization phenomenon. Thus, it has been proposed that insulin, via its internalization or its degradation products[149] or the insulin receptor,[150] might well be its own "second messenger." This hypothesis appears to be in accord with the demonstration of insulin-specific receptors at various sites within the cell, such as the Golgi apparatus, nuclear membranes, and the endoplasmic reticulum.[52,67,151–154]

Although the specificity of the various intracellular insulin-binding sites has been adequately proven, there are quite substantial functional differences from the plasma membrane receptors.[52,155] Although binding to nuclear membranes is similar to that of plasma membranes as regards regulation

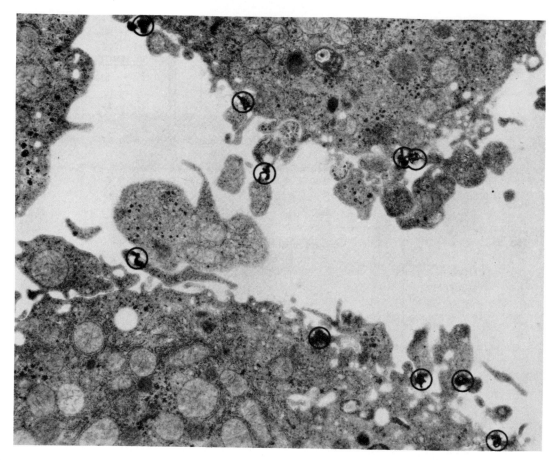

Fig. 6–9. Thin section of rat hepatocyte with developed autoradiography grains (circles) following 4 minutes of incubation of freshly isolated cells at 20°C with ^{125}I-insulin at physiologic concentrations. The labeled material can be both qualitatively and quantitatively localized to the plasma membrane of the hepatocytes. (Reprinted from Gorden et al.[67] by permission of the authors and publisher.)

by insulin and the presence of multiple orders of binding sites, differences appear in other respects. Whereas binding to plasma membranes is characterized by a pH optimum of 7.8 to 8.0, inhibition by antisera, negative cooperativity and salt dependence, such is not the case with nuclear membranes.

Pending further experimentation, one can only speculate as to the possibility of a direct insulin action on intracellular structures (without a mediator system), inducing metabolic actions such as the synthesis of glycogen, proteins or certain nucleotides. On the other hand, the internalization of insulin together with its receptor might be an important step in the process of degradation of the hormone; and it appears to be involved in the mechanism of "down-regulation" of the receptor number.

INSULIN DEGRADATION

Another feature of the interaction of insulin with its target cells which might be closely related to

both receptor binding and internalization of the hormone, is the degradation of insulin. Of several potential insulin degrading enzyme systems, the glutathione-insulin-transferase[156,157] and an insulin-specific protease[158,159] have been considered of definitive physiologic importance. The association of both these enzyme complexes with lysosomal cell fractions of rat liver,[160] as well as the autoradiographically demonstrated concentration of ^{125}I-tracer at lysosomal structures after exposure of the cell to ^{125}I-insulin,[67,161] have suggested that the lysosomes are an important site of insulin degradation. Thus, at least part of the insulin degradation process appears to be secondary to its internalization. Insulin bound to liver cell surface receptors is also subject to degradation.[162] Such a hormone degradation at the cell surface could be induced by:

1. a receptor-mediated cleavage of insulin subsequent to its association to the specific receptor, or

2. the activity of cell surface proteases unrelated to the insulin receptor, or

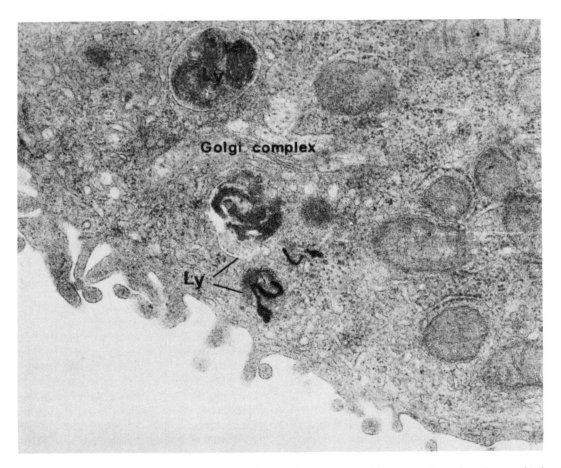

Fig. 6–10. Thin section of rat hepatocyte with developed autoradiography grains following prolonged incubation of isolated cells with 125I-insulin. "Ly" refers to lysosome-like structures in which grains have been shown to localize preferentially. (Reprinted from Gorden et al.[67] by permission of the authors and publisher.)

3. activities of enzymes leaked from the cells.

Freychet et al.[163] and Gammeltoft and Gliemann[164] observed certain basic discrepancies between characteristics of the cell surface capacities to bind insulin and to degrade the hormone, suggesting that insulin binding and degradation are unrelated. In contrast, the results of studies of Terris and Steiner[162] disclosed that a first-order relationship exists between the rates of insulin binding and its degradation by isolated hepatocytes. These observations have been confirmed by the demonstration of receptor-mediated degradation both in liver cell membranes and in isolated adipocytes.[165–167] On this basis, Steiner[149] concluded that both interactions of insulin with its receptor (i.e., its binding and its degradation) are closely related. At present, a relationship between insulin action and its subsequential degradation appears to be a plausible hypothesis. Indeed, binding to the cell surface might be the primary interaction of insulin with its target cell, followed by both the induction of metabolic actions and by the degradation of the hormone.

NET INSULIN ACTION AT THE TARGET ORGANS

Effect of Insulin on Transmembrane Transport Processes. Among the first actions of insulin at the target cell are its effects on transport processes across the cell surface membranes. These predominantly rapid effects of insulin include the modulation of transmembrane fluxes of both charged and neutral substances, i.e., hexoses, amino acids, cations and anions.[31] Of all these insulin actions, the stimulation of glucose uptake in skeletal muscle and in adipose tissue has been most extensively studied.[168]

The Hexose Transport Processes. More than 30 years ago, Levine and his colleagues[169,170] reported that the stimulation of glucose utilization in vivo was related to a stimulation of transmembrane transport of hexoses into the cell rather than an acceleration of glucose metabolism. More recently, the mechanism of action of insulin upon the flux of hexoses across cellular surface membranes has been most extensively studied in (rat) adipocytes or fat cell membranes (after preincubation of the intact cells with insulin), using non-metabolizable sugars such as 2-deoxy-glucose. While this action of insulin has been characterized as an increase in the facilitated diffusion of glucose, the molecular biology of the phenomenon remains poorly understood.

Three different hypotheses have been proposed, each supported by the results of several studies:

1. Insulin increases the number of basal glucose transport sites.

2. Insulin creates additional glucose transport sites and mechanisms which are different from the existing ones.

3. According to a third as yet purely speculative hypothesis, insulin might alter the existing glucose transport mechanisms in a way that makes them both more efficient and faster without increasing their number per cell surface area.

Most available evidence appears to indicate that the K_m of glucose uptake rates remains unaltered, whereas the V_{max} of the process can be increased severalfold by insulin.[122] This observation tends to favor the second hypothesis above. Studies by Whitesell and Gliemann,[171] Amatruda and Finch,[172] and Czech[173] indicate that these newly formed transport carriers (sites) induced by insulin vary from the basal ones in that they react differently to certain modulators, such as changes in pH or temperature and certain non-specific inhibitors. In contrast, Olefsky[174] and Ludvigsson and Jarett[175,176] suggest that, according to the first hypothesis, these new transport sites observed in intact adipocytes and in fat cell membranes, are similar or identical to the basic transport sites with regard to their susceptibility to changes in pH, their energy of activation characteristics, etc. Furthermore, it has been suggested that the effect of insulin in forming or uncovering additional transport sites depends on a stable alteration at the cell surface membrane (unaltered by the removal of specifically bound insulin) which may involve the formation of disulfide bonds.[173,177] Kinetic analyses demonstrate that the activation of glucose transport mechanisms in rat adipocytes represent an extremely rapid process, being effective within 20 to 30 seconds after exposure to insulin at physiologic temperatures. In addition to this rapid effect of insulin on hexose transport, Olefsky and Kobayashi[178] demonstrate that insulin is also an important long-term regulator of the number of glucose transport sites at the adipocyte membrane.

As to the mechanism of the rapid formation of new transport sites by insulin, several studies have indicated that its actions depend on the presence of Ca^{++} and Mg^{++} ions[176] in the environment of intact rat adipocytes. It is of note that only insulin action on glucose transport, and not the insulin binding process or other metabolic effect of insulin (such as the inhibition of lipolysis) was affected by the removal of divalent cations from the plasma membrane and from the medium.[179,180] On the other hand, several reports have indicated that the action of insulin on hexose transport may be linked to the availability of endogenous adenosine triphosphate (ATP). In fact, it has been suggested that the stimulation of glucose uptake may be connected with ATP utilization and thus, energy-requiring.[181] Wicklmayr et al.[182] have proposed that the liberation of kinins is involved in insulin action on glucose uptake into resting skeletal muscle.

More recently, studies by Suzuki and Kono[183] have offered a more detailed insight into the mechanism of the insulin-induced stimulation of glucose transport in adipocytes. Using a cell-free system prepared from rat fat cells, these authors observed that two separate glucose transport activities exist; the first is associated with the plasma cell membrane; the second is located intracellularly, possibly at the Golgi apparatus. The K_m and several other characteristics of these two transport sites have been shown to be similar if not identical. Subsequently, it was demonstrated that insulin might translocate intracellular glucose transport activities to the cell membrane, thus uncovering the total glucose-transmembrane transport activity of the cell. According to this hypothesis,[183] insulin makes glucose transport activity (which has been stored intracellularly) available by inducing its translocation to the cell membrane. These observations have been confirmed by an apparent translocation of cytochalasin-B-binding activities from intracellular to plasma membrane fractions as reported by Cushman and Wardzala.[184] This might explain the rapid increase in V_{max} for glucose transport (at unaltered K_m) induced by insulin. Furthermore, this model can easily explain the energy dependence of the process. Pending further confirmatory observations, the insulin-induced translocation of intracellularly stored glucose transport sites to the membrane represents a most attractive hypothesis for the mechanism of insulin action on hexose transmembrane transport. This hypothetically exocytotic translocation of glucose transport activity may be initiated or coupled to the endocytotic internalization of insulin or the insulin receptor complex.[183]

Possibly related to the direct stimulatory effect of insulin on glucose uptake into muscle cells, Berger et al.[184a] have described the phenomenon of a possible effect of insulin with respect to the exercise-induced augmentation of muscular glucose uptake (Fig. 6–11). In a number of studies in dia-

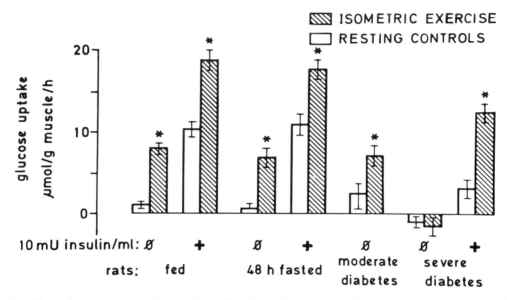

Fig. 6–11. Effects of strenuous isometric exercise and insulin on glucose uptake of isolated perfused skeletal muscle of fed and 48-hour fasted rats; moderately diabetic (blood glucose 20.9 ± 2.8 mmol/L; blood ketone bodies 1.7 ± 0.4 mmol/L); and severely diabetic (blood glucose 23.4 ± 1.5 mmol/L, blood ketone bodies 6.0 ± 0.2 mmol/L) rats. Asterisks indicate difference from resting controls is statistically significant (p < 0.05). (Adapted from Berger et al.[184a])

betic patients, this phenomenon has been shown to be of considerable clinical relevance.[184b,184c]

Electrolyte Transport Processes. Even in the early years of the therapeutic use of insulin, its effect in lowering circulating levels of potassium and phosphate was well known clinically.[185,185a] However, the effects of insulin on various electrolyte transport processes, independent of its metabolic effects, have been described in detail.[186]

Insulin increases the net inflow of K^+ into the cytoplasm of hepatocytes, adipocytes and muscle cells and of the perfused human forearm,[187] probably for the most part by inhibiting the cellular efflux of potassium ions. Even more marked effects are reported for the insulin action on sodium transport. Marked stimulation of Na^+ efflux, independent of its action on glucose transport, has been described in several tissues. In fact, the positive effect of insulin on the Na^+-K^+ ATPase activity appears to be generally accepted.[118] However, both the mechanism of action and the physiologic significance of these insulin effects on monovalent cation fluxes await clarification.

In addition, insulin has been shown to alter transmembrane potential differences, to increase the "short-circuit current" across the membrane, and to induce hyperpolarization in certain cells.[188,189] It remains unclear whether the alteration of ion fluxes is the primary event.[121,186,190] In any case, these effects of insulin occur rapidly and are thought to represent an initial primary action of insulin on the cell membranes. Zierler[186] has suggested that insulin decreases the cell membrane permeability to

sodium and potassium via the induction of structural changes within the membrane layers. At present, there is only incomplete evidence that these electrochemical phenomena of hyperpolarization do occur in vivo. Even less clearly supported is the claim that insulin stimulates the flow of water into muscle cells. Possibly, this phenomenon is caused by the increased inflow of hexoses and other metabolites under the influence of insulin. In a number of studies, insulin was shown to increase circulating Ca^{++} levels and the efflux of Ca^{++} from certain tissues.[118,121,186] More detailed information has been reported with regard to the stimulation of the influx of inorganic phosphates into various cell types under the influence of insulin. It has been suggested that this action of insulin is based on stimulation of an energy-requiring transport mechanism possibly related to the activity of the sodium/potassium pump.[143]

Amino Acid Transport Process. The stimulation of amino acid uptake by insulin due to an augmentation of the active transmembrane transport mechanism has been demonstrated in various muscle cell preparations.[191–196] These observations have, however, been limited to certain amino acids, most often alpha-amino-isobutyric acid (AIB). Insulin does stimulate the transport of some, but by no means all, amino acids.[197] In studies using the perfused rat hindquarter and the human forearm, it was shown that the new efflux of amino acids was substantially inhibited by insulin.[198,199] More detailed studies of transmembrane amino acid influx into the cells have been complicated by the complexity of the various transport systems and hypothetical carriers of differing specificity. On the other hand, the intracellular amino acid pool is influenced by a great many factors, so that the actual measurement of amino acid influx rates becomes quite difficult. Thus, results of detailed studies relating amino acid transport rates as stimulated by insulin to intracellular protein metabolism are, at present, not available.

INTRACELLULAR EFFECTS OF INSULIN

In addition to the various biologic actions of insulin on transmembrane transport processes, a number of intracellular effects of insulin have been characterized that cannot be ascribed to the stimulation of rates of substrate uptake into the target cells. These intracellular effects include: the stimulation of lipid, glycogen and protein synthesis; the inhibition of lipolysis and proteolysis; and the nuclear transcription of RNA, as well as the replication of DNA, etc. It is beyond the scope of this chapter to describe all of these in detail. Only a few examples and their respective mechanisms will be mentioned.

In general, the mechanisms of these intracellular effects of insulin seem to involve the alteration of cytosolic and mitochondrial enzyme activities. Whereas many of these activities have been reported to change under the influence of insulin, *direct* actions of insulin on these events have rarely been proven. In most cases, insulin appears to alter the activity of these enzyme complexes via hypothetical second messengers or via changes in ambient or intracellular metabolite and substrate concentrations. Most detailed information is available with respect to insulin action on the enzymatic systems involved in glycogen metabolism. This complicated system[120,200] is subject to regulatory influences of insulin at several points. In fact, the stimulatory action of insulin on glycogen synthesis in various tissues was among the first metabolic actions of the hormone studied in detail. Interestingly, this effect of insulin is independent of its action on glucose transport into the cell and unrelated to levels of glucose phosphate in tissue.[201,202] This suggests a direct effect of insulin on intracellular (cytosolic) hormone activities.

In subsequent in vitro studies it was shown that insulin:

1. activated the glycogen synthase activity, the rate-limiting enzyme in the pathway from glucose-6-phosphate to glycogen,[144,203] and
2. inactivated glycogen phosphorylase activity.

As in other biologic systems, it was found that two synthase forms of different activity exist and that insulin shifted to the steady state between these two forms toward the metabolically active form, thus increasing the total glycogen-synthase activity of the cytosol.[120] For some time a fall in cyclic AMP levels was believed to be the messenger of insulin in order to induce changes in glycogen synthase activity (see above). Subsequently, a clearcut diversity of changes in cyclic AMP levels and glycogen-synthase levels was described for many tissues.[120]

The mechanism by which insulin affects the glycogen synthase and glycogen phosphorylase activities remains unresolved. However, it continues to be an attractive hypothesis that insulin might affect the phosphoenzyme systems, the phosphatases, and the kinases, in order to induce activity or inactivation of the enzymatic systems involved in glycogen breakdown and glycogen synthesis (see above). Again, it is unknown whether these effects of insulin are due to alterations in metabolite, substrate or hypothetical second messenger concentrations at the site of the hormones or to direct hormone action. However, via the regulation of phosphorolysis-dephosphorolysis cycles and apart from glycogen synthase and phosphorylase, insulin might modify a whole host of enzyme activities and complexes (e.g., acetyl CoA carboxylase, glycerol-3-phosphateacyl-transferase, HMG-CoA reductase, the hormone sensitive lipase, cholesterol esterase, tyrosine hydrolase and pyruvate dehydrogenase, etc.).[120] In addition, insulin may also increase enzyme activities by stimulation of de novo enzyme protein synthesis, as has been suggested for the activation of hexokinase II.[196,204]

Direct or indirect actions of insulin on intracellularly located enzyme systems might also be involved in its stimulatory effect on protein synthesis since the insulin-induced acceleration of protein synthesis[193] is not necessarily dependent on the stimulation of transmembrane amino acid transport processes and the subsequent formation of aminoacyl-tRNA.[205] In contrast, insulin appears to activate protein synthesis in muscle at various intracellular enzymatic levels, depending on the nature of the muscle investigated.[206] In perfused heart and skeletal muscle, insulin appears to stimulate peptide-chain initiation. The reduction of protein synthesis in mixed skeletal muscle tissue of insulin-deficient rats is associated with a reduced number of ribosomes and a decrease in their translational efficiency.[206] Nevertheless, in various muscular tissues such as the heart and red fiber type muscles, processes of peptide-chain initiation are maintained in diabetes. This is probably due to the ''insulin-like'' effects of fatty acids and other non-carbohydrate substrates on certain steps of protein synthesis. In contrast, the reversible decrease of albumin and possibly other hepatic protein synthesis in the liver of insulin-deficient rats, appear to be mediated by a decreased availability of translatable mRNA.[206,207] According to Jefferson,[206,207] the insulin-induced stimulation of peptide-chain initiation in muscle might involve an inhibition of a protein-kinase system, similar to the mechanism of the action of insulin on glycogen synthase.

Insulin-induced inhibition of proteolysis—an effect which might likewise involve a direct or indirect inhibition of lysosomal proteases[208]—remains at present incompletely understood.[206] It has been suggested recently that the underlying mechanism involves a phosphorylation-dephosphorylation cycle.[196] A stimulatory effect of insulin on the biosynthesis of various nucleic acids, such as RNA, has been shown in the isolated rat diaphragm.[209] It remains unclear, however, whether the increased formation of RNA in muscle in vitro that is due to insulin is a consequence of de novo synthesis of mRNA or of an accelerated translation of preformed mRNA. Volfin and Hanoue[210] and Peterson[196] have recently reviewed the various actions of insulin on the metabolism of nucleic acids.

As a last example of intracellular insulin effects, the inhibition of lipolysis[211] will be briefly discussed. The decrease of triglyceride hydrolysis in adipose tissue by physiologic amounts of insulin has been demonstrated in numerous systems in vivo and in vitro.[211-214] In fact, the regulation of fat depot mobilization by insulin is of major importance for the overall energy metabolism of the organism. Again the underlying mechanism—i.e., the inhibition of the hormone-sensitive triglyceride lipase of adipocytes by insulin—might be mediated by phosphorolysis-dephosphorolysis cycles. Quite in contrast, insulin has been shown to stimulate the lipoprotein lipase which regulates the cleavage and thus the uptake of triglycerides from the circulation into adipose tissue.[214] The enzyme is probably synthesized in adipocytes and is subsequently transferred to the inner surface of adipose tissue capillaries. The lipoprotein lipase activity of fatty fibroblasts can be stimulated by insulin in vitro; this effect is sustained and it occurs only after 4 hours of incubation.[215]

Additional effects of insulin on the metabolism of adipose tissue include the stimulation of fatty acid synthesis and the fatty acid reesterfication process.[214] Direct action of insulin unrelated to transport processes might, at least in part, be involved in the mechanism of these insulin effects on adipocytes.

These and many other effects of insulin may involve the interaction of insulin with intracellular enzyme systems. As opposed to the rapid effects of insulin on transport processes, these generally slower effects of insulin seem to be mediated by a postreceptor information transfer system which might be a second messenger, an insulin-degradation product, the insulin-receptor complex, insulin itself or a hypothetical group of substances, such as the "insulin mediator" proposed by Larner et al.[144]

ADDITIONAL EFFECTS OF INSULIN

Insulin as Growth Factor. The overall anabolic effect of insulin as presented by von Mehring and Minkowski[216] has in recent years been characterized in more detail. Insulin induces both a stimulation of protein synthesis and a restriction of proteolysis. The mechanism of these effects of insulin involves almost every step in protein metabolism,[206] including the possibility that insulin might be instrumental in modifying gene expression. Possibly in addition to these protein-anabolic effects, insulin appears to have growth-promoting activities, which include the stimulation of DNA and RNA synthesis, bone collagen synthesis and sulfur incorporation into cartilage. In a series of recent studies, these growth-promoting activities of insulin have been investigated in tissue cultures by comparing them to the effect of a group of polypeptides which have been summarized as insulin-like growth factors[8] or somatomedins. This group includes substances such as the two insulin-like growth factors, IGF I and IGF II, somatomedin A, somatomedin C, the multiplication-stimulating activity (MSA) and possibly others. IGF I and IGF II have been characterized as components of NSILAs: they share many homologous amino acid sequences with insulin but they differ in their dependence on growth hormone levels.[217]

The common denominator of all these various insulin-like growth factors or somatomedins is their promotion of cellular growth processes, namely the initial phases and the maintenance phase of the fully differentiated state. The effect of somatomedin on the maturation and specialization phases of cell growth remains at present disputed. In addition, all somatomedins have been shown to exert the full spectrum of the acute metabolic effects of insulin, such as stimulation of transport processes, antilipolysis, etc. On the other hand, insulin has been reported to be active as a maintenance growth factor, whereas its potency as a mitotic factor is at present uncertain.[2] In general, insulin is substantially more potent with respect to these acute metabolic effects while the insulin-like growth factors are more potent concerning the chronic growth effects.[218,219] As for insulin, specific cell surface receptors have been described for various insulin-like growth factors. Furthermore, it has been shown that cross-affinity exists between insulin and somatomedins and their respective receptors. King et al.[220] have presented evidence that acute metabolic effects of both insulin and the somatomedins are mediated by the insulin receptor, and that the higher affinity of insulin to this receptor correlates with the higher biologic potency of insulin. The growth-promoting effects of both the insulin-like growth factors and insulin appear to be mediated by the growth factor receptor. At this receptor, both the affinity and the biologic effect of somatomedins were superior to similar functions of insulin.

According to a hypothesis put forward by Froesch et al.[221,222] insulin and certain insulin-like growth factors which may be related by evolutionary links,[217] act in vivo in a complementary fashion on anabolic growth processes (Fig. 6–12). Insulin acts predominantly by stimulating glucose, fat and protein storage via interaction with its receptors in liver, muscle, heart and adipocytes. On the other hand, the insulin-like growth factor(s) promote the growth of fibroblasts, chondrocytes, etc., via interaction with their specific receptors. Whether the cross-affinity shown in vitro is a physiologically relevant mechanism in fostering anabolic reactions (such as acromegaloid growth associated with certain cases of hyperinsulinemia),[223] or whether it is merely a phylogenetic atavism, remains to be elucidated by further studies.

Insulin Effect on the Immune Response. Clinically diabetes mellitus is related to increased susceptibility to infectious disease and possibly to autoimmune reactions. This association has been interpreted repeatedly as a possible sign of altered immune response in diabetic patients and/or as an indication that insulin affects the immune system.

Recently, a number of studies have concentrated upon the various immunologic functions in relationship to insulin and insulin-deficient states.[224] Several cellular immune responses have been found to be diminished in insulin-dependent diabetes. In particular, several T-lymphocyte functions, such as the generation of cytotoxic cells after activation[225] and the immune responses to allografts,[226,227] appear to be disturbed in association with insulin deficiency.

Strom et al.[228] have demonstrated that insulin increases the capacity of cytotoxins to destroy their target cells. It is of note that resting T-lymphocytes appear to be both insensitive to insulin and free of insulin receptors. It is only after activation (e.g., by an allograft, by mitogenic stimulation, etc.) that the T-lymphocytes display insulin-binding sites.[224,229] The mechanism by which the activation of the resting T-lymphocytes generates both specific insulin receptors at the cell surface and the cytotoxic functions of the activated cells (which in turn can be stimulated by insulin), remains to be elucidated. It appears at present plausible, however, that the presence of adequate amounts of insulin is necessary for the optimal function of effector T-lymphocytes. This receptor-mediated interaction of insulin with the activated T-lymphocytes might well be necessary to ensure a normal immune response. On the other hand, it might, in part, be on the basis of this mechanism that the patient with poorly controlled diabetes is prone to develop infectious diseases.

Various Other Effects of Insulin. A number of

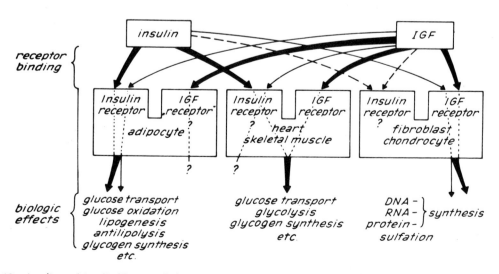

Fig. 6–12. Insulin and insulin-like growth factors (IGF) appear to have evolved from a common precursor. According to the hypothesis presented in this figure, the two hormones have a complementary anabolic action that is mediated by the insulin and/or IGF receptors according to the various tissues. (Reprinted from Froesch et al.[221] by permission of the authors and publisher.)

postulated insulin effects on various functions of the gastrointestinal tract, such as the influence on gastric secretion and motility, have subsequently been shown to be secondary to insulin-induced hypoglycemia.[230] It has been suggested repeatedly that insulin plays an important role in the development of exocrine pancreatic tissue. Such a hypothetical action of insulin might explain the apparent fibrosis of acinar pancreatic tissue and the decrease in amylase secretion rates associated with insulin deficiency.[230] Possibly related to the capacity of insulin as a growth-promoting factor (see above), it has been demonstrated to accelerate wound healing processes. On the other hand, this effect of insulin could be due to its stimulation of glucose uptake by skin tissues.[231]

Insulin appears to be of specific importance in the development and the functioning of the lactating mammary gland, probably due to its stimulatory actions on cell growth, protein synthesis, and membrane transport processes. Conflicting results have been reported with respect to the effect of insulin on the growth of malignant tumor cells, probably associated with differences in the organ from which the cells were obtained.[230]

SUMMARY

Rapid advances in methodology over the past 2 decades have resulted in considerable progress in our understanding of the mechanism of the metabolic actions of insulin. It has been possible to characterize partially the interaction of insulin with its target cell in relation to the biologic effects of the hormone. Thus, the binding of the insulin molecule to specific receptor structures at the cell surface, appears to represent a prerequisite for any insulin effect. In no experimental system can insulin exert any effect unless intact plasma membranes or certain membrane fractions are present. Furthermore, insulin actions—even intracellular "late" effects of this hormone[150]—can be abolished by the binding of insulin receptor antibodies to the cell surface insulin receptor. Thus, the interaction of insulin with its receptor (which is as yet only incompletely characterized chemically) initiates the subsequent actions of the hormone. These actions can be differentiated roughly as rapid effects on transmembrane transport processes and as generally somewhat slower intracellular effects of insulin.

The sensitivity of the various cell reactions to insulin can, in part, be regulated at the receptor level; high ambient insulin levels induce a "down-regulation" of receptors associated with a decrease in insulin sensitivity. In other cases, decreased insulin responsiveness of the cells is not related to a disturbance of the insulin-receptor interaction, but

rather a consequence of an intracellular postreceptor defect of glucose metabolism. The formation of the insulin receptor complex may be followed by its internalization and the subsequent degradation of insulin. The physiologic significance of these phenomena is at present unclear. The signals initiated by the insulin receptor interaction, to both the transmembrane transport processes and the intracellular sites of insulin action remain hypothetical. Clearly, some second messengers or insulin mediators and the activity of phosphorylation-dephosphorylation cycles, i.e., protein kinase phosphorylase oscillations, are involved in some of these processes.

Various states of decreased insulin sensitivity and/or insulin resistance have been found to be associated with pathologic insulin receptor interactions or with postreceptor defects. In certain cases, these discoveries have been helpful in the formulation of appropriate and rational therapeutic approaches. Because of the many aspects of insulin action on different metabolic pathways and fluxes in various organs of the body, future research will discover additional mechanisms of action rather than provide a uniform concept for the functional interaction of insulin with its target cells.

REFERENCES

1. Soeldner, J.S.: Insulin in diabetes—applied physiology. In: A. Marble, P. White, R.F. Bradley, L.P. Krall (Eds.): Joslin's Diabetes Mellitus, 11th Ed. Philadelphia, Lea & Febiger. 1971, pp 99-138.
2. Hall, K., Sara, V., Enberg, G., Fryklund, L: Somatomedins. In: W.K. Waldhäusl (Ed.): Diabetes 1979. Internat. Cong. Series No. 500. Amsterdam, Excerpta Medica, 1980, pp. 249–253.
3. Vallance-Owen, J., Lilley, M.D.: An insulin antagonist associated with plasma-albumin. Lancet 1:804, 1961.
4. Froesch, E.R., Schlumpf, U., Heimann, R., et al.: Purification procedures for NSILA-s. Adv. Metab. Disorders 8:203, 1975.
5. Froesch, E.R., Zapf, J., Meuli, C., et al.: Biological properties of NSILA-s. Adv. Metab. Disorders 8:211, 1975.
6. Froesch, E.R., Schlumpf, U., Heimann, R., et al.: Physiologic and pharmacologic significance as an insulinlike hormone and as a growth-promoting hormone. Adv. Metab. Disord. 8:237, 1975.
7. Poffenbarger, P.L.: Nonsuppressible insulin-like proteins in health and disease. In: M.P. Cohen and F.P. Foa (Eds.): Special Topics in Endocrinology and Metabolism. New York, Allen R. Liss. 1979, pp. 110–140.
8. Cüppers, H.J., Poffenbarger, P.L., Berger, M., et al.: Hormonal and metabolic studies in four patients with fibrosarcoma-associated hypoglycemia: elevation of plasma NSILP concentrations. In: D. Andreani, P.J. Lefebvre, V. Marks (Eds.): Current Views on Hypoglycemia and Glucagon. London, Academic Press. 1980, pp. 173–181.
9. Gorden, P., Hendricks, C.M., Roth, J.: Circulating proinsulin-like component in man: increased proportion in hypoinsulinemic states. Diabetologia 10:469, 1974.
10. Heding, L.G.: Specific and direct radioimmunoassay for human proinsulin in serum. Diabetologia 13:467, 1977.

11. Yalow, R.S., Berson, S.A.: Assay of plasma insulin in human subjects by immunological methods. Nature *184*:1648, 1959.

12. Izzo, J.L.: Pharmacokinetics of insulin. In: A. Hasselblatt, F.R. von Bruchhausen (Eds.): Handbook of Experimental Pharmacology. Insulin Part 2, Vol. 32. Berlin, Springer-Verlag. 1975, pp. 195–248.

13. Halban, P.A., Berger, M., Offord, R.E.: Distribution and metabolism of intravenously injected tritiated insulin in rats. Metabolism *28*:1097, 1979.

14. Sönksen, P.H., Tompkins, C.V., Srivastava, M.C., Nabarro, J.D.N.: A comparative study on the metabolism of human insulin and porcine proinsulin in man. Clin. Sci. Mol. Med. *45*:633, 1973.

15. Stein, O., Gross, J.: The localization and metabolism of I^{131} insulin in the muscle and some other tissues of the rat. Endocrinology *65*:707, 1959.

16. Navalesi, R., Pilo, A., Ferrannini, E.: Kinetic analysis of plasma insulin disappearance in nonketotic diabetic patients and in normal subjects. A tracer study with I^{125} insulin. J. Clin. Invest. *61*:197, 1978.

17. Berger, M., Halban, P.A., Müller, W.A., et al.: Mobilization of subcutaneously injected tritiated insulin in rats. Diabetologia *15*:133, 1978.

18. Berger, M., Halban, P.A., Assal, J-P.: Pharmacokinetics of subcutaneously injected tritiated insulin: effects of exercise. Diabetes *28* (Suppl. 1):53, 1979.

19. Halban, P.A., Berger, M., Gjinavci, A.: Pharmacokinetics of subcutaneously injected semisynthetic tritiated insulin in rats. In: R.E. Offord and C. diBello (Eds.): Semisynthetic Peptides and Proteins. London, Academic Press. 1978, pp. 237–246.

20. O'Brien, J.P., Sharpe, A.R., Jr.: The influence of renal disease on the insulin I^{131} disappearance curve in man. Metabolism *16*:76, 1976.

21. Bajaj, J.S., Bansal, D.D.: Insulin degradation. In: J.S. Bajaj (Ed.): Insulin and Metabolism. Amsterdam. Elsevier/North Holland, Excerpta Medica, 1977, pp. 52–72.

22. Waddell, W.R., Sussman, K.E.: Plasma insulin after diversion of portal and pancreatic venous blood to vena cava. J. Appl. Physiol. *22*:808, 1967.

23. Paulsen, E.P., Courtney, J.W. III, Duckworth, W.C.: Insulin resistance caused by massive degradation of subcutaneous insulin. Diabetes *28*:640, 1979.

24. Berger, M., Cüppers, H.J., Halban, P.A., Offord, R.E.: The effect of aprotinin on the absorption of subcutaneously injected regular insulin in normal subjects. Diabetes *29*:81, 1980.

25. Müller, W.A., Taillens, C., Lereret, S., et al.: Resistance against subcutaneous insulin successfully managed with aprotinin. Lancet *1*:1245, 1980.

25a.Kahn, C.R.: The insulin receptor and insulin: the lock and key to diabetes. Clin. Res. *31*:326, 1983.

26. Baxter, J.D., Funder, J.W.: Hormone receptors. N. Engl. J. Med. *301*:1149, 1979.

27. Stadie, W.C., Haugaard, N., Vaughan, M.: The quantitative relation between insulin and its biological activity. J. Biol. Chem. *200*:745, 1953.

28. Fong, C.T.O., Silver, L., Popenoe, E.A., Debons, A.F.: Some observations on insulin-receptor interaction. Biochim. Biophys. Acta *56*:190, 1962.

29. Garratt, C.J., Cameron, J.S., Menzinger, G.: The association of I^{131}-iodo-insulin with rat diaphragm muscle and its effect on glucose uptake. Biochim. Biophys. Acta *115*:179, 1966.

30. Stadie, W.C., Haugaard, N., Marsh, J.B., Hills, A.G.: The chemical combination of insulin with muscle (diaphragm) of normal rat. Am. J. Med. Sci. *218*:265, 1949.

31. Pilkis, S.J., Park, C.R.: Mechanism of action of insulin. Ann. Rev. Pharmacol. *14*:365, 1974.

32. Pastan, I., Roth, J., Macchia, V.: Binding of hormone to tissue: the first step in polypeptide hormone action. Proc. Natl. Acad. Sci. USA *56*:1802, 1966.

33. Cuatrecasas, P.: Interaction of insulin with the cell membrane: the primary action of insulin. Proc. Natl. Acad. Sci. USA *63*:450, 1969.

34. Butcher, R.W., Crofford, O.B., Gammeltoft, S., et al.: Insulin activity: the solid matrix. Science *182*:396, 1973.

35. Bergeron, J.J.M., Levine, G., Sikstrom, R., et al.: Polypeptide hormone binding sites *in vivo*: initial localization of ^{125}I-labelled insulin to hepatocyte plasmalemma as visualized by electron microscope radioautography. Proc. Natl. Acad. Sci. USA *74*:5051, 1977.

36. Jarett, L., Smith, R.M.: Electron microscopic demonstration of insulin receptors on adipocyte plasma membranes utilizing a ferritin-insulin conjugate. J. Biol. Chem. *249*:7024, 1974.

37. Jarett, L., Smith, R.M.: Ultrastructural localization of insulin receptors on adipocytes. Proc. Natl. Acad. Sci. USA *72*:3526, 1975.

38. Jarett, L., Smith, R.M.: The natural occurrence of insulin receptors in groups on adipocyte plasma membranes as demonstrated with monomeric ferritin-insulin. J. Supramol. Struct. *6*:45, 1977.

39. Orci, L., Rufener, C., Malaisse-Lagae, F., et al.: A morphological approach to surface receptors in islets and liver cells. Isr. J. Med. Sci. *11*:639, 1975.

40. Freychet, P., Roth, J., Neville, D.M., Jr: Monoiodoinsulin: demonstration of its biological activity and binding to fat cells and liver membranes. Biochem. Biophys. Res. Commun. *43*:400, 1971.

41. Freychet, P., Roth, J., Neville, D.M., Jr.: Insulin receptors in the liver: specific binding of [^{125}I] insulin to the plasma membrane and its relation to insulin bioactivity. Proc. Natl. Acad. Sci. USA *68*:1833, 1971.

42. Halban, P.A., Offord, R.E.: The preparation of a semisynthetic tritiated insulin with a specific radioactivity of up to 20 curies per millimole. Biochem. J. *151*:219, 1975.

43. Kahn, C.R.: Membrane receptors for hormones and neurotransmitters. J. Cell. Biol. *70*:261, 1976.

44. Olefsky, J.M., Ciaraldi, T.P.: The insulin receptor: basic characteristics and its role in insulin resistant states. In: M. Brownlee (Ed.): Handbook of Diabetes. Vol. II. Islet Cell Function/Insulin Action. New York, Garland Press. 1980, pp. 73–116.

45. Roth, J., Kahn, C.R., Lesniak, M.A., et al.: Receptors for insulin, NSILA-s, and growth hormone: applications to disease states in man. Rec. Prog. Horm. Res. *31*:95, 1975.

46. Muggeo, M., Ginsberg, B.H., Roth, J., et al.: The insulin receptor in vertebrates is functionally more conserved during evolution than insulin itself. Endocrinology *104*:1393, 1979.

47. DeMeyts, P.: Cooperative properties of hormone receptors in cell membranes. J. Supramo. Struct. *4*:241, 1976.

48. Olefsky, J.M., Chang, H.: Insulin binding to adipocytes. Evidence for functionally distinct receptors. Diabetes *27*:946, 1978.

49. Maturo, J.M. III, Hollenberg, M.D.: Insulin receptor: interaction with non-receptor glycoprotein from liver cell membranes. Proc. Natl. Acad. Sci. USA *75*:3070, 1978.

50. Krupp, M.N., Livingston, J.N.: Insulin binding to solubilized material from fat cell membranes: evidence for two binding species. Proc. Natl. Acad. Sci. USA *75*:2593, 1978.

51. Pollet, R.J., Standaert, M.L., Haase, B.A.: Insulin bind-

ing to the human lymphocyte receptor. J. Biol. Chem. *252*:5828, 1977.

52. Goldfine, I.D.: Insulin receptors and the site of action of insulin. Life Sciences *23*:2639, 1978.

53. Kono, T., and Barham, F.W.: The relationship between the insulin-binding capacity of fat cells and the cellular response to insulin. J. Biol. Chem. *246*:6210, 1971.

54. Olefsky, J.M.: The effects of spontaneous obesity on insulin binding, glucose transport, and glucose oxidation by isolated rat adipocytes. J. Clin. Invest. *57*:842, 1976.

54a. Olefsky, J.M.: Insulin resistance and insulin action. An *in vitro* and *in vivo* perspective. Diabetes *30*:148, 1981.

55. Olefsky, J.M.: The insulin receptor: its role in insulin resistance of obesity and diabetes. Diabetes *25*:1154, 1976.

56. Olefsky, J.M., Johnson, J., Liu, F., et al.: The effects of acute and chronic dexamethasone administration on insulin binding to isolated rat hepatocytes and adipocytes. Metabolism *24*:517, 1975.

57. Gliemann, J., Gammeltoft, S., Vinten, J.: Time course of insulin-receptor binding and insulin-induced lipogenesis in isolated rat fat cells. J. Biol. Chem. *250*:3368, 1975.

58. Kahn, C.R.: Role of insulin receptors in insulin-resistant states. Metabolism *29*:455, 1980.

59. Olefsky, J.M.: Effect of dexamethasone on insulin binding, glucose transport, and glucose oxidation of isolated rat adipocytes. J. Clin. Invest. *56*:1499, 1975.

60. Catt, K.J., Dufau, M.L.: Peptide hormone receptors. Ann. Rev. Physiol. *39*:529, 1977.

61. Cuatrecasas, P.: Membrane receptors. Ann. Rev. Biochem. *43*:169, 1974.

62. Jacobs, S., Schechter, Y., Bissell, K., Cuatrecasas, P.: Purification and properties of insulin receptors from rat liver membranes. Biochem. Biophys. Res. Commun. *77*:981, 1977.

63. Lang, U., Kahn, C.R., Chrambach, A.: Characterization of the insulin receptor and insulin-degrading activity from human lymphocytes by quantitative polyacrylamide gel electrophoresis. Endocrinology *106*:40, 1980.

64. Ginsberg, D.H., Kahn, C.R., Roth, J., DeMeyts, P.: Insulin-induced dissociation of its receptor into subunits: possible molecular concomitant of negative cooperativity. Biochem. Biophys. Res. Commun. *73*:1068, 1976.

64a. Kasuga, M., Karlsson, F.A., Kahn, R.C.: Insulin stimulates the phosphorylation of the 95,000-Dalton subunit of its own receptor. Science *215*:185, 1982.

65. Schlessinger, J., Schechter, Y., Cuatrecasas, P., et al.: Quantitative determination of the lateral diffusion coefficients of the hormone-receptor complexes of insulin and epidermal growth factor on the plasma membrane of cultured fibroblasts. Proc. Natl. Acad. Sci. USA *75*:5353, 1978.

66. Kahn, C.R., Baird, K.L., Jarrett, D.B., Flier, J.S.: Direct demonstration that receptor cross-linking or aggregation is important in insulin action. Proc. Natl. Acad. Sci. USA *75*:4209, 1978.

67. Gorden, P., Carpentier, J-L., Freychet, P., Orci, L.: Internalization of polypeptide hormones. Mechanism, intracellular localization and significance. Diabetologia *18*:263, 1980.

68. Pezzino, V., Vigneri, R., Pliam, N.B., Goldfine, I.D.: Rapid regulation of plasma membrane insulin receptors. Diabetologia *19*:211, 1980.

69. Bar, R.S., Gorden, P., Roth, J., et al.: Fluctuations in the affinity and concentration of insulin receptors on circulating monocytes of obese patients. Effects of starvation, refeeding and dieting. J. Clin;. Invest. *58*:1123, 1976.

70. Kolterman, O.G., Saekow, M., Olefsky, J.M.: The effects of acute and chronic starvation on insulin binding to isolated human adipocytes. J. Clin. Endocrin. Metab. *48*:836, 1979.

71. Beck-Nielsen, H., Pedersen, O.: Diurnal variations in insulin binding to human monocytes. J. Clin. Endocrinol. Metab. *47*:385, 1979.

72. Insel, J.R., Kolterman, O.G., Saekow, M., Olefsky, J.M.: Short-term regulation of insulin receptor affinity in man. Diabetes *29*:132, 1980.

73. Bar, R.S., Gorden, P., Roth, J., Siebert, C.W.: Insulin receptors in patients with insulinomas: changes in receptor affinity and concentration. J. Clin. Endocrin. Metab. *44*:1210, 1977.

74. Gavin, J.R. III, Roth, J., Neville, D.M., Jr., et al.: Insulin-dependent regulation of insulin receptor concentrations: a direct demonstration in cell culture. Proc. Natl. Acad. Sci. USA *71*:84, 1974.

75. Marshall, S., Olefsky, J.M.: Effects of insulin incubation on insulin binding, glucose transport, and insulin degradation by isolated rat adipocytes. Evidence for hormone-induced desensitization at the receptor and post-receptor level. J. Clin. Invest. *66*:763, 1980.

76. Hepp, K.D.: Studies on the mechanism of insulin action: basic concepts and clinical implications. Diabetologia *13*:177, 1977.

77. Wachslicht-Rodbard, H., Gross, H.A., Rodbard, D., et al.: Increased insulin binding to erythrocytes in anorexia nervosa. Restoration to normal with refeeding. N. Engl. J. Med. *300*:882, 1979.

78. Misbin, R.I., Pulkkinen, A.J., Lofton, S.A., Merimee, T.J.: Ketoacids and the insulin receptor. Diabetes *27*:539, 1978.

79. Muggeo, M., Bar, R.S., Roth, J., et al.: The insulin resistance of acromegaly: evidence for two alterations in the insulin receptor on circulating monocytes. J. Clin. Endocrinol. Metab. *48*:17, 1979.

80. Kahn, C.R., Goldfine, I.D., Neville, D.M., Jr., DeMeyts, P.: Alterations in insulin binding induced by changes *in vivo* in the levels of glucocorticoids and growth hormone. Endocrinology *103*:1054, 1978.

80a. Bachmann, W., Böttger, I., Haslbeck, M., Mehnert, H.: Extrapancreatic action of sulphonylureas: effect of gliquidone on insulin and glucagon binding to rat liver plasma membranes. Eur. J. Clin. Invest. *9*:411, 1979.

80b. Holle, A., Mangels, A., Dreyer, M., et al.: Biguanide treatment increases the number of insulin-receptor sites on human erythrocytes. N. Engl. J. Med. *305*:563, 1981.

81. Ip, C., Tepperman, H.M., Holohan, R., Tepperman, J.: Insulin binding and insulin response of adipocytes from rats adapted to fat feeding. J. Lipid Res. *17*:588, 1976.

82. Olefsky, J.M., Saekow, M.: The effects of dietary carbohydrate content on insulin binding and glucose metabolism by isolated rat adipocytes. Endocrinology *103*:2252, 1978.

83. Muggeo, M., Bar, R.S., Roth, J.: Change in affinity of insulin receptors following oral glucose in normal adults. J. Clin. Endocrinol. Metab. *44*:1206, 1977.

84. Pederson, O., Beck-Nielsen, H., Heding, L.G.: Increased insulin receptors after exercise in patients with insulin-dependent diabetes mellitus. N. Engl. J. Med. *302*:886, 1980.

85. Berger, M., Berchtold, P.: Effect of exercise in obese diabetics. In: P. Björntorp, M. Cairella, A.N. Howard (Eds.): Recent Advances in Obesity Research. III. London, F. Libbey, 1981, pp. 341–342.

86. Helderman, J.H., Raskin, P.: The T lymphocyte insulin receptor in diabetes and obesity: an intrinsic binding defect. Diabetes *29*:551, 1980.

87. Olefsky, J.M., Reaven, G.M.: Insulin binding in diabetes. Relationship with plasma insulin levels and insulin sensitivity. Diabetes 26:680, 1977.

88. Soll, A.H., Kahn, C.R., Neville, D.M., Jr., Roth, J.: Insulin receptor deficiency in genetic and acquired obesity. J. Clin. Invest. 56:769, 1975.

89. Kahn, C.R., Neville, D.M., Jr., Roth J.: Insulin-receptor interaction in the obese-hyperglycemic mouse. A model of insulin resistance. J. Biol. Chem. 248:244, 1973.

90. Harrison, L.C., Martin, F.T.R., Melick, R.A.: Correlation between insulin receptor binding in isolated fat cells and insulin sensitivity in obese human subjects. J. Clin. Invest. 58:1435, 1976.

91. DeFronzo, R.A., Soman, V., Sherwin, R.S., et al.: Insulin binding to monocytes and insulin action in human obesity, starvation and refeeding. J. Clin. Invest. 62:204, 1978.

92. Beck-Nielsen, H.: The pathogenic role of an insulin-receptor defect in diabetes mellitus of the obese. Diabetes 27:1175, 1978.

93. Archer, J.A., Gorden, P., Roth, J.: Defect in insulin binding to receptors in obese man. Amelioration with caloric restriction. J. Clin. Invest. 55:166, 1975.

94. Wigand, J.P., Blackard, W.G.: Down-regulation of insulin receptors in obese man. Diabetes 28:287, 1979.

95. Misbin, R.I., O'Leary, J.P., Pulkkinen, A.: Insulin receptor binding in obesity: a reassessment. Science 205:1003, 1979.

96. Amatruda, J.M., Livingston, J.N., Lockwood, D.H.: Insulin receptor: role in the resistance of human obesity to insulin. Science 188:264, 1975.

97. DePirro, R., Fusco, A., Lauro, R., et al.: Erythrocyte insulin receptors in non-insulin-dependent diabetes mellitus. Diabetes 29:96, 1980.

98. Robinson, T.J., Archer, J.A., Gambhir, K.K., et al.: Erythrocytes: a new cell type for the evaluation of insulin receptor defects in diabetic humans. Science 205:200, 1979.

99. Olefsky, J.M., Reaven, G.M.: Decreased insulin binding to lymphocytes from diabetic subjects. J. Clin. Invest. 54:1323, 1974.

100. Olefsky, J.M., Reaven, G.M.: Effects of sulfonylurea therapy on insulin binding to mononuclear leukocytes of diabetic patients. Am. J. Med. 60:89, 1976.

101. DeFronzo, R.A.: Pathogenesis of glucose intolerance in uremia. Metabolism 27:1866, 1978.

101a. DePirro, R., Lauro, R., Testa, I., et al.: Decreased insulin receptors but normal glucose metabolism in Duchenne muscular dystrophy. Science 216:311, 1982.

102. Beck-Nielsen, H., Pedersen, O., Lindskov, H.O.: Normalization of the insulin sensitivity and the cellular insulin binding during treatment of obese diabetics for one year. Acta Endocr. 90:103, 1979.

103. Beck-Nielsen, H., Pedersen, O., Sørensen, N.S.: Effects of dietary changes on cellular insulin binding and in vivo insulin sensitivity. Metabolism 29:482, 1980.

104. Flier, J.S., Kahn, C.R., Roth, J., Bar, R.S.: Antibodies that impair insulin receptor binding in an unusual diabetic syndrome with severe insulin resistance. Science 190:63, 1975.

105. Flier, J.S., Kahn, C.R., Jarrett, D.B., Roth, J.: Characterization of antibodies to the insulin receptor: a cause of insulin-resistant diabetes in man. J. Clin. Invest. 58:1442, 1976.

106. Flier, J.S., Kahn, C.R., Roth, J.: Receptors, antireceptor antibodies and mechanisms of insulin resistance. N. Engl. J. Med. 300:413, 1979.

107. Bar, R.S., Muggeo, M., Kahn, C.R., et al.: Characterization of insulin receptors in patients with the syndromes of insulin resistance and acanthosis nigricans. Diabetologia 18:209, 1980.

108. Oseid, S., Beck-Nielsen, H., Pedersen, O., Søvik, O.: Decreased binding of insulin to its receptor in patients with congenital generalized lipodystrophy. N. Engl. J. Med. 296:245, 1977.

108a. Bar, R.S., Levis, W.R., Rechler, M.M., et al.: Extreme insulin resistance in ataxia telangiectasia. Defect in affinity of insulin receptors. N. Engl. J. Med. 298:1164, 1978.

109. Czech, M.P.: Cellular basis of insulin insensitivity in large rat adipocytes. J. Clin. Invest. 57:1523, 1976.

110. Kemmer, F.W., Berger, M., Herberg, L., et al.: Glucose metabolism in perfused skeletal muscle. Demonstration of insulin resistance in the obese Zucker rat. Biochem. J. 178:733, 1979.

111. LeMarchand-Brustel, Y., Jeanrenaud, B., Freychet, P.: Insulin binding and effects in isolated soleus muscle of lean and obese mice. Am. J. Physiol. 234:E348, 1978.

112. Crettaz, M., Prentki, M., Zaninetti, D., Jeanrenaud, B.: Insulin resistance in soleus muscle from obese Zucker rats. Involvement of several defective sites. Biochem. J. 186:525, 1980.

113. Crettaz, M., Jeanrenaud, B.: Postreceptor alterations in the states of insulin resistance. Metabolism 29:467, 1980.

114. Jeanrenaud, B.: Hyperinsulinemia in obesity syndromes: its metabolic consequences and possible etiology. Metabolism 27(Suppl. 2):1881, 1978.

115. Ogilvie, R.F.: Sugar tolerance in obese subjects: a review of 65 cases. Quart. J. Med. 28:345, 1935.

116. Berger, M., Muller, W.A., Renold, A.E.: Relationship of obesity to diabetes. Some facts, many questions. In: H.M. Katzen, R.J. Mahler (Eds.): Advances in Modern Nutrition. Vol. 2: Diabetes, Obesity and Vascular Disease. Washington, Hemisphere Publishing Co. 1978, pp. 211–228.

117. Kolterman, O.G., Insel, J., Saekow, M., Olefsky, J.M.: Mechanisms of insulin resistance in human obesity. Evidence for receptor and postreceptor defects. J. Clin. Invest. 65:1272, 1980.

118. Czech, M.P.: Second messengers. In: M. Brownlee (Ed.): Handbook of Diabetes Mellitus. Vol. II. Islet Cell Function/ Insulin Action. New York, Garland Press, 1980, pp. 117–149.

119. Gavryck, W.A., Moore, R.D., Thompson, R.C.: Effect of insulin upon membrane-bound (Na+—K+) ATPase extracted from frog skeletal muscle. J. Physiol. 252:43, 1975.

120. Jungas, R.L.: Action of insulin enzymes. In: M. Brownlee (Ed.): Handbook of Diabetes Mellitus. Vol. II. Islet Cell Function/Insulin Action. New York, Garland Press, 1980, pp. 151–195.

121. Czech, M.P.: Molecular basis of insulin action. Ann. Rev. Biochem. 46:359, 1977.

122. Czech, M.P. Insulin action and the regulation of hexose transport. Diabetes 29:399, 1980.

123. Clausen, T.: Calcium, glucose transport and insulin action. In: G. Semenza, E. Carafoli (Eds.): Biochemistry of Membrane Transport. Berlin, Springer-Verlag, 1977, pp. 481–499.

124. Clausen, T.: The role of calcium in the action of insulin. In: FEBS Federation of European Biochemical Societies, 11th Meeting. Copenhagen 1977. Symposium A4. Membrane Proteins. 1977, pp. 229–238.

125. Exton, J.H., Lewis, S.B., Ho, R.H., et al.: The role of cyclic AMP in the interaction of glucagon and insulin in the control of liver metabolism. Ann. N.Y. Acad. Sci. 185:85, 1971.

126. Butcher, R.W., Baird, C.E., Sutherland, E.W.: Effects of lipolytic and antilipolytic substances and adenosine

3′,5′-monophosphate levels in isolated fat cells. J. Biol. Chem. 243:1705, 1968.

127. Jungas, R.L.: Role of cyclic 3′,5′-AMP in the response of adipose tissue to insulin. Proc. Natl. Acad. Sci. USA 56:757–763, 1966.

128. Siddle, K., Kane-Maguire, B., Campbell, A.K.: The effects of glucagon and insulin on adenosine 3′,5′-cyclic monophosphate concentrations in an organ culture of mature rat liver. Biochem. J. 132:765, 1973.

129. Zinman, B., Hollenberg, C.H.: Effect of insulin and lipolytic agents on rat adipocyte low K_m cyclic adenosine 3′,5′-monophosphate phosphodiesterase. J. Biol. Chem. 249:2182, 1974.

130. House, P.D.R., Poulis, P., Weidemann, M.J.: Isolation of a plasma-membrane subfraction from rat liver containing an insulin-sensitive cyclic AMP phosphodiesterase. Eur. J. Biochem. 24:429, 1972.

131. Kono, T., Robinson, F.W., Sarver, J.A.: Insulin-sensitive phosphodiesterase. Its localization, hormonal stimulation, and oxidative stabilization. J. Biol. Chem. 250:7826, 1974.

132. Manangiello, V., Vaughan, M.: An effect of insulin on cyclic adenosine 3′,5′-monophosphate phosphodiesterase activity in fat cells. J. Biol. Chem. 248:7164, 1973.

133. Loten, E.G., Assimacopoulos-Jeannet, F.D., Exton, J.H., Park, C.R.: Stimulation of a low K_m phosphodiesterase from liver by insulin and glucagon. J. Biol. Chem. 253:746, 1978.

134. Solomon, S.S., Palazzolo, M., King, L.E.: Cyclic nucleotide phosphodiesterase. Insulin activation detected in adipose tissue by gel electrophoresis. Diabetes 26:967, 1977.

135. Marx, J.L.: Calmodulin: a protein for all seasons. Science 208:274, 1980.

136. Klee, C.B., Crouch, T.H., Richmann, P.G.: Calmodulin. Ann. Rev. Biochem. 49:489, 1980.

137. Fain, J.N.: Effects of menadione and Vitamin K_5 on glucose metabolism, respiration, lipolysis, cyclic 3′,5′-adenylic acid accumulation, and adenyl cyclase in white fat cells. Mol. Pharmacol. 7:465, 1971.

138. Fain, J.N.: Insulin as an activator of cyclic AMP accumulation in rat fat cells. J. Cyclic. Nucleo. Res. 1:359, 1975.

139. Jarett, L., Steiner, A.L., Smith, R.M., Kipnis, D.M.: The involvement of cyclic AMP in the hormonal regulation of protein synthesis in rat adipocytes. Endocrinology 90:1277, 1972.

140. Siddle, K., Hales, C.N.: The relationship between the concentration of adenosine 3′,5′-cyclic monophosphate and the antilipolytic action of insulin in isolated rat fat cells. Biochem. J. 142:97, 1974.

141. Goldberg, N.D., Villar-Palasi, C., Sasko, H., Larner, J.: Effect of insulin treatment on muscle 3′,5′-cyclic adenylate levels in vivo and in vitro. Biochim. Biophys. Acta 148:665, 1967.

142. Nuttall, F.Q., Gannon, M.C., Corbett, V.A., Wheeler, M.P.: Insulin stimulation of heart glycogen synthase D phosphatase (protein phosphatase). J. Biol. Chem. 251:6724, 1976.

143. Walaas, O., Walaas, F. Grønnerød, O.: Molecular events in the action of insulin on cell metabolism. The significance of cyclic AMP dependent protein kinases. Acta Endocrin. (Suppl.) 77:93, 1974.

144. Larner, J., Galasko, G., Cheng, K., et al.: Generation by insulin of a chemical mediator that controls protein phosphorylation and dephosphorylation. Science 206:1408, 1979.

145. Cheng, L., Galasko, G., Huang, L., et al.: Studies on the insulin mediator. II. Separation of two antagonistic biologically active materials from fraction II. Diabetes 29:659, 1980.

146. Jarett, L., Seals, J.R.: Pyruvate dehydrogenase activation in adipocyte mitochondria by an insulin-generated mediator from muscle. Science 206:1407, 1979.

147. Carpentier, J.L., Gorden, P., Freychet, P., et al.: Binding, internalization and lysosomal association of ^{125}I-insulin in isolated rat hepatocytes. Experientia 34:936, 1978.

148. Carpentier, J.L., Gorden, P., Amherdt, M., et al.: ^{125}I-insulin binding to cultured human lymphocytes. Initial localization and fat of hormone determined by quantitative electron microscopic autoradiography. J. Clin. Invest. 61:1057, 1978.

149. Steiner, D.F.: Insulin today (The Banting Memorial Lecture, 1976). Diabetes 26:322, 1976.

150. Van Obberghen, E., Spooner, P.M., Kahn, C.R., et al.: Insulin-receptor antibodies mimic a late insulin effect. Nature 280:500, 1979.

151. Posner, B.I., Josefsberg, Z., Bergeron, J.J.M.: Intracellular polypeptide hormone receptors. Characterization of insulin binding sites in Golgi fractions from the liver of female rats. J. Biol. Chem. 253:4067, 1978.

152. Goldfine, I.D., Smith, G.J.: Binding of insulin to isolated nuclei. Proc. Natl. Acad. Sci. USA 73:1427, 1976.

153. Goldfine, I.D., Smith, G.J., Wong, K.Y., Jones, A.L.: Cellular uptake and nuclear binding of insulin in human cultured lymphocytes: evidence for potential intracellular sites of insulin action. Proc. Natl. Acad. Sci. USA 74:1368, 1977.

154. Bergeron, J.J.M., Posner, B.I., Josefsberg, Z., Sikstrom, R.: Intracellular polypeptide hormone receptors. The demonstration of specific binding sites for insulin and human growth hormone in Golgi fractions isolated from the liver of female rats. J. Biol. Chem. 253:4058, 1978.

155. Posner, B.I., Raquidan, D., Josefsberg, A., Bergeron, J.M.: Different regulation of insulin receptors in intracellular (Golgi) and plasma membranes from livers in obese and lean mice. Proc. Natl. Acad. Sci. USA 75:3302, 1978.

156. Varandani, P.T.: Insulin degradation: I. Purification and properties of glutathione-insulin transhydrogenase of rat liver. Biochim. Biophys. Acta 286:126, 1972.

157. Varandani, P.T.: Insulin degradation: X. Identification of insulin degrading activity of rat liver plasma membrane as glutathione-insulin transhydrogenase. Biochem. Biophys. Res. Commun. 55:689, 1973.

158. Duckworth, W.C., Heinemann, M., Kitabchi, A.E.: Purification of insulin-specific protease by affinity chromatography. Proc. Natl. Acad. Sci. USA 69:3698, 1972.

159. Brush, J.S.: Purification and characterization of a protease with specificity for insulin from rat muscle. Diabetes 20:140, 1971.

160. Grisolia, S., Wallace, R.: Insulin degradation by lysosomal extracts from rat liver; model for a role of lysosomes in hormone degradation. Biochem. Biophys. Res. Comm. 70:22, 1976.

161. Gorden P., Carpentier, J-L., Freychet, P., et al.: Intracellular translocation of iodine-125-labelled insulin: direct demonstration of isolated hepatocytes. Science 200:782, 1978.

162. Terris, S., Steiner, D.F.: Binding and degradation of ^{125}I-insulin by rat hepatocytes. J. Biol. Chem. 250:8389, 1975.

163. Freychet, P., Kahn, C.R., Roth, J., Neville, D.M., Jr.: Insulin interactions with liver plasma membranes. Independence of binding of the hormone and its degradation. J. Biol. Chem. 247:3953, 1972.

164. Gammeltoft, S., Gliemann, J.: Binding and degradation

of ^{125}I-labelled insulin by isolated rat fat cells. Biochim. Biophys. Acta 320:16, 1973.

165. Gliemann, J., Sonne, O.: Binding and receptor-mediated degradation of insulin in adipocytes. J. Biol. Chem. 253:7857, 1978.

166. Kahn, C.R., Baird, K.: The fate of insulin bound to adipocytes. J. Biol. Chem. 253:4900, 1978.

167. Dial, L.K., Miyamoto, S., Arquilla, E.R.: Modulation of ^{125}I-insulin degradation by receptors in liver plasma membranes. Biochem. Biophys. Res. Commun. 74:545, 1977.

168. Morgan, H.E., Neeley, J.R.: Insulin and membrane transport. In: N. Freinkel, D.F. Steiner (Eds.): Handbook of Physiology. Section 7: Endocrinology. Vol. 1. Endocrine Pancreas. Washington, Am. Physiol. Society, 1972, pp. 323–331.

169. Levine, R., Goldstein, M.S., Klein, S.F., Huddlestun, B.: The action of insulin on the distribution of galactose in eviscerated nephrectomized dogs. J. Biol. Chem. 179:985, 1949.

170. Levine, R., Goldstein, M.S., Huddlestun, B., Klein, S.F.: Action of insulin on the "permeability" of cells to free hexoses, as studied by its effect on the distribution of galactose. Am. J. Physiol. 163:70, 1950.

171. Whitesell, R.R., Gliemann, J.: Kinetic parameters of transport of 3-0-methylglucose and glucose in adipocytes. J. Biol. Chem. 254:5276, 1979.

172. Amatruda, J.M., Finch, E.D.: Modulation of hexose uptake and insulin action by cell membrane fluidity. J. Biol. Chem. 254:2619, 1979.

173. Czech, M.P.: Differential effects of sulfhydryl reagents on activation and deactivation of the fat cell hexose and transport system. J. Biol. Chem. 251:1164, 1976.

174. Olefsky, J.M.: Mechanisms of the ability of insulin to activate the glucose transport system in rat adipocytes. Biochem. J. 172:137, 1978.

175. Ludvigsen, C., Jarett, L.: A kinetic analysis of D-glucose transport by adipocyte plasma membranes. J. Biol. Chem. 254:1444, 1979.

176. Ludvigsen, C., Jarett, L.: A comparison of basal and insulin stimulated glucose transport in rat adipocyte plasma membranes. Diabetes 29:373, 1980.

177. Mukherjee, S.P., Lynn, W.S.: Reduced nicotinamide adenine dinucleotide phosphate oxidase in adipocyte plasma membrane and its activation by insulin. Possible role in the hormone's effects on adenylate cyclase and the hexose monophosphate shunt. Arch. Biochem. Biophys. 184:69, 1977.

178. Olefsky, J.M., Kobayashi, M.: Ability of circulating insulin to chronically regulate the cellular glucose transport system. Metabolism 27:1917, 1978.

179. Akhtar, R.A., Perry, M.C.: Insulin action in isolated fat cells: I. Effects of divalent cations on the stimulation by insulin of glucose uptake. Biochim. Biophys. Acta 585:107, 1979.

180. Akhtar, R.A., Perry, M.C.: Insulin action in isolated fat cells. II. Effects of divalent cations on stimulation by insulin of protein synthesis, on inhibition of lipolysis by insulin, and on the binding of ^{125}I-labeled insulin to isolated fat cells. Biochim. Biophys. Acta 585:117, 1979.

181. Gould, M.K.: Multiple roles of ATP in the regulation of muscle sugar transport. Trends in Biochem. Sci. 4:10 (Jan.) 1979.

182. Wicklmayr, M., Dietze, G., Mayer, L., et al.: Evidence for an involvement of kinin liberation in the priming action of insulin on glucose uptake into skeletal muscle. FEBS Letter 98:61, 1979.

183. Suzuki, K., Kono, T.: Evidence that insulin causes translocation of glucose transport activity to the plasma membrane from an intracellular storage site. Proc. Natl. Acad. Sci. USA 77:2542, 1980.

184. Cushman, S.W., Wardzala, L.J.: Potential mechanism of insulin action on glucose transport in the isolated rat adipose cell. J. Biol. Chem. 255:4758, 1980.

184a. Berger, M., Hagg, S.A., Ruderman, N.B.: Glucose metabolism of perfused skeletal muscle. Interaction of insulin and exercise on glucose uptake. Biochem. J. 146:231, 1975.

184b. Berger, M., Berchtold, P., Cüppers, H.J., et al.: Metabolic and hormonal effects of muscular exercise in juvenile type diabetes mellitus. Diabetologia 13:355, 1977.

184c. Berger, M., Christacopoulos, P., Wahren, J. (Eds.): Diabetes and Exercise. Bern, Switzerland, Huber-Verlag, 1982.

185. Harrop, G.A., Jr. Benedict, E.M.: The participation of inorganic substances in carbohydrate metabolism. J. Biol. Chem. 59:683, 1924.

185a. Kerr, S.E.: Effect of insulin and of pancreatectomy on distribution of phosphorus and potassium in blood. J. Biol. Chem. 78:35, 1928.

186. Zierler, K.L.: Insulin, ions, and membrane potentials. In: N. Freinkel, D.F. Steiner (Eds.): Handbook of Physiology. Section 7. Endocrinology. Vol. 1. Endocrine Pancreas. Washington, Amer. Physiological Society, 1972, pp. 347–368.

187. Andres, R., Baltzan, M.A., Cader, G., Zierler, K.L.: Effect of insulin on carbohydrate metabolism and on potassium in the forearm of man. J. Clin. Invest. 41:108, 1962.

188. Zierler, K.L.: Hyperpolarization of muscle in a glucose-free environment. Am. J. Physiol. 197:524, 1959.

189. Zierler, K.L.: Effect of insulin on potassium efflux from rat muscle in the presence and absence of glucose. Am. J. Physiol. 198:1066, 1960.

190. Moore, R.D., Rabovsky, J.L.: Mechanism of insulin action on resting membrane potential of frog skeletal muscle. Am. J. Physiol. 236:C249, 1979.

191. Kipnis, D.M., Noall, M.W.: Stimulation of amino acid transport by insulin in the isolated rat diaphragm. Biochim. Biophys. Acta 28:226, 1958.

192. Akedo, H., Christensen, H.N.: Nature of insulin action on amino acid uptake by the isolated diaphragm. J. Biol. Chem. 237:118, 1962.

193. Renold, A.E.: The mechanism of insulin action: attempt at synthesis. In: E.F. Pfeiffer (Ed.): Handbuch des Diabetes mellitus, Vol. I. Munich, J.F. Lehmanns Verlag, 1969, pp. 553–596.

194. Riggs, T.R., McKirahan, K.J.: Action of insulin on transport of L-alanine into rat diaphragm in vitro. Evidence that the hormone affects only one neutral amino acid transport system. J. Biol. Chem. 248:6450, 1973.

195. Farfel, Z., Karlish, S., Prives, J.: A transient increase in amino acid transport modulated by insulin in differentiating muscle cells. J. Cell Physiol. 98:279, 1979.

196. Peterson, D.T.: Effect of diabetes, insulin and glucagon on the translation process and ribosomal proteins. In: M. Brownlee (Ed.): Handbook of Diabetes. Vol. IV. Biochemical Pathology. New York, Garland Press, 1980, pp. 179–230.

197. Manchester, K.L.: The control by insulin of amino acid accumulation in muscle. Biochem. J. 117:457, 1970.

198. Ruderman, N.B., Berger, M.: The formation of glutamine and alanine in skeletal muscle. J. Biol. Chem. 249:5500, 1974.

199. Pozefsky, T., Felig, P., Tobin, J.D., et al.: Amino acid balance across tissue of the forearm in postabsorptive man. Effects of insulin at two dose levels. J. Clin. Invest. 48:2273, 1969.

200. Nimmo, H.G., Cohen, P.: Hormonal control of protein phosphorylation. Adv. Cyclic Nucleotide Res. 8:145, 1977.

201. Beloff-Chain, A., Cantanzaro, R., Chain, E.B., et al.: The influence of insulin on carbohydrate metabolism in the isolated diaphragm muscle of normal and alloxan diabetic rats. Proc. R. Soc. Lond. 143:481, 1955.

202. Steiner, D.F., Williams, R.H.: Some observations concerning hepatic glucose 6-phosphate content in normal and diabetic rats. J. Biol. Chem. 234:1342, 1959.

203. Villar-Palasi, C., Larner, J.: Insulin-mediated effect on the activity of UDPG-glycogen transglucosylase of muscle. Biochim. Biophys. Acta 39:171, 1960.

204. Krahl, M.E.: Effects of insulin on synthesis of specific enzymes in various tissues. In: I.B. Fritz (Ed.): Insulin Action. New York, Academic Press, 1972, pp. 461–486.

205. Wool, J.G.: Effects of insulin on cellular protein synthesis. In: A. Hasselblatt, F.R. Bruchhausen (Eds.): Insulin. Part II. Berlin, Springer Verlag, 1975, pp. 268–302.

206. Jefferson, L.S.: Role of insulin in the regulation of protein synthesis. Lilly Lecture 1979. Diabetes 29:487, 1980.

207. Jefferson, L.S., Flaim, K.E., Peavy, D.E.: Effect of insulin on protein turnover. In: M. Brownlee (Ed.): Handbook of Diabetes Mellitus. Vol. IV. Biochemical Pathology. New York, Garland Press, 1980, pp. 133–177.

208. Dahlman, B., Reinauer, H.: Purification and some properties of an alkaline proteinase from rat skeletal muscle. Biochem. J. 171:803, 1978.

209. Wool, I.G.: Insulin and incorporation of radioactivity into nucleic acid fraction of isolated diaphragm. Am. J. Physiol. 199:719, 1960.

210. Volfin, P., Nanoune, J.: Effect of insulin in nucleic acids, nucleotides and cyclic AMP. In: A. Hasselblatt, F.V. Bruchhausen (Eds.): Insulin, Part II. Berlin, Springer Verlag, 1975, pp. 303–327.

211. Berger, M.: Investigations on lipolysis of human adipose tissue in vitro. Thesis. Düsseldorf University, West Germany, 1969.

212. Gries, F.A.: Hormonal control of human adipose tissue metabolism in vitro. Hormone Metab. Res. 2(Suppl. 2):167, 1970.

213. Gries, F.A., Berger, M., Oberdisse, K.: Untersuchungen zum antihipolytischen Effekt des Insulins am menschlichen Fettgewebe in vitro. Diabetologia 4:262, 1968.

214. Jungas, R.L.: Metabolic effects on adipose tissue in vitro. In: A. Hasselblatt, F.R. Bruchhausen (Eds.): Insulin, Part II. Berlin, Springer-Verlag, 1975, pp. 371–412.

215. Spooner, P.M., Chernick, S.S., Garrison, M.M., Scow, R.O.: Development of lipoprotein lipase activity and accumulation of triacylglycerol in differentiating 3T3-L1 adipocytes. Effects of prostaglandin F_{2a}, 1-methyl-3-isobutylxanthine, prolactin, and insulin. J. Biol. Chem. 254:1305, 1979.

216. von Mehring, J., Minkowski, O.: Diabetes mellitus nach Pancreasextirpation. Arch. Path. Pharmak. 26:371, 1890.

217. Humbel, R.E., Andres, R.Y., Ernest, C., et al.: Insulin-like growth factors: homology to insulin. In: W.K. Waldhäusl (Ed.): Diabetes 1979. Internat. Congr. Series No. 500. Amsterdam, Excerpta Medica, 1980, pp. 254–258.

218. Zapf, J., Rinderknecht, R.E., Humbel, R.E., and Froesch, E.R.: Nonsuppressible insulin-like activity (NSILA) from human serum: recent accomplishments and their physiologic implications. Metab. 27:1803, 1978.

219. Zapf, J., Schoenle, E., and Froesch, E.R.: Insulin-like growth factors I and II: some biological actions and receptor binding characteristics of two purified constituents of nonsuppressible insulin-like activity of human serum. Eur. J. Biochem. 87:285, 1978.

220. King, G.L., Kahn, C.R., Rechler, M.M., Nissley, S.P.: Direct demonstration of separate receptors for growth stimulating and metabolic activities of insulin and multiplication-stimulating activity (an insulinlike growth factor) using antibodies to the insulin receptor. J. Clin. Invest. 66:130, 1980.

221. Froesch, E.R., Schoenle, E., Walter, H., Zapf, J.: Nonsuppressible insulin-like activity of serum: properties of IGF I and IGF II, the serum binding protein and NSILA levels in health and disease. In: W.K. Waldhäusl (Ed.): Diabetes 1979. Internat. Congr. Series No. 500. Amsterdam, Excerpta Medica, 1980, pp. 259–265.

222. Zapf, J., Rinderknecht, E., Humbel, R.E., Froesch, E.R.: Insulin-like growth factors from human serum. In: M. Brownlee (Ed.): Handbook of Diabetes Mellitus. Vol. I. Etiology/Hormone Physiology. New York, Garland Press, 1980, pp. 261–295.

223. Flier, J.S., Young, J.B., Landsberg, L.: Familial insulin resistance with acanthosis nigricans, acral hypertrophy and muscle cramps. N. Engl. J. Med. 303:970, 1980.

224. Strom, T.B., Helderman, J.H.: Role of insulin in development and modulation of the immune response. In: M. Brownlee (Ed.): Handbook of Diabetes Mellitus. Vol. II. Islet Cell Function/Insulin Action. New York, Garland Press, 1980, pp. 197–216.

225. Fernandes, G., Handwerger, B.S., Yunis, E.J., Brown, D.M.: Immune response in the mutant diabetic C57 BL/Ks-db mouse. Discrepancies between in vitro and in vivo immunological assays. J. Clin. Invest. 61:243, 1978.

226. Mahmoud, A.A.F., Rodman, H.M., Mandel, M.A., and Warren, K.S.: Induced and spontaneous diabetes mellitus and suppression of cell mediated immunologic responses. Granuloma formation, delayed dermal reactivity, and allograft rejection. J. Clin. Invest. 57:362, 1976.

227. Friedman, E.A., Beyer, M.M.: Immune competence of the streptozotocin-induced diabetic rat. I. Absent second-set skin allograft response. Transplantation 24:367, 1977.

228. Strom, T.B., Bear, R.A., and Carpenter, C.B.: Insulin-induced augmentation of lymphocyte-mediated cytotoxicity. Science 187:1206–1208, 1975.

229. Helderman, J.H., Strom, T.B.: Specific insulin binding site on T and B lymphocytes as marker of cell activation. Nature 274:62, 1978.

230. Bruchhausen, F.R.: Action of insulin on some other organs and on differentiation. In: A. Hasselblatt, F.R. Bruchhausen (Eds.): Insulin, Part II. Berlin, Springer-Verlag, 1975, pp. 435–495.

231. Ziboh, V.A., Wright, R., Hsia, S.L.: Effects of insulin on the uptake and metabolism of glucose by rat skin in vitro. Arch. Biochem. Biophys. 146:93, 1971.

7 Animal Models of Diabetes Mellitus

John P. Mordes and Aldo A. Rossini

POLYURIA, POLYDIPSIA, MELITURIA

This syndrome has been recognized for millennia. However, neither the passage of time, the discovery of insulin, nor the study of countless patients has yielded a cure for diabetes. Many distinct diabetic syndromes are now recognized, but the inheritance, etiology, physiology, therapy, and prevention of each remain poorly understood. Given both the number and complexity of these problems, diabetes research has come to rely heavily on the study of hyperglycemic animals. The use of animals rather than human subjects has many advantages.

The genetics of diabetes, for example, are extraordinarily complex. Inheritance is polygenic, exhibits variable penetrance, and is susceptible to environmental influence. In human populations these factors are difficult to study and impossible to control. Family histories tend to be inaccurate and include only a few generations. People marry and remarry; most couples have few children; families move and break up. In contrast, the animal colony permits clarification of the genetics of some forms of diabetes. Accurate genealogies can be maintained and many generations studied in a relatively short period of time. The knowledge that a certain percentage of animals will reliably develop diabetes becomes a powerful tool in the study of preventive therapies for the disease. The animal colony also permits study of the interaction of heredity and environmental factors such as diet, drugs, toxins, and infectious agents.

Diabetes may occur acutely, but it is also a chronic disease with late vascular sequelae. Understanding it fully will require metabolic, histologic, and immunologic studies at many stages of the illness. No diabetic patient, however, can provide such extensive material, particularly at the time of onset when it would be of paramount interest. The anatomic location of the pancreas is an obvious problem for researchers. The lifespan of the human is another problem; it is difficult to study the natural history of diabetes in subjects who might outlive their investigator.

Lastly, there are ethical impediments to the study of human diabetes. Provocation of the disease is obviously not permissible in humans, but constitutes a fruitful line of animal research. As a corollary, new therapeutics to prevent or reverse the disease must first be tested in animals.

The advantages of animal models are, of course,

balanced by limitations. No animal model of diabetes corresponds perfectly to human diabetes. The pathophysiology of most animal diabetic syndromes is poorly understood and difficult to relate to human data. The clinical course of animals with these syndromes may be variable and unpredictable. The vascular sequelae of animal diabetes syndromes have also proven difficult to study. Nonetheless, much of our hope for future progress in diabetes research rests with animals, and in this chapter we hope to summarize both the promise and the limitations of this approach.

Spontaneous hyperglycemic syndromes have long been recognized in mammalian species. Leblanc[1] documented the occurrence of diabetes in animals in 1861. Diabetic cats,[2] tree shrews,[3] and ground squirrels[4] have been found, as have diabetic pigs, horses, apes, sheep and goats.[5] Isolated cases of diabetes have been reported in a fox,[6] a dolphin,[5] antelopes,[7] and a hippopotamus.[5] While these observations attest to the phylogenetic exuberance of diabetes, the same limitations which impede the study of the disease in humans apply to most of these species as well. The data gathered from the larger mammals are so inchoate as to be of limited value.

From the standpoint of efficiency and cost, the small laboratory rodent is the most satisfactory animal in which to study diabetes. Not only do several species become spontaneously hyperglycemic, but some are amenable as well to the experimental induction of diabetes. Costs are reasonable, generation times short, and litters large. In addition, the genetics and environment of such animals are controllable. These rodents, along with a few primates, constitute the major focus of this chapter.

In this review, we are indebted to earlier writers, especially Cameron et al.,[5] Herberg and Coleman,[8] Like,[9] Renold,[10] and others.[11,12]

CLASSIFICATION

It must be remembered that diabetes-like syndromes in animals are *not* the same as diabetes in humans. The human system of classification itself leaves much to be desired, and animal syndromes simply do not fit neatly into a human framework.

Table 7–1 presents one useful system for classifying the animal models of diabetes. Certain features of the table deserve comment. First, the commonest and most extensively studied diabetic syndromes in animals correspond to the commonest form of human diabetes: obesity-related, noninsulin-deficient, noninsulin-dependent diabetes (NIDDM). The table includes one well-known strain, the Zucker or fatty rat, *(fa/fa)*[13] which exhibits hyperinsulinemia, insulin resistance, and obesity, but not basal hyperglycemia. While it is

Table 7–1. Animal Diabetic Syndromes

I. OBESE NONINSULIN-DEFICIENT ANIMAL SYNDROMES
   Obese mouse (*ob/ob*)
   Diabetes mouse (*db/db*)*
   Obese Yellow mouse (A^vy)
   Yellow-KK mouse
   KK mouse
   Wellesley hybrid mouse (C3hf × I)
   NZO mouse
   DBM mouse
   PBB/Ld mouse
   Spiny mouse (*Acomys cahirinus*)*
   Zucker fatty rat (*fa/fa*)
   BHE rat
   Sand rat (*Psammomys obesus*)*
   Tuco-tuco (*Ctenomys talarum*)
   Djungarian hamster (*Phodopus sungorus*)

II. NON-OBESE ANIMALS
   BB rat
   Chinese hamster (*Cricetulus griseus*)*
   Celebese black ape (*Macaca nigra*)
   Rhesus monkey (*Macaca mulatta*)
   South African hamster (*Mystromys albicaudatus*)
   Guinea pig
   NOD mouse
   Rhesus monkey (*Macaca mulatta*)

III. EXPERIMENTAL DIABETES
   A. Hypothalamic Diabetes
   B. Viral Diabetes
   C. Chemically-Induced Diabetes
       1. Irreversible Beta Cytotoxic Agents
       2. Reversible Beta Cytotoxic Agents
   D. Contra-Insulin Hormones

*A small number of these animals become terminally ketotic and possibly insulin dependent. The typical syndrome is noninsulin requiring.

glucose intolerant when stressed,[14] it is more appropriately viewed as a model of obesity and will not be discussed. The same holds true of the BHE rat.[15,16] Animals with insulin deficiency and true insulin-dependent diabetes (IDDM) are uncommon. *Lean* noninsulin-deficient diabetic animals are also found infrequently.

Some animals are difficult to classify and illustrate the limitations of our knowledge of both human and animal diabetes. The sand rat, spiny mouse, Chinese hamster, Tuco-tuco, and C57BL/KsJ *db/db* mouse can all become ketotic but as a rule are not insulin dependent. Ten percent of South African hamsters with basal hyperglycemia become insulin dependent. In such instances the question arises as to whether there exist various syndromes of differing etiology or one syndrome of varying severity. Classification is arbitrary in these cases.

It can be seen that there are elements in all of these models that correspond to a degree with human IDDM and NIDDM. It may be asked if there are also models of other types of human diabetes as defined in Chapter 15. Unfortunately, there exist few counterparts.

There is no satisfactory model of "gestational diabetes" although there are indications that one might exist among rhesus monkeys.[17-19a] "Previous abnormality of glucose tolerance" does not have a precise correspondence among animals. Many animals with carbohydrate intolerance exhibit either a spontaneous permanent remission or remission of variable duration induced by dietary restriction. Whether some of the former group might develop diabetes again if appropriately stressed is unknown.

"Potential diabetes" as empirically defined for *human* diabetes implies only the possibility of the development of diabetes. There are, however, four rodent species in which progression to frank diabetes can be predicted with absolute certainty. These four (the *mdb* mouse, the obese yellow (A^{vy}) mouse, the yellow-KK mouse, and the offspring of two ketotic Chinese hamsters) thus have a much better defined "potential" for developing diabetes than any human. Additionally, most rodent colonies inbred for diabetic syndromes yield a relatively stable incidence of carbohydrate intolerance. The percentages for some single gene mutations follow simple Mendelian rules. Even animals whose diabetic syndromes are polygenic or exhibit variable penetrance often yield a stable incidence of disease, as in the case of the BB rat and Chinese hamster.

The animal counterpart of human "diabetes in association with other conditions" is experimentally induced diabetes. In both humans and animals, diabetes can be induced by drugs, contrainsulin hormones, and streptozotocin. Other forms of experimental diabetes in animals—viral, chemical, and hypothalamic—have also been studied intensively.

Table 7-1 is not intended to be exhaustive, and animals in which diabetes occurs only sporadically or which have not been studied in detail will not be discussed. Finally, we again stress that any correspondences and analogies to human diabetes are just that: similarities useful for directing our thinking. The reader should not be misled into believing that the correspondences between animal and human diabetes are exact.

GENETICS

The inheritance of several diabetic syndromes in animals is presented in Table 7-2. It is noteworthy that such syndromes are heritable in several ways. Single gene mutations facilitate genetic manipulation of the model and offer an opportunity to identify single metabolic defects leading to diabetes. Unfortunately, single gene inheritance is not comparable to human inheritance, and one of the

Table 7-2. Genetics of Spontaneously Hyperglycemic Animals

SINGLE GENE MUTANTS	
Obese mouse (*ob/ob*)	(Autosomal Recessive)
Diabetes mouse (*db/db*)	(Autosomal Recessive)
Obese yellow mouse (A^{vy})	(Autosomal Dominant)
POLYGENIC INHERITANCE	
Chinese hamster	
NZO mouse	
KK mouse (one component dominant, penetrance influenced by recessive modifiers)	
Djungarian hamster	
South African hamster	
Pbb/Ld mouse	
HYBRIDS	
Wellesley hybrid mouse (C3Hf × I)	
UNKNOWN HEREDITY WITH MAJOR ENVIRONMENTAL COMPONENT	
Sand rat	
Spiny mouse	
Tuco-tuco	
UNKNOWN	
BB rat	
Celebese ape (*Macaca nigra*)	
Rhesus monkey (*Macaca mulatta*)	
Japanese Wistar rat	

most instructive lessons of the single gene mutations is in the illustration of the importance of the "normal" nondiabetic genetic background of the host.

Table 7-3 contrasts the diabetic syndromes observed with the obese (*ob*) and diabetes (*db*) mutations of the mouse.[20-22] When bred on the C57BL/6J background, syndromes of mild hyperglycemia with extreme obesity develop. When either gene is placed on the C57BL/KsJ background, however, the animal develops severe hyperglycemia with marked insulin deficiency and beta cell atrophy. Clearly the nature of the diabetic syndrome is modified by as yet undefined factors in the genetic background. In this instance the genetic modifiers that ameliorate the syndrome are dominant to the factors permissive to it.[23] These data imply that even when heritable as a single recessive gene, the expression of diabetes is perhaps always modified by other genes present in the host. Table 7-3 also points out Coleman's observation that the clinical expression of another diabetic syndrome, that of the obese yellow mouse, appears to be independent of genetic background.[24] Even in this instance, however, subtle effects of differing background genomes on the enzymatic characteristics of yellow mice have been identified.[25]

An animal that extends the observations made in mice is the Chinese hamster whose genetics are detailed in Table 7-4. This one species yields an entire spectrum of diabetic syndromes ranging from ketosis to minimal glycosuria.[26] At least four genes

Table 7–3.   Effect of Genetic Background on Diabetes*

Diabetic Gene	Background Genome	
	C57BL/6J	C57BL/KsJ
Obese (ob) and Diabetes (db)	Mild diabetes Severe obesity Chronic hyperinsulinemia	Severe diabetes Mild obesity Transient hyperinsulinemia followed by decreasing plasma insulin Beta cell degeneration
Obese Yellow (A^vy)	Moderate obesity Minimal diabetes Mild islet hyperplasia	Same as on BL/6J background

*Modified from Coleman and Hummel[20]

Table 7–4.   Genetics of the Chinese Hamster*

Incidence of Diabetes in Offspring of Various Matings

	% Diabetic Offspring		
	Ketotic	Nonketotic	Total
Ketotic × ketotic	54	46	100
Ketotic × nonketotic	16	43	59
Ketotic × trace glyco-suric	14	27	41
Ketotic × nondiabetic	6	18	24

*Adapted from Gerritsen et al.[27] Used by permission of the authors and publisher.

have been implicated,[27–29] and there is obvious genetic dose dependence in this form of diabetes. The progeny of two ketotic parents are all diabetic but with varying severity of diabetes. The progeny of less severely ill parents are less often diabetic. Whether the diabetes in the Chinese hamster represents a single syndrome of varying severity or a number of distinct syndromes remains to be clarified.

Other genetic investigations have revealed four species whose diabetic potential can be identified in the euglycemic state with absolute certainty: (1) the offspring of two ketotic Chinese hamsters, (2) the obese yellow (A^vy) mouse with dominant inheritance, (3) the yellow-KK hybrid mouse and (4) the *mdb* mouse. This last represents a cross of the C57BL/KsJ *db/+* with the C57BL/6J *m/m,* an animal displaying a recessive gray coat color early in life.[30] By careful manipulation over several generations, double homozygotes *(db/db m/m)* were created. These could be identified with certainty by their gray coat color as early as 10 days of age, long before the clinical appearance of diabetes. These prediabetic animals obviously do not correspond exactly to human "potential" diabetics, but do afford an opportunity to study some forms of "prediabetes" efficiently and in detail.

OBESE NON-INSULIN-DEFICIENT SPONTANEOUS ANIMAL SYNDROMES

As is the case in humans, the commonest form of diabetes in animals is that associated with obesity. Despite this gross similarity, we stress that there is no precise correspondence of NIDDM models to their human counterpart. One glaring discrepancy is the relative magnitude of obesity observed in these hyperglycemic rodents; it is generally far in excess of the degree of obesity commonly seen in human noninsulin-dependent diabetics. The poorly understood occurrence of ketonuria in the absence of fasting or insulin dependence is another discrepancy. Nonobese, non-insulin-dependent hyperglycemic animals are also difficult to analyze in terms of their relevance to human disease. This nonobese group contains the only extensively studied diabetic primate, the Celebese ape *(Macaca nigra).*

The Obese Mouse

Perhaps the best studied of all animals with diabetes, the obese *(ob/ob)* mouse arose as a spontaneous mutation at the Jackson Laboratory in 1949.[31] Inheritance is autosomal recessive. The homozygous animal is characterized by obesity, hyperglycemia, and hyperinsulinemia, but the severity of the syndrome observed, as with the diabetic *(db/db)* mouse, is dependent on the genetic background. A much more severe syndrome is found on the C57BL/KsJ as opposed to the C57BL/6J background [20,24] (Table 7–3). Ketosis is observed only in the C57BL/KsJ strain late in the course of the illness. The data recounted here, unless otherwise noted, pertain to the C57BL/6J, a less severely ill animal.

The obesity of the C57BL/6J *ob/ob* mouse is apparent in relation to heterozygotes at a weight of about 30 g, but increased adiposity[32] and fat cell size[8] have been reported in animals 10 to 14 days of age. Fat cell numbers are also increased.[33] Even at 30 g, the relative proportion of body weight represented by fat is increased when compared with controls. Mature animals may weigh 90 g with over 90% of excess weight in the form of fat.[34]

The etiology of the obesity is uncertain, but probably is not due to primary hyperphagia. Obese animals can be fed a restrictive diet sufficient to lower their weight to that of lean littermates and prolong their lifespan.[35] Nonetheless, the proportion of body weight represented by fat remains 2 to 3 times greater in the *ob/ob* animal than in the littermate.[36,37] Considerable data also indicate that the obesity may not be simply secondary to hyperinsulinemia.[38–43] Obesity persists even in the absence of hyperinsulinemia as shown in the *ob/ob* mouse treated with streptozotocin.[38,44] The obese mouse thus appears to exhibit a true "metabolic" rather than a primary "regulatory" defect in control of appetite.

Metabolic studies have revealed increased lipid synthesis in both liver and adipose tissue.[45–53] In fed animals, oxidation of free fatty acids to ketones is diminished.[53,54] While the obese mouse does shift to ketone body oxidation when deprived of food and can survive prolonged fasting,[55] hepatic lipogenesis nonetheless remains elevated even in the fasted state.[56,57] Both acetone metabolism[58] and lipoprotein lipase levels[59] are increased. The animal is probably not hypothyroid[8,60] despite earlier evidence to the contrary.[61] The primary metabolic defect in the obese mouse remains unproven, but it may be a disorder of lipogenesis originating in altered insulin, fatty acid,[49] or glycerol metabolism.[5,62,63] Compounding such metabolic derangements may also be a defect in thermoregulation resulting in decreased thermal energy expenditure.[64] Extending this observation are reports of decreased activity of sodium-potassium ATPase in *ob/ob* mice.[65–67]

Frank diabetes in the obese mouse occurs somewhat after the onset of obesity, although insulin resistance is the earliest detected metabolic abnormality.[68] Clinically the syndrome progresses through three phases.[69] First is a dynamic phase characterized by hyperglycemia, hyperinsulinemia, and increasing weight beginning at 1 month of age. Histologically the beta cell shows marked degranulation. In the second or transitional phase there is improvement of glucose tolerance and normalization of circulating insulin levels. This begins to occur when the mice weigh about 50 g. In the third and final static phase, blood glucose and insulin levels return to near normal. This recovery from the diabetic component of the *ob/ob* syndrome is accompanied by hyperplasia and regranulation of beta cells[70,71] (Fig. 7–1)

Insulin resistance is marked and creates major demands on the beta cell.[72–76] Decreases in insulin receptors on renal,[77] adipose,[78] and liver cells,[77,79–81] as well as lymphocytes[81,82] have been observed. The insulin molecule produced by the obese mouse is biochemically normal,[83] and its beta cells demonstrate a normal biphasic response to glucose when perifused.[84] In isolated islets, however, increased sensitivity to both glucose and fasting has been reported.[85] Glycolytic and gluconeogenic enzymes are elevated in the liver of *ob/ob* mice, but the changes are quantitatively similar to those observed in mice rendered obese by intraperitoneal injections of goldthioglucose known to produce hypothalamic lesions.[86] Whether these increased activities represent a primary derangement, or are secondary to obesity or cerebral disease, is unclear.

Several hormones have been implicated in the syndrome of the obese mouse, but none convincingly. Despite suggestions that growth hormone might play a role,[87–89] plasma levels have been found to be equal in both obese mice and lean controls.[90] The obese mouse does have elevated circulating corticosteroids,[91] and adrenalectomy reduces both glucose and insulin levels.[92] It is reported by one group to lose weight after adrenalectomy.[93] Others report persistent obesity despite adrenalectomy[92] or hypophysectomy.[94]

That there may be some other humoral factor or defect associated with the *ob/ob* syndrome is suggested by two lines of evidence. Strautz[95] implanted into obese mice the islets of normal littermates and reported reversal of the syndrome. The transplanted islets were encased in a filter permitting transfer of small molecules. Strautz inferred a deficiency of some humoral factor of islet origin, but confirmation of this report is still lacking.

Several investigators have created parabiotic pairs of mice by fashioning a cutaneous bridge between two animals along the abdomen.[96–100] Pairs of normal mice show no ill effect of their union and cross-circulate 1 to 2% of their blood volume hourly. When two obese mice are put in parabiotic union, neither is affected. When an obese mouse is joined to a lean littermate, the former eats less and gains weight less rapidly. When in parabiosis with a diabetic *(db/db)* mouse of the same genetic background, the obese mouse becomes completely anorectic and starves to death. These data imply that the obese mouse possesses a receptor for some factor that it fails to produce, a factor possessed in normal quantity by the lean littermate and in excess by the diabetes mouse. Identification and further characterization of this hypothetical factor or factors are lacking. That cholecystokinin might be one such factor was suggested by the much reduced concentrations of this peptide found in the brains of homozygous obese mice when compared to heterozygous or wild-type littermates.[101] There is also

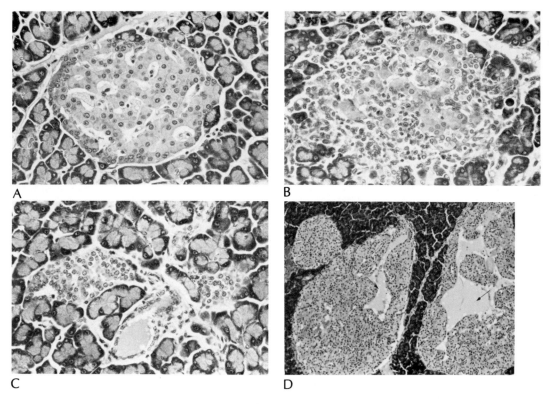

Fig. 7–1. Islet Histopathology in Animals. A. *A Normal Pancreatic Islet.* From a BB rat. Hematoxylin and eosin, ×300. B. *Pancreatic Insulitis.* Pancreatic islet from a BB rat at the onset of hyperglycemia. Hematoxylin and eosin stained section demonstrating insulitis with mononuclear leukocytes permeating and surrounding the islet, ×300. Similar insulitis is seen after multiple dose streptozotocin administration and in the EMC virus model. C. *An Endstage Islet.* Pancreatic islet from a BB rat with advanced diabetes and ketoacidosis. The islet is very small and consists entirely of non-beta cells. Inflammatory cells are absent; there is no fibrosis. Hematoxylin and eosin, ×300. A similar picture is seen after the administration of alloxan and single dose streptozotocin. D. *Hyperplastic Islets.* Islets of an older Wellesley hybrid mouse showing beta cell hyperplasia. Hematoxylin and eosin, ×70. Arrows indicate areas of cystic degeneration characteristic of markedly enlarged islets. A similar picture is seen in the islets of Toronto-KK mice and *ob/ob* mice. With permission of Arthur A. Like, from unpublished material.

a widespread disorder of somatostatin in the *ob/ob* mouse, with greatly reduced quantities found in the pancreas, but increased amounts in the hypothalamus.[102] Lastly, pancreatic polypeptide (PP) is also a suspect factor. One group has reported reduced numbers of PP cells in the islets of the obese mouse together with reversal of its obesity following parenteral administration of bovine PP.[103] This report is as yet unconfirmed, and is at variance with a report of elevated PP levels in the *ob/ob* mouse pancreas by radioimmunoassay.[104] In addition, it has been found that pharmacologic doses of PP cause diarrhea in *ob/ob* mice, making it unlikely that the peptide is purely an anorectic agent in these animals.[105]

A final curious observation on the obese mouse concerns its level of activity. Compared to lean littermates the *ob/ob* mouse is less active as early as 2 weeks of age, prior to the onset of diabetes or obesity,[106] and it remains less active even after

dieting and weight reduction.[107] The implications of this observation for the obese human diabetic are as yet unclear but certainly intriguing.

The Diabetic Mouse

Diabetes *(db)* is a single gene mutation first observed in the mouse at the Jackson Laboratory in the C57BL/KsJ strain.[108] On this background the gene produced marked hyperglycemia, hyperphagia, obesity, and beta cell atrophy. Several alleles producing identical syndromes have been described.[21,109] The previously described mouse mutation designated adipose *(ad)*[110,111] is in fact another allele of *db*.[8] When transferred to the C57BL/6J background, the expression of the diabetes gene is essentially identical to that of the obesity *(ob)* gene. In this section we discuss principally the more severely diabetic phenotype, the C57BL/KsJ *db/db*.

Inheritance of the diabetes syndrome is autosomal recessive with complete penetrance; heterozygotes, although lean, are mildly hyperinsulinemic.[112] Hyperinsulinemia occurs as early as 10 days of age. It has been suggested[30] that the hyperinsulinemia reflects early insulin resistance, but this is not proven. The early phase of hyperinsulinemia is followed, in fact, by a mild hypoglycemia.[30] By 4 weeks of age, however, db/db animals are clearly hyperglycemic, hyperinsulinemic, and hyperphagic. During the early phase of hyperinsulinemia with hypoglycemia, islets are degranulated and give autoradiographic evidence of increased DNA synthesis.[113,114] In the early hyperglycemic phase of the syndrome, progressive degranulation of beta cells occurs[113,115] with further augmentation of DNA synthesis.[114] The C57BL/KsJ db/db thereafter remains markedly hyperglycemic with reduced DNA synthesis until death.[114] Typically, the animals become hypoinsulinemic, begin to lose weight at 4 to 5 months of age, and live less than a year. Glucagon levels remain high and nonsuppressible throughout the hyperglycemic phase of the disease.[116] Histologically, beta cell loss, increased A and D cell numbers, and ductal ingrowth are the major findings. The severe diabetes syndrome terminates in ketosis,[117] but in general the diabetic mouse is rarely absolutely insulin deficient. Insulitis is not observed in the diabetic mouse on either the C57BL/6J or the C57BL/KsJ background but anti-islet immunity has been detected.[117a]

The etiology of the syndrome has not been clearly established. Initial investigations noted several metabolic defects consistent with insulin insensitivity in the periphery: decreased binding to hepatocytes,[81] lifelong increased nonsuppressible gluconeogenesis,[118,119] and failure of exogenous insulin to ameliorate the syndrome.[118] Subsequently, studies in the pre-weaning misty diabetic mouse led Coleman to postulate the primary defect to be insulin hypersecretion.[30] Early hyperinsulinemia due to dysregulation produces hypoglycemia not explained by the insulin insensitivity hypothesis. Hypoglycemia, according to Coleman, may in turn result in hyperphagia, obesity, and stimulation of still greater hyperinsulinemia. The cycle is interrupted only when the number of beta cells fails to meet increasing metabolic demands; hyperglycemia then ensues.

Another possible defect is one of glucagon metabolism. The db/db mouse exhibits hyperglucagonemia that is non-suppressible by conventional techniques.[116] As in the ob/ob mouse, there is extensive maldistribution of somatostatin in the db/db mouse[102] which is of uncertain relevance to the syndrome.

Parabiosis of the diabetic animal with normal littermates produces death of the lean partners from starvation.[97] These experiments suggest that both the diabetic animal and lean littermate possess some humoral satiety factor to which the diabetic animal cannot respond. Interestingly, lesions of the ventromedial hypothalamic "satiety center" of db/db mice prevent the development of hyperglycemia and pancreatic degranulation, but not the obesity or hyperphagia.[120] A defect in this center may be present in db/db mice.

That hyperphagia alone is not the answer to the riddle of the db/db syndrome is suggested by the observation that blood glucose and insulin do not normalize when the animals are dieted.[121] In addition, pair feeding of C57BL/6J db/db mice to lean siblings fails to prevent obesity. Cox and Powley[122] fed diabetic mice precisely the same amount of food at exactly the same time as lean controls for 6 weeks. At the end of that time the db/db mice weighed 42% more than controls, all of the excess weight being fat (Table 7–5). Recently, however, it has been reported that high protein intake can modify the syndrome.[123]

The DBM Mouse

The DBM mouse is an outcross of the diabetic (db/db) mouse.[124,125] It resulted from breeding a diabetic mouse on a C57BL/KsJ background and a misty (m/m) mouse on a C57BL/6J background. It is not to be confused with the C57BL/KsJ db/db m/m inbred strain developed by Coleman.[8,30] The distinction is of some importance since, as noted earlier, the severity of the db/db phenotype is dependent on the genetic background. Data derived from the outcrossed DBM of undefined background are therefore difficult to interpret.

These animals share many features of the db/db mouse and other obese rodents.[124–126] They develop hyperinsulinemia and hyperglycemia at a time when the beta cell displays degranulation and decreased insulin content. Subsequently beta cell hyperplasia develops and blood glucose and insulin normalize. Circulating cortisol is somewhat elevated in the DBM mouse,[127] but the pathogenesis of the syndrome is not known.[125]

Sand Rats (Psammomys obesus)

Sand rats are desert rodents closely related to hamsters and gerbils. Animals studied have come from Egypt and Israel. They are uniquely equipped for their native environments, surviving on desert vegetation. In the wild state, or when fed their naturally occurring vegetable diet in captivity, these animals are lean, euglycemic, and somewhat hypometabolic.[128] Diabetes in wild or food restricted sand rats has not been noted.

When allowed free access to laboratory chow,

Table 7–5.   Contrasting Effects of Diet on Animal Models of Diabetes

	Diet	Weight	Carcass Fat	Plasma Insulin	Hyperglycemia
Non-ketotic Chinese hamster (230)	Restricted	lean	normal	normal	absent
	Unrestricted	lean	normal	↑	present
Wellesley hybrid mouse (C3Hf × I) (191)	Restricted	lean	normal	normal	absent
	Unrestricted	obese	↑	↑	present
Diabetes (db/db) (121, 122)	Restricted	42% greater than controls*	↑ *	↑ †	mild
	Unrestricted	grossly obese*	↑ ↑ *	↓ †	severe
Sand rat (Psammomys obesus) (128–134)	Natural	lean	normal	normal	absent
	Laboratory	obese	↑ ↑	↓ ‡	mild

*C57BL/6J db/db (122)
†C57BL/KsJ db/db (121) over 3 months of age
‡Ketotic sand rat only

several extraordinary changes occur. About one-third of the animals become hyperphagic, hyperinsulinemic, and at least mildly hyperglycemic.[129–133] With time most animals become obese and severely hyperglycemic. Insulin resistance is marked.[131,134–136] At the cellular level dietary abundance produces islet enlargement, beta cell degranulation, glycogen infiltration, and increased protein synthesis.[132,137,138] Euglycemic and intermittently hyperglycemic animals generally show normal or increased amounts of pancreatic insulin.[131,132,134] In vitro studies show pancreatic insulin release in the sand rat to be 5 to 25 times that observed in other diabetic rodents.[139] A small number of these animals have developed frank beta cell necrosis and lethal diabetic ketoacidosis.[140] In these animals pancreatic insulin is decreased.[138] Insulitis is not observed.

Interestingly, the development of ketosis has been highly unpredictable. Nearly all of the first group of these animals studied at the Joslin Research Laboratories in 1966 became severely ketotic[140] with histologic evidence of beta cell degeneration and necrosis.[138] However, later shipments of animals from the Middle East and animals bred in captivity have failed to develop predictable ketosis.[141]

The sand rat is similar to the Chinese hamster in exemplifying a diabetic syndrome extending along a spectrum of beta cell insufficiency to beta cell death. The ketotic sand rat is dramatic in its demonstration of the role of metabolic-dietary stress in uncovering a genetic predisposition to a lethal diabetic syndrome (Table 7–5).

The obese sand rat is among the animals which exemplify the concept of diabetes as the expression of a "thrifty" genotype.[142,143] According to this theory a tendency to diabetes may have afforded an evolutionary survival advantage to certain species. Since insulin is anabolic, favoring the synthesis of glycogen, protein, and lipid, an animal with a capacity for high insulin output and efficient caloric storage would be well adapted to an environment where calories were scarce. Super-efficient sequestration of calories would confer an advantage to such animals as the sand rat. That advantage in the natural habitat becomes a liability only when overwhelmed by an unnatural dietary abundance. The same phenomenon may apply to db/db and to ob/ob mice. Not only are homozygotes capable of prolonged fasting, but lean heterozygotes as well appear to share an enhanced resistance to starvation.[144]

Spiny Mice (Acomys cahirinus)

Spiny "mice" are rodents related to mice but taxonomically distinct. Their natural habitat is the Middle East. They have been studied most extensively in the laboratories of Renold in Geneva[117,145,146] and of Shafrir and Gutman in Jerusalem.

Glycosuria occurred in about 40% of animals studied prior to 1965. In the majority of cases, somewhat over 85%, these animals remained either intermittently or persistently hyperglycemic without ketosis.[10] On average, the animals were mildly obese, although the incidence of obesity observed declined with time.[10] Among animals studied in the late 1960s plasma insulin levels correlated with weight suggesting that excessive weight gain might be secondary to hyperinsulinemia.[147] Histopathologically the diabetes of the spiny mouse is characterized initially by beta cell hyperplasia and an increase in pancreatic immunoreactive insulin; the hyperplasia may be extraordinary with islets comprising 15 to 25% of pancreatic mass.[145,146,148] Plasma insulin levels tend to be minimally elevated, but only briefly. Studies both in vivo and in isolated islets have suggested a defect in the release of insulin in response to glucose, particularly in the early phase of secretion.[84,149–151] Why a certain number of the first animals studied progressed to ketoacidosis and insulin dependence in the context of massive islet hypertrophy and hyperplasia is unclear. It has been shown, however, that the development of ketosis was preceded by an increase in plasma insulin followed by a decrease in both pancreatic and plasma insulin.[5] Although it was initially reported that the islets of spiny mice lacked innervation,[152] neuronal terminations in the pancreata of these animals have now been identified.[153] Other potential pathogenic mechanisms include alteration or decrease in islet cell microtubular protein[154] and decreased production of cyclic AMP during the early phase of stimulated insulin release.[155]

The development of ketosis was facilitated by caloric abundance in early life, but the incidence of ketosis has fallen with time despite unchanging conditions of housing and nutrition, and despite the persistence of abnormal pancreatic islets, both biochemically and histologically.[155]

The KK Mouse

The KK mouse is a mildly obese diabetic animal originally raised in Japan.[156,157] Subsequent grafting of the syndrome to the C57BL/6 mouse yielded an inbred variant called the Toronto-KK mouse.[158] Transfer of the Yellow (A^y) gene to the KK produced the yellow-KK.[159,160] The genetics of the KK mouse are not completely understood. Initially deemed polygenic,[161] it has more recently been regarded as the result of a single dominant gene with reduced penetrance mediated by recessive modifiers.[29]

Diminished glucose tolerance and hyperphagia are noted at about 2 months of age in both yellow and Toronto-KK mice.[162,163] This same syndrome also develops in the Japanese-KK mouse but only when fed a high calorie diet, thus making this animal useful in the study of the development of carbohydrate intolerance.[161,164] Maximal blood glucose concentrations are observed between 4 and 9 months of age[162,165] at which time insulin resistance is prominent.[158,165,166] By 1 year of age hyperglycemic animals go into remission with normalization of blood glucose and insulin occurring prior to reduction in food intake and body weight.[162] The beta cells of the KK mouse display hyperplasia, hypertrophy, and degranulation in proportion to the animal's hyperglycemia.[165]

The genesis of the syndrome is in dispute. Iwatsuka[166] noted that the insulin resistance of the Japanese KK was independent of cell size. He postulated a genetic defect in insulin sensitivity leading to both chronically elevated blood glucose and persistently increased lipogenesis. Appel et al.,[167] however, found that insulin failed to suppress gluconeogenesis in the KK mouse. They postulated that unimpeded glucose production caused a chronically increased glucose load and secondary hyperinsulinemia with attendant obesity. Hyperphagia is also a common feature of all KK strains, and the syndrome may be controlled and reversed with diet.[158] The possibility of a primary disorder of appetite in the KK mouse has not been excluded.

The Yellow Mouse

The yellow mouse was described by Lataste[168] in 1884. The original dominant allele designated A^y was found to be lethal when homozygous.[169,170] Two further mutations which arose at the Jackson Laboratory proved to be viable when homozygous and are designated A^{vy}, or viable yellow[171] and A^{iy}, or intermediate yellow. These mice are characterized by mild glucose intolerance and obesity.

While fasting blood glucose levels are equal in obese yellow mice and controls, feeding reveals the former to be glucose intolerant.[172,173] Histologically, both hypertrophy and hyperplasia of beta cells are observed.[174] Hyperinsulinemia is also present; its degree varies with the coat color, being highest in the phenotypically pure yellow mouse.[175,176]

Obesity in this mouse is also greatest in the pure yellow variant.[175] It is greater in males than females,[172,177,178] and appears to be affected by the background genome as well.[25] The obesity is hypertrophic in character.[179] Younger mice are hyperphagic[180] while older ones eat less and lose weight.[178,181] Obesity shortens the lifespan of obese yellow mice when compared to lean littermates.[182] As in the case of the obese mouse, parabiosis of an obese yellow mouse heterozygote (A^y/a) to a non-yellow, results in amelioration of obesity.[173] Abnormalities of fat cells[183] and adrenal function[174] have also been demonstrated. Adrenalectomy reportedly prevents obesity[174] and hyperadrenocorticism may bear on its pathogenesis. The absence of growth hormone does not affect development of the syndrome, however.[184]

The Yellow KK Mouse

Offspring of a cross between yellow (A^y) and Toronto KK mice uniformly develop diabetes and obesity.[160] Animals become hyperinsulinemic by 2 months of age and hyperglycemic by 3 months of age.[185] Insulin levels may be high, over 4000 μU/

ml.[185] These animals exhibit hyperadrenocorticism and adrenal hyperplasia, but such changes follow the development of diabetes and are thought not to be the cause of the diabetic syndrome.[186]

The PBB/Ld Mouse

This animal is a recently described, inbred model of obesity and diabetes.[187,188] Its inheritance may be polygenic. It is characterized by decreased glucose tolerance, hyperinsulinemia, adipocyte hyperplasia, and hyperlipidemia. Islets show little, if any, light microscopic pathology.

The Wellesley Hybrid Mouse (C3hf x I)

This mouse was developed at Wellesley College as a cross of the inbred I and C3Hf lines during the course of cancer studies.[189] About 50% of males and 5% of females develop at least intermittent glycosuria. The animals are also moderately obese with hyperglycemia and hyperinsulinemia in proportion to obesity.[190] The syndrome is entirely reversible with dietary restriction[190,191] (Table 7–5). Histopathologically, obese hyperglycemic animals show markedly enlarged islets (Fig. 7–1) comprised mostly of beta cells actively synthesizing insulin.[192,193]

The NZO Mouse

The New Zealand Obese (NZO) mouse was developed by Bielschowsky and Bielschowsky.[194] Its mode of inheritance is not well understood but is probably polygenic. The NZO syndrome is similar to that of other obese rodents; the animals are grossly overweight,[10,69] mildly hyperglycemic[195] and mildly hyperinsulinemic.[83] The hyperglycemia is more pronounced in males than females.[196] The most distinctive clinical feature of the syndrome is monotonic progression of both obesity and glucose intolerance with age.[69] Neither remission nor ketoacidosis is observed. Insulin secretion in response to common stimuli is abnormal, predominantly in the early phase.[197–199] In contrast to other obese diabetic rodents, NZO mice respond to long-term administration of sulfonylurea with increased insulin secretion and a fall in blood glucose.[200] Dietary restriction also improves insulin secretion.[201] Gluconeogenic enzyme activity is chronically elevated[202] and is not insulin suppressible,[202,203] a pattern common to most obese rodents. Insulin sensitivity is also diminished.[195,204] Pathologically, islet tissue shows only mild hyperplasia of beta cells.[195]

The obesity of this animal is marked; it may weigh as much as 100 g. As with other obese mice, the proportion of fat in NZO animals remains elevated even after weight reduction.[205] In contrast to the hypertrophic and hyperplastic obesity of the *ob/ob* mouse, adipose tissue of the NZO is predominantly hypertrophic. If fed a high fat diet when young, however, the NZO does develop adipose hyperplasia as well.[206] The etiology of this syndrome is unknown. A generalized syndrome of autoimmunity has recently been described in this animal, but its relationship to the diabetes is unclear.[207] It has been reported that either islet transplantation[208,209] or parenteral administration of pancreatic polypeptide[210] can reverse both the obesity and the carbohydrate intolerance. These reports remain to be confirmed.

The Tuco-tuco (Ctenomys talarum)

Tuco-tucos are burrowing rodents from Argentina. Wise and his colleagues[211,212] found that these animals exhibit both hyperglycemia and ketosis, but they are not insulin dependent. Insulin levels have not been measured. While lean in the wild, the animals tend to become obese in captivity. Blood glucose correlates with body weight.[212] It is speculated that both dietary abundance and enforced inactivity are important factors in the development of the obesity in these animals.[14] Histologically, islets tend to be degranulated and hyperplastic in hyperglycemic animals, but data are few.[212] The most striking pathologic finding is an extraordinary frequency of cataracts which appears to correlate with elevated blood glucose levels.[211,212]

The Djungarian Hamster (Phodopus sungorus)

Djungarian hamsters are obese rodents bred by Herberg and her colleagues.[14,213,214] The animals that are glycosuric are also hyperglycemic, hyperinsulinemic, and hypertriglyceridemic. Their islets show both hypertrophy and hyperplasia. The beta cells of non-glycosuric animals show diminished responsiveness to glucose, while in glycosuric animals stimulated insulin secretion is exaggerated. Inheritance appears to be polygenic. Most, but not all, animals are obese.

SPONTANEOUS SYNDROMES IN NON-OBESE ANIMALS

The BB Rat

The heritable diabetic syndrome of the BB rat was noted as a spontaneous mutation in the Wistar rat at the Bio-Breeding Laboratory in Canada.[215–217] The BB rat diabetes syndrome is characterized by absolute insulin deficiency and several other unique features which make its analogy to human IDDM relatively close. As bred at the University of Massachusetts in Worcester, about 30% of BB rats become glucose intolerant; another 30% develop frank ketoacidosis. The ketotic syndrome is lethal within 1 to 2 weeks unless treated with insulin. The time at which diabetes develops is relatively consistent, between 60 and 120 days of age. Diabetes occurs equally in both sexes, obesity is absent, and the frequency of diabetes has increased with inbreeding. Inheritance is unknown, but the working hypothesis is that transmission is autosomal recessive with variable penetrance. Several genes appear to be involved. The syndrome almost never remits spontaneously.[217a,217b]

The metabolic defects of the diabetic BB rat are similar to those seen in humans with IDDM: insulin deficiency; increased plasma glucagon and somatostatin; elevated levels of glucose, free fatty acids, and branched-chain amino acids; and absence of insulin response to arginine and tolbutamide.[215] Histopathologically the pancreata of diabetics display an intense insulitis. Animals at an early stage of their illness, at the very first manifestation of glycosuria, show small islets, reduced beta cell numbers, and striking infiltration of the islets with lymphocytes and macrophages (Fig. 7–1). At the end stage of the disease, islets are small and composed exclusively of A, D, and PP cells.[215] Insulitis precedes diabetes by 2 to 3 weeks.[215a]

This sequence of initial insulitis progressing to frank beta cell destruction is consonant with our present understanding of the pathology of human IDDM.

The BB rat offers an opportunity to study in detail the early phase of insulin-deficient diabetes and, in particular, the roles of infection and autoimmunity. To test the possibility of an infectious etiology for the diabetes of this animal, BB rats have been raised in a sterile environment. Under carefully maintained gnotobiotic conditions it was possible to exclude both viral and bacterial pathogens on the basis of negative cultures, stains, and complement fixation titers. Despite the sterility of the environment, the expected percentage of rats nonetheless become diabetic.[218] Histologically the pancreata of these animals showed either typical insulitis or end stage islets. This experiment implies that infection is not a prerequisite for the development of the BB rat syndrome and suggests a genetically mediated pathogenesis. Additional studies have shown that dietary manipulation, castration, hypophysectomy, nicotinamide, and stress do not alter the incidence of diabetes.[218a]

The role of the immune system in the pathogenesis of diabetes has been studied intensively in the BB rat. Thyroid, gastric parietal cell, splenic lymphocyte, and smooth muscle autoantibodies have been detected in these animals.[218b,218c] Islet cell surface antibodies in a radio-ligand assay using protein

A have been found.[218d] They may be complement-fixing and cytolytic.[218g]

Marked lymphopenia has been observed in the peripheral blood of BB rats,[217b,218e] particularly involving helper T-cell subsets.[218f] However, subsequent studies also suggest depression in suppressor T-lymphocyte subsets.[218e]

Immune interventions have been reported to alter both the course and incidence of BB diabetes. Acutely diabetic rats and non-diabetic littermates were given either rabbit anti-rat lymphocyte serum (ALS), 500 rads of whole body irradiation, or no treatment.[219] Normalization of glycemia occurred in 36% of ALS treated rats and 13% of irradiated animals, but in none of the untreated controls. Histologically partial reversal of insulitis was noted. In addition, the nondiabetic littermates given treatment failed to develop hyperglycemia in expected numbers, suggesting that some susceptible animals had been protected from the disease. More recent studies have indicated that neonatal thymectomy[220] and cyclosporin[220a,220b] prevent the development of diabetes in BB rats.

Transplantation of neonatal bone marrow from another strain of rat also prevents diabetes in susceptible BB rats.[220c] It has further been shown that whole blood transfusions not only prevent diabetes in BB rats, but also restore the depressed concanavalin A responsiveness of BB rat lymphocytes towards normal.[220d] T-lymphocytes may be the protective component of the transfusions.[220f]

Passive transfer of insulitis from acutely diabetic BB rats into nude mice has been reported.[220e] However, it has not been confirmed in other studies.[221]

Recently it has been demonstrated that concanavalin A treated splenic cells from diabetic rats can be used to transfer BB diabetes to nondiabetic recipients.[222] These studies all lend strength to the autoimmune hypothesis of the pathogenesis of BB rat diabetes.

Glucose intolerant but noninsulin-dependent BB rats have also been studied. Initial pathologic observations indicate that 57% of glucose-intolerant rats display some degree of insulitis regardless of whether or not they progress to ketoacidosis.[218] A number of nondiabetic but glucose-intolerant BB rats undergo spontaneous normalization of glucose tolerance, though the precise figure is as yet unknown. Lymphocyte thyroiditis also occurs in the BB rat.[222a]

The Chinese Hamster (Cricetulus griseus)

The Chinese hamster has been studied extensively for nearly 2 decades, primarily by Gerritsen and his collaborators.[26,223–229] With successive inbred generations, onset of diabetes has become relatively predictable at 2 to 3 months of age, though glycosuria may appear at up to 15 months of age.[223] About 50% of diabetic hamsters die within 14 months, whereas the normal lifespan is well over 2 years.[26,223] The earliest clinical manifestation in the prediabetic population (which may be identified precisely in the case of offspring of two ketotic parents) is hyperphagia.[230] Interestingly, despite the ingestion of 27% more food these prediabetic animals remain lean.[231] They exhibit normal caloric retention, with decreased absorption of fat and increased excretion of carbohydrates in urine and feces.[224] Hyperphagia is speculated to be the primary metabolic derangement in this form of animal diabetes.[26] Dietary restriction during the weaning period, particularly restriction of fat, can ameliorate the hyperglycemia and preclude the development of ketosis.[230] Prolonged food restriction produces clinically normal hamsters[230] (Table 7–5).

The development of glycosuria at 2 to 3 months of age is reflected pathologically in degranulation of the beta cells.[223,224,232] With time, beta cell numbers fall, and both pancreatic and circulating insulin decline.[223,224,233] Morphologic studies by electron microscopy reveal multiple alterations of the beta cell.[234,235] Alpha cells also undergo change characterized by lysosomal digestion of secretory granules.[227] In contrast to human IDDM, however, insulitis, total absence of beta cells, and absolute insulin deficiency have not been observed. Supplemental insulin delivered by infusion pumps ameliorates the diabetic syndrome substantially.[236] Mortality among ketotic hamsters is most frequently due to urinary tract disease.[26,237]

The question arises as to whether the ketotic and nonketotic forms of diabetes in Chinese hamsters represent different syndromes or segments of the spectrum of one disease. The answer is not clear. The capacity for beta cell hypertrophy and hyperplasia in response to beta cell loss could determine the amount of available insulin and the nature of the syndrome. Both the greater cell loss in ketotic animals and the marked islet hyperplasia of hyperglycemic hamsters in remission[226,235] are consonant with this simple algebraic view. On the other hand, some animals have glucose intolerance despite a normal plasma insulin level, suggesting defects in insulin action or hepatic glucose output.[238] In addition, certain islet abnormalities including reduced insulin stores[228,239] and decreased glucose responsiveness[229] have been noted and favor other diabetogenic mechanisms. Thus, genetic defects in cell replication, metabolism, and responsiveness may all play a role.

The Japanese Wistar Rat (The Goto Rat)

In Japan another diabetic syndrome of the Wistar rat has been recognized.[240,241] In contrast to the BB rat, these animals do not become insulin dependent nor do they develop insulitis. Pathologically, their islets show hydropic degeneration and vacuolization. A curious unconfirmed study reports amelioration of this syndrome by "islet activating protein," a substance obtained from culture medium in which are grown Bordetella pertussis bacteria.[242] The meaning of this observation remains obscure.

The Celebese Ape (Macaca nigra)

Macaca nigra, often called the Celebese black ape, has been studied by Howard and his colleagues.[243–249] It is the only subhuman diabetic primate as yet studied systematically. The genetics of the syndrome are unknown, but the prevalence of glucose intolerance in the Howard colony is about 50%.[245] The animals are lean; hyperglycemia is mild; ketosis is not observed. Onset occurs in juvenile apes but details of the epidemiology are yet to be defined. The few available examples of pancreatic histology reveal beta cell degranulation without insulitis.[249] The most striking pathologic feature is the presence of extensive amyloid infiltration of the islets.[243,245,246] The relationship of this nonobese, nonketotic diabetic syndrome to the human is unknown. Its pathologic situation may correlate with the occasional observation of amyloid in the human diabetic pancreas.

Other Primates

No well documented cases of gestational diabetes have been reported, but the literature does strongly suggest the occurrence of this syndrome in the monkey. Both DiGiacomo et al.[17] and Valerio et al.[18] noted hyperglycemia in female rhesus monkeys (Macaca mulatta) which had previously delivered infants of excessive birthweight. Possible worsening of diabetes during a subsequent pregnancy has been reported.[19,19a] Studies of the diabetic rhesus are continuing.[250–253] Diabetes in the squirrel monkey has also been reported.[254]

The Diabetic Guinea Pig

A colony of guinea pigs with a high incidence of hyperglycemia has been developed by Munger and his associates.[255–258] These are lean animals which develop moderate hyperglycemia but never become ketoacidotic. Pathologically the beta cells show fatty change, glycogen infiltration, and possible inclusion bodies, but no insulitis.[255] Interest has been focused on the possibility of an infectious etiology.[255] Normal animals placed in proximity to hyperglycemic animals become glycosuric with regularity. As yet, however, there is neither proof of an infectious agent nor detailed analysis of the metabolic derangement.

The South African Hamster (Mystromys albicaudatus)

The South African hamster, also known as the African White Tailed Rat, is a nonobese rodent studied by Stuhlman and his colleagues.[259,260] Approximately 50% of the animals in their colony develop hyperglycemia. About 10% develop severe hyperglycemia (up to 2300 mg/dl), with ketosis and death within 2 months if untreated.[261] Pathologically, the beta cells of hyperglycemic animals show only hyperplasia and glycogen deposition; those of severely hyperglycemic ketotic animals show degranulation, changes of cytoplasmic structures, nuclear pyknosis, and necrosis.[262,263] Insulitis has not been described. While the animals are not obese, blood sugar levels correlate positively with weight.[264]

The Nonobese Diabetic ("NOD") Mouse

Also called the Tochino mouse, this is a newly discovered insulin deficient animal from Japan. These mice are derived from the CTS strain. They are lean, ketosis prone, and appear to develop pancreatic insulitis. About 80% of males and 20% of females are affected.[265] Interestingly, nicotinamide ameliorates this syndrome,[265a] which appears to have multiple immunologic abnormalities.[265b]

Other Animals

Isolated and unconfirmed reports of severe diabetes, in some instances accompanied by post-mortem findings suggestive of insulitis, exist for the antelope,[7] ground squirrel,[4] and rhesus monkey.[12] The nature of the underlying diabetes in dogs and cats has not been studied systematically. Only rare reports, such as one of a diabetic cat,[2] suggest insulin deficiency with possible insulitis. Spontaneous diabetes in the dog is a hypoinsulinemic, ketosis prone disease requiring insulin therapy in those cases where it has been studied. The etiology is not clear. Both selective islet destruction and severe pancreatitis have been implicated.[266]

EXPERIMENTAL DIABETES

Diabetes both in humans and animals may be provoked by stress, infection, or toxins. Certain other manipulations, including pancreatectomy,[267] and lesioning of the central nervous system, can also produce diabetes. In the majority of cases the agents used to produce experimental diabetes in animals are not thought to play a major role in human pathophysiology. Nonetheless the ensuing animal syndromes mimic the human disease and thus merit close attention.

Contra-Insulin Hormones

Epinephrine, glucagon, glucocorticoids, and growth hormone all have an effect antagonistic to insulin. When present in excess, either as a physiologic response to stress or as a pathologic consequence of tumor or other metabolic derangement, glucose tolerance is reduced and hyperglycemia may ensue. Epinephrine and glucagon exert the same contra-insulin effect in animals as in humans when administered in excess. Studies have reported the induction of hyperglycemia and beta cell hyperplasia in mice,[268] rabbits,[269,270] rats,[271–273] guinea pigs,[274,275] and monkeys,[276,277] following exposure to hydrocortisone or ACTH.

Hypothalamic Diabetes

Hypothalamic lesions can cause obesity both in animals[278] and in humans.[279] Some humans with hypothalamic obesity have both insulin resistance and noninsulin-dependent diabetes mellitus. The severity of the diabetes, however, tends to be in proportion to the obesity.[279] The best studied animal model of this syndrome is the rat or mouse with lesions of the ventromedial nuclei (VMH) of the hypothalamus. These lesions may be either electrolytic or chemical, the latter being easily inducible only in the mouse by means of goldthioglucose,[280,281] a toxin whose uptake into the hypothalamus is insulin-dependent.[282] Adult rats subject to VMH lesions become obese, hyperglycemic, hyperinsulinemic, and insulin resistant.[283] In these rats, both growth hormone[284] and thyroid[285] levels are reduced. Most interestingly, if *weanling* rats are subjected to the same lesion, a different syndrome ensues in which are observed: (1) hyperinsulinemia but not hyperglycemia and (2) an increase in carcass fat without obesity or hyperphagia.[284,286] VMH lesioning in the diabetic mouse also prevents hyperglycemia, but not obesity.[120] The ventromedial hypothalamic syndrome in the rat can be abolished by subdiaphragmatic vagotomy.[287] Curiously VMH lesioning appears to protect against the development of seizures following insulin-induced hypoglycemia in mice.[288] An intriguing report is that of passive transfer of an appetite suppressant factor from the serum of goldthioglucose-lesioned mice to normal mice.[289] This report is consonant with the results of parabiosis experiments using *db/db* mice discussed earlier, but is as yet unconfirmed. The factor has not been identified.

Virus-Induced Diabetes

The temporal relationship of viral syndromes and onset of human IDDM, and the demonstration of Coxsackie B4 virus in the islets of a boy who died

Table 7–6. Viral Diabetes in Animals*

Virus	Type	Species	Comment
Encephalomyocarditis (EMC)	RNA	Mouse	Produces beta cell degranulation and necrosis with subsequent hyperglycemia. Pancreatic acinar cells also affected. A-cells functionally abnormal.[291–298b]
Coxsackie B	RNA	Mouse	Focal exocrine pancreatic inflammation.[306] Necrotizing exocrine lesions.[307,308] Fine structural alterations of beta cells without necrosis or hyperglycemia.[301–305] P14 passaged in B-cell culture produces mononuclear cell infiltration and islet disruption.[308,308a]
Mumps	RNA	Monkey	Beta cell infection documented in vitro only.
Foot-and-Mouth Disease	RNA	Cattle	Almost total islet cell necrosis with round cell infiltration.[290b]
		Mice	Beta cell degranulation and subcellular changes, especially in mitochondria.[290c]
		Guinea Pigs	Alterations in pancreatic zymogen tissue.[290d,290e]
Venezuelan Equine Encephalitis	RNA	Mice	Beta cell degranulation and subcellular changes, especially in mitochondria.[300a]
		Hamsters	Focal acinar necrosis.[300b]
		Monkey	No histologic changes within 10 months after inoculation.[300c]
Rubella	RNA	Rabbits	Beta cell degranulation and changes in subcellular organelles.[300d]
Reovirus (Type 3)	RNA	Mice	Focal to extensive islet cell necrosis with infiltration of islets by inflammatory cells.[300e]
C-Type Virus induced by multidose streptozotocin	RNA	CD-1 Mouse	Insulitis.[322,330–334]
Spontaneous (transmissible agent) diabetes mellitus		Guinea Pig	Degranulation of beta cells and cytoplasmic inclusions with sparing of A and D cells.[255,256]

*Modified from Rayfield and Seto[290a]

with acute onset IDDM,[290] have rekindled interest in animal models of virus-related diabetes. The role of viruses in the pathogenesis of animal diabetes, however, remains uncertain in all but a few instances. While viral particles have been described in several spontaneously diabetic animals, most notably *db/db* mice,[113] no animal models are of proven viral etiology. Most documented viral diabetes syndromes in animals are associated with generalized illnesses including rubella, encephalitis, myocarditis, and foot-and-mouth disease.[290b–290e] The majority are RNA viruses and all are highly species specific. The best studied models of viral animal diabetes are listed with references in Table 7–6.

The M variant of the encephalomyocarditis (EMC) virus of mice is one of the most important viral animal models.[291–298] Injection of this virus into certain strains of adult male mice causes non-insulin-dependent diabetes in about 40% of the animals. The occurrence of diabetes correlates with the ability of the beta cell to support viral replication. Histologic examination of the islets shows typical insulitis, which in turn has suggested that a cell-mediated immune response may play an important role in this form of beta cell destruction.

Supporting this hypothesis is the observation that irradiation of infected mice reduces the magnitude of subsequent hyperglycemia. The EMC syndrome also highlights the importance of the background genome in the development of diabetes, since it is both strain- and sex-specific.[299,300]

With the exception of the Type C virus seen following multiple-dose streptozotocin administration (to be discussed below), no other viruses are associated with the intense insulitis seen with EMC viral infections. The Coxsackie B virus, clearly implicated in at least one case of fatal human diabetes,[290] produces only fine structural alterations of beta cells in animals[301–305] while causing pronounced exocrine pancreatic lesions.[306–308] The diabetogenicity of several viruses in animals has been increased by serial passage in tissue culture, possibly by selecting organisms adapted to growth in beta cells. The hyperglycemia of the guinea pig was mentioned previously as possibly of infectious origin.

Chemical Agents Capable of Inducing Diabetes

The use of chemical agents to produce diabetes permits detailed study of the biochemical, hor-

Table 7–7. Chemical Agents Capable of Inducing Diabetes

A. Irreversible Beta-Cytotoxic Agents

Alloxan
Streptozotocin
Diphenylthiocarbazine
Oxine-9-hydroxyquinolone
Vacor

B. Reversible Beta-Cytotoxic Agents

6-Aminonicotinamide
L-Asparaginase
Azide
Cyanide
Cyproheptadine
Dehydroascorbic Acid
Fluoride
Iodoacetate
Phenytoin
Malonate
Thiazides
2-Deoxyglucose
Mannoheptulose

C. Other Agents

Anti-insulin antibodies
Somatostatin
Catecholamines
Glucocorticoids
Glucagon

Table 7–8. Species Susceptibility to the Beta-Cytotoxic Effects of Alloxan and Streptozotocin

	Streptozotocin	Alloxan
Man	?	+
Monkey	+	+
Dog	+	+
Cat	−	+
Rat	+	+
Mouse	+	+
Lamb/Sheep	+	+
Chinese Hamster	+	?
Hamster	?	+
Rabbit	±	+
Spiny Mouse	−	?
Mini Pig	+	?
Turtle	?	+
Pigeon	?	+
Fish	−	?
Guinea Pig	±	−
Chicken	−	−

monal, and morphologic events that occur during and after the induction of a diabetic state. Several classes of agents produce such effects. First are the cell-specific toxins which destroy beta cells and cause a primary insulin-deficient state. Second are those agents which act on the beta cell, but do not destroy it. A third class increases endogenous insulin requirements, stresses the pancreas, and secondarily produces diabetes. This last group includes the contra-insulin hormones previously discussed, as well as anti-insulin antibodies. Compounds that have been studied are listed in Table 7–7.

The two agents that have been most extensively studied and have yielded the vast majority of information pertinent to human diabetes are alloxan and streptozotocin. Both are beta cytotoxins which, in diabetogenic doses, are relatively free of nonspecific toxic effects. As was the case regarding spontaneous and viral diabetes in animals, the effectiveness of these diabetogenic chemical agents is highly dependent on the age, sex, and species of the recipient. In contrast to most other chemical agents capable of inducing diabetes, there is a wide margin of safety with these two compounds. The effective diabetogenic dose (ED_{50}) is 4 to 5 times lower than the lethal dose (LD_{50}).

Table 7–8 lists those species that are susceptible to the diabetogenic effects of alloxan and streptozotocin. Both sexes are susceptible. In most animals the toxicity of both compounds seems specific for the beta cell exclusively. Only in the Chinese hamster is there a suggestion that streptozotocin may cause alpha cell damage.[309] Table 7–9 lists some of the characteristics of these two widely used compounds. Readers interested in other diabetogenic agents are referred to Dulin and Soret,[310] Fischer and Rickert,[311] Okamoto,[312] and Rerup.[313]

Alloxan. Alloxan was first noted to have diabetogenic activity by Dunn in the course of studies on the effect of uric acid derivatives on the kidney following trauma.[314] Its mechanism of action is not known. Hypotheses have included chelation of intracellular zinc, Strecker reactions (alpha amino acid deamination and decarboxylation), deletion of sulfhydryl groups, and interference with various enzyme systems.[313] A major shortcoming of all of these hypotheses is their inability to account for the lack on toxicity in non-beta cells. Available evidence indicates that the initial effect of alloxan is mediated through some form of membrane interaction on the surface of the beta cell. Autoradiographic studies using ^{14}C alloxan reveal a high affinity on the drug for islet cell membranes.[315] Evidence has also been advanced for membrane permeability changes that could lead to necrosis,[316,317] but a definitive explanation for the highly specific toxicity of alloxan is lacking.

Following administration of alloxan to a susceptible animal, a slight fall in blood glucose occurs, followed by mild hyperglycemia within 1 to 4 hours. About 4 to 8 hours after administration, hypoglycemia recurs, probably as a result of the release of stored insulin by dying beta cells. Within 24 to 48 hours permanent hyperglycemia is established. Histopathologically, reduction of beta cell

Table 7–9. Characteristics of Alloxan and Streptozotocin

	Alloxan	Streptozotocin
Chemical Name	2,4,5,6-tetraoxy-hexahydropyrimidine	2-deoxy-2-(3-methyl-3-nitrosourea)-D-glucopyranose
Most Effective Route of Administration	I.V.	I.V. or I.P.
Circulatory Half-Life	1 minute	15 minutes; metabolites probably longer
Effect of Fasting on Diabetogenic Activity	↑ Sensitivity	Little effect
Potentiators of the Diabetogenic Effect	Hypoglycemia	None Known
Agents Protective Against Diabetogenicity:		
Glucose	+++	±
Nicotinic acid	++	−
Nicotinamide	+++	+++
3-0-methylglucose	++++	++++
2-deoxyglucose	−	++
D-Mannose	+	−
Glutathione	++++	−
Superoxide dismutase	≥ +	≥ +

numbers with sparing of other islet components is noted; insulitis is not observed.

Two interesting features of the alloxan model deserve further comment. One is the ability of certain sugars to protect an animal against its effects. When given before alloxan, glucose and to a lesser degree fructose and mannose can prevent or ameliorate the subsequent hyperglycemia.[318–321] More recently it has been shown that the protection afforded by sugars is highly stereospecific, being greater for alpha anomers.[321,322] Certain enzymes including superoxide dismutase and catalase are also protective.[323] The second noteworthy feature is the absence of alloxan toxicity in the guinea pig. It has been noted that the guinea pig beta cell lacks zinc, and it may well be that interference with zinc metabolism is important for the mechanism of action of alloxan.

Streptozotocin. Streptozotocin, an N-nitroso derivative of D-glucosamine, was initially isolated from cultures of *Streptomyces achromogenes,* but subsequently has been synthesized in the laboratory.[324] Like alloxan, streptozotocin is a relatively selective beta cytotoxin in certain animal species, causing an initial triphasic glucose response and then permanent diabetes. Cell membrane binding is again the likely first step in the pathologic process. In the case of streptozotocin, the alpha anomer of the glucosamine moiety has been shown to render the compound more cytotoxic than the beta anomer, suggesting that the drug's toxicity is mediated through specific recognition by some receptor on the beta cell.[325] It has further been suggested that the glucose component of streptozotocin enhances its uptake into the beta cell where the cytotoxicity of the nitrosourea moiety can be con-

centrated.[326–328] Removal of the glucose moiety renders the compound much less specifically toxic for beta cells;[310] substitution of galactose for glucose also decreases its effectiveness.[311] Within the beta cell streptozotocin is believed to reduce levels of nicotine adenine dinucleotide (NAD) by both decreasing its synthesis and increasing its breakdown.[328] Nicotinamide protects animals against the cytotoxicity of both streptozotocin and alloxan. Histopathologically, beta cell necrosis without insulitis is routinely observed.[310,329] As is the case with alloxan, certain carbohydrates have the ability to protect the beta cell against streptozotocin, but among them only 3-0-methyl glucose protects equally well against both.[329]

Streptozotocin-induced Insulitis. An important advance in the study of streptozotocin has come with the development of multidose administration at the Joslin Diabetes Center. If a single small sub-diabetogenic dose of streptozotocin is given to an animal, histologic study of the islets 72 hours later will show only mild alterations.[329] However, if the compound is given in multiple small doses (no one of which alone would be diabetogenic) it will produce in mice pancreatic insulitis with progression to nearly complete beta cell destruction and severe diabetes.[322,330–332] The effect is both sex[333] and strain[334] dependent. A most interesting facet of this syndrome, in addition to the presence of insulitis, is the induction of Type C virus in outbred CD-1 mice. Within 1 week of completing five intraperitoneal injections of streptozotocin, electron microscopy reveals both spherical and cylindrical Type C virus particles. Identification of the virus is confirmed by the observation of virus specific antigens within beta cells. Time course studies indicate that virus induction probably precedes insulitis by 2 days, and that insulitis is always accompanied by virus-containing islet cells. Multidose streptozotocin diabetes is not always accompanied by Type C virus induction, however. Administration to C57BL/KsJ mice produces insulitis and diabetes with Type A virus induction.[331] Alloxan, administered similarly, produces none of these effects.

The multi-dose method of inducing insulitis with streptozotocin suggests that an immune process, perhaps cell-mediated, may be a factor in this variety of toxic diabetes. The possibility of involvement of the immune system is best supported by the attenuation of the syndrome by immunosuppressive agents[335,335a] and antibodies.[335b] Other studies, however, suggest that insulitis may be the consequence rather than the cause of beta cell destruction in this model.[335c-335e] Currently the interrelationship of the drug, the immune system, and the induction of Type C viruses is not understood.

Other Possible Chemically Induced Diabetic Syndromes. A number of nonpharmacologic toxins have been implicated in human diabetes, most notably the rodenticide Vacor which on several occasions has been ingested either inadvertently or with suicidal intent.[336,337] Vacor has proven difficult to study in animals because of its low margin of safety, the ED_{50} for producing diabetes being nearly the LD_{50} for the compound. Preliminary data, however, appear to confirm its diabetogenicity in animals.[338]

Another unusual animal diabetes syndrome possibly due to a toxin is that of the Japanese carp.[339,340] Reportedly, when fed ''rancid'' foods, these carp develop a syndrome known as Sekoke disease. It is characterized by hyperglycemia and possibly ketosis, with beta cell degranulation and vacuolization. Since the initial studies of this most unusual form of animal diabetes, however, little new information has been forthcoming. While it is believed that an oxidized saury oil may be the toxin involved,[341] it has not been possible to exclude simple dietary overabundance as a cause of diabetes in these commercially bred fish.

COMPLICATIONS OF DIABETES MELLITUS IN ANIMALS

We present a separate section on the complications of diabetes, in part because of the limited information available from the animal models we have presented. What secondary pathology is observed is sometimes subject to markedly conflicting interpretation.

In general, macrovascular pathology, arteriosclerosis and its typical cerebral, coronary, and peripheral consequences, are not marked in the animals we have discussed. The only notable exception is *Macaca nigra* in which an excess of atherosclerosis is observed.[249] This situation is due both to the relative resistance of many animal species, particularly rodents, to atherosclerotic change, and also to the limited lifespan of these diabetic animals, which precludes the observation of indolent pathologic processes. In the aorta of the diabetic Chinese hamster, there are alterations of glucose metabolism[342] and ultrastructural changes of endothelium, elastin, and media consistent with early atheromatous pathology.[343] Cholesterol levels in diabetic hamsters may be elevated but are often normal.[344] Electron microscopic studies of this hamster[345] have also revealed degenerative vascular and neuronal abnormalities of the brain. In contrast, *ob/ob* mice rendered hypercholesterolemic by diet show no evidence of atherosclerosis.[346] There is a single report of gangrene of extremities in KK mice, but this has not been proven to relate to arterial pathologic condition.[347] Capillary basement membrane thickening has been reported in the South African hamster[260] and Chinese hamster.[348]

Various forms of renal disease have been documented in animals with diabetes-like syndromes.[349] Mesangial matrix and basement membrane changes have been observed in Chinese hamsters,[350] alloxan diabetic rats,[351] diabetic mice,[352] and spiny mice.[353] In all instances, however, basement membrane thickening has been found to correlate closely with the age of the animal. Infiltration of tubular epithelium with glycogen is seen in Chinese hamsters,[354,355] spiny mice,[353] KK mice,[347] and alloxan diabetic rats.[351] Dilatation and coalescence of glomerular capillaries are also marked in diabetic animals, but frank glomerulosclerosis has not been documented. It has been claimed that glomerulosclerosis is present in the South African hamster,[356] the alloxan diabetic monkey,[357] the diabetic dog,[358] and the KK mouse.[347] More recent studies in the KK mouse, however, have attributed the pathological picture in that animal to amyloidosis.[359] Rats made diabetic with streptozotocin were followed for 6 months and have revealed glomerular basement membrane disorder. Furthermore, histologic examination following normalization of glucose levels gave evidence that these structural basement abnormalities were a consequence of the metabolic disturbances of the diabetes.[360-362]

The vascular substrate of human diabetic retinopathy has been studied in many animals, particularly following chemical induction of diabetes.[363] Up to 4 years may be required for the development of retinopathy in dogs,[364-366] while typical proliferation, microaneurysms, exudates, and hemorrhages can be seen in rats diabetic for 1- to 6-months.[367–369] Evidence suggestive of capillary pathology[370] along with increased intracellular glycogen[354] has been found in the Chinese hamster.

Cataracts have been described in sand rats,[137] Tuco-tucos,[211,212] rhesus monkeys,[251] and streptozotocin diabetic rats.[371] Increased polyol activity has been documented in streptozotocin diabetic rats,[372] and in both the lens and sciatic nerve of the Chinese hamster.[373] Consistent with this last observation in the diabetic hamster is evidence of both peripheral myelin degeneration,[374] and multiple abnormalities of pelvic visceral nerves which may account for its neurogenic bladder.[237] Additional evidence of neuropathy has been documented in streptozotocin and alloxan diabetic rats,[372,375–377a] *db/db* mice,[377b] and the BB rats.[377c]

Miscellaneous observations have also been made of testicular abnormalities in diabetic Chinese hamsters[378] and obese mice;[379] amyloidosis in *Macaca nigra*,[245,246] KK mice,[359] and obese mice;[379] alterations of articular cartilage in Chinese hamsters;[380] and glycogenolysis in the kidney[381] and myocardium[145] of spiny mice. These last observations on spiny mice are somewhat doubtful, however, because they have also been reported in euglycemic animals.[353] Lastly, human data now indicate the importance of nonenzymatic glycosylation of proteins as a critical aspect of late diabetic disease. It has been shown that the marker of this process in humans, hemoglobin A_{Ic}, is also elevated in several hyperglycemic rodents including the *db/db* mouse,[382] the Celebese ape,[382a] and other inbred strains treated with streptozotocin at the Joslin Research Laboratories.[383]

REFERENCES

1. Leblanc, U.: Du diabete chez les animaux. Clinique Vétérinaire. Lyon. 1861, pp. 225–273.
2. Gepts, W., Toussaint, D.: Spontaneous diabetes in cats and dogs. A pathological study. Diabetologia *3*:249, 1967.
3. Rabb, G.B., Getty, R.E., Williamson, W.M., Lombard, L.S.: Spontaneous diabetes mellitus in tree shrews, *Urogale everetti*. Diabetes *15*:327, 1966.
4. Stuhlman, R.A., Wagner, J.E., Garro, F.M., Musacchia, X.J.: Diabetes mellitus in the 13-lined ground squirrel (Citellus tridecemlineatus). Lab. Animal Sci. *27*:477, 1977.
5. Cameron, D., Stauffacher, W., Renold, A.E.: Spontaneous hyperglycemia and obesity in laboratory rodents. In: R.O. Greep, E.B. Astwood, D.F. Steiner, N. Freinkel, S.R. Geiger (Eds.): Handbook of Physiology. Sec. 7. Endocrine, Vol. 1. Endocrine Pancreas. Washington, American Physiology Society, 1972, pp. 611–625.
6. Fox, H.: Disease in Captive Wild Mammals and Birds. Philadelphia, J.B. Lippincott Co., 1923, pp. 39–40, 412–414.
7. van der Gaag, I., Borst, G.H.A., Vroege, C.: Diabetes mellitus with pancreatic atrophy in antelopes in the Amsterdam Zoo. Zbl. Vet. Med. *20*:834, 1973.
8. Herberg, L., Coleman, D.L.: Laboratory animals exhibiting obesity and diabetes syndromes. Metabolism. *26*:59, 1977.
9. Like, A.A.: Spontaneous diabetes in animals. In: B.W. Volk, K.F. Wellman (Eds.): The Diabetic Pancreas, New York, Plenum, 1977, pp. 381–423.
10. Renold, A.E.: Spontaneous diabetes and/or obesity in laboratory rodents. In R. Levine, R. Luft (Eds.): Advances in Metabolic Disorders. New York, Academic Press Inc., 1968, Vol. 3, pp. 49–84.
11. Lage, A.L., Mordes, J.P., Rossini, A.A.: Animal models of diabetes mellitus. Comp. Pathol. Bull. *12*:1, 1980.
12. Mordes, J.P., Rossini, A.A.: Animal models of diabetes mellitus. Am. J. Med. *70*:353, 1981.
13. Bray, G.A.: The Zucker-fatty rat: a review. Fed. Proc. *36*:148, 1977.
14. Herberg, L.: Spontaneously hyperglycemic laboratory animals—models of human diabetes syndrome? Horm. Metab. Res. *11*:323, 1979.
15. Berdanier, C.D.: Metabolic abnormalities in BHE rats. Diabetologia *10*:691, 1974.
16. Berdanier, C.D.: The BHE strain of rat: an example of the role of inheritance in determining metabolic controls. Fed. Proc. *35*:2295, 1976.
17. DiGiacomo, R.F, Myers, R.E., Rivera-Baez, L.: Diabetes mellitus in a rhesus monkey (Macaca mulatta): a case report and literature review. Lab. Animal Sci. *21*:572, 1971.
18. Valerio, D.A., Miller, R.L., Innes, J.R.M., et al.: Macaca Mulatta: Management of a Laboratory Breeding Colony. New York, Academic Press Inc., 1969, p. 101.
19. Valerio, D.A., Valerio, M.G., Ulland, B.M., Innes, J.R.M.: Clinical conditions and diseases encountered in a large simian colony. In: Proc. 3rd Int. Congr. Primat. Zurich, 1970, Vol. II, Basel, Karger, 1971, pp. 205–212.
19a. Hamilton, C.L., Ciaccia, P.: The course of development of glucose intolerance in the monkey (Macaca mulatta). J. Med. Primatol. 7:165, 1978.
20. Coleman, D.L., Hummel, K.P.: The influence of genetic background on the expression of the obese *(ob)* gene in the mouse. Diabetologia *9*:287, 1973.
21. Hummel, K.P., Coleman, D.L., Lane, P.W.: The influence of genetic background on expression of mutations at the diabetes locus in the mouse. I. C57BL/KsJ and C57BL/6J strains. Biochem. Genet. *7*:1, 1972.
22. Boquist, L., Hellman, B., Lernmark, Å., Täljedal, J-B.: Influence of the mutation "Diabetes" on insulin release and islet morphology in mice of different genetic backgrounds. J. Cell Biol. *62*:77, 1974.
23. Coleman, D.L., Hummel, K.P.: Influence of genetic background on the expression of mutations at the diabetes locus in the mouse. II. Studies on background modifiers. Isr. J. Med. *11*:708, 1975.
24. Coleman, D.L.: Obese and diabetes: two mutant genes causing diabetes-obesity syndromes in mice. Diabetologia *14*:141, 1978.
25. Wolff, G.L., Pitot, H.C.: Influence of background genome on enzymatic characteristics of yellow ($A^y/-A^{vy}-$) mice. Genetics *73*:109, 1973.
26. Gerritsen, G.C., Johnson, M.A., Soret, M.G., Schultz, J.R.: Epidemiology of Chinese hamsters and preliminary evidence for genetic heterogeneity of diabetes. Diabetologia *10*:581, 1974.
27. Gerritsen, G.C., Needham, L., Schmidt, F.L., Dulin, W.E.: Studies on the prediction and development of diabetes in offspring of diabetic Chinese hamsters. Diabetologia *6*:159, 1970.
28. Butler, L.: The inheritance of diabetes in the Chinese hamster. Diabetologia *3*:124, 1967.

29. Butler, L., Gerritsen, G.C.: A comparison of the modes of inheritance of diabetes in the Chinese hamster and the KK mouse. Diabetologia 6:163, 1970.

30. Coleman, D.L., Hummel, K.P.: Hyperinsulinemia in pre-weaning diabetes (db) mice. Diabetologia 10:607, 1974.

31. Ingalls, A.M., Dickie, M.M., Snell, G.D.: Obese, a new mutation in house mouse. J. Hered. 41:317, 1950.

32. Thurlby, P.L., Trayhurn, P.: The development of obesity in pre-weanling obob mice. Br. J. Nutr. 39:397, 1978.

33. Herberg, L., Gries, F.A., Hesse-Wortmann, C.H.: Effect of weight and cell size on hormone-induced lipolysis in New Zealand obese mice and American obese hyperglycemic mice. Diabetologia 6:300, 1970.

34. Bates, M.W., Nauss, S.F., Hagman, N.C., Mayer, J.: Fat metabolism in three forms of experimental obesity. I. Body composition. Am. J. Physiol. 180:301, 1955.

35. Lane, P.W., Dickie, M.M.: The effect of restricted food intake on the life span of genetically obese mice. J. Nutr. 64:549, 1958.

36. Alonso, L.G., Maren, T.H.: Effect of food restriction on body composition of hereditary obese mice. Am. J. Physiol. 183:284, 1955.

37. Chlouverakis, C.: Induction of obesity in obese-hyperglycaemic mice on normal food intake. Experientia 26:1262, 1970.

38. Boozer, C.N., Mayer, J.: Effects of long-term restricted insulin production in obese-hyperglycemic (genotype ob/ob) mice. Diabetologia 12:181, 1976.

39. Genuth, S.M. Przybylski, R.J., Rosenberg, D.M.: Insulin resistance in genetically obese hyperglycemic mice. Endocrinology 88:1230, 1971.

40. Westman, S.: Development of obese-hyperglycaemic syndrome in mice. Diabetologia 4:141, 1968.

41. Joosten, H.F.P., van der Kroon, P.H.W.: Enlargement of epididymal adipocytes in relation to hyperinsulinemia in obese hyperglycemic mice (ob/ob). Metabolism 23:59, 1974.

42. Chlouverakis, C., Dade, E.F., Batt, R.A.L.: Glucose tolerance and time sequence of adiposity, hyperinsulinemia and hyperglycemia in obese hyperglycemic mice (ob/ob). Metabolism 19:687, 1970.

43. Genuth, S.M.: Effect of high fat vs high carbohydrate feeding on the development of obesity in weanling ob/ob mice. Diabetologia 12:155, 1976.

44. Loten, E.G., Rabinovitch, A., Jeanrenaud, B.: In vivo studies on lipogenesis in obese hyperglycaemic (ob/ob) mice: possible role of hyperinsulinaemia. Diabetologia 10:45, 1974.

45. Christophe, J., Winand, J., Furnelle, L., Wodon, C.: 7-day time study of the lipids labelled in vivo in normal and obese-hyperglycaemic (O-H) Bar Harbor Mice. Diabetologia 8:53, 1972.

46. Guggenheim, K., Mayer, J.: Studies of pyruvate and acetate metabolism in the hereditary obesity-diabetes syndrome of mice. J. Biol. Chem. 198:259, 1952.

47. Hughes, A.M., Tolbert, B.M.: Oxidation of acetate, glucose or glycine to carbon dioxide in mice exhibiting the hereditary obesity syndrome. J. Biol. Chem. 231:339, 1958.

48. Hollifield, G., Parson, W., Ayers, C.R.: In vitro synthesis of lipids from C-14 acetate by adipose tissue from four types of obese mice. Am. J. Physiol. 198:37, 1960.

49. Renold, A.E., Christophe, J., Jeanrenaud, B.: The obese hyperglycemic syndrome in mice. Metabolism of isolated adipose tissue in vitro. Am. J. Clin. Nutr. 8:719, 1960.

50. Christophe, J., Jeanrenaud, B., Mayer, J., Renold, A.E.: Metabolism in vitro of adipose tissue in obese-hyperglycemic and goldthioglucose-treated mice. I. Metabolism of glucose. J. Biol. Chem. 236:642, 1961.

51. Christophe, J., Jeanrenaud, B., Mayer, J., Renold, A.E.: Metabolism in vitro of adipose tissue in obese-hyperglycemic and goldthioglucose-treated mice. II. Metabolism of pyruvate and acetate. J. Biol. Chem. 236:648, 1961.

52. Hellman, B., Larsson, S., Westman, S.: Influence of glucose on the in vitro acetate metabolism in the epididymal adipose tissue of obese-hyperglycemic mice. Med. Exp. 7:39, 1962.

53. Assimacopoulos-Jeannet, F., Singh, A., LeMarchand, E.G., et al.: Abnormalities in lipogenesis and triglyceride secretion by perfused livers of obese-hyperglycaemic (ob/ob) mice: relationship with hyperinsulinaemia. Diabetologia 10:155, 1974.

54. Stein, J.M., Bewsher, P.D., Stowers, J.N.: The metabolism of ketones, triglyceride and monoglyceride in livers of obese hyperglycaemic mice. Diabetologia 6:570, 1970.

55. Cuendet, G.S., Loten, E.G., Cameron, D.P., et al.: Hormone-substrate responses to total fasting in lean and obese mice. Am. J. Physiol. 228:276, 1975.

56. Mayer, J., Hagman, N.C., Marshall, N.B., Stoops, A.J.: Fat metabolism in three forms of obesity. V. Hepatic lipogenesis in vitro. Am. J. Physiol. 181:501, 1955.

57. Bates, M.W., Zomzely, C., Mayer, J.: Fat metabolism in three forms of experimental obesity. IV. "Instantaneous" rates of lipogenesis in vivo. Am. J. Physiol. 181:187, 1955.

58. Coleman, D.L.: Acetone metabolism in mice: increased activity in mice heterozygous for obesity genes. Proc. Natl. Acad. Sci. 77:290, 1980.

59. Rath, E.A., Hems, D.A., Beloff-Chain, A.: Lipoprotein lipase activities in tissues of normal and genetically obese (ob/ob) mice. Diabetologia 10:261, 1974.

60. Ohtake, M., Bray, G.A., Azukuzawa, M.: Studies on hypothermia and thyroid function in the obese (ob/ob) mouse. Am. J. Physiol. 233:R110, 1977.

61. Joosten, H.F.P., van der Kroon, P.H.W.: Role of the thyroid in the development of the obese-hyperglycemic syndrome in mice (ob/ob). Metabolism 23:425, 1974.

62. Treble, D.H., Mayer, J.: Glycerolkinase activity in white adipose tissue of obese-hyperglycaemic mice. Nature 197:363, 1963.

63. Lochaya, S., Hamilton, J.C., Mayer, J.: Lipase and glycerokinase activities in the adipose tissue of obese hyperglycaemic mice. Nature 197:182, 1963.

64. Trayhurn, P., James, W.P.T.: Thermoregulation and nonshivering thermogenesis in the genetically obese (ob/ob) mouse. Pflügers Archiv 373:189, 1978.

65. York, D.A., Bray, G.A., Yukimura, Y.: An enzymatic defect in the obese (ob/ob) mouse: loss of thyroid-induced sodium and potassium adenosinetriphosphatase. Proc. Natl. Acad. Sci. 75:477, 1978.

66. Lin, M.H., Romsos, D.R., Akera, T., Leveille, G.A.: Na+, K+-ATPase enzyme units in skeletal muscle from lean and obese mice. Biochem. Biophys. Res. Comm. 80:398, 1978.

67. Flier, J.S., Usher, P., DeLuise, M.: Effect of sucrose over-feeding on Na, K-ATPase-mediated 86Rb uptake in normal and ob/ob mice. Diabetes 30:975, 1981.

68. Westman-Naeser, S.: The obese hyperglycaemic syndrome in young ob/ob mice. Diabetologia 8:49, 1972.

69. Herberg, L., Major, E., Hennings, U., et al.: Differences in the development of the obese-hyperglycemic syndrome in ob/ob and NZO mice. Diabetologia 6:292, 1970.

70. Gepts, W., Christophe, J., Mayer, J.: Pancreatic islets in mice with the obese hyperglycemic syndrome. Lack of effect of carbutamide. Diabetes 9:63, 1960.

71. Westman, S.: The endocrine pancreas of old obese-hyperglycemic mice. Acta Soc. Med. Upsal. 73:81, 1968.

72. Mayer, J., Bates, M.W., Dickie, M.M.: Hereditary diabetes in genetically obese mice. Science *113*:746, 1951.

73. Mayer, J., Russell, R.E., Bates, M.W., Dickie, M.M.: Metabolic, nutritional and endocrine studies of the hereditary obesity-diabetes syndrome of mice and mechanism of its development. Metabolism *21*:921, 1953.

74. Westman, S.: Metabolic studies of the obese-hyperglycaemic syndrome in mice. In: Proceedings of the VIth Congress of the International Diabetes Foundation, Stockholm. Amsterdam, Excerpta Medica International Congress Series No. 172, 1967, pp. 827–832.

75. Westman, S., Hellerström, C., Coore, H.C., Herbai, G.: Aspects of insulin resistance and insulin turn-over in mice with the obese-hyperglycaemic syndrome. Diabetologia *5*:58, 1969.

76. Batt, R., Miahle, P.: Insulin resistance of the inherently obese mouse, *ob/ob*. Nature *212*:289, 1966.

77. Chang, K.J., Huang, D., Cuatrecasas, P.: The defect in insulin receptors in obese-hyperglycemic mice: a probable accompaniment of more generalized alterations in membrane glycoproteins. Biochem. Biophys. Res. Commun. *64*:566, 1975.

78. Freychet, P., Laudat, M.H., Laudat, P., et al.: Impairment of insulin binding to the fat cell plasma membrane in the obese hyperglycemic mouse. FEBS Lett. *25*:339, 1972.

79. Kahn, C.R., Neville, D.M., Jr., Gorden, P., et al.: Insulin receptor defect in insulin resistance: studies in the obese hyperglycemic mouse. Biochem. Biophys. Res. Commun. *48*:135, 1972.

80. Kahn, C.R., Neville, D.M., Jr., Roth, J.: Insulin-receptor interaction in the obese-hyperglycemic mouse. J. Biol. Chem. *248*:244, 1973.

81. Soll, A.H., Kahn, C.R., Neville, D.M., Jr., Roth, J.: Insulin receptor deficiency in genetic and acquired obesity. J. Clin. Invest. *56*:769, 1975.

82. Soll, A.H., Goldfine, I.D., Roth, J., Kahn, C.R.: Thymic lymphocytes in obese *(ob/ob)* mice. A mirror of the insulin receptor defect in liver and fat. J. Biol. Chem. *249*:4127, 1974.

83. Stauffacher, W., Lambert, A.E., Vecchio, D., Renold, A.E.: Measurements of insulin activities in pancreas and serum of mice with spontaneous ("obese" and "New Zealand obese") and induced (goldthioglucose) obesity and hyperglycemia, with considerations on the pathogenesis of the spontaneous syndrome. Diabetologia *3*:230, 1967.

84. Rabinovitch, A., Gutzeit, A., Kikuchi, M., et al.: Defective early phase insulin release in perifused isolated pancreatic islets of spiny mice (Acomys cahirinus). Diabetologia *11*:457, 1975.

85. Lavine, R.L., Voyles, N., Perrino, P.V., Recant, L.: Functional abnormalities of islets of Langerhans of obese hyperglycemic mouse. Am. J. Physiol. *233*:E86, 1977.

86. Seidman, I., Horland, A.A., Teebor, G.W.: Glycolytic and gluconeogenic enzyme activities in the hereditary obese-hyperglycemic syndrome and in acquired obesity. Diabetologia *6*:313, 1970.

87. Hellerström, C., Westman, S., Herbai, G., et al.: Pathogenetic aspects of the obese-hyperglycemic syndrome in mice (genotype *ob/ob*): II. Extrapancreatic factors. Diabetologia *6*:284, 1970.

88. Herbai, G., Westman, S., Hellerström, C.: The growth hormone dependent incorporation of sulphate into the costal cartilage of obese-hyperglycemic mice of different ages. Acta Endocrinol. (Kbh) *64*:415, 1970.

89. Stauffacher, W., Crofford, O.B., Jeanrenaud, B., Renold, A.E.: Comparative studies of muscle and adipose tissue metabolism in lean and obese mice. Ann. N.Y. Acad. Sci. *131*:528, 1965.

90. Roos, P., Martin, J.M., Westman-Naeser, S., Hellerström, C.: Immunoreactive growth hormone levels in mice with the obese-hyperglycemic syndrome (genotype *ob/ob*). Hormone Metab. Res. *6*:125, 1974.

91. Naeser, P.: Function of the adrenal cortex, in obese-hyperglycaemic mice (gene symbol *ob*). Diabetologia *10*:449, 1974.

92. Naeser, P.: Effects of adrenalectomy on the obese-hyperglycemic syndrome in mice (gene symbol *ob*). Diabetologia *9*:376, 1973.

93. Solomon, J., Mayer, J.: The effect of adrenalectomy on the development of the obese-hyperglycemic syndrome in *ob/ob* mice. Endocrinology *93*:510, 1973.

94. Plocher, T.A., Powley, T.L.: Maintenance of obesity following hypophysectomy in the obese-hyperglycemic mouse (ob/ob). Yale J. Biol. Med. *50*:291, 1977.

95. Strautz, R.L.: Studies of hereditary-obese mice *(ob/ob)* after implantation of pancreatic islets in Millipore filter capsules. Diabetologia *6*:306, 1970.

96. Hausberger, F.X.: Parabiosis and transplantation experiments in hereditarily obese mice. Anat. Rec. *130*:313(Abstr.), 1958.

97. Coleman, D.L., Hummel, K.P.: Effects of parabiosis of normal with genetically diabetic mice. Am. J. Physiol. *217*:1298, 1969.

98. Chlouverakis, C.: Insulin resistance of parabiotic obese-hyperglycemic mice *(ob/ob)*. Horm. Metab. Res. *4*:143, 1972.

99. Coleman, D.L.: Effects of parabiosis of obese with diabetes and normal mice. Diabetologia *9*:294, 1973.

100. Haessler, H.A., Crawford, J.D.: Alterations in the fatty acid composition of depot fat associated with obesity. Ann. N.Y. Acad. Sci. *131*:476, 1965.

101. Straus, E., Yalow, R.S.: Cholecystokinin in the brains of obese and nonobese mice. Science *203*:68, 1978.

102. Patel, Y.C., Cameron, D.P., Stefan, Y., et al.: Somatostatin: widespread abnormality in tissues of spontaneously diabetic mice. Science *198*:930, 1977.

103. Malaisse-Lagae, F., Carpentier, J.L., Patel, Y.C., et al.: Pancreatic polypeptide: a possible role in the regulation of food intake in the mouse. Hypothesis. Experientia *33*:915, 1977.

104. Gingerich, R.L., Gersell, D.J., Greider, M.H., et al.: Elevated levels of pancreatic polypeptide in obese-hyperglycemic mice. Metabolism *27*:1526, 1978.

105. Mordes, J.P., Eastwood, G.L., Loo, S., Rossini, A.A.: Pancreatic polypeptide causes diarrhea and weight loss in obese mice but not in lean littermates. Peptides (Fayetteville) *3*:873, 1982.

106. Joosten, H.F.P., van der Kroon, P.H.W.: Growth pattern and behavioral traits associated with the development of the obese-hyperglycemic syndrome in mice *(ob/ob)*. Metabolism *23*:1141, 1974.

107. Clark, L.D., Gay, P.E.: Activity and body weight relationships in genetically obese animals. Biol. Psychiat. *4*:247, 1972.

108. Hummel, K.P., Dickie, M.M., Coleman, D.L.: Diabetes, a new mutation in the mouse. Science *153*:1127, 1966.

109. Staats, J.: Diabetes in the mouse due to two mutant genes. A bibliography. Diabetologia *11*:325, 1975.

110. Falconer, D.S., Isaacson, J.H.: Adipose, a new inherited obesity of the mouse. J. Hered. *50*:290, 1959.

111. Bulfied, G.: Genetic control of metabolism: Enzyme studies of the obese and adipose mutants in the mouse. Genet. Res. *20*:51, 1972.

112. Chick, W.L., Lavine, R.L., Like, A.A.: Studies on the diabetic mutant mouse: V. Glucose tolerance in mice

homozygous and heterozygous for the diabetes (db) gene. Diabetologia 6:257, 1970.

113. Like, A.A., Chick, W.L.: Studies in the diabetic mutant mouse: II. Electron microscopy of pancreatic islets. Diabetologia 6:216, 1970.

114. Chick, W.L., Like, A.A.: Studies in the diabetic mutant mouse. III. Physiological factors associated with alterations in beta cell proliferation. Diabetologia 6:243, 1970.

115. Like, A.A., Chick, W.L.: Studies in the diabetic mutant mouse. I. Light microscopy and radioautography of pancreatic islets. Diabetologia 6:207, 1970.

116. Laube, H., Fussgängen, R.D., Maier, V., Pfeiffer, E.F.: Hyperglucagonemia of the isolated perfused pancreas of diabetic mice (db/db). Diabetologia 9:400, 1973.

117. Stauffacher, W., Orci, L., Cameron, D.P., et al.: Spontaneous hyperglycemia and/or obesity in laboratory rodents: an example of the possible usefulness of animal disease models with both genetic and environmental components. Recent Progr. Horm. Res. 27:41, 1971.

117a. Debray-Sachs, M., Dardenne, M., Sai, P., et al.: Anti-islet immunity and thymic dysfunction in the mutant C57BL/KsJ db/db mouse. Diabetes 32:1048, 1983.

118. Coleman, D.L., Hummel, K.P.: Studies with the mutation, diabetes, in the mouse. Diabetologia 3:238, 1967.

119. Chang, A.Y., Schneider, D.I.: Abnormalities in hepatic enzyme activities during development of diabetes in Db mice. Diabetologia 6:274, 1970.

120. Coleman, D.L., Hummel, K.P.: The effects of hypothalamic lesions in genetically diabetic mice. Diabetologia 6:263, 1970.

121. Wyse, B.M., Dulin, W.E.: The influence of age and dietary conditions on diabetes in the Db mouse. Diabetologia 6:268, 1970.

122. Cox, J.E., Powley, T.L.: Development of obesity in diabetic mice pair-fed with lean siblings. J. Comp. Physiol. Psychol. 91:347, 1977.

123. Leiter, E.H., Coleman, D.L., Eisenstein, A.B., Strack, I.: Dietary control of pathogenesis in C57BL/KsJ db/db diabetes mice. Metabolism 30:554, 1981.

124. Chick, W.L., Like, A.A.: Studies in the diabetic mutant mouse: IV. DBM, a modified diabetic mutant produced by outcrossing of the original strain. Diabetologia 6:252, 1970.

125. Gunnarson, R.: Function of the pancreatic B-cell during the development of hyperglycaemia in mice homozygous for the mutations "diabetes" (db) and "misty" (m). Diabetologia 11:431, 1975.

126. Cameron, D., Stauffacher, W., Amherdt, M., et al.: Kinetics of immunoreactive insulin release in obese hyperglycemic laboratory rodents. Endocrinology 92:257, 1972.

127. Naeser, P.: Adrenal function in the diabetic mutant mouse (gene symbol dbm). Acta Physiol. Scand. 98:395, 1976.

128. Frenkel, G., Kraicer, P.F.: Metabolic pattern of sand rats (Psammomys obesus) and rats during fasting. Life Sci. 11:209, 1972.

129. Schmidt-Nielsen, K., Haines, H.B., Hackel, D.B.: Diabetes mellitus in the sand rat induced by standard laboratory diets. Science 143:689, 1964.

130. Haines, H.B., Hackel, D.B., Schmidt-Nielsen, K.: Experimental diabetes mellitus induced by diet in the sand rat. Amer. J. Physiol. 208:297, 1965.

131. Hackel, D.B., Frohman, L., Mikat, E., et al.: Effect of diet on the glucose tolerance and plasma insulin levels of the sand rat (Psammomys obesus). Diabetes 15:105, 1966.

132. Malaisse, W.J., Like, A.A., Malaisse-Lagae, F., et al.: Insulin secretion in vitro by the pancreas of the sand rat (Psammomys obesus). Diabetes 17:752, 1968.

133. Hahn, H-J., Köhler, E., Hahn von Dorsche, H., et al.: Insulin secretion of isolated islets of sand rats (Psammomys obesus) during adaptation in captivity. Endokrinologie (Leipzig) 66:348, 1975.

134. Miki, E., Like, A.A., Steinke, J., Soeldner, J.S.: Diabetic syndrome in sand rats. II. Variability and association with diet. Diabetologia 3:135, 1967.

135. De Fronzo, R., Miki, E., Steinke, J.: Diabetic syndrome in sand rats. III. Observations on adipose tissue and liver in the non-diabetic stage. Diabetologia 3:140, 1967.

136. Hackel, D.B., Mikat, E., Lebovitz, H.E., et al.: The sand rat (Psammomys obesus) as an experimental animal in studies of diabetes mellitus. Diabetologia 3:130, 1967.

137. Hackel, D.B., Schmidt-Nielsen, K., Haines, H.B., Mikat, E.: Diabetes mellitus in the sand rat (Psammomys obesus). Pathologic studies. Lab. Invest. 14:200, 1965.

138. Like, A.A., Miki, E.: Diabetic syndrome in sand rats. IV. Morphologic changes in islet tissue. Diabetologia 3:143, 1967.

139. Lebovitz, H.E., White, S., Mikat, E., Hackel, D.B.: Control of insulin secretion in the Egyptian sand rat (Psammomys obesus). Diabetologia 10:679, 1974.

140. Miki, E., Like, A.A., Soeldner, J.S., et al.: Acute ketotic-type diabetic syndrome in sand rats (Psammomys obesus) with special reference to the pancreas. Metabolism 15:749, 1966.

141. Rice, M.G., Robertson, R.P.: Reevaluation of the sand rat as a model for diabetes mellitus. Am. J. Physiol. 239:E340, 1980.

142. Neel, J.V.: Diabetes mellitus: a "thrifty" genotype rendered detrimental by "progress". Am. J. Human Genet. 14:353, 1962.

143. Cahill, G.F., Jr.: Pathophysiology of diabetes. Med. Clin. N. Am. 49:881, 1965.

144. Coleman, D.L.: Obesity genes: beneficial effects in heterozygous mice. Science 203:663, 1979.

145. Gonet, A.E., Stauffacher, W., Pictet, R., Renold, A.E.: Obesity and diabetes mellitus with striking congenital hyperplasia of the islets of Langerhans in spiny mice (Acomys cahirinus). I. Histologic findings and preliminary metabolic observations. Diabetologia 1:162, 1965.

146. Gonet, A.E., Renold, A.E.: Polynésie et macronésie Langerhansiennes avec obésité chez la souris à piquants (Acomys). Schweiz. Med. Wschr. 97:735, 1966.

147. Stauffacher, W., Orci, L., Amherdt, M., et al.: Metabolic state, pancreatic insulin content and B-cell morphology of normoglycemic spiny mice (Acomys cahirinus): Indications for an impairment of insulin secretion. Diabetologia 6:330, 1970.

148. Pictet, R., Orci, L., Gonet, A.E., et al.: Ultrastructural studies of the hyperplastic islets of Langerhans of spiny mice (Acomys cahirinus) before and during development of hyperglycaemia. Diabetologia 3:188, 1967.

149. Gutzeit, A., Rabinovitch, A., Studer, P.P., et al.: Decreased intravenous glucose tolerance and low plasma insulin response in spiny mice (Acomys cahirinus). Diabetologia 10:667, 1974.

150. Gutzeit, A., Rabinovitch, A., Karakash, C., et al.: Evidence for decreased sensitivity to glucose of isolated islets from spiny mice (Acomys cahirinus). Diabetologia 10:661, 1974.

151. Cameron, D.P., Stauffacher, W., Orci, L., et al.: Immunoreactive insulin secretion in the acomys cahirinus. Diabetes 21:1060, 1972.

152. Orci, L., Lambert, A.E., Amherdt, M., et al.: The autonomous nervous system and the B-cell: Metabolic and morphologic observations made in spiny mice (Acomys cahirinus) and in cultured fetal rat pancreas. Acta Diabet. Lat. 7(Suppl. 1):184, 1970.

153. Hahn von Dorsche, H., Krause, R., Fehrman, P., Sulzmann, R.: The verification of neurones in the pancreas of spiny mice *(Acomys cahirinus)*. Endokrinologie (Leipzig)*67*:115, 1976.

154. Malaisse-Lagae, F., Ravazzola, M., Amherdt, M., et al.: An apparent abnormality of the B-cell microtubular system in spiny mice *(Acomys cahirinus)*. Diabetologia *11*:71, 1975.

155. Rabinovitch, A., Gutzeit, A., Grill, V., et al.: Defective insulin secretion in the spiny mouse *(Acomys cahirinus)*: Possible value in the study of the pathophysiology of diabetes. Israel J. Med. *11*:730, 1975.

156. Nakamura, M.: A diabetic strain in the mouse. Proc. Japan Acad. *38*:348, 1962.

157. Kondo, K., Nozawa, K., Tomita, T., Ezaki, K.: Inbred strains resulting from Japanese mice. Bull. Exp. Anim. 6:107, 1957.

158. Dulin, W.E., Wyse, B.M.: Diabetes in the KK mouse. Diabetologia 6:317, 1970.

159. Iwatsuka, H., Shino, A., Suzuoki, Z.: General survey of diabetic features of yellow KK mice. Endocrinol. Jpn. *17*:25, 1970.

160. Butler, L.: The inheritance of glycosuria in the KK and A^y mouse. Can. J. Genet. Cytol. *14*:265, 1972.

161. Nakamura, M., Yamada, K.: A further study of the diabetic (KK) strain of mouse. F$_1$ and F$_2$ offspring of the cross between KK and C57BL. Proc. Japan Acad. *39*:489, 1963.

162. Wyse, B.M., Dulin, W.E.: Further characterization of diabetes-like abnormalities in the T-KK mouse. Diabetologia *10*:617, 1974.

163. Penhos, J.C., Wu, C.H., Camerini-Davalos, R.A.: Effect of several hormones on the tolerance to glucose in the nondiabetic stage of KK mice. J. Exp. Zool. *171*:209, 1969.

164. Furuno, K., Arakawa, M., Shino, A., Suzuoki, Z.: Induction of overt diabetes in KK mice by dietary means. Endocrinol. Jpn. *17*:477, 1971.

165. Nakamura, M., Yamada, K.: Studies on a diabetic *(KK)* strain of the mouse. Diabetologia 3:212, 1967.

166. Iwatsuka, H., Taketomi, S., Matsuo, T., Suzuoki, Z.: Congenitally impaired hormone sensitivity of the adipose tissue of spontaneously diabetic mice, KK. Validity of thrifty genotype in KK mice. Diabetologia *10*:611, 1974.

167. Appel, M.C., Chang, A.Y., Dulin, W.E.: Diabetes in the Toronto-KK hybrid mouse. Abnormalities in liver and pancreatic islets of Langerhans. Diabetologia *10*:625, 1974.

168. Lataste, F.: Trois questions. Bull. Scient. du dip du Nord *16*:364, 1884–1885.

169. Danforth, C.H.: The interaction of genes in development. Proc. Soc. Exp. Biol. and Med. *24*:69, 1926.

170. Danforth, C.H.: Hereditary adiposity in mice. J. Hered. *18*:153, 1927.

171. Dickies, M.M.: A new viable yellow mutation in the house mouse. J. Hered. *53*:84, 1962.

172. Carpenter, K.J., Mayer, J.: Physiologic observations on yellow obesity in the mouse. Am. J. Physiol. *193*:499, 1958.

173. Weitze, M.: Hereditary adiposity in mice and the cause of this anomaly. Thesis. Store Nordiske Videnskabsboghandel, Copenhagen, 1940.

174. Hausberger, F.X., Hausberger, B.C.: The etiologic mechanism of some forms of hormonally induced obesity. Am. J. Clin. Nutr. 8:671, 1960.

175. Wolff, G.L.: Genetic modification of homeostatic regulation in the mouse. Am. Naturalist *105*:241, 1971.

176. Wolff, G.L.: Body composition and coat color correlation in different phenotypes of "Viable Yellow" mice. Science *147*:1145, 1965.

177. Castle, W.E.: Influence of certain color mutations on body size in mice, rats, and rabbits. Genetics 26:177, 1941.

178. Dickies, M.M., Woolley, G.W.: The age factor in weight of yellow mice. J. Hered. *37*:365, 1946.

179. Johnson, P.R., Hirsch, J.: Cellularity of adipose depots in six strains of genetically obese mice. J. Lipid. Res. *13*:2, 1972.

180. Dickerson, G.E., Gowen, J.W.: Hereditary obesity and efficient food utilization in mice. Science *105*:496, 1947.

181. Hollifield, G., Parson, W.: Food drive and satiety in yellow mice. Am. J. Physiol. *189*:36, 1957.

182. Silberberg, R., Silberberg, M., Riley, S.: Lifespan of "yellow" mice fed enriched diets. Am. J. Physiol. *181*:128, 1955.

183. Soret, M.G., Kupiecki, F.P., Wyse, B.M.: Epididymal fat pad alterations in mice with spontaneous obesity and diabetes and with chemically induced obesity. Diabetologia *10*:639, 1974.

184. Wolff, G.L.: Hereditary obesity and hormone deficiencies in yellow dwarf mice. Am. J. Physiol. *209*:632, 1965.

185. Appel, M.C.: Characterization of diabetes mellitus in the Yellow-KK mouse. Thesis. University of Minnesota, 1977.

186. Appel, M.C., Schibly, B.A., Kamara, J.A., Sorenson, R.L.: Adrenal gland involvement in mice with hereditary obesity and diabetes mellitus. Diabetologia *16*:391, 1979.

187. Hunt, C.E., Lindsey, J.R., Walkley, S.U.: Animal models of diabetes and obesity, including the PBB/Ld mouse. Fed. Proc. *35*:1206, 1976.

188. Walkley, S.U., Hunt, C.E., Clements, L.S., Lindsey, J.R.: Description of obesity in the PBB/Ld mouse. J. Lipid Res. *19*:335, 1978.

189. Jones, E.E.: Spontaneous hyperplasia of the pancreatic islets associated with glyosuria in hybrid mice. In: S.E. Brolin, B. Hellman, H. Knutson (Eds.): The Structure and Metabolism of the Pancreatic Islets. Proceedings of the 3rd International Symposium, August, 1963, Oxford, Pergamon, 1964, pp. 189–191.

190. Cahill, G.F., Jr., Jones, E.E., Lauris, V., et al.: Studies on experimental diabetes in the Wellesley hybrid mouse. II. Serum insulin levels and response of peripheral tissues. Diabetologia 3:171, 1967.

191. Gleason, R.E., Lauris, V., Soeldner, J.S.: Studies on experimental diabetes in the Wellesley hybrid mouse. III. Dietary effects and similar changes in a commercial Swiss-Hauschka strain. Diabetologia 3:175, 1967.

192. Like, A.A., Jones, E.E.: Studies on experimental diabetes in the Wellesley hybrid mouse. IV. Morphologic changes in islet tissue. Diabetologia 3:179, 1967.

193. Like, A.A., Steinke, J., Jones, E.E., Cahill, G.F., Jr.: Pancreatic studies in mice with spontaneous diabetes mellitus. Am. J. Path. *46*:621, 1965.

194. Bielschowsky, M., Bielschowsky, F.: A new strain of mice with hereditary obesity. Proc. Univ. Otago Med. Sch. *31*:29, 1953.

195. Bielschowsky, M., Bielschowsky, F.: The New Zealand strains of obese mice. Their response to stilboestrol and to insulin. Aust. J. Exp. Biol. Med. Sci. *34*:181, 1956.

196. Crofford, O.B., Davis, C.K.: Growth characteristics, glucose tolerance and insulin sensitivity of New Zealand obese mice. Metabolism *14*:271, 1965.

197. Cameron, D.P., Opat, F., Insch, S.: Studies of immunoreactive insulin secretion in NZO mice *in vivo*. Diabetologia *10*:649, 1974.

198. Larkins, R.G., Martin, F.I.R.: Selective defect in insulin release in one form of spontaneous laboratory diabetes. Nature (New Biol) *235*:86, 1972.

199. Larkins, R.G.: Defective insulin secretion in the NZO mouse. *In vitro* studies. Endocrinology *93*:1052, 1973.

200. Borglund, E., Brolin, S.E., Ohlsson, A.: On the long-term effects of chlorpentazide in mice with hereditary hyperglycemia (NZO). In: International Diabetes Federation, Stockholm, 1967. Amsterdam. Excerpta Medica International Congress Series No. 172, 1969, pp. 747–753.

201. Larkins, R.G.: Defective insulin secretory response to glucose in the New Zealand obese mouse. Improvement with restricted diet. Diabetes *22*:251, 1973.

202. Rudorff, K.H., Huchzermeyer, H., Windeck, R., Staib, W.: Über den Einfluss von Insulin auf die Alanin-gluconeogenese in der isoliert perfundierten Leber von New Zealand obese Mice. Eur. J. Biochem. *16*:481, 1970.

203. Huchzermeyer, H., Rudorff, K.H., Staib, W.: Tierexperimentelle Untersuchungen zum Problem der Insulin-Resistenz bei Adipositas und Diabetes mellitus. Pathogenese des fettsüchtig-hyperglykämischen Syndrome. Z. Klin. Chem. Klin. Biochem. *11*:249, 1973.

204. Kamioka, T.: Untersuchungen des Glukose und Fettstoffwechsels bei hereditär fettsuchtigen under hyperglykämischem Mäusen. II. Glukose und Fettstoffwechsel bei New Zealand Obese (NZO) Mäusen. Folia Endocrinol. Jpn. *41*:148, 1965.

205. Purves, E.C.: The endocrine status of obese mice. Thesis. Univ. of Otago, New Zealand, 1964.

206. Herberg, L., Doeppen, W., Major, E., Gries, F.A.: Dietary-induced hypertrophic-hyperplastic obesity in mice. J. Lipid Res. *15*:580, 1974.

207. Melez, K.A., Harrison, L.C., Gilliam, J.N., Steinberg, A.D.: Diabetes is associated with autoimmunity in the New Zealand obese (NZO) mouse. Diabetes *29*:835, 1980.

208. Gates, R.J., Hunt, M.I., Smith, R., Lazarus, N.R.: Return to normal of blood glucose, plasma insulin and weight gain in New Zealand obese mice after implantation of islets of Langerhans. Lancet *2*:567, 1972.

209. Gates, R.J., Hunt, M.I., Lazarus, N.R.: Further studies on the amelioration of the characteristics of New Zealand obese (NZO) mice following implantation of islets of Langerhans. Diabetologia *10*:401, 1974.

210. Gates, R.J., Lazarus, N.R.: The ability of pancreatic polypeptides (APP and BPP) to return to normal the hyperglycaemia, hyperinsulinaemia and weight gain of New Zealand obese mice. Hormone Res. *8*:189, 1977.

211. Wise, P.H., Weir, B.J., Hime, J.M., Forrest, E.: Implications of hyperglycaemia and cataract in a colony of Tuco-tucos (Ctenomys talarum). Nature (London) *219*:1374, 1968.

212. Wise, P.H., Weir, B.J., Hime, J.M., Forrest, E.: The diabetic syndrome in the Tuco-tuco (Ctenomys talarum). Diabetologia *8*:165, 1972.

213. Voss, K.M., Herberg, L., Kern, H.F.: Fine structural studies of the islets of Langerhans in the Djungarian hamster (Phodopus sungorus). Cell Tissue Res. *191*:333, 1978.

214. Herberg, L., Buchanan, K.D., Herbertz, L.M., et al.: The Djungarian Hamster—a laboratory animal with inappropriate hyperglycemia. Comp. Biochem. Physiol. *65A*:35, 1980.

215. Nakhooda, A.F., Like, A.A., Chappel, C.I., et al.: The spontaneously diabetic Wistar rat. Metabolic and morphologic studies. Diabetes *26*:100, 1977.

215a.Logothetopoulos, J., Valiquette, N., Madura, E., Cvet, D.: The onset and progression of pancreatic insulitis in the overt, spontaneously diabetic, young adult BB rat studied by pancreatic biopsy. Diabetes *33*:33, 1984.

216. Nakhooda, A.F., Wei, C-N., Like, A.A., Marliss, E.B.:

The spontaneously diabetic Wistar rat (the "BB" rat): the significance of transient glycosuria. Diabete et Metabolisme (Paris) *4*:255, 1978.

217. Nakhooda, A.F., Like, A.A., Chappel, C.I., et al.: The spontaneously diabetic Wistar rat (the "BB" rat). Diabetologia *14*:199, 1978.

217a.Butler, L., Guberski, D.L., Like, A.A.: Genetic analysis of the BB/W diabetic rat. Can. J. Genet. Cytol. *25*:7, 1983.

217b.Guttmann, R.D., Colle, E., Michel, F., Seemayer, T.: Spontaneous diabetes mellitus syndrome in the rat. II. T lymphopenia and its association with clinical disease and pancreatic lymphocytic infiltration. J. Immunol. *130*:1732, 1983.

218. Rossini, A.A., Williams, R.M., Mordes, J.P., et al.: Spontaneous diabetes in the gnotobiotic BB/W rat. Diabetes *28*:1031, 1979.

218a.Rossini, A.A., Mordes, J.P., Gallina, D.L.: Hormonal and environmental factors in the pathogenesis of BB rat diabetes. Metabolism *32*(Suppl. 1):33, 1983.

218b.Elder, M., MacLaren, N., Riley, W., McConnell, T.: Gastric parietal cell and other autoantibodies in the BB rat. Diabetes *31*:313, 1982.

218c.Like, A.A., Butler, L., Williams, R.M., et al.: Spontaneous autoimmune diabetes mellitus in the BB rat. Diabetes *31*(Suppl. 1):7, 1982.

218d.Dyrberg, T., Nakhooda, A.F., Baekkeskov, S., et al.: Islet cell surface antibodies and lymphocyte antibodies in the spontaneously diabetic BB Wistar rat. Diabetes *31*:278, 1982.

218e.Jackson, R., Rassi, N., Crump, T., et al.: The BB diabetic rat: profound T-cell lymphocytopenia. Diabetes *30*:887, 1981.

218f.Poussier, P., Nakhooda, A.F., Falk, J.A., et al.: Lymphopenia and abnormal lymphocyte subsets in the "BB" rat: relationship to the diabetic syndrome. Endocrinology *110*:1825, 1982.

218g.Martin, D., Logothetopoulos, J.: Complement-fixing islet cell antibodies in the spontaneously diabetic BB rat. Diabetes *33*:93, 1984.

219. Like, A.A., Rossini, A.A., Appel, M.C., et al.: Spontaneous diabetes mellitus: reversal and prevention in the BB/W rat with antiserum to rat lymphocytes. Science *206*:1421, 1979.

220. Like, A.A., Kislauskis, E., Williams, R.M., Rossini, A.A.: Neonatal thymectomy prevents spontaneous diabetes mellitus in the BB/W rat. Science *216*:644, 1982.

220a.Laupacis, A., Stiller, C.R., Gardell, C., et al.: Cyclosporin prevents diabetes in BB Wistar rats. Lancet *1*:10, 1983.

220b.Like, A.A., Anthony, M., Guberski, D.L., Rossini, A.A.: Spontaneous diabetes in the BB/W rat: effects of glucocorticoids, cyclosporin A, and antiserum to rat lymphocytes. Diabetes *32*:326, 1983.

220c.Naji, A., Silvers, W.K., Bellgrau, D., Barker, C.F.: Spontaneous diabetes in rats: destruction of islets is prevented by immunological tolerance. Science *213*:1390, 1981.

220d.Rossini, A.A., Mordes, J.P., Pelletier, A.M., Like, A.A.: Transfusion of whole blood prevents diabetes mellitus in the BB/W rat. Science *219*:975, 1983.

220e.Nakhooda, A.F., Sima, A.A.S., Poussier, P., Marliss, E.B.: Passive transfer of insulitis from the "BB" rat to the nude mouse. Endocrinology *109*:2264, 1981.

220f.Mordes, J.P., Woda, B.A., Like, A.A., et al.: Lymphocyte transfusions prevent diabetes in the Bio Breeding/Worcester [BB/W] rat. Diabetologia *25*:182, 1983.

221. Rossini, A.A., Mordes, J.P., Pelletier, A.M., Like,

A.A.: Failure to transfer diabetes or insulitis in the BB rat. Metabolism *32*(Suppl 1):80, 1983.

222. Koevary, S., Rossini, A.A., Stoller, W., et al.: Passive transfer of diabetes in the BB rat. Science *220*:727, 1983.

222a Sternthal, E., Like, A.A., Sarantis, K., Braverman, L.E.: Lymphocytic thyroiditis and diabetes in the BB/W rat. A new model of autoimmune endocrinopathy. Diabetes *30*:1058, 1981.

223. Schmidt, F.L., Leslie, L.G., Schultz, J.R., Gerritsen, G.C. Epidemiologic studies of the Chinese hamster. Diabetologia *6*:154, 1970.

224. Gerritsen, G.C., Blanks, M.C.: Characterization of Chinese hamsters by metabolic balance, glucose tolerance, and insulin secretion. Diabetologia *10*:493, 1974.

225. Luse, S.A., Caramia, F., Gerritsen, G., Dulin, W.E.: Spontaneous diabetes mellitus in the Chinese hamster: an electron microscopic study of the islets of Langerhans. Diabetologia *3*:97, 1967.

226. Like, A.A., Gerritsen, G.C., Dulin, W.E., Gaudreau, P.: Studies in the diabetic hamster: light microscopy and autoradiography of pancreatic islets. Diabetologia *10*:501, 1974.

227. Orci, L., Stauffacher, W., Dulin, W.E., et al.: Ultrastructural changes in A-cells exposed to diabetic hyperglycaemia. Observations made on pancreas of Chinese hamsters. Diabetologia *6*:199, 1970.

228. Malaisse, W., Malaisse-Lagae, F., Gerritsen, G.C., et al.: Insulin secretion *in vitro* by the pancreas of the Chinese hamster. Diabetologia *3*:109, 1967.

229. Grodsky, G.M., Frankel, B.J., Gerich, J.E., Gerritsen, G.C.: The diabetic Chinese hamster: *In vitro* insulin and glucagon release; the "chemical diabetic"; and the effect of diet on ketonuria. Diabetologia *10*:521, 1974.

230. Gerritsen, G.C., Blanks, M.C., Miller, R.L., Dulin, W.E.: Effect of diet limitation on the development of diabetes in prediabetic Chinese hamsters. Diabetologia *10*:559, 1974.

231. Gerritsen, G.C., Blanks, M.C.: Preliminary studies on food and water consumption of prediabetic Chinese hamsters. Diabetologia *6*:177, 1970.

232. Carpenter, A-M., Gerritsen, G.C., Dulin, W.E., Lazarow, A.: Islet and beta cell volumes in offspring of severely diabetic (ketotic) Chinese hamsters. Diabetologia *6*:168, 1970.

233. Sims, E.A.H., Landau, B.R.: Diabetes mellitus in the Chinese hamster. I. Metabolic and morphologic studies. Diabetologia *3*:115, 1967.

234. Orci, L., Amherdt, M., Malaisse-Lagae, F., et al.: Morphological characterization of membrane systems in A- and B-cells of the Chinese hamster. Diabetologia *10*:529, 1974.

235. Like, A.A., Gerritsen, G.C., Dulin, W.E., Gaudreau, P.: Studies in the diabetic Chinese hamster: electron microscopy of pancreatic islets. Diabetologia *10*:509, 1974.

236. Frankel, B.J., Schmid, F.G., Grodsky, G.M.: Effect of continuous insulin infusion with an implantable seven-day minipump in the diabetic Chinese hamster. Endocrinology *104*:1532, 1979.

237. Dail, W.G., Jr., Evan, A.P., Gerritsen, G.C., Dulin, W.E.: Abnormalities in pelvic visceral nerves. A basis of neurogenic bladder in the diabetic Chinese hamster. Investigative Urology *15*:161, 1977.

238. Gerritsen, G.C., Dulin, W.E.: Characterization of diabetes in the Chinese hamster. Diabetologia *3*:74, 1967.

239. Chang, A.Y., Schneider, D.I.: Meatabolic abnormalities in the pancreatic islets and livers of the diabetic Chinese hamster. Diabetologia *6*:180, 1970.

240. Yamamoto, H.: Electron microscopic studies of the pan-creatic islets and some other organs in experimental congenital diabetic rats. Endocrinol. Jap. *18*:375, 1971.

241. Goto, Y., Kakizaki, M., Toyota, T., et al.: Spontaneous diabetes produced by repeated selective breeding of normal Wistar rats. In: Ninth Congress of the International Diabetes Federation. Amsterdam. Excerpta Medica Congress Series No. 413, 1977, pp. 703–710.

242. Toyota, T., Kakizaki, M., Kimura, K., et al.: Islet activating protein (IAP) derived from the culture supernatant fluid of Bordetella pertussis: effect on spontaneous diabetic rats. Diabetologia *14*:319, 1978.

243. Howard, C.F., Jr.: Diabetes in *Macaca nigra;* metabolic and histologic changes. Diabetologia *10*:671, 1974.

244. Howard, C.F., Jr.: Spontaneous diabetes in *Macaca nigra.* Diabetes *21*:1077, 1972.

245. Howard, C.F., Jr.: Correlations of serum triglyceride and prebetalipoprotein levels to the severity of spontaneous diabetes in *Macaca nigra.* J. Clin. Endocrinol. Metab. *38*:856, 1974.

246. Howard, C.F., Jr.: Insular amyloidosis and diabetes mellitus in *Macaca nigra.* Diabetes *27*:357, 1978.

247. Howard, C.F., Jr.: Phenotypic expression of diabetes mellitus in a closed breeding colony of *Macaca nigra.* In: R. Bogart (Ed.): Genetics Lectures, Vol. 5. Corvallis, Oregon University Press, 1977, pp. 67–88.

248. Howard, C.F., Jr.: Basement membrane thickness in muscle capillaries of normal and spontaneously diabetic *Macaca nigra.* Diabetes *24*:201, 1975.

249. Howard, C.F., Jr.: The relationship of diet and atherosclerosis in diabetic *Macaca nigra.* In: C. Sirtori, G. Ricci, S. Gorini (Eds.): Diet and Atherosclerosis. New York, Plenum, 1975, pp. 13–31.

250. Widness, J.A., Susa, J.B., Garcia, J.F., et al.: Increased erythropoiesis and elevated erythropoietin in infants born to diabetic mothers and hyperinsulinemic rhesus fetuses. J. Clin. Invest. *67*:637, 1981.

251. Farnsworth, P.N., Burke, P.A., Wagner, B.J., et al.: Diabetic cataracts in the rhesus monkey lens. Metab. Pediatr. Ophthalmol. *4*:31, 1980.

252. Hamilton, C.L., Ciaccia, P.: The course of development of glucose intolerance in the monkey *(Macaca mulatta).* J. Med. Primatol. *7*:165, 1978.

253. Lockwood, D.H., Hamilton, C.L., Livingston, J.N.: The influence of obesity and diabetes in the monkey on insulin and glucagon binding to liver membranes. Endocrinology *104*:76, 1979.

254. Davidson, I.W.F., Lang, C.M., Blackwell, W.L.: Impairment of carbohydrate metabolism of the squirrel monkey. Diabetes *16*:395, 1967.

255. Munger, B.L., Lang, C.M.: Spontaneous diabetes mellitus in guinea pigs. The acute cytopathology of the islets of Langerhans. Lab. Invest. *29*:685, 1973.

256. Lang, C.M., Munger, B.L.: Diabetes mellitus in the guinea pig. Diabetes *25*:434, 1976.

257. Balk, M.W., Lang, C.M., White, W.J., Munger, B.L.: Exocrine pancreatic dysfunction in guinea pigs with diabetes mellitus. Lab. Invest. *32*:28, 1975.

258. Lang, C.M., Munger, B.L., Rapp, F.: The guinea pig as an animal model of diabetes mellitus. Lab. Anim. Science *27*:789, 1977.

259. Stuhlman, R.A.: The genetic mode of transmission of spontaneous diabetes mellitus in *Mystromys albicaudatus.* M.S. Thesis. University of Missouri, Columbia, 1971.

260. Yesus, Y.W., Esterly, J.A., Stuhlman, R.A., Townsend, J.F.: Significant muscle capillary basement membrane thickening in spontaneously diabetic *Mystromys albicaudatus.* Diabetes *25*:444, 1976.

261. Stuhlman, R.A., Srivastava, P.K., Schmidt, G., et al.:

Characterization of diabetes in South African hamsters *(Mystromys albicaudatus)*. Diabetologia *10*:685, 1974.

262. Goeken, J.A., Packer, J.T., Rose, S.D., Stuhlman, R.A.: Structure of the islets of Langerhans: pathological studies in normal and diabetic *Mystromys albicaudatus*. Arch. Path. *93*:123, 1972.

263. Stuhlman, R.A., Packer, J.T., Doyle, R.E., et al.: Relationship between pancreatic lesions and serum glucose values in *Mystromys albicaudatus*. Lab. Anim. Science *25*:168, 1975.

264. Stuhlman, R.A., Packer, J.T., Doyle, R.E.: Spontaneous diabetes mellitus in *Mystromys albicaudatus*: repeated glucose values from 620 animals. Diabetes *21*:715, 1972.

265. Makino, S., Kunimoto, K., Muraoka, Y., et al.: Breeding of a non-obese diabetic strain of mice. Experimental Animals (Jikken Dobutsu) *29*:1, 1980.

265a.Yamada, K., Nonaka, K., Hanafusa, T., et al.: Preventive and therapeutic effects of large-dose nicotinamide injections on diabetes associated with insulitis: an observation in non-obese diabetic (NOD) mice. Diabetes *31*:749, 1982.

265b.Shigeki, K., Satoh, J., Fujiya, H., et al.: Immunologic aspects of the nonobese diabetic (NOD) mouse: abnormalities of cellular immunity. Diabetes *32*:247, 1983.

266. Kramer, J.W., Nottingham, S., Robinette, J., et al.: Inherited, early onset, insulin-requiring diabetes mellitus of keeshond dogs. Diabetes *29*:558, 1980.

267. Von Mehring, J., Minkowsky, O.: Diabetes Mellitus nach Pancreasextirpation. Naunyn Schmiedebergs Arch. Exp. Path. Pharmak. *26*:371, 1890.

268. Hausberger, F.X., Ramsay, A.J.: Islet hypertrophy in obesity of mice bearing ACTH-secreting tumors. Endocrinology *65*:165, 1959.

269. Abelove, W.A., Paschkis, K.E.: Comparison of the diabetogenic action of cortisone and growth hormone in different species. Endocrinology *55*:637, 1954.

270. Lazarus, S.S., Bencosme, S.A.: Alterations of pancreas during cortisone diabetes in rabbits. Proc. Soc. Exp. Biol. Med. *89*:114, 1955.

271. Franckson, J.R.M., Gepts, W., Bastenie, P.A., et al.: Observations sur le diabete steroide experimental du rat. Acta Endocrinol. *14*:153, 1953.

272. Baker, B.L.: A comparison of the histological changes induced by experimental hyperadrenalcorticalism and inanition. Rec. Progr. Horm. Res. *7*:331, 1951.

273. Cavellero, C., Mosca, L.: Mitotic activity in the pancreatic islets of the rat under pituitary growth hormone and adrenocorticotropic hormone treatment. J. Pathol. Bacteriol. *66*:147, 1953.

274. Kern, H., Logothetopoulos, J.: Steroid diabetes in the guinea pig: studies on islet cell ultrastructure and regeneration. Diabetes *19*:145, 1970.

275. Hausberger, F.X., Ramsay, A.J.: Steroid diabetes in guinea pigs. Effects of cortisone administration on blood and urinary glucose, nitrogen excretion, fat deposition and the islets of Langerhans. Endocrinology *53*:423, 1953.

276. Like, A.A., Chick, W.L.: Pancreatic beta cell replication induced by glucocorticoids in subhuman primates. Am. J. Pathology *75*:329, 1974.

277. Riviere, M., Combescot, C.H.: Sur le conditionement de certaines transformations langerhansiennes chez le singe. C. Rend. Soc. Biol. *148*:93, 1954.

278. Hetherington, A.W., Ranson, S.W.: Hypothalamic lesions and adiposity in the rat. Anat. Record *78*:149, 1940.

279. Bray, G.A., Gallagher, T.F., Jr.: Manifestations of hypothalamic obesity in man: a comprehensive investigation of eight patients and a review of the literature. Medicine *54*:301, 1975.

280. Marshall, N.B., Barnett, R.J., Mayer, J.: Hypothalamic lesions in goldthioglucose injected mice. Proc. Soc. Exp. Biol. Med. *90*:240, 1955.

281. Debons, A.F., Krimsky, I., Maayan, M.L., et al.: Goldthioglucose obesity syndrome. Fed. Proc. *36*:143, 1977.

282. Debons, A.F., Krimsky, I., From, A., Cloutier, R.J.: Rapid effects of insulin on the hypothalamic satiety center. Am. J. Physiol. *217*:1114, 1969.

283. Hales, C.N., Kennedy, G.C.: Plasma glucose, nonesterified fatty acid and insulin concentrations in hypothalamic-hyperphagic rats. Biochem. J. *90*:620, 1964.

284. Frohman, L.A., Bernardis, L.L.: Growth hormone and insulin levels in weanling rats with ventromedial hypothalamic lesions. Endocrinology *82*:1125, 1968.

285. Hinman, D.J., Griffith, D.R.: Effects of ventromedial hypothalamic lesions on thyroid secretion rate in rats. Horm. Metab. Res. *5*:48, 1973.

286. Frohman, L.A., Bernardis, L.L., Schnatz, J.D., Burek, L.: Plasma insulin and triglyceride levels after hypothalamic lesions in weanling rats. Am. J. Physiol. *216*:1496, 1969.

287. Powley, T.L., Opsahl, C.A.: Ventromedial hypothalamic obesity abolished by subdiaphragmatic vagotomy. Am. J. Physiol. *226*:25, 1974.

288. Kellar, K.J., Langley, A.E., Marks, B.H., O'Neill, J.J.: Ventral medial hypothalamus: involvement in hypoglycemic convulsions. Science *187*:746, 1975.

289. Riestra, J.L., Skowsky, W.R., Martinez, I., Swan, L.: Passive transfer of an appetite suppressant factor. Proc. Soc. Exp. Biol. Med. *156*:236, 1977.

290. Yoon, J-W., Austin, M., Onodera, T., Notkins, A.L.: Virus-induced diabetes mellitus. Isolation of a virus from the pancreas of a child with diabetic ketoacidosis. N. Engl. J. Med. *300*:1173, 1979.

290a.Rayfield, E.J., Seto, Y.: Viruses. In: M. Brownlee (Ed.): Handbook of Diabetes Mellitus. Vol. I., Etiology/Hormone Physiology. New York, Garland STPM Press, 1981, pp. 95–120.

290b.Barboni, E., Manocchio, I.: Alterazionia pancreatiche in bovino con diabete mellito post-aftoso. Arch. Vet. Ital. *13*:477, 1962.

290c.Platt, H.: The occurrence of pancreatic lesions in adult mice infected with the virus of FMD. Virology *9*:484, 1959.

290d.Platt, H.: A study of the pathological changes produced in young mice by the virus of foot-and-mouth disease. J. Pathol. Bacteriol. *72*:299, 1956.

290e.Platt, H.: Observations on the pathology of experimental foot-and-mouth disease in the adult guinea pig. J. Pathol. Bacteriol. *76*:119, 1958.

291. Boucher, D.W., Notkins, A.L.: Virus-induced diabetes mellitus. I. Hyperglycemia and hypoinsulinemia in mice infected with encephalomyocarditis virus. J. Exp. Med. *137*:1226, 1973.

292. Craighead, J.E., McLane, M.F.: Diabetes mellitus: induction in mice by encephalomyocarditis virus. Science *162*:913, 1968.

293. Craighead, J.E., Steinke, J.: Diabetes mellitus-like syndrome in mice infected with encephalomyocarditis virus. Am. J. Pathol. *63*:119, 1971.

294. Hayashi, K., Boucher, D.W., Notkins, A.L.:Virus-induced diabetes mellitus. II. Relationship between beta cell damage and hyperglycemia in mice infected with encephalomyocarditis virus. Am. J. Pathol. *75*:91, 1974.

295. Munterfering, H.: Zur Pathologie des Diabetes mellitus der veissen Maus bei der EMC-Virusinfektion: Histologische, elektron-mikroskopische und quantativ morphologische Befunde an den Langerhannschen Inseln. Virchows Arch. (Pathol. Anat.) A *356*:207, 1972.

296. Wellman, K.F., Amsterdam, D., Brancato, P., Volk, B.W.: Fine structure of pancreatic islets of mice infected with the M variant of the encephalomyocarditis virus. Diabetologia 8:349, 1972.

297. Petersen, K-G., Heilmeyer, P., Kerp, L.: Synthesis of proinsulin and large glucagon immunoreactivity in isolated Langerhans islets from EMC-virus infected mice. Diabetologia 11:21, 1975.

298. Craighead, J.E.: The role of viruses in the pathogenesis of pancreatic disease and diabetes mellitus. Prog. Med. Virol. 19:161, 1975.

298a. Wilson, G.L., Bellomo, S.C., Craighead, J.E.: Effect of interferon on encephalomyocarditis virus infection of cultured mouse pancreatic B cells. Diabetologia 24:38, 1983.

298b. Buschard, K., Hastrup, N., Rygaard, J.: Virus-induced diabetes mellitus in mice and the thymus-dependent immune system. Diabetologia 24:42, 1983.

299. Yoon, J-W., Notkins, A.L.: Virus-induced diabetes mellitus. VI. Genetically determined host differences in the replication of encephalomyocarditis virus in pancreatic beta cells. J. Exp. Med. 143:1170, 1976.

300. Boucher, D.W., Hayashi, K., Rosenthal, J., Notkins, A.L.: Virus induced diabetes mellitus. III. Influence of the sex and strain of the host. J. Infect. Dis. 131:462, 1975.

300a. Rayfield, E.J., Seto, Y., Goldberg, S.L., et al.: Venezuelan encephalitis virus-induced alterations in carbohydrate metabolism in genetically diabetic mice. Diabetes 28:799, 1979.

300b. Rayfield, E.J., Gorelkin, L., Curnow, R.T., Jahrling, P.B.: Virus-induced pancreatic disease by Venezuelan encephalitis virus: alterations in glucose tolerance and insulin release. Diabetes 25:623, 1976.

300c. Rayfield, E.J., Bowen, G.S.: The evolution of Venezuelan encephalitis virus-induced carbohydrate abnormalities in rhesus monkeys. Clin. Res. 25(Abstr.):398A, 1977.

300d. Menser, M.A., Forrest, J.M., Bransby, R.D.: Rubella infection and diabetes mellitus. Lancet 1:57, 1978.

300e. Onodera, T., Jenson, A.B., Yoon, J.-W., Notkins, A.L.: Virus-induced diabetes mellitus: reovirus infection of pancreatic B cells in mice. Science 201:529, 1978.

301. Burch, G.E., Tsui, C-Y., Harb, J.M., Colcolough, H.L.: Pathologic findings in the pancreas of mice infected with Coxsackie virus B4. Arch. Intern. Med. 128:40, 1971.

302. Tsui, C-Y, Burch, G.E., Harb, J.M.: Pancreatitis in mice infected with Coxsackie virus B1. Arch. Pathol. 93:397, 1972.

303. Harrison, A.K., Bauer, S.P., Murphy, F.A.: Viral pancreatitis: ultrastructural pathological effects of Coxsackie virus B3 infection in newborn mouse pancreas. Exp. Mol. Pathol. 17:206, 1972.

304. Coleman, T.J., Gamble, D.R., Taylor, K.W.: Diabetes in mice after Coxsackie B4 virus infection. Br. Med. J. 3:25, 1973.

305. Coleman, T.J., Taylor, K.W., Gamble, D.R.: The development of diabetes following Coxsackie B virus infection in mice. Diabetologia 10:755, 1974.

306. Kibrick, S., Benirschke, K.: Severe generalized disease (encephalohepatomyocarditis) occurring in the newborn period and due to infection with Coxsackie virus, group B; evidence of intrauterine infection with this agent. Pediatrics 22:857, 1958.

307. Pappenheimer, A.M., Kunz, L.J., Richardson, S.: Passage of Coxsackie virus (Connecticut-S strain) in adult mice with production of pancreatic disease. J. Exp. Med. 94:45, 1951.

308. Vizoso, A.D., Sanders, F.K.: Alteration of the pathogenicity of some group B Coxsackie viruses under different conditions of passage. I. Virus type 4. Acta Virol. (Praha) 8:38, 1964.

308a. Yoon, J.-W., Onodera, T., Notkins, A.L.: Virus-induced diabetes mellitus. XV. Beta cell damage and insulin-dependent hyperglycemia in mice infected with Coxsackie virus B4. J. Exp. Med. 148:1068, 1978.

309. Wilander, E.: Streptozotocin-diabetes in the Chinese hamster. Long-term effects on the light microscopic structure of the pancreatic islet tissue, liver and kidney. Acta Pathol. Microbiol. Scand. 82:767, 1974.

310. Dulin, W.E., Soret, M.G.: Chemically and hormonally induced diabetes. In: B.W. Volk, K.F. Wellman (Eds.): The Diabetic Pancreas. New York, Plenum, 1977, pp. 425–465.

311. Fischer, L.J., Rickert, D.E.: Pancreatic islet-cell toxicity. CRC Critical Reviews in Toxicology 3:231, 1975.

312. Okamoto, K.: Experimental production of diabetes. In: M. Ellenberg, H. Rifkin (Eds.): Diabetes Mellitus, Theory and Practice. New York, McGraw-Hill Book Co., 1970, pp. 230–255.

313. Rerup, C.C.: Drugs producing diabetes through damage of the insulin secreting cells. Pharmacol. Rev. 22:485, 1970.

314. Dunn, J.S., Sheehan, H.L., McLetchie, N.G.B.: Necrosis of islets of Langerhans produced experimentally. Lancet 1:484, 1943.

315. Landau, B.R., Renold, A.E.: The distribution of alloxan in the rat. Diabetes 3:47, 1954.

316. Watkins, D., Cooperstein, S.J., Lazarow, A.: Effect of alloxan on permeability of pancreatic islet tissue in vitro. Am. J. Physiol. 207:436, 1964.

317. Watkins, D., Cooperstein, S.J., Lazarow, A.: Effect of alloxan on islet tissue permeability; protection and reversal by sugars. Am. J. Physiol. 224:718, 1973.

318. Bhattacharya, G.: Protection against alloxan diabetes by mannose and fructose. Science 117:230, 1953.

319. Carter, W.J., Younathan, E.S.: Studies on protection against the diabetogenic effect of alloxan by glucose. Proc. Soc. Exp. Biol. Med. 109:611, 1962.

320. Rossini, A.A., Berger, M., Shadden, J., Cahill, G.F., Jr.: Beta cell protection to alloxan necrosis by anomers of D-glucose. Science 183:424, 1974.

321. Rossini, A.A., Arcangeli, M.A., Cahill, G.F., Jr.: Studies of alloxan toxicity on the beta cell. Diabetes 24:516, 1975.

322. Rossini, A.A., Like, A.A., Chick, W.L., et al.: Studies of streptozotocin-induced insulitis and diabetes. Proc. Natl. Acad. Sci. USA. 74:2485, 1977.

323. Fischer, L.J., Hamburger, S.A.: Inhibition of alloxan action in isolated pancreatic islets by superoxide dismutase, catalase, and a metal chelator. Diabetes 29:213, 1980.

324. Herr, R.R., Eble, T.E., Bergy, M.E., Jahnke, H.K.: Isolation and characterization of streptozotocin. Antibiot. Annu. 7:236, 1959–60.

325. Rossini, A.A., Like, A.A., Dulin, W.E., Cahill, G.F., Jr.: Pancreatic beta cell toxicity by streptozotocin anomers. Diabetes 26:1120, 1977.

326. Schein, P.S., Loftus, S.: Streptozotocin: depression of mouse liver pyridine nucleotides. Cancer Res. 28:1501, 1968.

327. Wilander, E., Gunnarson, R.: Diabetogenic effects of N-nitrosomethylurea in the Chinese hamster. Acta Pathol. Microbiol. Scand. Sect. A 83:206, 1975.

328. Gunnarson, R., Berne, C., Hellerström, C.: Cytotoxic effects of streptozotocin and N-nitrosomethylurea on the pancreatic B-cell with special regard to the role of nicotinamide-adenine dinucleotide. Biochem. J. 140:487, 1974.

329. Ganda, O.P., Rossini, A.A., Like, A.A.: Studies on streptozotocin diabetes. Diabetes 25:595, 1976.
330. Like, A.A., Rossini, A.A.: Streptozotocin-induced pancreatic insulitis: new model of diabetes mellitus. Science 193:415, 1976.
331. Appel, M.C., Rossini, A.A., Williams, R.M., Like, A.A.: Viral studies in streptozotocin-induced pancreatic insulitis. Diabetologia 15:327, 1978.
332. Like, A.A., Appel, M.C., Williams, R.M., Rossini, A.A.: Streptozotocin-induced pancreatic insulitis in mice. Morphologic and physiologic studies. Lab. Invest. 38:470, 1978.
333. Rossini, A.A., Williams, R.M., Appel, M.C., Like, A.A.: Sex differences in the multiple-dose streptozotocin model of diabetes. Endocrinology 103:1518, 1978.
334. Rossini, A.A., Appel, M.C., Williams, R.M., Like, A.A.: Genetic influence of the streptozotocin-induced insulitis and hyperglycemia. Diabetes 26:916, 1977.
335. Rossini, A.A., Williams, R.M., Appel, M.C., Like, A.A.: Complete protection from low-dose streptozotocin-induced diabetes in mice. Nature (London) 276:182, 1978.
335a. Paik, S.G., Blue, M.L., Fleischer, N., Shin, S-I.: Diabetes susceptibility of BALB/cBOM mice treated with streptozotocin. Inhibition by lethal irradiation and restoration by splenic lymphocytes. Diabetes 31:808, 1982.
335b. Kiesel, U., Kolb, H.: Suppressive effect of antibodies to immune response gene products on the development of low-dose streptozotocin-induced diabetes. Diabetes 32:869, 1983.
335c. Leiter, E.H., Beamer, W.G., Shultz, L.D.: The effect of immunosuppression on streptozotocin-induced diabetes in C57BL/KsJ mice. Diabetes 32:148, 1983.
335d. Leiter, E.H.: Multiple low-dose streptozotocin-induced hyperglycemia and insulitis in C57BL mice: influence of inbred background, sex, and thymus. Proc. Natl. Acad. Sci. USA 79:630, 1982.
335e. Bonnevie-Neilsen, V., Steffes, M.W., Lernmark, Å.: A major loss in islet mass and β-cell function precedes hyperglycemia in mice given multiple low doses of streptozotocin. Diabetes 30:424, 1981.
336. Prosser, P.R., Karam, J.H.: Diabetes mellitus following rodenticide ingestion in man. J.A.M.A. 239:1148, 1978.
337. Miller, L., Stokes, J.D., Siepipol, C.: Diabetes mellitus and autonomic dysfunction after Vacor rodenticide ingestion. Diabetes Care 1:73, 1978.
338. Rossini, A.A., Mordes, J.P.: Unpublished data.
339. Yokote, M.: Sekoke disease, spontaneous diabetes in carp, Cyprinus carpio, found in fish farms. I. Pathological study. Bulletin Freshwater Fisheries Research Laboratory (Japan) 20:38, 1970.
340. Yokote, M.: Sekoke disease, spontaneous diabetes found in fish farms. II. Some metabolic aspects. Bulletin Japanese Society Scientific Fisheries 36:1214, 1970.
341. Yokote, M.: Written communication. May 20, 1979.
342. Chobanian, A.V., Gerritsen, G.C., Brecher, P.I., McCombs, L.: Aortic glucose metabolism in the diabetic Chinese hamster. Diabetologia 10:589, 1974.
343. McCombs, H.L., Gerritsen, G.C., Dulin, W.E., Chobanian, A.V.: Morphologic changes in the aorta of the diabetic Chinese hamster. Diabetologia 10:601, 1974.
344. Chobanian, A.V., Gerritsen, G.C., Brecher, P.I., Kessler, M.: Cholesterol metabolism in the diabetic Chinese hamster. Diabetologia 10:595, 1974.
345. Luse, S.A., Gerritsen, G.C., Dulin, W.E.: Cerebral abnormalities in diabetes mellitus: an ultrastructural study of the brain in early onset diabetes mellitus in the Chinese hamster. Diabetologia 6:192, 1970.
346. Yen, T.T., Allan, J.A., Pearson, D.V., Schinitsky, M.R.:

347. Dissociation of obesity, hypercholesterolemia and diabetes from atherosclerosis in ob/ob mice. Experientia 33:995, 1977.
347. Camerini-Davalos, R.A., Oppermann, W., Mittl, R., Ehrenreich, T.: Studies of vascular and other lesions in KK mice. Diabetologia 6:324, 1970.
348. Diani, A.R., Weaver, E.A., Gerritsen, G.C.: Capillary basement membrane thickening associated with the small intestine of the ketonuric Chinese hamster. Lab. Invest. 44:388, 1981.
349. Mauer, S.M., Steffes, M.W., Brown, D.M.: Animal models of diabetic nephropathy. Adv. Nephr. 8:23, 1979.
350. Shirai, T., Welsh, G.W., Sims, E.A.H.: Diabetes mellitus in the Chinese hamster. II. The evolution of renal glomerulopathy. Diabetologia 3:266, 1967.
351. Ørskov, H.T., Olsen, T.S., Nielsen, K., et al.: Kidney lesions in rats with severe long-term diabetes. I. Influence of age, alloxan damage, and insulin administration. Diabetologia 1:172, 1965.
352. Like, A.A., Lavine, R.L., Poffenbarger, P.L., Chick, W.L.: Studies in the diabetic mutant mouse. VI. Evolution of glomerular lesions and associated proteinuria. Am. J. Path. 66:193, 1972.
353. Orci, L., Stauffacher, W., Amherdt, M., et al.: The kidney of spiny mice (Acomys cahirinus): electron microscopy of glomerular changes associated with aging and tubular glycogen accumulation during hyperglycemia. Diabetologia 6:343, 1970.
354. Soret, M.G., Dulin, W.E., Matthews, J., Gerritsen, G.C.: Morphologic abnormalities observed in retina, pancreas and kidney of diabetic Chinese hamsters. Diabetologia 10:567, 1974.
355. Lawe, J.E.: Renal changes in hamster with hereditary diabetes mellitus. Arch. Path. 73:166, 1962.
356. Riley, T., Stuhlman, R.A., Van Peenen, H.J., et al.: Glomerular lesions of diabetes mellitus in Mystromys albicaudatus. Arch. Path. 99:167, 1975.
357. Gibbs, G.E., Wilson, R.B., Gifford, H.: Glomerulosclerosis in the long-term alloxan diabetic monkey. Diabetes 15:258, 1966.
358. Bloodworth, J.M.B.: Experimental diabetic glomerulosclerosis. II. The dog. Arch. Path. 79:113, 1965.
359. Soret, M.G., Peterson, T., Wyse, B., et al.: Renal amyloidosis in KK mice that may be misinterpreted as diabetic glomerulosclerosis. Arch. Path. Lab. Med. 101:464, 1977.
360. Fox, C.J., Darby, S.C., Ireland, J.T., Sonksen, P.H.: Blood glucose control and glomerular capillary basement membrane thickening in experimental diabetes. Br. Med. J. 2:605, 1977.
361. Mauer, S.M., Sutherland, D.E.R., Steffes, M.W., et al.: Pancreatic islet transplantation. Effects on the glomerular lesions of experimental diabetes in the rat. Diabetes 23:748, 1974.
362. Steffes, M.W., Brown, D.M., Mauer, S.M.: Diabetic glomerulopathy following unilateral nephrectomy in the rat. Diabetes 27:35, 1978.
363. Caird, F.I., Pirie, A., Ramsell, T.G.: Diabetes and the Eye. Oxford. Blackwell Scientific Publications. 1968.
364. Engerman, R.L., Bloodworth, J.M.B.: Experimental diabetic retinopathy in dogs. Arch. Ophthal. 73:205, 1965.
365. Häusler, H.R., Sibay, T.M., Campbell, J.: Retinopathy in a dog following diabetes induced by growth hormone. Diabetes 13:122, 1964.
366. Sibay, T.M., Hausler, H.R.: Eye findings in two spontaneously diabetic related dogs. Am. J. Ophthal. 63:289, 1967.
367. Toussaint, D.: Lesions retiniennes au course de diabete

alloxanique chez le rat. Bull. Soc. Belg. Ophthal. *143*:648, 1966

368. Agrawal, P.K., Agrawal, L.P., Tandon, H.D.: Experimental diabetic retinopathy in albino rats. Orient. Arch. Ophthal. *4*:68, 1966.

369. Sosula, L., Beaumont, P., Hollows, F.C., Jonson, K.M.: Dilation and endothelial proliferation of retinal capillaries in streptozotocin diabetic rats: quantitative electron microscopy. Invest. Ophthal. *11*:926, 1972.

370. Federman, J.L., Gerritsen, G.C.: The retinal vasculature of the Chinese hamster: a preliminary study. Diabetologia *6*:186, 1970.

371. Leuenberger, P., Cameron, D., Stauffacher, W., et al.: Ocular lesions in rats rendered chronically diabetic with streptozotocin. Ophthal. Res. *2*:189, 1971.

372. Gabbay, K.H.: The sorbitol pathway and the complications of diabetes. N. Engl. J. Med. *288*:831, 1973.

373. Holcomb, G.N., Klemm, L.A., Dulin, W.E.: The polyol pathway for glucose metabolism in tissues from normal, diabetic, and ketotic Chinese hamsters. Diabetologia *10*:549, 1974.

374. Schlaepfer, W.W., Gerritsen, G.C., Dulin, W.E.: Segmental demyelination in the distal peripheral nerves of chronically diabetic Chinese hamsters. Diabetologia *10*:541, 1974.

375. Eliasson, S.G.: Nerve conduction changes in experimental diabetes. J. Clin. Invest. *43*:2353, 1964.

376. Eliasson, S.G.: Properties of isolated nerve fibers from alloxanized rats. J. Neurol. Neurosurg. Psychiat. *32*:525, 1969.

377. Lovelace, R.E.: Experimental neuropathy in rats made diabetic with alloxan. Electroenceph. Clin. Neurophysiol. *25*:399, 1968.

377a. Vlassara, H., Brownlee, M., Cerami, A.: Excessive nonenzymatic glycosylation of peripheral and central nervous system myelin components in diabetic rats. Diabetes *32*:670, 1983.

377b. Sharma, A.K., Thomas, P.K., Gabriel, G., et al.: Peripheral nerve abnormalities in the diabetic mutant mouse. Diabetes *32*:1152, 1983.

337c. Sima, A.A.F., Thibert, P.: Proximal motor neuropathy in the BB-Wistar rat. Diabetes *31*:784, 1982.

378. Sirek, O.V., Sirek, A.: The colony of Chinese hamsters of the C.H. Best Institute. Diabetologia *3*:65, 1967.

379. Hellman, B.: Some metabolic aspects of the obese-hyperglycemic syndrome in mice. Diabetologia *3*:222, 1967.

380. Silberberg, R., Gerritsen, G., Hasler, M.: Articular cartilage of diabetic Chinese hamsters. Arch. Path. Lab. Med. *100*:50, 1976.

381. Orci, L., Stauffacher, W.: Glycogenosomes in renal tubular cells of diabetic animals. J. Ultrastructure Res. *36*:499, 1971.

382. Koenig, R.J., Cerami, A.: Synthesis of hemoglobin A_{1c} in normal and diabetic mice: potential model of basement thickening. Proc. Natl. Acad. Sci. USA *72*:3687, 1975.

382a. Howard, C.F., Jr.: Correlations of hemoglobin A_{1c} and metabolic status in nondiabetic, borderline diabetic, and diabetic *Macaca nigra*. Diabetes *31*:1105, 1982.

383. Soeldner, J.S.: Personal communication.

8 Hormone-Fuel Interrelationships in Normal, Fasting, and Diabetic Man

Thomas T. Aoki

In order to more fully appreciate the disordered hormone-fuel-tissue interrelationships that exist in diabetic patients, a reasonably clear understanding of these same relationships in normal subjects is essential. In this brief presentation, we will first consider the fuel depots of a normal individual, and then review those mechanisms currently thought to be responsible for the distribution and utilization of various fuels (carbohydrate, lipid, protein) in normal, fasting, and diabetic man.

FUEL DEPOTS

In a normal 70-kg individual (Fig. 8-1) there are approximately 300 g of mobilizable carbohydrate, primarily in the form of blood glucose and liver glycogen, available for general use. There are an additional 400 to 500 g of carbohydrate in the form of muscle glycogen; however, this is not readily available to the rest of the body and, for practical purposes, can be used only by muscle during periods of exercise. Thus, readily available quantities of blood glucose and liver glycogen can furnish approximately 1200 calories or one half day's supply of energy in a normal subject. It should be pointed out that for every gram of liver or muscle glycogen, an additional 2 to 3 ml of water are required in order to store this particular fuel. Hence, the energy density of this substrate is relatively low.

In the same normal individual, there are approximately 6 kg of protein representing approxi-

mately 25,000 calories. However, virtually all of this tissue is in the form of functional structures such as muscle, enzymes, and albumin. For this reason, a normal individual cannot sustain a loss in total body protein of greater than 2 kg without becoming so weak that breathing and coughing become extremely difficult, leading to atelectasis and the development of pneumonia. In addition, approximately 3 to 4 ml of water are required to accompany each gram of protein retained. Hence, like carbohydrate, protein is low in terms of energy density.

In contrast to both carbohydrate and protein, adipose tissue is only 10% water by weight. Thus, 1 g of adipose tissue yields close to the theoretical 9 calories obtained by the oxidation of 1 g of pure triglyceride. Since even a normal adult has approximately 15 kg of adipose tissue (representing

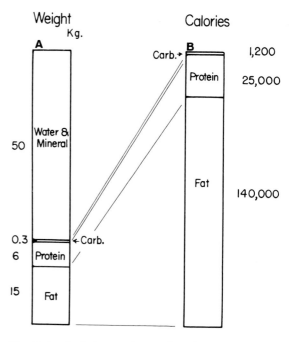

Fig. 8-1. Fuel depots of normal 70-kg man. A loss of greater than 2 kg of the approximately 6 kg of body protein results in significant impairment in the functioning of this individual. (Used with permission of authors and publishers.[71])

120 to 140,000 calories), it is clear that adipose tissue represents the primary source of mobilizable and expendable energy in most persons.

From the foregoing, it should be obvious that the rate-limiting fuel in man is protein, which in normal individuals is already fulfilling a functional role. Extensive dissolution of this particular tissue for energetic purposes can lead only to impaired functioning of the individual and, in primitive societies, to decreased survival. As we shall see later, the human body appears to recognize the necessity for minimizing the loss of muscle protein tissue under even the most adverse conditions.

THE METABOLISM OF FASTING MAN

In order to gain a clearer understanding of hormone-fuel-tissue interrelationships in normal subjects, it has been extremely profitable to examine these interrelationships in individuals undergoing a prolonged therapeutic fast for weight reduction. Unlike postabsorptive subjects, fasting subjects enter a metabolically steady state which permits close analysis of the changes—and their ramifications—in protein, lipid, and carbohydrate metabolism following the introduction of a given metabolic challenge. From these studies, a clearer understanding has gradually evolved of how man is able to maximally utilize his most abundant energy stores (i.e., adipose tissue) while simultaneously defending his relatively meager caloric store of body protein. The mechanisms activated by starving man, and the impairment of these same mechanisms in diabetic patients, will be discussed.

Participants in these studies were overweight (>100% over ideal body weight) but otherwise normal individuals (intravenous glucose tolerance test, a biochemical screening profile, and normal T_3, T_4, and TSH levels). Following admission to the Clinical Research Center at the Brigham and Women's Hospital and after completion of an equilibration period of 4 to 7 days (2500 calorie balanced diet), these individuals were fasted for 6 to 8 weeks. During the fast, they ingested daily tablets containing 17 mEq each of sodium chloride and potassium chloride and at least 2 liters of water. After approximately 3 weeks on this regimen, they entered a metabolically steady state (Figs. 8–2 to 5). In this situation, daily oscillations in concentration of substrates and hormones are minimal.

During a fast, a number of changes are seen in both blood and urine. As shown in Figure 8–2, serum insulin levels decline rapidly, reaching a nadir at about 3 to 5 days and remaining at this level for the duration of the fast. Triiodothyronine (T_3) levels also gradually decline.[1-3] In contrast, plasma glucagon levels peak on days 3 to 5[4] and then decline somewhat, but remain elevated for the

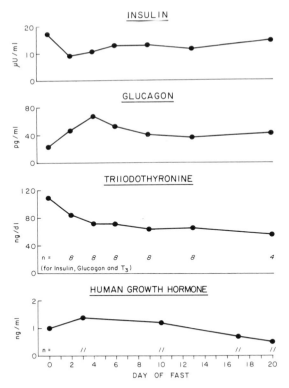

Fig. 8–2. Changes in circulating hormone levels during the performance of a fast. Note the decline in circulating insulin levels, the increase in plasma glucagon levels by the third to fifth day, and the fall in T_3 levels during the performance of the fast. Serum growth hormone levels do not change significantly. (Used with permission of authors and publishers.[72])

duration of the fast. Growth hormone levels do not change appreciably during the starvation regimen.[5]

Blood glucose levels (Fig. 8–3) decline from approximately 5 mM/L (90 mg/dl) to 3.5 mM/L (63 mg/dl) within the first 3 to 5 days. Plasma free fatty acids rise, reaching levels as high as 2 mM/L. Levels of the ketoacids β-hydroxybutyric and acetoacetic acids rise from approximately .05 mM/L to as high as 5 to 6 mM/L of β-hydroxybutyric and 1 mM of acetoacetic acid per liter of blood. Despite the gradual increase of circulating levels of these fuels, maximal rates of hepatic ketoacid production (100 to 150 g/day) are reached within 1 to 2 days.[6]

Approximately 100 to 150 mM/day of β-hydroxybutyric and acetoacetic acids combined are produced by days 5 to 7 in excess of metabolic needs. This excess is promptly excreted in the urine (Fig. 8–4), which necessitates a concomitant increased excretion of ammonia nitrogen to titrate the increased organic acid load. Figure 8–5 demonstrates total nitrogen excretion in overweight but otherwise normal subjects undergoing a therapeutic fast. It is readily seen that initially the primary

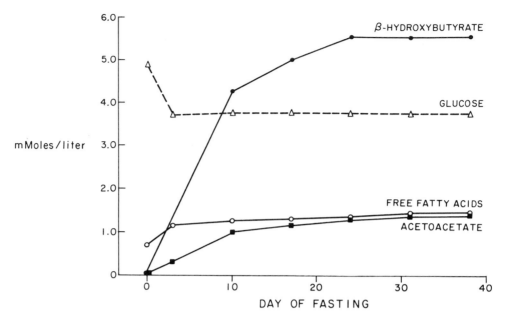

Fig. 8–3. Changes in substrate levels during the performance of a fast. Blood glucose levels decline within three days, while blood β-hydroxybutyric and acetoacetic acid increase significantly and peak at day 21. Levels of plasma free fatty acid, the primary fuel of both postabsorptive and fasting individuals, increase promptly and peak as high as 2000 μEq/l during the fasting period. (Used with permission of authors and publishers.[71])

nitrogenous component in the urine is in the form of urea, with only a small amount of ammonia being excreted each day. (It should be pointed out that urinary urea nitrogen excretion is an index of hepatic gluconeogenesis, while ammonia nitrogen excretion is an indicator of renal ammoniagenesis and gluconeogenesis.) With progression of a therapeutic fast, and the increased ketoacid production by the liver in response to falling insulin levels and rising levels of free fatty acids in plasma, there is a growing need to titrate the small but significant amount of ketoacids excreted in the urine, using ammonia nitrogen derived primarily from glutamine.[7] Thus late in the fast, glucose production by the liver is equal to or less than that produced by the kidney. However, the liver is now producing ketoacids at the same daily rate at which it had previously produced glucose.[6]

Hormone-fuel interrelationships change rapidly when the fasting period is extended beyond 3 to 5 days to greater than 3 to 6 weeks. Figure 8–6 depicts some of the changes that occur in briefly (1 to 3 days) fasted individuals. The primary fuel of these individuals, as in postabsorptive man, is fatty acids. The process of ketogenesis shown is stimulated by elevated levels of free fatty acids (and low insulin levels); ketogenesis supplies the needed energy for hepatic gluconeogenesis, a process by which amino acids derived primarily from muscle are converted to glucose. This utilization of

muscle[8] and perhaps splanchnic bed protein stores[2] is necessitated by the relatively slow increase in circulating ketoacid levels early in the therapeutic fast. With decreased utilization of the ketoacids by peripheral tissues,[9] circulating levels of this fat-derived glucose-equivalent fuel rise and the need for hepatic gluconeogenesis greatly decreases, as suggested by Figure 8–5.

Figure 8–7 is a representation of the metabolic changes in individuals who have undergone a much more sustained fast (6 to 8 weeks in duration). Note that protein mobilization and utilization are remarkably curtailed in such individuals. It was subsequently demonstrated[8] that this marked diminution in hepatic gluconeogenesis was due primarily to a decrease in amino acid release from muscle bed, and hence a decrease in substrate for hepatic gluconeogenesis. This adaptation was made possible by increased hepatic ketoacid production which, in turn, was able to supply to brain an adipose tissue-derived fuel in the form of β-hydroxybutyric and acetoacetic acids, that was water-soluble, calorically equivalent to glucose, and easily able to cross the blood-brain barrier.

With the foregoing in mind, attention was then directed toward characterizing and elucidating the mechanisms involved in the many adaptations seen in human subjects undergoing therapeutic fasts. As we shall see later, and germane to diabetic subjects in particular, the body of a fasting individual is

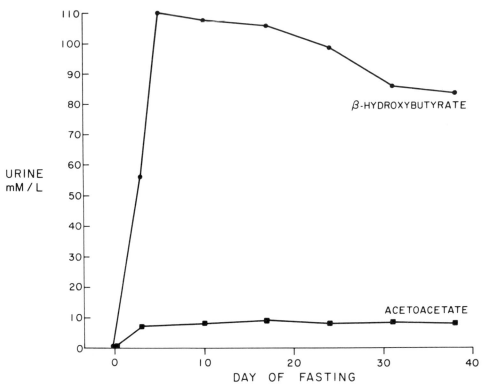

Fig. 8–4. Urinary excretion of β-hydroxybutyric and acetoacetic acids increases to a peak at day 7 to 10 of the fasting period. The gradual decline late in the fast may represent increased utilization of these fuels, which are calorically equivalent to glucose and do not require insulin in order to penetrate the blood-brain barrier. (Used with permission of authors and publishers.[71])

primarily concerned with defending its relatively meager stores of body protein. Over the years, this laboratory has sought to determine what roles various hormones play in the regulation of the metabolism of such tissues as muscle, adipose tissue, liver, and kidney—roles which permit overweight subjects to safely survive a sustained fast.

The Role of Hormones

Cortisol,[10] glucagon,[4,11] and human growth hormone[12] do not account for the adaptive changes observed during fasting. However, the actions of two hormones, insulin and triiodothyronine, do appear to permit overweight subjects to safely sustain a prolonged fast.

As pointed out previously, serum insulin levels decline (Fig. 8–2) during the initial phase of a fast, and remain at this lower level for the duration of the starvation period. At first glance it would seem somewhat paradoxical that a hormone that is importantly involved in the adaptation to fasting would decline. However, there appears to be good evidence suggesting that muscle tissue of prolonged fasted individuals becomes more sensitive to the effects of insulin.[13,14]

Perhaps of greater relevance is the observation that when 20 units of crystalline zinc insulin are infused over 24 hours into individuals who have starved for 4 to 6 weeks, circulating glucose levels decline rather rapidly from approximately 50 mg/dl down to as little as 15 mg/dl. Since the brains of these individuals are utilizing the ketoacids to meet 60 to 80% of their fuel requirements,[15] the fall in blood glucose level should not and does not result in symptomatic hypoglycemia[16] (Fig. 8–8). Note that during the 24-hour infusion of insulin into these fasted individuals, β-hydroxybutyric and acetoacetic acid levels do not change significantly. In contrast, blood glucose levels decline swiftly. Note also that plasma free fatty acid levels, which are elevated at the start of the study, do not fall during the insulin infusion. This is in marked contrast to postabsorptive individuals in whom a rather precipitous fall in plasma free fatty acid level follows insulin administration.[17] Also of interest is a small but significant transient decline in urinary urea nitrogen excretion. Taken as a whole, these data suggest that the infusion of small quantities of insulin into fasted individuals is able to further decrease the release of amino acids from muscle of individ-

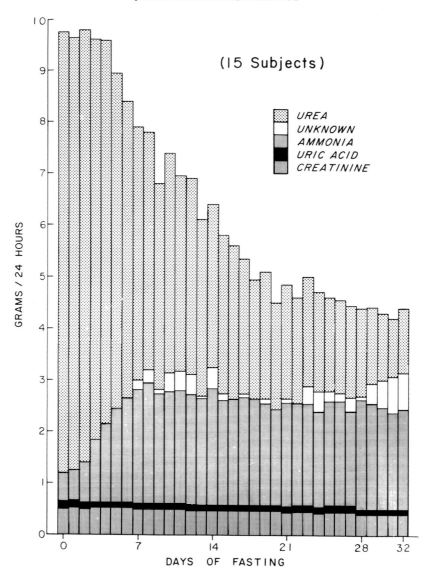

Fig. 8–5. Urinary nitrogen excretion during the performance of a fast. Note that the primary nitrogenous component in the postabsorptive period is urea, a splendid indicator of hepatic gluconeogenesis. After 7 to 10 days of the fast, ammonia nitrogen excretion—an equally good indicator of renal ammoniagenesis and renal gluconeogenesis—increases and remains elevated for the duration of the fast. (Used with permission of authors and publishers.[72])

uals already maximally conserving protein, resulting in a concomitant decline in hepatic gluconeogenesis as reflected by a decrease in urinary urea nitrogen excretion. Thus, insulin's role in affecting nitrogen metabolism in fasting individuals seems to be assured.

Even more persuasive is the observation that when physiologic quantities of insulin are infused into postabsorptive forearm muscle bed, amino acid release from forearm muscle bed is remarkably attenuated.[17] Indeed, in another study, infusion of similar quantities of insulin into forearm muscle bed of normal postabsorptive individuals resulted in an increase in uptake of glutamate by this tissue.[18]

In the early 1920s, a number of investigators began to study the metabolic consequences of thyroxine administration on fuel homeostasis in general and nitrogen metabolism in particular. It was quickly discovered that this hormone was capable of increasing the basal metabolic rate, as well as increasing nitrogen breakdown in man.[19] In the past several years, a number of studies have been performed in order to determine the mechanism by which thyroid hormone in general, and T_3 in particular, is capable of exerting relatively profound effects on nitrogen metabolism. As noted earlier, T_3 levels decline during a sustained fast. It has been reported[2] that the administration of 15 μg of T_3

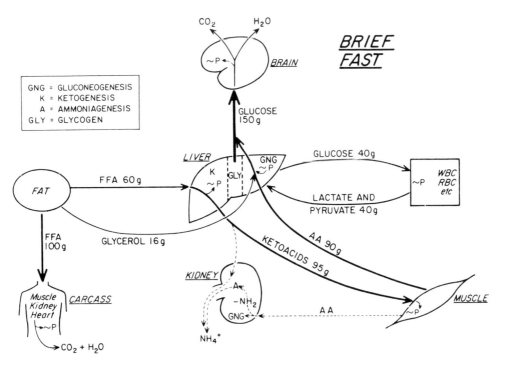

Fig. 8–6. A schematic representation of the changes that occur during the performance of a brief (1 to 3 day) fast. Early in the fast, ketoacid production by the liver results in the transport of ketoacid to muscle and subsequent utilization of this fuel by that tissue. Approximately 90 g of amino acid, as evidenced by urinary nitrogen excretion (Fig. 8–5), are mobilized and converted by the liver into glucose which is ultimately oxidized to CO_2 and H_2O by brain. Another 40 g of glucose are produced each day from lactate and pyruvate which are derived from glycolysis taking place in red and white blood cells and renal medulla. The lactate and pyruvate are subsequently transported to the liver and converted back to glucose, using hepatic energy in part derived from hepatic ketogenesis. Also, small amounts of ketoacids are being lost in the urine which necessitates a concomitant utilization of small amounts of glutamine to titrate that organic acid load.

every 6 hours for 2 days to overweight but otherwise normal individuals who had fasted for 3 weeks, resulted in the restoration of circulating T_3 levels back to postabsorptive concentrations. Importantly, there was a marked increase in both urinary urea (hence, hepatic gluconeogenesis) and ammonia (and, hence renal ammoniagenesis and gluconeogenesis) nitrogen excretion. In addition, it was observed that plasma free fatty acid levels increased significantly, as did blood glycerol levels, indicating that lipolysis had been stimulated. Urinary 3-methylhistidine excretion was monitored, but did not increase significantly until 5 days after the start of the investigation, suggesting that muscle proteolysis, of which 3-methylhistidine excretion in urine is an indicator,[20–23] occurred only secondarily, presumably to replete diminished or somewhat depleted splanchnic stores of protein. Thus the initial loss of nitrogen was almost entirely due to dissolution of splanchnic protein. The effect on adipose tissue still remains to be elucidated.

Increased urinary excretion of β-hydroxybutyric and acetoacetic acids was also observed during the course of the above investigation.[2] This increased organic acid load required increased renal ammo-niagenesis from glutamine, and, as might be expected, there was increased glutamine release from forearm muscle bed at this time of heightened renal ammonia production. Thus, directly or indirectly, T_3 had relatively profound effects on overall fuel homeostasis, and on nitrogen metabolism in particular.

The decline in T_3 levels during the fast is also accompanied by a fall in the respiratory quotient (ratio of CO_2 production to oxygen consumption), as well as a decrease of approximately 20% in the basal metabolic rate. Presumably, the fall in T_3 is due to a decrease in dietary carbohydrate and/or the change from a mixed carbohydrate-protein-lipid fuel economy to one almost exclusively based on lipid.

Glucagon, a hormone secreted by the alpha cells of the pancreas, is not currently considered an essential hormone with respect to fuel regulation in man. In part, this view stems from the observation that glucagon administration is not required for maintenance of apparently normal hormone-fuel interrelationships in patients who have undergone total pancreatectomy. However, this conclusion must be tempered by the discovery that cells similar

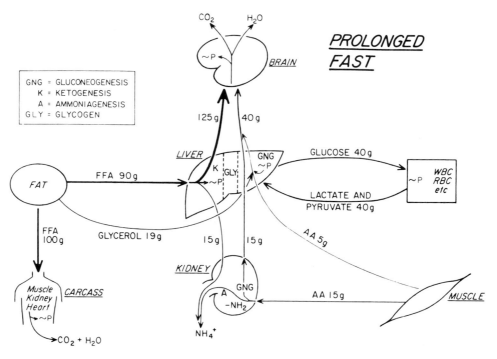

Fig. 8–7. A schematic representation of the changes that occur during the performance of a prolonged (5 to 6 weeks) fast. Note that in contrast to Figure 8–6, amino acid release from muscle is dramatically diminished to about 20 g/day. Free fatty acids remain the primary fuel, while ketoacid utilization by brain increases to approximately 100 to 125 g/day.

to the α-cells appear to be present in different parts of the GI tract. Nevertheless, some findings from investigations of fasting subjects suggest that glucagon may have an important, but as yet not appreciated, role in fuel homeostasis.

In subjects undergoing therapeutic starvation, plasma glucagon levels have been found to rise during days 3 to 6 of the fast (Fig. 8–2), and to decline thereafter though remaining at higher than postabsorptive levels for the duration of the fasting period. At first investigators were puzzled to find that this hormone, which was known to be a potent stimulator of hepatic gluconeogenesis, was elevated at a time when its levels apparently should have been reduced in order to conserve nitrogen. (Parenthetically, the elevated glucagon levels may be secondary to the elevated levels of glycine and threonine found in fasting subjects. Both amino acids are potent stimulators of the α-cell.[24]) As noted previously, however, protein utilization is largely determined by the rate of release of amino acids from muscle, and not by the activities of the liver itself. Thus, it could be persuasively argued that the primary purpose of the elevated plasma glucagon levels in fasting subjects is to maintain at optimal levels hepatic enzymes involved in amino acid trapping and gluconeogenesis. This sequence is especially important since the primary

stimulus for glucagon secretion in normal man is a protein meal.

Finally, when physiologic quantities of this hormone are infused into prolonged fasted individuals, urinary urea nitrogen secretion diminishes during the course of the infusion and for several days thereafter.[4,11] These data suggest that glucagon may be able to spare nitrogen by a direct effect on both liver and muscle. Much more work is needed in this area to confirm or deny the role of this hormone in overall hormone-fuel homeostasis in fasting subjects.

The Possible Role of Tissue Redox State

It has been previously noted that serum insulin levels decline during a fast, largely reflecting a decrease in incoming carbohydrate. Also, insulin is preeminent in its capacity to diminish amino acid release from forearm muscle bed of both prolonged fasted and postabsorptive individuals. However, it has been difficult to reconcile the fall in insulin levels during a fast when one might reasonably predict that levels of this hormone would remain at postabsorptive levels or actually increase. Because of this incongruity, a nonhormonally-based mechanism was considered that would perhaps complement the insulin-based process limiting amino acid release from forearm muscle.

As noted earlier, arterial lactate levels do not

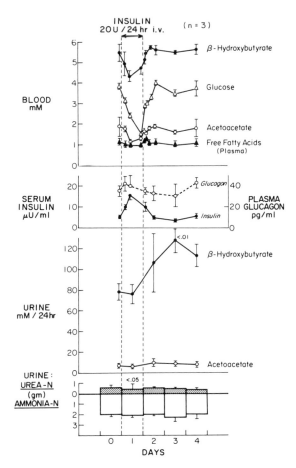

Fig. 8–8. Changes in blood and urine in fasted individuals (4 to 6 weeks) following the infusion of insulin (20 units/24 hours). Note the fall in blood glucose concentrations coincident with a slight fall in β-hydroxybutyric and acetoacetic acid levels. Free plasma fatty acid levels do not change significantly. There is a small but significant decline in urinary urea nitrogen excretion indicating that amino acid mobilization and utilization have decreased. (Used with permission of authors and publishers.[14])

Table 8–1. Blood β-Hydroxybutyrate/ Acetoacetate and Lactate/Pyruvate Ratios Before and After Passage Through Various Tissues of Fasting Human Subjects

Tissue	Vessel	Ratio
		β-OH/ACAC*
Muscle	Artery	$3.49 \frac{(5.291)}{1.515}$
	Vein	$4.00 \frac{(5.378)}{1.345}$
Splanchnic Bed + Kidney	Artery	$4.56 \frac{(6.480)}{1.420}$
	Hepatic Vein	$4.26 \frac{(6.815)}{1.600}$
	Renal Vein	$4.23 \frac{(6.210)}{1.467}$
Brain	Artery	$5.70 \frac{(6.670)}{1.170}$
	Jugular Vein	$5.97 \frac{(6.630)}{1.110}$
		L/P†
Muscle	Artery	$14.0 \frac{(.533)}{.038}$
	Vein	$19.2 \frac{(.613)}{.032}$

*β-OH = β-hydroxybutyrate, ACAC = Acetoacetate values in mM.
†L = Lactate. P = Pyruvate values in mM.
Adapted from Aoki, Finley, and Cahill, by permission of the authors and publishers.[60]

change significantly during a fast.[25] In contrast, arterial pyruvate levels decline significantly. For this reason, there is an increase in the arterial lactate:pyruvate ratio. It could reasonably be concluded that the total body "cytosolic compartment" of prolonged fasted man, as reflected by the arterial lactate:pyruvate ratio, is in a more reduced state than in the postabsorptive individual. If a similar analysis of the arterial β-hydroxybutyrate:acetoacetate ratio is conducted, it would be reasonable to surmise that the entire "mitochondrial compartment" of prolonged fasted individuals is in a reduced state, compared to postabsorptive subjects, the enzyme for this interconversion being mitochondrial as against lactate dehydrogenase which is cytosolic.

One further major assumption can be made:If one knows the arterial β-hydroxybutyrate:acetoacetate and lactate:pyruvate ratios (i.e., the ratios before they enter a given tissue bed), then the directional change of the ratios after passing through a given tissue (e.g., muscle) should reflect the redox state of that tissue.

A number of studies performed at the Joslin Research Laboratory were reviewed with the above assumptions in mind. These are summarized in Table 8 1.[25] Note that the β-hydroxybutyrate:acetoacetate ratio increases after passing across forearm muscle bed of prolonged fasted individuals. A similar increase in this ratio is not seen after it passes through splanchnic bed, kidney, or brain. A significant increase in the lactate:pyruvate ratio is seen after passage across forearm muscle bed of prolonged fasted subjects. These data suggest that muscle is the most reduced of the various tissues surveyed in fasting individuals.

But what is the significance of this observation

concerning muscle redox state and amino acid release from forearm muscle bed? To answer these questions, a number of other investigations previously performed were reviewed and are summarized in Figure 8–9. Note that the arterial-deep venous (A-DV) β-hydroxybutyrate:acetoacetate ratio difference across forearm muscle bed in postabsorptive individuals indicates that this tissue is in a relatively oxidized state compared to that in fasting man; however, note also that there is a large and significant excretion of urinary urea nitrogen. Following a 21-day fast, the arterial-deep venous β-hydroxybutyrate:acetoacetate ratio difference suggests that muscle has become much more reduced (more negative) and is associated with a significant diminution in urinary urea nitrogen excretion, indicating a curtailment of hepatic gluconeogenesis.

As noted previously, when 0.1 mg of glucagon per 24 hours × 4 days is infused into prolonged fasted individuals, the β-hydroxybutyrate:acetoacetate ratio increases (becomes more negative) across forearm muscle bed. Note the significant diminution in urinary urea nitrogen excretion, indicating a significant reduction in hepatic gluconeogenesis.

Again alluding to a study previously described,

when 20 units of crystalline zinc insulin were infused into 7 prolonged fasted individuals over a 24-hour period, there was a significant increase in the β-hydroxybutyrate:acetoacetate ratio. This observation suggests that muscle has become significantly more reduced compared to control values. In addition, there was a modest but significant diminution in urinary nitrogen excretion.

However, the most dramatic change in the β-hydroxybutyrate:acetoacetate ratio was observed in an individual who had been fasted for 6 weeks and then fed a 200-gm broiled ground sirloin meal while undergoing a forearm study. There was a dramatic increase in the β-hydroxybutyrate:acetoacetate ratio across the forearm muscle bed 2 hours after the ingestion of this meal. In addition, and coincident in time, there was a most remarkable uptake of amino acids across the forearm muscle bed.[26]

Thus, it would appear that a more reduced state of forearm muscle bed is associated with a diminution in release and/or increased uptake of amino acids by that tissue, as well as a significant diminution in urinary urea nitrogen excretion reflecting diminished hepatic gluconeogenesis. However, would a change from a more reduced state of muscle to a more oxidized state be reflected by an

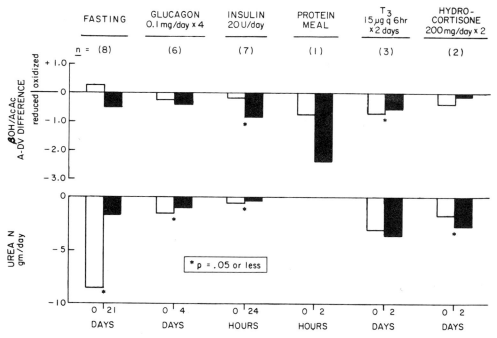

Fig. 8–9. Arterial-deep venous β-hydroxybutyric acid/acetoacetic acid differences across forearm muscle in various nutritional and experimental states. In the postabsorptive state, muscle is in a more oxidized state, and this is associated with increased urinary nitrogen excretion. However, after a 21-day fast, muscle has become significantly more reduced and urinary urea nitrogen excretion is diminished. Following the infusion of glucagon, insulin, or the ingestion of a protein meal, muscle becomes significantly more reduced, and urinary urea nitrogen excretion diminishes. In contrast, when T_3 or hydrocortisone hemisuccinate is administered, muscle becomes significantly more oxidized, and there is an increase in urinary nitrogen excretion. (Used with permission of authors and publishers.[73])

increase in amino acid release from forearm muscle bed, together with increases in urinary urea nitrogen excretion and hepatic gluconeogenesis? Fortunately, two studies shed some light on this possibility. In the first study,[2] which was described in detail above, 15 μg of triiodothyronine were administered every 6 hours over a 2-day period to prolonged fasted individuals. A significant diminution in the β-hydroxybutyrate:acetoacetate ratio across forearm muscle bed was observed, indicating that muscle had become more oxidized. In addition, a significant increase in urinary urea nitrogen excretion was noted. In the second study, 200 mg of hydrocortisone hemisuccinate was infused over a 24-hour period × 2 days in two prolonged fasted individuals. The arterial β-hydroxybutyrate:acetoacetate ratio was diminished (less negative) after passage through forearm muscle bed, indicating that this tissue had become more oxidized. In addition, there was a significant increase in urinary urea nitrogen excretion.

More recently, we have had an opportunity to infuse insulin into the forearm muscle bed of prolonged fasted individuals over a 2-hour period.[27] Thirty minutes after the start of the infusion, the subjects were asked to exercise their forearms while using a calibrated dynamometer. (They exerted a 10-kg pull on this device for a 5-second period, followed by a 5-second rest period; the entire sequence was repeated over the next 15 minutes.) The intraforearm insulin level achieved was approximately 70 μU/ml.

Blood flow measured by capacitance plethysmography[28–30] increased significantly in the exercised forearm and remained elevated above basal levels for the remainder of the study. The A-DV β-hydroxybutyrate:acetoacetate ratio differences indicated that muscle was reduced at the start of the study and became noticeably more oxidized (less negative) immediately after the exercise period. The A-DV ratio difference subsequently returned to control values after 2 hours. Of great interest, the resting total nitrogen release from forearm muscle bed, which before the test was approximately 300 nM/100 ml forearm/minute, changed little during the exercise sequence. However, an increase in alanine flux from the forearm muscle bed was observed. Subsequently, nitrogen efflux gradually approached zero and then changed to a highly significant uptake across forearm muscle bed at 2 hours.

These preliminary studies suggest that a strong association exists between a more reduced state of muscle and diminished release of amino acids and/or uptake by that tissue. In contrast, the change from a more reduced state to a more oxidized state appears to be associated with increased release of amino acids from forearm muscle bed and increased urinary urea nitrogen excretion. Thus, it now appears that insulin, triiodothyronine, and tissue redox state are important determinants of amino acid mobilization in prolonged fasted man.

The Role of Substrates on Nitrogen Metabolism in Postabsorptive Man

A study performed at this laboratory on postabsorptive individuals suggested that substrate concentrations as well as physical activity might play important roles in the regulation of amino acid mobilization. In this study, a double forearm procedure[31] was used in which a catheter was inserted into the radial artery of one arm. Separate catheters were then inserted into each antecubital vein in a retrograde direction. Blood flow in both forearms was measured by capacitance plethysmography. Pediatric blood pressure cuffs were applied to each wrist and inflated to 300 mm Hg 1 minute prior to blood sampling at 0, 30, 45, 60, 75, 90, 120, and 150 minutes in order to isolate the hand from the sampling circuit. Blood pressure cuffs were also transiently applied to both upper arms and inflated to 40 mm Hg only during the blood flow determinations.

Six normal postabsorptive individuals were studied, using the double forearm procedure, in order to ascertain the impact of a 14.7 g L-leucine meal on forearm muscle metabolism. Forty-five minutes following the consumption of the test meal, they began to exercise one forearm using the calibrated dynamometer in the fashion previously described. Peak arterial blood leucine levels approximating 1.5 mM/L were achieved during the study, and were associated with large uptakes of leucine across forearm muscle bed.

Glutamine efflux increased significantly thereafter in both dominant and nondominant forearms, clearly exceeding the nitrogen taken up as leucine by forearm muscle bed. Alanine efflux in the nondominant, nonexercised forearm muscle bed did not change significantly during the entire study. In addition, no change in alanine efflux was observed in the dominant forearm muscle bed until completion of the exercise sequence. No change was noted in ammonia efflux in either the dominant or the nondominant arm.

At rest, there was an efflux of nitrogen from both forearms in these postabsorptive individuals. Within 30 minutes, this efflux quickly changed to a large uptake of nitrogen, primarily due to leucine entry into both forearm muscle beds. However, prior to the initiation of the exercise sequence at 45 minutes, the nitrogen uptake had changed back to a net release from both forearms. A massive efflux of nitrogen was observed from the nonexercised forearm muscle bed at 75 and 90 minutes, clearly exceeding leucine uptake and glutamine release from that forearm. In addition, an even greater loss of nitrogen was observed in the exercised dominant forearm muscle bed. These data suggest that the ingestion of ~10 mM of L-leucine by postabsorptive individuals has a net catabolic effect on forearm muscle metabolism.

In *summary:* (1) Insulin appears to be a major determinant of amino acid efflux from forearm muscle bed in both postabsorptive and prolonged fasted individuals. (2) The decrease in levels of triiodothyronine during the performance of a prolonged fast appears to be a most important adaptation which permits the conservation of nitrogen manifested by fasting individuals. (3) The redox state of muscle tissue appears to play an important role in the regulation of amino acid mobilization in fasting individuals. A more reduced state of muscle appears to be associated with diminished release of amino acid from forearm muscle bed, while a more oxidized state appears to be associated with an increase in amino acid mobilization from that same tissue. (4) Substrate concentrations, e.g., leucine, may also have a direct role in amino acid mobilization to and from muscle. The ingestion of 10 mM of L-leucine by six normal postabsorptive individuals results in a pronounced leucine uptake by and glutamine efflux from exercised and nonexercised forearm muscle beds. In addition, this meal appears to trigger a massive and unexpected release of nitrogen from forearm muscle bed, indicating net forearm muscle catabolism.

METABOLIC CHANGES FOLLOWING INGESTION OF FOOD

Protein Meals and Normal Man

With this background of possible mechanisms involved in the regulation of fuel metabolism in general, and nitrogen metabolism in particular, we will now consider the metabolic changes in normal subjects by the ingestion of a protein meal.[32] When 200 g of broiled ground sirloin were ingested by four normal postabsorptive individuals, systemic levels of the branched chain amino acids increased significantly over baseline (Fig. 8–10). Indeed, analysis of A-DV amino acid differences across forearm muscle bed of these individuals revealed that the branched chain amino acids were preferentially removed by forearm muscle tissue. The other amino acids present in the meal were removed by the splanchnic bed, presumably liver. The branched chain amino acids apparently were able to make their way through the splanchnic bed because the liver does not possess the enzymatic ma-

chinery capable of initiating the oxidation of these amino acids.

Circulating levels of triglycerides increased during the study, reflecting the presence of saturated fats in the ingested meal and/or synthesis of low-density lipoproteins in liver (Fig. 8–11). Note also that serum insulin levels increased only modestly, while plasma glucagon levels almost doubled. (It should also be pointed out that when rat livers are perfused with glucagon, thereby initiating hepatic proteolysis, those amino acids which are not readily oxidized by the liver, including the branched chain amino acids, are released into the perfusate.[33]) Thus, the increase in systemic levels of the branched chain amino acids in particular may reflect a selective redirection of incoming branched chain amino acids to those tissues most capable of oxidizing them, namely muscle.

The above investigation is especially instructive for several reasons. First, glucagon levels increase significantly following the ingestion of the protein meal. It is tempting to ascribe this increase to the alpha cell stimulation provided by elevated levels of the branched chain amino acids. However, it has been shown that the branched chain amino acids are relatively poor stimulators of the alpha cell.[24] Indeed, in the study[31] previously alluded to in which 6 normal postabsorptive individuals ingested 10 mM of L-leucine, plasma glucagon levels did not increase significantly. Thus, in all probability the increase in levels of this hormone was probably due to stimuli other than amino acids.

It is especially noteworthy that uptake of amino acids by forearm muscle bed was largely restricted to that of the branched chain amino acids. That is, when normal postabsorptive individuals (whose nitrogen stores are already at an optimum) ingest a protein meal, amino acid uptake by forearm muscle bed is restricted to that of the branched chain amino acids. It is not clear why the branched chain amino acids are selectively removed by this tissue. However, unlike liver, muscle is fully capable of deaminating and oxidizing these amino acids.[34] In contrast, branched chain amino acid uptake by forearm muscle, appears to proceed with relatively tiny increments in insulin levels. Ultimately, the branched chain amino acids may represent an alternative aminated fatty acid equivalent for oxidative purposes in muscle.

Glucose Meals and Normal Man

When overweight but otherwise normal subjects ingest 37.5 g of glucose every 6 hours for 7 days,[13] with these meals representing their sole caloric intake, a number of interesting events take place as documented in blood and urine tests (Fig. 8–12). First, corroborating the observation made by Gam-

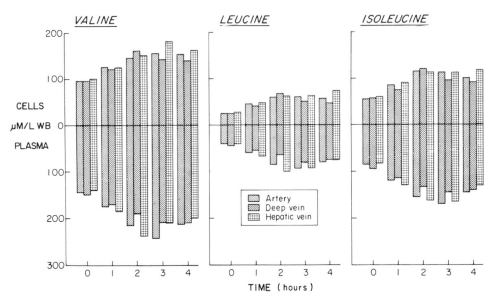

Fig. 8–10. Shortly after the ingestion of a protein meal, systemic concentrations of the branched chain amino acids valine, leucine, and isoleucine increase significantly. They are subsequently removed, primarily by muscle. (Used with permission of authors and publishers.[32])

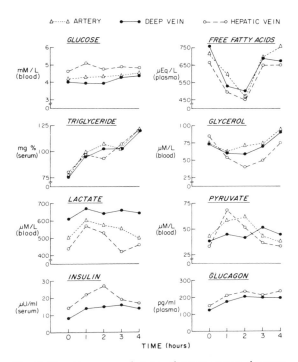

Fig. 8–11. Hormone-substrate changes across forearm muscle and splanchnic bed in 4 normal individuals following the ingestion of a protein meal. (Used with permission of authors and publishers.[32])

ble over 30 years ago,[35] there is a notable diminution in urinary nitrogen excretion, indicating that hepatic gluconeogenesis has been significantly curtailed. In addition, urinary ammonia nitrogen excretion does not increase, as one would expect in individuals undergoing total starvation (Fig. 8–5).

In view of our previous discussion, both of these observations taken together suggest that a sizable amount of body protein, especially that of muscle, is conserved by the simple expedient of taking small quantities (50 to 100 g) of glucose by mouth. Nevertheless, the body, apparently aware that hypocaloric quantities of glucose are being ingested, initiates those changes which will lead to the gradual increase in circulating levels of the primary fuel (i.e., fatty acids) of both postabsorptive and fasting individuals. Thus, serum insulin levels (Fig. 8–2) gradually decline, together with the fall in circulating blood glucose levels. In addition, there is a small but gradual increase in concentrations of plasma free fatty acids and β-hydroxybutyric and acetoacetic acids. Even more striking changes are seen between the plasma amino acid patterns obtained on days 0 and 7 of the study. Note that in the postabsorptive state, plasma alanine levels are approximately 380 μM/L (Fig. 8–13). After 7 days on this regimen, plasma alanine levels have declined significantly, and glycine and threonine levels have begun to rise. The importance of these observations is that the body is apparently capable of monitoring the amount of its caloric intake, as well as the type—an ability underscored by the following study.

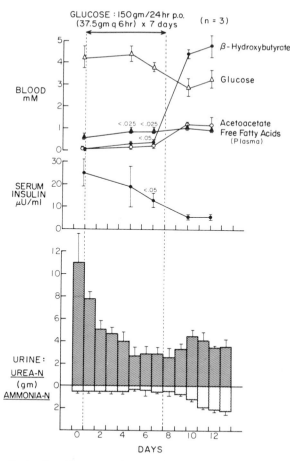

Fig. 8–12. Hormone-substrate changes in overweight but otherwise normal individuals subsisting on 37.5 g of glucose every 6 hours for 7 days. Note the dramatic decrease in urinary urea nitrogen excretion and a gradual fall in blood glucose and circulating insulin levels. There is a small but significant rise in plasma free fatty acids and β-hydroxybutyric acid levels. (Used with permission of authors and publishers.[13])

When the above experiment is repeated in individuals who have fasted for 3 weeks, even more dramatic changes in both blood and urine are observed (Fig. 8–14). First, urinary urea nitrogen excretion is minimal, indicating marked curtailment of hepatic gluconeogenesis. In contrast, urinary ammonia nitrogen excretion is at its maximum due to the need to titrate the increased organic acid load represented by β-hydroxybutyric and acetoacetic acids. It would be reasonable to assume that if hepatic ketogenesis could be curtailed, renal ammoniagenesis would be obviated and even more nitrogen could be conserved. Thus, the ingestion of 150 g of glucose per day (37.5 g every 6 hours × 7 days) results in no further diminution of hepatic gluconeogenesis, as reflected by urinary urea nitrogen excretion, but does result in a sharp cur-

tailment of hepatic ketogenesis. In consequence, renal ammoniagenesis is obviated and returns to basal levels of approximately .5 g/day. Thus, the ingestion of 150 g of glucose per day results in the saving of approximately 14 g of protein each day. Note, however, that plasma free fatty acid levels, the primary fuel of the rest of the body, did not change. Thus, the body is capable of recognizing that only 600 calories in the form of glucose have been ingested; however, since this amount is not enough to meet the total energy requirements of the body, free fatty acids must continue to be mobilized, and adipose tissue in particular must continue to be relatively resistant to the effects of insulin.

Turning now to studies in which isocaloric quantities of glucose are infused into normal subjects,[36] even more interesting observations become manifest. Five normal subjects were placed on a diet in which they ingested 700 g of carbohydrates a day. On the fourth and final day of this study, however, the 700 g of carbohydrate was administered in the form of a glucose infusion. Prior to the completion of this infusion, each subject underwent renal and hepatic vein catheterization combined with a forearm study. It was determined subsequently that total nitrogen release from forearm was reduced by approximately 50%. There was a significant increase in plasma triglyceride release from the splanchnic bed ($-2 \pm .7$ vs -18 ± 1.6 mg/dl). Both arterial-hepatic and venous differences of blood β-hydroxybutyric acid (-66 vs. -4 μM/L) and acetoacetic acid (-37 vs -6 μM/L) decreased to a great extent. Concomitant with the falling ketoacid production by the liver, β-hydroxybutyric acid removal by the kidney decreased by 16 μM to 2 μM/min, and acetoacetic acid removal changed from an uptake of 1 to a net production of 2 μM/min. Glutamine release from forearm muscle bed did not change noticeably from the postabsorptive state. Similarly, glutamine extraction by the kidney also proceeded and was not significantly altered. Of interest, urinary ammonia nitrogen excretion changed little whereas renal vein ammonia levels increased. Thus, it appeared that there was an obligate removal of glutamine by the kidney with the ammonia so generated being added to the venous blood leaving that tissue. In summary, the provision of 700 g of carbohydrate to normal subjects influences the metabolic activities of a number of organs including muscle, gut, liver, and kidney. Different metabolic fuels including fat, carbohydrate, and proteins are similarly affected.

Protein Meals and Diabetic Man

As might be anticipated, amino acid metabolism in diabetic subjects becomes progressively more

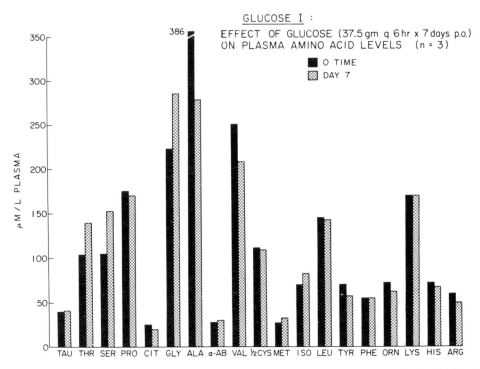

Fig. 8–13. Changes in circulating plasma amino acid levels in overweight but otherwise normal individuals subsisting on 37.5 g of glucose every 6 hours for 7 days. Note the decrease in plasma alanine and a significant increase in threonine and circulating glycine levels. These changes are consistent with the gradual adaptation to the fasting state. (Used with permission of authors and publishers.[13])

disordered as glucose homeostasis becomes more deranged. The reverse, however, is equally true. Thus, the use of an artificial β-cell device, or the judicious use of an insulin pump, can quickly restore circulating levels of amino acids, lipids, and glucose to normal concentrations.[37] However, in the postabsorptive state in general, circulating concentrations of the branched chain amino acids are elevated, and alanine levels are relatively depressed in diabetic patients compared to normal subjects. At present, it is not clear why circulating concentrations of the branched chain amino acids are elevated. The elevation may reflect increased muscle degradation followed by the removal of the glucogenic amino acids by the liver and kidney. Alternatively, it may reflect increased hepatic proteolysis with retention of the glucogenic amino acids and the release of those amino acids not readily oxidized by the liver, including the branched chain amino acids, lysine, and phenylalanine. The decrease in alanine concentrations is currently thought to be attributable primarily to increased fractional extraction of this amino acid by the liver of diabetic subjects.[38]

Of interest, branched chain amino acid oxidation by muscle of diabetic animals is increased significantly compared to controls.[39] However, enhanced branched chain amino acid oxidation in this experimental situation is reversed by the administration of insulin to the diabetic animal[39,40] but not by the addition of insulin to incubated muscle taken from a diabetic animal.[40]

Following the ingestion of a protein meal by diabetics, Wahren et al.[41] found splanchnic release of amino acids to be comparable to that observed in a control group. In contrast to the control group, however, arterial concentrations of the branched chain amino acids were significantly greater in the diabetic subjects. In addition, these amino acids, in contrast to the control group, were being removed by muscle only at the 60-minute sampling. The investigators concluded that these observations were most likely the result of insulin deficiency. In addition to the changes in branched chain amino acid removal by muscle of diabetic subjects, the same investigators also observed an increase in alanine release from muscle, compared to controls. They concluded that this failure to reduce alanine output reflected ongoing protein catabolism and branched chain amino acid oxidation due to insulin deficiency. However, it should also be observed that glucose concentrations in diabetic subjects are markedly elevated, and the alanine release from muscle of these patients may be derived primarily

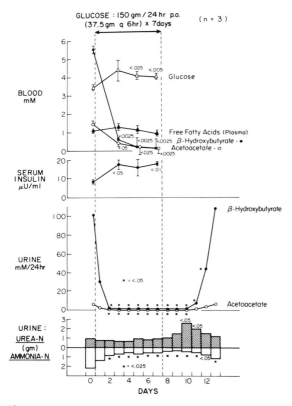

Fig. 8–14. Hormone-substrate changes in individuals who have fasted for 3 weeks and who then ingest 37.5 g of glucose every 6 hours for 7 days. Note the dramatic decrease in ammonia nitrogen excretion coincident with a remarkable decline of urinary excretion of the ketoacids, β-hydroxybutyric and acetoacetic acids. Note once again that despite the sizable increase in circulating insulin levels, plasma free fatty acid levels remain elevated. (Used with permission of authors and publishers.[13])

from glucose. This possibility is especially important in view of the fact that in diabetic subjects, the ingestion of a protein meal results in a 150% increase in splanchnic glucose production.[41] This increased hepatic glucose production is probably a consequence of a deficiency of insulin availability together with a significant rise in plasma glucagon concentration, the latter being exaggerated in diabetic subjects. This increase in glucose production is relatively transient, lasting 60 to 90 minutes following ingestion of the meal. Compounding this problem is the failure of the peripheral tissues, primarily muscle, to promptly remove the excess glucose produced.

Dietary Glucose Processing in Normal and Diabetic Man

In normal man, shortly after the ingestion of a 100 g glucose meal, absorption of this fuel from the stomach and small intestine commences and large quantities of it are transported, in the com-

pany of markedly elevated levels of insulin, via the portal vein to the liver. Approximately 50 to 60%[42] of the glucose load stops in the liver where it is oxidized or converted into fat or glycogen and the remainder passes through the liver into the systemic circulation.

In contrast, in poorly regulated type I diabetic individuals, less than 25% of the ingested glucose load is retained by the liver while approximately 70% passes through this organ and into the systemic circulation.[43] These observations underscore (1) the primary role of the liver in the maintenance of glucose homeostasis after the ingestion of carbohydrate-containing meals and (2) the inability of conventional insulin regimens to significantly improve the demonstrably impaired glucose processing (oxidation, storage, conversion to other fuels) capability of this organ in such patients.

Thus, the route and pattern of insulin delivery are apparently critical factors with respect to activation and maintenance of hepatic glucose processing. Since insulin is not required for glucose entry into the hepatocyte,[44] the site of modulation may be the initial conversion of glucose to glucose-6-phosphate, a step mediated by insulin-dependent glucokinase, hexokinase, and possibly to the phosphotransferase activity of glucose-6-phosphatase.[45,46]

Glucokinase is present in human liver and is generally considered to be the enzyme responsible for the initial phosphorylation of glucose.[47,48] The activity of this enzyme is increased in the presence of insulin[49] and decreased in its absence.[49,50] In addition, its high Km (10 to 20 mM)[47,48] gives it an important regulatory role vis à vis portal glucose concentrations after a glucose meal. In contrast, the livers of diabetic animals lack significant glucokinase activity, and presumably for this reason are unable to participate in the processing of the elevated portal venous glucose concentrations[44,49] attendant to the ingestion of meals containing significant amounts of carbohydrate.

In contrast to glucokinase, hepatic hexokinase activity is low even in normal liver[45,51] and is not increased by insulin. In addition, due to its low Km (10^{-5} mM), this enzyme cannot have an important regulatory role with respect to glucose concentrations seen in human portal or systemic venous blood.

Glucose-6-phosphate[52] was once thought to be a hydrolase found only in liver and kidney. More recently, however, this enzyme has been found in the mucosa of the small intestine, pancreas, adrenals, testes, brain, spleen, and lung.[45,52–54] In liver, 80 to 85% of the activity of this enzyme is found in the endoplasmic reticulum with only 15 to 19% found in the nuclear membrane.[55] This enzyme is unique in that it (1) can degrade glucose-6-phosphate and (2) has been reported to have the capacity to form glucose-6-phosphate in amounts that exceed by more than 50% its capacity to degrade this intermediate.[45,51,53,54,56,57]

In summary, it would appear that in normal liver, insulin-dependent glucokinase, and to a lesser extent hexokinase and possibly the phosphotransferase activity of glucose-6-phosphatase, all contribute to the formation of glucose-6-phosphate. Based upon both experimental and clinical observations, it would appear that in poorly regulated insulin-dependent diabetic patients glucokinase activity (and probably other hepatic enzymes involved in the processing of ingested fuels) is markedly decreased, and it is primarily because of this diminution of activity of glucokinase (and related enzyme(s)) that incoming glucose enters the liver via the portal vein, and surges through the liver into the systemic circulation following the ingestion of a glucose meal. A small amount of glucose may be phosphorylated, perhaps attributable to insulin-independent hexokinase and the phosphotransferase activity of glucose-6-phosphatase.

CLINICAL OBSERVATIONS AND IMPLICATIONS: THE SLEEPING LIVER HYPOTHESIS

The experimental data in the preceding section and the observation that 3 to 4 days of aggressive pursuit of elevated glucose levels with large and frequent insulin injections are required to improve glucose control in type I diabetic patients have led this unit to postulate a deficiency in hepatic glucokinase (and related fuel-processing enzymes) activity as the fundamental cause of the hyperglycemia of diabetes that is especially marked following the ingestion of carbohydrate-containing meals. Further support for this concept of a metabolically dormant hepatic glucose processing system stems from animal studies showing that many hours of insulin administration are required to restore the activity of hepatic glucokinase (and probably other fuel processing enzymes) once it has fallen due to insulin lack. Thus, frequent injections of reasonably large amounts of insulin (15 to 30 U) especially before and after meals for several days would be and are in fact needed to partially restore glucose control presumably via increased activity of hepatic glucose processing enzymes. Unfortunately, after some semblance of control is achieved, current clinical practice directs the physician to then place the diabetic patient on single or split doses of insulin (NPH + CZI), a practice which should and apparently does result in a rapid fall (24 to 48 hours) in the activity of hepatic glu-

cose processing enzymes. As a consequence, following discharge, the patient rapidly goes out of control again.

The above "sleeping liver" hypothesis is clinically testable. An artificial β-cell unit could track glucose concentrations and respond quickly to any changes in blood glucose levels by initiating and maintaining an insulin infusion under appropriate conditions imposed upon the instrument by the operator of the device. With such an instrument, rapid increases in circulating insulin concentrations could be achieved systemically.

In order to monitor the physiologic efficacy of the artificial β-cell, using the technique of indirect calorimetry,[44,58-65] hepatic carbohydrate oxidation was measured following the ingestion of a glucose meal. (The instrument used for this purpose is the Beckman Metabolic Measurement Cart (MMC) which is capable of measuring CO_2 production and oxygen consumption at the bedside.) Of historic interest, in 1912, F. Benedict and E.P. Joslin[66] published a study on the metabolism of diabetic patients using both direct and indirect calorimetry and showed that 1) the two techniques are equivalent and 2) diabetic subjects could not oxidize carbohydrate. Since the ratio of CO_2 production to oxygen consumption accurately reflects the fuel being oxidized,[59] it is possible, using indirect calorimetry, to calculate the rates at which carbohydrate, fat, and protein are being oxidized in mg/min in the basal state, after meals, and during exercise.

With the above instruments, we have determined that it is possible to restore the glucose processing capability (oxidation, storage) of an insulin-dependent diabetic subject to the extent that he/she is able to handle a 100 g glucose load in a near normal fashion (Fig. 8–15) and that the artificial β-cell unit alone is currently capable of accomplishing this feat within 72–96 hours.[67] It also appears that restoration of glucose homeostasis is an *inducible* phenomenon (Fig. 8–16) presumably due to increased synthesis of those enzymes involved in glucose processing.[67]

Of potentially great importance, we have studied over 50 Type I diabetic patients on a variety of therapeutic regimens including single and split insulin injection regimens, pre-meal injections of regular insulin coupled with a single NPH injection, and over 20 patients on the insulin pump, and none of these patients was found to be capable of normally processing a 100-g glucose load. In addition, based upon a number of inferences derived from euglycemic clamp studies[68,69] as well as our own work, we have concluded that the organ primarily affected by artificial β-cell directed insulin therapy is the liver. Strong support for this hy-

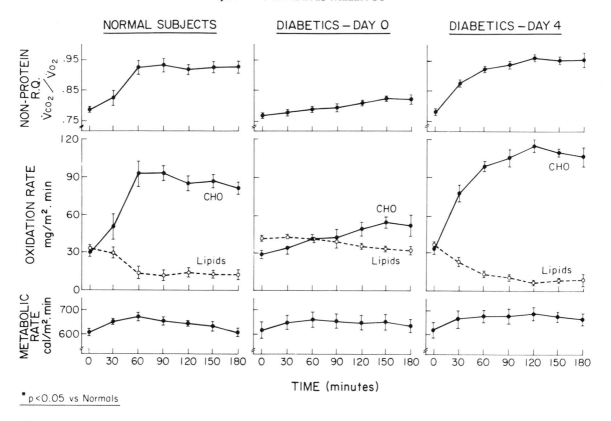

Fig. 8–15. Non-protein respiratory quotients (npRQ), carbohydrate (CHO) and lipid oxidation rates, and metabolic rates of normal subjects and diabetic patients on Day O (conventional insulin therapy) and on Day 4 (after 72 hours on artificial β-cell), before (0 time = postabsorptive state) and during the 3-hour oral 100 g glucose tests. (Used with permission of authors and publishers.[67])

pothesis derives from the observation in Type I diabetic subjects, following ingestion of a 100-g glucose meal, that the forearm glucose uptake is not significantly different, whether determined prior to or after 72 hours on the artificial beta cell unit, and indeed does not differ significantly from that of normal subjects.[70] The data indicate that portal instillation of insulin is not a necessary prerequisite for the reestablishment of normal (presumably hepatic) glucose processing and is clearly not required for normalization of muscle glucose clearance.[70] In addition, the data suggest that peripheral administration of insulin, intravenously (other than by artificial β-cell) or subcutaneously, is potentially capable of maintaining if not actually normalizing glucose processing, on an outpatient basis, in the insulin-dependent diabetic patient. The "sleeping liver" hypothesis which attributes the severe glucose intolerance in conventional insulin-treated Type I diabetic subjects, to a marked but reversible reduction in hepatic dietary glucose processing, appears to be promising both with respect to future research and the care of the diabetic subject.

The implications of the above are many. For

example, it suggests that the achievement of near normal fasting blood glucose, hemoglobin A_{Ic}, and postprandial glucose concentrations in Type I diabetic patients using multiple insulin injections may be accomplished without hepatic participation. That is, current conventional insulin therapy results in muscle sequestration of glucose that has surged through the liver into the systemic circulation. Thus, the diabetic patient on conventional insulin therapy is required to estimate precisely the amount of insulin required to sequester in muscle that dietary carbohydrate which has escaped from his/her liver. It is therefore not surprising that attempts to achieve near normal fasting blood glucose levels via multiple insulin injection regimens are associated with frequent daily episodes of hypoglycemia.

In summary, fuel homeostasis in fasting, normal, and diabetic man is primarily a function of a number of hormones, the nutritional state, tissues, tissue sensitivity to hormones, and physical activity, all operating more or less simultaneously and in interaction with one another. At present, insulin appears to be pre-eminent in this theoretical concept, with glucagon playing a lesser role. Glucose

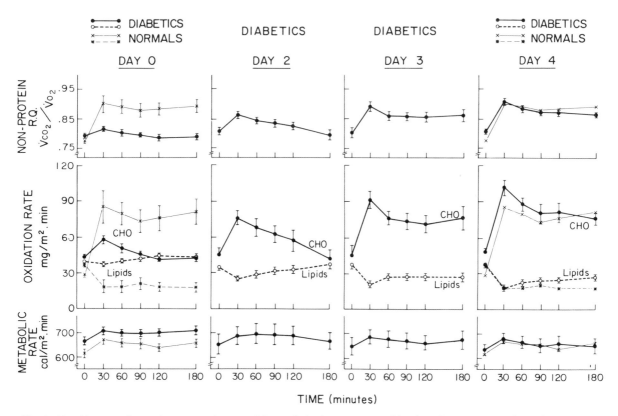

Fig. 8–16. Non-protein respiratory quotients (npRQ), carbohydrate (CHO) and lipid oxidation rates, and metabolic rates of normal subjects and diabetic patients on Day O and on Days 2, 3 and 4, during the mixed meal studies. (Used with permission of authors and publishers.[67])

utilization by peripheral tissues, primarily muscle, is chiefly a function of both glucose concentration and insulin levels, while hepatic glucose production (gluconeogenesis and/or glycogenolysis) and sequestration (glycogen, oxidation, fat synthesis) are directed by both insulin and glucagon. Insulin, however, is the primary modulator of amino acid uptake of the liver and by muscle. In addition, this hormone is dominant with respect to the direction of glucose to fat synthesis.

REFERENCES

1. Portnay, G.I., O'Brian, J.T., Bush, J., et al.: The effect of starvation on the concentration and binding of thyroxine and triiodothyronine in serum and on the response to TRH. J. Clin. Endocrinol. Metab. *39*:191, 1974.
2. Vignati, L., Finley, R.J., Hagg, S., Aoki, T.T.: Protein conservation during prolonged fast: a function of triiodothyronine levels. Trans. Assoc. Am. Physicians *91*:169, 1978.
3. Vagenakis, A.G., Burger, A., Portnay, G.I., et al.: Diversion of peripheral thyroxine metabolism from activating to inactivating pathways during complete fasting. J. Clin. Endocrinol. Metab. *41*:191, 1975.
4. Marliss, E.B., Aoki, T.T., Unger, R.H., et al.: Glucagon levels and metabolic effects in fasting man. J. Clin. Invest. *49*:2256, 1970.
5. Owen, O.E., Felig, P., Morgan, A.P., et al.: Liver and kidney metabolism during prolonged starvation. J. Clin. Invest. *48*:574, 1969.
6. Reichard, G.A., Jr., Owen, O.E., Haff, A.C., et al.: Ketone-body production and oxidation in fasting obese humans. J. Clin.Invest. *53*:508, 1974.
7. Pitts, R.F.: Renal production and excretion of ammonia. Am. J. Med. *36*:720, 1964.
8. Felig, P., Pozefsky, T., Marliss, E., Cahill, G.F., Jr.: Alanine: key role in gluconeogenesis. Science *167*:1003, 1970.
9. Owen, O.E., Reichard, G.A., Jr.: Human forearm metabolism during progressive starvation. J. Clin. Invest. *50*:1536, 1971.
10. Owen, O.E., Cahill, G.F., Jr.: Metabolic effects of exogenous glucocorticoids in fasted man. J. Clin. Invest. *52*:2596, 1973.
11. Aoki, T.T., Müller, W.A., Brennan, M.F., Cahill, G.F., Jr.: Effect of glucagon on amino acid and nitrogen metabolism in fasted man. Metabolism *23*:805, 1974.
12. Felig, P., Marliss, E.B., Cahill, G.F., Jr.: Metabolic response to human growth hormone during prolonged starvation. J. Clin. Invest. *50*:411, 1971.
13. Aoki, T.T., Müller, W.A., Brennan, M.F., Cahill, G.F., Jr.: Metabolic effects of glucose in brief and prolonged fasted man. Am. J. Clin. Nutr. *28*:507, 1975.
14. Aoki, T.T., Cahill, G.F., Jr.: Metabolic effects of insulin, glucagon, and glucose in man: clinical application. In: L.J. DeGroot, G.F. Cahill, Jr., W.D. Odell, et al. (Eds.): Endocrinology, Vol. 2. New York, Grune & Stratton, 1979, pp. 1843–1854.
15. Owen, O.E., Morgan, A.P., Kemp, H.G., et al.: Brain metabolism during fasting. J. Clin. Invest. *46*:1589, 1967.

16. Drenick, E.J., Alvarez, L.C., Tamasi, G.C., Brickman, A.S.: Resistance to symptomatic insulin reactions after fasting. J. Clin. Invest. 51:2757, 1972.

17. Pozefsky, T., Felig, P., Tobin, J.D., et al.: Amino acid balance across tissues of the forearm in postabsorptive man. Effects of insulin at two dose levels. J. Clin. Invest. 48:2273, 1969.

18. Aoki, T.T., Brennan, M.F., Müller, W.A., et al.: Effect of insulin on muscle glutamate uptake. Whole blood versus plasma glutamate analysis. J. Clin. Invest. 51:2889, 1972.

19. Deuel, H.J., Jr., Sandiford, K., Sandiford, I., Boothby, W.M.: Deposit protein: the effect of thyroxine on the deposit protein after reduction of the nitrogen excretion to a minimal level by a prolonged protein-free diet. J. Biol. Chem. 67:XXIII, 1926.

20. Johnson, P., Perry, S.V.: Biological activity and the 3-methylhistidine content of actin and myosin. Biochem. J. 119:293, 1970.

21. Young, V.R., Alexis, S.D., Baliga, B.S., Munro, H.N.: Metabolism of administered 3-methylhistidine. Lack of muscle transfer ribonucleic acid charging and quantitative excretion as 3-methylhistidine and its N-acetyl derivative. J. Biol. Chem. 247:3592, 1972.

22. Young, V.R., Haverberg, L.N., Bilmazes, C., Munro, H.N.: Potential use of 3-methylhistidine excretion as an index of progressive reduction in muscle protein catabolism during starvation. Metabolism 22:1429, 1973.

23. Long, C.L., Haverberg, L.N., Young, V.R., et al.: Metabolism of 3-methylhistidine in man. Metabolism 24:929, 1975.

24. Rocha, D.M., Faloona, G.R., Unger, R.H.: Glucagon-stimulating activity of twenty amino acids in dogs. J. Clin. Invest. 51:2346, 1972.

25. Aoki, T.T., Toews, C.J., Rossini, A.A., et al.: Glucogenic substrate levels in fasting man. Adv. Enzyme Regul. 13:329, 1975.

26. Aoki, T.T., Müller, W.A., Brennan, M.F., Cahill, G.F., Jr.: Blood cell and plasma amino acid levels across forearm muscle during a protein meal. Diabetes 22:768, 1973.

27. Finley, R.J., Vignati, L., Aoki, T.T.: Effects of insulin and exercise on forearm metabolism in fasting man. Clin. Res. 26:414A, 1978.

28. Figar, S.: Electrocapacitance plethysmography. Physiol. Bohemoslov. 8:275, 1950.

29. Wood, J.R., Hyman, C.: A direct reading capacitance plethysmograph. Med. Biol. Eng. 8:59, 1970.

30. Wenger, C.B., Roberts, M.F., Stolwijk, J.A., Nadel, E.R.: Forearm blood flow during body temperature transients produced by leg exercise. J. Appl. Physiol. 38:58, 1975.

31. Aoki, T.T., Brennan, M.F., Fitzpatrick, G.F., Knight, D.: Glutamine efflux from normal forearm following leucine meals. Clin. Res. 26:410A, 1978.

32. Aoki, T.T., Brennan, M.F., Müller, W.A., et al.: Amino acid levels across normal forearm muscle and splanchnic bed after a protein meal. Am. J. Clin. Nutr. 29:340, 1976.

33. Mallette, L.E., Exton, J.H., Park, C.R.: Effects of glucagon on amino acid transport and utilization in the perfused rat liver. J. Biol. Chem. 244:5724, 1969.

34. Goldberg, A.L., Odessey, R.: Oxidation of amino acids by diaphragms from fed and fasted rats. Am. J. Physiol. 223:1384, 1972.

35. Gamble, J.L.: Physiological information gained from studies on the life raft ration. Harvey Lect. 42:247, 1946–1947.

36. Finley, R.J., Aoki, T.T., Beckmann, C., et al.: Mechanisms of protein sparing in carbohydrate loaded man. Surg. Forum 30:76, 1979.

37. Santiago, J.V., Clemens, A.H., Clarke, W.L., Kipnis, D.M.: Closed-loop and open-loop devices for blood glu-cose control in normal and diabetic subjects. Diabetes 28:71, 1979.

38. Wahren, J., Felig, P., Cerasi, E., Luft, R.: Splanchnic and peripheral glucose and amino acid metabolism in diabetes mellitus. J. Clin. Invest. 51:1870, 1972.

39. Buse, M.G., Herlong, H.F., Weigand, D.A.: The effect of diabetes, insulin, and the redox potential on leucine metabolism by isolated rat hemidiaphragm. Endocrinology 98:1166, 1976.

40. Buse, M.G., Biggers, J.F., Drier, C., Buse, J.F.: The effect of epinephrine, glucagon and the nutritional state on the oxidation of branched chain amino acids and pyruvate by isolated hearts and diaphragms of the rat. J. Biol. Chem. 248:697, 1973.

41. Wahren, J., Felig, P., Hagnefeldt, L.: Effect of protein ingestion on splanchnic and leg metabolism in normal man and patients with diabetes mellitus. J. Clin. Invest. 57:987, 1976.

42. Felig, P., Wahren, J., Hendler, R.: Influence of oral glucose ingestion on splanchnic glucose and gluconeogenic substrate metabolism in man. Diabetes 24:468, 1975.

43. Perley, M.J., Kipnis, D.M.: Plasma insulin responses to oral and intravenous glucose: studies in normal and diabetic subjects. J. Clin. Invest. 46:1954, 1967.

44. Cahill, G.F., Jr., Ashmore, J., Earle, A.S., Zottu, S.: Glucose penetration into liver. Am. J. Physiol. 192:491, 1958.

45. Nordlie, R.C.: Metabolic regulation by multifunctional glucose-6-phosphatase. In B.L. Horecker, E.R. Stadtman, (Eds.): Current Topics in Cellular Regulation. Vol. 8. New York, Academic Press, 1974, pp. 33–117.

46. Arion, W.J., Wallin, B.K., Lange, A.J., and Ballas, L.M.: On the involvement of a glucose 6-phosphate transport system in the function of microsomal glucose 6-phosphatase. Mol. Cell. Biochem. 6:75, 1975.

47. Pilkis, S.J.: Identification of human hepatic glucokinase and some properties of the enzyme (33396). Proc. Soc. Exper. Biol. Med. 129:681, 1968.

48. Storer, A.C. and Cornish-Bowden, A.: Kinetics of rat liver glucokinase. Biochem. J. 159:7, 1976.

49. Cahill, G.F., Jr., Ashmore, J., Renold, A.E., Hastings, A.B.: Blood glucose and the liver. Am. J. Med. 26:264, 1959.

50. Ruderman, N.B., Lauris, V.: Effect of acute insulin deprivation on rat liver glucokinase. Diabetes 17:611, 1968.

51. Nordlie, R.C.: Multifunctional hepatic glucose-6-phosphatase and the "tuning" of blood glucose level. TIBS 1:199, 1976.

52. Anchors, J.M., Karnovsky, M.L.: Purification of cerebral glucose-6-phosphatase. An enzyme involved in sleep. J. Biol. Chem. 250:6408, 1975.

53. Lygre, D.G., Nordlie, R.C.: Phosphohydrolase and phosphotransferase activities of intestinal glucose-6-phosphatase. Biochem. 7:3219, 1968.

54. Colilla, W., Jorgenson, R.A., Nordlie, R.C.: Mammalian carbamyl phosphate: glucose phosphotransferase and glucose-6-phosphate phosphohydrolase: extended tissue distribution. Biochim. Biophys. Acta 377:117, 1975.

55. Gunderson, H.M., Nordlie, R.C.: Carbamyl phosphate: glucose phosphotransferase and glucose-6-phosphate phosphohydrolase of nuclear membrane. Interrelationships between membrane integrity, enzymic latency, and catalytic behavior. J. Biol. Chem. 250:3552, 1975.

56. Alvares, F.L., Nordlie, R.C.: Glucose uptake by perfused livers from fed and fasted normal rats: involvement of phosphotransferase activities of glucose-6-phosphatase in regulation of blood glucose levels. Fed. Proc. 34:881, 1975.

57. Alvares, F.L., Nordlie, R.C.: Glucose uptake and phos-

phorylation by livers isolated from alloxan-diabetic rats and perfused in the presence of 3-mercaptopicolinate; involvement of synthetic activities of glucose-6-phosphatase. Fed. Proc. *35*:1397, 1976.

58. DuBois, E.F.: Clinical calorimetry. A graphic representation of the respiratory quotient and the percentage of calories from protein, fat and carbohydrate. J. Biol. Chem. *59*:43, 1924.

59. Lusk, G.: Animal calorimetry. Analysis of the oxidation of mixtures of carbohydrate and fat. A correction. J. Biol. Chem. *59*:41, 1924.

60. Michaelis, A.M.: Clinical calorimetry. A graphic method of determining certain numerical factors in metabolism. J. Biol. Chem. *59*:51, 1924.

61. Wilder, R.M.: Calorimetry. The basis of the science of nutrition. Arch. Intern. Med. *103*:146, 1959.

62. Gomez, F., Jéquier, E., Chabot, V., et al.: Carbohydrate and lipid oxidation in normal human subjects: its influence on glucose tolerance and insulin response to glucose. Metabolism *21*:381, 1972.

63. Felber, J.P., Magnenat, G., Casthelaz, M., et al.: Carbohydrate and lipid oxidation in normal and diabetic subjects. Diabetes *26*:693, 1977.

64. Felber, J.P., Jéquier, E.: Oxydation des glucides et des lipides dans le diabete. Journ. Annu. Diabetol. Hotel Dieu (Paris), 239, 1978.

65. Durnin, J.V.: Indirect calorimetry in man; a critique of practical problems. Proc. Nutr. Soc. *37*:5, 1978.

66. Benedict, F.G. and Joslin, E.P.: A study of metabolism in severe diabetes. Carnegie Inst. Washington Publ. No. 176, 1912.

67. Foss, M.C., Vlachokosta, F.V., Cunningham, L.N., Aoki, T.T.: Restoration of glucose homeostasis in insulin-dependent diabetic subjects: an inducible process. Diabetes *31*:46, 1982.

68. DeFronzo, R.A., Jacot, E., Jéquier, E., et al.: The effect of insulin on the disposal of intravenous glucose: results from indirect calorimetry and hepatic and femoral venous catheterization. Diabetes *30*:1000, 1981.

69. DeFronzo, R.A., Simonson, D., Ferraninni, E.: Hepatic and peripheral insulin resistance: a common feature of Type 2 (non-insulin-dependent) and Type 1 (insulin-dependent) diabetes mellitus. Diabetologia *23*:313, 1982.

70. Aoki, T.T., Vlachokosta, F.V., Foss, M.C., Meistas, M.T.: Evidence for restoration of hepatic glucose processing in type I diabetes mellitus. J. Clin. Invest. *71*:837, 1983.

71. Cahill, G.F., Jr., Aoki, T.T.: How metabolism affects clinical problems. Medical Times *98*:106, (Oct.) 1970.

72. Aoki, T.: Metabolic adaptations to starvation, semi-starvation, and carbohydrate restriction. In: N. Selvey, P.L. White (Eds.): Nutrition in the 1980's: Constraints on Our Knowledge. New York, Alan R. Liss, Inc., 1981, pp. 161–177.

73. Aoki, T.T., Finley, R.J., Cahill, G.F., Jr.: The redox state and regulation of amino acid metabolism in man. Biochem. Soc. Symp. *43*:17, 1978.

9 Hormones Affecting the Secretion and Actions of Insulin

Om P. Ganda

During the past decade, tremendous advances have taken place in the field of several hormones affecting the secretion and/or action of insulin. Within the islet itself, besides insulin and glucagon, at least two distinct peptides (somatostatin and human pancreatic polypeptide (hPP)) have been identified in discrete cell types (D, PP respectively) and extensively investigated. This chapter will begin with a detailed account of the pathophysiology of glucagon and deal with the current understanding of the importance of somatostatin and hPP. Other candidate hormones involved in the gastro-entero-pancreatic system will be reviewed, as will the significance of certain hormones common to such divergent locations as the nervous system, gut, and the islets. In the latter section, the role of counter-regulatory hormones including growth hormone, glucocorticoids, and catecholamines, as well as glucagon in the maintenance of glucose homeostasis, will be discussed. Finally, the preliminary but potentially important data regarding prolactin and prostaglandins, as they relate to islet physiology, will be summarized.

GLUCAGON

The term "glucagon" was coined in 1923 by Murlin and co-workers, who clearly demonstrated a hyperglycemic effect of certain pancreatic extracts in dogs.[1] Similar results were observed independently by Collip[2] and others. However, almost half a century after its discovery, little was known regarding the regulation and physiologic significance of glucagon secretion due to lack of suitable methodology for its measurement. Although a specific radioimmunoassay was first developed by the pioneering work of Unger and co-workers in the early 1960s,[3] it was not until several years later that the initial studies in man could be carried out with confidence.[4] During the past 10 to 15 years, however, a vast amount of knowledge has accrued in regard to our current concepts of the role of glucagon in human pathophysiology. Also, in the past decade, the availability of somatostatin, a tetradecapeptide originally isolated from the hypothalamus and subsequently identified in the D cells of the pancreatic islets, has resulted in rapid strides in the understanding of the relative importance of insulin and glucagon in glucose homeostasis.

Characterization of Circulating Glucagon

The alpha, or A, cells of the pancreatic islets of Langerhans secrete glucagon, a hormone of major biologic significance in man, which is composed of a single strand of 29 amino acids with a molecular weight of 3,485. However, a small amount of glucagon is also secreted by the extra-pancreatic alpha cells present in the gastrointestinal tract. Although these alpha cells are immunohistochemically and ultrastructurally similar to the pancreatic alpha cells, the relative contribution and significance of this source to the total circulating glucagon in man remains uncertain. The true glucagon must be distinguished from another more abundant, glucagon-like immunoreactivity (GLI), largely from the gastrointestinal tract of many species but which markedly differs from the "pancreatic" glucagon in physico-chemical and biologic characteristics.[5-7]

Some evidence suggests a common origin of pancreatic glucagon and all of the known glucagon-like polypeptides from a 100 amino-acid precursor, termed glycentin (~12,000-dalton). According to a recently proposed nomenclature,[7] the term "immunoreactive glucagon (IRG)" should be employed for the polypeptides which react with both C- and N- terminal specific glucagon antibodies whereas those which react only with N- terminal specific antibodies should be called "glucagon-like immunoreactivity (GLI)." Small quantities of IRG components in the gut and of GLI components in the pancreas have been shown to exist in various species. In addition, Lawrence and her associates have described the presence of a glucagon-like material in the submaxillary salivary glands of various animals and man, the precise nature of which remains to be determined.[8]

Like insulin, glucagon is primarily removed and degraded by the liver and kidney, disappearing from the circulation with a half-life of about 10 minutes. Recent studies of Jaspan et al.[6] have shown that the liver is the major site for the extraction of the 3,500-dalton glucagon, whereas the 9,000-dalton proglucagon is primarily removed by the kidney. This accounts for the fact that proglucagon is the major component increased in renal failure, a situation analogous to the relative handling of insulin and proinsulin by the liver and kidney, respectively. The heterogeneity of circulating human glucagon has recently been well documented.[6,7,9] At least four discrete fractions of IRG can be recognized by the so-called glucagon-specific antisera (Table 9–1). The 3,500 molecular fraction is believed to be the true glucagon, and this is the fraction which is most responsive to various stimulating factors, e.g., arginine and hypoglycemia, and inhibitors, e.g., hyperglycemia and somatostatin. The IRG fraction of approximately 9000 molecular weight is the probable glucagon precursor, proglucagon, which is increased in patients with renal failure,[6] glucagonoma,[10,11] and familial hyperglucagonemia.[12,13] The largest fraction referred to as the "big plasma glucagon", or 'interference factor',[14] is biologically inactive and is the major contributor of the circulating glucagon of familial hyperglucagonemia, an autosomal dominant disorder.[12,13] The physiologic significance of this large molecular weight IRG remains obscure.

Regulation of Secretion in Normal Man

The physiologic control of glucagon secretion has been reviewed in detail by Unger[15,16] and by Gerich et al.[17] In health, the regulation of insulin and glucagon secretion is intimately governed by nutrient, autonomic, and perhaps hormonal factors with the ultimate goal of a fine tuning of glucose homeostasis. The pancreatic A and B cells, along with the somatostatin-secreting D cells, may also be regulated by a direct cell-to-cell (paracrine) communication through the gap junctions[17a] which are presumed to be of sufficient size to permit transport of energy intermediates.

Substrates. In general, the hormonal output of A and B cells is primarily governed by the prevailing arterial glucose concentration, the latter overriding the influence of other stimulators and inhibitors of islet cell function. This makes teleologic sense since the fuel demands of the central nervous system have to take precedence and any threat of neuroglucopenia is to be averted. Thus, glucagon secretagogues are more effective when hyperglycemia is not present and insulin secretagogues, other than glucose, are more effective in the absence of impending hypoglycemia.

Glucose. Carbohydrate ingestion is well known to be a most potent stimulus for prompt increase in insulin secretion and a concomitant suppression of glucagon. On a molar basis, glucose has been shown to be a more effective inhibitor of A cells, than a stimulator of B cells. In vitro, the threshold, half-maximum, and maximum responses of the A cells to glucose occur at approximately 2.5, 5.0, and 10.0 mM glucose, whereas the corresponding values for the stimulation of insulin secretion are 4.5, 8.0, and 25.0 mM.[17] In "in-vivo" situations, the islet cell secretions are markedly influenced by the antecedent diet, i.e., the nutritional status of an individual, so that at any given time, the insulin-glucagon (I/G) molar ratio, rather than the prevailing absolute concentrations of either hormone, might be a more important determinant of normal glucose homeostasis.[18] Thus, total starvation or a

Table 9–1.   Heterogeneity of Circulating "Pancreatic" Glucagon (IRG) in Man*

	Fractions			
	A	B	C	D
Molecular Weight	~160,000 ("Big" Glucagon)	~9000 (?Proglucagon)	~3500	<2000
Bioactivity	?	?	+ +	0
Degradation site	?	Kidney	Liver & Kidney	?
Proportion of total:				
Normals	30–80%	Trace	15–60%	Trace
Diabetes	<30%	10%	>50%	Trace
Renal Failure	~10%	50–70%	~20%	Trace
Glucagonoma	5–10%	~25% (10–90)	~70%	
Familial hyperglucagonemia	←————————→		Trace	Trace

*Adapted from refs. 6, 7, and 9.

The relative proportion and significance of a 4500 dalton glucagon-like (GLI) fraction, claimed to share the bioactivity of IRG, needs further clarification.

carbohydrate-restricted diet result in a low I/G molar ratio, a situation promoting gluconeogenesis, whereas intravenous glucose infusion, providing surplus carbohydrate calories, causes an augmented I/G molar ratio, allowing complete suppression of hepatic glucose output.

Amino acids. Unlike glucose, a mixture of amino acids or a protein meal stimulates both insulin and glucagon. In general, the secretion of glucagon is stimulated more than that of insulin in individuals on a balanced diet or a carbohydrate-restricted diet. The amino acid-induced glucagon rise, thus, is a protective mechanism against aminogenic hypoglycemia which may otherwise result due to insulin secretion following a pure protein meal. If, however, carbohydrate is ingested or infused simultaneously with the protein meal, the I/G molar ratio increases up to 6 fold, with almost complete suppression of glucagon, in order to facilitate the disposition of amino acids toward protein synthesis—the so-called 'protein-sparing' action of glucose.

Individual amino acids vary in their relative capacity to elicit glucagon vs insulin secretion, some being completely inactive. Arginine[4] and alanine[19,20] are potent stimulators of glucagon secretion and both are used as tests for evaluation of alpha cell function. Arginine and leucine are potent stimulators of insulin secretion but alanine is ineffective in this regard.

Fat. The ingestion of long-chain triglycerides may stimulate glucagon secretion,[21] although this has not been confirmed by others.[17] Elevation and lowering of free fatty acids (FFA) within the physiologic range have been shown to result in suppression and stimulation of glucagon, respectively, in man,[22] as long as these alterations are not accompanied by changes in glucose and insulin. The role

of lipids and their intermediates, e.g., free fatty acids and ketone bodies, in the physiologic regulation of insulin and glucagon secretion requires further studies.

Neural Factors. Several recent in vitro and in vivo experiments indicate a significnt modulating effect of both sympathetic and parasympathetic nervous system on the islet cell function. Earlier work has documented an inhibition of insulin secretion and augmentation of glucagon secretion by epinephrine. Beta adrenergic stimulation specifically augments basal glucagon secretion and alpha adrenergic stimulation is inhibitory.[23,24] L-Dopa has been shown to stimulate glucagon release in man.[25] These effects of adrenergic receptors are surprisingly similar to those for insulin secretion. It has been postulated that B cells may have predominantly alpha adrenergic, and A cells a higher beta adrenergic receptor concentration. The effects of the parasympathetic system are less well studied. Stimulation of the vagus appears to provoke both insulin and glucagon release; these effects are probably mediated via certain gastrointestinal factors (vide infra).

Hormonal Regulation. Various hormones, e.g., growth-hormone and corticosteroids, may influence glucagon secretion indirectly via other effects. However, somatostatin (somatotropin release-inhibiting factor, SRIF) has been shown to inhibit directly the secretion of insulin and glucagon in many species including man.[26,27] Furthermore, it has been established that the pancreatic islet D cells secrete somatostatin in significant quantities. Based on this evidence, it is possible that the secretions of the pancreatic A, B, and D cells may be intimately governed by a "paracrine" feedback system within the islets.[28] The mechanisms underlying, and the factors affecting, the inter-hormonal relationship, of these three major islet hormones, in various metabolic settings are currently under intensive scrutiny (vide infra).

Exercise. Besides starvation and protein ingestion, another physiologic stimulus for glucagon surge is exercise.[29,30] The progressive augmentation of glucagon release in this setting is related to the intensity and duration of exercise. The mechanism underlying this phenomenon is probably multifactorial, including increased adrenergic discharge, and hyperaminoacidemia. The hyperglucagonemia of exercise is a desirable signal to help maintain glucose homeostasis, in the presence of increased peripheral glucose utilization, by inducing compensatory increase in hepatic glucose output via glycogenolysis.

Metabolic Effects of Glucagon

Recently there has been a renewed interest in the better understanding of the physiologic effects of glucagon on the intermediary metabolism, primarily because of the availability of somatostatin. The latter has provided a tool which permits creating experimental situations with combined deficiency of both insulin and glucagon in in vivo situations or an isolated deficiency of either of these by replacing the other hormone. Several elegant studies during the past several years have helped clarify the relative importance of insulin versus glucagon in various metabolic situations. In general, insulin and glucagon appear to have biologically opposite actions on several metabolic functions, predominantly at the hepatic level.[15,31,32] A higher glucagon to insulin molar ratio is specifically conducive to catabolic events, i.e., glycogenolysis, gluconeogenesis, lipolysis and ketogenesis. In contrast, a high insulin to glucagon molar ratio would promote glycogenesis, lipogenesis and protein synthesis, events geared to anabolic processes (Table 9–2). A second rule of action is as follows: in normal situations, the effects of ambient concentrations of insulin predominate so that the responses to physiologic concentrations of glucagon are attenuated, whereas in the presence of absolute or relative insulin deficiency, the effects of glucagon are accentuated.

Carbohydrate Metabolism. The primary effect of glucagon is to increase the activity of adenylate cyclase in liver by binding to a specific membrane receptor-site, and thereby increasing hepatic cyclic AMP concentration.[33,34] The net effect is increased hepatic glucose output via reciprocal alteration in the activities of phosphofructokinase-2 and fructose biphosphatase-2, thereby stimulating the phosphorylase system and increasing glycogen breakdown, as well as by decreased activity of the glycogen synthetase system.[35,36,36a] Glucagon also

Table 9–2. Metabolic Effects of Insulin vs Glucagon in Man

Site	Effect	Insulin	Glucagon
Liver	Glycogenolysis	↓	↑
	Glycogenesis	↑	↓
	Gluconeogenesis	↓	↑
	Ketogenesis	?	↑
	VLDL Synthesis	↑	↓
Muscle	Protein Synthesis	↑	0
	Proteolysis	↓	?
Adipose Tissue	Lipolysis	↓	?
	Lipogenesis	↑	0

↑ = Stimulation, ↓ = Inhibition, 0 = No effect

stimulates gluconeogenesis from precursors, e.g., glycerol, lactate, and amino acids, via activation of several key gluconeogenic regulatory enzymes, phosphoenolpyruvate kinase and fructose 1,6-biphosphatase, again via critical alterations in the hepatic levels of fructose 2,6-biphosphate.[36a]

Some controversy exists in regard to the role of glucagon in the maintenance of glucose homeostasis in normal man. Studies, employing somatostatin, have clearly shown that glucagon has a significant role in the maintenance of basal hepatic glucose output in postabsorptive man.[37,38] On the other hand, several lines of evidence tend to undermine the importance of ambient glucagon concentrations in normal man in affecting moment to moment glycemic excursions. Felig and co-workers have shown that when glucagon is infused in normal subjects so as to produce distinct hyperglucagonemia and an increase in glucagon-insulin molar ratio to several times the basal level, no significant alteration in glucose tolerance is produced.[39] Furthermore, their data indicate that glucagon has only transient effects on hepatic glucose output in the presence of normal insulin secretion.[40] Similarly, Tasaka et al.[41] monitored the glucose, insulin and glucagon levels over a 24-hour period, in normal subjects and found the expected excursions in the levels of glucose and insulin with meals, whereas glucagon levels revealed no remarkable variations throughout the 24-hour period.

Protein Metabolism. The key role of insulin in stimulating muscle protein synthesis and probably in inhibiting protein degradation is well established.[42] However, the role of glucagon, if any, on these processes is poorly understood. Although glucagon is a potent stimulator of gluconeogenesis by acting directly on the liver, it seems to be devoid of direct effects on muscle protein balance in physiologic concentrations in normal man. In carefully conducted studies across the human forearm, Pozefsky et al.[43] found no significant effect of glucagon on either the uptake or the release of amino acids, glucose, lactate and acetoacetate by the skeletal muscle in either the postabsorptive state or after 60 hours of fast. This was despite the fact that glucagon infusion lasting 2 hours resulted in its supraphysiologic concentrations. Marliss et al.[44] infused glucagon into 4-to-6 week fasted subjects at varying dose levels. Although physiologic increments in glucagon levels over 24 to 48 hours resulted in a significant reduction in plasma concentrations of threonine, serine, and glycine, in the absence of changes in blood glucose or insulin, this was not accompanied by an increased hepatic amino acid utilization since urinary urea nitrogen failed to rise, but actually declined. These results were later confirmed by Aoki et al.[45] who also observed a decline of circulating alanine and glutamine levels, despite significant prolongation of radiolabeled alanine in the circulation of subjects after prolonged starvation.

The extraction of amino acids by the liver for gluconeogenesis is probably influenced by physiologic concentrations of glucagon. Acute glucagon deficiency induced by somatostatin infusion (with insulin replacement), and chronic glucagon deficiency due to pancreatectomy, are both associated with hyperaminoacidemia and decreased urinary urea nitrogen.[46] These abnormalities are corrected by restoring physiologic glucagon levels, suggesting an important role of glucagon in the mediation of gluconeogenesis from amino acids.[46]

Lipid Metabolism. The classic studies of Heimberg et al.[47] have established a pronounced ketogenic effect of glucagon on the liver, in the absence of an increased uptake of free fatty acids (FFA). Administration of pharmacologic amounts of glucagon have been shown to augment lipolysis and ketogenesis in man. However, such studies are difficult to interpret because of known effects of pharmacologic amounts of glucagon in stimulating catecholamine and growth-hormone secretion. Glucagon is known to stimulate lipolysis in adipose tissue from a number of species. Isolated human adipose tissue, however, is poorly responsive.[48] In most of the studies in which glucagon was shown to be lipolytic in man, non-physiologic concentrations of glucagon were achieved[49,50] with rare exceptions.[51] In studies of glucagon infusion across the forearm, no significant gradient of FFA, glycerol, or acetoacetate existed across the adipose tissue.[43] Thus, the evidence for glucagon-induced lipolysis in man is rather flimsy. Even where demonstrable, the lipolytic effects of glucagon are exquisitely sensitive to suppressive effects of insulin.[49,51]

In pharmacologic doses, glucagon has been shown to exert a hypotriglyceridemic effect in normal subjects, despite a simultaneous stimulation of insulin release.[50,52,53] The mechanism of this effect is uncertain, although one important factor might be the diversion of FFA in liver from very low density lipoprotein (VLDL) synthesis to the ketogenic pathway.

Glucagon and Insulin Secretion. Samols et al.[54] demonstrated a direct betacytotropic effect of glucagon. Several investigators have since utilized this action of glucagon in the evaluation of beta cell function. The mechanism of insulin secretory response to glucagon is distinct from that resulting in response to glucose and has been found to be preserved in early stages of both Types I and II diabetes when the response to glucose is impaired.[53,55,55a] In non-diabetic individuals, glucose[55-58] or tolbutamide[56] potentiate the insulin secretory response to glucagon. The C-peptide response to glucagon has been used in the assessment of residual B-cell function in diabetics of recent onset.[59]

The stimulatory effects of glucagon on insulin secretion led Samols et al.[60] to postulate the existence of a glucagon-insulin feedback loop system in the regulation of the secretion of these hormones. However, it is not certain whether the local concentration of glucagon in the islets has significant effects on insulin secretion under physiologic circumstances.

Electrolyte Balance. Glucagon may have important physiologic influence on the regulation of electrolyte balance. This has been borne out by the studies in which sodium balance has been studied during prolonged starvation. During the first few days of a fast, a paradoxical state of "pseudohypoaldosteronism" ensues during which an increased rate of aldosterone secretion is accompanied by distal tubular insensitivity to mineralocorticoids with consequent natriuresis.[61] With continued fasting, however, this tubular refractoriness is reversible and sodium conservation spontaneously resumes. The maximal mineralocorticoid refractoriness during the initial several days of starvation coincides with the peak rise in glucagon concentration. Similarly, carbohydrate refeeding during this period will inhibit glucagon secretion, with return of the distal tubular sensitivity to mineralocorticoid.[62] Thus, under certain situations, glucagon excess or deficiency may induce states of mineralocorticoid antagonism, or hypersensitivity.

The relative impact of glucagon lack vs insulin secretion in explaining the phenomenon of "refeeding edema" which is seen in the early stages of post-starvation, refeeding, or insulin treatment, is not yet fully understood. Similarly, studies employing somatostatin indicate a more important role for insulin than for glucagon secretion in modulating sodium and potassium balance in normal man.[63]

A-Cell Function in Diabetes. That A-cell dysfunction exists in diabetes is well recognized. Beginning with the earliest work of Unger and his associates, several reports have confirmed the presence of an absolute or relative hyperglucagonemia in insulin-dependent (Type I) as well as in non-insulin-dependent (Type II) diabetes.[4,5,64–66] Patients with poorly controlled or unstable diabetes,[67] particularly those in ketoacidosis,[68] reveal the greatest elevations of glucagon concentrations.

The nature of the A-cell abnormality in diabetes is characterized by a hyperresponsiveness to amino acids, e.g., arginine, alanine, and protein-meals[4,17,19,65,66] even in the presence of hyperglycemia;[69] as well as a lack of suppression with glucose.[4,16] Glucose alone may paradoxically cause further elevation of glucagon levels.[64] That the A cells in diabetes are uniquely "blind" to glucose is supported by the additional observations of Gerich et al.[70] that, unlike in normal subjects, hypoglycemia fails to stimulate A cells, while the response to arginine stimulation in the same patients was exaggerated. Furthermore, a lack of A-cell responsiveness to hyperglycemia persists despite long-term restoration of euglycemia by insulin infusion therapy.[70a] This failure to respond to hypoglycemia in the diabetics is not secondary to an impaired secretion of, or responsiveness to, catecholamines as might be suspected.[71] Further evidence for a selective impairment of recognition of glucose by the A-cells in diabetes comes from the demonstration that the suppression of the A-cells by other agents, e.g., free fatty acids, may be normal.[72]

Three Controversial Issues Regarding the Role of Glucagon in Diabetes

Despite universal acceptance of the fact that alpha cell function is impaired in diabetes, three main issues are surrounded by considerable controversy and must be resolved before one can accept diabetes to be a 'bihormonal' disorder as proposed by Unger.[5] Some of the details of the current controversy have recently been reviewed.[15,72a,73]

Is A-Cell Dysfunction a Primary or a Secondary Defect? The demonstration of A-cell in sensitivity to both hyper and hypoglycemia as alluded to above, suggests a primary abnormality consisting of a selective impairment of A-cell glucoreceptor. On the other hand, it may be argued that the A-cell defect is secondary to insulin lack or hyperglycemia itself since hyperglucagonemia readily occurs in experimental animals following beta cell destruction by alloxan or streptozotocin and, in fact, is reversible by insulin administra-

tion.[74] However, it has been contended that the hyperglucagonemia of human insulin-dependent diabetes is not as readily reversible, even with supraphysiologic doses of insulin, as in experimental animals, unless insulin concentrations are acutely raised.[75] On the other hand, recent work with long-term, near-normal glucoregulation achieved by an open-loop continuous insulin infusion system has been shown to result in normalization of glucagon levels during 24-hour monitoring.[76] Thus, the diabetic A-cell abnormalities may indeed result primarily from insulin lack. As hypothesized by Unger,[72a] it may be the loss of the intra-islet insulin secretion that results in the loss of "glucose-sensing" function of the A cells in insulin-dependent diabetes. Nevertheless, this mechanism will not explain the hyperresponsiveness of A cells in non-insulin-dependent diabetes with normal or increased β-cell and insulin content of the islets. What influence the islet somatostatin secretion might exert in such a situation remains to be studied.

There is a paucity of information on the A-cell response to various regulatory factors in true "prediabetic" individuals or in "early" (borderline) diabetics. In one recent study of persons in the pre-Type I diabetic phase, a blunted A-cell response to arginine was found.[77] This suggests that during insulitis there is a functional defect of A-cells with subsequent restoration of function when overt diabetes develops. Additional studies of A-cell function in nondiabetics with subsequent development of diabetes in the same persons will undoubtedly be of interest in this regard.

Is Glucagon Essential in the Pathogenesis of Diabetes? Considerable controversy exists on this question. Since hyperglucagonemia is commonly observed in diabetes of "genetic" or "experimental" type, Unger and Orci have proposed an essential role for glucagon in the pathogenesis of the diabetic syndrome.[78] It has been claimed that this hypothesis is supported by several observations, such as experimental studies demonstrating lack of severe hyperglycemia and hyperketonemia in the absence of glucagon[73,79] and the reversal of diabetes in pancreatectomized dogs by glucagon-suppression induced by somatostatin.[80]

While it is generally agreed that a relative glucagon excess would potentiate the effects of insulin-deficiency in the augmentation of hyperglycemia and hyperketonemia, other evidence would weaken the concept of the essentiality of glucagon in the development of diabetes itself. Perhaps the strongest argument comes from the pancreatectomized human model, where in contrast to the situation in pancreatectomized dogs, an absence of pancreatic glucagon has been shown by several investigators to exist in the presence of diabetes.[81,81a,82] In studies of Barnes et al.,[82] ketoacidosis was shown to develop after withdrawal of insulin, in the absence of glucagon in the four patients studied, albeit the glycemia and ketonemia achieved were significantly less severe than in similarly studied juvenile-type diabetics. Others, however, have shown that the pancreatic glucagon (~3500 dalton) can be demonstrated in such patients but the significance of these relatively small amounts of glucagon remains uncertain.[82a,82b,83] Thus, unlike dogs, human diabetics may not secrete significant amounts of glucagon from extrapancreatic sources; yet diabetes and ketonemia can develop, even though of less severity and magnitude. The glucagon secretion in patients with chronic pancreatitis and diabetes secondary to hemochromatosis has been reported with variable results; reduced, normal, and increased levels have been found.[84-92] These inconsistencies are, at least partly, explained by the methodologic differences in glucagon measurements.[7] Similarly, the relationship and the significance of this with a recently described 4,500-dalton GLI in pancreatectomized man[7] is uncertain and requires further work.

Olefsky et al.[93] compared glucagon levels in patients with mild to moderately severe, non-insulin-dependent diabetes characterized by adequate insulin reserve and relative insulin resistance. No differences in the plasma glucagon levels were found among these diabetics and the healthy controls. Thus glucagon does not appear to be necessary for the insulin resistance commonly incriminated in the pathogenesis of non-insulin-dependent diabetes. In glucagonoma syndrome, marked elevations of glucagon, in the presence of insulin, are accompanied by only mild hyperglycemia.[12]

Finally, chronic glucagon deficiency, such as that encountered in the human somatostatinoma syndrome,[94] does not prevent the development of diabetes, again exonerating glucagon from an "essential" role in the pathogenesis of diabetes in this experiment of nature wherein insulin deficiency occurs in combination with the absence of glucagon.

Effect of Glucagon Suppression on the Control of Diabetes. Whether the suppression of glucagon might help improve control of diabetes is another issue surrounded by considerable controversy, largely because of the conflicting evidence regarding the importance of hyperglucagonemia in the hyperglycemia of uncontrolled diabetes. In normal persons and in non-insulin-dependent diabetics, glucagon infusions over several hours, varying its concentrations to ranges seen in uncontrolled diabetes, seem not to have significant effects on ambient glucose levels or glucose tolerance.[39] It

has been proposed that as long as insulin is available, the effects of glucagon on hepatic glucose output are transient, lasting no more than 30 to 60 minutes, despite ongoing hyperglucagonemia.[95] On the other hand, intermittent elevations in glucagon concentrations have been shown to significantly augment hepatic glucose output, and this may mimic the in-vivo situation in the diabetic more closely.[15]

Administration of somatostatin in normal subjects and in maturity-onset (Type II) diabetics worsens the glucose tolerance since suppression of glucagon is accompanied by a concomitant suppression of insulin secretion.[95-98] However, in insulin-dependent diabetics, particularly in those with negligible insulin reserve associated with unstable diabetes, Unger and co-workers have put forth strong arguments in favor of beneficial effects of glucagon suppression, as opposed to conventional treatment with insulin alone.[73,99] There is no doubt that in such diabetics, excessive glucagon secretion has a considerable role in maintaining persistent hyperglycemia and hyperketonemia[66,100] and that an augmented sensitivity to ketogenic effects of glucagon exists in the presence of insulin deficiency.[101] Similar argument has been put forth for elevated growth hormone in juvenile diabetics.[102] Raskin and Unger[99] and Gerich[103] have shown that glucagon suppression induced by somatostatin infusion in juvenile-type diabetics, along with insulin treatment, markedly improves diabetes control, compared with insulin alone. These results have been challenged by the studies of Felig et al.,[95,104] and of Clarke et al.[105] who failed to show an appreciable worsening of the control of diabetes in the insulin-dependent diabetics by raising glucagon levels to a supraphysiologic range by continuous infusions of glucagon. Part of the inconsistency in these results may lie in the fact that somatostatin-induced effects may be dependent upon its additional, poorly understood, metabolic consequences (e.g., interference with nutrient absorption[95] and perhaps direct hepatic effects), rather than upon glucagon suppression itself. The latter has not thus far been shown conclusively.

SOMATOSTATIN

Somatostatin, a tetradecapeptide, was isolated and synthesized in 1973 after many years of extensive search for hypothalamic factor(s) regulating pituitary growth hormone secretion.[106,107] Soon after its discovery, Koerker et al.[26] reported significant inhibitory effects of somatostatin on insulin and glucagon secretion in baboons, associated with a decline in blood glucose levels. This observation of the potent inhibitory effects of somatostatin on the endocrine pancreas has been confirmed in nor-

Table 9–3. Biologic Actions of Somatostatin in Man

I. *Endocrine:*

	Inhibition	No Inhibition
Pituitary	GH	FSH
	TSH	LH
		HPr*
		ACTH*
Pancreatic	Insulin	
	Glucagon	
	HPP	
G.I. Tract	Gastrin	
	CCK-PZ	
	Secretin	
	VIP	
	GIP	
Adrenal		Cortisol
		Aldosterone
		Catecholamines
Parathyroid	? Calcitonin	PTH
Kidney	Renin	

II. *Non-Endocrine:*

	Inhibits or Prevents
Stomach	HCl
	Pepsin
	Gastric motility
Intestine	Nutrient Absorption
	Motility
Pancreas (exocrine)	Bicarbonate & enzyme release
Gallbladder	Contractility
Splanchnic Vessels	Blood Flow
Hemopoietic	? Platelet aggregation
Liver	?

*Except in some patients with pituitary tumor.

mal and in diabetic persons by several investigators.[27,108–111] Further explosion of interest in relation to the possible role of somatostatin in glucose homeostasis ensued when it was shown that this peptide is widely distributed not only in the nervous system but also in the D cells of the gastrointestinal tract and pancreatic islets.[112–116] Recently, larger molecular-weight peptides of the somatostatin family have been characterized.[116a] Somatostatin-28 is an amino-terminal-extended peptide that appears to be even more potent than somatostatin-14 at certain sites.[116a]

Biologic Actions

The precise role of somatostatin in human physiology remains uncertain. However, the administration of synthetic somatostatin results in a wide variety of endocrine as well as of non-endocrine effects[107,116,117] as summarized in Table 9–3. In addition to the inhibition of growth hormone (GH) and thyrotropin (TSH) from the anterior pituitary, and of all other known hormones from the endocrine pancreas (insulin, glucagon and human pan-

creatic polypeptide), a number of important inhibitory actions on both endocrine and exocrine secretions of the gastrointestinal tract are noteworthy. Furthermore, somatostatin has been shown to impair nutrient absorption from the gut, probably via a combination of effects including a reduction of splanchnic blood flow as well as diminished gastric, intestinal and gallbladder motility.[118,119] Interestingly, no direct effects of somatostatin on the liver have thus far been clearly demonstrable albeit this area requires further work. The possible effects of long-term administration of somatostatin on hemostasis have been controversial. Earlier work in baboons suggested a thrombocytopenic effect and a bleeding tendency following chronic, repeated infusions of somatostatin.[120] Subsequently, a detailed investigation in human subjects revealed no significant effects on several indices of coagulation as well as of platelet function despite infusions of somatostatin lasting several hours.[121] In fact, recent preliminary studies have shown somatostatin to be efficient in the control of acute bleeding in peptic ulcer disease.[122,123]

Regulation of Secretion

In contrast to a great deal of information available regarding the biologic effects of somatostatin, much less is known about the physiologic regulation and significance of somatostatin in normal man. The main obstacles underlying the paucity of data in this regard are the relatively short half-life of somatostatin (<4 minutes) in the circulation and the lack of sensitive methods for its measurement in plasma. The available data in various species including man indicates an extreme variability of somatostatin levels in different laboratories,[124–127a] reflecting the lack of standardization of its assay.[127b] The bulk of available information regarding the factors affecting its secretion has been derived from "in-vitro" experimental situations. Studies of Ipp et al.[128] and Weir et al.,[129] using isolated perfused canine pancreas have suggested a number of secretagogues for somatostatin, including glucose, arginine, leucine, vasoactive intestinal polypeptide (VIP), and pancreozymin-cholecystokinin, in this respect resembling the situation with insulin secretion. Interestingly, glucagon and tolbutamide also stimulated immunoreactive somatostatin in these studies. In contrast, in two preliminary reports concerning measurement of somatostatin in human plasma, arginine was shown to produce disparate results on somatostatin secretion.[124,125] Whether this discrepancy is due to immunoassay differences or other factors, remains to be resolved. Finally, variable effects on somatostatin secretion from different anatomic sites is suggested by another preliminary report which showed an inhibitory effect of insulin on the release of somatostatin from the pancreas and antrum of the intact dog but not from the gastric fundus.[130]

Morphometric studies of endocrine cells have revealed an increase in the number of D as well as A cells in the B-cell-deficient rat[131-133] and monkey.[134] However, the relevance of this finding and its significance need further work in relation to the human diabetic syndrome, since the scant data on the circulating levels of somatostatin in this regard are controversial.[116a,127b]

During the past several years, attention has been focused on the possibility of somatostatin-producing cells being governed by a "paracrine" regulation.[28,117] Morphologic studies have shown a characteristic distribution of various types of endocrine cells within the islets and anatomic junctional complexes between adjacent islet cells.[135] Moreover, the somatostatin-containing cells in the gastric antrum have been shown to have long, nonluminal processes which terminate in gastrin-producing G cells and in the other effector cells.[136] Such observations support the hypothesis[117,135] that certain widely distributed "hormones" such as somatostatin might more importantly exert their influence via a "paracrine" effect on neighboring cells within an organ than via the "endocrine effects," thus obviating the need for release into the circulation and transport to other organs as necessary prerequisites for the physiologic role of such peptides.

In view of the many inhibiting effects of somatostatin in various tissues, it seems plausible that its cellular mechanism of action involves a step common to several secretory processes. Two such possibilities receiving considerable support from various studies are (a) an inhibition at the level of cyclic AMP or at a step distal to cyclic AMP[107,117] and (b) an inhibition of Ca^{++} transport as suggested by studies using a calcium ionophore.[137]

Therapeutic Potential of Somatostatin in Diabetes

A major impact of the discovery and synthesis of somatostatin has been the availability of a research tool for exploring the relative roles of insulin and glucagon in the pathophysiology of diabetes as discussed above. The potential efficacy of somatostatin as an adjunct in the treatment of Type I (insulin-dependent) diabetes[99-103] and the controversy surrounding this issue have been presented above (see last section under "Glucagon"). In the Type II diabetic, the use of somatostatin seems clearly unjustified and may even worsen the metabolic control by inhibiting the preserved B cell function.[95-98] Before an approach to the treatment of Type I diabetes is undertaken, we need (a) a

long-acting preparation as well as (b) an analog of somatostatin preferably free of numerous undesirable effects, e.g., inhibitory effects on the gastrointestinal system and, in juvenile age group, inhibition of GH. The use of protamine zinc (PZ) suspensions, similar to those used for insulin, might facilitate the first goal.[138] Current efforts toward the synthesis of somatostatin analogs with greater potency against glucagon and less gastrointestinal effects are in progress. Two such analogs are [D-cys[14]]-somatostatin and [D-Trp[8], D-Cys[14]]-somatostatin.[139] Both, however, are also more potent inhibitors of GH than the natural somatostatin. More recently, an interesting glucagon-selective analog, des-Ala[1], Gly[2] [His[4,5]-D-Trp[8]]-somatostatin (Wy-41,747), has been developed which is also relatively long-acting.[140] Another long-acting octapeptide analog (Des AA[1,2,4,5,12,13] D-Trp[8]) has been developed and found to be effective in patients with islet-cell tumors for up to 24 hours following a single injection in initial trials.[141] An orally effective analogue has been reported by Veber et al.[141b] Further studies with such compounds are awaited and probable effects at other sites need to be carefully evaluated.

HUMAN PANCREATIC POLYPEPTIDE (hPP)

Human pancreatic polypeptide is a strand of 36 amino acids localized to a discrete cell-type (PP) in the human endocrine pancreas, distinct from A, B and D cells.[142] In contrast to insulin and glucagon which are detected in higher concentrations in the body and tail of the pancreas, hPP is found largely in the regions of the uncinate process and the head of the pancreas,[143] suggesting a different mode of its embryogenesis. In contrast to several other gut hormones, no significant concentration of hPP have been detected in the human gastrointestinal tract or other tissues, including brain.

Physiologic Regulation and Actions

The knowledge about the role of hPP in human physiology is at present quite limited.[144] Recent availability of radioimmunoassay has indicated an appreciable increase in the basal plasma levels with advancing age. The secretion of hPP can be stimulated by practically all nutrients but is most marked after protein ingestion. In addition, hypoglycemia has been shown to be a potent stimulus for hPP release,[144,145] probably a vagal effect. A number of neural and hormonal factors probably mediate the release of hPP, since the intravenous infusion of nutrients including glucose, lipid and amino acids results in no appreciable increase in blood levels of hPP, whereas infusions of any of several gut hormones, e.g., secretin, cholecystokinin, cerulin, or pentagastrin stimulates and somatostatin inhibits hPP secretion. Cholinergic agents have been shown to stimulate and atropine to inhibit the release of hPP.[146-148]

Administration of bovine PP to normal subjects has been shown to result in a significant suppression of exocrine pancreatic and biliary secretions, suggesting either independent effects or a common effect via an action on gallbladder motility.[149] Secretions of gastrin, gastric acid and pepsin, and islet hormones appear not to have been affected by PP.

Clinical Implications

Any alterations in circulating hPP levels should be interpreted with caution and keeping in view the known increases with age and renal failure.[144,150] Striking increases in the levels of plasma hPP and high tumor concentrations have been reported in up to 50% of patients with various types of islet-cell tumors including insulinomas, glucagonomas, gastrinomas, and the watery-diarrhea syndrome due to VIP-secreting tumors.[151,152] PP cells have also been detected in otherwise "nonfunctioning" tumors although the significance of this finding has been uncertain in view of the lack of clinical symptoms in such patients.[144] The earlier suggestion that increased hPP level may be a tumor-maker for patients with gastrinomas (Zollinger-Ellison syndrome) has not been confirmed.[153] At present, it remains to be seen if serial estimations of hPP in certain patients with malignant islet-cell tumors would be helpful in following the response to surgical treatment or chemotherapy, as has been suggested by some. Similarly, raised levels of hPP may help screen the family members of some patients with M.E.N. (multiple endocrine neoplasia) syndromes.[154] Conversely, a reduced hPP release following secretin administration has been shown in patients with chronic pancreatitis, indicating a diminished endocrine cell mass.[148]

Studies of Floyd et al.[154] have revealed elevated plasma levels of hPP in insulin-treated diabetics (both juvenile and maturity-onset types) but not in mild, non-insulin treated diabetics. It was further suggested from their studies that the increased hPP levels may correlate with the degree of severity of diabetes and that the levels may return toward a normal range by improved control. In this regard, however, it should be noted that significant levels of circulating antibody to PP have been shown in a majority of patients treated with insulin due to contaminant PP in various insulin preparations. The assay of PP in such patients may be, therefore, somewhat unreliable because of methodologic problems. However, studies in a spontaneously diabetic mutant mice strain (C57 BL/6ks) have documented an increase in the islet PP cell population in the presence of severe B cell deficiency.[155]

An effect of hPP in the regulation of satiety and appetite control has been suggested by the reports of a diminished hPP response to meals in obese subjects.[156,157] These results are in keeping with the earlier reports of a diminished number of PP-secreting cells and low plasma PP levels in genetically obese mice. The significance of the observed alterations in islet morphology and hPP secretion in obesity as well as in the diabetic clearly requires further work.

GUT HORMONES

A number of years ago it was reported that the magnitude of insulin release following an oral glucose load is much greater than that following an intravenous glucose infusion, despite comparable blood glucose levels.[158,159] During the past decade, a number of interesting observations have been made in an effort to understand the nature and properties of the putative "gut factor(s)" (or hormones) mediating an augmented insulin response to various ingested substances.[160-163] It has become increasingly clear that a variety of hormones released from the gastrointestinal tract during the digestive phase serve not only in the digestive function and exocrine secretion but, in addition, regulate the release of islet hormones, primarily insulin. The precise role and the relative importance of each of the putative gut hormones of the so-called gastro entero-pancreatic axis (Table 9-4) are still incompletely understood. However, it appears that more than one hormone is involved, depending upon the nature of the ingested nutrient and other factors.[161,163] For example, gastric inhibitory polypeptide (GIP) appears to be a major candidate involved after glucose or lipid ingestion (Table 9-5). On the other hand, the release of a different gut-hormone, e.g., cholecystokinin (CCK), may be more important following protein ingestion.[163-165] The functional overlap between groups of gut hormones may be partly explained by a common phylogenetic origin and consequent chemical structural similarities, e.g., between GIP, secretin, VIP and glucagon, and between gastrin and cholecystokinin.

It has been postulated that one or more of the gut factors may also be responsible for certain extra-pancreatic effects, e.g., mediation of insulin action on the liver in facilitating glucose uptake[166] or modulating the peripheral effects of insulin on lipolysis.[161]

Secretin

Since its discovery in 1902, speculations have been made regarding the possible influence of se-

Table 9–4. Nomenclature of Gastro-Entero-Pancreatic System

Cell	Product	Presence in		
		Pancreas	G.I. Tract	Nervous System
P	? Bombesin	+ *	+	+
EC	Serotonin, substance P	+	+	+
	? Motilin			
D₁	V.I.P.-like	+	+	+
PP	Pancreatic Polypeptide	+	+ *	
D	Somatostatin	+	+	+
B	Insulin	+		+
A	Glucagon	+	+	?
G	Gastrin	+ *	+	+
S	Secretin		+	
I	Cholecystokinin		+	+
K	GIP		+	
N	Neurotensin	+ *	+	+
L	Enteroglucagon-Glycentin		+	
X	Unknown		+	
?	Enkephalin	+	+	+
?	Corticotropin (ACTH)-like	+	+	+
?	TRH†	+	+	+

*Not detected in man.
†Thyrotropin-releasing hormone.
Adapted and updated from 1977 Lausanne Classification[160] and Guillemin, R.[192]

Table 9–5. Gut-Factors Released by Enteric Signals

	Glucose	Amino Acids	Fat
GIP	+	+	+
CCK	0	+	+
Gastrin	0	?	0
Secretin	0	?	0
VIP	0	0	?
Glycentin	0	?	?

+ = Release, 0 = No effect, ? = Uncertain. See text for details. Adapted from ref. 163.

cretin on islet hormone secretion. Secretin is a 27 amino-acid polypeptide, produced by the S cells of the upper small intestine. Studies in the past employed impure preparations and pharmacologic amounts of secretin, leading to the suggestion of an insulinotropic effect. Recent studies employing pure preparations and sensitive radioimmunoassays have, however, revealed no increment of insulin release following either intravenous secretin infusion or intraduodenal acid infusion, a well known secretagogue for endogenous secretin release.[167,168] Oral glucose has been shown not to result in secretin release.[169] However, Lerner has reported that in maturity-onset diabetics with diminished or absent acute insulin response to intravenous glucose, secretin infusion results in a significant insulin out-

put and augments the insulin response to an intravenous glucose infusion.[170] The levels of secretin in plasma were not measured in Lerner's studies and may well have been much higher than those seen in physiologic circumstances in view of the dose of secretin used. However, it must be pointed out that elevated levels of plasma secretin have been reported by other investigators, in patients with untreated, maturity-onset diabetes, and positively correlated with fasting blood glucose levels.[171] Whether there is indeed a feedback regulation between insulin secretion and secretin release in diabetes, has not been studied. Thus, based on available evidence, a physiologic role for secretin in islet regulation cannot be established.

Cholecystokinin (CCK) and Gastrin

A 33 amino-acid polypeptide, cholecystokinin (CCK), like secretin, has not proved to be an important mediator of endocrine pancreas secretion. It is secreted in response to protein ingestion and fat, but not carbohydrate, and was initially thought to represent an important gut signal for protein or amino-acid-induced betacytotropic effect. However, since most of the CCK preparations have been found to contain GIP (see below), the role of CCK per se remains dubious.[160,163] Understanding of the role of CCK has been limited until recently because of the lack of a reliable radioimmunoassay for this hormone. One interesting observation made by several investigators concerns its possible effect on appetite regulation and the control of satiety. Experiments in rhesus monkeys and other species have suggested a decrease in food intake following intravenous or intraperitoneal injections of CCK.[172,173] These observations are similar to those made with intraventricular injections of cerulin, a decapeptide which shares structural homology with CCK. In addition, a markedly reduced content of immunoreactive CCK has been demonstrated in brain extracts from hyperphagic, genetically obese mice, compared with their non-obese litter-mates or normal mice.[174] The mechanism of the regulation of satiety by the CCK or CCK-like peptides released from the gut, is under investigation.

Gastrin is another important gut hormone from a metabolic point of view inasmuch as it shares several amino acid residues with CCK. Like CCK, it has received considerable attention as a likely signal for oral amino-acid-induced beta-cytotropic effect.[175] However, the effects seen with gastrin are often relatively modest and poorly sustained unless pharmacologic doses are employed.[160]

Gastric Inhibitory Polypeptide (GIP)

GIP is currently thought to be the most important "gut hormone" responsible for mediating the entero-insular effects following ingestion of various types of nutrients. It is a 43 amino-acid polypeptide which was originally isolated from crude preparations of cholecystokinin-pancreozymin. During the past several years, extensive studies have been carried out with this compound and reviewed elsewhere by Brown and co-workers.[176,177] The source of GIP in various species, including man, has been localized in the well-defined K cells of upper small intestine.[160] The development of a specific radioimmunoassay has made possible a spate of studies pertaining to the regulation of GIP secretion in healthy as well as in diabetic subjects.

GIP has been clearly shown to be insulinotropic in normal man in several studies.[177] This effect is dependent upon the prevailing blood glucose concentrations with a threshold glucose level of 5.5 mM (100 mg/dl). GIP is released in response to oral glucose, lipid (triglyceride), or protein (amino acids) ingestion. The insulinotropic effect in normal subjects is magnified by the induction of hyperglycemia. Glucose-induced increase in GIP is inhibited by acetylcholine, isoproterenol as well as epinephrine in dogs,[178] suggesting a modulation by the autonomic nervous system. In patients with reactive hypoglycemia following vagotomy, exaggerated early GIP and insulin responses have been observed, suggesting a possible role of neural factors in mediating the "late phase" of the dumping syndrome.[179] In the presence of low glucose concentrations, GIP has also been shown to be "glucagonotropic" in isolated perfused pancreas preparations.[179] A feedback control of GIP by insulin in normal subjects is suggested by the blunted increment of GIP levels in response to oral fat by the simultaneous infusion of glucose.[177]

A number of reports have shown abnormalities of GIP secretion in patients with obesity and/or maturity-onset (Type II) diabetes.[180-185] While fasting GIP levels been shown to be normal in non-obese diabetics, the post-glucose levels are exaggerated in the presence of a somewhat diminished insulin response, suggesting a relative insensitivity of B cells to GIP.[181,182] Moreover, a paradoxical increase in glucagon levels was seen in such patients, commensurate with the peak GIP response[182] raising the possibility of a stimulation of the islet A cells by GIP in contrast to normals. The triglyceride-induced GIP response was found to be normal in a group of non-insulin-dependent diabetics.[186]

Studies of Ebert et al.[185] and Willms et al.[184] have dealt with the impaired feedback control of GIP secretion in obesity. When compared to the responses in normal weight controls, these investigators reported an exaggerated secretion of GIP in obese subjects following oral glucose, a mixed

test meal, or fat ingestion, and an incomplete suppression following an intravenous glucose infusion administered after an oral fat challenge.[185] However, the abnormalities were restored toward normal following reduced caloric intake or starvation. In one study on insulin-requiring, severe diabetics (mean fasting blood glucose = 262 mg/dl), the secretion of GIP in response to oral glucose was found to be significantly impaired and there was little evidence of suppression of GIP by exogenous insulin infusion in both diabetics and normal controls.[187] The question of feedback control of GIP by insulin, therefore, remains unsettled.

In addition to the effects of GIP on the pancreas, indirect evidence indicates that GIP may also have certain peripheral effects. In preliminary studies, GIP was found to inhibit glucagon binding and cyclic AMP generation in rat adipocytes.[188] In another study, an antilipolytic effect of GIP has been further suggested by a stimulation of lipoprotein lipase activity in cultured mouse pre-adipocytes.[189] Additional studies are in progress to explore the possibility of a role for GIP in the adipose tissue metabolism and triglyceride clearance in man.

Finally, as discussed by Creutzfeldt,[163] it should be re-emphasized that GIP is probably not capable of eliciting all the effects ascribed to a putative "gut hormone" even though evidence thus far is lacking for a significant role of several other gut hormones (gastrin, CCK, secretin, VIP, glucagon-glycentin) studied. The insulinotropic effect of "gut factor" is reduced but not abolished, despite complete neutralization of GIP by GIP antiserum.[163] Similarly, Ganda and colleagues observed an enhancement of intravenous glucose disposal, when preceded by oral ingestion of certain non-glucose hexoses such as mannose and fructose, in the absence of a significant release of GIP.[190]

PEPTIDES COMMON TO NERVOUS SYSTEM, GUT, AND ISLETS

During the past several years, an exciting new era in the field of neuroendocrinology has begun with the demonstration of a variety of peptides common to various locations in the central nervous system, gastrointestinal tract and endocrine pancreas (Table 9–4). A precedent for the existence of a peptide in such diverse locations was first shown in the case of substance P in the report of von Euler and Gaddum in 1931, a finding which remained dormant for a number of years.[191] This 11 amino-acid peptide, originally described to have hypotensive and smooth-muscle stimulating properties, has subsequently been claimed to be primarily involved with sensory neurotransmission. In 1979, it was shown to inhibit insulin release from the pancreas.[191] While the relevance of various peptides now known to be present in the nervous system and gut (including pancreas) is far from clear, a number of provocative studies are currently in progress in order to clarify their significance in human physiology and disease. Perhaps most importantly, these peptides serve a neurotransmitter function in the nervous system by specific "peptidergic" pathways, whereas a "paracrine" function is subserved in relation to various endocrine secretory cells in the gut and pancreas.[192-194] These may indeed be more important functions of such peptides in contrast to a less important "hormonal" role.

Perhaps the best studied peptide in this family, from the point of view of glucose metabolism, is somatostatin (discussed above). The following account relates to some of the pertinent studies regarding a few other peptides of probable importance in this context.

Enkephalins and Endorphins

The fascinating story of the "endorphin" family of peptides began during the past decade with the demonstration of receptors for opium alkaloids in brain.[195,196] This was soon followed by two fundamental observations. One was the isolation and characterization of two pentapeptides, leuenkephalin and met-enkephalin[197] and the other was the discovery of several polypeptide (α,β,γ, and δ) endorphins from the porcine brain.[198] Each of these substances avidly binds to the opiate receptors. The entire sequence of met-enkephalin and the endorphins (including the most potent β-endorphin) is contained in the 91 amino-acid polypeptide, β-lipotropin, which had been earlier isolated from the pituitary.[199] However, later work has revealed that even β-lipotropin is derived from a much larger, 31,000 molecular weight, glycoprotein molecule, proopiomelanocortin (POMC), which also contains the sequence for ACTH and α-MSH (melanocyte-stimulating hormone).[200] From the evolutionary viewpoint, the presence of endorphins and other POMC-derived peptides has been traced back to various nonvertebrate species, including earthworms and insects.[194]

The clinical significance of enkephalins and endorphins is presently under intensive scrutiny.[194,201] A number of key roles for these compounds have been claimed and some of them subsequently refuted in the literature. Nevertheless, there seems to be a growing consensus that these substances are intimately involved in certain neuropsychiatric processes including the phenomena of pain perception, drug addiction and behavior. Furthermore, several interesting reports have recently drawn attention to the possible role of the members of "endorphin" family in metabolic regulation:

(a) Polak et al.[202] have shown a significant content of enkephalin-like immunoreactivity in human gastric antrum, upper small intestine, and pancreas.

(b) In genetically obese mice and rats, a 2- to 3-fold elevated concentration of β-endorphin has been demonstrated in the pituitary and in plasma.[203] This has been associated with a 14-fold elevation of pituitary ACTH content in the obese mice, which is in keeping with the observation of a common precursor for β-endorphin and ACTH and with their known concomitant release from the pituitary.[204] Furthermore, the hyperphagia in the obese animals was inhibited by the administration of naloxone, a specific antagonist to opiates.

(c) In experiments employing isolated, perfused canine pancreas, studies in Unger's laboratory have shown a prompt inhibition of somatostatin release by morphine or β-endorphin, followed by a release of insulin and glucagon.[205] These effects were antagonized by the addition of naloxone to the perfusate. In human studies, two groups of investigators[206a,206b] have shown acute release of insulin and glucagon in normal subjects, along with a significant rise in blood glucose levels. These effects could not, however, be blocked by naloxone.[206b] Somewhat contradictory results were observed in a rat islet cell culture system, wherein the addition of enkephalins was shown to inhibit the secretion of insulin and glucagon, while morphine enhanced the release of both hormones.[206]

(d) Stubbs et al.[207] have studied the effects of intravenous administration of a long-acting enkephalin analog, [D-Ala,[2] MePhe,[4] Met (o) ol] enkephalin (DAMME), in normal men. There was a significant rise in levels of growth-hormone and prolactin, and a significant fall in FSH, LH, ACTH and cortisol; no significant effects were observed on the levels of gastrin, VIP, insulin and glucagon. The latter findings are at variance with the results in isolated perfused pancreas and the islet cell culture system described above.

(e) In another interesting study in normal subjects, Nakao et al.[208] have shown a marked increase in the plasma levels of β-endorphin levels following insulin-induced hypoglycemia.

(f) A phenomenon of chlorpropamide alcohol-induced facial flushing has been considered a possible genetic marker for non-insulin-dependent (Type II) diabetes. Leslie and Pyke[209] have shown that this phenomenon can be reproduced by the enkephalin analog, DAMME, and blocked by prior administration of naloxone. Based on this and other[209a] evidence, it has been suggested that a subgroup with non-insulin-dependent diabetes associated with chlorpropamide-alcohol flushing phenomenon may likewise be hypersensitive to endogenous opiates.

These various studies underscore the need for further work in exploring the significance of opiate receptors and the physiologic relevance of endogenous enkephalin-like substances in human gut and pancreas.

Neurotensin

Neurotensin is a 13 amino-acid peptide, isolated and characterized by Carraway and Leeman.[210] It has been localized in the N cells of human intestine and is widely distributed in brain. The receptors for neurotensin are distinct from those for endorphins; its actions are not blocked by naloxone. Its properties are somewhat similar to substance P in causing vasodilation, hypotension and increased vascular permeability. Intravenous infusion of neurotensin in healthy subjects leads to a significant decrease of gastric acid and pepsin output as well as to delayed gastric emptying.[211]

Administration of neurotensin in experimental studies has been shown to have metabolic effects, e.g., hyperglycemia, hyperglucagonemia, and variable effects on insulin secretion, the last-named depending upon the experimental animal.[212] In the dog, the effects of neurotensin are blocked by somatostatin.[212] Immunoreactive neurotensin has been detected in normal pancreas in several animal species and preliminary data suggest a persistently increased content in the pancreas of insulinopenic C57BL/KsJ mutant mice, but not of the mice with C57BL/6J background.[213]

A few patients with pancreatic diarrhea (Verner-Morrison syndrome) have been reported to have severalfold elevation in plasma neurotensin levels, in association with elevated PP and VIP levels, as well as glucose intolerance.[213a]

Corticotropin (ACTH)

ACTH-like immunoreactivity and its presence in discrete cells of the gastro-entero-pancreatic system have been confirmed in a study by Larsson et al.[214] As in brain, the gut ACTH-like molecule and enkephalin probably originate from a common precursor in the same cells. Preliminary evidence indicates that ACTH-peptide (1–39) or the ACTH-like intermediate peptide, CLIP (18–39) may stimulate insulin release. The combined presence of immunoreactive ACTH, β-lipotropin, α-endorphin and β-endorphin in a human pancreatic islet cell carcinoma, presenting as the ectopic ACTH syndrome, further supports the common origin of these peptides.[215]

GROWTH HORMONE

A relationship between the anterior pituitary and diabetes mellitus was first shown by the classic experiments of Houssay and Biosatti and of Young, using crude pituitary extracts.[216,217] Subsequently, it was demonstrated by Ikkos and Luft that the administration of growth hormone resulted in a marked deterioration of metabolic control in diabetic individuals.[218] Arguments, pro and con, have been put forth by a number of investigators regarding the possible roles of growth hormone (GH) in (a) the etiology of human diabetes, (b) the metabolic control of diabetes, and (c) the development of chronic complications including microangiopathy and macroangiopathy.[219–221]

Physiologic Secretion and Actions of Growth Hormone

Growth hormone is secreted as a single strand of 191 amino acids. Growth hormone does not possess a tissue specificity since it acts on a variety of organs and cell types. However, it is clearly species-specific.

A number of physiologic factors affect the secretion of GH in a normal person.[222] The stimuli for the release of GH include hypoglycemia, sleep, muscular exercise, stress, and amino acids, while hyperglycemia is a potent suppressor of its release.

Employing human forearm technique, Zierler and co-workers, in a series of elegant experiments, showed the diabetogenic effects of acute increments of GH to occur via (a) an inhibition of glucose uptake by the skeletal muscle and the adipose tissue and (b) an augmentation of lipolysis.[223] Whether a significant lipolytic effect is seen during physiologic circumstances in normal individuals has not always been confirmed.[224] As regards in vivo glucose tolerance, physiologic increments of circulating GH (30 to 40 ng/ml) result in an early but transient insulin-like effect comprising a diminished glucose production and enhanced peripheral glucose clearance. However, this is subsequently followed by effects antagonistic to insulin, leading to hyperglycemia.[225] The diabetogenic effects of physiologic increments in growth hormone are primarily exerted via peripheral, rather than hepatic, effects and at the post-receptor, rather than at the receptor, level.[225,226] Chronic administration of GH resulting in permanent diabetes in dogs is accompanied by eventual exhaustion of pancreatic B cells.[227]

The interpretation of various in vitro studies dealing with GH is surrounded by considerable uncertainty because of evidence that the in vivo effects of GH may be mediated via the generation of a family of agents, termed somatomedins, in response to this hormone in liver.[228] These include somatomedin A, B, and C; insulin-like growth factors (IGF-I, IGF-II) and multiplication stimulating activity (MSA). In contrast, evidence reviewed elsewhere suggests that at least some of the effects of GH may be elicited directly by physiologic concentrations of GH, independent of somatomedin generation.[229] This view is further supported by the demonstration of the receptors for GH in a variety of tissues, e.g., cultured human lymphocytes.[230]

Growth Hormone and Diabetes

Hansen and co-workers convincingly showed that the circulating GH levels were elevated in uncontrolled diabetics, both insulin-dependent and non-insulin-dependent.[231–233] Furthermore, they showed a greater diurnal fluctuation in serum GH concentrations and a hypersecretory response to exercise in the poorly controlled diabetics. Similar observations of an absolute or relative (inappropriate) increase of GH secretion have been confirmed by others.[234–236] That an increased GH secretion pattern is a consequence of the underlying metabolic state rather than an independent factor in the pathogenesis of diabetes is suggested by the normalization of this abnormality by meticulous control of hyperglycemia.[231,237]

The implications of long-term elevation in GH levels in a diabetic individual are of considerable interest. Osterby et al.[238] have shown an enhanced basement membrane thickening induced by GH injections in streptozotocin-diabetic rats. Passa et al. found a significantly greater release of GH in diabetics with proliferative retinopathy, compared with those without retinopathy and non-diabetic controls, following exercise of similar extent.[239] A blunted or absent GH secretion has been suggested as a cause for the relative lack of severe retinopathy in patients with diabetes secondary to hemachromatosis[240] and in sexual ateliotic dwarfs with diabetes.[241] While these observations are in keeping with the reported beneficial effects of pituitary ablation on the clinical course of diabetic retinopathy,[219,242] it is of interest to recall the well-known paucity of clinical microvascular complications in patients with acromegaly who demonstrate such high GH concentrations. Perhaps the best explanation would invoke a permissive role for GH in the presence of other metabolic hormonal factors in the pathogenesis of diabetic microangiopathy.

Arguments for and against a potential role of GH in the pathogenesis of macrovascular complications of diabetes are discussed in Chapter 11.

GLUCOCORTICOIDS

It has been known for a long time that glucocorticoids antagonize the actions of insulin.[243] The spectrum of insulin insensitivity in patients with Cushing's syndrome and the insulin hypersensitivity in Addison's disease is clinically well recognized. Cahill[244] has reviewed extensive evidence for the diverse metabolic actions of glucocorticoids on liver, adipose tissue and muscle. In the liver, glucocorticoids appear to accelerate reactions at every rate-limiting step in the sequence of events leading to gluconeogenesis. Some of these crucial loci are (a) hepatic uptake of amino acids, (b) activation of pyruvate carboxylase in generating pyruvate from amino acid precursors, and (c) activation of phosphoenolpyruvate carboxykinase, the unidirectional rate-limiting enzyme in the initiation of the cascade of glucogenesis from pyruvate. Glucocorticoids, paradoxically, stimulate glycogen deposition and in this respect resemble the action of insulin. In fact, some evidence suggests that the glycogen-synthesizing effect of glucocorticoids may be mediated by insulin rather than by the direct effect of glucocorticoids.

At the level of adipose tissue and muscle, the main effect of glucocorticoids involves an antagonism of insulin-induced glucose uptake via complex interaction with insulin receptors leading to diminished receptor affinity as well as post-receptor defects.[244a,244b] In addition, glucocorticoids appear to exert a "permissive effect" on lipolysis by promoting the activation of cyclic AMP-dependent hormone-sensitive lipase in the adipose tissue of several species. However, the net clinical effect of glucocorticoid excess in man is generally not fat mobilization but a relocation of fat depots, resulting in typical truncal obesity. The clinical effects of hypercortisolism clearly depend upon the consequent secondary hyperinsulinism while the unique pattern of fat redistribution remains unexplained. Relatively little is known about the actions of glucocorticoids on protein metabolism. Several in vitro studies have shown an augmentation of proteolysis in skeletal muscle with perhaps a decreased incorporation of amino acids in muscle protein synthesis.

In the normal person, increments of plasma cortisol within the physiologic range result acutely in a mild increase of glucose levels secondary to a diminished glucose clearance rate, as well as in a significant increase in blood ketone and branched-chain amino acid levels.[245] These changes are accompanied by no significant alterations in serum insulin, or glucagon levels, or in insulin receptors. However, the effects of chronic administration of glucocorticoids in normal subjects with intact islet reserve generally are fully compensated by increased insulin release so that the net effects observed may be minimal or absent. The spectrum of diverse clinical manifestations of glucocorticoid excess in a patient with Cushing's syndrome is largely dependent upon the endogenous B-cell reserve. However, an increased sensitivity to physiologic hypercortisolemia has been shown in juvenile diabetes despite normalization of blood glucose levels.[246]

An indirect diabetogenic effect of pharmacologic administration of glucocorticoids involves a stimulation of glucagon secretion.[247,248] Glucocorticoid treatment was shown to induce an augmented A-cell responsiveness both in the basal state and following protein ingestion or amino acid infusion in these studies. This effect may be mediated indirectly via hyperaminoacidemia brought about by augmented proteolysis, and perhaps by other factors such as decreased islet glucose utilization. Finally, other studies[249] indicate an increase in hepatic glucagon receptors induced by dexamethasone, thus promoting its diabetogenic effects by an enhanced sensitivity to glucagon.

CATECHOLAMINES

The availability of assays for the separate determinations of epinephrine (E) and norepinephrine (NE) has rekindled interest in the interrelationship between catecholamines, insulin secretion and metabolic actions of these hormones in normal subjects and in diabetics. Christensen[250] has reviewed evidence for elevated catecholamine concentrations in uncontrolled diabetes, particularly of NE.

The activity of the sympathetic nervous system depends upon several factors in an individual including stress, exercise, hypoglycemia, autonomic neuropathy and drugs affecting the sympathetic system.[251,251a] Landsberg and co-workers[251] have documented that the regulation of epinephrine secretion from the adrenal medulla is governed by mechanisms other than those for norepinephrine release from the sympathetic nerve endings. For example, fasting inhibits and carbohydrate feeding stimulates NE turnover without significantly affecting E secretion. Based on this and other evidence, they have proposed that during fasting, suppression of sympathetic activity diminishes metabolic activity and calorie expenditure, whereas during overfeeding, the converse occurs. Furthermore, it was shown that hypoglycemia results in catecholamine (predominantly epinephrine) surge from the adrenal medulla, with an inhibition of NE release from sympathetic nerve endings, again suggesting a dichotomous control over these two components of the sympathetic system.[252] Employing glucose clamp techniques, Rowe et al.[253] have shown a stimulation of sympathetic activity in man by insulin, as reflected by NE levels, which was independent of changes in blood glucose levels. These studies underscore the differences in the relative importance of E and NE in exerting metabolic and cardiovascular effects.

Actions of Catecholamines

Catecholamines, acting via adrenergic receptors, produce their effects on several loci in metabolic pathways.[254] The classical effect of epinephrine in enhancing hepatic glucose production via glycogenolysis results from at least two different mechanisms: (a) a β-adrenergic effect via cyclic AMP, and perhaps more importantly, (b) an α-adrenergic, Ca^{++}-dependent but cyclic AMP-independent mechanism.[254a] Recent evidence, however, suggests an important beta-adrenergic mechanism in the diabetic.[255] Muscle glycogenolysis, on the other hand, is provoked only by β-adrenergic stimulation. This may explain the occurrence of clinical hypoglycemia in some patients with β-adrenergic blockade, when hepatic glycogen reserves have been depleted. In vitro studies of Garber et al. have revealed a significant inhibition of the release of gluconeogenic amino acids (alanine and glutamine) in response to β-adrenergic agonists.[255a] Similar hypoaminoacidemia in response to epinephrine infusion was observed in normal and Type I diabetic subjects, although the effects on individual amino acids were different in that they were most pronounced in the branched-chain amino acids.[255b] Therefore, the physiologic relevance of the effects of catecholamines on muscle protein balance requires further elaboration. Finally, stimulation of lipolysis by catecholamines appears also to be a predominantly β-adrenergic effect.

A number of experiments have been performed to study the possible adrenergic regulation of islet hormone secretion. Robertson et al.[256,257] have provided evidence suggesting an inhibition of basal insulin secretion by α-adrenergic stimulation or by β-adrenergic blockade. In addition, they have postulated that excessive endogenous alpha adrenergic activity may contribute to the defective glucose-stimulated insulin secretion in maturity-onset type diabetics. However, the role of catecholamines in the physiologic regulation of insulin secretion and in the pathogenesis of diabetes remains controversial.[254] Regarding the pancreatic A-cell, both α and β adrenergic stimulation have been shown to augment glucagon secretion,[23,258] although the relative importance of α and β sympathetic vs the parasympathetic tone in maintaining basal glucagon release, remains uncertain.

Many of the biologic actions of catecholamines alluded to above occur with pharmacologic amounts of these agents. Studies in normal subjects with physiologic infusions of epinephrine have indicated only a transient stimulation of hepatic glucose output and a sustained inhibition of peripheral glucose uptake.[259,260] The latter effect is mediated via β-adrenergic stimulation in muscle.[251a,261] Norepinephrine was found to be devoid of a significant hyperglycemic effect and the effects of epinephrine were not mediated via glucagon hypersecretion. The effects of epinephrine in this regard may be of additional significance in diabetic patients since in these subjects, an exaggerated responsiveness of liver to epinephrine, similar to that for cortisol, has been demonstrated even after prior normalization of blood glucose control with insulin.[246] Moreover, an exaggerated epinephrine release in the diabetic may occur under special circumstances (e.g., during exercise), as compared to non-diabetic individuals.[262]

Although the role of catecholamines in the regulation of islet hormone secretion remains unproven, patients with pheochromocytoma with combined excess of E and NE frequently reveal a marked suppression of glucagon secretion as well as inappropriately low insulin levels in the presence of hyperglycemia, although the basal concentrations of both insulin and glucagon were normal in a series of seven patients.[263]

ROLE OF COUNTER-REGULATORY HORMONES IN GLUCOSE HOMEOSTASIS

In the normal human, blood glucose homeostasis is finely regulated by the presence of a negative feedback loop between the liver and beta cells.[264] In addition, a major factor controlling the hepatic glucose efflux in health is the ambient blood glucose concentration itself.[265] Because of these regulatory mechanisms, factors potentially capable of disrupting glucose homeostasis via counter-regulatory hormones such as glucagon, catecholamines, growth-hormone and cortisol during certain situations in life, (e.g., starvation, hypoglycemia, "stress," trauma, acute illness, and exercise,) are offset primarily by appropriate readjustment of insulin secretion.[42,266] However, in the diabetic individual with relatively fixed insulin availability, one or more of these counter-regulatory hormones assume a much more significant role in altering the metabolic milieu in the above situations (Table 9–6). The relative roles of these and other factors remain subjects of intensive investigation in two clinical settings: (a) the recovery from hypoglycemia and (b) the pathogenesis of acute worsening of diabetes control and consequent diabetic ketoacidosis.

Recovery from Hypoglycemia

In normal individuals, insulin-induced hypoglycemia does not result in a significant release of counter-regulatory hormones until a critically low blood glucose concentration is reached, suggesting a direct effect of hypoglycemia in stimulating he-

patic glucose output.[267] However, in later stages, a concerted increase in the secretion of all of the counter-regulatory hormones including epinephrine, glucagon, cortisol and growth-hormone may play a role in supporting glucose production by liver.[267] Rizza et al. employed somatostatin to induce a combined deficiency of growth-hormone and glucagon, and further induced a combined α- and β-adrenergic blockade during insulin-induced hypoglycemia in normal subjects.[268] Their results indicate a more important role for glucagon in maintaining normal glucose homeostasis, and for the adrenergic mechanisms, if glucagon deficiency is present. In contrast, in diabetic subjects, the response of pancreatic A cells to hypoglycemia is known to be markedly impaired or absent,[70,71] so that epinephrine, cortisol, and growth hormone are of greater significance. Moreover, a rapid decline of glycemia within the physiologic range may be sufficient to elicit a significant release of counter-regulatory hormones in the diabetic,[269] and the tissue responsiveness to these hormones may be exaggerated.[246] The latter has been postulated as a possible explanation for "rebound hyperglycemia" or Somogyi effect, although this concept has not been supported by others, who claim free insulin levels as a more critical determinant of this phenomenon.[270]

Finally, it should be remembered that patients with diabetic autonomic neuropathy may be particularly vulnerable to frequent, disabling consequences of hypoglycemia when both glucagon and epinephrine release are blunted. This again points to the crucial role of these two hormones in recovery from hypoglycemia.[270a]

The Genesis of Ketoacidosis

High plasma concentrations of one or more of the counter-regulatory hormones have been reported in patients in diabetic ketoacidosis. However, the significance and relative roles of these hormones in the pathogenesis of ketoacidosis remain controversial.[271–273] Barnes et al.[274] have reported evidence for the contribution of growth hormone and cortisol in the evolution of this process although previous studies showed neither of these to be important.[273] An important role of cortisol in mediating the insulin resistance associated with ketoacidosis has, however, been suggested by Ginsberg.[275] Schade and Eaton have championed the view that an elevated level of at least one of the four counter-regulatory hormones is essential in the pathogenesis of ketoacidosis in addition to the presence of a relative insulin deficiency,[272,276] and that the latter alone is not sufficient. Their studies reveal a temporal relationship between the rise in plasma levels of each of these hormones and the devel-

Table 9–6.   The Major Sites of Actions of Counter-Regulatory Hormones

	Liver		Muscle		Adipose Tissue	
	Glycogen[a]	Gluconeogenesis	Glucose uptake	Amino Acid release	Glucose uptake	Lipolysis
Growth Hormone	+	+	–	?	–	+
Glucocorticoids	+	+	–	+	–	+[b]
Epinephrine	–	+	–	–[c]	?	+
Glucagon	–	+	0	?	0	?

[a]Net effect on glycogen content via glycogen synthesis or glycogenolysis.
[b]A permissive role (see text for details).
[c]A β-adrenergic effect, common to several β-adrenergic agonists.
+ = Stimulation or increase; – = inhibition or decrease; 0 = no effect; ? = uncertain

opment of ketoacidosis. However, since insulin deficiency was prevented in these studies by a continuous insulin infusion, the data presented do not rule out a primary role for insulin deficiency in the pathogenesis of diabetic ketoacidosis.

PROLACTIN

Prolactin, a poorly understood pituitary hormone, has become a focus of increasing interest within the last decade since the availability of sensitive immunoassays for its determination. Hyperprolactinemic states have been found to be associated with disorders of the reproductive system in both sexes. However, the precise physiologic role of prolactin in the human remains elusive.[277]

Among the various physiologic factors known to augment prolactin secretion, insulin-induced hypoglycemia has been shown to result in a significant release of prolactin in normal subjects, similar to the responses of thyrotropin-releasing hormone (TRH) or chlorpromazine. In fact, hypoglycemia has been suggested as a provocative test for prolactin release.[278] In addition to a number of neuropharmacologic factors affecting prolactin secretion, certain dietary factors may, either directly or indirectly, modify the prolactin response. In this regard, it is of interest that prolactin release following insulin-induced hypoglycemia, is impaired in the presence of massive obesity.[279]

A role of prolactin in the pathogenesis of human diabetogenic syndrome has been suggested by the studies of Landgraf et al.[280] These investigators studied the blood glucose and insulin levels during oral glucose tolerance tests in 26 patients with prolactin-secreting pituitary tumors. The basal glucose and insulin levels were similar to those of control subjects despite chronic, endogenous hyperprolactinemia. However, the glucose tolerance was significantly impaired and was accompanied by a relative peripheral insulin insensitivity as reflected by the associated hyperinsulinemia. On the other hand, the 24-hour plasma prolactin pattern in a group of relatively stable, insulin-dependent (juvenile) diabetics was found to be identical to that in normal controls,[281] suggesting a normal regulation of secretion in such diabetics. In contrast, elevated plasma concentrations of prolactin have been reported in diabetics in ketoacidosis[282] but this finding could not be confirmed by others,[283] even after stimulation with TRH. Further studies are clearly required in the delineation of aberrations, if any, of prolactin secretion in both IDDM and NIDDM.

The relationship of prolactin with the control of diabetes and with the complications of diabetes also requires further work, since the data available thus far are controversial. For instance, in patients with diabetic retinopathy, prolactin levels have been reported to be impaired in one study[284] but normal in another.[285] The significance of such observations, therefore, remains dubious.

PROSTAGLANDINS

During the past several years, considerable interest has been generated in prostaglandin metabolism and its relationship with islet physiology, particularly in regard to its significance in the pathogenesis of NIDDM.[286] It has been known for many years that large doses of salicylates, a well-recognized inhibitor of prostaglandin E (PGE), may result in a significant improvement of hyperglycemia. Field et al. reported an augmentation of glucose-induced insulin secretion in healthy persons and in mild diabetics by sodium salicylate administration.[287]

Studies by Robertson and co-workers[286,288] have further characterized the role of prostaglandins in the defective recognition of glucose by the B-cell in diabetes. Their results show an inhibition of the acute insulin secretory response to glucose in normal and in diabetic subjects by PGE infusion, and an augmented response by infusion of the prostaglandin-inhibitor, sodium salicylate. Similar observations have been made by others in normal subjects and in diabetics.[289,290] Employing pancreatic monolayer cultures, Braaten et al.[291] showed a direct effect of salicylates and indomethacin in augmenting insulin secretion. Metz et al. have sown that the salicylate-induced beta-cytotropic effect is accompanied by an inhibition of PGE release from the islet cells.[292] Furthermore, it has been shown that PGE inhibition also improves the glucose potentiation of the arginine-induced acute insulin release in diabetics but not in normals.[293]

Discrepant results have, however, been observed by other investigators. Some studies have shown a stimulation, rather than an inhibition, by PGE of the insulin release in vitro.[294] In support of this, indomethacin was found to blunt the insulin secretion in the basal state as well as following glucose or glucagon infusion in normal subjects.[295] Furthermore, neither exogenous PGE_2, nor several PGE inhibitors including aspirin, ibuprofen and sulfinpyrazone resulted in any significant changes in basal or glucose-stimulated insulin release or in glucose tolerance in other studies.[296] Robertson has attempted to reconcile these discrepancies by alluding to several methodologic differences in various studies, and by pointing to other effects of certain agents such as indomethacin.[297]

The effects of prostaglandins on A-cell secretion are not well investigated. The available evidence remains inconclusive, some studies showing a stimulation and others, an inhibition or no effect.[286,294,296]

The purported role of endogenous prostaglandins in mediating defective glucose recognition by islet cells in human diabetes clearly requires additional work in light of the controversial results obtained by different investigators.

Certain prostaglandin derivatives may have additional metabolic effects at a peripheral level. An important interaction with insulin appears to exist in adipose tissue. Considerable evidence indicates that PGE_2 and PGI_2 are produced by adipocytes, and modulate the lipolytic activity in response to the sympathetic nervous system on the one hand and insulin on the other.[298] PGE_2 may be a physiologically important inhibitor of lipolysis.[298] It has been proposed that elevated circulating concentrations of PGE_2 and PGI_2 in diabetic ketoacidosis[299] might mediate some of the symptoms of this disorder in man.[300]

The postulated role of prostaglandins in the pathogenesis of macrovascular complications of diabetes via their effects on platelet-vessel wall interaction is reviewed in Chapter 11.

REFERENCES

1. Murlin, J.R., Clough, H.D., Gibbs, C.B.F., Stokes, A.M.: Aqueous extracts of pancreas. I. Influence on the carbohydrate metabolism of depancreatized animals. J. Biol. Chem. 56:253, 1923.
2. Collip, J.B.: Delayed manifestation of the physiological effects of insulin following administration of certain pancreatic extracts. Am. J. Physiol. 63:391, 1923.
3. Unger, R.H., Eisentraut, A.M., McCall, M.S., Madison, L.L.: Measurement of endogenous glucagon in plasma and the influence of blood glucose concentration upon its secretion. J. Clin. Invest. 41:682, 1962.
4. Unger, R.H., Aguilar-Parada, E., Müller, W.A., Eisentraut, A.M.: Studies of pancreatic alpha cell function in normal and diabetic subjects. J. Clin. Invest. 49:837, 1970.
5. Unger, R.H.: Diabetes and the alpha cell. The Banting Memorial Lecture 1975. Diabetes 25:136, 1976.
6. Jaspan, J., Rubenstein, A.H.: Circulating glucagon. Plasma profiles and metabolism in health and disease. Diabetes 26:887, 1977.
7. Conlon, J.M.: The glucagon-like polypeptides—order out of chaos? Diabetologia 18:85, 1980.
8. Lawrence, A.M., Tan, S., Hojvat, S., Kirsteins, L.: Salivary gland hyperglycemic factor: an extrapancreatic source of glucagon-like material. Science 195:70, 1976.
9. Valverde, I., Villanueva, M.L., Lozano, I., Marco, J.: Presence of glucagon immunoreactivity in the globin fraction of human plasma ("big plasma glucagon"). J. Clin. Endocrinol. Metab. 39:1090, 1974.
10. Valverde, I., Lemon, H.M., Kessinger, A., Unger, R.H.: Distribution of plasma glucagon immunoreactivity in a patient with suspected glucagonoma. J. Clin. Endocrinol. Metab. 42:804, 1976.
11. Weir, G.C., Horton, E., Aoki, T.T., et al.: Secretion by glucagonomas of a possible glucagon precursor. J. Clin. Invest. 59:325, 1977.
12. Palmer, J.P., Werner, P.L., Benson, J.W., Ensinck, J.W.: Dominant inheritance of large molecular weight immunoreactive glucagon (IRG). J. Clin. Invest. 61:763, 1978.
13. Boden, G., Owen, O.E.: Familial hyperglucagonemia—an autosomal dominant disorder. N. Engl. J. Med. 296:534, 1977.
14. Weir, G.C., Knowlton, S.D., Martin, D.B.: High molecular weight glucagon-like immunoreactivity in plasma. J. Clin. Endocrinol. Metab. 40:296, 1975.
15. Unger, R.H.: Glucagon and the A cell. Physiology and pathophysiology. N. Engl. J. Med. 304:1518, 1575, 1981.
16. Unger, R.H.: Alpha- and beta-cell interrelationships in health and disease. Metabolism 23:581, 1974.
17. Gerich, J.E., Charles, M.A., Grodsky, G.M.: Regulation of pancreatic insulin and glucagon secretion. Ann. Rev. Physiol. 38:353, 1976.
17a. Orci, L.: The microanatomy of the islets of Langerhans. Metabolism 25(Suppl. 1):1303, 1976.
18. Müller, W.A., Faloona, G.R., Unger, R.H.: The influence of the antecedent diet upon glucagon and insulin secretion. N. Engl. J. Med. 285:1450, 1971.
19. Müller, W.A., Faloona, G.R., Unger, R.H.: The effect of alanine on glucagon secretion. J. Clin. Invest. 50:2215, 1971.
20. Rossini, A.A., Aoki, T.T., Ganda, O.P., et al.: Alanine-induced amino acid interrelationships. Metabolism 24:1185, 1975.
21. Böttger, I., Dobbs, R., Faloona, G.R., Unger, R.H.: The effects of triglyceride absorption upon glucagon, insulin, and gut glucagon-like immunoreactivity. J. Clin. Invest. 52:2532, 1973.
22. Gerich, J.E., Langlois, M., Schneider, V., et al.: Effects

of alterations of plasma free fatty acid levels on pancreatic glucagon secretion in man. J. Clin. Invest. 53:1284, 1974.

23. Gerich, J.E., Langlois, M., Noacco, C., et al.: Adrenergic modulation of pancreatic glucagon secretion in man. J. Clin. Invest. 53:1441, 1974.

24. Samols, E., Stagner, J., Weir, G.: Presynaptic dopaminergic modulation of pancreatic insular secretions. Diabetes 28:371, 1979.

25. Rayfield, E.J., George, D.T., Eichner, H.L., Hsu, T.H.: L-Dopa stimulation of glucagon secretion in man. N. Engl. J. Med. 293:589, 1975.

26. Koerker, D.J., Ruch, W., Chideckel, E., et al.: Somatostatin:hypothalamic inhibitor of the endocrine pancreas. Science 184:482, 1974.

27. Mortimer, C.H., Tunbridge, W.M.G., Carr, D., et al.: Effects of growth-hormone release-inhibiting hormone on circulating glucagon, insulin, and growth hormone in normal, diabetic, acromegalic, and hypopituitary patients. Lancet 1:697, 1974.

28. Unger, R.H., Orci, L.: Possible roles of the pancreatic D-cell in the normal and diabetic states. Diabetes 26:241, 1977.

29. Böttger, I., Schlein, E.M., Faloona, G.R., et al.: The effect of exercise on glucagon secretion. J. Clin. Endocrinol. Metab. 35:117, 1972.

30. Wahren, J., Felig, P., Hagenfeldt, L.: Physical exercise and fuel homeostasis in diabetes mellitus. Diabetologia 14:213, 1978.

31. Mackrell, D.J., Sokal, J.E.: Antagonism between the effects of insulin and glucagon on the isolated liver. Diabetes 18:724, 1969.

32. Parrilla, R., Goodman, M.N., Toews, C.J.: Effect of glucagon:insulin ratios on hepatic metabolism. Diabetes 23:725, 1974.

33. Liljenquist, J.E., Bomboy, J.D., Lewis, S.B., et al.: Effect of glucagon on net splanchnic cyclic AMP production in normal and diabetic men. J. Clin. Invest. 53:198, 1974.

34. Hendy, G.N., Tomlinson, S., O'Riordan, J.L.H.: Impaired responsiveness to the effect of glucagon on plasma adenosine 3':5'-cyclic monophosphate in normal man. Europ. J. Clin. Invest. 7:155, 1977.

35. Exton, J.H.: Gluconeogenesis. Metabolism 21:945, 1972.

36. Pilkis, S.J., Park, C.R., Claus, T.H.: Hormonal control of hepatic gluconeogenesis. Vitamins and Hormones 36:383, 1978.

36a. Hers, H-G., Van Schaftingen, E.: Fructose 2-biphosphate 2 years after its discovery. Biochem. J. 206:1, 1982.

37. Cherrington, A.D., Chiasson, J-L., Liljenquist, J.E., et al.: The role of insulin and glucagon in the regulation of basal glucose production in the postabsorptive dog. J. Clin. Invest. 58:1407, 1976.

38. Liljenquist, J.E., Mueller, G.L., Cherrington, A.D., et al.: Evidence for an important role of glucagon in the regulation of hepatic glucose production in normal man. J. Clin. Invest. 59:369, 1977

39. Sherwin, R.S., Fisher, M., Hendler, R., Felig, P.: Hyperglucagonemia and blood glucose regulation in normal, obese and diabetic subjects. N. Engl. J. Med. 294:455, 1976.

40. Felig, P., Wahren, J., Hendler, R.: Influence of physiologic hyperglucagonemia on basal and insulin-inhibited splanchnic glucose output in normal man. J. Clin. Invest. 58:761, 1976.

41. Tasaka, Y., Sekine, M., Wakatsuki, M., et al.: Levels of pancreatic glucagon, insulin and glucose during twenty-

four hours of the day in normal subjects. Horm. Metab. Res. 7:205, 1975.

42. Cahill, G.F., Jr.: Physiology of insulin in man. Diabetes 20:785, 1971.

43. Pozefsky, T., Tancredi, R.G., Moxley, R.T., et al.: Metabolism of forearm tissues in man. Studies with glucagon. Diabetes 25:128, 1976.

44. Marliss, E.B., Aoki, T.T., Unger, R.H., et al.: Glucagon levels and metabolic effects in fasting man. J. Clin. Invest. 49:2256, 1970.

45. Aoki, T.T., Müller, W.A., Brennan, M.F., Cahill, G.F., Jr.: Effect of glucagon on amino acid and nitrogen metabolism in fasting man. Metabolism 23:805, 1974.

46. Boden, G., Master, R.W., Rezvani, I., et al.: Glucagon deficiency and hyperaminoacidemia after total pancreatectomy. J. Clin. Invest. 65:706, 1980.

47. Heimberg, M., Weinstein, I., Kohout, M.: The effects of glucagon, dibutyryl cyclic adenosine 3',5'-monophosphate, and the concentration of free fatty acid on hepatic lipid metabolism. J. Biol. Chem. 244:5131, 1969.

48. Björntorp, P., Karlsson, M., Hoyden, A.: Quantitative aspects of lipolysis and reesterification in human adipose tissue in vitro. Acta. Med. Scand. 185:89, 1969.

49. Liljenquist, J.E., Bomboy, J.D., Lewis, S.B., et al.: Effects of glucagon on lipolysis and ketogenesis in normal and diabetic man. J. Clin. Invest. 53:190, 1974.

50. Schade, D.S., Eaton, R.P.: Modulation of fatty acid metabolism by glucagon in man. I. Effects in normal subjects. Diabetes 24:502, 1975.

51. Gerich, J.E., Lorenzi, M., Bier, D.M., et al.: Effects of physiologic levels of glucagon and growth hormone on human carbohydrate and lipid metabolism. Studies involving administration of exogenous hormone during suppression of endogenous hormone secretion with somatostatin. J. Clin. Invest. 57:875, 1976.

52. Amatuzio, D.S., Grande, F., Wada, S.: Effect of glucagon on the serum lipids in essential hyperlipemia and in hypercholesterolemia. Metabolism 11:1240, 1962.

53. Ganda, O.P., Smith, T.N., Gleason, R.E.: Delineation of metabolic aberration in non-diabetic offspring of conjugal diabetic parents (ODP): differential responsiveness to IV glucose (G), glucagon (Gn), and tolbutamide (T). Diabetes 24(Suppl. 2):433, 1975. (Abstract)

54. Samols, E., Marri, G., Marks, V.: Promotion of insulin secretion by glucagon. Lancet 2:415, 1965.

55. Simpson, R.G., Benedetti, A., Grodsky, G.M., et al.: Early phase of insulin release. Diabetes 17:684, 1968.

55a. Ganda, O.P., Srikanta, S., Brink, S.J., et al.: Differential sensitivity to B-cell secretagogues in "early" type I diabetes mellitus. Diabetes 33:516, 1984.

56. Ryan, W.G., Nibbe, A.F., Schwartz, T.B.: Beta-cytotrophic effects of glucose, glucagon, and tolbutamide in man. Lancet 1:1255, 1967.

57. Oakley, N.W., Harrigan, P., Kissebah, A.H., et al.: Factors affecting insulin response to glucagon in man. Metabolism 21:1001, 1972.

58. Josefsberg, Z., Flatau, E., Doron, M., Laron, Z.: The influence of oral glucose loading on the insulin response to I.V. glucagon in children and adolescents. Metabolism 25:277, 1976.

59. Faber, O.K., Binder, C.: C-peptide response to glucagon: a test for the residual B-cell function in diabetes mellitus. Diabetes 26:605, 1977.

60. Samols, E., Tyler, J.M., Marks, V.: Glucagon-insulin interrelationships. In: P-J. LeFebvre, R.H. Unger (Eds.): Glucagon: Molecular Physiology, Clinical and Therapeu-

tic Implications. Oxford, England. Pergamon Press, 1972, pp. 151–173.

61. Boulter, P.R., Spark, R.F., Arky, R.A.: Dissociation of the renin-aldosterone system and refractoriness to the sodium-retaining action of mineralocorticoid during starvation in man. J. Clin. Endocrinol. Metab. 38:248, 1974.

62. Spark, R.F., Arky, R.A., Boulter, P.R., et al.: Renin, aldosterone and glucagon in the natriuresis of fasting. N. Engl. J. Med. 292:1335, 1975.

63. DeFronzo, R.A., Sherwin, R.S., Dillingham, M., et al.: Influence of basal insulin and glucagon secretion on potassium and sodium metabolism. Studies with somatostatin in normal dogs and in normal and diabetic human beings. J. Clin. Invest. 61:472, 1978.

64. Buchanan, K.D., McCarroll, A.M.: Abnormalities of glucagon metabolism in untreated diabetes mellitus. Lancet 2:1394, 1972.

65. Wise, J.K., Hendler, R., Felig, P.: Evaluation of alpha-cell function by infusion of alanine in normal, diabetic and obese subjects. N. Engl. J. Med. 288:487, 1973.

66. Gerich, J.E., Lorenzi, M., Karam, J.H., et al.: Abnormal pancreatic glucagon secretion and postprandial hyperglycemia in diabetes mellitus: JAMA 234:159, 1975.

67. Reynolds, C., Molnar, G.D., Horwitz, D.L., et al.: Abnormalities of endogenous glucagon and insulin in unstable diabetes. Diabetes 26:36, 1977.

68. Müller, W.A., Faloona, G.R., Unger, R.H.: Hyperglucagonemia in diabetic ketoacidosis. Am. J. Med. 54:52, 1973.

69. Raskin, P., Aydin, I., Yamamoto T., Unger, R.H.: Abnormal alpha-cell function in human diabetes: the response to oral protein. Am. J. Med. 64:988, 1978.

70. Gerich, J.E., Langlois, M., Noacco, C., et al.: Lack of glucagon response to hypoglycemia in diabetes: evidence for an intrinsic pancreatic alpha cell defect. Science 182:171, 1973.

70a.Bergenstal, R.M., Polonsky, K.S., Pons, G., et al.: Lack of glucagon response to hypoglycemia in Type I diabetics after long-term optimal therapy with a continuous subcutaneous insulin infusion pump. Diabetes 32:575, 1983.

71. Benson, J.W., Jr., Johnson, D.G., Palmer, J.P., et al.: Glucagon and catecholamine secretion during hypoglycemia in normal and diabetic man. J. Clin. Endocrinol. Metab. 44:459, 1977.

72. Gerich, J.E., Langlois, M., Noacco, C., et al.: Comparison of the suppressive effects of elevated plasma glucose and free fatty acid levels on glucagon secretion in normal and insulin-dependent diabetic subjects. Evidence for selective alpha-cell insensitivity to glucose in diabetes mellitus. J. Clin. Invest. 58:320, 1976.

72a.Unger, R.H.: Insulin-glucagon relationships in the defense against hypoglycemia. The Berson Memorial Lecture. Diabetes 32:575, 1983.

73. LeFebvre, P-J., Luyckx, A.S.: Glucagon and diabetes: a reappraisal. Diabetologia a16:347, 1979.

74. Braaten, J.T., Faloona, G.R., Unger, R.H.: The effect of insulin on the alpha-cell response to hyperglycemia in long-standing alloxan diabetes. J. Clin. Invest. 53:1017, 1974.

75. Yamamoto, T., Raskin, P., Aydin, I., Unger, R.: Effects of insulin on the response of immunoreactive glucagon to an intravenous glucose load in human diabetes. Metabolism 28:568, 1979.

76. Raskin, P., Pietri, A., Unger, R.H.: Changes in glucagon levels after four to five weeks of glucoregulation by portable insulin infusion pumps. Diabetes 28:1033, 1979.

77. Ganda, O.P., Srikanta, S., Gleason, R.E., et al.: Lack of A-cell hyperresponsiveness in early phase of Type I diabetes. Int. Cong. Endocrinol. Quebec, 1984, p. 613.

78. Unger, R.H., Orci, L.: The essential role of glucagon in the pathogenesis of diabetes mellitus. Lancet 1:14, 1975.

79. Gerich, J.E., Lorenzi, M., Bier, D., et al.: Prevention of human diabetic ketoacidosis by somatostatin. Evidence for an essential role of glucagon. N. Engl. J. Med. 292:985, 1975.

80. Dobbs, R., Sakurai, H., Sasaki, H., et al.: Glucagon: role in the hyperglycemia of diabetes mellitus. Science 187:544, 1975.

81. Müller, W.A., Brennan, M.F., Tan, M.H., Aoki, T.T.: Studies of glucagon secretion in pancreatectomized patients. Diabetes 23:512, 1974.

81a.Tiengo, A., Bessioud, M., Valverde, I., et al.: Absence of islet alpha cell function in pancreatectomized patients. Diabetologia 22:25, 1982.

82. Barnes, A.J., Bloom, S.R., Alberti, K.G.M.M., et al.: Ketoacidosis in pancreatomized man. N. Engl. J. Med. 296:1250, 1977.

82a.Boden, G.: Extrapancreatic glucagon in human subjects. In: R.H. Unger, L. Orci (Eds.): Glucagon, Physiology, Pathophysiology, and Morphology of the Pancreatic A-cells. New York, Elsevier, 1981, p. 349.

82b.Holst, J.J., Pedersen, J.H., Baldiserra, F., Stadil, F.L.: Circulating glucagon after total pancreatectomy in man. Diabetologia 25:396, 1983.

83. Werner, P.L., Palmer, J.P.: Immunoreactive glucagon responses to oral glucose, insulin infusion and deprivation, and somatostatin in pancreatectomized man. Diabetes 27:1005, 1978.

84. Persson, I., Gyntelberg, F., Heding, L.G., Boss-Nielsen, J.: Pancreatic-glucagon-like immunoreactivity after intravenous insulin in normals and chronic-pancreatitis patients. Acta. Endocrinol. 67:401, 1971.

85. Vinik, A.I., Kalk, W.J., Jackson, W.P.U.: A unifying hypothesis for hereditary and acquired diabetes. Lancet 1:485, 1974.

86. Donowitz, M., Hendler, R., Spiro, H.M., et al.: Glucagon secretion in acute and chronic pancreatitis. Ann. Intern. Med. 83:778, 1975.

87. Kalk, W.J., Vinik, A.I., Paul, M., et al.: Immunoreactive glucagon responses to intravenous tolbutamide in chronic pancreatitis. Diabetes 24:851, 1975.

88. Lassman, M.N., Genel, M., Wise, J.K., et al.: Carbohydrate homeostasis and pancreatic islet cell function in thalassemia. Ann. Intern. Med. 80:65, 1974.

89. Ganda, O.P., Soeldner, J.S., Goldstein, H.H., et al.: Lack of alpha-cell hyperresponsiveness in diabetes secondary to hemachromatosis. Clin. Res. 25:391A, 1977.

90. Passa, P., Luyckx, A.S., Carpentier, J.L., et al.: Glucagon secretion in diabetic patients with idiopathic haemochromatosis. Diabetologia 13:509, 1977.

91. Müller, W.A., Berger, M., Cüppers, H.J., et al.: Plasma glucagon in diabetes of haemachromatosis: too low or too high? Gut 20:200, 1979.

92. Nelson, R.L., Baldus, W.P., Rubenstein, A.H., et al.: Pancreatic alpha-cell function in diabetic hemochromatotic subjects. J. Clin. Endocrinol. Metab. 49:412, 1979.

93. Olefsky, J.M., Sperling, M.A., Reaven, G.M.: Does glucagon play a role in the insulin resistance of patients with adult non-ketotic diabetes? Diabetologia 13:327, 1977.

94. Ganda, O.P., Weir, G.C., Soeldner, J.S., et al.: "Somatostatinoma": A somatostatin-containing tumor of the endocrine pancreas. N. Engl. J. Med. 296:963, 1977.

95. Felig, P., Wahren, J., Sherwin, R., Hendler, R.: Insulin, glucagon, and somatostatin in normal physiology and diabetes mellitus. Diabetes 25:1091, 1976.

96. Waldhäusl, W., Bratusch-Marrain, P., Dudczak, R., et al.: The diabetogenic action of somatostatin in healthy subjects and in maturity-onset diabetics. J. Clin. Endocrinol. Metab. 44:876, 1977.

97. Tamborlane, W.V., Sherwin, R.S., Hendler, R., Felig, P.: Metabolic effects of somatostatin in maturity-onset diabetes. N. Engl. J. Med. 297:181, 1977.

98. Christensen, S.E., Hansen, Aa. P., Lundbaek, K.: Somatostatin in maturity-onset diabetes. Diabetes 27:1013, 1978.

99. Raskin, P., Unger, R.H.: Hyperglucagonemia and its suppression. Importance in the metabolic control of diabetes. N. Engl. J. Med. 299:433, 1978.

100. Gerich, J.E., Lorenzi, M., Schneider, V., et al.: Effects of somatostatin on plasma glucose and glucagon levels in human diabetes mellitus. Pathophysiologic and therapeutic implications. N. Engl. J. Med. 291:544, 1974.

101. Schade, D.S., Eaton, R.P.: Glucagon regulation of plasma ketone body concentration in human diabetes. J. Clin. Invest. 56:1340, 1975.

102. Christensen, S.E., Hansen, Aa.P., Weeke, J., Lundbaek, K.: 24-hour studies of the effects of somatostatin on the levels of plasma growth hormone, glucagon, and glucose in normal subjects and juvenile diabetics. Diabetes 27:300, 1978.

103. Gerich, J.E.: Metabolic effects of long-term somatostatin infusion in man. Metabolism 25 (Suppl. 1):1505, 1976.

104. Sherwin, R.S., Felig, P.: (Letter to the Editor) Hyperglucagonemia in diabetes. N. Engl. J. Med. 299:1366, 1978.

105. Clarke, W.L., Santiago, J.V., Kipnis, D.M.: The effect of hyperglucagonemia on blood glucose concentrations and on insulin requirements in insulin-requiring diabetes mellitus. Diabetes 27:649, 1978.

106. Brazeau, P., Vale, W., Burgus, R., et al.: Hypothalamic polypeptide that inhibits the secretion of immunoreactive pituitary growth hormone. Science 179:77, 1973.

107. Guillemin, R., Gerich, J.E.: Somatostatin: physiological and clinical significance. Ann. Rev. Med. 27:379, 1976.

108. Alberti, K.G.M.M., Christensen, N-J., Christensen, S.E., et al.: Inhibition of insulin secretion by somatostatin. Lancet 2:1299, 1973.

109. Hall, R., Besser, G.M., Schally, A.V., et al.: Action of growth-hormone-release inhibitory hormone in healthy men and in acromegaly. Lancet 2:581, 1973.

110. Yen, S.S.C., Siler, T.M., DeVane, G.W.: Effect of somatostatin in patients with acromegaly: suppression of growth hormone, prolactin, insulin, and glucose levels. N. Engl. J. Med. 290:935, 1974.

111. Gerich, J.E., Lorenzi, M., Schneider, V., et al.: Inhibition of pancreatic glucagon responses to arginine by somatostatin in normal man and in insulin-dependent diabetics. Diabetes 23:876, 1974.

112. Luft, R., Efendic, S., Hökfelt, T., et al.: Immunohistochemical evidence for the localization of somatostatin-like immunoreactivity in a cell population of pancreatic islets. Med. Biol. 52:428, 1974.

113. Dubois, M.P.: Immunoreactive somatostatin is present in discrete cells of the endocrine pancreas. Proc. Natl. Acad. Sci. 72:1340, 1975.

114. Polak, J.M., Pearse, A.G.E., Grimelius, L., et al.: Growth-hormone release-inhibiting hormone in gastrointestinal and pancreatic D cells. Lancet 1:1220, 1975.

115. Arimura, A., Sato, H., Dupont, A., et al.: Somatostatin: abundance of immunoreactive hormone in rat stomach and pancreas. Science 189:1007, 1975.

116. Reichlin, S., Saperstein, R., Jackson, I.M.D., et al.: Hypothalamic hormones. Ann. Rev. Physiol. 38:389, 1976.

116a.Reichlin, S.: Somatostatin. N. Engl. J. Med. 309:1495, 1556, 1983.

117. Luft, R., Efendic, S., Hökfelt, T.: Somatostatin—both hormone and neurotransmitter? Diabetologia 14:1, 1978.

118. Wahren, J., Felig, P.: Influence of somatostatin on carbohydrate disposal and absorption in diabetes mellitus. Lancet 2:1213, 1976.

119. Schusdziarra, V., Zyznar, E., Rouiller, D., et al.: Splanchnic somatostatin: a hormonal regulator of nutrient homeostasis. Science 207:530, 1980.

120. Koerker, D.J., Harker, L.A., Goodner, C.J.: Effects of somatostatin on hemostasis in baboons. N. Engl. J. Med. 293:476, 1975.

121. Mielke, C.H., Jr., Gerich, J.E., Lorenzi, M., et al.: The effect of somatostatin on coagulation and platelet function in man. N. Engl. J. Med. 293:480, 1975.

122. Limberg, B., Kommerell, B.: Somatostatin after failure of cimetidine for acute bleeding ulcers. Lancet 2:1361, 1979.

123. Kayasseh, L., Gyr, K., Keller, U., et al.: Somatostatin and cimetidine in peptic-ulcer haemorrhage. A randomised controlled trial. Lancet 1:844, 1980.

124. Hirsch, H.J., Gabbay, K.H.: Radioimmunoassay of somatostatin-like immunoreactivity (SLI) in human plasma. Diabetes 27 (Suppl. 2):441, 1978.

125. Saito, H., Ogawa, T., Ishimaru, K., et al.: Plasma somatostatin in normal and diseased states. In: Program and abstracts of the Sixth International Congress of Endocrinology. Canberra, Union Offset, 1980, p. 247.

126. Kronheim, S., Berelowitz, M., Pimstone, B.L.: The characterization of somatostatin-like immunoreactivity in human serum. Diabetes 27:523, 1978.

127. Zyznar, E.S., Pietri, A.O., Harris, V., Unger, R.H.: Evidence for the hormonal status of somatostatin in man. Diabetes 30:883, 1981.

127a.Mackes, K., Itoh, M., Greene, K., Gerich, J.: Radioimmunoassay of human plasma somatostatin. Diabetes 30:728, 1981.

127b.Vinik, A.I., Shapiro, B., Glaser, B., Wagner, L.: Circulating somatostatin in primates. In: S.L. BLoom, J.M. Polak (Eds.): Gut Hormones. 2nd Ed. Edinburgh, Churchill, Livingstone, 1981, p. 371.

128. Ipp, E., Dobbs, R.E., Arimura, A., et al.: Release of immunoreactive somatostatin from the pancreas in response to glucose, amino acids, pancreozymin-cholecystokinin, and tolbutamide. J. Clin. Invest. 60:760, 1977.

129. Weir, G.C., Samols, E., Loo, S., et al.: Somatostatin and pancreatic polypeptide secretion. Effects of glucagon, insulin and arginine. Diabetes 28:35, 1979.

130. Rouiller, D., Schusdziarra, V., Unger, R.H.: Effect of insulin upon pancreatic and gastric release of somatostatin-like immunoreactivity. Diabetes 28:352, 1979.

131. Orci, L., Baetens, D., Rufener, C., et al.: Hypertrophy and hyperplasia of somatostatin-containing D cells in diabetes. Proc. Natl. Acad. Sci. 73:1338, 1976.

132. McEvoy, R., Hegre, O.D.: Morphometric quantitation of the pancreatic insulin-, glucagon-, and somatostatin-positive cell populations in normal and alloxan-diabetic rats Diabetes 26:1140, 1977.

133. Patel, Y.C., Cameron, D., Bankier, A., et al.: Changes in somatostatin concentration in pancreas and other tissues

of streptozotocin-diabetic rats. Endocrinology *103*:917, 1978.

134. Jones, C.W., Reynolds, W.A., Hoganson, G.E.: Streptozotocin diabetes in the monkey. Plasma levels of glucose, insulin, glucagon, and somatostatin, with corresponding morphometric analysis of rat endocrine cells. Diabetes 29:536, 1980.

135. Orci, L., Unger, R.H.: Functional subdivision of islets of Langerhans and possible role of D cells. Lancet 2:1243, 1975.

136. Larsson, L-I, Goltermann, N., de Magistris, L., et al.: Somatostatin cell processes as pathways for paracrine secretion. Science 205:1393, 1979.

137. Griffey, M.A., Conaway, H.H., Harshfield, D.L., Whitney, J.E.: Effect of somatostatin on insulin secretion induced by ionophore. Pro. Soc. Exp. Biol. Med. *154*:198, 1977.

138. Martin, J.B., Renaud, L.P., Brazeau, P., Jr.: Pulsatile-growth hormone secretion: suppression by hypothalamic ventromedial lesions and by long-acting somatostatin. Science *186*:538, 1974.

139. Brown, M., Rivier, J., Vale, W.: Somatostatin: analogs with selected biological activities. Science *196*:1467, 1977.

140. Lien, E., Sarantakis, D.: Effect of a long-acting glucagon selective somatostatin analogue on plasma glucose, insulin and glucagon levels in the anesthetized rat during arginine infusion. Diabetologia *17*:59, 1979.

141. Long, R.G., Barnes, A.J., Adrian, T.E., et al.: Suppression of pancreatic endocrine tumour secretion by long-acting somatostatin analogue. Lancet 2:764, 1979.

141a. Veber, D.F., Holly, F.W., Nutt, R.F., et al.: Highly active cyclic and bicyclic somatostatin analogues of reduced ring size. Nature 280:512, 1979.

142. Pelletier, G.: Identification of four cell types in the human endocrine pancreas by immunoelectron microscopy. Diabetes 26:749, 1977.

143. Gersell, D.J., Gingerich, R.L., Greider, M.H.: Regional distribution and concentration of pancreatic polypeptide in the human and canine pancreas. Diabetes 28:11, 1979.

144. Floyd, J.C., Jr.: Human pancreatic polypeptide. J. Clin. Endocrinol. Metab. 8:379, 1979.

145. Levitt, N.S., Vinik, A.I., Sive, A.A., et al.: Impaired pancreatic polypeptide responses to insulin-induced hypoglycemia in diabetic autonomic neuropathy. J. Clin. Endocrinol. Metab. 50:445, 1980.

146. Schwartz, T.W., Holst, J.J., Fahrenkrug, J., et al.: Vagal, cholinergic regulation of pancreatic polypeptide secretion. J. Clin. Invest. *61*:781, 1978.

147. Taylor, I.L., Feldman, M., Richardson, C.T., Walsh, J.H.: Gastric and cephalic stimulation of human pancreatic polypeptide release. Gastroenterology 75:432, 1978.

148. Glaser, B., Vinik, A.I., Sive, A.A., Floyd, J.C., Jr.: Plasma human pancreatic polypeptide responses to administered secretin: effects of surgical vagotomy, cholinergic blockade, and chronic pancreatitis. J. Clin. Endocrinol. Metab. 50:1094, 1980.

149. Greenberg, G.R., McCloy, R.F., Adrian, T.E., et al.: Inhibition of pancreas and gallbladder by pancreatic polypeptide. Lancet 2:1280, 1978.

150. Boden, G., Master, R.W., Owen, O.E., Rudnick, M.R.: Human pancreatic polypeptide in chronic renal failure and cirrhosis of the liver: role of kidney and liver in pancreatic polypeptide metabolism. J. Clin. Endocrinol. Metab. *51*:573, 1980.

151. Larsson, L-I., Schwartz, T., Lundquist, G., et al.: Occurrence of human pancreatic polypeptide in pancreatic endocrine tumors. Possible implications in the watery diarrhea syndrome. Am. J. Pathol. 85:675, 1976.

152. Polak, J.M., Bloom, S.R., Adrian, T.E., et al.: Pancreatic polypeptide in insulinomas, gastrinomas, vipomas, and glucagonomas. Lancet *1*:328, 1976.

153. Taylor, I.L., Walsh, J.H., Rotter, J., Passaro, E., Jr.: Is pancreatic polypeptide a marker for Zollinger-Ellison syndrome? Lancet *1*:845, 1978.

154. Floyd, J.C., Jr., Fajans, S.S., Pek, S., Chance, R.E.: A newly recognized pancreatic polypeptide; plasma levels in health and disease. Rec. Prog. Horm. Res. *33*:519, 1977.

155. Baetens, D., Stefan, Y., Ravazzola, M., et al.: Alteration of islet cell population in spontaneously diabetic mice. Diabetes 27:1, 1978.

156. Marco, J., Zulueta, M.A., Correas, I., Villanueva, M.L.: Reduced pancreatic polypeptide secretion in obese subjects. J. Clin. Endocrinol. Metab. 50:744, 1980.

157. Lassman, V., Vague, P., Vialettes, B., Simon, M-C.: Low plasma levels of pancreatic polypeptide in obesity. Diabetes 29:428, 1980.

158. McIntyre, N., Holdsworth, C.D., Turner, D.S.: New interpretation of oral glucose tolerance. Lancet 2:20, 1964.

159. Perley, M.J., Kipnis, D.M.: Plasma insulin responses to oral and intravenous glucose: studies in normal and diabetic subjects. J. Clin. Invest. 46:1954, 1967.

160. S.R. Bloom (Ed.): Gut Hormones. London, Churchill Livingstone, 1978.

161. K.D. Buchanan (Ed.): Gastrointestinal hormones. General concepts. J. Clin. Endocrinol. Metab. 8:249, 1979.

162. Walsh, J.H., Tompkins, R.K., Taylor, I.L., et al.: Gastrointestinal hormones in clinical disease: recent developments. Ann. Intern. Med. 90:817, 1979.

163. Creutzfeldt, W.: The incretin concept today. Diabetologia *16*:75, 1979.

164. Turner, R.C., Mann, J.I., Simpson, R.D., et al.: Fasting hyperglycemia and relatively unimpaired meal responses in mild diabetics. Clin. Endocrinol. 6:253, 1977.

165. Moxley, R.T., Lockwood, D.H., Amatruda, J.M., et al.: Loss of insulin response to ingested amino acids after jejunoileal bypass surgery for morbid obesity. Diabetes 27:78, 1978.

166. DeFronzo, R., Ferrannini, E., Wahren, J., Felig, P.: Lack of a gastrointestinal mediator of insulin action in maturity-onset diabetes. Lancet 2:1077, 1978.

167. Fahrenkrug, J., Schaffalitzky de Muckadell, O.B., Kühl, C.: Effect of secretin on basal- and glucose-stimulated insulin secretion in man. Diabetologia *14*:229, 1978.

168. Brodows, R.G., Chey, W.Y.: Physiological doses of secretin do not stimulate acute insulin release. J. Clin. Endocrinol. Metab. 50:603, 1980.

169. Boden, G., Essa, N., Owen, O.E., Reichle, F.A.: Effects of intraduodenal administration of HCl and glucose on circulating immunoreactive secretin and insulin concentrations. J. Clin. Invest. 53:1185, 1974.

170. Lerner, R.L.: Augmented insulin response to glucose after secretin priming in diabetic subjects. J. Clin. Endocrinol. Metab. 48:462, 1979.

171. Trimble, E.R., Buchanan, K.D., Hadden, D.R., Montgomery, D.A.D.: Secretin: high plasma levels in diabetes mellitus. Acta Endocrinol. 85:799, 1977.

172. Antin, J., GIbbs, J., Holt, J., et al.: Cholecystokinin

elicits the complete behavioral sequences of satiety in rats. J. Comp. Physiol. Psych. 89:784, 1975.

173. Gibbs, J., Falasco, J.D., McHugh, P.R.: Cholecystokinin-decreased food intake in rhesus monkeys. Am. J. Physiol. 230:15, 1976.

174. Straus, R., Yalow, R.S.: Cholecystokinin in the brains of obese and non-obese mice. Science 203:68, 1979.

175. Rehfeld, J.F., Holst, J.J., Kühl, C.: The effect of gastrin on basal and amino-acid stimulated insulin and glucagon secretion in man. Eur. J. Clin. Invest. 8:5, 1978.

176. Brown, J.C., Dryburgh, J.R., Ross, S.A., Dupré, J.: Identification and actions of gastric inhibitory polypeptide. Rec. Prog. Horm. Res. 31:487, 1975.

177. Brown, J.C., Otte, S.C.: GIP and the entero-insular axis. Clin. Endocrinol. Metab. 8:365, 1979.

178. Williams, R.H., Biesbroeck, J.: Gastric inhibitory polypeptide and insulin secretion after infusion of acetylcholine, catecholamines, and gut hormones. Proc. Soc. Exp. Biol. Med. 163:39, 1980.

179. Thomford, N.R., Sirinek, K.R., Crockett, S.E., et al.: Gastric inhibitory polypeptide. Response to oral glucose after vagotomy and pyloroplasty. Arch. Surg. 109:177, 1974.

180. Crockett, S.E., Cataland, S., Falko, J.M., Mazzaferri, E.L.: The insulinotropic effect of endogenous gastric inhibitory polypeptide in normal subjects. J. Clin. Endocrinol. Metab. 42:1098, 1976.

181. Crockett, S.E., Mazzaferri, E.L., Cataland, S.: Gastric inhibitory polypeptide (GIP) in maturity-onset diabetes mellitus. Diabetes 25:931, 1976.

182. Ross, S.A., Brown, J.C., Dupré, J.: Hypersecretion of gastric inhibitory polypeptide following oral glucose in diabetes mellitus. Diabetes 26:525, 1977.

183. May, J.M., Williams, R.H.: The effect of endogenous gastric inhibitory polypeptide on glucose-induced insulin secretion in mild diabetes. Diabetes 27:849, 1978.

184. Willms, B., Ebert, R., Creutzfeldt, W.: Gastric inhibitory polypeptide (GIP) and insulin in obesity: II. Reversal of increased response to stimulation by starvation or food restriction. Diabetologia 14:379, 1978.

185. Ebert, R., Frerichs, H., Creutzfeldt, W.: Impaired feedback control of fat induced gastric inhibitory polypeptide (GIP) secretion by insulin in obesity and glucose intolerance. Eur. J. Clin. Invest. 9:129, 1979.

186. Ross, S.A., Dupré, J.: Effects of ingestion of triglyceride or galactose on secretion of gastric inhibitory polypeptide and on responses to intravenous glucose in normal and diabetic subjects. Diabetes 27:327, 1978.

187. Reynolds, C., Tronsgard, N., Gibbons, E., et al.: Gastric inhibitory polypeptide response to hyper- and hypoglycemia in insulin-dependent diabetics. J. Clin. Endocrinol. Metab. 49:255, 1979.

188. Dupré, J., Greenidge, N., McDonald, T.J., et al.: Inhibition of actions of glucagon in adipocytes by gastric inhibitory polypeptide. Metabolism 25:1197, 1976.

189. Eckel, R.H., Fujimoto, W.Y., Brunzell, J.D.: Gastric inhibitory polypeptide. Enhanced lipoprotein lipase activity in cultured preadipocytes. Diabetes 28:1141, 1979.

190. Ganda, O.P., Soeldner, J.S., Gleason, R.E., et al.: Metabolic effects of glucose, mannose, galactose and fructose in man. J. Clin. Endocrinol. Metab. 49:616, 1979.

191. Lancet Editors: Substance P. Lancet 2:1067, 1976.

192. Guillemin, R.: Peptides in the brain; the new endocrinology of the neuron. Science 202:390, 1978.

193. Hökfelt, T., Johansson, O., Ljungdahl, Å., et al.: Peptidergic neurones. Nature 284:515, 1980.

194. Krieger, D.T.: Brain peptides: what, where and why? Science 222:975, 1983.

195. Pert, C.B., Snyder, S.H.: Opiate receptor:demonstration in nervous tissue. Science 179:1011, 1973.

196. Snyder, S.H.: Opiate receptors in the brain. N. Engl. J. Med. 296:266, 1977.

197. Hughes, J., Smith, T.W., Kosterlitz, H.W., et al.: Identification of two related pentapeptides from the brain with potent opiate agonist activity. Nature 258:577, 1975.

198. Ling, N., Burgus, R., Guillemin, R.: Isolation, primary structure, and synthesis of α-endorphin, and γ-endorphin, two peptides of hypothalamic-hypophysial origin with morphinomimetic activity. Proc. Natl. Acad. Sci. 73:3042, 1976.

199. Li, C.H.: Lipotropin, a new active peptide from pituitary glands. Nature 201:924, 1964.

200. Krieger, D.T., Liotta, A.S.: Pituitary hormones in brain: where, how, and why? Science 205:366, 1979.

201. Bunney, W.E., Jr., Pert, C.B., Klee, W., et al.: Basic and clinical studies of endorphins. Ann. Intern. Med. 91:239, 1979.

202. Polak, J.M., Bloom, S.R., Sullivan, S.N., et al.: Enkephalin-like immunoreactivity in the human gastrointestinal tract. Lancet 1:972, 1977.

203. Margules, D.L., Moisset, B., Lewis, M.J., et al.: β-endorphin is associated with overeating in genetically obese mice (ob/ob) and rats (fa/fa). Science 202:988, 1978.

204. Guillemin, R., Vargo, T., Rossier, J., et al.: β-endorphin and adrenocorticotropin are secreted concomitantly by the pituitary gland. Science 197:1367, 1977.

205. Ipp, E., Dobbs, R., Unger, R.H.: Morphine and β-endorphin influence the secretion of the endocrine pancreas. Nature 276:190, 1978.

206. Kanter, R.A., Ensinck, J.W., Fujimoto, W.Y.: Disparate effects of enkephalin and morphine upon insulin and glucagon secretion by islet cell cultures. Diabetes 29:84, 1980.

206a. Reid, R.L., Yen, S.S.C.: B-endorphin stimulates the secretion of insulin and glucagon in humans. J. Clin. Endocrinol. Metab. 52:592, 1981.

206b. Feldman, M., Kiser, R.S., Unger, R.H., Li, C.H.: Beta-endorphin and the endocrine pancreas. Studies in healthy and diabetic human beings. N. Engl. J. Med. 308:349, 1983.

207. Stubbs, W.A., Delitala, G., Jones, A., et al.: Hormonal and metabolic responses to an enkephalin analogue in normal man. Lancet 2:1225, 1978.

208. Nakao, K., Nakai, Y., Jingami, H., et al.: Substantial rise of plasma β-endorphin levels after insulin-induced hypoglycemia in human subjects. J. Clin. Endocrinol. Metab. 49:838, 1979.

209. Leslie, R.D.G., Pyke, D.A.: Sensitivity to enkephalin as a cause of non-insulin dependent diabetes. Lancet 1:341, 1979.

209a. Mason, J.S., Heber, D.: Endogenous opiates modulate insulin secretion in flushing noninsulin-dependent diabetics. J. Clin. Endocrinol. Metab. 54:693, 1982.

210. Carraway, R., Leeman, S.E.: The amino acid sequence of a hypothalamic peptide, neurotensin. J. Biol. Chem. 250:1907, 1975.

211. Blackburn, A.M., Fletcher, D.R., Bloom, S.R., et al.: Effect of neurotensin on gastric function in man. Lancet 1:987, 1980.

212. Ukai, M., Inoue, I., Itatsu, T.: Effect of somatostatin on

neurotensin-induced glucagon release and hyperglycemia. Endocrinology *100*:1284, 1977.

213. Berelowitz, M., Frohman, L.A.: Immunoreactive neurotensin in the pancreas of genetically obese and diabetic mice. A longitudinal study. Diabetes *32*:51, 1983.

213a. Shulkes, A., Boden, R., Cook, I., et al.: Characterization of a pancreatic tumor containing vasoactive intestinal peptide, neurotensin, and pancreatic polypeptide. J. Clin. Endocrinol. Metab. *58*:41, 1984.

214. Larsson, L-I.: Corticotropin-like peptides in central nerves and in endocrine cells of gut and pancreas. Lancet *2*:1321, 1977.

215. Orth, D.N., Guillemin, R., Ling, N., Nicholson, W.E.: Immunoreactive endorphins, lipotropins, and corticotropins in a human non-pituitary tumor: evidence for a common precursor. J. Clin. Endocrinol. Metab. *46*:849, 1978.

216. Houssay, B.A., Biosatti, A.: La diabetes pancreatica de los perros hipofisoprivos. Rev. Soc. Argent. Biol. *6*:251, 1930.

217. Young, F.G.: The relation of the anterior pituitary gland to carbohydrate metabolism. Br. Med. J. *2*:393, 1939.

218. Ikkos, D., Luft, R.: Aspects of metabolic action of human growth hormone. In: G.E.W. Wolstenholme, C.M. O'Connor (Eds.): Human Pituitary Hormones. Vol. 13. London, Ciba Foundation Colloquia on Endocrinology, 1960, pp. 106–134.

219. Luft, R., Guillemin, R.: Growth-hormone and diabetes in man. Old concepts-new implications. Diabetes *23*:783, 1974.

220. Spiro, R.G.: Search for a biochemical basis of diabetic microangiopathy. Claude Bernard Lecture. Diabetologia *12*:1, 1976.

221. Lundbaek, K.: Growth-hormone's role in diabetic microangiopathy. Diabetes *25*(Suppl. 2):845, 1976.

222. Roth, J., Glick, S.M., Cuatrecasas, P., Hollander, C.S.: Acromegaly and other disorders of growth hormone secretion. Ann. Intern. Med. *66*:760, 1967.

223. Zierler, K.L., Rabinowitz, D.: Roles of insulin and growth-hormone on studies of forearm metabolism in man. Medicine *42*:385, 1963.

224. Fineberg, S.E., Merimee, T.J.: Acute metabolic effects of human growth hormone. Diabetes *23*:499, 1974.

225. Rizza, R.A., Mandarino., L.J., Gerich., J.E.: Effects of growth hormone on insulin action in man. Mechanisms of insulin resistance, impaired suppression of glucose production, and impaired stimulation of glucose utilization. Diabetes *31*:663, 1982.

226. Bratusch-Marrain, P.R., Smith, D., DeFronzo, R.A.: The effect of growth hormone on glucose metabolism and insulin secretion in man. J. Clin. Endocrinol. Metab. *55*:973, 1982.

227. Pierluissi, J., Campbell, J.: Metasomatotrophic diabetes and its induction: basal insulin secretion and insulin release responses to glucose, glucagon, arginine and meals. Diabetologia *18*:223, 1980.

228. Van Wyk, J.J., Underwood, L.E.: Relation between growth hormone and somatomedin. Ann. Rev. Med. *26*:427, 1975.

229. Golde, D.W., Herschman, H.R., Lusis, A.J., Groopman, J.E.: Growth factors. Ann. Intern. Med. *92*:650, 1980.

230. Lesniak, M.A., Gorden, P.: Growth hormone receptors. In: G.S. Levey (Ed.): Hormone-Receptor Interaction: Molecular Aspects. Modern Pharmacology-Toxicology. Vol. 9. New York, Marcel Dekker, 1976, pp. 201–219.

231. Hansen, Aa.P.: Normalization of growth hormone hyperresponse to exercise in juvenile diabetics after "normalization" of blood sugar. J. Clin. Invest. *50*:1806, 1971.

232. Johansen, K., Hansen, Aa.P.: Diurnal serum growth hormone levels in poorly and well-controlled juvenile diabetics. Diabetes *20*:239, 1971.

233. Hansen, Aa.P.: Abnormal serum growth hormone response to exercise in maturity-onset diabetics. Diabetes *22*:619, 1973.

234. Vigneri, R., Squatrito, S., Pezzino, V., et al.: Growth hormone levels in diabetes. Correlation with the clinical control of the disease. Diabetes *25*:167, 1976.

235. Merimee, T.J., Fitzgerald, C.R., Gold, L.A., McCourt, J.P.: Characteristics of growth hormone secretion in clinically stable diabetes. Diabetes *28*:308, 1979.

236. Hayford, J.T., Danney, M.M., Hendrix, J.A., Thompson, R.G.: Integrated concentration of growth hormone in juvenile-onset diabetes. Diabetes *29*:391, 1980.

237. Tamborlane, W.V., Sherwin, R.S., Koivisto, V., et al.: Normalization of the growth hormone and catecholamine response to exercise in juvenile-onset diabetic subjects treated with a portable insulin infusion pump. Diabetes *28*:785, 1979.

238. Østerby, R., Seyer-Hansen, K., Gundersen, H.J.G., Lundbaek, K.: Growth hormone enhances basement membrane thickening in experimental diabetes. A preliminary report. Diabetologia *15*:487, 1978.

239. Passa, P., Gauville, C., Canivet, J.: Influence of muscular exercise on plasma level of growth hormone in diabetics with and without retinopathy. Lancet *2*:72, 1974.

240. Passa, P., Rousselie, F., Gauville, C., Canivet, J.: Retinopathy and plasma growth hormone levels in idiopathic hemochromatosis with diabetes. Diabetes *26*:113, 1977.

241. Merimee, T.J.: A follow-up study of vascular disease in growth-hormone-deficient dwarfs with diabetes. N. Engl. J. Med. *298*:1217, 1978.

242. Ray, B.S., Pazianos, A.G., Greenberg, E., et al.: Pituitary ablation for diabetic retinopathy. I. Results of hypophysectomy (a ten-year evaluation). J.A.M.A. *203*:79, 1968.

243. Long, C.N.H., Katzin, B., Fry, E.G.: The adrenal cortex and carbohydrate metabolism. Endocrinology *26*:309, 1940.

244. Cahill, G.F., Jr.: Action of adrenal cortical steroids on carbohydrate metabolism. In: N.P. Christy (Ed.): The Human Adrenal Cortex. New York, Harper & Row, 1971, pp. 205–239.

244a. Kahn, C.R., Goldfine, J.D., Neville, D.M., Jr., DeMeyts, P.: Alterations in insulin binding induced by changes in vivo in the levels of glucocorticoids and growth hormone. Endocrinology *103*:1054, 1978.

244b. Yasuda, K., Hines, E., III, Kitabchi, A.E.: Hypercortisolism and insulin resistance: comparative effects of prednisone, hydrocortisone, and mexamethasone on insulin binding of human erythrocytes. J. Clin. Endocrinol. Metab. *55*:910, 1982.

245. Shamoon, H., Soman, V., Sherwin, R.S.: The influence of acute physiological increments of cortisol on fuel metabolism and insulin binding to monocytes in normal humans. J. Clin. Endocrinol. Metab. *50*:495, 1980.

246. Shamoon, H., Hendler, R., Sherwin, R.S.: Altered responsiveness to cortisol, epinephrine, and glucagon in insulin-infused juvenile-onset diabetics. A mechanism for diabetic instability. Diabetes *29*:284, 1980.

247. Marco, J., Calle, C., Román, D., et al.: Hyperglucagonism induced by glucocorticoid treatment in man. N. Engl. J. Med. *288*:128, 1973.

248. Wise, J.K., Hendler, R., Felig, P.: Influence of glucocorticoids on glucagon secretion and plasma amino acid concentrations in man. J. Clin. Invest. *52*:2774, 1973.

249. Soman, V., Oertel, L., Felig, P.: Modulation of hepatic glucagon receptors by dexamethasone: cellular mecha-

nism of glucocorticoid-induced hypersensitivity to glucagon. Clin. Res. 27:377A, 1979.

250. Christensen, N.J.: Catecholamines and diabetes mellitus. Diabetologia 16:211, 1979.

251. Landsberg, L., Young, J.B.: Fasting, feeding and regulation of the sympathetic nervous system. N. Engl. J. Med. 298:1295, 1978.

251a. Cryer, P.E.: Physiology and pathophysiology of the human sympathoadrenal neuroendocrine system. N. Engl. J. Med. 303:436, 1980.

252. Rappaport, E.B., Young, J.B., Landsberg. L.: Dissociation of sympathetic nervous system (SNS) and adrenal medullary responses to 2-deoxy-D-glucose (2-DG). Clin. Res. 28:403A, 1980.

253. Rowe, J.W., Young, J.B., Minaker, K.L., et al.: Effect of insulin and glucose infusions on sympathetic nervous system activity in normal man. Diabetes 30:219, 1981.

254. Day, J.L.: The metabolic consequences of adrenergic blockade: a review. Metabolism 24:987, 1975.

254a. Strickland, W.G., Blackmore, P.F., Exton, J.H.: The role of calcium in alpha-adrenergic inactivation of glycogen synthase in rat hepatocytes and its inhibition by insulin. Diabetes 29:617, 1980.

255. Shamoon, H.: β-adrenergic blockade inhibits the hepatic response to epinephrine in diabetic but not in normal humans. Diabetes 29(Suppl. 2):20A, 1980.

255a. Garber, A.J., Karl, I.E., Kipnis, D.M.: Alanine and glutamine synthesis and release from skeletal muscle. IV. β-adrenergic inhibition of amino acid release. J. Biol. Chem. 251:851, 1976.

255b. Shamoon, H., Jacob, R., Sherwin, R.S.: Epinephrine-induced hypoaminoacidemia in normal and diabetic human subjects. Effect of beta blockade. Diabetes 29:875, 1980.

256. Robertson, R.P.: Adrenergic modulation of basal insulin secretion in man. Diabetes 22:1, 1973.

257. Robertson, R.P., Halter, J.B., Porte, D., Jr.: A role for alpha-adrenergic receptors in abnormal insulin secretion in diabetes mellitus. J. Clin. Invest. 57:791, 1976.

258. Asplin, C.M., Werner, P., Hollander, P., Palmer, J.P.: The differential effect of the autonomic nervous system on insulin and glucagon secretion during glucopenia. Program. 62nd Annual Meeting of the Endocrine Society. June 18–20, 1980, p. 269.

259. Sacca, L., Morrone, G., Cicala, M., et al.: Influence of epinephrine, norepinephrine, and isoproterenol on glucose homeostasis in normal man. J. Clin. Endocrinol. Metab. 50:680, 1980.

260. Hamburg, S., Hendler, R., Sherwin, R.S.: Influence of small increments of epinephrine on glucose tolerance in normal humans. Ann. Intern. Med. 93:566, 1980.

261. Chiasson, J-L., Shikama, H., Exton, J.H.: Dual effect of epinephrine on glucose clearance in skeletal muscle. Diabetes 29(Suppl. 2):16A, 1980.

262. Gustafson, A.B., Kalkhoff, R.K.: Plasma epinephrine disturbances in diabetic subjects during isometric exercise. Diabetes 29(Suppl. 2):40A, 1980.

263. Hamaji, M.: Pancreatic α- and β-cell function in pheochromocytoma. J. Clin. Endocrinol. Metab. 49:322, 1979.

264. Lang, D.A., Matthews, D.R., Peto, J., Turner, R.C.: Cyclic oscillations of basal plasma glucose and insulin concentrations in human beings. N. Engl. J. Med. 301:1023, 1979.

265. Liljenquist, J.E., Mueller, G.L., Cherrington, A.D., et al.: Hyperglycemia per se (insulin and glucagon withdrawn) can inhibit hepatic glucose production in man. J. Clin. Endocrinol. Metab. 48:171, 1979.

266. Aoki, T.T., Cahill, G.F., Jr.: Metabolic effects of insulin,

glucagon, and glucose in man: clinical applications. In: L.J. DeGroot (Editor-in-chief): Endocrinology Vol. III. New York, Grune & Stratton, 1979, pp. 1843–1854.

267. Sacca, L., Sherwin, R., Hendler, R., Felig, P.: Influence of continuous physiologic hyperinsulinemia on glucose kinetics and counterregulatory hormones in normal and diabetic humans. J. Clin. Invest. 63:849, 1979.

268. Rizza, R.A., Cryer, P.E., Gerich, J.E.: Role of glucagon, catecholamines, and growth hormone in human glucose counterregulation. Effects of somatostatin and combined α- and β-adrenergic blockade on plasma glucose recovery and glucose flux rates after insulin-induced hypoglycemia. J. Clin. Invest. 64:62, 1979.

269. DeFronzo, R.A., Hendler, R., Christensen, N.: Stimulation of counterregulatory hormonal responses in diabetic man by a fall in glucose concentration. Diabetes 29:125, 1980.

270. Gale, E., Kurtz, A., Tattersall, R.: The myth of rebound hyperglycemia. Diabetes 28:349, 1979.

270a. Cryer, P.E., Gerich, J.E.: Relevance of glucose counterregulatory systems to patients with diabetes: critical roles of glucagon and epinephrine. Diabetes Care 6:95, 1983.

271. Foster, D.W., McGarry, J.D.: The metabolic derangements and treatment of diabetic ketoacidosis. N. Engl. J. Med. 309:159, 1983.

272. Schade, D.S., Eaton, R.P.: The controversy concerning counterregulatory hormone secretion. A hypothesis for the prevention of diabetic ketoacidosis? Diabetes 26:596, 1977.

273. Kreisberg, R.A.: Diabetic ketoacidosis: new concepts and trends in pathogenesis and treatment. Ann. Intern. Med. 88:681, 1978.

274. Barnes, A.J., Kohner, E.M., Bloom, S.R., et al.: Importance of pituitary hormones in aetiology of diabetic ketoacidosis. Lancet 1:1171, 1978.

275. Ginsberg, H.N.: Investigation of insulin resistance during diabetic ketoacidosis: role of counterregulatory substances and effect of insulin therapy. Metabolism 26:1135, 1977.

276. Schade, D.S., Eaton, R.P.: The temporal relationship between endogenously secreted stress hormones and metabolic decompensation in diabetic man. J. Clin. Endocrinol. Metab. 50:131, 1980.

277. Frantz, A.G.: Prolactin. N. Engl. J. Med. 298:201, 1978.

278. Woolf, P.D., Lee, L.A., Leebaw, W.F.: Hypoglycemia as a provocative test of prolactin release. Metabolism 27:869, 1978.

279. Kopelman, P.G., White, N., Pilkington, T.R.E., Jeffcoate, S.L.: Impaired hypothalamic control of prolactin secretion in massive obesity. Lancet 1:747, 1979.

280. Landgraf, R., Landgraf-Leurs, M.M.C., Weissmann, A., et al.: Prolactin: a diabetogenic hormone. Diabetologia 13:99, 1977.

281. Hanssen, K.F., Christensen, S.E., Hansen, Aa.P., et al.: Plasma prolactin in juvenile diabetics. 24-h studies with somatostatin. Diabetologia 15:369, 1978.

282. Hanssen, K.F., Torjesen, P.A.: Increased serum prolactin in diabetic ketoacidosis: correlation between serum sodium and serum prolactin concentration. Acta Endocrinol. 85:372, 1977.

283. Naeije, R., Badawi, M., Vanhaelst, L., et al.: Prolactin response to TRH in diabetic ketoacidosis. Diabetologia 16:381, 1979.

284. Hunter, P.R., Anderson, J., Lunn, T.A., et al.: Letter: Diabetic retinopathy and prolactin. Lancet 1:1237, 1974.

285. Harter, M., Balarac, N., Pourcher, Ph., et al.: Letter: Diabetic retinopathy and prolactin. Lancet 2:961, 1976.

286. Robertson, R.P.: Prostaglandins as modulators of pancreatic islet function. Diabetes 28:943, 1979.

287. Field, J.B., Boyle, C., Remer, A.: Effect of salicylate

infusion on plasma-insulin and glucose tolerance in healthy persons and mild diabetics. Lancet *1*:1191, 1967.

288. Robertson, R.P., Chen, M.: A role for prostaglandin E in defective insulin secretion and carbohydrate intolerance in diabetes mellitus. J. Clin. Invest. *60*:747, 1977.

289. Micossi, P., Pontiroli, A.E., Baron, S.H., et al.: Aspirin stimulates insulin and glucagon secretion and increases glucose tolerance in normal and diabetic subjects. Diabetes *27*:1196, 1978.

290. Gugliano, D., Torella, R.: Prostaglandin E inhibits glucose-induced insulin secretion in man. Prostaglandins Med. *1*:165, 1978.

291. Braaten, J.T., Siddiqui, Y., Andreadis, C., Posnaski, W.J.: Influence of inhibitors of prostaglandin (PG) synthesis on insulin secretion in superfused pancreatic monolayer cell cultures. Diabetes *28*:405, 1979.

292. Metz, S., Robertson, R.P., Fujimoto, W.: Sodium salicylate augments glucose recognition and insulin secretion and inhibits prostaglandin synthesis in pancreatic monolayer cultures. Clin. Res. *28*:400A, 1980.

293. McRae, J., Robertson, R.P.: A role for prostaglandin

(PG) E in defective glucose potentiation of a nonglucose insulin secretagogue in diabetics. Diabetes *29*(Suppl. 2):9A, 1980.

294. Pek, S., Tai, T-Y., Elster, A.: Stimulatory effects of prostaglandins E-1, E-2, and F-2-alpha on glucagon and insulin release in vitro. Diabetes *27*:801, 1978.

295. Topol, E., Brodows, R.G.: Effects of indomethacin on acute insulin release in man. Diabetes *29*:379, 1980.

296. Brodows, R.G.: Acute alterations in prostaglandin status fail to influence insulin secretion in man. Diabetes *29* (Suppl. 2):9A, 1980.

297. Robertson, R.P.: Hypothesis. PGE, carbohydrate homeostasis, and insulin secretion. A suggested resolution of the controversy. Diabetes *32*:231, 1983.

298. Axelrod, L., Levine, L.: Arachidonic acid derivatives (PGE$_2$ and PGI$_2$) produced by adipocytes modulate sympathetic nervous system activity. Diabetes *29*(Suppl. 2):54A, 1980.

299. Axelrod, L., Levine, L.: Plasma prostaglandin levels in rats with diabetes mellitus and diabetic ketoacidosis. Diabetes *31*:994, 1982.

300. Axelrod, L.: Personal communication.

10 Microvascular Disease and Related Abnormalities: Their Relation to Control of Diabetes

Michael Brownlee

It is estimated that 60 million people worldwide are afflicted with diabetes mellitus.[1] It is reasonably definite that 3 to 4 million persons in the United States are under treatment with insulin or oral agents and perhaps another 3 million treated with diet alone; in addition to these 6 to 7 million, there may be an additional 4 or more million with varying degrees of asymptomatic glucose intolerance. Although conventional treatment with diet, insulin, and oral hypoglycemic agents has been extraordinarily successful in ameliorating insulin deficiency and prolonging life, it has been unable to prevent the development of chronic complications affecting the vascular and nervous systems. On the bright side, the recent revival of interest in attempts to maintain "strict" control with multiple injections of insulin daily or the use of insulin "pumps," has given renewed hope that the maintenance of normoglycemia insofar as safe and practicable, may prevent, postpone, or minimize complications which take such a great toll in morbidity and mortality.

Retinal capillary damage resulting in edema, new vessel formation, and hemorrhage makes blindness 25 times more prevalent in diabetics than in the normal population. Cataracts appear earlier in life and seem to progress more rapidly in diabetic than in nondiabetic persons. Chronic renal failure with proteinuria, resulting from glomerular capillary damage secondary to basement membrane thickening, is 17 times more prevalent. Axonal dwindling and segmental demyelination in the diabetic peripheral nerves, are associated with a high incidence of motor, sensory, and autonomic impairments, including a 40% rate of impotence among male diabetics. Because of increased atheromata in medium and large arteries, diabetics have a 2-fold greater risk of coronary artery disease and stroke than the normal population, and a 3- to 4-fold greater risk of symptomatic peripheral arterial disease. Amputation due to gangrene is several times more frequent in diabetics than in nondiabetics. It has been estimated that on the average, the expected life span of diabetics is only two-thirds that of nondiabetics.[2]

In the past, knowledge about diabetic complications was largely limited to descriptions of morphologic changes and clinical manifestations. However, in the last decade physiologic and biochemical studies have provided a great deal of new information about microangiopathy and diabetic complications.[2a,2b] In this chapter, much of this rapidly accumulating information is summarized and critically examined from the standpoint of actual relation to diabetes. One must recognize that, despite the large volume of data now available,[2c] the exact cause of microangiopathy remains unclear so that some of the following discussion must deal with reasonable hypotheses. Some of the topics receive attention in other chapters, but from a somewhat different point of view.

INTRODUCTION

It has been observed that the dilatation of retinal veins in diabetic patients can be reversed by good metabolic control.[3] Since dilatation of these vessels is postulated to be an autoregulatory mechanism that occurs in response to local hypoxia, it has been suggested that relative tissue hypoxia may play a role in the pathogenesis of certain diabetic complications.[4] This concept, which was originally based on reports of the presence of diabetic-like retinal lesions in such disorders as macroglobulinemia, sickle cell anemia, severe heart disease with cyanosis, and cystic fibrosis, has gained credibility as the result of more recent laboratory observations that have confirmed abnormalities predisposing to decreased tissue oxygenation in diabetic persons.

Since relative tissue hypoxia may play a role in the pathogenesis of several diabetic complications, hematologic abnormalities that could result in decreased tissue oxygenation are discussed first. These include: increased erythrocyte aggregation and microviscosity and decreased deformability; increased levels of non-enzymatically glycosylated hemoglobins that have altered oxygen affinities; decreased effective levels of 2,3,-diphosphoglycerate; platelet function abnormalities, including increased adhesiveness, enhanced sensitivity to aggregating agents, and accelerated synthesis of thrombogenic prostaglandin derivatives; plasma protein abnormalities resulting in increased blood viscosity; accelerated fibrinogen consumption; reduced levels of antithrombin III; increased levels of von Willebrand factor (VWF); and decreased fibrinolysis.

Glucose has been found to alter a variety of proteins in vivo in addition to the hemoglobin molecule. Increased formation of these glycoproteins in tissues not requiring insulin for glucose transport could be a causative factor in certain diabetic complications.

A considerable amount of research effort has been focused on microvascular disease in the diabetic kidney. Early changes in renal function and structure that may play some part in the pathogenesis of diabetic renal disease include: increased filtration rate and filtration fraction; augmented excretion of urinary albumin and other proteins; increased accumulation of mesangial actomyosin-like material; persistence of certain extravasated serum proteins within glomerular basement membrane; diminished localized mechanisms for clearing mesangial macromolecules; and increased renal size, glomerular tuft volume, capillary luminal volume, and capillary filtration surface area. However, the relationship between these early changes and the development of the renal disease characteristic of chronic diabetes has as yet not been determined. Continual thickening of the glomerular basement membrane over many years ultimately leads to progressive occlusion of the glomerular capillaries and chronic renal failure. This chapter reviews information that has been obtained during recent years on the chemical characterization of glomerular basement membrane and the changes in composition that occur in the basement membrane of diabetic patients. Also discussed are biosynthetic studies demonstrating that increased synthesis is a major factor in the excessive accumulation of glomerular basement membrane in diabetic individuals.

There is less information at present about the causes of microvascular disease in the retina. Regional ischemia appears to be central to the development of diabetic retinopathy, and may be exacerbated by an early, persistent increase in retinal capillary permeability, alterations in endothelial and mural cell structure, and, perhaps, by thickening of the basement membrane.

It has been suggested that abnormal growth hormone secretion, which has been noted in some diabetic patients, may contribute in various ways to the development of microangiopathy. The evidence supporting this theory, as well as conflicting data, will be evaluated.

Diabetic neuropathy is characterized by various structural changes that are associated with reduced sensory function and motor nerve conduction velocities: decreased number of intramembranous particles on the myelin surface; endoneurial edema, resulting in shrinkage of axons and Schwann cells; increased permeability of nodal gap substance; basement membrane thickening in the intra- and perineural vessels; axonal degeneration; and segmental demyelination. Particularly important in the pathogenesis of diabetic neuropathy are certain biochemical alterations in the diabetic nerve: changes in the composition and rate of synthesis of various myelin lipid and protein components; increased activity of the polyol pathway; decreased concentration and rate of synthesis of myoinositol and phosphatidylinositol; and diminished axoplasmic transport of choline acetylase, acetylcholinesterase, norepinephrine, and several glycoproteins.

In the final section of this chapter, the relationship between the degree of clinical metabolic dysfunction and the development of diabetic complications, is explored. The basic conclusion that emerges is that insulin deficiency and its metabolic consequences, notably chronic hyperglycemia, are the primary causes of diabetic complications.

HEMATOLOGIC ABNORMALITIES

In Table 10–1 are listed the various hematologic abnormalities associated with diabetes. Most of these are discussed either in this chapter or in Chapter 37 to which the reader is referred.

Erythrocytes

Red Blood Cell Aggregation. It has been argued that increased aggregation of red blood cells, which has been observed in the blood of diabetic patients, may contribute to obliterative microvascular changes in the retina.[5-7] The finding that washed red blood cells from both diabetics and nondiabetics aggregate in plasma from diabetic patients but not in plasma from normal subjects suggests that increased erythrocyte aggregation may be due to increased levels of certain plasma proteins rather than to changes in the erythrocytes themselves.[6,7] Although there is a correlation between the abnormal red cell aggregation in diabetes and the degree of glycohemoglobin elevation,[8] there is no direct evidence at present to support the asser-

Table 10–1. Hematologic Abnormalities Associated with Diabetes

White blood cells
1. Decreased chemotaxis
2. Decreased diapedesis
3. Decreased phagocytosis
4. Decreased bactericidal activity
5. Decreased cell-mediated immunity

Red blood cells
1. Increased aggregation
2. Decreased deformability
3. Decreased oxyhemoglobin dissociation curve P_{50}

Platelets
1. Increased platelet adhesion
2. Increased platelet aggregation (ADP, epinephrine, arachidonic acid)
3. Increased PGE_2-like material in platelets (ADP, epinephrine, collagen, arachidonic acid)

Whole blood
1. Increased whole blood and plasma viscosity
2. Increased fibrinogen, haptoglobin
3. Increased vWF activity (other clotting factors, e.g. V)
4. Increased alpha 2-macroglobulin, alpha l-antiprotease
5. Decreased antithrombin III (AOD)
6. Increased CH50, C_1S, C_3, C_4 (complement system)
7. Increased fibrinogen, alpha 2-macroglobulin turnover
8. Decreased fibrinolysis
   a. decreased spontaneous blood fibrinolytic activity
   b. decreased plasminogen activator release
   c. decreased fibrinolytic response to venous occlusion

tion that increased aggregation plays a role in the development of microvascular sequelae.

Erythrocyte Deformability. This abnormality, as determined by the ability of red cells to pass through 5 micron pores, is significantly decreased in diabetic individuals.[9] This observation has been verified in studies using a different technique in which pressure is measured while single red cells are moved in a cyclic standard velocity pattern in micropipettes.[10,11] The ratio of mean pressure in diabetics to that in normal subjects averaged 1.51. Since erythrocytes must often travel through capillaries that are much smaller than their own diameter, this decreased deformability might seriously hamper rapid and homogeneous perfusion within the microcirculation. Although the cause of this reduced deformability is unknown, its correlation with the degree of control of diabetes[9-11] suggests that metabolic factors may play a major role. One such factor may be the higher degree of erythrocyte membrane microviscosity observed in diabetic patients whose fasting blood glucose is greater than 140 mg/dl.[12] This increased microviscosity may perhaps be due to increased glycosylation of membrane proteins.[13] The deformability characteristics of diabetic red blood cells may also be adversely affected by decreases in sialic acid and cholesterol content, which have been observed in red blood cells of chronically diabetic rats[14] and humans,[15] and by membrane-bound hemoglobin molecules, which have been found in human diabetic erythrocyte membranes.[16] The possible role of other cell surface changes in causing altered functional properties is discussed below.

Leukocytes

Numerous functional abnormalities in both polymorphonuclear leukocytes and lymphocytes have been demonstrated in diabetic patients.[17,18] Polymorphonuclear leukocytes from patients with poorly-controlled diabetes exhibit various impairments in host defense response: defective granulocytic adherence, chemotaxis, phagocytosis, and intracellular bactericidal activity.[17,19] All of these impairments can be reversed or ameliorated by tighter diabetic control. Lymphocytes from juvenile-onset diabetics in poor control demonstrate a diminished proliferative response to mitogen stimulation and a decrease in T- and B-cell surface membrane markers,[18] which are rapidly normalized by 5 days of optimal blood glucose control using an external artificial pancreas. Although the clinical significance and relevance to microangiopathy of these abnormalities in leukocyte cell surface are unclear at present, similar alterations in the surfaces of other cells from diabetic persons could have important implications.

Cell Surface Changes. Current theories of cell surface organization suggest that changes in the mobility and distribution as well as in the chemical composition of plasma membrane components may significantly alter cell function.[20,21] Changes in the cell surface may, in part, be responsible for alterations in a variety of cellular properties that have been observed in diabetes, which, in turn, may play a role in the development of chronic complications including microangiopathy. This new and relatively unexplored area has great potential for the further elucidation of the pathophysiology of diabetic complications.

Studies of lectin binding have demonstrated significant reductions in plasma membrane receptors for these molecules in the liver cells of diabetic rats. There was a 20 to 25% reduction in the binding of concanavalin A and ricin,[22] reflecting an apparent decrease in plasma membrane glycoprotein carbohydrate content.[23] There was also a 50% decrease in the binding of desialylated thyroxine-binding globulin,[22] an interaction that depends on membrane sialic acid residues. The fact that this reduction in the binding of desialylated thyroxine-binding globulin is much greater than the reported decrease in sialic acid in these membranes[14] suggests that either the sialic acid content of this specific receptor is selectively reduced, or that the structure or mobility of receptor components on the membrane surface is altered. The occurrence of extensive changes in cell-surface glycoproteins in this animal model of diabetes is also suggested by alterations in lectin binding to plasma membrane components of various molecular weights that have been separated by SDS polyacrylamide gel electrophoresis.[24] It is conceivable that such alterations could influence a variety of cellular properties, including erythrocyte aggregation, deformability, and permeability; electrical resistance; and the binding properties of mitogen, hormone, and lipoprotein receptors.

Although the chemical basis for the observed alterations in diabetic cell surfaces is not clearly understood, both insulin deficiency and secondary metabolic and hormonal changes could alter the synthesis of macromolecules in certain tissues. Post-synthetic chemical modification resulting from abnormally elevated substrate levels may also play a role in causing cell-surface changes, as suggested in the following discussion of glycosylated hemoglobins.

Hemoglobin Glycosylation and Oxygenation

It has long been appreciated that normal hemolysates contain several minor hemoglobins in addition to the single major hemoglobin, HbA_o. These minor hemoglobin species account for 5 to 10% of the total hemoglobin content in normal adult erythrocytes. Patients with inadequately controlled diabetes may exhibit 2- to 3-fold elevations in three of these minor hemoglobins: HbA_{1a}, HbA_{1b}, and HbA_{1c},[25] thereby reflecting the degree of hyperglycemia. Recently, HbA_{1a} has been separated into two distinct components: HbA_{1a1} and HbA_{1a2}.[26] It has been proposed that all four of these negatively-charged minor hemoglobins are glycosylated, with carbohydrate present on the beta chain.[27] Glucose has been shown to react with the NH_2-terminal of the beta chain of HbA_{1c}, the most abundant of the glycosylated hemoglobins, by means of a Schiff-base and an Amadori rearrangement to form a 1-amino, 1-deoxyfructose derivative.[28] Presumably, the carbohydrate moieties of the other minor glycohemoglobins attach to the protein via analogous ketoamine linkages. It has been found that a significant portion of HbA_o is also glycosylated[29] and glucose-ketoamine linkages have been identified on the N-terminus of the alpha chain as well as on several lysine residues in both the alpha and beta chains. Studies in diabetic subjects have shown increases of glycosylated HbA_o comparable to those of HbA_{1c}.[29,30] See Fig. 10–1 and Table 10–2.

HbA_{1a1} and HbA_{1a2} contain phosphate in addition to carbohydrate.[27] The finding that synthetic glycohemoglobin, formed by incubating HbA_o with glucose-6-phosphate, co-chromatographs with HbA_{1a2} has led to the assumption that phosphorylated sugars are the source of this phosphate in vivo. The structures of minor hemoglobins other than HbA_{1c} have not yet been described.

The minor glycosylated hemoglobins have unique functional properties that are significantly different from those of HbA_o. In comparison to HbA_o, HbA_{1a1} and HbA_{1a2} have low oxygen affinities whereas HbA_{1b} has a high affinity and HbA_{1c}, a moderately high affinity.[31] While the removal of organic phosphate increases the oxygen affinities of HbA_{1b} and HbA_{1c} and also that of HbA_o, the affinities of HbA_{1a1} and HbA_{1a2} remain low. The oxygen affinities of HbA_{1b} and HbA_{1c} are substantially reduced by the addition of organic phosphate, although to a much lesser degree than that of HbA_o. In contrast, the addition of organic phosphate essentially has no effect on the affinities of HbA_{1a1} and HbA_{1a2}. These alterations in the oxygen-binding properties of the glycohemoglobins may be explained in part by the location of their carbohydrate moieties, which prevents the binding of organic phosphates such as 2,3-diphosphoglycerate (2,3-DPG). The fact that HbA_{1a1} and HbA_{1a2} contain covalently bound organic phosphate could account for their persistently low oxygen affinities in the absence of added phosphate.

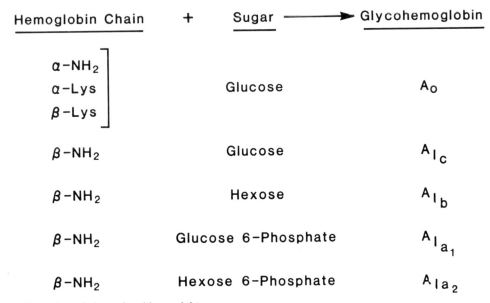

Fig. 10–1.   Formation of glycosylated hemoglobins.

The organic phosphate 2,3-DPG (which is derived from red blood cell glucose metabolism) is thought to play an important role in the regulation of oxygen exchange by hemoglobin in vivo. Increased 2,3-DPG levels lower hemoglobin oxygen affinity, thus increasing the release of oxygen to tissues. However, even in the presence of high concentrations of organic phosphate, all of the glycohemoglobins are still 50% saturated with oxygen at partial pressures where little HbA$_o$ remains oxygenated.[31] In diabetics, the combination of a relative deficiency of 2,3-DPG and elevated glycohemoglobin levels during periods of change in blood glucose level[32,33] may result in decreased oxygen delivery to critical tissues. Blood from ambulatory diabetic children actually does show increased hemoglobin oxygen affinity,[34] but the clinical relevance of this phenomenon has not yet been determined. It has been reported that pronounced hyperlipoproteinemia accentuates the impairment of oxygen delivery to tissues.[35]

Glycohemoglobin biosynthesis occurs in vivo during the whole life-span of the red blood cell (approximately 120 days) via post-synthetic non-enzymatic glycosylation of HbA$_o$. The rate of formation of glycohemoglobin is proportional to the integrated concentration of blood glucose.[28,36–38] Glycohemoglobin levels in diabetic patients correlate linearly with the peak, or with the area under the curve of the glucose tolerance test,[39] and glycohemoglobin concentrations gradually decrease as glycemic control is improved.[40] The decline in glycohemoglobin levels reflects the normal destruction of red cells and the slow reversibility of non-enzymatic glycosylation. In tissue proteins with longer half-lives, however, glycosylation mirrors the true chemical equilibrium. Covalent modification of such proteins by glucose could be a factor in the pathogenesis of diabetic complications.[41] This hypothesis is supported directly by the results of studies of lens crystallins in which high glucose concentrations enhanced the non-enzymatic glycosylation of the lysine residues of lens proteins both in vitro and in vivo. Crystallins modified in this way by glucose showed a greater susceptibility to sulfhydryl oxidation, which produces high-molecular-weight aggregates linked by disulfide bonds. The opalescence of these aggregates in solution is similar to that observed in diabetic cataracts, which suggests that analogous mechanisms may contribute to their clinical formation.[41,42,42a]

Reports of increased non-enzymatic glycosylation in renal glomerular proteins and in peripheral nerve myelin proteins isolated from diabetic animals,[43,43a] suggest that this mechanism may also be involved in the development of diabetic nephropathy and neuropathy. Non-enzymatic glycosylation of erythrocyte membrane proteins occurs to a greater degree in diabetics than in normal subjects and this may be associated with the decreased deformability discussed earlier.[13] Human albumin has been shown to undergo non-enzymatic glycosylation both in vitro and in vivo.[44] The level of glycosylated albumin in diabetic patients has been reported to average more than double that of normal controls.[45–47] Similarly, other serum proteins undergo non-enzymatic glycosylation in vitro and in vivo, both in animals and in man.[48,49] The level

Table 10-2. Nonenzymatic Glycosylation of Proteins*

Protein	Function	Glycosylation Site	Carbohydrate
Red cell membranes	hemoglobin regulation	lysine (lys)	ketoamine
Hemoglobin	O_2 transport		
$\quad$ A$_{1c}$	"	N-term valine B chain	1-deoxy-fructose
$\quad$ A$_o$ heterogeneous	"	unspecific, lys ($\alpha + \beta$), N-term-α chain	glucose
Peripheral nerve myelin	nerve conductivity	lys	ketoamine ϵ-hexitolyl-lysine
Tubulin	axonal transport	lys	ketoamine
Crystallins α, β, γ	transmission of light	lys	ϵ-hexitolyl-lysine
Albumin	transport	lys-189	glucose, ketoamine
Low density lipoprotein	lipid transport	lys	glucose, ketoamine
Collagen	tissue structure	lys-OH-lys	ϵ-hexitolyl-lysine ϵ-hexitolyl-OH-lys ketoamine
Glomerular basement membrane	renal filtration barrier	lys	ϵ-hexitolyl-lysine

*Modified from Monnier et al.[42a]

of these glycoproteins is elevated in diabetics in proportion to the degree of hyperglycemia. Currently, studies are seeking to determine whether similar glycosylated derivatives are present in other tissues subject to diabetic complications.

For a discussion of the practical use of HbA$_1$ and A$_{1c}$ in evaluating the degree of control of diabetes, see Chapters 16, 19, and 24.

Platelets

Platelets from diabetic subjects have been reported to exhibit various functional and biochemical abnormalities, including increased platelet adhesion, greater sensitivity to several aggregating agents, and accelerated synthesis of thrombogenic prostaglandin derivatives. These findings have prompted speculation that abnormalities in platelet behavior may play a role in the development of obliterative microvascular disease in diabetes.[50]

It should be noted, however, that proliferative retinopathy has developed in patients who have defects of platelet function such as von Willebrand's disease. This suggests that diabetic platelet-rich plasma prepared for in-vitro assay may have been artifactually enriched with a subpopulation of more reactive platelets due to other blood factors that affect the conditions of assay which employ centrifugation.[51] Moreover, the non-physiologic laboratory assay conditions under which platelets have been studied prevent these data from being directly extrapolated to the intact organism. As yet, no convincing evidence has been presented to support in vivo platelet dysfunction.[52]

Participation of platelets in clot formation begins with their adhesion to exposed subendothelial components of the blood vessel wall. Although several investigators have observed increased platelet adhesiveness in diabetic patients,[53] adhesion assays utilizing a rotating glass bulb or glass beads in a column are notorious for being difficult to perform and imprecise.[54] Proper interpretation of published data is made even more difficult by the fact that fibrinogen and other plasma proteins known to be elevated in diabetes, influence the results of these assays. Along these lines, it is interesting to note that the addition of glucose in vitro increases the adhesion of both normal and diabetic platelets.[55] Adhesion experiments using a physiologic substrate such as basement membrane might result in more relevant data for this important aspect of platelet physiology.[56]

After platelets adhere to the exposed subendothelium, they undergo aggregation, a process which has both a surface and an intracellular component. The surface reaction, the so-called primary wave of aggregation, occurs in response to low concentrations of such stimuli as adenosine diphosphate (ADP) and epinephrine, and is reversible. At higher concentrations of these stimuli, and in the presence of collagen, platelets undergo irreversible aggregation and, at the same time, release stored intracellular thrombogenic substances. This irreversible reaction is the secondary wave of aggregation. Increased second-phase aggregation has been observed in diabetics in response to ADP, epinephrine, arachidonic acid, and collagen.[53,57-62] Increased release of platelet factors 3 and 4, two accelerators of the coagulation process, has also been reported in various subgroups of diabetic patients during the secondary wave of aggregation.[54] Results obtained in individual diabetic patients range from normal to extremely abnormal, and there appears to be no clear-cut association between abnormalities of second-phase aggregation and the class of diabetes. However, there may well be a good correlation between this value and the level of hyperglycemia, since increased second-phase aggregation can be corrected by strict diabetic control, as confirmed by blood glucose determinations near mealtimes, by degree of glycosuria, and by HbA$_{1c}$ assays.[63] Plasma factors that enhance ADP-induced platelet aggregation have been observed in 50% of unselected male diabetics,[64] and the initial characterization of this activity has recently been carried out.[65] The failure of other groups[57,66] to confirm ADP-induced platelet hyperaggregation has been attributed to methodologic differences.[64] Levels of plasma beta thromboglobulin, a platelet-specific protein that is released during the aggregation process, are also elevated in diabetics.[67]

Increased aggregation of diabetic platelets may be mediated by alterations in the activities of thromboxane synthetase in platelets and of prostacyclin synthetase in blood vessel endothelial cells. Thromboxane synthetase converts the cyclic endoperoxide prostaglandins G$_2$ and H$_2$ to thromboxanes A$_2$ and B$_2$, both of which are potent stimulators of platelet clumping and arterial constriction. Prostacyclin synthetase transforms these same endoperoxides to prostacyclin, a compound which blocks the effect of the thromboxanes.[68] Because the thromboxanes and prostacyclin have diametrically opposing actions, it is thought that the balance between the two processes may determine the formation of the platelet plug. Drugs that inhibit prostaglandin synthesis have been shown to reverse the enhanced second-phase aggregation of diabetic platelets.[59] Moreover, platelets from diabetic patients exhibit increased synthesis of prostaglandin-E-like material in response to several aggregating agents; the rate and extent of metabolism of arachidonic acid to prostaglandin-E-like material is significantly greater in diabetics than in nondiabetic controls.[69] ADP-induced biosynthesis of thromboxane A$_2$ is also enhanced in diabetic platelets.[70] There was a significantly higher net synthesis of prostaglandins in whole blood obtained from diabetic children.[71] Some preliminary studies indicate that the degree of thromboxane B$_2$ synthesis is directly proportional to the plasma glucose level at the time of the study.[64] However, other workers[72] have found no difference in thromboxane B$_2$ synthesis between diabetics and normal subjects. Together, these findings suggest that increased synthesis of prostaglandins may, in part, mediate the abnormal aggregation response of diabetic platelets. In addition, marked decreases in prostacyclin activity have been observed in tissues of diabetic animals and man.[73-75] Prostacyclin levels were less than one-half of normal in both aorta and renal cortex of diabetic experimental animals.[73,74] Insulin treatment restored these values to normal.[76] Similar reductions in prostacyclin levels have been observed in venous tissue from juvenile-onset diabetics.[75] Plasma concentrations of the prostacyclin metabolite, 6-keto-PGF$_1\alpha$, are unchanged in diabetic tissues, however.[72,77]

Increased amounts of lipid phosphorus, together with alterations in the fatty acid pattern of various phospholipids, have been reported in diabetic platelets.[78] Phosphorylation of endogenous platelet proteins is also enhanced in some diabetic patients.[79] Diabetic platelets have also been shown to exhibit increased myosin-adenosine triphosphatase activity.[80] However, at present, the significance of these findings is unclear.

PLASMA PROTEINS

Various plasma protein abnormalities have been reported in diabetes. Particular attention has been focused on proteins which contribute to plasma viscosity, as well as those which are involved in the formation and dissolution of blood clots. Although it has been postulated that alterations in these processes might play a role in the pathogenesis of diabetic vasculopathy, as yet there has been no direct evidence to support this theory. Nevertheless, a significant association has been noted between the diabetic state and several factors that could interfere with microcirculatory flow.

Levels of the blood glycoproteins fibrinogen, haptoglobin, beta-lipoprotein, ceruloplasmin, and alpha$_2$-macroglobulin have been shown to be elevated in diabetic patients.[81-83] These increases in glycoproteins, particularly fibrinogen and haptoglobin, cause plasma viscosity to rise by as much as 16% at low shear-rates, thus increasing the flow resistance of whole blood.[83-86] Increased fibrinogen and alpha$_2$-globulin levels also foster enhanced red cell aggregation.[6,7] Although diabetics who have either proliferative retinopathy or nephropathy show the most striking increases in plasma viscosity and erythrocyte aggregation,[6,7,83-85] this association most likely reflects the greater degree of hyperglycemia in these patients. Decreases in these elevated blood glycoprotein levels correlate with the use of regular insulin[81] and with the normalization of blood glucose values.[82] Glycoprotein levels are most significantly correlated with the presence or absence of recent hypoglycemic symptoms. Patients reporting hypoglycemia have a significantly lower level of all the glycoproteins studied thus far. The association of near-normal glycoprotein values with recent hypoglycemic symptoms (an indicator of short-term blood glucose control), rather than with hemoglobin A_{1c} levels (a measure of integrated glycemic control over several weeks),[66] suggests that alterations in plasma glycoproteins of diabetics occur fairly rapidly.

Increases in coagulation factors VIII and V have also been reported in diabetes.[87] This observation has prompted speculation that a hypercoagulable state might be involved in the evolution of diabetic vascular complications. Strong support for this hypothesis has come from recent studies of fibrinogen survival and turnover rate in diabetic patients.[88] These studies demonstrated a reduction in the survival of autologous radioiodinated fibrinogen in adult-onset diabetes, indicating that consumption of fibrinogen increases at hyperglycemic levels commonly observed in outpatients. Once euglycemia was achieved, this abnormality was rapidly normalized. Although the administration of antiplatelet agents during the hyperglycemic period did not restore fibrinogen survival, the infusion of heparin normalized the fibrinogen kinetics of hyperglycemic patients. This finding suggests that thrombin coagulation factors XI, IX, X, and/or the alpha globulin antithrombin III may be involved in decreasing fibrinogen survival in diabetics.

Antithrombin III plays an important regulatory role in hemostasis by adsorbing thrombin released during clot formation and by inhibiting its effect on fibrinogen. Deficiencies of this protein have been reported in maturity-onset diabetics, and may contribute to a hypercoagulable state.[89–91] Increased antithrombin III levels have been observed in juvenile diabetics, however.[92] There are no published studies as yet showing a correlation between antithrombin III levels and blood glucose values. Turnover data to differentiate the relative roles of synthetic versus degradative defects are also currently unavailable. Finally, the effect of nonenzymatic glycosylation on bioactivity is still unknown.

The glycoprotein plasma cofactor of platelet function, von Willebrand factor (vWF), may play an important role in the platelet abnormalities that have been observed in diabetics (discussed in detail above). Elevated levels of vWF, believed to play a role in both the adhesion and aggregation of platelets, have been reported in diabetic patients, and these increases correlated with the degree of platelet aggregation in at least one study.[57,62,93–96] Enhanced vWF activity, in turn, appears to be promoted by growth hormone[59,97] and may be inhibited by insulin.[98] Studies of spontaneous and high cholesterol diet-induced arteriosclerosis in pigs have provided indirect evidence that increases in vWF contribute to the development of diabetic vascular disease. Significant arteriosclerotic plaques developed in 1 to 3 years in normal animals but not in those with homozygous von Willebrand's disease (i.e., lacking vWF). Similar results were obtained when the pigs were fed diets high in cholesterol.[99]

In addition to increased plasma viscosity and coagulability, changes in the fibrinolytic system may contribute to the pathogenesis of diabetic vasculopathy. Blood fluidity is maintained not only by the carefully regulated activity of coagulation factors, but also by the precise coordination of humoral factors, which remove fibrin deposited in blood vessels. An activator substance must be released from vascular endothelium in order for plasmin, the enzyme that digests fibrin, to be converted from its inactive circulating precursor, plasminogen. The fibrinolytic activity of diabetic blood is significantly below normal,[100] and the fibrinolytic response to venous occlusion is also diminished, perhaps due to decreased release of plasminogen activator.[101] These abnormalities are most marked in diabetics who have retinopathy, although no systematic attempt has been made to determine whether these findings correlate with the degree of hyperglycemia. The elevations in serum protease inhibitors such as alpha-2-macroglobulin that have been reported to occur in diabetics may also contribute to the decreased degradation of fibrin and other proteins.[102] Recent histologic studies suggest that fibrin deposition may play a role in the development of microvascular damage in diabetics.[103,104]

The alterations in levels and/or activities of plasma proteins that are associated with hyperglycemia may provide further illustrations of overutilization of glucose in diabetes. The enhanced availability of sugar-nucleotide precursors of glycoproteins may preferentially stimulate their synthesis.[105] The rate of protein secretion in isolated, perfused livers from diabetic rats is only one-third that in livers from nondiabetic rats, while glycoprotein production is twice as great.[106] This may be the result of either increased synthesis of new glycoproteins or enhanced glycosylation of existing proteins.

Circulating plasma proteins may also undergo further glycosylation via a non-enzymatic reaction comparable to the glycosylation of hemoglobin. Glycosylation of each of the major molecular weight classes of serum protein results when human serum is incubated with glucose. In addition, glycosylated albumin has been isolated and quantitated from both normal and diabetic human serum.[44–47] Diabetic plasma contains higher levels of these glycoproteins, since their rate of formation is a function of the ambient glucose concentration.[48,49,107] Since the carbohydrate moiety of vWF is the most important determinant of its interaction with platelets,[108] and the carbohydrate moiety of clotting factor V is crucial to its role in coagulation,[109] it is conceivable that enhanced glycosylation of such proteins could increase their biologic activity. Changes in type and/or quantity may also be partly responsible for the altered pattern of plasma protein degradation observed in diabetics. Ordinarily, there is a general correlation between isoelectric points of serum proteins and their rates of degradation. However, this relationship is abolished in diabetic animals.[110] Further study is necessary to elucidate the biochemical mechanisms by which hyperglycemia causes these abnormalities in plasma proteins.

For further discussion of blood changes in diabetes from a somewhat different perspective, see Chapter 37.

CATARACTS

Cataract, opacification of the ocular lens, is more prevalent and occurs at an earlier age in diabetics than in the normal population. The development of cataracts is especially rapid in a number of experimental diabetic animals, and, occasionally, in severe juvenile-onset diabetics. The biochemical mechanisms underlying the formation of nondiabetic cataracts have been studied in both humans and experimental animals. Dische and Zil[111] were the first to observe that there was a greater number of disulfide bonds in the proteins of human cataractous lenses than in normal lens proteins, which reflects markedly increased sulfhydryl oxidation. A number of other investigators have since confirmed the association between increased disulfide bonds and cataract formation in humans and have also demonstrated this relationship in animals.[112-116] Since disulfide bonds can act as intermolecular cross-links, it has been suggested that these bonds are involved in the polymerization of lens proteins to high molecular weight aggregates. Based on theoretic considerations, Benedek[117] has proposed that cataracts may result from the scattering of light produced by protein aggregates with molecular weights over 50×10^6 daltons. The molecular weights of aggregates found in human cataracts, as well as in lenses of normal, older subjects, range from 50×10^6 to 200×10^6 daltons.[118,119]

Lenses from diabetic and galactosemic rats contain similar disulfide-bonded high-molecular-weight protein aggregates that are capable of scattering light.[120] It has been suggested that the increased tendency of lens proteins to undergo sulfhydryl oxidation, which is due to enhanced non-enzymatic glycosylation, may facilitate the formation of these high-molecular-weight aggregates.[41,42] The lens, like other tissues subject to diabetic complications, does not require insulin for glucose transport. As a result, hyperglycemia would increase glucose concentration within the lens.

Increased levels of aldoses and ketoses would cause more frequent interactions with amino groups of lens proteins which, in turn, would lead to enhanced formation of stable Amadori or Heyns rearrangement products similar to that observed with hemoglobin A_{1c}. These altered lens proteins form disulfide bonds more readily than do normal lens proteins. Since there is little or no replacement of the major lens proteins (α, β, and γ crystallins,) during the life-span of the individual, the total amount of glycosylated protein in the lens would increase continually over time. It has also been suggested that the yellow-brown pigments found in lens proteins from human cataracts represent further rearrangements of the sugar-protein adducts, analogous to the thoroughly investigated non-enzymatic browning that develops in stored foods.[121] Other long-lived proteins, such as collagen, would also be expected to accumulate browning products.

van Heyningen and Kinoshita and colleagues have explored another mechanism that may be involved in the pathogenesis of diabetic cataract.[122-124] In the lens, the enzyme aldose reductase catalyzes the reduction of aldoses such as glucose and galactose to their corresponding sugar alcohols. Since polyols do not readily diffuse across cell membranes, elevated amounts of glucose in the diabetic lens would result in an intracellular accumulation of sorbitol. It is thought that the accumulation of polyol within the cells produces osmotic swelling and eventually disrupts cell architecture. An associated abnormality in electrolyte transport leads to an influx of sodium ions, which is believed to increase edema and thus accelerate lens opacification. Thus far, the strongest evidence in support of this hypothesis is the finding that several drugs which significantly inhibit aldose reductase retard the development of cataracts in diabetic and galactosemic rats.[125-127]

For a discussion of cataracts from a clinical standpoint, see Chapter 29.

DIABETIC NEPHROPATHY

Functional and Morphologic Changes

The renal disease associated with chronic diabetes is manifested clinically by continuous proteinuria and a decreasing glomerular filtration rate (GFR). There is a correlation between the severity of these clinical features and the degree of glomerular basement membrane (GBM) thickening. The width of GBM in diabetics is normal at the onset of the disease but after several years of sustained metabolic derangement, it becomes increasingly thicker.[128,129] This continual thickening over many years causes progressive occlusion of glomerular capillaries, leading to chronic renal failure. Thus, the accumulation of basement membrane material that has altered filtration properties constitutes the ultimate structural and functional abnormality underlying diabetic nephropathy. Although a great deal of information has been obtained about the biochemistry of GBM (see below), the progression of events from abnormal glucose homeostasis to the late manifestations of diabetic renal disease has not yet been elucidated.

Certain studies have characterized early functional and morphologic changes in diabetes, some of which may contribute to the development of diabetic renal disease. Glomerular filtration rate and filtration fraction (GFR/renal plasma flow) rise at the onset of diabetes, and are normalized by intensive insulin treatment.[130] Soon after the onset of diabetes, excretion of urinary proteins that have molecular weights ranging from 44,000 to 150,000 daltons also increases significantly.[131] Excretion rates of urinary albumin are elevated in newly-diagnosed, poorly-controlled juvenile diabetics; these may be normalized by strict blood glucose control.[130] Similar changes have been observed both in diabetic rats[132,133,133a] and longer-duration insulin-dependent human diabetics who have no clinical manifestations of renal disease.[133b] Such patients also excrete abnormally large amounts of albumin in response to exercise,[130] when there is a higher glomerular filtration pressure. The amount of albumin excreted becomes progressively larger with increasing duration of diabetes.[134]

Renal clearance of neutral dextran polymer is similarly elevated in newly-diagnosed juvenile diabetics, and returns to normal after several weeks of effective insulin therapy.[130,135] Since the clearance of high-molecular-weight dextran is not markedly increased, it is unlikely that alterations in renal function reflect changes in the size-selective properties of the glomerular filtration barrier. Rather, these alterations appear to be due primarily to increased filtration pressure across the glomerulus.[130,135,136] The pronounced increase in actomyosin-like material in the mesangium, which is specific for diabetes,[137,138] may be a contributing factor, since contractile proteins in the mesangium may play an important role in regulating glomerular blood flow and ultrafiltration.[139]

Interrupting glomerular blood flow for short periods in normal rats causes a marked increase in glomerular permeability.[140] If permeability is significantly influenced by hemodynamic factors, the hematologic abnormalities in diabetes that favor microvascular stasis (discussed earlier) might induce intermittent changes in permeability in a non-homogeneous pattern that is consistent with the characteristics of diabetic glomerulopathy. Since fixed negative charges in the glomerular capillary wall also markedly influence glomerular permeability to anionic serum proteins,[141] decreased sialic acid in diabetic glomeruli[142] might also allow increased passage of appropriately charged serum components. Whatever the mechanism of increased glomerular permeability in diabetes may be, immunohistochemical studies have shown that several serum proteins are present in glomerular and muscle capillaries and in muscle basement membranes of diabetics. The immunofluorescent pattern for IgG, albumin, and fibrin was the same as that observed using heterologous antibasement membrane antiserum which indicates the presence of these proteins in the basement membranes.[143] The rapid accumulation of such extravasated serum proteins could provide an explanation for the remarkable rate of structural changes that occur early in the course of human and experimental diabetes. A few weeks after the acute onset of the disease, there are significant increases in renal size, glomerular tuft volume, capillary luminal volume, and capillary filtration surface area.[134,144–146] Many of these abnormalities can be reversed by appropriate insulinization.

Isotransplantation of the kidneys from rats that have been diabetic for 6 months into normal rats causes IgG, IgM, and C3 to disappear from the mesangium and halts glomerular mesangial thickening.[147] Glomerular basement membrane (GBM) thickness is unchanged, however,[148] reflecting the slow GBM turnover rates.[149] The accumulation of serum proteins or their degradation products in the glomerulus as a result of increased glomerular permeability, together with excess fibrin due to decreased fibrinolysis (discussed above), may contribute to the capillary occlusion and progressive glomerular dropout characteristic of chronic diabetes. Non-enzymatically glycosylated plasma proteins (also discussed above) may play a particularly important role in this process, especially if enhanced glycosylation decreases the susceptibility of these proteins to proteolysis.[150] A connection between plasma protein glycosylation and diabetic renal disease is suggested by a report that repeated intravenous injection of glycosylated plasma proteins resulted in glomerular basement membrane thickening in nondiabetic animals.[151]

Expansion of ''basement membrane-like'' mesangial matrix material seems to inhibit localized mechanisms for clearing mesangial macromolecules.[152,153] Such mesangial dysfunction leads to a more rapid thickening of the GBM in nondiabetic animals.[154] Although GBM thickening occurs before mesangial changes in juvenile diabetics,[128] the resulting mesangial damage may ultimately contribute to the long-term accumulation of proteins in the diabetic glomerulus.

Basement Membrane Chemistry and Metabolism

Chemical Characterization of Glomerular Basement Membrane (GBM). During the past 2 decades, much information has been obtained about the chemical structure of normal GBM. Although much of the basic structural research was done on bovine GBM, compositional studies performed in several mammalian species have produced similar findings.[149,155,156] Basement membrane is composed of collagen-like glycoprotein material, which is especially rich in the amino acids glycine, hydroxyproline, and hydroxylysine. However, this collagen-like material clearly differs from fibrillar collagen, in that it contains 3 times as much hydroxylysine and large amounts of half-cystine, as well as having a significant carbohydrate content.[105] A recent analysis of the C1q component of complement has shown that the amino acid composition of this soluble serum protein is similar to that of basement membrane.[157] The sugar constituents of the basement membrane are divided between two distinct types of carbohydrate units.[158] The first type is a complex asparagine-linked heteropolysaccharide that contains galactose, mannose, fucose, sialic acid, and glucosamine on relatively more polar, less collagen-like portions of the peptide chain. These heteropolysaccharide units are not unique to basement membrane, having been described in various other glycoproteins.[159] The second type of carbohydrate unit is comprised of a glucose-galactose disaccharide unit attached to hydroxylysine. The ratio of the number of the two carbohydrate units in basement membrane is 1:10. Hydroxylysine is formed by the enzymatic hydroxylation of lysine residues that are already incorporated in nascent or released polypeptides; 80% of this hydroxylysine is then linked to galactose, and, afterwards, to glucose by sequential sugar transferases to form the disaccharide-hydroxylysine complex[160] (See Fig. 10–2).

After its disulfide cross-links are reduced, basement membrane can be solubilized in sodium dodecylsulfate (SDS) or urea and then separated into a large number of components ranging in molecular weight from 25,000 to more than 200,000 daltons.[161-163] The amino acid and carbohydrate composition of these subunits varies considerably.

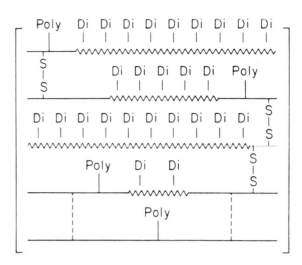

Fig. 10–2. Schematic representation of a section of glomerular basement membrane, showing the relation of the disaccharide (Di) and heteropolysaccharide (Poly) units to each other and to the peptide chain. (From Spiro[160] with permission from author and publisher).

Some of these subunits are rich in collagen-like amino acids, whereas others contain more polar amino acids such as half-cystine, tyrosine, and aspartic acid. Most of these subunits contain the two types of carbohydrate units, but in different proportions. This compositional heterogeneity occurs even in material of the same molecular size. Although the reason for this subunit polydispersity is unknown, it has been demonstrated that these various polypeptides do not result from proteolytic cleavage of a high-molecular-weight component during membrane isolation.[164,165] Instead, they may be the products of limited physiologic in vivo proteolytic digestion of a smaller number of large basement membrane subunits.[105] It has been proposed that basement membrane is composed mainly of three α1 collagen chains, and should therefore be designated "Type IV" collagen. However, since such material represents less than 2% of purified glomerular basement membrane after pepsin digestion, this proposed model cannot be correct.[166]

Compositional Changes in Diabetic GBM. Several groups of investigators have performed compositional studies on human GBM from normal and diabetic subjects.[167-170] Beisswenger and Spiro were the first to demonstrate an increase in basement membrane protein in glomeruli from patients with chronic diabetes who showed histologic evidence of nephropathy. In addition, the composition of this material was found to be distinctly different from that of normal basement membrane.[155,171,172] When compared with normal GBM, membrane from diabetics showed an increase in hydroxylysine content and a proportional decrease in lysine content, such that the sum of the two was constant. Diabetic membrane also exhibited elevations in glucose and galactose, reflecting a rise in hydroxylysine-linked disaccharide residues. In addition, there were smaller, yet significant, increases in hydroxyproline and glycine, as well as decreases in valine and tyrosine. These results suggest that there is an increase in hydroxylysine-rich subunits composed of collagen-like amino acids in the diabetic basement membrane. Canivet et al. have subsequently confirmed these findings[170] (See Table 10–3).

Although these alterations were not observed in two other studies,[168,169] a significant reduction in the half-cystine and sialic acid content of diabetic glomerular basement membrane was noted. Canivet et al. also observed decreases in half-cystine and sialic acid content.[170] These apparent discrepancies among studies may be explained by important differences, in both the technique for preparing basement membrane and in the diabetic kidneys chosen for study.

Biosynthesis and Degradation of GBM. The compositional abnormalities discussed above may be responsible in part, for the altered filtration properties of the diabetic GBM that eventually result in clinically significant, continuous, and nonselective proteinuria. It has been proposed that increased glycosylation might interfere with polypeptide packing and/or hydroxylysine-derived cross-link formation which, in turn, might lead to an increased effective pore size of the basement membrane.

The proteinuria associated with diabetic renal disease almost certainly is due to alterations in the structures of the GBM and perhaps other components of the glomerular filtration barrier. However, the progressive decrease in glomerular filtration rate (GFR) with chronic renal failure is caused by the accumulation of excessive amounts of basement membrane material, which results in glomerular capillary occlusion. This excessive accumulation of GBM in diabetics may reflect an increase in the synthesis of basement membrane, a decrease in degradation, or a combination of the two. There may be an increase in the synthesis of all subunits of basement membrane or, alternatively, there may be a relative overproduction of only certain basement membrane components. Similarly, degradation of the basement membrane may be uniform and nonspecific, or it may affect selected portions only. If such differential subunit effects do occur, they may account for the qualitative, as well as quantitative changes in diabetic GBM. Compositional analysis, however, would be a relatively insensitive method for detecting these alterations.

Metabolic studies of GBM have of necessity been restricted to animals. Although some investigators have questioned the appropriateness of the rat model,[173] recent studies have demonstrated that there are increases in protein content and protein/DNA ratio in the kidneys of experimentally diabetic rats, as well as significant thickening of the GBM.[174–178] There is a highly significant, positive correlation between these abnormalities and the degree of hyperglycemia. Kidney ribosome preparations from rats rendered diabetic with alloxan, streptozotocin, or anti-insulin serum, incorporate amino acids into protein at a greater rate than do kidney ribosomes from normal rats.[179] This finding suggests that diabetes results in increased synthesis of kidney proteins.

Biosynthetic Enzyme Activities. Studies of enzymes involved in the formation of the hydroxylysine-linked disaccharide units of GBM provide indirect evidence for accelerated GBM biosynthesis in diabetic kidneys. These units are synthesized by a series of specific enzymatic, postribosomal steps. In the first step, lysine residues that have already been incorporated into the newly synthesized peptide chains are hydroxylated.[160] There is evidence to suggest that the activity of lysyl hydroxylase is increased in the soluble fraction of kidney homogenates from diabetic animals, and is normalized by prior insulin therapy.[180,181]

After the hydroxylation of lysine, the synthesis of hydroxylysine-linked disaccharide units is completed through the sequential participation of two highly specific glycosyltransferases. The first is a galactosyltransferase whose function is limited to transferring galactose from the activated sugar UDP-galactose to hydroxylysine in high-molecular-weight components.[182] The second is a glucosyltransferase, which acts only to transfer glucose from UDP-glucose to hydroxylysine-linked galactose.[183] Both galactosyltransferase and glucosyltransferase have been thoroughly investigated in the rat renal cortex, utilizing "glucose-free" and "disaccharide-free" GBM as the enzyme substrates. The activity of the specific basement membrane glucosyltransferase varies markedly with the age of the animals, reaching a peak at 9 days and then decreasing rapidly as the rat matures.[183] Spiro and Spiro found that the activity of this enzyme is significantly greater in the renal cortex from rats diabetic for 1 to 5 months than from age-matched normal controls; this difference widens with increasing duration of the disease. Following treatment of the animal with insulin, the enzyme activity level falls to normal if done in earlier, but not in later, stages of diabetes. Simultaneous measurements of glucosyltransferase activity in several other tissues of diabetic rats show no abnormalities.[184] Moreover, activity of another renal glyco-

Table 10–3.   Compositional Changes in Diabetic Glomerular Basement Membrane

	Increased	Decreased	Reference Nos.
Hydroxylysine	+		(151, 169, 171, 172)
Lysine		−	(151, 171)
Glucose-galactose disaccharide	+		(151, 171)
Hydroxyproline	+		(151, 168, 169, 171)
Glycine	+		(151, 168, 169, 171, 172)
Half-cystine		−	(168, 169, 172)
Sialic acid		−	(169, 172)
Heparan sulfate		−	(202a)

syltransferase involved in the synthesis of the basement membrane heteropolysaccharide unit is also not abnormal. The increase in glucosyltransferase activity observed in the kidneys of diabetic animals probably reflects a specific increase in GBM synthesis.

This finding was questioned by another group of investigators,[185] who found no changes in renal glucosyltransferase activity in rats after either 4 or 12 weeks of streptozotocin-induced diabetes, although only three animals diabetic for 12 weeks, were studied. However, other workers[186] have subsequently confirmed that glucosyltransferase activity is increased in the renal cortex from diabetic rats (See Table 10–3).

Amino Acid Incorporation. While studies of glucosyltransferase activity provide indirect evidence to support the theory that glomerular basement membrane synthesis is accelerated in diabetes, investigations of amino acid incorporation into glomerular proteins furnish more direct evidence. Several studies of basement membrane biosynthesis in both normal and diabetic animals have utilized incubations of isolated rat glomeruli.[187–191] However, these studies must be interpreted cautiously because of serious problems inherent in the metabolic properties of these preparations.

Price and Spiro have performed in vivo studies of normal glomerular basement membrane turnover,[149] utilizing injected tracer doses of tritiated amino acids. Basement membrane turnover rates were ascertained from the decay in the specific activity of a number of incorporated amino acids. Data from studies of proline and hydroxyproline indicate that the turnover rate of GBM is extremely slow compared with that of other glomerular proteins, and approaches the turnover rate of fibrillar collagen. Additional data from the specific activity of other amino acids suggest that GBM polypeptide components with different compositions may have different turnover rates.

Brownlee and Spiro[192] have extended these analyses to include comparative data from diabetic and normal rats by utilizing injected tracer doses of tritiated proline. In this in vivo animal experiment, radioactivity was incorporated into the basement membrane of both normal and diabetic rats at a slow rate. There was a period of near-constant specific activity of proline and hydroxyproline after maximum incorporation was reached. However, the specific activity of both these amino acids in the diabetic basement membrane was nearly twice that observed in normal basement membrane. These findings are consistent with the accelerated rates of GBM polypeptide synthesis and proline-hydroxylation in diabetes, and provide the most direct evidence to date in support of this hypothesis.

Pathogenesis of Basement Membrane Changes in Diabetes. The following considerations provide a conceptual framework for understanding the alterations in basement membrane synthesis that develop in diabetes. Only certain tissues need insulin for the intracellular transport of glucose.[193] Other tissues, including those of the kidney, do not. Due to hyperglycemia, there is an elevated glucose concentration within the cells of such tissues. High glucose concentrations in glomerular cells could have two significant effects on basement membrane synthesis: First, since glycosylation of hydroxylysine in the peptide chain is a postribosomal synthetic step, availability of sugar substrate may well be an important rate-limiting factor in the regulation of basement membrane disaccharide synthesis.[194] The increased levels of the activated sugar [uridine diphosphate glucose (UDPG)], in the renal cortex of diabetic rats are consistent with this theory.[195]

Second, in addition to augmenting the synthesis of disaccharide units, high glucose concentrations may also directly influence the synthesis and secretion of the peptide portion of basement membrane. The data derived from diabetic rats discussed above support this concept. Additional confirmation of this effect of hyperglycemia on disaccharide synthesis comes from in vitro studies of collagen secretion by human skin fibroblasts.[196] Cells incubated in a high glucose medium secreted more collagen than those growing in glucose at a physiologic concentration. Amino acid analysis of the extracted collagen indicated that each sample of the high glucose medium contained twice as much hydroxyproline as the physiologic glucose medium. Isotope incorporation studies confirmed that incubating fibroblasts in a medium equivalent to a plasma glucose concentration of 300 mg/dl produces increased collagen synthesis.

The conclusion that can be drawn from the preceding discussion is that increased synthesis plays a central role in the excessive accumulation of GBM in the diabetic kidney. While there may also be decreased degradation of GBM, at present there is no direct evidence to support this. However, the findings of a decrease in glomerular beta-glycosidase activities[197,198] and the presence of urinary glomerular basement membrane-like protein[199] in diabetic rats, do suggest that decreased glycoprotein catabolism may, in fact, be involved in the accumulation of GBM. Since increased glycosylation may also decrease the susceptibility of glycoproteins to proteolysis,[150] increased synthesis of disaccharide units or non-enzymatic glycosylation may also alter the degradation of basement membrane peptides. The elevation of serum protease inhibitors associated with diabetes may also contribute to this process.[102]

Glomerular Proteoglycans

Of great interest and importance are studies of proteoglycans in diabetic nephropathy. These heteropolysaccharide polymers may help to organize the quaternary structure of collagen, influence glomerular permeability, exert an antithrombotic effect, and possibly bind certain macromolecules such as circulating immune complexes.[200] The recent localization of proteoglycans at the interface between cell-surface membranes and the GBM[201,202,202a] suggests that quantitative or qualitative alterations in these molecules may play a role in the pathologic processes that initiate diabetic nephropathy. As was discussed earlier, glomerular permeability to anionic serum proteins is markedly affected by fixed negative charges in the glomerular capillary wall.[141] Since proteoglycans are highly charged polyanions, diabetes-induced alterations in these molecules could well result in the development of the proteinuria characteristic of diabetic nephropathy. It is also possible that increased synthesis of proteoglycans and the deposition of these polyanions next to or within the GBM could contribute to the glomerulosclerosis associated with progressive renal failure in diabetes. Most samples of proteoglycans isolated from the renal cortexes of a heterogeneous group of human diabetics exhibited slight increases in the percentage of heparan sulfate, and varying increases in hyaluronic acid, depending on the degree of histologic abnormality.[203] Analyses of proteoglycans extracted from glomerular and/or GBM preparations might be

more meaningful than those performed on renal cortex homogenates, however, since diabetic nephropathy is primarily a glomerular disease. Significant glomerular changes might otherwise be masked by dilution from other locations, or might be artificially suggested by altered proteoglycans in nonglomerular extracellular matrix.

For further discussion of diabetic nephropathy, see Chapter 30.

DIABETIC RETINOPATHY

Regional ischemia appears to be a central mechanism in the pathogenesis of diabetic retinopathy.[204–206] Initially, there is a compensatory increase in both the volume of retinal blood and segmental retinal blood flow, accompanied by autoregulatory dilatation of retinal blood vessels.[205,207] As background retinopathy progresses, there is a corresponding further increase in retinal blood flow,[207] although this process may ultimately aggravate regional hypoperfusion by shunting red blood cells through some capillaries and only plasma through others (so-called skimming). Eventually, gradual, focal occlusion of capillaries limits the autoregulatory response. At first, retinal hypoxia, inadequately compensated for by increased blood flow, results in the formation of microaneurysms. As the severity of retinal hypoxia increases, new vessel formation ensues.[207–209]

In the early stages of diabetes, prior to the development of significant capillary occlusion, the autoregulatory dilatation of retinal vessels can be rapidly reversed by adequate insulin therapy.[3] This early, reversible retinal ischemia in the diabetic probably is the result of certain major pathophysiologic processes. Within days after the onset of diabetes, there is a breakdown of the blood-retinal barrier, which is detectable clinically by vitreous fluorophotometry.[210–213] The severity of this breakdown in diabetics correlates with the degree of metabolic control, as well as with the duration of the disease.[211] Early in the course of diabetes, this increased capillary permeability can be significantly reduced by normalization of blood glucose levels with insulin.[212,213]

It appears that the morphologic basis for these alterations in permeability is a diabetes-induced opening in the endothelial cell tight junctions.[214] Another factor that may contribute to the breakdown of the blood-retinal barrier is decreased active transport of osmotically-active substances from the extravascular to the intravascular space, since diabetes results in a decreased number of micropinocytotic vesicles in capillary endothelial cells.[215] These functional abnormalities of endothelial cells may, in turn, be magnified by selective loss of accompanying pericytes, possibly as the result of polyol-induced toxicity (discussed in the section on neuropathy below).[216]

Eventually, increased retinal capillary permeability results in the clinical manifestations of intraretinal edema and hard exudate formation. Before these changes can be detected clinically, however, accumulation of fluid in the retina may significantly impair oxygen diffusion. Increased polyol pathway activity (see below), which in the lens is associated with fluid accumulation, might intensify intraretinal edema. It is also possible that intraretinal edema and increased capillary extravasation are caused by a simple Starling mechanism, since decreases in intraocular pressure occur with elevations in blood glucose,[217] and asymmetric diabetic retinopathy has been associated with asymmetry in intraocular tensions.[218] Removal of edema fluid from the retina may also be impeded, since thickening of basal membrane[219] creates a greater barrier to diffusion at the pigment epithelial cell layer.

In addition to increased capillary permeability and the resulting intraretinal edema, reversible diabetic hematologic abnormalities may also contribute to early diabetic retinal ischemia. These hematologic abnormalities discussed in detail above would tend to produce reductions in oxygen delivery to retinal tissue per unit of blood flow. The increased oxygen affinity of the diabetic red cell may result in hypoxia at the venous end of the capillary bed, even in the presence of normal arterial oxygen pressure. Hyperviscosity due to elevated levels of plasma proteins such as fibrinogen may cause microvascular "sludging" which would decrease local blood flow and increase intracapillary pressure, thus facilitating leakage of serum contents into the tissue space. Increased platelet and red cell aggregability, decreased erythrocyte deformability, enhanced coagulability, and decreased fibrinolysis would all produce qualitatively similar effects, some of which would be additive, and others, possibly synergistic.

Although increased capillary permeability as well as the above-mentioned hematologic abnormalities can be reversed to a certain degree by insulin treatment, they may be contributing factors in the gradual development of irreversible capillary occlusion. Extravasated growth-promoting substances from plasma may play a role in the thickening of retinal capillary basement membrane.[220,221] Endothelial cell proliferation and swelling may result from local hypoxia.[205,206,222] These structural alterations in capillary basement membrane and endothelial cells would tend to decrease the size of capillary lumina, further reducing local blood flow and exacerbating any already-existing regional ischemia. In addition, increased capillary basement

membrane thickening would limit the autoregulatory response of retinal blood vessels to intermittent hypoxia. Ultimately, progressive capillary occlusion and intensifying regional ischemia would result in microaneurysms, cotton-wool spots, and neovascularization.

Panretinal photocoagulation has been shown to be beneficial in treating proliferative diabetic retinopathy.[223] It has been speculated that this partial destruction of the retina may decrease its oxygen demands and thereby reduce the degree of ischemia. See also Chapter 29.

ROLE OF GROWTH HORMONE

It has been proposed that abnormal growth hormone secretion, which has been observed in some diabetic patients, may contribute in various ways to the development of microangiopathy.[224] Mean 24-hour growth hormone levels in ambulatory juvenile diabetics have been reported to average 3 times those of normal subjects.[225,226] However, subsequent investigators found no differences in 24-hour serum growth hormone levels between obese, maturity-onset diabetics and obese nondiabetics,[227] nor between clinically stable non-obese diabetics and weight-matched controls.[228] It has been reported also that diabetics with proliferative retinopathy have a markedly enhanced growth hormone response to insulin-induced hypoglycemia[229] and to exercise[230] as compared to diabetics without retinopathy. However, it is likely that these variations in growth hormone response merely reflect differing levels of diabetic control among these groups, since the degree of growth hormone elevation correlates with the level of hyperglycemia.[231]

During a 10-year follow-up period, no retinopathy was observed in a group of glucose-intolerant, growth hormone-deficient dwarfs, matched for sex, age, and duration of diabetes, with a group of diabetics without such deficiency.[232–234] Although these observations suggest that increases in growth hormone may play a role in the pathogenesis of diabetic microangiopathy, this theory would seem to be invalidated by the report of a diabetic patient, deficient in growth hormone, who had severe nephropathy, neuropathy, and retinopathy.[235] Persons with excess growth hormone as in acromegaly, but no diabetes, do not develop diabetic tissue changes.

Serum levels of somatomedins (proteins which mediate the growth-promoting actions of growth hormone) are decreased in both diabetic animals and humans.[236–239] There is an inverse correlation between hemoglobin A_{1c} levels and serum somatomedin activity.[239] Levels of a somatomedin inhibitor may also be increased in diabetes.[240–242] Since insulin facilitates growth hormone-mediated somatomedin release by the liver,[243] the increased growth hormone levels observed in some diabetics may merely represent compensatory adjustments to alterations in somatomedin levels.

The renal mesangial cell dysfunction characteristic of diabetic rats can be duplicated experimentally by administering growth hormone to normal animals.[244] Administration of growth hormone also produced a 2½ times greater increase in glomerular basement membrane thickness in the kidneys of diabetic rats.[175] Supplementing normal serum with growth hormone in vitro causes aortic smooth-muscle cell proliferation to be significantly enhanced.[245] Further investigation is needed to elucidate such processes.

DIABETIC NEUROPATHY

Morphologic and Functional Changes

Numbness and paresthesias are the most common symptoms of peripheral neuropathy in the diabetic person. These symptoms are believed to be the clinical manifestations of changes in nerve electrophysiology, and to reflect altered morphologic and biochemical properties of the axon and the myelin sheath.[246] Alterations in nerve electrophysiology can be detected in the majority of diabetic animals and humans, even in the absence of clinically apparent symptoms. Decreased sensory and motor nerve conduction velocities are found in untreated, newly diagnosed diabetics,[247,248] and similar abnormalities rapidly develop in animals rendered diabetic.[249] Treatment to correct glucose intolerance improves nerve function in both animals and humans.[247,249–251] Decreased conduction velocity in myelinated neurons is thought to be caused by diminished internodal resistance, which would reduce current density at the nodes and delay excitation.[252,253] Such alterations in internodal resistance could be produced by changes in myelin composition, as discussed below. Paranodal separation of myelin lamellae,[254] due perhaps to accumulation of interlamellar fluid,[255] could also reduce internodal resistance and nerve conduction velocity. Alterations in axon structure and/or metabolism may result in other electrophysiologic and clinical abnormalities.

Morphologic studies of peripheral nerves from diabetics characteristically show segmental demyelination.[256] The extent and degree of this pathologic finding in rats are directly correlated with the severity and duration of hyperglycemia.[257,258] Segmental demyelination either may reflect primary metabolic impairment of Schwann cells or, alternatively, may be secondary to prior axonal dysfunction.[256,258] In either case, loss of myelin would contribute to the slowing of nerve conduction velocity.

A long time before segmental demyelination can be demonstrated histologically in diabetic animals, it is possible to detect alterations in the internodal myelin membrane structure via freeze-fracture electron microscopy.[259] When nerve conduction velocity first becomes impaired, significant reductions in the number of intramembranous particles can be observed on both the inner and outer myelin surfaces of diabetic nerves. Insulin treatment prevents both the alteration in myelin structure and the decreased rate of nerve conduction.[259]

Endoneurial edema with resultant shrinkage of axons and Schwann cells is another morphologic alteration that develops early in the peripheral nerves of diabetic rats.[260] Increased water content in the endoneurial space of diabetic nerves produces a 30% decrease in Schwann cell volume. Although this fluid accumulation could have deleterious effects on endoneurial capillary blood flow, as yet there has been no evidence of such adverse consequences. It has been suggested that increased endoneurial fluid in the nerves of diabetic rats is due to a greater permeability of endoneurial vessels,[261] but this concept has not been substantiated by subsequent investigations. Therefore, it seems unlikely that extravasation of protein into the endoneurial space is a factor in the pathogenesis of diabetic neuropathy.[262,263] It has also been suggested that the permeability of nodal gap substance is increased in the diabetic nerve.[264] Since nodal gap substance prevents the diffusion of potassium ions away from the node, increases in this material could result in alterations in membrane resting potential or ion conductances. If these alterations, in turn, led to excessive generation of action potentials in sensory nerves, paresthesias might be expected to occur.

Recent quantitative electromyographic studies have also demonstrated that there is extensive axonal dysfunction in diabetic patients.[265] Axonal degeneration, the morphologic basis for this functional abnormality, has been observed in both diabetic humans and animals.[258,260,266–268] Loss of large and small myelinated and unmyelinated fibers is evident in patients with diabetic neuropathy early in the course of the disease. Although this finding suggests that loss of axon fibers may be an important factor in the development of peripheral nerve dysfunction, it has been shown, based on calculations of fiber diameter, that 20 to 30% decreases in conduction velocity are primarily the result of causes other than fiber loss.[266] Axonal degeneration and decreased diameter of myelinated axons have also been noted in diabetic rats.[258,260,269,270] Fewer such structural alterations are found in insulin-treated diabetic animals than in untreated animals.

In addition to the abnormalities in myelin and axons discussed above, alterations in neuronal vasculature also occur in diabetes. Nerves from diabetic patients and rats have been reported to exhibit marked thickening of basement membranes surrounding intra- and perineural vessels.[258,266,268,271] Frequently there is also hyperplasia of endothelial cells in small vessels, and in some cases, these excess cells completely occlude the vessel lumen.[271] A series of biopsies of sural nerves from diabetic patients with clinical and electrophysiologic evidence of neuropathy showed fibrin deposition in the microvasculature.[104] These abnormalities in the microvasculature of peripheral nerves may diminish blood flow through small vessels which, in turn, may result in regional ischemia or microinfarcts that could contribute to neuronal dysfunction and degeneration.

Biochemical Alterations

Myelin Composition. By dry weight, 75% of peripheral nerve is composed of myelin. For this reason, the composition and rate of synthesis of myelin in diabetics have been the focus of much attention in the search for the biochemical basis of peripheral neuropathy. Myelin is a complex lipid composed of triglyceride, sphingomyelin, cholesterol, cerebrosides, and proteins. There have been reports of abnormalities in almost all of these components in diabetics,[272,273] in association with decreased nerve conduction velocity. Decreased triglyceride levels have been observed in diabetic sciatic nerves,[272] and are perhaps the result of defective incorporation of acetate into fatty acids.[274] These alterations may be due to a reversible 70% decrease in the activity of the enzyme, acetic thiokinase.[274] There is a decrease in the amount of cerebrosides synthesized in diabetes, as well as a change in the type of cerebrosides produced, with a marked reduction in the incorporation of saturated fatty acids.[275]

No compositional alterations have been observed in myelin protein of diabetics, but the total amount of protein in peripheral nerve myelin from diabetic patients is significantly reduced.[276] This may be due either to altered protein synthesis or degradation. The rate at which amino acids are incorporated into some myelin proteins has been found to be decreased in diabetic animals,[277] while the activities of two peripheral nerve proteinases seem to be enhanced.[276] However, the importance of these findings is unclear, since peripheral nerve myelin from animals with experimental diabetes is less susceptible to proteolytic digestion.[278] Since glycosylation appears to result in a decreased rate of proteolysis

of ribonuclease B relative to the nonglycosylated ribonuclease A,[150] in diabetes there may be an alteration in the carbohydrate content of myelin that alters myelin degradation. It has been speculated that the localization of myelin glycoproteins to the external surface of the myelin sheath enhances their potential role in specific interactions in the process of myelination or myelin maintenance.[279] However, no specific analyses of the carbohydrate and glycopeptide contents of diabetic peripheral nerve myelin have yet been performed.

The relative contributions of these individual abnormalities to diabetic neuropathy are unknown. However, together they produce major physicochemical changes which result in abnormal peripheral myelin sedimentation and electrophoretic patterns in human diabetic nerves.[280] The relationship between these changes and altered nerve conduction velocities in diabetics has yet to be elucidated.

Sorbitol Pathway. The Schwann cell sheath and certain other mammalian tissues are unique in their ability to synthesize free (nonphosphorylated) fructose for a variety of metabolic uses.[281] This biosynthetic pathway, termed the sorbitol pathway, consists of two reactions: (1) glucose is reduced to its corresponding sugar alcohol, sorbitol, by the enzyme aldose reductase, with reduced nicotinamide-adenine dinucleotide phosphate (NADPH) as the electron-donating coenzyme; and (2) the sorbitol molecule is oxidized to fructose by the enzyme sorbitol dehydrogenase and nicotinamide-adenine dinucleotide (NAD^+). Several tissues of diabetic animals and humans, including the lens, retina, arterial wall, erythrocytes, and Schwann cell sheath have been reported to have significantly increased concentrations of both sorbitol and fructose[216,281-285] (See Fig 10–3).

The activity of the sorbitol pathway is controlled by the ambient glucose concentration in those tissues that do not require insulin for glucose transport, such as the nerve,[286] since the Km for aldose reductase is within the range of physiologic glucose concentrations.[287] Increased activity of the sorbitol pathway has been implicated in the pathogenesis of neuropathy in acute diabetic cataracts, diabetic macrovascular disease, and diabetic peripheral neuropathy.[282,287,288] Hyperglycemia and the resultant increased sorbitol pathway activity are associated with decreased oxygen uptake in the peripheral nerves of diabetic animals.[289,290] It is conceivable that this impaired tissue oxygen delivery may play a role in the development of neurologic dysfunction. Increased sorbitol pathway activity in diabetic nerves may also contribute to the accumulation of endoneurial fluid discussed in the previous section. Insulin treatment returns the ac-

$$\text{Glucose} + \text{NADPH} \xrightarrow[\substack{\text{Aldose} \\ \text{reductase}}]{} \text{Sorbitol} + \text{NADP}$$

$$\text{Sorbitol} + \text{NAD} \xrightarrow[\substack{\text{Sorbitol} \\ \text{dehydrogenase}}]{} \text{Fructose} + \text{NADH}$$

Fig. 10–3. The sorbitol pathway.

tivity of the sorbitol pathway toward normal[291] and prevents the slowing of nerve conduction in diabetic animals.[249,282] Although the administration of an aldose reductase inhibitor also prevents the accumulation of sorbitol in the sciatic nerves of diabetic animals,[292] these compounds have not yet demonstrated any sustained beneficial effects on nerve conduction velocity in diabetes.

Myoinositol. Myoinositol, one of the cyclic nonreducing isomers of glucose, may play an important role in such nerve cell functions as the transport of electrolytes and amino acids and the transmission of nerve impulses. Recent findings suggest that alterations in the metabolism of this axon phospholipid precursor may be responsible for some of the functional abnormalities seen in diabetics with peripheral neuropathy.[249,256,293] The myoinositol content of sciatic nerve is decreased in severely diabetic animals.[249,294] There are also reductions in the content and rate of synthesis of phosphatidylinositol from myoinositol,[294–296] as well as decreases in the activities of CDP-diglyceride-inositol transferase and phosphatidylinositol 4-phosphate kinase in diabetic sciatic nerves.[297,298] When dietary supplementation restores nerve myoinositol content to normal, conduction velocity increases.[249,294,299] However, because these observations have not been confirmed in animals with less severe diabetes, their specific relevance to human diabetic neuropathy is unclear.

There is a marked increase in urinary myoinositol excretion, as well as an apparent decrease in intracellular transport of myoinositol in uncontrolled human diabetics.[293] Appropriate insulin treatment corrects these abnormalities.[249,293] The decreased motor conduction velocity and vibratory perception threshold in symptomatic or asymptomatic diabetic patients were not affected by dietary myoinositol supplementation,[300–302] although sensory nerve conduction velocity may have improved slightly.[300,301] The clinical significance of these observations has not yet been determined.

Axoplasmic Transport. Many enzymes and substrates used for the synthesis of neurotransmitters in the nerve axon actually originate in the neuronal cell body. From here they are transported via axoplasmic flow to distal locations. Recently, it has been suggested that decreased axoplasmic transport of certain critical proteins may cause peripheral nerve dysfunction in diabetes.[303,304] There are marked reductions in both fast and slow axonal flow in diabetic rats. The rate of acetylocholinesterase transport is decreased by 32%, and the rate of choline acetylase transport in cholinergic neurons by 41%.[303] There is a similar reduction in axoplasmic transport of noradrenaline in noradrenergic neurons.[304] Retrograde axonal flow of transported glycoproteins is also decreased early in diabetes.[305] These changes could have adverse effects on action potential regeneration at the synapse, which could result in decreases in propagated conduction velocity. Insulin treatment effectively reverses all of the observed decreases in axoplasmic transport.

See Chapter 31 for further discussion of diabetic neuropathy.

DIABETIC COMPLICATIONS AND THE DEGREE OF METABOLIC DYSFUNCTION

The foregoing discussions have detailed evidence from a variety of morphologic, physiologic, and biochemical studies which strongly implicate insulin deficiency and its metabolic sequelae in the pathogenesis of diabetic complications. From such data alone, however, it is difficult to draw clinically valid conclusions as to whether diabetic control is effective in preventing these complications. Dogs rendered diabetic develop retinal microaneurysms, hemorrhages, and exudates, as well as diffuse glomerulosclerosis with typical nodular lesions.[306,307] Good control of hyperglycemia with insulin inhibits the development of these lesions.[308–310] In spontaneously diabetic Macaca nigra, the degree of atherosclerosis is directly proportional to the severity of the hyperglycemia and insulin deficiency.[311] However, the clinical relevance of these findings is unclear since the diabetes-like lesions in these animals are similar but not identical to those seen in man.

The assumption implicit in the previous discussions is that perfect metabolic control of diabetes, although extremely difficult or impossible to achieve at present, would prevent the development of diabetic complications. Do the levels of excellent diabetic control which can be attained with current therapies (multiple doses of insulin daily or the use of insulin "pumps") approximate normal glucose homeostasis sufficient to favorably alter the long-term clinical course of the disease? Clinical studies that would conclusively answer this question are difficult to design and execute, due to formidable methodologic problems.[312] Nevertheless, the available clinical data strongly confirm the effectiveness of excellent control.

Retrospective Clinical Studies. In a review of the world literature in 1964, encompassing over 300 publications on this topic, Knowles found that 51 of 85 studies gave results interpreted as showing a correlation between the degree of diabetic control and the development of complications; results in 26 led to the opposite conclusion, and those of 8 were regarded as inconclusive.[313] However, in 40 studies, the data were insufficient to support the claims of the authors. The remaining 45 studies did not randomly allocate treatment and used unacceptable measures of diabetic control. In 39 of these, descriptions of the methods used to interpret the results were unsatisfactory.[314] Thus, it was not possible to make a final critical appraisal of the consensus at that time.

Most clinical studies have been retrospective in nature. One of the largest was a Joslin Clinic study involving 451 patients who had become diabetic before the age of 20 and who had had the disease for 10 to 36 years.[315] Only one of the 101 patients with diabetic nephropathy was in the group who had achieved excellent or good control. In patients with diabetes of 20 years' duration or more, nephropathy was present in 3% of those in the excellent/good group, compared with 32% of those in the fair/poor control group. Similarly, the incidence of grade 3 retinopathy (on a scale of 4) was 3% of the patients who had had diabetes for 20 or more years and who were in excellent or good control, and 31% in those with diabetes of similar duration who were in fair or poor control. There was no evidence of grade 4 (proliferative) retinopathy in the excellent/good control group. Other retrospective studies have demonstrated a significant diminution of motor nerve conduction velocity in poorly-controlled diabetics.[250] There is a close relationship between the degree of this impairment in conduction velocity and the levels of fasting plasma glucose and glycosylated hemoglobin.[248] Thickness of muscle capillary basement membrane (MCBM) is normal in juvenile diabetics who have been extremely well controlled for 5 to 20 years, while increased MCBM thickness is evident in diabetics after less than 5 years of poor control.[316]

Some retrospective studies have not found any relationship between diabetic control and the incidence of complications.[317,318] However, the criteria used to define "good control" in these studies are similar to those established for the "fair control" groups in other studies, which perhaps obscures the real difference between excellent/good and fair/poor control groups. Attempts to compare the conclusions reached by institutions that have different therapeutic philosophies have been seriously undermined by the failure to differentiate between clinic patients as a whole and the subgroup of excellent/good control patients.

It has been suggested that persons with one type of diabetes may be able to achieve good control more easily than those with another type, and hence any observed correlation between the degree of diabetic control and the incidence of complications may, in fact, reflect the heterogeneous nature of the disease rather than differences in control.[319] On the other hand, since most of the measures of diabetic control do not adequately reflect the degree of minute-to-minute metabolic regulation, the failure to observe such correlations may be due simply to the insensitivity of the variable chosen to measure diabetic control. Both of these difficulties might be avoided by replacing the independent variable "degree of control" with "therapeutic regimen."

One large retrospective study which has a direct bearing on this issue compared all diabetics diagnosed in Malmö, Sweden, from 1922 to 1935 with those diagnosed from 1936 to 1945.[320] The former group was given multiple daily injections of short-acting insulin and was placed on a strict dietary regimen. The latter group primarily received a single daily injection of longer-acting insulin coupled with a less precise dietary program. All of the patients from both groups had been diabetic for more than 15 years. Even though the 1936–1945 group had had diabetes for 8.6 fewer years than the 1922–1935 group, the single injection group had more than a 6-fold greater incidence of grades 3 and 4 retinopathy and nearly a 2-fold greater incidence of nephropathy than those observed in the multiple injection group. Retrospective analyses confirm that the great majority of diabetic patients surviving for 20 to 40 years[321] and for 40 years or more[322,323] have also received multiple daily insulin injections for most of their diabetic lives.

All the retrospective studies discussed up to this point support the contention that better insulinization decreases the occurrence of diabetic complications. However, these conclusions have been based on data characterizing the available survivors of an undefined initial study population. More valid information would be obtained if such studies included in their analyses deaths occurring prior to the study and possible transfers from one initial cohort to another. In one large retrospective study that does consider these factors, relatively well-controlled juvenile diabetics survived significantly longer than moderately- or poorly-controlled patients.[324] In fact, survival of the well-controlled group was not significantly different from that of the general population.

Prospective Clinical Studies. Many of the problems in design inherent in retrospective analyses can be avoided by prospective clinical studies, which have provided important new information about the relationship between diabetic control and complications. In one 20-year prospective study, mortality of patients who were poorly controlled was 2.5 times that of patients who achieved better control.[325] A prospective study undertaken by Kohner et al.[326] evaluated the relationship between the progression of established diabetic retinopathy and the degree of diabetic control achieved during the study period. Only patients in "very good" control seemed to be protected against a worsening of microaneurysms, hemorrhages, and new vessel formation. Similarly, Miki et al.[327] found that over a 6-year period established retinopathy was 3 times more likely to progress in patients with poor control than in patients with good control.

The conclusions of one randomized, prospective study comparing the effects of single- and multiple-dose daily insulin regimens on the progression of retinopathy in insulin-dependent diabetics have generated a great degree of controversy. Patients who received multiple insulin injections were said to have a slower increase in the development of microaneurysms than patients given single insulin injections, despite the fact that there were only minimal differences in mean urinary glucose excretion and fasting blood glucose levels between the two groups.[328] However, a subsequent analysis of the published data[329] raised questions about the statistical significance of these conclusions. Later follow-up data from the original study appeared to reconfirm the previously published results.[330] Other prospective studies have reported an association between very good diabetic control and decreases in the frequency, degree, and progression of proteinuria in diabetic patients.[331,332] Proteinuria wors-

ened in only 9% of the good control group during a 6-year period, compared with 22% of the poor-control group.

The largest, most comprehensive prospective investigation of the relationship between diabetic control and long-term complications included 4400 patients observed between 1947 and 1973.[333-336] Close to 2800 of these patients were followed continuously from the time that diabetes was diagnosed, thereby permitting both the incidence and prevalence of specific complications to be ascertained. This study is unique in fulfilling virtually all of the design prerequisites for deriving valid conclusions from the data obtained.[335] The study found a strong correlation between the incidence and prevalence of complications and the known duration but not the inherent severity of diabetes. Rather, a higher prevalence and incidence of neuropathy, retinopathy, and nephropathy were associated with poor control, assessed cumulatively over the years. Furthermore, the annual rate of occurrence of these complications was clearly and separately related to the diabetic control achieved during the preceding year, regardless of the prior degree of control.

This study, together with the others discussed in this chapter, offers compelling evidence for the need to maintain blood glucose levels of diabetic patients as close to normal as possible. At present, the most effective regimens for achieving this therapeutic goal utilize multiple daily insulin injections in conjunction with home self-monitoring of blood glucose.[337] Ongoing research efforts are attempting to develop methods for delivering insulin which will simulate normal physiology even more closely.[338-341] See Chapter 19 for further discussion.

REFERENCES

1. Johnson, I.S.: Human insulin from recombinant DNA technology. Science *219*:632, 1983.
2. Crofford, O.: Diabetes Data. DHEW Pub. No. (NIH) 78–1468. Bethesda, National Diabetes Data Group. 1977. pp. 8–11.
2a. Brownlee, M., Cerami, A.: The biochemistry of the complications of diabetes mellitus. Ann. Rev. Biochem. *50*:385, 1981.
2b. Alberti, K.G.M.M., Press, G.M.: The biochemistry of the complications of diabetes mellitus. In: H. Keen, J. Jarrett (Eds.): Complications of Diabetes. 2nd Ed. London, Edward Arnold, Ltd., 1982, pp. 231–271.
2c. D.E. McMillan, J. Ditzel (Eds.): Proceedings of a conference on diabetic microangiopathy. (Introduction and 16 papers with index.) Diabetes *32*(Suppl. 2):1–104, (June) 1983.
3. Ditzel, J.: Functional microangiopathy in diabetes mellitus. Diabetes *17*:388, 1968.
4. Ditzel, J., Standl, E.: The problem of tissue oxygenation in diabetes mellitus. I. Its relation to the early functional changes in the microcirculation of diabetic subjects. Acta Med. Scand. *578* (Suppl.):49, 1975.
5. Little, H.L., Sacks, A.H., Krupp, M., et al.: Abnormal

hemorrheology in the pathogenesis of diabetic microangiopathy. Cong. Int. Diab. Fed. 8th, *280*:176, 1973.

6. Little, H., Sacks. A., Vassiliadis, A., Greer, R.: Current concepts on pathogenesis of diabetic retinopathy: a dysproteinemia. Tr. Am. Ophth. Soc. *75*:397, 1977.
7. Little, H.L., Sacks, A.: Role of abnormal blood rheology in the pathogenesis of diabetic retinopathy. Tr. Am. Acad. Ophth. Otol. *83*:522, 1977.
8. Paulsen, E.: Discussion of papers presented by Drs. Colwell and Waitzman. Metabolism *28* (Suppl. 1):407, 1979.
9. Schmid-Schönbein, H., Volger, E.: Red-cell aggregation and red-cell deformability in diabetes. Diabetes *25* (Suppl. 2):897, 1976.
10. McMillan, D.E., Utterback, N.G., La Puma, J.: Reduced erythrocyte deformability in diabetes. Diabetes *26* (Suppl. 1):369, 1977.
11. McMillan, D.E., Utterback, N.G., La Puma, J.: Reduced erythrocyte deformability in diabetes. Diabetes *27*:895, 1978.
12. Baba, Y., Kai, M., Kamada, T., et al.: Higher levels of erythrocyte membrane microviscosity in diabetes. Diabetes *28*:1138, 1979.
13. Miller, J.A., Gravallese, E., Bunn, H.F.: Nonenzymatic glycosylation of erythrocyte membrane proteins. Relevance to diabetes. J. Clin. Invest. *65*:896, 1980.
14. Chandramouli, V., Carter, J.R., Jr.: Cell membrane changes in chronically diabetic rats. Diabetes *24*:257, 1975.
15. Baba, Y., Kai, M., Setoyama, S., Otsuji, S.: The lower levels of erythrocyte surface electric charge in diabetes mellitus. Clin. Chim. Acta *84*:247, 1978.
16. Paulsen, E.P., Koury, M.: Hemoglobin A₁c levels in insulin-dependent and -independent diabetes mellitus. Diabetes *25* (Suppl. 2):890, 1976.
17. Bagdade, J.D., Stewart, M., Walters, E.: Impaired granulocyte adherence. A reversible defect in host defense in patients with poorly controlled diabetes. Diabetes *27*:677, 1978.
18. Selam, J.L., Clot, J., Andary, M., Mirouze, J.: Circulating lymphocyte subpopulations in juvenile insulin-dependent diabetics. Correction of abnormalities by adequate blood glucose control. Diabetologia *16*:35, 1979.
19. Nolan, C.M., Beaty, H.N., Bagdade, J.D.: Further characterization of the impaired bactericidal function of granulocytes in patients with poorly controlled diabetes. Diabetes *27*:889, 1978.
20. Edelman, G.M.: Surface modulation in cell recognition and cell growth. Some new hypotheses on phenotypic alteration and transmembranous control of cell surface receptors. Science *192*:218, 1976.
21. Nicolson, G.L., Poste, G.: The cancer cell: dynamic aspects and modifications in cell-surface organization. N. Engl. J. Med. *295*:197, 1976.
22. Chandramouli, V., Williams, S., Marshall, J.S., Carter, J.R., Jr.: Cell surface changes in diabetic rats. Studies of lectin binding to liver cell plasma membranes. Biochim. Biophys. Acta *465*:19, 1977.
23. Chandramouli, V., Lundt, B., Carter, J.R., Jr.: Isolation of major cell-surface glycoproteins from normal and diabetic rat-liver membranes. FEBS Letts. *104*:309, 1979.
24. Carter, J.R., Jr., Chandramouli, V.: Glycoprotein changes in liver plasma membranes from diabetic rats. Diabetes *26* (Suppl. 1):366, 1977.
25. Trivelli, L.A., Ranney, H.M., Lai, H.-T.: Hemoglobin components in patients with diabetes mellitus. N. Engl. J. Med. *284*:353, 1971.
26. McDonald, M.J., Shapiro, R., Bleichman, M.: Glycosylated minor components of human adult hemoglobin. Purification, identification and partial structural analysis. J. Biol. Chem. *253*:2327, 1978.
27. Shapiro, R., McManus, M., Garrick, L., et al.: Nonenzymatic glycosylation of human hemoglobin at multiple sites. Metabolism *28*:427, 1979.
28. Koenig, R.J., Blobstein, S.H., Cerami, A.: Structure of carbohydrate of hemoglobin A₁c. J. Biol. Chem. *252*:2992, 1977.
29. Bunn, H.F., Shapiro, R., McManus, M.: Structural heterogeneity of human hemoglobin A, due to nonenzymatic glycosylation. J. Biol. Chem. *254*:3892, 1979.
30. Gabbay, K.H., Sosenko, J.M., Banuchi, G.A., et al.: Glycosylated hemoglobins: increased glycosylation of hemoglobin A in diabetic patients. Diabetes *28*:337, 1979.
31. McDonald, M.J., Bleichman, M., Bunn, H.F., Noble, R.W.: Functional properties of the glycosylated minor components of human adult hemoglobin. J. Biol. Chem. *254*:702, 1979.
32. Standl, E., Kolb, H.J.: 2,3-Diphosphoglycerate fluctuations in erythrocytes reflecting pronounced blood glucose variations. *In vivo* and *in vitro* studies in normal, diabetic and hypoglycemic subjects. Diabetologia *9*:461, 1973.
33. Ditzel, J., Jaeger, P., Standl, E.: An adverse effect of insulin on the oxygen-release capacity of red blood cells in nonacidotic diabetics. Metabolism *27*:927, 1978.
34. Ditzel, J.: Improved erythrocytic oxygen release following a dietary supplement of calcium diphosphate to diabetic and healthy children. Diabetologia *10*:363, 1974.
35. Ditzel, J., Dyerberg, J.: Hyperlipoproteinemia, diabetes, and oxygen affinity of hemoglobin. Metabolism *26*:141, 1977.
36. Bunn, H.F., Gabbay, K.H., Gallop, P.M.: The glycosylation of hemoglobin: relevance to diabetes mellitus. Science *200*:21, 1978.
37. Bunn, H.F., Haney, D.N., Gabbay, K.H., Gallop, P.M.: Further identification of the nature and linkage of the carbohydrate in hemoglobin A₁c. Biochem. Biophys. Res. Commun. *67*:103, 1975.
38. Stevens, V.J., Vlassara, H., Abati, A., Cerami, A.: Nonenzymatic glycosylation of hemoglobin. J. Biol. Chem. *252*:2998, 1977.
39. Koenig, R.J., Peterson, C.M., Kilo, C., et al.: Hemoglobin A₁c as an indicator of the degree of glucose intolerance in diabetes. Diabetes *25*:230, 1976.
40. Koenig, R.J., Peterson, C.M., Jones, R.L., et al.: Correlation of glucose regulation and hemoglobin A₁c in diabetes mellitus. N. Engl. J. Med. *295*:417, 1976.
41. Cerami, A., Stevens, V.J., Monnier, V.M.: Role of nonenzymatic glycosylation in the development of the sequelae of diabetes mellitus. Metabolism *28* (Suppl. 1):431, 1979.
42. Stevens, V.J., Rouzer, C.A., Monnier, V.M., Cerami, A.: Diabetic cataract formation: potential role of glycosylation of lens crystallins (nonenzymatic glycosylation/sulfhydryl oxidation). Proc. Natl. Acad. Sci. USA *75*:2918, 1978.
42a. Monnier, V.M., Cerami, A.: Nonenzymatic glycosylation and browning in diabetes and aging. Studies on lens proteins. Diabetes *31* (Suppl. 3):57, 1982.
43. Chang, A.Y., Noble, R.E.: Estimation of HbA₁c-like glycosylated proteins in the kidneys of streptozotocin-diabetic and control rats. Diabetes *28*:408, 1979.
43a. Vlassara, H., Brownlee, M., Cerami, A.: Nonenzymatic glycosylation of peripheral nerve protein in diabetes mellitus. Proc. Natl. Acad. Sci. USA *78*:5190, 1981.
44. Day, J.F., Thorpe, S.R., Baynes, J.W.: Nonenzymatically glycosylated albumin; *in vitro* preparation and isolation from normal human serum. J. Biol. Chem. *254*:595, 1979.

45. Dolhofer, R., Wieland, O.H.: Glycosylation of serum albumin: elevated glycosyl-albumin in diabetic patients. FEBS Letts. *103*:282, 1979.
46. Gundersen, H.J., Mogensen, C.E., Seyer-Hansen, K., et al.: Early and late changes in the diabetic kidney. Adv. Neph. *8*:43, 1979.
47. Dolhofer, R., Wieland, O.H.: Increased glycosylation of serum albumin in diabetes mellitus. Diabetes *29*:417, 1980.
48. McFarland, K.F., Catalano, E.W., Day, J.F., et al.: Nonenzymatic glycosylation of serum proteins in diabetes mellitus. Diabetes *28*:1011, 1979.
49. Yue, D.K., Morris, K., McLellan, S., Turtle, J.R.: Glycosylation of plasma protein and its relation to glycosylated hemoglobin in diabetes. Diabetes *29*:296, 1980.
49a. Goldstein, D.E., Parker, K.M., England, J.D., et al.: Clinical application of glycosylated hemoglobin measurements. Diabetes *31* (Suppl. 2):70, 1982.
50. Harrison, H.E., Reece, A.H., Johnson, M.: Effect of insulin treatment on prostacyclin in experimental diabetes. Diabetologia *18*:65, 1980.
51. Bern, M.M. (Moderator): Discussion of papers presented by Drs. Colwell and Waitzman. Metabolism *28* (Suppl. 1):407, 1979.
52. Abrahamsen, A.: Platelet survival studies in man with special reference to thrombosis and atherosclerosis. Materials and methods. Scand. J. Hematol. *1* (Suppl. 3):9, 1968.
53. Colwell, J.A., Halushka, P.V., Sarji, K.E., Sagel, J.: Platelet function and diabetes mellitus. Med. Clin. N. Am. *62*:753, 1978.
54. Bern, M.M.: Platelet functions in diabetes mellitus. Diabetes *27*:342, 1978.
55. Bridges, J.M., Dalby, A.M., Miller, J.H.D., Weaver, J.A.: An effect of D-glucose on platelet stickiness. Lancet *1*:75, 1965.
56. Freytag, J.W., Dalrymple, P.N., Maguire, M.H., et al.: Glomerular basement membrane. Studies on its structure and interaction with platelets. J. Biol. Chem. *253*:9069, 1978.
57. Bensoussan, D., Levy-Toledano, S., Passa, P., et al.: Platelet hyperaggregation and increased plasma level of von Willebrand factor in diabetics with retinopathy. Diabetologia *11*:307, 1975.
58. Dobbie, J.G., Kwaan, H.C., Colwell, J.A., Suwanwela, N.: Role of platelets in pathogenesis of diabetic retinopathy. Arch. Ophthalmol. *91*:107, 1974.
59. Colwell, J.A., Halushka, P.V., Sarji, K., et al.: Altered platelet function in diabetes mellitus. Diabetes *25* (Suppl. 2):826, 1976.
60. Heath, H., Brigden, W.D., Canever, J.V., et al.: Platelet adhesiveness and aggregation in relation to diabetic retinopathy. Diabetologia *7*:308, 1971.
61. Sagel, J., Colwell, J.A., Crook, L., Laimins, M.: Increased platelet aggregation in early diabetes mellitus. Ann. Intern. Med. *82*:733, 1975.
62. Sarji, K.E., Nair, R.M.G., Chambers, A.L., et al.: Increased levels of von Willebrand factor (vWF) and platelet aggregation in diabetes mellitus. Diabetes *24* (Suppl. 1):398, 1975.
63. Peterson, C.M., Jones, R.L., Koenig, R.J., et al.: Reversible hematologic sequelae of diabetes mellitus. Ann. Intern. Med. *86*:425, 1977.
64. Colwell, J.A., Nair, R.M.G., Halushka, P.V., et al.: Platelet adhesion and aggregation in diabetes mellitus. Metabolism *28* (Suppl. 1):394, 1979.
65. Nair, R.M.G., Van Zile, J., Johnson, J., et al.: Potentiation of platelet aggregation and secretion by purified diabetic plasma factors. Diabetes *28*:385, 1979.

66. Coller, B.S., Frank, R.N., Milton, R.C., Gralnick, H.R.: Plasma cofactors of platelet function: correlation with diabetic retinopathy and hemoglobins A$_{1c}$. Studies in diabetic patients and normal persons. Ann. Intern. Med. *88*:311, 1978.
67. Borsey, D.Q., Dawes, J., Fraser, D.M., et al.: Plasma beta-thromboglobulin in diabetes mellitus. Diabetologia *18*:353, 1980.
68. Marx, J.L.: Blood clotting: the role of the prostaglandins. Science *196*:1072, 1977.
69. Halushka, P.V., Lurie, D., Colwell, J.A.: Increased synthesis of prostaglandin-E-like material by platelets from patients with diabetes mellitus. N. Engl. J. Med. *297*:1306, 1977.
70. Ziboh, V.A., Maruta, H., Lord, J.: Increased biosynthesis of thromboxane A$_2$ by diabetic patients. Eur. J. Clin. Invest. *9*:223, 1979.
71. Chase, H.P., Williams, R.L., Dupont, J.: Increased prostaglandin synthesis in childhood diabetes mellitus. J. Pediatr. *94*:185, 1979.
72. German, G.A., Stampfer, H.G.: Hypothalamic releasing factor for reactive depression. Lancet *2*:789, 1979.
73. Harrison, H.E., Reece, A.H., Johnson, M.: Decreased vascular prostacyclin in experimental diabetes. Diabetologia *15*:(Abstr.) 237, 1978.
74. Idem. Life Sci. *23*:351, 1978.
75. Silberbauer, K., Schernthaner, G., Sinzinger, H., et al.: Decreased vascular prostacyclin in juvenile-onset diabetes (Letter). N. Engl. J. Med. *300*:366, 1979.
76. Haft, D.E., Reddi, A.S.: Glycosyltransferase activity in kidney fractions of normal and streptozotocin-diabetic rats. Biochim. Biophys. Acta *584*:1, 1979.
77. Davis, T.M.E., Mitchell, M.D., Dornan, T.L., Turner, R.C.: Plasma 6-keto-PGF$_{1a}$ concentrations and diabetic retinopathy. Lancet *1*:373, 1980.
78. Nordöy, A., Rödset, J.M.: Platelet phospholipids and their function in patients with juvenile diabetes and maturity onset diabetes. Diabetes *19*:698, 1970.
79. Kranias, G., Kranias, E., Dobbie, G.J., Jungmann, R.A.: Human platelet protein kinases in diabetic retinopathy. FEBS Letts. *92*:357, 1978.
80. Muhlrad, E., Eldor, A., Bar-On, H., Kahane, I.: The distribution of platelet contractile proteins in normal and streptozotocin-diabetic rats. Thromb. Res. *14*:621, 1979.
81. Mitchell, A.A.: Relation between insulin-induced hypoglycemia and serum haptoglobin level. A report from the Boston Collaborative Drug Surveillance Program, Boston University Medical Center. Diabetes *23*:151, 1974.
82. Jonsson, A., Wales, J.K.: Blood glycoprotein levels in diabetes mellitus. Diabetologia *12*:245, 1976.
83. Barnes, A.J., Locke, P., Scudder, P.R., et al.: Is hyperviscosity a treatable component of diabetic microcirculatory disease? Lancet *2*:789, 1977.
84. McMillan, D.E.: Disturbance of serum viscosity in diabetes mellitus. J. Clin. Invest. *53*:1071, 1974.
85. McMillan, D.E.: Two roles for plasma fibrinogen in the production of diabetic microangiopathy. Diabetes *24* (Suppl. 2):438, 1975.
86. Lowe, G.D.O., Lowe, J.M., Drummond, M.M., et al.: Blood viscosity in young male diabetics with and without retinopathy. Diabetologia *18*:359, 1980.
87. Egebert, O.: The blood coagulability in diabetic patients. J. Clin. Lab. Med. *15*:833, 1963.
88. Jones, R.L., Peterson, C.M.: Reduced fibrinogen survival in diabetes mellitus. A reversible phenomenon. J. Clin. Invest. *63*:485, 1979.
89. Banerjee, R.N., Sahni, A.L., Kumar, V., Arya, M.: Antithrombin III deficiency in maturity onset diabetes mellitus

and atherosclerosis. Thromb. Diath. Haemorrh. *31*:339, 1974.

90. Monnier, L., Follea, G., Mirouze, J.: Antithrombin III deficiency in diabetes mellitus: influence on vascular degenerative complications. Horm. Metab. Res. *10*:470, 1978.

91. Gandolfo, G.M., de Angelis, A., Torresi, M.V.: Determination of antithrombin III activities by different methods in diabetic patients. Haemostasis *9*:15, 1980.

92. Corbella, E., Miragliotta, G., Masperi, R., et al.: Platelet aggregation and antithrombin III levels in diabetic children. Haemostasis 8:30, 1979.

93. Almér, L-O, Pandolfi, M., Österlin, S.: The fibrinolytic system in patients with diabetes mellitus with special reference to diabetic retinopathy. Ophthalmologica, Basel *170*:353, 1975.

94. Pandolfi, M., Almér, L-O., Holmberg, L.: Increased von Willebrand antihaemophilic factor A in diabetic retinopathy. Acta Ophthalmol. *52*:823, 1974.

95. Lufkin, E.G., Fass, D.N., O'Fallon, W.M., Bowie, E.J.W.: Increased von Willebrand factor in diabetes mellitus. Metabolism *28*:63, 1979.

96. Gensini, G.F., Abbate, R., Favilla, S., Neri Serneri, G.G.: Changes of platelet function and blood clotting in diabetes mellitus. Thromb. Haemostas. *42*:983, 1979.

97. Sarji, K.E., Levine, J.A., Nair, R.M.G., et al.: Relation between growth hormone levels and von Willebrand factor activity. J. Clin. Endocrinol. Metab. *45*:853, 1977.

98. Graves, J.M., Colwell, J.A., Nair, R.M.G., Sarji, K.E.: The effect of oral glucose on von Willebrand factor activity in normal and diabetic subjects. Clin. Endocrinol. *6*:437, 1977.

99. Fuster, V., Bowie, E.J.W., Lewis, J.C., et al.: Resistance to arteriosclerosis in pigs with von Willebrand's disease. Spontaneous and high cholesterol diet-induced arterio sclerosis. J. Clin. Invest. *61*:722, 1978.

100. Almér, L-O., Nilsson, I.M.: On fibrinolysis in diabetes mellitus. Acta Med. Scand. *198*:101, 1975.

101. Almér, L-O., Pandolfi, M.: Fibrinolysis and diabetic retinopathy. Diabetes *25* (Suppl. 2):807, 1976.

102. Brownlee, M.: α 2-macroglobulin and reduced basement membrane degradation in diabetes. Lancet *1*:779, 1976.

103. Cameron, J.S., Ireland, J.T., Watkins, P.J.: The kidney and renal tract. In: H. Keen, J. Jarrett (Eds.): Complications of Diabetes. London, Edward Arnold Ltd., 1975, p. 120.

104. Timperley, W.R., Ward, J.D., Preston, F.E., et al.: Clinical and histological studies in diabetic neuropathy. A reassessment of vascular factors in relation to intravascular coagulation. Diabetologia *12*:237, 1976.

105. Spiro, R.G.: Search for a biochemical basis of diabetic microangiopathy. Diabetologia *12*:1, 1976.

106. Bar-On, H., Berry, E., Ziv, E.: Glycoprotein synthesis by isolated perfused livers from diabetic and nondiabetic rats. Diabetologia *13*:380, 1977.

107. Day, J.F., Ingebretsen, C.G., Ingebretsen, W.R., Jr., et al.: Nonenzymatic glycosylation of serum proteins and hemoglobin: response to changes in blood glucose levels in diabetic rats. Diabetes *29*:524, 1980.

108. Gralnick, H.R., Coller, B.S., Sultan, Y.: Carbohydrate deficiency of the Factor VIII/von Willebrand factor protein in von Willebrand's disease variants. Science *192*:56, 1976.

109. Saraswathi, S., Colman, R.W.: Role of galactose in bovine factor V. J. Biol. Chem. *250*:8111, 1975.

110. Dice, J.F., Walker, C.D., Byrne, B., Cardiel, A.: General characteristics of protein degradation in diabetes and starvation (protein catabolism/protein molecular size/protein isoelectric point/glycoproteins). Proc. Natl. Acad. Sci. USA *75*:2093, 1978.

111. Dische, Z., Zil, H.: Studies on the oxidation of cysteine to cystine in lens proteins during cataract formation. Am. J. Ophthalmol. *34* No. 5, Part II:104, 1951.

112. Pirie, A.: Color and solubility of the proteins of human cataracts. Invest. Ophthalmol. *7*:634, 1968.

113. Harding, J.J.: Disulphide cross-linked protein of high molecular weight in human cataractous lens. Exp. Eye Res. *17*:377, 1973.

114. Dilley, K.J.: The proportion of protein from the normal and cataractous human lens which exists as high molecular weight aggregates *in vitro*. Exp. Eye Res. *20*:73, 1975.

115. Truscott, R.J.W., Augusteyn, R.C.: The state of sulfhydryl groups in normal and cataractous human lenses. Exp. Eye Res. *25*:139, 1977.

116. Takemoto, L.J., Azari, P.: Isolation and characterization of covalently linked, high molecular weight proteins from human cataractous lens. Exp. Eye Res. *24*:63, 1977.

117. Benedek, G.B.: Theory of transparency of the eye. Appl. Ophthalmol. *10*:459, 1971.

118. Jedziniak, J.A., Kinoshita, J.H., Yates, E.M., et al.: On the presence and mechanism of formation of heavy molecular weight aggregates in human normal and cataractous lenses. Exp. Eye Res. *15*:185, 1973.

119. Jedziniak, J.A., Kinoshita, J.H., Yates, E.M., Benedek, G.B.: The concentration and localization of heavy molecular weight aggregates in aging normal and cataractous human lenses. Exp. Eye Res. *20*:367, 1975.

120. Monnier, V.M., Stevens, V.J., Cerami, A.: Nonenzymatic glycosylation of hemoglobin and lens crystallins. In: S.K. Srivastava (Ed.): Red Blood Cell and Lens Metabolism. v. 9. New York, Elsevier/North Holland Pub. Co., 1980, p. 465.

121. Reynolds, T.M.: Chemistry of nonenzymic browning. II. Adv. Food Res. *14*:167, 1965.

122. Van Heyningen, R.: The sorbitol pathway in the lens. Exp. Eye Res. *1*:396, 1962.

123. Kinoshita, J.H., Merola, L.O., Dikmak, E.: Osmotic changes in experimental galactose cataracts. Exp. Eye Res. *1*:405, 1962.

124. Obazawa, H., Merola, L.O., Kinoshita, J.H.: The effects of xylose on the isolated lens. Invest. Ophthalmol. *13*:204, 1974.

125. Kinoshita, J.H.: Mechanisms initiating cataract formation. Proctor Lecture. Invest. Ophthalmol. *13*:713, 1974.

126. Varma, S.D., Mikuni, I., Kinoshita, J.H.: Flavonoids as inhibitors of lens aldose reductase. Science *195*:1215, 1975.

127. Dvornik, D., Gabbay, K.H., Kinoshita, J.H., et al.: Polyol accumulation in galactosemic and diabetic rats: control by an aldose reductase inhibitor. Science *182*:1146, 1973.

128. Østerby, R.: Diabetic glomerulopathy. A quantitative electron microscopic study of the initial phases. In: R.R. Rodriguez and J. Vallance-Owen (Eds.): Proceedings of the Seventh Congress of the International Diabetes Federation. Buenos Aires, 23–28 August, 1970. Amsterdam, Excerpta Medica, 1971, pp. 793—803.

129. Østerby, R.: Kidney structural abnormalities in early diabetes. In: R.A. Camerini-Davalos, H.S. Cole (Eds.): Vascular and Neurological Changes in Early Diabetes. New York, Academic Press, 1973, pp. 323–340.

130. Mogensen, C.E.: Renal function changes in diabetes. Diabetes *25* (Suppl. 2):872, 1976.

131. Schnider, S., Aronoff, S.L., Tchou, P., et al.: Urinary protein excretion in prediabetic (PD), normal (N), and diabetic (D) Pima Indians and normal Caucasians (NC) (Abstr.). Diabetes *26* (Suppl. 1):362, 1977.

132. Mauer, S.M., Brown, D.M., Matas, A.J., Steffes, M.W.: Effects of pancreatic islet transplantation on the increased urinary albumin excretion rates in intact and uninephrectomized rats with diabetes mellitus. Diabetes 27:959, 1978.

133. Rasch, R.: Prevention of diabetic glomerulopathy in streptozotocin-diabetic rats by insulin treatment. The mesangial regions. Diabetologia 17:243, 1979.

133a. Rasch, R.: Prevention of diabetic glomerulopathy in streptozotocin diabetic rats by insulin treatment. Albumin excretion. Diabetologia 18:413, 1980.

133b. Viberti, G.C., Pickup, J.C., Jarret, R.J., Keen, H.: Effect of control of blood glucose on urinary excretion of albumin and B₂ microglobulin in insulin-dependent diabetes. N. Engl. J. Med. 300:638, 1979.

134. Mogensen, C.E., Østerby, R., Gundersen, H.J.G.: Early functional and morphologic vascular renal consequences of the diabetic state. Diabetologia 17:71, 1979.

135. Parving, H-H., Rutili, F., Granath, K., et al.: Effect of metabolic regulation on renal leakiness to dextran molecules in short-term insulin-dependent diabetes. Diabetologia 17:157, 1979.

136. Hostetter, T.H., Fray, J.L., Brenner, B.M., Green, A.A.: Glomerular dynamics in rats with diabetes mellitus. Kidney Int. 14:725, 1978.

137. Scheinman, J.I., Fish, A.J., Michael, A.F.: The immunohistopathology of glomerular antigens. The glomerular basement membrane, collagen, and actomyosin antigens in normal and diseased kidneys. J. Clin. Invest. 54:1144, 1974.

138. Scheinman, J.I., Steffes, M.W., Brown, D.M., Mauer, S.M.: The immunohistopathology of glomerular antigens. III. Increased mesangial actomyosin in experimental diabetes in the rat. Diabetes 27:632, 1978.

139. Deen, W.M., Robertson, C.R., Brenner, B.M.: Glomerular ultrafiltration. Fed. Proc. 33:14, 1974.

140. Ryan, G.B., Karnovsky, M.J.: Distribution of endogenous albumin in the rat glomerulus: role of hemodynamic factors in glomerular barrier function. Kidney Int. 9:36, 1976.

141. Bennett, C.M., Glassock, R.J., Chang, R.L.S., et al.: Preselectivity of the glomerular capillary wall. Studies of experimental glomerulonephritis in the rat using dextran sulfate. J. Clin. Invest. 57:1287, 1976.

142. Westberg, N.G.: Biochemical alterations of the human glomerular basement membrane in diabetes. Diabetes 25 (Suppl. 2):920, 1976.

143. Cohn, R.A., Mauer, S.M., Barbosa, J., Michael, A.F.: Immunofluorescence studies of skeletal muscle extracellular membranes in diabetes mellitus. Lab. Invest. 39:13, 1978.

144. Kroustrup, J.P., Gundersen, H.J.G., Østerby, R.: Glomerular size and structure in diabetes mellitus. III. Early enlargement of the capillary surface. Diabetologia 13:207, 1977.

145. Rasch, R.: Prevention of diabetic glomerulopathy in streptozotocin diabetic rats by insulin treatment, kidney size and glomerular volume. Diabetologia 13:207, 1977.

146. Østerby, R., Gundersen, H.J.G.: Fast accumulation of basement membrane material and the rate of morphological changes in acute experimental diabetic glomerular hypertrophy. Diabetologia 18:493, 1980.

147. Lee, C.S., Mauer, S.M., Brown, D.M., et al.: Renal transplantation in diabetes mellitus in rats. J. Exp. Med. 139:793, 1974.

148. Steffes, M.W., Brown, D.M., Basgen, J.M., et al.: Glomerular basement membrane thickness following islet transplantation in the diabetic rat. Lab. Invest. 41:116, 1979.

149. Price, R.G., Spiro, R.G.: Studies on the metabolism of the renal glomerular basement membrane. Turnover measurements in the rat with the use of radio labeled amino acids. J. Biol. Chem. 252:8597, 1977.

150. Birkeland, A.J., Christensen, T.B.: Resistance of glycoproteins to proteolysis ribonuclease, A and B compared. J. Carbohydrates, Nucleosides, Nucleotides 2:83, 1975.

151. McVerry, B.A., Hopp, A., Fisher, C., Huehns, E.R.: Production of pseudodiabetic renal glomerular changes in mice after repeated injections of glycosylated proteins. Lancet 1:738, 1980.

152. Mauer, S.M., Steffes, M.W., Michael, A.F., Brown, D.M.: Studies of diabetic nephropathy in animals and men. Diabetes 25 (Suppl. 2):850, 1976.

153. Mauer, S.M., Steffes, M.W., Chern, M., Brown, D.M.: Mesangial uptake and processing of macromolecules in rats with diabetes mellitus. Lab. Invest. 41:401, 1979.

154. Romen, W., Morath, R.: Diffuse glomerulosclerosis—a dysfunction of the mesangium? A morphometric study of the rat's kidney. Virchow. Arch. B Cell Path. 31:205, 1979.

155. Beisswenger, P.J., Spiro, R.G.: Studies on the human glomerular basement membrane. Composition, nature of the carbohydrate units and chemical changes in diabetes mellitus. Diabetes 22:180, 1973.

156. Sato, T., Spiro, R.G.: Studies on the subunit composition of the renal glomerular basement membrane. J. Biol. Chem. 251:4062, 1976.

157. Reid, K.B.M.: A collagen-like amino acid sequence in a polypeptide chain of human Clq (a subcomponent of the first component of complement). Biochem. J. 141:189, 1974.

158. Spiro, R.G.: Studies on the renal glomerular basement membrane. Nature of the carbohydrate units and their attachment to the peptide portion. J. Biol. Chem. 242:1923, 1967.

159. Spiro, R.G.: Glycoproteins. Adv. Protein Chem. 27:349, 1973.

160. Spiro, R.G.: Biochemistry of the renal glomerular basement membrane and its alterations in diabetes mellitus. N. Engl. J. Med. 288:1337, 1973.

161. Hudson, B.G., Spiro, R.G.: Studies on the native and reduced alkylated renal glomerular basement membrane. Solubility, subunit size, and reaction with cyanogen bromide. J. Biol. Chem. 247:4229, 1972 (Abstr.).

162. Hudson, B.G., Spiro, R.G.: Fractionation of glycoprotein components of the reduced alkylated renal glomerular basement membrane. J. Biol. Chem. 247:4239, 1972. (Abstr.)

163. Cohen, M.P., Klein, C.V: Glomerulopathy in rats with streptozotocin diabetes. Accumulation of glomerular basement membrane analogous to human diabetic nephropathy. J. Exp. Med. 149:623, 1979.

164. Cohen, M.P., Klein, C.V.: Evidence for heterogeneous origin of glomerular basement membrane. Biochem. Biophys. Res. Comm. 77:1326, 1977.

165. Freytag, J.W., Ohno, M., Hudson, B.G.: Bovine renal glomerular basement membrane. Assessment of proteolysis during isolation. Biochem. Biophys. Res. Comm. 72:796, 1976.

166. Spiro, R.G.: Nature of the glycoprotein components of basement membranes. Ann. N.Y. Acad. Sci. 312:106, 1978.

167. Beisswenger, P.J., Spiro, R.G.: Human glomerular basement membrane: chemical alterations in diabetes mellitus. Science 168:596, 1970.

168. Kefalides, N.A.: Biochemical properties of human glomerular basement membrane in normal and diabetic kidneys. J. Clin. Invest. 53:403, 1974.

169. Westberg, N.G., Michael, A.F.: Human glomerular basement membrane: chemical composition in diabetes mellitus. Acta Med. Scand. *194*:39, 1973.

170. Canivet, J., Cruz, A., Moreau-Lalande, H.: Biochemical abnormalities of the human diabetic glomerular basement membrane. Metabolism *28*:1206, 1979.

171. Beisswenger, P.J.: Specificity of the chemical alteration in the diabetic glomerular basement membrane. Diabetes *22*:744, 1973.

172. Spiro, R.G.: Investigations into the biochemical basis of diabetic basement membrane alterations. Diabetes *25* (Suppl. 2):909, 1976.

173. Klein, L., Yoshida, M., Miller, M.: Does experimental diabetes in the rat produce basement-membrane (BM) thickening in renal glomeruli? Diabetes *26* (Suppl.1):361, 1977.

174. Fox, C.J., Darby, S.C., Ireland, J.T., Sönksen, P.H.: Blood glucose control and glomerular capillary basement membrane thickening in experimental diabetes. Br. Med. J. *2*:605, 1977.

175. Østerby, R., Seyer-Hansen, K., Gundersen, H.J.G., Lundbaek, K.: Growth hormone enhances basement membrane thickening in experimental diabetes. A preliminary report. Diabetologia *15*:487, 1978.

176. Seyer-Hansen, K.: Renal hypertrophy in experimental diabetes: relation to severity of diabetes. Diabetologia *13*:141, 1977.

177. Yagihashi, S., Goto, Y., Kakizaki, M., Kaseda, N.: Thickening of glomerular basement membrane in spontaneously diabetic rats. Diabetologia *15*:309, 1978.

178. Rasch, R.: Prevention of diabetic glomerulopathy in streptozotocin diabetic rats by insulin treatment. Glomerular basement membrane thickness. Diabetologia *16*:319, 1979.

179. Peterson, D.T., Greene, W.C., Reaven, G.M.: Effect of experimental diabetes mellitus on kidney ribosomal protein synthesis. Diabetes *20*:649, 1971.

180. Khalifa, A., Cohen, M.P.: Glomerular protocollagen lysyl-hydroxylase activity in streptozotocin diabetes. Biochim. Biophys. Acta *386*:332, 1975.

181. Cohen, M., Khalifa, A.: Effect of diabetes and insulin on rat renal glomerular protocollagen hydroxylase activities. Biochim. Biophys. Acta *496*:88, 1977.

182. Spiro, R.G., Spiro, M.J.,: Studies on the biosynthesis of the hydroxylysine-linked disaccharide unit of basement membranes and collagens. II. Kidney galactosyltransferase. J. Biol. Chem. *246*:4910, 1971.

183. Spiro, M.J., Spiro, R.G.: Studies on the biosynthesis of the hydroxylysine-linked disaccharide unit of basement membranes and collagens. I. Kidney glucosyltransferase. J. Biol. Chem. *246*:4899, 1971.

184. Spiro, R.G., Spiro, M.J.: Effect of diabetes on the biosynthesis of the renal glomerular basement membrane. Studies on the glucosyltransferase. Diabetes *20*:641, 1971.

185. Risteli, J., Koivisto, V.A., Akerblom, H.K., Kivirikko, I.I.: Intracellular enzymes of collagen biosynthesis in rat kidney in streptozotocin diabetes. Diabetes *25*:1066, 1976.

186. Guzdek, A., Sarnecka-Keller, M., Dubin, A.: The activities of perfused livers of control and streptozotocin diabetic rats in the synthesis of some plasma proteins and peptides. Horm. Metab. Res. *11*:107, 1979.

187. Beisswenger, P.J.: Glomerular basement membrane. Biosynthesis and chemical composition in the streptozotocin diabetic rat. J. Clin. Invest. *58*:844, 1976.

188. Cohen, M.P., Vogt, C.: Evidence for enhanced basement membrane synthesis and lysine hydroxylation in renal glomerulus in experimental diabetes. Biochem. Biophys. Res. Comm. *49*:1542, 1972.

189. Cohen, M.P., Vogt, C.A.: Collagen synthesis and secretion by isolated rat renal glomeruli. Biochim. Biophys. Acta *383*:78, 1975.

190. Grant, M.E., Harwood, R., Williams, I.F.: The biosynthesis of basement membrane collagen by isolated rat glomeruli. Eur. J. Biochem. *54*:531, 1975.

191. Grant, M.E., Harwood, R., Williams, I.F.: Proceedings: Increased synthesis of glomerular basement membrane collagen in streptozotocin diabetes. J. Physiol. (London) *257*:56P, 1976.

192. Brownlee, M., Spiro, R.G.: Glomerular basement membrane metabolism in the diabetic rat: in vivo studies. Diabetes *28*:121, 1979.

193. Spiro, R.G.: Glycoproteins and diabetic microangiopathy. In: A. Marble, P. White, R.F. Bradley, L.P. Krall (Eds.): Joslin's Diabetes Mellitus, 11th ed., Philadelphia, Lea & Febiger, 1971, pp. 146–156.

194. Rasio, E., Bendayan, M.: Le métabolisme du tissu capillaire et ses anomalies au cours du diabète. Diabète et Metabolisme *4*:57, 1978.

195. Sochor, M., Baquer, N.Z., McLean, P.: Glucose overutilization in diabetes: evidence from studies on the changes in hexokinase, the pentose phosphate pathway and glucuronate-xylulose pathway in rat kidney cortex in diabetes. Biochem. Biophys. Res. Comm. *86*:32, 1979.

196. Villee, D.B., Powers, M.L.: Effect of glucose and insulin on collagen secretion by human skin fibroblasts *in vitro*. Nature *268*:156, 1977.

197. Chang, A.Y.: Acid glycohydrolase in Chinese hamster with spontaneous diabetes. I. Depressed levels of renal L-galactosidase and B-galactosidase. Biochim. Biophys. Acta *522*:491, 1978.

198. Fushimi, H., Tarui, S.: B-glycosidases and diabetic microangiopathy. I. Decreases of B-glycosidase activities in diabetic rat kidney. J. Biochem. *79*:265, 1976.

199. Weil, R., III, Nozawa, M., Koss, M., et al.: The kidney in streptozotocin diabetic rats. Arch. Pathol. Lab. Med. *100*:37, 1976.

200. Lindahl, U., Hook, M.: Glycosaminoglycans and their binding to biological macromolecules. Ann. Rev. Biochem. *47*:385, 1978.

201. Kanwar, Y.S., Farquhar, M.G.: Presence of heparan sulfate in the glomerular basement membrane. Proc. Natl. Acad. Sci. *76*:1303, 1979.

202. Kanwar, Y.S., Farquhar, M.G.: Isolation of glucosaminoglycans (heparan sulfate) from glomerular basement membranes. Proc. Natl. Acad. Sci. *76*:4493, 1979.

202a. Parthasarathy, N., Spiro, R.G.: Effect of diabetes on the glycosaminoglycan component of the human glomerular basement membrane. Diabetes *31*:738, 1982.

203. Berenson, G.S., Ruiz, H., Dalferes, E.R., Jr., Dugan, F.A.: Acid/mucopolysaccharide changes in diabetic kidneys. Diabetes *19*:161, 1970.

204. Goldberg, M.F.: The role of ischemia in the production of vascular retinopathies. In: J.R. Lynn, W.B. Snyder, A. Vaiser (Eds.): Diabetic Retinopathy. New York, Grune & Stratton, 1974, pp. 47–63.

205. Kohner, E.M.: The problems of retinal blood flow in diabetes. Diabetes *25* (Suppl. 2):839, 1976.

206. Kohner, E.M., Oakley, N.W.: Diabetic retinopathy. Metabolism *24*:1085, 1975.

207. Cunha-vaz, J.G., Fonseca, J.R., de Abreu, J.R.F., Lima, J.J.P.: Studies on retinal blood flow. II. Diabetic retinopathy. Arch. Ophthalmol. *96*:809, 1978.

208. Cunha-vaz, J.G.: Pathophysiology of diabetic retinopathy. Br. J. Ophthalmol. *62*:351, 1978.

209. Kohner, E.M.: Diabetic retinopathy. Clin. Endocrinol. Metab. *6*:345, 1977.

210. Cunha-vaz, J.G., de Abreu, J.R.F., Campos, A.J., Figo, G.M.: Early breakdown of the blood-retinal barrier in diabetes. Br. J. Ophthalmol. *59*:649, 1975.

211. Cunha-vaz, J.G., Fonseca, J.R., Abreu, J.R.F., Ruas, M.A.: Detection of early retinal changes in diabetes by vitreous fluorophotometry. Diabetes *28*:16, 1979.

212. Waltman, S., Krupin, T., Hanish, S., et al.: Alteration of the blood-retinal barrier in experimental diabetes mellitus. Arch. Ophthalmol. *96*:878, 1978.

213. Scharp, D., Krupin, T., Waltman, S., et al.: Relationship of abnormal insulin release to fluorophotometry in experimental diabetes. Diabetes *27*:435, 1978.

214. Wallow, I.H.L., Engerman, R.L.: Permeability and patency of retinal blood vessels in experimental diabetes. Invest. Ophthalmol. Vis. Sci. *16*:447, 1977.

215. Østerby, R., Gundersen, H.J.G., Christensen, N.J.: The acute effect of insulin on capillary endothelial cells. Diabetes *27*:745, 1978.

216. Buzney, S.M., Frank, R.N., Varma, S.D., et al.: Aldose reductase in retinal mural cells. Invest. Ophthalmol. Vis. Sci. *16*:392, 1977.

217. Raman, P.G., Jain, S.C.: Changes in intraocular tension in overt diabetes. (Abstr. 251). J.S. Bajaj (Ed.): Current Topics in Diabetes Research. Abstracts, IX Congress of the International Diabetes Federation. New Delhi, India. International Congress Series No. 400, 1976, p. 124.

218. Duane, T.D., Behrendt, T., Field, R.A.: New vascular pressure ratios in diabetic retinopathy. In: M.F. Goldberg, S.L. Fine (Eds.): Symposium on the Treatment of Diabetic Retinopathy. Washington, D.C., U.S. Public Health Service Publ. #1890, 1968, pp. 657–663.

219. Steffes, M.W., Brown, D.M., Mauer, S.M.: Bruch's membrane in experimentally induced diabetes mellitus in rats. Clin. Res. *24*:584A, 1976.

220. Papachristodoulou, D., Heath, H.: Ultrastructural alterations during the development of retinopathy in sucrose-fed and streptozotocin-diabetic rats. Exp. Eye Res. *25*:371, 1977.

221. Sosula, L.: Capillary radius and wall thickness in normal and diabetic rat retinae. Microvasc. Res. *7*:274, 1974.

222. Sosula, L., Beaumont, P., Hollows, F., Jonson, K.M.: Dilatation and endothelial proliferation of retinal capillaries in streptozotocin-diabetic rats: quantitative electron microscopy. Invest. Ophthal. *11*:926, 1972.

223. Diabetic Retinopathy Study Research Group: Preliminary report on effects of photocoagulation therapy. Am. J. Ophthalmol. *81*:383, 1976.

224. Navalesi, R., Pilo, A., Vigneri, R.: Growth hormone kinetics in diabetic patients. Diabetes *24*:317, 1975.

225. Johansen, K., Hansen, A.P.: High 24-hour level of serum growth hormone in juvenile diabetics. Br. Med. J. *2*:356, 1969.

226. Lundbaek, K., Jensen, V.A., Olsen, T.S., et al.: Diabetes, diabetic angiopathy, and growth hormone. Lancet *2*:131, 1970.

227. Kjeldsen, H., Hansen, A.P., Lundbaek, K.: Twenty-four hour serum growth hormone levels in maturity-onset diabetics. Diabetes *24*:977, 1975.

228. Merimee, T.J.: Characteristics of growth hormone secretion in clinically stable diabetes. Diabetes *28*:308, 1979.

229. Beaumont, P., Schofield, P.J., Hollows, F.C., Williams, J.F.: Growth hormone, sorbitol, and diabetic capillary disease. Lancet *1*:579, 1971.

230. Passa, P., Gauville, C., Canivet, J.: Influence of muscular exercise on plasma level of growth hormone in diabetics with and without retinopathy. Lancet *2*:72, 1974.

231. Vigneri, R., Squatrito, S., Pezzino, V., et al.: Growth hormone levels in diabetes. Correlation with the clinical control of the disease. Diabetes *25*:167, 1976.

232. Merimee, T.J., Hall, J.G., Rimoin, D.L., et al.: Sexual ateliotic dwarfism and diabetes mellitus. (Abstr. #185). J. Clin. Invest. *48*:58a, 1969.

233. Merimee, T.J., Siperstein, M.D., Hall, J.D., Fineberg, S.E.: Capillary membrane structure: a comparative study of diabetics and sexual ateliotic dwarfs. J. Clin. Invest. *49*:2161, 1970.

234. Merimee, T.J.: A follow-up study of vascular disease in growth-hormone-deficient dwarf with diabetes. N. Engl. J. Med. *298*:1217, 1978.

235. Rabin, D., Bloomgarden, Z., Feman, S., Davis, T.: Nephropathy, neuropathy, and retinopathy in a patient with post-pancreatectomy diabetes and growth hormone deficiency (Abstr.). Diabetes *28*:412, 1979.

236. Phillips, L.S., Young, H.S.: Nutrition and somatomedin. II. Serum somatomedin activity and cartilage growth activity in streptozotocin diabetic rats. Diabetes *25*:516, 1976.

237. Yde, H.: The growth hormone dependent sulfation factor in serum from patients with various types of diabetes. Acta Med. Scand. *186*:293, 1969.

238. Baxter, R.C., Brown, A.S., Turtle, J.R.: Decrease in serum receptor-reactive somatomedin in diabetes. Horm. Metab. Res. *11*:216, 1979.

239. Winter, R.J., Phillips, L.S., Klein, M.N., et al.: Somatomedin activity and diabetic control in children with insulin-dependent diabetes. Diabetes *28*:952, 1979.

240. Phillips, L.S., Belosky, D.C., Young, H.S., Reichard, L.A.: Nutrition and somatomedin. VI. Somatomedin activity and somatomedin inhibitory activity in sera from normal and diabetic rats. Endocrinology *104*:1519, 1979.

241. Phillips, L.S., Vassilopoulou-Sellin, R., Reichard, L.A.: Nutrition and somatomedin. VIII. The "somatomedin inhibitor" in diabetic rat serum is a general inhibitor of growing cartilage. Diabetes *28*:919, 1979.

242. Phillips, L.S., Belosky, D.C., Reichard, L.A.: Nutrition and somatomedin. V. Action and measurement of somatomedin inhibitor(s) in serum from diabetic rats. Endocrinology *104*:1513, 1979.

243. Daughaday, W.H., Phillips, L.S., Mueller, M.C.: The effects of insulin and growth hormone on the release of somatomedin by the isolated rat liver. Endocrinology *98*:1214, 1976.

244. Wardle, E.N.: Mesangial cell dysfunction detected by accumulation of aggregated protein in rats with streptozotocin induced diabetes. Biomedicine *23*:299, 1975.

245. Ledet, T.: Growth hormone stimulating the growth of arterial medial cells *in vitro*. Absence of effect of insulin. Diabetes *25*:1011, 1976.

246. Moorhouse, J.A.: Diabetic peripheral neuropathy. In: S.S. Fajans (Ed.) Diabetes Mellitus. DHEW Publ. No. (NIH) 76-854. Bethesda, Md., National Institutes of Health, 1976, pp. 243–255.

247. Ward, J.D., Fisher, D.J., Barnes, C.G., et al.: Improvement in nerve conduction following treatment in newly diagnosed diabetes. Lancet *1*:428, 1971.

248. Graf, R.J., Halter, J.B., Halar, E., Porte, D., Jr.: Nerve conduction abnormalities in untreated maturity-onset diabetes: relation to levels of fasting plasma glucose and glycosylated hemoglobin. Ann. Intern. Med. *90*:298, 1979.

249. Greene, D.A., De Jesus, P.V., Jr., Winegrad, A.I.: Effects of insulin and dietary myoinositol on impaired peripheral motor nerve conduction velocity in acute streptozotocin diabetes. J. Clin. Invest. *55*:1326, 1975.

250. Gregersen, G.: Diabetic neuropathy: influence of age, sex,

metabolic control, and duration of diabetes on motor conduction velocity. Neurology *17*:972, 1967.

251. Graf, R., Halter, J., Pfeifer, M., Halar, E.: The influence of glycemic control on nerve conduction abnormalities in diabetics. (Abstr.). Diabetes *28*:387, 1979.

252. Eliasson, S.G.: Properties of isolated nerve fibres from alloxanized rats. J. Neurol. Neurosurg. Psych. *32*:525, 1969.

253. McDonald, W.I.: The effects of experimental demyelination on conduction in peripheral nerve: a histological and electrophysiological study. II. Electrophysiological observations. Brain *86*:501, 1963.

254. Babel, J., Bischoff, A., Spoendlin, H.: Atlas of Normal and Pathologic Anatomy. St. Louis, C.V. Mosby Co., 1970.

255. Thomas, P.K.: The morphological basis for alterations in nerve conduction in peripheral neuropathy. Proc. R. Soc. Med. *64*:295, 1971.

256. Clements, R.S., Jr.: Diabetic neuropathy—new concepts of its etiology. Diabetes *28*:604, 1979.

257. Chopra, J.S., Sawhney, B.B., Chakravorty, R.N.: Pathology and time relationship of peripheral nerve changes in experimental diabetes. J. Neur. Sci. *32*:53, 1977.

258. Yagihashi, S., Kudo, K., Nishihira, M.: Peripheral nerve structures of experimental diabetic rats and the effect of insulin treatment. Tohoku J. Exp. Med. *127*:35, 1979.

259. Fukuma, M., Carpentier, J-L., Orci, L.: An alteration in internodal myelin membrane structure in large sciatic nerve fibers in rats with acute streptozotocin diabetes and impaired nerve conduction velocity. Diabetologia *15*:65, 1978.

260. Jakobsen, J.: Peripheral nerves in early experimental diabetes. Expansion of the endoneurial space as a cause of increased water content. Diabetologia *14*:113, 1978.

261. Seneviratne, K.N.: Permeability of blood nerve barriers in the diabetic rat. J. Neurol. Neurosurg. Psych. *35*:156, 1972.

262. Jakobsen, J., Malmgren, L., Olsson, Y.: Permeability of the blood-nerve barrier in the streptozotocin-diabetic rat. Exp. Neurol. *60*:277, 1978.

263. Sima, A.A.F., Robertson, D.M.: The perineurial and blood-nerve barriers in experimental diabetes. Acta Neuropathologica *44*:189, 1978.

264. Seneviratne, K.N., Weerasuriya, A.: Nodal gap substance in diabetic nerve. J. Neurol. Neurosurg. Psych. *37*:502, 1974.

265. Hansen, S., Ballantyne, J.P.: Axonal dysfunction in the neuropathy of diabetes mellitus: a quantitative electrophysiological study. J. Neurol. Neurosurg. Psych. *40*:555, 1977.

266. Behse, F., Buchthal, F., Carlsen, F.: Nerve biopsy and conduction studies in diabetic neuropathy. J. Neurol. Neurosurg. Psych. *40*:1072, 1977.

267. Sima, A.A., Robertson, D.M.: Peripheral neuropathy in the diabetic mutant mouse. An ultrastructural study. Lab. Invest. *40*:627, 1979.

268. Yagihashi, S., Matsunaga, M.: Ultrastructural pathology of peripheral nerves in patients with diabetic neuropathy. Tohoku J. Exp. Med. *129*:357, 1979.

269. Jakobsen, J.: Axonal dwindling in early experimental diabetes. I. A study of cross sectioned nerves. Diabetologia *12*:539, 1976.

270. Jakobsen, J.: Axonal dwindling in early experimental diabetes. II. A study of isolated nerve fibers. Diabetologia *12*:547, 1976.

271. Timperly, W.R., Williams, E., Ward, J.D., Preston, F.E.: Abnormalities of small blood vessels in diabetic neuropathy. Diabetologia *13*:437, 1977.

272. Pratt, J.H., Berry, J.F., Kaye, B., Goetz, F.C.: Lipid class and fatty acid composition of rat brain and sciatic nerve in alloxan diabetes. Diabetes *18*:556, 1969.

273. Spritz, N., Singh, H., Marinan, B.: Decrease in myelin content of rabbit sciatic nerve with aging and diabetes. Diabetes *24*:680, 1975.

274. Field, R.A.: Altered nerve metabolism in diabetes. Diabetes *15*:696, 1966.

275. Eliasson, S.G.: Lipid synthesis in peripheral nerve from alloxan diabetic rats. Lipids *1*:237, 1966.

276. Palo, J., Reske-Nielsen, E., Riekkinen, P.: Enzyme and protein studies of demyelination in diabetes. J. Neurol. Sci. *33*:171, 1977.

277. Spritz, N., Singh, H., Marinan, B.: Metabolism of peripheral nerve myelin in experimental diabetes. J. Clin. Invest. *55*:1049, 1975.

278. Spritz, N., Singh, H., Marinan, B., Silberlicht, I.: Effect of experimental diabetes on the susceptibility of myelin proteins to proteolysis. Diabetes *30*:292, 1981.

279. Poduslo, J.F., Quarles, R.H., Brady, R.O.: External labeling of galactose in surface membrane glycoproteins of the intact myelin sheath. J. Biol. Chem. *251*:153, 1976.

280. Palo, J., Savolainen, H., Haltia, M.: Proteins of peripheral nerve myelin in diabetic neuropathy. J. Neurol. Sci. *16*:193, 1972.

281. Ludvigson, M.A., Sorenson, R.L.: Immunohistochemical localization of aldose reductase in the rat. Diabetes *27*:463, 1978.

282. Gabbay, K.H.: The sorbitol pathway and the complications of diabetes. N. Engl. J. Med. *288*:831, 1973.

283. Heath, H., Hamlett, Y.C.: The sorbitol pathway: effect of streptozotocin induced diabetes and the feeding of a sucrose-rich diet on glucose, sorbitol and fructose in the retina, blood and liver of rats. Diabetologia *12*:43, 1976.

284. Winegrad, A.I., Morrison, A.D., Clements, R.S., Jr.: Polyol pathway in aorta. In: R.A. Camerini-Davalos, H.S. Cole (Eds.): Vascular and Neurological Changes in Early Diabetes. New York, Academic Press, 1973, pp. 117–124.

285. Malone, J.I., Knox, G., Benford, S.: Red cell sorbitol, an indicator of diabetic control. Diabetes *28*:386, 1979.

286. Gonzalez, A.M., Sochor, M., Hothersall, J.S., McLean, P.: Effect of experimental diabetes on the activity of hexokinase in rat lens: an example of glucose overutilization in diabetes. Biochem. Biophys. Res. Comm. *84*:858, 1978.

287. Winegrad, A.I., Clements, R.S., Morrison, A.D.: Pathophysiology. A polyol pathway and diabetic complications. In: S.S. Fajans, K.E. Sussman (Eds.): Diabetes Mellitus: Diagnosis and Treatment. Vol. III. New York, American Diabetes Association, 1971, pp. 269–273.

288. Ludvigson, M.A., Sorenson, R.L.: Immunohistochemical localization of aldose reductase. I. Enzyme purification and antibody preparation—localization in peripheral nerve, artery, and testis. Diabetes *29*:438, 1980.

289. Winegrad, A.I., Morrison, A.D., Clements, R.S., Jr.: The polyol pathway: a model for biochemical mechanisms by which hyperglycemia may contribute to the pathogenesis of the complications of diabetes mellitus. In: Proc. VIII Congr. Int. Diab. Fed., 1973, pp. 387–395.

290. Greene, D., Winegrad, A.: Effects of alloxan diabetes on peripheral nerve metabolism. (Abstr.). Diabetes *28*:388, 1979.

291. Gabbay, K.H.: Hyperglycemia, polyol metabolism, and complications of diabetes mellitus. Ann. Rev. Med. *26*:521, 1975.

292. Peterson, M.J., Sarges, R., Aldinger, C.E.: Inhibition on polyol pathway activity in chronically diabetic and galactosemic rats by the aldose reductase inhibitor CP-45,634. Diabetes *28*:367, 1979.

293. Clements, R.S., Jr., Reynertson, R.: Myoinositol metabolism in diabetes mellitus. Effect of insulin treatment. Diabetes 26:215, 1977.

294. Palmano, K.P., Whiting, P.H., Hawthorne, J.N.: Free and lipid myo-inositol in tissues from rats with acute and less severe streptozotocin-induced diabetes. Biochem. J. 167:229, 1977.

295. Clements, R.S., Estes, T., Stockard, R.: Abnormal myoinositol and phosphatidylinositol metabolism in diabetic rat nerve. Clin. Res. 26:789A, 1978.

296. Ho, P.C., Feman, S.S., Stein, R.S., McKee, L.C.: Proliferative diabetic retinopathy in patients with defects of platelet function. Am. J. Ophthalmol. 88:37, 1979.

297. Whiting, P.H., Palmano, K.P., Hawthorne, J.N.: Enzymes of myo-inositol and inositol lipid metabolism in rats with streptozotocin-induced diabetes. Biochem. J. 179:549, 1979.

298. Clements, R.S., Jr., Stockard, C.R.: Abnormal sciatic nerve myo-inositol metabolism in the streptozotocin-diabetic rat. Effect of insulin treatment. Diabetes 29:227, 1980.

299. Jeffreys, J.G.R., Palmano, K.P., Sharma, A.K., Thomas, P.K.: Influence of dietary myoinositol on nerve conduction and inositol phospholipids in normal and diabetic rats. J. Neurol. Neurosurg. Psych. 41:333, 1978.

300. Clements, R.S., Jr., Vourganti, B., Juba, T.: Dietary myo-inositol intake and peripheral nerve function in diabetic neuropathy. Metabolism 28 (Suppl. 1):477, 1979.

301. Clements, R., Vourganti, B., Darnell, B., Oh, S.: Effect of low and high dietary myoinositol (MI) content upon nerve conduction velocities (NCV's) in neuropathic diabetes. (Abstr.) Diabetes 27:436, 1978.

302. Gregersen, G., Børsting, H., Theil, P., Servo, C.: Myoinositol and function of peripheral nerves in human diabetics. Acta Neurol Scand. 58:241, 1978.

303. Schmidt, R.E., Matschinsky, F.M., Godfrey, D.A., et al.: Fast and slow axoplasmic flow in sciatic nerve of diabetic rats. Diabetes 24:1081, 1975.

304. Giachetti, A.: Axoplasmic transport of noradrenaline in the sciatic nerves of spontaneously diabetic mice. Diabetologia 16:191, 1979.

305. Jakobsen, J., Sidenius, P.: Decreased axonal flux of retrogradely transported glycoproteins in early experimental diabetes. J. Neurochem. 33:1055, 1979.

306. Bloodworth, J.M.B., Jr., Engerman, R.L., Davis, M.D.: Pathology of diabetic microangiopathy. In: R.R. Rodriguez, J. Vallance-Owen (Eds.): Proc. VII Congress of International Diabetes Federation. Amsterdam, Excerpta Medica, 1971, pp. 804–819.

307. Engerman, R.L., Davis, M.D., Bloodworth, J.M.B., Jr.: Retinopathy in experimental diabetes. Its relevance to diabetic retinopathy in man. In: R.R. Rodriguez, J. Vallance-Owen (Eds.): Proc. VII Congress of International Diabetes Federation. Amsterdam, Excerpta Medica, 1971, pp. 261–267.

308. Bloodworth, J.M.B., Jr., Engerman, R.L.: Diabetic microangiopathy in the experimentally diabetic dog and its prevention by careful control with insulin. Diabetes 22 (Suppl. 1):290, 1973.

309. Engerman, R.L., Bloodworth, J.M.B.: Role of diabetes control in microvascular disease. W.J. Malaisse, J. Pirart, J. Vallance-Owen (Eds.): Abstracts of Proc. VIII Congress of International Diabetes Federation. Amsterdam, Excerpta Medica, 1973, p. 188.

310. Engerman, R., Bloodworth, J.M.B., Jr., Nelson, S.: Relationship of microvascular disease in diabetes to metabolic control. Diabetes 26:760, 1977.

311. Howard, C.F., Jr.: Aortic atherosclerosis in normal and spontaneously diabetic Macaca nigra. Atherosclerosis 33:479, 1979.

312. Kaplan, M.H., Feinstein, A.R.: A critique of methods in reported studies of long-term vascular complications in patients with diabetes mellitus. Diabetes 22:160, 1973.

313. Knowles, H.C.: The problem of the relation of the control of diabetes to the development of vascular disease. Trans. Am. Clin. Climatol. Assoc. 76:142, 1964.

314. Ricketts, H.T.: The influence of diabetic control on angiopathy. In: B.S. Leibel, G.A. Wrenshall (Eds.): On the Nature and Treatment of Diabetes. Amsterdam, Excerpta Medica, 1965, pp. 588–600.

315. Keiding, N.R., Root, H.F., Marble, A.: Importance of control of diabetes in prevention of vascular complications. J.A.M.A. 150:964, 1952.

316. Jackson, R., Guthrie, R., Esterly, J., et al.: Muscle capillary basement membrane changes in normal and diabetic children. (Abstr.). Diabetes 24 (Suppl. 1):400, 1975.

317. Downie, E., Martin, F.I.R.: Vascular disease in juvenile diabetic patients of long duration. Diabetes 8:383, 1959.

318. Knowles, H.C., Guest, G.M., Lampe, J., et al.: The course of juvenile diabetes treated with unmeasured diet. Diabetes 14:239, 1965.

319. Bondy, P.K., Felig, P.: Relation of diabetic control to development of vascular complications. Med. Clin. N. Am. 55:889, 1971.

320. Johnsson, S.: Retinopathy and nephropathy in diabetes mellitus. Comparison of the effects of two forms of treatment. Diabetes 9:1, 1960.

321. Ryan, J.R., Balodimos, M.C., Chazan, B.I., et al.: Quarter Century Victory Medal for diabetes: a follow-up of patients one to 20 years later. Metabolism 19:493, 1970.

322. Oakley, W.G., Pyke, D.A., Tattersall, R.B., Watkins, P.J.: Long-term diabetes. A clinical study of 92 patients after 40 years. Q. J. Med. 43:145, 1974.

323. Deckert, T., Poulsen, J.E., Larsen, M.: Prognosis of diabetics with diabetes onset before the age of thirty-one. I. Survival, causes of death, and complications. Diabetologia 14:363, 1978.

324. Deckert, T., Poulsen, J.E., Larsen, M.: Prognosis of diabetics with diabetes onset before the age of thirty-one. II. Factors influencing the prognosis. Diabetologia 14:371, 1978.

325. Goodkin, G.: Mortality factors in diabetes. A 20-year mortality study. J. Occup. Med. 17:716, 1975.

326. Kohner, E.M., Fraser, T.R., Joplin, G.F., Oakley, N.W.: The effect of diabetic control on diabetic retinopathy. M.F. Goldberg, S.L. Fine (Eds.): Symposium on the Treatment of Diabetic Retinopathy. U.S. Public Health Service Publication #1890. Washington, D.C., 1968, pp. 119–128.

327. Miki, E., Fukuda, M., Kuzuya, T.: Relation of the course of retinopathy to control of diabetes, age, and therapeutic agents in diabetic Japanese patients. Diabetes 18:773, 1969.

328. Job, D., Eschwege, E., Guyot-Argenton, C., et al.: Effect of multiple daily insulin injections on the course of diabetic retinopathy. Diabetes 25:463, 1976.

329. Ashikaga, T., Borodic, G., Sims, E.A.H.: Multiple daily insulin injections in the treatment of diabetic retinopathy. The Job study revisited. Diabetes 27:592, 1978.

330. Eschwege, E., Job, D., Guyot-Argenton, C., et al.: Delayed progression of diabetic retinopathy by divided insulin administration: a further follow-up. Diabetologia 16:13, 1979.

331. Miki, E., Kuzuya, T., Ide, T., Nakao, K.: Frequency, degree, and progression with time of proteinuria in diabetic patients. Lancet 1:922, 1972.

332. Takazakura, E., Nakamoto, Y., Hayakawa, H., et al.: Onset and progression of diabetic glomerulosclerosis. A prospective study based on serial renal biopsies. Diabetes 24:1, 1975
333. Lauvaux, J.P., Vassart, G., Pirart, J.: Development and evolution of nervous and vascular complications in the course of diabetes: a prospective study. I. Material and methods. Effect of duration of diabetes. Abstracts of Proc. VIII Congress of International Diabetes Federation. Amsterdam, Excerpta Medica, 1973, pp. 189–190.
334. Lauvaux, J.P., Vassart, G., Pirart, J.: Development and evolution of nervous and vascular complications in the course of diabetes: a prospective study. II. Diabetic retinopathy. Relation to sex, age, severity of diabetes and degree of control. Abstracts of Proc. VIII Congress of International Diabetes Federation. Amsterdam, Excerpta Medica, 1973, p. 185.
335. Pirart, J.: Diabetes mellitus and its degenerative complications: A prospective study of 4,400 patients observed between 1947 and 1973. (Part 1). Diabetes Care 1:168, 1978.
336. Pirart, J.: Diabetes mellitus and its degenerative complications: A prospective study of 4,400 patients observed between 1947 and 1973. (Part 2). Diabetes Care 1:252, 1978.
337. Multiple authors: Symposium on home blood glucose monitoring. (26 articles). Diabetes Care 3:57–186, 1980.
338. Raskin, P.: Treatment of diabetes mellitus. The future. Metabolism 28:780, 1979.
339. Santiago, J.V., Clemens, A.H., Clarke, W.L., Kipnis, D.M.: Closed-loop and open-loop devices for blood glucose control in normal and diabetic subjects. Diabetes 28:71, 1979.
340. J.S. Skyler (Ed.): Symposium on insulin delivery devices. Diabetes Care 3:253, 1980.
341. J. Brown (Ed.): Proceedings of a conference on pancreas transplantation. Toward transplantation of the human pancreas. Diabetes 29 (Suppl. 1):1, 1980.

ADDENDUM

Interest in the important area covered by this chapter continues to run high, resulting in a constant stream of publications. The following references hopefully will assist the reader to keep abreast of developing knowledge. For convenience, they are listed according to the topics discussed in the text.

HEMATOLOGIC ABNORMALITIES

Erythroyctes

Carandente, O., Colombo, R., Girardi, A.M., et al.: Role of red cell sorbitol as determinant of reduced erythrocyte filtrability in insulin-dependent diabetics. Acta Diabetol. Lat. 19:359, 1982.

Juhan, I., Vague, P., Buonocore, M., et al.: Abnormalities of erythrocyte deformability and platelet aggregation in insulin-dependent diabetics corrected by insulin in vivo and in vitro. Lancet 1:535, 1982.

Kamada, T., Otsuji, S.: Lower levels of erythrocyte membrane fluidity in diabetic patients; a spin label study. Diabetes 32:585, 1983.

Bryszewska, M., Leyko, W.: Effect of insulin on human erythrocyte membrane fluidity in diabetes mellitus. Diabetologia 24:311, 1983.

Hemoglobin Glycosylation and Oxygenation

Samaja, M., Melotti, D., Carenini, A., Pozza, G.: Glycosylated haemoglobins and the oxygen affinity of whole blood. Diabetologia 23:399, 1982.

Williams, S.K., Devenny, J.J., Bitensky, M.W.: Micropinocytic ingestion of glycosylated albumin by isolated microvessels: Possible role in pathogenesis of diabetic microangiopathy. Proc. Natl. Acad. Sci. USA 78:2393, 1981.

Schleicher, E., Deufel, T., Wieland, O.H., et al.: Non-enzymatic glycosylation of human serum lipoproteins. Elevated ε-lysine glycosylated low-density lipoprotein in diabetic patients. FEBS Lett. 129:1, 1981.

McVerry, B.A., Thorpe, S., Joe, F., et al.: Non-enzymatic glucosylation of fibrinogen. Haemostasis 10:261, 1981.

Brownlee, M., Vlassara, H., Cerami, A.: Nonenzymatic glycosylation reduces the susceptibility of fibrin to degradation by plasmin. Diabetes 32:680, 1983.

Schleicher, E., Scheller, L., Wieland, O.H.: Quantitation of lysine-bound glucose of normal and diabetic erythrocyte membranes by HPLC analysis of furosine [ε-N (L-furoyl-methyl)-L-lysine]. Biochem. Biophys. Res. Commun. 99:1011, 1981.

Williams, S.K., Howarth, N.L., Devenny, J.J., Bitensky, M.W.: Structural and functional consequences of increased tubulin glycosylation in diabetes mellitus. Proc. Natl. Acad. Sci. USA 79:6546, 1982.

Vlassara, H., Brownlee, M., Cerami, A.: Excessive nonenzymatic glycosylation of peripheral and central nervous system myelin components in diabetic rats. Diabetes 32:670, 1983.

Rosenberg, H., Modrak, J.B., Hassing, J.M., et al.: Glycosylated collagen. Biochem. Biophys. Res. Commun. 91:498, 1979.

Schnider, S.L., Kohn, R.R.: Glucosylation of human collagen in aging and diabetes mellitus. J. Clin. Invest. 66:1179, 1980.

Cohen, M.P., Urdanivia, E., Surma, M, Wu, V-Y.: Increased glycosylation of glomerular basement membrane collagen in diabetes. Biochem. Biophys. Res. Commun. 95:765, 1980.

Schnider, S.L., Kohn, R.R.: Effects of age and diabetes mellitus on the solubility and nonenzymatic glucosylation of human skin collagen. J. Clin. Invest. 67:1630, 1981.

Vogt, B.W., Schleicher, E.D., Wieland, O.H.: ε-Aminolysine-bound glucose in human tissues obtained at autopsy. Diabetes 31:1123, 1982.

Bassiouny, A.R., Rosenberg, H., McDonald, T.L.: Glucosylated collagen is antigenic. Diabetes 32:1182, 1983.

Yue, D.K., McLennan, S., Delbridge, L., et al.: The thermal stability of collagen in diabetic rats: correlation with severity of diabetes and non-enzymatic glycosylation. Diabetologia 24:282, 1983.

Yue, D.K., McLennan, S., Turtle, J.R.: Non-enzymatic glycosylation of tissue protein in diabetes in the rat. Diabetologia 24:377, 1983.

Brownlee, M., Pongor, S., Cerami, A.: Covalent attachment of soluble proteins by nonenzymatically glycosylated collagen. Role in the in situ formation of immune complexes. J. Exp. Med. 158:1739, 1983.

Brownlee, M., Vlassara, H., Cerami, A.: Nonenzymatic glycosylation and the pathogenesis of diabetic complications. Ann. Intern. Med. In press. 1984.

Platelets

Ishibashi, T., Tanaka, K., Taniguchi, Y.: Platelet aggregation and coagulation in the pathogenesis of diabetic retinopathy in rats. Diabetes 30:601, 1981.

Halushka, P.V., Rogers, R.C., Loadholt, C.B., Colwell,

J.A.: Increased platelet thromboxane synthesis in diabetes mellitus. J. Lab. Clin. Med. 97:87, 1981.

Halushka, P.V., Mayfield, R., Wohltmann, H.J., et al.: Increased platelet arachidonic acid metabolism in diabetes mellitus. Diabetes 30 (Suppl. 2):44, 1981.

Davi, G., Rini, G.B., Averna, M., et al.: Thromboxane B2 formation and platelet sensitivity to prostacyclin in insulin-dependent and insulin-independent diabetics. Thromb. Res. 26:359, 1982.

Betteridge, D.J., El Tahir, K.E.H., Reckless, J.P.D., Williams, K.I.: Platelets from diabetic subjects show diminished sensitivity to prostacyclin. Eur. J. Clin. Invest.12:395, 1982.

Jeremy, J.Y., Mikhailidis, D.P., Dandona, P.: Simulating the diabetic environment modifies in vitro prostacyclin synthesis. Diabetes 32:217, 1983.

Jones, R.L., Paradise, C., Peterson, C.M.: Platelet survival in patients with diabetes mellitus. Diabetes 30:486, 1981.

Ek, I., Thunell, S., Blombäck, M.: Enhanced in vivo platelet activation in diabetes mellitus. Scand. J. Haematol. 29:185, 1982.

Davi, G., Rini, G.B., Averna, M., et al.: Enhanced platelet release reaction in insulin-dependent and insulin-independent diabetic patients. Haemostasis 12:275, 1982.

Porta, M., Peters, A.M., Cousins, S.A., et al.: A study of platelet-relevant parameters in patients with diabetic microangiopathy. Diabetologia 25:21, 1983.

Mordes, D.B., Lazarchick, J., Colwell, J.A., Sens, D.A.: Elevated glucose concentrations increase Factor VIIIR: Ag levels in human umbilical vein endothelial cells. Diabetes 32:876, 1983.

Voisin, P.J., Rousselle, D., Streiff, F., et al.: Reduction of beta-thromboglobulin levels in diabetics controlled by artificial pancreas. Metabolism 32:138, 1983.

Berry, E.M., Ziv, E., Bar-On, H.: Protein and glycoprotein synthesis and secretion by the diabetic liver. Diabetologia 19:535, 1980.

Borkenstein, M.H., Muntean, W.E.: Elevated Factor VIII activity and Factor VIII-related antigen in diabetic children without vascular disease. Diabetes 31:1006, 1982.

Sowers, J.R., Tuck, M.L., Sowers, D.K.: Plasma antithrombin III and thrombin generation time: correlation with hemoglobin A₁ and fasting serum glucose in young diabetic women. Diabetes Care 3:655, 1980.

Brownlee, M., Vlassara, H., Cerami, A.: Inhibition of heparin-catalyzed human antithrombin III activity by nonenzymatic glycosylation: possible role in fibrin deposition in diabetes. Diabetes 33:532, 1984.

Patrassi, G.M., Vettor, R., Padovan, D., et al.: Contact phase of blood coagulation in diabetes mellitus. Eur. J. Clin. Invest. 12:307, 1982.

Paisey, R.B., Harkness, J., Hartog, M., Chadwick, T.: The effect of improvement in diabetic control on plasma and whole blood viscosity. Diabetologia 19:345, 1980.

Smokovitis, A., Auerswald, W., Binder, B.R.: The effect of alloxan-induced diabetes on tissue plasminogen activator activity and plasmin inhibition in the rat. Thromb. Res. 23:421, 1981.

CATARACTS

Kasai, K., Nakamura, T., Kase, N., et al.: Increased glycosylation of proteins from cataractous lenses in diabetes. Diabetologia 25:36, 1983.

Gonzalez, A-M., Sochor, M., McLean, P.: The effect of an aldose reductase inhibitor (Sorbinil) on the level of metabolites in lenses of diabetic rats. Diabetes 32:482, 1983.

DIABETIC NEPHROPATHY

Functional and Morphologic Changes

Parving, H.H., Viberti, G.C., Keen, H., et al.: Hemodynamic factors in the genesis of diabetic microangiopathy. Metabolism 32:943, 1983.

Michels, L.D., Davidman, M., Keane, W.F.: Glomerular permeability to neutral and anionic dextrans in experimental diabetes. Kidney Int. 21:699, 1982.

Myers, B.D., Winetz, J.A., Chui, F., Michaels, A.S.: Mechanisms of proteinuria in diabetic nephropathy: a study of glomerular barrier function. Kidney Int. 21:633, 1982.

Herlihy, W.G., Nordquist, J.A., Mandal, A.K., Llach, F.: Diabetic nephropathy associated with fibrin formation. Hum. Pathol. 12:658, 1981.

Mauer, S.M., Steffes, M.W., Connett, J., et al.: The development of lesions in the glomerular basement membrane and mesangium after transplantation of normal kidneys to diabetic patients. Diabetes 32:948, 1983.

Michael, A.F., Brown, D.M.: Increased concentration of albumin in kidney basement membranes in diabetes mellitus. Diabetes 30:843, 1981.

Mauer, S.M., Steffes, M.W., Brown, D.M.: The kidney in diabetes. Am. J. Med. 70:603, 1981.

Basement Membrane Chemistry and Metabolism

Kefalides, N.A.: Basement membrane research in diabetes mellitus. Coll. Relat. Res. 1:295, 1981.

Sternberg M., Andre, J., Peyroux, J.: Inhibition of the α-glucosidase specific for collagen disaccharide units in diabetic rat kidney by in vivo glucose levels: possible contribution to basement membrane thickening. Diabetologia 24:286, 1983.

Glomerular Proteoglycans

Brown, D.M., Klein, D.J., Michael, A.F., Oegema, T.R.: ³⁵S-glycosaminoglycan and ³⁵S-glycopeptide metabolism by diabetic glomeruli and aorta. Diabetes 31:418, 1982.

Rohrbach, D.H., Hassell, J.R., Kleinman, H., Martin, G.R.: Alterations in the basement membrane (heparan sulfate) proteoglycan in diabetic mice. Diabetes 31:185, 1982.

Kjellen, L., Bielfeld, D., Hook, M.: Reduced sulfation of liver heparan sulfate in experimentally diabetic rats. Diabetes 32:337, 1983.

Saraswathi, S., Vasan, N.S.: Alterations in the rat renal glycosaminoglycans in streptozotocin-induced diabetes. Biochim. Biophys. Acta 755:237, 1983.

Kanwar, Y.S., Rosenzweig, L.J., Linker, A., Jakubowski, M.L.: Decreased de novo synthesis of glomerular proteoglycans in diabetes: biochemical and autoradiographic evidence. Proc. Natl. Acad. Sci. USA 80:2272, 1983.

DIABETIC RETINOPATHY

Ishibashi, T., Tanaka, K., Taniguchi, Y.: Disruption of blood-retinal barrier in experimental diabetic rats: an electron microscopic study. Exp. Eye Res. 30:401, 1980.

Porta, M., Townsend, C., Clover, G.M., et al.: Evidence for functional endothelial cell damage in early diabetic retinopathy. Diabetologia 20:597, 1981.

Naeser, P., Andersson, A.: Effects of pancreatic islet implantation on the morphology of retinal capillaries in alloxan diabetic mice. Acta Ophthalmol (Copenh.) 61:38, 1983.

Ernest, J.T., Goldstick, T.K., Engerman, R.L.: Hyperglycemia impairs retinal oxygen autoregulation in normal and diabetic dogs. Invest. Ophthalmol. Vis. Sci. 24:985, 1983.

ROLE OF GROWTH HORMONE

Ledet, T.: Diabetic macroangiopathy and growth hormone. Diabetes 30 (Suppl. 2):14, 1981.

Merimee, T.J., Zapf, J., Froesch, E.R.: Insulin-like growth factors. Studies in diabetics with and without retinopathy. N. Engl. J. Med. *309*:527, 1983.

DIABETIC NEUROPATHY

Morphologic and Functional Changes

Williams, E., Timperley, W.R., Ward, J.D., Duckworth, T.: Electron microscopical studies of vessels in diabetic peripheral neuropathy. J. Clin. Pathol. *33*:462, 1980.

Johnson, P.C., Brendel, K., Meezan, E.: Human diabetic perineurial cell basement membrane thickening. Lab. Invest *44*:265, 1981.

Sugimura, K., Dyck, P.J.: Sural nerve myelin thickness and axis cylinder caliber in human diabetes. Neurology *31*:1087, 1981.

Mattingly, G.E., Fischer, V.W.: Peripheral neuropathy following prolonged exposutre to streptozotocin-induced diabetes in rats: a teased fiber study. Acta Neuropathol. *59*:133, 1983.

Biochemical Alterations

Myelin Composition

Palo, J., Reske-Nielsen, E., Riekkinen, P.: Biochemical studies of CNS and PNS in human and experimental diabetes. Adv. Exp. Med. Biol. *100*:479, 1978.

Brown, M.J., Iwamori, M., Kishimoto, Y., et al.: Nerve lipid abnormalities in human diabetic neuropathy: a correlative study. Ann. Neurol. *5*:245, 1979.

Baughman, S., Felten, S.Y., Lee, W., et al.: The effect of diabetes on leucine and fucose incorporation into PNS myelin proteins. Horm. Metab. Res. *13*:331, 1981.

Spritz, N., Singh, H., Marinan, B., Silberlicht, I.: Effect of experimental diabetes on the susceptibility of myelin proteins to proteolysis. Diabetes *30*:292, 1981.

Bell, M.E., Peterson, R.G., Eichberg, J.: Metabolism of phospholipids in peripheral nerve from rats with chronic streptozotocin-induced diabetes: increased turnover of phosphatidylinositol -4,5-biphosphate. J. Neurochem. *39*:192, 1982.

Chez, M.G., Peterson, R.G.: Altered metabolic incorporation of fucose and leucine into PNS myelin of 25-week-old diabetic (C57BL/Ks [db/db]) mice: effects of untreated diabetes on nerve metabolism. Neurochem. Res. *8*:465, 1983.

Sorbitol Pathway

Judzewitsch, R.G., Jaspan, J.B., Polonsky, K.S., et al.: Aldose reductase inhibition improves nerve conduction velocity in diabetic patients. N. Engl. J. Med. *308*:119, 1983.

Myoinositol

Clements, R.S., Jr., Stockard, C.R.: Abnormal sciatic nerve myo-inositol metabolism in the streptozotocin-diabetic rat: effect of insulin treatment. Diabetes *29*:227, 1980.

Natarajan, V., Dyck, P.J., Schmid, H.H.: Alterations of inositol lipid metabolism of rat sciatic nerve in streptozotocin-induced diabetes. J. Neurochem. *36*:413, 1981.

Greene, D.A., Lewis, R.A., Lattimer, S.A., Brown, M.J.: Selective effects of myo-inositol administration on sciatic and tibial motor nerve conduction parameters in the streptozotocin-diabetic rat. Diabetes *31*:573, 1982.

Mayhew, J.A., Gillon, K.R.W., Hawthorne, J.N.: Free and lipid inositol, sorbitol and sugars in sciatic nerve obtained post-mortem from diabetic patients and control subjects. Diabetologia *24*:13, 1983.

Gregersen, G., Bertelsen, B., Harbo, H., et al.: Oral supplementation of myoinositol: effects on peripheral nerve function in human diabetics and on the concentration in plasma, erythrocytes, urine and muscle tissue in human diabetics and normals. Acta Neurol. Scand. *67*:164, 1983.

Greene, D.A., Lattimer, S.A.: Impaired rat sciatic nerve sodium-potassium adenosine triphosphatase in acute streptozotocin diabetes and its correction by dietary myo-inositol supplementation. J. Clin. Invest. *72*:1058, 1983.

Greene, D.A.: Metabolic abnormalities in diabetic peripheral nerve: relation to impaired function. Metabolism *32* (Suppl. 1):118, 1983.

Gillon, K.R.W., Hawthorne, J.N.: Transport of myo-inositol into endoneurial preparation of sciatic nerve from normal and streptozotocin-diabetic rats. Biochem. J. *210*:775, 1983.

Finegold, D., Lattimer, S.A., Nolle, S., et al.: Polyol pathway activity and myo-inositol metabolism: a suggested relationship in the pathogenesis of diabetic neuropathy. Diabetes *32*:988, 1983.

Axoplasmic Transport

Jakobsen, J., Sidenius, P.: Decreased axonal transport of structural proteins in streptozotocin diabetic rats. J. Clin. Invest. *66*:292, 1980.

Bisby, M.A.: Axonal transport of labeled protein and regeneration rate in nerves of streptozotocin-diabetic rats. Exp. Neurol. *69*:74, 1980.

Sidenius, P., Jakobsen, J.: Retrograde axonal transport. A possible role in the development of neuropathy. Diabetologia *20*:110, 1981.

Jakobsen, J., Brimijoin, S., Skau, K., et al.: Retrograde axonal transport of transmitter enzymes, fucose-labeled protein, and nerve growth factor in streptozotocin-diabetic rats. Diabetes *30*:797, 1981.

Sidenius, P.: The axonopathy of diabetic neuropathy. Diabetes *31*:356, 1982.

Sidenius, P., Jakobsen, J.: Reversibility and preventability of the decrease in slow axonal transport velocity in experimental diabetes. Diabetes *31*:689, 1982.

Tomlinson, D.R., Gillon, K.R.W., Smith, M.G.: Axonal transport of noradrenaline and noradrenergic transmission in rats with streptozotocin-induced diabetes. Diabetologia *22*:199, 1982.

Mayer, J.H., Tomlinson, D.R.: Prevention of defects of axonal transport and nerve conduction velocity by oral administration of myo-inositol or an aldose reductase inhibitor in streptozotocin-diabetic rats. Diabetologia *25*:433, 1983.

DIABETIC COMPLICATIONS AND THE DEGREE OF METABOLIC DYSFUNCITON

West, K.M., Erdreich, L.J., Stober, J.A.: A detailed study of risk factors for retinopathy and nephropathy in diabetes. Diabetes *29*:501, 1980.

West, K.M., Ahuja, M.M.S., Bennett, P.H., et al.: Interrelationships of microangiopathy, plasma glucose and other risk factors in 3583 diabetic patients: a multinational study. Diabetologia *22*:412, 1982.

Dornan, T.L., Ting, A., McPherson, C.K., et al.: Genetic susceptibility to the development of retinopathy in insulin-dependent diabetics. Diabetes *31*:226, 1982.

Ganda, O.P., Williamson, J.R., Soeldner, J.S., et al.: Muscle capillary basement membrane width and its relationship to diabetes mellitus in monozygotic twins. Diabetes *32*:549, 1983.

Barnett, A.H., Spiliopoulos, A.J., Pyke, D.A., et al.: Muscle capillary basement membrane in identical twins discordant for insulin-dependent diabetes. Diabetes *32*:557, 1983.

Porte, D., Jr., Graf, R.J., Halter, J.B., et al.: Diabetic neuropathy and plasma glucose control. Am. J. Med. *70*:195, 1981.

Graf, R.J., Halter, J.B., Pfeifer, M.A., et al.: Glycemic control and nerve conduction abnormalities in non-insulin-dependent diabetic subjects. Ann. Intern. Med. *94*:307, 1981.

White, N.H., Waltman, S.R., Krupin, T., Santiago, J.V.: Reversal of abnormalities in ocular fluorophotometry in insulin-dependent diabetes after five to nine months of improved metabolic control. Diabetes *31*:80, 1982.

Steno Study Group: Effect of 6 months of strict metabolic control on eye and kidney function in insulin-dependent diabetics with background retinopathy. Lancet *1*:121, 1982.

Lauritzen, T., Frost-Larsen, K., Larsen, H.-W., et al.: Effect of 1 year of near-normal blood glucose levels on retinopathy in insulin-dependent diabetics. Lancet *1*:200, 1983.

Forst-Larsen, K., Christiansen, J.S., Parving, H.-H.: The effect of strict short-term metabolic control on retinal nervous system abnormalities in newly diagnosed Type I (insulin-dependent) diabetic patients. Diabetologia *24*:207, 1983.

Holman, R.R., Dornan, T.L., Mayon-White, V., et al.: Pre-

vention of deterioration of renal and sensory-nerve function by more intensive management of insulin-dependent diabetic patients. A two-year randomised prospective study. Lancet *1*:204, 1983.

Viberti, G.C., Bilous, R.W., Mackintosh, D., et al.: Long term correction of hyperglycaemia and progression of renal failure in insulin-dependent diabetes. Br. Med. J. *286*:598, 1983.

Cataland, S., D'Orisio, T.M.: Diabetic nephropathy. Clinical course in patients treated with the subcutaneous insulin pump. J.A.M.A. *249*:2059, 1983.

Agardh, C.D., Rosen, I., Schersten, B.: Improvement of peripheral nerve function after institution of insulin treatment in diabetes mellitus. A case-control study. Acta Med. Scand. *213*:283, 1983.

Raskin, P., Pietri, A.O., Unger, R., Shannon, W.A., Jr.: The effect of diabetic control on the width of skeletal-muscle capillary basement membrane in patients with Type I diabetes mellitus. N. Engl. J. Med. *309*:1546, 1983.

11 Pathogenesis of Macrovascular Disease Including the Influence of Lipids

Om P. Ganda

"Does an excess of fat in the diet lead to arteriosclerosis? I believe the chief cause of premature development of arteriosclerosis in diabetes, save for advancing age, is an excess of fat, an excess of fat in the body (obesity), an excess of fat in the diet, and an excess of fat in the blood. With an excess of fat diabetes begins and from an excess of fat diabetics die, formerly of coma, recently of arteriosclerosis."

Elliott P. Joslin, 1927[1]

While the exact role of fat and other factors in the diet and in the blood of the diabetic may still be controversial, few authorities will dispute the clairvoyance of Dr. Joslin's statement, made at a time when insulin had just begun to make increased longevity possible for the diabetic. Today, the macrovascular complications, originating from atherosclerosis, account for the majority of fatalities in the diabetic population.[2,3]

Most authorities would agree that atherosclerosis tends to occur at an earlier age and with greater severity in the diabetic than in the nondiabetic population, matched for other variables. The evidence for this conclusion is primarily derived from the extensive analyses of the autopsy data summarized by Warren, LeCompte, and Legg,[4] by Robertson and Strong,[5] and in Chapters 10, 12, and 14 of this book. However, the incidence of atherosclerosis according to clinical studies has some limitations in accurate diagnosis, particularly when the disease is asymptomatic. In the 1975 report of the National Commission on Diabetes, West[6] extensively reviewed clinical and autopsy statistics from the world literature. He concluded that heart attacks or strokes are about twice as likely in persons with overt diabetes as in the general population; gangrene is at least 5 times as likely. In persons with known diabetes, macrovascular disease accounts for about 75% of all deaths, mainly expressing itself as cardiovascular disease.[2,3,6] Moreover, despite evidence of striking heterogeneity in the etiology of diabetes (see Chapter 2), the increased propensity to macrovascular complications is not restricted to any one type of diabetes, e.g. insulin-dependent vs noninsulin-dependent. However, unlike the microvascular complications which occur more frequently in insulin-dependent (Type I) diabetics, the macrovascular complications are more frequently observed in noninsulin-dependent (Type II) diabetics in the 5th to 7th decades of life. According to the Joslin Clinic experience, clinically significant atherosclerotic lesions in older patients are frequently unrelated to the duration or severity of overt diabetes. In fact, such lesions may be the presenting feature in individuals who may have had relatively mild diabetes in the form of impaired glucose tolerance ("chemical" diabetes) for an uncertain duration. This view is supported by the results of studies by Pirart,[7] and of several epidemiologic surveys including those from Framingham,[8,9] Tecumseh,[10] and Bedford and Whitehall.[11,12] On the other hand, in insulin-dependent diabetics, evidence of accelerated atherosclerosis can be documented frequently after 10 to 15 years of diabetes, when compared with age and sex-matched controls.[13]

A peculiar feature of the incidence of atherosclerosis in the diabetic is its striking prevalence in diabetic women, including those who are premenopausal. In the Framingham study, no premenopausal woman in a cohort of 2873 non-diabetic women develped myocardial infarction or died of coronary heart disease after 24 years of follow-up. However, there was a striking increase of these events after menopause.[14] In contrast, the morbidity and mortality from atherosclerotic events in all diabetic women were equal to or greater than in diabetic men.[9] Similar results have been reported from the Joslin Clinic experience.[15-17]

The term arteriosclerosis, as employed in the literature, includes atherosclerosis, characterized by the fatty intimal plaque, as well as diffuse intimal fibrosis, regarded as similar or identical to atherosclerosis.[4] In this review, both of these will be referred to collectively as atherosclerosis. Another macrovascular lesion, well known as Mönckeberg sclerosis, is a fairly common roentgenographic and histopathologic finding, characterized by calcific deposits in the media of muscular arteries of the legs and occasionally of visceral and coronary arteries.[4,18] Although increased in diabetics, Mönckeberg's sclerosis does not by itself involve the intima and therefore does not result in luminal narrowing or ischemia. Its cause is unknown and its course is benign. This entity has been reviewed by Lachman et al.[18]

Several recent reviews have dealt with the pathogenesis of atherosclerosis in the diabetic human.[3,19-22,460] Over the past decade, a number of significant observations have been made in the epidemiology of atherosclerosis around the world and in understanding various risk factors or protective factors in the pathogenesis of human atherosclerosis. In addition, important insights have been gained from experimental models of atherosclerosis, especially in primates,[23,24] which may have considerable relevance to the human pathology. The diabetic human, in addition to being suscep-tible to any one or a combination of pathogenetic factors operative in the nondiabetic, is at particular disadvantage because of at least three additional influences unique to the diabetic state: (1) associated presence of microangiopathy; (2) hyperglycemia and its direct or indirect consequences; and (3) hormonal aberrations underlying the altered metabolic/biochemical state, either as a cause or an effect of diabetes. Finally, the superimposed multiplicity of factors (e.g. hypertension, hyperlipidemia and hypercoagulability) which occur with an increased frequency, not generally seen in such co-dominance in the nondiabetic, make the diabetic more vulnerable. This review will begin with the recent progress in the theories of atherogenesis, followed by a brief description of each of the the pathogenetic factors, with particular reference to the diabetic.

THEORIES REGARDING THE PATHOGENESIS OF ATHEROSCLEROSIS

The subject of cellular mechanisms in the pathogenesis of atherosclerosis was extensively explored in several symposia[25-27a] and reviews.[28-32] Two early hypotheses explaining atherogenesis have withstood the test of time. The first was the "thrombogenic" theory put forth by Rokitansky in 1852, and later modified by Duguid in 1946 and Duguid and Robertson in 1957.[33] The second, namely the "insudative" or "imbibition" hypothesis, was the result of Virchow's pioneering work in 1856. This theory also was later modified by Aschoff in 1924, by Anitschkow in 1933 and by Mustard and Packham in 1975.[34]

The response-to-injury hypothesis of Virchow has received increasing attention in recent years.[29,30,34,35] According to Ross and co-workers, the key event in the initiation and perpetuation of the fibrous plaque, the pathognomonic lesion of atherosclerosis, is the proliferation of the smooth muscle cell in the arterial wall.[36] This event is followed by two other fundamental sequelae: deposition of intracellular and extracellular lipid, and accumulation of extracellular matrix components including collagen, elastic fibers and proteoglycans. According to this hypothesis, a disruption of the endothelial barrier of the arterial intima is a sine qua non for the proliferation of the arterial smooth muscle cell. Such disruption, leading to focal desquamation and increased endothelial permeability, has been shown to occur experimentally by virtually any form of injury to endothelium including mechanical,[29,35] chemical,[37] and immune[38] mechanisms. Furthermore, in vitro experiments have suggested that a platelet factor may be required in order to trigger the smooth muscle proliferation. The nature of this non-dialyzable, heat-stable, mitogenic factor, which apparently is liberated during the "release-reaction," is being characterized.[38a] Recent evidence suggests that low-density lipoproteins in serum also have a definite role in cell proliferation. Other macromolecules as yet unidentified, may also be involved. Regardless of the stimulus for proliferation, the smooth muscle cells, once in intima, are responsible for the synthesis and deposition of other components of extracellular matrix, i.e., collagen, elastic fibers and glycosaminoglycan.

From the postulated sequence of events in the hypothesis of Ross and co-workers, it is conceivable that in the initial stages of the genesis of the fibrous plaque, the entire process might be subject to repair and regression, unless the injury to the endothelium continues unabated or is repetitive.[39,40] Various "risk factors" (discussed below) may affect the balance between the injury and repair, and ultimately the net outcome.

Of the various risk factors in the pathogenesis of atherosclerosis, the role of hyperlipidemia, particularly an increased body pool of low density lipoprotein (LDL) has received the most attention for two reasons. The studies of Ross and Harker[30] have established that not only is the deposition of lipids in the smooth muscle cell the hallmark of atheromatous lesions, but in addition, LDL may produce the primary endothelial injury that initiates and perpetuates the process. Secondly, the elegant studies of Goldstein and Brown[41,42] have clearly established the molecular mechanism underlying one prototype entity of premature atherosclerosis, namely familial hypercholesterolemia, an autosomal dominant disorder secondary to LDL receptor defect. Their work has shown the presence of a high affinity, surface receptor system that regulates the binding, internalization, and degradation of cholesterol in the body. Once the LDL levels in extracellular fluid (lymph) exceed a critical concentration, the process of endothelial desquamation may set in, particularly in the presence of other synergistic factors such as increased shear stress in hypertension and perhaps hormonal dysfunction.

A number of physicochemical and enzymatic mechanisms probably mediate the final development of a positive cholesterol balance in the arterial smooth muscle cell.[31,43] Among other factors, lysosomal enzymes may be intimately involved in the intralysosomal accumulation or release of cholesterol and other macromolecules. Wolinsky[44] has put forth a unifying concept which states that multiple factors such as hypercholesterolemia, hypertension and diabetes may act in concert in diminishing the activity of acid hydrolases. Interestingly, in rats rendered insulin-deficient by streptozotocin or alloxan, the activities of acid cholesteryl esterase

could be restored by optimal control of diabetes with insulin treatment.[45] Evidence of a low acid cholesteryl esterase activity was also recently demonstrated in patients with premature coronary artery disease.[46] Moreover, cholesteryl ester deposition may perpetuate further injury to the vessel wall by activating complement pathway.[47]

Two other hypotheses concerning atherogenesis should be mentioned. Benditt and Benditt[48,49] have provided evidence for a monoclonal origin of the arterial smooth muscle cell that may result in its proliferation. Their hypothesis is supported by the work of Pearson et al.[50] who have shown the presence of a single G-6-PD isoenzyme in the plaques of black women heterozygous for X-linked G-6-PD, whereas all normal tissues revealed both A and B isoenzymes. Thus, according to this theory, the atherosclerotic lesions are neoplastic rather than hyperplastic, as suggested by Ross and Glomset.[36] Finally, another hypothesis, put forth by Martin, Osburn, and Sprague[51] is based simply on the finite replicative ability of the aging cells in culture, as shown by Hayflick[52] and others. Their theory states that atherogenesis is a paradoxical function of declining stem cell activity in the arterial media. This hypothesis thus reflects a phenomenon of the aging process which has received considerable attention in the pathogenesis of atherosclerosis.[53] One of the components in this theory is the secretion of substances termed "chalones"—by arterial smooth muscle cells—which inhibit the replication of stem cells in forming new smooth muscle cells. The precise nature and regulation of chalones remain to be determined. However, this is an attractive hypothesis since it has been suggested that in diabetes, there may exist a primary cellular abnormality which results in decreased life-span of cells of various tissues,[54,55] with perhaps diminished response-to-injury in the arterial wall as well. However, the age-related effects clearly must be modulated by environmental influences, e.g., other risk factors.

LIPOPROTEIN METABOLISM AND ATHEROGENESIS

The role of lipids as fuel and in the synthesis and integrity of cell membranes in the body is well recognized.[56] The lipids (cholesterol, triglycerides, phospholipids) are transported in human plasma as macromolecular complexes with specific proteins, thus forming lipoproteins. Over the past decade, there has been a burgeoning of interest in the significance of lipids and lipoprotein metabolism in the context of atherogenesis. Since the delineation of various types of human lipoproteins by Barr, Goffman, and their associates about 3 decades ago,[57,58] our understanding of the structure and metabolism of lipoproteins has advanced tremendously.[59–66] In addition, studies of large kindreds with diverse types of hyperlipidemic states have led to the recognition of various genetic models of hyperlipidemia in man, thus resulting in newer classifications,[65,67–69] and extending the original phenotypic classification proposed by Fredrickson, Levy and Lees in 1967.[70]

Great interest in studies related to lipids was stimulated in the early 1950s when investigators noted that premature atherosclerosis is related to altered concentrations of certain plasma lipoproteins.[57,58] Subsequent confirmation of the significance of hyperlipidemia came from various epidemiologic observations. In addition, the family studies of Goldstein et al. revealed that levels of plasma cholesterol and/or triglycerides were elevated in approximately 50% of the survivors of premature myocardial infarction, i.e., men before age 50 years and women before age 60 years.[71] More recently interest has been rekindled in the hitherto dormant studies of Barr et al. in 1951[57] concerning an inverse correlation of high density lipoprotein (HDL) with cardiovascular disease. An explosion of studies ensued in which the mechanism of this protective effect of HDL has been investigated.[72,73] In addition to the extensive literature concerning circulating lipoproteins, an increased concentration of phospholipids in plasma has recently been reported in patients with premature atherosclerosis.[74]

Nomenclature and Classification of Lipoproteins

The human lipoproteins provide an efficient mechanism for transporting water-insoluble lipid moieties in circulation. Each lipoprotein is composed of a non-polar lipid core, consisting of cholesterol ester and triglyceride, surrounded by a monolayer membrane of polar lipids (free cholesterol and phospholipids) in combination with specific proteins (apoproteins). The ultracentrifugal and electrophoretic characteristics and fractional composition of the four major human lipoproteins are shown in Table 11–1.

1. Chylomicrons. The largest and least dense particles, the chylomicrons, are synthesized in the small intestine. Their major function is the transporting of exogenous (dietary) fat as triglyceride. In normal man, they are cleared from the circulation within a few hours. They are catabolized, mainly by hydrolysis, under the influence of a triglyceride lipase located at the capillary endothelium in adipose tissue and muscle. Triglyceride lipase (or lipoprotein lipase) is often referred to as "postheparin lipolytic activity" (PHLA). This includes a hepatic lipase, also released by heparin.

Several techniques have been developed to dissociate the lipoprotein lipase of extrahepatic origin from the hepatic lipase.[75–77]

2. Very Low-Density Lipoproteins (VLDL). Human Very-Low Density Lipoproteins consist of endogenous triglyceride in combination with cholesterol, and are mainly of hepatic origin. VLDL composition depends upon the particle size; the proportion of triglyceride and apoprotein C varies directly, and that of apo B and total protein varies inversely with the size of the VLDL particle. A smaller fraction of VLDL also arises from the intestine.

The mechanisms controlling the synthesis and regulation of VLDL are not completely understood. Depending upon the availability of free fatty acids, the synthesis of VLDL is increased in the presence of excessive carbohydrate and the process is undoubtedly under hormonal regulation.[78–80]

VLDL and chylomicrons probably share a common saturable catabolic pathway; however, the clearance of VLDL is probably less efficient than that of chylomicrons.[81] A VLDL remnant formed by partial hydrolysis of VLDL in peripheral tissues results in the cholesterol-enriched intermediate density lipoprotein (IDL), a process in which HDL plays a crucial role, as discussed below.

3. Low-Density Lipoprotein (LDL). LDL in man is considered to be largely a breakdown product of VLDL metabolism. LDL constitutes about 50% of plasma lipoprotein mass in the normal human and carries about 75% of circulating cholesterol.

Peripheral tissues[82] appear to be a major site for LDL catabolism, although newer techniques estimate some degradation in the liver as well.[43,83] Experimental depletion of plasma cholesterol leads to a severalfold increase in the rate of cholesterol synthesis in several extrahepatic sites.[84] These observations support the hypothesis of a receptor-mediated control of LDL regulation.[42,82]

4. High-Density Lipoprotein (HDL). HDL is the most dense lipoprotein because 50% of its mass is protein. It carries about 15 to 20% of total circulating cholesterol. It is synthesized in the liver, as well as in the human intestinal tract.[85] HDL from the normal human can be subdivided into fractions of density 1.063 to 1.120 (HDL_{2a} and HDL_{2b}) and 1.120 to 1.210 (HDL_3). The HDL_2 concentrations are generally about twice as high in premenopausal females as in males and may reflect more accurately the protective role of HDL in atherogenesis.[86,87] Newly synthesized (nascent) HDL particles carry mainly unesterified cholesterol and undergo a number of critical changes in the periphery as discussed below.

Apoproteins. The major apoprotein constituents

Table 11–1.   Major Lipoproteins of Human Plasma

	Chylomicrons	Very Low Density Lipoproteins (VLDL)	Low Density Lipoproteins (LDL)	High Density Lipoproteins (HDL)
Particle size (Å)	750–12,000	300–700	180–300	50–120
Density[1] (g/ml)	<0.95	0.95–1.006	1.006–1.063	1.063–1.210
(Sf)	>400	20–400	0–20	0–9[2]
Electrophoretic migration	Origin	Pre-beta	Beta	Alpha
Composition (%)				
Cholesterol	3–7	20–30	51–58	18–25
Triglyceride	80–95	50–65	4–10	3–7
Phospholipid	3–6	15–20	18–24	24–32
Protein	1–2	6–10	18–22	45–55
Apoproteins				
Major	B-48, C, A-I	B-100, C, E	B-100	A-I, A-II
Minor	A-II, E[3], PRP[4]	A-I, A-II, D[5]	C	C, D, E
Origin	Intestine	Liver, Intestine	End Product of VLDL	Intestine, liver

[1]Estimated by ultracentrifugation. Sf is the corrected flotation rate at d = 1.063, expressed in Svedbergs, except[2], at d = 1.210
[3]Also called ARP (arginine-rich protein, [4]proline-rich protein, [5]Also called "thin-line" protein or Apo A-III.

of human lipoproteins are being extensively studied. The two major proteins in HDL, A-I and A-II, exist in a ratio of 3:1. Apo A-I activates lecithin-cholesterol acyltransferase (LCAT), the key enzyme involved in the formation of HDL cholesterol esters by catalyzing the reaction: lecithin + cholesterol → cholesterol ester + lysolecithin.[88] Apoprotein B-100 is the major protein of LDL and also comprises 20 to 35% of total protein content of VLDL. Apo B-100 is responsible for the recognition of LDL by its receptor. The Apo-B, synthesized by the intestine (Apo B-48), is the one contained in chylomicrons and chylomicron-remnants. Apo B-48 is recognized by a distinct remnant receptor in liver.[82] Apoprotein C is a family of three well-characterized subunits, Apo C-I, Apo C-II, and Apo C-III, based on their migration on polyacrylamide gel electrophoresis. The Apo C-III further consists of three subspecies (Apo-C$_0$, C-III$_1$, and C-III$_2$). Apo C constitutes about 40 to 50% of VLDL protein and about 5% of HDL protein. Apo C-II has been shown to be a physiologic stimulator of lipoprotein lipase, but not of hepatic lipase; in contrast, Apo C-III might be an inhibitor of the lipoprotein lipase. With the availability of techniques for measuring these apoprotein constituents, newer mechanisms of hyperlipidemia are being revealed. For example, it has been proposed that a deficiency of Apo C-II, or a relative excess of Apo C-III, might account for a resistance to the lipoprotein lipase activation and thus result in certain states of endogenous hypertriglyceridemia.[89–93] Also, a severe deficiency of Apo C-II has been described in a patient with marked hypertriglyceridemia;[94] the deficiency was shown to be transmitted as a familial trait.[95]

Apo E, also termed the "arginine-rich" protein (ARP), is found in chylomicrons, VLDL and HDL. The precise role of Apo E is unknown but it is thought to play an important part in cholesterol transport. Apo E is increased in the "broad-beta" disease, a disorder characterized by a cholesterol-enriched VLDL with beta mobility on electrophoresis.[96] More specifically, this disorder has been shown to be characterized by an inherited deficiency of Apo E-3 subfraction.[97] Furthermore, Mahley et al.[98] have shown an increase in the Apo E content of HDL, accounting for the appearance of a cholesterol-enriched HDL, termed HDL$_c$, following increased consumption of dietary cholesterol in animals and in man. This HDL$_c$ lacks APO-A and competes for LDL binding sites in cultured fibroblasts. The increased binding was correlated with the increase in Apo E content of the HDL$_c$.

Lipoprotein Metabolism and Interconversions

The first step in the series of complex degradative steps of lipoprotein interconversion involves the breakdown of triglyceride-rich chylomicrons and VLDL by the lipolytic enzymes (vide supra). This results in the formation of an intermediate density lipoprotein (IDL) in the density range of 1.006 to 1.019. During this process of IDL formation, the Apo C and Apo E are transferred to HDL. The chylomicron remnant and IDL are triglyceride-poor but enriched in cholesterol and Apo B. The further interactions and fate of these particles in the formation and disposal of LDL are not well understood but HDL plays an important role. This has been the focus of attention since accumulating evidence indicates a role of HDL in the prevention of cholesterol deposition in peripheral tissues. According to one attractive scheme outlined by Hamilton[99] and by Tall and Small,[73] the nascent HDL is secreted by the liver as a discoidal particle, containing mostly phospholipids. In the blood or in the periphery, the discoidal HDL picks up free cholesterol from the cell membranes and from remnant particles and IDL. The LCAT system, intimately involved in this process, generates cholesteryl esters in the HDL from these lipids and converts them into spherical shape. Each of these cholesteryl ester-enriched particles, HDL and remnant, may then be recognized by the hepatocyte receptors leading to uptake, degradation, and finally biliary excretion of cholesterol. A preferential utilization of free cholesterol from high density lipoproteins for biliary cholesterol secretion has been demonstrated in man.[100] In familial[88] or acquired[101] LCAT deficiency, most HDL particles remain disk shaped and the cholesterol remains unesterified.[88,99,101] Similarly, in Tangier disease, a disorder characterized by virtual absence of normal HDL,[64,102,103] the metabolism of chylomicrons and VLDL remnants is impaired and marked accumulation of cholesteryl esters results in several organs.[64,104] The similarities in the manifestations of LCAT deficiency and Tangier disease further support the concept of these pathways in the mobilization of cholesterol from the periphery.[64,73,105]

The pioneering work of Goldstein and Brown in cultured fibroblast, lymphocyte and other models has established the presence of a specific LDL receptor pathway.[41,42,106] According to this hypothesis, LDL-cell interaction involves binding at a cell surface receptor site which specifically recognizes Apo B-100 and Apo-E.[82] This is followed by internalization and lysosomal degradation. The free cholesterol thus released intracellularly leads to: (1) suppression of hydroxymethylglutaryl (HMG)-CoA reductase, thus suppressing cholesterol synthesis, and (2) stimulation of cholesterol esterification by activating the acyl CoA:cholesterol acyl transferase (ACAT) enzyme system. These events lead to inhibition of LDL receptor when a critical concentration of intracellular cholesterol is available. The interactions of HDL and its subtypes with the LDL receptor are poorly understood.[87] However, in cultured human fibroblasts, HDL somehow reduces the binding of LDL, thereby reducing the internalization and degradation of LDL.[107] In cultured human arterial cells, a competition of HDL with LDL binding sites has also been shown.[108–110] Presence of high-affinity binding sites specific for HDL have been demonstrated on human fibroblasts as well as smooth muscle cells.[110a]

Familial Hyperlipoproteinemias

Based on 90 percentile limits of plasma total cholesterol and triglycerides levels (Table 11–2), and lipoprotein patterns, Fredrickson et al.[70] class-

ified hyperlipidemia into five major groups, a terminology that soon became commonplace in the lipid literature. Each type of hyperlipoproteinemia could be primary or secondary to an underlying illness. Fredrickson Type II, originally synonymous with familial hypercholesterolemia, was later subdivided into Types IIa and IIb, depending upon whether or not triglycerides are simultaneously increased. Type IIb thus resembles Type IV (familial hypertriglyceridemia), except that LDL cholesterol is also increased. The latter can be easily calculated in most situations (triglyceride concentration <400 mg/dl), once HDL-cholesterol is known:[111] LDL cholesterol = total cholesterol − (triglyceride/5 + HDL-cholesterol).

The extensive genetic studies of Goldstein et al.[71,112] have uncovered the presence of three major autosomal dominant forms of hyperlipidemia in the families of survivors of myocardial infarction: familial hypercholesterolemia, familial hypertriglyceridemia, and familial combined hyperlipidemia. Both Fredrickson's phenotypic and Goldstein's genotypic classifications have considerable overlap in presentation, but taken together, they provide a helpful approach in the study of hyperlipidemias (Table 11–3).

Familial Lipoprotein Lipase Deficiency (Type I Hyperlipoproteinemia). This disorder, typically beginning in childhood, is characterized by absence of lipoprotein lipase activity, and is inherited as an autosomal recessive trait. Interestingly, this disorder is not associated with any increase in atherosclerosis, although few if any of the patients studied were over 50 years of age.

Familial Hypercholesterolemia (Type II Hyperlipoproteinemia). This is the most extensively studied type of lipid disorder; it has a well-established relationship with premature atherosclerosis in direct correlation with a single or double dose of the abnormal gene.[42,65,113,114] The basic defect in this disorder has been shown conclusively to be a deficient or defective receptor for LDL, which is associated with defective catabolism of LDL and increased cellular cholesterol biosynthesis.

Familial Dysbetalipoproteinemia (Type III Hyperlipoproteinemia). A rare disorder, this entity is characterized by hypercholesterolemia and hypertriglyceridemia associated with (a) the presence of an abnormal VLDL with beta mobility on electrophoresis and (b) an increased content of cholesteryl ester and Apo E in VLDL.[115–117] Recent work has indicated an inherited deficiency of Apo E-3 in these families.[97] Coronary and peripheral atherosclerosis is frequent. Approximately 25% of affected individuals have associated glucose intolerance.

Familial Hypertriglyceridemia (Type IV Hy-

Table 11–2   Mean and Range (5th–90th Percentile) for Plasma Lipid Concentrations (mg/dl) in the United States White Population*

Age (yr.)	Total Cholesterol		Total Triglycerides		HDL-Cholesterol	
	Male	Female	Male	Female	Male	Female
0–19	155(115–185)	160(120–190)	65(30–100)	70(35–105)	50(30–70)	55(35–70)
20–29	175(130–215)	165(125–210)	100(40–165)	90(40–115)	45(30–65)	55(35–80)
30–39	195(140–245)	175(130–225)	140(50–235)	95(40–160)	45(30–65)	55(35–80)
40–49	210(155–255)	200(145–245)	150(55–250)	105(45–180)	45(30–65)	60(35–85)
50–59+	210(160–260)	225(155–275)	140(60–220)	120(55–195)	42(30–65)	60(35–90)

*Based on more than 60,000 participants in Lipid Research Clinic (LRC) Prevalence Study.[110b] For HDL-cholesterol, 95th percentile limit is shown, based on LRC as well as Fredrickson data.[65]

Table 11–3.   Classification of Hyperlipoproteinemias Based on Phenotypic and Genotypic Characteristics

Genetic Disorder	Elevated Lipoprotein	Plasma Lipids Cholesterol	Plasma Lipids Triglyceride	Lipoprotein Pattern	Frequency*
Familial lipoprotein lipase deficiency	Chylomicrons	N, ↑	↑ ↑ ↑	I	
Familial hypercholesterolemia	LDL	↑ ↑	N, ↑	IIa, rarely IIb	1:500
Familial dysbetalipoproteinemia	Beta VLDL	↑ ↑	↑ ↑	III	1:10,000
Familial hypertriglyceridemia	VLDL	N, ↑	↑ ↑	IV	1:500
Familial combined hyperlipidemia	LDL, VLDL	N, ↑	N, ↑	IIa, IIb, IV, rarely V	1:250
Familial Type V hyperlipoproteinemia	VLDL, Chylomicrons	↑	↑ ↑ ↑	V	

*In general population.
↑ = slight elevation; ↑ ↑ = moderate elevation; ↑ ↑ ↑ = marked elevation (see text for details). N = normal.
Adapted from refs. 65, 71, 112.

perlipoproteinemia). In the kindreds studied by Goldstein et al.,[113] familial hypertriglyceridemia was about as frequent as familial hypercholesterolemia. In these families, cholesterol levels are normal or moderately increased, commensurate with the cholesterol contribution by VLDL. The prevalence of atherosclerosis in this form of hyperlipidemia remains controversial. In one study, the frequency of myocardial infarction in living hyperlipidemic relatives with familial hypertriglyceridemia was no different than in the normolipidemic controls.[118] It is recognized that a major problem in identifying familial hypertriglyceridemia as a "risk factor" might be the genetic heterogeneity and the existence of hypertriglyceridemia as a part of other disorders such as familial combined hyperlipidemia, Type III and IV disorders as well as its frequent association with underlying secondary conditions, e.g., diabetes.

Familial Combined Hyperlipidemia. This newly discovered genetic hyperlipidemia is now thought to be more frequent than familial hypercholesterolemia and familial hypertriglyceridemia combined.[65,113] The description of this monogenic disorder most clearly underscores the limitation of Fredrickson's classification in studying familial transmission since these individuals can present as Type IIa, IIb, IV or V, as the varied expression of the same genetic mutation. This entity is clearly

associated with premature atherosclerosis, and diabetes is common in some families. No defect of LDL receptor has been found in this disorder, unlike the situation in familial hypercholesterolemia.

Type V Hyperlipoproteinemia. Patients with Type V hyperlipoproteinemia have marked triglyceridemia (usually greater than 1000 mg/dl) due to increased concentrations of chylomicrons and VLDL.[65,119] The levels of triglycerides are quite variable and are modified by associated factors such as obesity, alcohol, diet, drugs and diabetes. The prevalence of atherosclerosis in many kindreds with primary Type V hyperlipoproteinemia is not increased.[119] Affected relatives are either Type V, or more commonly Type IV, and often fluctuate between Types V and IV, depending upon the environmental (e.g. dietary) influences. Many Type V individuals may belong to the category of familial combined hyperlipidemia.

A history of premature atherosclerosis in a family may alert one to early recognition and treatment of hyperlipidemia during childhood.[120,121] Recent extensive studies have indicated that children of parents with high cholesterol or triglyceride levels are two to three times more likely to have their respective lipid levels above the 95th percentile of pediatric population.[122]

Familial Lipoproteinemic Disorders with Protection Against Atherosclerosis. In certain familial disorders of lipoprotein metabolism, a low prevalence of atherosclerosis has been documented.

1. Hyper-alpha-lipoproteinemia. Glueck and others[64,123] have recently described aggregation of individuals with high levels of HDL in certain families. The longevity in such kindreds is significantly prolonged and the incidence of atherosclerotic events decreased. This entity seems to be transmitted as an autosomal dominant disorder and the affected individuals reveal mildly elevated cholesterol levels within the normal distribution of LDL and VLDL.

2. Hypo-beta-lipoproteinemia. This familial disorder is also characterized by increased longevity and lowered incidence of atherosclerosis. Glueck et al.[123] have described 18 kindreds in detail and shown a markedly reduced LDL-cholesterol, and LDL-cholesterol to HDL-cholesterol ratio in the affected members. Striking absence of atherosclerotic lesions has been documented in such individuals.[124]

HYPERLIPIDEMIA IN DIABETES

Hyperlipidemia as a metabolic abnormality is frequently associated with diabetes. Its prevalence is variable, depending on the type and severity of diabetes, glycemic control, nutritional status, age, and other factors. Because of this, estimates of its prevalence have ranged from about 20 to 70%. In a statistical sense, the most characteristic lipid abnormality in the diabetic is hypertriglyceridemia, with or without associated increase in plasma cholesterol.[20,66,125-135] Virtually any lipoprotein phenotype may be encountered in a diabetic patient. However, the most common forms are Types IV > IIb > V > IIa, the isolated hypercholesterolemia being uncommon. However, it is most important not to be complacent about a "normal" level of cholesterol (within 90 percentile of general population range, Table 11–2), or of LDL-cholesterol, since there is overwhelming evidence indicating an increased risk of atherosclerotic disease with increasng levels of cholesterol within the normal range.[136,137] In the Framingham Study, for example, the risk of myocardial infarction over a 14-year period, in men prospectively followed from 30 to 49 years of age, was 4-fold greater in those with total cholesterol of 250 or higher, than in those with a level of 193 or lower.[136] This may be of particular concern in the diabetic who is often concurrently besieged with other atherogenic factors.

LDL Metabolism in Diabetes

Using tracer-labeled VLDL and LDL, Kissebah et al.[138] have found an increased LDL turnover in adult-onset diabetics, even when the fraction of total flux of VLDL converted to LDL is lower than normal. It has therefore been postulated that an increase in the turnover of LDL could be an important factor in the deposition of lipid-rich material in the arterial walls. Bennion and Grundy[139] have shown that improved control of diabetes results in diminished cholesterol synthesis, although the effects of insulin and diabetes control on total sterol balance remain somewhat controversial[140] and require further investigation.

Insulin may also have important effects on HMG-CO A reductase, the key rate-limiting enzyme in LDL metabolism. However, divergent results have been noted in the few studies available thus far.[141,142] Similarly, the effects of insulin deficiency or insulin excess on LDL composition have not been well studied, although altered triglyceride/cholesterol ratio has been noted in patients with inadequately controlled diabetes.

In preliminary studies, no defects in LDL receptor binding was found in skin fibroblasts from diabetics.[143] However, when the interaction of fibroblasts from normal individuals with the LDL isolated from diabetics was studied, a significant impairment was observed in diabetic LDL internalization and degradation.[143a] Furthermore, two recent lines of evidence might explain the increased atherogenicity of diabetic lipoproteins, even when the absolute concentrations of LDL-cholesterol or total cholesterol are not strikingly elevated. First, elegant studies by Mahley and co-workers have revealed that diets high in cholesterol and saturated fats induce the synthesis of cholesterol-rich Apo-E containing β-VLDL particles which interact with macrophages and transform them into lipid-laden foam cells in the arterial wall.[144] The β-VLDL is thus highly atherogenic, similar to the chylomicron-remnant particle, which is also produced in excess following a cholesterol-rich diet,[145] and may be involved in the increased production of foam cells. Therefore, dietary manipulation in the diabetic could result in major alterations in the intermediary lipoprotein interconversions without substantial changes in total cholesterol levels. Secondly, in vitro studies have shown that chemical modifications of the LDL particle itself, e.g., acetylation, might result in its increased incorporation in the arterial wall via a receptor-independent pathway. A similar mechanism has been proposed, particularly in the diabetic, by the demonstration of non-enzymatic glycosylation of LDL in vitro.[146] The critical range of glycemia sufficient to induce LDL glycosylation in vivo remains to be determined and would obviously be of great interest.

Triglyceride Metabolism in Diabetes

Insulin plays a critical role in the production and clearance of triglycerides in the diabetic. Nikkilä,[131] Howard,[147] and Reavan[148] have reviewed evidence for various mechanisms involved in the development of hypertriglyceridemia in the diabetic state. Most of the diabetic patients are found to have variable combinations of triglyceride overproduction or underutilization and part of the discrepancies in results from various investigators can be attributed to differences in methodology.[149]

In severe insulin deficiency, lipoprotein-lipase (LPL) activity, frequently estimated as post-heparin lipolytic activity (PHLA) is markedly impaired,[66,131,150] resulting in the syndrome of "diabetic lipemia."[150a] Insulin treatment promptly restores the activity of LPL in such a situation, with rapid decrease in plasma triglycerides. On the other hand, LPL activity is relatively intact in mild to moderately severe, noninsulin-requiring diabetics.[131,150] In such diabetics, endogenous triglyceride (VLDL) synthesis is enhanced,[151] particularly in the presence of obesity and adequate amounts of insulin. A combination of overproduction and under-utilization is not uncommon, however, in moderately severe, untreated diabetes with gross elevations of triglycerides, and subtle abnormalities of triglyceride clearance have been found even in the absence of severe insulin deficiency.[151,152]

Patients with impaired glucose tolerance ("chemical" diabetes) frequently manifest a constellation of endogenous hypertriglyceridemia, obesity, and hyperinsulinism.[66,153] However, attempts to correlate hypertriglyceridemia with adiposity and hyperinsulinism have by no means yielded a clear relationship. Hyperinsulinism and increased triglyceride levels are often present in the absence of obesity[154,155] and moderate degrees of obesity have been shown not to affect VLDL triglyceride kinetics in patients whose triglyceride levels vary over a wide range.[156] However, in most situations in which hypertriglyceridemia and mild glucose intolerance co-exist, a close correlation between VLDL production rate and plasma triglyceride levels can be shown, indicating relatively intact clearance mechanisms.[151,156,157] Despite frequent co-existence of hypertriglyceridemia and diabetes, the results of the genetic studies of Brunzell et al.[158] do not indicate any evidence of increased risk of diabetes in kindreds with familial hypertriglyceridemia.

While the significance of LDL in premature atherosclerosis seems well established, the role of endogenous triglycerides or VLDL remains somewhat controversial. Prospective epidemiologic studies from Sweden,[159] Finland,[160] and Michigan[161] suggested an additional risk from serum triglycerides. Similarly, familial combined hyperlipidemia was twice as frequent as familial hypercholesterolemia in the survivors of myocar-

dial infarction studied by Goldstein et al.[113] In diabetics, Albrink's observations over 30 years (1931–1961) suggested a marked increase in macrovascular disease in the years 1951–1961 compared to the previous years. This was accompanied by the trend toward increasing triglyceride levels.[126] Moreover, in a study of 101 diabetic patients, matched for age and sex, Santen et al.[129] concluded that atherosclerosis could be better recognized clinically by levels of triglyceride than by those of cholesterol; 50% of diabetics with atherosclerosis had elevated triglyceride levels, compared with 15% of those without atherosclerosis and 19% of controls. On the other hand, in angiographically documented coronary artery disease patients, Type IV hyperlipoproteinemia was the commonest lipoprotein abnormality in one study,[162] but in others,[137,163,164] it was less strikingly, or not at all, associated with severe coronary atherosclerosis. However, it must be pointed out that these studies and another prospective study which, after multilogistic analysis, failed to reveal a risk association with triglycerides,[165] were done without particular reference to diabetes. There may be other factors, such as altered lipoprotein composition, which should be considered in the diabetic. In streptozotocin-induced diabetic rats, striking alterations in apoprotein composition of various lipoproteins have been described.[166] Schonfeld et al.[132] have described increased triglyceride content of LDL and HDL in normolipidemic as well as hyperlipidemic diabetics. The significance of these alterations in apoproteins and lipoprotein composition remains to be determined. In this regard, of particular interest is the observation that a subgroup of patients with endogenous hypertriglyceridemia might be identifiable on the basis of increased apoprotein B levels.[166a] Such individuals with elevated Apo B might be at increased risk, regardless of the relative circulating levels of triglycerides.

HDL and Diabetes

Observations made some three decades ago by Barr et al.[57] and Nikkilä[167] and more recently in epidemiologic studies in Hawaiian Japanese,[168] Framingham,[169,170] other American populations,[171] Tromsø,[172] and Israeli populations,[173] have strongly suggested an inverse correlation of HDL-cholesterol level with the development of ischemic heart disease. Other investigators have shown a similar protective effect of HDL, as reflected by direct measurement of the plasma concentrations of apoprotein A-I and A-II.[174–176] Most of these studies have revealed the inverse relationship of HDL with atherosclerosis to be independent of other lipid abnormalities. Low levels of HDL have also been described in large series of patients with peripheral vascular disease,[177] ischemic cerebrovascular disease,[178] and angiographically defined coronary artery disease.[179,180] Also, in a large kindred with familial hypercholesterolemia,[181] the HDL-cholesterol levels were low and independently correlated with coronary heart disease.

In view of the known interaction of HDL with catabolism of chylomicrons and VLDL, and of the inverse correlation of triglycerides with HDL-cholesterol,[169,182] it is of interest that although patients with Type I or V hyperlipoproteinemia are the ones with lowest HDL-cholesterol levels,[182,183] marked reductions of triglyceride levels achieved after treatment of such patients were not accompanied by appreciable increase in HDL-cholesterol Apo A-1 levels.[183,184,185] A similar lack of improvement in HDL-cholesterol was observed in Type IV hyperlipidemic persons.[186] Despite the explosion of studies demonstrating a significanat role of HDL in the pathogenesis of atherosclerosis, some investigators have maintained that the observed association could be a by-product of the "atherogenic process rather than its cause."[105,187] Nevertheless, the availability of HDL-cholesterol estimation has clearly shown the fallacy of estimating only total cholesterol and the lack of strong correlations between total cholesterol and atherosclerosis in many earlier studies. Similarly, studies of lipid profiles in children[188,189] and elderly subjects[190] have indicated the "benign" nature of "hypercholesterolemia" in many children who have elevated HDL-cholesterol levels. Interesting results from the Bogalusa heart study[191] indicate that children with higher HDL-cholesterol have lower LDL-cholesterol and blood pressure, and less obesity. The ranges of HDL-cholesterol levels up to age 60 are indicated in Table 11–2.

The resurgence of interest in HDL-cholesterol metabolism in relation to atherosclerosis has led to several studies in diabetic subjects during the past several years. Many reports now indicate an overall reduction in HDL-cholesterol levels in diabetic patients. One important finding emerging from several studies is that diabetic women generally have a greater lowering of HDL-cholesterol levels than diabetic men, compared with nondiabetic controls.[192–194] This may partly explain the relative increase in coronary heart disease in diabetic women compared to that in diabetic men, as observed in the Framingham and other studies.[8,192] Another important observation has been that the low HDL-cholesterol levels reported in the diabetics[192,193,195–200] are confined particularly to noninsulin-dependent diabetics.[193,194,198,200–202] In some studies, insulin-dependent diabetics of either sex were found to have normal or significantly higher levels of HDL-cholesterol than the non-dia-

betic controls,[134,203] a finding apparently not associated with an unfavorable apoprotein composition of HDL in the former.[204] On the other hand, low levels of HDL-cholesterol in Type II diabetes may be accompanied by triglyceride-enriched HDL particles.[461]

In a study of 165 diabetic outpatients at the Joslin Clinic, HDL-cholesterol was lower in non-insulin-dependent diabetics and normal in the insulin-dependent diabetics of both sexes, while total cholesterol was similar in the two groups.[193] These observations can be at least partly explained by the known inverse correlation of HDL-cholesterol with adiposity and triglyceride levels,[169,170,182] and its positive correlation with lipoprotein lipase activity.[203] Non-insulin-dependent diabetic patients, whether under treatment with diet alone or with diet and oral hypoglycemic agents, are more likely to be obese and hypertriglyceridemic. Further studies on HDL metabolism are clearly needed since in some studies, low HDL-cholesterol was observed in the diabetics treated with oral hypoglycemic agents but not in those treated with diet alone.[198,202] However, the findings were not confirmed by others.[462] As suggested,[201] it would be premature to suggest that the lowering of HDL-cholesterol by sulfonylureas might explain the alleged accelerated ischemic heart disease,[198,205] a controversy which remains unsettled.[206,207]

Another important issue concerns the relationship of HDL-cholesterol to the control of hyperglycemia. In some studies, HDL-cholesterol or LDL/HDL cholesterol ratios have been shown to be inversely correlated with prevailing blood glucose levels[195,196] or with the glycosylated hemoglobin level, as an index of blood glucose control.[196,198,198a] However, this has not been confirmed by others.[200,208,209] Interestingly, in insulin-dependent diabetics, prospective studies with insulin infusion pumps have revealed a rise in HDL-cholesterol levels after several months of euglycemia.[210,211] These differences can probably be explained by the heterogeneity in the patient population and the possible effects of treatment itself in altering HDL turnover. Further work is required before resolving this question, with careful comparison of diabetics before and after control.

Factors Affecting HDL Metabolism. In addition to the genetic factors which are undoubtedly important, a number of other variables can favorably or adversely affect HDL metabolism.[20,212] These are summarized in Table 11–4. The roles of several important aspects of diabetes treatment (e.g., diet) are not well understood; these are obviously of great significance in interpretation of data dealing with the purported relationship be-

Table 11–4. Certain Common Factors Affecting HDL-Cholesterol Levels

Factor	Effect	Reference
1. Obesity	Decrease	72,169,170,193
2. Diet		
a. High carbohydrate	Decrease	215
b. High P:S ratio	Decrease	217
	Increase	216
c. Vegetarian	Increase	218,219
3. Alcohol (moderate)	Increase	220–222
4. Physical activity	Increase	232–234,333
5. Smoking	Decrease	235
6. Drugs		
a. Estrogen	Increase	225,228
b. Progestins	Decrease	225–228
c. Androgens	Decrease	212,231
d. Clofibrate	No change	238
e. Gemfibrozil	Increase	238a
f. Probucol	Decrease	238b
g. Nicotinic acid	Increase	215
h. Dilantin	Increase	236,237
i. β-blockers	Decrease	240,241
7. Uremia	Decrease	243–246

tween HDL and the control of diabetes. Moreover, changes in total HDL-cholesterol may not always reflect favorable effects in relation to various subfractions of HDL, and the relative importance of these subfractions (HDL$_2$, HDL$_3$) awaits clarification.[86,87,213,214] In most situations, the HDL-cholesterol levels are simultaneously influenced by multiple factors. In addition to the known inverse association of HDL-cholesterol with obesity and hypertriglyceridemia, high carbohydrate diets tend to sharply reduce HDL-cholesterol via enhanced degradation.[215] High cholesterol diets are associated with variable changes, the most important of which are the synthesis of an abnormal HDL particle, enriched with Apo E[98] and of β-VLDL particles, as discussed above.[144] A low fat diet with an increased polyunsaturated/saturated fatty acid (P:S) ratio resulted in a 20% increase in HDL-cholesterol in an Oslo study;[216] however, in another study, HDL-cholesterol and Apo A-I syntheses were markedly reduced (out of proportion to decline in total cholesterol) by a "metabolic" diet containing a P:S ratio of 4:1, a ratio rarely practical in real life.[217] Vegetarian diets have been shown to result in increased HDL-cholesterol[218] or an increased HDL/LDL cholesterol ratio.[218,219] Also, alcohol in moderate amounts has been shown to raise HDL-cholesterol levels.[220–222] However, this must be considered in light of its effect on raising VLDL,[223] particularly in hypertriglyceridemic individuals such as diabetics or those with familial hypertriglyceridemia.[224] Oral contraceptives have been shown to affect HDL-cholesterol, depending upon the formulation,[225] since estrogens raise and certain progestins lower HDL-cholesterol.[226–229]

The effects of androgens on lipid metabolism have been extensively investigated.[230] The few studies of their impact upon HDL metabolism suggest a lowering effect.[212,231] Several studies have shown a salutary effect of physical activity on HDL,[232–234] although the degree and frequency of activity needed, remain to be established. Smoking has been shown to adversely affect HDL-cholesterol.[235] The effects of drugs are poorly studied but would undoubtedly be revealing. A few reports have shown decreased catabolism of HDL by treatment with nicotinic acid[215] and increased HDL-cholesterol levels in chronic dilantin users.[236,237] Clofibrate has been found to cause no effects[238] or an increase[239] in HDL-cholesterol. Gemfibrozil, a potent triglyceride-lowering agent, is associated with considerable increase in HDL-cholesterol levels in most individuals.[238a] A major concern with probucol, an LDL-lowering agent, has been its significant adverse effect in reducing HDL-cholesterol and apoprotein A–1 levels.[238b] Propranolol and other β-blockers have been reported to result in a significant decrease in HDL-cholesterol or HDL/LDL cholesterol ratio.[240,241] Chronic uremia, a well known predisposing factor in accelerated atherosclerosis[242] and germane to the diabetic with microangiopathy, is frequently associated with markedly reduced HDL-cholesterol levels[243–245] and altered apoprotein composition.[246] The low HDL-cholesterol in uremia cannot be fully accounted for by elevated VLDL levels, another hallmark of this condition,[247–250] most likely due to a reduced clearance of endogenous triglycerides in uremic patients.[251,252] The low HDL-cholesterol of uremia is not reversible with dialysis.

Treatment of Lipid Disorders

The premise that reduction of plasma lipids in patients with hyperlipidemia would result in a reduction in the severity of atherosclerosis (the "fat-atherosclerosis" or simply, "lipid hypothesis") has been controversial.[253–256] Mann,[254] one of its strongest opponents, has presented vehemently his view that anti-atherogenic diets are futile in the lowering of lipids and in the prevention of progression of atherosclerotic events. This has led to a strong rebuttal in favor of the hypothesis, by the Nutrition Committee of the American Heart Association.[255] As pointed out by Dawber,[256] "it is not reasonable to expect that changes in dietary intake after 40 to 50 years on a diet high in fat and cholesterol would produce dramatic results."

Despite some suggestions to the contrary,[254,257] most evidence suggests that differences in cholesterol levels are at least partially explained by differences in diet,[258,259] and that the emphasis on changes in diet and life style has indeed reduced the incidence of coronary[260] and cerebrovascular disease[261] in the general population over the past 2 decades. Additional evidence suggests that the initiation of plasma lipid lowering in childhood might be more efficacious in retarding atherogenesis than intervention in later years of life.[255] Strong epidemiologic evidence from Framingham and elsewhere[170,253] leaves no doubt that the levels of lipids in the general population in the Western World are too high[43] and that a distinction must be made between "normal" levels and "desirable" levels. In several animal species, absence of atherosclerosis correlates with low cholesterol levels,[262] and in the human, the levels at birth (about 50 mg/dl) approximate those which, once exceeded, would saturate LDL receptors on peripheral cells. This would be particularly crucial in individuals with multiple risk factors, a point central to the cumulative atherogenic potential of various risk factors.[263-266]

Prevention Trials

Numerous clinical trials of lipid-lowering (chiefly cholesterol-lowering) through diet or drug intervention, have been conducted throughout the world. Most of these have dealt with secondary, and a few with primary, prevention, and were summarized by Davis and Havlik[268] and by Borhani.[269] Some of the larger series on dietary prevention were the Los Angeles Veterans Administration study,[270] the Oslo diet-heart study,[271] and the Finnish diet study.[272] The degrees of cholesterol lowering in most studies were rather modest (10 to 15%) and the results equivocal or negative, when subjected to rigorous statistical analysis.[268] Of the various drug trials,[268] the largest were the Coronary Drug Project (CDP) in U.S.A.,[273] and the WHO trial.[274,275] In the CDP study, a secondary prevention trial using clofibrate, no significant effect could be shown on overall mortality or new coronary events. In the WHO study, a primary prevention trial conducted in three European centers— Edinburgh, Prague and Budapest—involving about 15,000 healthy men, clofibrate was shown to result in about 20% reduction in the incidence of myocardial infarction. However, the total mortality in the clofibrate group was significantly increased. Of particular concern was an increase in deaths from cancer in various organs. However, a similar trend toward increase in cancer was also reported in at least two dietary prevention trials.[270,271] This intriguing association between cancer and cholesterol-lowering by diet or clofibrate, needs careful scrutiny, especially in view of other studies showing an inverse correlation between blood cholesterol and colon cancer.[276] However, this latter association is probably multifactorial.[277] The applicability

of the WHO trial in individual situations cannot be inferred from this wide-scale community trial. Another crucial issue is that clofibrate is not the drug of choice for cholesterol-lowering,[278,279] and other drugs or drug combinations might be better indicated.

Perhaps the most conclusive and convincing evidence to date in favor of the lipid hypothesis comes from the Lipid Research Clinics' (LRC) primary preventive trial with diet and cholestyramine involving 12 centers in this country.[279a,279b] This protocol enrolled 35- to 59-year-old men with primary Type II hyperlipoproteinemia who were normotensive, non-diabetic, and asymptomatic for coronary artery disease. In this study, a total of 3806 men were randomized into a placebo and a cholestyramine group, each group also receiving a diet plan providing a modest reduction in saturated fat and cholesterol. After a mean follow-up on these regimens for 7.4 years, the cholestyramine group showed a mean reduction in total and LDL cholesterol of 13.4% and 20.3%, respectively, a significantly greater reduction for each than the placebo group. In the cholestyramine group, the "definite" coronary mortality declined by 24% and non-fatal myocardial infarction by 19%. The incidence rates of other cardiovascular events, including angina, coronary by-pass surgery, and positive exercise tests, were also significantly reduced. Furthermore, there was a strong correlation between the extent of decline in total or LDL-cholesterol levels and the incidence of coronary events.[279b] The HDL-cholesterol remained almost unchanged so that HDL/total cholesterol ratios, on the average, rose by 21% in the first year and by 12% by the end of the study.

In the LRC study, no increase in the incidence of cancer was found but the participants would need to be monitored for several additional years in order to be completely certain of this possibility. Most importantly, the LRC study provides the most valuable and strongest support for the etiologic role of LDL cholesterol in the pathogenesis of coronary artery disease as well as for reversibility of this pathogenic process by treatment.

Treatment of Hyperlipidemia in Diabetes

The principles of dietary and drug treatment of hyperlipidemia have been reviewed elsewhere.[280-284] In the diabetic, control of hyperglycemia and treatment of frequently underlying factors (e.g. obesity, renal disease, hypothyroidism, alcohol abuse), will often mitigate the severity of hyperlipidemia. The residual hyperlipidemia frequently reflects a primary lipid disorder.

Diet Treatment. Diet modification remains the cornerstone of treatment and must be attempted rigorously before drug intervention. Hypertriglyceridemia, presenting as Type IV, V, IIb, or rarely Type I, requires treatment with a diet which is of low fat content when chylomicrons are present, and/or low in refined sugars and hypocaloric when due to endogenous VLDL excess. Hypercholesterolemia, defined as levels above the 90th percentile of normal population, is not as common as hypertriglyceridemia in the diabetic. Nevertheless, since the diabetic is subject to other risk factors (e.g., hypertension, smoking, obesity), every attempt must be made to maintain the LDL cholesterol in low-normal range and below the mean cholesterol levels seen in those with no other risk factors. To meet this goal, careful diet modifications (Table 11–5) should include a low-cholesterol diet with increased polyunsaturated:saturated fatty acid (P:S) ratio and a restriction of total fat intake to 25 to 30% of total calories. This dietary modification, resulting in an increased proportion of calories from carbohydrates (50 to 55%), would not result in adverse effects on glycemic control, as long as complex carbohydrates are consumed.[282] Some investigators have reported further reductions in cholesterol levels with adjuncts such as soybean protein.[285] Such reports are encouraging since even rigorous attempts at lowering cholesterol often achieve only a modest reduction of 15 to 20%, attesting to the pronounced ability of the body's cholesterol synthesis mechanism to compensate for any reduction in the cholesterol pool.[114,286]

Although the beneficial effect of increased P:S ratio (above 1.0) of fats is well documented, the mechanism of this approach remains controversial and is poorly understood. One exciting suggestion is that the unsaturation of fatty acyl chains of lipoproteins might increase the fluidity of the LDL moiety which could affect the rate at which these particles are deposited or removed from the arterial wall.[31,287] Thus, dietary manipulation may work by altering physical properties of lipoproteins. Whatever the mechanism, striking reversals in diet-induced atherosclerosis have been achieved in experimental situations by substituting polyunsaturated for saturated fat.[288] The potential toxicity of excessive polyunsaturated fats[289] is not yet confirmed.

Other dietary factors that have been incriminated in hyperlipidemia and/or the development of atherosclerosis include increased sucrose consumption,[290,291] low fiber content of diet,[292,293] soft vs. hard water,[294] and vitamin E.[295,296] None of these appears to have a significant impact by itself.[297,298] Initial trials of high fiber diets have suggested significant improvement in plasma triglyceride levels[299,300] and in HDL/LDL cholesterol ratio.[300] However, the results are often variable in individuals and the effect of fiber supplementation on lipid metabolism needs elucidation. Data in man regarding the role of vitamin C[301] are inconclusive.

Drug Therapy. Patients with hyperlipidemia should be treated with drugs after careful consideration of side effects and only after satisfactory compliance to diet has produced inadequate results. The most frequently employed drugs are clofibrate, nicotinic acid, and bile acid sequestrants (cholestyramine and colestipol). A number of clinical trials have documented the efficacy of bile acid sequestrants in lowering LDL-cholesterol by 15 to 30%. In one recent trial, 5 years of treatment with cholestyramine resulted in significant retardation of angiographically defined coronary lesions.[301a] During the past few years, fairly good results have been obtained with probucol, a cholesterol-lowering agent with uncertain mode of action, but which differs from that of cholestyramine.[238b,302,303] In a study by Kuo et al.,[303] combined treatment with diet and probucol resulted in mean cholesterol reductions of about 40% (total and LDL). This was accompanied by a decrease in size of xanthomata and in stabilization of atherosclerotic lesions as seen on angiography. However, a potentially untoward effect, namely, decreased HDL-cholesterol, is of main concern.[238b] No studies in diabetic patients with this drug are yet available. Combination of drugs (e.g., cholestyramine or colestipol with nicotinic acid) can achieve further reduction of cholesterol levels, particularly in refractory patients with familial hyperlipidemia.[304,305]

The mechanisms of action and potential side effects of more commonly used hypolipidemic drugs are summarized in Table 11–6. Newer drugs under trial in various forms of hyperlipidemia include

Table 11–5. A Comparison of "Traditional" American Diet and Revised Dietary Goals

	Current Diet	Dietary Goals
Cholesterol (mg/day)	750	100–200
Fat (% total calories)	40	25–30
Saturated (%)	15–20	10
Polyunsaturated (%)	5–7	10
P:S ratio	0.4	1.3
Vegetable fat (% fat)	38	75
Animal fat (% fat)	62	25
Protein (% total calories)	15	15
Vegetable protein (% protein)	32	56
Animal protein (% protein)	68	44
Carbohydrate (% total calories)	40–45	55–60
Starch* (% calories)	22	40–45
Sucrose (% calories)	15	5–10
Crude fiber (g)	2–3	12–15

*including other complex carbohydrates.
Adapted from Connor, W.E.[282]

Table 11-6.   Pharmacology of Commonly Used Drugs for Hyperlipidemias

Drug	Mechanism(s) of Action	Indication	Dose	Side Effects
Cholestyramine or Colestipol	↑ Catabolism of LDL	↑ LDL (Type II)	4–8 g qid 5–10 g tid	Constipation, steatorrhea, pancreatitis (rare)
Probucol	Uncertain	↑ LDL (Type II)	250–500 mg bid	Diarrhea, flatulence, vent. arrhythmia
Clofibrate	↓ VLDL synthesis ↑ FFA oxidation ↑ LPL (PHLA) ?	↑ VLDL, IDL (Type III, IV, V)	1.0 g bid	Gallstones, nausea, antidiuresis, PVC's, Abn LFT, Myositis, Phlebitis
Gemfibrozil	↓ VLDL synthesis ↓ Lipolysis ↑ VLDL clearance	↑ VLDL, IDL (Type III, IV, V)	600 mg bid	Skin rash, dizziness, ↓ Glucose tolerance
Nicotinic acid	↓ Lipolysis ↓ Synthesis of VLDL, LDL ↑ VLDL catabolism	↑ VLDL, ↑ IDL (Type III, IV, V, II)	100 mg tid 1–3 g tid	Flushing, pruritus, Nausea, diarrhea ↑ Uric acid, ↓ Glucose tolerance
D-Thyroxine	↑ LDL catabolism	↑ LDL, ↑ IDL (Type II, III)	2–4 mg bid	CHD worsening

chenodeoxycholic acid,[306] carnitine,[307] and compactin.[308] The last-named is of particular interest, since it is the first available agent which has potent effects on inhibition of cholesterol biosynthesis via antagonism of HMG-CoA reductase, the rate limiting enzyme. In later studies in Japan, compactin was able to reduce total LDL-cholesterol by more than 25% in patients with familial hypercholesterolemia.[309] In those studies, the HDL-cholesterol was not lowered and no other adverse effects were observed. In a subsequent study, a combination of cholestyramine and compactin was shown to result in as much as 35 to 40% reduction in LDL-cholesterol, the most dramatic results yet with a drug combination, as regards LDL-cholesterol.[309a]

A recently introduced agent, gemfibrozil, is highly effective in lipid disorders characterized by hypertriglyceridemia.[238a] It primarily lowers triglycerides while raising HDL-cholesterol. Further experience with this agent will surely be forthcoming.

HYPERTENSION

The role of hypertension as a major factor in the intimal injury and initiation of atherosclerosis is well established.[310] One poorly understood aspect is the particular susceptibility of the cerebrovascular system to the atherogenic effects of hypertension. The mechanisms of hypertension in the diabetic are discussed at length in Chapter 28.

Despite the general impression that the incidence of hypertension is increased in the diabetic, this association remains somewhat controversial.[3,19,20] The factors which have resulted in uncertainty regarding a significant association between the two, include a lack of well-matched controls for obesity, age and sex, lack of standardization of blood pressure measurements, and different definitions of hypertension itself. An increased incidence of hypertension has been reported in many large series of patients[8,19,311,312] but not in others.[313,314]

In an unselected but representative diabetic population, Bryfogle and Bradley[311] found hypertension in 20%, increasing to 41%, of patients over 50 years of age. The incidence in men and women younger than 50 was equal, but above this age it was greater in women, the ratio being 2.6 to 1. Similarly, higher systolic blood pressure was noted in the Framingham study in women diabetics in particular, compared with age and sex-matched controls,[8] although this did not account for much of the excess rate of macrovascular disease. On the other hand, Goodkin,[315] in a 20-year survey, found a much higher mortality in diabetics than in nondiabetics with comparable degrees of hypertension, suggesting a worse prognostic significance of hypertension in the diabetic. In a recent long-term study of juvenile-onset Type I diabetics, followed for 40 years after the onset of diabetes, deaths due to coronary heart disease as well as to renal disease were strongly related to hypertension.[316]

Certain endocrinopathies may present with both hypertension and diabetes (e.g., pheochromocytoma, Cushing's syndrome and primary hyperaldosteronism), although these disorders are rare and do not account for increased prevalence of hypertension in most surveys of diabetic patients.

CIGARETTE SMOKING

A pronounced effect of smoking on the pathogenesis of atherosclerosis is firmly established. A positive association between cigarette smoking and coronary heart disease persists even after every additional variable is accounted for.[317,318] Friedman et al.[318] reported smoker-to-nonsmoker mortality ratios, crude and adjusted respectively, to be 4.7 and 3.6 for coronary heart disease. Moreover, data from the Framingham Study[319] and those of Bain et al.[317] have emphasized that those who smoke more than 40 cigarettes a day could halve their risk of death from coronary heart disease by reducing their tobacco consumption to between 20 to 40 cigarettes a day and lower the risk even further by reducing to less than 20 cigarettes a day.

Although some of the adverse cardiovascular effects of smoking are mediated via nicotine, the principal unfavorable consequence of smoking is probably an increased concentration of carboxyhemoglobin and resultant tissue hypoxia. Carboxyhemoglobin has been shown to impair directly the hepatic metabolism of lipoprotein remnants.[320] The resulting remnant particle accumulation simulates Type III hyperlipoproteinemia, a lipid disorder with a well-known association with atherogenesis.[65,117] Additional mechanisms contributing to the atherogenic response to smoking include increased endothelial permeability in response to carbon monoxide-induced hypoxia, resulting in increased lipid uptake,[321] and increased platelet adhesiveness.[322] Finally, hypoxia has been shown to have a stimulating effect on the proliferation of cultured human arterial smooth cell.[323]

In the diabetic population, smoking undoubtedly may play a role in the accelerated atherogenesis, since additional factors are already present which might promote tissue hypoxia, by shifting the oxyhemoglobin dissociation curve to the left. These additional factors include reduced 2,3-diphosphoglycerate (2,3 DPG),[324,325] hyperlipoproteinemia,[326] and increased glycosylated hemoglobin.[327,328] Furthermore, the effects of smoking on increased platelet adhesiveness[322] are superimposed on the already altered platelet function in the diabetic (see below).

Whether the incidence of smoking per se is different in diabetics with macrovascular disease has not been well studied, but it does not appear to be appreciably different from that in nondiabetics.[19]

PHYSICAL ACTIVITY

The influence of physical fitness as an independent risk factor on the development of atherogenesis has long been debated and is still unproven.[297,328a] In the extensive studies of Morris et al.[329] of 16,882 male civil servants in Britain, 11% of men with documented ischemic heart disease were engaged in "vigorous" physical activities compared with 26% of controls. They estimated that the relative risk of developing coronary disease was about one-third in vigorously active men as compared to men who were not so active. Interestingly, the smoking habits of the men in two groups were similar. A similarly striking protective effect of vigorous exercise was seen in a long-term prospective study of 6351 U.S. longshoremen.[330] The age-adjusted coronary death rates for the "high-activity" category in that study were about half of those for "medium" and "low" categories. The studies by Brunner et al.[331] of several thousand men and women, aged 40 to 64, living in Israeli collective settlements (Kibbutzim) under uniform environmental conditions, have shown a marked protective effect of physical activity in both the primary and secondary prevention of ischemic heart disease.

The protective effect of exercise against atherosclerosis probably involves the reduction of other risk factors in physically active people, e.g., hypertension, hyperlipidemia, obesity, smoking and glucose intolerance.[332] A number of recent studies have shown increased HDL-cholesterol with exercise,[232–234] probably due to stimulation of lipoprotein lipase activity in adipose tissue and in skeletal muscle, and the concomitant rapid turnover of triglyceride-rich lipoprotein.[333] In persons with mild, maturity-onset diabetes, studies of physical conditioning carried out at the Joslin Clinic[334] and elsewhere[335] have shown improvement in plasma lipids and glucose tolerance with enhanced sensitivity to endogenous insulin. Further studies of exercise therapy in different types and severities of diabetes will clearly be important. The non-insulin-dependent diabetic, with a constellation of increased adiposity, hyperlipidemia and insulin-insensitivity, can benefit immensely from an exercise program, since the capacity for carbohydrate storage in the sedentary state is clearly limited.[336] Moreover, effects of exercise are short-lived,[334] and chronic adaptation requires sustained physical conditioning.

SEX AND SEX HORMONES

The relative biologic immunity of non-diabetic, pre-menopausal women[14] to atherosclerosis has led to a search for the mechanisms for this protection.

It has been suggested that the favorable status of women before menopause might be related to a protective effect of estrogens. An increase in HDL-cholesterol with the use of estrogens[225,228] has been invoked as one of the possible mechanisms. In a recent study, administration of a natural estrogen to hypercholesterolemic (Type II), postmenopausal women was shown to decrease LDL cholesterol and increase HDL-cholesterol.[337] Women with normal lipid levels were not studied.

On the other hand, several lines of evidence argue against this explanation. In the Coronary Drug Project,[273] the use of estrogen in men was associated with worsening of coronary disease and the incidence of myocardial infarction was increased in young women on oral contraceptives.[338] In the Lipid Research Clinic Program, hypercholesterolemia was up to 3 times more common and hypertriglyceridemia was up to 5 times more common in young women on oral contraceptives than in non-users.[339] Thus, the effects of estrogen in the pre-menopausal women are different from those in the post-menopausal women as studied by Tikkanen et al.[337] Furthermore, studies of Phillips[340,341] and Entrican et al.[342] have consistently revealed either raised plasma estrogen levels or elevated estradiol to testosterone ratio in men with documented myocardial infarction at a young age. Interestingly, in the studies of Phillips, the estradiol to testosterone ratio showed a positive correlation with glucose and insulin responses during oral glucose tolerance tests, thus explaining the abnormal glucose tolerance and insulin secretion frequently encountered in men with premature atherosclerosis.[341] These findings are supported by the recent demonstration of elevated estradiol levels in men with coronary artery disease in the Framingham Study, who also had significantly elevated blood glucose levels in comparison to those of controls with no evidence of coronary disease.[342a]

Taken together, from the evidence summarized, the role of estrogen or other sex hormones in the pathogenesis of atherosclerosis remains controversial, and other factors might be operative in the protection against atherosclerosis in the non-diabetic, pre-menopausal women.[343] It has been postulated that estrogens could have a protective effect on the early stages of smooth-muscle cell proliferation and a later stimulating effect on the formation of atheromatous plaque and mural thrombosis.[344] In any case, other as yet unidentified factors must influence the lack of protection against atherosclerosis in diabetic women and accelerated atherogenesis in the diabetic in general.

OBESITY

Epidemiologic evidence, using multivariate analyses, suggests only a minor additional risk due to obesity, when other risk factors are taken into account.[297,345] This is true also in the non-insulin-dependent (Type II) diabetic in whom obesity is prevalent. However, there is evidence for higher mortality in obese female diabetics, from acute myocardial infarction, suggesting a "larger infarction" in such patients.[346] Cramer et al.[347] studied relationship of several factors with atherosclerosis in 224 patients undergoing coronary angiography and found no relation between adiposity and coronary lesions. Similar lack of association was seen in Dupont company employees studied by Pell and D'Alonzo,[348] in the Framingham Study,[345] in the Swedish prospective study,[159] and in several other prospective studies.[297] The association of obesity with hypertension seems to be more significant and this could be an important factor in those studies where obesity and hypertension may not have been analyzed separately. The reversible nature of mild hypertension with weight loss has been re-emphasized in other large-scale studies.[349,350] Obesity is also frequently associated with hyperlipidemia and low HDL-cholesterol levels.[72,169,170] Thus most of the evidence would suggest that obesity by itself is not a major risk factor but is an important underlying factor in a large proportion of diabetics in relation to other risk factors, e.g., hypertension and dyslipidemia.

STRESS AND PERSONALITY

In recent years, increasing attention has been devoted to the interaction between stress, behavioral patterns and atherogenesis. Several important observations reviewed by Jenkins et al.,[351] Glass[352] and Rosenman[353] suggest that neuropsychologic aberrations play an important role in the development and, perhaps more so in the clinical expression of human atherosclerosis.

In an animal model,[354] Gutstein et al. have shown the development of coronary lesions, morphologically resembling human atheroma, by sustained electrical stimulation of the lateral hypothalamus over prolonged periods. Such lesions appeared in the absence of changes in lipids or blood pressure. Based on such observations, many investigators have expressed skepticism over the role of other risk factors since abnormalities of various risk factors, e.g. hyperlipidemia, hypertension, smoking, and diabetes may not always be impressive in patients with proven clinical evidence of atherosclerosis.[352,353,355,356] Rosenman[353] has provided a unifying concept that these risk factors may be of much more ominous significance in individuals with Type A rather than Type B personality, as regards incidence and severity, as well as recurring events of atherosclerosis. The major facets of a Type A behavior pattern are (1) a chronic sense of urgency and (2) enhanced aggressiveness, drive and competitive hostility. Type A individuals are chronically impatient, work-oriented, and preoccupied with deadlines. Other features include alertness, restlessness, tenseness of facial muscles and explosive speech. In contrast, Type B behavior pattern is characterized by the absence of pressing conflict with time or other persons, no chronic sense of urgency or impatience, and a more relaxed pace of activity. Biochemical correlates of Type A personality are exemplified by enhanced catecholamine responses to various stimuli.[357] Although increased concentrations of catecholamines[358] and associated metabolic changes[359] have been documented in patients hospitalized for acute myocardial infarction,[358] the significance of these findings in the pathogenesis of atherosclerosis remains to be critically examined.

The significance of behavior patterns deserves emphasis as an additional factor in the diabetic, tantamount to other risk factors. A detailed screening of personality patterns in Joslin Clinic patients with long-standing diabetes, revealed important differences between those developing vascular complications and those free of such complications.[360] Such observations underscore the need for early personality screening and appropriate therapy to help diabetic patients adapt to stress.[361,361a]

GENETIC AND RACIAL FACTORS IN ATHEROGENESIS

Genetic factors in atherosclerotic disease are intimately intertwined with the genetic control of some of the key risk factors (e.g. hyperlipoproteinemia, hypertension and diabetes). For example, several types of familial disorders of hyperlipoproteinemia with increased propensity for atherosclerosis are inherited, either as monogenic mutant genes or in a more complex polymorphic transmission.[69,362] Rapacz[362] has reviewed evidence for a positive correlation between an immunogenetically defined LP system and arterial lipidosis in swine fed a high fat diet. Similarly, studies in the squirrel monkey by Clarkson et al.[23] have shown that the response of plasma cholesterol to diet in hypo- and hyper-responder monkeys is genetically determined. A polymorphism also might explain the marked differences in atherosclerotic deposition in various types of blood vessels in the body, i.e., coronary vs. peripheral. In current studies, the polymorphism of DNA sequences flanking the insulin gene on chromosome 11 is being investigated. In a few reports, an insertion sequence in the DNA region flanking the insulin gene has been shown to confer greater risk of coronary atherosclerosis.[362a] Such studies of the genetic basis of atherosclerosis need to be pursued.

Whether genetic factors unique for atherosclerosis per se govern its development was the subject of a task force of the National Heart and Lung Institute.[363] Even in studies utilizing the monozygotic twin model, considerable difficulty exists in segregating the genetic vs. environmental risk factors. Further work is needed in this direction. At present, overwhelming evidence suggests that genetic factors in the inheritance of atherosclerosis are most likely determined by the sum of the genetic expressions of various underlying causative or protective mechanisms.

Apart from genetic factors, certain racial characteristics in the pathogenesis of atherosclerosis are noteworthy. One of the best examples is the unique protection of the Masai of East Africa who have persistently low levels of LDL-cholesterol and extreme paucity of atherosclerosis at autopsy despite a diet in which 66% of calories are provided as fat.[364] One of the protective mechanisms in this tribe seems to be a highly efficient negative feedback control of endogenous cholesterol biosynthesis to compensate for the influx of dietary cholesterol. Similarly, although the Bantu have as much diabetes as the white people in Cape Town, their incidence of ischemic heart disease is low and not entirely explained by differences in diet and obesity.[365] West[366] has reviewed extensive data on tribes of American Indians such as the Pimas, who are known to have one of the highest incidences of diabetes in the world. The markedly low incidence of atherosclerosis in these tribes as compared to Caucasians, despite comparable incidence of microangiopathy, is at least partly explained by their lower levels of plasma lipids, which are comparable to the levels seen in nondiabetic American Indians.

The vascular complications of diabetes in the Japanese typify an interesting dichotomy between diet and distribution of atherosclerotic lesions.[367] Although the traditional Japanese diet, high in carbohydrate and low in fat, appears to be favorable for protection against coronary disease and peripheral vascular disease, cerebrovascular disease is the most frequent vascular cause of death. On the other hand, epidemiologic studies comparing the Japanese in Hiroshima with the Hawaiian Japanese and Hawaiian Caucasians have shown that ischemic heart disease is a much more frequent cause for mortality in the Japanese diabetics in Hawaii (equivalent to Caucasians) than in Hiroshima.[368] These differences are in large part explained by the changing diet, lifestyles, and urbanization of Hawaiian Japanese.

With rare racial exceptions, it appears that atherosclerosis is an event markedly influenced by nutritional status, being universally present in overnourished and rare in non-overnourished peoples. It seems to be largely independent of ethnic origin.[369] This generalization is validated by the increasing incidence of atherosclerosis in Yemenite Jews, American Indians and Japanese.

FACTORS UNIQUE TO DIABETIC VASCULAR DISEASE

Disturbances of Coagulability, Platelet Function and Hemorrheology

Several lines of evidence indicate disorders of blood coagulability, viscosity and other rheologic disturbances in the diabetic. The cause-effect relationship of hematologic disturbances with atherosclerosis is presently under intensive scrutiny.

1. Defects in Coagulation and Blood Flow. The thrombogenic theory of atherosclerosis, as proposed by Rokitansky and others, was supported by earlier studies in which a diminished rate of fibrinolysis was observed in a group of diabetics, when compared with age-matched controls.[376] More recently, only non-insulin requiring diabetics were found to have decreased fibrinolysis.[371,372] However, others found fibrinolytic activity to be normal[373] or even increased.[374] On the other hand, serum fibrinogen levels have been reported to be increased in diabetics with cardiovascular disease; elevated fibrinogen levels may sometimes predict subsequent atherosclerotic events.[11,375] Interestingly, fibrinogen levels have been found to correlate with degree of diabetes control, as indicated by the glycosylated hemoglobin levels.[376] Recently, a provocative mechanism for reduced fibrinolysis in diabetes has been proposed based on evidence for impaired degradation of fibrin by plasmin due to glycosylation of fibrin itself.[376a] The implications of these studies and their relationship with diabetic complications require further work.

Abnormalities in coagulation factors V, VII, and X have also been demonstrated in diabetes but the specificities of these changes were not well studied.[19] The role of increased blood viscosity due to a number of factors including reduced red cell deformability, increased red cell aggregation, and resultant blood flow changes may also be of considerable significance.[376b,376c]

2. Platelet Function in Diabetes Mellitus. Alterations in platelet function in the diabetic have received increasing attention in recent years.[377,378] Platelets are known to play a key role in the development of atherosclerosis as well as in its thromboembolic complications.[379] In animal experiments, endothelial injury has been shown to be a most potent stimulus for platelet adhesion and aggregation at the site of injury, resulting in release of platelet-derived growth factors[138a] which pro-

voke smooth muscle cell proliferation. Recent studies have confirmed that in diabetes, with or without vascular disease, platelet adhesiveness and response to several aggregating agents is enhanced.[378,380,381] Several studies have revealed that increased platelet sensitivity is correlated with elevated levels of von Willebrand factor (vWF) activity (and Factor VIII antigen) in the diabetic plasma.[376,382–384] The vWF is produced by the vascular endothelial cell. In a pig model studied by Fuster et al.,[385] absence of vWF is associated with striking resistance to atherosclerosis despite a high cholesterol diet which resulted in severe atherosclerotic plaques in control pigs without von Willebrand disease. The activity of vWF is highly dependent upon the carbohydrate content of this glycoprotein,[386] but the structure of vWF in diabetic patients has not yet been studied. Despite the persuasive evidence of abnormal platelet function in the diabetic patients,[387] it must be pointed out that other investigators have found no appreciable differences in platelet aggregation in diabetics with coronary artery disease, compared to non-diabetic controls with coronary artery disease.[388] Such studies underscore the need for well-matched nondiabetic controls with comparable vascular disease. Furthermore, it should be recalled that enhanced platelet sensitivity in the diabetic may result from other concomitants well known to be associated with this phenomenon, e.g., hyperbetalipoproteinemia,[389] hypertension, reduced erythrocyte deformability[376b] and smoking.[322,378]

3. Prostaglandin Interactions with Platelets and Vessel Wall. Prostaglandins are a family of a large variety of vasoactive agents, with a wide spectrum of other actions. Their role in the pathogenesis of thrombosis and atherosclerosis has recently become a focus of increasing attention.[389a] As discussed by Moncada and Vane,[390] the prostaglandin pathway in platelets and in vessel wall initially involves the release of arachidonic acid from membrane phospholipids by the enzyme phospholipase A_2, which can be activated by a variety of hormonal, mechanical, and chemical stimuli. Once released, the arachidonic acid is rapidly converted to cyclic endoperoxides, PGG_2 and PGH_2, under the effect of an enzyme, cyclooxygenase (PG synthetase). These unstable prostaglandins are further broken down to a variety of stable compounds, including PGE_2, $PGF_2\alpha$ and PGD_2. More importantly, PGG_2 and PGH_2 are also transformed into either prostacyclin (PGI_2) in the vessel wall or into thromboxane A_2 (TXA_2) in the platelets (Fig. 11–1). PGI_2 generation is the physiologic defense against platelet aggregation which is stimulated by TXA_2. The mediation of these anti- or pro-aggregant effects is brought about by the reciprocal changes in platelet cyclic AMP levels. TXA_2 is also a vasoconstrictor and PGI_2 a vasodilator. The close contact of platelets and vessel wall thus results in an intimate interaction between the two; the relative imbalance between the formation of PGI_2 and TXA_2 is of crucial significance in platelet aggregation and release phenomena.

Whereas several drugs such as aspirin, indomethacin, and sulfinpyrazone[390–392] have been shown to retard experimental atherogenesis by inhibiting a rate limiting step (cyclooxygenase) in the prostaglandin cascade, a more desirable approach might be to inhibit TXA_2 generation selectively, without affecting vascular PGI_2 synthesis. A prototype drug, imidazole, is an example of an effective thromboxane synthetase inhibitor.[393] Whether such a drug will indeed be effective remains to be shown.[393a] Another possibility involves use of agents which would directly stimulate platelet cAMP generation, e.g., dipyridamole, which inhibits phosphodiesterase in platelets. The extent to which the intake of certain dietary polyunsaturated fatty acids, such as W-3vs W-6 fatty acids, might affect the relative synthesis of vasoactive prosta-

glandins, is obviously an important question which requires urgent scrutiny.[393a,394]

Several studies have revealed an increased synthesis of TXA_2 or an elevated ratio of thromboxane to prostacyclin synthesis in the diabetic rat models[395,396] and the restoration of prostacyclin pathway by insulin, but others have failed to confirm this finding.[397] Halushka et al.[398] have reported that the platelets from patients with diabetes produce increased amounts of PGE-like material and that this could be an important mechanism for hypersensitivity to platelet aggregation in diabetes. Moreover, recently the same group of investigators have demonstrated an increased synthesis of TXA_2 by the platelets of diabetic patients with apparently no clinical evidence of macrovascular disease.[399] Similarly, elevated concentrations of factor VIII activity were demonstrable in Type I diabetic children with a short duration of diabetes, supporting the possibility that endothelial injury may indeed precede the platelet abnormalities.[400] Such studies are obviously provocative and if confirmed, will provide additional biochemical basis for disturbed platelet-vessel wall interaction in the explanation

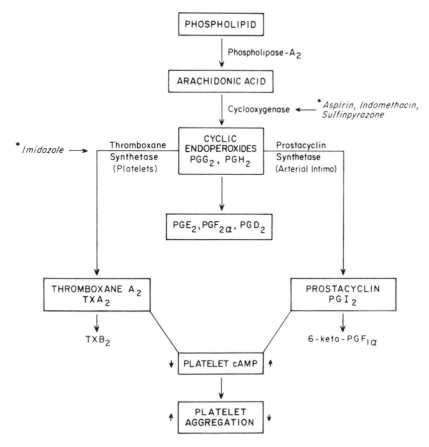

Fig. 11–1.   Prostaglandin-platelet-vessel wall interaction.
*Indicates drugs effective in the inhibition of enzymes shown. (Adapted from Moncada, S., and Vane, J.R.[390])

of enhanced vulnerability of the diabetic to vaso-occlusive disease.[401]

In addition to the effects of prostaglandins upon platelet aggregation, these agents may have significant effects on arterial smooth muscle cell proliferation.[402] Another possible interaction between atherogenic TXA_2 and anti-atherogenic PGI_2 may involve their reciprocal inhibition or activation of lysosomal cholesterol ester hydrolase activity,[24] which may have profound influence on the lipid deposition in arterial wall (vide supra).[402]

Hyperglycemia

As noted above, multilogistic analyses of various risk factors in the development of coronary artery disease in diabetics in the Framingham Study[8] led to the conclusion that a "unique" factor must be invoked to explain the increased morbidity in such individuals. The possibility that long-term hyperglycemia itself may be atherogenic has by no means been ruled out, although the mechanism of a direct or indirect interaction of hyperglycemia with blood vessel wall is a moot point.[460]

In a classic study by Kingsbury,[403] an extensive analysis was carried out concerning glucose tolerance in relation to clinical and arteriographic findings in 338 surgical patients with symptomatic peripheral vascular disease. A progressive worsening of glucose tolerance was observed to be associated with worsening vascular occlusion, categorized as "slight," "moderate" and "extensive." Moreover, repeat glucose tolerance tests after several months revealed further worsening of glucose tolerance in the "extensive" group but not in the "slight" or "moderate" group. Epidemiologic studies from Tecumseh,[161] Whitehall, England,[19,405] and Busselton, Australia[404] point toward apparently mild but statistically significant hyperglycemia as a harbinger of coronary heart disease in people followed prospectively; albeit a direct cause and effect relationship cannot be deduced from such evidence.

Several indirect clues suggest that hyperglycemia has a role in the development of tissue hypoxia which, in concert with a pre-existing adverse metabolic milieu, could be a significant factor in the perpetuation of the atherogenic process. The increased activity of the polyol (sorbitol) pathway in the diabetic[406] has been shown to result in increased cell water content and impaired oxygenation in the arterial wall.[407] Uncontrolled hyperglycemia may further accentuate impaired tissue oxygen delivery by reduced 2,3-DPG levels,[324,325] if not well compensated,[408] and by increasing glycosylated hemoglobin levels[327] over prolonged periods. This may be an important contributory mechanism, even in persons with relatively mild

diabetes.[409] Preliminary experiments with cultured human skin fibroblasts and arterial smooth muscle cell indicate a direct stimulating effect of glucose and sorbitol on cell proliferation, an effect not seen with equimolar concentrations of sucrose or mannitol.[410] Furthermore, high concentrations of glucose inhibit the replication of cultured human endothelial cells, indicating a direct, damaging effect of hyperglycemia on endothelial repair.[410a]

Microangiopathy

It has long been postulated that microvascular lesions (i.e. lesions of arterioles, capillaries and venules) play a possible role in the production of atherosclerotic lesions.[411] Nonatheromatous microvascular lesions involving the intramural coronary arteries of the diabetic have been described by Blumenthal et al.[412] and Crall et al.[13] The thickness of coronary walls was observed by Goodale and others to be 10 to 15% greater in the diabetic patient than in nondiabetic individuals.[413] A greater prevalence of congestive heart failure in diabetics has received increased attention; the increase in prevalence is not explained by coronary artery occlusion or other forms of heart disease.[414] Several reports suggest the presence of a form of "cardiomyopathy" in some diabetic patients who have no evidence of significant coronary occlusive disease.[415,416] Although abnormalities of small arteries or capillaries have been postulated in such patients,[417,418] most evidence indicates that these abnormalities alone would be insufficient to explain the observed states of myocardial dysfunction.[419,420]

In any case, the speculation that microangiopathy of coronary vasculature accounts for the increased severity of the atherosclerotic process per se, requires further study. However, it seems clear that disease in small blood vessels may intensify disease in larger vessels by impairing microcirculatory blood flow and/or by involvement of vasa vasorum in the larger muscular arteries. Whether or not the small blood vessels are themselves at fault in the pathogenesis of macrovascular disease, they may account for direct impairment of nutrition in tissues and the hindrance to the development of adequate collateral circulation.

To what extent and by what mechanism the microangiopathy of other vital organs, particularly the kidney, might influence the atherosclerotic process, is another important aspect of the interaction of these complex diabetic processes. Accelerated atherosclerosis has been well documented in the presence of azotemic renal disease,[242] and is undoubtedly provoked by multiple concurrent mechanisms affecting blood pressure, lipid metabolism, hormonal alterations, and other biochemical alterations in the presence of uremia. Despite some ongoing controversy,[421] increasing clinical and experimental data point to a marked dependence of microangiopathic complications upon the degree of diabetic control as recently reviewed by Spiro[422] and by Tchobroutsky.[423]

Hormonal Alterations

A number of provocative experimental studies have revealed that various hormones play important mediating roles in the pathogenesis of atherosclerosis. Evidence for the potential role of sex hormones was discussed above.

1. Insulin. Considerable controversy exists concerning the role of insulin in the development of atherosclerosis; experimental evidence has been presented for both a protecting and a promoting influence. Stout[424,425] has reviewed several lines of evidence incriminating hyperinsulinism in promoting atheroma formation. Insulin, in supraphysiologic doses, has been shown to stimulate arterial smooth muscle cell proliferation and enhance the synthesis of cholesterol and other lipids, and to inhibit lipolysis in the arterial wall tissue.[424] Moreover, it has been suggested that insulin might inhibit hydrolysis of cholesterol ester in the arterial smooth muscle cell, thus accelerating lipid deposition.[426] The presence of high-affinity insulin receptors on cultured endothelial as well as smooth muscle cells of bovine aorta has been demonstrated.[426a] On the other hand, Wolinsky et al.[45] have presented findings of reduced cholesterol acid hydrolase activity in alloxan diabetic rats, with reversal of these changes by insulin administration. Furthermore, there is evidence for decreased arterial wall mucopolysaccharides in the presence of insulin deficiency which would also link atherogenic events with insulin deficiency rather than insulin excess.[427]

Fraser et al.[428] have shown a relative insulinopenia in persons with mild diabetes and macrovascular disease when compared to similar diabetics without large vessel involvement. Epidemiological studies from Finland in non-diabetic men,[429] on the other hand, have incriminated hyperinsulinemia as a risk factor in a prospective study of coronary heart disease. Needless to say, based on other evidence for and against the role of insulin in atherogenesis, the findings of the prospective Finnish study are challenging, and need to be pursued. A number of factors in the non-insulin-requiring diabetic—such as obesity, hypertriglyceridemia, and nutritional factors—might be associated with endogenous hyperinsulinism. Additional long-term prospective studies, taking into account all other risk factors, are required to resolve the question.

2. Growth Hormone and Growth Factors.

The role of growth hormone (GH) in the development of atherosclerosis has been suspected from the results of various studies. Sexual ateliotic dwarfs with monotropic deficiency of growth hormone are resistant to atherosclerosis, even though their incidence of diabetes is increased.[430] Carefully designed studies by Hansen et al.[431,432] and Vigneri et al.[433] have clearly shown increased GH secretion, in both fasting and stimulated states, in uncontrolled insulin-dependent as well as non-insulin-dependent diabetics. "Tight" control of diabetes often resulted in normalization of growth hormone levels in these studies. The interesting experimental work of Ledet with rabbit aortic medial cell cultures has shown a stimulation of growth and cell proliferation in the presence of human GH-containing serum from young diabetic subjects.[434,435] Moreover, the effect seen with diabetic serum was greater than that with normal human serum; the addition of GH antiserum suppressed these stimulatory effects.[434]

Taken together, these observations appear to support an important permissive effect of GH in atherogenesis. Since many of the actions of GH are mediated in vivo through the generation of "somatomedins," it is of interest that the synthesis of somatomedin and similar growth factors has been found to be impaired in the presence of uncontrolled diabetes.[436,437] However, a direct effect of growth hormone on the arterial wall, as suggested by studies of Ledet, cannot as yet be ruled out.

A number of other growth factors[438] are known to exist—e.g., epidermal growth factor (urogastrone), fibroblast growth factor, nerve growth factor, insulin-like growth factors (IGF I, IGF II), non-suppressible insulin-like proteins, etc. Since many of these poorly studied factors may have important growth-promoting activities, further elucidation of their mechanism of action is awaited. Fibroblast growth factor has been shown to be mitogenic for vascular endothelium.[438] The relationship (or influence), if any, of these growth factors with the platelet-derived growth factor[38a,439] is unknown.

3. Catecholamines. The interrelationship of catecholamines with neural and metabolic factors may contribute importantly to the pathogenesis of atherosclerosis in the diabetic.[440] Christensen[441] has shown elevated levels of catecholamines in the uncontrolled diabetic patient, with return toward normal after control of diabetes. In view of the known increase of catecholamine turnover in the presence of stress and the impact of personality pattern on the evolution and expression of atheroma in the human,[351–353] catecholamines probably do play a significant role in the progression of atherosclerosis in the diabetic. Catecholamines might also mediate the increased prevalence of hypertension in some diabetics. Landsberg and co-workers have reported evidence for augmented activity of the sympathetic nervous system by carbohydrate overconsumption[442] and directly by insulin.[443] These observations may be of particular relevance in the pathogenesis of Type II diabetes in the obese as well as in the process of atherogenesis.

OTHER CONSIDERATIONS

Trace Elements

Klevay[444,445] has championed the view that one of the crucial determinants underlying the pathogenesis of atherosclerosis is a relative deficiency of copper or a high ratio of zinc to copper in the diet.[445] According to this hypothesis, an imbalance in copper and zinc metabolism results in decreased activity of lysyloxidase at a young age, causing decreased cross-linking of connective tissue in the coronary arteries. In addition, relative or absolute copper or chromium deficiency have also been linked with subsequent development of hypercholesterolemia.[444,446] Another hypothesis suggests de-

velopment of premature atherosclerosis due to prenatal deficiency of vitamin B_6.[447] This, too, remains conjectural.

Virus and Auto-Immunity in Atherosclerosis?

Another provocative etiologic factor suggested in the pathogenesis of atherosclerosis is the viral hypothesis. Burch[448] has described a number of instances in the literature where viral antigens were isolated from the arterial tissues of victims of premature atherosclerosis. In exciting studies by Fabricant et al.[449,450] with Marek's disease herpes virus (MDV) in the chicken, only those chickens which were inoculated with MDV, whether hyper- or normocholesterolemic, developed lesions resembling human atheroma, as compared to controls. In light of the "monoclonal" mutation theory of Benditt and Benditt,[48,49] "virus-induced" lesions could provide a plausible mechanism for the mutation of underlying arterial smooth muscle cell growth. The role of other metabolic factors, e.g., hyperlipidemia, could conceivably be facilitated by such cofactors. An increased prevalence of auto-immune disease documented in certain patients with coro-

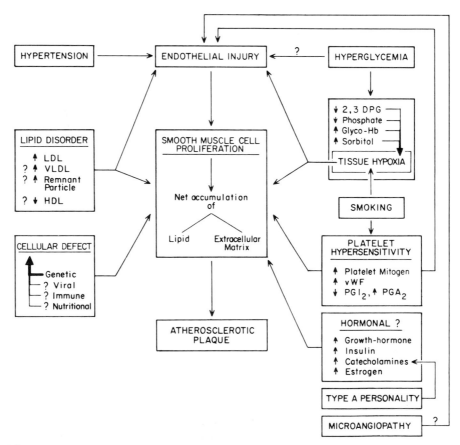

Fig. 11–2. Schematic representation of some of the salient atherogenic events in the diabetic. (From Ganda[20])

nary heart disease[451,452] might also be explained by an underlying viral interaction.

There appears to be little doubt that the process of atherogenesis is a highly complex series of events, regulated by an array of intricate genetic and environmental influences. The interactions of some of the salient atherogenic processes are depicted in Figure 11–2.

Atherosclerosis is a prototype among the diseases which become increasingly prevalent with the process of aging itself.[453,454] However, growing interest in gerontology suggests that the intrinsic biologic events are highly modified by "environmental factors that require long periods of exposure or have long latent periods before they become clinically evident."[454] Inasmuch as glucose intolerance itself becomes increasingly prevalent with aging,[455] and is associated with decreased cellular life span,[54,55] the effect of this disease entity synergizes with all the other environmental factors operating in the nondiabetic individual. Despite some argument to the contrary, there is overwhelming evidence that beside other environmental influences, nutritional factors are of paramount importance in the initiation as well as perpetuation of atherosclerotic plaque formation as an index of the aging process.[456] In early stages, the development of the atheromatous plaque may be amenable to regression and reversal by proper intervention.[39,40,301a,303,456,457,458] The inclement effects of nutritional and other environmental factors are intimately governed by the hormonal regulation of cell growth,[459] an exciting area of current research, particularly germane to diabetes.

REFERENCES

1. Joslin, E.P: Arteriosclerosis and diabetes. Ann. Clin. Med. 5:1061, 1927.
2. Marble, A.: Late complications of diabetes. A continuing challenge. Diabetologia 12:193, 1976.
3. West, K.M.: Epidemiology of Diabetes and its Vascular Lesions. New York, Elsevier, 1978.
4. Warren, S., LeCompte, P.M., Legg, M.A.: Arteriosclerosis in diabetes mellitus. In: Warren, S., Le Compte, P.M., Legg, M.A.: The Pathology of Diabetes Mellitus, 4th Ed. Philadelphia, Lea & Febiger, 1966, pp. 178–187.
5. Robertson, W.B., Strong, J.P.: Atherosclerosis in persons with hypertension and diabetes mellitus. Lab. Invest. 18:538, 1968.
6. West, K.: Report of workgroup on macrovascular disease. In: Report of the National Commission on Diabetes, Vol. 3, Part 2. DHEW Publication (NIH) 76–1022, 1976. pp. 35–77.
7. Pirart, J.: Diabetes mellitus and its degenerative complications: a prospective study of 4,400 patients observed between 1947 and 1973. Diabetes Care 1:168; 252, 1978.
8. Garcia, M.J., McNamara, P.M., Gorton, T., Kannel, W.B.: Morbidity and mortality in diabetes in the Framingham population. Sixteen year follow-up study. Diabetes 23:105, 1974.
9. Kannel, W.B., McGee, D.L.: Diabetes and cardiovascular disease. The Framingham study. J.A.M.A. 241:2035, 1979.
10. Ostrander, L.D., Jr., Lamphiear, D.E., Block, W.D.: Biochemical precursors of atherosclerosis. Studies in apparently healthy men in a general population. Tecumseh, Mich. Arch. Intern. Med. 134:224, 1974.
11. Keen, H.: Glucose intolerance, diabetes mellitus and atherosclerosis: prospects for prevention. Postgrad. Med. J. 52:445, 1976.
12. Keen, H., Jarrett, R.J., Alberti, K.G.M.M.: Diabetes mellitus: a new look at diagnostic criteria. Diabetologia 16:283, 1979
13. Crall, F.V., Jr., Roberts, W.C.: The extramural and intramural coronary arteries in juvenile diabetes mellitus: analysis of nine necropsy patients aged 19 to 38 years with onset of diabetes before age 15 years. Am. J. Med. 64:221, 1978.
14. Gordon, T., Kannel, W.B., Hjortland, M.C., McNamara, P.M.: Menopause and coronary heart disease. The Framingham study. Ann. Intern. Med. 89:157, 1978.
15. Entmacher, P.S., Root, H.F., Marks, H.H.: Longevity of diabetic patients in recent years. Diabetes 13:373, 1964.
16. Bradley, R.F., Partamian, J.O.: Coronary heart disease in the diabetic patient. Med. Clin. N. Am. 49:1093, 1965.
17. Kessler, I.I.: Mortality experience of diabetic patients. A 26-year follow-up study. Am. J. Med. 51:715, 1971.
18. Lachman, A.S., Spray, T.L., Kerwin, D.M., et al.: Medial calcinosis of Mönckeberg. A review of the problem and description of a patient with involvement of peripheral visceral and coronary arteries. Am. J. Med. 63:615, 1977.
19. Jarrett, R.J., Keen, H., Chakrabarti, R.: Diabetes, hyperglycemia and arterial disease. In: H. Keen, J. Jarrett (Eds.): Complications of Diabetes. 2nd Ed. London, Edward Arnold, Ltd., 1982, pp. 179–203.
20. Ganda, O.P.: Pathogenesis of macrovascular disease in the human diabetic. Diabetes 29:931, 1980.
21. Colwell, J.A., Lopes-Virella, M., Halushka, P.V.: Pathogenesis of atherosclerosis in diabetes mellitus. Diabetes Care 4:121, 1981.
22. G.M. Reaven, G. Steiner (Eds.): Proceedings of a conference on diabetes and atherosclerosis. Diabetes 30 (Suppl. 2):1–104, 1981.
23. Clarkson, T.B., Prichard, R.W., Bullock, B.C., et al.: Pathogenesis of atherosclerosis; some advances from using animal models. Exp. Mol. Path. 24:264, 1976.
24. Kottke, B.A., Subbiah, M.T.R.: Pathogenesis of atherosclerosis. Concepts based on animal models. Mayo Clin. Proc. 53:35, 1978.
25. R.A. Camerini-Davalos, E.L. Bierman, W., Redisch, D.B. Zilversmit (Eds.): Atherogenesis. Ann. N.Y. Acad. Sci. 275:1–390, 1976.
26. A.B. Chandler, K. Eurenius, G.C. McMillan, et al. (Eds.): The Thrombotic Process in Atherogenesis. Adv. Exp. Med. Biol. Vol. 104, 1978.
27. H.J. Day, B.A. Molony, E.E. Nishizawa, R.H. Rynbrandt (Eds.): Thrombosis; Animal and Clinical Models. Adv. Ex. Med. Biol. Vol. 102, 1978.
27a. D.E. McMillan, J. Ditzel (Eds.): Proceedings of a Conference on Diabetic Microangiopathy (Kroc Foundation). Diabetes 32 (Suppl. 2):1–104, 1983. (16 papers)
28. Walton, K.W.: Pathogenetic mechanisms in atherosclerosis. Am. J. Cardiol. 35:542, 1975.
29. Ross, R., Glomset, J.A.: The pathogenesis of atherosclerosis. N. Engl. J. Med. 295:369; 420, 1976.
30. Ross, R., Harker, L.: Hyperlipidemia and atherosclerosis. Science 193:1094, 1976.
31. Small, D.M.: Cellular mechanisms for lipid deposition in atherosclerosis. N. Engl. J. Med. 297:873; 924, 1977.

32. Woolf, N.: Thrombosis and atherosclerosis. Br. Med. Bull. *34*:137, 1978.

33. Duguid, J.B., Robertson, W.B.: Mechanical factors in atherosclerosis. Lancet *1*:1205, 1957.

34. Mustard, J.F., Packham, M.A.: The role of blood and platelets in atherosclerosis and the complications of atherosclerosis. Thromb. Diath. Haemorrh. *33*:444, 1975.

35. Moore, S.: Responses of the arterial wall to injury. Diabetes *30* (Suppl. 2):8, 1981.

36. Ross, R., Glomset, J.A.: Atherosclerosis and the arterial smooth muscle cell. Proliferation of smooth muscle is a key event in the genesis of the lesions of atherosclerosis. Science *180*:1332, 1973.

37. Mudd, S.H., Levy, H.L.: Disorders of transsulfuration. In: J.B. Stanbury, J.B. Wyngaarden, D.S. Fredrickson (Eds.): Metabolic Basis of Inherited Disease, 4th Ed. New York, McGraw-Hill Book Co., 1978. pp. 458–503.

38. Minick, C.R.: Immunologic arterial injury in atherogenesis. Ann. N.Y. Acad. Sci. *275*:210, 1976.

38a. Antoniades, H.N., Hunkapiller, M.W.: Human platelet-derived growth factor (PDGF): amino-terminal amino acid sequence. Science *220*:963, 1983.

39. Wissler, R.W., Vesselinovitch, D.: Evidence for prevention and regression of atherosclerosis in man and experimental animals at the arterial level. In: G. Schettler, A. Weizel (Eds.): Proceedings of the Third International Symposium on Atherosclerosis. Berlin, Springer Verlag, 1974. pp. 747–750.

40. G. Schettler, E. Stange, R.W. Wissler (Eds.): Atherosclerosis—Is It Reversible? Berlin, Springer-Verlag, 1978. pp. 1–101.

41. Goldstein, J.L., Brown, M.S.: Lipoprotein receptors: genetic defense against atherosclerosis. Clin. Res. *30*:417, 1982.

42. Goldstein, J.L., Brown, M.S.: Atherosclerosis: the low-density lipoprotein receptor hypothesis. Metabolism *26*:1257, 1977.

43. Brown, M.S., Kovanen, P.T., Goldstein, J.L.: Regulation of plasma cholesterol by lipoprotein receptors. Science *212*:628, 1981.

44. Wolinsky, H., Fowler, S.: Participation of lysosomes in atherosclerosis. N. Engl. J. Med. *299*:1173, 1978.

45. Wolinsky, H., Goldfischer, S., Capron, L., et al.: Hydrolase activities in the rat aorta. I. Effects of diabetes mellitus and insulin treatment. Circ. Res. *42*:821, 1978.

46. Stark, R.M., Brewer, H.B.: Reduced acid cholesterol esterase activity in premature coronary artery disease. Clin. Res. *27*:489, 1979.

47. Greenberg, C.S., Hammerschmidt, D.E., Craddock, P.R., et al.: Atheroma cholesterol activates complement and aggregates polymorphonuclear neutrophil leukocytes: possible role in myocardial infarct extension and in cholesterol embolization syndrome. Clin. Res. *27*:509A, 1979.

48. Benditt, E.P., Benditt, J.M.: Evidence for a monoclonal origin of human atherosclerotic plaques. Proc. Natl. Acad. Sci. USA *70*:1753, 1973.

49. Benditt, E.P.: Implications of the monoclonal character of human atherosclerotic plaques. Am. J. Path. *86*:693, 1977.

50. Pearson, T.A., Kramer, E.C., Solez, K., Heptinstall, R.H.: The human atherosclerotic plaque. Am. J. Path. *86*:657, 1977.

51. Martin, G., Ogburn, C., Sprague, C.: Senescence and vascular disease. Adv. Exp. Med. Biol. *61*:163, 1975.

52. Hayflick, L.: The cell biology of human aging. N. Engl. J. Med. *295*:1302, 1976.

53. Bierman, E.L., Ross, R.: Aging and atherosclerosis. Atherosclerosis Reviews. *2*:79, 1977.

54. Vracko, R., Benditt, E.P.: Manifestations of diabetes mellitus: their possible relationships to an underlying cell defect. A review. Am. J. Pathol. *75*:204, 1974.

55. Goldstein, S., Moerman, E.J., Soeldner, J.S., et al.: Diabetes mellitus and genetic prediabetes. Decreased replicative capacity of cultured skin fibroblast. J. Clin. Invest. *63*:358, 1979.

56. Masoro, E.J.: Lipids and lipid metabolism. Ann. Rev. Physiol. *39*:301, 1977.

57. Barr, D.P., Russ, E.M., Eder, H.A.: Protein-lipid relationship in human plasma. II. In atherosclerosis and related conditions. Am. J. Med. *11*:480, 1951.

58. Gofman, J.W., Rubin, L., McGinley, J.P., Jones, H.B.: Hyperlipoproteinemia. Am. J. Med. *17*:514, 1954.

59. Eisenberg, S., Levy, R.I.: Lipoprotein metabolism. Adv. Lipid Res. *13*:1, 1975.

60. Fisher, W.R., Truitt, D.H.: The common hyperlipoproteinemias. An understanding of disease mechanisms and their control. Ann. Intern. Med. *85*:497, 1976.

61. Jackson, R.L., Morrisett, J.D., Gotto, A.M., Jr.: Lipoproteins and lipid transport: structural and functional concepts. In: B.M. Rifkind, R.I. Levy (Eds.): Hyperlipidemia, Diagnosis and Therapy. New York, Grune & Stratton, 1977, pp. 1–16.

62. Faergeman, O.: Metabolism of plasma lipoproteins. Acta Med. Scand. Suppl. *614*:1, 1977.

63. Smith, L.C., Pownall, H.J., Gotto, A.M., Jr.: The plasma lipoproteins: structure and metabolism. Ann. Rev. Biochem. *47*:751, 1978.

64. Herbert, P.N., Gotto, A.M., Fredrickson, D.S.: Familial lipoprotein deficiency (Abetalipoproteinemia, hypobetalipoproteinemia, and Tangier disease). In: J.B. Stanbury, J.B. Wyngaarden, D.S. Fredrickson (Eds.): Metabolic Basis of Inherited Disease, 4th Ed. New York, McGraw-Hill Book Co., 1978, pp. 544–588.

65. Fredrickson, D.S., Goldstein, J.L., Brown, M.S.: The familial hyperlipoproteinemias. In: J.B. Stanbury, J.B. Wyngaarden, D.S. Fredrickson (Eds.): Metabolic Basis of Inherited Disease. 4th Ed. New York, McGraw-Hill Book Co., 1978, pp. 604–655.

66. Brunzell, J.D., Chait, A., Bierman, E.L.: Pathophysiology of lipoprotein transport. Metabolism *27*:1109, 1978.

67. Havel, R.J.: Classification of the hyperlipidemias. Ann. Rev. Med. *28*:195, 1977.

68. Glueck, C.J.: Classification and diagnosis of hyperlipoproteinemia. In: B.M. Rifkind, R.I. Levy (Eds.): Hyperlipidemia, Diagnosis and Therapy. New York, Grune & Stratton, 1977, pp. 17–39.

69. Murphy, E.A., Kwiterovich, P.O.: Genetics of hyperlipoproteinemias. In: B.M. Rifkind, R.I. Levy (Eds.): Hyperlipidemia, Diagnosis and Therapy. New York, Grune & Stratton, 1977, pp. 217–247.

70. Fredrickson, D.S., Levy, R.I., Lees, R.S.: Fat transport in lipoproteins—an integrated approach to mechanisms and disorders. N. Engl. J. Med. *276*:34; 94; 148; 215; 273, 1967.

71. Goldstein, J.L., Hazzard, W.R., Schrott, H.G., et al.: Hyperlipidemia in coronary heart disease. I. Lipid levels in 500 survivors of myocardial infarction. J. Clin. Invest. *52*:1533, 1973.

72. Miller, N.E.: The evidence for the antiatherogenicity of high density lipoprotein in man. Lipids *13*:914, 1978.

73. Tall, A.R., Small, D.M.: Plasma high-density lipoproteins. N. Engl. J. Med. *299*:1232, 1978.

74. Gershfeld, N.L.: Selective phospholipid adsorption and atherosclerosis. Science *204*:506, 1979.

75. Krauss, R.M., Levy, R.I., Fredrickson, D.S.: Selective measurement of two lipase activities in postheparin

plasma from normal subjects and patients with hyperlipoproteinemia. J. Clin. Invest. 54:1107, 1974.

76. Huttunen, J.K., Ehnholm, C., Nikkila, E.A., Ohta, M.: Effect of fasting on two postheparin plasma triglyceride lipases and triglyceride removal in obese subjects. Europ. J. Clin. Invest. 5:435, 1975.

77. Glueck, C.J.: Editorial. Postheparin lipoprotein lipases. N. Engl. J. Med. 292:1347, 1975.

78. DenBesten, L., Reyna, R.H., Connor, W.E., Stegnik, L.D.: The different effects on the serum lipids and fecal steroids of high carbohydrate diets given orally or intravenously. J. Clin. Invest. 52:1384, 1973.

79. Nestel, P.J.: Triglyceride turnover in man. Effects of dietary carbohydrate. Prog. Biochem. Pharmacol. 8:125, 1973.

80. Reaven, G.M., Lerner, R.L., Stern, M.P., Farquhar, J.W.: Role of insulin in endogenous hypertriglyceridemia. J. Clin. Invest. 46:1756, 1967.

81. Grundy, S.M., Mok, H.Y.: Chylomicron clearance in normal and hyperlipidemic man. Metabolism 25:1225, 1976.

82. Brown, M.S., Goldstein, J.L.: Lipoprotein receptors in the liver. Control signals for plasma cholesterol traffic. J. Clin. Invest. 72:743, 1983.

83. Carew, T.E., Pittman, R.C., Steinberg, D.: Tissue sites of degradation of native and reductively methylated (^{14}C) sucrose-labelled low density lipoprotein in rats. J. Biol. Chem. 257:8001, 1982.

84. Andersen, J.M., Dietschy, J.M.: Cholesterogenesis: derepression in extrahepatic tissues with 4-aminopyrazolo [3,4-d] pyrimidine. Science 193:903, 1976.

85. Johansson, C., Rössner, S., Walldius, G.: HDL secretion from human intestinal tract. Lancet 1:324, 1978.

86. Anderson, D.W.: HDL cholesterol: the variable components. Lancet 1:819, 1978.

87. Daerr, W.H., Gianturco, S.H., Patsch, J.R., et al.: Different effects of high density lipoprotein subclasses on 3-hydroxy-3 methylglutaryl coenzyme A reductase in normal human fibroblasts. Clin. Res. 27:437A, 1979.

88. Gjone, E., Norum, K.R., Glomset, J.A.: Familial lecithin: cholesterol acyltransferase deficiency. In: J.B. Stanbury, J.B. Wyngaarden, D.S. Fredrickson (Eds.): Metabolic Basis of Inherited Disease, 4th Ed. New York, NcGraw-Hill Book Co., 1978, pp. 589–603.

89. Kashyap, M.L., Srivastava, L.S., Chen, C.Y., et al.: Radioimmunoassay of human apolipoprotein C II. A study in normal and hypertriglyceridemic subjects. J. Clin. Invest. 60:171, 1977.

90. Carlson, L.A., Ballantyne, D.: Changing relative proportions of apolipoproteins CII and CIII of very low density lipoproteins in hypertriglyceridaemia. Atherosclerosis 23:563, 1976.

91. Montes, A., Knopp, R.H.: Lipid metabolism in pregnancy. IV. C apoprotein changes in very low and intermediate density lipoproteins. J. Clin. Endocrin. Metab. 45:1060, 1977.

92. Stocks, J., Holdsworth, G., Galton, D.: Hypertriglyceridaemia associated with an abnormal triglyceride-rich lipoprotein carrying excess apolipoprotein C-III-2. Lancet 2:667, 1979.

93. Kashyap, M.L., Hynd, B.A., Robinson, K., Gartside, P.S.: Abnormal preponderance of sialylated apolipoprotein CIII in triglyceride-rich lipoproteins in Type V hyperlipoprotcinemia. Metabolism 30:111, 1981.

94. Breckenridge, W.C., Little, J.A., Steiner, G., et al.: Hypertriglyceridemia associated with deficiency of apolipoprotein C-II. N. Engl. J. Med. 298:1265, 1978.

95. Cox, D.W., Breckenridge, W.C., Little, J.A.: Inheritance

96. Kushwaha, R.S., Hazzard, W.R., Wahl, P.W., Hoover, J.J.: Type III hyperlipoproteinemia: diagnosis in whole plasma by apolipoprotein-E immunoassay. Ann. Intern. Med. 87:509, 1977.

97. Havel, R.J., Kotite, L., Vigne, J-L., et al.: Radioimmunoassay of human arginine-rich apolipoprotein, apoprotein E-3. Concentrations in blood plasma lipoproteins as affected by apoprotein E-3 deficiency. J. Clin. Invest. 66:1351, 1980.

98. Mahley, R.W., Innerarity, T.L., Bersot, T.P., et al.: Alterations in human high-density lipoproteins, with or without increased plasma cholesterol, induced by diets high in cholesterol. Lancet 2:807, 1978.

99. Hamilton, R.L.: Hepatic secretion and metabolism of high-density lipoproteins. In: J.M. Dietschy, A.M. Gotto, Jr., J.A. Ontko (Eds.): Disturbances in Lipid and Lipoprotein Metabolism. Bethesda, Am. Physiol. Soc. 1978, pp. 155–171.

100. Schwartz, C.C., Halloran, L.G., Vlahcevic, Z.R., et al.: Preferential utilization of free cholesterol from high-density lipoproteins for biliary cholesterol secretion in man. Science 200:62, 1978.

101. Turner, P., Miller, N., Chrystie, I., et al.: Splanchnic production of discoidal plasma high-density lipoprotein in man. Lancet 1:645, 1979.

102. Schaeffer, E.J., Blum, C.B., Levy, R.I., et al.: Metabolism of high density lipoprotein apolipoproteins in Tangier disease. N. Engl. J. Med. 299:905, 1978.

103. Glickman, R.M., Green, P.H.R., Lees, R.S., Tall, A.: Apoprotein A-1 synthesis in normal intestinal mucosa and in Tangier disease. N. Engl. J. Med. 299:1424, 1978.

104. Herbert, P.N., Forte, T., Heinen, R.J., Fredrickson, D.S.: Tangier disease. One explanation of lipid storage. N. Engl. J. Med. 299:519, 1978.

105. Cramp, D.G., Tickner, T.R., Wills, M.R.: Controlled storage of biological energy: the role of plasma lipoproteins. Lancet 2:176, 1976.

106. Brown, M.S., Goldstein, J.L.: Expression of the familial hypercholesterolemia gene in heterozygotes: mechanism for a dominant disorder in man. Science 185:61, 1974.

107. Miller, N.E., Weinstein, D.B., Carew, T.E., et al.: Interaction between high density and low density lipoproteins during uptake and degradation by cultured human fibroblasts. J. Clin. Invest. 60:78, 1977.

108. Bierman, E.L., Albers, J.J.: Lipoprotein uptake by cultured human arterial smooth muscle cells. Biochem. Biophys. Acta 388:198, 1975.

109. Carew, T.E., Koschinsky, T., Hayes, S.B., Steinberg, D.: A mechanism by which high density lipoprotein may slow the atherogenic process. Lancet 1:1315, 1976.

110. Stein, O., Stein, Y.: High density lipoproteins reduce the uptake of low density lipoproteins by human endothelial cells in culture. Biochem. Biophys. Acta 431:363, 1976.

110a. Oram, J.F., Brinton, E.A., Bierman, E.L.: Regulation of high-density lipoprotein receptor activity in cultured human skin fibroblasts and human arterial smooth muscle cells. J. Clin. Invest. 72:1611, 1983.

110b. Rifkind, B.M., Segal, J.: Lipid Research Clinics program reference values for hyperlipidemia and hypolipidemia. J.A.M.A. 250:1869, 1983.

111. Friedewald, W.T., Levy, R.I., Fredrickson, D.S.: Estimation of the concentration of low-density lipoprotein cholesterol in plasma, without use of the preparative ultracentrifuge. Clin. Chem. 18:499, 1972.

112. Goldstein, J.L., Schrott, H.G., Hazzard, W.R., et al.: Hyperlipidemia in coronary heart disease. II. Genetic analysis of lipid levels in 176 families and delineation of

a new inherited disorder, combined hyperlipidemia. J. Clin. Invest. *52*:1544, 1973.

113. Goldstein, J.L., Brown, M.S.: Familial hypercholesterolemia. A genetic regulatory defect in cholesterol metabolism. Am. J. Med. *58*:147, 1975.

114. Sodhi, H.S., Mason, D.T.: New insights into the homeostasis of plasma cholesterol. A time for changing concepts. Am. J. Med. *63*:325, 1977.

115. Kushwaha, R.S., Hazzard, W.R., Gagne, C., et al.: Type III hyperlipoproteinemia: paradoxical hypolipidemic response to estrogen. Ann. Intern. Med. *87*:517, 1977.

116. Levy, R.I., Morganroth, J.: Familial Type III hyperlipoproteinemia. Ann. Intern. Med. *87*:625, 1977.

117. Mishkel, M.A., Crowther, S.M.: Broad beta disease: clinical and diagnostic characteristics. Cardiovasc. Med. *3*:957, 1978.

118. Brunzell, J.D., Schrott, H.G., Motulsky, A.G., Bierman, E.L.: Myocardial infarction in the familial forms of hypertriglyceridemia. Metabolism *25*:313, 1976.

119. Greenberg, B.H., Blackwelder, W.C., Levy, R.I.: Primary Type V hyperlipoproteinemia. A descriptive study in 32 families. Ann. Intern. Med. *87*:526, 1977.

120. Goldstein, J.L., Albers, J.J., Schrott, H.G., et al.: Plasma lipid levels and coronary heart disease in adult relatives of newborns with normal and elevated cord blood lipids. Am. J. Human. Genet. *26*:727, 1974.

121. Glueck, C.J., Fallat, R.W., Tsang, R., Buncher, C.R.: Hyperlipidemia in progeny of parents with myocardial infarction before age 50. Am. J. Dis. Child. *127*:70, 1974.

122. Morrison, J.A., Kelly, K.A., Mellies, M.J., et al.: Parent-child association at upper and lower ranges of plasma cholesterol and triglyceride levels. Pediatrics *62*:468, 1978.

123. Glueck, C.J., Gartside, P., Fallat, R.W., et al.: Familial hypobeta and familial hyperalpha lipoproteinemia. J. Lab. Clin. Med. *88*:941, 1976.

124. Kahn, J.A., Glueck, C.J.: Familial hypobetalipoproteinemia. Absence of atherosclerosis in a postmortem study. J.A.M.A. *240*:47, 1978.

125. New, M.I., Roberts, T.N., Bierman, E.L., Reader, G.G.: The significance of blood lipid alterations in diabetes mellitus. Diabetes *12*:208, 1963.

126. Albrink, M.J., Lavietes, P.H., Man, E.B.: Vascular disease and serum lipids in diabetes mellitus. Observations over thirty years (1931–1961). Ann. Intern. Med. *58*:305, 1963.

127. Chance, G.W., Albutt, E.C., Edkins, S.M.: Serum lipids and lipoproteins in untreated diabetic children. Lancet *1*:1126, 1969.

128. Wilson, D.E., Schreibman, P.H., Day, V.C., Arky, R.A.: Hyperlipidemia in an adult diabetic population. J. Chronic Dis. *23*:501, 1970.

129. Santen, R.J., Willis, P.W., III, Fajans, S.S.: Atherosclerosis in diabetes mellitus. Correlations with serum lipid levels, adiposity, and serum insulin level. Arch. Intern. Med. *130*:833, 1972.

130. Lewis, B., Mancini, M., Mattock, M., et al.: Plasma triglyceride and free fatty acid metabolism in diabetes mellitus. Europ. J. Clin. Invest. *2*:445, 1972.

131. Nikkilä, E.A.: Triglyceride metabolism in diabetes mellitus. Prog. Biochem. Pharmacol. *8*:271, 1973.

132. Schonfeld, G., Birge, C., Miller, J.P., et al.: Apolipoprotein B levels and altered lipoprotein composition in diabetes. Diabetes *23*:827, 1974.

133. Kaufmann, R.L., Assal, J. Ph., Soeldner, J.S., et al.: Plasma lipid levels in diabetic children. Effect of diet restricted in cholesterol and saturated fats. Diabetes *24*:672, 1975.

134. Sosenko, J.M., Breslow, J.L., Miettinen, O.S., Gabbay, K.H.: Hyperglycemia and plasma lipid levels. A prospective study of young insulin-dependent diabetic patients. N. Engl. J. Med. *302*:650, 1980.

135. Simpson, R.W., Mann, J.I., Hockaday, T.D.R., et al.: Lipid abnormalities in untreated maturity-onset diabetics and the effect of treatment. Diabetologia *16*:101, 1979.

136. Kannel, W.B., Castelli, W.P., Gordon, T., McNamara, P.M.: Serum cholesterol, lipoproteins and the risk of coronary heart disease. The Framingham Study. Ann. Intern. Med. *74*:1, 1971.

137. Cohn, P.F., Gabbay, S.I., Weglicki, W.B.: Serum lipid levels in angiographically defined coronary artery disease. Ann. Intern. Med. *84*:241, 1976.

138. Kissebah, A.H., Alfarsi, S., Evans, D.J., Adams, P.W.: Integrated regulation of very low density lipoprotein triglyceride and apolipoprotein-B kinetics in non-insulin-dependent diabetes mellitus. Diabetes *31*:217, 1982.

139. Bennion, L.J., Grundy, S.M.: Effects of diabetes mellitus on cholesterol metabolism in man. N. Engl. J. Med. *296*:1365, 1977.

140. Saudek, C.D., Brach, E.L.: Cholesterol metabolism in diabetes. I. The effect of diabetic control on sterol balance. Diabetes *27*:1059, 1978.

141. Saudek, C.D., Eder, H.A.: Lipid metabolism in diabetes mellitus. Am. J. Med. *66*:843, 1979.

142. Saudek, C.D., Young, N.L.: Cholesterol metabolism in diabetes mellitus. The role of diet. Diabetes *30* (Suppl. 2):76, 1981.

143. Chait, A., Bierman, E.L., Albers, J.J.: Low density lipoprotein receptor activity in skin fibroblasts cultured from diabetic donors. Diabetes *28*:914, 1979.

143a. Lopes-Virella, M.F., Sherer, G.K., Lees, A.M., et al.: Surface binding, internalization and degradation by cultured human fibroblasts of low density lipoproteins isolated from Type I (insulin-dependent) diabetic patients: changes with metabolic control. Diabetologia *22*:430, 1982.

144. Mahley, R.W.: Cellular and molecular biology of lipoprotein metabolism in atherosclerosis. Diabetes *30* (Suppl. 2):60, 1981.

145. Zilversmit, D.B.: Atherogenesis: a postprandial phenomenon. Circulation *60*:473, 1979.

146. Gonen, B., Baenziger, J., Schonfeld, G., et al.: Nonenzymatic glycosylation of low density lipoproteins in vitro. Effects on cell-interactive properties. Diabetes *30*:875, 1981.

147. Howard, C.F., Jr.: Diabetes and lipid metabolism in nonhuman primates. Adv. Lipid Res. *13*:91, 1975.

148. Reaven, G.M., Greenfield, M.S.: Diabetic hypertriglyceridemia. Evidence for three clinical syndromes. Diabetes *30* (Suppl. 2):66, 1981.

149. Kaye, J.P., Galton, D.J.: Triglyceride-production rates in patients with type IV hypertriglyceridaemia. Lancet *1*:1005, 1975.

150. Nikkila, E.A., Huttunen, J.K., Enholm, C.: Postheparin plasma lipoprotein lipase and hepatic lipase in diabetes mellitus. Relationship to plasma triglyceride metabolism. Diabetes *26*:11, 1977.

150a. Chait, A., Brunzell, J.D.: Severe hypertriglyceridemia: role of familial and acquired disorders. Metabolism *32*:209, 1983.

151. Abrams, J.J., Ginsberg, H., Grundy, S.M.: Metabolism of cholesterol and plasma triglycerides in nonketotic diabetes mellitus. Diabetes *31*:903, 1982.

152. Brunzell, J.D., Porte, D., Jr., Bierman, E.L.: Reversible abnormalities in postheparin lipolytic activity during the late phase of release in diabetes mellitus. Metabolism *24*:1123, 1975.

153. Bagdade, J.D., Bierman, E.L., Porte, D., Jr.: Influence of obesity on the relationship between insulin and triglyceride levels in endogenous hypertriglyceridemia. Diabetes *20*:664, 1971.

154. Bernstein, R.S., Grant, N., Kipnis, D.M.: Hyperinsulinemia and enlarged adipocytes in patients with endogenous hyperlipoproteinemia without obesity or diabetes mellitus. Diabetes *24*:207, 1975.

155. Ganda, O.P., Gleason, R.E.: Hypertriglyceridemia: a frequent concomitant of "abnormal" glucose tolerance in non-obese adults. Diabetes *26* (Suppl. 1):398, 1977.

156. Reaven, G.M., Bernstein, R.M.: Effect of obesity on the relationship between very low density lipoprotein production rate and plasma triglyceride concentration in normal and hypertriglyceridemic subjects. Metabolism *27*:1047, 1978.

157. Robertson, R.P., Gavareski, D.J., Henderson, J.D., et al.: Accelerated triglyceride secretion. A metabolic consequence of obesity. J. Clin. Invest. *52*:1620, 1973.

158. Brunzell, J.D., Hazzard, W.R., Motulsky, A.G., Bierman, E.L.: Evidence for diabetes mellitus and genetic forms of hypertriglyceridemia as independent entities. Metabolism *24*:1115, 1975.

159. Böttiger, L.E., Carlson, L.A.: Risk factors for ischemic vascular death for men in the Stockholm prospective study. Atherosclerosis *36*:389, 1980.

160. Pelkonen, R., Nikkila, E.A., Koskinen, S., et al.: Association of serum lipids and obesity with cardiovascular mortality. Brit. Med. J. *2*:1185, 1977.

161. Ostrander, L.D., Jr., Lamphiear, D.E., Block, W.D., et al.: Physiological variables and diabetic status. Findings in Tecumseh, Michigan. Arch. Intern. Med. *140*:1215, 1980.

162. Salel, A.F., Riggs, K., Mason, D.T., et al.: The importance of type IV hyperlipoproteinemia as a predisposing factor in coronary artery disease. Am. J. Med. *57*:897, 1974.

163. Bloch, A., Dinsmore, R.E., Lees, R.S.: Coronary arteriographic findings in Type II and Type IV hyperlipoproteinaemia. Lancet *1*:928, 1976.

164. Miller, N.E., Hammett, F., Saltissi, S., et al.: Relation of angiographically defined coronary artery disease to plasma lipoprotein subfractions and apolipoproteins. Br. Med. J. *282*:1741, 1981.

165. Wilhelmsen, L., Wedel, H., Tibblin, G.: Multivariate analysis of risk factors for coronary heart disease. Circulation *48*:950, 1973.

166. Bar-On, H., Roheim, P.S., Eder, H.A.: Serum lipoproteins and apolipoproteins in rats with streptozotocin-induced diabetes. J. Clin. Invest. *57*:714, 1976.

166a.Sniderman, A.D., Wolfson, C., Teng, B., et al.: Association of hyperapobetalipoproteinemia with endogenous hypertriglyceridemia and atherosclerosis. Ann. Intern. Med. *97*:833, 1982.

167. Nikkilä, E.A.: Letter. Serum high-density-lipoprotein and coronary heart disease. Lancet *2*:320, 1976.

168. Rhoads, G.G., Gulbrandsen, C.L., Kagan, A.: Serum lipoproteins and coronary heart disease in a population study of Hawaii Japanese men. N. Engl. J. Med. *294*:293, 1976.

169. Gordon, T., Castelli, W.P., Hjortland, M.C., et al.: High-density lipoprotein as a protective factor against coronary heart disease. The Framingham Study. Am. J. Med. *62*:707, 1977.

170. Kannel, W.B., Castelli, W.P., Gordon, T.: Cholesterol in the prediction of atherosclerotic disease. New perspectives based on the Framingham Study. Ann. Intern. Med. *90*:85, 1979.

171. Castelli, W.P., Doyle, J.T., Gordon, T., et al.: HDL cholesterol and other lipids in coronary heart disease. The cooperative lipoprotein phenotyping study. Circulation *55*:767, 1977.

172. Miller, N.E. Førde, O.H.., Thelle, D.S., Mjøs, O.D.: The Tromsø heart study. High-density lipoprotein and coronary heart disease: a prospective case-control study. Lancet *1*:965, 1977.

173. Goldbourt, U., Medalie, J.H.: High-density lipoprotein cholesterol and incidence of coronary heart disease; the Israeli Ischemic Heart Disease Study. Am. J. Epidemiol. *109*:296, 1979.

174. Berg, K., Børrescn, A-L, Dahlen, G.: Serum high-density-lipoprotein and atherosclerotic heart disease. Lancet *1*:499, 1976.

175. Albers, J.J., Cheung, M.C., Hazzard, W.R.: High-density lipoproteins in myocardial infarction survivors. Metabolism *27*:479, 1978.

176. Avogaro, P., Bon, G.B., Cazzolato, G., Quinci, G.B.: Are apolipoproteins better discriminators than lipids for atherosclerosis? Lancet *1*:901, 1979.

177. Bradby, G.V.H., Valente, A.J., Walton, K.W.: Serum high-density lipoproteins in peripheral vascular disease. Lancet *2*:1271, 1978.

178. Rössner, S., Kjellin, K.G., Mettinger, K.L., et al.: Normal serum cholesterol but low HDL-cholesterol concentration in young patients with ischemic cerebrovascular disease. Lancet *1*:577, 1978.

179. Pearson, T.A., Bulkley, B.H., Achuff, S.C., et al.: The association of low levels of HDL cholesterol and arteriographically defined coronary artery disease. Am. J. Epidemiol. *109*:285, 1979.

180. Zampogna, A., Luria, M.H., Manubens, S.J., Luria, M.A.: Relationship between lipids and occlusive coronary artery disease. Arch. Intern. Med. *140*:1067, 1980.

181. Streja, D., Steiner, G., Kwiterovich, P.O., Jr.: Plasma high-density lipoproteins and ischemic heart disease. Studies in a large kindred with familial hypercholesterolemia. Ann. Intern. Med. *89*:871, 1978.

182. Schaeffer, E., Levy, R.I., Anderson, D.W., et al.: Plasma triglycerides in regulation of HDL-cholesterol levels. Lancet *2*:391, 1978.

183. Glueck, C.J., Stein, E.A., Kashyap, M.L., Steiner, P.M.: Persistent hypoalphalipoproteinemia during therapy of familial Type V hyperlipoproteinemia. Clin. Res. *27*:680A, 1978.

184. Herbert, P.N., Henderson, L.O.: Plasma-triglycerides do not regulate high-density lipoprotein concentrations. Lancet *1*:1368, 1979.

185. Falko, J.M., Witztum, J.L., Schonfeld, G., Bateman, J.: Dietary treatment of Type V hyperlipoproteinemia fails to normalize low levels of high-density lipoprotein cholesterol. Ann. Intern. Med. *91*:750, 1979.

186. Witztum, J.L., Dillingham, M.A., Giese, W., et al.: Normalization of triglycerides in type IV hyperlipoproteinemia fails to correct low levels of high-density-lipoprotein cholesterol. N. Engl. J. Med. *303*:907, 1980.

187. Cramp, D.G., Tickner, T.R.: Lipoproteins and atheroma. (letter). Lancet *2*:1086, 1977.

188. Morrison, J.A., de Groot, I., Kelly, K.A., et al.: High and low density lipoprotein cholesterol levels in hypercholesterolemic school children. Lipids *14*:99, 1979.

189. Glueck, C.J., Kelly, K., Mellies, M.J., et al.: Hypercholesterolemia and hyper-α-lipoproteinemia in school children. Pediatrics *62*:478, 1978.

190. Nicholson, J., Gartside, P.S., Siegel, M., et al.: Lipid and lipoprotein distributions in octo- and nonagenarians. Metabolism *28*:51, 1979.

191. Berenson, G.S., Srinivasan, S.R., Frerichs, R.R., Webber, L.S.: Serum high density lipoprotein and its rela-

tionship to cardiovascular disease risk factor variables in children—the Bogalusa heart study. Lipids *14*:91, 1979.

192. Gordon, T., Castelli, W.P., Hjortland, M.C., et al.: Diabetes blood lipids, and the role of obesity in coronary heart disease risk for women. The Framingham Study. Ann. Intern. Med. *87*:393, 1977.

193. Ganda, O.P., Hayes, E.J., Soeldner, J.S., et al.: Alterations in high-density lipoprotein cholesterol (HDL-c) and its relationship to control of diabetes (DM). Program, 10th Congress of the International Diabetes Federation. Vienna, Austria, Sept. 9–14, 1979, p. 72.

194. Beach, K.W., Brunzell, J.D., Conquest, L.L., Strandness, D.E.: The correlation of arteriosclerosis obliterans with lipoproteins in insulin-dependent and non-insulin-dependent diabetes. Diabetes *28*:836, 1979.

195. Lopes-Virella, M.F.L., Stone, P.G., Colwell, J.A.: Serum high density lipoprotein in diabetic patients. Diabetologia *13*:285, 1977.

196. Lopes-Virella, M.F., Wohltmann, H.J., Loadholt, C.B., Buse, M.G.: Plasma lipids and lipoproteins in young insulin-dependent diabetic patients: relationship with control. Diabetologia *21*:216, 1981.

197. Reckless, J.P.D., Betteridge, D.J., Wu, P., et al.: High-density and low-density lipoproteins and prevalence of vascular disease in diabetes mellitus. Br. Med. J. *1*:883, 1978.

198. Calvert, G.D., Graham, J.J., Mannik, T., et al.: Effects of therapy on plasma-high-density lipoprotein-cholesterol concentrations in diabetes mellitus. Lancet *2*:66, 1978.

198a.Schmitt, J.K., Poole, J.R., Lewis, S.B., et al.: Hemoglobin A$_1$ correlates with the ratio of low- to high-density lipoprotein cholesterol in normal weight Type II diabetics. Metabolism *31*:1084, 1982.

199. Howard, B.V., Savage, P.J., Bennion, L.J., Bennett, P.H.: Lipoprotein composition in diabetes mellitus. Atherosclerosis *30*:153, 1978.

200. Stanton, K.: HDL cholesterol in diabetes and heart disease. Lancet *2*:638, 1978.

201. Stalenhoef, A.F.H., Demacker, P.N.M., Lutterman, J.A., van't Laar, A.: High-density lipoprotein and maturity-onset diabetes. Lancet *1*:325, 1978.

202. Lisch, H-J., Sailer, S.: Lipoprotein patterns in diet, sulphonylurea and insulin treated diabetics. Diabetologia *20*:118, 1981.

203. Nikkilä, E.A., Hormila, P.: Serum lipids and lipoproteins in insulin-treated diabetes. Demonstration of increased high density lipoprotein concentrations. Diabetes *27*:1078, 1978.

204. Eckel, R.H., Albers, J.J., Cheung, M.C., et al.: High density lipoprotein composition in insulin-dependent diabetes mellitus. Diabetes *30*:132, 1981.

205. Bar-On, H., Landau, D., Berry, E.: Serum-high-density-lipoprotein and University Group Diabetes Program results. Letter. Lancet *1*:761, 1978.

206. Kolata, G.B.: Controversy over study of diabetes drugs continues for nearly a decade. Science *203*:896, 1979.

207. Whitehouse, F.W., Arky, R.A., Bell, D.I., et al.: Policy statement: The UGDP controversy. Diabetes *28*:168, 1979.

208. Boucher, B.J., Yudkin, J.: Diabetic control and HDL cholesterol levels. Lancet *2*:269, 1978.

209. Elkeles, R.S., Wu, J., Hambley, J.: Haemoglobin A$_1$, blood glucose, and high-density-lipoprotein cholesterol in insulin-requiring diabetics. Lancet *2*:547, 1978.

210. Dunn, F.L., Pietri, A., Raskin, P.: Plasma lipid and lipoprotein levels with continuous subcutaneous insulin infusion in Type I diabetes mellitus. Ann. Intern. Med. *95*:426, 1981.

211. Falko, J.M., O'Dorisio, T.M., Cataland, S.: Improvement of high-density lipoprotein-cholesterol levels. Ambulatory Type I diabetics treated with the subcutaneous insulin pump. J.A.M.A. *247*:37, 1982.

212. Witztum, J., Schonfeld, G.: High density lipoproteins. Diabetes *28*:326, 1979.

213. Johansson, B.G., Nilsson-Ehle, P.: Alcohol consumption and high-density lipoprotein. N. Engl. J. Med. *298*:633, 1978.

214. Durrington, P.: HDL cholesterol in diabetes mellitus. Lancet *2*:206, 1978.

215. Blum, C.B., Levy, R.I., Eisenberg, S., et al.: High density lipoprotein metabolism in man. J. Clin. Invest. *60*:795, 1977.

216. Hjermann, I., Enger, S.C., Helgeland, A., et al.: The effect of dietary changes on high density lipoprotein cholesterol. The Oslo study. Am. J. Med. *66*:105, 1979.

217. Shepherd, J., Packard, C.J., Patsch, J.R., et al.: Effect of dietary polyunsaturated and saturated fat on the properties of high density lipoproteins and the metabolism of apolipoprotein A-I. J. Clin. Invest. *61*:1582, 1978.

218. Burslem, J., Schonfeld, G., Howald, M.A., et al.: Plasma apoprotein and lipoprotein lipid levels in vegetarians. Metabolism *27*:711, 1978.

219. Sacks, F.M., Castelli, W.P., Donner, A., Kass, E.H.: Plasma lipids and lipoproteins in vegetarians and controls. N. Engl. J. Med. *292*:1148, 1975.

220. Castelli, W.P., Doyle, J.T., Gordon, T., et al.: Alcohol and blood lipids. The cooperative lipoprotein phenotyping study. Lancet *2*:153, 1977.

221. Yano, K., Rhoads, G.G., Kagan, A.: Coffee, alcohol and risk of coronary heart disease among Japanese men living in Hawaii. N. Engl. J. Med. *297*:405, 1977.

222. Hulley, S.B., Cohen, R., Widdowson, G.: Plasma high-density lipoprotein cholesterol level. Influence of risk factor intervention. J.A.M.A. *238*:2269, 1977.

223. Ginsberg, H., Olefsky, J., Farquhar, J.W., Reaven, G.M.: Moderate ethanol ingestion and plasma triglyceride levels. A study in normal and hypertriglyceridemic persons. Ann. Intern. Med. *80*:143, 1974.

224. Mendelson, J.H., Mello, N.K.: Alcohol-induced hyperlipidemia and beta lipoproteins. Science *180*:1372, 1973.

225. Shelton, J.D., Petitti, D.: Formulation-dependent effect of oral contraceptives on HDL-cholesterol. Lancet *2*:677, 1978.

226. Arntzenius, A.C., van Gent, C.M., van der Voort, H., et al.: Reduced high-density lipoprotein in women aged 40–41 using oral contraceptives. Consultation Bureau Heart Project. Lancet *1*:1221, 1978.

227. Roösner, S.: Lowering of HDL cholesterol by oral contraceptives. Lancet *2*:269, 1978.

228. Bradley, D.D., Wingerd, J., Petitti, D.B., et al.: Serum high-density lipoprotein cholesterol in women using oral contraceptives, estrogens and progestins. N. Engl. J. Med. *299*:17, 1978.

229. Hirvonen, E., Mälkönen, M., Manninen, V.: Effects of different progestogens on lipoproteins during postmenopausal replacement therapy. N. Engl. J. Med. *304*:560, 1981.

230. Enholm, C., Huttunen, J.K., Kinnunen, P.J., et al.: Effect of oxandrolone treatment on the activity of lipoprotein lipase, hepatic lipase, and phospholipase Al of human postheparin plasma. N. Engl. J. Med. *292*:1314, 1975.

231. Solyom, A.: Effect of androgens on serum lipids and lipoproteins. Lipids *7*:135, 1972.

232. Cantwell, J.D.: Running. J.A.M.A. *240*:1409, 1978.

233. Wood, P.D., Haskell, W., Klein, H., et al.: The distribution of plasma lipoproteins in middle-aged male runners. Metabolism *25*:1249, 1976.

234. Miller, N.E., Rao, S., Lewis, B., et al.: High-density lipoprotein and physical activity. Lancet *1*:111, 1979.

235. Hulley, S., Ashman, P., Kuller, L., et al.: HDL-cholesterol levels in the Multiple Risk Factor Intervention Trial by the MRFIT Research Group[1,2]. Lipids *14*:119, 1979.

236. Nikkilä, E.A., Kaste, M., Ehnholm, C., Viikari, J.: Increase of serum high-density lipoprotein in phenytoin users. Br. Med. J. *2*:99, 1978.

237. Henry, D., Bell, G.D, Glithero, P.: Plasma high-density lipoproteins. N. Engl. J. Med. *300*:797, 1979.

238. Manninen, V., Mälkönen, M., Tuomilehto, J.: Hypolipidaemic agents: What are they good for? (Letter). Lancet *2*:1281, 1977.

238a. Samuel, P.: Effect of gemfibrozil on serum lipids. Am. J. Med. *74* (Suppl. 5A):23, 1983.

238b. Glueck, C.J.: Colestipol and probucol: treatment of primary and familial hypercholesterolemia and amelioration of atherosclerosis. Ann. Intern. Med. *96*:475, 1982.

239. Goldberg, A.P., Applebaum-Bowden, D.M., Bierman, E.L., et al.: Increase in lipoprotein lipase during clofibrate treatment of hypertriglyceridemia in patients on hemodialysis. N. Engl. J. Med. *301*:1073, 1979.

240. Leren, P., Foss, P.O., Helgeland, A., et al.: Effect of propranolol and prazosin on blood lipids. The Oslo study. Lancet *2*:4, 1980.

241. Day, J.L., Metcalfe, J., Simpson, C.N.: Adrenergic mechanisms in control of plasma lipid concentrations. Br. Med. J. *284*:1145, 1982.

242. Lindner, A., Charra, B., Sherrard, D.J., Scribner, B.H.: Accelerated atherosclerosis in prolonged maintenance hemodialysis. N. Engl. J. Med. *290*:697, 1974.

243. Bagdade, J.D., Albers, J.J.: Plasma high-density lipoprotein concentrations in chronic-hemodialysis and renal-transplant patients. N. Engl. J. Med. *296*:1436, 1977.

244. Brunzell, J.D., Albers, J.J., Haas, L.B., et al.: Prevalence of serum lipid abnormalities in chronic hemodialysis. Metabolism *26*:903, 1977.

245. Levine, J., Falk, B., Henriquez, M., et al.: High-density lipoproteins—correlation with cardiovascular disease in hemodialysis patients. Trans. Am. Soc. Artif. Organs *24*:43, 1978.

246. Rapoport, J., Aviram, M., Chaimovitz, C., Brook, J.G.: Defective high-density lipoprotein composition in patients on chronic hemodialysis. A possible mechanism for accelerated atherosclerosis. N. Engl. J. Med. *299*:1326, 1978.

247. Bagdade, J.D., Porte, D., Jr., Bierman, E.L.: Hypertriglyceridemia. A metabolic consequence of chronic renal failure. N. Engl. J. Med. *279*:181, 1968.

248. Gutman, R.A., Shalhoub, R.J., Wade, A.D., et al.: Hypertriglyceridemia in chronic nonnephrotic renal failure. Am. J. Clin. Nutr. *26*:165, 1973.

249. Daubresse, J.C., Lerson, G., Plamteux, G., et al.: Lipids and lipoproteins in chronic uremia. A study of the influence of regular haemodialysis. Europ. J. Clin. Invest. *6*:159, 1976.

250. Ganda, O.P., Aoki, T.T., Soeldner, J.S., et al.: Hormone-fuel concentrations in anephric subjects. Effect of hemodialysis (with special reference to amino acids). J. Clin. Invest. *57*:1403, 1976.

251. Murase, T., Cattran, D.C., Rubenstein, B., Steiner, G.: Inhibition of lipoprotein lipase by uremic plasma, a possible cause of hypertriglyceridemia. Metabolism *24*:1279, 1975.

252. Mordasini, R., Frey, F., Flury, W., et al.: Selective deficiency of hepatic triglyceride lipase in uremic patients. N. Engl. J. Med. *297*:1362, 1977.

253. Ahrens, E.H.: The management of hyperlipidemia: whether, rather than how. Ann. Intern. Med. *85*:87, 1976.

254. Mann, G.V.: Diet-heart: end of an era. N. Engl. J. Med. *297*:644, 1977.

255. Glueck, C.J., Mattson, F., Bierman, E.l.: Diet and coronary heart disease: another view. N. Engl. J. Med. *298*:1471, 1978.

256. Dawber, T.R.: Annual discourse—unproved hypothesis. N. Engl. J. Med. *299*:452, 1978.

257. Nichols, A.B., Ravenscroft, C., Lamphiear, D.E., Ostrander, L.D., Jr.: Independence of serum lipid levels and dietary habits. The Tecumseh study. J.A.M.A. *236*:1948, 1976.

258. Joossens, J.V., Brems-Heyns, E., Claes, J.H., et al.: The pattern of food and mortality in Belgium. Lancet *1*:1069, 1977.

259. Shekelle, R.B., Shryock, A.M., Paul, O., et al.: Diet, serum cholesterol, and death from coronary heart disease. The Western Electric Study. N. Engl. J. Med. *304*:65, 1981.

260. Walker, W.J.: Changing United States life-style and declining vascular mortality: cause or coincidence? (Editorial). N. Engl. J. Med. *297*:163, 1977.

261. Levy, R.I.: Stroke decline: implications and prospects. N. Engl. J. Med. *300*:490, 1979.

262. Mills, G.L., Taylaur, C.E.: The distribution and composition of serum lipoproteins in eighteen animals. Comp. Biochem. Physiol. *40B*:489, 1971.

263. Keys, A., Aravanis, C., Blackburn, H., et al.: Probability of middle-aged men developing coronary heart disease in five years. Circulation *45*:815, 1972.

264. Salel, A.F., Fong, A., Zelis, R., et al.: Accuracy of numerical coronary profile. Correlation of risk factors with arteriographically documented severity of atherosclerosis. N. Engl. J. Med. *296*:1447, 1977.

265. Gordon, T., Castelli, W.P., Hjortland, M.C., et al.: Predicting coronary heart disease in middle-aged and older persons. The Framingham Study. J.A.M.A. *238*:497, 1977.

266. Logan, R.L., Riemersma, R.A., Thomson, M., et al.: Risk factors for ischaemic heart disease in normal men aged 40. Edinburgh-Stockholm study. Lancet *1*:949, 1978.

267. Williams, P., Robinson, D., Bailey, A.: High-density lipoprotein and coronary risk factors in normal men. Lancet *1*:72, 1979.

268. Davis, C.E., Havlik, R.J.: Clinical trials of lipid lowering and coronary artery disease prevention. In: B.M. Rifkind, R.I. Levy (Eds.): Hyperlipidemia—Diagnosis and Therapy. New York, Grune & Stratton, 1977, pp. 79–92.

269. Borhani, N.O.: Primary prevention of coronary heart disease: a critique. Am. J. Cardiol *40*:251, 1977.

270. Dayton, S., Pearce, M.L., Hashimoto, S., et al.: A controlled clinical trial of a diet high in unsaturated fat in preventing complications of atherosclerosis. Circulation *39,40* (Suppl. 2):1, 1969.

271. Miettinen, M., Turpeinen, O., Karvonen, M.J., et al.: Effect of cholesterol-lowering diet on mortality from coronary heart-disease and other causes. A twelve-year clinical trial in men and women. Lancet *2*:835, 1972.

272. Leren, P.: The effect of plasma cholesterol-lowering diet in male survivors of myocardial infarction. Acta Med. Scand. *466* (Suppl.):1, 1966.

273. The Coronary Drug Project Research Group: Clofibrate and niacin in coronary heart disease. J.A.M.A. *231*:360, 1975.

274. Report from the Committee of Principal Investigators: A co-operative trial in the primary prevention of ischaemic heart disease using clofibrate. Brit. Heart J. *40*:1069, 1978.

275. Oliver, M.F.: Cholesterol, coronaries, clofibrate and death. N. Engl. J. Med. 299:1360, 1978.

276. Rose, G., Blackburn, H., Keys, A., et al.: Colon cancer and blood-cholesterol. Lancet 1:181, 1974.

277. Williams, R.R., Sorlie, P.D., Feinlieb, M., et al.: Cancer incidence by levels of cholesterol. J.A.M.A. 245:247, 1981.

278. Lees, R.S.: Clofibrate and atherosclerosis. N. Engl. J. Med. 300:491, 1979.

279. Ganda, O.P.: Cholesterol, coronaries, clofibrate and death. (Letter) N. Engl. J. Med. 300:497, 1979.

279a.Lipid Research Clinics Program: The Lipid Research Clinics coronary primary prevention trial results. I. Reduction in incidence of coronary heart disease. J.A.M.A. 251:351, 1984.

279b.Lipid Research Clinics Program: The Lipid Research Clinics coronary primary prevention trial results. II. The relationship of reduction in incidence of coronary heart disease to cholesterol lowering. J.A.M.A. 251:365, 1984.

280. E. Levy (Ed.): Hyperlipoproteinemia: dietary and pharmacologic intervention. Am. J. Med. 74 (Suppl. 5A):1–36, 1983.

281. Yeshurun, D., Gotto, A.M., Jr.: Drug treatment of hyperlipidemia. Am. J. Med. 60:379, 1976.

282. Connor, W.E., Connor, S.L.: Dietary treatment of hyperlipidemia. In: B.M. Rifkind, R.I. Levy (Eds.): Hyperlipidemia, Diagnosis and Therapy. New York, Grune & Stratton, 1977, pp. 281–326.

283. Hunninghake, D.B., Probstfield, J.L.: Drug treatment of hyperlipoproteinemia. In: Ibid. pp. 327–362.

284. D. Kritchevsky, R. Paoletti, W.L. Holmes (Eds.): Drugs, lipid metabolism, and atherosclerosis. Adv. Exp. Med. Biol. 109:1, 1978.

285. Sirtori, C.R., Agradi, E., Conti, F., et al.: Soybean-protein diet in the treatment of Type II hyperlipoproteinemia. Lancet 1:275, 1977.

286. Deckelbaum, R.J., Lees, R.S., Small, D.M., et al.: Failure of complete bile diversion and oral bile acid therapy in the treatment of homozygous familial hypercholesterolemia. N. Engl. J. Med. 296:465, 1977.

287. Soutar, A.: Does dietary fat influence plasma lipoprotein structure? Nature 273:11, 1978.

288. Mahley, R.W., Nelson, A.W., Ferrans, V.J., Fry, D.L.: Thrombosis in association with atherosclerosis induced by dietary perturbations in dogs. Science 192:1139, 1976.

289. Pinckney, E.R.: The potential toxicity of excessive polyunsaturates. Do not let the patient harm himself. Am. Heart J. 85:723, 1973.

290. Yudkin, J., Morland, J.: Sugar intake and myocardial infarction. Am. J. Clin. Nutr. 20:503, 1967.

291. Ahrens, R.A.: Sucrose, hypertension, and heart disease: an historical perspective. Am. J. Clin. Nutr. 27:403, 1974.

292. Trowell, H.C.: Dietary fiber hypothesis of the etiology of diabetes mellitus. Diabetes 24:762, 1975.

293. Mendeloff, A.I.: Dietary fiber and human health. N. Engl. J. Med. 297:811, 1977.

294. Neri, L.C., Johansen, H.L.: Water hardness and cardiovascular mortality. Ann. N.Y. Acad. Sci. 304:203, 1978.

295. Shute, W.D., Taub, H.J.: Vitamin E for Ailing and Healthy Hearts. New York, Pyramid Books, 1972.

296. Hodges, R.E.: Vitamin E and coronary heart disease. J. Am. Diet. Assoc. 63:638, 1973.

297. Keys, A.: Coronary heart disease—the global picture. Atherosclerosis 22:149, 1975.

298. Nuttall, F.Q., Gannon, M.C.: Sucrose and disease. Diabetes Care 4:305, 1981.

299. Jenkins, D.J.A.: Dietary fibre, diabetes, and hyperlipidaemia. Lancet 2:1287, 1979.

300. Simpson, H.C.R., Simpson, R.W., Lousley, S., et al.: A high carbohydrate leguminous fibre diet improves all aspects of diabetic control. Lancet 1:1, 1981.

301. Cerna, O., Ginter, E.: Blood lipids and Vitamin C status. (Letter). Lancet 1:1055, 1978.

301a.Brensike, J.F., Levy, R.I., Kelsey, S.F., et al.: Effect of therapy with cholestyramine on progression of coronary arteriosclerosis: results of the NHLBI Type II coronary intervention study. Circulation 69:313, 1984.

302. Murphy, B.F.: Probucol (Lorelco) in treatment of hyperlipidemia. J.A.M.A. 238:2537, 1977.

303. Kuo, P.T., Hayase, K., Kostis, J.B., Moreyra, A.E.: Use of combined diet and colestipol in long term (7–7½ years) treatment of patients with Type II hyperlipoproteinemia. Circulation 59:199, 1979.

304. Kane, J.P., Malloy, M.J., Tun, P., et al.: Normalization of low-density-lipoprotein levels in heterozygous familial hypercholesterolemia with a combined drug regimen. N. Engl. J. Med. 304:251, 1981.

305. Illingworth, D.R., Phillipson, B.E., Rapp, J.H., Connor, W.E.: Colestipol plus nictoinic acid in treatment of heterozygous familial hypercholesterolemia. Lancet 1:296, 1981.

306. Miller, N.E., Nestel, P.J.: Triglyceride-lowering effect of chenodeoxycholic acid in patients with endogenous hypertriglyceridemia. Lancet 2:929, 1974.

307. Maebashi, M., Kawamura, N., Sati, M., et al.: Lipid-lowering effect of carnitine in patients with Type IV hyperlipoproteinemia. Lancet 2:805, 1978.

308. Betteridge, D.J., Krone, W., Reckless, J.P.D., Galton, D.J.: Compactin inhibits cholesterol synthesis in lymphocytes and intestinal mucosa from patients with familial hypercholesterolemia. Lancet 2:1342, 1978.

309. Mabuchi, H., Haba, T., Tatami, R., et al.: Effects of an inhibitor of 3-hydroxy-3-methylglutaryl coenzyme A reductase on serum lipoproteins and ubiquinone-10 levels in patients with familial hypercholesterolemia. N. Engl. J. Med. 305:478, 1981.

309a.Mabuchi, H., Sakai, T., Sakai, Y., et al.: Reduction of serum cholesterol in heterozygous patients with familial hypercholesterolemia. Additive effects of compactin and cholestyramine. N. Engl. J. Med. 308:609, 1983.

310. Hollander, W.: Role of hypertension in atherosclerosis and cardiovascular disease. Am. J. Cardiol. 38:786, 1976.

311. Bryfogle, J.W., Bradley, R.F.: The vascular complications of diabetes mellitus. A clinical study. Diabetes 6:159, 1957.

312. Pell, S., d'Alonzo, C.A.: Some aspects of hypertension in diabetes mellitus. J.A.M.A. 202:104, 1967.

313. Freedman, P., Moulton, R., Spencer, A.G.: Hypertension and diabetes mellitus. Quart. J. Med. 27:293, 1958.

314. Pyke, D.A.: Arterial disease and diabetes. In: W.G. Oakley, D.A. Pyke, K.W. Taylor (Eds.): Clinical Diabetes and its Biochemical Basis. Oxford, Blackwell, 1968, pp. 506–541.

315. Goodkin, G.: Mortality factors in diabetes. A 20-year mortality study. J. Occup. Med. 17:716, 1975.

316. Christlieb, A.R., Warram, J.H., Krolewski, A.S., et al.: Hypertension: the major risk factor in juvenile-onset insulin-dependent diabetics. Diabetes 30 (Suppl. 2):90, 1981.

317. Bain, C., Hennekens, C.H., Rosner, B., et al.: Cigarette consumption and deaths from coronary heart disease. Lancet 1:1087, 1978.

318. Friedman, G.D., Dales, L.G., Ury, H.K.: Mortality in middle aged smokers and non-smokers. N. Engl. J. Med. 300:213, 1979.

319. Gordon, T., Kannel, W.B., McGee, D., Dawber, T.R.: Death and coronary attacks in men after giving up cigarette

smoking. A report from the Framingham Study. Lancet 2:1345, 1974.

320. Topping, D.L., Dwyer, T., Weller, R.A.: Peripheral vascular disease in cigarette smokers and impaired hepatic metabolism of lipoprotein remnants. Lancet 2:1327, 1977.

321. Sarma, J.S.M., Tillmanns, H., Ikeda, S., Bing, R.J.: The effect of carbon monoxide on lipid metabolism of human coronary arteries. Atherosclerosis 22:193, 1975.

322. Topping, D.L.: Metabolic effects of carbon monoxide in relation to atherogenesis. Atherosclerosis 26:129, 1977.

323. Bierman, E.L., Albers, J.J.: Lipoprotein uptake and degradation by human arterial smooth muscle cells in tissue culture. Ann. N.Y. Acad. Sci. 275:199, 1976.

324. Ditzel, J., Standl, E.: The problem of tissue oxygenation in diabetes mellitus. Acta Med. Scand. (Suppl.)578:59, 1975.

325. Ditzel, J.: Oxygen transport impairment in diabetes. Diabetes 25 (Suppl. 2):832, 1976.

326. Ditzel, J., Dyerberg, J.: Hyperlipoproteinemia, diabetes, and oxygen affinity of hemoglobin. Metabolism 26:141, 1977.

327. Bunn, H.F., Gabbay, K.H., Gallop, P.M.: The glycosylation of hemoglobin; relevance to diabetes mellitus. Science 200:21, 1978.

328. Gonen, B., Rubenstein, A.H.: Haemoglobin Al and diabetes mellitus. Diabetologia 15:1, 1978.

328a. Eichner, E.R.: Exercise and heart disease. Epidemiology of the "exercise hypothesis." Am. J. Med. 75:1008, 1983.

329. Morris, J.N., Chave, S.P.W., Adam, C., et al.: Vigorous exercise in leisure-time and the incidence of coronary heart disease. Lancet 1:333, 1973.

330. Paffenbarger, R.S., Hale, W.E.: Work activity and coronary heart mortality. N. Engl. J. Med. 292:545, 1975.

331. Brunner, D., Manelis, G., Modan, M., Levin, S.: Physical activity at work and the incidence of myocardial infarction, angina pectoris and death due to ischemic heart disease: an epidemiological study in Israeli collective settlements (Kibbutzim). J. Chr. Dis. 27:217, 1974.

332. Cooper, K.H., Pollock, M.L., Martin, R.P., et al.: Physical fitness levels vs selected coronary risk factors. A cross-sectional study. J.A.M.A. 236:166, 1976.

333. Nikkilä, E.A., Taskinen, M-R., Rehunen, S., Härkönen, M.: Lipoprotein lipase activity in adipose tissue and skeletal muscle of runners: relation to serum lipoproteins. Metabolism 27:166, 1978.

334. Ruderman, N.B., Ganda, O.P., Johansen, K.: The effect of physical training on glucose tolerance and plasma lipids in maturity-onset diabetes. Diabetes 28 (Suppl. 1):89, 1979.

335. Saltin, B., Lindgärde, F., Houston, M., et al.: Physical training and glucose tolerance in middle-aged men with chemical diabetes. Diabetes 28 (Suppl. 1):30, 1979.

336. Björntorp, P., Sjostrom, L.: Carbohydrate storage in man: speculations and some quantitative considerations. Metabolism 27:1853, 1978.

337. Tikkanen, M.J., Nikkilä, E.A., Vartiainen, E.: Natural estrogen as an effective treatment for Type II hyperlipoproteinemia in postmenopausal women. Lancet 2:490, 1978.

338. Mann, J.I., Inman, W.H.W., Thorogood, M.: Oral contraceptive use in older women and fatal myocardial infarction. Brit. Med. J. 2:445, 1976.

339. Wallace, R.B., Hoover, J., Sandler, D., et al.: Altered plasma-lipids associated with oral contraceptive or oestrogen consumption. The Lipid Research Clinic Program. Lancet 2:11, 1977.

340. Phillips, G.B.: Relationship between serum sex hormones and glucose, insulin, and lipid abnormalities in men with myocardial infarction. Proc. Natl. Acad. Sci. USA 74:1729, 1974.

341. Phillips, G.B.: Sex hormones, risk factors and cardiovascular disease. Amer. J. Med. 65:7, 1978.

342. Entrican, J.H., Beach, C., Carroll, D., et al.: Raised plasma oestradiol and oestrone levels in young survivors of myocardial infarction. Lancet 2:487, 1978.

342a. Phillips, G.B., Castelli, W.P., Abbott, R.D., McNamara, P.M.: Association of hyperestrogenemia and coronary heart disease in men in the Framingham cohort. Am. J. Med. 74:863, 1983.

343. Waldron, I.: Why do women live longer than men? J. Hum. Stress 2:2, 1976.

344. Oestrogens and atheroma. Lancet 2:508, 1978.

345. Gordon, T., Kannel, W.B.: The effects of overweight on cardiovascular diseases. Geriatrics 28:80, 1973.

346. Tansey, M.J.B., Opie, L.H., Kennelly, B.M.: High mortality in obese women diabetics with acute myocardial infarction. Br. Med. J. 1:1624, 1977.

347. Cramer, K., Paulin, S., Werkö, L.: Coronary angiographic findings in correlation with age, body weight, blood pressure, serum lipids and smoking habits. Circulation 33:888, 1966.

348. Pell, S., d'Alonzo, C.A.: Acute myocardial infarction in a large industrial population—report of a 6-year study of 1356 cases. J.A.M.A. 105:831, 1963.

349. Reisin, E., Abel, R., Modan, M., et al.: Effect of weight loss without salt restriction on the reduction of blood pressure in overweight hypertensive patients. N. Engl. J. Med. 298:1, 1978.

350. Tobian, L.: Hypertension and obesity. N. Engl. J. Med. 298:46, 1978.

351. Jenkins, C.D., Zyzanski, S.J., Rosenman, R.H.: Risk of new myocardial infarctions in middle-aged men with manifest coronary heart disease. Circulation 53:342, 1976.

352. Glass, D.C.: Stress, behavior patterns, and coronary disease. Am. Sci. 65:177, 1977.

353. Rosenman, R.H.: Role of Type A behavior pattern in the pathogenesis of ischemic heart disease, and modification for prevention. Adv. Cardiol. 25:35, 1978.

354. Gutstein, W.H., Harrison, J., Parl, F., et al.: Neural factors contribute to atherogenesis. Science 199:449, 1978.

355. Corday, E., Corday, S.R.: Editorial. Prevention of heart disease by control of risk factors: the time has come to face the facts. Am. J. Cardiol. 35:330, 1975.

356. Werkö, L.: Risk factors and coronary heart disease—facts or fancy? Am. Heart J. 91:87, 1976.

357. Friedman, M., Byers, S.O., Diamant, J., Rosenman, R.: Plasma catecholamine response of coronary-prone subjects (Type A) to a specific challenge. Metabolism 24:205, 1975.

358. Christensen, N.J., Videbaek, J.: Plasma catecholamines and carbohydrate metabolism in patients with acute myocardial infarction. J. Clin. Invest. 54:278, 1974.

359. Opie, L.H., Tansey, M., Kennelly, B.M.: Proposed metabolic vicious circle in patients with large myocardial infarcts and high plasma-free-fatty-acid concentrations. Lancet 2:890, 1977.

360. Murawski, B.J., Chazan, B.I., Balodimos, M.C., Ryan, J.R.: Personality patterns in patients with diabetes mellitus of long duration. Diabetes 19:259, 1970.

361. Hauser, S.T., Pollets, D.: Psychological aspects of diabetes mellitus: a critical review. Diabetes Care 2:227, 1979.

361a. Jacobson, A.M., Hauser, S.T.: Behavioral and psychological aspects of diabetes. In: M. Ellenberg, H. Rifkin (Eds.): Diabetes Mellitus. Theory and Practice, 3rd Ed. New York, Medical Examination Publishing Co., Inc., 1983, pp. 1037–1052.

362. Rapacz, J.: Lipoprotein immunogenetics and atherosclerosis. Am. J. Med. Genet. *1*:377, 1978.

362a.Mandrup-Poulsen, T., Owerbach, D., Mortensen, S.A., et al.: DNA sequences flanking the insulin gene on chromosome 11 confer risk of atherosclerosis. Lancet *1*:250, 1984.

363. Task force on genetic factors in atherosclerotic disease. Report from the National Heart and Lung Institute DHEW Publ. (NIH) 76–922, 1975.

364. Biss, K., Ho, K-J., Mikkelson, B., et al.: Some unique biologic characteristics of the Masai of East Africa. N. Engl. J. Med. *284*:694, 1971.

365. Jackson, W.P.U.: Epidemiology of diabetes in South Africa. Adv. Metab. Dis. *9*:111, 1978.

366. West, K.M.: Diabetes in American Indians. Adv. Metab. Dis. *9*:29, 1978.

367. Goto, Y.: Vascular complications in diabetes in Japan. Adv. Metab. Dis. *9*:167, 1978.

368. Kawate, R., Miyanishi, M., Yamakido, M., Nishimoto, Y.: Preliminary studies of the prevalence and mortality of diabetes mellitus in Japanese of Japan and on the Island of Hawaii. Adv. Metab. Dis. *9*:201, 1978.

369. Cahill, G.F., Jr.: "Health" Steak. New Engl. J. Med. *288*:415, 1973.

370. Fearnley, G.R., Chakrabarti, R., Avis, P.R.D.: Blood fibrinolytic activity in diabetes mellitus and its bearing on ischaemic heart disease and obesity. Brit. Med. J. *1*:921, 1963.

371. Farid, N.R., Anderson, J., Martin, A., Weightman, D.: Letter: Fibrinolytic activity and treatment of diabetes. Lancet *1*:631, 1974.

372. Jones, R.L., Peterson, C.M.: The fluid phase of coagulation and the accelerated atherosclerosis of diabetes mellitus. Diabetes *30* (Suppl. 2):33, 1981.

373. Tanser, A.R.: Fibrinolytic response of diabetics and non-diabetics to adrenaline. J. Clin. Pathol. *20*:231, 1967.

374. Cash, J.D., McGill, R.C.: Fibrinolytic response to moderate exercise in young male diabetics and non-diabetics. J. Clin. Pathol. *22*:32, 1969.

375. Wardle, E.N., Piercy, D.A., Anderson, J.: Some chemical indices of diabetic vascular disease. Postgrad. Med. J. *49*:1, 1973.

376. Coller, B.S., Frank, R.N., Milton, R.C., Gralnick, R.: Plasma cofactors of platelet function: correlation with diabetic retinopathy and hemoglobin A_{1c}. Studies in diabetic patients and normal persons. Ann. Intern. Med. *88*:33, 1978.

376a.Brownlee, M., Vlassara, H., Cerami, A.: Nonenzymatic glycosylation reduces the susceptibility of fibrin to degradation by plasmin. Diabetes *32*:680, 1983.

376b.Juhan, I., Vague, Ph., Buonocore, M.: Abnormalities of erythrocyte deformability and platelet aggregation in insulin-dependent diabetics corrected by insulin in vivo and in vitro. Lancet *1*:535, 1982.

376c.McMillan, D.E.: The effect of diabetes on blood flow properties. Diabetes *32*(Suppl.2):56, 1983.

377. Mustard, J.F., Packham, M.D.: Platelets and diabetes mellitus. (Editorial). N. Engl. J. Med. *297*:1345, 1977.

378. Bern, M.B.: Platelet functions in diabetes mellitus. Diabetes *27*:342, 1978.

379. Mustard, J.F., Packham, M.A., Kinlough-Rathbone, R.l.: Platelets and thrombosis in the development of atherosclerosis and its complications. Adv. Exp. Med. Biol. *102*:7, 1978.

380. Peterson, C.M., Jones, R.L., Koenig, R.J., et al.: Reversible hematologic sequelae of diabetes mellitus. Ann. Intern. Med. *86*:425, 1977.

381. Colwell, J.A., Halushka, P.V., Sarji, K.E., Sagel, J.: Platelet function and diabetes mellitus. Med. Clin. N. Am. *62*:753, 1978.

382. Bensoussan, D., Levy-Toldano, S., Passa, P., et al.: Platelet hyperaggregation and increased plasma level of von Willebrand factor in diabetics with retinopathy. Diabetologia *11*:307, 1975.

383. Colwell, J.A., Halushka, P.V., Sarji, K., et al.: Altered platelet function in diabetes mellitus. Diabetes 25 (Suppl. 2):826, 1976.

384. Lufkin, E.G., Fass, D.N., O'Fallon, W.M., Bowie, E.J.W.: Increased von Willebrand factor in diabetes mellitus. Metabolism *28*:63, 1979.

385. Fuster, V., Bowie, E.J.W., Lewis, J.C.: Resistance to arteriosclerosis in pigs with von Willebrand's disease. Spontaneous and high cholesterol diet-induced arteriosclerosis. J. Clin. Invest. *61*:722, 1978.

386. Gralnick, H.R., Coller, B.S., Sultan, Y.: Carbohydrate deficiency of the factor VIII/von Willebrand factor protein in von Willebrand's disease variants. Science *192*:56, 1976.

387. Colwell, J.A., Winocour, P.D., Halushka, P.V.: Do platelets have anything to do with diabetic microvascular disease? Diabetes *32*(Suppl. 2):14, 1983.

388. Davis, J.W., Phillips, P.E., Yue, K.T.N., et al.: Platelet aggregation. Adult-onset diabetes mellitus and coronary artery disease. J.A.M.A. *239*:732, 1978.

389. Carvalho, A.C.A., Colman, R.W., Lees, R.S.: Clofibrate reversal of platelet hypersensitivity in hyperbetalipoproteinemia. Circulation *50*:570, 1974.

389a.Pitt, B., Shea, M.J., Romson, J.L., Lucchesi, B.R.: Prostaglandins and prostaglandin inhibitors in ischemic heart disease. Ann. Intern. Med. *99*:83, 1983.

390. Moncada, S., Vane, J.R.: Arachidonic acid metabolites and the interactions between platelets and blood-vessel walls. N. Engl. J. Med. *300*:1142, 1979.

391. Pick, R., Chediak, J., Glick, G.: Aspirin inhibits development of coronary atherosclerosis in cynomolgus monkeys (Macaca Fascicularis) fed an atherogenic diet. J. Clin. Invest. *63*:158, 1979.

392. The Anturane Reinfarction Trial Research Group: Sulfinpyrazone in the prevention of cardiac death after myocardial infarction. The Anturane Reinfarction Trial. N. Engl. J. Med. *298*:289, 1978.

393. Needleman, P., Wyche, A., Raz, A.: Platelet and blood vessel arachidonate metabolism and interactions. J. Clin. Invest. *63*:345, 1979.

393a.Majerus, P.W.: Arachidonate metabolism in vascular disorders. J. Clin. Invest. *72*:1521, 1983.

394. Needleman, P., Raz, A., Minkes, M.S., et al.: Triene prostaglandins: prostacyclin and thromboxane biosynthesis and unique biological properties. Proc. Nat. Acad. Sci. *76*:944, 1979.

395. Harrison, H.E., Reece, A.H., Johnson, M.: Effect of insulin treatment on prostacyclin in experimental diabetes. Diabetologia *18*:65, 1980.

396. Rogers, S.P., Larkins, R.G.: Production of 6-oxo-prostaglandin F1α by rat aorta. Influence of diabetes, insulin treatment, and caloric deprivation. Diabetes *30*:935, 1981.

397. Davis, T.M.E., Mitchell, M.D., Turner, R.C.: Prostacyclin and thromboxane metabolites in diabetes. Lancet *2*:789, 1979.

398. Halushka, P.V., Lurie, D., Colwell, J.A.: Increased synthesis of prostaglandin-E-like material by platelets from patients with diabetes mellitus. N. Engl. J. Med. *297*:1306, 1977.

399. Halushka, P.V., Mayfield, R., Wohltmann, H.J., et al.: Increased platelet arachidonic acid metabolism in diabetes mellitus. Diabetes *30* (Suppl. 2):44, 1981.

400. Berkenstein, M.H., Muntean, W.E.: Elevated factor VIII activity and factor VIII-related antigen in diabetic children without vascular disease. Diabetes *31*:1006, 1982.

401. Waitzman, M.B.: Proposed metabolic dysfunctions in diabetic microthromboses and microangiopathy. Metabolism *28* (Suppl.1):401, 1979.

402. Huttner, J.J., Gwebu, E.T., Panganamala, R.V., et al.: Fatty acids and their prostaglandin derivatives: inhibitors of proliferation in aortic smooth muscle cells. Science *197*:289, 1977.

403. Kingsbury, K.J.: The relation between glucose tolerance and atherosclerotic vascular disease. Lancet *2*:1374, 1966.

404. Welborn, T.A., Wearne, K.: Coronary heart disease incidence and cardiovascular mortality in Busselton with reference to glucose and insulin concentrations. Diabetes Care *2*:154, 1979.

405. Keen, H., Jarrett, R.J., Fuller, J.H., McCartney, P.: Hyperglycemia and arterial disease. Diabetes *30* (Suppl. 2):49, 1981.

406. Gabbay, K.H.: The sorbitol pathway and the complications of diabetes. N. Engl. J. Med. *288*:831, 1973.

407. Morrison, A.D., Clements, R.S., Jr., Winegrad, A.I.: Effects of elevated glucose concentrations on the metabolism of the aortic wall. J. Clin. Invest. *51*:3114, 1972.

408. Kanter, Y., Bessman, S.P., Bessman, A.N.: Red cell 2,3-diphosphoglycerate levels among diabetic patients with and without vascular complications. Diabetes *24*:724, 1975.

409. Ditzel, J., Nielsen, N.V., Kjaergaard, J-J.: Hemoglobin A_{1c} and red cell oxygen release capacity in relation to early retinal changes in newly discovered overt and chemical diabetics. Metabolism *28* (Suppl. 1):440, 1979.

410. Turner, J.L., Bierman, E.L.: Effects of glucose and sorbitol on proliferation of cultured human skin fibroblasts and arterial smooth-muscle cells. Diabetes *27*:583, 1978.

410a. Stout, R.W.: Glucose inhibits replication of cultured human endothelial cells. Diabetologia *23*:436, 1982.

411. Winternitz, M.C., Thomas, R.M., LeCompte, P.M.: The Biology of Arteriosclerosis. Springfield, Charles C Thomas, 1938.

412. Blumenthal, H.T., Alex, M., Goldenberg, S.: A study of lesions of the intramural coronary artery branches in diabetes mellitus. Arch. Path. *70*:13, 1960.

413. Goodale, F., Daoud, A.S., Florentin, R., et al.: Chemicoanatomic studies of arteriosclerosis and thrombosis in diabetics. I. Coronary arterial wall thickness, thrombosis, and myocardial infarcts in autopsied North Americans. Exp. Molec. Path. *1*:353, 1962.

414. Kannel, W.B., Hjortland, M., Castelli, W.P.: Role of diabetes in congestive heart failure: the Framingham Study. Am. J. Cardiol. *34*:29, 1974.

415. Hamby, R.I., Zoneraich, S., Sherman, L.: Diabetic cardiomyopathy. J.A.M.A. *229*:1749, 1974.

416. Regan, T.J., Lyons, M.M., Ahmed, S.S., et al.: Evidence for cardiomyopathy in familial diabetes mellitus. J. Clin. Invest. *60*:884, 1977.

417. Sanderson, J.E., Brown, D.J., Rivellese, A., Kohner, E.: Diabetic cardiomyopathy? An echocardiographic study of young diabetics. Br. Med. J. *1*:404, 1978.

418. Rubler, S.: Cardiac manifestations of diabetes mellitus. Cardiovasc. Med. *2*:823, 1977.

419. Regan, T.J., Weisse, A.B.: The question of cardiomyopathy in diabetes mellitus. Ann. Intern. Med. *89*:1000, 1978.

420. Ledet, T., Neubauer, B., Christensen, N.J., Lundbaek, K.: Diabetic cardiopathy. Diabetologia *16*:207, 1979.

421. Siperstein, M.D., Foster, D.W., Knowles, H.C., Jr., et al.: Control of blood glucose and diabetic vascular disease. (Editorial). N. Engl. J. Med. *296*:1060, 1977.

422. Spiro, R.G.: Search for a biochemical basis of diabetic microangiopathy. Diabetologia *12*:1, 1976.

423. Tchobroutsky, G.: Relation of diabetic control to development of microvascular complications. Diabetologia *15*:143, 1978.

424. Stout, R.W.: The relationship of abnormal circulating insulin levels to atherosclerosis. Atherosclerosis *27*:1, 1977.

425. Stout, R.W.: Diabetes and atherosclerosis—the role of insulin. Diabetologia *16*:141, 1979.

426. Grant, N.: Insulin and atherosclerosis. N. Engl. J. Med. *300*:679, 1979.

426a. King, G.L., Buzney, S.M., Kahn, C.R., et al.: Differential responsiveness to insulin of endothelial and support cells from micro- and macrovessels. J. Clin. Invest. *71*:974, 1983.

427. Brosnan, M.E., Sirek, O.V., Sirek, A., Przybylska, K.: Effect of pancreatectomy, with and without hypophysectomy, and of insulin treatment on the composition of canine aorta. Diabetes *22*:397, 1973.

428. Fraser, R., Lowy, C., Elkeles, R.S., et al.: Insulin, glucose and lipid levels in mild diabetics in relation to complications. In: R.A. Camerini-Davalos, H.S. Cole (Eds.): Vascular and Neurological Changes in Early Diabetes. New York, Academic Press, 1973, pp. 83–93.

429. Pyörälä, K.: Relationship of glucose tolerance and plasma insulin to the incidence of coronary heart disease. Results from two population studies in Finland. Diabetes Care *2*:131, 1979.

430. Merimee, T.J.: A follow-up study of vascular disease in growth-hormone-deficient dwarfs with diabetes. N. Engl. J. Med. *298*:1217, 1978.

431. Hansen, A.P.: Normalization of growth hormone hyperresponse to exercise in juvenile diabetics after "normalization" of blood sugar. J. Clin. Invest. *50*:1806, 1971.

432. Hansen, A.P.: Abnormal serum growth-hormone response to exercise in maturity-onset diabetics. Diabetes *22*:619, 1973.

433. Vigneri, R., Squatrito, S., Pezzino, V., et al.: Growth hormone levels in diabetes. Correlation with the clinical control of the disease. Diabetes *25*:167, 1976.

434. Ledet, T.: Growth hormone antiserum suppresses the growth effect of diabetic serum. Studies on rabbit aortic medial cell cultures. Diabetes *26*:798, 1977.

435. Ledet, T.: Diabetic macroangiopathy and growth hormone. Diabetes *30* (Suppl. 2):14, 1981.

436. Yde, H.: The growth hormone dependent sulfation factor in serum from patients with various types of diabetes. Acta Med. Scand. *186*:293, 1969.

437. Tamborlane, W.V., Hintz, R.L., Bergman, M., et al.: Insulin-infusion-pump treatment of diabetes. Influence of improved metabolic control on plasma somatomedin levels. N. Engl. J. Med. *305*:303, 1981.

438. Gospodarowicz, D., Valodavsky, I., Greenburg, G., et al.: Studies on atherogenesis and corneal transplantation using cultured vascular and corneal endothelia. Rec. Prog. Horm. Res. *35*:375, 1979.

439. Ross, R.: Platelet cell proliferation and atherosclerosis. Metabolism *28* (Suppl. 1):410, 1979.

440. Christensen, N.J.: Catecholamines and diabetes mellitus. Diabetologia *16*:211, 1979.

441. Christensen, N.J.: Plasma norepinephrine and epinephrine in untreated diabetics, during fasting and after insulin administration. Diabetes *23*:1, 1974.

442. Landsberg, L., Young, J.B.: Fasting, feeding and regulation of the sympathetic nervous system. N. Engl. J. Med. *298*:1295, 1978.

443. Rowe, J.W., Young, J.B., Minaker, K.L., et al.: Effect of insulin and glucose infusions on sympathetic nervous system activity in normal man. Diabetes *30*:219, 1981.

444. Klevay, L.M.: Coronary heart disease: the zinc/copper hypothesis. Am. J. Clin. Nutr. *28*:764, 1975.

445. Klevay, L.M., Allen, K.G.D.: Vitamin B_6, copper, and atherosclerosis. (Letter). Lancet *1*:1209, 1977.

446. Mertz, W.: Trace minerals and atherosclerosis. Fed. Proc. *41*:2807, 1982.

447. Levene, C.I., Murray, J.C.: The aetiological role of maternal Vitamin B_6 deficiency in the development of atherosclerosis. Lancet *1*:628, 1977.

448. Burch, G.E.: Editorial: Viruses and arteriosclerosis. Am. Heart J. *87*:407, 1974.

449. Fabricant, C.G., Fabricant, J., Litrenta, M.M., Minick, C.R.: Virus-induced atherosclerosis. J. Exp. Med. *148*:335, 1978.

450. Fabricant, C.G.: Herpesvirus-induced atherosclerosis. Diabetes *30* (Suppl. 2):29, 1981.

451. Anon: Thyroiditis, autoimmunity, and coronary risk factors. Lancet *2*:173, 1977.

452. Davies, D.F.: Immunological aspects of atherosclerosis. Proc. Nutr. Soc. *35*:293, 1976.

453. Rowe, J.W.: Clinical research on aging. Strategies and directions. N. Engl. J. Med. *297*:1332, 1977.

454. Blumenthal, H.T.: Aging: biologic or pathologic? Hosp. Practice *13*:127, 1977.

455. Andres, R.: Aging and diabetes. Med. Clin. N. Am. *55*:835, 1971.

456. Harman, D.: The aging process. Proc. Nat. Acad. Sci. *78*:7124, 1981.

457. Crawford, D.W., Blankenhorn, D.H.: Regression of atherosclerosis. Ann. Rev. Med. *30*:289, 1979.

458. Duffield, R.G.M., Lewis, B., Miller, N.E., et al.: Treatment of hyperlipidaemia retards progression of symptomatic femoral atherosclerosis. A randomized controlled trial. Lancet *2*:639, 1983.

459. Holley, R.W.: Control of growth of mammalian cells in cell culture. Nature *258*:487, 1975.

460. Ruderman, N.B., Haudenschild, C.: Diabetes as an atherogenic factor. Prog. Cardiovasc. Dis. *26*:373, 1984.

461. Biesbroeck, R.C., Albers, J.J., Wahl, P.W., et al.: Abnormal composition of high density lipoproteins in non-insulin-dependent diabetics. Diabetes *31*:126, 1982.

462. Greenfield, M.S., Doberne, L., Rosenthal, M., et al.: Lipid metabolism in non-insulin-dependent diabetes mellitus. Effect of glipizide therapy. Arch. Intern. Med. *142*:1498, 1982.

12 Onset, Course, Complications, and Prognosis of Diabetes Mellitus

Andrzej S. Królewski, James H. Warram, and
A. Richard Christlieb

Diabetes is a truly chronic disease, one in which the course evolves over many years or even decades. The complications and associated morbidity are varied in nature, some unique to diabetes but others similar or identical to forms of morbidity occurring in non-diabetic individuals. This poses special methodologic problems in the study of the determinants of these various outcomes as well as the overall prognosis. As pointed out by Mac-Mahon and Pugh[1] in their description of the aims of epidemiology, methods recently developed to study the determinants of the incidence of disease are equally suited to the study of the clinical course of established disease.

> While most epidemiologic work is directed towards elucidating causal factors [of the incidence of disease], the same methods are used in studies that seek to identify factors related to the course of a disease once established. Thus it is useful to know how the duration of a disease and the probability of the various possible outcomes (recovery, death, specific complications, etc.) vary by age, sex, geography, and so on. Such information is useful not only for prognostic purposes but also in stimulating hypotheses as to what specific factors may be more directly involved in determining the course of a disease in an individual.

To describe the natural history of diabetes, the indices of frequency described in Chapter 2 are used. The best measures are incidence rates of specific outcomes, such as diabetic ketoacidosis (DKA) or the first evidence of coronary artery disease (CAD). However, for late complications, prevalence rates are often the only measure available in the literature.

There are several types of epidemiologic strategies for studying the natural history of diabetes. The easiest and most frequently used approach is a cross-sectional survey. The prevalences of specific complications are ascertained among patients with diabetes at a particular point in time, and the findings are analyzed according to such characteristics as sex, age at examination, duration of diabetes, type of treatment, etc. As discussed in Chapter 2, prevalence rates are an ambiguous measure of the frequency of a condition's occurrence since a low prevalence rate might equally well result from unsuccessful management of the condition (affected patients being removed from the population by death) as from a low incidence rate.

A more informative approach is a cohort study which permits the calculation of incidence and cumulative incidence rates. The main feature of such a study is the follow-up of a group of patients from some logical starting point, the onset of diabetes for example, through some chosen interval of time. The study may be conducted prospectively or retrospectively, and the required duration of follow-up depends upon the end-points which are under consideration. A modification of this approach, a prospective cohort study with random assignment of therapeutic regimens, is the familiar clinical trial which permits the assessment of particular methods of intervention on the course of diabetes.

A third approach is a case-control study. Its main feature is the identification of a group of diabetics with a particular complication (cases) and another group (controls) which can be considered a representative sample of the larger population of diabetics which supplied the cases. The histories of the two groups, obtained by medical record review, questionnaire, interview, or examination, are compared to determine factors which are different for the two groups. For a concise, but more detailed, description of these epidemiologic methods, see textbook of MacMahon and Pugh.[1]

In evaluating any investigation of the clinical course of diabetes or in trying to reconcile studies with different findings, careful consideration should be given to two sources of error: the process of selecting patients for study and the techniques of measuring the condition of interest.

The selection process is the sequence of steps involved in bringing the study subjects to the attention of the investigators. For example in a clinic or hospital, the patients most readily available may be those with diabetes which is difficult to manage and requires frequent medical attention. Another example of selection is represented by studies of patients with diabetes of long duration. They have been selected by virtue of surviving the mortality which removed from observation some of their less fortunate counterparts. Volunteers, on the other hand, may select themselves for participation (or non-participation) because of conscious or unconscious awareness of some morbid condition. The common feature of all of these examples is that patients with the clinical condition under investigation and patients without it do not have an equal chance to be studied. These selection processes can have enormous influence on the rates obtained, whether they are incidence, prevalence or mortality rates. Recall that each type of rate is obtained by dividing the number of afflicted individuals by the number of individuals at risk of the affliction. The selection process can give an erroneous count of either number.

The second major source of error is the measurement technique used to ascertain the presence of an end-point. Thus the accuracy and reproducibility of the method applied must have been determined and described in detail. Errors of measurement technique affect only the number of afflicted individuals which are identified rather than the number at risk.

The following section will consider the natural history of diabetes separately for insulin-dependent (IDDM) and noninsulin-dependent diabetes (NIDDM). In reviewing the literature on natural history, some choices have been made. In general, data of the Joslin Diabetes Center which have already been published as well as special analyses for this chapter have been selected preferentially.

NATURAL HISTORY OF INSULIN-DEPENDENT DIABETES (IDDM)

Clinical Manifestation

There is a consensus that the underlying morphologic process responsible for the development of IDDM is a selective destruction of the beta cells of the pancreas (see Chapter 14). Unfortunately, there is no direct method of observing the process or measuring the amount of destruction. Clinical manifestation occurs only after the loss of beta cells is substantial and insulin secretion is inadequate for the body's needs. Situations involving stress such as puberty, trauma or infections temporarily increase the demand for insulin, probably through increased resistance to its effects,[2-4] and may precipitate the clinical onset of IDDM at an earlier point in time. So far there have been no population-based studies describing the circumstances surrounding the clinical onset of IDDM, the forms of clinical manifestation, or levels of insulin secretory capacity at the time of diagnosis.

The available data regarding clinical manifestation of diabetes among children and adolescents were derived from observations in clinics or hospitals, and the referral of patients to such facilities may have involved some selectivity. Thus data from different sources are not necessarily comparable.[5-7] All of the reports, however, have shown a wide spectrum of disease as measured by the presence of diabetic ketoacidosis (DKA), acetonuria, and hyperglycemia at diagnosis. Data reviewed at the Joslin Clinic[8] on 315 patients aged 0 to 20 years, who were Massachusetts residents and referred to the clinic in 1939, 1949 and 1959 within a year of diagnosis, indicated that 23 (7.3%) of them had impaired glucose tolerance (IGT) or NIDDM and during subsequent years did not require treatment with insulin. Among the remainder, 127 were already being treated with insulin at the time of referral, and 165 started insulin treatment on the first or a subsequent visit to the Joslin Clinic. In the group who arrived without previous treatment, 10% were in DKA, 49% had significant acetonuria and 15% had minor acetonuria, while the remaining 26% had hyperglycemia and glycosuria without acetonuria. All those treated with insulin remained on insulin thereafter except for a few who were able to discontinue it after several years and were subsequently managed with oral agents or diet.

Studies of C-peptide secretion in newly diagnosed, juvenile-onset diabetics have indicated that a substantial proportion were secreting endogenous insulin, and that the residual secretion varied considerably from person to person.[9-13] (For a review see ref. 14.) Since the groups that have been studied came from clinic populations, mild cases may have been under-represented relative to their occurrence in the general population. Therefore, in a population-based study the proportion of juvenile-onset IDDM with significant secretion of endogenous insulin might be higher than found in these studies.

In considering the clinical presentation of IDDM among adults, one finds a situation quite different from that among children and adolescents. The proportion of adults with newly diagnosed diabetes who require insulin from the start is quite small (see Chapter 2). Furthermore, according to studies conducted in Copenhagen,[15] and Rochester, Minnesota,[16] only one-third of those started on insulin had ketonuria at diagnosis. The available data on C-peptide secretion in insulin-treated patients with adult-onset diabetes indicate that many of them secrete insulin.[17–20] On the other hand, some patients with NIDDM progress over the years to IDDM. In Copenhagen the incidence rate of this phenomenon was 2.5 per 100,000 per year in the adult population.[15] This was one-fourth the incidence rate of new IDDM in the same population. Since the number of patients with NIDDM in Copenhagen was not known, this incidence rate cannot be expressed as the risk of progressing from a state of having NIDDM to a state of having IDDM. In a study at the Joslin Clinic,[21,22] the incidence rate of changing treatment from diet or oral agents to insulin was relatively high, particularly five and more years after the diagnosis of diabetes (Fig. 12–9). However, it is not known how many of these individuals have true IDDM.

Another issue in the clinical presentation of IDDM is the duration of time between the onset of destruction of beta cells and the diagnosis of the disease. This period consists of two components: the symptomatic period and an interval preceding symptoms during which the process was "silent"—the latent period.

The duration of the symptomatic period for about 4000 patients in the British voluntary registry of juvenile-onset diabetes[23] is shown in Figure 12–1. A sudden onset of symptoms less than 4 weeks before diagnosis was reported by 70%, but the 30% who had a longer duration of symptoms included 10% with a duration longer than 3 months and some for 4 years. The same pattern was found in an older group of newly diagnosed insulin-requiring diabetics in Edinburgh.[24] One must remember that the duration of symptoms is a subjective variable which may be underestimated, particularly in recalling health events which happened months or years previously. (For an overview of this problem see ref. 25.) Thus, it is possible that symptoms lasted much longer, particularly if they were intermittent and did not interfere with daily activities.

Regarding the latent period, there are several pieces of evidence indicating that it can have a long duration. One study found that adult women with newly diagnosed IDDM frequently gave a history of delivering large babies in the years prior to diagnosis, some as many as five years before.[26] Other

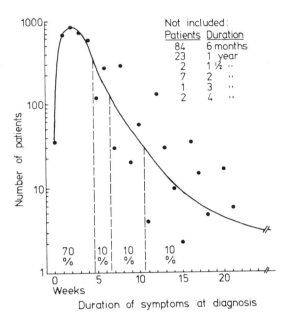

Fig. 12–1. Duration of diabetic symptoms as of the date of diagnosis of diabetes in 4088 patients aged 0 to 15 years. (From ref. 23 with permission of author and publisher)

investigators have observed asymptomatic patients with IGT who developed IDDM months to years later.[27] Moreover, islet cell antibodies have been demonstrated in sera obtained years before the onset of IDDM in secondary cases in families of patients with IDDM.[28–30]

In summary, there is evidence that the process of destruction of beta cells in IDDM may begin months or even years before the disease is diagnosed. If any of the patients who become insulin-requiring after many years of treatment of overt diabetes with oral agents and diet have true IDDM, this could be the strongest evidence that the process may be very long indeed. Additionally, there is a broad spectrum in the severity of the clinical presentation of IDDM. Perhaps this spectrum is a result of various forms of intercurrent stress bringing the process to light at different stages.

Clinical Course

The clinical course of IDDM has changed dramatically since the introduction of insulin to clinical practice early in this century. Although the effect of insulin on prognosis was profound, the fate of patients before the insulin era was not always rapid deterioration and death. Based on the experience of Dr. Elliott P. Joslin between 1898 and 1919, it has been possible to compute survival rates for patients with onset under age 20 (virtually all cases would be considered IDDM by present criteria of classification) according to time elapsed since onset of diabetes. As can be seen in Figure

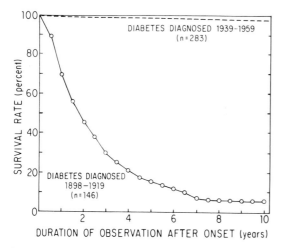

Fig. 12–2. Survival during the first 10 years of diabetes in two periods: before the discovery of insulin (1898–1922) and after introduction of long-acting insulin and antibiotics (1939–1970). Note that in the latter period, 10-year survival was nearly 100%. All patients were first seen within 1 year of symptoms. Common closing date for life table analysis of survival during the earlier period was July 1, 1922; for the later, April 1, 1970. (Unpublished data of the Joslin Clinic; see refs. 31 and 37)

12–2, a substantial number of patients were able to survive in the pre-insulin era for several years after the clinical onset of disease; median survival was 20 months. Deaths were mainly due to diabetic ketoacidosis, but there are no data to explain why, in the absence of exogenous insulin, the expected manifestation of insulin dependence was delayed several years in some of these patients.

Perhaps this variability in fate reflected various degrees of residual beta-cell function at the time of clinical onset of IDDM. One possibility is that some patients manifested their diabetes early in the course of a progressive destruction of the beta cells and then entered a "remission phase".[7,32,33] Several years of further beta cell destruction may have passed before reaching a level of endogenous insulin which was inadequate for preventing ketoacidosis. Another possibility is that the initial process which was destroying the beta cells did not persist, and in some patients a residual beta cell mass remained. Relative insulinopenia and hyperglycemia may then have been responsible for a progressive increase in peripheral insulin resistance,[34–36] eventually leading to ketoacidosis. One cannot exclude that both mechanisms were operating.

Also shown in Figure 12–2 are survival rates during the first 10 years of diabetes for patients with juvenile-onset, insulin-dependent diabetes diagnosed in 1939, 1949, and 1959 at the Joslin Clinic.[37] All deaths which characterized the experience before 1919 were eliminated. Almost all

patients survived ten years regardless of the year of diagnosis, age at onset, or sex.

The improvement in survival rates, however, did not mean that the severe metabolic complications were eliminated. A study called "Natural History of Diabetes Mellitus" was conducted at the Joslin Clinic in the 1960s. Five cohorts of diabetics, who were first seen at the clinic within 1 year of their diagnosis in 1939, 1944, 1949, 1954 and 1959 were traced to 1963.[38] A cross-sectional study was performed in a systematic sample of survivors in 1964–65.[39] Every effort was made to examine all patients selected for the study regardless of whether they were still in the care of Joslin physicians or that of other physicians. The reported occurrences of ketoacidosis in juvenile-onset diabetics during the 5 years preceding the survey yielded an incidence rate of 13/1000 person-years among men and 23/1000 person-years among women (additional details regarding DKA in that study are shown in Tables 12–1 and 12–3 which appear later in this chapter).

In Rochester, Minnesota, where hospital records from the period 1924–1976 were used as the source of information, the incidence of severe ketoacidosis was 13.4/1000 person-years among patients with diabetes diagnosed before the age of 30.[40] Again the rate was higher for women than men. In a study of the population of Rhode Island,[41] the incidence of severe ketoacidosis was 53/1000 diabetics per year among those under age 15, and 11/1000 and 3/1000 diabetics per year among those age 15 to 44 and 45 or more, respectively. The rates were higher among women than men in this study also.

Another issue regarding diabetic ketoacidosis is whether all patients with IDDM have the same risk of developing this metabolic complication. Is it only a matter of exposure time and the occurrence of suitable environmental circumstances, or is there a distinct subset of these patients who are particularly vulnerable to ketoacidosis because of some inherent characteristic? Although there is evidence from clinical practice that the latter may be true, the question has not been examined adequately. In the extensive study by Knowles et al.,[6] 31% of 108 juvenile-onset diabetics never had ketoacidosis and another 30% had only one episode despite a long period of observation. Knowles also reported that the incidence of ketoacidosis was highest in the age group 15 to 20 and decreased with duration of diabetes. This observation agrees with data in Table 12–1. Gottlieb[42] reported the results of a survey of 267 juvenile-onset diabetics diagnosed at the Joslin Clinic between 1928 and 1939 and surviving until 1968, the year of study. In contrast to the results of Knowles, she found only 15% had not had ketoacidosis during 25 or more years of diabetes.

The availability of improved preparations of insulin and growing awareness of the late complications of diabetes have led an increasing number of physicians to change therapeutic goals from prevention of ketoacidosis and glycosuria to striving for normal blood glucose levels. Unfortunately, this goal is not easily achieved and, at present, seems impossible in many instances. In Table 12–1 are data from the Joslin Clinic study previously described concerning the control of diabetes in juvenile-onset patients in 1964–65.[39] A post-prandial blood glucose in excess of 200 mg/dl was found in 39%, and a similar percentage had significant glycosuria (3 g/dl or more in a single urine specimen) or acetonuria. The proportion with poor control decreased with attained age. Only 46% of the patients were free of both indicators of poor control. These results are only a little better than data reported by others.[6,43,44]

Poor control of blood glucose is also characteristic of adult-onset IDDM. The WHO-Multinational Study of the Vascular Complications of Diabetes[45] obtained data on the fasting levels of blood glucose among insulin-treated diabetics aged 35 to 54 years, most of whom had the onset of diabetes as adults. Mean values of fasting blood glucose in the populations studied in nine centers around the world are presented in Table 12–2 according to duration of diabetes. Except for Tokyo, the mean values are in the range 200 to 300 mg/dl. No values for glycosylated hemoglobin were available.

In the earlier discussion of DKA, the issue of whether all patients with IDDM have the same risk of developing DKA was considered. Similar questions can be raised with regard to control as assessed by blood glucose. Is there a distinguishable subgroup which consistently manifests poor control? How large might this group be? If present, this would suggest that these individuals have a type of diabetes which is inherently difficult to control. Alternatively, is the glycemic pattern generally inconsistent over time in most individuals? This would suggest that lack of control is largely the result of external circumstances, including factors which influence adherence to a prescribed treatment plan.

The data on control presented so far were derived from cross-sectional surveys in which a single determination of blood glucose (together with acetone and sugar in urine) was performed for each individual. One blood glucose value is an imprecise estimate of that individual's usual level of control and gives no indication of how variable that level might be. Unfortunately, those who carried out the few long-term studies of groups of patients with IDDM have not published quantitative data regarding control which was analyzed separately for individuals. Thus, we do not have a description of how much patients differ in their usual level of control, how unstable an individual's levels is, or how it changes with age.

In the previously mentioned survey conducted at the Joslin Diabetes Center in 1964–65,[39] patients aged 15 to 44 at the time of examination were questioned regarding their effort to control blood glucose levels. Fifteen percent reported that they performed daily urine tests and either weighed or measured their food. Another 45% took less care with their diet but still performed daily urine tests. The remaining 40% tested the urine less frequently, many of them weekly or monthly, and some never tested it. In Table 12–3 are shown indicators of the control of diabetes according to the level of effort expended to control blood glucose. There were no significant differences among the groups although patients who reported the greatest effort tended to have the worst indices of diabetic control. Due to the emphasis on patient education at the Joslin Clinic, one can assume that most of these patients had knowledge of standard techniques for controlling diabetes. It is unlikely, therefore, that

Table 12–1.   Prevalence and Incidence Rates of Indicators of Poor Control of Diabetes in a Sample of Patients with Juvenile Onset Diabetes 5 to 25 Years after Diagnosis according to Age at Examination. (Adapted from unpublished Joslin data, ref. 39)

Age at Examination in Years	No. of Patients Examined*	Postprandial Measurements (prevalence rates in percent)			Self-reported Coma during Previous 5 Years (incidence rate per 1000 person-years)
		Blood Glucose ≥200 mg/dl	Glycosuria ≥3 g/dl	Acetonuria†	
5–14	52	52	48	42	15
15–24	98	37	43	42	29
25–34	97	38	34	37	16
35–44	50	32	30	32	12
Total	297	39	39	39	20

*78.8% of the patients invited for the study participated.
†Includes trace and significant acetonuria.

Table 12–2. Mean Values of Fasting Plasma Glucose among Insulin-Treated Diabetics Aged 35 to 54 Years in 9 Populations. (Adapted from data in ref. 45)

	Fasting Plasma Glucose (mean in mg/dl)	
	Duration of Diabetes in years	
Population	7–13	14+
London	308	308
Switzerland	196	207
Warsaw	260	262
Berlin (GDR)	198	225
New Delhi	247	200
Tokyo	166	172
Havana	198	215
Oklahoma Indians	226	249
Pima Indians	267	271

the finding of large variability in patient behavior can be attributed to differences in knowledge. Symptoms of hyperglycemia, particularly if they interfere with daily activities, are another factor which might have affected patient behavior. Perhaps a patient with unstable diabetes would be prompted to expend more effort to control hyperglycemia than a patient with easy-to-control diabetes. It is conceivable that the outcome would be similar levels of control despite different levels of effort as was found in this study. This explanation is in accordance with the observation in other diseases that adherence to therapy is correlated with severity of symptoms (for reviews see refs. 46 and 47.) If true for diabetes, it would be evidence for heterogeneity in IDDM with regard to its controllability.

Complications of IDDM

Prolongation of life in IDDM due to the availability of insulin and antibiotics revealed health problems other than ketoacidosis and infections. The pathologic changes in both small and large blood vessels have become the most devastating complications of diabetes.

The increasing importance of these complications, particularly among patients with juvenile-onset diabetes, has been presented in several publications which describe the experience of the Joslin Clinic.[48–54] Unfortunately, these reports used various definitions for end-points and presented the results in such a way that it is impossible to make comparisons among the studies. Moreover, bias due to referral to the clinic of patients with complications was not controlled or even assessed. The first attempt to overcome these problems was the previously described study of the "Natural History of Diabetes Mellitus" conducted in the 1960s at the Joslin Clinic.[39] Table 12–4 shows the prevalence rates of certain complications according to the duration of diabetes in a systematic sample of patients with diabetes diagnosed before age 21. The prevalence of hypertension and renal and eye complications increased with duration of diabetes. The prevalence of retinopathy was essentially the same for males and females while proteinuria and hypertension were more prevalent among males than females. Different results were described in some earlier Joslin reports,[52] but it is not possible to assess whether the differences represent changes over time or that earlier studies were biased. Even this cross-sectional study was biased due to early mortality in the 1939 and 1944 cohorts. These issues are rarely taken into account in cross-sectional

Table 12–3. Age-Adjusted Prevalence and Incidence Rates† of Indicators of Control of Diabetes in a Sample of Patients with Juvenile Onset Diabetes aged 15 to 44 at Examination According to Effort Spent to Control Blood Glucose. (Adapted from unpublished Joslin data, ref. 39)

	Effort Spent to Control Blood Glucose*		
Indicator of Control of Diabetes	Large (n = 36)	Moderate (n = 110)	Small (n = 99)
Postprandial measurements (prevalence rates in percent)			
acetonuria‡	43	38	37
glycosuria ≥3 g/dl	36	36	34
blood glucose ≥200 mg/dl	34	42	29
none of the above	46	45	53
Self-reported coma during previous 5 years (incidence rates per 1000 person-years)	26	19	18

*Large = daily urine testing and weighing or measuring food, Moderate = daily, and Small = less frequent urine testing
†Age-adjusted to the age distribution of the total study group
‡Includes trace and significant acetonuria

Table 12–4.   Prevalence Rates (percent) of Certain Complications in a Sample of Patients with Juvenile-Onset Diabetes (diagnosis before age 21) According to Sex and Duration of Diabetes. (Adapted from unpublished Joslin data, ref. 39)

Complications		5 years (n = 80)[a]	10 & 15 years (n = 121)[a]	20 & 25 years (n = 97)[a]
		Duration of Diabetes		
Retinopathy[b]	M	0	58	78
	F	10	48	85
Proliferative retinopathy[c]	M	0	12	29
	F	0	6	27
Proteinuria ≥20 mg/dl[d]	M	2	20	39
	F	3	12	18
Blood pressure 160/95 mm	M	2	11	24
Hg or more[e]	F	3	2	19

[a]Participation rates for the examination were 82.3%, 80.1%, 75.2% in group with diabetes for 5 years, 10 and 15 years, and 20 and 25 years, respectively.
[b]Standard ophthalmologic examination through dilated pupils (background and proliferative).
[c]Presence of retino-blindness and/or fibrous tissue in the retina or in vitreous; and/or new vessels.
[d]The salicylsulfonic acid method was used.
[e]Using a standard cuff after the patient had been supine for at least 10 minutes.

studies, and they cannot be overcome by improvements in the techniques of measuring end-points or by statistical analysis.[55]

To avoid the limitations of cross-sectional studies, one must examine the development of late complications of diabetes by applying a cohort approach. The best study of this type was the follow-up of a cohort of juvenile-onset diabetics which was conducted by Knowles et al.[6,56,57] They found that retinopathy and protcinuria bcgan to appeai after 10 years of diabetes and leveled off after 30 years. Between the 10th and 30th years of diabetes, about 45% of the cohort developed proliferative retinopathy and the same number developed persistent proteinuria (Fig. 12–3). This gave an incidence rate of 2.25% per year in the population of patients with diabetes of 10 or more years' duration. In Figure 12–3 are shown also the cumulative incidence rates for blindness and renal fail-

ure, the major consequences of small vessel disease.

In a recently completed cohort study conducted at the Joslin Diabetes Center,[8] similar results were found regarding the incidence of proliferative retinopathy. Nephropathy, assessed by the occurrence of persistent proteinuria and hypertension, was less frequent than in the study of Knowles. The incidence of this complication was found to be dependent on attained age rather than on the duration of diabetes. Moreover, the incidence of nephropathy had declined over time in that the 1949 cohort had a lower cumulative incidence rate by age 50 than the 1939 cohort. A cohort study of diabetic complications among juvenile-onset diabetics in France,[58] revealed that only 15% of the patients developed persistent proteinuria and hypertension during 25 years of diabetes, a figure much lower than that in Knowles' study. Because the French

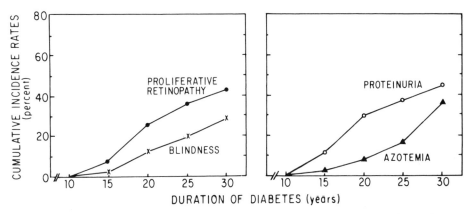

Fig. 12–3.   Cumulative incidence rates of specified forms of microvascular complications according to duration of juvenile-onset diabetes. (Adapted from ref. 56)

study involved a cohort diagnosed between 1950 and 1960, one might consider these data as evidence of a further decline in the incidence of diabetic nephropathy among juvenile-onset diabetics.

As another end-point in cohort studies, deaths due to specified causes can be considered. This approach is particularly useful for studying the occurrence of complications such as renal failure and coronary heart disease. Unfortunately, the published data regarding specific causes of death in juvenile-onset diabetes are not adequate for informative comparisons. The authors have mainly presented proportional mortality. These might be of value for clinical purposes, such as appraising the importance of some complication relative to other causes of death, but they cannot be used for population comparisons.[54,59,60] In a recent study at the Joslin Diabetes Center, it was possible to examine mortality in a quantitative manner in an inception cohort of 292 insulin-dependent diabetics who had been followed 20 to 40 years.[61] Mortality was found to depend more on attained age than duration of diabetes. The death rates from renal failure and coronary disease both rose abruptly at around age 35, regardless of the age at onset of diabetes. Almost 47% of the group died of these two complications by age 54 (Fig. 12–4). When the sexes were examined separately, renal failure was found to be more common among men. This finding is in agreement with the earlier evidence that persistent proteinuria was more frequent in men than in women. Both sexes experienced similar mortality due to coronary heart disease, which was much higher than that in the general population.

The occurrence of diabetic complications among adult-onset IDDM is much more difficult to evaluate. In most of the literature, IDDM and NIDDM

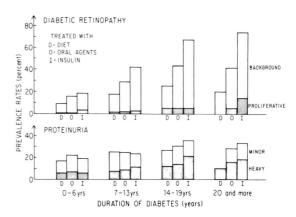

Fig. 12–5. Prevalence rates of two microvascular complications in patients aged 35–54 (pooled results from 9 study populations) according to the duration of diabetes and method of treatment. (Adapted from ref. 45)

have been lumped together. The first study which examined the occurrence of microangiopathic complications among adult-onset, insulin-requiring diabetics from a population point of view was the WHO-Multinational Study on Vascular Complications of Diabetes. It was a cross-sectional study conducted among representative samples of diabetic patients aged 35 to 54 from 14 populations around the world. The selection process was designed to limit the bias introduced by referral of patients to specialists.[62] In a report on selected findings in nine centers,[45] some confirmation of the earlier observations on microvascular complications in IDDM can be found in the relationship between their occurrence and the type of diabetes as indicated by treatment (Fig. 12–5). Prevalence rates of retinopathy increased sharply with the duration of diabetes, particularly among insulin-treated patients. However, the increase of prevalence rates for proliferative retinopathy was only modest. When the prevalence of proteinuria was considered, the type of hypoglycemic treatment was not as important as it had been for retinopathy. Moreover, there was not as sharp an increase in the prevalence of nephropathy with duration of diabetes.

In Figure 12–6 are shown, for eight of the centers, the prevalence rates of proteinuria and proliferative retinopathy among patients with diabetes for 14 or more years, regardless of type of treatment. Considerable variation in the occurrence of each complication is seen, but proteinuria and retinopathy do not vary in parallel. The proportion of patients treated with insulin in each center is also shown. It happens that the centers with the highest prevalence of proteinuria also have the highest proportion of patients with NIDDM. Thus, if the prevalence rates were analyzed for only those being

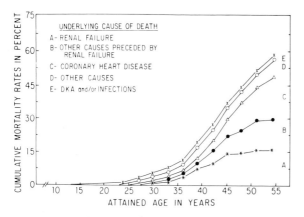

Fig. 12–4. Cumulative mortality rates due to specified causes during 40 years of follow-up of a cohort of patients with onset of IDDM before age 21. (Unpublished data of the Joslin Clinic; see ref. 61)

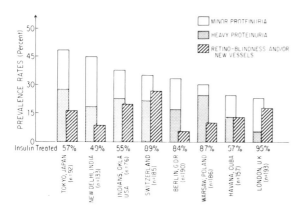

Fig. 12–6. Prevalence rates of proteinuria and proliferative retinopathy after 14 or more years of diabetes in patients aged 35 to 54 in 8 countries. (Adapted from refs. 45, 62, and 63 with permission of authors.)

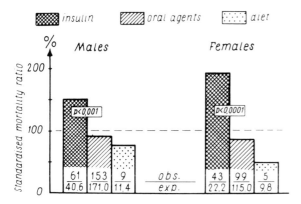

Fig. 12–7. Standardized mortality ratios for deaths due to all causes in a cohort of 5210 newly diagnosed patients with adult-onset diabetes followed for 1 to 10 years (average 4.2) according to type of treatment prescribed at diagnosis. Obs = observed number; Exp = expected number. (Reproduced with permission of publisher from ref. 64)

treated with insulin, one would find even larger differences among centers. These may result from differences in policies regarding the control of diabetes, or they may be due to differences in certain environmental factors. Further, these are prevalence rates from cross-sectional studies, and the differences could reflect peculiarities in the selection process in various centers. This last problem can be solved only through a cohort approach.

There are a few cohort studies of IDDM with adult-onset, but cause-specific mortality rather than morbidity has been used as the end-point. In Warsaw a cohort of 5210 patients with newly diagnosed diabetes between the ages of 30 and 68 were followed an average of 4.5 years.[64] Males experienced mortality 31% higher than the general population, and females a similar excess of 27%. When mortality was analyzed according to the type of initial

treatment of diabetes, those patients treated with insulin had the highest mortality while those treated with diet had the lowest (Fig. 12–7). The excess of deaths among insulin-treated women was mainly due to coronary and cerebrovascular causes, while among insulin-treated men, causes other than cardiovascular diseases were responsible. Similar results regarding mortality from cardiovascular diseases according to type of diabetes management were found in the small group of diabetics in the Framingham Heart Study.[65] A population study of mortality in Edinburgh also showed higher mortality in patients treated with insulin than in those treated with diet or oral agents. Regardless of sex, the higher mortality in the insulin-treated patients was due to genitourinary diseases, ketoacidosis, hypoglycemia and, among women, circulatory and respiratory diseases as well. The patients treated with insulin, however, had significantly longer known duration of diabetes at the beginning of the observation than the other treatment groups.[66]

In summary, through use of the new classification of diabetes, IDDM emerges as a disease with a high frequency of microangiopathic complications. This is perhaps due not only to the accumulation over years or decades of the effects of metabolic disturbances of diabetes, but also to the interaction of these disturbances with aging processes and perhaps some environmental factors as well. This last issue deserves much more attention and further study. IDDM is also characterized by early and high morbidity and mortality due to cardiovascular causes, particularly among women. It remains unknown whether or not this increased occurrence of atherosclerosis is due to the diabetic milieu alone interacting with an aging process, or due additionally to an interaction of these metabolic disturbances with the background risk factors prevalent in the general population in which the diabetics were born.

NATURAL HISTORY OF NON-INSULIN-DEPENDENT DIABETES (NIDDM)

Clinical Manifestation

In contrast to IDDM, there is no agreement as to the nature of the lesion responsible for the development of NIDDM in adults. Abnormalities in both insulin secretion and insulin action have been demonstrated, but there is continuing debate as to which of these is the primary and which the secondary phenomenon (for a review see ref. 67). Regardless of its identity, the process is a slowly evolving one which is first detectable as abnormality in glucose tolerance only after a glucose challenge. In 1961, Conn and Fajans wrote, ''Presently all experts agree that a diagnosis of diabetes mellitus can be made on a completely asymptomatic patient on the basis of a carefully performed glucose tolerance test.''[68] That belief was shaken in the late 1960s and subsequently as reports from several prospective studies changed this deterministic picture of the evolution of glucose intolerance to diabetes into a much more probabilistic one.[69–74] The best designed and executed of these prospective studies was the follow-up of 241 individuals with blood glucose values between 120 to 199 mg/dl 2 hours after an oral glucose load in the Bedford Survey.[73] During 10 years of observation, 15% of the original group worsened to diabetes, 22.8% remained glucose intolerant, and the majority rapidly recovered or were only temporarily intolerant. The levels of post-glucose hyperglycemia and obesity at the baseline examination were the best predictors of progression to diabetes. Curiously, obesity was also a predictor of returning to normoglycemia.

In other studies, post-glucose hyperglycemia and obesity at baseline were good predictors of worsening to overt diabetes, but the proportions progressing were a little higher than in the Bedford Study.[69,70,72,74] Little significance should be attached to these differences since the authors used various definitions of overt diabetes and different procedures for identifying study patients. The important and consistent finding, however, was that impaired glucose tolerance was a dynamic process, as were perhaps, its determinants such as insulin resistance or insulin secretory capacity. Progression to significant post-prandial or fasting hyperglycemia was infrequent.

Once significant fasting hyperglycemia is present, patients commonly have symptoms but these are not as specific or severe as those typical of the onset of IDDM in juveniles. Consequently, diabetes in these individuals can remain undetected since they may not seek medical care. Several population surveys have found previously undetected fasting hyperglycemia of significant degree in about 0.3% of those screened.[75–77] Symptoms were minor or absent; therefore, it is unknown how long the patients would have remained undiagnosed before seeking medical care, or if all of them would ever have been diagnosed in the absence of screening.

Some clinical characteristics of patients with newly diagnosed diabetes in the Rochester Study in Minnesota[78] are summarized in Table 12–5. Only one-quarter of the patients reported typical symptoms of hyperglycemia. While some of these patients would be classified by current criteria as having impaired glucose tolerance (IGT) rather than diabetes, their exclusion would have raised the percentage with symptoms only a little.[16] An-

other feature of newly diagnosed adult-onset diabetes is the frequent presence of obesity. In the Rochester Study, about 40% of all newly diagnosed patients had significant obesity despite the weight loss which was frequently reported for the period before diagnosis.

Figure 12–8 shows the distribution of Body Mass Index (BMI)* among all patients who came (within 1 year of diagnosis) to the Joslin Clinic in the years 1957 to 1963 and were age 40 or over.[21,22] According to the new recommendations on the classification of diabetes, males with a BMI above 27 and females above 25 should be considered obese individuals.[79] By these standards, 37% of the males and 63.5% of the females were obese on their first visit to the Joslin Clinic.

In summary, NIDDM seems to be a slowly developing disease with a long pre-clinical phase. Its pre-clinical manifestation, post-glucose hyperglycemia, is nonspecific since a substantial number of such individuals revert to normoglycemia or remain for many years without progression to diabetes. Only 2%, approximately, of individuals with impaired glucose tolerance progress to overt diabetes per year. The determinants of this progression (as well as the associated pathologic events) are unknown, except that obesity is a significant risk factor. More information on these determinants and a more specific test for early diagnosis of NIDDM

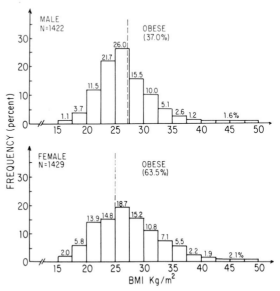

Fig. 12–8. Distribution of patients with adult-onset diabetes according to Body Mass Index at diagnosis. Unpublished data from the Joslin Clinic for all patients first seen between 1957 and 1963 who were over the age of 40 and came to the Clinic within 1 year of diagnosis of diabetes. (see refs. 21 and 22)

---

*Body Mass Index = weight/height^2 measured in kg/m^2.

Table 12–5. Prevalence Rates (percent) of Selected Clinical Characteristics in Newly Diagnosed Adult-Onset Diabetes in the Population of Rochester, Minnesota (Adapted from ref. 78)

History and Examination Findings	Age at Diagnosis in Years				
	30–39 (n = 61)	40–49 (n = 130)	50–59 (n = 259)	60–69 (n = 302)	70 + (n = 285)
Family history*	41	46	46	40	36
Glycosuria	50	47	61	56	57
Polyuria, Polydipsia	26	30	32	28	25
Weight loss	23	23	22	22	24
Relative weight ≥1.25†	40	42	49	41	33

*History of diabetes in parents, siblings, or children
†Ratio of actual to ideal weight was determined for medium frame from Metropolitan Life Insurance tables

are needed before attempts can be made to retard the development of NIDDM.

A separate issue is the number of individuals with significant hyperglycemia who remain undiagnosed in the community. Their number will depend upon the frequency of physician contacts for other medical problems or periodic check-ups. Before consideration can be given to the question of whether a screening program to detect them is justified, more knowledge regarding two issues is required: (a) If left undetected, does the prolonged exposure of their beta cells to hyperglycemia lead to irreversible damage that will increase their chance of requiring insulin? (b) If left undetected, are the pathogenetic mechanisms leading to complications initiated irreversibly?

Clinical Course

A small fraction of adult-onset diabetics are truly insulin-dependent from the onset of the disease (see Chapter 2); however, a larger fraction of them are insulin-treated from the beginning. Perhaps those who remain with undetected hyperglycemia for a long time are more likely to require insulin from the beginning.[80] In the previously cited study of diabetics age 40 and over who came to the Joslin Clinic within 1 year of diagnosis in the years 1957 to 1963,[21,22] the initial treatment was diet alone for 30%, oral agents for 40% and insulin for 30% (Table 12–6). In the last group 75% remained on insulin throughout the 12-year follow-up.

No population-based study of newly diagnosed NIDDM has been conducted which is analogous to the previously mentioned Bedford Study of impaired glucose tolerance (IGT).[73] Thus, we do not know what proportion of NIDDM can revert to IGT or even normal glucose tolerance nor what proportion evolve to IDDM, although both directions of progression have been observed. Modification of diet and reduction of weight have been shown in clinical studies to diminish insulin resistance, restore beta cell responsiveness to glucose and improve control of glycemia,[81–87] and in some pa-

tients, to permit discontinuation of treatment.[88] The University Group Diabetes Program (UGDP) demonstrated that dietary restriction was sufficient to lower fasting glycemia for almost 2 years in a selected group of patients.[89,90] In that interval, glycemia returned to the baseline value and subsequently deteriorated further in the diet-treated group, as well as in the groups treated with tolbutamide or a standard dose of insulin. This deterioration was, apparently, more evident in some patients than in others. For example, 27% of the patients treated with diet had fasting blood glucose values below 150 mg/dl throughout the period of study and 37% almost always had fasting glucose levels above 150 mg/dl. The remainder presumably accounted for much of the trend. Unfortunately, the UGDP report does not describe the characteristics of this deterioration, in particular its relation to baseline values for fasting blood glucose.

Figure 12–9 shows data from the Joslin Clinic on the deterioration of hyperglycemia among adult-onset diabetics. The previously described group of patients from the years 1957 to 1963[21,22] (see Table 12–6) were followed for 12 years and changes of treatment from diet or oral agents to insulin were recorded. During the first 3 years changes from the initial type of treatment were few, but by the 12th year of diabetes, 35% of those treated with oral agents and 15% of those treated with diet had become insulin-requiring. Within each of these groups the likelihood of this change may have been related to the level of hyperglycemia at diagnosis, as was found for the progression of IGT to NIDDM, but in this analysis the initial level was not taken into account. Furthermore, the nature of the insulin requirement is unclear; does it represent insulin-dependency?

In a prospective study of 160 newly diagnosed adult-onset diabetics, the patients were classified according to the presence of islet cell antibodies.[91] During 3.5 years of observation, 86% of those with antibodies became insulin-requiring, while this occurred in only 18% of those without antibodies.

Table 12–6.   Type of Treatment Prescribed at First Visit to Joslin Clinic in 3040 Adult-Onset Diabetics who came to the Clinic within One Year of Diagnosis of Diabetes According to Age at Diagnosis (Unpublished Joslin data, refs. 21,22)

| Initial Treatment | Age at Diagnosis of Diabetes | | | | |
	40–49 Percent	50–59 Percent	60–69 Percent	70 and more Percent	All ages Percent
Diet only	34.9	28.1	27.4	25.7	28.9
Oral agents	29.2	37.6	45.4	48.5	39.9
Insulin	35.9	34.3	27.3	25.8	31.2
Total	100.0	100.0	100.0	100.0	100.0
Number	619	1037	932	452	3040

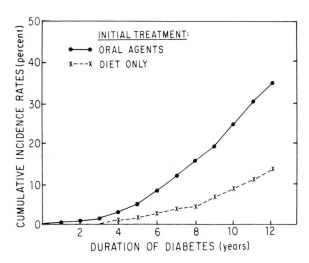

Fig. 12–9. Cumulative incidence rates of commencing treatment with insulin among patients with adult-onset diabetes treated initially with oral hypoglycemic agents or diet only. (Unpublished data of the Joslin Clinic; see refs 21 and 22)

However, based on the early timing of these changes of treatment from oral agents to insulin, this mechanism does not seem to relate to the pathogenesis of the events described in the Joslin Clinic data which occurred primarily after 5 years. Instead, it should be considered as evidence that some adult-onset IDDM develops very gradually and may not require insulin at the time of diagnosis.

Turning to glycemic control in adult-onset diabetes, one finds that there have not been any population-based studies. However, for the Diabetes Natural History Study, conducted at the Joslin Clinic in 1964–65, a systematic sample of patients with adult-onset diabetes of 5 to 25 years' duration was examined.[39] A post-prandial blood glucose above 200 mg/dl was found in 30%, significant glycosuria in 18.9% and acetonuria in 18.1% (Table 12–7). Although patients with more severe diabetes are somewhat over-represented in the sample from the Joslin Clinic, these results show that uncontrolled glycemia is common in adult-onset

diabetes. When the analysis was performed separately for those treated with oral agents or diet, 18% had high post-prandial hyperglycemia, 10% had significant glycosuria, and 12% had trace or significant acetonuria. The UGDP reports also provide this type of information.[89,90] During 10 years of follow-up, "good" control of hyperglycemia (75% of visits with FBG < 150 mg/dl) was achieved in only 42% of those treated with an insulin dose which was varied according to need while 20% had "poor" control (75% of visits with FBG > 150 mg/dl). It is noteworthy that in a similar group of patients treated with diet alone, "good" control was achieved by only 25% while 45% had "poor" control. One must remember, however, that according to the new criteria, the UGDP population included a substantial number of patients with IGT rather than diabetes. Moreover, the patients were sufficiently motivated to participate in a clinical trial. Thus, one cannot generalize directly to all NIDDM patients the levels of glycemic control achieved in that study. Presumably, in the general population of NIDDM patients, control of hyperglycemia can only be worse than that in the UGDP study.

As was discussed earlier, a substantial proportion of patients are obese at the time of diagnosis of diabetes and weight reduction should be considered a major therapeutic goal as well as control of hyperglycemia. In Table 12–8 is presented the distribution of a sample of adult-onset diabetics according to their Body Mass Index (BMI in kg/m²) at diagnosis of diabetes and again 5 to 25 years later. The data are from the previously described Diabetes Natural History Study conducted at the Joslin Clinic in 1964–65.[39] BMI was grouped into three categories: thin (less than 22.5), normal weight to moderate obesity (22.5 to 27.4) and obese (more than 27.5). As can be seen, 54% of the patients who were thin at diagnosis remained so, while 37% gained a moderate amount of weight and 9% became obese. In the group with normal weight or moderate obesity at diagnosis, most did not change weight categories and as many became

Table 12-7. Prevalence Rates (percent) of Indicators of Control of Diabetes in a Sample of 408 Patients with Adult-Onset Diabetes 5 to 25 Years after Diagnosis According to Age at Examination. (Adapted from unpublished Joslin data, ref. 39)

Age at Examination in Years	No. of Patients Examined*	Postprandial Measurements		
		Blood Glucose ≥200 mg/dl	Glycosuria ≥3 g/dl	Acetonuria†
30–39	56	39	39	32
40–49	70	31	24	23
50–59	92	26	16	20
60–69	93	33	16	15
70–79	97	25	8	8
Total	408	30	18	18

*74.6% of patients invited for the study participated
†Includes trace and significant acetonuria

Table 12-8. Distribution of 381 Patients with Adult-Onset Diabetes According to Body Mass Index (BMI) at Diagnosis of Diabetes and 5 to 25 Years Later. (Adapted from unpublished Joslin Data, ref. 39)

BMI (kg/m²) at Diagnosis (1939–1959)	No. of Patients	BMI (kg/m²) in 1964–65			
		Less than 22.5 Percent	22.5–27.4 Percent	27.5 or more Percent	Total Percent
Less than 22.5	140	54	37	9	100
22.5–27.4	145	13	72	15	100
27.5 or more	96	1	22	77	100

obese as became thin. Similarly, patients obese at diagnosis mostly remained obese. Among the UGDP treatment groups, the group treated with diet alone lost a little weight and did not regain it, while the insulin-treated groups actually became a little heavier during the 10-year observation period.[90]

In summary, hyperglycemia increases in many patients with NIDDM to the point that treatment with insulin is required, typically 5 or more years after onset. There are no data on how many of these patients become insulin-dependent or what mechanisms are responsible for the worsening of hyperglycemia. One can speculate that deterioration may be an intrinsic characteristic in some types of diabetes determined genetically and expressed as part of the aging process. Alternatively, patient or physician behavior may be responsible through diminishing attention to planning and/or executing treatment. Another possibility is that hyperglycemia itself may initiate a vicious circle of increasing insulin resistance and diminishing insulin responsiveness to glucose.[92] If true, deterioration could be prevented only by early diagnosis and normalization of glycemia. Unfortunately, there is no evidence that conventional methods of treatment have achieved normoglycemia in a majority of patients.

Complications of NIDDM

Although patients with NIDDM are less likely to experience the acute metabolic complications of

diabetes than patients with IDDM, their vulnerability to late vascular complications, particularly macroangiopathy, is not correspondingly reduced. Some basic characteristics of the occurrence of retinopathy, nephropathy and large vessel disease in patients with diabetes diagnosed after age 30 are presented in the following sections. This use of age at diagnosis as a criterion for distinguishing NIDDM from IDDM is an approximation which is necessary, given the data available. However, it does introduce some bias in the results for conditions that have different frequencies in the two types of diabetes. Microangiopathy, for example, is common in IDDM and will be found with a slightly higher frequency in a group of adult-onset diabetics than it would be in a group consisting only of NIDDM.

Retinopathy. Prevalence rates for retinopathy in the sample of patients with adult-onset diabetes who were examined at the Joslin Clinic in 1964–65 for the Diabetes Natural History Study[39] and in Oklahoma Indians with diabetes[93] are presented in Figure 12–10. In both studies, physicians used comparable criteria for a diagnosis of retinopathy. Prevalence rates of background retinopathy were similar in the two populations and increased significantly with duration of diabetes. Proliferative retinopathy also increased with duration but was relatively rare. It was a little less frequent in Joslin Clinic patients with diabetes of long duration than in the Indians.

A population-based, cross-sectional study of retinopathy was conducted among participants in the Framingham Heart Study. It yielded prevalence rates similar to the other studies even though much more sensitive and specific diagnostic procedures were used.[94] Prevalence rates for retinopathy among diabetics in that population rose from 5% among those with diabetes less than 5 years to 30, 45, and 62% among those with duration of diabetes 5 to 9 years, 10 to 14 years, and 15 or more years, respectively. It is noteworthy that changes in the retina, characteristic of diabetes, were found in 0.8% of persons without diabetes. An Australian study of retinal changes showed that prevalence rates of various types increased with age, even in those examined at the time of diagnosis of diabetes,[95] as well as with duration of diabetes at examination. For example in the age group 50 to 59, over 20% of newly diagnosed diabetics already had diabetic retinopathy while almost no one in the age group 20 to 30 had these changes at the diagnosis of diabetes.

Prospective observations of the development of diabetic retinopathy in NIDDM are limited to short-duration studies. The baseline level of hyperglycemia appears to have significant impact on the development of retinal changes. During 6 years of observation, few patients with IGT developed diabetic retinopathy, while 20 to 30% of those with significant fasting or post-challenge hyperglycemia did.[96-98] Furthermore, the risk increased with the severity of hyperglycemia.[99] These observations are in agreement with the results of the WHO-Multinational Study on Vascular Complications of Diabetes in which the prevalence of retinopathy correlated with the severity of diabetes, as measured by the type of treatment (Fig. 12–5).

In summary, background retinopathy appears to be a frequent complication of NIDDM which is closely related to the severity and duration of diabetes. Although more descriptive data from prospective studies are needed, the severe forms of retinal changes, such as proliferative retinopathy, appear to be infrequent in NIDDM.[100] The increasing prevalence of pre-existing retinal changes with increasing age at diagnosis of diabetes has implications for hypotheses regarding the pathogenesis of NIDDM as well as diabetic retinopathy. This relationship could be explained by an aging process which increases the vulnerability of retinal vessels to hyperglycemia, or by an increase with age in the delay between the unrecognized onset of hyperglycemia and the diagnosis of diabetes.

Nephropathy. In the following review, only clinically manifest diabetic nephropathy will be considered, i.e., proteinuria and renal failure as early and late manifestations, respectively. Although not specific for diabetic nephropathy, proteinuria (which may be intermittent initially but later becomes persistent) is the best indicator of its presence (see also Chapter 30). Prevalence rates of proteinuria in patients with adult-onset diabetes

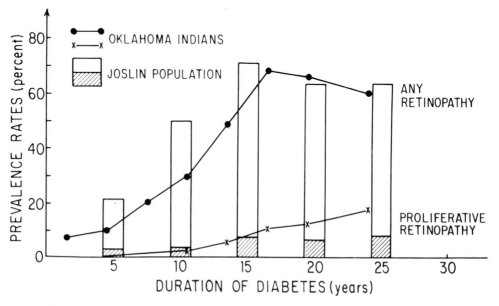

Fig. 12–10. Prevalence rates of retinopathy according to duration of diabetes in a sample of patients of the Joslin Clinic with adult-onset diabetes in comparison with Oklahoma Indians with diabetes. The Joslin sample consisted of patients first seen at the Clinic between 1939 and 1959, within 1 year of diagnosis, and surviving 5 to 25 years of diabetes. (Adapted from ref. 93 and unpublished data of the Joslin Clinic; see ref. 39)

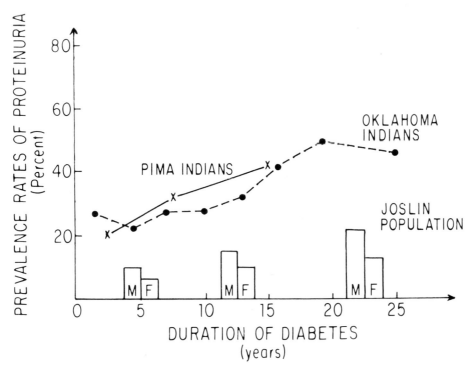

Fig. 12–11. Prevalence rates of proteinuria according to duration of diabetes in a sample of patients (see Table 12–7) of the Joslin Clinic with adult-onset diabetes in comparison with Oklahoma and Pima Indians. The Joslin sample is the same as described for Figure 12–10. For the Joslin Clinic study, the criterion for proteinuria was a urine protein of 20 mg/dl or greater in a single, postprandial urine sample; see refs. 93 and 101 for details of the criteria used in the studies of Indians.

are shown in Figure 12–11, according to duration of diabetes. The data are from three studies, one the previously described Diabetes Natural History Study conducted at the Joslin Clinic in 1964–65[39] and two studies of Indians with diabetes in Oklahoma[93] and Arizona.[101] In the Joslin Clinic population, where prevalence rates were lower than among Indians, males had higher rates than females, but the sexes were equally affected in the Indian studies. Figure 12–6 also showed variability among populations, but the causes of these differences are unknown.

There are only two prospective studies of the incidence of diabetic nephropathy in NIDDM. During 6 years' observation of a group of adult-onset diabetics in Japan, 12% developed persistent proteinuria.[102] In contrast, only 4% of the patients in the UGDP study developed nephropathy (defined as proteinuria of 1.0 g or more per 24 hours) in 10 years of observation. If persistent proteinuria was considered sufficient for a diagnosis of nephropathy, the cumulative incidence became 9.2%.[89,90] Since the UGDP participants included a substantial number of patients with IGT, the cumulative incidence of proteinuria would have been higher if the analysis had been limited to those meeting the newly proposed criteria for NIDDM.

Another approach to assessing the magnitude and importance of renal complications in NIDDM is to examine mortality due to renal failure in a population of adult-onset diabetics. Preliminary results regarding mortality due to renal failure are available from such a study in progress at the Joslin Clinic of the pattern of survival in diabetes.[103] A systematic sample of diabetics residing in Massachusetts who came to the Joslin Clinic within 5 years of their diagnosis between 1923 and 1960 have been traced until their death or until 1977. For deceased patients, all available information regarding causes of death was collected and classified according to the primary cause by one of three physicians. Results for patients aged 40 to 54 at their first visit to the clinic are shown in Figure 12–12. Death due to renal failure by age 75 occurred in 7.4% of the men and 7.6% of the women. The cumulative mortality rates for renal failure among those with diabetes diagnosed between 1945 and 1960 were about the same as for those diagnosed earlier, between 1922 and 1944.

In summary, clinically manifest diabetic nephropathy is an infrequent complication of NIDDM in the population of white Massachusetts residents who come to the Joslin Clinic, but it may contribute more significantly to the health problems of other

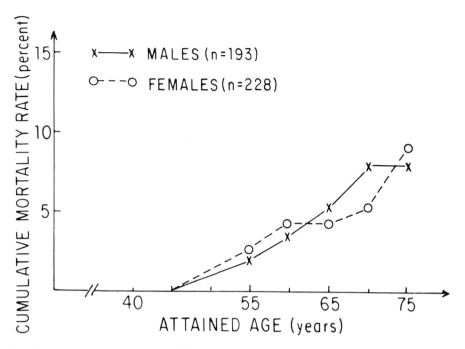

Fig. 12–12. Cumulative mortality rates for renal failure among patients of the Joslin Clinic according to attained age. (Data are for patients who were Massachusetts residents, came to the Clinic between 1923 and 1960, were aged 40 to 54 years, and had diabetes diagnosed less than 5 years before first visit; see ref. 103).

diabetic populations such as American Indians,[93,101] Blacks,[104,105] or Japanese.[102,106] Studies are needed to clarify the role of socio-economic conditions in the etiology of renal failure in diabetes.[107] Regarding this issue, there are two separate problems for consideration. First is the influence of race and socio-economic conditions on the incidence of new cases of proteinuria, and second, their influence on progression of proteinuria to renal failure and death. A factor which accelerates progression of established disease may have no role or a different role in the etiology of the disease. A possible example is suggested by the hypothesis that a high-protein diet accelerates progression of nephropathy to renal failure,[108] although the populations with a high or low prevalence of nephropathy in Tables 12–6 and 12–11 do not appear to be those with correspondingly high- or low-protein consumption.

Macroangiopathy. Coronary heart disease (CHD) and other large vessel diseases have long been observed clinically to occur earlier and with greater frequency in patients with diabetes than in the general population (see also Chapters 11 and 27). Over the years, considerable laboratory and epidemiologic evidence has accumulated to confirm this clinical impression (for an extensive review see ref. 109). In the discussion which follows, the major issues to be considered in research into the causes of excess cardiovascular disease in

adult-onset diabetes will be reviewed and highlighted with some basic descriptive data.

Evidence of an etiologic link between CHD and NIDDM is found in their aggregation within families. Patients with adult-onset NIDDM reported having a parent with CHD or hypertension more often than insulin-treated patients or non-diabetic controls.[110] In another study, children whose parents had heart attacks or diabetes were heavier and had different lipid and lipoprotein profiles than children without this background.[111] Significant interrelationships among variables such as blood glucose, blood pressure, lipids and obesity have also been demonstrated within individuals.[112–114] Another type of evidence for this link is the observation that patients with CHD[115] or peripheral vascular disease[116,117] had a higher risk of developing diabetes subsequently than individuals without vascular disease. The risk of developing NIDDM has also been shown to be related to blood pressure level.[115,116,118] These interrelationships suggest the existence of an earlier factor in the causal process which is common to all of these conditions. Obesity is one possible candidate since it predisposes to hypertension[118–122] and is a known risk factor for NIDDM (see Chapter 2). It has been postulated that hyperinsulinemia, which is characteristic of obesity and may precede the clinical onset of NIDDM,[67] can be responsible for the initiation of hypertension.[123,124] Moreover, large prospective studies have found that an elevated insulin level is a risk factor for CHD,[125–127] and it is postulated that hyperinsulinemia may be an independent risk factor for atherosclerosis.[128]

An implication of this discussion is that cardiovascular risk factors, as well as cardiovascular diseases, should be present in excess at the time of diagnosis of NIDDM. Confirmation of this can be seen in several population-based studies.[114,129–133]

After clinically manifest diabetes develops, risk factors for cardiovascular disease are further increased. Adult-onset diabetics typically have elevated cholesterol levels accompanied by other changes in lipid profiles (see ref. 134). Moreover, hyperglycemia itself may accelerate progression of atherosclerosis,[135] and some authors suggest that the microangiopathic complications promote the development of CHD and other large vessel complications.[136] Finally, the unknown factor(s) which protect non-diabetic women from CHD are overcome in diabetic women so that their risk of CHD is equal to, or greater than, that of men.

In view of these relationships between diabetes and CHD risk factors, an excess frequency of atherosclerotic complications in adult-onset diabetes is not unexpected. Incidence rates for coronary heart disease, atherosclerotic brain infarction, and peripheral vascular disease during 24 years of observation of the Framingham population are shown separately for diabetics and non-diabetics in Figure 12–13. Diabetic men as well as women had incidence rates for atherosclerotic complications several times higher than those for nondiabetics. In addition, diabetics may survive these events less well than nondiabetics. For example, diabetics have twice the mortality of nondiabetics during an episode of acute myocardial infarction.[137–140] A similar relationship may exist for survival following a stroke, but that event has not been investigated in diabetics as thoroughly as myocardial infarction.

Both the higher incidence rate for these events and their higher fatality have the effect of increasing the mortality rate for arteriosclerotic complications in diabetes. Mortality rates, then, can be considered as integrated indices of the two processes, high incidence and high case-fatality, and are useful for descriptive purposes.

Cumulative mortality rates are available from the study in progress at the Joslin Clinic on the pattern of survival in diabetes, mentioned previously in the description of mortality due to renal failure. Preliminary results for patients aged 40 to 54 at their first visit to the Joslin Clinic are shown in Figure 12–14. Cumulative mortality rates for all causes and for CHD, specifically, were computed using life table techniques, separately for patients who

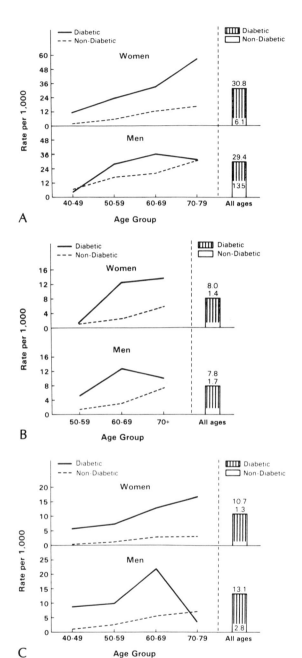

Fig. 12–13. Average annual incidence of coronary heart disease (panel A), atherothrombotic brain infarction (panel B) and peripheral vascular disease (panel C) in diabetics and non-diabetics during 24 years of observation of the Framingham Study Population according to age and sex. (Reproduced from ref. 133 with permission of the author and publisher)

came to the Joslin Clinic between 1923 and 1944 and for those who came between 1945 and 1960. In both groups, CHD accounted for most of the mortality, but it was significantly lower in the group with more recently diagnosed diabetes. When the trend in mortality rates was examined separately for men and women, the decline was found to have been mainly among men; that among women was small.[141] The trend for diabetic males was quite similar to that for CHD mortality among men in the general population, but the lack of a distinct trend among diabetic females does not agree with the trend for women in the general population where there has been a significant decline in CHD mortality for women as well as men.[142]

Other causes of death, represented by the vertical distance between the curves for CHD mortality and for mortality due to all causes, have also declined in the group with more recently diagnosed diabetes. To find out which causes were responsible for this decline, cause-specific mortality rates were calculated for each group and are shown in Table 12–9. Coma, tuberculosis, and stroke were eliminated or significantly reduced as causes of death in the group that came to the clinic after 1945.

To illustrate the magnitude of cardiovascular mortality in diabetes, CHD mortality for the group of patients who came to the clinic after 1945 was compared to the CHD mortality experienced by the Framingham Heart Study population (Table 12–10). Among males who were 40 to 54 years of age at the time of their first visit to the clinic, 42% were dead from CHD and 23% dead from other causes by age 70. Among nondiabetic individuals of similar age in Framingham, 23% were dead from CHD and 9% from other causes. Thus, only 35% of the diabetic men were alive while 68% of the Framingham men were alive. The differences for women were even more striking. Among females who were age 40 to 54 at the time of diagnosis of diabetes, 39% were dead from CHD and 16% from other causes by age 70. For nondiabetic women in Framingham the percentages were 10% for CHD and 8% for other causes. Thus, only 45% of the diabetic women were alive as compared to 82% in Framingham. Although many studies have shown an excess mortality due to CHD in diabetics relative to nondiabetics,[59,64–66,144] this observation in the Joslin Clinic population is the first with long enough follow-up to demonstrate so clearly the enormity of the excess, particularly among women. For them, CHD is the most important health problem.

In summary, cardiovascular diseases emerge as the major causes of premature mortality in NIDDM. There are at least three components contributing to the excess macroangiopathy seen in diabetics as compared to nondiabetics: (a) cardiovascular diseases are already present in excess at the time of diagnosis of diabetes; (b) the incidence rate of atherosclerotic diseases in diabetics is several times that found in nondiabetics; and (c) the probability of surviving once the disease is established is lower for diabetics than nondiabetics. In terms of mechanisms, aggregation of several risk factors for cardiovascular disease is already evident

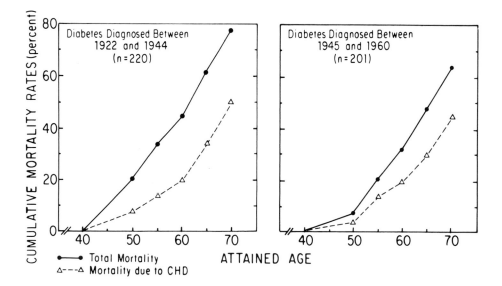

Fig. 12–14. Cumulative mortality rates for all causes and for CHD in patients with diabetes who came to the Joslin Clinic in two time periods: 1923–1944 and 1945–1960. (Data are for patients who were Massachusetts residents, aged 40 to 54 years and had diabetes diagnosed less than 5 years before first visit; ref. 103)

Table 12–9.   Cause-Specific Mortality Rates per 1000 Person-Years in Patients of the Joslin Clinic† According to Age at Death and Year of Diagnosis of Diabetes (Unpublished Joslin data, ref. 103)

Causes of Death	Mortality Rate before Age 65 Year of Diagnosis of Diabetes		Mortality Rate between Age 65 and 74 Year of Diagnosis of Diabetes	
	1923–1944	1945–1959	1923–1944	1945–1959
Coma	1.9	0	1.7	0
Tuberculosis	2.3	0	0	0
Other infections	1.5	1.2	6.7	6.0
Renal failure	1.9	2.3	5.0	3.0
Stroke	6.0	3.1	25.2	9.1
Coronary heart disease	19.2	17.3	65.5	54.5
Other vascular	1.5	1.2	3.4	3.0
Cancer	4.9	4.6	8.4	9.1
Other causes	4.1	3.5	1.7	7.6
All causes	43.3	33.2	117.6	93.9
Total Deaths	115	86	70	62
Person years	2655	2595	595	660

†A systematic sample of patients who were Massachusetts residents, came to the clinic in the period 1923–1944 (N = 220) or 1945–1960 (N = 201), were aged 40 to 54 and had diabetes diagnosed less than 5 years before first visit. The sample was followed until 1977.

Table 12–10.   Cumulative Mortality by Age 70 (%) in Patients of the Joslin Clinic and in the Framingham Population. (Adapted from ref. 143 and unpublished Joslin data, ref. 103)

Status by Age 70		Joslin Population†	General Population‡
MALES			
	Dead due to:		
	CHD	44	25
	Other causes	24	12
	Alive	32	63
	Total	100	100
		(n = 104)	(n = 1153)
FEMALES			
	Dead due to:		
	CHD	42	12
	Other causes	18	9
	Alive	40	79
	Total	100	100
		(n = 97)	(n = 1394)

†A representative sample of patients who were Massachusetts residents, came to the clinic in the period 1945–1960, were aged 40–54 and had diabetes diagnosed less than 5 years before first visit. The sample was followed until 1977.
‡A random sample of Framingham population aged 40 to 54 followed from 1949 to 1973.

in NIDDM even at the time of diagnosis of diabetes. Once diabetes is established, the levels of risk factors increase and perhaps interact with some unknown diabetic factor(s) to augment their effect in ways as yet unknown. From this perspective on the problem of arteriosclerosis in diabetes, the recently published findings of the WHO Multinational Study on Vascular Diseases in Diabetes are particularly interesting. If diabetic factors are of major importance, then similar frequencies of arterial disease would be expected in diabetics regardless of their country of origin, yet the prevalence rates of macrovascular complications in the centers participating in that study varied widely.[63,145] Since these data are from cross-sectional studies in each country, one must consider

them as preliminary. Also, one should recall that the major impact of diabetes on the risk of cardiovascular disease appeared to occur long after the onset of diabetes. Most of the WHO study patients had diabetes of short duration and the vascular conditions which they manifested may reflect the frequency of vascular disease in the source populations rather than the impact of diabetes.

PROGNOSIS IN DIABETES MELLITUS

The last issue for consideration regarding the natural history of diabetes is prognosis: How does diabetes affect longevity? The discussion in the preceding section of specific causes of mortality (acute complications, renal failure, and coronary artery disease) is useful for studying the pathogenesis of complications, but it presents a fragmentary, incomplete picture of prognosis. From a pragmatic viewpoint, the age at death is the primary fact of interest, and the specific cause a secondary concern. Furthermore, there are technical difficulties with cause-specific mortality. Ideas about causation of death are arbitrary in many instances and are influenced by observer biases and changing criteria. In contrast, deaths from all causes combined are rarely a matter for dispute.

Comparisons will be made with general population data, so a brief review of the pattern of survival in the general population is useful at this point. After high mortality during the first year of life, the proportion surviving remains almost constant until about age 35 for men and age 40 for women, at which time rising mortality rates again equal and then surpass the level characteristic of the first year of life. In each decade thereafter, survival declines progressively more rapidly so that half of the men remain alive at age 72, and half of the women at age 80. The age at which half of a population is still alive is called the *median survival age,* or equivalently, median age at death. In a sense, median survival age can be thought of as the "typical" age at death and, as such, is a useful benchmark for comparisons. A statistic frequently quoted for populations is the "expectation of life." While median survival age is not precisely the same, it has the same interpretation as "expectation of life," and is readily obtainable from the type of follow-up study to be described in the following paragraphs if the follow-up interval is long enough. In assessing prognosis, examination of the whole survival curve is more informative than any single summary figure, but when brevity is essential, median survival age is a reasonable substitute.

A standard technique for examining survival patterns in chronic diseases is life table analysis,[146] which yields the proportion of a population with the disease who survive at each anniversary after the diagnosis. Diabetes may be diagnosed at any age, and the prognosis can be expected to depend very much on the age at diagnosis, just as prognosis in the general population depends on age. In order to see the influence of age, it is useful to examine survival according to attained age as well as duration of diabetes. This requires calculating survival in subgroups with the same age at diagnosis. For the figures which follow, age at diagnosis was grouped into 20-year intervals to simplify presentation. This was achieved by modifying the life table technique so that those diagnosed later than the start of the interval did not enter the calculations until their actual age at diagnosis.

Each figure includes a survival curve based on the 1950 United States life table for whites of the same sex and starting age for the particular range of onset ages.[147] Since the deaths in the studies to be described took place during 6 decades, the specific magnitude of a difference between a diabetic group and this single standard for the general population does not have a literal interpretation. Rather, it is the pattern of differences between specific age groups and the single standard which is of interest.

Diabetes Diagnosed Before Age 30

Diabetes which is clinically manifest before the age of 30 is predominantly insulin-dependent or Type I. Valid studies of prognosis in IDDM have been few. However, there have been a number of other types of studies which yield statistics which the unwary might mistakenly believe relate to prognosis. Unfortunately, the statistics that they yield give an unjustifiably grim impression about survival after the diagnosis of diabetes. Therefore, it is important to point out the misinterpretation of these statistics.

One type of study has been that of deceased patients. In these studies, the average duration of diabetes was calculated for the deceased, and that statistic used to examine time trends or age differences. Under the circumstances that existed before insulin became available, most patients with IDDM died within 2 years, and the average duration of diabetes for deceased patients was a reasonable representation of their prognosis. Once insulin became available, however, most of these young patients survived for decades. Under this new set of circumstances, the deceased were a minority and their duration of diabetes no longer represented the whole group. All of the years of duration experienced by the survivors, and all of the years that they will experience before they die were not included in the average duration for the deceased.

The second type of statistic which can be misleading is the standardized mortality ratio (SMR) which is simply the number of deaths observed in a population divided by the number of deaths expected in that population if it had experienced the mortality rates of the general population. Unlike the previous case, the SMR is legitimate for certain purposes, e.g., testing whether there are excess deaths in a study population. However, it is not useful as a descriptive statistic because, in general, comparisons cannot be made among SMRs. The reasons are technical and will not be discussed here; it is sufficient to say that an SMR of 300% does not necessarily imply poorer survival than an SMR of 150%. Another difficulty wth SMRs is well illustrated by mortality studies among young diabetics in which it gives the impression that a large number of deaths occur before the age of 40. As pointed out earlier, general population mortality rates between ages 5 and 40 are low. Studies of diabetics in this age range give SMRs of 300 to 500% even though few diabetics die at these ages. The problem arises because even a small number of deaths is a large percentage increase over the tiny number of deaths expected in the general population at these ages. One can avoid being misled by an SMR by examining the magnitude of the difference between the observed and expected numbers of deaths as well as the ratio.

The most straightforward method for studying prognosis is to identify a cohort of all newly diagnosed patients from some period in the past and then trace all of them to determine who has died and who remains alive. Alternative approaches are available but they will give incorrect results if there has been a change in prognosis over time, and they are more vulnerable to selection biases than the cohort approach.

A cohort study of patients who first visited the Joslin Clinic between 1923 and 1960 is being conducted to determine the pattern of survival in diabetes.[103] Preliminary data are available for follow-up through 1977, giving a minimum follow-up interval of 27 years and a maximum of 55 years. From previous studies at the Joslin Diabetes Center,[37,61] it is known that there is little excess mortality during the first 25 years of diabetes among those with onset before age 20. The explanation for this is evident from the data regarding complications presented in the preceding section. The fatal complications, renal failure and coronary heart disease, appear in number only after age 35, regardless of whether diabetes was diagnosed at age 9 or 19. Therefore, survival is examined here in terms of attained age rather than duration of diabetes so that the pattern of these significant events is more clearly presented.

Survival according to attained age for those with onset before age 30 is shown in Figure 12–15 for females and males separately. While few deaths had occurred by age 25, diabetic survival was already appreciably below that of the general population by age 30, and after age 35 diabetic survival decreased rapidly so that survival at age 50 was only 52% for women and 46% for men. Starting from age 10 in the general population, 93% of women and 91% of men survived to age 50. Although the diabetic women were not followed long enough to observe the median survival age, it appears unlikely that it would be more than 52 years for this study sample. Median survival age for women in the general population surviving from age 10 was 77 years; thus, typical survival for diabetic women was about 25 years less than that

for the general population. Median survival age for diabetic males was 47 as compared to 71 for the males in the general population. In terms of the number of years lost, relative to the general population, the impact of diabetes was enormous. A particularly notable result was that the survival curves for the two sexes were almost identical. The survival advantage seen for women in the general population was greatly diminished in this diabetic population.

An additional aspect of this study was the possibility to examine changes in survival pattern over time. For this purpose, the group was divided into those diagnosed in years 1922 to 1944 and those diagnosed 1945 to 1960. Since the survival patterns were the same for the two sexes, they have been combined to avoid small numbers. In the pre-1945 period, 58% of the patients survived to age 40 and the median survival age was 44, whereas in the post-1945 period, 80% survived to age 40 and the follow-up period was too short to determine median survival age. The explanation for this substantial improvement is not clear. As expected, deaths due

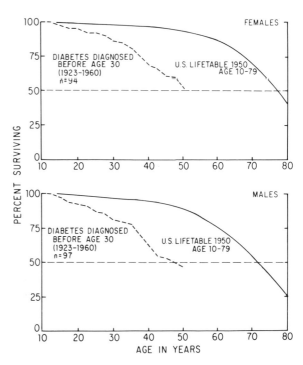

Fig. 12–15. Prognosis in diabetes diagnosed before age 30: Cumulative survival rates according to sex and attained age in comparison with sex specific survival rates from age 10 to 79 in the general population, based on the United States Life Table for 1950 for whites. Patients were white residents of Massachusetts first seen at the Joslin Clinic between 1923 and 1960, with a duration of diabetes less than 5 years at the time of first visit. Follow up was to 1977. (Unpublished data of the Joslin Clinic; ref. 103)

to the acute complications and infections were virtually eliminated, but their disappearance is insufficient to explain the magnitude of improvement which occurred. As noted in the previous section, there has been some decline in deaths due to renal failure as well. However, when renal deaths were also eliminated in the calculation of survival rates, those diagnosed after 1945 still showed significantly better survival than the pre-1945 cohort.

There have been only two other studies with long-term follow-up of young diabetics. One was the study by Knowles in Cincinnati[56,57] and the most recent report was a Danish study.[60] Since neither of these studies followed cohorts of patients from the diagnosis of diabetes, selection bias could have affected the findings. While this may not have been a significant issue in the Cincinnati study since most patients were identified soon after age 15, one cannot assess the impact of this bias on the results of the Danish study since the patients were ascertained at many ages, often long after the diagnosis of diabetes.

Diabetes Diagnosed After Age 30

Diabetes occurring after age 30 is typically less difficult to manage than diabetes with onset in youth, but the prognosis is not necessarily correspondingly better. The Diabetes Natural History Study, conducted at the Joslin Clinic in the early 1960s, traced patients from the diagnosis of diabetes in 5 time periods (1939, 1944, 1949, 1954 and 1959) through 1963.[38] Life table methods were then used to calculate survival rates according to age at diagnosis. The 25-year survival rates were found to decrease as age at diagnosis increased.

The following figures are the result of a new analysis of the data from the Natural History Study. Survival of these patients in terms of duration of diabetes is presented separately for females and males in Figure 12–16. In these figures, patients have been grouped according to age at diagnosis of diabetes in 20-year intervals, beginning with age 30 instead of age 20 as in the earlier publication. There is a clear pattern of progressively poorer prognosis as age at diagnosis increases. This indicates that the effects of diabetes on survival are not strong enough to overwhelm the significant effect of age itself on prognosis. A detailed comparison of the figures for males and females shows that the survival patterns for the two sexes are nearly identical. A similar lack of a sex difference in prognosis was observed in insulin-dependent diabetes and is strikingly different from the large sex difference seen in the general population. Hypotheses about the pathogenetic mechanisms leading to premature death in diabetes must include a specific interaction of diabetes with whatever fac-

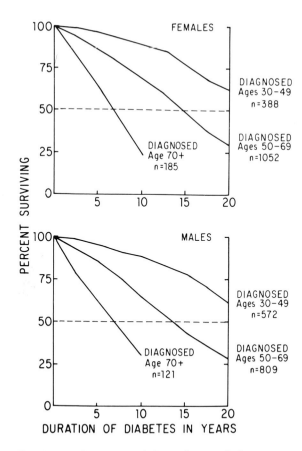

Fig. 12–16. Prognosis in diabetes diagnosed after age 30: Cumulative survival rates according to sex, age at diagnosis of diabetes and duration of diabetes. Patients were white residents of Massachusetts first seen in 1939, 1944, 1949 and 1959 within 1 year of diagnosis and followed to 1963. (Reanalysis of data in ref. 38)

tors are responsible for greater longevity in nondiabetic women.

The interaction of diabetes with aging processes can be seen more clearly if survival is plotted against attained age as was done in the figures for diabetes diagnosed before age 30. In panel A of Figure 12–17, survival of patients diagnosed between ages 30 and 49 is shown separately for females and males. Sex-specific survival for the United States white population for the comparable ages is again shown for comparison. For males there was no excess mortality until after age 50, but for females there was a noticeable excess mortality before age 45. None of these deaths among women was directly related to pregnancy or childbirth, and the significance of this finding remains uncertain. After age 50, survival for both sexes declined rapidly so that median survival was reached at age 65 for women and 66 for men. This is 12 years earlier than the general population for

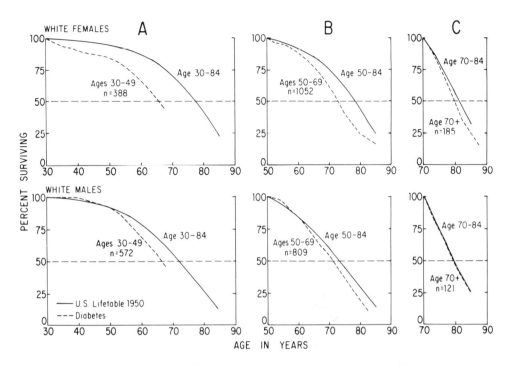

Fig. 12–17. Prognosis in diabetes diagnosed after age 30: Cumulative survival rates according to sex, age at diagnosis of diabetes and attained age in comparison with age and sex specific survival rates in the general population, based on the United States Life Table for 1950 for whites. The patient sample was the same as described for Figure 12–16. (Reanalysis of data in ref. 38)
Panel A: Diabetes diagnosed between ages 30 and 49.
Panel B: Diabetes diagnosed between ages 50 and 69.
Panel C: Diabetes diagnosed after age 70.

women and 5 years earlier for men. This difference is due to different survival patterns for the two sexes in the general population used for comparison; for diabetics there was no sex difference after age 50.

Figure 12–17, panel B, presents similar data for patients diagnosed between ages 50 and 69. Diabetic females reached median survival age by age 72, 5 years before females in the general population while diabetic males reached median survival by 71, only 2 years before males in the general population.

Figure 12–17, panel C, shows that median survival for female diabetics diagnosed after age 70 was only 2 years younger than the general population, while for males, there was no difference between the survival of diabetics and the general population.

In summary, survival for the two sexes was similar, but since women in the general population survived longer than males, this represented a greater impact of diabetes on women than men. In both sexes, the reduction in median survival age associated with diabetes diminished steadily with increasing age at diagnosis.

In order to determine whether there has been any change in survival over time, the data of the previously described study of the pattern of survival were examined for these same age groups. Median survival ages for those diagnosed after 1945 were only slightly greater than those diagnosed before 1945 (4 years for those 30 to 49 at diagnosis, 3 years for those 50 to 69, and 2 years for those over 70). These were small changes in comparison with those seen for patients with onset before age 30.

Data from survival studies of adult diabetics were compiled by Entmacher in 1976.[148] Unfortunately, the data available at that time do not permit useful comparisons with the data of the Joslin Clinic because the survival rates have not been calculated separately according to age at diagnosis. Subsequently, three studies have been published, and while the follow-up intervals were short, their findings do permit interesting comparisons with the data of the Joslin Clinic. Two from Europe are population-based. One presents 5- and 8-year survival rates for all diabetics (age 30 to 69) in Warsaw, Poland, diagnosed between 1963 and 1970.[64] Age at diagnosis was grouped in 10-year intervals, and the survival rates were almost identical to the

Joslin Clinic results except for better survival among women diagnosed after age 50 in Warsaw (87.4% at 8 years as compared to 77.9%). The second reports 10-year survival rates for all diabetics (age 40–79) diagnosed in 1966 in the Urfurt District of the German Democratic Republic.[149] The rates for women were almost identical to the earlier data from the Joslin Clinic, but survival rates for men diagnosed after age 50 were worse (53.6% as compared to 64.5%). The University Group Diabetes Program (UGDP) recently published 13-year survival rates for three of the treatment groups followed in that study from 1961 to 1975.[90] Because of the nature of that clinical trial, insulin-requiring patients were excluded. For the three groups combined, survival rates were 76.2% for women and 66.3% for men. These rates are 8% higher for women and 5% higher for men than the rates from the Joslin Clinic adjusted to the age distribution of the total UGDP population. There were differences among these studies with regard to diagnostic criteria, age distribution, race, time of study, the management of diabetes, as well as many other factors.

None of these recent studies had a follow-up interval long enough to obtain a complete picture of overall survival. Even 13 years is not sufficient to observe the majority of deaths in the study group except in the oldest age categories, where the impact of diabetes on longevity is least. The comparisons might tell quite a different story once the majority of deaths have occurred. Also, presentation of survival rates in terms of attained age rather than duration of diabetes might be more discriminating in detecting differences in survival pattern.

Interpopulation comparisons are a valuable epidemiologic strategy for gaining knowledge of the relative contributions of environmental and genetic factors affecting survival in diabetes. In particular they provide a unique opportunity for the study of the pathogenesis of fatal complications such as renal failure and cardiovascular disease. The extent to which the impact of these complications on diabetic populations varies in parallel with renal and vascular disease in the corresponding nondiabetic populations is an indication of the contribution of population characteristics relative to that of the metabolic disturbances of diabetes. Concurrent studies using a common protocol are needed to acquire informative interpopulation comparisons. Equally important is the requirement that the follow-up interval be long enough to observe a substantial portion of the deaths in the study groups rather than merely the early deaths. Only then can the importance of various factors be assessed.

REFERENCES

1. MacMahon, B., Pugh, T.F.: Epidemiology, Principles and Methods. Boston, Little, Brown & Co., 1970, pp. 1–16 and 103–300.
2. Deibert, D.C., DeFronzo, R.A.: Epinephrine-induced insulin resistance in man. J. Clin. Invest. 65:717, 1980.
3. MacGorman, L.R., Rizza, R.A., Gerich, J.E.: Physiological concentrations of growth hormone exert insulin-like and insulin antagonistic effects on both hepatic and extrahepatic tissues in men. J. Clin. Endocrinol. Metab. 53:556, 1981.
4. Rizza, R., Mandarino, L., Westland, R., et al.: Growth hormone induced insulin resistance in man; postreceptor impairment in hepatic and peripheral tissue sensitivity to insulin. Diabetes 30 (Suppl. 1):10A, 1981.
5. Danowski, T.S.: Diabetes Mellitus with Emphasis on Children and Young Adults. Baltimore, Williams & Wilkins, 1957, pp. 126–142.
6. Knowles, H.C., Jr., Guest, G.M., Lampe, J., et al.: The course of juvenile diabetes treated with unmeasured diet. Diabetes 14:239, 1965.
7. White, P., Graham, C.A.: The child with diabetes. In: A. Marble, P. White, R.F. Bradley and L.P. Krall (eds.): Joslin's Diabetes Mellitus. 11th ed., Philadelphia, Lea & Febiger, 1971, pp. 339–360.
8. Krolewski, A.S., Warram, J.H., Christlieb, A.R., et al.: Is diabetic microangiopathy a homogenous entity? An epidemiological observation of three inception cohorts of juvenile onset insulin dependent diabetics for 20–40 years. (Unpublished manuscript).
9. Block, M.B., Rosenfield, R.L., Mako, M.E., et al.: Sequential changes in beta-cell function in insulin treated diabetic patients assessed by C-peptide immunoreactivity. N. Eng. J. Med. 288:1144, 1973.
10. Ludvigsson, J., Heding, L.G.: Beta-cell function in children with diabetes. Diabetes 27 (Suppl. 1):230, 1978.
11. Mirel, R.D., Ginsberg-Fellner, F., Horwitz, D.L., et al.: C-peptide reserve in insulin-dependent diabetes. Comparative responses to glucose, glucagon and tolbutamide. Diabetologia 19:183, 1980.
12. Heding, L.G., Ludvigsson, J., Kasperska-Czyzykowa, T.: B-cell secretion in non-diabetics and insulin-dependent diabetics. Acta Med. Scand. Suppl. 656:5, 1981.
13. Rjasanowski, I., Michaelis, D., Besch, W.: Follow-up study of C-peptide secretion in newly diagnosed diabetic children. Diabetologia 23:196, 1982. (Abstr.).
14. Madsbad, S.: Prevalence of residual B cell function and its metabolic consequences in type 1 (insulin-dependent) diabetes. Diabetologia 24:141, 1983.
15. Christau, B., Molbak, A.G.: Incidence of insulin dependent diabetes mellitus in groups older than 30 years. Abstract presented at 16th Annual Meeting of European Diabetes Epidemiology Study Group, 1981, Vesegrad, Hungary. See also Diabetologia 23:160, 1982.
16. Milton, L.J., Palumbo, P.J., Chu, C.: Incidence of diabetes mellitus by clinical type. Diabetes Care 6:75, 1983.
17. Faber, O.K., Binder, C.: B-cell function and blood glucose control in insulin dependent diabetics within the first month of insulin treatment. Diabetologia 13:263, 1977.
18. Hendriksen, C., Faber, O.K., Drejer, J., et al.: Prevalence of residual B-cell function in insulin treated diabetics evaluated by the plasma C-peptide response to intravenous glucagon. Diabetologia 13:615, 1977.
19. Madsbad, S., Faber, K.O., Binder, C., et al.: Prevalence of residual beta-cell function in insulin dependent diabetics in relation to age at onset and duration of diabetes. Diabetes 27 (Suppl. 1):262, 1978.
20. Garcia-Webb, P., Bonser, A., Welborn, T.A.: Correlation between fasting serum C-peptide and B cell insulin secretory capacity in diabetes mellitus. Diabetologia 22:296, 1982.
21. Kanarek, P.H.: Investigation of an exponential model for assessing survival in diabetic population. Doctoral dissertation. Harvard University, Cambridge, 1973.
22. Kanarek, P.H., Balodimos, M.C., Marble, A.: Survival and causes of death among diabetic patients treated with

insulin, tolbutamide, or diet alone. Unpublished manuscript.

23. Gamble, D.R.: Seed and soil; infection and susceptibility. In: H. Keen, J.C. Pickup and C.V. Talwalkar (eds.): Epidemiology of Diabetes and Its Vascular Complications. Proceedings of Satellite Meeting of IXth IDF Meeting, Bombay 1976, London, International Diabetes Federation, 1978, pp. 15–18.

24. Gray, R.S., Duncan, L.J.P., Clark, B.F.: Seasonal onset of insulin dependent diabetes in relation to sex and age at onset. Diabetologia 17:29, 1979.

25. Cannell, C.F., Marquis, K.H., Laurent, A.: A summary of studies of interviewing methodology. National Center for Health Statistics. Series 2, No. 69, U.S. DHEW Publication No. (HRA) 77-1343, 1977.

26. Steel, J.M., Gray, R.S., Clarke, B.F.: Obstetric history of diabetes: its relevance to the aetiology of diabetes. Br. Med. J. 1:1303, 1979.

27. Rosenbloom, A.L., Hunt, S.S., Rosenbloom, E.K., et al.: Ten-year prognosis of impaired glucose tolerance in siblings of patients with insulin-dependent diabetes. Diabetes 31:385, 1982.

28. Gorsuch, A.N., Spencer, K.M., Lister, J., et al.: Evidence for a long prediabetic period in Type I (insulin dependent) diabetes mellitus. Lancet 2:1363, 1981.

29. Betterle, C., Zanette, F., Tiengo, A., et al.: Five year follow-up of non-diabetes with islet cell antibodies. Lancet 1:284, 1982.

30. Srikanta, S., Ganda, O.P., Eisenbarth, G.S., Soeldner, J.S.: Islet cell antibodies and beta-cell function in monozygotic triplets and twins initially discordant for type I diabetes mellitus. N. Engl. J. Med. 308:322, 1983.

31. Krolewski, A.S., Warram, J.H., Christlieb, A.R.: Evidence of heterogeneity of IDDM based on the follow-up of untreated cases. Diabetes 33 (Suppl. 1): 92A, 1984.

32. Park, B.N., Soeldner, J.S., Gleason, R.E.: Diabetes in remission. Insulin secretory dynamics. Diabetes 23:616, 1974.

33. Heinze, E., Beischner, W., Keller, L., et al.: C-peptide secretion during the remission phase of juvenile diabetes. Diabetes 27:670, 1978.

34. DeFronzo, R.A., Hendler, R., Simonson, D.: Insulin resistance is a prominent feature of insulin-dependent diabetes. Diabetes 31:795, 1982.

35. DeFronzo, R.A., Ferrannini, E.: Influence of plasma glucose and insulin concentration on plasma glucose clearance in man. Diabetes 31:683, 1982.

36. Clark, A., Bown, E., King, T., et al.: Islet changes induced by hyperglycemia in rats. Effect of insulin or chlorpropamide therapy. Diabetes 31:319, 1982.

37. Christlieb, A.R., Warram, J.H., Krolewski, A.S., et al.: Hypertension: The major risk factor in juvenile-onset insulin-dependent diabetics. Diabetes 30 (Suppl. 2):90, 1981.

38. Hirohata, T., MacMahon, B., Root, H.F.: The natural history of diabetes. I. Mortality. Diabetes 16:875, 1967.

39. Root, H.F., Gorman, C.K., Szabo, A.J., et al.: The natural history of diabetes. II. Morbidity due to micro and macrovascular complications. Unpublished data.

40. Johnson, D.D., Palumbo, P.J., Chu, Ch.: Diabetic ketoacidosis in a community-based population. Mayo Clin. Proc. 55:83, 1980.

41. Faich, G.A., Fishbein, H.A., Ellis, S.E.: The epidemiology of diabetic acidosis: A population-based study. Am. J. Epidemiol. 117:551, 1983.

42. Gottlieb, M.S.: Diabetes in offspring and siblings of juvenile and maturity-onset type diabetics. J. Chron. Dis. 33:331, 1980.

43. Malone, J.I., Hellrung, J.M., Malphus, E.W., et al.: Good diabetic control—a study in mass delusion. J. Pediatr. 88:943, 1976.

44. Goldstein, D.E., Walker, B., Rawlings, S.S., et al.: Hemoglobin Alc levels in children and adolescents with diabetes mellitus. Diabetes Care 3:503, 1980.

45. West, K.M., Ahuja, M.M.S., Bennett, P.H., et al.: Interrelationship of microangiopathy, plasma glucose and other risk factors in 3583 diabetic patients: A multinational study. Diabetologia 22:412, 1982.

46. Blackwell, B.: Drug therapy: patient compliance. N. Engl. J. Med. 289:249, 1973.

47. Becker, M.H.: Understanding patient compliance: the contributions of attitudes and other psychosocial factors. In: S.J. Cohen (ed.): New Directions in Patient Compliance. Lexington, D.C. Heath and Company, 1979, pp. 1–31.

48. Millard, E.B., Root, H.F.: Degenerative vascular lesions and diabetes mellitus. Am. J. Dig. Dis. 15:41, 1948.

49. Mann, G.V., Gardner, C., Root, H.F.: Clinical manifestations of intercapillary glomerulosclerosis in diabetes mellitus. Am. J. Med. 7:3, 1949.

50. Root, H.F., Sinden, R.H., Zanca, R.: Factors in the rate of development of vascular lesions in the kidneys, retinae and peripheral vessels of the youthful diabetic. Am. J. Dig. Dis. 17:179, 1950.

51. Keiding, N., Root, H.F., Marble, A.: Importance of control of diabetes in prevention of vascular complications. J.A.M.A. 150:964, 1952.

52. White, P.: Natural course and prognosis of juvenile diabetes. Diabetes 5:445, 1956.

53. White, P.: Childhood diabetes. Its course and influence on second and third generations. Diabetes 9:345, 1960.

54. Paz-Guevara, A.T., Tah-Hsiung, White, P.: Juvenile diabetes mellitus after forty years. Diabetes 24:559, 1975.

55. Palmberg, P., Smith, M., Waltman, S., et al.: The natural history of retinopathy in insulin dependent juvenile-onset diabetes. Ophthalmology 88:613, 1981.

56. Knowles, H.C., Jr.: Long term juvenile diabetes mellitus and unmeasured diet. In: R.R. Rodriguez and J. Vallance-Owen (eds.): Diabetes. Proceedings of the 7th Congress of IDF, Buenos Aires, 1970, Amsterdam, Excerpta Medica, 1971, pp. 209–215.

57. Knowles, H.C., Jr.: Long term juvenile diabetes treated with unmeasured diet. Trans. Assoc. Am. Phys. 84:95, 1971.

58. Lestradet, H., Papoz, L., DeMenibus, Cl.H., et al.: Long-term study of mortality and vascular complications in juvenile-onset (Type I) diabetes. Diabetes 30:175, 1981.

59. Marks, H.H., Krall, L.P.: Onset, course, prognosis and mortality in diabetes mellitus. In: A. Marble, P. White, R.F. Bradley and L.P. Krall (eds.): Joslin's Diabetes Mellitus. 11th ed., Philadelphia, Lea & Febiger, 1971, pp. 209–254.

60. Deckert, T., Poulsen, J.E., Larsen, M.: Prognosis of diabetics with diabetes onset before the age of thirty-one. I. Survival, causes of death, and complicatons. Diabetologia, 14:363, 1978.

61. Krolewski, A.S., Warram, J.H., Christlieb, A.R., et al.: The changing natural history of nephropathy in type I diabetes. Submitted for publication.

62. Report of the WHO Multinational Study of Vascular Disease in Diabetics; based upon the meeting of investigators held in Bern, Switzerland, 3–8 September 1979. Geneva, World Health Organization, NCD/OND/79.4.

63. The World Health Organization Multinational Study of Vascular Disease in Diabetics: Prevalence of small vessel and large vessel disease in diabetic patients from fourteen centers. Submitted for publication.

64. Krolewski, A.S., Czyzyk, A., Janeczko, D., et al.: Mortality from cardiovascular disease among diabetics. Diabetologia 13:345, 1977.

65. Garcia, M.J., McNamara, P.M., Gordon, T., et al.: Morbidity and mortality in diabetics in the Framingham population. Sixteen year follow-up study. Diabetes 23:105, 1974.

66. Shenfield, G.M., Elton, R.A., Bhalla, I.P., et al.: Dia-

betic mortality in Edinburgh. Diabete Metab. 5:149, 1979.

67. DeFronzo, R.A., Ferrannini, E., Koivisto, V.: New concepts in the pathogenesis and treatment of noninsulin-dependent diabetes mellitus. Am. J. Med. 74(Jan. Suppl.):52, 1983.

68. Conn, J.W., Fajans, S.S.: The prediabetic state. Am. J. Med. 31:839, 1961.

69. O'Sullivan, J.B., Mahan, C.M.: Prospective study of 352 young patients with chemical diabetes. N. Engl. J. Med. 278:1038, 1968.

70. Fitzgerald, M.G., Malins, J.: Ten year follow-up report on the Birmingham Diabetes Survey of 1961. Br. Med. J. 2:35, 1976.

71. Jarrett, R.J., Keen, H., Fuller, J.H., et al.: Worsening to diabetes in men with impaired glucose tolerance. Diabetologia 16:25, 1979.

72. Sartor, G., Schersten, B., Carlstrom, S., et al.: Ten year follow-up of subjects with impaired glucose tolerance. Prevention of diabetes by tolbutamide and diet regulation. Diabetes 29:41, 1980.

73. Keen, H., Jarrett, R.J., McCartney, P.: The ten year follow-up of the Bedford Survey (1962–1972); glucose tolerance and diabetes. Diabetologia 22:73, 1982.

74. Tanaka, S., Fujii, S., Seki, J., et al.: Longitudinal study of chemical diabetes in an urban population in Japan. In: J.S. Melish, J. Hanna, S. Baba (eds.): Genetic Environmental Interaction in Diabetes Mellitus. Amsterdam, Excerpta Medica, 1982, pp. 64–69.

75. Diabetes Survey Working Party: A diabetes survey. Br. Med. J. 1:1497, 1962.

76. Munke, A.: A mass survey to trace previously unknown diabetes mellitus. A preliminary report. Acta Med. Scand. 176:169, 1964.

77. Brandt, L., Norden, A., Schersten, B., et al.: A diabetes detection campaign in Southern Sweden: Results of 69,000 examinations. Acta Med. Scand. 176:555, 1964.

78. Palumbo, P.J., Labarth, D.R.: The incidence of diabetes mellitus in Rochester, Minnesota, 1945–1969. In: R. Levine and R. Luft (eds): Advances in Metabolic Disorders. New York, Academic Press, 1978, pp. 13–28.

79. National Diabetes Data Group: Classification and diagnosis of diabetes mellitus and other categories of glucose intolerance. Diabetes 28:1039, 1979.

80. Manservigi, D., Samori, G., Graziani, R., et al.: Impaired glucose tolerance and clinical diabetes: A 6-year follow-up of screened versus non-screened subjects. Diabetologia 23:185, 1982.

81. Hadden, D.R., Montgomery, D.A.D., Skelly, R.J., et al.: Maturity-onset diabetes mellitus: response to intensive dietary management. Br. Med. J. 3:376, 1975.

82. Doar, J.W.H., Thompson, M.E., Wilde, C.E., et al.: Influence of treatment with diet alone on oral glucose-tolerance test and plasma sugar and insulin levels in patients with maturity onset diabetes mellitus. Lancet 1:1263, 1975.

83. Perkins, J.R., West, T.E.T., Sönksen, D.H., et al.: The effects of energy and carbohydrate restriction in patients with chronic diabetes mellitus. Diabetologia 13:607, 1977.

84. Savage, P.J., Bennion, L.H., Flock, E.V., et al.: Diet-induced improvement of abnormalities in insulin and glucagon secretion and in insulin receptor binding in diabetes mellitus. J. Clin. Endocrinol. Metab. 48:999, 1979.

85. Savage, P.J., Bennion, L.J., Bennet, P.H.: Normalization of insulin and glucagon secretion in ketosis-resistant diabetes mellitus with prolonged diet therapy. J. Clin. Endocrinol. Metab. 49:830, 1979.

86. Stanik, S., Marcus, R.: Insulin secretion improves following dietary control of plasma glucose in severely hyperglycemic obese patients. Metabolism 29:346, 1980.

87. Beck-Nielsen, H., Pederson, O., Sorensen, N.S.: Effects of dietary changes on cellular insulin binding and in vivo insulin sensitivity. Metabolism 29:482, 1980.

88. Pirart, J., Lavaux, J.P.: Remission in diabetes. In: E.F. Pfeiffer (ed.): Handbook of Diabetes Mellitus. vol. II, Munich, J. Lehmann, 1971, pp. 443–502.

89. Klimt, C.R., Knatterud, G.L., Meinert, C.L., Prout, T.E.: The University Group Diabetes Program: A study of the effects of hypoglycemic agents on vascular complications in patients with adult-onset diabetes. I. Design, methods and baseline characteristics. Diabetes 19 (Suppl. 2):747, 1970.

90. Knatterud, G.L., Klimt, C.R., Goldner, M.G., et al.: The University Group Diabetes Program. Effects of hypoglycemic agents on vascular complications with adult-onset diabetes. VIII. Evaluation of insulin therapy: Final report. Diabetes 31 (Suppl. 5):1, 1982.

91. Irvine, W.J., Sawers, J.S.A., Feek, C.M., et al.: The value of islet-cell antibody in predicting secondary failure of oral hypoglycemic agent therapy in diabetes mellitus. J. Clin. Lab. Immunol. 2:23, 1979.

92. Skyler, J.S. (Editorial): Type II diabetes: toward improved understanding and rational therapy. Diabetes Care 5:447, 1982.

93. West, K.M., Erdreich, L.J., Stober, J.A.: A detailed study of risk factors for retinopathy and nephropathy in diabetes. Diabetes 29:501, 1980.

94. Leibowitz, The Framingham Eye Study. V. Diabetic retinopathy. Surv. Ophthalmol. 24: (Suppl. May-June) 401, 1980.

95. Mitchell, P.: The prevalence of diabetic retinopathy: A study of 1300 diabetics from Newcastle and the Hunter Valley. Aust. J. Ophthalmol. 8:241, 1980.

96. Jarrett, R.J., Keen, H.: Hyperglycemia and diabetes mellitus. Lancet 2:1009, 1976.

97. Al Sayegh, H., Jarrett, R.J.: Oral glucose tolerance tests and the diagnosis of diabetes. Results of a prospective study based on the Whitehall Survey. Lancet 2:431, 1979.

98. Pettitt, D.J., Knowler, W.C., Lisse, J.R., et al.: Development of retinopathy and proteinuria in relation to plasma glucose concentrations in Pima Indians. Lancet 2:1050, 1980.

99. Miki, E., Fukuda, M., Kuzuya, T., et al.: Relation of the course of retinopathy to control of diabetes, age, and therapeutic agents in diabetic Japanese patients. Diabetes 18:773, 1969.

100. Aiello, L.M., Rand, L.I., Briones, J.C., et al.: Diabetic retinopathy in Joslin Clinic patients with adult-onset diabetes. Ophthalmology 88:619, 1981.

101. Kamenetzky, S.A., Bennett, P.H., Dippe, S.E., et al.: A clinical and histologic study of diabetic nephropathy in the Pima Indians. Diabetes 23:61, 1974.

102. Miki, E., Kuzuya, T., Ide, T., et al.: Frequency, degree, and progression with time of proteinuria in diabetic patients. Lancet 1:922, 1972.

103. Warram, J.H., Marble, A., Krolewski, A.S.: Pattern of survival in patients with diabetes mellitus diagnosed after 1922. Unpublished data.

104. Easterling, R.E.: Racial factors in the incidence and causation of end-stage renal disease. Trans. Soc. Artif. Intern. Organs 23:28, 1977.

105. Rostand, S.G., Kirk, K.A., Rutsky, E.A., et al.: Racial differences in the incidence of treatment for end-stage renal disease. N. Engl. J. Med. 306:1276, 1982.

106. Hirata, Y., Mihara, T.: Principal causes of death among diabetic patients in Japan from 1968 to 1970. In: S. Baba, Y. Goto, and I. Fukui, eds.: Diabetes mellitus in Asia. Amsterdam, Excerpta Medica, 1976, pp. 91–97.

107. Light, G., Barker, C.O., Wilber, J.A.: Diabetic nephropathy—Georgia. MMWR 30:296, 1981.

108. Brenner, B.M., Meyer, T.W., Hostetter, T.H.: Dietary protein intake and the progressive nature of kidney disease: The role of hemodynamically mediated glomerular injury in the pathogenesis of progressive glomerular scle-

rosis in aging, renal ablation, and intrinsic renal disease. N. Engl. J. Med. *307*:652, 1982.

109. West, K.M.: Epidemiology of diabetes and its vascular lesions. New York, Elsevier North-Holland, Inc., 1978, pp. 353–401.
110. Krolewski, A.S., Czyzyk, A., Kopczynski, J., et al.: Prevalence of diabetes mellitus, coronary heart disease and hypertension in the families of insulin dependent and insulin independent diabetics. Diabetologia *21*:520, 1981.
111. Blonde, C.V., Webber, L.S., Foster, T.A., Berenson, G.S.: Parental history and cardiovascular disease risk factor variables in children. Prevent. Med. *10*:25, 1981.
112. Voors, A.W., Radhakrishnamurthy, B., Srinivasan, S.R., et al.: Plasma glucose level related to blood pressure in 272 children, ages 7–15 years, sampled from a total biracial population. Am. J. Epidemiol. *113*:347, 1981.
113. Ostrander, L.D., Lamphiear, D.E.: Coronary risk factors in a community. Findings in Tecumseh, Michigan. Circulation *53*:152, 1976.
114. Wingard, D.L., Barrett-Connor, E., Criqui, H., Suarez, L.: Clustering of heart disease risk factors in diabetic compared to nondiabetic adults. Am. J. Epidemiol. *117*:19, 1983.
115. Ipsen, J., Clark, T.W., Elsom, K.O., et al.: Diabetes and heart disease: periodic health examination programs. Am. J. Public Health *59*:1595, 1969.
116. Medalie, J.H., Papier, C.M., Coldbourt, U., et al.: Major factors in the development of diabetes mellitus in 10,000 men. Arch. Intern. Med. *135*:811, 1975.
117. Wilson, P.W., McGee, D.L., Kannel, W.B.: Obesity, very low density lipoproteins, and glucose intolerance over fourteen years. The Framingham Study. Am. J. Epid. *114*:697, 1981.
118. Dunn, J.P., Ipsen, J., Elsom, K.O., et al.: Risk factors in coronary artery disease, hypertension and diabetes. Am. J. Med. Sci. *259*:309, 1970.
119. Kannel, W.B., Brand, N., Skinner, J.J., et al.: The relation of adiposity to blood pressure and development of hypertension. The Framingham Study. Ann. Intern. Med. *67*:48, 1967.
120. Ashley, F.W., Kannel, W.B.: Relation of weight change to changes in atherogenic traits: The Framingham Study. J. Chron. Dis. *27*:103, 1974.
121. Noppa, H.: Body weight change in relation to incidence of ischemic heart disease and change in risk factors for ischemic heart disease. Am. J. Epidemiol. *111*:693, 1980.
122. Dyer, A.R., Stamler, J., Shekelle, B., et al.: Relative weight and blood pressure in four Chicago eidemiologic studies. J. Chron. Dis. *35*:897, 1982.
123. DeFronzo, R.A.: The effect of insulin on renal sodium metabolism. A review with clinical implications. Diabetologia *21*:165, 1981.
124. Björntorp, P.: Hypertension in obesity. Acta Med. Scand. *211*:241, 1982.
125. Pyorala, K.: Relationship of glucose tolerance and plasma insulin to the incidence of coronary heart disease; results from two population studies in Finland. Diabetes Care *2*:131, 1979.
126. Welborn, T.A., Wearne, K.: Coronary heart disease incidence and cardiovascular mortality in Busselton with reference to glucose and insulin concentrations. Diabetes Care *2*:154, 1979.
127. Ducimetiere, P., Eschwege, E., Papoz, L., et al.: Relationship of plasma insulin levels to the incidence of myocardial infarction and coronary heart disease mortality in a middle-age population. Diabetologia *19*:205, 1980.
128. Stout, R.W.: Hyperinsulinaemia as an independent risk factor for atherosclerosis. Int. J. Obes. *6* (Suppl. 1):111, 1982.
129. Ostrander, L.D., Francis, T., Hayner, N.S., et al.: The

relationship of cardiovascular disease to hyperglycemia. Ann. Intern. Med. *62*:1188, 1965.
130. Keen, H., Rose, G., Pyke, D.A., et al.: Blood-sugar and arterial disease. Lancet *2*:505, 1965.
131. Herman, J.B., Medalie, J.H., Goldbourt, U.: Differences in cardiovascular morbidity and mortality between previously known and newly diagnosed adult diabetics. Diabetologia *13*:229, 1977.
132. Kannel, W.B., McGee, D.L.: Diabetes and glucose tolerance as risk factors for cardiovascular disease: The Framingham Study. Diabetes Care *2*:120, 1979.
133. Dawber, T.R.: Diabetes and cardiovascular disease. In: T.R. Dawber: The Framingham Study. The Epidemiology of Atherosclerotic Disease. Cambridge, Harvard University Press, 1980, pp. 190–201.
134. Goldberg, R.B.: Lipid disorders in diabetes. Diabetes Care *4*:561, 1981.
135. Winegrad, A.I., Morrison, A.D., Clements, R.S.: Polyol pathway activity in aorta. In: R.A. Camerini-Davalos and H.S. Cole (eds.): Vascular and Neurological Changes in Early Diabetes. New York, Academic Press, 1973, pp. 117–124.
136. Yodaiken, R.E.: The relationship between diabetic capilaropathy and myocardial infarction. A hypothesis. Diabetes *25* (Suppl. 2):928, 1976.
137. Henning, R.: Swedish cooperative CCU study, part 2: The short term prognosis. Acta Med. Scand. Suppl. *586*:18, 1975.
138. Soler, N., Bennett, M., Lamb, P., et al.: Coronary care for myocardial infarction in diabetics. Lancet *1*:475, 1974.
139. Tansey, J.J.B., Opie, L.H., Kennelly, B.: High mortality in obese women diabetics with acute myocardial infarction. Br. Med. J. *1*:1624, 1977.
140. Czyzyk, A., Krolewski, A.S., Szablowska, S., et al.: Clinical course of myocardial infarction among diabetic patients. Diabetes Care *3*:526, 1980.
141. Warram, J.H., Marble, A., Conlon, T.P.: Is cardiovascular mortality declining in diabetes? Diabetes *31* (Suppl. 2):89A, 1982.
142. Patrick, C.H., Palesch, Y.Y., Feinleib, M., et al.: Sex differences in declining cohort death rates from heart disease. Am. J. Public Health *72*:161, 1982.
143. Sorlie, P.: Cardiovascular diseases and death following myocardial infarction and angina pectoris: Framingham study, 20-year follow-up. Sec. 32. In: W.B. Kannel and T. Gordon: The Framingham Study. An epidemiological investigation of cardiovascular disease. D.H.E.W. Publication No. (NIH) 77-1247, 1977.
144. Jarrett, R.J., McCartney, P., Keen, H.: The Bedford Survey: Ten year mortality rates in newly diagnosed diabetics, borderline diabetics and normoglycaemic controls and risk indices for coronary heart disease in borderline diabetes. Diabetologia *22*:79, 1982.
145. West, K.M., Ahuja, M.M.S., Bennett, P.H., et al.: The role of circulating glucose and triglyceride concentrations and their interactions with other "risk factors" as determinants of arterial disease in nine diabetic population samples from the WHO Multinational Study. Diabetes Care *6*:361, 1983.
146. Merrell, M., and Shulman, L.E.: Determination of prognosis in chronic disease, illustrated by systemic lupus erythematosus. J. Chron. Dis. *1*:12, 1955.
147. United States Life Tables 1949–51, Vital Statistics-Special Reports, Vol. 41, No. 1, U.S. Public Health Service, National Office of Vital Statistics, pp. 28-29.
148. Entmacher, P.S.: Endocrine and Metabolic Diseases. In: Singer, R.B., and Levinson, L. (eds.): Medical Risks. Lexington, D.C. Heath and Company, 1976, pp. 165–172.
149. Panzram, G., and Zabel-Langhennig, R.: Prognosis of diabetes mellitus in a geographically defined population. Diabetologia *20*:587, 1981.

13 Diabetes Mortality from Vital Statistics

Paul S. Entmacher, Leo P. Krall, and
Stanley N. Kranczer

Chapters 2 and 12 of this book present data regarding the natural history of diabetes as analyzed by epidemiologic methods. It has seemed desirable, however, also to prepare this chapter in which conventional statistics compiled from death certificates are used as the basis for discussion. Their inadequacies, chiefly the failure to mention diabetes on the death certificate, are well known. However, since data of this type are commonly cited in publications throughout much of the world, one would be remiss in not including them in this text, despite numerous irregularities in the method of acquiring them.

If a person dies of an acute myocardial infarction brought about because of occlusive vascular disease due to atherosclerosis after 40 years of diabetes, the acute myocardial infarction is listed as the cause often without any mention of diabetes as either an underlying or contributing cause.

In a 1945–70 study of the course of 1470 residents of Rochester, Minnesota, with known diabetes, Palumbo et al.[1] found that of the 510 deaths diabetes was not recorded anywhere on the death certificates in two-thirds of the cases. It was reported as the underlying cause in only 7% and as a contributing or "other" cause in 25%. In Pennsylvania, Tokuhata and co-workers[2] estimated that about 16.9% of all decedents were known diabetics, although in only 8.6% was diabetes mentioned at all (2.2% as underlying and 6.4% as contributing cause). In the United States as a whole, data for 1978 indicated that only 26% of the deaths in which diabetes did appear on the death certificate were assigned to that disease.[3]

Apparently the situation in other countries is about the same, although customs vary. In 1980, the World Health Organization (WHO) Expert Committee on Diabetes Mellitus stated that "Only 10–20% of the death certificates of diabetics assign diabetes as the underlying cause of death, even though mortality rates are excessive by a factor of 2–3 in diabetics."[4] There is a difference also between countries simply because of changes in coding procedures to conform with the WHO Classification Convention. However, in spite of the efforts of WHO and appropriate agencies in the United States and other countries, reporting according to death certificates is still spotty.

Although the obtaining of data from death certificates is an extremely variable and inexact science, it is still so widely used in much, if not most, of the world that it is important at least to present what data there are, hoping that more modern and scientific methods, as espoused elsewhere in this volume, will give more precision to the discovering of how many diabetics lived and died in this world. Epidemiology no longer simply counts bodies, but also tries to answer the how, when, and why regarding morbidity and mortality. It attempts to discover trends and from them determine what caused people to behave as they did in life and, indeed, until death.

CURRENT MORTALITY STATISTICS FOR THE UNITED STATES

In 1981 the estimated number of deaths from diabetes was 34,750. This corresponds to a mortality rate of 15.2/100,000 population and results in its being ranked seventh among the leading causes of death in the United States. Although mortality from diabetes accounts for only 1.7% of all deaths in the U.S.A., it is implicated as a contributory cause in a substantial proportion of deaths from other diseases, particularly those of the cardiovascular-renal system and is especially associated with deaths in the elderly population.

The number of deaths ascribed to diabetes, as shown in Table 13–1, has not changed much in the last few years. In 1980, diabetes accounted for 34,230 deaths, approximately the same as in 1981 and about 1000 more than the 33,192 in 1979. Moreover, in 1978, the last year for which detailed final data are available, 33,841 deaths were due to diabetes. Although the recent data indicate that mortality from diabetes may have leveled off, past history reveals that deaths ascribed to diabetes have been steadily increasing up until 1972, reaching a record of 38,674 in that year and then gradually declining to 32,989 in 1977.

Table 13–1 lists the number and percentage of deaths from diabetes by age, race, and sex. Of the deaths due to diabetes, only 5% occurred under the age of 45, whereas almost 90% were recorded at ages 55 and older. The table also shows that among females other than white, the relative number of deaths due to diabetes as a percentage of all causes of death, is greater than in any of the other groups and that the percentage among white females is next highest. In 1980, among females of races other than white, the percentage was 3.3 and among white females, 2.1. In each instance these percentages are roughly twice those of their male counterparts; there is only a slight difference between white and all other males. It is of interest that among white persons, a greater percentage of diabetes deaths occur at the older ages than is true for nonwhites. Also apparent is the fact that among females, the percentage of deaths occurring at ages 75 and over is much larger than for corresponding males.

Mortality from Ten Leading Causes of Death

Table 13–2 presents the number of deaths and death rates attributed to the 10 leading causes of death in the United States for 1979 through 1981. As is shown, cardiovascular and malignant diseases are by far the most prevalent causes of mortality, followed by accidents. In 1979, the Ninth International Classification of Diseases was instituted, resulting in a reclassification with more deaths due to the chronic obstructive pulmonary diseases and as a consequence, placing this disease category in 5th place. Pneumonia and influenza are next in rank order, and diabetes now is listed as the 7th leading cause of death. It is not unreasonable to combine diseases of the heart and cerebrovascular diseases in one cardiovascular category, thus making diabetes the 6th leading cause of death, and if accidents are excluded and only diseases are considered, diabetes would rise into 5th place.

The relative ranking of mortality from diabetes varies somewhat by sex.

Trends in Age-Adjusted Death Rates, 1900–1980

Significant changes have been occurring in the pattern of mortality from diabetes. As shown in Table 13–3, the peak age-adjusted mortality rate in the period since 1950 was recorded in 1968, namely, 14.7/100,000. Thereafter, the rate has gradually declined, reaching 9.9/100,000 in 1980, or a decrease of one-third. Also evident from the table are the divergent trends in the death rate by sex. During the 1950s, the age-adjusted mortality rate for total females, initially significantly higher than for males, gradually diminished, whereas among males there was virtually no improvement. In the mid- and late 1960s, mortality rates for males rose somewhat but those for females were for the most part level. The narrowing of the gap in sex differential accelerated in the 1970s so that starting in 1977, females began experiencing a more favorable mortality rate. It is of interest that this crossover occurred earlier among Whites, namely in 1972, and has not occurred at all among persons of all other races. All nonwhite females still record higher mortality than males; in fact, they experience the highest mortality of any group. Table 13–3 also shows that for both sexes combined, mortality among persons of all other races is consistently higher than that for Whites. Furthermore, whereas the mortality for Whites started to decline after 1968, the decline for Nonwhites did not start until several years later. From the mid-1960s until 1979, the mortality rate for Nonwhites was generally more than twice that of the white population.

Figure 13–1 depicts in graphic form the trends in age-adjusted death rates from 1950 to 1980 by race and sex. During the 1950s and 1960s, the mortality rate for Whites fluctuated in a narrow range while that for persons of all other races increased significantly. The precipitous drop which occurred in the 1970s was more pronounced for Nonwhites, thereby offsetting the sharp rise before then.

As already noted, the age-adjusted mortality rate for total persons in 1980 was estimated at 9.9/100,000 population, or two-thirds of the crude death rate of 15.1/100,000. The trends in the crude and age-adjusted death rates from diabetes for the period 1900 to 1980 are shown in Figure 13–2.

Table 13–1.   Number and Percentage of Deaths from Diabetes by Age, Race, and Sex, United States, 1978, 1979, and 1980*

Age	Number of Deaths			Percent of All Causes			Percent of All Ages		
	1978	1979	1980*	1978	1979	1980*	1978	1979	1980*
				Total Persons					
All Ages	33,841†	33,192†	34,230	1.8	1.7	1.7	100.0	100.0	100.0
Under 25	190	227	144	0.2	0.2	0.1	0.6	0.7	0.4
25–44	1,484	1,417	1,671	1.4	1.3	1.5	4.4	4.3	4.9
45–54	2,227	2,057	2,275	1.6	1.5	1.7	6.6	6.2	6.6
55–64	5,563	5,537	5,486	1.9	1.9	1.9	16.4	16.4	16.0
65–74	9,629	9,398	9,772	2.1	2.1	2.1	28.4	28.3	28.6
75 +	14,743	14,550	14,882	1.8	1.8	1.7	43.6	43.8	43.5
				White Male					
All Ages	11,846†	11,688†	12,015	1.3	1.3	1.3	100.0	100.0	100.0
Under 25	66	81	55	0.1	0.1	0.1	0.6	0.7	0.5
25–44	631	613	723	1.2	1.1	1.3	5.3	5.3	6.0
45–54	945	796	880	1.3	1.1	1.3	8.0	6.8	7.3
55–64	2,177	2,212	2,187	1.4	1.4	1.4	18.4	18.9	18.2
65–74	3,559	3,521	3,649	1.5	1.5	1.5	30.0	30.1	30.4
75 +	4,467	4,464	4,521	1.3	1.3	1.3	37.7	38.2	37.6
				White Female					
All Ages	16,453†	15,936†	16,533	2.1	2.1	2.1	100.0	100.0	100.0
Under 25	84	94	59	0.3	0.3	0.2	0.5	0.6	0.4
25–44	478	442	530	1.8	1.7	2.0	2.9	2.8	3.2
45–54	697	648	725	1.7	1.7	1.9	4.3	4.1	4.4
55–64	2,170	2,097	2,098	2.4	2.4	2.3	13.2	13.1	12.7
65–74	4,347	4,165	4,367	2.8	2.7	2.7	26.4	26.1	26.4
75 +	8,674	8,486	8,754	2.0	2.0	1.9	52.7	53.3	52.9
				All Other Male					
All Ages	2,064	2,107†	2,122	1.5	1.6	1.5	100.0	100.0	100.0
Under 25	17	26	14	0.1	0.2	0.1	0.8	1.2	0.7
25–44	208	188	215	1.2	1.1	1.2	10.1	8.9	10.1
45–54	246	271	292	1.5	1.7	1.8	11.9	12.9	13.8
55–64	487	487	469	1.9	1.9	1.7	23.6	23.1	22.1
65–74	619	612	618	2.1	2.1	2.0	30.0	29.1	29.1
75 +	487	522	514	1.6	1.8	1.5	23.6	24.8	24.2
				All Other Female					
All Ages	3,478†	3,461	3,560	3.4	3.4	3.3	100.0	100.0	100.0
Under 25	23	26	16	0.2	0.3	0.2	0.7	0.8	0.4
25–44	167	174	203	1.9	2.0	2.3	4.8	5.0	5.7
45–54	339	342	378	3.3	3.4	3.6	9.7	9.9	10.6
55–64	7290	741	732	4.3	4.5	4.1	21.0	21.4	20.6
65–74	1,104	1,100	1,138	4.8	4.7	4.6	31.7	31.8	32.0
75 +	1,115	1,078	1,093	3.3	3.2	3.0	32.1	31.1	30.7

*1980—Estimated.
†Includes small number of deaths with age not stated.
Source: Computed by the Statistical Bureau of the Metropolitan Life Insurance Company, based on data from the Division of Vital Statistics, National Center for Health Statistics and the Bureau of the Census.

Both the crude and age-adjusted mortality rates have greatly declined since 1968 with the disparity between the rates holding at about 5/100,000. The difference in the death rates, with the crude rate being higher, has steadily widened to this level since 1949 when the gap was about 2/100,000. Prior to this date, rates are not comparable with current figures because of the significant changes in coding procedures instituted by the Fifth Revision of the International Classification of Causes of Death. In the early and mid-1940s, the age-adjusted mortality rate was also lower than the crude rate, but this was not the case in the years prior to 1940. As Figure 13–2 clearly shows, the level of the age-adjusted mortality rate varied for the most part between 2 and 4/100,000 higher than that for the crude rate. Also evident are the sharp rise in this period for both measures of diabetes mortality and the diminishing of the differences between them in the mid- and late 1930s.

Age-Specific Death Rates by Race and Sex

Both the crude and age-adjusted death rates in 1980 by race and sex are shown in Table 13–4.

Table 13–2. Mortality from Ten Leading Causes of Death* United States, 1979, 1980, and 1981

Cause of Death (Ranked as per 1981)	Number of Deaths	1979 Death Rate/100,000		Number of Deaths	1980 Death Rate/100,000		Number of Deaths	1981 Death Rate/100,000	
		Crude	Age-Adjusted†		Crude	Age-Adjusted†		Crude	Age-Adjusted†
Diseases of heart	733,235	333.1	203.5	763,060	335.9	201.3	759,100	330.6	196.4
Malignant neoplasms‡	403,395	183.3	133.2	414,320	182.4	131.6	422,720	184.3	132.0
Cerebrovascular diseases	169,488	77.0	42.5	170,420	75.0	40.7	164,330	71.7	38.5
Accidents and adverse effects	105,312	47.8	43.7	106,550	46.9	42.4	102,130	44.5	40.4
Chronic obstructive pulmonary disease and allied conditions	49,933	22.7	14.9	55,810	24.6	15.8	59,870	26.1	16.7
Pneumonia and influenza	45,030	20.5	11.4	52,720	23.2	12.4	54,420	23.7	12.4
Diabetes mellitus	33,192	15.1	10.0	34,230	15.1	9.9	34,750	15.2	9.9
Chronic liver disease and cirrhosis	29,720	13.5	12.2	31,330	13.8	12.5	29,520	12.9	11.5
Atherosclerosis	28,801	13.1	5.7	29,830	13.1	5.7	28,750	12.5	5.2
Suicide	27,206	12.4	11.9	28,290	12.5	12.0	28,100	12.3	11.7

*Figures for "Certain conditions originating in the perinatal period" are not included.
  Deaths are coded according to the 9th Revision. Numbers and rates of death for 1980 and 1981 are provisional.
†Adjusted on basis of age distribution of the United States total population, 1940.
‡Including neoplasms of lymphatic and hematopoietic tissues.
Source: Reports of the Division of Vital Statistics, National Center for Health Statistics.

The crude death rate from diabetes is highest for nonwhite females, closely followed by that for white females. The lowest crude death rates are found among white males and are somewhat higher for all other males, but they are still lower than those for females. The higher crude death rates among females reflect the greater prevalence of diabetes in females as well as their greater longevity and the fact that most deaths among diabetics occur at the older ages. Greater longevity may also explain why white males have higher crude death rates than all other males.

When adjustment is made for the differences in the age distributions of the population, white death rates become much lower than their crude death rates. Among persons of all other races, age adjustment does not affect the values nearly as much. The comparison of the age-adjusted death rates reveals that they are much lower for Whites than all others. As described previously, in recent years among Whites, the age-adjusted death rate is greater for males than for females and the reverse is true among persons of all other races. Among females, the age-adjusted death rate for all other races is over twice as great as for white females and for males the excess is more than three-fifths.

Also presented in Table 13–4 are age-specific death rates which clearly indicate that the major concentration of mortality from diabetes is in middle and later years of life. In 1980, for the population as a whole, the death rates were less than 1/100,000 in the age groups under 25 years. They increased gradually to 10.0/100,000 at ages 45 to 54, and there was a more rapid acceleration at the older ages.

While the general pattern of increasing death rates is similar for all race and sex groups, among nonwhite males and females there is an earlier rise in death rates as compared to white males and females. For example, in 1980 at ages 35 to 44, the death rate for nonwhite females was 7.8 as compared to 2.6 for white females. The corresponding rate for nonwhite males was 9.2 and for white males, 4.0. At ages 45 to 54, nonwhite females had a rate of 25.1, compared to 7.1 for white females, and nonwhite males had a rate of 23.6, compared to 9.0 for white males. Comparison of the death rates by race for each sex showed that Nonwhites had greater death rates than did the white population. The data for 1978 and 1979 show a mortality pattern similar to that for 1980, except at the oldest ages for males.

Change in Age-Specific Death Rates, 1967–68 to 1977–78

When one compares the relative change in age-specific death rates by race and sex for the decade between 1967–68 and 1977–78 (Table 13–5), it is evident that all categories showed a fall in mortality but the percentage of such was substantially larger for females with the age-adjusted rate declining by about one-third as compared to approximately one-fifth for males. A detailed examination reveals that the relative decline generally diminished with advance in age. Among Whites under age 25, the rates for males fell by at least half and the decline was almost as pronounced among females. At ages 25 to 44, males continued to experience sharper declines than females, but thereafter the declines

Table 13–3. Age-Adjusted* Death Rates per 100,000 from Diabetes Mellitus, by Race and Sex, United States, 1950 to 1980

Year	Total, All Races			White			All Other		
	Both Sexes	Male	Female	Both Sexes	Male	Female	Both Sexes	Male	Female
1950	14.3	11.4	17.1	13.9	11.3	16.4	17.2	11.8	22.6
1951	14.2	11.3	16.9	13.9	11.2	16.4	16.6	11.8	21.3
1952	14.1	11.5	16.4	13.8	11.5	15.8	16.5	11.5	21.5
1953	13.9	11.2	16.3	13.5	11.2	15.6	17.2	11.3	22.9
1954	13.1	10.9	15.2	12.8	10.9	14.5	16.4	11.3	21.2
1955	13.0	10.9	14.8	12.6	10.9	14.1	16.5	11.2	21.6
1956	13.0	11.0	14.8	12.6	10.9	14.0	17.1	11.7	22.2
1957	13.2	11.1	15.2	12.7	10.9	14.3	18.2	12.5	23.6
1958	13.0	11.3	14.6	12.5	11.1	13.6	18.8	13.0	24.3
1959	13.0	11.3	14.5	12.4	11.0	13.5	19.4	14.1	24.2
1960	13.6	12.0	15.0	12.8	11.6	13.7	21.6	16.1	26.8
1961	13.3	11.7	14.6	12.5	11.4	13.3	21.0	14.9	26.7
1962	13.5	12.3	14.5	12.5	11.8	13.1	21.8	16.1	27.1
1963	13.8	12.4	14.9	12.7	11.9	13.3	23.1	16.6	29.1
1964	13.5	12.4	14.4	12.5	11.8	12.9	23.6	17.6	29.0
1965	13.5	12.5	14.4	12.5	11.9	12.9	23.6	18.1	28.6
1966	13.9	12.8	14.6	12.7	12.3	13.0	24.8	18.3	30.5
1967	13.7	12.9	14.4	12.7	12.4	12.8	24.5	18.5	29.7
1968	14.7	14.0	15.3	13.4	13.2	13.5	28.0	21.3	33.7
1969	14.5	13.6	15.1	13.2	12.8	13.3	27.7	21.3	33.2
1970	14.1	13.5	14.4	12.9	12.7	12.8	25.2	20.4	29.3
1971	13.8	13.2	14.2	12.4	12.4	12.4	27.5	21.7	32.4
1972	13.6	13.2	13.9	12.2	12.3	12.1	26.0	21.2	30.1
1973	13.2	12.9	13.3	11.8	12.0	11.6	25.3	21.1	28.6
1974	12.5	12.2	12.7	11.4	11.5	11.2	23.4	18.8	27.1
1975	11.6	11.4	11.6	10.4	10.7	10.2	21.7	17.9	24.6
1976	11.1	10.9	11.1	10.0	10.2	9.7	21.0	17.5	23.7
1977	10.4	10.5	10.3	9.4	9.8	9.0	19.5	16.3	22.0
1978	10.4	10.5	10.3	9.4	9.8	9.1	19.0	16.3	21.0
1979	10.0	10.2	9.8	9.0	9.5	8.6	18.5	16.2	20.3
1980 Est.	9.9	10.2	9.7	9.0	9.5	8.5	18.0	15.9	19.4

*Adjusted on basis of age distribution of the United States total population, 1940.
Source: Computed by the Statistical Bureau of the Metropolitan Life Insurance Company, based on data from the Division of Vital Statistics, National Center for Health Statistics.

were higher among females. Among nonwhite persons, the death rates at ages under 25 are relatively small and with the exception of the apparent rise in male mortality during the decade at ages under 1, males experienced larger relative declines than did females. Past age 25, however, larger mortality declines were reported in females of all other races than in their male counterparts. In fact, mortality rates among males of all other races aged 75 and over increased between 1967–68 and 1977–78.

In 1977 to 1978, at all ages, mortality among white males was higher than among white females. At ages under 25 there were minor differences in their rates. On the other hand, between ages 25 to 74, the mortality rate among white males was greater than among white females. For ages 75 and over, females recorded higher death rates. An entirely different picture is presented by persons of other races. For all ages combined, higher mortality was recorded in females than in males. At

ages under 45, age-specific mortality rates were generally higher among males, but at ages 45 and over, the period of life when mortality from diabetes takes its greatest toll, the death rate among females was higher than for males and in some cases, quite markedly so.

Mortality for Separate Racial Groups Other than White, 1969–71 and 1976

A separate tabulation of mortality by sex for races other than white is shown in Table 13–6. The data presented are for 1976 (the latest available) and for 1969–71. As is evident, there are marked differences in the mortality between the groups. Mortality among Blacks is significantly higher than for persons of all other Nonwhite races combined. For the most part, the latter group is composed of Indians, Japanese, Chinese and other Asians. In 1976, the age-adjusted mortality rate for Blacks was almost twice as large as for persons of all other

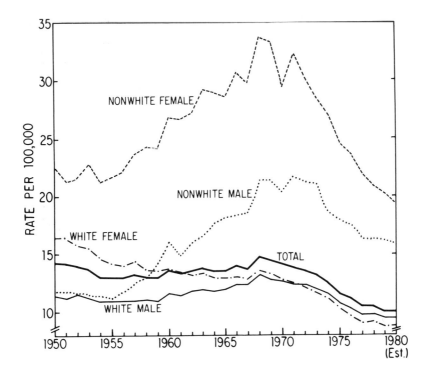

Fig. 13–1. Age-adjusted* death rates from diabetes mellitus in the United States, 1950 to 1980.
*Based on age distribution of the United States total population, 1940.

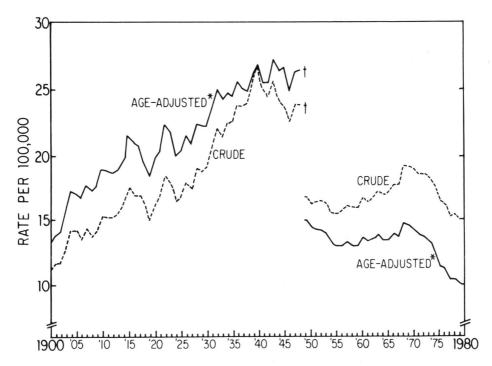

Fig. 13–2. Trend in crude and age-adjusted* death rates from diabetes mellitus: death-registration United States, 1900 to 1932, and United States, 1933 to 1980.
*Based on age distribution of the United States total population, 1940.
†Break in comparability.

Table 13–4. Death Rates per 100,000 from Diabetes Mellitus by Age, Race, and Sex, United States, 1978, 1979, and 1980

Age	Total Persons	White		All Other	
		Male	Female	Male	Female
All Ages			1978		
Crude					
Revised*	15.2	12.7	16.7	14.4	22.0
NCHS	15.5	12.9	17.0	14.7	22.5
Age-Adjusted†	10.4	9.8	9.1	16.3	21.0
Under 15	0.1	0.1‡	0.1	0.1‡	0.2‡
15–24	0.3	0.3	0.4	0.4‡	0.5‡
25–34	1.7	1.7	1.3	3.6	2.4
35–44	3.8	3.7	2.7	9.7	6.5
45–54	9.6	9.5	6.6	19.7	23.4
55–64	26.9	24.6	22.1	52.1	66.6
65–74	64.5	60.9	57.0	95.2	134.1
75–84	145.5	134.9	141.6	164.0	258.3
85+	211.9	208.5	220.2	128.2	191.7
All Ages			1979		
Crude					
Revised*	14.8	12.4	16.1	14.4	21.4
NCHS	15.1	12.6	16.4	14.7	21.9
Age-Adjusted†	10.0	9.5	8.6	16.2	20.3
Under 15	0.1	0.1‡	0.1	0.1‡	0.2‡
15–24	0.4	0.4	0.4	0.7‡	0.5‡
25–34	1.5	1.5	1.2	2.7	1.9
35–44	3.6	3.6	2.3	9.1	7.2
45–54	9.0	8.1	6.3	21.4	23.3
55–64	26.4	24.7	21.2	50.9	66.0
65–74	61.5	58.9	53.5	91.5	129.3
75–84	140.4	133.9	135.5	164.2	231.5
85+	199.3	193.2	204.0	154.2	204.5
All Ages			1980§		
Crude	15.1	12.6	16.5	14.0	21.3
Age-Adjusted†	9.9	9.5	8.5	15.9	19.4
Under 15	0.1	0.1‡	0.1	0.1‡	0.2‡
15–24	0.2	0.2	0.2	0.3‡	0.2‡
25–34	1.7	1.7	1.5	2.8	2.1
35–44	4.0	4.0	2.6	9.2	7.8
45–54	10.0	9.0	7.1	23.6	25.1
55–64	25.2	23.9	20.3	46.7	59.4
65–74	62.4	59.6	54.7	93.2	129.6
75–84	126.1	121.9	122.7	140.4	181.3
85+	221.1	211.4	221.7	221.3	288.3

*Based on population estimates which take 1980 Census figures into account.
†Adjusted on basis of age distribution of the United States total population, 1940.
‡Less than 20 deaths.
§Estimated.
Source: Computed by the Statistical Bureau of the Metropolitan Life Insurance Company, based on data from the Division of Vital Statistics, National Center for Health Statistics and the Bureau of the Census.

nonwhite races. Among males, the rate among Blacks was about 70% larger and among females it was 85% greater. The disparity among females was approximately of the same magnitude in 1969 to 1971, but for males the differences between the racial groups doubled in the intervening years. Age-specific mortality rates for black males, while declining between 1969–71 and 1976, did not fall as rapidly as for males of other nonwhite races, thus producing a substantial race disparity. On the other hand, for females, the mortality rate among black women decreased much faster than for their

male counterparts, thus closing the gap in race differences for mortality.

The last period for which a mortality breakdown of the category of persons of all other races is available is 1959–61. Data (not shown here) from that analysis showed that the Chinese had the highest age-adjusted mortality rate from diabetes, followed by that for Blacks and then for Indians. Mortality among Japanese was less than half that for Chinese and Blacks and they were the only major racial group to experience lower diabetes death rates than Whites. Among males, Chinese

Table 13–5.   Death Rates per 100,000 and Percent Change from Diabetes Mellitus by Age, Race, and Sex, United States, 1967–68 and 1977–78

Age	Average Annual Death Rate per 100,000			Average Annual Death Rate per 100,000		
	1967–68	1977–78	Percent Change 1967–68 to 1977–78	1967–68	1977–78	Percent Change 1967–68 to 1977–78
	White Male			White Female		
All Ages*	12.8	9.8	− 23.4	13.2	9.1	− 31.1
Under 1	0.5	0.1	− 80.0	0.6	0.3	− 50.0
1–4	0.2	0.1	− 50.0	0.2	0.1	− 50.0
5–14	0.2	0.1	− 50.0	0.3	0.2	− 33.3
15–24	0.6	0.3	− 50.0	0.7	0.4	− 42.9
25–34	2.6	1.6	− 38.5	2.0	1.3	− 35.0
35–44	5.3	3.6	− 32.1	3.3	2.7	− 18.2
45–54	11.7	9.4	− 19.7	9.1	6.6	− 27.5
55–64	33.7	24.9	− 26.1	31.1	21.8	− 29.9
65–74	83.0	61.8	− 25.5	95.0	57.6	− 39.4
75–84	157.6	132.9	− 15.7	189.7	141.3	− 25.5
85 +	240.5	206.1	− 14.3	266.9	213.9	− 19.9
	All Other Male			All Other Female		
All Ages*	19.9	16.3	− 18.1	31.7	21.5	− 32.2
Under 1	0.2	0.8	30.0	0.4	0.4	†
1–4	—	0.2	†	0.1	0.1	†
5–14	0.2	0.1	− 50.0	0.3	0.2	− 33.3
15–24	1.1	0.4	− 63.6	1.2	0.7	− 41.7
25–34	5.0	3.3	− 34.0	4.6	2.2	− 52.2
35–44	10.5	9.3	− 11.4	12.1	6.9	− 43.0
45–54	27.5	20.9	− 24.0	40.2	24.2	− 39.8
55–64	62.0	51.3	− 17.3	117.9	71.9	− 39.0
65–74	136.2	95.9	− 29.6	222.0	135.7	− 38.9
75–84	133.0	160.2	20.5	205.7	249.8	21.4
85 +	118.0	139.8	18.5	182.8	193.6	5.9

*Adjusted on basis of age distribution of the United States total population, 1940.
†Less than 0.05.
Source: Reports of the Division of Vital Statistics, National Center for Health Statistics.

had by far the highest mortality, whereas among females, Blacks experienced the highest death rates. Black and Indian female mortality was higher than that of males; there was little variation among the Japanese, but among the Chinese, the rate for males was higher.

Geographic Variations

Diabetes is characterized by considerable variations in mortality from one area of the United States to another. Table 13–7 presents both crude and age-adjusted death rates due to diabetes for the nine geographic divisions of the country and for each state for the period 1969–71 and the year 1977. In both of these time periods, mortality from diabetes as measured by the crude death rates was highest in the Middle Atlantic and the East North Central States, and lowest in the Pacific and Mountain States. In every region of the country there was a significant drop in crude death rates in the interval from 1969–71 to 1977. In general, residents of the Southern and Western areas of the country fared better than persons dwelling in the Northeast and North Central areas. In 1969–71,

the same pattern existed when mortality was measured by age-adjusted rates. The highest age-adjusted death rates were found in the East North Central and Middle Atlantic States, while the lowest rates were in the Pacific and Mountain States.

On a state by state basis, in 1977, mortality was highest in Rhode Island followed by that in Louisiana, Delaware, Indiana, Ohio, Pennsylvania, and New York—all with death rates of 18.0/100,000 or higher. The lowest rates (Alaska is excluded because of the small number of deaths) were reported in Colorado, Hawaii, California, Arizona, Oregon, Minnesota, New Mexico, and Montana—with mortality rates of less than 12.0/100,000.

Further analysis of geographic disparities are presented in Tables 13–8 and 13–9. These tables show the trend in diabetes mortality for white males and white females aged 45 to 74 between 1959–61, 1969–71 and 1975. Because rates based on small numbers of deaths are difficult to evaluate, no death rates are shown for states with fewer than 20 deaths. In 1975, mortality from diabetes among white males aged 45 to 74 averaged 27/100,000 population for the nation as a whole, compared

Table 13–6. Death Rates per 100,000 from Diabetes Mellitus by Age, Race, and Sex, United States, 1969–71 and 1976

Age	1969–71				1976			
	Total	White	Black	All Other	Total	White	Black	All Other
	Total Persons							
All ages, crude	18.9	18.2	24.7	13.6	16.1	15.4	21.7	10.4
Age-adjusted*	14.0	12.7	26.3	15.7	11.0	10.0	21.6	11.7
45–74, age adjusted*	36.0	31.7	80.1	46.3	27.7	24.1	63.2	34.5
45–54	12.8	10.3	37.2	17.6	9.8	7.9	27.8	8.0
55–64	36.2	30.7	92.5	49.5	28.4	24.0	72.8	42.0
65–74	92.0	85.2	164.1	110.7	70.0	63.7	133.6	86.7
75 +	199.6	198.8	213.9	172.0	170.0	166.7	218.0	126.5
	Male							
All ages, crude	15.8	15.6	18.1	14.2	13.4	13.1	16.4	9.7
Age-adjusted*	13.4	12.6	20.3	15.3	10.8	10.2	17.9	10.4
45–74, age-adjusted*	34.3	31.8	59.3	44.4	27.5	25.1	52.2	28.3
45–54	13.2	11.5	30.7	16.0	10.0	8.4	25.5	6.8
55–64	34.8	31.8	65.5	47.5	28.3	25.4	59.2	31.3
65–74	84.7	81.3	118.4	108.6	68.9	65.3	105.6	75.4
75 +	182.9	184.0	169.9	174.7	157.1	157.1	164.0	124.5
	Female							
All ages, crude	21.8	20.7	30.8	13.0	18.6	17.7	26.5	10.9
Age adjusted*	14.5	12.8	31.1	16.0	11.1	9.8	24.5	13.2
45–74, age-adjusted*	37.4	31.4	97.4	48.6	27.7	23.2	72.1	41.5
45–54	12.4	9.1	42.8	18.9	9.6	7.4	29.7	8.9
55–64	37.5	29.7	115.3	53.4	28.4	22.7	84.3	53.0
65–74	97.8	88.3	200.3	113.0	70.8	62.5	154.9	101.7
75 +	210.3	208.1	245.2	163.1	177.5	172.2	252.8	128.3

*Adjusted on basis of age distribution of the United States total population, 1940.
Source: Computed by the Statistical Bureau of the Metropolitan Life Insurance Company, based on data from the Division of Vital Statistics, National Center for Health Statistics.

with 32/100,000 in 1969–71 and 29/100,000 a decade earlier. Among white females, the corresponding death rates were 24/100,000 in 1975, 31/100,000 in 1969–71 and 36/100,000 in 1959–61. During the period under review, the sex differential in mortality reversed from a 7/100,000 advantage in favor of white males in 1959–61 to a 1/100,000 advantage in favor of females in 1969–71, which widened to 3/100,000 by 1975.

In 1975 the highest mortality from diabetes among white men aged 45 to 74 (33 deaths/100,000 population) was recorded in the East North Central States. As shown in Table 13–8, the states in this geographic division also experienced the highest mortality in 1969–71 and 1959–61. On the other hand, the lowest death rates from diabetes among males were registered in the Pacific States—20/100,000 population in 1975, 25/100,000 in 1969–71 and 19/100,000 a decade earlier.

The mortality pattern was similar for white women aged 45 to 74. As shown in Table 13–9, in 1959–61 the highest death rate from diabetes among white women (46/100,000 population) was recorded in the East North Central and Middle Atlantic States; this rate was substantially higher than the comparable rates for white men in these areas.

By 1969–71, the mortality rates among white females had declined to 38/100,000 in the East North Central States and to 35/100,000 in the Middle Atlantic division—the same rates experienced by males in these states. White females residing in the Pacific States have consistently registered the most favorable mortality in the period under review. Since 1969–71, they have enjoyed a slight advantage in mortality over white males in the Pacific States.

Among males at ages 45 to 74 combined, the age-adjusted death rates from diabetes in 1975 ranged from a high of 47/100,000 in Delaware to a low of 18/100,000 in Arizona. In Delaware and in 7 other states (New Hampshire, South Carolina, Ohio, Louisiana, Michigan, Maryland, and New Mexico), death rates from diabetes were at least 25% above the national average. On the other hand, death rates at least 25% below that for the nation as a whole were recorded in Arizona, Oregon, California, Oklahoma, Idaho, and Virginia. Among women, the death rate at these ages was highest (36/100,000) in New Hampshire. Other states where death rates exceeded the national average by 25% or more included Michigan, Kentucky, Ohio, Arkansas, Indiana, West Virginia, and Lou-

Table 13–7. Death Rates per 100,000 from Diabetes Mellitus by Region and State, United States, 1969–71 and 1977

Region and State	1969–71 Crude	1969–71 Age-Adjusted*	1977 Crude	Region and State	1969–71 Crude	1969–71 Age-Adjusted*	1977 Crude
United States	18.8	14.1	15.0				
New England	20.2	13.6	16.0	South Atlantic			
Middle Atlantic	21.8	15.1	17.9	Delaware	24.8	22.0	18.7
East North Central	21.1	16.1	17.0	Maryland	20.8	18.5	14.9
West North Central	19.8	12.7	15.4	District of Columbia	25.0	21.2	17.6
South Atlantic	17.9	14.4	14.9	Virginia	13.7	12.4	12.1
East South Central	18.5	14.4	15.4	West Virginia	18.8	13.0	17.4
West South Central	17.9	14.3	13.9	North Carolina	17.0	15.4	14.6
Mountain	14.1	11.9	11.1	South Carolina	19.3	19.2	15.9
Pacific	13.4	10.4	10.3	Georgia	16.5	15.5	13.8
				Florida	18.9	11.1	15.9
New England							
Maine	20.3	13.2	13.2	East South Central			
New Hampshire	21.8	15.2	17.4	Kentucky	20.7	15.1	17.2
Vermont	16.9	11.8	13.2	Tennessee	15.7	12.3	12.7
Massachusetts	20.4	13.3	16.8	Alabama	18.7	14.9	16.9
Rhode Island	28.3	18.2	19.4	Mississippi	20.1	16.2	15.2
Connecticut	17.4	12.6	14.3				
				West South Central			
Middle Atlantic				Arkansas	18.0	11.9	14.0
New York	20.6	14.2	18.0	Louisiana	23.9	21.3	18.8
New Jersey	21.2	15.5	17.3	Oklahoma	17.9	11.6	14.3
Pennsylvania	24.2	16.3	18.1	Texas	15.9	13.4	12.2
East North Central				Mountain			
Ohio	22.0	17.0	18.2	Montana	17.1	11.9	11.5
Indiana	20.5	15.6	18.5	Idaho	16.7	12.5	12.9
Illinois	17.7	13.3	15.4	Wyoming	13.5	9.9	12.6
Michigan	24.4	20.2	17.6	Colorado	11.9	9.7	9.2
Wisconsin	20.9	14.3	15.2	New Mexico	14.9	14.9	11.3
				Arizona	13.2	10.9	11.0
West North Central				Utah	15.6	14.9	12.6
Minnesota	16.4	11.1	11.3	Nevada	14.2	14.3	12.1
Iowa	20.3	12.1	16.1				
Missouri	22.9	14.8	17.9	Pacific			
North Dakota	17.9	12.1	14.9	Alaska	2.9†	6.7†	2.3†
South Dakota	17.9	11.8	16.1	California	12.9	10.1	10.0
Nebraska	19.0	11.8	13.7	Hawaii	14.0	16.5	9.5
Kansas	20.2	12.7	17.1	Oregon	14.2	9.6	11.2
				Washington	16.2	12.0	12.4

*Adjusted on basis of age distribution of the United States total population, 1940.
†Less than 10 deaths.
Source: Computed by the Statistical Bureau of the Metropolitan Life Insurance Company, based on data from the Division of Vital Statistics, National Center for Health Statistics.

isiana. The lowest mortality among women (14/100,000 population) was recorded in Florida. Death rates of less than 25/100,000 were also reported in Arizona, Connecticut, South Dakota, California, and Minnesota.

For the most part, states with high mortality rates from diabetes in 1975 also reported high rates during 1969–71 and 1959–61. During these periods mortality among white males was substantially above the national average in Delaware, Michigan, Rhode Island, and Ohio. The lowest rates in the earlier period were generally recorded in Colorado, Wyoming, Oregon, California, North Dakota, Virginia, and West Virginia. Among women this pattern was not quite so pronounced.

Mortality from diabetes rises sharply with advance in age and is heavily concentrated at the older ages. For the groups here considered, diabetes death rates among white males in 1975 more than doubled with each 10-year advance in age and the rate at ages 65 to 74 was about 7 times that at ages 45 to 54. Essentially the same pattern was noted among females although the progression was more pronounced. At the younger ages the death rates from diabetes for both men and women were relatively low in 1975; more than two-thirds of the states reported fewer than 20 deaths in this age group. However, at ages 55 to 64, mortality from diabetes reached a much higher level, while the highest death rates occurred at ages 65 to 74.

Table 13–8.　Regional Trend in Mortality from Diabetes, White Males Aged 45–74, United States, 1959–61, 1969–71, and 1975

| | Death Rate per 100,000 | | | | | | | | | | | |
| | 1959–61 | | | | 1969–71 | | | | 1975 | | | |
Area	Ages 45–74*	Ages 45–54	Ages 55–64	Ages 65–74	Ages 45–74*	Ages 45–54	Ages 55–64	Ages 65–74	Ages 45–74*	Ages 45–54	Ages 55–64	Ages 65–74
United States	29	11	30	73	32	11	32	81	27	10	27	69
New England	33	12	33	83	34	14	33	88	30	9	32	78
Maine	28	†	25	77	29	†	28	73	33	†	†	87
New Hampshire	39	†	36	92	36	†	31	106	44	†	†	118
Vermont	21	†	†	60	36	†	†	92	†	†	†	†
Massachusetts	32	12	33	77	35	14	34	86	30	10	30	79
Rhode Island	44	†	40	135	44	18	42	109	31	†	†	†
Connecticut	33	11	35	82	32	12	30	82	25	†	29	69
Middle Atlantic	33	12	34	84	35	12	35	88	28	10	29	69
New York	31	11	31	80	33	13	33	85	29	11	31	69
New Jersey	35	12	33	92	35	11	37	91	27	10	25	72
Pennsylvania	36	13	40	87	37	13	38	91	26	9	28	67
East North Central	35	12	36	89	38	13	38	100	33	11	33	85
Ohio	41	14	41	106	41	13	40	110	39	12	40	103
Indiana	35	12	37	88	37	12	37	99	29	9	32	71
Illinois	26	10	26	61	31	12	33	74	27	10	25	70
Michigan	44	12	44	119	48	16	45	130	36	12	38	93
Wisconsin	31	12	33	73	36	13	36	92	30	11	25	84
West North Central	26	10	27	65	29	10	28	75	25	8	23	69
Minnesota	27	13	25	61	28	12	24	70	22	†	22	54
Iowa	26	11	24	63	27	11	27	65	27	†	24	72
Missouri	27	9	31	65	32	9	34	85	28	†	26	84
North Dakota	22	†	†	55	24	†	†	85	†	†	†	†
South Dakota	24	†	22	59	29	†	26	71	†	†	†	†
Nebraska	30	11	26	83	32	13	29	83	23	†	†	51
Kansas	25	†	27	67	26	9	26	68	28	†	22	88
South Atlantic	26	10	28	63	30	11	32	75	27	10	28	65
Delaware	46	†	55	99	45	†	†	132	47	†	†	†
Maryland	35	9	36	96	39	10	38	112	35	11	41	82
District of Columbia	23	†	†	†	37	†	†	†	†	†	†	†
Virginia	22	9	21	56	24	8	25	61	20	†	20	54
West Virginia	23	12	24	51	24	9	26	59	25	†	24	56
North Carolina	28	12	29	66	34	13	34	85	31	9	30	83
South Carolina	31	11	34	72	43	14	45	113	40	20	37	93
Georgia	27	11	27	64	34	13	35	83	28	†	29	70
Florida	23	9	24	56	26	9	29	60	23	9	23	55
East South Central	23	10	21	57	29	10	30	74	28	12	29	63
Kentucky	24	11	19	62	33	11	38	82	30	14	33	66
Tennessee	22	11	23	49	25	10	25	59	26	13	28	54
Alabama	23	7	22	63	29	8	28	79	29	†	35	68
Mississippi	21	†	20	53	30	13	25	79	24	†	†	70
West South Central	26	10	25	69	29	11	29	72	25	9	24	67
Arkansas	22	†	21	59	25	12	21	62	24	†	†	57
Louisiana	33	9	27	101	39	14	38	101	37	14	38	88
Oklahoma	25	11	23	60	28	10	26	73	19	†	22	37
Texas	26	10	26	66	28	11	29	67	25	8	21	74
Mountain	22	8	23	56	26	10	24	70	24	10	22	59
Montana	26	†	30	69	29	†	32	70	22	†	†	†
Idaho	20	†	†	62	27	†	24	69	20	†	†	†
Wyoming	23	†	†	†	20	†	†	†	†	†	†	†
Colorado	19	7	19	48	19	†	17	54	25	†	†	72
New Mexico	26	†	†	77	31	18	25	72	34	†	†	†
Arizona	18	†	21	46	28	13	24	71	18	†	†	42
Utah	23	†	24	59	34	†	31	93	25	†	†	†
Nevada	31	†	†	†	32	†	†	98	33	†	†	†
Pacific	19	7	21	47	25	9	24	65	20	7	18	53
Washington	25	11	25	58	30	13	28	77	24	†	27	56
Oregon	18	8	17	45	23	7	24	58	19	†	23	46
California	18	6	20	45	24	8	24	63	19	7	16	54
Alaska	†	†	†	†	†	†	†	†	†	†	†	†
Hawaii	†	†	†	†	32	†	†	†	†	†	†	†

*Adjusted on the basis of age distribution of the United States total population, 1940.
†Fewer than 20 deaths; rate not computed.
Source: Computed by the Statistical Bureau of the Metropolitan Life Insurance Company, based on data from the Division of Vital Statistics, National Center for Health Statistics.

Table 13–9. Regional Trend in Mortality from Diabetes, White Females Aged 45–74, United States, 1959–61, 1969–71, and 1975

	Death Rate per 100,000											
	1959–61				1969–71				1975			
Area	Ages 45–74*	Ages 45–54	Ages 55–64	Ages 65–74	Ages 45–74*	Ages 45–54	Ages 55–64	Ages 65–74	Ages 45–74*	Ages 45–54	Ages 55–64	Ages 65–74
United States	36	9	36	104	31	9	30	88	24	7	23	68
New England	39	8	39	114	32	9	31	90	24	8	20	71
Maine	36	†	35	101	35	†	33	95	25	†	†	59
New Hampshire	41	†	51	109	42	18	52	87	36	†	†	117
Vermont	36	†	37	100	28	†	34	50	28	†	†	†
Massachusetts	34	7	33	101	31	8	30	87	25	9	19	76
Rhode Island	62	15	59	183	47	11	35	153	26	†	†	92
Connecticut	43	9	42	128	28	7	27	79	17	†	19	45
Middle Atlantic	46	10	47	133	35	10	32	103	26	7	25	76
New York	37	8	37	108	31	9	28	90	24	6	24	67
New Jersey	51	10	53	148	36	9	32	107	27	7	25	81
Pennsylvania	58	13	59	165	42	11	39	122	29	7	26	87
East North Central	46	11	46	133	38	11	34	109	29	8	28	83
Ohio	54	12	54	155	42	12	38	121	32	8	31	93
Indiana	45	12	47	124	39	11	37	108	31	10	31	84
Illinois	34	9	32	99	31	11	28	84	24	6	23	71
Michigan	59	13	59	172	45	12	35	142	34	10	33	96
Wisconsin	42	10	43	118	33	9	31	91	23	†	22	68
West North Central	30	7	29	90	30	9	29	81	23	7	21	64
Minnesota	32	6	30	96	25	8	22	69	18	†	15	46
Iowa	29	9	27	80	29	9	25	83	25	†	26	67
Missouri	31	6	31	92	36	11	37	93	24	†	23	69
North Dakota	28	†	29	84	28	†	30	85	†	†	†	†
South Dakota	23	†	†	80	26	†	33	55	17	†	†	†
Nebraska	32	†	27	97	27	9	24	73	27	†	†	77
Kansas	31	8	30	89	30	9	28	86	26	†	32	74
South Atlantic	28	7	29	76	27	8	27	72	21	7	20	56
Delaware	61	†	60	183	58	†	61	165	†	†	†	†
Maryland	49	9	52	140	41	10	36	123	27	†	21	88
District of Columbia	14	†	†	43	21	†	†	48	†	†	†	†
Virginia	25	7	24	70	22	6	21	65	22	†	24	55
West Virginia	36	9	39	98	37	13	39	90	31	†	31	85
North Carolina	25	5	24	74	29	8	29	77	22	†	21	59
South Carolina	28	†	29	77	36	10	35	101	29	†	25	83
Georgia	22	7	26	53	28	10	29	70	24	†	21	64
Florida	22	8	23	53	18	6	19	47	14	†	14	38
East South Central	28	7	26	79	30	8	30	83	26	9	26	69
Kentucky	36	10	33	106	35	9	36	98	34	12	32	89
Tennessee	22	7	22	61	27	8	28	74	21	†	20	61
Alabama	25	7	25	68	29	6	27	87	26	†	30	65
Mississippi	24	†	21	80	27	10	27	69	23	†	†	51
West South Central	31	8	31	86	32	10	31	86	27	8	29	71
Arkansas	24	†	19	72	27	†	29	78	32	†	35	73
Louisiana	43	10	44	122	40	12	40	109	31	†	26	89
Oklahoma	26	6	28	70	24	7	22	67	19	†	25	46
Texas	30	8	30	85	33	11	32	88	27	8	29	73
Mountain	28	7	27	79	27	7	26	75	21	8	20	55
Montana	30	†	29	93	21	†	†	62	†	†	†	†
Idaho	35	†	31	107	29	†	28	82	21	†	†	†
Wyoming	27	†	†	86	23	†	†	†	†	†	†	†
Colorado	23	8	21	63	24	7	21	72	25	†	23	62
New Mexico	30	†	32	76	37	†	42	98	22	†	†	†
Arizona	27	†	30	70	21	†	27	50	15	†	†	40
Utah	30	†	26	94	33	†	29	111	24	†	†	77
Nevada	28	†	†	†	33	†	†	116	†	†	†	†
Pacific	23	7	23	62	23	7	22	62	18	6	17	50
Washington	30	7	30	86	28	10	25	75	24	†	19	74
Oregon	28	8	27	75	22	7	23	56	21	†	†	63
California	21	7	21	55	22	6	21	60	17	6	17	44
Alaska	†	†	†	†	†	†	†	†	†	†	†	†
Hawaii	72	†	†	†	38	†	†	†	†	†	†	†

*Adjusted on the basis of age distribution of the United States total population, 1940.
†Fewer than 20 deaths; rate not computed.
Source: Computed by the Statistical Bureau of the Metropolitan Life Insurance Company, based on data from the Division of Vital Statistics, National Center for Health Statistics.

Table 13–10. Death Rates per 100,000 from Diabetes Mellitus in Metropolitan and Non-Metropolitan Counties, by Race and Sex, United States, 1969–71

Race and Sex	Metropolitan	Non-Metropolitan
Total Persons	17.7	21.5
White male	14.5	17.9
White female	19.7	23.1
All other male	15.9	21.6
All other female	25.9	36.9

Source: Computed by the Statistical Bureau of the Metropolitan Life Insurance Company, based on data from the Division of Vital Statistics, National Center for Health Statistics.

At ages 65 to 74, the highest death rate from diabetes among white males in 1975 was recorded in the East North Central States—85/100,000—followed by a rate of 78/100,000 in New England. The lowest rate was recorded in the Pacific States—53/100,000. Death rates per 100,000 ranged from 37 in Oklahoma and 42 in Arizona to 118 in New Hampshire and 103 in Ohio. Among white women aged 65 to 74, the mortality rate from diabetes was lowest in the Pacific States—50/100,000—and highest in the East North Central States, 83/100,000. The death rates by states varied from 38/100,000 in Florida to 117 in New Hampshire.

Comparison of Diabetes Mortality in Metropolitan and Non-Metropolitan Counties, 1969–71

A comparison of mortality differences in 1969–71 between the population residing in metropolitan counties with that dwelling in non-metropolitan counties is shown in Table 13–10. A metropolitan county is defined as one which is included in a Standard Metropolitan Statistical Area (SMSA). In 1970, in order to qualify for inclusion, the county must either have had at least one city with 50,000 or more inhabitants or twin cities satisfying this criteria, or be a contiguous county essentially metropolitan in character and socially and economically integrated with the central city. The data in the table reveal that the mortality rate for all persons in metropolitan counties was about four-fifths that of the population in non-metropolitan counties. This differential is approximately the same for white males and white females but among persons of all other races, the mortality advantage for those living in metropolitan areas is more pronounced—their mortality is less than three-quarters that of their non-metropolitan counterparts. Females of all other races fare the poorest in both metropolitan and non-metropolitan counties. Their death rate from diabetes is about 1.5 times that for all persons in metropolitan counties and 1.7 times that of the overall figure in non-metropolitan counties.

Standard Metropolitan Statistical Areas (SMSAs)

For the most part, the data in Table 13–11 reinforce the prior findings that diabetes mortality is higher in the North and North Central parts of the country than in the South and West. For example, for SMSAs with over 1,000,000 inhabitants in 1970, death rates of around 20/100,000 were usually found in the large population areas in the North and North Central regions. On the other hand, the rates were much lower for the SMSAs in the South and West. Some notable exceptions were Minneapolis-St. Paul in the North Central region and New Orleans, Baltimore, Tampa-St. Petersburg, and Miami SMSAs in the South. The markedly low death rates in some of the California SMSAs may be attributed to the ethnic composition of their population. Among the SMSAs with 1970 population between 500,000 and 1,000,000, some exceptions to the general regional pattern were also found. Specifically, notable disparities occurred in Rochester and Syracuse in the North and Omaha in the North Central region of the country. In the South, Louisville, San Antonio, Birmingham, and Fort Lauderdale-Hollywood recorded relatively high mortality.

Seasonal Variation

It is apparent from Table 13–12 that mortality from diabetes has a well-defined seasonal pattern. For the years under review, deaths from diabetes were more frequently reported in the winter months, especially January and February, and were least prevalent in the late summer months. In fact, on a month-to-month basis, mortality generally followed a consistent trend, being highest in the beginning of the year, steadily declining to a low in September, and then gradually rising again. In 1978 there were some slight deviations from this pattern, especially in July. The distinct seasonality of diabetes mortality may be somewhat attributed to a similar, although more marked pattern of deaths from influenza and pneumonia. In addition, diabetes is linked to cardiovascular-renal diseases, which exhibit a comparable seasonal picture.

INTERNATIONAL COMPARISONS OF DIABETES

In any effort to compare mortality in one country with that in another, several important factors must be taken into account. As mentioned earlier, especially with the use of data from death certificates,

Table 13–11.   Death Rates from Diabetes Mellitus in Standard Metropolitan Statistical Areas with Populations of 500,000 or More by Region, United States, 1969–71

SMSAs of 1,000,000 or Over	Death Rate per 100,000	SMSAs of 500,000 to 999,999	Death Rate per 100,000
North		**North**	
Boston, Mass.	23.6	Albany-Schenectady-Troy, N.Y.	23.7
Buffalo, N.Y.	19.1	Allentown-Bethlehem-Easton, Pa.-N.J.	21.3
Newark, N.J.	22.9	Hartford, Conn.	20.3
New York, N.Y.	21.6	Jersey City, N.J.	32.1
Paterson-Clifton Passaic, N.J.	18.9	Providence-Pawtucket-Warwick, R.I.-Mass.	26.3
Philadelphia, Pa.-N.J.	20.6	Rochester, N.Y.	14.2
Pittsburgh, Pa.	22.9	Springfield-Chicopee-Holyoke, Mass.-Conn.	20.6
		Syracuse, N.Y.	16.1
South		**South**	
Atlanta, Ga.	13.8	Birmingham, Ala.	19.8
Baltimore, Md.	26.6	Fort Lauderdale-Hollywood, Fla.	18.0
Dallas, Tex.	12.1	Fort Worth, Tex.	13.3
Houston, Tex.	11.4	Greensboro-Winston-Salem-High Point, N.C.	12.5
Miami, Fla.	19.5	Jacksonville, Fla.	16.3
New Orleans, La.	31.3	Louisville, Ky.-Ind.	20.9
Tampa-St. Petersburg, Fla.	20.7	Memphis, Tenn.-Ark.	14.4
Washington, D.C.-Md.-Va.	12.9	Nashville-Davidson, Tenn.	10.9
		Norfolk-Portsmouth, Va.	11.1
North Central		Oklahoma City, Okla.	13.3
Chicago, Ill.	17.4	Richmond, Va.	15.6
Cincinnati, Ohio-Ky.-Ind.	18.9	San Antonio, Tex.	20.7
Cleveland, Ohio	21.5		
Detroit, Mich.	24.9	**North Central**	
Indianapolis, Ind.	17.4	Akron, Ohio	17.5
Kansas City, Mo.-Kans.	17.1	Columbus, Ohio	18.8
Milwaukee, Wis.	18.1	Dayton, Ohio	18.0
Minneapolis-St. Paul, Minn.	12.5	Gray-Hammond-East Chicago, Ind.	20.4
St. Louis, Mo.-Ill.	22.2	Grand Rapids, Mich.	16.9
		Omaha, Nebr.-Iowa	14.9
West		Toledo, Ohio-Mich.	23.1
Anaheim-Santa Ana-Garden Grove, Calif.	4.5	Youngstown-Warren, Ohio	24.1
Denver, Colo.	9.4		
Los Angeles-Long Beach, Calif.	15.1	**West**	
Portland, Oreg.-Wash.	13.3	Honolulu, Hawaii	12.3
San Bernardino-Riverside-Ontario, Calif.	12.1	Phoenix, Ariz.	13.2
San Diego, Calif.	9.0	Sacramento, Calif.	12.2
San Francisco-Oakland, Calif.	12.2	Salt Lake City, Utah	14.8
San Jose, Calif.	10.0		
Seattle-Everett, Wash.	14.3		

Source: Computed by the Statistical Bureau of the Metropolitan Life Insurance Company, based on data from the Division of Vital Statistics, National Center for Health Statistics.

international differences in coding practices, diagnostic procedures and quality of medical care are among the most essential of these factors. Since diabetes is a disease with significant complications, studies have shown that different methods of handling mortality data result in substantial variations between countries in the proportion of deaths of diabetics ascribed to diabetes. In addition, it is difficult to make meaningful comparisons between a large country with a heterogeneous population like the United States and smaller countries with more homogenous populations such as the Scandinavian countries. The regional variations within the United States are as great or greater than many of the international differences.

Table 13–13 gives crude death rates by sex for 1977–78 and for a decade earlier. It also gives age-adjusted death rates for 1977–78. The inclusion of age-adjusted mortality rates in the table enables valid comparisons to be made between countries because adjustments are made for differences in the age composition in each country. Analysis of crude death rates between 1967–68 and 1977–78 permits the trend in mortality for a particular country to be determined.

As is evident, there are significant variations in mortality rates. Age-adjusted mortality rates range from a high of 18.1/100,000 population in Greece to a low of 3.5/100,000 in Northern Ireland. Again, it is advisable that caution be used when viewing

Table 13–12. Seasonal Variation in Mortality from Diabetes Mellitus, Deaths in Each Month, Adjusted for Length of Month, Expressed as Percentage of Annual Number of Deaths, Total Persons, United States, 1959–61, 1969–71, 1977, and 1978

Month	Percent of Annual Rate			
	1959–61	1969–71	1977	1978
January	108.9	113.8	113.7	122.2
February	110.0	109.2	108.2	111.7
March	103.7	104.0	107.1	105.9
April	100.6	100.3	103.5	97.9
May	99.0	98.2	99.1	96.9
June	97.5	96.9	97.4	92.5
July	94.0	95.9	97.1	96.3
August	91.6	91.7	88.9	90.9
September	90.9	89.5	88.7	91.3
October	97.0	94.4	92.4	96.4
November	98.6	101.3	95.5	95.7
December	108.6	105.3	108.6	102.5

Source: Reports of the Division of Vital Statistics, National Center for Health Statistics.

the differences in mortality rates between countries because the apparent substantial disparities that are evident may be in major part due to methodologic procedures. Next in rank order of mortality were Chile, the Federal Republic of Germany, Egypt, and the United States, all with age-adjusted death rates of above 10/100,000. On the other hand, low mortality was reported in Norway, the Philippines, England and Wales, Denmark, and the Netherlands; the death rates in these countries were less than 7/100,000.

Among both males and females there was essentially no difference in the ranking of the countries; however, there is considerable variation in each country between the sexes. Over the years the gap between male and female mortality has considerably narrowed; formerly death rates were much higher among females than among males. In more than half of the 21 countries presented in the table, male mortality was higher than that for females. In Sweden the male mortality exceeded that for females by the largest relative margin, while Hungary reported the greatest differential where female mortality exceeded male mortality.

In the decade between 1967–68 and 1977–78, whereas diabetes mortality decreased in the United States and 9 other countries shown in the table, there were increases in 11 countries. The Netherlands and Northern Ireland showed the greatest relative decreases, almost 40%, while Israel and Greece had increases of almost 65%, and Hungary had an increase of about 58%. In addition, there were substantial increases in Yugoslavia, Japan, Chile, the Philippines, and Norway.

In general, the percentage changes in the 10 years were greater among females. The only countries that experienced significant deviations in the relative numbers were England and Wales, France, and Scotland. Among males in England and Wales, mortality from diabetes increased by 24.6%, while among females the increase was only 3.5%. In France there was a 0.8% decrease for males in the decade compared to a decrease of 5.2% for females. Scotland was the only country with a different direction in the change in mortality for each sex; males experienced a 12.1% increase, while females had a 13.8% decline.

Age-Adjusted Death Rates in Various Countries by Age and Sex, 1977–78

Mortality rates from diabetes in different countries varied considerably by age and these figures are presented in Table 13–14. The data for each broad age group have been age-adjusted to facilitate international comparisons. Death rates for ages under 25 are not presented because the numbers are small but they have been utilized in calculating the age-adjusted rate for all ages. At ages 25 to 44, diabetes has not yet become a major cause of death, as is reflected by mortality rates that for the most part are less than 2/100,000 population. Only in Scotland, the United States, Denmark, Egypt, and Sweden are the rates higher and even then they do not exceed 4/100,000. For this age group the mortality rate among males was greater than that for females in every country in the table with the sole exception of Israel where the female rate was twice that for males.

Among persons aged 45 to 64, the rate for both sexes combined ranged from a low of 3.1/100,000 in Northern Ireland to a high of 25.5/100,000 in Egypt. Death rates of less than 10/100,000 occurred in 8 other countries and, in addition to Egypt, only in Greece and Chile was mortality higher than 20/100,000. In this age bracket, greater mortality rates were reported in females than in males in 6 countries—Israel, Greece, Hungary, the Netherlands, Northern Ireland, and Scotland. The largest sex disparity occurred in Northern Ireland where the female mortality rate was double that for males. On the other hand, in Sweden the male rate was almost two-thirds larger than that for females. It should be noted that for each sex no country reported a diabetes death rate at ages 45 to 64 of 30/100,000 or higher.

In 1977–78, among persons 65 years of age and over, the sex disparity in mortality rates in favor of females shown at the younger ages reversed. In 15 of the 20 countries for which data are available, male mortality was lower than that for females. The countries where female mortality was lower

DIABETES MORTALITY FROM VITAL STATISTICS

Table 13–13. Average Annual Death Rates per 100,000 from Diabetes Mellitus in Various Countries by Sex, 1967–68 and 1977–78

Country	Total Crude 1967–68	Total Crude 1977–78	Total % change 1967–68 to 1977–78	Total Age-Adjusted* 1977–78	Male Crude 1967–68	Male Crude 1977–78	Male % change 1967–68 to 1977–78	Male Age-Adjusted* 1977–78	Female Crude 1967–68	Female Crude 1977–78	Female % change 1967–68 to 1977–78	Female Age-Adjusted* 1977–78
Americas												
United States	18.5	15.4	−16.8	10.4	15.6	13.1	−16.0	10.5	21.3	17.6	−17.4	10.3
Canada	13.6	12.7	−6.6	9.5	12.0	11.4	−5.0	10.0	15.2	14.0	−7.9	9.1
Chile[a]	7.9	10.7	35.4	14.2	7.3	9.9	35.6	14.8	8.5	11.5	35.3	13.7
Africa												
Egypt[b]	6.1[e]	6.8	11.5	11.0	6.2[e]	6.9	11.3	11.4	6.0[e]	6.7	11.7	10.6
Asia												
Israel	5.1	8.4	64.7	7.9	4.5	7.3	62.2	7.1	5.7	9.5	66.7	8.6
Japan	6.2	8.5	37.1	7.1	6.1	8.2	34.4	7.8	6.3	8.7	38.1	6.5
Philippines[c]	2.1	2.7	28.6	5.0	2.1	2.7	28.6	4.8	2.1	2.8	33.3	5.3
Europe												
Austria	20.8	17.5	−15.9	8.8	14.5	12.2	−15.9	8.2	26.4	22.2	−15.9	8.9
Denmark	13.0	10.9	−16.2	6.2	11.4	9.5	−16.7	6.5	14.5	12.4	−14.5	6.0
England & Wales[a]	9.1	10.2	12.1	5.4	6.9	8.6	24.6	5.8	11.3	11.7	3.5	5.1
France[c]	17.4	16.7	−4.0	9.4	13.3	13.2	−0.8	9.2	21.2	20.1	−5.2	9.4
Germany, Fed. Rep.[d]	22.9	27.3	19.2	13.6	16.4	19.8	20.7	13.2	28.8	34.2	18.8	13.7
Greece	19.3	31.7	64.2	18.1	15.6	25.6	64.1	16.4	22.9	37.5	63.8	19.5
Hungary	9.7	15.3	57.7	9.0	5.9	10.1	71.2	7.1	13.2	20.2	53.0	10.3
Netherlands	17.8	11.0	−38.2	6.9	11.6	7.9	−31.9	6.0	23.9	14.1	−41.0	7.6
Northern Ireland[a]	8.8	5.5	−37.5	3.5	6.2	4.4	−29.0	3.6	11.2	6.5	−42.0	3.5
Norway	7.0	8.7	24.3	4.5	6.3	7.6	20.6	4.9	7.6	9.9	30.3	4.1
Scotland	13.1	12.4	−5.3	7.3	9.1	10.2	12.1	7.4	16.7	14.4	−13.8	7.2
Sweden	18.6	16.1	−13.4	7.6	16.1	14.5	−9.9	8.3	21.1	17.8	−15.6	6.8
Switzerland	20.8	19.0	−8.7	9.9	15.6	14.5	−7.1	9.5	25.7	23.1	−10.1	6.9
Yugoslavia[a]	6.2	8.7	40.3	7.5	4.9	6.7	36.7	6.6	7.4	10.8	45.9	8.1

*Adjusted on basis of age distribution of the United States total population, 1940.
[a] 1976 and 1977.
[b] 1974 and 1975.
[c] 1975 and 1976.
[d] Includes West Berlin.
[e] 1970 and 1971.

Source: Computed by the Statistical Bureau of the Metropolitan Life Insurance Company, based on data from the Division of Vital Statistics, National Center for Health Statistics, Statistics Canada, and World Health Statistics Annual.

Table 13–14. Age-Adjusted* Death Rates from Diabetes Mellitus in Various Countries by Age, and Sex, 1977–78

| | Death Rates per 100,000 | | | | | | | | | | | |
| | Total | | | | Male | | | | Female | | | |
Country	All Ages	25–44	45–64	65 & Over	All Ages	25–44	45–64	65 & Over	All Ages	25–44	45–64	65 & Over
Americas												
United States	10.4	2.6	16.7	90.9	10.5	3.0	17.4	88.4	10.3	2.2	16.0	92.4
Canada	9.5	1.8	12.1	94.8	10.0	2.3	13.6	94.6	9.1	1.3	10.7	94.9
Chile[a]	14.2	1.7	24.0	128.2	14.8	1.8	25.4	133.6	13.7	1.6	22.8	124.8
Africa												
Egypt[b]	11.0	3.4	25.5	66.4	11.4	4.1	27.0	63.0	10.6	2.7	24.0	69.1
Asia												
Israel	7.9	0.5	10.7	81.4	7.1	0.3	10.6	72.2	8.6	0.6	10.8	90.1
Japan	7.1	1.2	9.9	67.9	7.8	1.6	11.8	71.9	6.5	0.9	8.2	65.3
Philippines.[c]	5.0	0.9	8.8	NA	4.8	1.1	9.2	NA	5.3	0.7	8.4	NA
Europe												
Austria	8.8	1.7	10.5	89.5	8.2	2.2	11.9	75.0	8.9	1.2	9.3	97.4
Denmark	6.2	2.6	8.7	53.7	6.5	3.4	9.9	49.2	6.0	1.8	7.5	56.8
England & Wales[a]	5.4	1.2	7.2	51.3	5.8	1.5	8.3	51.6	5.1	0.8	6.2	51.1
France[c]	9.4	1.1	10.5	92.3	9.2	1.4	12.4	88.3	9.4	0.7	8.6	94.5
Germany, Fed. Rep.[d]	13.6	1.5	15.7	145.3	13.2	1.9	18.1	130.0	13.7	1.1	13.8	153.1
Greece	18.1	1.3	21.9	194.8	16.4	1.6	20.7	171.6	19.5	1.1	22.9	213.0
Hungary	9.0	1.2	12.5	89.0	7.1	1.2	11.5	63.7	10.3	1.1	13.3	106.1
Netherlands	6.9	1.0	8.8	70.5	6.0	1.2	8.1	57.7	7.6	0.7	9.4	79.5
Northern Ireland[a]	3.5	1.0	3.1	37.4	3.6	1.7	1.9	38.1	3.5	0.3	4.2	37.3
Norway	4.5	1.5	5.2	43.5	4.9	2.3	6.2	42.0	4.1	0.6	4.1	44.4
Scotland	7.3	2.1	10.5	63.9	7.4	2.4	10.2	65.3	7.2	1.9	10.9	62.9
Sweden	7.6	3.4	8.1	70.5	8.3	4.9	10.0	68.3	6.8	2.0	6.2	71.5
Switzerland	9.9	1.1	9.2	111.5	9.5	1.3	10.6	102.0	9.9	1.0	7.9	117.1
Yugoslavia[a]	7.5	1.3	12.4	66.6	6.6	1.5	12.7	51.4	8.1	1.0	12.1	77.5

*Adjusted on basis of age distribution of the United States total population, 1940.
[a] 1976 and 1977.
[b] 1974 and 1975.
[c] 1975 and 1976.
[d] Includes West Berlin.
NA: Not available.
Source: Computed by the Statistical Bureau of the Metropolitan Life Insurance Company, based on data from the Division of Vital Statistics, National Center for Health Statistics, Statistics Canada, and World Health Statistics Annual.

than male were Chile, Japan, England and Wales, Northern Ireland, and Scotland. No data are available in this age group for the Philippines. For males, death rates of around 50 or less/100,000 were reported in England and Wales, Yugoslavia, Denmark, Norway, and Northern Ireland. The highest death rate among males in the age category occurred in Greece where the rate was 171.6/100,000. Rates exceeding 100/100,000 were also present in Chile, Federal Republic of Germany, and Switzerland. Greece also reported the highest mortality among females, namely, 213/100,000. With the exclusion of Hungary, the same nations that experienced high male mortality recorded high female mortality.

English Studies of Mortality by Social Class of Occupation and Sex

For over 100 years, the Office of the Registrar General of England and Wales has periodically published studies of occupational mortality. The latest of these reports is based on registered deaths during 1970 to 1972 and the 1971 census. Although the report contains statistics for specific occupations, the number of deaths from diabetes is small and unless the data are grouped, statistically significant results are not attainable.

Table 13–15 shows that among men and married women who were classified according to their husband's occupation, the most favorable mortality ratios were found in the professional group and the ratios tended to increase as the occupations became less skilled. Since the occupational groupings reflect socio-economic status, the data show that the lower socio-economic groups have a higher mortality than the higher socio-economic groups. The trends for the two time periods shown in the table are similar.

Among single women the pattern is quite different. Of particular note was the higher mortality among single women who were professionals as compared to professional men and women who were married to professionals. Among single women there was a lower mortality ratio in Social Class II and the ratios then tend to increase in Social Classes III, IV, and V, with the exception of Class V in the period 1970–72 when there was a decrease, the significance of which is not clear.

SIGNIFICANCE OF THE DATA PRESENTED

Although it is difficult to determine firm reasons for much of the data, blemished as they are by inconsistencies of methods of gathering vital statistics around the world, nonetheless they provide much material for discussion and perhaps stimulation for further studies and comparisons. Death, after all, is a most definitive end-point and a most decisive fact even though the reasons for its occurrence may often be in the realm of speculation.

There are several intriguing facts concerning the data presented. There is reaffirmation of the belief that although the reported mortality from diabetes, per se, accounts for only 1.7% of all deaths in the United States, it is so closely associated with deaths from other diseases such as those affecting the cardiovascular and renal systems that it may rank as high as third as the basic or underlying cause of death.

Other data indicate that deaths from diabetes have leveled off and indeed are declining (Fig. 13–1). Why? There may be many explanations but the simplest conjecture would be that far fewer diabetic patients die from acute causes plainly related to diabetes (ketoacidotic coma, diabetic gangrene, etc.). Instead, they are increasingly dying from cardiovascular-renal causes and cancer, all of which occur at older ages, and usually are listed as dying from the more obvious disease. The data shown in Figure 13–1 are quite remarkable when contrasted with those in a similar figure providing the same type of information in the 11th edition of this book. At that point in time, age-adjusted death rates for diabetes were at their zenith. In the late

Table 13–15. Standardized Mortality Ratios for Diabetes Mellitus, at Ages 15 to 64 Years by Social Class of Occupation and Sex, England and Wales, 1959–63† and 1970–72‡

Social Class		Men		Married Women*		Single Women	
		1959–63	1970–72	1959–63	1970–72	1959–63	1970–72
I.	Professional, etc.	81	84	43	61	100	92
II.	Intermediate occupations	103	93	67	59	83	59
III.	Non-manual skilled	} 100	111	} 95	66	} 80	63
III.	Manual skilled		98		120		133
IV.	Partly skilled	98	111	121	143	114	137
V.	Unskilled	122	128	183	189	173	114

*Classified according to husband's occupation.
Source: †The Registrar General's Decennial Supplement, England and Wales, Occupational Mortality, 1961, Her Majesty's Stationery Office, London, 1971.
‡The Registrar General's Decennial Supplement, England and Wales, Occupational Mortality, 1971–72, Her Majesty's Stationery Office, London, 1978.

Table 13–16.　Percentage Distribution of Causes of Death Among 34,499 Diabetic Patients Dying in Specified Periods Between 1897 and 1979* (Experience of the Joslin Clinic)

Cause of Death	Pre-Insulin Era		Insulin Era					
	1897 to 5/31/14	6/1/14 to 8/6/22	8/7/22 to 12/31/36	1/1/37 to 12/31/43	1/1/44 to 12/31/49	1/1/50 to 12/31/59	1/1/60 to 12/31/68	1/1/69 to 7/31/79
All Causes:	100.0	100.0	100.0	100.0	100.0	100.0	100.0	100.0
Diabetic Coma: Total	63.8	41.5	8.3	2.8	1.7	1.0	1.1	1.2
a. Ketoacidotic	—	—	—	—	—	—	—	1.0
b. Hyperosmolar	—	—	—	—	—	—	—	0.2
Insulin (hypoglycemic) Reaction	0.0	0.0	0.2	0.3	0.2	0.2	0.3	0.4
Cardiorenal-vascular	17.5	24.6	54.4	65.7	71.3	76.7	77.0	75.6
Arteriosclerotic: Total	17.5	24.3	54.0	65.3	70.7	76.0	76.0	74.1
Cardiac	6.1	9.9	29.8	41.1	47.2	50.6	53.7	54.5
Renal: Total	3.4	3.8	4.8	4.6	5.8	9.0	8.1	7.0
Diabetic Nephropathy	—	—	—	—	—	5.2	5.5	5.4
Cerebral	2.8	4.9	9.3	11.8	12.8	12.9	12.4	11.1
Gangrene	3.7	4.2	8.0	5.3	2.9	2.0	1.0	0.9
Other Arteriosclerotic (including generalized)	1.5	1.4	2.1	2.5	2.0	1.5	0.8	0.6
Other Cardio-Vascular Disease	0.0	0.4	0.4	0.5	0.7	0.8	1.0	1.5
Infections: Total	12.3	17.6	17.7	12.6	7.6	5.7	5.3	4.3
Pneumonia	4.3	7.7	6.0	5.6	3.6	2.7	3.0	2.8
Gallbladder	0.0	0.5	0.5	0.6	0.3	0.3	0.2	0.1
Appendicitis	0.6	0.4	0.6	0.5	0.1	0.1	—	0.1
Kidney, acute	0.0	0.1	0.9	0.9	0.7	0.7	0.7	0.0
Abscesses	1.8	2.4	2.4	1.3	0.2	0.1	0.2	0.0
Other Infections	0.6	1.6	2.4	1.5	0.9	1.2	1.1	1.2
Tuberculosis	4.9	4.9	4.1	2.2	1.7	0.6	0.1	0.0
Cancer	1.5	3.8	8.7	9.0	9.7	10.5	10.5	12.0
Accident	0.0	0.8	2.0	1.9	2.1	1.9	1.8	1.7
Cirrhosis of the Liver	0.0	0.4	0.6	0.9	1.2	1.0	1.3	1.2
Suicide	0.3	0.2	0.7	0.6	0.6	0.3	0.3	0.5
Other Causes	2.1	4.7	4.9	2.7	2.9	2.1	2.1	2.4
"Diabetes" and Unknown	2.5	6.7	3.0	3.5	2.6	0.6	0.3	0.5
Number of deaths	326	843	4160	3641	4154	9925	7160	4290

*Deaths reported up to 7/31/79.
Note: Figures for 1950 and later are not strictly comparable with those for earlier periods because of changes in the basis of classification.

1960s a downward trend began which continues quite remarkably.

Some of the other data are not surprising although the reason for their occurrence is a matter for conjecture. In the nonwhite racial groups, that mortality among Blacks is significantly higher than that among Indians, Japanese, Chinese or other ethnic classes is known but not understood. Economic advantages or disadvantages and access to necessary medical care may be factors, but this is difficult to prove. Why, for example, should mortality among those U.S.A. residents of Japanese ancestry be only half that of the Chinese? Is it heredity, dietary factors or some other influence? The geographic variations in mortality rates are interesting. Judging from vital statistics, people living in the Southern and Western parts of the United States fared much better than those in other areas as to both crude and age-adjusted death rates. This is difficult to understand. Is it due to climate? Or does it reflect differences in types of persons, ancestry, life style, or type of medical care and recording of deaths? Of possible relevance is the fact that, in general, many of the older population live in the warmer climates.

Just as the seasonal patterns may seem to influence the onset of diabetes in juveniles, deaths from diabetes in the general population are most prevalent in the winter months. Here a common assumption is that illnesses common in winter weather play a major role. The fact that the most favorable mortality rates are found in the professional groups and that the rates tend to increase as occupations become less skilled is not surprising and is consistent with data from previous editions. The tendency is to believe that those in the more skilled occupations possess superior knowledge and health awareness as well as better access to medical care, but why the increased mortality from diabetes among single women who were professionals as compared to professional men and women married to professionals? These data provoke further study; it is from conjecture and the constant seeking for further information that progress is made in the understanding of all chronic diseases including diabetes.

Probably the most interesting information comes to physicians in answer to age-old questions concerning how diabetics fare over the long span of many decades. One suspects that the causes of death have changed and that acute deaths are slowly diminishing. Table 13–16, which presents the percentage distribution of principal causes of death

among 34,499 diabetic patients dying in specified periods between 1897 and July 13, 1979, is quite remarkable. It is an extension of data found in the prior edition of this book which ended with statistics from 1968. One can argue that this information is not complete and that it has a built-in bias since it reflects only the experience of Joslin Clinic patients and largely the hospital experience from the New England Deaconess Hospital. Nevertheless, it is a long-term record of the lives and deaths of a large series of patients from the same group in whom comparisons can be made over decades. Deaths from ketoacidotic coma, for example, have stabilized, while there has been a small increase in those from hyperosmolar coma. This probably was true for many years, but only recently has it been succinctly defined. Deaths ascribed to insulin (hypoglycemic) reactions have increased although minutely. Cardiovascular deaths reached their apex 2 decades ago and now, while still high, have dropped somewhat, in keeping with the trend in the general population, possibly due to better care. The renal death rate is decreasing, although slowly; one hopes and presumes that this improvement also is because of better treatment. Fatal acute infections such as pneumonia and those involving the gallbladder continue to decrease in number, and death from tuberculosis, still the scourge of developing nations, has literally disappeared in this study group. Since everyone eventually dies from some cause, cancer, most often found in older age groups, has increased.

One can argue about the complete validity of this type of information, but if it encourages those with diabetes, knowing that they are indeed living longer and better, and if it shows that the most recent experience of one large group has improved when compared to statistical data concerning the same group over a period embracing close to a century, then this chapter will have been useful.

REFERENCES

1. Palumbo, P.J., Elveback, L.R., Chu, C-P., et al.: Diabetes mellitus: Incidence, prevalence, survivorship, and causes of death in Rochester, Minnesota 1945–1970. Diabetes 25:566, 1976.
2. Tokuhata, G.H., Miller, W., Digon, E., et al.: Diabetes mellitus: an undetermined health problem. J. Chron. Dis. 28:23, 1975.
3. Dr. Maureen Harris, National Diabetes Data Group, National Institutes of Health, Bethesda, Maryland. Personal communication.
4. World Health Organization: Footnote to Annex 3, In: WHO Expert Committee on Diabetes Mellitus, 2nd Report. Technical Report Series #646. Geneva, World Health Organization, 1980, p. 73.

14 The Pathology of Diabetes Mellitus

Merle A. Legg and Sami J. Harawi

Diabetes mellitus, a disease with an extraordinarily diverse pathology, with a range of anatomic lesions that is hard to duplicate by any other disease, and with a long history of known related lesions, still is a disease with many puzzles in correlating the anatomic and the clinical. The pancreas is the logical first organ to study in diabetes because it is the source of insulin. Hyalinization of the islets of Langerhans was described in 1901[1] but it is still not certain how this peculiar deposit of an amyloid variant comes about nor is it limited to the diabetic. Nevertheless, great strides in information about the endocrine pancreas have been taken since the last edition of this book. Some observations of previous years have been modified as the result of studies made possible by new tools such as immunocytochemistry and some previous observations are more understandable because of additional new information. Statements made in previous editions of this book are still true, namely, that there is no consistent anatomic lesion found at autopsy on diabetic patients, but there are some distinctive abnormalities which provide a solid basis for the pathophysiology and clinical features of diabetes.[2] The diverse lesions are not limited to the pancreas but are systemic. The autopsy is not less but more important than before in the study of diabetes as the knowledge of pancreatic biology increases and as new modes of therapy such as renal and pancreatic transplants and laser photocoagulation in diabetic retinopathy are employed.

In a brief summary such as this, the discussion and weighing of references to studies must be kept to the summary level. More detailed reporting and discussion are in the monograph by Warren, LeCompte and Legg,[3] the more recent and extensive review by Bloodworth and Greider,[4] and the monographs edited by Volk and Wellman[5] and Cooperstein and Watkins.[5a]

PANCREAS

Normal Pancreas

There is such a wide range of variation in the normal pancreas that it is difficult to define the abnormal. In the normal human adult it weighs on the average about 95 g with a range of 60 to 160 g. Some of the variability of the weight of the normal dissected pancreas depends on the amount of loose connective tissue and fat both within the septa between lobules and on the surface of the gland. The average weight of the pancreas at birth is 2.6 g. The pancreas consists of a head, body, and tail as a single structure but aberrant pancreatic tissue may be found in the gastric antrum, the wall of the duodenum, the jejunum, Meckel's diverticulum, and in certain other sites including the gallbladder.

Embryology. The development of the pancreas has been studied not only in animals, but also in human embryos and fetuses.[6-9] The pancreas develops from two buds of the endoderm; the dorsal evagination occurs before the ventral. The ventral bud is a branch of the liver bud, from which arise the liver, bile ducts, and gallbladder. The dorsal bud grows toward the spleen and forms the duct of Santorini, while the ventral bud forms the uncinate process and the duct of Wirsung. The buds fuse and the ducts usually fuse; ducts form the ductules. The outpouching is rather similar to that in the formation of the lung. The primitive epithelial cells rest in a single layer on a basal lamina surrounded by a cap of mesenchymal cells. The branching and budding of ductules progress until the intralobular ductules are formed and from these are developed both the acini and the islets of Langerhans. The adult form of the pancreas is already apparent at about 14 weeks. Robb noted human islets developing at 10 to 16 weeks.[7] A (alpha) and B (beta) cells may be seen early in fetal life but with more A cells than in the post-natal pancreas.

Rutter also observed differentiation of pancreatic primordia isolated in tissue culture and found that both endocrine and exocrine cells developed.[8] Because of the interest in the dispersed endocrine system, the similarity in appearance of the cells and the common capacity of amine precursor uptake and decarboxylation (APUD) in a large number of endocrine organs and tissue, the idea of an APUD system including the pancreatic endocrine cells has been suggested as has the thought that the cells are derived from the neural crest.[10-13] However, from the above embryologic observations and some elegant experiments involving removal and transplantation of embryonic neural crests, the more reliable conclusion seems to be that the islet tissue is of endodermal origin and that the islet tissue has a ductular cell ancestor.[14] This explanation of the islet origin facilitates the understanding of the intimate relationship between ductules and islet tissue and the apparent new formation of islets from ductules sometimes seen in both diabetic (Fig. 14–1) and nondiabetic pancreases and the occurrence of ductular components in islet cell neoplasms.

Islet Size and Distribution. Most but not all of the cells of the endocrine pancreas are clustered in islands of cells as described by Langerhans in 1869.[15] The size of the individual normal islets varies considerably: while most islets measure from 75 to 175 μm in diameter, islets as large as 300 μm in diameter cannot be considered abnormal.

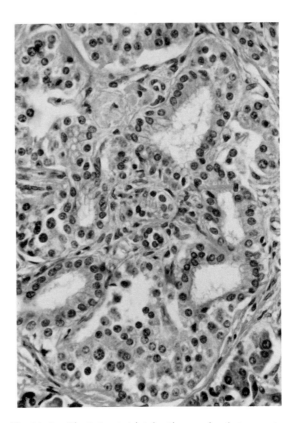

Fig. 14–1. The intimate islet-ductile complex that suggests new formation of islet tissue from ductular progenitor cells, recapitulating islet embryogenesis. The patient was a 73-year-old obese woman who had had diabetes mellitus for 5 years and who died with cirrhosis of the liver. H & E × 400. (#238470).

The number of islets is also extremely variable in the normal pancreas. In a 1913 study of normal human pancreases, Clark found from 250,000 to 1,750,000 islets.[16] Estimates of the number of islets from a few sections of the pancreas may be quite misleading since there is great variation in the distribution of islets from pancreas to pancreas. Although islets usually are more common in the tail of the pancreas than in the remainder of the organ, there are exceptions. Of the various methods which have been used for the estimation of number and size of islets, probably the most accurate are those of Ogilvie,[17] Hellman and associates,[18] and Gepts.[19] Because of the distribution problem and the variation in size and shape of the islets, any accurate estimation of total islet number and volume requires a great deal of time and meticulous technique. Thus, such studies have been practical only in small series of patients.

Pancreatic Endocrine Cells. The cell population of the islets includes at least 8 different cells or cells that produce at least 8 different secretory products, although not all can be demonstrated con-

Table 14–1.   Pancreatic Endocrine Cells

Cell	Secretory Product
A	Glucagon
B	Insulin
D	Somatostatin
D₁	Vasoactive intestinal polypeptide (VIP)
EC	5-hydroxytryptamine or 5-hydroxytryptophane
G	Gastrin
P	Bombesin
PP	Pancreatic polypeptide

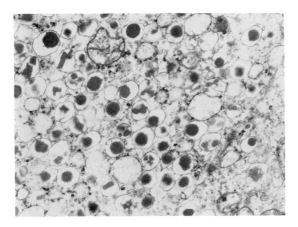

Fig. 14–2. The range of appearance of B cell granules in a normal islet of Langerhans. The crystalloid rectangular granules, which represent insulin, are specific. Electron micrograph with Karnovsky's fixative, prepared by Dr. M. Federman. × 20,000.

sistently in normal human adult islets of Langerhans. In Table 14–1 is a listing of pancreatic endocrine cells derived from the Lausanne classification.[20] One might add other cells since they have occurred in pancreatic endocrine tumors and some have found such cells in normal pancreases.[21,22] Adrenocorticotropin-secreting cells and calcitonin-secreting cells are examples. It is clear also that the interrelationships among the pancreatic endocrine cells are much more complex than the simple insulin-glucagon relationship of only a few years ago. Furthermore, many of the cells are scattered through the mucosa of the gastrointestinal tract and some in the bronchial mucosa.

Relatively simple staining techniques for the islet cells were, and still are, useful for identifying beta (B) cells, using Gomori's aldehyde fuchsin[23] and chrome alum hematoxylin phloxine[24] methods and modifications of them.[25] These techniques are inadequate for identifying most of the other cells and their products (See Plate IA).* Immunocytochem-

*All color plates will be found in a separate signature in the center of the book.

istry and extraction and chemical analysis are the techniques that have opened the door to the diversity of cells and their secretory products.[26–28] The immunoperoxidase technique is the most widely used because of its availability for previously fixed and paraffin-embedded tissue (See Plate IB).

The B cell granules stain deep purple with the aldehyde fuchsin stain and the Gomori trichrome counterstain; the A cells stain red and the D cells a clear, pale blue. With the chrome alum hematoxylin phloxine stain, the B granules are blue-gray and those of the A cells and certain other cells, particularly D cells, red. With immunocytochemistry, the B granules were labeled for insulin first with immunofluorescent techniques and then with immunoperoxidase techniques.[29–31] The B granules in man are distinctive when studied by electron microscopy. Some are sharply defined rectangular granules floating in a larger saccule and others are variations between this specific form and round to irregular granules but still with a clearly crystalloid structure[32,33] (Fig. 14–2). The arrays of rough endoplasmic reticulum common to polypeptide hormone-secreting cells are prominent in B cells as well. The estimation of B granule content in the pancreas provides a quick estimate of pancreatic insulin. The A cells in electron micrographs have double-contoured granules with a central dense core and a paler aura more completely filling the membrane-bound secretory granule 200 to 450 nm (nanometers) in diameter[32,33] (Fig. 14–3). The dense core of the A cell granule reacts as glucagon with immunocytochemical techniques, while the paler aura has been shown by immuno-electron-microscopy to contain glicentin, a glucagon precursor.[33a] The B cells are 3 to 8 times as numerous as A cells and comprise 60 to 70% of the total islet cell population.[33,34]

Using the Hellerström-Hellman technique, one can identify the black-stained granules of the D cells.[4,35] In electron micrographs, the D granules are relatively large (mean diameter of 375 nm), finely granular and fill the limiting membrane of the secretory granule[33] (Fig. 14–4). These granules are not as distinctive as those of A and B cells; this helps to explain the confusion in identification of the cell in relationship to its secretory product, particularly as a source of tumors. It is clear now that the D cells secrete somatostatin.[33,36] They form a small minority (2 to 8%) of the normal islet population. The micro-universe of just these three cell types, A, B, and D, becomes clear when one considers the interactions of the respective three hormones: glucagon, insulin, and somatostatin. By transmission electron microscopy and freeze-fracture techniques, gap junctions have been demonstrated between islet cells.[33a] Peptide messengers

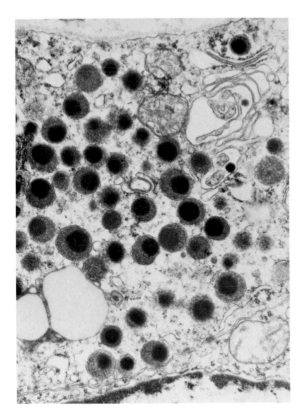

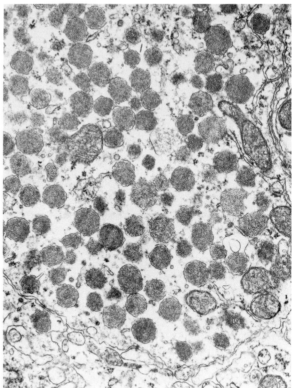

Fig. 14–3. The distinctive double contour secretory granules of normal A cells of the islet of Langerhans. Electron micrograph with Karnovsky fixative, prepared by Dr. M. Federman. ×20,000.

Fig. 14–4. D cell granules of a normal islet of Langerhans. Electron micrograph with Karnovsky fixative, prepared by Dr. M. Federman. ×20,000.

seem to pass from one cell to its neighbor through these intercellular gaps, a phenomenon referred to as paracrine secretion. As part of its generalized inhibitory action, somatostatin inhibits both glucagon and insulin.[35] The paracrine inhibitory action of somatostatin seems to play an important role in maintaining optimal glucose homeostasis.[35]

Of the other cell types included in the endocrine pancreas and listed in Table 14–1, the PP cells are particularly abundant in the pancreases of human fetuses and newborns but are much less frequent in adult pancreases.[33] They can be identified by using the immunoperoxidase technique for pancreatic polypeptide and less reliably by electron microscopy.[37] The PP cells are found outside, as well as within, the islets of Langerhans, as part of duct epithelium and seem to be much more frequent in the head of the pancreas.[33,38] In electron micrographs, the secretory granules of PP cells are small, 80 to 200 nm, vary in shape from round to ovoid to irregular, and have a narrow or imperceptible clear zone between the granule and the membrane.[33,37,39] Although the functional significance of pancreatic polypeptide is not entirely clear, the cells appear frequently as a component of islet cell tumors of different types and sometimes as the predominant cell.[32]

The D_1, EC, and G cells which produce respectively, vasoactive intestinal polypeptide (VIP), serotonin and related products, and gastrin have not been demonstrable consistently in normal human adult pancreases although they have been important as islet tumor cells.[32] The granule ultrastructure of some of the cells is not distinctive enough for reliable classification on that basis alone.

The islets of Langerhans are well supplied with blood vessels providing wide anastomosing sinusoids for a rich blood flow about the islet cells. The interstitial tissue is usually scant. Numerous fine, non-myelinated nerve fibers surround and extend into islets and seem to be not only sympathetic, but also parasympathetic in origin. However, nerve endings in human islets are found rarely if at all.[33]

Changes in the Islets of Langerhans in Diabetes

Since the B cells of the islets of Langerhans clearly produce insulin and since the estimation of the quantity of B secretory granules provides an estimate of pancreatic insulin, a logical study to perform in an autopsy on a diabetic patient is to determine whether the number of B granules is sufficient to control normal carbohydrate metabolism. The presence of seemingly adequate secretory granules does not exclude the possibility of diabetes since there could still be defects in secretion, barriers to the transport of insulin, lack of insulin receptors on target cell membranes and other mechanisms beyond the adequate production of insulin within the B cell. The islet lesions in patients with insulin-dependent, compared with those in non-insulin-dependent, diabetes tend to fall into different groups, although there is some overlap and there is a wide range in the appearance of the islets.

Hyalinization. The longest known and most frequently found lesions of the islets is *hyalinization*. It is seen in about 30% of diabetic subjects who come to autopsy (See Plate IC).[40] Although it is one of the typical lesions of diabetes, it is not pathognomonic of the disease, since hyalinization occurs with increasing frequency with age and has been reported in 10% of nondiabetics over 50 years of age.[41] The deposition of hyaline material varies in extent from one islet to another in the same pancreas, ranging from minimal to almost complete replacement of the islet. Furthermore, there may be areas of the pancreas in which the islets are involved, even severely involved, while in other parts of the organ there is no discernible involvement of the islets. The material is deposited between the islet cells and the capillaries in contact with the capillary walls but not in the capillary basement membrane.[41] The material is less dense than the smudgy material in the small blood vessel walls of diabetic microangiopathy and is much less intensely stained with the periodic acid-Schiff technique which, together with the separation from the basement membrane, clearly separate the material from the lesion of diabetic microangiopathy. Despite the resemblance to amyloid, many attempts to identify the material as amyloid have been frustrated by the inconstancy of the substance in taking the amyloid stains.[41] Nevertheless, the fact that it does stain often with amyloid stains plus the demonstration by Lacy that the material has the thin fibrils and periodicity which resemble those of amyloid in fine structural studies, are persuasive in classifying the material as amyloid. Westermark found fine differences in the ultrastructure of the fibrils from that of other amyloid.[42] Clearly there does not seem to be any relationship between the presence of islet amyloid and the ordinary forms of amyloidosis.[41] Amyloid does occur in islet tumors. One might also speculatively compare islet amyloid with the isolated amyloid of the small cerebral vessels in the aged or of the isolated myocardial amyloid in the same age group.

Hyalinization of the islets is rare in insulin-dependent diabetes. It is particularly likely to be present in older individuals with diabetes of long duration and appears to be more closely related to the age of the patient than to duration or severity of diabetes. In our laboratory, it occurred in only 1 of 81 patients whose diabetes appeared before the age of 20 and was of 10 or more years' duration. On the other hand, hyalin was present in 44 of 86 persons with diabetes of similar duration, but who were 61 years of age or older.[43]

The exact significance of hyalinization or amyloid deposition in the islets is still unknown but it seems unlikely to be the basic defect in the production of diabetes. In some instances the hyaline deposits seem to be crowding out the islet cells, resulting in pyknotic, poorly granulated B cells with extensive involvement of islets, seemingly an obvious reason for insufficient insulin (Fig. 14–5). Such severe and extensive involvement is rare, however, and there are many instances in which there is still abundant B cell granulation in well-hyalinized islets. Some evidence suggests that the hyaline material develops from degenerating B

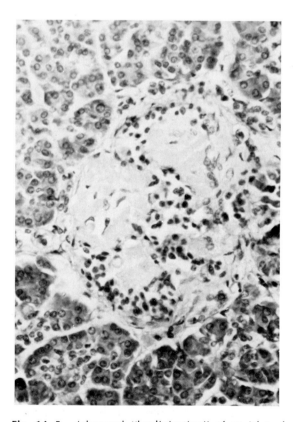

Fig. 14–5. Advanced "hyalinization" of an islet of Langerhans. The amorphous amyloid has compressed the pyknotic islet cells and replaced most of the islet. The patient was a 67-year-old man who had had diabetes mellitus for 13 years. H & E ×400 (#240405).

cells.[44] The hyalin may represent an associated phenomenon rather than either a cause or effect of diabetes. It is possible that the hyalin acts as a barrier between well-granulated B cells and capillaries. In view of the presence of the same material in insulin-producing islet tumors (amyloid may also be seen in other islet tumors), hyalin may be related to the production of excessive or abnormal insulin or to a local reaction to insulin (or other hormones).

B Cell Degranulation. A reduction in B cell granulation in the absence of other apparent change in the islets is a frequent finding in diabetes and is usually referred to as "degranulation of beta (B) cells" (See Plate ID). In Bell's series of 995 diabetic autopsies, decreased granulation of some degree was found in all patients under 20 years of age, in 79.5% of those between 20 and 40, in 48.2% of those between 40 and 60, and in 33.6% of those over 60 years of age.[44] In contrast, Bell found degranulation of B cells in only 2 of 250 nondiabetics. In our own laboratory, 43 of 223 diabetic pancreases showed decreased B granulation. The two series are not comparable since Bell included all kinds of islet lesions in which B cell granulation was decreased while Warren, LeCompte, and Legg[3] referred to decreased B cell granulation in the absence of other lesions, thus excluding hyalinization, hydropic change, shifts in cell ratios, etc. A reduction in B granulation seems to offer a simple and ready explanation for a lack of insulin. However, its interpretation in a specific case must be dealt with cautiously, especially when a number of other factors are not known. Decreased granulation can be produced experimentally with later return to normal granulation by such contrasting mechanisms as glucose loading, tolbutamide administration, and long-term insulin administration. Furthermore, the estimation of the adequacy of B cell granulation is somewhat subjective unless degranulation is marked. Continued stimuli of the sort just mentioned may result in progression to more permanent injury such as hydropic degeneration, glycogen infiltration, and necrosis.[4]

In the pancreas of the patient who has died after having had the juvenile-onset type of diabetes (IDDM) for 20 or 30 years, the changes in the islets are usually quite different from those described above. The pancreas is small and the islets are reduced in number, sometimes so severely reduced that they are hard to find. In addition, the islets are small with small, pyknotic-appearing cells, often in cords and often with a compressed or distorted outline of the islet instead of the normal rounded configuration. The cells do not stain for B granules and so they have been referred to as "atrophic" or "undifferentiated" islets of

Langerhans.[45] With immunocytochemical techniques, the cells appear to be mostly PP cells secreting pancreatic polypeptide and in fact there is an increase in PP cells dispersed through the exocrine pancreas[45] (See Plate IE). In some of the patients studied by Gepts and DeMey, there were prominent A cells with glucagon secretion, so prominent that they thought there might be a true, rather than just apparent, hyperplasia of A cells.[46] In another report, Gepts et al. observed D cells with somatostatin secretion as well as A cells in the long-term juvenile type of diabetes.[47]

Insulitis. The characteristic lesion of the pancreas in the patient with recently developed IDDM (acute or recent onset) is *insulitis,* in which there is infiltration of the islets by lymphocytes, plasma cells, and/or histiocytes.[45–49] It is not consistently present in acute onset juvenile diabetes but it is the most frequent finding in such patients. The occasional series of such patients reported without insulitis is hard to understand, except statistically.[50] In most patients, Gepts and DeMey found that B cells were still present in pancreases with insulitis, often partly obscured by the inflammatory reaction and often with evidence of hyperactivity, but with a reduced number of cells.[45] In contrast, the A and D cells were numerous. In a second stage group, patients with juvenile diabetes of one-half to 10 years' duration had greatly decreased or absent B cells but still many A and D cells as well as an increased number of PP cells. In 2 of 14 cases, there were absent A cells. Gepts and DeMey suggested that the injury to islets resulting in insulitis stimulates regenerative activity of islet cells with fairly good A cell and D cell response but that in diabetes of longer duration, a more abnormal regeneration from ductular cells producing PP cells takes over.[46] Such an hypothesis ties together the range of changes from insulitis with remaining B cells to small islets composed mostly of PP cells.

The reason for the development of insulitis may not be a single one or else it might be a common pathway arrived at by different routes. The type of mononuclear inflammatory cells in insulitis (occasionally polymorphonuclear leukocytes and eosinophils may be present as well) tempts one to think of an autoimmune reaction comparable to lymphocytic thyroiditis or to the immune reaction in transplant rejection. Renold and others did demonstrate insulitis following both heterologous and homologous insulin injection in cows.[51,52] Such experimental evidence supports the autoimmune concept. However, some viral diseases in man and those produced experimentally in animals result in insulitis. Mumps pancreatitis has long been suggested and the viruses implicated experimentally and clinically include encephalomyocarditis virus, group B Coxsackie viruses, and cytomegalovirus.[53–56] Perhaps the insulitis is an autoimmune reaction following the initial injury to the islets or perhaps it is all due to direct viral injury. It does not seem likely, however, that a large number of patients with IDDM owe their disease to viral infection.

Hydropic Change. In our experience, hydropic change of islet cells is an infrequent lesion in the human diabetic pancreas; it can be simulated by autolysis. The B granules disappear and are replaced by vacuoles which coalesce, resulting in a cell largely replaced by watery fluid. While mild degrees of hydropic change are reversible, more advanced degrees result in atrophy and disappearance of the cell.[4,45] Some cells with the appearance of hydropic change contain large amounts of glycogen in the cleared cytoplasm.[57] The glycogen-containing cells seem to be related to hyperglycemia and the high glycogen content is reversible.[45] Hydropic change is also found more frequently in patients whose islets have been "overstrained" and who have severe diabetic symptoms. It has been found in nondiabetic patients, although rarely.[58] It has been also produced experimentally in animals and in tissue culture of islet cells.[50]

Fibrosis. Another long-recognized lesion of the islets in the human diabetic pancreas is fibrosis, a change found in 13% of the diabetic pancreases in our laboratory. The range of fibrosis is variable from islet to islet and the severity within an islet ranges from minimal interstitial fibrosis to complete replacement of the islet. Fibrosis seems to relate to the older age group and to vascular disease.[4]

Quantitative Changes. The quantitative changes within the endocrine pancreas are difficult to study because of the problems referred to above and because of the wide range of normal in the number and size of islets and their dispersal through the pancreas. It is possible, however, to assess the ratios of cells by using reasonable samples of the pancreas to represent head, body, and tail. The ratio studies of large series were done with granule stains and not the more recent immunocytochemical techniques and so they were most accurate in terms of the number of B cells relative to other cells (See Plate lF). In the group reported by Warren, LeCompte, and Legg, 38 of 223 consecutive diabetic pancreases studied showed *islet ratio changes* in which the ratio of B cells to other cells was less than 3:1.[59] Since the demonstration of the true identity of the cells in the "atrophic, undifferentiated" islets of the juvenile diabetic (see above), it seems quite likely that the cell ratio changes described as A:B cell ratios are not that simple. Nevertheless, it does appear possible that

a patient could have an absolute increase in A cells with excess circulating glucagon, but as a diffuse process (not a neoplasm), such must be rare.

In view of the presently recognized diversity of cells in the endocrine pancreas, the quantitative studies of *islet mass* and *beta cell mass* by Gepts and by Maclean and Ogilvie, respectively, seem more crude now, despite the painstaking effort they required.[19,60] Nevertheless, the total B cell mass alone seems a significant figure. Gepts found a mean total weight of islet tissue of 1.358 g in 31 nondiabetic pancreases and 0.765 g in 28 diabetic pancreases.[19] He computed the B cell mass as 0.754 g in the nondiabetics and 0.301 g in the diabetics. Maclean and Ogilvie with a different technique compared islet B cell mass in 30 persons with long-term diabetes with that in 30 nondiabetics. In the diabetics, they computed 0.22 g of B cells compared to 0.64 g in nondiabetics.[60]

Hypertrophy and Hyperplasia. *Hypertrophy of islets* does occur in diabetics, although in less than 5% of autopsied cases, using a diameter of 400 μm as the threshold in considering an islet hypertrophied. When the phenomenon is observed, it is usually seen in scattered islets and not as a general picture. The normal arrangement of cells may be preserved, there may be a coiling ribbon pattern of cells, and there may or may not be changes in cell ratios. Hypertrophy of islets is a common change, however, in infants born of diabetic mothers.[61]

Hyperplasia is related to hypertrophy of the islets since there is usually an actual increase in the number of cells in such instances and perhaps should be the term used instead of hypertrophy. It is frequently assumed that hyperinsulinism may result from diffuse islet hyperplasia, but this is difficult to prove and in our own experience, is rare. It seems likely that most such instances are the result of wishful explanation of otherwise unexplained hypoglycemia. The best evidence for hypersecretion by hypertrophic or hyperplastic islets is in the infants of diabetic mothers in whom the islets typically average more than normal size and often are several times normal size.[61] The presumption has been that the hyperplasia is a compensatory one in response to the hyperglycemia of the mother, although the evidence for poor control of diabetes was not consistently present. With the use of glycosylated hemoglobin values, it is now possible to estimate more accurately the consistency of control in the pregnant diabetic woman.

Hyperplasia of islets has been reported in diabetic patients who have received tolbutamide therapy.[62] According to studies by Potet and co-workers, the non-neoplastic islets in patients with the Zollinger-Ellison syndrome are increased in size

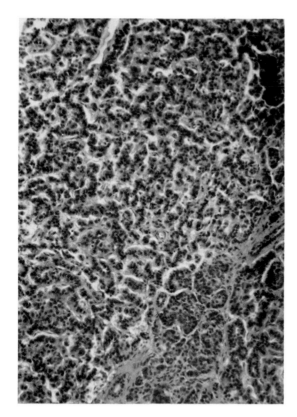

Fig. 14–6. Unusual islet hyperplasia, leaving only the exocrine pancreatic tissue in the right lower corner of the picture. The patient was a 68-year-old obese man with diabetes for 9 years who was treated by diet and, for the last year of his life, tolbutamide. H & E ×150 (#191943).

and show an increase in the percentage of non-B cells.[63] We have observed such a phenomenon in some patients with the Zollinger-Ellison syndrome but have found normal background islets in others.[39] Nesidioblastosis is a term that has been used to indicate widespread proliferation of islet tissue from ductules, although it has also been used less properly to indicate islet tumors as well. It does seem to be the basic lesion in some cases of infants with neonatal hypoglycemia.[64]

Tumors of the Islets of Langerhans. In 1854 autopsies on diabetic patients, Warren, LeCompte, and Legg found 18 islet cell tumors, including 2 carcinomas, a frequency which was not significantly different from their finding of 24 tumors, also including 2 carcinomas, in 2708 autopsied nondiabetic patients.[65] Those tumors were reported in 1966, well before the era of immunocytochemistry and have not been studied retrospectively. There are four kinds of islet cell tumors that can produce a clinical picture of diabetes, namely those whose secretion is respectively glucagon, somatostatin, vasoactive intestinal polypeptide (VIP), or adrenocorticotropin (ACTH). However, each of

these tumors usually has a specific set of other symptoms and signs that make diagnosis easier; such tumors provide a source of reversible diabetes.

Other Pancreatic Changes

In the normal pancreas there is relatively little fibrous tissue in the septa between the lobules and only a delicate basement membrane between the acini and islets. A relatively common finding in the pancreas of diabetics is *fibrosis,* either interlobular or interacinar or both. At times the fibrosis is associated with lymphocytic and histiocytic infiltration and may well represent the end-stage of chronic pancreatitis. The fibrosis may vary from small foci to almost complete replacement of acinar tissue. There is no constant relationship between acinar fibrosis and islet lesions. Often the islets are left apparently intact in a sea of fibrous tissue with the acinar tissue replaced.

Fibrosis may be the result of infection, an attack of acute hemorrhagic pancreatitis, the end-stage of

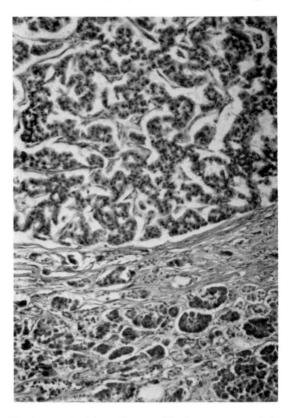

Fig. 14–7. An islet cell tumor fills the upper part of the picture. When this tumor was studied in 1963, no specific granules were found. Modern immunocytochemical techniques should clarify the cell type and secretory products of such tumors. The tumor is from the pancreas of a 79-year-old man who had had diabetes mellitus for 22 years and who died with arteriosclerotic heart disease. H & E ×150 (#225510).

chronic pancreatitis, duct obstruction by calculi or tumor, arteriosclerosis, or cystic fibrosis. Usually the relationship of fibrosis either to the diabetic state or to another cause cannot be defined in an individual instance. There is evidence, however, that patients with cystic fibrosis usually develop diabetes if there is a familial history of that disease.[66] Farber found no significant alterations in the islets in cases of cystic fibrosis.[67] Bloodworth reported that in patients with cystic fibrosis who reached adulthood, the frequency of diabetes was 20 times that in the general population.[4] Partly because of the degree of preservation of the pancreas in such patients, he suggested that there is a parallel inheritance of diabetes and cystic fibrosis. We have not studied the islets of a series of patients with cystic fibrosis.

Fatty infiltration of the pancreas is rather common in diabetic individuals. It is also frequent in obese persons and it seems to be related to fat storage rather than to diabetes per se.

Arteriosclerosis, being a prominent problem in diabetic patients, might be considered to be the source of pancreatic lesions. However, the increase in arteriosclerosis in the rest of the body is not equally reflected in the pancreas. Warren, LeCompte, and Legg reported severe arteriosclerosis in only 7.4% of their diabetic autopsy series.[68] The arteriosclerosis seems to be a result rather than the cause of the diabetes (see below).

Acute pancreatitis occasionally is a causative factor in diabetes. Hyperglycemia frequently occurs during the acute attack. In a review, Wellmann and Volk found reported incidences of hyperglycemia in various series ranging from 4.4 to 79% of patients during an attack of acute pancreatitis.[69] The hyperglycemia is transient, however, and generally subsides if the patient survives the acute pancreatitis. In the same review, though, different series reported permanent diabetes in from 1.4 to 31% of the patients who recovered. Complicating the relationship is the apparent increased incidence of acute pancreatitis in diabetic persons.

Chronic pancreatitis (chronic recurrent pancreatitis and chronic calcifying pancreatitis) seems to be followed by an increased incidence of diabetes.[69-71] Many series are cited by Wellmann and Volk with the majority reporting one third to one half of patients with chronic pancreatitis to have diabetes.[69] They also point out not only the preservation of islets in chronic pancreatitis, but also that some even show hypertrophy, hyperplasia or neoformation of islets. Although the diabetes in such patients tends to be mild, in some persons there are wide swings with hypoglycemia more frequent than ketoacidosis.

Other kinds of inflammation occur in the pan-

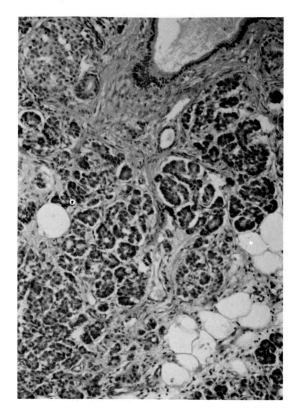

Fig. 14–8. Early stage of chronic pancreatitis with mild duct cell hyperplasia, partial fibrosis replacement of acinar tissue, and a remaining islet of Langerhans in the left upper corner. Same patient as in Figure 14–1. H & E ×150 (#238470).

creas: e.g., abscess formation, tuberculosis, and syphilis. All are infrequent and appear to have little or no relationship to diabetes.

Carcinoma of the pancreas was more frequently observed in the diabetic autopsy series of Warren, LeCompte, and Legg than in the nondiabetic population.[68] Others have noted increased pancreatic carcinoma in patients with diabetes.[4,39,72] However, some recent prospective epidemiologic studies of pancreatic cancer have not supported this increase. MacMahon and others found a relationship to coffee drinking and Lin and Kessler noted that this extended to the decaffeinated variety.[73,74] Since there is such extensive reserve in the endocrine pancreas, a carcinoma would need to replace most of the pancreatic tissue, either directly or indirectly, in order to cause diabetes by loss of islet tissue. Carcinoma of the pancreas seldom replaces the larger part of the pancreatic tissue but frequently obstructs the ducts in the head of the pancreas to produce pancreatitis.

Size of Pancreas in Diabetes. Because of the great variation in size of the normal pancreas and because it is difficult to determine accurately the *total pancreatic mass* without meticulous removal of peripancreatic and interlobular fat, figures on total pancreatic weight or size in the diabetic arc unreliable. Most investigators, however, have reported that the average weight of the pancreas in diabetes is lower than the normal, particularly with the juvenile diabetic population.

Total pancreatectomy in man leads to a diabetic state with an insulin requirement of about 40 units per day.[75,76] It is usually stated that removal of 90 to 95% of the pancreas is necessary to produce diabetes.

KIDNEY

Certain renal glomerular lesions in diabetic patients are among the most specific pathologic changes in the disease. Other renal lesions seem to be accentuated in the presence of diabetes, but are by no means limited to this disease. Renal lesions in the diabetic may involve the glomeruli, tubules, interstitial tissue, and blood vessels, but the most characteristic and significant changes are in the glomeruli.

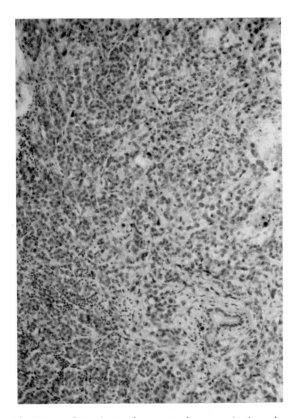

Fig. 14–9. Extensive replacement of pancreatic tissue by a poorly differentiated adenocarcinoma of the pancreas. A few acini can be seen in the flood of tumor cells and a remaining small ductule in the right lower corner. The patient was a 57-year-old man who had had diabetes for 8 years. H & E ×150 (#220345).

Glomerulus: Structure and Function

The normal glomerulus is a filtering device consisting of numerous capillary loops covered by a reflected epithelium of mesodermal origin with the parietal component of the epithelium forming Bowman's capsule. The capillary loops are arranged in small lobules budding from a central axis in the glomerulus. Between the fenestrated endothelial cells and the foot processes of the epithelial cells (podocytes) is the glomerular basement membrane apparently composed of components from both the endothelial cell and the epithelial cell. The endothelial cells, basement membrane, and epithelial cells thus form the filtration membrane but, because of the fenestrations of the endothelial cells and the spaces between the foot processes of the epithelial cells, the basement membrane provides the only consistent barrier.[77–83]

In addition to these cells of the filtration membrane, a third type of cell is the mesangial cell, which is in intimate relationship both to the endothelium and basement membrane and is located mainly in the central stalk of each glomerular lobule.[77–79] The name is used as an analogy to the mesentery of the bowel. The mesangial cells have both phagocytic and fibroblastic properties. Bloodworth considers the mesangial cells to be specialized pericytes and totally within the confines of the capillary basement membrane.[4] Others refer to the mesangial cells as modified smooth muscle cells.[84] It seems that there are at least two types of cells in the mesangium:[80] (1) Predominant is a stellate, contractile cell which has receptors for vasoactive hormones such as angiotensin II,[84a] and which appears to be responsible for the synthesis of the mesangial proteins;[84] and (2) the other cell type is predominantly phagocytic and has been well documented in the rat.[84b]

The two important determinants of filtration through the glomerular capillary wall are the molecular radius of a substance and its charge.[80] The polyanionic proteoglycans—in particular heparan sulfate—present in the glomerular filter are key elements of selective diffusion of molecules across the filter.[85,85a] Perfusion of rat kidneys with polycations modifies considerably (but reversibly) both the structure and function of the glomerular filter with effacement of foot processes.[85]

Glomerular Lesions in Diabetes

There are three glomerular lesions of particular interest in the diabetic kidney: (1) nodular glomerulosclerosis, the classic Kimmelstiel-Wilson lesion; (2) diffuse glomerulosclerosis; and (3) the "exudative" lesion.[86] All three involve accumulation of material that stains strongly with the periodic acid-Schiff (PAS) method, and each involves one or more components of the glomerulus (See Plate IIA).

Nodular Glomerulosclerosis. The nodular lesion typically is a round hyaline mass centrally located in a peripheral glomerular lobule with the patent, often dilated, capillary running over its surface. In contrast, the outer wall of the capillary is usually remarkably thin. The nodule stains strongly with the PAS method and is composed of glycoprotein and other protein, possibly with changes of amino acid content, and probably other carbohydrates and lipids, all of which appear as basement membrane-like dense material in and around mesangial cells, as viewed in electron micrographs.[87] The lesion, then, consists of nodular accumulations of basement membrane-like material in the mesangium[88,89] (See Plate IIB). The number of mesangial nuclei in the nodules varies from almost none to numerous. Bloodworth concluded that there are at least two types of nodules and suggests that some nodules may form from obstructed capillary microaneurysms in glomerular loops with mesangial organization.[4,90] The nodule eventually appears as a rounded laminated mass when stained with the PAS or siver reticulum stain. Nodular glomerulosclerosis is a lesion nearly pathognomonic of diabetes.

The main differential problems are with lobular glomerulonephritis. By light microscopy these diabetic glomerular nodules may resemble those in the lobular variant of membranoproliferative glomerulonephritis.[90a] Amyloid stains, immunofluorescence, and electron microscopy easily distinguish these entities from each other.

In our experience, about 25% of diabetics have the nodular lesion at autopsy, but seldom if ever as an isolated renal glomerular lesion.[87] It is more likely to be seen in association with juvenile-type, insulin-dependent diabetes of long duration than with non-insulin-dependent diabetes. Although it seems unlikely that such focal lesions in glomeruli are important in terms of glomerular function, if the filtering membrane-clearing function of mesangial cells is important, the nodules might have functional significance.[81,88]

Diffuse Glomerulosclerosis. This is a combination of more diffuse deposits in the mesangial matrix.[4,90-93] It, rather than the nodular lesion, has been thought to be more closely associated with the clinical syndrome which includes proteinuria and renal failure.[94] The diffuse lesions are not morphologically so distinctive as the nodular lesion, but they can be clearly separated from membranous glomerulonephritis and disseminated lupus erythematosus by electron microscopy and immunofluorescent techniques. While it is often assumed that

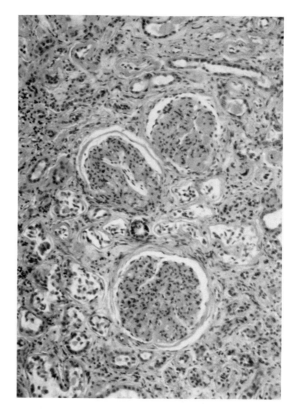

Fig. 14–10. Advanced diabetic nephropathy causing the death of the patient. There are interstitial, tubular, and vascular changes as well as the obvious glomerular sclerosis. The patient, a 58-year-old woman with diabetes for 25 years, also had severe retinopathy and peripheral neuropathy. H & E × 150 (#190281).

the diffuse change is the initial one and that it progresses to the nodular lesion, Kimmelstiel believed that the two lesions developed quite differently.[89] Martinez-Hernandez and Amenta consider the mesangial matrix to be specialized basement membrane of the mesangial cell and conclude that the basic mechanisms are the same in producing diffuse basement membrane thickening, diffuse mesangial thickening, and nodular mesangial deposits in diabetes.[84] We have already referred to Bloodworth's findings of two different routes by which nodular lesions develop.[4,90] The problem is that the basic mechanism by which diabetic glomerulosclerosis develops is still not clear or at least not agreed upon. Cotran[94a] reviewed the clinical and the experimental data linking different types of glomerulosclerosis to a hyperfiltration state in the kidney. Mesangial cells have contractile properties that seem to be important in regulating glomerular blood flow. Recent experiments[94b] show that insulin is necessary for the contractility of these mesangial cells. Thus glomerulosclerosis in the insulin-dependent diabetic might result from a state of increased glomerular blood flow.

Because basement membrane thickening, and sometimes mesangial deposits, have been reported in prediabetic persons, the possibility must be considered that the diffuse glomerular lesions may not be dependent on disturbed carbohydrate metabolism, at least as reflected in abnormal blood glucose levels.[95-97] Most recent reviews, however, return to the view that the glomerular lesions depend on altered carbohydrate metabolism and that basement membrane thickening is the initial lesion.[4,84,90,98-100] Results of biochemical studies of the thickened basement membrane and the mesangial deposits do not agree on the altered amino acid and glycoprotein content.[85a,99,101-103a] The lack of agreement on morphometric studies has hampered the discussion on the development of renal glomerular basement membrane thickening. Gundersen and others point out the increased glomerular size followed by basement membrane thickening as early lesions occurring with the development of altered carbohydrate metabolism.[98] Another factor that can be used as evidence that the defect in carbohydrate metabolism is basic in the production of diabetic glomerulosclerosis, is the development of the lesions in renal transplants given to diabetic patients.[104] A report of the resolution of glomerulopathy upon transplantation of the kidneys of a Type I diabetic to two nondiabetics is instructive in that respect.[104a]

Exudative Lesions. Another glomerular change often found in diabetes is the exudative lesion, a lesion which can be duplicated experimentally.[86,87,105] Typically, the lesions show homogeneous deposits of brightly acidophilic, glossy material having a spherical or drop-like shape. They may occur in glomerular tufts as globoid masses, as cap-like plaques over a glomerular loop or attached to Bowman's capsule, often with capsular adhesions in the latter instance.[4] The lesions contain lipid, sometimes sufficient to produce a somewhat bubbly appearance in the otherwise homogeneous material. Fibrin and immunoglobulins are also present.[4] Exudative lesions should be clearly separated from nodular glomerulosclerosis. They are completely non-specific for diabetes, occurring also in glomerulonephritis and in disseminated lupus erythematosus.[4]

Renal Vascular Changes

There is a close association between renal glomerular and vascular lesions. Both atherosclerosis and arteriolosclerosis are prominent in the renal changes of diabetes. The arteriolosclerosis is similar qualitatively to that in nondiabetics, although perhaps has more distinctly segmental hyaline thickening of arteriolar walls progressing to occlu-

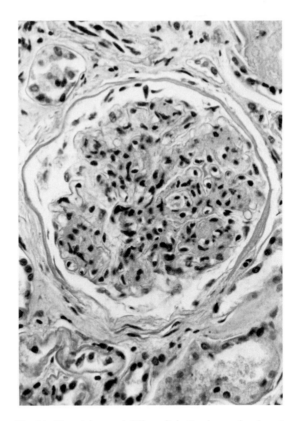

Fig. 14–11. Advanced diffuse diabetic glomerulosclerosis with extensive diffuse mesangial deposits and basement membrane thickening. Same patient as Figures 14–10 and 14–12. Periodic acid-Schiff and hematoxylin. × 400 (#190281).

sion of the vessel. A significant difference is that both the afferent and efferent arterioles are involved in the diabetic in contrast to the involvement of afferent arterioles only in essential hypertension.[106] Arteriolosclerosis may occur in the diabetic in the absence of hypertension. In general, renal artery atherosclerosis occurs at younger ages and with greater severity in diabetics than in nondiabetics, just as is true with atherosclerosis elsewhere in the body.

The renal glomerular and arteriolar lesions of diabetes tend to occur more frequently and severely in the insulin-dependent type of diabetes. Most patients with life-threatening diabetic renal disease are the long-term insulin-dependent diabetics with onset early in life.[87] The lesions do occur in the non-insulin-dependent diabetic, however, and may be severe. Bloodworth subclassifies the lesions of diabetic glomerulosclerosis as benign or slowly developing and accelerated or malignant, with 11% of adult diabetics developing the accelerated form.[4]

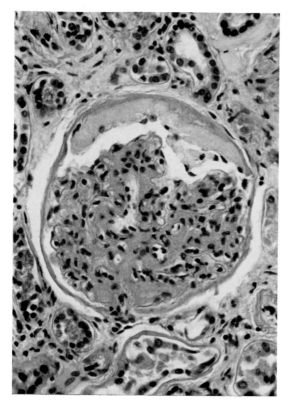

Fig. 14–12. Advanced diffuse diabetic glomerulosclerosis with large, crescentric capsular droplet at the top of the glomerulus. Same patient as Figures 14–10 and 14–11. Periodic acid-Schiff and hematoxylin. ×400 (#190281).

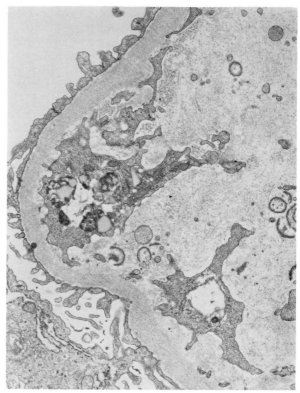

Fig. 14–13. Electron micrograph of diabetic glomerulosclerosis with thickening of the basement membrane to the left and deposits in the mesangial cells to the right. Karnovsky fixative. Prepared by Dr. M. Federman. ×4,400.

Renal Tubules

Thickening of the basement membrane of the renal tubules is often seen in conjunction with diabetic glomerular lesions. It is a non-specific change, however, being found in conditions other than glomerulosclerosis, such as pyelonephritis.

A rather common finding in the tubular epithelium of diabetic patients dying in a period of poor diabetic control or in acidosis, is a vacuolization due to glycogen, the Armanni-Ebstein lesion (See Plate IIC). While this change is not specific for diabetes or due to the diabetic state directly, it does seem to be directly related to glycosuria.[87] It is a reversible change of no apparent clinical significance but of considerable forensic significance. The glycogen vacuoles should not be confused with the vacuoles that are caused by hypokalemia. In severe acidosis, there may be potassium depletion and hypokalemic nephropathy. Thus the vacuoles due to potassium depletion are likely to occur in the same diabetic population as glycogen deposition, particularly during the treatment of diabetic ketoacidosis with insufficient potassium replacement. The hypokalemic vacuoles occur in various

locations in the tubule, but most consistently in the collecting tubules, and are not PAS- or fat-positive.[107] The glycogen vacuoles are not as discrete as those associated with hypokalemia, often being more like a clearing of the cytoplasm. They are PAS-positive, and occur most prominently in the cells of the straight descending part of the proximal tubule and often on into the loop of Henle.[108]

Pyelonephritis

The pyelonephritis occurring in diabetes is no different pathologically from that in nondiabetics. Although most observers state that there is an increased frequency of the disease in diabetics,[109,110] the true incidence is difficult to determine because of unreliable criteria for the consistent diagnosis of pyelonephritis, particularly when the disease is chronic. In the older figures of our laboratory, pyelonephritis was an infrequent cause of death in diabetes, but a rather common complication, with the incidence being 33% in males and 40% in females as determined in 351 diabetic autopsy studies.[87] If more strict criteria were used, such as demanding the demonstration of microorganisms and/or correlation with an active febrile course clinically, the

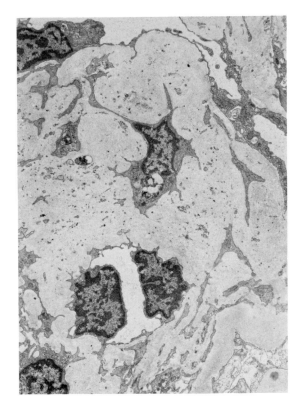

Fig. 14–14. Electron micrograph of Kimmelstiel-Wilson nodule of diabetic nephropathy with the mesangial deposits focally fusing with the thickened basement membrane. Same patient as Figure 14–13. Karnovsky fixative. Prepared by Dr. M. Federman. ×10,500.

incidence would be much lower. Pyelonephritis, when it occurs, is often associated with the renal complex of diabetic nephropathy. The decrease in pyelonephritis associated with diabetes in recent years may be real or an artifact of classification.

Necrotizing Renal Papillitis

Renal papillary necrosis has been a lesion particularly associated with diabetes mellitus, but much less so in recent years.[111,112] It is characterized by necrosis of about two-thirds of a renal pyramid, including the papillary projection of the pyramid into its respective calyx. In most cases, the majority of the pyramids of a kidney are involved. The process may be unilateral or bilateral. In general, acute pyelonephritis is present with some associated ischemia. In spite of the infarct-like appearance of the lesion, the precarious blood supply of the papillae, and the experimental evidence for ischemia as a strong factor in the pathogenesis of the lesion, clinically ischemia alone does not seem to result in papillary necrosis.[113] Excessive phenacetin ingestion, particularly common in Europe, has been correlated with a high rate of renal papillary

necrosis.[112] Urinary tract obstruction, infection, diabetes mellitus, and interstitial nephritis are the background factors associated with necrotizing papillitis. In our own series of diabetic autopsies, necrotizing papillitis is distinctly and increasingly uncommon. In some patients, the passage of necrotic renal papillae in the urine has promoted a clear-cut clinical diagnosis.

Infections of the Lower Urinary Tract. These are frequent in diabetic patients and may in part reflect the neurogenic bladder of diabetic neuropathy (See Chapter 36).

THE EYES AND DIABETES

Although a variety of changes in different parts of the eye have been related to diabetes, by far the most significant lesions occur in the retina. Diabetic retinopathy is now one of the most important causes of visual loss in the United States, the most important cause of new ("legal") blindness.[114,115]

Diabetic Retinopathy

The retinal changes closely related to diabetes include some features which are quite distinctive. The most important of these is the microaneurysm, a lesion described in 1888 but forgotten until rediscovery in 1944.[116,117] Retinal microaneurysms are best studied histologically with techniques by which most of the retinal vasculature is visualized, such as the earlier flat retinal preparation of Friedenwald and the later preparations of Kuwabara and Cogan, who used trypsin to digest away the other retinal elements, leaving exposed the entire vascular system of the retina.[118,119] The minute aneurysms, which vary from 20 to 150 μm in diameter, are outpouchings of capillary or arteriolar or, less often, venular, walls and occur most frequently in the posterior region of the retina in the inner nuclear layer. The aneurysms progress to develop a thick wall, staining intensely with the PAS stain. They often contain a large amount of lipid (See Plate IID). Thrombosis, as well as rupture or leakage, may take place, resulting in hemorrhages which may extend to the vitreous, exudates, edema, and other degenerative changes.[120] Many of the previously described retinal "punctate hemorrhages" are actually microaneurysms.

Various theories have been proposed to explain the pathogenesis of microaneurysms. It has been suggested that the aneurysms may be secondary to venous stasis, hyaline and proliferative lesions of retinal veins, kinks of capillary walls, abortive myovascular changes, intervascular fibrous bands, or damage to the capillary wall from the disturbed carbohydrate metabolism. Cogan and associates emphasized the importance of the "mural cell" in the walls of retinal capillaries, focally present outside the layer of endothelial cells.[121] Mural cells are similar in some respects to pericytes and to the mesangial cells of the renal glomerulus. They postulated that in diabetes there is a loss of mural cells with a resultant weakening or loss of tone of the capillary wall and the development of the microaneurysm. At the same time the endothelial cells proliferate to form the aneurysms and thick arteriovenous shunts, bypassing segments of acellular capillary network. Others have noted similar findings, sometimes emphasizing more the importance of early basement membrane thickening of the capillary or occlusion of the capillary lumen.[4,115,122,123]

Arteriolosclerosis of hyaline type occurs commonly with retinopathy, may be an essential feature for its development, and is comparable to that in the kidney and elsewhere. The exudates of diabetic retinopathy are composed of dense, acidophilic material which stains brightly with the PAS method and usually contains some lipid. The exudates and hemorrhages appear first in the inner (or vitreous side) retinal layers, but in more advanced cases, may extend throughout all layers with considerable disruption of normal architecture as well as extending into the vitreous (See Plate IIE). Different forms of degenerative lesions have been described and given distinctive names—"microspheres," "cytoid bodies," and "pseudocysts."[124] Loss of retinal neurons occurs and is massive in late stages of diabetic retinopathy. With extensive hemorrhage and tissue destruction, large clusters of foamy histiocytes may appear. As hemorrhage occurs into the vitreous, neovascularization develops, organization occurs, and retinal separation may develop. The end stage is retinitis proliferans with a vascularized, scarred retina and organization extending into the vitreous. Macular degeneration, perhaps only edema at first, may be an early lesion[125] (See Plate IIF). Retinal vascular changes may develop early in the course of diabetes.[123] In a combined study of diabetic retinas at autopsy from our laboratory, by far the majority had some of the lesions of diabetic retinopathy, often in the absence of demonstrable renal glomerular lesions.[120]

Cataracts

The relation of cataracts to diabetes has long been controversial. In 1935 Waite and Beetham[125] in a large clinical study noted no significant difference in the frequency of "senile" cataracts between diabetic and nondiabetic patients. They did find floccular cataracts in 11 (3.7%) of 297 patients with juvenile-onset diabetes, a frequency much greater than that today due presumably to the overall improvement in the treatment of diabetes in the past half-century.

Cerami et al. have shown experimentally that

with hyperglycemia, glycosylation of the lens occurs, making the lens more susceptible to sulfhydryl oxidation and the formation of opalescence.[126]

For an extensive clinical discussion of ocular manifestations in diabetes, see Chapter 29.

THE NERVOUS SYSTEM

Neural syndromes of several types are so common in diabetes that some authors report that nearly all diabetic patients exhibit neural dysfunction of some degree if nerve conduction defects are included.[4,127,128] The relationship of the syndromes to poor carbohydrate control varies, but in some groups, improvement in the neurologic signs and symptoms follows institution of good diabetic control. The implication is obvious that the neural lesions in some instances are neither large nor permanent. It is not strange, therefore, that the correlation of anatomic lesions with the clinical syndromes has been difficult.

Diabetic Peripheral Neuropathy

This common neural syndrome of diabetes is associated with pain, paresthesias which are usually symmetrical, and loss of vibration sense in the feet and legs. In more advanced cases, anesthesia may be complete enough to allow the development of Charcot joints in the foot and ankle.[4,128,129] Although the study of Woltman and Wilder early in the insulin era related the changes to vascular insufficiency of peripheral nerves,[130] later workers could not correlate large or small blood vessel disease and peripheral neuropathy.[130–132] More recent summaries include more than one basis for neuropathy but generally conclude that except for mononeuropathies, the lesions are metabolically based rather than vascular.[4,128,129] However, the subject is still an open one (See discussion in Chapter 31).

Experimental evidence clearly relates certain neuropathies to reversible metabolic pathways and hyperglycemia, and the sorbitol or polyol pathway has been implicated.[133,134,134a] Patchy demyelinization and variable loss of axons are the most consistent findings in peripheral nerves and often there is some lower segment posterior column degeneration of mild degree in the spinal cord. Thomas and Lascelles emphasized segmental demyelinization of peripheral nerves as the first significant lesion in peripheral diabetic neuropathy.[135] Such changes are so difficult to demonstrate that it is often easier to see the peripheral results than the nerve injury itself. The most easily demonstrated change of this type is a motor unit type of skeletal muscle atrophy, since some motor nerve fibers are involved in addition to sensory nerves, also suggesting more nerve injury such as loss of axons. The loss of axons clearly occurs and there is disagreement as to whether demyelinization or axon loss occurs first or independently.[4,128,136]

Diabetic Amyotrophy

This is the name given to the syndrome of asymmetrical proximal muscle atrophy, weakness, and pain most often seen in elderly patients with uncontrolled diabetes.[137] The thigh muscles and pelvic girdle are more often involved than the shoulder girdle. Partly because the spinal fluid protein is usually elevated, it was thought at first that the lesion was in the spinal cord. It is clear now that although there may be some radiculopathy, the lesion is not of the spinal cord but must occur either in the motor nerves, perhaps the motor end plates, or in the muscle fibers.[128,138,139] The evidence presently favors a motor neuropathy.[128] The characteristic pathologic picture is atrophy of single muscle fibers without respect to motor units. Beading and reduction in the motor end plates have been demonstrated in patients with diabetic amyotrophy as well as in persons having alcoholic neuritis.[140] Raff and Asbury have concluded, however, that diabetic amyotrophy is a mononeuropathy multiplex due to small infarcts in myelinated nerves.[141] The syndrome tends to slowly improve with good control of diabetes.

Mononeuropathy and Mononeuropathy Multiplex

These represent discrete lesions of single nerves and, as just suggested, tend to be due to ischemic lesions of the nerves, although perhaps not exclusively so.[4,128] The peripheral nerves most frequently involved are the ulnar, median, radial, femoral, sciatic, and peroneal.[128] Raff and Asbury included the cranial nerve palsies in the same group. The oculomotor nerve is the one most frequently involved.[129,141]

Autonomic Neuropathy

Clinical neural syndromes involving the autonomic system include vasomotor and sudomotor disturbances, postural hypotension, pupillary abnormalities, paresis of the urinary bladder, gastroparesis, "diabetic diarrhea," and possibly Charcot joint. Anatomic lesions to correlate well with the distressing clinical pictures are not demonstrable. Martin concluded that the nonmyelinated fibers in peripheral nerves are particularly susceptible to degeneration.[142] Olsson and Sourander reported axon loss and segmental demyelination.[143] Hydropic vacuolization in the cytoplasm of sympathetic ganglion cells in diabetics is more marked, occurs at earlier ages, and has been prominent in some pa-

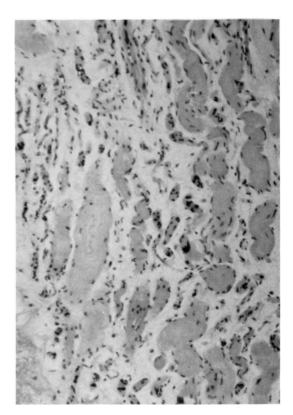

Fig. 14–15. Motor unit atrophy of skeletal muscle, the picture often seen with peripheral diabetic neuropathy. Motor units to the left and in the center of the field are severely atrophic. The specimen is from the less ischemic muscle from the amputated leg of a diabetic patient with a gangrenous foot. H & E ×150 (#229529).

tients with the autonomic syndrome.[143a] However, a few such vacuoles are commonly found in the sympathetic ganglia of the elderly, whether diabetic or not.

Spinal Cord Involvement

Pure spinal cord syndromes are rare, although it has been difficult to separate peripheral neuropathy and diabetic amyotrophy from spinal cord involvement, mainly because of the commonly found high spinal fluid protein in these syndromes and because of the frequent, mild, posterior column changes associated with peripheral diabetic neuropathy.[131] "Pseudotabes diabetica" is the extreme example of marked posterior column degeneration, but this is rare.[144] Mild involvement of the posterior columns is much more common, however, and may be related to the "cord bladder" in the diabetic. Other columns may be involved as well. Scattered shrinkage and loss of anterior horn neurons have been reported.[145,146]

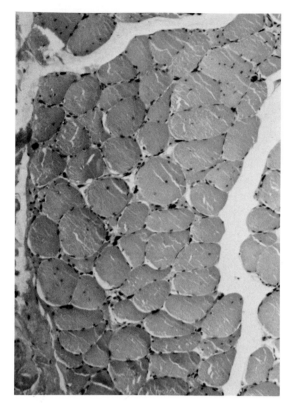

Fig. 14–16. Single fiber muscle, the characteristic lesion of diabetic amyotrophy. In the cross section, single, markedly atrophic fibers are surrounded by large, preserved fibers. The specimen is a muscle biopsy of the vastus of the thigh from a 51-year-old diabetic man with amyotrophy. H & E ×150 (#236026).

Brain and Cranial Nerves

Although the most frequent changes in the brain are *cerebral infarction* or *hemorrhage* secondary to vascular disease, these disorders are relatively less frequent than other types of vascular disorders in the diabetic. Some have reported degeneration of ganglion cells, demyelinization and loss of axons in cerebrum, mid-brain, and cerebellum with calcinosis in small blood vessel walls.[4,145] There are no distinctive changes in the brains of diabetics other than the abnormal glycogen deposits seen in some patients dying of diabetic coma. The cranial nerve palsies have been mentioned already. *Hypoglycemic coma* is a significant threat to the brain, resulting in patchy neuron necrosis first in the cerebral cortex and then in lower centers. This may develop into larger foci of necrosis in the most severe cases.[147]

To supplement this relatively brief discussion, see Chapter 31.

CARDIOVASCULAR DISEASE

The increased frequency and severity of arteriosclerosis of muscular and larger arteries in the diabetic have been accepted by most investigators for a long time. The importance of these changes to the survival of the diabetic patient increased steadily until in the years 1948 to 1980, vascular disease accounted for well over half of the deaths in our diabetic autopsy series. More recently, there has been some decrease in vascular deaths with an increase of cancer deaths. If a pathologist were to classify the problem eras of diabetes through the years, the diabetic coma years were superseded by the infection era and now we are in the era of vascular disease with cancer increasing.

Arteriosclerosis includes *atherosclerosis*, characterized by the intimal plaque, *medial calcification* or Mönckeberg sclerosis with its deposits of calcium in the media, and *diffuse intimal fibrosis* which many regard as similar or identical to atherosclerosis.

Medial calcification in muscular arteries, or *Mönckeberg's calcific medial sclerosis*, is a process that is independent of atherosclerosis but that may occur concomitantly. Calcium is deposited first in small granules in the stroma of the muscular media and may progress to fairly solid calcific and bony rings which are striking in roentgenograms. Although the early occurrence of this lesion in diabetes is common, it is not distinctive of that disease and it does not encroach upon the vessel lumen.

Blumenthal, Goldenberg, et al.[147a] in the 1950s and 60s described lesions in the smaller arteries (20–100 Å) of diabetic patients which consisted of nonatheromatous endothelial cell proliferations with a reticulated network of fibrils between the cells. There were similar fibrils between the fibers of the muscularis. Electron microscopy reveals the fibrils to be thickened basement membranes. There has been no general acceptance of the endothelial proliferative lesions as distinct for diabetes. Most reports indicate that their incidence is quite low and that they are seen just as frequently in non-diabetics.[147b]

Atherosclerosis

Atherosclerosis tends to occur at an earlier age and with greater severity in the diabetic than in the nondiabetic.[148] Although there has never been shown any convincing qualitative difference between atherosclerosis in the nondiabetic and in the diabetic, various studies have reported unconfirmed differences such as more lecithin and cephalin in diabetic coronary arteries,[149] more ash, calcium, and cholesterol in diabetic brachial arteries,[150] and more mucopolysaccharides in diabetic atheromas.[151,151a] Despite an enormous amount of investigation, the pathogenesis of the disease is not entirely clear and in fact, there may well be a different balance of factors involved in different cases.[152-154] In a succinct statement introducing a summary article on atherosclerosis, Ross and Harker stated, "The lesions of atherosclerosis are characterized by intimal proliferation of smooth muscle cells, accumulation of large amounts of connective tissue matrix including collagen elastic fibers, and proteoglycans, and deposition of intra- and extracellular lipid. Many factors are involved in this process."[154] Endothelial injury and lipid deposition seem to be ubiquitous components of atherosclerosis.

The quantitative association of atherosclerosis with diabetes mellitus is firmly established, despite the difficulty in understanding atherosclerosis itself. The association accounts for the disproportionately high incidence of gangrene of the lower extremities and for coronary heart disease, the most important cause of death in diabetic patients.[155] An unexpected finding is the decrease in proportion of deaths due to arteriosclerotic heart disease in the diabetic autopsy population in our laboratory in the most recent years (1964 to 1980) compared to the previous period (1948 to 1964), a shift from 42 to 35% (Table 14–2). The figures are crude and do not take into account variables that might explain the difference. In an autopsy study of 12 consecutive patients age 35 or younger who had died of myocardial infarcts, we found that 11 had had diabetes; in our autopsy population, 20% are diabetic patients. Not only do myocardial infarcts tend to occur at an earlier age in diabetics than in nondiabetics, they also occur more commonly in women with diabetes. Stearns, Schlesinger, and Rudy found that significant atherosclerosis was twice as common in diabetic males in comparison to nondiabetic males and in females more than 40 years old, 8 times as frequent in diabetics as in nondiabetics.[156] In a review of 50,000 autopsy reports, Clawson and Bell found that fatal coronary artery disease was twice as frequent in diabetic males and 3 times as frequent in diabetic females as in the nondiabetic subjects.[157] In the Framingham study, glucose intolerance was one of the five factors identified as contributing to a high risk of cardiovascular disease.[158]

Gangrene of the Lower Extremities. This is still a major problem in the diabetic population although, apart from infection, seldom the cause of death. The most important basis for gangrene is atherosclerosis of the muscular arteries of the leg and foot. However, the common diabetic gangrene of a toe often has a component of infection and osteomyelitis and may have a background of neurotrophic changes. One also cannot ignore the interplay of disease in arterioles and capillaries (diabetic microangiopathy) which will be discussed below.

One of the interesting features in the association of atherosclerosis with diabetes is the lack of uniformity of involvement throughout the arterial system. In the autopsy series shown in Table 14–2, the number of deaths due to cerebral infarcts is not much different from what one would expect in the general population (See also Chapter 11 on Macrovascular Disease).

Diabetic Microangiopathy

This term usually includes arteriolosclerosis and thickening of capillary walls and sometimes even some involvement of venular walls. The arteriolosclerosis of diabetes refers to fairly concentric hyaline thickening of arteriolar walls, a prominent component of diabetic nephropathy, which also affects organs other than the kidney. In the diabetic, it appears as a segmental process which does not appear qualitatively different from that seen in essential hypertension. As noted earlier, a distinctive feature is that both the afferent and efferent arterioles may be involved in the kidney in contrast to the afferent arterioles only in essential hypertension.[106] Prominent sites for its appearance, usually in conjunction with diabetic nephropathy, are the pancreas, retina, and the pericapsular zone of the adrenal glands. In patients who have died of diabetic nephropathy, the arteriolosclerosis of the pancreas is usually striking and probably produces, by ischemia, the patches of acinar degeneration often seen in the centers of lobules in the pancreases of such patients. The report of Fagerberg emphasized arteriolosclerosis as a more generalized change in diabetes.[159]

Fagerberg also drew attention to capillary wall changes and there is no reasonable separation of the capillary wall changes from arteriolosclerosis. After Aagenaes and Moe described in the skin of diabetics a thickening of the capillary walls by material that stained intensely with the PAS technique, similar changes were found in capillaries elsewhere.[160] Most reports have considered the capillary wall thickening to be of the basement membrane of the capillary. Banson and Lacy reported capillary basement membrane thickening in the skin of the toes in 16 of 18 diabetics in comparison to 4 of 17 nondiabetics.[161] The average basement membrane thickness as measured in electron micrographs was 5900 Å in nondiabetics and 13,300 Å in the diabetics. Siperstein and co-workers studied capillary basement membranes in skeletal muscle biopsies and found basement membranes

Table 14–2.   Causes of Death in 2897 Diabetics upon Whom Autopsies were Performed

	to 1924		1924 to 1930		1930 to 1937		1937 to 1948		1948 to 1964		1964 to 1980		Total	
	No.	%	No.	%	No.	%	No.	%	No.	%	No.	%	No.	%
Total cases	105		157		224		332		1036		1043		2897	
A. Coma present	66	62	32	20	29	13	9	3	18	2	9	1	163	6
B. Coma absent	39	38	125	80	195	87	323	97	1018	98	1034	99	2734	94
1. Cardiovascular lesions	13	33	41	33	71	36	143	44	653	64	502	48	1423	52
a. Aneurysm	0		0		1		1		6		8			
b. Cardiac	7		27		49		117		438		367			
c. Cerebral	2		5		12		10		71		44			
d. Gangrene	4		6		1		0		2		1			
e. Mesenteric	0		0		6		2		6		3			
f. Renal disease, vascular*	0		3		2		13		126		56			
g. Miscellaneous	0		0		0		0		4		23			
2. Renal disease, nonvascular	0		2		2		1		1		2			
3. Infections	20	51	54	43	60	30	79	24	88	9	123	12	424	16
a. Gas gangrene	1		1		0		0		0		1			
b. Meningitis	0		2		2		2		0		2			
c. Multiple abscesses	3		7		2		3		2		0			
d. Pericarditis	0		2		4		0		1		0			
e. Peritonitis	1		6		5		9		3		4			
f. Pneumonia														
(1) Bronchial	4		12		9		13		37		58			
(2) Lobar	2		4		2		2		0		1			
g. Pyelonephritis†	0		1		1		11		21		8			
h. Rheumatic fever‡	0		0		1		1		5		9			
i. Septicemia	3		12		30		35		10		11			
j. Syphilis	0		1		0		0		0		0			
k. Tuberculosis	6		5		4		2		0		2			
l. Empyema	0		1		0		1		0		0			
m. Endocarditis	—		—		—		—		8		3			
n. Other infections	—		—		—		—		1		24			
4. Cancer	0	0	13	10	26	13	42	13	143	14	256	25	480	18
5. Hemochromatosis	1		1		2		3		9		4			
6. Cirrhosis of liver (not hemochromatosis)	—		—		—		—		12		23			
7. Pulmonary embolism§	0		4		12		17		20		30			
8. Insulin reaction (hypoglycemia)	0		0		3		1		13		2			
9. Peptic ulcer (duodenal and gastric)	—		—		—		—		11		27			
10. Accident	0		1		1		0		2		1			
11. Pancreatitis	—		—		—		—		3		2			
12. Other causes	5		9		18		17		45		53			
13. Undetermined	0		0		0		20		18		11			

From Warren, LeCompte, and Legg: Ref. 3, with extension and modifications.
*Includes intercapillary glomerulosclerosis.
†Includes necrotizing renal papillitis.
‡Includes old valvular lesions.
§Includes infarcts.
—Prior to 1948 listed under "other causes."

thicker than 1325 Å in 98% of diabetic patients in contrast to 8% of nondiabetics.[162]

Since the measurements of capillary basement membranes and many of the capillary studies have been done by electron microscopy, one should keep in mind the restricted area sampled in such studies and the problem of artifacts, as emphasized by Kimmelstiel mainly in reference to the renal glomerular capillaries.[92,93] Some of the capillary wall thickening is visible by light microscopy, however, particularly since the material stains well with the PAS technique. We have observed such capillary wall thickening by light microscopy in both diabetics and "prediabetics" (children with two diabetic parents) in biopsy tissue from the ear lobe, gingiva, and skin of the flank. That the lesion is not qualitatively distinctive is evident in that we have observed similar capillary wall thickening in biopsy specimens of the skin from nondiabetic patients with chronic skin disease. Bercovici and collaborators first called attention to capillary wall thickening in nondiabetics with dermatoses.[163]

Some workers have noted that the thickened basement membrane enveloped the capillary pericytes. Friederici and associates separated the capillary wall into a true inner basement membrane and an outer layer of basement membrane-like material which was more variable than the inner one.[164] They could find no significant difference between capillary basement membrane thickness in diabetics compared to nondiabetics.

While the work of Kilo, Vogler, and Williamson confirmed the statistical significance of skeletal muscle capillary basement membrane thickening in diabetes, their data show a positive correlation with age and the known duration of hyperglycemia.[165] Basement membrane thickening was present in 63% of the diabetics over the age of 50 and in 25% of those under the age of 50 who had had the disease for 4 years or less. The incidence increased to 93% in those who had had diabetes for 20 years or longer. Muscle capillary basement membrane thickening is usually not present in newly diagnosed juvenile diabetes.[166]

The metabolic hypothesis for the development of diabetic microangiopathy is supported by the following evidence: (1) The clinical experience that diabetic nephropathy and retinopathy increase in frequency and severity with longer duration of diabetes;[165,167] (2) Electron microscopic studies of the glomerular basement membrane;[168] (3) The fact that diabetic nephropathy develops in a normal kidney transplanted in a diabetic subject;[104] (4) Biochemical data;[169] (5) Animal experimental data;[100,170,171] (6) Occurrence of basement membrane thickening in patients with secondary diabetes, e.g., hemochromatosis and chronic pancreatitis.[172,173]

See also Chapter 10 on "Microvascular Disease and its Relation to Control of Diabetes."

The contradictory results obtained in the studies on the skeletal muscle capillary basement membrane thickening seem due to several factors: (1) heterogeneity of patient population as to type of diabetes and the ages of diabetics and controls; (2) the regional variations in muscle capillary basement membrane thickness; (3) the focal and segmental nature of the lesion and the restricted sample of electron microscopy; and (4) differences in tissue preparation and techniques in measuring the basement membrane width. In a 2-year study, Raskin et al. reported that there was a significant decrease in the width of skeletal muscle capillary basement membrane of Type I diabetics on continuous subcutaneous insulin infusion as compared to controls receiving conventional treatment.[173a] There is as yet no convincing evidence, however, that strict euglycemia will influence retinal and glomerular microangiopathy.[173b]

Though thickened, the basement membrane is more permeable in the diabetic.[174,174a] This increased permeability has important clinical applications in detecting early microangiopathy. It accounts for the leakage of fluorescein during retinal angiography, the earliest sign of diabetic retinopathy. Increased permeability of the glomerular filter leads to microalbuminuria, an early sign of diabetic nephropathy. Clinical studies on diabetics reveal that microalbuminuria predicts clinical proteinuria and early mortality.[174b,174c]

Whether there is additional myocardial disease that is not directly attributable to atherosclerosis is not clear, although the involvement of the heart by diabetic microangiopathy seems well established.[175,176] Electron microscopic morphometric studies on myocardial biopsies taken during heart surgery showed a statistically significant thickening of the capillary basement membrane in 8 patients with overt diabetes.[177] The basal laminar thickness of 1113 Å in the myocardial capillaries is thinner than that reported in other tissues. Factor and others reported perfusion studies of the myocardial microcirculation of diabetic hearts and described saccular and fusiform microaneurysms in 3 of the 6 cases in contrast to none of the eight control subjects.[178]

Some diabetic patients appear to succumb to heart disease without morphologic evidence of significant vascular disease. Regan and others considered the presence of conspicuous PAS-positive material in the interstitium of the left ventricle as an important extravascular finding in nine such patients with heart failure.[179] The patients did not have significant coronary artery obstruction in either extramural or intramural components. Myocardial hypertrophy is more common in the diabetic patient than in the nondiabetic, and there is increased myocardial glycogen content.

For clinical aspects of "The Heart and Diabetes," see Chapter 27.

ENDOCRINE GLANDS

Overactivity of some endocrine glands, particularly as the result of secreting tumors, may produce hyperglycemia and thus, at least, reversible diabetes. In the pancreas itself there may appear four different *islet cell tumors* that produce clinical diabetes in contrast to only one kind that produces hypoglycemia, the insulin-producing B cell tumors.[39] The A cell tumors producing glucagon, the ACTH-producing islet cell carcinomas, the D cell somatostatin-producing tumors, and the vasoactive intestinal-polypeptide-producing tumors of the Verner-Morrison syndrome—all result in hyperglycemia. The mechanisms are self-evident except in the Verner-Morrison syndrome in which hypokalemia is the key defect interfering with insulin secretion.

Rarely *Schmidt's syndrome* of coexistent adrenal and thyroid disease has been reported as associated with diabetes.[180] The hyperglycemia of *Cushing's syndrome* and the use of cortisone in the experimental production of diabetes, with or without administration of growth hormone, makes it imperative that the adrenal glands be carefully studied in autopsies performed on diabetics. One might expect the *adrenal cortex* to have an increased prevalence of adenoma and hyperplasia in the diabetic autopsy population. Such has not been the case. Of a series of 1036 autopsies performed on diabetics in our laboratory, only 38 (3.7%) of the subjects had significant adrenal cortical nodules. Of these, 6 had a total adrenal mass twice the normal size or larger. Two had characteristic Cushing's syndrome.

In the 1960s, Conn described a syndrome of hypertension, impaired carbohydrate metabolism, and hypokalemia attributable to *primary aldosteronism*.[181] At that time it was stated that one-half of patients with primary aldosteronism had impaired glucose tolerance of the diabetic type. However, depending on criteria used, the percentage of abnormal tests is much lower. In these patients, if an adrenal cortical tumor is present, its removal relieves the carbohydrate defect as well as the aldosteronism. When impaired carbohydrate metabolism is observed in primary aldosteronism, potassium loading restores normal glucose tolerance. It seems clear from the available data in our own material and from those of others, that adrenal cortical hyperfunction seldom provides the basis for the diabetic state.[182]

Diabetes and *Addison's disease* may occur together, usually with the diabetes preceding Addison's disease. Solomon and associates collected reports of 113 such cases.[180] The patients have unusually sensitive responses to insulin. There is nothing distinctive about the pathology when the diseases occur together.

Hyperglycemia has been reported to occur in from 11 to 66⅔% of individuals with *pheochromocytoma*, the only adrenal medullary lesion with such an association.[183,184] Removal of the pheochromocytoma may completely relieve the diabetes, or at least ameliorate it.

Some relationship between *pituitary* function and diabetes has long been noted. Anterior pituitary extracts or growth hormone injections experimentally produce hyperglycemia, both degranulation and hydropic change of islet B cells, and sometimes permanent diabetes.[185,186] In acromegaly, diabetes occurs in at least 10% of the subjects and in some series, considerably more.[187] In the general diabetic autopsy population, no consistent change in cell types of the anterior pituitary has been found and pituitary tumors related to hyperglycemia are rare indeed.

Houssay observed long ago that extirpation of the pituitary ameliorated the diabetic state in animals and made them unusually sensitive to insulin.[188] The Houssay phenomenon may occur spontaneously in human diabetics. We have observed only one such patient upon whom an autopsy was performed—a woman with Sheehan's syndrome whose insulin requirement dropped from 88 units a day to none at all for a short period and then returned to 18 units a day at the time of death 5 years later. The anterior lobe had been almost completely destroyed (Fig. 14–17). Although damage sufficient to produce the Houssay phenomenon rarely occurs spontaneously, small pituitary infarcts occur 3 times as often in diabetics as in nondiabetics.[189,190] Incomplete ablation of the pituitary was used for a time in the 1960s with some success to arrest the progression of diabetic retinopathy.[190a] In such patients, the Houssay phenomenon was observed in varied degree, depending inversely on the mass of surviving pituitary anterior lobe. An instructive finding in that respect is the absence of microangiopathy in growth-hormone-deficient dwarfs with diabetes.[190b]

The *gonads* show no consistent changes in diabetes. There seems to be a greater frequency of hypofunction of the ovaries, some of which may be secondary to pituitary changes. Ovarian cortical stromal hyperplasia has been associated with endometrial carcinoma and diabetes.[191]

Hyperthyroidism may result in hyperglycemia and glycosuria. Experimentally, diabetes has been produced by giving thyroid extract to animals whose pancreases have been partially removed.[192] This experiment, other experimental evidence, and clinical experience suggest that the increased metabolism of hyperthyroidism exposes a relative insulin deficiency which might otherwise have remained latent.

No *thymic* changes have been related to diabetes except for the occurrence of Cushing's syndrome in patients with the carcinoid tumor of the thymus.[193]

Secondary chief cell hyperplasia of the *parathyroids* occurs in patients with advanced diabetic nephropathy as a reflection of disturbed calcium and phosphorus metabolism, but no parathyroid changes are directly related to the diabetic state.

No change has been found in the *pineal* body.

MISCELLANEOUS TISSUES AND ORGANS

Many other organs and tissues of the body in addition to those described above are involved in

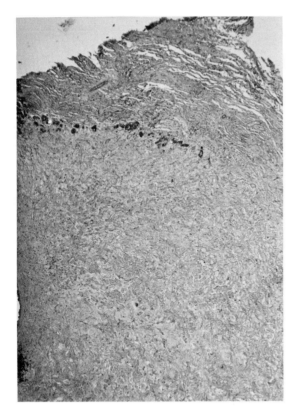

Fig. 14–17. A thin rim of anterior pituitary cells near the top is the only residual tissue, with fibrous replacement of the rest of the anterior pituitary in this example of Sheehan's syndrome. The patient, a 35-year-old woman with diabetes for 20 years, demonstrated the Houssay phenomenon after the necrosis of her pituitary gland. H & E ×40 (#198586).

diabetes, some of them because of microangiopathy, some because of neuropathy, and some because of the end results of actual carbohydrate and fat metabolism. Only a few of the changes are distinctive and so only brief consideration will be given to the majority.

Digestive Tract

The *liver* is important in carbohydrate metabolism and normally may contain a reservoir of about 400 g of glycogen.[194] In diabetics, particularly in those with poor control, hepatic glycogen is often considerably decreased. As the cytoplasmic glycogen decreases, the intranuclear glycogen tends to increase.[195] Glycogen infiltration of hepatic cell nuclei is a finding not limited to diabetes, however. In some cases, particularly in the recovery period following diabetic ketoacidosis, hepatomegaly due to increased hepatic glycogen has been reported.[196] However, the enlargement of the liver commonly found in diabetics is due to fat. According to one report, fatty change of the liver occurred in 48% of diabetics.[194] Most workers conclude that there

is a higher frequency of portal cirrhosis in diabetic patients than in nondiabetics, but the proportion of diabetics reported with *portal cirrhosis* varies from 2.9 to 32.3%.[197] With such a wide diversity in numbers, it seems evident that other factors are involved. In our diabetic autopsy subjects, the incidence of cirrhosis has decreased in recent years but has never been an important cause of death. The cirrhosis of hemochromatosis is a special circumstance that will be considered below.

The effect of diabetes on the *biliary tract* is reflected by an increased frequency of both cholecystitis and cholelithiasis in the diabetic. Most of the stones are composed predominantly of cholesterol.[198]

Although various gastrointestinal syndromes occur in association with diabetes, there are no histologic changes distinctive of this disease. Marked gastric dilation occurs with diabetic ketoacidosis, but there is no demonstrable basic anatomic lesion. The hemorrhage which may accompany the acidosis in these cases seems to be due to diffuse capillary bleeding in the gastric mucosa. Diabetic diarrhea is apparently really part of the diabetic autonomic neuropathy; there are no jejunal villous changes comparable to those of the spruce-celiac syndrome.

See also Chapter 40, "The Digestive System and Diabetes."

Hemochromatosis

In a short summary of the pathology of diabetes mellitus, hemochromatosis must be considered only briefly, with emphasis on the more generally accepted pathologic aspects. For more extensive general discussions, see the classic early monograph by Sheldon,[199] later publications of others,[200–202] and Chapter 40 of this book.

Pathologically, hemochromatosis is characterized by the deposition of iron pigment in excessive amounts both in connective tissue and epithelial cells, especially of the liver, pancreas, gastrointestinal tract, endocrine glands, choroid plexus, and the dermis. In the liver and pancreas, cell injury and fibrosis are present. In contrast, the deposition of iron pigment from excessive breakdown of hemoglobin, as in hemolytic anemias, or from multiple transfusions, affects chiefly the reticuloendothelial system. It should be pointed out, however, that the distinction between severe hemosiderosis and idiopathic hemochromatosis is not sharply drawn, either pathologically or clinically, and the experimental evidence is contradictory.

The high concomitance of diabetes and hemochromatosis has long been known and this, plus the characteristic skin pigmentation, is the basis of the term "bronze diabetes." In our own autopsy cases, diabetes usually followed the appearance of hemochromatosis, but in some instances the opposite appeared to be true.

The liver cirrhosis, which is a basic element in hemochromatosis, has a finely nodular pattern. The pigment is found in hepatic cells, bile duct cells, Kupffer cells, and in the dense fibrous zones. In a review series, hepatic carcinoma, usually hepatocellular carcinoma, has been reported in 18.9% of patients with hemochromatosis.[203]

In the pancreas, the pigment is most densely deposited in the duct cells, acinar cells, and stroma, with the islet cells least involved (Fig. 14–18). Extensive atrophy of exocrine tissue may occur with associated marked fibrosis. In contrast, the islets of Langerhans are prominent, large, and cellular. The presence of mitoses in islet cells may be a reflection of the association found by LeCompte and Merriam of islet cell mitoses with liver disease in general.[204] Although McGavran and Hartroft noted that the islet iron seemed more prominent in B cells than in others, we have found that the B cells may be nearly completely degranulated in the presence of scant iron.[205]

Although nodular diabetic glomerulosclerosis (the Kimmelstiel-Wilson lesion) is rarely found in hemochromatosis patients with diabetes, it has been reported.[206] A curious diffuse membrane thickening of renal glomeruli may be seen.[202] Pigment is seldom noted in the kidney, but sloughed renal tubular cells containing iron, if found in the urine, may provide a diagnostic aid.

In diagnosis, the best screening tests are those of plasma iron and iron binding capacity. Usually the former is greater than 200 μg/dl and transferrin saturation is greater than 70%. Since the skin pigment responsible for the bronze appearance is more often increased melanin than dermal iron, a skin biopsy often is not adequate for the diagnosis. Much more reliable material for the histologic confirmation of the diagnosis may be obtained by biopsy of the liver.

Hemochromatosis patients may die as the result of the disease with the most common modes being congestive heart failure related to myocardial iron deposition, cirrhosis with esophageal varices, and hepatocellular carcinoma. With present-day wide use of venesection and chelating agents, cardiac deaths are less common than formerly.

Skin and Skeletal Muscle

For a complete listing and discussion of skin lesions associated with diabetes or seen frequently or coincidentally with diabetes, see Chapter 38.

Changes in skeletal muscle in diabetes may assume three basic patterns: (1) the motor unit or neural type of muscle atrophy found in peripheral

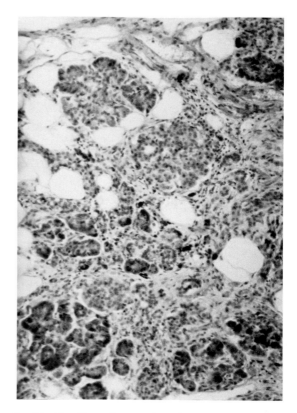

Fig. 14–18. Hemochromatosis with extensive fibrous replacement of acinar tissue of the pancreas but with two islets of Langerhans relatively intact. The black smudgy material is iron-containing pigment. The patient was a 54-year-old woman who had carbohydrate intolerance in the last 6 months of her life. H & E ×150 (#216765).

diabetic neuropathy, (2) single fiber muscle atrophy of diabetic amyotrophy, and (3) ischemic atrophy (see above section on neuropathy). Motor unit muscle atrophy consists of shrinkage of the muscle fibers supplied by damaged nerves, and therefore the unit involved is the cluster of muscle fibers supplied by one nerve fiber. In single fiber muscle atrophy, individual muscle fibers shrink markedly while maintaining myofibrils and intact cross-striations.[139] Ischemic atrophy is much more variable, ranging from large areas of irregular shrinkage and swelling of fibers with increased stroma, to granular degeneration and finally, frank necrosis. Patients with poorly controlled diabetes tend to have decreased muscle glycogen.[207]

Other Tissues

A relatively common enigmatic finding in male diabetics is calcification of the muscularis of the *vas deferens*[208] (See Chapter 32). Merriam and Sommers reported that diabetic women frequently had dense hyaline material around *mammary ducts* and that the ultraviolet absorption pattern was similar to that of diabetic glomerulosclerosis.[209]

INFANTS OF DIABETIC MOTHERS

At the Joslin Clinic in the early years of the insulin era from 1924 to 1938, among 128 viable (28 weeks' gestation) pregnancies of diabetic mothers, the fetal survival was only 54%. With improved treatment, this was raised to 90% among 1119 pregnancies in the period from 1958 to 1974. By 1979, fetal survival had improved to 98%, and accompanying this during the years 1975 to 1979 maternal survival was 100% (see Table 33–1). By 1979, the frequency of the common distressing problems of the infants had decreased to the extent that it was approaching that of infants of nondiabetic mothers. These difficulties had included excessive perinatal mortality, generalized macrosomia ("big babies"), respiratory distress syndrome, hypocalcemia, hyperbilirubinemia, and hypoglycemia. All of these complications persist today but to a substantially smaller degree. However, congenital malformations still are considerably more common than in infants of nondiabetic mothers. In the current Joslin Clinic experience, malformations occur to the extent of 9% major and 5% minor. The major anomalies include congenital heart disease, neural tube defects, and other conditions which are either incompatible with life as anencephaly, or are life-threatening or disabling.

The cause of the problems which beset the infant of the diabetic mother seems to involve various factors. The improvement noted above has resulted from successful attempts to correct identifiable influences. As for the congenital malformations, the thought has arisen that they may reflect the abnormal metabolism of the mother and that by consistent and meticulous control of hyperglycemia, they might be avoided. Since the congenital defects probably have their beginning in early embryogenesis, exploratory attempts have been, and are being made in various centers, including the Joslin Diabetes Center,[210] to strive to maintain a normal or nearly normal plasma glucose in the diabetic woman, beginning at the earliest possible time, even at, or prior to, the time of conception, continuing such meticulous control at least during the first trimester, but hopefully also through pregnancy.

Reports to date have been favorable. For example, in December, 1981, Jovanovic, Druzin, and Peterson[211] reported success in maintaining near euglycemia in 52 women in whom meticulous treatment was instituted prior to the 12th week of pregnancy. The results in the admittedly small study group were most gratifying. There were no major or minor congenital anomalies, no bilirubin value above 12 mg/dl, no hematocrit higher than 65%, and no instance of respiratory disease. Similar results were reported by Fuhrmann[212] of the German Democratic Republic. The attempt there was made to initiate normoglycemic treatment as soon as possible after conception by means of multiple doses of insulin daily, hospital and home blood glucose monitoring, and hospitalization if difficulties arose in the control of diabetes and, in any case, from the 32nd week of pregnancy on. There were no congenital anomalies in 110 infants of diabetic mothers in whom strict metabolic control had been instituted prior to conception. In 228 infants whose mothers had received strict metabolic control from the 10th to 16th week of pregnancy on, there were 18 anomalies (7.9%).

In the Joslin Clinic experience thus far, the results have likewise been favorable. In the better controlled half of a study group, the congenital anomaly rate was 3% (quite close to that in infants of nondiabetic mothers), whereas in the less well-controlled group, the rate was 22%, and in this group were most of the major defects and all of the deaths.[210]

Fortunately, not nearly as many infants of diabetic mothers reach the pathologist as before. However, a summary of findings in the past and continuing to some extent today, is appropriate. Most obvious is the increased body weight and length probably due to the excessive fetal production of insulin with its growth hormone effect, in response to the hyperglycemia of the mother. Other than the brain, there is generalized organomegaly. The placenta tends to be large. In the pancreas, hypertrophy and hyperplasia of the islets may be striking, mainly of the B cells, so that such infants may have twice the normal islet tissue[61,213,214] (Fig. 14–19). There is clear evidence of the increased B cell function: (1) such pancreases have been found to have increased insulin content;[215] (2) the infants have high plasma insulin levels;[216] (3) following a brief period of hyperglycemia after birth, neonatal hypoglycemia may be present for as much as ten days;[61] and (4) glucose injection into the umbilical vein of such infants produces an insulin response several times normal.[217] Maternal periods of hyperglycemia seem the best basis for explaining the islet cell hyperplasia in the infant.[214]

The association of the respiratory distress syndrome of infancy with maternal diabetes is an important one and in the past was the basis of from one-sixth to one-half neonatal deaths.[218] This hyaline membrane disease seems to be another expression of the prematurity of the infant with insufficiently developed surfactant. The histologic appearance is one of general atelectasis with some alveolar ducts and antra distended with air and lined by the hyaline membrane of dense acidophilic material.

Other reported changes are glycogen infiltration of renal tubules, growth of follicles in the ovary, decidual change of the endometrium, hyperplasia of testicular Leydig cells, and extramedullary hematopoiesis in the spleen and liver (probably attributable to the prematurity).[61] None of these changes occurs consistently (See also Chapter 33).

DIABETES AND INFECTION

Although many have accepted the conclusion that infections are common in diabetes and that diabetics are more susceptible to infection than are nondiabetics, there is much basis for doubt that persons with well-controlled diabetes are less resistant to infection than are normal persons. It is true that there is increased difficulty in the clinical control of diabetes during an active infection, and this imprints the episode indelibly on the physician's memory. It is clear from Table 14–1 that infection in the modern era is not a major cause of death, in contrast to the period from 1924 to 1948. Various reasons have been given for diabetics to be more susceptible to infection than is the general population: (1) increased sugar content of blood and tissues (probably not a direct cause); (2) decreased effectiveness of leukocytes in combatting infection (see Chapters 36 and 37); and (3) lowered state of cellular nutrition[219] (an ill-defined term).

There are several facets of infection in diabetes that deserve further examination. One is the occurrence of pyelonephritis, necrotizing renal papillitis, and lower urinary tract infections, which are discussed above with the renal lesions. Another is the frequent initiation of a process in the toes following minor injury that results in gangrene. This is often a complex of infection, ischemia, and neurotrophic changes. A third facet is the occasional production of so much gas by nonclostridial gram-negative organisms, e.g., *E. coli,* in infections of diabetics that, prior to bacteriologic studies, a diagnosis of gas gangrene often has been made. The fourth is the occasional appearance of fungal infections in diabetic patients (Fig. 14–20). There is good experimental evidence that the acutely diabetic animal is more susceptible to low-virulence fungal infections than are other animals.[220]

For consideration of infection in greater detail, see Chapter 36.

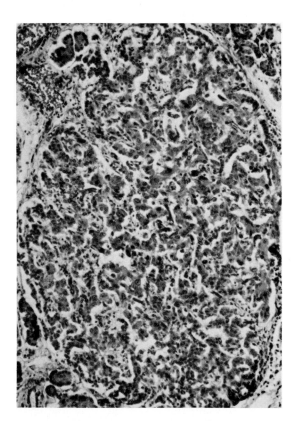

Fig. 14–19. Hyperplastic islet of Langerhans from infant born of diabetic mother. H & E ×150 (#32024).

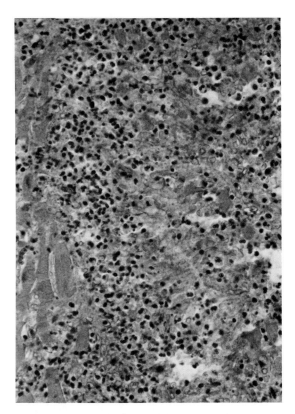

Fig. 14–20. Myocardial abscess due to *Aspergillus.* Hyphae can be discerned in the center and to the right in the picture. The 71-year-old man with 22 years of diabetes also had pancreatic carcinoma. H & E ×400 (#195372).

CANCER AND DIABETES

A relationship between cancer and diabetes has been suggested many times, not only as the total incidence, but also as individual types of cancer occurring in diabetic patients.[221] Unfortunately it is difficult to develop statistics in a control series that would be identical to those of any diabetic series. In contrast to reports in the older literature (See Chapter 42), the results of more recent surveys, including that of the Joslin Clinic as studied by Kessler,[222] show that the total incidence of cancer and cancer deaths in diabetics is not significantly different from that of nondiabetics. As may be seen in Table 14–2, it is clear that the relative proportion of deaths due to cancer in our autopsy series increased from 14% in 1948 to 1964 to 25% in 1964 to 1980. This may be biased by two factors: (1) the New England Deaconess Hospital is both a cancer and a diabetes center; and (2) cancer seems to have "taken up the slack" of the reduction in deaths from cardiovascular disease from 64 to 48% in the two periods concerned. The most frequent sites of the 256 cancer deaths were: lung, 46; hematopoietic system, 38; pancreas, 34; colon, 29; breast, 18; stomach, 10; ovary, 9; liver, 8; urinary bladder, 8; biliary tree, 7; esophagus, 6; and endometrium, 6.

Three cancers have led to discussions regarding possible association with diabetes. The first is *carcinoma of the pancreas,* which accounts for 11.9% of all cancer deaths in the diabetic autopsy population. In our series, the frequency of pancreatic carcinoma (of all types) is about 3 times as great in diabetics as in nondiabetics. No particular histologic type of pancreatic cancer seems to be incriminated in this increased prevalence. As was pointed out previously, there are four islet cell tumors that can produce diabetes but they are rare.[39] Perhaps one-third of the persons with pancreatic carcinoma and diabetes have signs of the malignancy prior to the onset of clinical symptoms of diabetes; in those persons, actual destruction of pancreatic tissue could conceivably account to some extent for the diabetes in such patients. Others have reported a relationship between diabetes and pancreatic carcinoma, but some prospective epidemiologic studies have failed to show such an association.[39,72,223–227]

Conflicting evidence is even more difficult to unscramble with *endometrial carcinoma* and diabetes. In some reported series of endometrial carcinoma, from 9 to 11% of the patients were diabetics.[228] In the autopsy series and in incidence overall, our figures do not support a major association.[221] Endometrial carcinoma is a disease of post-menopausal women, a time in life when carbohydrate intolerance is highly prevalent.

The marked increase in incidence of *hepatic carcinomas* in patients with hemochromatosis has been noted under the earlier discussion of hepatic disease and this component explains the increase in hepatic cancer deaths.

For additional discussion regarding cancer and diabetes, see Chapter 42.

HYPOGLYCEMIA

Hypoglycemia may be caused by medication, organic disease, functional imbalances, or factitious intent. The differential diagnosis is well summarized in several excellent reviews[228–231] and in Chapters 15, 31, and 43. The discussion here is limited to hypoglycemia associated with anatomic changes.

Islet Cell Tumors

Insulin-secreting beta-cell tumors are the most important cause of organic hypoglycemia. They may occur at any age and are slightly more frequent in women than in men (60%).[39,232,233] The tumors occur in any part of the pancreas, but also in the wall of the duodenum, adjacent to the pancreas, in the hilus of the spleen, and in the gastrosplenic ligament. Islet tumors vary from pale tan, or pale gray-white, to deep red and hemorrhagic; the last-named is undoubtedly due to the rich vascular supply that lends itself to angiographic localization. Most of the benign tumors are less than 2.0 cm in diameter, roughly spherical, and sharply demarcated. Less than 10% consist of more than one tumor and/or the multiple endocrine adenoma syndrome.[39,233] The clearly malignant islet cell tumors are generally larger than 2.0 cm, poorly defined, and have mitoses, pleomorphism, and other features common to malignant tumors. However, there is an intermediate group of well-differentiated but poorly demarcated tumors in which the predictability of behavior is risky.[39] About 75% of insulin-producing tumors are benign.

Microscopically, the typical islet cell tumor shows cells growing in a serpentine fashion, in solid nests or cords with a vascular stroma. The fine, stippled chromatin pattern of the nucleus is typical. B granules can be identified by special stains or by electron microscopy. Immunoperoxidase or immunofluorescent techniques label the insulin in the secretory granules. It is now clear that most islet cell tumors secrete more than one hormone, although one hormone dominates the clinical picture and the immunocytochemistry.[39,233–236] The amount of extractable insulin from B cell tumors is less per weight of tissue in carcinomas than in adenomas.[237] In some islet tumors there are ductular or even acinar components, reminiscent of the embryology of the pancreas.

Islet cell tumors are uncommon in diabetic patients but, as discussed above, there are four kinds that can produce reversible diabetes. Other islet tumors are not logically included in this report.[39] When an insulin-producing tumor develops in a diabetic, amelioration of the diabetes usually occurs.[238]

Although it would seem logical that islet cell hyperplasia should cause hyperinsulinism, the only circumstances in which this has been shown clearly is in nesidioblastosis and in transient neonatal hypoglycemia of infants.[39,213]

Large extrapancreatic tumors have been associated with hypoglycemia.[147,231,239,240] Usually such tumors are large, cellular, spindle-cell sarcomas. In most instances they occur in the retroperitoneum, pelvis, or lower mediastinum. No islet cells can be demonstrated in the tumors and, with few exceptions, no significant insulin or insulin-like activity can be extracted from the tumor.[241–243] Removal of the tumor stops the hypoglycemic episodes; recurrence or growth of metastases corresponds with resumption of hypoglycemia. It seems most likely that the tumor produces a peptide or protein with non-suppressible insulin-like activity.[244] A variety of tumors has been reported to be associated with hypoglycemia. In addition to the sarcomas, these are hepatocellular carcinomas and adrenocortical carcinomas as well as a sprinkling of other carcinomas and some lymphomas.[244] The mechanism of hepatocellular carcinoma is probably different, especially since hypoglycemia is likely to occur with severe hepatocellular disease, including hepatitis, cirrhosis, fatty change, and glycogenesis.[229]

Decreased function of the anterior pituitary because of destructive lesions of that body has been referred to above in relationship to diabetes, but may also result in hypoglycemia in nondiabetics.[188,189,245] The hypoglycemia related to brain lesions is usually referable to hypothalamic injury, and so is comparable to pituitary destruction.[229] Congenital adrenal hypoplasia is the most prominent adrenal basis for hypoglycemia.[229]

Although some reports of pancreatic studies in idiopathic hypoglycemia of infants blame islet hyperplasia, in the cases that we have studied and in most cases reported, islet hyperplasia has not been present.[246] Rosenbloom and Sherman have related this syndrome to a family history of diabetes.[247] In the leucine-induced hypoglycemia cases, few good pancreatic studies have been reported, but partial B cell degranulation has been observed in some.[147,148]

The results of hypoglycemia are demonstrable in the brain when the blood glucose reaches sufficiently low levels. Hypoglycemic brain lesions are basically neuron necrosis, occurring most prominently in the cerebral cortex. However, in more severe cases these also involve the lower centers and expand to become larger zones of patchy necrosis resembling micro-infarcts.[147,249–251]

Autopsy Diagnosis of Diabetes and Hypoglycemia

At times it may become important for legal or other reasons to establish at autopsy a diagnosis of diabetes mellitus, or conversely, hypoglycemia as a cause of death in the absence of sufficient clinical information. A distinct impediment to such studies is the very rapid change in blood glucose after death, due partly to glucose breakdown and more strikingly, to liver glycogenolysis. Blood from the right side of the heart is therefore of little use even within a few hours of death because of the rapid rise to levels of 300 mg/dl or more. More valid levels for longer periods of time can be obtained by the use of cerebrospinal fluid or the vitreous of the eye.

Since many diabetics die without anatomic changes pathognomonic of diabetes mellitus, the establishment of the diagnosis solely on autopsy grounds, therefore, may be impossible. There are anatomic lesions that give strong evidence for diabetes mellitus, the single most important of which is nodular intercapillary glomerulosclerosis. In the presence of this lesion, together with retinal aneurysms and some islet beta cell granule reduction, a strongly presumptive diagnosis of diabetes mellitus can be made. Other relatively helpful lesions are well-defined diffuse intercapillary glomerulosclerosis, arteriolosclerosis of both afferent and efferent arterioles of renal glomeruli, glycogen infiltration of renal tubules, the other features of diabetic retinopathy, marked hyalinization of islets of Langerhans, and the presence of the distinctive atrophic undifferentiated islets of many growth-onset diabetics.

The autopsy diagnosis of hypoglycemia cannot be made without corroborating history or unequivocally low glucose levels from spinal fluid and/or vitreous within a few hours of death. Neuron necrosis in the brain is not diagnostically specific, but is supportive evidence whenever there has been time in life for it to develop.

CAUSES OF DEATH

Table 14–2 lists the causes of death in 2897 diabetics upon whom autopsies were performed, and points up the changes during the years in response to therapy. It is clear that the present problems in extending the survival of patients with diabetes are vascular disease and particularly arteriosclerotic heart disease.

REFERENCES

1. Opie, E.L.: On the relation of chronic interstitial pancreatitis to the islands of Langerhans and to diabetes mellitus. J. Exp. Med. 5:397, 1901.
2. Meissner, W.A., Legg, M.A: The pathology of diabetes. In: A. Marble, P. White, R.F. Bradley, L.P. Krall (Eds.): Joslin's Diabetes Mellitus, 11th ed. Philadelphia, Lea & Febiger, 1971, p. 157.
3. Warren, S., LeCompte, P.M., Legg, M.A.: The Pathology of Diabetes Mellitus, 4th ed. Philadelphia, Lea & Febiger, 1966.
4. Bloodworth, J.M.B., Jr., Greider, M.H.: The endocrine pancreas and diabetes mellitus. In: J.M.B. Bloodworth, Jr. (Ed.): Endocrine Pathology, General and Surgical, 2nd ed. Baltimore, Williams & Wilkins Co., 1982, pp. 556–721.
5. B.W. Volk, K.F. Wellmann (Eds.): The Diabetic Pancreas. New York, Plenum Press, 1977.
5a. S.J. Cooperstein, D. Watkins (Eds.): The Islets of Langerhans. Biochemistry, Physiology, and Pathology. New York, Academic Press, 1981.
6. Like, A.A., Orci, L.: Embryogenesis of the human pancreatic islets: a light and electron microscopic study. Diabetes 21:511, 1972.
7. Robb, P.: The development of the islets of Langerhans in the human faetus. Q. J. Exper. Physiol. 46:335, 1961.
8. Rutter, W.J.: The development of the endocrine and exocrine pancreas. In: P.J. Fitzgerald, A.B. Morrison (Eds.): The Pancreas. Baltimore, Williams & Wilkins Co., 1980, pp. 30–38.
9. White, T.T.: Surgical anatomy of the pancreas. In: L.D. Carey (Ed.): The Pancreas. St. Louis, C.V. Mosby Co., 1973, pp. 3–16.
10. Pearse, A.G.E.: The gut as an endocrine organ. Br. J. Hosp. Med. 11:697, 1974.
11. Pearse, A.G.E.: The APUD cell concept and its implications in pathology. In: S.C. Sommers (Ed.): Pathology Annual. New York, Appleton-Century-Crofts, 1974, pp. 27–41.
12. Pearse, A.G.E., Polak, J.M., Heath, C.M.: Development, differentiation and derivation of the endocrine polypeptide cells of the mouse pancreas. Immunofluorescence, cytochemical and ultrastructural studies. Diabetologia 9:120, 1973.
13. Pearse, A.G.E., Polak, J.M.: The diffuse endocrine system and the APUD concept. In: S.R. Bloom (Ed.): Gut Hormones. New York, Churchill-Livingston, 1978, pp. 33–39.
14. LeDouarin, H.M.: The embryological origin of the endocrine cells associated with the digestive tract: experimental analysis based on the use of a stable cell marking technique. In: S.R. Bloom (Ed.): Gut Hormones. New York, Churchill-Livingston, 1978, pp. 49–56.
15. Langerhans, P.: Beiträge zur mikroskopischen Anatomie der Bauchspeicheldrüse. Inaugural Dissertation. Berlin, Gustav Lange, 1869.
16. Clark, E.: The number of islands of Langerhans in the human pancreas. Anat. Anz. 43:81, 1913.
17. Ogilvie, R.F.: Quantitative estimation of pancreatic islet tissue. Q. J. Med. 6:287, 1937.
18. Hellman, G., Petersson, B., Hellerström, C.: The growth pattern of the endocrine pancreas in mammals. In: S.F. Brolin, B. Hellman, H. Knutson (Eds.): Structure and

Metabolism of the Pancreatic Islets. New York, The Macmillan Co., 1964.
19. Gepts, W.: Contribution à l'étude morphologique des ilots de Langerhans au course du diabète. Étude des variations quantitative des differents constituents insulaires. Ann. Soc. Roy. Sci. Med. Natur. (Brux.) 10:5, 1957.
20. Solcia, F., Polak, J.M., Pearse, A.G.E., et al.: Lausanne 1977 classification of gastroenteropancreatic endocrine cells. In: S.R. Bloom (Ed.): Gut Hormones. New York, Churchill-Livingston, 1978, pp. 40–48.
21. Larsson, L-I.: Corticotropin-like peptides in central nerves and in endocrine cells of gut and pancreas. Lancet 2:1321, 1977.
22. Galmiche, J.P., Chayvalle, J.A., Dubois, P.M., et al.: Calcitonin-producing pancreatic somatostatinoma. Gastroenterol. 78:1577, 1980.
23. Gomori, G.: Aldehyde-fuchsin: a new stain for elastic tissue. Am. J. Clin. Pathol. 20:665, 1950.
24. Gomori, G.: A differential stain for cell types in the pancreatic islets. Am. J. Clin. Pathol. 15:497, 1939.
25. Warren, S., LeCompte, P.M., Legg, M.A.: Autopsy and staining methods. Ref. 3. Appendix A. pp. 499–511.
26. Bussolati, G., Capella, C., Vassallo, G., Solcia, A.E.: Histochemical and ultrastructural studies on pancreatic A cells. Evidence for glucagon and non-glucagon components of the A granule. Diabetologia 7:181, 1971.
27. Lacy, P.E.: Electron microscopic identification of different cell types in the islets of Langerhans of the guinea pig, rat, rabbit and dog. Anat. Rec. 128:255, 1957.
28. Orci, L.: The microanatomy of the islets of Langerhans. Metabolism 25 (Suppl. 1):1303, 1976.
29. Lacy, P.E., Davies, J.: Preliminary studies on the demonstration of insulin in the islets by the fluorescent antibody technic. Diabetes 6:354, 1957.
30. Lacy, P.E.: Electron microscopy of the beta cell of the pancreas. Am. J. Med. 31:851, 1961.
31. DeLellis, R.A., Sternberger, L.A., Mann, R.B., et al.: Immunoperoxidase technics in diagnostic pathology. Report of a workshop sponsored by the National Cancer Institute. Am. J. Clin. Pathol. 71:483, 1979.
32. Lacy, P.E.: Electron microscopy of the islets of Langerhans. Diabetes 11:509, 1962.
33. Warren, S., LeCompte, P.M., Legg, M.A.: The Pathology of Diabetes Mellitus, 4th ed. Philadelphia, Lea & Febiger, 1966, pp. 19–52.
33a. Unger, R.H., Orci, L.: Glucagon and the A cell. Physiology and pathophysiology. N. Engl. J. Med. 304:1518, 1575, 1981.
34. Creutzfeldt, W.: Endocrine tumors of the pancreas: clinical, chemical and morphological findings. In: P.J. Fitzgerald, A.B. Morrison (Eds.): The Pancreas. Baltimore, Williams & Wilkins Co., 1980, pp. 208–230.
35. Orci, L., Baetens, D., Dubois, M.P., et al.: Evidence of the D-cell of the pancreas secreting somatostatin. Horm. Metab. Res. 7:400, 1975.
35a. Reichlin, S.: Somatostatin. N. Engl. J. Med. 309:1495, 1556, 1983.
35b. Gerich, J.E.: Somatostatin and diabetes. Am. J. Med. 70:619, 1981.
36. Larsson, L.-I., Sundler, F., Håkanson, R.: Pancreatic polypeptide. A postulated new hormone: identification of its cellular storage site by light and electron immunocytochemistry. Diabetologia 12:211, 1976.
37. Baetens, D., Stefan, Y., Ravazzola, M., et al.: Alterations of islet cell populations in spontaneously diabetic mice. Diabetes 27:1, 1978.
38. Volk, B.W., Wellmann, K.F.: Quantitative studies on the islets of non-diabetic patients. In: B.W. Volk, K.F. Well-

mann (Eds.): The Diabetic Pancreas. New York, The Plenum Press, 1977, pp. 121–128.

39. Legg, M.A., Khettry, U.: The pancreas and extrahepatic biliary system. In: S.G. Silverberg (Ed.): Principles and Practice of Surgical Pathology. New York, John Wiley and Sons, 1983, pp. 1017–1050.

40. Volk, B.W., Wellmann, K.F.: Idiopathic diabetes. In: B.W. Volk, K.F. Wellmann (Eds.): The Diabetic Pancreas. New York, The Plenum Press, 1977, pp. 231–260.

41. Lacy, P.E.: Pancreatic beta cell. In: Ciba Foundation Colloquia on Endocrinology: Etiology of Diabetes Mellitus and its Complications. 15:75, 1964.

42. Westermark, P.: Amyloid of human islets of Langerhans. II. Electron microscopic analysis of isolated amyloid. Virchows Arch. (Pathol. Anat.) 373:61, 1977.

43. Westermark, P.: Fine structure of islets of Langerhans in insular amyloidosis. Virchows Arch. (Pathol. Anat.) 359:1, 1973.

44. Bell, E.T.: The incidence and significance of degranulation of the beta cells in the islets of Langerhans in diabetes mellitus. Diabetes 2:125, 1953.

45. LeCompte, P.M., Gepts, W.: The pathology of juvenile diabetes. In: B.W Volk, K.F. Wellmann (Eds.): The Diabetic Pancreas. New York, Plenum Press, 1977, pp. 325–363.

46. Gepts, W., De Mey, J.: Islet cell survival determined by morphology. An immunocytochemical study of the islets of Langerhans in juvenile diabetes mellitus. Diabetes 27 (Suppl. 1):251, 1978.

47. Gepts, W., De Mey, J., Marichal-Pipeleers, M.: Hyperplasia of "pancreatic polypeptide" cells in the pancreas of juvenile diabetes. Diabetologia 13:27, 1977.

48. Warren, S.: The pathology of diabetes in children. J.A.M.A. 88:99, 1927.

49. Gepts, W.: Pathologic anatomy of the pancreas in juvenile diabetes mellitus. Diabetes 14:619, 1965.

50. Junker, K., Egberg, J., Kromann, H., Nerup, J.: An autopsy study of the islets of Langerhans in acute-onset juvenile diabetes mellitus. Acta Pathol. Microbiol. Scand. 85:699, 1977.

51. Renold, A., Soeldner, J.S., Steinke, J.: Immunological studies with homologous and heterologous pancreatic insulin in the cow. In: Ciba Foundation Colloquia on Endocrinology: Etiology of Diabetes Mellitus and Its Complications. 15:122–139, 1964.

52. LeCompte, P.M., Steinke, J.: Changes in the islets of Langerhans in cows injected with heterologous and homologous insulin. Diabetes 15:586, 1966.

53. Craighead, J.E.: Viral diabetes. In: B.W Volk, K.F. Wellmann (Eds.): The Diabetic Pancreas. New York, The Plenum Press. 1977, pp. 467–488.

54. Craighead, J.E.: The role of viruses in the pathogenesis of pancreatic disease and diabetes mellitus. Prog. Med. Virol. 19:161, 1975.

55. Craighead, J.E.: Viral diabetes mellitus in man and experimental animals. Am. J. Med. 70:127, 1981.

56. Hultquist, G., Nordvall, S., Sundström, C.: Insulitis in cytomegalovirus infection in a newborn infant. Uppsala J. Med. Sci. 78:139, 1973.

57. Toreson, W.E.: Glycogen infiltration (so-called hydropic degeneration) in the pancreas in human and experimental diabetes mellitus. Am. J. Pathol. 27:327, 1951.

58. Gomori, G.: The histology of the normal and diseased pancreas. Bull. N.Y. Acad. Med. 21:99, 1945.

59. Warren, S., LeCompte, P.M., Legg, M.A.: The Pathology of Diabetes Mellitus, 4th Ed. Philadelphia, Lea & Febiger, 1966, p. 62 (Table 6).

60. Maclean, N., Ogilvie, R.F.: Quantitative estimation of the pancreatic islet tissue in diabetic subjects. Diabetes 4:367, 1955.

61. Warren, S., LeCompte, P.M., Legg, M.A.: The Pathology of Diabetes Mellitus, 4th Ed. Philadelphia, Lea & Febiger, 1966, pp. 413–418.

62. Bloodworth, J.M.B., Jr.: Morphologic changes associated with sulfonylurea therapy. Metabolism 12:287, 1963.

63. Potet, F.-G., Bader, J.-P., Martin, E., Lambling, A.: Etude histologique des ilots de Langerhans non tumoraux dans le syndrome de Zollinger-Ellison. Technique et resultats. Arch. Anat. Pathol. (Paris) 13:206, 1965.

64. Heitz, P.U., Klöppel, G., Häcki, W.H., et al.: Nesidioblastosis: the pathologic basis of persistent hyperinsulinemic hypoglycemia in infants. Morphologic and quantitative analysis of seven cases based on specific immunostaining and electron microscopy. Diabetes 26:632, 1977.

65. Warren, S., LeCompte, P.M., Legg, M.A.: The Pathology of Diabetes Mellitus, 4th Ed. Philadelphia, Lea & Febiger, 1966, p. 383.

66. Rosann, R.C., Schwachman, H., Kulczvcki, L.L.: Diabetes mellitus and cystic fibrosis of the pancreas. Laboratory and clinical observations. Am. J. Dis. Child. 104:625, 1962.

67. Farber, S.: Pancreatic function and disease in early life; pathologic changes associated with pancreatic insufficiency in early life. Arch. Pathol. 37:238, 1944.

68. Warren, S., LeCompte, P.M., Legg, M.A.: The Pathology of Diabetes Mellitus, 4th Ed. Philadelphia, Lea & Febiger, 1966, p. 106.

69. Wellmann, K.F., Volk, B.W.: Pancreatitis, pancreatic lithiasis, and diabetes mellitus. In: B.W Volk, K.F. Wellmann (Eds.): The Diabetic Pancreas. New York, Plenum Press. 1977, pp. 291–309.

70. Comfort, M.W., Gambill, E.E., Baggenstoss, A.H.: Chronic relapsing pancreatitis; a study of twenty-nine cases without associated disease of the biliary or gastrointestinal tract. Gastroenterology 6:239, 376, 1946.

71. Maimon, S.N., Kirsner, J.B., Palmer, W.L.: Chronic recurrent pancreatitis: a clinical study of twenty cases. Arch. Intern. Med. 81:56, 1948.

72. Volk, B.W., Wellmann, K.F.: Cancer and diabetes. In: B.W Volk, K.F. Wellmann (Eds.): The Diabetic Pancreas. New York, Plenum Press. 1977, pp. 311–316.

73. MacMahon, B., Yen, S., Trichopoulos, D., et al.: Coffee and cancer of the pancreas. N. Engl. J. Med. 304:630, 1981.

74. Lin, R.S., Kessler, I.I.: A multifactorial model for pancreatic cancer in man. Epidemiologic evidence. J.A.M.A. 245:147, 1981.

75. Priestley, J.T., Comfort, M.W., Sprague, R.G.: Total pancreatectomy for hyperinsulinism due to islet cell adenoma: follow-up report five and one-half years after operation, including metabolic studies. Ann. Surg. 130:211, 1949.

76. Ricketts, H.T., Brunschwig, A., Knowlton, K.: Diabetes in a totally depancreatized man. Proc. Soc. Exper. Biol. Med. 58:254, 1945.

77. Suzuki, Y.: An electron microscopy of the renal differentiation. II. Glomerulus. Keio. J. Med. 8:129, 1959.

78. Yamada, E.: The fine structure of the renal glomerulus of the mouse. J. Biophys. Biochem. Cytol. 1:551, 1955.

79. Suzuki, Y., Churg, J., Grishman, E., et al.: The mesangium of the renal glomerulus. Electron microscopic studies of pathologic alterations. Am. J. Pathol. 43:555, 1963.

80. Robbins, S.L., Cotran, R.S.: The kidney. In: Pathologic Basis of Disease. 2nd Ed. Philadelphia, W.B. Saunders Co., 1979, pp. 1115–1118.

81. Farquhar, M.G.: The primary glomerular filtration barrier—basement membrane or epithelial slits? (Editorial). Kidney Int. 8:197, 1975.

82. Brenner, B.M., Hostetter, T.H., Humes, H.D.: Molecular basis of proteinuria of glomerular origin. N. Engl. J. Med. 298:826, 1978.

83. Venkatachalam, M.A., Rennke, H.G.: The structural and molecular basis of glomerular filtration. Circ. Res. 43:337, 1978.

84. Martinez-Hernandez, A., Amenta, P.S.: The basement membrane in pathology. Lab. Invest. 48:656, 1983.

84a. Ausiello, D.A., Kreisberg, J.I., Roy, C., Karnovsky, M.J.: Contraction of cultured rat glomerular cells of apparent mesangial origin after stimulation with angiotensin II and arginine vasopressin. J. Clin. Invest. 65:754, 1980.

84b. Schreiner, G., Cotran, R.S.: Localization of an Ia-bearing glomerular cell in the mesangium. J. Cell Biol. 94:483, 1982.

85. Seiler, M.W., Rennke, H.G., Venkatachalam, M.A., et al.: Pathogenesis of polycation-induced alterations ("fusion") of glomerular epithelium. Lab. Invest. 36:48, 1977.

85a. Parthasarathy, N., Spiro, R.G.: Effect of diabetes on the glycosaminoglycan component of the human glomerular basement membrane. Diabetes 31:738, 1982.

86. Kimmelstiel, P., Wilson, C.: Intercapillary lesions in the glomeruli of the kidney. Am. J. Pathol. 12:83, 1936.

87. Warren, S., LeCompte, P.M., Legg, M.A.: The Pathology of Diabetes Mellitus, 4th Ed. Philadelphia, Lea & Febiger, 1966, pp. 211–217.

88. Farquhar, M.G., Palade, G.E.: Functional evidence for the existence of a third cell type in the renal glomerulus. Phagocytosis of filtration residues by a distinctive "third" cell. J. Cell. Biol. 13:55, 1962.

89. Kimmelstiel, P.: Diabetic nephropathy. In: F.K. Mostofi, D.E. Smith (Eds.): The Kidney. Baltimore, Williams & Wilkins Co., 1966, p. 226.

90. Bloodworth, J.M.B., Jr.: A re-evaluation of diabetic glomerulosclerosis 50 years after the discovery of insulin. Hum. Pathol. 9:439, 1978.

90a. Heptinstall, R.H.: Diabetes mellitus and gout. In: R.H. Heptinstall (Ed.): Pathology of the Kidney, 3rd Ed. Boston, Little, Brown and Co., 1983, pp. 1399–1400.

90b Morel-Maroger, L., Verroust, P., Preus'Homme, J.-P.: Glomerular lesions in plasma dyscrasias. In: S. Rosen (Ed.): Pathology of Glomerular Dissease. New York, Churchill Livingstone, 1983, pp. 207–217.

91. Fahr, T.: Über glomerulosklerose. Virchow Arch. (Pathol. Anat.) 309:16, 1942.

92. Osawa, G., Kimmelstiel, P., Seiling, V.: Thickness of glomerular basement membranes. Am. J. Clin. Pathol. 45:7, 1966.

93. Kimmelstiel, P., Osawa, G., Beres, J.: Glomerular basement membrane in diabetics. Am. J. Clin. Pathol. 45:21, 1966.

94. Gellman, D.D., Pirani, C.C., Soothill, J.F., et al.: Diabetic nephropathy: a clinical and pathologic study based on renal biopsies. Medicine 38:321, 1959.

94a. Cotran, R.S.: Glomerulosclerosis in reflux nephropathy. Kid. Int. 21:528, 1982.

94b. Kreisberg, J.I.: Insulin requirement for contracture of cultured rat glomerular mesangial cells in response to angiotensin II: possible role for insulin in modulating glomerular hemodynamics. Proc. Natl. Acad. Sci. 79:4190, 1982.

95. Daysog, A., Jr., Dobson, H.L., Brennan, J.C.: Renal glomerular and vascular lesions in prediabetes and in diabetes mellitus: a study based on renal biopsies. Ann. Intern. Med. 54:672, 1961.

96. Rosenbaum, P., Kattine, A.A., Gottsegen, W.L.: Diabetic and prediabetic nephropathy in childhood. Am. J. Dis. Child. 106:83, 1963.

97. Camerini-Davalos, R.A., Caulfield, R.A., Rees, S.B., et al.: Preliminary observations on subjects with prediabetes. Diabetes 12:508, 1963.

98. Gundersen, H.J., Mogensen, C.E., Seyer-Hansen, K., et al.: Early and late changes in diabetic kidney. Adv. Nephrol. 8:43, 1979.

99. Spiro, R.G.: Search for a biochemical basis of diabetic microangiopathy. Diabetologia 12:1, 1976.

100. Mauer, S.M., Steffes, M.W., Brown, D.M.: Animal models of diabetic nephropathy. Adv. Nephrol. 8:23, 1979.

101. Canivet, J., Cruz, A., Moreau-Lalande, H.: Biochemical abnormalities of the human diabetic glomerular basement membrane. Metabolism 28:1206, 1979.

102. Kefalides, N.A.: Biochemical properties of human glomerular basement membrane in normal and diabetic kidneys. J. Clin. Invest. 53:403, 1974.

103. Westberg, N.G., Michael, A.F.: Human glomerular basement membrane: chemical composition in diabetes mellitus. Acta Med. Scand. 194:39, 1973.

103a. Wahl, P., Deppermann, D., Hasslacher, C.: Biochemistry of glomerular basement membrane of the normal and diabetic human. Kid. Int. 21:744, 1982.

104. Mauer, S.M., Barbosa, J., Vernier, R.L., et al.: Development of diabetic vascular lesions in normal kidneys transplanted into patients with diabetes mellitus. N. Engl. J. Med. 295:916, 1976.

104a. Abouna, G.M., Al-Adnani, M.S., Kremer, G.D., et al.: Reversal of diabetic nephropathy in human cadaveric kidneys after transplantation into non-diabetic recipients. Lancet 2:1274, 1983.

105. Bloodworth, J.M.B., Jr.: Experimental diabetic glomerulosclerosis. II. The dog. Arch. Pathol. 79:113, 1965.

106. Bell, E.T.: Renal vascular disease in diabetes mellitus. Diabetes 2:376, 1953.

107. Oliver, J., MacDowell, M., Welt, L.G., et al.: The renal lesions of electrolyte imbalance. I. The structural alterations in potassium-depleted rats. J. Exper. Med. 106:563, 1957.

108. Ritchie, S., Waugh, D.: The pathology of Armanni-Ebstein diabetic nephropathy. Am. J. Pathol. 33:1035, 1957.

109. Baldwin, A.D., Root, H.F.: Infections of the upper urinary tract in the diabetic patient. N. Engl. J. Med. 223:244, 1940.

110. Kleeman, S.E.T., Freedman, L.R.: The finding of chronic pyelonephritis in males and females at autopsy. N. Engl. J. Med. 263:988, 1960.

111. Robbins, S.L., Mallory, G.K., Kinney, T.D.: Necrotizing renal papillitis: a form of acute pyelonephritis. N. Engl. J. Med. 235:885, 1946.

112. Harvald, B.: Renal papillary necrosis. A clinical survey of sixty-six cases. Am. J. Med. 35:481, 1963.

113. Beswick, I.P., Schatzki, P.F.: Experimental renal papillary necrosis. Arch. Pathol. 69:733, 1960.

114. Mooney, A.J.: Diabetic retinopathy—a challenge. Br. J. Ophthalmol. 47:513, 1963.

115. Kohner, E.M.: Diabetic retinopathy. Clin. Endocrinol. Metab. 6:345, 1977.

116. Nettleship, E.: Chronic retinitis, with formation of blood vessels in the vitreous in a patient with diabetes; one eye lost by results of chronic iritis accompanied by the formation of large vessels in the iris. Trans. Ophthalmol. Soc. U.K. 8:159, 1888.

117. Ballantyne, A.J., Lowenstein, A.: Diseases of the retina.

I. The pathology of diabetic retinopathy. Trans. Ophthalmol. Soc. U.K. *63*:95, 1944.

118. Friedenwald, J.S.: Diabetic retinopathy. Am. J. Ophthalmol. *33*:1187, 1950.

119. Kuwabara, T., Cogan, D.G.: Studies of retinal vascular patterns. I. Normal architecture. Arch. Ophthalmol. *64*:904, 1960.

120. Warren, S., LeCompte, P.M., Legg, M.A.: In: The Pathology of Diabetes Mellitus, 4th Ed. Philadelphia, Lea & Febiger, 1966, pp. 250–258.

121. Cogan, D.G., Toussaint, D., Kuwabara, T.: Retinal vascular patterns. IV. Diabetic retinopathy. Arch. Ophthalmol. *66*:366, 1961.

122. Merin, S., Ber, I., Ivry, M.: Retinal ischemia (capillary nonperfusion) and retinal neovascularization in patients with diabetic retinopathy. Ophthalmologica (Basel) *177*:140, 1978.

123. Malone, J.I., Van Cader, T.C., Edwards, W.C.: Diabetic vascular changes in children. Diabetes 26:673, 1977.

124. Toussaint, D., Cogan, D.G., Kuwabara, T.: Extravascular lesions of diabetic retinopathy. Arch. Ophthalmol. *67*:42, 1962.

125. Waite, J.H., Beetham, W.P.: The visual mechanism in diabetes mellitus (a comparative study of 2,002 diabetics and 458 non-diabetics for control.) N. Engl. J. Med. *212*:367, 429, 1935.

126. Cerami, A., Stevens, V.I., Monnier, V.M.: Role of nonenzymatic glycosylation in the development of the sequelae of diabetes mellitus. Metabolism 28 (Suppl. 1):431, 1979.

127. Logothetis, J., Baker, A.B.: Neurologic manifestations in diabetes mellitus. Med. Clin. North Am. *47*:1459, 1963.

128. Thomas, P.K., Ward, T.D.: Diabetic neuropathy. In: H. Keen, J. Jarrett (Eds.): Complications of Diabetes. Chicago, Yearbook Medical Publishers, Inc., 1975, pp. 151–177.

129. Colby, A.O.: Neurologic disorders of diabetes mellitus. Parts I and II of a two-part review. Diabetes *14*:424, 516, 1965.

130. Woltman, H.W., Wilder, R.M.: Diabetes mellitus. Pathologic changes in the spinal cord and peripheral nerves. Arch. Intern. Med. *44*:576, 1929.

131. Dolman, C.L.: The morbid anatomy of diabetic neuropathy. Neurol. *13*:135, 1963.

132. Greenbaum, D., Richardson, P.C., Salmon, M.V., Urich, H.: Pathological observations on six cases of diabetic neuropathy. Brain 87:201, 1964.

133. Yagihashi, S., Nishihara, M., Baba, M.: Morphometrical analysis of the peripheral nerve lesions in experimental diabetes rats. Tahoku J. Exp. Med. *129*:139, 1979.

134. Gabbay, K.H.: Hyperglycemia, polyol metabolism and complications of diabetes mellitus. Annu. Rev. Med. 26:521, 1975.

135. Thomas, P.K., Lascelles, R.G.: The pathology of diabetic neuropathy. Q. J. Med. *35*:489, 1966.

136. Behse, F., Buchthal, F., Carlsen, F.: Nerve biopsy and conduction studies in diabetic neuropathy. J. Neurol. Neurosurg. Psychiatry *40*:1072, 1977.

137. Garland, H., Taverner, D.: Diabetic myelopathy. Br. Med. J. *1*:1405, 1953.

138. Garland, H.: Diabetic amyotrophy. Br. J. Clin. Pract. *15*:9, 1961.

139. Locke, S., Lawrence, D.G., Legg, M.A.: Diabetic amyotrophy. Am. J. Med. *34*:775, 1963.

140. Coërs, C., Hildebrand, J.: Latent neuropathy in diabetes and alcoholism: electromyographic and histological study. Neurol. *15*:19, 1965.

141. Raff, M.C., Asbury, A.K.: Ischemic mononeuropathy and mononeuropathy multiplex in diabetes mellitus. N. Engl. J. Med. *279*:17, 1968.

142. Martin, M.M.: Involvement of autonomic nerve-fibres in diabetic neuropathy. Lancet *1*:560, 1953.

143. Olsson, Y., Sourander, P.: Changes in the sympathetic nervous system of diabetes mellitus. A preliminary report. J. Neurovisceral Rel. *31*:86, 1968.

143a. Warren, S., LeCompte, P.M., Legg, M.A.: The nervous system. In: The Pathology of Diabetes Mellitus, 4th Ed. Philadelphia, Lea & Febiger, 1966, pp. 269–283.

144. Griggs, D.F., Olsen, C.W.: Changes in spinal cord in diabetes mellitus; report of case with autopsy. Arch. Neurol. Psychiatry *38*:564, 1937.

145. DeJong, R.N.: CNS manifestations of diabetes mellitus. Postgrad. Med. *61*:101, 1977.

146. Ellenberg, M., Krainer, L.: Diabetic neuropathy; review of literature and a case report with post-mortem findings. Diabetes 8:279, 1959.

147. Warren, S., LeCompte, P.M., Legg, M.A.: In: The Pathology of Diabetes Mellitus, 4th Ed. Philadelphia, Lea & Febiger, 1966, p. 395.

147a. Goldenberg, S., Alex, M., Joshi, R.A., Blumenthal, H.T.: Nonatheromatous peripheral vascular disease of the lower extremity in diabetes mellitus. Diabetes 8:261, 1959.

147b. Bloodworth, J.M.B., Jr., Greider, M.H.: The endocrine pancreas and diabetes mellitus. In: J.M.B. Bloodworth, Jr. (Ed.): Endocrine Pathology. General and Surgical, 2nd Ed. Baltimore, Williams & Wilkins, 1982, p. 640.

148. LeCompte, P.M.: Vascular lesions in diabetes mellitus. J. Chron. Dis. *3*:178, 1955.

149. Lundbaek, K., Posborg-Petersen, V.: Lipid composition of diabetic and non-diabetic coronary arteries. Acta Med. Scand. *144*:354, 1953.

150. Hevelke, G.: Beiträge zur Funktion und Struktur der Gefässe. II. Angiochemische Gefässveränderungen beim Diabetes mellitus. Ztschr. Altenforsch 9:28, 1955.

151. Burstein, R., Soule, S.D., Blumenthal, H.T.: Histogenesis of pathological processes in placentas of metabolic disease in pregnancy. II. The diabetic state. Am. J. Obstet. Gynecol. *74*:6, 1957.

151a. Randerath, E., Diezel, P.B.: Vergleichende histochemische Untersuchungen der Arteriosklerose bei Diabetes mellitus und ohne Diabetes mellitus. Deutsch. Arch. Klin. Med. *205*:523, 1959.

152. Ross, R., Glomset, J.A.: The pathogenesis of atherosclerosis. (Second of two parts). N. Engl. J. Med. *295*:420, 1976.

153. Blumenthal, H.T., Hirata, Y., Owens, C.T., Berns, A.W.: A histo- and immunologic analysis of the small vessel lesion of diabetes in the human and in the rabbit. In: M.D. Siperstein, A.R. Colwell, Jr., K. Meyer (Eds.): Small Blood Vessel Involvement in Diabetes Mellitus. Washington, D.C., American Institute of Biological Sciences, 1964, p. 279.

153a. Walton, K.W.: Pathogenetic mechanisms in atherosclerosis. Am. J. Cardiol. *35*:542, 1975.

154. Ross, R., Harker, L.: Hyperlipidemia and atherosclerosis. Science *193*:1094, 1976.

155. Warren, S., LeCompte, P.M., Legg, M.A.: The Pathology of Diabetes Mellitus, 4th ed. Philadelphia, Lea & Febiger, 1966. A.: Arteriosclerosis in diabetes mellitus. pp. 178–187. B.: The heart. pp. 188–198. C. Diabetic angiopathy. pp. 310–332.

156. Stearns, S., Schlesinger, M.J., Rudy, A.: Incidence and clinical significance of coronary artery disease in diabetes mellitus. Arch. Intern. Med. *80*:463, 1947.

157. Clawson, B.J., Bell, E.T.: Incidence of fatal coronary

disease in nondiabetic and in diabetic persons. Arch. Pathol. 48:105, 1949.

158. Kannel, W.B., McGee, D., Gordon, T.: A general cardiovascular risk profile: The Framingham study. Am. J. Cardiol. 38:46, 1976.

159. Fagerburg, S.E.: Diabetic neuropathy: a clinical and histological study of the significance of vascular affections. Acta Med. Scand. 164 (Suppl. 345):9, 1959.

160. Aagenaes, Ö., Moe, H.: Light- and electron-microscopic study of skin capillaries of diabetics. Diabetes 10:253, 1961.

161. Banson, B.B., Lacy, P.E.: Diabetic microangiopathy in human toes, with emphasis on the ultrastructural change in dermal capillaries. Am. J. Pathol. 45:41, 1964.

162. Siperstein, M.B., Unger, R.H., Madison, L.L.: Studies of muscle capillary basement membranes in normal subjects, diabetic, and prediabetic patients. J. Clin. Invest. 47:1973, 1968.

163. Bercovici, E., Solomon, L.M., Beerman, H.: Microangiopathy in diabetes mellitus and nondiabetic dermatoses. Am. J. Med. Sci. 248:20, 1964.

164. Friederici, H.H.R., Tucker, W.R., Schwartz, T.B.: Observations on small blood vessels of skin in the normal and in diabetic patients. Diabetes 15:233, 1966.

165. Kilo, C., Vogler, N., Williamson, J.R.: Muscle capillary basement membrane changes related to aging and to diabetes mellitus. Diabetes 21:881, 1972.

166. Williamson, J.R., Kilo, C.: Current status of capillary basement-membrane disease in diabetes mellitus. Diabetes 26:65, 1977.

167. Williamson, J.R., Kilo, C.: Basement-membrane thickening and diabetic microangiopathy. Diabetes 25:925, 1976.

168. Østerby, R.: Morphometric studies of the peripheral glomerular basement membrane in early juvenile diabetes. I. Development of initial basement membrane thickening. Diabetologia 8:86, 1972.

169. Spiro, R.G.: Biochemistry of the renal glomerular basement membrane and its alterations in diabetes mellitus. N. Engl. J. Med. 288:1337, 1973.

170. Goldstein, J.L., Brown, M.S.: The low density lipoprotein pathway and its relation to atherosclerosis. Annu. Rev. Biochem. 46:897, 1977.

171. Chandramouli, V., Carter, J.R., Jr.: Cell membrane changes in chronically diabetic rats. Diabetes 24:257, 1975.

172. Ennis, G., Miller, M., Unger, F.M., Unger, L.: Intercapillary glomerulosclerosis in diabetes secondary to chronic relapsing pancreatitis. Diabetes 18 (Suppl. 1):333, 1969.

173. Wellmann, K.F., Volk, B.W.: Nodular intercapillary glomerulosclerosis in diabetes secondary to chronic calcific pancreatitis. Diabetes 25:713, 1976.

173a.Raskin, P., Pietri, A.O., Unger, R., Shannon, W.A., Jr.: The effect of diabetic control on the width of skeletal muscle capillary basement membrane in patients with Type I diabetes mellitus. N. Engl. J. Med. 309:1546, 1983.

173b.Siperstein, M.D.: Diabetic microangiopathy and the control of blood glucose (Editorial). N. Engl. J. Med. 309:1577, 1983.

174. Alpert, J.S., Coffman, J.D., Balodimos, M.C., et al.: Capillary permeability and blood flow in skeletal muscle of patients with diabetes mellitus and genetic prediabetes. N. Engl. J. Med. 286:454, 1972.

174a.Bollinger, A., Frey, J., Jäger, K., et al.: Patterns of diffusion through skin capillaries in patients with long-term diabetes. N. Engl. J. Med. 307:1305, 1982.

174b Viberti, G.C., Hill, R.D., Jarrett, R.J., et al.: Microal-
buminuria as a predictor of clinical nephropathy in insulin-dependent diabetes mellitus. Lancet 1:1430, 1982.

174c.Mogensen, C.E.: Microalbuminuria predicts clinical proteinuria and early mortality in maturity-onset diabetes. N. Engl. J. Med. 310:356, 1984.

175. Ledet, T.: Diabetic cardiopathy. Acta Pathol. Microbiol. Scand. 84:421, 1976.

176. Crall, F.V., Roberts, W.C.: The extramural and intramural coronary arteries in juvenile diabetes mellitus: analysis of nine necropsy patients aged 19 to 38 years with onset of diabetes before age 15 years. Am. J. Med. 64:221, 1978.

177. Fischer, V.W., Barner, H.B., Leskiw, M.L.: Capillary basal laminar thickness in diabetic human myocardium. Diabetes 28:713, 1979.

178. Factor, S.M., Okun, E.M., Minase, T.: Capillary microaneurysms in the human diabetic heart. N. Engl. J. Med. 302:384, 1980.

179. Regan, T.J., Lyons, M.M., Ahmed, S.S., et al.: Evidence for cardiac myopathy in familial diabetes mellitus. J. Clin. Invest. 60:885, 1977.

180. Solomon, N., Carpenter, C.C.J., Bennett, I.L., Jr., Harvey, A.M.: Schmidt's syndrome (thyroid and adrenal insufficiency) and coexistent diabetes mellitus. Diabetes 14:300, 1965.

181. Conn, J.W.: Hypertension, the potassium ion and impaired carbohydrate intolerance. N. Engl. J. Med. 273:1135, 1965.

182. Neville, A.M., Symington, T.: The pathology of primary aldosteronism. Cancer 19:1854, 1966.

183. Eisenberg, A.A., Wallenstein, H.: Pheochromocytoma of suprarenal medulla (paraganglioma); clinicopathologic study. Arch. Pathol. 14:818, 1932.

184. Gifford, R.W., Jr., Kvale, W.F., Maher, F.T., et al.: Clinical features, diagnosis and treatment of pheochromocytoma: a review of seventy-six cases. Mayo Clin. Proc. 39:281, 1964.

185. Houssay, B.A., Foglia, V.G., Smyth, F.S., et al.: The hypophysis and secretion of insulin. J. Exper. Med. 75:547, 1942.

186. Volk, B.W., Lazarus, S.S.: Ultrastructure of pancreatic B cells in severely diabetic dogs. Diabetes 13:60, 1964.

187. Coggeshall, C., Root, H.F.: Acromegaly and diabetes mellitus. Endocrinol. 26:1, 1940.

188. Houssay, B.A.: Carbohydrate metabolism. N. Engl. J. Med. 214:971, 1936.

189. Frey, H.M.: Spontaneous pituitary destruction in diabetes mellitus. J. Clin. Endocrinol. 19:1642, 1959.

190. Warren, S., LeCompte, P.M., Legg, M.A.: The Pathology of Diabetes Mellitus, 4th ed. Philadelphia, Lea & Febiger, 1966, pp. 340, 342–344.

190a.Fager, C.A., Rees, S.B., Bradley, R.F.: Surgical ablation of the pituitary in the treatment of diabetic retinopathy. J. Neurosurg. 24:727, 1966.

190b.Merimee, T.J.: A follow-up study of vascular disease in growth-hormone-deficient dwarfs with diabetes. N. Engl. J. Med. 298:1217, 1978.

191. Sommers, S.C., Meissner, W.A.: Endocrine abnormalities accompanying human endometrial cancer. Cancer 10:516, 1957.

192. Houssay, B.A.: Other hormones. In: R.H. Williams (Ed.): Diabetes. New York, Paul B. Hoeber, Inc., 1960, p. 233.

193. Rosai, J., Levine, G.D.: Tumors of the thymus. In: Atlas of Tumor Pathology. Washington, D.C., Armed Forces Institute of Pathology, 1976, pp. 167–181.

194. Eppinger, H.: Die Leberkrankheiten. Vienna, Julius Springer, 1937, p. 40.

195. Bogoch, A., Caselman, W.G.B., Kaplan, A., Bockus,

H.L.: Studies of hepatic function in diabetes mellitus, portal cirrhosis and other liver diseases. A correlation of clinical, biochemical and liver needle biopsy findings. I. Diabetes mellitus. Am. J. Med. *18*:354, 1955.

196. Vallance-Owen, J.: Liver glycogen in diabetes mellitus. J. Clin. Pathol. *5*:42, 1952.

197. Kalk, H.: The relationship between fatty liver and diabetes mellitus. German Med. Monthly *5*:81, 1960.

198. Feldman, M., Feldman, M., Jr.: The incidence of cholelithiasis, cholesterolosis, and liver disease in diabetes mellitus. An autopsy study. Diabetes *3*:305, 1954.

199. Sheldon, J.H.: Haemochromatosis. London, Oxford University Press, 1935.

200. Pollycove, M.: Hemochromatosis. In: J.B. Stanbury, J.B. Wyngaarden, D.S. Fredrickson (Eds.): Metabolic Basis of Inherited Disease. 4th ed. New York, McGraw-Hill Book Co., 1978, pp. 1127–1164.

201. Volk, B.W., Wellmann, K.F.: Hemochromatosis and diabetes. In: B.W. Volk, K.F. Wellmann (Eds.): The Diabetic Pancreas. New York, Plenum Press, 1977, pp. 317–324.

202. Warren, S., LeCompte, P.M., Legg, M.A.: The Pathology of Diabetes Mellitus, 4th ed. Philadelphia, Lea & Febiger, 1966, pp. 364–373.

203. Warren, S., Drake, W.L., Jr.: Primary carcinoma of the liver in hemochromatosis. Am. J. Pathol. *27*:573, 1951.

204. LeCompte, P.M., Merriam, J.C., Jr.: Mitotic figures and enlarged nuclei in the islands of Langerhans in man. Diabetes *11*:35, 1962.

205. McGavran, M.H., Hartroft, W.S.: The predilection of pancreatic beta cells for pigment deposition in hemochromatosis and hemosiderosis. Sci. Proc. Am. Assoc. Pathol. Bacteriol., Am. J. Pathol. *32*:631, 1956. (Abstr.)

206. Becker, D., Miller, M.: Presence of diabetic glomerulosclerosis in patients with hemochromatosis. N. Engl. J. Med. *263*:367, 1960.

207. Bergstrom, J., Hultman, E., Roch-Norlund, A.E.: Muscle glycogen in juvenile diabetes before and during treatment with insulin. Nature *198*:97, 1963.

208. Marks, J.H., Ham, D.P.: Calcification of vas deferens. Am. J. Roentgenol. *47*:859, 1942.

209. Merriam, J.C., Jr., Sommers, S.C.: Mammary periductal hyalin in diabetic women. Report of twenty cases. Lab. Invest. *6*:412, 1957.

210. Hiller, E., Hare, J.W., Cloherty, J.P., et al.: Elevated maternal hemoglobin A_{1c} in early pregnancy and major congenital anomalies in infants of diabetic mothers. N. Engl. J. Med. *304*:1331, 1981.

211. Jovanovic, L., Druzin, M., Peterson, C.M.: Effect of euglycemia on the outcome of pregnancy on insulin-dependent diabetic women as compared with normal control subjects. Am. J. Med. *71*:921, 1981.

212. Fuhrmann, K.: Diabetic control and outcome in the pregnant patient. In: C.M. Peterson (Ed.): Diabetic Management in the 80's. The Role of Home Blood Glucose Monitoring and New Insulin Delivery Systems. New York, Praeger Publishers, 1982, pp. 66–79.

213. D'Agostino, A.N., Bahn, R.C.: A histopathologic study of the pancreas of infants of diabetic mothers. Diabetes *12*:327, 1963.

214. Wellmann, K.F., Volk, B.W.: The islets of infants of diabetic mothers. In: B.W. Volk, K.F. Wellmann (Eds.): The Diabetic Pancreas. New York, Plenum Press, 1977, pp. 365–380.

215. Steinke, J., Driscoll, S.G.: The extractable insulin content of pancreas from fetuses and infants of diabetic and control mothers. Diabetes *14*:573, 1965.

216. Stimmler, L., Brazie, J.V., O'Brien, D.: Plasma-insulin levels in the newborn infants of normal and diabetic mothers. Lancet *1*:137, 1964.

217. Baird, J.D., Farquhar, J.W.: Insulin-secreting capacity in newborn infants of normal and diabetic women. Lancet *1*:71, 1962.

218. Driscoll, S.G., Benirschke, K., Curtis, G.W.: Neonatal deaths among infants of diabetic mothers. Post-mortem findings in ninety-five infants. Am. J. Dis. Child. *100*:818, 1960.

219. Warren, S., LeCompte, P.M., Legg, M.A.: Diabetes and infection. In: The Pathology of Diabetes Mellitus, 4th ed. Philadelphia, Lea & Febiger, 1966, pp. 167–177.

220. Elder, T.D., Baker, R.D.: Pulmonary mucormycosis in rabbits with alloxan diabetes; increased invasiveness of fungus during acute toxic phase of diabetes. Arch. Pathol. *61*:159, 1956.

221. Warren, S., LeCompte, P.M., Legg, M.A.: Cancer and diabetes. In: The Pathology of Diabetes Mellitus, 4th ed. Philadelphia, Lea & Febiger, 1966, pp. 434–439.

222. Kessler, I.I.: Mortality experience of diabetic patients: a twenty-six year follow-up study. Am. J. Med. *51*:715, 1971.

223. Fraumeni, J.F., Jr.: Cancers of the pancreas and biliary tract: epidemiological considerations. Cancer Res. *35*:3437, 1975.

224. Malagaleda, J.R.: Pancreatic cancer. An overview of epidemiology, clinical presentation, and diagnosis. Mayo Clin. Proc. *54*:459, 1979.

225. Wynder, E.L.: An epidemiological evaluation of the causes of cancer of the pancreas. Cancer Res. *35*:2228, 1975.

226. Bell, E.T.: Carcinoma of the pancreas. I. A clinical and pathologic study of 690 necropsied cases. II. The relation of carcinoma of the pancreas to diabetes mellitus. Am. J. Pathol. *33*:499, 1957.

227. Green, R.C., Jr., Baggenstoss, A.H., Sprague, R.G.: Diabetes mellitus in association with primary carcinoma of the pancreas. Diabetes *7*:308, 1958.

228. Hertig, A.T., Sommers, S.C.: Genesis of endometrial carcinoma. I. Study of prior biopsies. Cancer *2*:946, 1949.

229. F.J. Service (Ed.): Hypoglycemic Disorders. Boston, G.K. Hall Medical Publishers, 1983.

230. D. Andreani, P. Lefebvre, V. Marks (Eds.): Hypoglycemia. Proceedings of the European Symposium, Rome. Stuttgart, Georg Thieme Publishers, 1976.

231. V. Marks, F.C. Rose (Eds.): Hypoglycemia, 2nd Ed. Oxford, Blackwell Scientific Publications, 1981.

232. Howard, J.M., Moss, N.H., Rhoads, J.E.: Hyperinsulinism and islet cell tumors of the pancreas. With 398 recorded tumors. Int. Abstracts Surg. *90*:417, 1950.

233. Stefanini, P., Carboni, M., Patrassi, N., et al.: Beta-islet cell tumors of the pancreas: results of a study on 1,067 cases. Surgery *75*:597, 1974.

234. Larsson, L.-I., Grimelius, L., Häkonson, R., et al.: Mixed endocrine pancreatic tumors producing several peptide hormones. Am. J. Pathol. *79*:271, 1975.

235. Heitz, P., Kasper, M., Polak, J.M., Klöppel, G.: Pancreatic endocrine tumors: Immunocytochemical analysis of 125 tumors. Human Pathol. *13*:263, 1982.

236. Mukai, K., Grotting, J.C., Grider, M.H., Rosai, J.: Retrospective study of 77 pancreatic endocrine tumors using the immunoperoxidase method. Am. J. Surg. Pathol. *6*:387, 1982.

237. Steinke, J., Soeldner, J.S., Renold, A.E.: Measurement of small quantities of insulin-like activity with rat adipose tissue. IV. Serum insulin-like activity and tumor insulin content in patients with functioning islet-cell tumors. J. Clin. Invest. *42*:1322, 1963.

238. Gittler, R.D., Zucker, G., Eisinger, R., Stoller, N.: Ame-

lioration of diabetes mellitus by an insulinoma. N. Engl. J. Med. *258*:932, 1958.

239. Kahn, C.R.: The riddle of tumour hypoglycemia revisited. Clin. Endocrinol. Metab. *91*:335, 1980.

240. Laurent, J., Debry, G., Floquet, J.: Hypoglycaemic Tumours. Amsterdam, Excerpta Medica, 1971.

241. Steinke, J., Soeldner, J.S., Renold, A.E.: Insulin-like activity of extracts from large sarcomatous tumors associated with hypoglycemia. J. Clin. Invest. *41*:1403, 1962.

242. Field, J.B., Keen, H., Johnson, P., Herring, B.: Insulin-like activity of nonpancreatic tumors associated with hypoglycemia. J. Clin. Endocrinol. *23*:1229, 1963.

243. Unger, R.H.: The riddle of tumor hypoglycemia. (Editorial). Am. J. Med. *40*:325, 1966.

244. Sommers, S.C., Gould, V.E.: Endocrine activities of tumors (ectopic hormones). In: J.M.B. Bloodworth, Jr. (Ed.): Endocrine Pathology, General and Surgical, 2nd Ed. Baltimore, Williams & Wilkins Co., 1982, pp. 221–243.

245. Sheehan, H.L., Sommers, V.K.: The syndrome of hypopituitarism. Q.J. Med. *18*:319, 1949.

246. Haworth, J.C., Coodin, F.J.: Idiopathic spontaneous hypoglycemia in children. Report of seven cases and review of the literature. Pediatrics *25*:748, 1960.

247. Rosenbloom, A.L., Sherman, L.: The natural history of idiopathic hypoglycemia of infancy and its relation to diabetes mellitus. N. Engl. J. Med. *274*:815, 1966.

248. Cochran, W.A., Payne, W.W., Simpkiss, M.J., Woolf, L.I.: Familial hypoglycemia precipitated by amino acids. J. Clin. Invest. *35*:411, 1956.

249. Baker, A.B.: Cerebral damage in hypoglycemia. Am. J. Psychiatr. *96*:109, 1939.

250. Lawrence, R.D., Meyer, A., Nevin, S.: The pathological changes in the brain in fatal hypoglycemia. Q. J. Med. *11*:181, 1942.

251. Hoff, E.C., Grenell, R.G., Fulton, J.F.: Histopathology of the central nervous system after exposure to high altitudes, hypoglycemia and other conditions associated with central anoxia. Medicine *24*:161, 1945.

15 Diagnosis and Classification of Diabetes Mellitus and the Nondiabetic Meliturias

Alexander Marble and B. Dan Ferguson

In recent decades, the results of studies both in the clinic and laboratory have demonstrated amply that the complex condition of diabetes mellitus is heterogeneous in cause and type.[1] Over the years this has led to a consideration of classification by groups of knowledgeable workers with the goal of developing an international agreement as to diagnostic procedures, criteria, and terminology. In the past there has been great variation in each of these areas despite repeated efforts to reach a consensus.

For some years, the World Health Organization (WHO) has had an "Expert Committee on Diabetes Mellitus" which in 1965 published a report which contained a classification of patients according to age of recognized onset.[2] At about this time, other organizations showed renewed interest in devising procedures that might be generally acceptable. In 1968, the Committee on Statistics of the American Diabetes Association made recommendations regarding the preparation of the patient for the oral glucose tolerance test (OGT), size of glucose load, etc.[2a] Diagnostic procedures in common usage and recognized as workable included: (1) the U.S. Public Health Service point method;[2b] (2) the widely used Fajans-Conn procedure;[2c] and the summation of fasting, 1, 2, and 3-hour plasma glucose values.[2a] Continuing its interest in this nagging problem, the Committee published in 1972 a call for criticisms and suggestions as to criteria of diagnosis and classification.[2d] Meanwhile, for some years workers in Europe, especially in the United Kingdom, continued to be concerned about differences of opinion with regard to classifying persons with impairment of glucose tolerance as found in population surveys. They sought a cut-off point above which the diagnosis of diabetes mellitus would be made and below which the specific diagnosis of impaired glucose tolerance (IGT) would apply. Over periods of 5 to 10 years or more, long-term longitudinal surveys were conducted in England to determine the relative risk of the later development of vascular and neurologic disease, particularly in those persons whose impaired glucose tolerance appeared to be in a borderline area between diabetes and IGT.

Among groups discussing the overall problem in 1978 were the European Society for the Study of Diabetes (EASD), meeting in Zagreb, Yugoslavia, and an International Work Group, convened in April at Bethesda, Maryland, under the sponsorship of the National Diabetes Data Group (NDDG) of the National Institutes of Health. The objective was to develop classification and diagnostic criteria which would reflect current knowledge regarding diabetes and, over time, reach an international agreement on terminology. Detailed reports were published in 1979 by the NDDG[3] and a somewhat different, abbreviated version in 1980 by the WHO Expert Committee[4] (Table 15–1).

RECOMMENDATIONS OF THE NATIONAL DIABETES DATA GROUP AND THE WORLD HEALTH ORGANIZATION

The recommendations of the NDDG, WHO, and EASD and the approval of the Australian Diabetes Society, and American Diabetes Association are meant to be tentative and subject to change with experience in their use and with increase in knowledge during the coming years. As Keen et al. stated in publishing the EASD suggestions regarding diagnostic standards, ''The numbers are neither sacrosanct nor eternal, but are for discussion.''[5] Constructive criticism such as that of O'Sullivan and Fajans[6] and Köbberling and Creutzfeldt[7] is desirable.

In the text which follows, a summary of the proposals will be presented and following that, the diagnostic procedures and criteria which are currently used at the Joslin Clinic. These are, of course, subject to modification.

Table 15–1. Proposed Classification of Diabetes Mellitus and Other Degrees of Glucose Intolerance

I. Clinical types

   1. Diabetes mellitus
       A. Type 1. Insulin-dependent
       B. Type 2. Noninsulin-dependent
           a. Nonobese
           b. Obese
       C. Other types including diabetes mellitus associated with certain conditions and syndromes:
           a. Pancreatic disease
           b. Disease of hormonal etiology
           c. Drug- or chemical-induced conditions
           d. Insulin receptor abnormalities
           e. Certain genetic syndromes
           f. Miscellaneous

   2. Impaired glucose tolerance
       A. Nonobese
       B. Obese
       C. Impaired glucose tolerance associated with certain condtions and syndromes

   3. Gestational diabetes

II. Normal glucose tolerance but substantially increased risk of developing diabetes

   1. Previous abnormality of glucose tolerance (formerly ''latent'' diabetes)
   2. Potential abnormality of glucose tolerance (formerly ''prediabetes'')

Adapted from 1980 report of the WHO Expert Committee[4]

Diagnostic Procedures and Criteria

Members of the NDDG recommended that the oral glucose tolerance test be standardized by using in adults 75 g of glucose and in children, 1.75 g/kg of body weight (up to a maximum of 75 g) given in water in a concentration no greater than 25 g/dl and drunk in about 5 minutes. The 75 g glucose load represents a compromise between the 100 g commonly used in the U.S.A. and 50 g given in certain other countries. The test is to be done after a fast of 10 to 16 hours following at least 3 days of a diet providing not less than 150 g of carbohydrate a day. The beginning of the drink is to be considered as zero time, blood samples are to be collected at 30-minute intervals for 2 hours, and glucose determined by a specific enzymatic method. In Table 15–2, adapted from the 1980 report of the WHO Expert Committee, are shown the values recommended for the diagnosis of diabetes mellitus and of ''impaired glucose tolerance'' in nonpregnant adults. Somewhat differing procedures were recommended for children and for women with gestational diabetes.

Diabetes in Childhood. The proposed diagnostic criteria for diabetes in children are the same as for nonpregnant adults. Those for impaired glucose tolerance are expressed somewhat differently and so are reprinted here in Table 15–3.[4] The 2-hour value as determined in capillary whole blood appears here as 140 mg/dl rather than 120 mg/dl.

In this connection, the report states that the diagnosis of diabetes in children may be made without a glucose tolerance test if classic symptoms are present together with a random plasma glucose greater than 200 mg/dl. Furthermore, diabetes may be considered present in asymptomatic children if during the oral glucose tolerance test both an elevated fasting and post-glucose values are obtained on more than one occasion.

As for the diagnosis of impaired glucose tolerance, two criteria must be met: The fasting blood glucose must be below the value that is diagnostic of diabetes and the value at 2 hours must be elevated.

It is emphasized that there should be a clear indication for performing a tolerance test in children without symptoms and without glycosuria. Exceptions might include those with diabetes in first degree relatives and, above all, the nondiabetic (as yet) member of an identical twin set of whom one has diabetes. In such special patients, yearly testing is indicated with blood drawn not only for glucose content but also for tests of islet cell antibodies, and serum should be kept frozen for future tests.[7a] If a tolerance test is carried out, emphasis

Table 15–2. Diagnostic Criteria for the Oral Glucose Tolerance Test in Non-Pregnant Adults* as Proposed by the National Diabetes Data Group[3]

	Glucose Concentration		
	Venous whole blood	Capillary whole blood	Venous plasma
Diabetes Mellitus			
A. Fasting	≥120 mg/dl (6.7 mmol/L)	≥120 mg/dl (6.7 mmol/L)	≥140 mg/dl (7.8 mmol/L)
B. 2 hours after glucose load†	≥180 mg/dl (10.0 mmol/L)	≥200 mg/dl (11.1 mmol/L)	≥200 mg/dl (11.1 mmol/L)
Impaired Glucose Tolerance (IGF)‡			
A. Fasting	<120 mg/dl (6.7 mmol/L)	<120 mg/dl (6.7 mmol/L)	<140 mg/dl (7.8 mmol/L)
B. ½, 1, or 1½ hrs after glucose load	≥180 mg/dl (10.0 mmol/L)	≥200 mg/dl (11.1 mmol/L)	≥200 mg/dl (11.1 mmol/L)
C. 2 hrs after glucose load	>120 but <180 mg/dl (>6.7 but <10.0 mmol/L)	>140 but <200 mg/dl (>7.8 but <11.1 mmol/L)	>140 but <200 mg/dl (>7.8 but <11.1 mmol/L)

Note: By dividing by 18, or multiplying by 0.055, values expressed in mg/dl may be converted to mmol/L. For ease of use, values are "rounded" to some degree.
*Glucose tolerance test is unnecessary in the presence of classic symptoms of diabetes mellitus together with unequivocal elevation on more than one occasion, of the plasma glucose equal to, or higher than, the above-cited values.
†Criteria apply also to any value obtained between fasting and 2 hours after glucose load.
‡For the diagnosis of IGT, the criteria in each of the three time intervals lists must be met.

Table 15–3. Diagnostic Criteria for Impaired Glucose Tolerance (IGT) in Children as Proposed by the National Diabetes Data Group*

	Glucose Concentration		
	Venous whole blood	Capillary whole blood	Venous plasma
A. Fasting	<120 mg/dl (6.7 mmol/L)	<120 mg/dl (6.7 mmol/L)	<140 mg/dl (7.8 mmol/L)
B. 2 hours after glucose load	>120 mg/dl (6.7 mmol/L)	>140 mg/dl (7.8 mmol/L)	>140 mg/dl (7.8 mmol/L)

*Two criteria must be met: the fasting glucose concentration must be below the value that is diagnostic of diabetes, and the glucose concentration 2 hours after an oral glucose challenge must be elevated.
Note: Criteria for diagnosis of overt diabetes are considered to be the same as for non-pregnant adults (see text).

is placed on the fasting value as a criterion for impaired glucose tolerance.

Classification

For many years, certain terms for the classes of diabetes have been in general use. Recognized for decades have been two main types of overt diabetes, namely that which has its onset chiefly in children, adolescents, and young adults in whom symptoms are severe and the overall course aggressive. Prior to the availability of insulin, such patients lived only weeks, months, or at most a few years after onset. In recent times, this has been spoken of as juvenile, growth-onset, or juvenile-onset type of diabetes. The other variety, which includes by far the greater proportion of diabetic patients, often has an insidious onset with relatively few or no symptoms, a much greater tendency to obesity, and is usually controllable by a restricted diet. Occurring chiefly in older persons, it has been called maturity-onset or maturity-onset type of diabetes.

These two groups are not clear-cut, however. A certain fraction, perhaps 15 to 20%, of persons with onset of diabetes after the age of 40 or 45 are either insulin-dependent or require treatment with insulin to allow an intake of food adequate to maintain satisfactory weight and strength. Furthermore, as pointed out by Tattersall and Fajans,[8] a small number, perhaps 5%, of people with onset of diabetes under the age of 30 have the less aggressive, adult-onset type of diabetes (Maturity Onset Diabetes in the Young or MODY). Finally, there are various other conditions with impaired glucose tolerance. In the following discussion the classification proposed by WHO and NDDG is made not according to age at onset or present age, but rather according to the type of diabetes. Certain insulin-taking persons may not be truly insulin-dependent.

Type I, Insulin-Dependent Diabetes Mellitus (IDDM). Patients with this type usually have a relatively abrupt onset of classic symptoms, insulinopenia which may become total or nearly total after some months or years, proneness to ketoacidosis, and aggressive character with dependence upon exogenous insulin for maintenance of health and of life itself. The onset is usually in childhood, adolescence, and young adult life, but as noted above, may occur later in life. Persons with Type I diabetes may have circulating islet-cell antibodies early in the course of the disease and, indeed, they may be present months or years prior to the appearance of glucose intolerance.[9] Autoimmunity may play a role. Certain histocompatibility antigens (HLA) on chromosome 6 may be present. This type of diabetes appears to be heterogeneous as to hereditary and environmental factors; as regards the latter, viral infections have been incriminated but not conclusively proved (see Chapters 2 and 4).

Type II, Non-insulin-Dependent Diabetes (NIDDM). This type often has an insidious onset with few or no classic symptoms of diabetes. In contrast to Type I, patients of this type are not dependent upon exogenous insulin for survival. Although the vast majority of patients develop the disease after the age of 45, as mentioned earlier, it may occur in adolescence or young adult life.[8] Patients with NIDDM do not develop ketoacidosis except under conditions of unusual stress such as febrile infections or following trauma. Plasma insulin levels may be normal, slightly or moderately below normal, or even increased in the presence of obesity or other complications in which insulin resistance may be a feature. They develop retinopathy and nephropathy although, taking all such patients into consideration, not to the degree that those with Type I do. They are prone to macroangiopathy of coronary, peripheral vascular, and cerebral types occurring at a frequency of 2 to 3 times that in the nondiabetic person. Patients with NIDDM may be divided into those who are *obese* (20% or more above ideal weight) or *non-obese;* the majority are obese. Hyperglycemia and glucose tolerance are improved by loss of weight and maintenance at the lower level attained. In persons with Type II diabetes, including those of the MODY group,[8] no characteristic pattern of HLA types has been noted; islet cell antibodies have not been demonstrated. Studies in identical twins indicate a much higher degree of concordance (95 + %) than in twin sets in which the onset of diabetes in the index twin is under the age of 40 years (about 40%), suggesting a stronger influence of heredity.[10]

Secondary Diabetes. Although the majority of patients seeking care from the physician will fall into one or the other of the main types of diabetes described above, diabetes forms a part of other conditions and syndromes of which certain examples are given below. For an elaboration of these, see the NDDG report[3] and the book edited by Podolsky and Viswanathan.[11]

Diseases of the Pancreas. These include transient diabetes of the newborn, surgical removal of more than nine tenths of the pancreas, pancreatitis, pancreatic calculi with fibrosis, cystic fibrosis, cancer of the pancreas, hemochromatosis, and toxic damage to the pancreas.

Hormonal Overactivity. In a wide variety of disturbances of endocrine organs, hyperglycemia may occur and require treatment. If the condition of the endocrine gland is one of hyperactivity and if appropriate treatment is possible against that, the diabetes may be cured. Instances of such over-activity include pheochromocytoma, acromegaly, Cushing's syndrome, glucagonoma, somatostatinoma, and aldosteronoma as well as medications such as somatotropin, glucocorticoids, progestins and estrogens (oral contraceptives), growth hormone, glucagon, epinephrine, etc.

Drug or Chemically Induced Conditions. An extremely wide variety of drugs and chemical agents may elevate the blood glucose or exacerbate an already established hyperglycemia. In most instances the chemical agents used as medicines have only a slight effect, but the more potent include the thiazides, diazoxide, and streptozotocin as well as some hormonally active agents listed in the preceding paragraph.

Insulin Receptor Abnormalities. These abnormalities include a defect in the receptor, congenital lipodystrophy, acanthosis nigricans associated with virilization, and antibodies to insulin receptor-associated immune disorders.

Genetic Syndromes. These consist of various conditions most of which are seen uncommonly by the average practitioner and which rarely cause difficulty in diagnosis and treatment, insofar as hyperglycemia is concerned. These include certain inborn errors of metabolism, insulin resistant syndromes, hereditary neuromuscular disorders, progeroid syndrome, syndromes with glucose intolerance secondary to obesity, cytogenetic disorders, and a miscellaneous group. For a complete listing of the conditions mentioned, see Chapters 24 and 42.

Impaired Glucose Tolerance (IGT). This diagnosis is suggested for those patients in whom the fasting plasma glucose level is lower than that required for the diagnosis of diabetes but in whom, during an oral glucose tolerance test, the 2-hour value lies between the normal and diabetic values ($\geq$ 140 and < 200 mg/dl) (See Table 15–2). Those who took part in the National Diabetes Data Group formulation of the proposed new classification had in mind that persons in this status would not receive the diagnosis of diabetes mellitus but would be put in this class because they are regarded at higher risk for the development of diabetes than persons in the general population. It was anticipated that only 1 to 5% of individuals with IGT would later progress to overt clinical diabetes per year, and that many might return to normal glucose tolerance spontaneously. Within the overall IGT class are those who are nonobese, obese, or who have certain associated conditions and syndromes such as those outlined above in the discussion of diabetes mellitus.

It is evident that most persons to be placed in the IGT class have in the past, and indeed in the present, been given by most clinicians the designation of chemical diabetes, glucose tolerance diabetes, borderline diabetes, or simply diabetes. The proponents of the new terminology give as the reason for their stand that the diagnosis of "diabetes" may well carry with it a stigma which will prevent the individual from getting or holding a job or from obtaining life insurance. To us, these arguments lack full validity. Many of the IGT results are found in older persons who are either employed already or have retired and, in any case, a letter or statement from a physician should serve to document the benign character of the condition. As for life insurance, when a company requires a glucose tolerance test, it is the company which makes the decision as to insurability according to its established standards. Finally, individuals with IGT need to be followed by longitudinal testing for not only 5, 10, or 20 years, but for as long as possible, depending upon the age of the person (and of the clinician or researcher!) at the time of the initial observation. Otherwise, statistics as to progression or nonprogression to overt diabetes or the development of one or more manifestations of diabetic micro- or macro-angiopathy are of limited value. Furthermore, an ideal study should comprise truly large numbers of people.

Early steps in this direction have been taken by O'Sullivan and Mahan as a result of the Oxford, Mass., survey;[12] in the United Kingdom in the Bedford,[13] Birmingham,[14] and Whitehall[15] studies; and in Denmark by Agner et al.[16] The results so far have in general shown that over a period of 10 to 17 years, definite, though relatively small, percentage of persons with "borderline" diabetes have a worsening of glucose tolerance and development of characteristic complications. On the other hand, in some persons there is improvement. In the Danish study, if IGT was present at age 70, the incidence of worsening to diabetes by age 80 years was 20%, whereas in control subjects, this

incidence was only 4% when normal glucose tolerance had been found at age 70. Obviously, the results of all investigations of the sort discussed in this paragraph are influenced greatly by the diagnostic standards used and the known variability of results of periodic glucose tolerance tests in the same individual with borderline values.[17]

Gestational Diabetes. This class is restricted to pregnant women in whom the onset or diagnosis of diabetes or impaired glucose tolerance occurs during pregnancy. Women known to be diabetic who become pregnant are not included. Following the termination of pregnancy, further studies must be carried out for purposes of re-classification.

The National Diabetes Data Group recommended that diagnostic procedures be modified somewhat in the case of pregnant women, following the methods and criteria suggested by O'Sullivan and Mahan[18] on the basis of their extensive long-term longitudinal study (Table 15–4). These workers gave 100 g of glucose in water, carried out the test for 3 hours, and used only whole venous blood for glucose determinations. Values for plasma and whole capillary blood were added by the National Diabetes Data Group and published in its report.[3] However, the figures listed in Table 15–4 are the published values of O'Sullivan and Mahan[18] for venous whole blood. Those for plasma and capillary blood were estimated by the writer and regarded as acceptable by O'Sullivan in personal communication.

Other Classes. *Previous Abnormality of Glucose Tolerance.* This designation has been suggested for those individuals who at the time of study have normal glucose tolerance but who in the past have had hyperglycemia due to diabetes or impaired glucose tolerance either spontaneously or in response to an identifiable stimulus. The term "latent" diabetes has in the past often been given to this group. Individuals assigned here would include: those shown to have gestational diabetes but following termination of pregnancy, have had normal results; erstwhile obese diabetics whose glucose tolerance has become normal after weight loss; transient hyperglycemia during myocardial infarction, trauma, infections, etc.

Potential Abnormality of Glucose Tolerance. This statistical risk group was designed to include persons who have never shown glucose intolerance but who are considered on the basis of general experience to be at greater risk than others in the population for the later development of either overt diabetes or impaired glucose tolerance. This category includes the monozygotic twin of a NIDDM patient; a parent, offspring, or sibling of a person with diabetes; obese persons, especially if close family members have diabetes; mothers of children

Table 15–4. Diagnostic Criteria for the Oral Glucose Tolerance Test in Gestational Diabetes* as Used by O'Sullivan and Mahan[11] for Venous Whole Blood (Values for Capillary and Venous Plasma Were Added by the Authors)

	Glucose Concentration†		
	Venous whole blood*	Capillary whole blood	Venous plasma
Fasting	90 mg/dl (5.0 mmol/L)	90 mg/dl (5.0 mmol/L)	105 mg/dl (5.8 mmol/L)
1 hour after glucose load	165mg/dl (9.2 mmol/L)	195 mg/dl (10.8 mmol/L)	190 mg/dl (10.6 mmol/L)
2 hours after glucose load	145 mg/dl (8.1 mmol/L)	165 mg/dl (9.2 mmol/L)	165 mg/dl (9.2 mmol/L)
3 hours after glucose load	125 mg/dl (7.0 mmol/L)	125 mg/dl (7.0 mmol/L)	145 mg/dl (8.1 mmol/L)

*Two or more of the above values must be met or exceeded following a 100 g glucose challenge.
†Values in this table are not those which appear in the report of the NDDG.[3] Those for venous whole blood appear in the article by O'Sullivan and Mahan.[11] Those for capillary whole blood and venous plasma have been supplied by the authors and approved by O'Sullivan (personal communication).

with a birth weight of 4 kg (9 lb) or more; and members of racial or ethnic groups who have been shown by studies to have a high prevalence of diabetes such as certain American Indian tribes.[18a]

Final Comment

The response of "diabetologists" the world over has in general been favorable to the proposed classification of diabetes and related conditions. The terms proposed are now in common usage. There are, and probably will continue to be, questions especially regarding borderline situations. Examples are (1) the difficulty in classifying the patient who needs insulin for good glycemic control but who, in the pre-insulin era, would have survived for years without succumbing to ketoacidosis (Someone has said facetiously that we need a Type I½); (2) the area between Type II diabetes and IGT—many believe that the criteria for inclusion of this area in the designation of Type II should be less strict; and (3) related to these matters is the criticism of Massari et al.[18b] who studied the results of oral glucose tolerance tests of 543 asymptomatic subjects. Massari et al. attempted to classify their findings according to WHO and NDDG standards, plus seven other published criteria. They interpreted their results as indicating "imprecision" when the proposed "new" criteria were applied; consequently, large percentages of the results were classified as "non-diagnostic" or otherwise "not classifiable." Their paper drew responses from Jarrett and Alberti[18c]; the latter defended strongly the WHO criteria.

Aside from terminology, there will undoubtedly continue to be disagreement, especially as regards borderline segments of the very large group of persons with IGT. Such disagreement will affect the epidemiologist doing population surveys much more than the clinician. Certainly after a period of trial of the proposed classification, the details should again be reviewed by an international study group about 10 years after the original publications.

JOSLIN CLINIC DIAGNOSTIC PROCEDURES

Although the diagnostic methods and standards proposed by the National Diabetes Data Group appear in general to be reasonable, those used currently at the Joslin Clinic differ to some extent; they are outlined stepwise below.

1. Determination of the amount of glucose in urine and blood in specimens obtained at random. Non-fasting values between 130 and 160 ($\geq$130-<160) mg/dl for venous whole blood or $\geq$150-<180 mg/dl for serum or plasma are considered suggestive but not definitive for diabetes.

2. If the results obtained on random samples are not conclusive, then the simplest procedure is to determine the amount of glucose in blood obtained 1 hour after food or glucose. If a meal is used, it should contain a liberal amount of carbohydrate including bread, potato, fruit, and a sweet dessert. In lieu of a meal, a modified oral glucose tolerance test may be carried out, regardless of the time of day, by giving 50 g of glucose in 250 ml of water and obtaining blood and urine samples 1 hour later. A whole blood glucose value of 160 mg/dl (plasma glucose 180 mg/dl) or higher is considered diagnostic of diabetes or impaired glucose tolerance subject to confirmation by other determinations.

3. If the results of both of these procedures are not conclusive, a formal glucose tolerance test is performed. It must be emphasized, however, that it is not logical to carry out such a test if levels of blood glucose already obtained have been definitely

JOSLIN'S DIABETES MELLITUS

diagnostic. Glucose tolerance tests may be carried out in one of three ways: (a) oral test; (b) intravenous test; and (c) steroid-primed oral test. The first two procedures are standard whereas the third remains confined to clinical research.

The results of any glucose tolerance test must be interpreted in terms of complications which might influence them. These include liver disease, thyrotoxicosis, pituitary or adrenal dysfunction, infections, especially if accompanied by fever, and subtotal gastrectomy. In most of these conditions, glucose tolerance is affected adversely. The effect of age, previous diet, physical activity, and other factors will be discussed later. For a more detailed and well-documented presentation, see the monograph by West.[19]

Oral Glucose Tolerance Test

After at least 3 days of an unrestricted diet or one containing at least 200 g of carbohydrate a day, the patient reports after an overnight fast of 10–12 hours. Smoking is not permitted. To be noted, however, is that Walsh et al.[20] concluded from their studies that cigarette smoking did not affect the blood glucose of habitual smokers. Water may be taken but other beverages (coffee, tea, etc.) are not allowed. Blood and urine specimens are obtained and the patient's height, weight, and body temperature are determined and recorded. If the patient has fever, the test is deferred until another time. Glucose is then given in the form of a sweetened drink. To adult patients, we give 100 g, preferably in a 20 to 25% solution in water. Since some patients may have difficulty in taking 400 to 500 ml of sweetened water, 200 ml of chilled 50% solution of glucose flavored with lemon juice and followed by 200 ml of plain water may be substituted. One may use a commercially prepared glucose solution, such as Dextol* (100 g glucose in 300 ml of water with a lemon-lime flavor) or similar flavored preparations (100 g glucose) such as Koladex.† Although the amount of glucose may be varied by giving 1.75 g/kg body weight, the standard dose of 100 g is simpler, works well, and has the advantage of the availability in the literature of a wealth of data obtained with this amount. For children and those weighing less than 100 lb (45 kg), 1 g/lb (or 1.75 g/kg) of body weight may be given (up to 100 g). Blood and urine samples are taken at ½, 1, 2, and 3 hours after the taking of glucose. As stated above, blood taken from a vein is preferable for diagnostic purposes. Capillary

blood may be necessary for small and fearful children, but if so, an effort should be made to take at least the 1- and 2-hour samples from a vein, since following glucose the capillary-venous difference is variable.

The diagnostic standards currently used by the Joslin Clinic are shown in Table 15–5. They are in general the same as those of Fajans and Conn.[21] In addition to a peak value of 160 mg/dl or higher, another abnormal value is required for diagnosis. Variations of the standard technique described above have been suggested and used. Many workers omit the taking of blood at the ½-hour interval and others take samples at 1½ or 2½ hours after glucose.

In Table 15–6 are shown the diagnostic criteria suggested by the United States Public Health Service[22] for use in glucose tolerance tests.

Rarely used now is the 1-hour, two-dose glucose tolerance test introduced by Exton and Rose.[23] It never won general acceptance and has been largely abandoned because it offers few or no advantages and has some disadvantages over the standard test.

If the oral glucose tolerance test gives equivocal, borderline, or inconsistent results, it should be re-

Table 15–5. Diagnostic Criteria for Diabetes Currently in Use at the Joslin Clinic Standard Oral Glucose Tolerance Test

Time	Blood Glucose Concentration in mg/dl		
	Venous whole blood	Capillary whole blood	Venous plasma
Fasting	110	110	125
Hours after 100 g glucose:			
One	160	180–200	180
Two	120	140–160	140
Three	110	110	125

To indicate diabetes, at least two values must equal or exceed the above.

Table 15–6. Diagnostic Criteria for Standard Oral Glucose Tolerance Test as Suggested by U.S. Public Health Service[22] (Venous Whole Blood)

Time	Diagnostic Values Blood Glucose in mg/100 ml	Points Allotted*
Fasting	110	1
Hours after glucose		
One	170	½
Two	120	½
Three	110	1

*The total of 2 points required for diagnosis is obtained when any 3 or more of the above values, or when the fasting and 3-hour combination, are met or exceeded.

*Scientific Products Division of American Hospital Supply Corporation, McGaw Park, Illinois, 60085.
†Custom Laboratories, Inc., Baltimore, Maryland, 21223.

peated, but not before at least a week has elapsed. If the test gives normal values and yet melituria persists, steps should be taken to identify the type of sugar excreted and the relationship to glycemia, as discussed later in this chapter.

Test Meals

A test meal of mixed nutrients would appear on first thought to be a good substitute for glucose in a tolerance test. It is more palatable and provides a stimulus to insulin response which is more familiar to the body. For rough testing it is, indeed, satisfactory, particularly if conclusive results are obtained. Usually blood glucose values are somewhat higher after glucose than after a comparable amount of carbohydrate in a test meal. Disadvantages include the difficulty in standardizing the composition of the meal as actually eaten and the relative paucity of values recorded in the literature.

Intravenous Glucose Tolerance Test

Although the standard oral glucose tolerance test is the most convenient one for routine use, at times determination of tolerance after an intravenous injection of glucose is desirable. This type of test is useful, particularly when the rate of absorption of glucose is disturbed by conditions such as thyrotoxicosis and postgastrectomy states, which favor rapid absorption, and hypothyroidism and malabsorption syndromes, in which absorption is slowed. Indeed there are those who regard the intravenous method as the one of choice in all situations. Apart from the conditions just named, however, the oral test would seem to be more physiologic since the sugar is presented to the body by a normal route and since there is opportunity for normal stimulation of insulin secretion by enzymes released from the upper bowel in response to food. In general, the oral test is more sensitive than the intravenous one.

The intravenous glucose tolerance test is performed by various methods. The one used in the Elliott P. Joslin Research Laboratory is described below.

Glucose in dosage of 0.5 g/kg of body weight is injected intravenously as a 25% solution within 1 to 3 minutes. Blood is collected every 10 minutes for 1 hour thereafter. Under these conditions, the level of blood glucose decreases from its height in an exponential manner and the glucose disappearance rate is calculated by the use of the formula: disappearance rate = $70 \div t\frac{1}{2}$ where $t\frac{1}{2}$ is the number of minutes required for the blood glucose to fall 50% from its level at 10 minutes. Normally, the rate (Kg value) exceeds 1.2% per

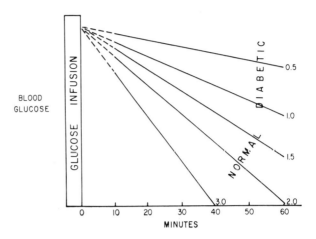

Fig. 15–1. Diagrammatic curves of blood glucose fall after administration of glucose intravenously during a tolerance test. The ranges for normal and diabetic responses are indicated.

minute. Values below 1% definitely indicate diabetes; those between 1.2 and 1.0 are regarded as borderline (Fig. 15–1).

FACTORS INFLUENCING RESULTS OF THE GLUCOSE TOLERANCE TEST

Many factors influence the outcome of glucose tolerance tests. Some of these warrant more detailed discussion. For extensive documentation, see the monograph by West.[19]

1. Previous Diet. Normal persons or animals who for long periods have fasted or have been kept on low carbohydrate diets may exhibit a diabetic type of response when challenged with a glucose load. In clinical work, preparation for the test should include a diet liberal in carbohydrate (200 to 300 g daily) including sweets and pastry for the 3 days just prior to the test. Although some evidence suggests that valid results may be expected if the individual has been taking as little as 125 g of carbohydrate daily together with adequate amounts of protein and calories,[24] a larger amount of at least 200 g per day is preferable.

2. Insulin and Oral Hypoglycemic Agents. In both people and animals, administration of insulin during the days just preceding a glucose tolerance test has been shown to cause a temporary decrease in glucose tolerance. Consequently, no such test for diagnostic purposes should be carried out unless the subject has received no insulin for a definite period of time, arbitrarily for 3 days for regular insulin and a week for insulin of intermediate or prolonged action. The same general principle applies to the previous administration of oral hypoglycemic agents. Should the oral agent be chlorpropamide (Diabinese), the interval should probably be even longer because of the long-continued action of this drug.

3. Physical Inactivity. Prolonged physical inactivity decreases carbohydrate tolerance. Consequently, the results of tolerance tests in elderly, bedridden patients are apt to show an unusually high percentage of abnormal results.

4. Infections. The deleterious effect of infections on diabetes is well known, especially those accompanied by fever. Glucose tolerance tests should not be performed for diagnostic purposes in persons who have signs or symptoms of an infection or who, on routine examination, have an elevation in body temperature. As a standard procedure, the body temperature should be measured and recorded at the beginning and end of each test.

5. Diseases and Abnormal States Other than Diabetes. The routine performance of glucose tolerance tests in certain segments of the population has long been a favorite project for clinical investigation. Consequently, the literature is replete with articles giving the results of studies carried out with persons of all types, ages, and diseases. In supposedly nondiabetic subjects with obesity, hyperthyroidism, acromegaly, hypertension, pregnancy, cancer, chronic neurologic diseases, cerebrovascular accidents, acute myocardial infarction, or various other conditions, a high percentage of abnormal results is commonly found. To attempt to analyze and discuss these findings in detail would not be profitable here, especially since the results obtained in any study must be viewed in the light of the effect of basic, nonspecific, modifying factors which have been mentioned, i.e., age, state of nutrition, physical activity, drugs taken previously, and previous diet. To all of these factors must be added the possibility of an underlying hereditary predisposition to reduced carbohydrate tolerance.

6. Drugs. A variety of drugs are known to decrease glucose tolerance and should be avoided at least 3 days before the test. These include benzothiadiazines, nicotinic acid, salicylates, steroids, and oral contraceptive agents (the last-named should be omitted for one cycle prior to the test).

7. Time of Day. The general consensus is that the glycemic response to glucose given orally is substantially higher in the afternoon than in the forenoon.[25] However, this diurnal variation has not been observed under all conditions. At any rate, in comparing the results of forenoon and afternoon tests, one must keep in mind such items as the length of the period of fasting prior to the test, the amount of glucose administered, and other factors which affect carbohydrate tolerance.

8. Age. The influence of the age of patients on sugar tolerance has long been recognized. Toler-

ance has been generally accepted to decrease as age advances. Interest in this subject has become heightened in the last 3 or 4 decades because of the results obtained on the routine testing of the population on a large-scale basis with consequent difficulty in interpreting the data. The conclusions reached have varied according to the conditions of study and the diagnostic criteria used, but the general truth has emerged that, in supposedly nondiabetic persons over the age of 50 years, the number of those with results in a range commonly accepted as diabetic runs as high as 30 to 50%, depending upon the actual age, physical status, etc. of the special groups tested. This has led to certain basic questions: To what extent should these persons be regarded as having diabetes? If diabetes is present, is this primary (hereditary) or secondary? If secondary, to what is the decreased carbohydrate tolerance due? Is the aging process responsible for the impaired tolerance and, if so, is vascular disease affecting the insular mechanism an important factor? To what extent are obesity and relative inactivity, both common in older persons, responsible for the decreasing carbohydrate tolerance? These provocative questions cannot be answered easily or definitely.

OTHER TOLERANCE AND RESPONSE TESTS

Various theoretical possibilities suggest themselves as to the cause of the impaired glucose tolerance found in elderly persons. Among these are the following: (a) decreased or delayed secretion or release of insulin from the pancreas; (b) increasing amounts of insulin antagonists with advancing age; (c) diminished sensitivity of the tissues to insulin, due to decreased number and/or affinity of insulin receptors; (d) physical inactivity, obesity, and concomitant other disease—all common in elderly persons.

Some of these possibilities have been subjected to study. Streeten and his associates[26] found that during oral glucose tolerance tests, 10 of 13 healthy individuals over 70 years of age had values which were abnormal by commonly used standards. When the studies were extended to include an analysis of "glucose disposal rates" and serum insulin-like activity levels after the intravenous administration of glucose, however, Streeten and co-workers concluded that the decreased glucose tolerance of elderly persons is due neither to retarded absorption of glucose given orally nor to impaired pancreatic secretion of insulin. In comprehensive 5-hour glucose tolerance tests, Zeytinoglu, Gherondache, and Pincus[27] found abnormal results in 72.5% of 40 persons aged 68 to 91 years. In addition to determining serum glucose, they followed the level of serum immunoreactive insulin

(IRI). They found that although the elderly subjects responded to glucose stimulation with an increase in serum IRI levels, the response was delayed and inappropriate in those persons in whom glucose values were abnormal.

These findings reported in the 1960s are consistent with the results of more recent studies as summarized by DeFronzo in a review article.[28] He concludes that tissue unresponsiveness to insulin is the primary reason why glucose tolerance decreases with age.

For a detailed and extensive discussion of the effect of age on carbohydrate tolerance, see the monograph by West[29] published in 1978.

Tolbutamide Response Test

After the administration to a nondiabetic person of the rapidly acting sulfonylurea compound, tolbutamide, the level of blood glucose falls promptly. With this in mind, a response test was designed to serve as an indicator of the ability of the pancreas of a given subject to respond to the stimulus. Patients with well-established insulin-dependent diabetes respond little, if at all, to tolbutamide, whereas those with the stable, adult-onset type of diabetes may show a response between that of the normal subject and the insulin-dependent diabetic.

As with glucose tolerance tests, the patient should have had a diet of at least 150 to 200 g of carbohydrate for 3 days prior to the test. On the day of the test, a blood specimen is obtained in the fasting state for glucose determination. Sodium tolbutamide (1.0 g dissolved in 20 mg of sterile water) is injected intravenously at a constant rate over a period of 2 to 3 minutes. Blood specimens are drawn at 20 and 30 minutes after the midpoint of the injection, and the level of blood glucose is determined in each. After the final sample is drawn, the patient is given orange juice or other carbohydrate-containing liquid, followed by a meal.

According to the criteria of Unger and Madison,[30] if the blood glucose value at 20 minutes is greater than 89%, and that at 30 minutes is greater than 76% of the pre-injection level, diabetes is considered to be present. If the value at 20 minutes is less than 75% of the initial value, diabetes may be assumed not to be present. Percentages falling in between these values suggest probable diabetes.

The tolbutamide response test may at times offer valuable supportive or accessory information helpful in diagnosis. It is less sensitive than the oral glucose tolerance test, however, and is not recommended as the sole test to be done, although in general the results are consistent with those of glucose tolerance tests. It is now used much less than formerly.

Steroid-Primed Oral Glucose Tolerance Test

As has been mentioned earlier, this test, introduced by Fajans and Conn[21] in 1954, is not a standard one. Originally it was thought to increase the sensitivity of the standard oral test and thereby disclose individuals who have a basic tendency to diabetes, although at the time of observation, give no evidence of glucose intolerance when glucose alone is used. Overall, however, it has seemed to some workers to be no more sensitive than the standard test in which glucose alone is given. For this reason, the steroid-primed test may be used only as an investigational procedure and its value even here has been questioned.[31]

Preparation for the test is the same as for the standard oral glucose tolerance test except that cortisone acetate in a dosage of 50 mg is given orally 8½ hours and again 2 hours prior to the administration of 100 g of glucose to patients weighing 160 lb (73 kg) or less. For persons of greater weight, a dosage of 62.5 mg of cortisone acetate instead of 50 mg is used at each of the two time intervals. (Some workers have used triamcinolone instead of cortisone.[32]) When whole venous blood is used, the criteria for a positive response to the test are a 1-hour level of 160 mg/dl or more, a 1½-hour level of 150 mg/dl or more, and a 2-hour level of 140 mg/dl or more. Fajans and Conn stipulate that these criteria apply only to otherwise healthy, ambulatory, nonpregnant individuals under the age of 45 years.

EVALUATION OF TOLERANCE AND RESPONSE TESTS

In the vast majority of patients studied in clinical practice by tolerance and response tests, the outcome is straightforward and leaves no doubt as to whether diabetes is or is not present. In a significant percentage of cases, however, equivocal, borderline, or inconstant results are obtained, or the blood glucose sequence does not follow a pattern which appears sensible. Such results suggest a laboratory error or a mixing of samples. In any case in which there is doubt, the tests should be repeated after a suitable interval, preferably not until a few or several days have elapsed. Some patients will be found to have consistently borderline results and with others the degree of reproducibility of results is not satisfactory. For these, repetitions of the test at least annually is wise so as to determine the course of the disorder and to be able to apply treatment when and if it is indicated.

The physician at present sees increasingly larger

numbers of patients in their 70s or older. In such an individual in whom, by random tests, an elevated postprandial whole blood glucose value (e.g., 160 to 170 mg/dl) is found despite the lack of diabetic symptoms and despite normal fasting and 2-hour blood glucose values after food or glucose ingestion, the question arises as to management. In such a person, the diagnosis of diabetes or impaired glucose tolerance may be made, but rigid treatment need not be applied. Often all that is necessary is to prescribe omission of sweets and pastries and to limit modestly other foods which are rich in simple carbohydrate. Calories should be restricted if obesity is present. Besides these measures, keeping the patient under observation and carrying out urine and blood tests periodically for an indefinite period are important. At long intervals, a formal glucose tolerance test may be performed to determine the status of the mild disorder of metabolism. To dismiss such a patient initially as not having any noteworthy abnormality is to encourage carelessness in terms of food intake and body weight.

The diagnosis of diabetes is a major event in the life of any person affected. It must be made only after consideration of data collected by trustworthy means. At the present time, the easiest and most reliable method of diagnosing diabetes is by determination of the blood glucose and, if necessary, by tests of carbohydrate tolerance. Fortunately, there is in the medical literature a vast amount of information regarding glucose tolerance tests acquired over many decades. With most patients who consult the physician, the diagnosis can be made easily and definitely because of characteristic symptoms, presence of glycosuria, and definitely elevated concentrations of glucose in the blood. In instances in which the diagnosis is in doubt, a glucose tolerance test usually gives definitive results. There are some patients in whom findings in sugar tolerance tests are borderline, variable from one test to another, and overall, not satisfying for a definite diagnosis of either diabetes or glucose intolerance. This problem is met only occasionally in clinical practice but fairly often in field projects in which entire populations are studied by means of glucose tolerance tests. In the latter situation, this is due to the greater difficulty encountered in setting up a suitable protocol and gaining examinee compliance.

Diagnostic standards may be set so low as to lack *specificity* or so high as to lack *sensitivity*. In other words, if standards are too low, some persons may be erroneously labeled "diabetic;" if they are too high, some with diabetes may escape diagnosis. Consequently, one must attempt to effect a workable compromise. In doubtful situations, tests

should be repeated periodically so that the true condition may become evident.

Despite its widespread use in the past and present, the worth of the oral glucose tolerance test has been questioned in recent years. Siperstein[33] has called it a pitfall in the diagnosis of diabetes and suggested that it be abandoned completely. Admittedly, it has its faults but at the present time it is the best tool available and, with all its imperfections, for many years it has served the patient, the clinician, and the investigator well.

GENERAL LABORATORY PROCEDURES

Although diabetes may be suspected because of characteristic symptoms, the disease often develops insidiously, particularly in the adult. Consequently, its detection depends upon the screening of all patients and even the supposedly healthy. Large surveys throughout the world have demonstrated the relatively high frequency of diabetes in the general population, particularly in certain racial groups.

A complete urine examination and blood glucose determination should be a part of every physical survey. Specimens of urine and blood secured within 1 or 2 hours after a meal liberal in carbohydrate are desirable, because in some subjects, fasting specimens or those obtained at 3 or more hours after eating may yield results within normal limits and glucose intolerance overlooked.

The diagnosis and successful treatment of diabetes depends more upon laboratory findings than in any other common disease. In the present day, the relationship of the clinical laboratory to the physician is influenced by various factors including: (1) automation of increasing numbers of procedures; (2) the high cost of laboratory tests; (3) quality assurance programs; and (4) methods of reporting, i.e., traditional vs. molecular (Systèmes International or S.I.) units.

Examination of the Urine for Sugar and Ketones

The Volume of Urine in a 24-Hour Period. In diabetic patients, the amount of urine excreted by the kidneys in 24 hours frequently parallels the quantity of sugar eliminated in the urine, but the relationship is by no means invariably close. Indeed, at times the amount may be within a normal range even though the urine contains a significant amount of sugar.

Wide-mouthed plastic containers of 2000 ml capacity, graduated at intervals of 50 ml, have replaced the glass bottles formerly used in diabetes units of hospitals and summer camps for diabetic children. If the container in which the 24-hour urine specimen is being collected cannot be kept in a cold place, a small amount of xylene or toluene should be added as a preservative.

Sugars in "Normal" Urine. The presence of sugar in the urine of presumably normal individuals was a subject of controversy among biochemists and physicians for many years. Clarification of the character of these sugars has been aided by specific enzymatic techniques for the determination of glucose. Using such a method, Froesch, Renold, and McWilliams[34] found that in 30 normal persons, the mean 24-hour excretion of glucose in the urine was only 72 mg (range, 16 to 132 mg). This made up only about one seventh of the total reducing substance; the non-glucose remainder had a mean value of 511 mg (range, 242 to 845 mg). Froesch and associates noted that the glucose excretion of nondiabetic individuals was relatively independent of the amount of carbohydrate in the diet, although after the administration of glucocorticoids there were significant increases.

Fine[35] obtained similar results for the 24-hour secretion of glucose. In 30 adults (excluding findings in 4 persons considered to have renal glycosuria), the mean value was 65 mg (range, 31.7 to 93 mg). However, Fine maintained, on the basis of rate of excretion, that the amount of glucose in the urine is related to carbohydrate intake. In 8 persons in whom the mean value for the fasting rate of excretion was 1.6 mg/hr, at $1\frac{1}{4}$ hours after the administration of 50 g of glucose, the mean rate increased to 4 mg/hr.

Thus it is possible for the presumed normal individual to show sugar in the urine which may be measured by specific and sensitive methods. However, the amount is so small as not to be detected by the qualitative methods commonly used by patients and clinicians.

Sugar in the Urine of a Diabetic Patient. Unless facilities exist either in the hospital or home for frequent determinations of the blood glucose, a precise evaluation of the degree of control of diabetes is difficult to obtain. However, much help may be obtained by determining the total quantity of sugar excreted in the urine in 24 hours. Joslin Clinic patients in the Diabetes Treatment Unit and the boys and girls attending summer camps have a 24-hour urine collection daily to be used as one guide in planning treatment. The total volume is recorded, the percentage of sugar is determined by a rapid, convenient method, and the number of grams excreted in the total collection is calculated. An excellent refinement of this is to collect in separate containers and test the urine voided during approximately each 6 hours of the 24-hour day (forenoon, afternoon, evening, and night) thereby obtaining detailed information about the degree of glycosuria at various times of the day and night (4-period test).

The amount of sugar excreted in 24 hours by the patient with insulin-dependent diabetes should be less than 20 g and, preferably, less than 10 g. However, the insulin-dependent patient with unstable diabetes under poor control, may excrete up to 100 g of glucose per day. Often, as the treatment program is changed in the Diabetes Treatment Unit, significant reductions in the 24-hour glycosuria are documented before there is appreciable change in the random blood glucose determinations.

The semi-quantitative tests for sugar in single specimens of urine are generally considered to be an indirect measure of the blood glucose. This is true, however, only when testing the second or third specimens taken several hours after the ingestion of a meal, since the first specimen contains sugar lost in the urine during the post-prandial rise. Three hours later, the blood glucose might be falling, but this would not be reflected by the first urine specimen. Even with the second specimen after food, there are instances of widely varying blood glucose levels in the face of a negative urine glucose test. There is a better correlation between the percent of glycosuria and the blood glucose in excess of 200 mg/dl. In younger individuals in whom there may be a significant glycosuria at relatively low blood glucose levels, a third urine specimen following food may be required. At best, these are rough indications of the ambient blood glucose and at times may be misleading.

Semi-quantitative Tests for Sugar. Nearly all of these tests have the advantage, except as stated above, of producing negative reactions unless sugar exists in important amounts.

Benedict's Test. This test is reliable, inexpensive (if the solution is made in large quantities), and easy for the layman to interpret results. It requires only a single alkaline copper solution which keeps indefinitely and is not reduced by creatinine or uric acid. Furthermore, it is not affected by temperature or humidity. Formerly a mainstay in guiding treatment, today it is used relatively little because of the availability and convenience of glucose-specific methods. However, the expense of test strips precludes extensive use by poor patients, especially in developing nations.[35a]

Various rapid methods have been devised to test the urine for sugar. Among these are Clinitest,*

---

*Ames Division, Miles Laboratories, Inc., Elkhart, Indiana 46515.

Clinistix,* Diastix,* Ketodiastix,* TesTape,† and Chemstrip uG‡ procedures.

Clinitest is a modification of Benedict's test employing a reagent tablet containing anhydrous copper sulfate, anhydrous sodium hydroxide, citric acid, and sodium bicarbonate. The standard technique calls for 5 drops of urine and 10 drops of water mixed in a test tube into which one reagent tablet is dropped. Heat is generated within the tube by contact of the tablet with the liquid, producing boiling that continues for a few seconds. The colors produced by varying amounts of sugar are roughly the same as those obtained in Benedict's test. The color scale permits the estimation of the approximate amount of sugar up to 2%. As the tablets attract moisture, their potency may diminish. It is important, therefore, that they be kept in a tightly stoppered container or purchased in sealed foil packages.

In a modification of the standard technique, 2 drops of urine and 10 drops of water are mixed and a tablet added. With this method, useful in patients with marked glycosuria, a special color chart is required with a scale ranging from 0 to 5%.

Glucose Oxidase Methods. TesTape, Clinistix, Diastix, and Chemstrip uG have the advantage of being specific for glucose. They are simple to use and the responses are ascertained quickly.

Using *TesTape*, a strip of test paper is dipped into urine and the change in color, if any, from the original yellow is noted after 1 minute. The presence of glucose is indicated by varying shades of green and blue, ranging from 0.1 to 2% or more. The percentages of glucose are estimated by matching the colors with the standard color chart. *Diastix*, a plastic strip with a light blue impregnated paper tip, is dipped into the urine. Glucose causes a change in color through shades of green and light brown to dark brown (0.1 to 2% or more).

Chemstrip uG. A plastic strip with a small piece of impregnated yellow paper on the tip is dipped into urine for 2 minutes, then removed and compared with the test colors on a chart. Changes from the original yellow are first to light green (0.1%), then through deep green to shades of blue (maximum, 5%).

Substances in Urine Causing Confusion in Testing for Sugar. Certain substances other than sugar may cause confusion in testing the urine. Of those which occur normally, creatinine and uric acid are the most common. More important are the growing number of drugs prescribed for various disease conditions. Many have been reported as interfering with both the copper reduction and the glucose oxidase methods, chiefly the former. In such instances, drugs have often been taken in quite large doses. Most common are falsely positive responses to Benedict's and/or Clinitest methods. Included in this group are the following antibiotics: cephalosporins, chloramphenicol, furazolidene, isoniazid, nalidixic acid, nitrofurantoin, paraminosalicylic acid, penicillin G, streptomycin, sulfonamides, and tetracycline. False positive tests have also been reported with the anti-inflammatory agents, phenacetin and salicylates. In addition, false positive tests to Benedict's and/or Clinitest methods have been reported for a variety of other drugs including methyldopa, ascorbic acid, levodopa, metaxalone, morphine, probenecid, iodinated radiographic contrast material, and vaginal powders if glucose or other reducing sugars have been added.

False negative tests by glucose oxidase methods have been reported for melluride, salicylates, ascorbic acid, levodopa, and phenazopyridin HCl. A false positive test to glucose oxidase has been reported as due to in-vitro contamination by hydrogen peroxide in a container for urine.

It must be emphasized that some of the reports vary, others appear to be inconsistent, and very often as stated above, interference occurs only when drugs have been given in large doses. Finally, the interference may consist not of producing the usual positive result in the case of copper reduction tests, but rather of production of a dark color as with certain of the cephalosporins. In the case of iodinated radiographic contrast material, a black color has been reported produced when the urine of the patient is tested with Benedict's solution. This is said to be inconsistent.

Tests for Ketone Bodies

At the present time, tests for acetoacetic (diacetic) acid and acetone in the urine are usually made quickly and conveniently by the use of special paper strips such as Ketostix. Alternatively, one may use the ferric chloride (Gerhardt) test or better, the sodium nitroprusside (Rothera) test. The procedures followed in these two tests may be found in clinical laboratory texts.

The ketone bodies include acetoacetic acid, acetone, and betahydroxybutyric acid. Acetoacetic acid occurs in the urine under the same conditions as acetone and it is rarely found except when associated with acetone. In freshly voided urine containing ketone bodies, the quantity of acetoacetic acid is 9 or 10 times that of acetone. The older the urine, the greater the relative proportion of acetone

---

*Ames Division, Miles Laboratories, Inc., Elkhart, Indiana 46515.

†Eli Lilly and Co., Indianapolis, Indiana 46285.

‡Bio-Dynamics, Inc., Indianapolis, Indiana 46250.

because of spontaneous degradation of acetoacetic acid. There is no quick and easy test for the third member of the trio, betahydroxybutyric acid.

It must be kept in mind that if a patient is taking salicylates, antipyrine, cyanates, or acetates, the ferric chloride test may give a response somewhat similar to that due to acetoacetic acid. However, there can be no question as to the cause of the positive test if one boils the solution for 2 minutes. Acetoacetic acid is unstable and any color it causes will disappear upon boiling, whereas the red color due to any of the drugs mentioned does not disappear on boiling ("drug reaction").

Examination of the Blood

The advent of mechanized, automated procedures for the determination of various constituents of the blood has caused a revolution in clinical laboratory work. On a single sample of blood with a minimal expenditure of time and effort, multiple determinations may be carried out at the present time. In the clinical laboratory of the Joslin Clinic, a Technicon AutoAnalyzer is used for the separate determination of blood glucose by a modification of Hoffman's alkaline ferricyanide method. This is done so that blood obtained at the beginning of the visit may be analyzed promptly, and the glucose concentration reported within 30 minutes to the physician and patient, thereby providing guidance as to any change in treatment. A Beckman ASTRA 4 (Automated Stat/Routine Analyzer) is used for the determination of sodium, potassium, chloride, CO_2, and creatinine. A Dupont instrument, ACA 4, is employed for general chemistry procedures apart from those just mentioned.

Rapid Blood Glucose Estimation. Patients in the hospital for vigorous treatment of diabetes may at times experience symptoms suggesting hypoglycemia. Since these are often of non-specific type, it is desirable to determine the blood glucose prior to giving carbohydrate. To avoid delay, a rapid test may be carried out on a drop of blood obtained by prick of a finger pad or ear lobe for use with reagent strips such as Dextrostix (Ames) or Chemstrip bG (Bio-Dynamics). Such may be done by a registered nurse or other trained staff member who is immediately available. These results are sufficiently accurate to determine whether the symptoms are due to hypoglycemia. Our impression is that visual inspection of the reagent strips is more satisfactory with Chemstrip bG than with Dextrostix.

More recently introduced are Visidex (Ames) test strips. A large drop of blood is required to cover the two reagent pads. Directions for tests are on the container. It is stated that levels of blood glucose ranging from 20 to 800 mg/dl may be estimated.

Self-Monitoring of Blood Glucose. Although knowledge of the blood glucose is helpful to any insulin-taking diabetic, it is imperative for those who are using insulin "pumps" (see Chapter 19) or are giving themselves multiple doses of insulin daily, often in changing amounts from day to day. Use of the reagent strips described above may suffice for reasonable accuracy, particularly if the Chemstrip bG and their respective color charts are used. Readings of Chemstrip bG may be made with a StatTek* reflectance meter, but with most people, visual estimation of the color chart yields values close to those obtained by standard laboratory procedures. Satisfactory accuracy with Dextrostix may be obtained by the use of a reflectance meter (Ames Eyetone, Dextrometer, or Glucometer). See reference 36 for papers prepared for a symposium on blood glucose self-monitoring.

Glycosylated Hemoglobin. It is well appreciated that single determinations of the blood glucose at periodic visits of the patient to the physician's office or out-patient department, furnish an incomplete idea of the long-term control of diabetes. One does better, of course, if the urine and blood are tested for sugar before each meal and at bedtime, thereby providing a profile of sorts. However, even this does not fill the need completely. Consequently, the discovery[37,38] that diabetic patients have elevated levels of hemoglobin A_1 (glycosylated hemoglobin) and particularly of hemoglobin A_{1c} (HbA_{1c}) was welcomed with satisfaction, as a means of evaluating the degree of control over an extended period.[39]

Glucose condenses with the N-terminal valine of the beta chain of hemoglobin ($A_{1a,1b,1c}$) to a degree determined by the level of plasma glucose in a two-stage chemical process. The first which results in an aldimine base is reversible, but the second involves rearrangement into a stable ketoamine. When the plasma glucose is chronically elevated, the degree of glycosylation provides an index as to the average glucose level over the half-life of erythrocytes, i.e., about 2 months.[40]

HbA_{1c} normally forms only 4 to 6% of the total hemoglobin. In the treatment of diabetes by conventional means, one aims for a value as close to normal as possible, but usually, perforce, must accept up to 8 or even 10%. Values above the latter figure are unacceptable, particularly in the range of 15 to 20%. One must admit, however, that in persons with highly unstable diabetes, this goal may be difficult to attain even with two injections daily of both regular and NPH insulins.[41]

Glycosylated hemoglobin moieties may be determined by ion exchange chromatography, affinity

---

*Bio-Dynamics, Inc., Indianapolis, Indiana 46250.

chromatography, radioimmunoassay, colorimetry, or isoelectric focusing. Currently in use in the Joslin Clinic laboratory is an agar gel electrophoretic method of measuring HbA_1 as described by Menard et al.[42] This electrophoretic method measures all the fast hemoglobins (i.e., HbA_{1a}, HbA_{1b}, and HbA_{1c}). This complex and rapid method shows a high degree of correlation with the more ambient high-performance liquid chromatography method, which is specific for HbA_{1c}. The electrophoretic method range of normality is 5.6 to 7.6%.

Blood Ketones. A semi-quantitative test for ketones in the blood may permit differentiation between ketosis and other forms of acidosis. Furthermore, the degree of response of a positive reaction serves as an indication of the severity of ketosis and a guide to treatment. A rough estimation of the amount of ketones in plasma or serum of patients with presumed or suspected ketoacidotic coma should invariably be carried out at once when the patient is first seen.

Method for Detection of Acetoacetic Acid and Acetone in the Blood. The blood is drawn into a syringe or tube containing a tiny amount of potassium oxalate, then centrifuged for 5 minutes at medium speed. The test is made on the plasma with as little delay as possible, since there may be some loss of acetone if the plasma is allowed to stand. If it must be kept for future testing, it should be placed in the refrigerator in a stoppered tube.

Dilutions of the plasma are made with water or saline solution so that one has 6 tubes containing the following:

Undiluted plasma
1:2 dilution—0.5 ml plasma + 0.5 ml water
1:4 dilution—0.5 ml plasma + 1.5 ml water
1:8 dilution—0.5 ml of 1:4 dilution + 0.5 ml water
1:16 dilution—0.5 ml of 1:4 dilution + 1.5 ml water
1:32 dilution—0.5 ml of 1:16 dilution + 0.5 ml water

In testing for acetoacetic acid and acetone, use is made of the Rothera nitroprusside reaction employing either Ketostix test strips or Acetest* (both Ames) crushed tablets. If the former is used, test strips are dipped into the plasma and dilutions. Changes in color (from light purple or lavender to deep purple) read in 15 to 30 seconds against a color chart as 0, 1+, 2+, 3+, or 4+. If Acetest tablets are used, 6 are placed in a row on a flat, white surface, 2 drops of each dilution are placed serially on a tablet and color changes read after 15 to 30 seconds (no longer).

---

*Ames Division, Miles Laboratories, Inc., Elkhart, Indiana 46515.

INTERNATIONAL SYSTEM OF UNITS
(Le Système International d'Unités)

For some years there has been a movement to urge the adoption of an international system of units for the expression of scientific values. Whereas at present in the United States, we are accustomed to stating the concentration of substances in body fluids in *mass* units per volume, e.g., milligrams per deciliter (mg/dl), a change would be made to express such in *molecular* units per volume, e.g., millimoles per liter (mmol/L). The advantages of using the International System (S.I.) would be uniformity throughout the world in reporting of laboratory values and the fact that chemical relationships between various substances would become more readily apparent.

The expression of values in S.I. units has been adopted to a greater or lesser degree in Europe, especially in Scandinavian countries, and to some extent in other countries including Canada, Japan, South Africa, Australia, and New Zealand. Most journals published outside the United States now use S.I. units in whole or in part. Some medical journals in the United States (e.g., J.A.M.A.) are printing S.I. units usually along with conventional values. However, acceptance has not been universal by any means. In addition to the fact that physicians would need to become accustomed to a new set of figures for almost all laboratory values, they have not thought that better diagnoses and/or treatment would result from the adoption of molecular units. However, as time brings familiarity, acceptance may well result gradually as it has in other countries.

In this book, values have been expressed in the familiar, conventional units except in the discussion of diagnosis at the beginning of this chapter. However, in Table 15–7 are shown values for selected blood serum constituents in both systems together with conversion factors.

As far as glucose is concerned, conversion is easily accomplished by multiplying the number of milligrams per deciliter by 0.0555 or by dividing by 18. Thus, a blood glucose of 90 mg/dl = 5 mmol/L. For additional information, see references 43, 44, and 45.

NONDIABETIC MELITURIAS

Nondiabetic melituria is a general term used to designate a variety of conditions in which, apart from diabetes mellitus, sugar of any variety appears in the urine in amounts large enough to give positive reactions in routine testing, particularly if an alkaline copper reduction method is used. Certain of the conditions represent ''inborn errors of metabolism'' inherited as a specific enzymatic defect.

Table 15–7.   Reference Values for Blood Serum or Plasma
Conventional vs. S I Units

Constituent	Conventional (mass/volume)	Conversion Factor	S I Units
Glucose	(Fasting) 70–115 mg/dl	0.0555	3.9–6.4 mmol/L
SGOT	7–40 m units/ml	1.0	7–40 m units/ml
LDH	100–225 m units/ml	1.0	100–225 m units/ml
Alk. phosphatase	(Adult) 30–115 m units/ml	—	30–115 m units/ml
Bilirubin (total)	0.2–1.2 mg/dl	17.1	3.4–20.5 μmol/L
Creatinine	(Adult) 0.7–1.4 mg/dl	88.4	61.9–123.8 μmol/L
Uric acid	(Females) 2.2–7.7 mg/dl	0.0595	0.13–0.46 mmol/L
	(Males) 3.9–9.0 mg/dl	0.0595	0.23–0.54 mmol/L
Urea nitrogen	10–26 mg/dl	0.714	7.1–18.6 mmol/L
Cholesterol	150–250 mg/dl	0.0259	3.9–6.5 mmol/L
Triglycerides	40–150 mg/dl	0.0114	0.45–1.71 mmol/L
Inorganic phosphorus	2.5–4.5 mg/dl	0.323	0.8–1.5 mmol/L
Calcium	8.5–10.5 mg/dl	0.25	2.1–2.6 mmol/L
Albumin	3.3–5.2 g/dl	10	33–52 g/L
Total protein	6.0–8.5 g/dl	10	60–85 g/L
Sodium	134–146 mEq/L	1.0	134–146 mmol/L
Potassium	3.6–5.2 mEq/L	1.0	3.6–5.2 mmol/L
Chloride	96–109 mEq/L	1.0	96–109 mmol/L
Carbon dioxide	23–33 mEq/L	1.0	23–33 mmol/L

Note: The conventional reference values (normal ranges) listed above are those in use at the Joslin Clinic. Except for those for cholesterol, they have been taken from Technicon Chart No. 017-0301-22, Technicon Instruments Corporation, 250 Ballard Vale Street, Wilmington, MA 01887. Conversion factors have been taken from the comprehensive list compiled by Conn.[33]

The majority, although not all, are benign, asymptomatic, and without known influence on life expectancy.

Judging from published reports, one gains the impression that, in the present day, melituria other than glucosuria is not being recognized as frequently as in the past. This would be expected because of the increasing tendency to use glucose oxidase methods which yield positive results only for glucose. Since special studies of nondiabetic melituria have not been carried on in recent years at the Joslin Diabetes Center, the discussion which follows will be presented in abbreviated form. For more extensive coverage, the reader is referred to other texts which describe the conditions in detail.[46]

Nondiabetic Glucosuria

Glucose may be found in the urine, almost always in small amounts, in a wide variety of conditions. No treatment is necessary, but pains should be taken to make certain that diabetes mellitus is not present and responsible for the glucosuria. Table 15–8 represents an attempt to classify the various situations in which glucose may be found in the urine apart from diabetes. As one scans the list, one notes that, in some instances, transient hyperglycemia reflecting some degree of glucose intolerance may be responsible. If so, the results of a glucose tolerance test would clarify the situation. In renal glucosuria, including the benign glucosuria of pregnancy, and in glucosuria following a chemical agent as phlorhizin, the mechanism is that of blocking the reabsorption of glucose by the renal tubules.

Renal Glucosuria. The term renal glucosuria is used to describe the condition in which glucose appears in the urine despite a normal blood glucose. If one defines the condition loosely, then it is quite common. However, if one uses strict criteria including: (1) constant glucosuria even in the fasting state; (2) lack of significant influence of the amount of dietary carbohydrate; (3) identification of glucose as the urinary sugar; and (4) evidence that the patient metabolizes carbohydrate normally, then renal glucosuria is uncommon. There is disagreement among those who have studied the matter as to whether or not renal glucosuria progresses over time to diabetes mellitus. In the Joslin Clinic experience, this has not taken place, although frequently diabetes has been present in the families of patients with renal glucosuria. In one of our patients, a male (J.C. 2165), sugar was first found in the urine when he was 10 years old. During the following 70 years, sugar was found in sizeable amounts in every specimen of urine examined and at times in quantities as great as 5% or more.

JOSLIN'S DIABETES MELLITUS

Table 15–8. Types of Nondiabetic Glucosuria

A. Renal glucosuria including benign glucosuria of pregnancy.

B. Glucosuria accompanying hyperactivity of endocrine glands other than the pancreas.
 1. In hyperthyroidism
 2. In hyperpituitarism
 3. In conditions in which the suprarenal glands are stimulated.

C. Glucosuria due to stimulation of intracranial centers.
 1. Piqûre diabètique of Claude Bernard.
 2. Brain tumors
 3. Cerebral hemorrhage
 4. Injuries of the skull

D. Alimentary glucosuria.
 1. Minimal glucosuria found by sensitive methods
 2. Glucosuria following prolonged starvation

E. Glucosuria accompanying infection, toxemias, anesthesia, and asphyxia.

F. Glucosuria in chronic or degenerative conditions.
 1. Vascular hypertension
 2. Chronic nephritis and nephrosis
 3. Chronic hepatic disease as cirrhosis of the liver
 4. Malignant disease

G. Glucosuria due to chemical agents.
 1. Phlorizin
 2. Poisoning as by heavy metals

Throughout his life, this patient restricted his diet little, if any. He died at the age of 80 years of bronchopneumonia and metastases from carcinoma of the prostate.

The concentration of glucose in the glomerular filtrate is normally the same as that in the plasma water. Glucose is reabsorbed in the proximal convoluted tubules, chiefly in their proximal portions. As the plasma glucose level increases, the amount of glucose absorbed by the tubules reaches a transfer maximum (Tm_G) which in the normal adult is about 300 to 350 mg per minute. When the arterial blood glucose exceeds a certain level (usually about 150 to 180 mg/dl) and the amount of glucose presented to the tubules for reabsorption is greater than the Tm_G, glucose appears in the urine. However, this concentration of blood glucose, spoken of loosely as the "renal threshold," is not rigidly fixed. Indeed, it is not the only factor concerned: changes in the glomerular filtration rate obviously alter the total quantity of glucose reaching the proximal tubules per unit of time and variations in the activity of tubules of individual nephrons influence the composite effect.

In renal glucosuria, it appears that various factors just mentioned may play a part with a majority of patients showing a decrease in Tm_G. Since the condition is benign and symptomless, few studies have been done in an attempt to discover any anatomic abnormality in the kidney. In a few patients, careful studies have shown structural defects in the

renal proximal convoluted tubules and, in others, no abnormalities have been noted. The pattern of inheritance has been variously interpreted as that of an autosomal dominant or autosomal recessive trait.

For a complete and detailed discussion of renal glucosuria, see the article by Krane.[47]

Renal Glucosuria of Pregnancy. Glucose is often found in the urine of pregnant women. In studies carried out in the past, a frequency ranging from 5.4 to 13.6% has been noted in routine testing and in practically all during a formal glucose tolerance test. It goes without saying that if significant glucosuria is found in routine testing, blood glucose determinations should be made at 1 hour after a meal liberal in carbohydrate, and in doubtful or borderline situations resort should be had to a formal glucose tolerance test. In this connection, it is worthwhile noting that sugar in the urine during pregnancy is practically always glucose except during the last stages when some lactose may be present.

Melituria Other than Glucosuria

Benedict's or other alkaline copper tests, including Clinitest, give positive results for all sugars which may be found in the urine. In the case of pentose, reduction of the copper solution takes place after a few hours at room temperature (i.e., without heating), and within 10 minutes at 50 to 60 ° C. Fructose (levulose), also a ketose, reduces Benedict's solution quickly at 50° C, but much more slowly than pentose at temperatures below 40° C. Like pentose and fructose, mannoheptulose reduces Benedict's solution without heating.

Since glucose oxidase tests are specific for glucose, other tests less well known to the clinician must be used for pentose and fructose: the Bial (orcinol-HCl) reaction is positive for pentose and the Seliwanoff (resorcinol-HCl), for fructose.

In order to obtain positive identification for pentose and fructose, one must turn to paper chromatography, and then to carry the study to its desirable end, one should enlist the aid of a chemist in obtaining characteristic osazone crystals with phenylhydrazine or methylphenylhydrazine (the latter in the case of fructose since fructose and glucose form the same osazone). The melting point of the crystals should be determined since in distinguishing between glucose and pentose, that of glucosazone (205° C) and of pentosazone (157° to 160° C) are quite different and distinctive.

For other tests, some specific for lactose and galactose, see standard texts of laboratory procedures. Of interest is the nonfermentable sugar, mannoheptulose, which may be found in the urine of certain persons following the ingestion of avocado.

For a listing of the meliturias other than glucosuria, see Table 15–9.

Chronic Essential Pentosuria.[48] Chronic essential pentosuria is a rare benign condition characterized by the constant excretion in the urine of small quantities (1 to 4 g daily) of a pentose, 1-xylulose. Most reported cases have occurred in Jews although some have been noted in members of Lebanese families. Although pentosuria was thought formerly to occur predominantly in males, it now appears that the sex distribution is about equal. The condition is harmless, asymptomatic, and has no relation to diabetes mellitus. No treatment is necessary.

Essential pentosuria is inherited as an autosomal recessive trait. The genetic defect is related to the metabolism of glycuronic acid. Normally, uronic acids are converted to a pentose, 1-xylulose, then to a sugar alcohol, xylitol, and finally, through a series of steps, to a hexose. In persons with pentosuria, the enzyme (*NADP-linked xylitol dehydrogenase) responsible for the conversion of 1-xylulose to xylitol is deficient[49] and, as a result, 1-xylitol accumulates and is excreted in the urine.

Essential pentosuria is to be distinguished from other pentosurias which are not genetic in nature. These include (1) alimentary pentosuria in which tiny amounts (less than 100 mg in 24 hours) of 1-arabinose and 1-xylose may appear in the urine following the ingestion of unusually large quantities of fruit such as plums, cherries, and grapes; (2) even smaller quantities of a pentose (d-ribose) may occur in the urine of healthy persons and of some with muscular dystrophy; (3) traces of d-ribulose and tiny quantities (up to 60 mg in 24 hours) of 1-xylulose and d-ribose may be found in the urine of normal persons.

From routine life insurance examinations, essential pentosuria is found in about 1 in 40,000 to 50,000 persons, whereas Hiatt[48] estimates that it is present in a ratio of about 1:2000 to 1:2500 among American Jews. The Joslin Clinic series, when first

reported in 1932,[49] consisted of 3 cases; by 1970 it included 12 patients. The number has not grown since because of change in laboratory procedures and the absence of any special project regarding the condition. All of our 12 patients were Jews ranging in age from 7 to 51 years at the time of the first discovery of melituria and all but 2 were males.

Lasker[50] found that most of the families of pentosurics living at the time of first study in New York City area came from locations of relatively limited extent in what is now East Germany and Poland. Cases have been reported in Israeli Jews who have migrated from Europe and in Lebanese living in Lebanon or South Africa. One case has been reported in an American Indian.

Fructosuria (Levulosuria).[51] Fructose is known to occur in the urine in association with three rare conditions: (1) essential fructosuria; (2) hereditary fructose intolerance; and (3) familial fructose and galactose intolerance. It may also be found in persons with advanced liver disease. The urine of normal individuals may contain traces of fructose but in amounts so small as not to give positive results with conventional tests. In each of the situations mentioned above, the fructosuria depends upon the ingestion of fructose and disappears when fructose is withheld from the diet.

Essential Fructosuria. Essential fructosuria is a benign asymptomatic condition which requires no treatment. Judging from published reports, it occurs rarely but the actual incidence probably is higher than one estimate of 1 in 130,000 persons in the general population. Fructose gives a positive result with alkaline copper tests, does not react with glucose oxidase, and is levorotatory. As with pentosuria, its discovery depends a great deal on the routine testing of all patients. This is not likely to be done except in a special project such as one at the Joslin Clinic in the 1930s when 4 cases were discovered in a relatively short period of time, perhaps fortuitously.[52] None has been found since, but this probably is because special attention has not been focused on the subject.

The metabolic defect in essential fructosuria is a deficiency of hepatic fructokinase, an enzyme which catalyzes the conversion of fructose to fructose 1-phosphate. Consequently, when fructose is ingested, it is metabolized incompletely with the result that a significant amount remains in the blood and fructose is excreted in the urine to the extent of 10 to 20% of the ingested amount. No treatment is required for essential fructosuria. This disorder is inherited as an autosomal recessive trait.

Hereditary Fructose Intolerance. In 1956 Chambers and Pratt,[53] and in 1957 more extensively, Froesch and associates,[54] described an un-

Table 15–9. Meliturias Other than Glucosuria

1. Chronic essential pentosuria
2. Fructosuria
   A. Essential
   B. Hereditary intolerance
      a. Fructose-1-phosphate aldolase deficiency
      b. Fructose-1-6-diphosphatase deficiency
3. Lactosuria
4. Galactosuria
5. Sucrosuria

---

*NADP = nicotinamide adenine dinucleotide phosphate.

common and hitherto unrecognized condition characterized by symptomatic hypoglycemia and vomiting shortly after the ingestion of fructose or fructose-containing foods. Hypoglycemia may lead occasionally to unconsciousnes. In small children with chronic fructose ''poisoning,'' there is failure to thrive, and findings include hepatomegaly, jaundice, proteinuria, and aminoaciduria. Cachexia may result in death. The fructose intolerance is considered to be an inborn error of metabolism, probably inherited as an autosomal recessive trait. The primary defect is a deficiency of the liver enzyme, fructose-1-phosphate aldolase. The accumulation of fructose-1-phosphate is thought to inhibit fructose phosphorylation by fructokinase with consequent fructosemia and fructosuria. The mechanism for the secondary hypoglycemia is not clear, although there is some evidence to suggest that hepatic glucose production or release is inhibited by the excess fructose-1-phosphate.

Treatment consists of elimination of fructose-containing foods from the diet. The prognosis is excellent if the condition is recognized early in infancy and fructose avoidance instituted. Froesch states that, in the natural course of events, older children and adults are apt to develop a strong aversion to sweets and fruit and thereby protect themselves. If fructose is not omitted from the diet, long-term effects may include hepatic damage and renal impairment.

Hereditary Fructose-1, 6-Diphosphatase Deficiency. This rare genetic disorder described first by Baker and Winegrad[55] is discussed by Froesch[54] together with the other inherited disturbances of fructose metabolism summarized above.

Lactosuria. Lactose in the urine may give rise to confusion in diagnosis following the performance of the Benedict or Clinitest procedures. Fortunately, the condition in which it characteristically occurs, namely, lactation, is known to the physician, and its presence at this time is not considered significant. It has also been found in the urine of nurslings. The concentration of lactose in the breast milk of lactating diabetic women is said to remain remarkably constant in spite of marked elevations or depressions of the blood glucose concentration.[56]

Lactose, like glucose, reduces copper, and is dextrorotatory, but it yields a characteristic osazone with phenylhydrazine and is not fermented by pure yeast. However, the osazone is difficult to obtain from the urine and ordinary yeast is not to be depended upon for the fermentation test. Rubner's test and the mucic acid test for lactose are described in clinical laboratory texts.

Galactosuria. Galactose is another sugar which reduces alkaline copper solutions. It is noteworthy because its presence in the urine is the result of an inherited error of metabolism, congenital galactosemia, which is not benign but fortunately is treatable. It occurs characteristically in infants and children and is manifested classically by an enlarged liver and spleen, cataracts, and mental retardation.[57] It is due to a congenital absence of a specific enzyme, galactose 1-phosphate uridyl transferase which, when normally present, catalyzes the conversion of galactose-1-phosphate to glucose-1-phosphate. When it is deficient, galactose-1-phosphate accumulates in the tissues including the liver, red blood cells, and lens of the eye. The mechanism by which this accumulation and subsequent enzyme (phosphoglucomutase) inhibition leads to hepatic fibrosis and central nervous system damage is not clear.

Shortly after birth, infants with this condition, on taking milk, develop vomiting and diarrhea. Nutrition becomes impaired, jaundice may develop, and hepatosplenomegaly may be noted. If the child continues to ingest milk, cataract formation and mental retardation may follow. If milk is omitted from the diet at an early enough stage, the abnormalities mentioned, other than mental retardation, may disappear. The infant and young child should be maintained on milk substitutes. Commonly used is Nutramigen (Mead Johnson and Co.), a casein hydrolysate. Soy milk formulas have also been used. After 5 or 6 years, foods containing galactose may usually be introduced to a small degree but it is best throughout life to restrict galactose.

The diagnosis, made presumptively on clinical grounds, is confirmed by demonstrating the absence of galactose-1-phosphate uridyl transferase in the patient's red blood cells or by using a simple chromatographic screening procedure for the detection of galactosemia in newborn infants.

Of interest are the studies of Engerman and Kern[58] who made normal dogs galactosemic by feeding a high galactose diet. Within 4 years, certain of the animals developed not only cataracts and neuropathy but also diabetes-like retinopathy. Blood levels of glucose remained normal although those of glycosylated hemoglobin were slightly elevated.

Gitzelmann and Illig[59] described another inherited disorder of galactose metabolism in which there is a deficiency of galactokinase with inability to phosphorylate galactose. Following the ingestion of lactose and galactose, there was a prolonged rise of blood galactose with the appearance of galactose and galacticol in the urine, but no change in the blood glucose and no rise in serum immunoreactive insulin.

Sucrosuria. Sucrose (cane sugar) is excreted in the urine promptly after intravenous administration, since under these conditions the body has no provision for hydrolyzing it to simple sugars. It is said that small amounts of sucrose may appear in the urine of normal individuals following the ingestion of a large amount of cane sugar. Endogenous sucrosuria has been reported rarely and, if such indeed exists, is difficult to explain. One must be on guard for factitious sucrosuria in which patients add cane sugar to the urine brought to the physician for examination, not realizing that sucrose will not reduce alkaline copper reagents or be detected by glucose oxidase tests. Unusually high specific gravity of the urine, as 1.070, alerts one to the possibility of the addition of sucrose to the urine.

REFERENCES

1. Fajans, S.S., Cloutier, M.C., Crowther, R.L.: Clinical and etiologic heterogeneity of idiopathic diabetes mellitus. Diabetes 27:1112, 1978.
2. WHO Expert Committee: Report on Diabetes Mellitus. WHO Technical Report Series, No. 310, Geneva, World Health Organization, 1965.
2a. Klimt, C.R. (Chairman): Committee on Statistics of the American Diabetes Association, June 14, 1968: Standardization of the oral glucose tolerance test. Diabetes 18:299, 1969.
2b. Wilkerson, H.L.C.: Diagnosis: oral glucose tolerance tests. In: T.S. Danowski (Ed.): Diabetes Mellitus, Diagnosis and Treatment. New York, American Diabetes Association, 1964, pp. 31–34.
2c. Fajans, S.S., Conn, J.W.: An approach to the prediction of diabetes mellitus by modification of the glucose tolerance test with cortisone. Diabetes 3:296, 1954.
2d. Meinert, C.L.: Standardization of the oral glucose tolerance test. Criticisms and suggestions invited. Diabetes 21:1197, 1972.
3. National Diabetes Data Group: Classification and diagnosis of diabetes mellitus and other categories of glucose intolerance. Diabetes 28:1039, 1979.
4. WHO Expert Committee: Second Report on Diabetes Mellitus. WHO Technical Report Series, No. 646, Geneva, World Health Organization, 1980.
5. Keen, H., Jarrett, R.J., Alberti, K.G.M.M.: Diabetes mellitus: a new look at diagnostic criteria. Diabetologia 16:283, 1979.
6. O'Sullivan, J.B., Fajans, S.S.: Selecting criteria for the diagnosis of "diabetes mellitus." Diabetes Care 3:565, 1980.
7. Köbberling, J., Creutzfeldt, W.: Diabetes mellitus: a new look at diagnostic criteria. Diabetologia 17:263, 1979.
7a. Srikanta, S., Ganda, P., Jackson, R.A.: Type I diabetes mellitus in monozygotic twins: chronic progressive beta cell dysfunction. Ann. Intern. Med. 99:320, 1983.
8. Tattersall, R.B., Fajans, S.S.: A difference between the inheritance of classic juvenile-onset and maturity-onset diabetes of young people. Diabetes 24:44, 1975.
9. Srikanta, S., Ganda, O.P., Eisenbarth, G.S., Soeldner, J.S.: Islet cell antibodies and beta cell function in monozygotic triplets and twins initially discordant for Type I diabetes mellitus. N. Engl. J. Med. 308:322, 1983.
10. Tattersall, R.B., Pyke, D.A.: Diabetes in identical twins. Lancet 2:1120, 1972.
11. S. Podolsky, M. Viswanathan (Eds.): Secondary Diabetes. The Spectrum of the Diabetic Syndromes. New York, Raven Press, 1980.
12. O'Sullivan, J.B., Mahan, C.M.: Blood sugar levels, glycosuria and body weight related to development of diabetes mellitus. The Oxford epidemiologic study 17 years later. JAMA 194:587, 1965.
13. Jarrett, R.J., Keen, H.: Hyperglycaemia and diabetes mellitus. Lancet 2:1009, 1976.
14. Birmingham Diabetes Survey Working Party: Ten-year follow-up report on Birmingham diabetes survey of 1961. Br. Med. J. 2:35, 1976.
15. Jarrett, R.J., Keen, H., Fuller, J.H., McCartney, M.: Worsening to diabetes in men with impaired glucose tolerance ("borderline diabetes"). Diabetologia 16:25, 1979.
16. Agner, E., Thorsteinsson, B., Eriksen, M.: Impaired glucose tolerance and diabetes mellitus in elderly subjects. Diabetes Care 5:600, 1982.
17. Kahn, C.B., Soeldner, J.S., Gleason, R.E., et al.: Clinical and chemical diabetes in offspring of diabetic couples. N. Engl. J. Med. 281:343, 1969.
18. O'Sullivan, J.B., Mahan, C.M.: Criteria for the oral glucose tolerance test in pregnancy. Diabetes 13:278, 1964.
18a. Bennett, P.H., Knowler, W.C.: Increasing prevalence of diabetes in the Pima (American) Indians over a ten-year period. In: W.K. Waldhäusl (Ed.): Diabetes, 1979. International Congress Series No. 500. Amsterdam, Excerpta Medica, 1980, p. 507.
18b. Massari, V., Eschwege, E., Valleron, A.J.: Imprecision of new criteria for the oral glucose tolerance test. Diabetologia 24:100, 1983.
18c. Jarrett, R.J., Alberti, K.G.M.M.: Diagnostic criteria (Separate letters to the editor). Diabetologia 25:451, 1983.
19. West, K.M.: Epidemiology of Diabetes and its Vascular Lesions. New York, Elsevier, 1978.
20. Walsh, C.H., Wright, A.D., Allbutt, E., Pollock, A.: The effect of cigarette smoking on blood sugar, serum insulin, and non-esterified fatty acids in diabetic and nondiabetic subjects. Diabetologia 13:491, 1977.
21. Fajans, S.S., Conn, J.W.: An approach to the prediction of diabetes mellitus by modification of the glucose tolerance test with cortisone. Diabetes 3:296, 1954.
22. Remain, Q.R., Wilkerson, H.L.C.: The efficiency of screening tests for diabetes. J. Chron. Dis. 13:6, 1961.
23. Exton, W.G., Rose, A.R.: The one-hour two-dose dextrose tolerance test. Am. J. Clin. Pathol. 4:381, 1934.
24. Wilkerson, H.L.C., Kaufman, M., et al.: Diagnostic evaluation of oral glucose tolerance tests in nondiabetic subjects after various levels of carbohydrate intake. N. Engl. J. Med. 262:1047, 1960.
25. Bowen, A.J., Reeves, R.L.: Diurnal variation in glucose tolerance. Arch. Intern. Med. 119:261, 1967.
26. Streeten, D.H.P., Gerstein, M.M., Marmor, B.M., Doisy, R.J.: Reduced glucose tolerance in elderly human subjects. Diabetes 14:579, 1965.
27. Zeytinoglu, I.Y., Gherondache, C.N., Pincus, G.: The process of aging: serum glucose and immunoreactive insulin levels during the oral glucose tolerance test. J. Am. Geriat. Soc. 17:1, 1969.
28. DeFronzo, R.A.: Glucose intolerance and aging. Diabetes Care 4:493, 1981.
29. West, K.M.: Epidemiology of Diabetes and its Vascular Lesions. New York, Elsevier, 1978, pp. 103–107.
30. Unger, R.H., Madison, L.L.: A new diagnostic procedure for mild diabetes mellitus. Evaluation of an intravenous tolbutamide response test. Diabetes 7:455, 1958.
31. West, K.M.: Epidemiology of Diabetes and its Vascular Lesions. New York, Elsevier, 1978, pp. 113–122.
32. Navarrete, V.N., Torres, I.H.: A triamcinolone-glucose tolerance test in the early diagnosis of diabetes. Diabetes 14:481, 1965.
33. Siperstein, M.D.: The glucose tolerance test: a pitfall in

the diagnosis of diabetes mellitus. Adv. Intern. Med. 20:297, 1973.

34. Froesch, F.A., Renold, A.E., McWilliams, N.B.: Specific enzymatic determination of glucose in blood and urine using glucose oxidase. Diabetes 5:1, 1956.

35. Fine, J.: Glucose content of normal urine. Br. Med. J. 1:1209, 1965.

35a. Lester, F.T.: Long-standing diabetes mellitus in Ethiopia: a survey of 105 patients. Diabetologia 25:222, 1983.

36. Symposium (9 articles): Blood Glucose Self-Monitoring. Diabetes Care 4:392–426, 1981.

37. Rabhar, S.: An abnormal hemoglobin in red cells of diabetics. Clin. Chim. Acta 22:296, 1968.

38. Bunn, H.S., Gabbay, K.H., Gallop, P.M.: The glycosylation of hemoglobin: relevance to diabetes mellitus. Science 200:21, 1978.

39. Gabbay, K.H., Sosenko, J.M., Banuchi, C.A., et al.: Glycosylated hemoglobins: increased glycosylation of hemoglobin A in diabetic patients. Diabetes 28:337, 1979.

40. Koenig, R.J., Cerami, A.: Hemoglobin A_{1c} and diabetes mellitus. Ann. Rev. Med. 31:29, 1980.

41. Goldstein, D.E., Walker, B., Rawlings, S.S., et al.: Hemoglobin A_{1c} levels in children and adolescents with diabetes mellitus. Diabetes Care 3:503, 1980.

42. Menard, L., Dempsey, M.E., Blankstein, L.A., et al.: Quantitative determination of glycosylated hemoglobin A_1 by agar gel electrophoresis. Clin. Chem. 26:1598, 1980.

43. Conn, R.B., Jr.: Laboratory reference values of clinical importance. In: Conn, H.F., Conn, R.B., Jr.: Current Diagnosis, 6th Ed. Philadelphia, W.B. Saunders Co., 1980, pp. 1154–1172.

44. Young, D.S.: S.I. units for clinical laboratory data. J.A.M.A. 240:1618, 1978.

45. Henry, J.B., Lehmann, H.P.: S.I. units. In: J.B. Henry et al. (Eds.): Clinical Diagnosis and Management by Laboratory Methods, 16th Ed. Philadelphia, W.B. Saunders Co., 1979, pp. 2083–2107.

46. Stanbury, J.B., Wyngaarden, J.B., Fredrickson, D.S. (Eds.): The Metabolic Basis of Inherited Disease, 4th Ed. New York, McGraw-Hill Book Co., 1978.

47. Krane, S.M.: Renal glycosuria. In: J.B. Stanbury, J.B. Wyngaarden, D.S. Fredrickson (Eds.): The Metabolic Basis of Inherited Disease, 4th Ed. New York, McGraw-Hill Book Co., 1978, pp. 1607–1617.

48. Hiatt, H.H.: Pentosuria. In: J.B. Stanbury, J.B. Wyngaarden, D.S. Fredrickson (Eds.): The Metabolic Basis of Inherited Disease, 4th Ed. New York, McGraw-Hill Book Co., 1978, pp. 110–120.

49. Marble, A.: Chronic essential pentosuria: a report of three cases. Am. J. Med. Sci. 183:827, 1932.

50. Lasker, M.: Mortality of persons with xyloketosuria; follow-up study of a rare metabolic anomaly. Human Biol. 27:294, 1955.

51. Wang, Y.M., van Eys, J.: The enzymatic defect in essential fructosuria. N. Engl. J. Med. 282:892, 1970.

52. Marble, A., Smith, R.M.: Essential fructosuria. J.A.M.A. 106:24, 1936.

53. Chambers, R.A., Pratt, R.T.C.: Idiosyncrasy to fructose. Lancet 2:340, 1956.

54. Froesch, E.R.: Essential fructosuria, hereditary fructose intolerance, and fructose-1, 6-diphosphatase deficiency. In: J.B. Stanbury, J.B. Wyngaarden, D.S. Fredrickson (Eds.): The Metabolic Basis of Inherited Disease, 4th Ed. New York, McGraw-Hill Book Co., 1978, pp. 121–136.

55. Baker, L., Winegrad, A.I.: Fasting hypoglycemia and metabolic acidosis associated with deficiency of hepatic fructose-1, 6-diphosphatase activity. Lancet 2:13, 1970.

56. Tolstoi, E.: Relationship of blood glucose in concentration of lactose in milk of lactating diabetic women. J. Clin. Invest. 14:863, 1935.

57. Felig, P.: Congenital galactosemia. In: P.K. Bondy and L.E. Rosenberg (Eds.): Metabolic Control and Disease, Philadelphia, W.B. Saunders Co., 1980, p. 369.

58. Engerman, R.L., Kern, T.S.: Experimental galactosemia produces diabetic-like retinopathy. Diabetes 31 (Suppl. 2):26A (Abstr.), 1982.

59. Gitzelmann, R., Illig, R.: Inability of galactose to mobilize insulin in galactokinase-deficient individuals. Diabetologia 5:143, 1969.

16 General Plan of Treatment

Alexander Marble, Allen P. Joslin, and Gisella G. Garan

Because of the varied types and manifestations of diabetes, treatment must be suited to the individual. However, it is essential that the physician have in mind a general plan together with the goals of treatment. To this end, the material in this chapter is presented in a general way; specifics are covered in the chapters that follow. The approach described refers particularly to the management of the patient who presents first in the physician's office or in an outpatient department, but the same general plan applies equally to the patient who is seen first as a hospital in-patient.

In the management of both acute and chronic diseases, the eventual aims of therapy consist ideally of providing a cure or, even better, a means of prevention. This is not possible with diabetes at present, although the words "prevention" and "cure" have been spoken more frequently with renewed hope in recent years. In the preceding chapters of this monograph, much evidence has been presented to suggest that if it were possible by treatment to bring about a state in which the abnormal metabolism is reversed and the blood glucose maintained constantly within normal limits, both acute and chronic complications might be prevented and might, if already present, be ameliorated in some instances. This, then, provides a rational basis for establishing a long-term goal toward which to work. The immediate aims of such therapy must, of course, be the overcoming of characteristic symptoms of diabetes and the correction of acidosis, if present.

For many years at the Joslin Clinic, the standards of control designed to evaluate effectiveness of treatment with diet alone or with oral hypoglycemic agents, have been as shown in Table 1 in Chapter 21. The values given there are for glucose both in whole venous blood and in plasma or serum; the latter values are about 15% higher than the former.

The most important guide expressed in the table is that in the fasting state and at 3 or more hours after food, the whole blood glucose should be no higher than 110 mg/dl (plasma or serum, 125 mg/dl). Many will argue that these standards are too lenient to protect the patient, whereas others will say that they are too strict to be realistic. From what is known today, it appears that ideally one should strive for euglycemia both fasting and even at one hour post-prandially, if one is to hope for the *best* protection of the patient with Type I diabetes. One knows that as far as the blood glucose alone is concerned, this can be accomplished with the Biostator glucose controller or to a remarkable degree by dedicated, intelligent patients using an insulin "pump" or multiple injections of insulin daily with guidance from frequent home blood glucose monitoring. However, the patient in daily life must not suffer frequent or severe hypoglycemic episodes. Until easier methods of treatment are available, perfect glycemic control will continue to be a challenge. With the individual patient, one must simply do the very best one can.

Zeal in treating the insulin-dependent patient is crucial. At the same time, one must not forget the vast army of people with Type II diabetes and impaired glucose tolerance; they also need and deserve the best possible treatment. Although not dependent on insulin for survival, many Type II patients benefit from treatment with insulin to promote health both in the present and future. Those with impaired glucose tolerance need careful periodic follow-up and advice as to diet and other measures to promote good general health including correcting obesity if present.

INITIATION OF TREATMENT

Once the diagnosis of diabetes has been made (see Chapter 15), the question arises as to whether treatment should be started in the physician's office (or outpatient clinic) or in a hospital. In either case, it is important that a detailed history be taken, a complete physical examination be made, and such laboratory studies be carried out as will be helpful in the management of the patient's problems, both diabetic and non-diabetic. The physician must be concerned with the treatment of the "whole person" and not simply of the diabetes. Physical and emotional problems often have little or no relation to diabetes and yet may be as important, or more important, to the patient's health and happiness. To the familiar items of diet, insulin, oral hypoglycemic agents and exercise, must be added the necessity of continuing education of the patient and his family regarding diabetes and its treatment.

History. Both initial and interval histories are best taken with the use of printed forms that are designed to make future reference and tabulation easy and remind the physician of specific points to cover. If patients are seen by appointment, it is helpful if they are sent a questionnaire to fill out in advance and bring to the first visit. This allows the prospective patient ample time for consultation at home with other members of the family regarding dates of onset of symptoms, diagnosis of diabetes, initiation of treatment (if the diabetes has been present for some time), family history in detail, dates of past illnesses and hospitalizations, as well as current medications (with name, strength and dosage). Without such a completed questionnaire, history-taking by the physician could be a tedious and time-consuming effort, with the recording of incomplete or inaccurate data.

Physical Examination. The complete physical examination should include, but not be limited to, ophthalmoscopic and neurologic examinations, blood pressure (sitting, lying and standing), thorough inspection of the feet, and palpation of the dorsalis pedis, posterior tibial, popliteal, and femoral pulses. Rectal and (in women) pelvic examinations should be carried out. Careful recording of the body weight and height is essential; in young patients, a standard chart should be started so that growth and development may be followed over the years and compared with values for nondiabetic children and adolescents (see Chapter 24).

Laboratory Studies. At the first visit, tests should include, as a bare minimum, a complete urine analysis, blood glucose determination, and complete blood count. In ordering other studies, the physician must consider the real need vs the cost to the patient. However, in most instances it is helpful to obtain blood for a "chemistry screening profile" with special attention to serum cholesterol, urea nitrogen and creatinine. If the patient is in the fasting state, determinations of serum triglycerides and the lipoprotein electrophoretic pattern may furnish valuable baseline information. Values for high density lipoprotein cholesterol (HDL) and glycosylated hemoglobin ($HgbA_1$) are of value but not critical at first visit. The physician may decide that an electrocardiogram and/or chest x-ray are advisable in certain patients. Regardless of what laboratory studies are done, it is important that facilities exist for the prompt determination of the amount of glucose in urine and blood so that the physician and patient may know these values during the first visit.

Education. After completion of the above, it is the responsibility of the physician to speak with the patient and members of the family (if present), to explain the findings and the treatment to be undertaken. Such treatment may consist of a restricted diet alone or diet plus an oral hypoglycemic agent or insulin. The patient should have time to ask questions. This may be regarded as the beginning of the patient's education. Instruction is then continued by a teaching nurse and/or Registered Dietitian and, for the initial visit, the teaching session may require an hour or more. Material must be presented simply and important points repeated to make sure that the patient or a responsible member of the family fully understands what has been said. With children, the responsibility will fall chiefly on the parents, and with elderly patients, often on a younger family member. Many patients with "new" diabetes are so upset emotionally that repetition is imperative. The teaching session should include: (1) a simple explanation as to the nature of diabetes and its course. The patient should be provided with a booklet or manual for reading and reference at home; (2) a demonstration of methods to test for sugar and acetone in the urine; (3) a detailed explanation of the diet that has been prescribed by the physician. The patient should be given a written outline of the meal plan, with details of the prescribed amounts for specific items in the various food groups (see Chapter 17 and Appendices B–E for details of the diabetic diet). It is important that the concept of food groups and exchanges be understood; (4) instruction in the use of insulin, if such has been prescribed. The goal is to teach the patient not only how to measure and inject insulin, but also how to make minor adjustments in dosage at home according to the general trend of the results of urine tests. Recognition and treatment of insulin reactions should be discussed, with additional instruction at later sessions; (5) rules regarding management of food, insulin, and urine testing on days of acute illness; and (6) a brief review of important items of hygiene, particularly in care of the teeth, skin and feet.

For a comprehensive discussion of the education of the diabetic patient, see Chapter 23.

FOLLOW-UP VISITS

At the initial visit the patient should be asked to report again shortly for further tests of glucose in blood and urine and for additional examination and instruction. The interval between visits may be as short as 1 or 2 weeks for patients newly started on insulin, or as long as 2 to 3 months for those whose treatment is diet alone or with an oral hypoglycemic agent. The patient should be told to feel free to phone or write the physician, teaching nurse, or dietitian if there are questions or if difficulties arise. A helpful aid in monitoring the effects of treatment is a printed form on which the patient records the results of urine tests taken at home before meals and at bedtime (see Fig. 1, Chapter 19) and mails or brings the report to the physician at the end of a week. Future visits to the physician's office or to the outpatient clinic are arranged at intervals of 1 to 6 months, as indicated for the individual patient.

At follow-up visits, it is desirable to suggest and teach selected patients the monitoring of blood glucose at home by means of test strips such as Dextrostix, Visidex or Chemstrip (with or without a reflectance meter). One may also at times obtain an index of long-term control by serial determinations of glycosylated hemoglobin (Hgb A_1 or A_{1c}).

The majority of patients who are not acutely ill with ketoacidosis, infection, or disabling complications, can be treated successfully in the physician's office or the outpatient clinic. A team approach is best in which physicians, dietitians, teaching nurses, psychiatric social workers, and laboratory and office personnel work together to inform, encourage, and motivate the patient. In no other disease is it so important for the patient to realize that he/she must take an active part in treatment and that consistent self-care will do much to govern the state of health in the future. The physician and other members of the team can outline the treatment program and monitor its results, but it is the patient and family who must attend to details of daily management. For some patients this is not a welcome responsibility, and at times it seems overwhelming to them, particularly when insulin injections are part of the program. Hostility, resentment and uncooperative behavior occur frequently, especially in adolescents. Thus, it is imperative to provide as much guidance, advice and encouragement as possible, both to the patient and the family.

EMOTIONAL ASPECTS

To live with a chronic illness is not easy. Any physician who cares for diabetic patients knows that the impact of having the disease is tremendous. The patient may not verbalize this at first, but often carries the memory of a close relative who had a leg amputated, became blind, or who perhaps had difficulty with pregnancies. The patient may be worried about not being able to continue at work; whether the employer should be told, risking the possibility of being overlooked for promotion, or worse yet, losing the job; or whether there will be an increase in the premium on the life insurance for which application has been made, or whether insurance will be refused. Recently graduated high school students who were star athletes may worry about whether they can get athletic scholarships at college or whether they will be able to participate in sports at all. Young women ask if they can look foward to marriage and having children. The business person who travels a great deal, not only in this country but also overseas, becomes concerned about the differences in food, the carrying of insulin and syringes, and how to allow for time zone differences. Elderly patients who already may have one or more chronic ailments such as heart disease, hypertension, and arthritis, become frightened and depressed by the added burden of diabetes and the implementation of dietary restriction, urine testing and, possibly, "one more pill" or insulin injections.

Some patients hide their condition, not only from their employers and co-workers but, in a few instances, from family members. Clearly, it is not in the best interest of the patient to be tempted with forbidden foods by well-meaning friends or to be subjected to a home environment that is not conducive to good diabetes care. In the event of hypoglycemia or impending ketoacidosis, a well-informed spouse, parent or co-worker can be of great help and can make sure that the patient receives proper care in the fastest possible way.

For a full discussion of these and related aspects of diabetes, see Chapters 24 (youth), 44 (psychosocial), and 45 (socio-economic).

TREATMENT IN THE HOSPITAL

There are two classes of patients whose initial treatment is best carried out in a hospital: (1) those who are in ketoacidosis; are acutely ill for other reasons; have conditions requiring surgery or other treatment not feasible in office or home; or who in emergencies, may enter the hospital without having been seen as an outpatient. Such patients need to be in a conventional general hospital. (2) Those ambulatory patients who have insulin-dependent diabetes of either recent or remote onset and, because of poor control of diabetes, require treatment and instruction under close observation. They are best cared for in a special unit which is part of or near a general hospital.

Diabetes Treatment Unit

Beginning in 1915, ambulatory diabetic patients were treated on an inpatient basis by the late Elliott P. Joslin and associates in cottages near the New England Deaconess Hospital. This innovative type of care has been continued in the 70 years since. In 1957 an area accommodating 40 patients was set aside in a permanent building connected with the Deaconess Hospital and administered as an integral part of the hospital. Currently, the enlarged Diabetes Treatment Unit (DTU) has a capacity for 70 patients. In the DTU, ambulatory patients wear street clothes, walk to a common dining room on the same floor, attend classes twice daily in a lecture hall or conference room on the same floor, and may exercise in a small gymnasium. They have easy access to physicians, dietitians and nurses, including those designated as teaching nurses, as well as to services and consultants in the main part of the hospital. The average length of stay is 7 to 8 days. Because less nursing care is required, costs in the DTU average only 60 to 65% of those in the main part of the hospital.

The DTU has been of special benefit in the treatment of children and adolescents with insulin-dependent diabetes. Of particular note is the child under 8 years of age with newly discovered diabetes. The mother accompanies the child and stays as a guest with the patient in a small private room. The mother, by attending special conferences and twice-daily lectures, learns how to care for the child at home. By this arrangement, mother and child are not separated and instruction of the mother can be more complete.

Since diabetes is a chronic disease for which there is no cure at present, and since diabetics have shared in the increased longevity enjoyed by persons in the general population, a patient and physician may establish a relationship which lasts for many years. It is not uncommon for physicians in a diabetic clinic to follow and care for a patient for 20 to 40 years or more. Accordingly, the first visit and the initial training of the patient are all-important. In the present day, the "diabetologist"—whether internist, pediatrician, or generalist—is often the primary physician to whom the patient looks for advice for any illness, whether related to diabetes or not. The physician's responsibility is great but the reward lies in the satisfaction of seeing patients with well-controlled diabetes lead long, useful and happy lives.

17 Dietary Management of Diabetes

Thomas M. Flood, Beverly N. Halford,
Ramachandiran Cooppan, and
Alexander Marble

Regulation of the type and quantity of food ingested is the basis of treatment for all patients with diabetes. This statement remains fundamentally as correct today as in the pre-insulin era when dietary restriction, often severe, was the only method of treatment available. Despite nearly unanimous support of this concept, the actual use of the diabetic diet in terms of physician-directed teaching and patient acceptance often is poor. The factors responsible for this failure have been summarized by West[1] in a classic review of the topic, and include: the composition of the diet in terms of ethnic, cultural, social, and personal preferences; a lack of self-discipline; a dislike of rigid meal schedules and of the amounts and types of foods prescribed; a misunderstanding on the part of both medical personnel and patient of the principles, priorities, or methods of diet therapy; and an inadequate system of patient education.

The topic of dietary management will be discussed as three closely interrelated areas: (a) philosophic and practical considerations designed to lead to the formation of clinical strategies; (b) specific nutritional recommendations, which encompass foodstuffs, formulas and other actual components of the diabetic diet; and (c) teaching of the patient and family. Obesity, a major problem for many diabetic patients, deserves special emphasis and therefore is covered not only in Chapter 18, but also discussed here briefly as it relates to the specifics of management.

Table 17–1 furnishes a guide to the terminology that in general will be employed in this chapter. Such definitions may be matters of semantics. However, if they present more clearly to the patient what is expected regarding types and quantities of various foods, times of eating, etc., it is more likely that the food plan will be followed.

Table 17–1. Glossary of Terms

1. Diet: What an individual actually eats.

2. Dietary prescription: Recommended food intake as to amounts of carbohydrate, protein, fat and calories.

3. Meal plan: A diabetic diet for normal weight individuals. Its use is preferred to avoid the hypocaloric implications of the word "diet."

4. Calculated meal plan: A diabetic diet which emphasizes precision in the timing of food intake with good continuity on a day-to-day basis as well as a major effort in calculating sizes of portions of food in the various groups by weighing, measuring, or carefully estimating. "Strict diet" or "rigid diet" are often used synonymously but also imply decreased food intake and are less desirable alternatives.

5. Free diet: Consumption of foodstuffs in a totally random fashion. May or may not include the use of concentrated carbohydrates.

PHILOSOPHIC AND PRACTICAL CONSIDERATIONS

Diagnosis

The diagnosis of diabetes is not always clear-cut, particularly in borderline situations, but it is obviously necessary before prescribing a diet. Chapter 15 provides an in-depth discussion of diagnostic standards and current thinking relative to classifying the diabetic state. If the diagnosis of overt diabetes is established, a dietary prescription becomes an intrinsic component of the treatment plan. The actual specifics of the diet depend upon a number of factors, the most important of which are the type of diabetes [insulin-dependent (Type I) or non-insulin-dependent (Type II)] and the patient's body habitus.

Most would agree that patients with impaired glucose tolerance ("chemical" diabetes) usually need little more than a common sense approach to weight control rather than a formal diet. Avoidance of sweets and pastries and modest restriction of concentrated carbohydrate hopefully may protect against not only transient episodes of slightly elevated blood glucose levels, but also against progression to overt diabetes.

Prior and potential abnormalities of glucose tolerance are two additional subcategories in which precise dietary prescriptions are not necessary.

Individualized Dietary Prescriptions

The chief characteristics which differentiate Type I and Type II diabetes are listed in Table 17–2. The major feature separating these two types of diabetes is the capacity for endogenous insulin production.

Persons with well-established *Type I diabetes* are unable to produce any significant amount of insulin. Excessive body weight is infrequent in this group at the onset of diabetes. A dietary prescription calling for a significantly reduced caloric intake (in comparison to calories consumed prior to developing diabetes) is a mistake and, in the long run, is doomed to failure. Assuming that the patient is not overweight, there are certain basic reasons why, within reason and judgment, the caloric intake prior to onset should be maintained for the newly diagnosed Type I diabetic patient. These are: (a) Hypocaloric diets are not necessary for optimal blood glucose control in the lean, insulin-dependent patient. (b) Normal weight patients will almost always abandon the prescribed diet if they are chronically hungry and therefore will consume inappropriate foods or eat at the wrong times, thereby doubly jeopardizing the efforts at controlling their disease. (c) Those few patients who do accept and follow a diet that is too low for their needs will, in time, lose lean body mass. To be sure, excessive weight gain may become a problem in later years and necessitate a reduction in calories prescribed and consumed.

Patients with *Type II diabetes* may be obese or non-obese. Those Type II patients who are truly lean (i.e., at or under their desirable body weight) need a diet which is approximately isocaloric with that prior to onset for all of the reasons cited earlier as applying to the Type I diabetic.

"Obesity" is obviously a continuum but it is most often, albeit arbitrarily, defined as being 20% or more in excess of average body weight or, less objectively, of "desirable" body weight as given in life insurance tables. There is unanimous agreement that caloric restriction and weight reduction represent an optimal initial treatment for obese individuals with Type II diabetes. With patients who are cooperative and compliant, it may serve in many as the only treatment needed to reduce the

Table 17–2. Contrasting Features of the Two Types of Overt Diabetes

	Type I (IDDM)	Type II (NIDDM)
Age	Young	Old
Body habitus	Non-obese	Obese
Characteristic symptoms of diabetes	Present; onset often rapid or sudden	Variable; onset often insidious
Ketones in urine at onset or diagnosis	Strongly positive	Absent to weakly positive
Endogenous insulin (by C-peptide assay)	Absent or extremely low, esp. 1 to 5 yr after onset	Present
Islet-cell antibodies	Present	Absent
HLA antigens	Increased association	No correlation
Clinical course	Difficult to control with conventional therapy	With patient cooperation, relatively easy to control

All of the characteristics listed in this table are relative. Clearly there are Type II diabetics who are not obese; not all Type I diabetics have islet cell antibodies at the time of diagnosis; etc. The table is a composite of those characteristics usually seen, and exceptions to one or more are common.

blood glucose level to normal. In the course of time, however, an oral agent or insulin may become necessary for some. The mechanism whereby caloric restriction and weight loss yield effective blood glucose control, will be discussed later in this chapter and in Chapter 18. The period of time during which a calorically restricted diet is needed may be short or long. If and when the compliant patient reaches desirable body weight, calories may be adjusted to permit weight maintenance.

DIETARY CONSIDERATIONS FOR NON-OBESE PATIENTS WITH TYPE I OR TYPE II DIABETES

Type I Diabetes

For the patient with insulin-dependent diabetes, even with the best conventional treatment now available, the control of diabetes rarely achieves completely the normal physiologic state. This will remain the case until there is generally available a more physiologic and acceptable means of delivering insulin.

It is true that the ideal may be approached closely by the meticulous patient who takes 2, 3, or more injections of insulin daily and carries out home monitoring of the blood glucose. In addition, the current widespread clinical trial of ''insulin pumps'' (see Chapter 19) is a step in the right direction. Furthermore, clinical and experimental evidence continues to accumulate in support of the thesis that obtaining the best possible blood glucose control may prevent, minimize, or postpone late complications of the vascular and nervous systems; a large number of authorities have endorsed this concept.[2,3] To this end, the physician must recognize and consider the benefits of a precise and uniform calculated meal plan, tailored for the individual diabetic.

The Diabetes Treatment Unit (DTU) of the New England Deaconess Hospital (see Chapter 16) admits hundreds of patients annually with unstable (''brittle'') diabetes, who give a clearcut history of poorly controlled diabetes. By careful attention to individualized meal plans, results of blood and urine tests in the DTU document greatly improved control of diabetes during the several days of admission. Quite often this is accompanied by a significant decrease in insulin dosage as compared to that used prior to admission. The same phenomenon may be seen less dramatically in the patient whose degree of control and habitual level of compliance at home have been better. Thus, improved control becomes a reflection of greater precision in compliance with the prescribed meal plan in which carbohydrate, protein, and fat are distributed in a balanced fashion. The provision of well-timed and

measured amounts of food, evenly distributed throughout the day, and consistently on a day-to-day basis, affords a smooth foundation for finding an insulin dosage that will minimize glycemic excursions.

A common and frustrating experience for both patient and physician is that of the person with inherently unstable diabetes who, having attained adequate regulation of diabetes during hospitalization, demonstrates once again overt evidence of poor control within days or weeks of returning home. This emphasizes the need for frequent follow-up visits to the physician, dietitian, and other members of the health team.

Type II Diabetes; Non-obese

Attributes of the meal plan such as those for patients with Type I diabetes are desirable for the management of many non-obese patients with Type II diabetes. These persons do have reserves of endogenous insulin and thus often have a greater degree of flexibility than the patient with typical Type I diabetes. They are not insulin-dependent in the strict sense of the term, but some may do better with an insulin dose which will permit a satisfying food intake. The level of precision needed for best regulation can usually be determined easily by comparing the results achieved in a controlled environment, such as the DTU, with what the patient accomplishes by self-management. Faced with results that do not measure up to expected or previously observed standards, the physician should be sure that the patient is really motivated to achieve maximum control, and insist upon compliance with the prescribed diet for at least a trial period of observation (1 to 2 weeks is usually sufficient). Following this, the physician should review the results and urge continued compliance if the expected improvement can be documented.

STEPS IN EFFECTIVE MEAL PLANNING

The First Interview

The process of developing a meal plan that is medically and nutritionally sound as well as one that will work, is basically the same for insulin-dependent and non-insulin-dependent diabetic patients. This should include the participation of the patient and, hopefully, a member of the family, preferably the one who prepares the meals. The meal plan is based on a prescription initiated by the physician, which specifies the amount of carbohydrate, protein, fat, and calories per day. These estimates are based on the patient's age, sex, occupation, height, present weight, and level of usual physical activity.

It is the responsibility of the physician to develop

a meal plan from the dietary prescription and to instruct the patient. However, some physicians may not have adequate dietary knowledge or have the time or opportunity to use such skills frequently enough to remain facile in this area. In any case, the physician should seek the aid of a Registered Dietitian, if available, who may personally or by supervision translate the dietary prescription into a meal plan appropriate for the individual. The dietitian* will take a detailed dietary history and survey the needs of the patient from the standpoint of the factors mentioned in the preceding paragraph as well as such matters as ethnic origin, likes and dislikes regarding food, etc. Table 17–3 provides an outline of the components of patient assessment. The information obtained will allow the dietitian

Table 17–3. Components of Patient Assessment

1. *Medical evaluation:* Identify those medical factors which have an impact on the dietary prescription. Review the problem list.
   Consider: Type of diabetes
   Weight, height history
   Growth curve
   Medications
   Insulin treatment
   Abnormal laboratory findings
   Significant physical findings
   Family history

2. *Nutritional assessment:* Identify the present nutritional status and factors which should be considered when developing a nutritional care plan.
   Evaluate the current dietary history and activity patterns.
   Consider: Average intake of: carbohydrate, protein, fat, and calories
   Saturated fat intake
   Nutritional density of intake
   Alcohol intake
   Food preferences/allergies
   Special needs, i.e., growth, stress
   Drug/diet interactions

3. *Educational assessment:* Identify preferred teaching methods, scope and level of proposed educational program.
   Consider: Motivational level
   Reading level
   Learning preferences
   Emotional status

4. *Evaluation of support systems available:* Identify significant problems the patient may encounter in implementing the dietary prescription.
   Consider: Facilities for food preparation
   Food budget
   Ethnic, cultural, social, religious background
   Life style
   Support available from family and others

*In this chapter wherever the word "dietitian" appears, it will be understood as "Registered Dietitian."

to establish goals and priorities which seem practicable in teaching the individual patient. It goes without saying that the dietitian must work in concert with the physician so that the originally estimated dietary prescription may be modified if necessary.

Teaching Nurses

For many years, patients of the Joslin Clinic benefited greatly by the presence of specially trained "Diabetes Teaching Nurses" who interviewed patients and their families, took dietary histories and translated the physician's prescription into definite meal and snack plans. At present, Teaching Nurses instruct patients in the measuring and injection of insulin, testing of urine for sugar, home monitoring of blood glucose, treatment of insulin reactions, care of the feet, and other measures important in the overall treatment of diabetes. Dietary management is now performed by Registered Dietitians both in the main part of the New England Deaconess Hospital and in its Diabetes Treatment Unit as well as in the Joslin Clinic office (for outpatients).

Dietary History

From the detailed record of the patient's usual food intake, the dietitian estimates the protein, carbohydrate, fat, and calories which have been consumed daily. The adequacy of these elements as well as that of vitamins and minerals, can be quickly appraised by the professional and in case of doubt, standard tables[4] may be consulted (see also Appendix A). Tables for average and desirable body weights (see Appendix F) are used to determine whether the patient is over- or underweight. Alternatively, an abbreviated method may be used to obtain a rough estimate of the number of calories needed per day as established by weight, age, and activity levels (Table 17–4); the total calories are broken down into carbohydrate, protein, and fat percentages. The American Diabetes Association guidelines call for 50 to 60% of total calories to be provided by carbohydrate, 20% protein, 30% fat (10% polyunsaturated, 10% monounsaturated, and 10% saturated fatty acids) per day.[5] At the Joslin Clinic the proportions are roughly the same, with somewhat less carbohydrate and a little more fat, namely 40 to 50% carbohydrate, 15 to 20% protein, and 30 to 40% fat with adjustment for individual needs. The calorie breakdown may now be translated into food exchanges and a calculated meal plan prepared.

In planning diets for diabetic patients, it is important not only to restrict total fat, but also to teach patients to select, whenever possible, those fats which are composed of unsaturated fatty acids,

Table 17–4. Abbreviated Method for Estimating Desirable Body Weight and Caloric Needs

	Men	Women
To estimate desirable body weight:		
Medium frame	5 ft = 106 lbs	5 ft = 100 lbs
	Plus 6 lbs for each additional inch.	Plus 5 lbs for each additional inch.
Small frame	Subtract 10%	Subtract 10%
Large frame	Add 10%	Add 10%
To estimate caloric needs:	Basal kilocalories = 10 × desirable body weight	
Add activity calories:	Sedentary - 3 × desirable body weight	
	Moderate - 5 × desirable body weight	
	Strenuous - 10 × desirable body weight	
To promote weight gain	Add 300–500 kcal/day	
To promote weight loss	Subtract 500 kcal/day = 1 lb loss per week	
	1000 kcal/day = 2 lb loss per week	
Nutrient needs of children	Estimate caloric requirement (see Chapter 24). Monitor growth curve (height/weight) for indication of growth status (e.g., Fig. 5 in Chapter 24).	

especially of the polyunsaturated type. Although the subject is controversial, one hopes thereby to exert a favorable influence in lowering the serum cholesterol and in preventing cardiovascular disease. In general, fats of vegetable origin are (mono- or poly-) unsaturated, whereas those of animal origin are saturated. Also, in general, animal fat is solid in texture; vegetable fat has a lower melting point and is therefore soft or liquid. Margarine made with corn, cottonseed, safflower, soy, or sunflower oil is rich in polyunsaturates and therefore desirable; it is marketed in relatively soft form in tubs. However, palm and coconut oils are saturated. If vegetable oil is hydrogenated, it becomes saturated; margarine made from this is firm and is sold in stick form.

In olive oil, avocado and in most nuts, the fat is primarily monounsaturated. Butter, bacon fat, cream, cream cheese, and lard are all high in saturated fat (see Appendix C, list 6).

For many diabetic patients, it is important to restrict sodium in the diet as part of the treatment of hypertension, congestive heart failure with edema, etc. Consequently, suggestions regarding the selection of foods for a ''no added salt'' diet are given in Appendix D.

EXCHANGE SYSTEMS OF MEAL PLANNING

With the foregoing as background, this and following sections will present the specifics of developing a program for teaching the individual patient. All dietary planning and instruction must, for the sake of simplicity, use a system which utilizes food groups and approximate equivalents. In this way the patient may learn readily how to select for a given meal the type and amount of food which conform to the diet plan and thereby promote variation and palatability.

The method of diet planning and patient education employed by the late Elliott P. Joslin in 1916 when the first edition of this book appeared, ac-

tually was an exchange system. This was, of course, somewhat modified in subsequent decades. This system was built around certain representative foods with nutritional values expressed per 30 g (1 ounce) portions or fractions or multiples of such. This was used in connection with tables in which were listed key items including milk, vegetables, fruit, bread, meat, and fats with a list of foods of approximate nutritional equivalence. The lists were so arranged as to show the amount which, in terms of carbohydrate, protein, fat, and calories, could be substituted for the key food. The amounts were expressed in metric and English equivalents as well as in household measures (see Appendix G, Tables 1–4).

The A.D.A. Exchange System

In 1950 a Joint Committee of the American Diabetes Association, the American Dietetic Association, and the Diabetes Section, U.S. Public Health Service, developed a simplified method of prescribing the diabetic diet. A booklet now entitled ''Exchange Lists for Meal Planning'' (with modifications) has been extensively used during 3 decades and many thousands of copies have been distributed. The brochure may be purchased from the American Diabetes Association, Inc., 2 Park Avenue, New York, NY 10016 or from the American Dietetic Association, 430 North Michigan Avenue, Chicago, IL 60611.

There can be no doubt that the A.D.A. diet plan has improved the standards of dietary treatment throughout the country. In this plan, foods are divided into six groups called ''exchange lists.'' Each food in a list contains roughly the same amount of carbohydrate, protein and fat as any other food in that list. Patients are instructed as to the number of exchanges to take from the various lists for the three main meals and between-meal snacks. They should receive as much detailed information regarding the diet as their intelligence and interest will allow. The lists and standard types and amounts of foods are given in Table 17–5.

The Present Joslin Clinic Procedures

The Joslin Clinic method as used currently is patterned closely after the A.D.A. plan except that it places somewhat greater emphasis on actual weights or measures of food and on teaching the calculation of diets to selected receptive patients. In Appendices B through E to be found at the end of this book are shown the following Joslin Clinic forms: Appendix B, a blank on which to record the meal plan for the individual patient; Appendix C, showing the 6 basic food lists and, in addition, lists 7, 8, and 9, giving, respectively, miscellaneous foods, a snack list which facilitates easy selection of combinations with varying fat content, a list of foods which may be taken freely in amounts appropriate to those in common usage; and, finally, Appendix D with a "no added salt" diets, and Appendix E providing additional guidelines for patients.

The use of exchange lists, whether A.D.A., Joslin Clinic, or other, simplifies meal planning for four reasons: (a) foods of similar nutritional composition and caloric content are grouped together; (b) they provide a system whereby meals can be planned to allow a variety of foods; (c) they represent a basic teaching tool that is applicable to most patients with diabetes; (d) they give the patient a flexible system applicable to nearly any eating situation, such as dinner parties, restaurant meals, and holidays.

Although the cooperative efforts of physicians, dietitians, and other trained professionals are universally recognized as invaluable in the handling of diabetic diets, unfortunately many patients have never received formal dietary instruction. A preprinted standard diet sheet handed to all patients is not a suitable approach to prescribing diets. Individually prepared meal plans should be presented and explained to the patient in detail.

One must teach a method of meal planning which is both understandable and practical for the individual patient. At the Joslin Clinic, most patients, especially those with hard-to-manage diabetes, traditionally have been taught that, for the first days or weeks, weighing or measuring of foods are the best methods for becoming familiar with sizes of portions prescribed. Initial *weighing* (on gram scales, adjustable for taring of the container) or careful *measuring* (using household articles such as cups, spoons, etc.) afford the best training for future estimation. Alternative methods must be used for those individuals whose intelligence, receptiveness, location at mealtimes or other practical considerations make *estimation* necessary at the start. Food models or pictures are helpful in this regard. During the training period, the patient (or person who will be preparing food for the patient) learns best if encouraged to participate in the selection of food and sizes of portions, rather than to observe passively the making of such decisions.

Keeping a Food Diary. The first month or so of following a meal plan is generally the time when new eating behaviors become established, especially for patients with newly diagnosed diabetes or those requiring radical changes in their eating habits. Careful monitoring of this critical period is essential, along with continued reinforcement and teaching. One method is that of encouraging the patient to keep a food diary for a week prior to the next medical visit. This allows the physician and dietitian to discover how the new meal plan is actually working, how fully the patient understands and applies the information received, and the ways in which the plan is medically effective. The entries provide a valuable day-by-day source of information, not only about eating patterns and problems arising therefrom, but also about the management of the diabetes itself, especially if this diary in-

Table 17–5. A.D.A. Exchange Lists

List	Exchange Lists	Food Type	Amount	Carbo-hydrates	Protein	Fat	kcalories
1	Milk[a]	Non-fat	1 cup	12	8	Trace	80
		Whole	1 cup	12	8	8	152
2	Vegetables[b]		½ cup	5	2	0	25
3	Fruit	Orange	1 small	10	0	0	40
4	Bread[c]	Bread	1 slice	15	2	0	70
5	Meat[d]	Meat, lean	1 ounce	0	7	3	55
6	Fat[e]	Margarine	1 teaspoon	0	0	5	45

[a]Figures for low fat (1 and 2%) are given in the booklet.
[b]Includes beets and carrots. Chicory, Chinese cabbage, endive, escarole, lettuce, parsley, radishes, and watercress may be used as desired. Starchy vegetables are regarded as bread exchanges.
[c]Includes starchy vegetables: corn, beans, parsnips, peas, potato, pumpkin, winter squash, sweet potato, and yams.
[d]Figures for medium and high fat meat are given in the booklet.
[e]Special attention is given as to whether the fat is of saturated, monounsaturated, or polyunsaturated type.

cludes information about urine or blood test results and any hypoglycemic episodes.

The Second Interview. The next interview concerning meal planning should coincide, if possible, with a visit to the physician so that information about the results of blood, urine and other tests may be used along with the experience of a month-long practice with new eating patterns. At this time, progress should be evaluated, both from the patient's own explanation and by examining the food diary kept by the patient. Follow-up interviews provide the physician and dietitian an opportunity to introduce more information. If instructions given at the original interview have been understood and followed, and if improvement is noted in the patient's condition, this would be the time to teach various "adaptation skills." These include how to select foods from restaurant menus, read labels in supermarkets, read recipes for gourmet or ethnic foods, etc., all in terms of their suitability for persons with diabetes. The second session is also a time to encourage the patient to begin setting long-term goals. This underscores for the patient the importance of personal participation in treatment. The more the patient takes part in planning, the greater are chances of adherence to the meal plan and of better self-care.

Opportunities for furthering education occur with each patient contact. Many individuals, despite participation in a quality training program will, over a period of time, experience a gradual erosion of compliance, due to complacency or boredom. In patients whose general health is good, lapse or inconsistency in compliance with the meal plan is the most common reason for suboptimal control of diabetes. Although positive urine tests and elevated blood glucose values may at times reflect a change in insulin requirement, more often they represent a lack of dietary compliance for which increase in the dose of insulin is not an effective solution. For those patients in whom the reason for deteriorating control is not clear, it is prudent and frequently effective to urge that they review and carefully enforce all aspects of the calculated meal plan before changing the insulin dose.

SPECIAL CONCERNS IN CHILDHOOD AND ADOLESCENCE

Nutrition Issues for Children

The child with diabetes presents the most compelling need for periodic revisions of the diet. These young patients require special attention from the physician and dietitian who must monitor growth carefully and balance insulin requirement, exercise, and food intake. The growing child requires not only adequate calories, but ample amounts of protein, vitamins, and minerals. Special attention needs to be paid to meat, fish, and poultry; to vegetables and fruit; and to milk and other dairy products. See Chapter 24 and Appendices C through E for further details.

Traditional diet prescriptions call for a base of 1000 calories with an additional 100 calories for each year of life. By this formula, the average 7-year-old child would be on a diet of 1700 kcal, a 13-year-old child, 2300 kcal, etc. It should be noted that these are averages; the actual meal plan must be flexible enough to allow for adjustment of several hundred calories in either direction to accommodate varying circumstances. Having established an appropriate meal plan, it is crucial to remember that this must be revised upward periodically in order to facilitate normal growth and development. This is accomplished by a symmetrical increase in the diet prescription every 1 to 2 years. Failure to make incremental increases is usually brought to the physician's attention by failure to grow and develop normally or by complaints of hunger from the child or parents.

It is important to have the diabetic child exposed to a variety of foods at home. This helps to assure nutritional balance and enables the child to have choices of foods which can lessen the feeling of deprivation of coveted foods as sweets and pastries, whereas nondiabetic children may eat what they want. In addition, the opportunity of choosing food helps the child begin to recognize the various effects foods have on metabolism, an important step in self-monitoring of diabetes. With more varied preferences, the child and parents can be more flexible, too, in traveling, visiting others, and eating out.

Mealtime when families are together has the potential for being a forum for pleasant conversation and happy sharing of experiences. Unfortunately, it can also be a stressful time and present hazards for the child or adult with diabetes. Children often express their concerns in the familiar routines of dawdling, "playing" with their food, and worse, failing to eat at all. Parents should be urged to keep meal-times as calm as possible and to encourage their children to eat fully, regularly, and happily.

Special Issues in Adolescence

The need for the balancing of food, insulin, and exercise continues through adolescence. Although this is true during all of life, the physician and dietitian must be particularly aware of metabolic changes in adolescent girls at menarche (see Chapter 24), which require monitoring of food intake to avoid excess weight gain. Also, there are special nutritional issues for adolescents in regard to their peers. Much of the teen-ager's social life revolves around food, often high in calories, and often eaten at irregular hours. The diabetic youngster is faced with a painful choice: maintain regular (diabetic) eating habits and appear "different" to peers, or disregard the meal plan and risk the consequences. Both physician and dietitian can provide valuable and essential help at this time by re-evaluating meal plans with the adolescent's participation and with an eye to incorporating as much flexibility as is medically advisable. Various restaurants, especially those in "fast-food" chains, cooperated in furnishing the nutritional composition of foods on the menu. With such data, the dietitian may prepare sheets listing the carbohydrate, protein, fat, and calorie content of sandwiches, pizzas, etc., so that patients may make the necessary adjustments in the calculated meal plan.

For further discussion regarding diets for children and adolescents, see Chapter 24.

NUTRITION AND SICK DAY MANAGEMENT

A patient may be unable to follow the regular meal plan during illness because of anorexia, nausea, vomiting, or general malaise. Should this happen, carbohydrates, certain minerals, and fluids should be replaced, at least in part, in an alternative meal plan developed especially for use on sick days. The amount of carbohydrate should be roughly equivalent to that specified in the regular meal plan. If the patient's illness prevents full replacement of the carbohydrate in the regular meal pattern, 50–75 g of carbohydrate should be taken at 6–8 hour intervals. Quick-acting, simple carbohydrates such as orange juice, regular ginger ale, etc., should be used instead of their sugarless substitutes. Sipping on fruit juice or a sweet soft drink throughout the day and sucking on hard candies may be helpful to protect against hypoglycemia. It is important during the illness to maintain an adequate intake of fluids including those containing carbohydrate. Electrolytes—sodium and potassium—may be lost during excess urination, vomiting, or sweating and may be replaced in part by taking broth.

Tables 17–6 and 17–7 give carbohydrate, protein, fat, and calorie values of simple foods and combinations which are suitable for a period of short-term or minor illness.

FACTORS MAKING DIABETES CONTROL DIFFICULT

Even highly motivated patients, who fully understand the role of the calculated meal plan and make a serious effort at remaining compliant, experience difficulties which may seem to be beyond their control but which simply reflect the realities of daily living. The in-hospital training period represents a controlled environment relatively free of demands, temptation, and ordinary stresses. Some of the more common situations which make precise compliance with a calculated meal plan difficult are listed below.

Occupation. Police and fire personnel, nurses, factory workers, and others whose employment may call for alternating work shifts, are in a difficult and challenging situation when they must also cope with the problem of insulin-dependent diabetes. Less dramatic examples include the office worker whose lunch is delayed by the urgency of a work assignment, the student who may have variable mealtimes due to course scheduling, or any individual who encounters an unexpectedly demanding situation that renders eating on time a practical impossibility. However, this problem can usually be handled satisfactorily if adequate amounts of food are always at hand—either at the place of work, in the car, or on the person.

Social Events. Restaurant dining or a pleasant evening with friends frequently creates a situation in which the evening meal is delayed. In addition, the patient may be exposed to a type or variety of food which makes meal plan compliance difficult. However, the well-trained and well-motivated patient usually handles such situations with no great difficulty. If a patient takes insulin before leaving home, knowing that there probably will be an hour or so before dinner is served, a small amount of carbohydrate, say the bread or equivalent portion of the usual dinner, may be taken shortly before leaving home. An approximate equivalent of this food should be omitted from the dinner unless hypoglycemia seems impending. Patients, especially those with unstable diabetes, should be encouraged to select foods which are simple and simply prepared when eating in restaurants. A suitable meal would be meat, poultry or fish, green salad, leafy green vegetables, modest amounts of bread or other complex carbohydrate foods, and (if available) fresh fruit in place of sweet dessert.

Changing Caloric Needs. Despite the emphasis on "precision" as a key to successful diet management, the insulin-dependent patient must be taught to cope with variability of expenditure of energy and caloric needs. Exercise, whether occupational or recreational, can result in hypoglycemic episodes unless one compensates by taking additional food or less insulin. Instructions regarding the type and amount of food needed to prevent undesirably low blood glucose levels is as crucial as is training regarding the type and amount of carbohydrate needed for treatment of an actual hypoglycemic episode.

At times, supplementary food is preferable to a

Table 17–6. Food Suggestions on Days of Illness

Food	Grams	House-hold Measures	CHO	PRO	Fat	kcal
1. Beverages						
Regular ginger ale	180	6 oz.	15	0	0	60
Regular cola drink	180	6 oz.	20	0	0	80
Grapefruit juice	150	5 oz.	10	0	0	40
Tomato juice	240	8 oz.	10	0	0	40
Cranberry juice	100	3.5 oz.	16	0	0	54
2. Broth, chicken or meat		Freely				
3. Hot cereal	120	½ cup	10	2.5	1	59
Milk, whole	120	½ cup	6	4	4	76
						Total: 135
4. Egg Nog						
Combine						
Egg	—	one	0	6	6	78
Milk	180	6 oz.	9	6	6	114
Saltines	15	6 oz.	11	2	1.5	66
Margarine	5	1 tsp.	0	0	4	36
						Total: 294
5. Dropped or scrambled egg on toast						
Egg	—	one	0	6	6	78
Bread	30	1 slice	15	2.5	0	70
Margarine	5	1 tsp.	0	0	4	36
Milk, whole	120	½ cup	6	4	4	76
						Total: 260
6. Creamed soup	150	5 oz.	15	7	5	133
Saltines	10	4	7	1	1	41
						Total: 177

decrease in insulin dosage and, in other situations, the reverse is true. Furthermore, both must be done prior to extreme exertion, as in mountain climbing or marathon running, when the insulin dose must be reduced and simple carbohydrate taken frequently during the exercise.

Economic Conditions. The balance sought in a calculated meal plan may prove to be a financial hardship. People in need often find it necessary to subsist on greater quantities of starch-rich foods and proportionately less protein and fat than would routinely be recommended. However, meal plans may provide much more complex carbohydrate than was previously assumed and still function as an efficient vehicle for control of diabetes as long as precision and consistency as well as caloric content are maintained. It is important that the planner be aware of the individual patient's food budget so that the meal plan selected is a fiscal reality for that patient.

Ethnic Habits. Studies of the eating habits of the people of the world reveal fascinating differences relating to types of food, timing of food intake, and other important variables. Dietary prescriptions must be flexible enough to take into account a person's background and life situation.

Working from this base, the calculated meal plan will be more acceptable.

Overinsulinization. Excessive zeal for diabetic control can cause both meal plan noncompliance and excessive weight gain. Frank hypoglycemic episodes require treatment with carbohydrate and thereby inadvertently increase caloric intake. Rebound hyperglycemia (Somogyi effect) can extend this phenomenon further if it is not appreciated, and may lead to additional increases in the insulin dose. Insulin may simply serve as an appetite stimulant for many individuals. Although they may not be symptomatic from hypoglycemia, they may be forced to eat increasingly large amounts to keep up with an inappropriately high insulin dose.

Boredom and Complacency. These are two common emotions which can lead to loss of compliance with the calculated meal plan. The patient with newly diagnosed Type I diabetes is usually quite compliant during the early period subsequent to the initial diagnosis and treatment. As time passes, attention to finer details of management tend to diminish. This is not surprising since the typical patient experiences no unpleasant symptoms unless the blood glucose falls to hypoglycemic levels or unless hyperglycemia is significant

Table 17–7.   Example of a Concentrated Diet for a Day of Minor Illness

	Household Measure	Weight (g)	Carbo-hydrate (g)	Protein (g)	Fat (g)	Calories
Breakfast						
Orange	small	100	10	0	0	40
Egg	1	50	0	6	6	78
Bread	1 large slice	30	15	3	0	72
Margarine	1 teaspoon	5	0	0	4	36
Milk	6 oz	180	9	6	6	114
Forenoon						
Orange	medium	150	15	0	0	60
Lunch						
Oatmeal (cooked)	½ cup	120	10	3	1	61
Milk	8 oz	240	12	8	8	152
Bread	1 large slice	30	15	3	0	72
Margarine	1 teaspoon	5	0	0	4	36
Orange	medium	150	15	0	0	60
Afternoon						
Crackers, 2 × 2½ in.	2	10	7	1	1	41
Margarine	1 teaspoon	5	0	0	4	36
Milk	6 oz	180	9	6	6	114
Supper						
Egg	1	50	0	6	6	78
Bread	1 large slice	30	15	3	0	72
Margarine	1 teaspoon	5	0	0	4	36
Milk	6 oz	180	9	6	6	114
Orange	medium	150	15	0	0	60
Bedtime						
Crackers, 2 × 2½ in.	2	10	7	1	1	41
Margarine	1 teaspoon	5	0	0	4	36
Milk	6 oz	180	9	6	6	114
Total			172	58	67	1523

Substitutions may be made according to principles previously outlined. Bread may be given as toast in amounts stated above. Fruit or fruit juice other than orange may be substituted in appropriate amounts (See Appendix G, Table 4).

The caloric content of milk and thereby the percentage of calories derived from fat may be decreased by using 1 or 2% fat or skim milk rather than whole milk.

and prolonged. A subjective state of well-being is an extremely basic immediate objective of treatment. Paradoxically, this very situation may allow a well-trained and compliant individual to drift into carelessness.

Serious Attitude Failure. Individuals who have habitually given evidence of self-destructive or anti-social behavior seldom, if ever, achieve the necessary compliance with a calculated meal plan. The basic problems of the alcoholic, the drug abuser, or the school dropout in trouble with the law, all require specific and intensive therapy in an attempt to correct these problems. Otherwise it may be unreasonable to expect these patients to adhere carefully to a calculated meal plan for the management of diabetes.

Less striking examples are even more common, e.g., there are patients who do not have the serious problems noted above but are simply not "health motivated." Despite exposure to an adequate training program and their statement that they understand the role and necessity for a calculated meal plan, they chronically fail in compliance. The precise reason may be obscure but this is unfortunately a common situation which will tax the physician's ability to serve as a motivating force.

Depression. Depression of both the reactive and endogenous varieties in patients is a common medical problem which can appear at any time in any age group. Intense, specific therapy may be necessary before the individual is able to resume the previous level of diabetes management. The calculated meal plan is especially vulnerable because some depressed patients eat poorly, whereas others find their only solace in food.

SPECIAL ASPECTS RELATING TO CARBOHYDRATE IN THE DIET

High Fiber Diets

Diets high in fiber are not new in the treatment of diabetes. In fact, in the pre-insulin days, leafy green vegetables were a mainstay, providing not only bulk and satiety, but in certain instances, considerable fiber. Other high-fiber foods which in the present day may be used, include bran, seeds, whole grain bread and cereals, dry kidney and lima beans, peas and fruit. Recent years have brought a revival of interest in these foods because of reports that high-fiber diets may promote reduction in blood glucose, cholesterol, and triglyceride levels.[5a,5b]

Anderson divides plant fibers into two types: (1) water-soluble (pectins, gums, certain hemicelluloses, and storage polysaccharides) and (2) water-insoluble (cellulose, lignin, and many hemicelluloses).[6] None of these is digestible by the human small intestine. Some, as wheat bran, increase fecal bulk and accelerate transit time in the bowel whereas others, as pectin, slow transit time and do not alter fecal weight. When the amount of plant fiber in the diet is increased moderately, patients usually have abdominal fullness for a few days and increased intestinal gas which is apt to persist. When large quantities of bran are taken, abdominal discomfort and diarrhea may occur.

From his experience with high-fiber, high-carbohydrate diets, Anderson[7] states that with lean diabetic patients, the results are best when the total calories per day are derived from 55 to 70% carbohydrate, (chiefly of complex type), 18% protein, and 12% fat, including 70 g of plant fiber per day. Over a period of time, the blood glucose, cholesterol, triglycerides, and insulin requirements fall. With obese patients he prescribes initial diets providing 600 to 1000 kcal/day of which 55% is furnished by carbohydrate, 25% by protein and 20% by fat with 40 g of plant fiber per 1000 calories. Modifications in the diet are made later, depending upon the short-term response.

Jenkins et al.[8] have reported success with the use of guar gum which becomes viscous when hydrated, either outside or within the stomach. To improve acceptance by patients, these workers have incorporated guar into a crisp bread.[9] It seems likely, however, that any widespread acceptance of high-fiber diets will depend on the use of more palatable common foods. In fact, Anderson et al.[7] conclude a review of the subject by recommending

"that any increase in plant fiber intake should be provided by minimally processed foods such as whole grains, legumes, and vegetables."

Although many clinicians today probably prescribe diets significantly higher in carbohydrate than was the case a decade or more ago, one wonders how many clinicians recommend a figure of 50% or more in terms of calories derived from carbohydrate. If 60% of a 2800-calorie diet were consumed as carbohydrate, 420 g of carbohydrate a day would be necessary. The sheer bulk of complex carbohydrates required to furnish this amount is great, even for the young person with Type I diabetes for whom it is intended. With all patients, both those patients with Type I and those with Type II diabetes, one must use foresight in prescribing diets in which more than 45 to 50% of calories are derived from carbohydrate. The problems are related not only to the bulk and unpleasant gastrointestinal symptoms often experienced with high fiber intake, but also include the tendency of many patients to regard the prescription of a high carbohydrate diet as license to venture into the area of sweets and pastries.

Glycemic Index

The term "glycemic index" has been applied to the degree of blood glucose response to the ingestion of specific carbohydrate foods in comparison with the response to a standard load, usually 50 g of glucose or, at times, 1 slice of bread. The indices were calculated by using the maximal rise in blood glucose or, more often, the area beneath the curve formed by the response of the blood value for a period usually of 2 to 4 hours. The results of studies have indicated that by no means do all starchy foods yield the same response. Using the glycemic index of glucose as 100%, indices above 70% have been obtained in normal persons with maltose, honey, potatoes (instant mashed), whole meal bread, white rice, corn flakes, carrots, and parsnips. At the other end of the scale, indices below 30% (indicative of slow digestion and absorption) included red kidney beans, lentils, soya beans and peanuts.

For the values obtained for other foods by Jenkins, et al.,[9a] see Appendix C–10 and *Diabetes Mellitus and Glycemic Responses to Different Foods: A Summary and Annotated Bibliography*, published by the American Dietetic Association.[9b]

Starch Blockers

From about 1980 to 1982, many "starch blocker" products were consumed, to the estimated extent of one million a day.[9c] Manufacturers stated that these starch blockers contained a "special legume protein concentrate" that would act as an inhibitor of salivary and pancreatic α-d-amylase, thereby preventing the digestion of starch. The tablets were promoted for the control of body weight without any restriction on the intake of starchy foods. However, when the preparation and its effects were subjected to critical study, it was found to contain variable amounts of amylase, trypsin inhibitor, and lectins. Lectin is known to be toxic in animals, presumably due to damage of the microvilli of the intestinal mucosa. Numerous persons taking the tablets experienced adverse reactions, most commonly nausea, vomiting, stomach pain, and diarrhea. Consequently in July 1982 the U.S. Food and Drug Administration (FDA) ordered the product removed from the market. Efforts by manufacturers to obtain a reversal of the FDA ban, on the basis that the preparation is a food substance rather than a drug and therefore is not under FDA jurisdiction, have been unsuccessful.[9d]

ALCOHOL

In Chapter 45, the general aspects of drinking alcoholic beverages by the diabetic are discussed at some length. Here only the effect of alcohol on nutrition and food intake will be included.

Ethyl alcohol, or ethanol, upon ingestion is absorbed quickly and unchanged from the gastrointestinal tract, about 20% from the stomach and the remainder from the upper bowel. It is absorbed directly into the blood stream and may be detected there within 5 minutes after ingestion. Absorption is slowed by the presence of food in the stomach. Less than 10% is lost through the lungs, skin, and kidneys. The remainder is metabolized by oxidation, chiefly in the liver, at a fixed rate of 5–10 ml/ hr. Depending on the quantity and rate consumed, ethanol accumulates in the blood stream since the rate of absorption usually exceeds that of oxidation. The first step in the metabolism of ethanol is accomplished by the action of alcohol dehydrogenase with the production of acetaldehyde which is then broken down by acetaldehyde dehydrogenase to carbon dioxide and water which are eliminated from the body, and to acetyl coenzyme-A, which is metabolized to fatty acid which is stored. Excessive drinking may lead to abnormal deposition of fat in the liver.[9e,9f]

The harmful effects of prolonged over-indulgence of alcohol, chiefly on the nervous system but also, in severe alcohol abuse, on the stomach, liver and pancreas, are universally acknowledged. Despite this, moderate or so-called "social drinking" is so widespread throughout the world today that the physician must face the probability that many patients will use alcohol to some extent.

Ethanol is not a true food and contains no carbohydrate, protein or fat. However, it yields 7 kcal/g and, if used, must be included in calculations of calories. Alcohol cannot be stored in the body or used in the replacement of destroyed tissue. Consequently, in the chronic alcoholic, if an adequate amount of protein is not consumed, a state of negative nitrogen balance will result.

Mixed drinks, liqueurs, and cordials have high carbohydrate value and should be avoided. "Hard" liquors (whiskey, gin, vodka, brandy, and rum), if consumed, should be taken with water or noncaloric soda. If wines are drunk as at a meal, they should be of the dry white type and amounts limited to 120 ml (4 oz). Beer, ale, and other malt liquors contain less alcohol than "hard" liquors but do provide additional calories in the form of carbohydrate. Consumption of a "6-pack" of beer (six 12-oz, or 360-ml cans) in an evening by a young person with insulin-dependent diabetes, may play havoc with control of blood glucose.

The use of alcohol and its implications should always be discussed when diabetic patients receive dietary instruction. They should know that alcohol itself does not raise the blood glucose but, on the other hand, may lower it to hypoglycemic levels if taken while fasting, and particularly after prolonged starvation. This is true especially in an individual with depleted glycogen reserves who has insulin available endogenously or from a prior injection. This comes about because of an inhibitory effect of alcohol on gluconeogenesis (see topic of hypoglycemia in Chapter 19).

SPECIAL FOODS AND SWEETENERS

Special foods are not necessary for patients with diabetes to achieve the recommended dietary objectives. These may be reached conveniently and at much less expense through enlightened choices of commonly available food items. The use of "dietetic" or "diabetic" candy, chocolates, cookies, etc., should be discouraged. Such products may contain little or no straight sugar but almost always have significant caloric value due to the basic ingredients. Another real difficulty is psychologic: patients are apt to take such items in addition to the prescribed type and amount of food rather than as substitutes. Furthermore, one piece of candy or one sweet cookie may call for another, and another, etc. The same human failing applies to nuts of various types; these are concentrated high-calorie foods which are difficult to work into a prescribed meal plan which one expects the patient to follow.

Supermarket shelves display hundreds of products containing sweetening agents, only one of which, saccharin, has no nutritive value. (Cyclamate, also calorie-free, is available in many countries other than the U.S.A.). Other sweeteners yield about 4 kcal/g. Of these, fructose and sorbitol may be tolerated by some patients in amounts up to 30 to 40 g/d. Finally, because of their marked sweetness, tiny amounts of xylitol, mannitol, and aspartame, suffice. The U.S. Food and Drug Administration (FDA) in 1978 published regulations requiring that a food labeled "low calorie" contain no more than 40 calories per average serving; that one called "reduced calorie" have a calorie content which is at least one-third lower than a similar food for which it can be substituted; and that a food cannot be labeled as for diabetic patients unless it is useful in the diet of such persons.[10] Actually, most health professionals would agree that no food should be labeled or advertised as special for diabetics, but rather that, in addition to calorie labeling as noted above, additives be listed on labels with amounts indicated in terms understandable to the consumer.

Wunschel and Sheikholislam[11] evaluated the role of "dietetic" foods in the treatment of diabetes and/or obesity. They concluded that the nutritional value of a majority of products labeled as "dietetic" was not different or better than that of regular products. The differences were related to increased cost, calories, and the substitution of other sweetening agents for sucrose. In their study, the only group of dietetic products with cost and calories less than the regular ones were puddings and gelatins. Leaving cost aside, however, there is nothing to indicate that sweetening agents other than straight glucose, sucrose and products made therefrom, have any deleterious effect when taken in sensible quantities, provided due allowance is made for the caloric value of the additive.

For more detailed discussions and other views regarding sweetening agents, see the group of articles published as a symposium.[12]

Fructose. The use of fructose (levulose) in the diet of diabetic patients has long been controversial. Fructose is found naturally in many fruits (2–6% of fresh edible portion) and vegetables, and its content in honey may be as high as 40%. In any discussion, one must keep in mind that sucrose (table sugar made from sugar cane or sugar beets) is composed of half fructose and half glucose. Fructose is said to be 80% sweeter than sucrose. It yields 3.75 kcal/g.

When fructose is ingested, it is absorbed slowly in the upper bowel largely unchanged; perhaps only about 10% is broken down there to glucose and lactate. It is carried by the portal vein to the liver where by far the larger part of its metabolism takes place. Liver cells are freely permeable to fructose without the aid of insulin. The break-down of fructose occurs chiefly by way of the fructose-1-phosphate pathway which is catalyzed by the enzyme fructokinase. This process is also not dependent

upon insulin, in contrast with the first steps in the metabolism of glucose which are insulin-dependent. The metabolism of fructose takes place rapidly with a half-life of about 18 minutes. Pursuing fructose metabolism further, fructose-1-phosphate is converted to glyceraldehyde and dihydroxyacetone phosphate. When adequate amounts of insulin are present, these are oxidized to pyruvate and finally to intermediates in the Krebs cycle. However, when the concentration of insulin is inadequate, glyceraldehyde and dihydroxyacetone phosphate are converted to glucose.[13]

As may be seen from the above, it is easy for fructose to be absorbed and its metabolism started in the liver without the aid of insulin. From that point on, insulin is necessary for complete, normal metabolism. It follows from this that if the diabetic patient is to include fructose in the diet plan, adequate amounts of insulin, either of endogenous or exogenous origin, must be present. In any case, fructose leaves the liver in the form of glucose, lactate, or other metabolites whence they may be utilized as such or converted to glycogen. The utilization of fructose other than by the liver is small and does not occur at all in the brain which contains no fructokinase. Consequently, the giving of fructose intravenously in hypoglycemic coma due to insulin is ineffective and may be detrimental.[14]

One must keep in mind that a goodly amount of fructose is included in the food intake of most persons, diabetic or nondiabetic. The actual amount depends upon the quantity of fruit and of sucrose in prepared foods. If fructose is used, 1 ounce (30 g) a day should be adequate as a sweetener and in the patient with well-controlled diabetes, this should pose no great problem. However, one must take into account the caloric value of nearly 4 kcal/g and this must be allowed for. The use of fructose in larger amounts than mentioned above should not be encouraged, particularly in patients whose control of diabetes is poor. All told, the advantages of using fructose as such in the diet are ultimately few.

Sorbitol. Sorbitol, a polyalcohol or "sugar alcohol," is present in certain plants, fruits, and seaweeds. It results from the hydrogenation of glucose. It is absorbed from the intestine more slowly than fructose so that osmotic diarrhea often occurs when sorbitol is taken daily in amounts greater than 30–40 g. Sorbitol is rapidly oxidized to fructose. At the present time it is often used in ice cream, chewing gum, and many prepared foods. The rationale for its use arises from the assumption that sorbitol dehydrogenation and fructose phosphorylation by the liver of a diabetic person proceed at a normal rate without the presence of insulin. Sorbitol yields 4 kcal/g and has little advantage over fructose. However, if it is used, one need not fear that it poses any special threat in the causation of neuropathy because following ingestion it is metabolized into fructose and then through the usual pathways.

Xylitol. The sweetness of xylitol, another sugar alcohol, is similar to that of fructose. After absorption from the bowel, it is taken up by the liver where it is broken down to trioses in the glycolytic pathway. As with certain other sweetening agents, it yields 4 kcal/g. It is said that of the nutritive preparations, it is the least likely to cause dental caries and from a medical standpoint, is preferable to the others in the manufacture of chewing gum. Xylitol is present naturally in many plants, including trees and in fruits as strawberries and raspberries. If xylitol is used as a sweetening agent, large amounts should be avoided because of the possibility of osmotic diarrhea. It has been reported as tumorigenic in animals but has not been shown to be so in humans.

Mannitol. This is another of the trio of sugar alcohols. Derived by reduction from fructose, it is a white crystalline sweet substance. In addition to its use commercially as a sweetening agent, as in chewing gum, it has been employed intravenously as an osmotic diuretic in patients with oliguria or anuria when other measures have failed.

Saccharin. The synthesis of saccharin was reported in 1880 by Fahlberg and Remsen working at Johns Hopkins University, and 5 years later a United States patent was awarded to Fahlberg for the manufacture of saccharin compounds. By the turn of the century, saccharin was in general although limited use. During both World Wars I and II, usage increased greatly due to the rationing and shortage of sucrose, especially in Europe.

During the 1960s and 1970s, there was a great increase in the demand of consumers for low-calorie products, especially beverages which, in recent years, have accounted for approximately ¾ of all saccharin consumed as a food additive in the United States. Saccharin is used widely in canned fruits, fruit preserves, salad dressings, and chewing gum. Tooth pastes, mouthwashes and drugs, both prescription and non-prescription, may contain saccharin. Saccharin has been used by many diabetic patients but by even greater numbers of nondiabetic persons who attempt to follow a diet reduced in calories in order to lose weight or prevent weight gain.

In 1949, there occurred the first long-term testing of saccharin in relation to possible causation of cancer. Six years later, the National Academy of Sciences reported that saccharin was safe for human consumption. However, in 1958, an important regulation came into effect by action of the Congress in including the now well-publicized "Delaney Clause" in an amendment to the Food, Drug and Cosmetic Act of 1938. This clause prohibits the sale of food additives if they have been found to be carcinogenic in animals or humans.

Prior to this, as indicated above, studies of saccharin had begun in experimental animals including rats, mice, hamsters, and monkeys. In 1977, Canadian workers issued a preliminary report of the results of experiments in rats which suggested a link between saccharin and carcinoma of the urinary bladder. Extremely high doses of saccharin given to two successive generations of rats were reported to result in the development of significantly more bladder tumors, both benign and malignant, in male animals than in control rats.[15] Following this report, unpublished at that time, the FDA in 1977 proposed a ban on the use of saccharin in foods. However, in October of that year, the Congress voted a moratorium on such ban for 18 months. At its expiration, futher legislation by the Congress extended the moratorium to June 30, 1981,[16] following which it was again extended until at least August, 1983. As of August 1984 the product is still available.

Although the subject is regarded by some as controversial, firm evidence is lacking to indicate that saccharin is carcinogenic in humans. In an article published by Kalkhoff and Levin in 1978,[17] comparing the results of 10 epidemiologic studies of artificial sweeteners, only the one by Howe and co-workers[18] indicated any statistical relationship in that there was a 1.6 risk ratio for men using saccharin as opposed to those never using this agent. In common with other studies, no risk was found for women. The work of Howe et al. has been criticized as regards methods and analyses.[19] The study of Kessler,[20] who failed to find a connection between diabetes and bladder cancer, is of special interest since it was a prospective study among 21,447 diabetic patients of the Joslin Clinic. The series was followed from 1930 to 1959 with no increased bladder cancer mortality during that period. It seems safe to draw a general conclusion, that until significant and trustworthy evidence is presented, saccharin is safe for human consumption.

Cyclamate. Cyclamate was discovered in 1937 by Sveda at the University of Illinois but it was not until 1950 that it was marketed under the trade name of Sucaryl (Abbott Laboratories). It became popular because it did not leave a bitter after-taste such as noted by many persons following the use of saccharin alone. In the 1960s, cyclamate was used widely, often along with saccharin, in low- or no-calorie soft drinks, canned fruit, etc., in addition to chewing gum, mouthwashes, tooth pastes, and other products. By 1967, 18,000,000 pounds of cyclamates were being used annually.

Following the passage of the Delaney Clause (see above discussion regarding saccharin) in 1958, the FDA placed cyclamate in the list of products "Generally Recognized as Safe" (GRAS). Seven years later, the FDA reported that there was no evidence that cyclamate was a hazard to health and in 1968 the National Academy of Sciences re-stated a former opinion that up to 5 g of cyclamate a day presented no hazard to adults. However, in 1969, studies at the Wisconsin Alumni Research Foundation were reported to show a significant frequency of bladder tumors in mice. A Canadian investigation resulted in finding tumors (50% of them cancerous) in the urinary bladder of second generation rats fed a mixture of cyclamate and saccharin in a ratio of 10:1 (used in many soft drinks at that time). Following this, cyclamate was removed from the GRAS list and in August, 1970, the FDA banned the use of cyclamate effective September 11, 1970. To date, efforts to have the ban lifted have been unsuccessful. Although the prohibition of the use of cyclamates in food products in the U.S.A. was followed by similar bans in some countries, the substance is still available in many others.

Aspartame. Aspartame is a dipeptide formed by a synthetic combination of two naturally occurring amino acids, L-aspartic acid and the methyl ester of phenylalanine. Although it yields 4 kcal/g, it is approximately 200 times sweeter than sucrose so that its caloric production creates no difficulties. It has no known effect on glucose tolerance.

In 1974 it was approved by the Food and Drug Administration (FDA) for use in the United States for cold breakfast cereals, chewing gum, dry bases for beverages, instant coffee and tea, gelatin products, puddings and fillings, non-dairy toppings, and as a table-top sweetener in powder and tablet form. However, final permission to market aspartame was not given until October, 1981 due to the time taken to carry out further studies of possible toxicity. In July, 1983 it was approved by the FDA for use additionally in liquid preparations as carbonated soft drinks.

Aspartame was developed by G.D. Searle and Co. of Chicago, and is sold by them under the brand names of NutraSweet and Equal. It loses its sweet taste if exposed to high temperatures as in cooking. Extensive testing has shown it to be non-toxic except in persons with the rare inherited disorder of phenylketonuria in which there is a marked reduction in phenylalanine hydroxylase activity. Although its general use is regarded by most authorities as safe,[20a] the controversy lingers. As of April 1984, the FDA had denied petitions to withdraw aspartame from the market.

REFERENCES

1. West, K.M.: Diet therapy of diabetes: An analysis of failure. Ann. Intern. Med. 79:425, 1973.
2. Cahill, G.F.,Jr., Etzwiler, D.D., Freinkel, N.: Blood glucose control in diabetes. Diabetes 25:237, 1976.
3. Editorial: "Control" and diabetic complications. Diabetes Care 1:204, 1978.
4. Food and Nutrition Board, National Academy of Sciences—National Research Council: Recommended Daily Dietary Allowances. Washington, D.C. 1979.
5. American Diabetes Association: Principles of nutrition and dietary recommendations for individuals with diabetes mellitus: 1979. Diabetes Care 2:520, 1979.
5a. Editorial: High carbohydrate, high-fibre diets for diabetes mellitus. Lancet 1:741, 1983.
5b. Diabetes Care and Education Practice Group: Fiber and the Patient with Diabetes Mellitus: A Summary and Annotated Bibliography. 2nd Ed. Chicago, American Dietetic Association, 1982.
6. Anderson, J.W.: Plant fiber treatment for metabolic diseases. In: M.P. Cohen and P.P. Foa (Eds.): Special Topics in Endocrinology and Metabolism, v. 2, New York, Alan R. Liss, 1981, pp. 2–42.
7. Anderson, J.W., Midgley, W.R., Wedman, B.: Fiber and diabetes. Diabetes Care 2:369, 1979. (See bibliography here for other papers.)
8. Jenkins, D.J.A., Wolever, T.M.S., Hockaday, T.D.R., et al.: Treatment of diabetes with guar gum. Lancet 2:779, 1977.
9. Jenkins, D.J.A., Wolever, T.M.S., Nineham, R., et al.: Guar crispbread in the diabetic diet. Br. Med. J. 2:1744, 1978.
9a. Jenkins, D.J.A.: Lente carbohydrate: A newer approach to the dietary management of diabetes. Diabetes Care 5:634, 1982.
9b. Diabetes Care and Education Practice Group: Diabetes Mellitus and Glycemic Responses to Different Foods: A Summary and Annotated Bibliography. Chicago, American Dietetic Association, 1983.
9c. Rosenberg, I.H.: Starch blockers—still no calorie-free lunch. N. Engl. J. Med. 307:1444, 1982.
9d. Liener, I.E., Donatucci, D.A., Tarcza, J.C.: Starch blockers: a potential source of trypsin inhibitors and lectins. Am. J. Clin. Nutr. 39:196, 1984. (See this article for further references.)
9e. McDonald, J.: Alcohol and diabetes. Diabetes Care 3:629, 1980.
9f. Kissin, B.: Alcohol abuse and alcohol-related illnesses. In: J.B. Wyngaarden, L.H. Smith Jr. (Eds.): Cecil Textbook of Medicine, 16th Ed. Philadelphia, W.B. Saunders Co., 1982, pp. 2016–2022.
10. U.S. Food and Drug Administration (1978): Code of Federal Regulations. Title 21—Food and Drugs, Section 101.9: Nutritional labelling of food. Washington, D.C., Office of the Federal Register. pp. 17–22.
11. Wunschel, I.M., Sheikholislam, B.M.: Is there a role for dietetic foods in the management of diabetes and/or obesity? Diabetes Care 1:247, 1978.
12. Select Committee on Sugar Substitutes, American Diabetes Association: Symposium on Sweeteners, Diabetes Care 1:209, 1978.
13. Koivisto, V.A.: Fructose as a dietary sweetener in diabetes mellitus. Diabetes Care 1:241, 1978.
14. Woods, H.F., Alberti, K.G.M.M.: Dangers of intravenous fructose. Lancet 2:1354, 1972.

15. Arnold, D.L., Moodie, C.A., Grice, H.C., et al.: Long-term toxicity of orthotoluenesulfonamide and sodium saccharin in the rat. Toxicol. Appl. Pharmacol. *52*:113, 1980.

16. National Health and Welfare Ministry (Canada): Restrictions on Saccharin in Drug Products. Ottawa, Bull. No. 100/77, 1977. (Quoted by National Cancer Institute, U.S.A.): Progress Report to the Food and Drug Administration concerning the National Bladder Cancer Study, 1980.

17. Kalkhoff, R.A., Levin, M.E.: The saccharin controversy. Diabetes Care *1*:211, 1978.

18. Howe, G.R., Burch, J.D., Miller, A.B., et al.: Artificial sweeteners and human bladder cancer. Lancet *2*:578, 1977.

19. Editorial: Bladder cancer and saccharin. Lancet *2*:592, 1977.

20. Kessler, I.J.: Cancer mortality among diabetics. J. Natl. Cancer Inst. *44*:673, 1970.

20a. Horwitz, D.L., Bauer-Nehrling, J.K.: Can aspartame meet our expectations? J. Am. Dietet. Assoc. *83*:142, 1983.

18 Obesity and Diabetes

Ramachandiran Cooppan and Thomas M. Flood

The relationship between obesity and diabetes has been noted for many years, even in the earliest descriptions of the disease. Today, the majority of patients over the age of 50 years with maturity-onset Type II (non-insulin-dependent) diabetes are overweight. In these individuals, excess weight is viewed as a factor in precipitating overt diabetes, especially in those predisposed by heredity.

In 1916 Dr. Elliott P. Joslin wrote that "No pre-existent abnormal condition has occurred more frequently among my diabetic patients than has obesity. Obesity affords a splendid opportunity for the physician in which to practice preventive medicine."[1] Throughout his long life, much of his effort both in prevention and treatment, was directed toward the avoidance or correction of obesity in his patients, through caloric restriction and exercise.

The details for the dietary treatment of diabetic patients are given in the preceding chapter. Considerations applicable to the obese patient, are presented here.

DEFINITION

If the desirable (or ideal) body weight for height and age (see Appendix F) is exceeded by 20% or more, obesity is said to exist. "Morbid" obesity is usually defined as a weight which is twice that of the desirable. Lesser degrees of overweight are harder to define. However, these standards for "ideal" weight are generally established by insurance groups and may not be representative of the whole population, because they are based on those insured persons who, by observation, showed the best survival. The extent of the problem of obesity is shown in the data collected by the United States Public Health Service, which indicate that 14% of men and 23.8% of women in the United States aged 20 years and older are 20% or more overweight.[2]

ETIOLOGY AND DEVELOPMENT

Overeating plays a dominant role in the etiology of obesity. Increased caloric intake combined with a more sedentary way of life has become the norm in many affluent Western societies. Other metabolic, genetic, neurologic, psychologic, and socioeconomic factors also play a role.

Animal studies have shown that in the development of obesity, fat cells undergo an increase in number as well as in size and lipid content. In obese humans, Hirsch and Knittle et al.[3,4] found that these individuals similarly have a greater *number of fat cells* with varying degrees of lipid content. It was also noted that, in general, those subjects with childhood obesity tended to have the greatest degree of fat cell hyperplasia (increased cell number). When obesity occurred during puberty or adolescence or in later life, *adipose cell hypertrophy* (increased cell size) made a greater contribution. This led to the hypothesis that once fat cells have increased in number, no change can be effected, other than decrease in size, no matter how much weight is lost by diet or other measures.

Knittle et al.[5] noted that after the age of 2 years, one can detect significant differences in adipose tissue growth and development between obese and non-obese children. Obese children have attained adult levels per fat cell size by 2 years of age, and thereafter enlarge the fat stores exclusively by increasing the number of fat cells. In non-obese children there is no major change in the fat depots until around puberty when both cell size and number increase. The underlying mechanism for this cell hyperplasia or hypertrophy is not known. Undoubtedly, increased caloric intake is of utmost importance, apart from the unknown contribution of genetic and hypothalamic influences. The tendency to obesity starts at this early stage of life and adds to the already frustrating problems of treating these individuals. Detailed reviews of the problem of obesity have been published by Mann[6] and Bray.[7] An analysis of hormonal and metabolic factors has been reviewed by Salans.[8]

ASSOCIATION OF OBESITY WITH OTHER DISEASES

Hypertension, diabetes, respiratory and gallbladder diseases are more frequently linked to those who are obese than to those in the nonobese general population.[6,9] In diagnosing hypertension in obese persons, it should be remembered that use of the standard blood pressure cuff may result in an error of 8 to 12 mm Hg in overestimating the pressure. The use of a 42 cm cuff bladder is recommended.

In the Framingham experience, persons who were 20% or more overweight developed high blood pressure 10 times more frequently than normal-weight individuals.[10] Furthermore, men whose weight remained at an appropriate level for age and height over a 20-year period of adult life, had only one-fifth as much hypertension in middle life as those who gained weight. The relationship of obesity to cerebrovascular disease is even more impressive. In the Evans County (Georgia, U.S.A.) prospective study,[11] neither obesity nor excess weight gain after age 20 years were associated with coronary heart disease, but both were linked with cerebrovascular disease. Overweight men at age 20 years who had later gained more than 30 pounds, had 3 times as much cerebrovascular disease as those with no weight gain. Whether this is due to the increase in blood pressure with obesity has not been definitely assessed. Of relevance in this regard is the well-known, frequent association of obesity with not only diabetes but also hypertension and increased levels of cholesterol and triglyceride in the blood. The possible interaction of one or more of these risk factors in the causation of atherosclerosis, e.g., cerebrovascular disease, must be considered (see Chapter 11).

INSULIN AND INSULIN RECEPTORS

In 1935 Ogilvie suggested that obesity might cause diabetes to emerge by overstimulating the pancreas, thereby leading to pancreatic exhaustion. This thought was based on observations of pancreatic hyperplasia in obesity.[12] Studies of forearm metabolism by Rabinowitz and Zierler gave results indicating the presence of insulin insensitivity in obese subjects.[13]

Since the development of the radioimmunoassay for insulin, the hyperinsulinism of the obese state has been repeatedly documented.[14-16] Basal levels of insulin are elevated and increase excessively after a glucose challenge. The insulin resistance in

this state has been found to be correlated with a decrease of insulin receptors on the fat cell.[17] These receptors serve two major functions. First, they allow the specific recognition of insulin molecules among the other circulating hormones, and second, they trigger a series of intracellular events resulting in increased transport of substrates or alterations of enzyme activity. The exact nature of the insulin receptor has not been fully elucidated but it is thought to be a glycoprotein. Apart from stimuli like exercise, pH, and food intake, the insulin molecule can "downregulate" its own receptor. In the presence of hyperinsulinemia, the number of receptors falls, leading to a state of insulin resistance.

It has been noted that with a low caloric diet, the number of receptors increases and the insulin levels decrease even before substantial weight loss occurs, suggesting that overeating rather than the mass of adipose tissue is responsible for the hyperinsulinism and insulin resistance.[18] This is in keeping with clinical observations that most obese patients consume diets rich in carbohydrates that stimulate excess insulin production.

In obese patients with diabetes, however, studies have shown that despite basal hyperinsulinemia, insulin levels do not increase following a glucose challenge to the same degree as in obese nondiabetics.[19,20] In the study by Genuth,[20] the 24-hour insulin production was calculated to be 31 units in nondiabetic persons of normal weight, 114 in obese nondiabetics, 14 units in thin adult diabetics, 46 units in obese adult diabetics, and 4 in juvenile diabetics. In addition, postprandial delivery of insulin in the obese, frankly diabetic person was only 25% of the daily total compared to 60% in normal and nondiabetic obese persons.

Given the fact that the majority of maturity-onset diabetic patients are overweight, one may view the chronic obese state in the genetically prone individual as a predisposing factor in precipitating the clinical syndrome. It is more likely to be the duration, rather than the degree, of obesity that leads to carbohydrate intolerance.[21]

DIAGNOSIS

The diagnosis of obesity is fairly obvious from inspection and consideration of height and body weight. For epidemiologic and other studies, improved indices of obesity have been sought. As mentioned earlier, height and weight tables for age and sex are mainly derived from insurance data and are useful for clinical assessment in office practice. The results of the test in which special calipers are used to measure triceps or subscapular skinfold thickness are said to correlate better with the assessment of total body fat. However, this test measures mainly subcutaneous fat and does not determine the fat in the other body locations. The study by Montoye gives a tabulation of the 20th, 50th, and 80th percentile levels for age and sex.[22] A useful measurement is the body mass index, which is calculated by dividing the weight (in kg) by the height (in meters squared). Indices of about 27 for men and 25 for women are equivalent to 120% of desirable body weight in each instance.

PREVENTION AND TREATMENT

The initial objective in dealing with any disease is prevention. With obesity, however, this is an elusive goal. If the data of Hirsch are accepted, then the problems start at infancy, and in those genetically predisposed, probably at conception. The most reasonable approach is to advise all members of families with strong diabetic backgrounds to guard against excessive weight gain. One has to contend with cultural, socioeconomic, and psychologic factors, all of which play a role in the development of obesity.

The treatment of the obese diabetic and the obese nondiabetic are, for practical purposes, the same initially. The desired objective is weight loss that will be gradual and sustained, using a hypocaloric diet as the first, and hopefully only, step in treatment.[23]

Unfortunately, the universal experience over the years has been that unless patients have unusual motivation, the percentage of those who do not regain the weight after a few or several years, is quite small.[24] This poor result has led to a great deal of frustration for physician and patient. It has produced numerous diet programs, some with poor nutritional principles and erroneous scientific bases. Furthermore, there are many publications in which methods for weight reduction are described with claims for success.

The results of the short-term study of Doar et al.[25] illustrated the value of treatment by diet alone. In 118 obese patients with newly diagnosed maturity-onset diabetes, there was an average reduction in the fasting plasma glucose from approximately 250 to 170 mg/dl within 2 months on a restricted diet. Random levels were below 140 mg/dl in 59% of the group. The mean weight loss in the two months was stated to be 5.1 ± 4.0 kg.

In the study by Berger et al.[26] that extended over 5 years, 35 of the 70 patients were excessively obese with subclinical diabetes. Their weight had not changed significantly; there was further deterioration of glucose tolerance, and overt diabetes developed in 10 of them. In the remaining 35 patients who had decreased their weight by 20%, the glucose tolerance became normal. There was a significant correlation between the weight loss and improved glucose tolerance. However, in those patients who, at the start of the study, were more than 100% overweight and who were more than 50 years old, there was no correlation between weight loss and increased glucose tolerance.

Protein Diets

Protein-Sparing Modified Fast. In 1976 Bistrian et al.[27] reported the use of a protein-sparing, modified fast (PSMF) in the treatment of obese diabetics. A diet was used that provided protein (1 to 1.5 g/kg/d) in the form of lean meat, supplemented with potassium, calcium, iron, and vitamins. Fluids were allowed ad libitum. In this study, 7 obese patients with maturity-onset diabetes, who received 30 to 100 units of insulin per day, were put on a PSMF diet which was discontinued after 0 to 19 days (mean, 6.5 days). Three patients showed a positive nitrogen balance despite the low caloric intake. Improvement was noted in the lipid profile, blood pressure, and carbohydrate metabolism. Of the 7 patients, 5 achieved weight losses of > 40 lb in an outpatient setting. At intervals of 5 to 12 months, substantial weight loss was maintained.

The rationale for the diet, as compared to others with a similar decrease in calories, was thought to be the marked lowering of serum insulin levels, thereby reducing the antilipolytic effect of insulin which might otherwise oppose the effects of treatment. Hirsch in a review[28] questions the validity of the diet. The study of Yang and van Itallie[29] showed that regardless of the nature of caloric intake, fat loss due to a hypocaloric diet is strictly proportional to the calorie deficit.

From the results of their study, Dehaven et al.[30] concluded that, compared with mixed diets, hypocaloric protein diets offered no advantages with respect to nitrogen metabolism and, in fact, resulted in greater sodium depletion, a decrease in sympathetic nervous system activity, and the development of orthostatic hypotension.

Liquid Protein Diets. The protein-sparing principle was further extended and popularized by Linn and Stuart in their book entitled "The Last Chance Diet Book."[30a] Here protein supplements were used with or without small amounts of carbohydrate. There was a tremendous increase in the use of liquid protein diets and with it came a series of unfortunate deaths.[31,31a] The quality of protein in these diets (not to be confused with the biologically high quality protein of PSMF) was lacking in certain essential amino acids and led to various electrolyte imbalances. As a result of these deaths, the Department of Food and Nutrition of the American Medical Association[31] expressed its concern and recommended that the diet not be used without proper medical supervision. In a concise and provocative editorial, Felig expressed skepticism with regard to the unique value of low protein diets in sustained weight loss and concern regarding the safety of such diets, especially those of the liquid protein type.[31a]

Other Methods of Weight Loss

Another approach to the patient with diabetes who is 50 lb or more overweight is used by Davidson.[32] Here a 1-week fast is initiated before the hypocaloric diet is used, and diuretic and insulin therapy are discontinued if appropriate. If weight loss is slower than predicted, then shorter fasts are used on an out- or in-patient basis.

Before considering diet treatment a failure, an adequate trial should be carried out. This usually takes 3 to 4 months. In those patients who remain hyperglycemic and symptomatic, oral hypoglycemic drugs may be used. Obese patients with long-duration, maturity-onset diabetes, often fail to respond to oral agents and require insulin treatment. The use of oral agents in short-term trials has been reported to result in increased activity of insulin receptors and a decrease in hyperglycemia.[33] The exact mechanism of this effect is not clear but recently Kolterman et al.[33a] have shown that glyburide (glibenclamide), a "second generation" sulfonylurea, increases adipocyte insulin binding after long-term (18 mos), but not after short-term (3 mos) treatment. They conclude that it acts not only by increasing the secretion of insulin but also, in long-term treatment, by increasing postreceptor function and reducing the basal output of glucose from the liver.

Treating the "Total" Patient

Besides the various physical difficulties attendant to diabetes, obese patients often have underlying psychologic problems. Hirsch, in his review,[28] refers to a study of Rand and Stunkard[34] in which 84 obese patients completed a questionnaire. Only 6% cited obesity as the reason why psychoanalytic treatment had been sought, whereas depression, anxiety, and other problems were the more common reasons given. Of these individuals, 19% lost 40 lb or more, and 54% lost 20 lb or more. Over the 4-year treatment period, the average weight loss was 21 lb. The exact mechanism of weight loss with psychoanalysis is not clearly known, but the findings in this study emphasize the need to consider the total patient as an individual and not to concentrate on the mass of adipose tissue alone.

Details about the use of jejuno-ileal bypass and of gastric stapling in "morbidly" obese persons are beyond the scope of this discussion, but may

be obtained in a recent review by Bray and Benfield.[35]

Team Approach

In summary, the treatment of the obese patient, diabetic or nondiabetic, remains a difficult problem that is increasing in magnitude. A team approach in a setting committed to this type of treatment is necessary for maximal success. However, this may involve the efforts of physicians, dietitians, teaching nurses, licensed nurse practitioners, clinical psychologists, social workers and psychiatrists, and in massively (morbidly) obese patients, the surgeon.

Admittedly, such a team is not available for most physicians. Nevertheless, with the aid of some ancillary personnel and a well-organized program in which patients are seen frequently, the physician may achieve a reasonably good success rate. To this end, in the section which follows, certain suggestions are offered.

PRACTICAL SUGGESTIONS FOR THE TREATMENT OF THE OBESE DIABETIC PATIENT

1. Explain the mechanism, in lay terms, whereby diet and weight loss represent specific therapy for lowering elevated blood glucose levels. The patient must be counseled as to how caloric restriction and weight reduction will have a specific impact on the elevated blood glucose. For certain individuals, an explanation of the role of cell receptors may be appropriate and effective. For many patients this may not be understood and a simpler explanation will be required.

2. Take a comprehensive diet history. One must ferret out those eating habits which may be responsible for obesity and draw attention to those areas in which change will be necessary. A few of the eating patterns that frequently contribute to obesity include: evening snacking, alcoholic beverages (often with extra food), emotional overeating, and meal skipping followed later by excessive intake. These may not be apparent if the diet history is taken in a superficial way. It helps to have the cooperation of the spouse or other family member.

3. Take a history of past dieting. Most obese individuals have previously made a serious effort to lose weight and have achieved transient success only later to regain what had been lost. It is helpful to know the answers to such questions as: What motivated you to lose weight at that time? Why do you think you then regained the weight? Did you attend any weekly group meetings for education and support? How reduced in calories did your diet have to be in order to achieve significant weight loss? The answer to this last question can be of great importance. For every fortunate individual who loses weight easily as soon as excessive food consumption is cut back, there are literally scores of others for whom weight loss is a slow and emotionally painful process. For many of them, the caloric deprivation they require to achieve continuing weight loss is significantly beyond that ordinarily needed.

4. Take a weight history. It is helpful to have certain bench mark statistics to identify patterns of weight gain and devise effective reduction strategies. Has the patient been overweight since childhood? The times most often associated with accelerated weight gain are puberty, adolescence, marriage, pregnancy, menopause, retirement, occupational change, disability and death of a family member. On the other hand, the history may reveal that the patient has simply been gaining weight steadily in linear fashion without any precipitating event. Knowing the weight at the time the patient achieved full linear growth can also be valuable in terms of setting an ultimate objective and defining ideal body weight.

5. Push hard, especially at the beginning. As previously stated, the initial blood glucose-lowering response to caloric restriction seems to be related to proliferation of insulin receptors at the cell surface (including as yet ill-defined post-receptor intracellular events). This is triggered by the sudden decrease in endogenous insulin production which accompanies a cutback in calories consumed.

Most patients with Type II diabetes will both tolerate and benefit from a brief period of extremely restricted dieting at the onset of therapy. The physician may gain cooperation in this venture by explaining that an important purpose in following a weight-reduction diet is to help their bodies become more sensitive to the action of insulin. There are no controlled studies of how long this period of very restricted diet should last or what, if any, level of caloric reduction is best suited to initiate cell receptor response. One may prescribe arbitrarily a daily intake in the range of 600 to 1000 calories (with appropriate vitamin and mineral supplements) which should be low enough to initiate an insulin receptor response and yet protect against ill effects.

A small number (perhaps 10 to 20%) of patients with newly diagnosed Type II diabetes will not respond to diet therapy alone but continue to show significant hyperglycemia even with careful adherence to the restriction of calories. Failure to achieve any drop in the blood glucose level, despite a history indicating careful cooperation, is not an absolute sign that diet alone will be insufficient

therapy. It should, however, alert the physician to those patients who will continue to require frequent follow-up and who may ultimately show an early need for oral hypoglycemic agents or insulin. On the other hand, documentation of a dramatic drop in the blood glucose provides strong impetus for both patient and physician to continue a conservative therapeutic plan that is obviously proving successful.

6. Be enthusiastic. Many diabetic patients have struggled with excess weight for years. The inability to diet successfully has become a pervasive symbol of failure. Now they are faced with the need to manage a serious chronic disease and yet the mechanism is one that has eluded them up to this point. That diabetes has appeared is not sufficient, of itself, to provide the motivation for weight loss. These patients need enthusiasm and support from their physicians to motivate them to embark on a radical change in their eating habits, with the assurance that success will yield a high probability of excellent control of diabetes.

7. Set realistic goals. Although weight loss is usually a slow process, many patients do not realize this and become discouraged. They should be advised that an ongoing weight reduction of 1 to 2 pounds a week is desirable as long as it can be maintained. Furthermore, they need to be warned that a rapid drop in weight, often seen in the first days after commencing a diet, represents fluid loss and that this rate will not be maintained.

Patients should be instructed to weigh themselves no more than once a week since daily weighing may lead to frustration because of variable results. By the same token, failure to reach the goal of 1 to 2 pounds a week is a signal that diet compliance is suboptimal, or the caloric intake is still too high for that individual.

The *total* weight loss projected should also be realistic and it is often effective to set a goal which falls short of desirable body weight. In general, the more overweight the patient, the less likely it is that the diet plan will be totally effective in shedding all the excess pounds. This is because the psychologic or social problems which led to the obesity tend to be greater in these patients. In addition, the longer time span needed to lose this amount of weight simply affords more time and opportunity for the diet to be abandoned. It is far more effective to suggest to a patient who needs to lose, say 100 lb (45 kg), that a loss of 25 to 50 lb (11 to 22 kg) within a shorter time be aimed for first. Many patients who succeed in such an initial effort are buttressed by a physical and psychologic sense of well-being. As a result, the physician can negotiate additional weight loss if the patient seems motivated to continue the diet.

8. Suggest the use of outside help. Patients embarking upon a serious attempt at weight loss need regular follow-up and every possible support. Busy physicians are frequently unable to see these patients often enough to provide this ongoing supervision. The results often fall far short of those achieved with regular follow-up by registered dietitians and legitimate private weight-loss groups. The obese Type II diabetic can derive the same benefits as those dieting for cosmetic reasons and should be encouraged to affiliate with one of these groups. This advice is especially germane for those patients who are not showing the expected progress toward the desired goal.

9. Encourage physical activity. An exercise program should be an integral part of the treatment plan for all obese Type II diabetics. It is true that exercise alone is not an effective means of losing weight since the caloric expenditure required to burn excess fat is enormous. However, physical activity is an excellent method of combating boredom and lassitude, feelings which often lead to excess food consumption. In addition, the physical and mental sense of well-being that frequently accompanies "getting into shape" provides another support for the dieting diabetic. Naturally, other medical problems which are so severe as to contraindicate even simple exercises, must be respected.

10. Avoid the premature use of oral hypoglycemic agents or insulin. Caloric restriction alone is the recommended treatment for all obese individuals with newly diagnosed Type II diabetes. Occasionally patients may present with such extreme hyperglycemia that a temporary course of insulin is helpful in providing relief of symptoms or protection against the potential development of hyperosmolar coma. However, all too often one observes the typical obese Type II diabetic patient presenting with only moderate hyperglycemia who has been committed immediately to oral agents or insulin. In the worst examples, this error is compounded by the use of such agents without any attempt to prescribe an appropriate diet concomitantly.

11. Avoid premature hospitalization. It may be argued that a period of training and intense support is of benefit to the newly diagnosed diabetic. While this is certainly true for the insulin-dependent patient, it is seldom necessary for the obese Type II patient who will be treated with diet alone. The training in diet and other educational benefits of hospitalization must be balanced against the real possibility that the response to diet alone may not be dramatically swift and in the hospital environment the urge to "do something" may be so strong that one does not give a conservative approach the time necessary to show the full effect of diet alone, as shown by the case history which follows.

> Mrs. C.P. (J.C. #125115), a 79-year-old obese woman, came to the Joslin Clinic with a 5-week history of polyuria and polydipsia. Earlier that day a blood glucose of 280 mg/dl had been found at a neighborhood health center. She was 58 in (147 cm) tall and weighed 180 lb (81.8 kg). A repeat blood glucose was 272 mg/dl. Urine and plasma were negative for ketones and the plasma bicarbonate was not decreased. General medical problems included osteoarthritis involving the hips and knees, and a history of congestive heart failure treated successfully with digitalis therapy.
>
> She was admitted to the Diabetes Treatment Unit where a 1000-calorie diet was instituted. After 5 days there had been no change in the blood glucose which ranged from 260 to 300 mg/dl fasting and 210 to 270 mg/dl at 3 hours after a meal. Despite the temptation to add an oral agent, therapy with diet alone was continued and she was discharged 2 days later with blood glucose values still elevated. By the time of the initial follow-up visit in 8 weeks, she had lost 20 lb. (9.1 kg) and the blood glucose was 130 mg/dl at 2¼ hr p.c. By continuing to follow a restricted diet, her weight stabilized at 140 lb (63.6 kg). All blood glucose values remained normal over the next 4 years. Thus, on Feb. 23, 1984, at 4 hours after breakfast, the blood glucose was 108 mg/dl.

To overcome obesity is a worthwhile goal for both diabetic and nondiabetic persons. In the diabetic person, it affords an extra benefit, that of making possible better control of the disorder by increasing the numbers of functioning insulin receptors. Therefore, the physician, with the full cooperation of the patient, must make whatever practical efforts are necessary to bring the patient's weight down to a suitable level.

REFERENCES

1. Joslin, E.P.: The Treatment of Diabetes Mellitus. Philadelphia, Lea & Febiger, 1916, p. 230.
2. Johnson, A.S.: Overweight adults 20–74 years of age, United States, 1971–74. Vital and Health Statistics. Advance Data No. 51. Hyattsville, Md., Public Health Service, DHEW.
3. Hirsch, J., Knittle, J.L.: Cellularity of obese and nonobese human adipose tissue. Fed. Proc. 29:1516, 1970.
4. Hirsch, J., Batchelor, B.R.: Adipose tissue cellularity in human obesity. Clin. Endocrinol. Metab. 5:299, 1976.
5. Knittle, J.L., Ginsberg-Fellner, F., Brown, R.E.: Adipose tissue development in man. Am. J. Clin. Nutr. 30:762, 1977.
6. Mann, G.V.: The influence of obesity on health. N. Engl. J. Med. 291:(two parts) 178 and 226, 1974.
7. Bray, G.A.: The Obese Patient. Vol. IX in the series: Major Problems in Internal Medicine. Philadelphia, W.B. Saunders Co., 1976.
8. Salans, L.B.: Obesity and the adipose cell. In: P.K. Bondy, L.E. Rosenberg (Eds.): Metabolic Control and Disease. Philadelphia, W.B. Saunders Co., 1980, p. 495.

9. Bortz, W.M.: Metabolic consequences of obesity. Ann. Intern. Med. *71*:833, 1969.

10. Kannel, W.B., Brand, N., Skinner, J.J.,Jr., et al.: The relation of adiposity to blood pressure and development of hypertension: The Framingham Study. Ann. Intern. Med. *67*:48, 1967.

11. Heyden, S., Hames, C.G., Bartel, A., et al.: Weight and weight history in relation to cerebrovascular and ischemic heart disease. Arch. Intern. Med. *128*:956, 1971.

12. Ogilvie. R.F.: Sugar tolerance in obese subjects. A review of sixty-five cases. Quart. J. Med. *28*:345, 1935.

13. Rabinowitz, D., Zierler, K.L.: Forearm metabolism in obesity and its response to intra-arterial insulin. Characterization of insulin resistance and evidence for adaptive hyperinsulinism. J. Clin. Invest. *41*:2173, 1962.

14. Karam, J.H., Grodsky, G.M., Forsham, P.H.: Excessive insulin response to glucose in obese subjects as measured by immunochemical assay. Diabetes *12*:197, 1963.

15. Perley, M.J., Kipnis, D.M.: Plasma insulin responses to oral and intravenous glucose studies in normal and diabetic subjects. J. Clin. Invest. *46*:1954, 1967.

16. Bagdade, J.D., Bierman, E.L., Porte, D.,Jr.: The significance of basal insulin level in the evaluation of the insulin response to glucose in diabetic and nondiabetic subjects. J. Clin. Invest. *46*:1549, 1967.

17. Archer, J.A., Gorden, P., Roth, J.: Defect in insulin binding to receptors in obese man: amelioration with calorie restriction. J. Clin. Invest. *55*:166, 1975.

18. Bar, R.S., Roth, J.: Insulin receptor status in disease states of man. Arch. Intern. Med. *137*:474, 1977.

19. Kipnis, D.M.: Insulin secretion in diabetes mellitus. Ann. Intern. Med. *69*:891, 1968.

20. Genuth, S.M.: Plasma insulin and glucose profiles in normal, obese and diabetic persons. Ann. Intern. Med. *79*:812, 1973.

21. Bierman, E.L. et al.: Obesity and diabetes. The odd couple. Am. J. Clin. Nutr. *21*:1434, 1968.

22. Montoye, H.J., Epstein, F.H., Kjelsberg, M.O.: The measurement of body fatness. A study in a total community. Am. J. Clin. Nutr. *16*:417, 1965.

23. Stone, D.B.: Treatment of the obese diabetic patient. Mod. Treatment *4*:1181, 1967.

24. Sohar, E., Sneh, E.: Follow-up of obese patients: 14 years after a successful reducing diet. Am. J. Clin. Nutr. *26*:845, 1973.

25. Doar, J.W.H., Thompson, M.E., Wilde, C.E., Sewell, P.F.J.: Influence of treatment with diet alone on oral glucose tolerance test and plasma sugar and insulin levels in patients with maturity onset diabetes mellitus. Lancet *1*:1263, 1975.

26. Berger, M., Baumhoff, E.E., Gries, F.A.: Gewichtsreduktion und Glucose-Intoleranz bei Adipositas: Deutsch. Med. Wochenschr. *101*:307,1976.

27. Bistrian, B.R., Blackburn, G.L., Flatt, J.P., et al.: Nitrogen metabolism and insulin requirements in obese diabetic adults on a protein sparing modified fast. Diabetes *25*:494, 1976.

28. Hirsch, J.: What's new in the treatment of obesity? In: N. Freinkel (Ed.): The Year in Metabolism. New York, Plenum, 1977, p. 169.

29. Yang, M.U., Van Itallie, T.B.: Composition of weight lost during short-term weight reduction: metabolic responses of obese subjects to starvation and low-calorie ketogenic and non-ketogenic diets. J. Clin. Invest. *58*:722, 1976.

30. DeHaven, J., Sherwin, R., et al.: Nitrogen and sodium balance and sympathetic nervous system activity in obese subjects treated with a low-calorie protein or mixed diet. N. Engl. J. Med. *302*:477, 1980.

30a.Linn, R., Stuart, S.L.: The Last Chance Diet Book. Secaucus, New Jersey, Lyle Stuart, 1976.

31. Protein diets. FDA Drug Bull. *8*:2, Jan.-Feb. 1978.

31a.Felig, P.: Four questions about protein diets (Editorial). N. Engl. J. Med. *298*:1025, 1978.

32. Davidson, J.K.: Symposium: Controlling diabetes mellitus with diet therapy. Postgrad. Med. *59*:114, 1976.

33. Olefsky, J.M., Reaven, G.M.: Effects of sulfonylurea therapy to mononuclear leukocytes of diabetic patients. Am. J. Med. *60*:89, 1976.

33a.Kolterman, O.G., Gray, R.S., Shapiro, G., et al.: The acute and chronic effects of sulfonylurea therapy in Type II diabetic subjects. Diabetes *33*:346, 1984.

34. Rand, C., Stunkard, A.J.: Obesity and psychoanalysis. Am. J. Psychiatry *135*:5, May, 1978.

35. Bray, G.A., Benfield, J.R.: Intestinal bypass for obesity: a summary and perspective. Am. J. Clin. Nutr. *30*:121, 1977.

19 Insulin in the Treatment of Diabetes

Alexander Marble

The first injection of insulin, as prepared by Banting and Best, given to a human diabetic patient, was administered to a 14-year-old boy at the Toronto General Hospital on January 12, 1922.[1,2] Although 63 years have elapsed since then, all too often insulin is not employed when needed or if taken, it is not used in a way and in such dosage as to yield optimal results. It is not uncommon for patients to be treated with diet alone or with oral hypoglycemic agents despite consistently poor results in the control of diabetes. Conversely, many patients are treated with insulin in the presence of obesity when the better policy would be to encourage loss of body weight by careful following of a hypocaloric diet.

It has been estimated that in 1980 about 1.3 million diabetic patients in the United States took insulin at least once a day, that approximately 1.8 million were treated with oral hypoglycemic agents, that another 3 million were managed by dietary restriction alone, and that perhaps an additional 4 million had varying degrees of glucose intolerance without being aware of such or without having been diagnosed as diabetic. These figures, except for those regarding insulin and oral compounds, are gross estimates because of the lack of firm data and the tremendous difficulty in acquiring such.

During the past decade, there has been a gratifying ferment of activity regarding insulin and methods of its delivery to the patient. Advances include:

(a) Development of purer forms of insulin resulting in decreased immunogenicity and reduction of the frequency of lipoatrophy at the sites of injection.

(b) Simplification and uniformity of strengths of insulin so that now all of the insulin used in Canada and 90% or more of that used in the United States is of U-100 strength. Production of U-80 strength has ceased, and discontinuance of U-40 strength is under consideration (not marketed now by some manufacturers).

(c) Development of improved syringes, including those for the accurate measurement of low doses. Widely used are disposable, plastic syringe-needle units packaged to preserve sterility. The use of these is admittedly more expensive than that of glass syringes which with proper care may be used almost indefinitely.

(d) Development of devices for the continuous delivery of insulin subcutaneously (or intravenously for short terms). However, for the present and for some time to come, insulin by subcutaneous injection at times and in amounts prescribed by the physician or selected by the patient will continue to be the standard method of delivery.

(e) Production of insulin of human formulation by biosynthetic (DNA) and semi-synthetic (chemical) methods.

INDICATIONS FOR INSULIN TREATMENT

The indications for treatment with insulin are given in Table 19–1. In young patients with Type I diabetes, these are usually plain and compelling because of symptoms. In patients with onset in middle or later life and not acutely ill, the best rule is: if, on a diet which is found necessary to maintain the strength and ideal or desirable weight of a given person, glycosuria and significant hyperglycemia persist, then insulin should be prescribed without hesitation. Exceptions may be made for those middle-aged and elderly patients in whom one or another of the oral hypoglycemic compounds may be effective.

If other measures of treatment are ineffective, no patient should be denied the benefit of insulin. Insulin has unique advantages: it meets a specific body lack, at least in patients with Type I (insulin-dependent) diabetes; it acts directly on metabolic processes, although admittedly in treatment it is not delivered first to the liver as is the case with endogenous insulin; and its dose may be graduated to suit individual needs. On the other hand, maturity-onset, *obese* patients with Type II (non-insulin-dependent) diabetes should not be treated with insulin unless symptomatic, or in special situations (surgery, fever, illness, etc.), or unless by diet and exercise, prolonged efforts fail to bring about weight reduction and control of diabetes. Current evidence and thinking indicate that in such patients the hyperglycemia and (often) insulin resistance are due to a decrease in the number and affinity of receptors on cell membranes and not basically to insulin lack. Reduction in body weight through dietary restriction is usually followed by an increase in receptors and fall in blood glucose.

Table 19–1. Indications For Insulin Treatment

1. All patients with insulin-dependent (Type I) diabetes including not only those with onset of diabetes in childhood or adolescence but also many patients below the age of 40 years and a substantial number, perhaps 10 to 15%, of older patients with onset above the age of 40.
2. Patients of any age who have ketoacidotic or hyperosmolar coma.
3. Almost all pregnant diabetic women.
4. Many patients of any age with hyperglycemia (though ordinarily not truly insulin-dependent) who have febrile illnesses, who are receiving glucocorticoids, or who are undergoing or have just undergone major surgery under general anesthesia. In such situations, treatment with insulin often may be discontinued when the effect of the metabolic insult has passed.

Considering the great benefit conferred, the complications of insulin treatment are of relatively small consequence. In time most patients become accustomed to the inconvenience and discomfort of daily injections. *Allergic skin responses* are usually mild and now much less common with the use of purified insulins. Hypersensitivity which manifests itself soon after initiation of treatment as redness, swelling and soreness at sites of injection, gradually disappears. In general, beef is more immunogenic than pork insulin. *Lipodystrophy*—atrophy and/or hypertrophy of subcutaneous fat—at sites of insulin injections has no serious import and is chiefly a cosmetic nuisance. Insulin atrophies occur more frequently in women and children than in adult males (see Chapters 24 and 38). Lipodystrophy has become much less common with the advent of insulins of greater purity. *Hypoglycemia* is an ever-present possibility, but its occurrence can be minimized by careful planning as to the type, amount and timing of the three variables: diet, insulin, and exercise.

Despite the availability of rapid, intermediate and slowly acting insulins, securing "ideal" control of diabetes is not possible with conventional methods, especially with patients with Type I (insulin-dependent) diabetes. "Ideal" control implies that insulin is available for use in the body in exactly the amount needed at any given moment. To maintain physiologic conditions and thus to mimic Nature is such a large order that it cannot be completely filled, although such can be approached closely with the use of a "closed-loop" bench-model apparatus (Biostator)* for short periods and "open-loop" insulin "pumps" for extended treatment. Nevertheless, if care is taken, good or even excellent control of blood glucose may be obtained in most adult patients with stable diabetes and in many patients, young and old, with unstable diabetes, especially if those in the latter group will accept two or more injections of insulin daily. In fact, on a short-term basis (24-hour periods) in a special in-patient study, Rizza, Gerich, and co-workers[3] found no significant difference in the ability of closed-loop insulin infusion, open-loop continuous subcutaneous insulin infusion (CSII), and multiple-dose conventional insulin treatment in bringing the blood glucose of 6 insulin-dependent diabetics to a level comparable to that of normal control subjects. However, as a result of a 2-month out-patient study of 5 cooperative adult patients with Type I diabetes, Nathan et al.[3a] concluded that pump therapy was more effective than intensified

---

*Biostator Glucose Controller, Life Sciences Instruments Division, Miles Laboratories, Elkhart, Indiana 46515

conventional treatment. Similar findings were reported by Buysschaert et al.[3b] and by Schiffrin and Belmonte.[3c]

TYPES OF INSULIN

The characteristics of market insulins are shown in simplied form in Table 19–2. Durations of effect as shown in the table are based on clinical impressions in non-fasting patients taking mixed diets, and differ from data obtained in fasting normal and diabetic patients and animals and from results of studies on patients maintained on continuous glucose infusions.[4] In any case, there is variation from subject to subject and in a given subject, from time to time. If insulins are arranged as to promptness of action and duration of effect, the order is: regular (crystalline), semi-lente, isophane (NPH), lente, ultralente, and protamine zinc. The lente family of insulins includes three members whose action is relatively rapid (semi-lente), intermediate (lente), and slow (ultralente).

All types of insulin are effective and lend themselves to various programs that will yield success. The selection of a given program depends upon the individual patient, the type of diabetes, and the experience and judgment of the physician. Lente and isophane (NPH—Neutral Protamine Hagedorn) insulins possess much the same rate of action and duration of effect; for all practical purposes, they may be used interchangeably. Theoretically, lente insulin is preferable since it contains no protamine or other added protein and therefore might be expected to provoke fewer allergic responses. This factor is not a matter of great practical importance since the vast majority of patients tolerate NPH insulin well.

Except for the regular type, all insulins are modified to delay absorption from a subcutaneous or intramuscular depot and thereby to achieve a relatively slow action of extended duration. These modifications are made by the addition of zinc or protamine or both, in the presence of a suitable buffer. Insulins are currently available in the U.S.A. in U-40 and U-100 strengths (respectively, 40 and 100 units/ml). Regular insulin may also be obtained in U-500 (and, by special arrangement, U-5000) strength for use in patients with high insulin requirements. Although U-40 strength is now used very little in the United States, it is greatly favored in many other countries. For patients receiving two varieties of insulin in the same injection, both must be of the same strength. To avoid confusion and error, a single-scale insulin syringe should be used. Patients requiring only small doses of insulin may measure this conveniently and accurately, in a U-100 syringe with a 0.5 ml capacity.

Market insulins from solely beef or pork, or combined beef and pork sources may be obtained, at least in certain types and strengths, depending upon the manufacturer. Insulin has been extracted from the pancreases of a wide variety of other animals including fish, but these preparations are not available commercially.

PURITY OF INSULIN

Starting with the earliest days of insulin, pharmaceutical houses have attempted to make a product as nearly "pure" as possible with the techniques available. This resulted in a preparation which in the late 60s was of a high degree of purity but which contained tiny quantities of proinsulin, desamido-insulin, glucagon, pancreatic polypeptide, somatostatin, etc. Up until 1972, insulins marketed in the United States contained proinsulin

Table 19–2. Characteristics of Market Insulins

Types and Actions	Appearance	Added Protein*	Zinc Content (mg/100 units)	Buffer†	Action (hours)‡	
					Peak	Duration
RAPID						
Regular (crystalline)	Clear	None	0.01 –0.04	None	2–4	5–7
Semilente	Turbid	None	0.2 –0.25	Acetate	2–8	12–16
INTERMEDIATE						
Isophane (NPH)	Turbid	Protamine	0.016–0.04	Phosphate	6–12	18–24
Lente	Turbid	None	0.2 –0.25	Acetate	6–12	18–24
SLOW						
Ultralente	Turbid	None	0.2 –0.25	Acetate	16–18	20–24
Protamine zinc	Turbid	Protamine	0.2 –0.25	Phosphate	14–20	24–36

*NPH insulin contains 0.5 mg, and protamine zinc 1.25 mg, respectively, of protamine per 100 units.
†At present all Novo preparations are neutral in reaction; Lilly insulins have a pH of 7.2.
‡Approximate figures, based on clinical impressions in non-fasting patients with insulin-dependent diabetes, eating a mixed diet and engaging in their usual activities. There is considerable variation from patient to patient and from time to time in the same patient.

(measured as an index of purity) to the extent of more than 10,000 parts per million (ppm). Beginning about 1970, Eli Lilly & Co. added gel-filtration chromatography to the process of purification and called the product "single peak" insulin (less than 3000 ppm of proinsulin). Further purification by ion-exchange chromatography resulted in "improved single-peak" insulin with a proinsulin content of less than 50 ppm. Currently commercial purified insulins in the United States contain 20 to 25 ppm of proinsulin and, in certain types, less than 10 ppm. This is stated to be roughly comparable to the "monocomponent" or "purified" insulin of Novo Laboratories (value quoted for proinsulin-like substances of 1 ppm) and to the "rarely immunogenic" insulin of Nordisk Laboratories.[5,6]

TRADE NAMES OF INSULIN

In the United States for many years, insulin has been made and marketed by Eli Lilly and Company (trade name, Iletin) and by E.R. Squibb and Sons (generic names used). Burroughs Wellcome Company originally developed globin zinc insulin but no longer carries this product, and Squibb discontinued its production during 1981. Novo Laboratories of Copenhagen, Denmark, entered the U.S.A. market in 1980. Their products (distributed by Squibb-Novo) bear the following trade names: Actrapid (pork regular); Semitard (pork semilente); Monotard (pork lente); Lentard (mixed beef and pork lente); and Ultratard (beef ultralente). In addition, Nordisk insulins are now available in the United States from Nordisk-USA, an affiliate of Nordisk-Gentofte, Denmark. Nordisk markets purified insulins in U-100 strengths as follows: Velosulin (regular), Insulatard (NPH), and Mixtard (pre-mixed 30% regular and 70% NPH).

HUMAN INSULIN

As a result of work for some years which culminated in the period from 1963 to 1966, insulin was synthesized chemically in Germany by Meienhofer,[6a] in China by Kung,[6b] and in the United States by Katsoyannis,[6c] together with their respective co-workers. This indicated that insulin with human formulation can be made; however, the procedure is technically difficult and expensive. Also, insulin can and has been extracted from the human pancreas if the organ is obtained before auto-digestion takes place. Obviously, these two sources of human insulin do not lend themselves to large-scale production.

Semi-Synthetic Human Insulin

In addition to the above, "semi-synthetic" human insulin may be made by enzymatic procedures to remove the amino acid alanine from the terminal position 30 in the B-chain of purified pork insulin, and then replacing it with threonine. This results in a product with an amino acid sequence identical to that of insulin of human origin. Semi-synthetic "human" insulin is produced and marketed by Novo Laboratories. Extensive trial with patients has indicated no difference in clinical effect between this product and purified pork insulin.[6d] On both theoretical grounds and past experience, this is what one would expect since dealanation of pork insulin without replacement by threonine does not alter clinical effectiveness. The supply of semi-synthetic insulin is limited only by that of pork insulin from which it is made.

Recombinant DNA (rDNA) Human Insulin

In the making of insulin with rDNA techniques by inserting human gene sequences into plasmids of Escherichia coli, there is separate production of the A and B chains with two fermentations and subsequent sulphur linkage of the chains by chemical means. An alternate method involving one fermentation, may be used to produce proinsulin which then can be cleaved to provide human insulin and C-peptide. This procedure has the advantage of making available a supply of proinsulin and C-peptide for research.

Early in 1979 Goeddel et al.[7] reported success in the preparation of small amounts of human insulin, using E. coli fermentation as just described. By the latter part of that year, Eli Lilly and Co. had worked out methods by which quantities of this biosynthetic human insulin (BHI) large enough for clinical trials became available. Work then proceeded rapidly both in the large-scale production of BHI and in clinical trials in diabetes centers throughout the world. Intense investigation in laboratories and clinics resulted in enough data so that by 1980, symposia on BHI were held in Europe. Articles summarizing these results occupied 125 pages in the March-April, 1981 issue of DIABETES CARE.[8] Additional data were summarized in a special supplement to that journal late in 1982.[9] In the same year the product was approved by the Food and Drug Administration for marketing in the United States.

The results of studies carried out by many investigators and clinicians throughout the world have indicated that BHI prepared by rDNA techniques is equivalent to pancreatic human insulin chemically and biologically.[10] It is free not only of pancreatic peptides but also has been found free of contaminants of bacterial origin. In its action, human insulin of rDNA origin is almost identical to that of purified pork insulin (PPI) although there has been some evidence that it is absorbed a little more rapidly than PPI and its duration of action may be slightly shorter.[9] After it has been used for 6 months, the rate and degree of antibody formation is about the same as with PPI.[10a] On the other hand, when patients who have been on PPI for 3 months and then changed to rDNA insulin, there is a decrease in insulin-binding globulin.[10b] All told, experience to date indicates that it is a safe and effective product.

Should patients under treatment with insulin of conventional origin be shifted to the new type? There would be nothing against doing so, but unless there were present certain complications as insulin allergy, lipodystrophy or resistance, not controlled by PPI, there would seem no urgent reason to do so. One, and perhaps the most important, advantage of insulin of rDNA origin is freedom from the necessity of obtaining insulin by extraction from pancreases of animals, almost entirely cattle and swine. Although by no means certain, a shortage of such pancreases is possible in view of the steady increase in the number of persons with diabetes, estimated by the National Diabetes Commission to be about 6% (600,000 new cases) per year in the United States alone. To be taken into account is the number of hogs and cattle brought to abattoirs and the number of pancreases made available commercially for insulin production which might be curtailed in a national emergency.

INITIATION OF TREATMENT WITH INSULIN

If a patient is acutely ill, markedly symptomatic, or lives at such a distance from the physician's office or out-patient department as to preclude frequent visits, treatment with insulin—if such is judged to be necessary—should be started in a hospital. Indeed, initial treatment under hospital conditions is advantageous for *all* patients with insulin-dependent diabetes if the hospital's facilities include provision for the patient to be physically active, for weighed or measured diets, for an intensive program of both individual and group instruction, and for testing for sugar in the urine and blood at frequent intervals (using mostly capillary blood samples). Concentrated treatment for a week under such conditions and the association with others having similar problems provide the patient with knowledge and confidence that are difficult to acquire by other means. The Joslin Clinic has used this principle of treatment for many years and is currently privileged to have available a special 70-bed section ("Diabetes Treatment Unit") for ambulatory in-patients at the New England Deaconess Hospital (See Chapter 16). However, it is possible to achieve excellent results on an outpatient basis

and, in fact, most older patients are, of necessity, treated in this way. The procedure described below is designed especially for the adult outpatient who is not acutely ill (See Chapter 24 for Diabetes in Youth). Treatment in the hospital follows the same general principles but progresses faster and the teaching aspect is intensified. For essentials of the initial visit, including history, physical examination, laboratory studies, etc., see Chapter 16.

For the average adult outpatient who is not acutely ill and for whom hospitalization is deemed unnecessary, the initial dose of lente (or NPH) insulin may be chosen arbitrarily as 12 to 16 units to be given daily before breakfast. Instructions are given to test the urine for sugar just before each of the three main meals and also at bedtime, and to keep a record of the results of the tests in tabular form on a suitably ruled sheet (Fig. 19–1) or in a notebook or Clinilog.* The patient is told that the best index of the effect of the lente (or NPH) insulin is the result of the test of urine voided *just before the evening meal*. Instructions are given to increase the dose of insulin, 2 units at a time, until the results of the tests of the before-supper specimen become satisfactory. Two or 3 days are allowed between successive increases to avoid overshooting the mark. Specimens to be tested should consist of *urine from a second or later voiding*, rather than from the first voiding following the taking of food (meal or snack).

At first the patient is seen frequently (at intervals of 1 to 4 weeks) so that progress may be evaluated and advice given to supplement the general directions outlined above. During the visits, urine and blood glucose determinations are made, as well as periodic tests of glycosylated hemoglobin in selected patients. Home blood glucose monitoring is encouraged when indicated.

PATTERNS OF RESPONSE TO INSULIN

Patients respond differently to insulin depending upon the character of their diabetes. This in turn may be related to their capacity for endogenous insulin production which in the truly insulin-dependent diabetic usually decreases steadily as months and years elapse from the time of onset (Table 19–3). When an insulin dose is found with which the results of urine tests (and blood glucose test, if available) in the late afternoon are satisfactory, then one turns attention to the outcome of tests of specimens obtained just before the noon meal. If these are not satisfactory, a dose of regular insulin before breakfast is added to the treatment

---

*Ames Division, Miles Laboratories, Inc., Elkhart, Indiana 46515

Patient's Full Name

Please insert
dates, giving
year, month
and day

Street

Body
Weight. . . . . lbs.
(State whether with
or without clothing)

City & State

REPORT OF URINE TESTS

DATE 19	Before breakfast	Before noon meal	Before supper	At bedtime	INSULIN							REMARKS
					AM				PM			
					R.I.	NPH	LENTE	ULTRA LENTE OR PZI	R.I.	NPH OR LENTE		

NPH–NPH insulin
RI=Regular or crystalline insulin
PZI=Protamine zinc insulin
L=Lente

JC 13

Mail or
bring to Dr. _____

Joslin Clinic
One Joslin Place, Boston, Ma. 02215

Fig. 19–1. Form used at Joslin Clinic for recording results of urine tests for sugar.

Table 19–3. Patterns of Response to Insulin

Pattern	Type of response	Treatment indicated	Time of key urine and/or blood test
I	Stable	Lente or NPH insulin before breakfast	Before supper
II	Early instability. Significant glycosuria in forenoon	Regular insulin along with lente or NPH before breakfast	Before noon meal
III	Increased instability. Unacceptably high fasting blood glucose.	Add small dose of lente or NPH at bedtime (or before supper)	Before breakfast
IV	Still greater instability with marked bedtime glycosuria.	Add regular insulin along with lente or NPH before supper	Bedtime and before breakfast

schedule. At the start, only 4 or 6 units are added. The regular insulin is drawn into the syringe first and followed by the lente (or NPH) type. Thus both types are given in a single injection made daily before breakfast immediately after the syringe has been loaded. If time has elapsed (as with ''pre-filled'' syringes) and a precipitate has formed, the syringe should be gently up-ended a couple of times and rolled between the palms so as to re-establish a uniform suspension. The syringe should not be shaken vigorously lest troublesome bubbles appear.

From this point on, adjustment of insulin dosage is relatively simple. The tests of before-supper urine specimens continue to serve as a guide to the dose of lente (or NPH) insulin, and the tests of specimens obtained before the noon meal act as a guide to the dose of regular insulin. Increases or decreases may be made, 1 or 2 units at a time, in the appropriate types of insulin. Changes should not be made daily but rather, over longer intervals according to the *general trend* of the outcome of the urine tests (or blood glucose determinations) at the times of day indicated. These trends are most easily and conveniently seen, as mentioned earlier, when the results of tests are tabulated, preferably in a notebook ruled for that purpose. The patient may not be able, or may not need, to test the urine before each meal every day, but the results of the tests that are carried out are entered in the appropriate blanks on the chart, and serve as a long-range guide.

In most adult patients who, despite the seemingly "mild" character of diabetes, require insulin for excellent control, it suffices to give 1 injection daily before breakfast. However, in certain of these patients and in the majority of youthful patients with well-established Type I diabetes, fasting (before-breakfast) hyperglycemia of unwanted degree may persist despite good results during the course of the day. This occurs presumably because of the lack or near-lack of endogenous insulin production. In this situation, the amount of insulin given before breakfast cannot be increased lest hypoglycemic attacks be provoked. Instead, a small amount of insulin is given in the latter part of the day, reducing correspondingly the amount given before breakfast (Pattern III in Table 19–3). This evening injection may be given before supper, but in most patients a small dose of lente (or NPH) insulin at bedtime proves to be the most convenient and satisfactory way to provide control of diabetes during the night. A starting dose might well be only 4 units with increases in increments of 1 unit at a time until the fasting blood glucose is brought to a satisfactory level. This program of a "split dose" of insulin has received worldwide use and acceptance in the last 25 years and, with dietary adjustment, is the best conventional method of treatment of patients having unstable ("brittle") diabetes.

As long as the results of tests before the three meals are satisfactory, the presence of small amounts of sugar in the urine at bedtime should not cause much concern. However, in those patients in whom the amount of sugar at bedtime is consistently large, the evening dose of insulin may be given before supper rather than at bedtime (Pattern IV in Table 19–3). This permits the use of a small amount of regular insulin to aid in the utilization of food eaten at the evening meal. An appropriate amount of lente (or NPH) insulin, given in the same syringe, can provide a sustained effect during the night. In some patients the results are better if an appropriate dose of regular insulin is given before supper and then a dose of lente (or NPH) insulin at bedtime.

The diet should be so planned that snacks providing 10 to 20 g of carbohydrate are taken regularly in the midafternoon and at bedtime. Snacks, usually smaller, may also be desirable in the mid-morning for those patients who have an unusually long interval between breakfast and the noon meal and who are quite active physically during the forenoon. The food value of all snacks is included in the total dietary prescription.

For many years it has been the custom at the Joslin Clinic to teach patients how to make minor adjustments in insulin dosage at home. This policy has been extraordinarily successful and has allowed interested, cooperative patients the means of achieving better and more consistent control of diabetes. Table 19–4 serves as a guide to adjustment of dosage.

REMISSION OF DIABETES

It is a common experience that following the initial adjustment of treatment with insulin and the establishment of a satisfactory dose, within days or weeks there may be a reduction in insulin requirement, necessitating gradual decrease in the prescribed dosage in order to avoid hypoglycemic episodes. At times, it may be possible or even necessary to lower the dose to such levels that insulin may be discontinued.

Such remissions, partial or complete, may occur in patients of all ages. In older persons, often the cause is evident such as the improvement of glucose tolerance with loss of weight in a previously obese person. Remissions are seen also with the correction of some complicating condition which has been responsible for the need for insulin, such as febrile illnesses, major surgery under anesthesia, acromegaly, hyperthyroidism, adrenal-cortical tumors, pheochromocytoma, etc.

In 1971, Pirart and Lauvaux of Brussels reported their experience with remission of diabetes.[11] They encountered 280 such patients among 3800 followed from 1950 to 1964. The total of 280 included 138 males and 142 females, chiefly in older age groups; of 138 patients whose remission came within the first year of diabetes, only 4 were 20 years of age or less at the time of remission. On the other hand, 124 experienced a remission at age 41 to 60 and 130 at age 61 or more. In 128 of their patients, remission lasted from 1 to 5 years. Obviously, the composition of the patient population and perhaps the definition of remission were different from those at the Joslin Clinic.

When we speak of remission, ordinarily we have in mind the situation of a truly insulin-dependent patient, usually a child, adolescent, or young adult. Here the decrease in insulin requirement after initial adjustment must be classed as idiopathic since the cause is not known for this "honeymoon" period in which it seems that the patient has regained to a considerable degree the capacity of endogenous insulin production. Unfortunately, the remission is a temporary state although, as noted above, it may occasionally last for several months or rarely even a few years. Except in extremely unusual

Table 19–4. Guide to Adjustment of Insulin Dose According to Outcome of Blood and Urine Glucose Tests

Insulin		Urine or blood glucose tests (or conversely, hypoglycemic reactions) serving as best indices of insulin dose			
Type	Time of Administration	Before Breakfast	Before Noon Meal	Before Supper	At Bedtime
Regular	Before breakfast		X		
Lente (or NPH)	Before breakfast			X	
Regular	Before supper				X
Lente (or NPH)	Before supper	X			
Lente (or NPH)	At bedtime	X			

situations, diabetes with its characteristic insulin lack always asserts itself again and the course from then on is that of insulin-dependent diabetes.

In some patients, there is, indeed, a great temptation to stop insulin entirely or to shift to treatment with a sulfonylurea. Indeed, over the years it has been done at times at the Joslin Clinic, but we prefer to continue insulin even though in token dosage of, say, only 1 to 4 units daily. The reasons for this policy are: (a) total discontinuance of insulin may give the impression to the patient and family that the diabetes has been cured; (b) by continuing a token dose of insulin on at least 2 or 3 days a week, the patient and family are reminded that diabetes is still present and will return in its usual form; and (c) if insulin is discontinued for a period of a few or several weeks, there is a considerable likelihood that on resuming injections, manifestations of skin allergy will occur with this challenging dose to a previously sensitized person, or, less commonly, insulin resistance due to antibody formation may appear. These tendencies may occur much less frequently in the future with the use of purified insulins or of biosynthetic and semisynthetic human insulins.

Jackson has long been a staunch advocate of early diagnosis and prompt treatment. He states that "most children in our clinic from stable homes who have received prompt treatment, have remained in partial remission not only for a few months as is commonly observed, but for several years."[12] During an extended period of partial remission, he and his associates found that children with normal growth and body build requiring less than about 0.6 U/kg/day usually have a measurable increase in C-peptide level after a glucose challenge and an essentially normal glycosylated hemoglobin. He states that, in contrast, most young children coming to his clinic 6 to 12 months after diagnosis and who have had delayed or inadequate replacement therapy, usually require 0.8 or more U/kg/day and have no measurable C-peptide levels before or after a glucose challenge.

For further comments regarding remissions, see Chapter 24.

OTHER INSULIN PROGRAMS

All varieties of insulin are effective and, with care, any type could be used alone with at least fair success if it were the only one available. However, due regard must be had for the rate of action and duration of effect of the insulin used and for the necessary adjustments to be made in the type, amount, and distribution of food. Some of the programs described below are uncommonly or rarely used at the Joslin Clinic but are outlined for the guidance of those who prefer them.

Regular Insulin. Regular insulin may be used as the sole type. Indeed, it has long been recognized that in patients with hard-to-manage diabetes, regular insulin given 2, 3 or more times a day, often yields better results than other plans of treatment.[12a] However, this program—the only one possible prior to 1937, when the first modified insulin was introduced—may not be the best one to prescribe for many patients because they forget or are reluctant to take more than 1 or 2 injections daily and are therefore insulin-deficient for a substantial part of each 24 hours. In the early days of insulin, this deficiency existed, particularly in children, adolescents, and others with unstable diabetes who, for adequate coverage, needed injections of regular insulin before each meal, at bedtime, and often at 2 AM. Pseudo-dwarfism, hepatomegaly and, at times, the complete Mauriac syndrome occurred in young patients, not necessarily due to a poor treatment plan but because the patient failed to take insulin the required number of times daily. These abnormalities practically disappeared as important complications of diabetes after depot insulins of prolonged action became available.[13] In recent years, there has been a revival of interest in regular insulin as the sole type used largely because of the gratifying results obtained in short-term studies with the Biostator and longer trials with an "open loop" insulin delivery system.

Globin Zinc Insulin. This type, discussed in

previous editions, is no longer available in the United States or elsewhere.

Protamine Zinc Insulin. Protamine zinc insulin (PZI) may be used before breakfast either alone or with accompanying *separate* injections of regular insulin provided overdosage is avoided. Since its action is a prolonged one, the best single guide to dosage is the urine or blood glucose test performed before breakfast on the day following the injection. Regardless of the degree of glycosuria or hyperglycemia during the daytime, the dosage of PZI must not be pushed beyond the point at which the blood glucose level the following morning is satisfactory. Larger amounts of PZI may well cause hypoglycemic reactions during the night. Any additional insulin effect during the daytime must be secured by the use of regular insulin in appropriate dosage. Often necessary is a dose of regular insulin before breakfast, administered by *separate injection* at the same time as the protamine zinc is given. In usual dosage the two types must *not* be given in the same syringe because the regular insulin would be converted to more PZI due to the excess of protamine contained in this type of modified insulin. In certain patients another dose of regular insulin must be given before the evening meal to prevent the occurrence of gross glycosuria during the evening.

At the Joslin Clinic PZI is no longer used except in a dwindling number of patients who have been taking this type for many years and seem to have done satisfactorily with it. This would appear to be the policy of most clinicians.

Insulin Mixtures. Before the introduction of isophane (NPH) insulin in 1950, quite wide use was made of insulin mixtures, i.e., mixtures of regular and protamine zinc insulin in the syringe or vial. These mixtures were usually in the proportion of 2:1 although they varied according to the needs of the individual patient. By mixing, in terms of units, an amount of regular insulin *larger* than that of the protamine zinc variety, both long-lasting effect and prompt action were obtained since the amount of regular insulin exceeded that which was bound and converted by the excess protamine in protamine zinc insulin. With the advent of NPH and later lente insulin, the need for 2:1 and similar mixtures disappeared.

Lente Insulins. Market lente insulin is a 70:30 mixture of ultralente and semilente insulins. Any other combination is possible, made either daily in the syringe or in advance in a vial, to produce an effect "tailor-made" for the individual. Semilente insulin may be mixed with lente insulin or the latter may be combined with ultralente insulin in varying proportions. Such combinations have not been used as widely in the United States as in certain other countries, probably because of the earlier introduction of NPH insulin to the United States and because of the ease with which desired effects may be produced by varying the amounts of regular and lente (or NPH) insulins given by single injection. With due regard to promptness and duration of action, semilente or ultralente may be used solely although usually they are combined with another member of the lente family.

TREATMENT OF UNSTABLE ("BRITTLE") DIABETES

In most diabetics the condition is in a form that is relatively stable. If these patients are cooperative and if reasonable care is used in planning treatment by means of diet and insulin or oral hypoglycemic agents, usually no great difficulty is encountered in maintaining satisfactory results in blood and urine tests without the risk of hypoglycemic reactions. In contrast, the diabetic state is controlled with great difficulty in certain other patients, particularly those with Type I diabetes in whom the onset of the disease is in childhood, adolescence, or early adult life. However, this unstable, labile, or "brittle" type of diabetes may occur in persons of any age. Patients of this group in whom the onset of diabetes takes place in middle or later life usually are not overweight but are lean and "ketosis-prone" in the same manner as are younger patients.

Persons with unstable diabetes are sensitive to insulin and to physical exertion; they readily develop hypoglycemic reactions which are often severe and at times lead to unconsciousness with or without convulsions; their blood glucose rises easily following ingestion of food or glucose as well as during infections and emotional stress; and, as stated previously, they have a tendency toward ketoacidosis and coma. Although in the minority when one considers all persons with diabetes, those with unstable diabetes loom large because of the difficult problems presented. The variability of the blood glucose and the frequent attacks of hypoglycemia are annoying to the patient and family and often frustrating to the physician.

In most persons with unstable diabetes it appears likely that little or no endogenous insulin is available so that contra-insulin hormones act more or less unopposed. The patient is therefore nearly or completely dependent on injected insulin. The normal homeostatic mechanism of increased release of insulin in response to a rising blood glucose is lacking and injected insulin obviously does not provide the automatic variability of response to the changing needs of the body.

Treatment, including adjustment of insulin dosage, follows the same general principles as those outlined in the preceding discussion. As applied specifically to patients with unstable diabetes, management is based on an attempt to secure uniformity and evenness of effect of the controllable factors which influence blood glucose, and should include: (1) distribution of food throughout the waking part of the day with routine between-meal snacks; (2) careful selection of the type or types of insulin, as well as the dosage, and time and frequency of administration; most patients will require insulin at least twice daily; and (3) reasonable uniformity in physical activity from day to day. Additional help may be obtained through home blood glucose monitoring and, in selected patients, trial of pump treatment.

Somogyi Effect

In any plan of treatment, effort must be made to avoid hypoglycemic reactions insofar as possible lest fluctuations in blood glucose be increased because of a "hyperglycemic rebound" (Somogyi effect) and all-too-frequent overdosage with glucose or food in the treatment of hypoglycemic attacks. If such a rebound is encountered, blood glucose values may be high temporarily. In this situation one should not "chase" the elevated blood glucose but allow the upset condition a day or two to become quiet. In this connection, one must keep in mind the possibility of episodes of hypoglycemia at night during sleep and unnoticed by the patient but demonstrated by nocturnal monitoring. The "rebound" is reflected in an elevation of the fasting blood glucose. In the present day, this situation is often over-diagnosed on inadequate evidence.[14] The commonest cause of an elevated fasting blood glucose level remains a lack of insulin.

We have found most workable a program which includes a dose of regular and lente (or NPH) insulin before breakfast and a second (usually smaller) dose of lente (or NPH), often with a small dose of regular insulin, before supper. Instead, in some patients a small dose of lente (or NPH) insulin (without regular insulin) at bedtime suffices and often is more convenient. At any time when two types of insulin are used, they are given in a single injection in the same syringe.

"Dawn Phenomenon"

Closely allied to the above situation is that in which the fasting blood glucose rises between 5 and 9 A.M. with no hypoglycemia during the night, as noted in hourly determinations of the blood glucose.[14a] The elevated value before breakfast is reflected in post-prandial hyperglycemia. Originally described in patients with Type I diabetes, it has been noted also in those with Type II diabetes[14b]

and in certain non-diabetic persons[14c] (in whom, however, the elevations of the blood glucose are smaller). In patients in whom the blood glucose is kept constant by means of closed-loop intravenous administration of insulin, the insulin requirements in the early morning hours are increased.

The cause of this phenomenon has been sought assiduously but not definitely established. Apparently it is not due to a surge of cortisol or growth hormone. The most tenable hypothesis appears to be that it is a variant of a circadian rhythm.

PRACTICAL POINTS IN THE USE OF INSULIN

Storage. Regular (crystalline) insulin will maintain its potency for months even at room temperature. The modified insulins with intermediate and long actions are quite stable, but less so than the regular type. Consequently, patients should be taught to keep a reserve supply of any insulin in the refrigerator (40°F; 4°C); for convenience, the bottle in current use may be kept at room temperature. The loss of potency of modified insulins unavoidably kept at temperatures consistently above 75°F (24°C) proceeds slowly enough that patients who are away from home or living under unusual conditions may be assured that practically all of the potency will be maintained for some weeks or months. Any loss in potency may be compensated for easily by slight increases in the number of units taken, depending, of course, upon the results of the day-by-day urine tests for sugar. One difficulty encountered in keeping suspensions such as NPH, protamine zinc, or the lente insulins at temperatures consistently above 75°F (24°C) lies in the tendency to clumping of the insulin-containing material which precipitates on standing. The larger particles so formed may be difficult to resuspend by shaking and, although they retain potency, the patient may have difficulty in securing a true aliquot and withdrawing a desired dose accurately.

When regular and NPH (or lente) are placed in the same syringe and allowed to stand, a variable amount of the regular may become bound to the intermediate type within the first 24 hours. From a practical standpoint, this has not seemed to be a significant problem in patients using pre-filled syringes.

Insulin should not be kept in the freezing compartment of a refrigerator or otherwise allowed to freeze. Should this happen inadvertently, the insulin should be discarded.

The storage of insulin during travel ordinarily presents no problem. Thermos bottles or special kits for cooling are rarely necessary. In most instances, even during the summer, the vials currently being used may be kept safely in a case or handbag. The traveler should carry insulin, syringe, and needles (or disposable syringe-needle units) in hand luggage and not in baggage to be shipped separately, lest loss or delay in transit separate the traveler from critically needed medication. When extended stops are made during prolonged travel, the insulin may be transferred to a refrigerator if available.

Sterilization of Equipment. In the United States at the present time, increasing use is being made of disposable, plastic syringe-needle units packaged so as to preserve sterility. They have the advantages not only of sterility and ready availability, but also those of consistent sharpness of needles and (with some brands) of no "dead space" in the syringe. Since they are more expensive than glass syringes, some have claimed that a given syringe-needle unit may be used for at least 3 times without acquiring infections.[15] Obviously, this depends upon the degree of care taken by the patient to preserve sterility.

The best method of sterilizing needles and glass syringes in the home is by boiling. For patients who are away from home, this may be difficult or impossible. Various traveling kits are on the market to meet this situation. Keeping the syringe and needle in alcohol (preferably isopropyl alcohol or, if not obtainable, 70% ethyl alcohol) is permissible provided that there has been prior sterilization of all equipment by boiling. Because of the time required for water sterilization, many patients while at home keep the syringe and needle under alcohol in a covered stainless steel or enamel container. After removing the syringe and needle from the alcohol and before loading the syringe with insulin, it is important to expel all traces of alcohol by motion of the plunger, because alcohol may alter the insulin and, in addition, may lead to irritation when introduced beneath the skin. At least once a week, the container, the syringe, and the needle should be sterilized by boiling and the used alcohol replaced by fresh.

Administration of Insulin

In teaching patients how to give insulin the rules and precautions common to any injection should be emphasized. In addition, certain special items are worthy of mention.

1. Loading the Syringe. In loading the syringe, the insulin vial should be held with its base down and air injected first. The amount of air should roughly equal the space which will be occupied by the volume of insulin to be withdrawn. This maneuver, designed to prevent the gradual production of a partial vacuum, is simple when only one type of insulin is being administered. If two varieties

of insulin are to be given in a single injection, special instructions are necessary. As an example, if 10 units of regular and 30 units of NPH insulin are to be given, the instructions are as follows: (a) mix gently but thoroughly the contents of the NPH vial (do not shake vigorously lest bubbles form!); (b) inject "30 units" of air into the NPH vial; (c) withdraw the needle; (d) inject "10 units" of air into the vial of regular insulin and withdraw 10 units of regular insulin into the syringe; (e) withdraw 30 units of NPH insulin into the syringe; (f) proceed with injection.

2. Site of the Injection. Patients should be taught that injections may be made beneath the skin over any part of the body. Areas such as the abdomen, upper arms, thighs, flanks, and upper buttocks in which the skin is loose and in which there is considerable subcutaneous fat are preferable because of ease of administration and less pain. An excellent site is the skin of the abdominal wall. This area is particularly desirable for patients, especially girls and women, who, even with "purified" insulin may develop atrophy of subcutaneous fat at sites of insulin injections. The atrophies which occur here are ordinarily not exposed to public view and the area is large enough to allow long-term use.

In any part of the body, sites of injection should be rotated in systematic fashion so that no one area 3 cm in diameter receives insulin oftener than every 3 or 4 weeks. In this way the skin will remain supple, the formation of scar tissue obviated, and a uniform absorption of insulin favored. We commonly prescribe hypodermic needles of 26 gauge and ½-inch length (25 to 27 gauge and ⅜ and ⅝ inch length are acceptable).

3. Making the Injection. In making the injection, patients are instructed as follows: (a) load the syringe; (b) rub a small area of skin gently with sterile cotton wet with alcohol; (c) pick up a sizeable fold of skin and subcutaneous tissue between the thumb and forefinger of one hand; (d) with the other hand, hold the loaded syringe as one would hold a pencil at an angle of about 20 to 30 degrees less than perpendicular; (e) push the needle swiftly through the skin up to the butt; (f) release pressure on the fold of skin and expel the insulin from the syringe gradually; (g) withdraw the needle swiftly; (h) dab the area of injection lightly with cotton, noting whether any insulin has leaked out through the track of the needle; (i) if using a glass syringe, rinse the barrel, plunger, and needle thoroughly under a cold water faucet; (j) place the syringe and needle in alcohol (isopropyl or 70% ethyl) in a covered container.

Use of Insulin by the Visually Impaired. Patients who live alone and are blind or have such reduced vision as to be unable to load a syringe accurately, even with a magnifying glass, present a problem in treatment. If available, a family member or friend should be taught to do this. Lacking this, the most workable plan is to arrange for a nurse, pharmacist, or other knowledgeable person to "pre-load" enough syringes to last 7 to 10 days. These are kept between clean cloths on a tray in a refrigerator (*not* the freezing compartment) from which the patient removes one daily and makes the injection. One's first thought is to question the bacteriologic safety of this procedure. However, with many patients so managed in the past several years, no case of infection has been reported.

Certain devices have been developed to aid visually impaired patients. These include (1) a tiny magnifying glass attached to a small clip so that the scale on the syringe may be read more easily; and (2) for patients with whom the above does not suffice, one may try using a small clip which may be attached to the syringe and set so that the plunger cannot be pulled out beyond the desired point.

EFFECT OF EXERCISE ON INSULIN DOSAGE

During a period of adjustment in the hospital, ambulatory diabetic patients should be encouraged to continue to be as active as their physical state and hospital conditions allow. A significant difference is usually noted between the insulin requirement of a patient who is resting in bed and one who is active physically. This difference is most apparent in diabetic children observed in summer camps. It is a common and striking finding that despite liberal diets, the diabetes in these children can be much better controlled with smaller doses of insulin than when the children are less active at home or in school. In the hospital, indoor facilities for exercise are desirable, especially in case of inclement weather. Patients at home should be encouraged to engage in physical activity regularly. Since most patients are middle-aged or elderly, such exercise may well consist of walking which, if the general physical condition permits, should be at a brisk, and not a sauntering pace.

In order for exercise to have its maximal effect, patients should be receiving an amount of insulin sufficient to control the diabetic condition. Patients who need insulin but do not receive it or receive only an inadequate amount, may actually experience increases in the blood glucose from physical exercise. This effect was common in patients with severe diabetes prior to the introduction of insulin in 1922.

Even for patients confined to bed, mild forms of exercise may often be possible. In addition to the beneficial effect upon the diabetes, muscular tone may be preserved. Patients long in bed because of slowly healing foot lesions can profit from arm exercises combined with mild leg activity as Buerger exercises (see Chapter 35).

The favorable effect of exercise must be borne in mind whenever insulin is prescribed. As a rule, the insulin requirement for patients outside the hospital is less than that in the hospital (assuming that the diet is the same). Consequently, the amount of insulin prescribed at discharge should usually be slightly less than that which the patient has been receiving in the hospital. Furthermore, if unusually strenuous exercise is planned at home on a given day, the patient should take slightly less insulin or more food than usual, lest a reaction ingloriously terminate a game of golf, a mountain climb, or a day of hard work. At times the reaction is not experienced until the day following unusual exercise.

It has been suggested that physical exercise after the subcutaneous injection of insulin into an exercising extremity may accelerate the rate of absorption of insulin. Corollary thinking is that injection into non-active parts of the body, as the abdominal wall, would help prevent hypoglycemia.[15a] However, in their studies Kemmer et al.[15b] found that acceleration of absorption did not occur during exercise although the expected lowering of the blood glucose took place. This occurred regardless of whether the insulin had been injected into a moving or resting limb. They suggest that the hypoglycemia was due to a "fixed hyperinsulinemic state" in the subjects. In interpreting their results it is important to keep in mind that the diabetic patients on the morning of the study received intermediate-acting insulin at 7:30. Breakfast began 30 minutes later. Regular insulin (Actrapid) was given at 9:00 AM followed by exercise 35 minutes later. It is obvious that results reported from investigations carried out regarding the effect of exercise, depend a great deal on the protocol and conditions of study.

For a detailed discussion of exercise in the treatment of diabetes, see Chapter 22.

INSULIN REQUIREMENTS DURING ACUTE ILLNESS

During an acute illness, especially if accompanied by fever, in most instances the patient has a greater insulin requirement than usual even though food intake may decrease because of anorexia, nausea or vomiting. At all times, the patient's inviolable rule must be: *Never omit insulin or decrease the dose unless tests made every 4 hours show the urine to be free from acetone and free from glucose or nearly so.* The following instructions are given to be used in case of illness:

1. Continue the usual pattern of insulin injec-

tions whether regular, lente, NPH or other modified type of insulin is being used.

2. Take the same amount of insulin as usual on arising, or, if overdosage seems a real possibility, reduce the dose by no more than 25%.

3. Test the urine at noon, 5 or 6 P.M., and at bedtime. If indicated, give additional regular insulin according to a schedule such as this:

If urine test (second specimen) shows: Give regular insulin, units	2% or more	½–1%	0–¼%
	10	6	0

The numerical scale must be adjusted to the age of the patient, type of illness and usual insulin requirement. It may range from 4-2-0 in children under 5 years, 6-4-0 in those 5 to 10 years, 10-6-0 in those 10 to 15 years old, and up to 12-8-0 in older patients. An alternate plan for additional insulin is to give 20% of the usual daily requirement of a given patient at the times indicated above. If other methods of urine testing (Testape, Diastix, etc.) are used, the results may be interpreted as strongly positive, moderately positive, slightly positive or negative, respectively.

If during an illness lasting more than a few days, the patient's tests show a consistent need for additional insulin during the day, the before-breakfast doses should be increased gradually to meet this requirement.

METHODS OF DELIVERY OF INSULIN

Jet Injection

In addition to the time-tested, familiar injection methods of insulin delivery, namely subcutaneously, intramuscularly, intravenously, and intraperitoneally, there are other routes which are possible. Thus, some 30 years ago Perkin et al.[16] reported results obtained with the use of a jet injector (Hypospray, then made by the R.P. Scherer Corporation, Detroit). Experience at the Joslin Clinic was not favorable enough over the years to bring about general adoption of this method. The chief disadvantages were cost, weight, large size, and difficulty encountered in using insulin mixtures of changing composition. Currently other types of jet injectors are being offered for sale including Syrijet (Mizzy, Inc., Clifton Forge, Virginia), Medijector (Derata Corp., Minneapolis, Minnesota) and Med-E-Jet (Med-E-Jet Corp., Cleveland, Ohio). We have not had experience with these devices but Danowski and Sunder have reported favorable results with the Syrijet.[17]

Other Routes

For some years after the discovery of insulin, studies were carried out to determine its effect when taken by mouth. The chief obstacle, of course, lies in the digestion and thereby loss of potency of insulin when exposed to the digestive juices. Various ways of protecting insulin, as by capsules, during its passage through the stomach and upper jejunum have shown that only a small and highly variable amount is absorbed, resulting in wastage of insulin. Trials with other routes including the use of rectal suppositories[18] and spray administration to the respiratory tract have been reported. Results to date with these unusual methods of giving insulin indicate that they are impractical. However, Moses and co-workers[19] have taken up anew the delivery of insulin by intra-nasal spray. They mixed insulin with 1% deoxycholate and reported efficacy and reproducibility by the use of this insulin-bile salt aerosol. In diabetic patients, serum insulin levels peaked by 10 minutes after spraying. These recent studies of Moses et al. call to mind other attempts over the decades since the discovery of insulin to secure effective and dependable absorption of insulin through various mucous membranes including the nose.[20,21] The considerable work done up until 1938 was summarized by Jensen in his monograph on insulin.[22]

With increasing acceptance of the concept that the vascular and neurologic complications of diabetes are due to the abnormal metabolism, great interest has been aroused in developing workable and acceptable methods of insulin delivery, designed to maintain the blood glucose consistently within a normal range. This can be accomplished to a considerable degree by the giving of multiple doses of regular insulin daily, varying the amount according to need as determined by frequent self-monitoring of the blood glucose (see further discussion later in this chapter). Obviously, for the patient this becomes a never-ending and time-consuming schedule which will be followed only by the most meticulous and dedicated person. Since this program consists in essence of an attempt to convert a diabetic into a non-diabetic individual insofar as possible, attention has been directed toward other ways of reaching the same goal. These efforts have included the items listed below.

Transplantation of the Pancreas

Although transplantation of the pancreas was carried out much earlier in animals, it was not until the late 1960s that the problem was tackled in a concerted fashion in human patients.[23] Much of the work in the U.S.A. in the last 15 years has been done at the Hospital of the University of Minnesota, and almost entirely with patients who had received a kidney transplant because of diabetic nephropathy, since these patients were already receiving immuno-suppressive therapy. As experience has been gained over the years, techniques, site of transplantation, amount of pancreas transplanted and other features of the procedure have been modified and improved.

For a detailed discussion of pancreas and islet tissue transplantation, see Chapter 20.

"Artificial Beta Cell"

Modern technology has made it possible to develop an apparatus such as the previously mentioned Biostator Glucose Controller which, when appropriately attached to the patient, can constantly determine and record the blood glucose which prompts a computer to stimulate a pump to release to the patient on a continuous basis, an amount of insulin appropriate to the needs of the moment. This, then, becomes indeed an "artificial beta cell." The apparatus is excellent for short-time studies (as in a Clinical Research Unit) or for treatment lasting only a few or several days. However, it is relatively large and applicable for use only at the laboratory bench or bedside.

Since miniaturization of apparatus has been accomplished and in widespread use for some years, both medically and nonmedically, it was natural that investigators should try to compress the elements of an artificial beta cell into a package small enough to be implanted under the skin as with a cardiac pacemaker. The key elements as outlined by Soeldner et al.[24] consist of a glucose sensor, power supply, computer, pump, and insulin reservoir, all miniaturized. It is generally agreed that current knowledge and techniques are available to produce and assemble all of these elements except a satisfactory glucose sensor. In fact, one development has been to implant only the insulin reservoir, power supply and transmitter with other elements packaged externally. Under the direction of a programmable computer, insulin is delivered from the reservoir continuously in appropriate amounts.[25]

The development of a satisfactory sensor has been the object of work for some years by Bessman et al.[26] in Los Angeles and Soeldner and associates[25] in Boston. Bessman and co-workers have used a glucose oxidase enzyme system, and Guyton, Soeldner, Giner et al. have developed a platinum catalytic electrode device[27] (See Fig. 19–2). The problems encountered have been formidable: not only must the sensor be biocompatible but it must respond also to glucose and not to the many substances in tissue fluids such as amino acids, urea, and uric acid, to say nothing of various drugs which the patient may be taking. Steady, albeit slow, progress in the development of the glucose sensor gives hope that in time success may be achieved.

Insulin Pumps (Open-Loop System)

The Biostator Glucose Controller and the hoped-for miniaturized beta cell described briefly in the preceding section represent closed-loop systems in which the plasma (or tissue fluid) glucose is, or would be, constantly determined and an appropriate amount of insulin continuously and automatically supplied to the body. At the present time, however, no such device is available for the long-term treatment of ambulatory patients with diabetes. Consequently, one must resort to an open-loop system using an infuser or "pump" in selected patients (Continuous Subcutaneous Insulin Infuser; CSII).

The first significant reports of open loop systems providing continuous subcutaneous delivery of insulin, were published by Pickup et al. in 1977 and 1978, who achieved normalization of blood glucose as well as other metabolites such as lactate and pyruvate.[28,29] In close proximity, Tamborlane and co-workers[30,31] also demonstrated that use of this system could normalize lipid and amino acid metabolism as well as blood glucose in patients with Type I diabetes. Interest in the pump quickly ran high, as indicated in the papers read in an early symposium sponsored by the Kroc Foundation, held in December, 1979.[32]

The insulin infuser in its simplest form consists essentially of a reservoir (syringe) containing a small amount (somewhat more than the anticipated need for 24 to 48 hours) of regular insulin; a small pump; an infusion rate selector by which the rate of release of insulin can be adjusted; a small rechargeable battery; and a small plastic catheter with attached needle which leads from the syringe to the place for subcutaneous delivery. Usually the pump is fastened to a belt or to clothing around the waist. At the Joslin Clinic, patients are instructed to change the syringe daily and the catheter, needle, and site of injection (usually the lower abdomen) every other day. It is helpful to have two batteries (plus a spare), alternating them daily so that one may be recharging while the other is in

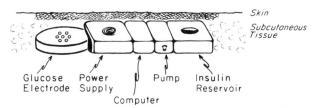

Fig. 19–2. Diagram of major components of an implantable "artificial beta cell." (Adapted from Soeldner[25] with permission of the author and publisher.)

use. These details of usage vary somewhat from clinic to clinic.

There is as yet no implantable automatic device for the continuous determination of glucose in blood or tissue fluid. This is done by the patient who, when a reading is desired, pricks a finger pad for a drop of blood and determines the glucose content by a glucose oxidase test strip such as Visidex (Ames) or Chemstrip-bG (Bio-Dynamics) used with or without a reflectance meter such as the Glucometer (Ames) or Accu-Chek (Bio-Dynamics). Patients are advised to determine the blood glucose level 2 to 4 times a day. The patient releases an extra amount (bolus) of insulin prior to a meal and smaller amounts before a snack. Otherwise, insulin is supplied constantly by the pump throughout the 24 hours in tiny amounts.

Treatment should be initiated under controlled conditions with or (usually) without the use of the Biostator, to determine the true insulin need for 24 hours and to teach the patient how to use the apparatus. The infusion rate selector is set so as to deliver automatically about one-half of the total daily requirement; the patient releases the rest periodically as just described. The continuous infusion is adjusted to result in blood glucose values in the range of 100 to 150 mg/dl fasting or 2 to 3 hours postprandially.

Improvements and refinements are constantly being made in the various pumps available, chiefly to make them smaller, more automatic, and "programmable" as regards time and rate of delivery of insulin, both continuously and in boluses. In view of the constant increase in the number of pumps on the market, it would not be profitable in this rapidly changing situation to describe and evaluate the present infusers individually. In general, designers and manufacturers are overcoming quite well the problems encountered with the early models.[33] Pumps are now available which are of light weight and small enough to be held easily in the palm of one's hand; some have program versatility, long-life batteries (up to 5 years), safety devices, etc.

In addition to the effects on carbohydrate, protein and fat metabolism, normalization of counterregulatory hormones has also been demonstrated. As is well known, uncontrolled diabetes is associated with superphysiologic responses of epinephrine, norepinephrine, growth hormone, cortisol and glucagon in addition to the normal secretory stimuli such as stress, exercise and hypoglycemia. Use of insulin pumps has been shown to modulate the secretory response of these counterregulatory hormones. Tamborlane et al.[34] demonstrated that with conventional therapy, plasma norepinephrine rose with exercise from 280 ± 21 to 1465 ± 450 pg/ml.

However, after only two weeks of control of diabetes using an open-loop insulin system, the same group of patients had a smaller increase of norepinephrine with a similar amount of exercise (296 ± 45 to 444 ± 71 pg/ml). In a similar study, Tamborlane also showed that after 14 days of control of blood glucose using open-loop insulin systems, the level of growth hormone following exercise decreased from 21.3 ± 5.2 ng/dl to 4.1 ± 1.6 ng/dl. Similar improvements in glucagon dynamics were demonstrated by Raskin et al.[35]

The Joslin Clinic experience with open loop pump therapy began in 1978 and, as of April 1984, more than 300 selected patients with Type I diabetes had been treated for variable periods in this manner, guided by initial hospitalization, frequent visits to the clinic, periodic monitoring of hemoglobin A_1 and/or A_{1c}, and home monitoring of blood glucose 2 to 4 times daily. At the beginning of treatment, patients were instructed to determine the blood glucose at least 4 times daily (before each of the three meals and bedtime snack, plus in some patients, at times another determination at about 3:00 AM). There has been considerable attrition due to rejection by certain patients of the rigorous schedule. In 1983, a study was made of a group of 73 patients who had been receiving pump therapy over a period of 6 to 24 months.[36] Of the 61 patients who had continued with such treatment, 75% reported a feeling of better general health and 85% had noted improvement in blood glucose values. Better psychological health, particularly a more hopeful attitude about the outcome and future of their diabetes, was reported in about 60%. The blood had been tested for glucose 2 or more times daily by over 75% of the patients.

In the course of trials over the years, one study was made to evaluate criteria for selection of patients.[37] This was done by comparing results in patients without significant impairment of renal or gastric function with those of another group with renal impairment and a third group with autonomic neuropathy. Following initial hospitalization for intensive training and dietary instruction, patients received CSII treatment for 3 to 11 months; during this period, monitoring of the blood glucose was done 2 to 4 times a day and determinations of the hemoglobin A_{1c} were carried out periodically. The results indicated that those patients with severe nephropathy or neuropathy presented greater problems in achieving glycemic control than those without such complications.

In another study reported in 1982,[38] 23 women with insulin-dependent diabetes were treated with CSII during the first trimester of pregnancy. In this group, the average duration of diabetes was 10 ± 7 years and the average age, 29 ± 4 years. They were hospitalized briefly at the initiation of special treatment which was carried out up to the 10th or 12th week of pregnancy. During the 4th to 6th week, the mean hemoglobin A_{1c} was 8.7% and in the period of 10 to 12 weeks, 7.2%. The mean daily blood glucose fell from 159 to 118 mg/dl. The daily insulin requirement remained the same, 43 vs 44 units daily, and reactions from insulin were essentially the same, 1.6 per week during the first period and 1.4 during the second. The conclusion was drawn that open-loop pump delivery was safe and effective in early pregnancy during which control is important but often difficult to obtain. However, apart from this special study, experience with large numbers of pregnant diabetic women treated aggressively but by more conventional means (insulin administration 2 to 4 times daily together with hemoglobin A_{1c} and home blood glucose monitoring) has given such good results as regards the outcome of pregnancy that pump treatment has not been continued routinely in pregnant women. However, a total of some 60 women have been treated in this fashion. One consideration is the cost of the pump, which at present is in the range of $1500–$2500, plus the weekly cost of care of the pump, supplies, etc. Patients in general have considered it not worthwhile for a period of only 3 months unless they have been women dedicated to the continued use of the pump following delivery. An additional problem has been the great difficulty of obtaining patients before or very shortly after conception which is considered a prerequisite for best results in the prevention of congenital defects.

Since the techniques of design and use of insulin pumps are still being developed and there are certain risks and disadvantages to using them, patient selection is critical. Indications for the use of insulin pumps at the present time fall into three main categories: (1) wide excursions of blood glucose on a daily basis despite optimal insulin and dietary regimens; (2) women with diabetes during the first trimester of pregnancy; (3) inability of the patient to eat meals on a routine basis either because of employment or life style. The first two indications are the more important ones; the last-named is less compelling. Patients chosen should be able to do home blood glucose monitoring, make decisions with regard to changes and timing of insulin dose based on the results, and be willing to maintain an appropriate dietary regimen. At the present time, contraindications to the use of the pump are: history of noncompliance regarding diet, insulin, and home monitoring; inadequate medical follow-up by the patient; inability to recognize hypoglycemic symptoms; significant complications of diabetes such as proliferative retinopathy, advanced renal disease, or severe autonomic neuropathy.

The major disadvantages of insulin pump therapy are related to the technical aspects of its use. Infections do occur at injection sites but they are not common and usually not severe. At times plugging of the catheter may occur or the connection between the catheter and the insulin reservoir may become loosened and insulin lost. Lack of care by the patient to insure an adequate insulin supply interrupts treatment. Fortunately, all of these potential hazards are preventible.

In a follow-up of an earlier report[39] of 11 deaths among pump-treated patients, in 1984 members of the Centers for Disease Control, together with other members of a study committee, identified 35 deaths among an estimated 3500 diabetic patients using pumps in the United States as of October 1982.[39a] They compared the actual number of deaths with that expected among comparable patients with Type I diabetes under conventional treatment. The observed number was not greater than the expected number. They judged that only 2 of the 35 deaths appeared unusual, one from hypoglycemia in a patient whose pump apparently malfunctioned and a second from bacterial endocarditis arising from a large, unrecognized abscess at the site of insertion of the catheter.

Certainly, no patient who is subject to insulin reactions without warning should be treated with the open-loop insulin pumps now available lest severe, or even fatal, hypoglycemia occur. For the same reason, overly zealous efforts to maintain the blood glucose always at a normal level should be discouraged. In commenting on this problem, Goldstein[39b] states that in his experience, many patients can safely keep the glycosylated hemoglobin as low as within 1 to 2 percent of the nondiabetic range.

It is obvious that the successful operation of an insulin pump requires an intelligent, reliable, and psychologically well-adjusted patient who is dedicated to the thought of keeping the blood glucose as close to normal as is feasible. The patient must then be kept under close supervision and, preferably, not live alone. For some, it may be more work than the injection of insulin in conventional fashion 3 or 4 times in 24 hours. Our experience thus far suggests that those patients whose unstable diabetes is so "brittle" that, despite 3 or 4 injections of insulin daily in conventional fashion, they still exhibit unpredictable swings in blood glucose, are not good candidates for successful pump treatment.

The larger question with regard to insulin delivery systems is whether they will have any impact in the prevention or reversal of the characteristic complications of Type I diabetes. Although there are some reports of short-term studies[40–42] which indicate that there may be some improvement in certain parameters, no long-term data are as yet available in this regard. Consequently, at the moment it is difficult to predict the future of open-loop systems in the treatment of insulin-dependent diabetes. However, since they are now being used with thousands of patients throughout the world, one can be sure that much will be learned in the years ahead.

DIABETES CONTROL AND COMPLICATIONS TRIAL

Because of the results obtained with the use of pumps or multiple doses of insulin daily, great interest has been aroused in the possibility of obtaining an answer to the long-debated question as to whether correction of the metabolic defect would prevent or minimize the late vascular and neurologic complications of diabetes. Although there is quite general agreement that maintenance of normoglycemia, if obtainable and safe, is desirable, certain questions arise. Among these is the question of feasibility: Can one reasonably expect that patients will be willing and able to follow a rigorous program of diet adherence, insulin pump therapy (or, alternatively, 3 or 4 insulin injections daily), close blood glucose monitoring at home or at work with several determinations daily, careful record keeping, and close contact with the physician and ancillary personnel over many years of time?

In an attempt to provide answers to these questions, which are literally of vital importance, beginning in March 1982 the National Institute of Arthritis, Diabetes, and Digestive and Kidney Diseases (NIADDK) of the National Institutes of Health (NIH) initiated a long-term study called the Diabetes Control and Complications Trial (DCCT).[42a] The project is divided into four phases: (1) a planning stage (6 to 12 months), (2) a feasibility study (2 years), (3) a full-scale clinical trial (7 to 10 years), and (4) data analysis and preparation of a report (1 year). For Phase 2, some 250 patients in 21 centers across the country were to be enrolled, and, if the results were encouraging, then Phase 3 would follow, with many additional patients to be added for the long clinical trial.

By 1984, Phase 2 was well underway, with more than 250 volunteer patients who were between the ages of 13 and 39 years, had had Type I diabetes for periods of time between 1 and 15 years, and who had no severe complications of diabetes.

The patients enrolled in the DCCT are divided randomly into two groups according to treatment: (1) standard and (2) experimental. Members of both groups receive excellent treatment. Those in the *standard* group will take one or two insulin injections daily, and will be expected to follow a meal plan, to do urine tests at home regularly, and to monitor blood glucose at home if time shows the diabetes cannot be controlled otherwise. The patient will receive thorough instruction regarding all elements of good diabetes control and will visit the medical center every 3 months for evaluation.

Members of the *experimental* group will follow the same general plan of treatment except that they will take insulin three or four times daily or use an insulin pump. They will monitor the blood glucose at home several times daily and report to the medical center weekly at first, and then, when the desired blood glucose level has been achieved, monthly.

Large-scale, multi-centered projects such as the DCCT are difficult to carry out and the results often are hard to interpret. Tchobroutsky et al.[42b] questioned the "cost-benefit" ratio of the project. However, all persons involved with diabetes and its treatment will look forward with great interest and hope to the outcome of this ambitious study.

BIOAVAILABILITY OF INSULIN

There is no question but that insulin "works" when injected subcutaneously, intramuscularly, intravenously, intraperitoneally, or by any method which permits absorption into the bloodstream. However, observation over many years both in people and animals have shown a good deal of variation in the plasma level of free insulin. Various questions arise: What percentage of the injected insulin actually becomes "free" in the blood stream and available for action on tissue cells? In view of the great importance of the liver in metabolism, what is the difference in effect of endogenous insulin which is transported directly to the liver through the portal vein and insulin given by conventional injection? What are the factors which result in a plasma-free insulin considerably lower in amount than that injected? As far as the last question is concerned, studies have given results which suggest various influences including binding of insulin by antibodies in plasma, excessive amounts of insulin antagonists as growth hormone and glucagon; abnormalities of insulin receptors including antibodies against receptors; and degradation by excessive enzyme action or sequestration of insulin at injection sites.

With regard to the degradation of insulin, Paulsen[43] reported the case of a diabetic girl in whom an enzyme appeared to degrade insulin at the site of subcutaneous injection. In this connection, the experience of Berger et al.[44] and of Freidenberg and colleagues[45] is enlightening. The latter group studied 5 female diabetics ranging from 14 to 31 years of age who required daily large amounts (2.5 to 30.0 U/kg body weight) of beef or pork insulin to avoid recurrent ketoacidosis. All responded to conventional doses (0.35 to 0.9 U/kg/day) if given intravenously. However, when aprotinin (a protease inhibitor) was added to regular pork insulin and the mixture given subcutaneously in dosage of 0.7–1.4 U/kg/day, plasma levels of free insulin rose and the blood glucose fell to a normal range. The results strongly suggest that in these patients, insulin injected subcutaneously was sequestered or degraded by tissue proteases. The authors regard the long-term safety and effectiveness of aprotinin as uncertain.

Galloway et al.[46] have looked into certain of these matters in nondiabetic subjects after injections of regular insulin alone and in combination with lente and NPH types. They found marked variation in results in serum insulin concentrations and blood glucose response, both among different subjects and in the same subject from time to time. There was slower absorption of insulin when preparations of higher strength (U-500, U-5000) were used. As for the site of injection, use of the deltoid and abdominal areas produced a significantly higher peak level of insulin than when the anterior thigh and buttock were used. The influence of depth of injection indicated that the deeper the intramuscular injection, the sooner the peak serum concentration was reached. Using mixtures of regular with lente and with NPH, they found that the ratio necessary for the regular:lente mixture to reach the peak serum insulin concentration was higher than that when the regular:NPH mixture was used.

CERTAIN COMPLICATIONS OF TREATMENT WITH INSULIN

Scar Tissue and Lipodystrophy. As stated previously, patients should be taught to vary the site of injection from day to day; a good rule is that no area 3 cm in diameter receive insulin oftener than once in 3 or 4 weeks. If insulin is injected daily into the same place, the skin and subcutaneous tissue may become thickened and scarred with the formation of "insulin lumps;" absorption of insulin from such an area may proceed at an unpredictably slower rate.

Another untoward effect of insulin administration is *lipodystrophy* which may take two forms: hypertrophy or atrophy, both of which are much less common with the present-day highly purified insulins. Hypertrophy of subcutaneous fat at the site of insulin injections may at times be unsightly but is not a source of complaint as often as are insulin atrophies. Formerly, atrophies occurred to a varying degree in about 50% of children who received insulin, in approximately 20% of adult females, and in 5% of adult males, but the frequency has become much less since the advent of

highly purified insulins. Insulin atrophies are of cosmetic importance only since no significant change occurs other than the disappearance of subcutaneous fat. If areas of fat atrophy are left alone and further injections at their sites are studiously avoided, restoration of adipose tissue may take place slowly over a year or two. Restoration of subcutaneous fat may be hastened in many patients by injection into the depths or the walls of the area of atrophy with the purer insulins which are now a standard market product (see Chapters 24 and 38 for additional information concerning lipodystrophy).

Antibodies to Insulin. It is well documented that practically all patients who receive insulin daily over a few or several weeks develop antibodies.[47] In this respect, insulin of pork origin is less immunogenic than that of beef origin, possibly because the former more nearly resembles human insulin in the type and location of the constituent amino acids. The simpler regular insulin is less immunogenic than NPH or even lente. Finally, the more highly purified insulins available today are less apt to produce antibodies than preparations of former days when small amounts of other substances, albeit usually related to insulin (proinsulin, desamido insulin, arginine insulin, etc.), were present. However, even highly purified porcine regular insulin possesses some degree of immunogenicity since insulin itself is a small protein.

Immune responses to insulin are due to the development of immunoglobulins, particularly skin sensitizing antibodies of the IgE class which mediate insulin allergy and neutralizing antibodies of the IgG group which are mediators of insulin resistance (See also Chapter 4).

Insulin Allergy. Since insulin from conventional sources is to the human body a foreign protein, it is not surprising that at the initiation of insulin treatment, many patients develop an allergic tissue response varying from slight redness, swelling, stinging, and itching to marked swelling, induration, and pain at the site of injections. This was much more common prior to the introduction of highly purified insulins.

Allergic reactions appear usually within 15 minutes to 2 hours after injection, although rarely a delayed response may occur. Milder degrees of response require no treatment and the patient may be reassured that usually the condition will gradually diminish as daily injections of insulin are continued. For more troublesome situations, symptomatic treatment such as cold compresses or the giving of an antihistamine preparation orally for several days will tide the patient over the annoying period. However, if insulin of combined beef-pork origin has been used, improvement may be expected in the majority of patients if a shift is made to purified pork insulin. Some patients who do not respond to this may do so if given insulin solely of bovine origin. With a few patients, in the end one must rely on desensitization either of spontaneous type or that provided as described below.

The variation in response to treatment programs probably is related in part to the fact that insulin allergy may be due either to impurities in the market preparation, (no longer an important factor), to hypersensitivity to the insulin molecule itself or to the fact that the patient has been sensitized by treatment with insulin some weeks, months or years in the past with then discontinuance of such therapy.

The above comments apply to local tissue responses. Much less common fortunately are systemic allergic reactions consisting of generalized urticaria and angioedema, and even rarer, anaphylactic shock. Desensitization is the treatment of choice and this is best carried out by the use of regular pork insulin. If the history indicates, however, that there is greater sensitivity to pork than to beef insulin, the latter should be tried in the desensitization process. This is started after the patient has received no insulin for at least 12 and preferably 24 to 48 hours. Antihistamines or steroids should not be used during the desensitization because of the possibility that their effect might mask an allergic reaction. Desensitization should be carried out under hospital conditions. If during the procedure a severe response occurs, epinephrine (1/1000 solution) should be given and this should be available at the bedside.

Desensitization is initiated by giving a tiny amount of insulin intradermally or subcutaneously and then increasing the amount step by step. For years at the Joslin Clinic, we made our own dilutions, but of convenience are the desensitization kits prepared by Eli Lilly and Company[5] and made available on request. The dilutions are so arranged that the first injection provides 1/1000 of a unit. Subsequent injections of 0.1 ml deliver 1/500, 1/250, 1/100, 1/50, 1/25, 1/10, 1/5, 1/2, and 1 unit. The first dilution may be prepared by mixing 0.1 ml of U_{100} insulin with 0.9 ml of saline solution, thereby resulting in 1/100 U/ml. The first injection of 0.1 ml therefore provides 1/1000 unit. It is suggested that the first 10 desensitizing doses should be given in an 0.1 ml amount every 30 minutes, injecting the first 3 dilutions intradermally and from then on, subcutaneously. If an allergic response occurs, one drops back 2 dilutions and then proceeds up the scale as before.

Using the procedures just outlined, Galloway and Bressler[5] found only 6 treatment failures in 129 patients (5%). If desensitization to pork regular insulin fails, one may try using insulin of beef origin. If this fails and if the patient truly has insulin-dependent diabetes, one may resort to antihistamines and/or steroids.

Following desensitization, one may continue to use regular insulin or may try shifting to an intermediate type which should be lente insulin to avoid introducing another protein, namely protamine, in NPH insulin. Always to be kept in mind is that in the course of time following initial desensitization, the patient may again exhibit an allergic reaction and require another desensitization procedure.

Insulin Edema. For years, the rapid appearance of edema, significant weight gain, abdominal bloating, and blurred vision have been observed in many diabetic patients when severe hyperglycemia and glycosuria are brought under control. These clinical events are most often noted during or after intensive treatment of patients with ketoacidosis or in patients in whom the diagnosis of diabetes has been made recently but who have had symptomatic diabetes for some time. They are particularly pronounced after insulin therapy—thus the term "insulin edema"—but have been noted following rapid improvement in uncontrolled diabetes brought about by diet or oral hypoglycemic agents. The edema disappears spontaneously after a number of days unless underlying renal or cardiac disease is present. Occasionally the temporary use of a diuretic may be indicated.

In patients recovering from ketoacidosis, the edema and other signs have been attributed to excessive water and sodium chloride therapy, particularly after treatment with physiologic saline solution. However, this explanation would obviously not account for the common occurrence of water accumulation in those not requiring water and electrolytes administered parenterally.

Saudek et al.[48] studied the effect of insulin treatment on sodium excretion in 6 patients with poorly controlled diabetes, one of whom had well-marked, and another mild, ketoacidosis. The remaining 4 patients had blood glucose values ranging from 211 to 398 mg/dl. All patients retained sodium when hyperglycemia was brought under control with insulin (mean positive sodium balance, 286 mEq in 3 days.) The peak weight gain (admission weight vs that after 2 to 4 days of treatment) ranged from 0.35 to 2.53 kg (0.77 to 5.57 lb) with a mean of 1.45 kg (3.19 lb). Edema was noted in the patient who had been definitely ketotic and semicomatose on admission and in the other who had been admitted in mild ketoacidosis. They concluded that sodium retention occurs regularly during insulin treatment of poorly controlled diabetes, whether ketoacidosis is present or not.

Insulin Resistance. Patients are encountered occasionally who require large amounts of insulin daily for control of hyperglycemia. Arbitrarily, "insulin resistance" is considered to be present in a clinical sense when 200 units or more are required daily for a period of 2 or 3 days or longer. Resistance may be classified as immunologic or non-immunologic. In the immunologic type, there are excessive amounts of circulating insulin antibodies which bind large amounts of the injected insulin, rendering it less active biologically.

Most persons develop antibodies to some degree after they have received injections of insulin for several weeks. The insulin-binding capacity is usually less than 10 units per liter of serum. In those few patients with immune insulin resistance and resulting high insulin requirement, insulin-binding capacities may range from 50 to over 5000 U/L. The insulin-neutralizing activity of the antibodies is associated with the globulin fractions, chiefly those of the IgG class, although IgM and IgD have been found in some patients with insulin resistance.

Insulin resistance of the immunologic type has become much less common with the introduction of highly purified insulins.

Non-immunologic insulin resistance has a variety of causes including (a) binding of insulin by protein apart from an antigen-antibody relationship;[49] (b) unresponsiveness of peripheral tissue despite an excess of insulin in the plasma,[50] due possibly to a decrease in the number and/or affinity of receptors on the surface of target cells, especially in obese individuals. Antibodies against receptors themselves have been incriminated; (c) presence in serum of increased amounts of insulin antagonists such as glucagon or growth hormone; (d) diabetic ketoacidosis or coma, representing a transient insulin resistance, at least when insulin is given subcutaneously; (e) other conditions including lipoatrophic diabetes, cirrhosis of the liver and hemochromatosis, infections, chronic lymphocytic leukemia, and hyperfunctioning of endocrine glands, as of the thyroid and adrenal cortex.

Treatment of insulin resistance varies according to the cause, and often more than one measure after another must be tried. Types of therapy successful in certain cases include:

(a) Use of purified pork insulin which may result in a lower insulin requirement, presumably because the tendency to antibody formation is much less than with insulin of beef origin. On the other hand, certain patients may be more tolerant of pure beef insulin. Some indication as to which is better borne may be obtained by skin tests.

(b) Treatment with prednisone or other immuno-suppressive agents, starting with high doses and tapering down gradually over a period of three or four weeks.

(c) Possible trial of sulfated insulin, used to some extent in Canada since 1964 and available in the United States as an investigational drug since 1968. In a report published in 1978, Davidson and DeBra[51] stated that treatment was successful in 34 of 35 patients, failing in only one person with lipoatrophic diabetes. By 1982, Davidson's group had treated "almost 100 patients with immunologic insulin resistance," finding that all who had insulin-binding antibody titers greater than 30 μ/L of serum, responded well.[52]

(d) Passage of time during which excellent control of diabetes is maintained. A clinical impression is that aggressive treatment over a period of months, satisfies the insulin requirement and corrects the insulin resistance in perhaps a third of patients.

(e) In obese patients, loss of body weight by reduction of calorie intake. This often results in an increase in cell receptors and reduction of insulin requirement.

(f) Trial of oral hypoglycemic agents in place of insulin. Success depends upon the ability of the patient's pancreas to produce endogenous insulin in adequate amounts.

For further discussion of insulin resistance, see Chapter 3.

HYPOGLYCEMIA DUE TO INSULIN

Insulin Reactions

Episodes of hypoglycemia due to insulin constitute one of the major problems in the treatment of diabetes. For a patient, perhaps following a traffic violation or an automobile accident, to be arrested and taken to jail on the presumption of drunkenness; for students to fail in written or oral examinations upon which important ratings depend; or for directors of large corporations to develop irritability, garrulousness, tremor, or somnolence at an annual meeting of their boards—are not matters of indifference. Fear of an "insulin reaction" is almost worse than the actual experience. Moreover, the dangers of a hypoglycemic reaction to the life and limb of both the patient and others nearby, especially on the highway, are by no means trifling.

If excellent glycemic control is to be attained, it is difficult to avoid occasional hypoglycemic episodes. However, it is imperative that diabetic patients avoid frequent or severe attacks. Not only are they inconveniencing and embarrassing to the patient, but also their occurrence reflects upon the ability of diabetic individuals as a group to take a normal part in everyday life. Frequent insulin reactions in one diabetic worker may discourage employers from hiring other diabetics. Also, there is the possibility that hypoglycemia induced by insulin may lead to hyperglycemia because homeostatic processes set in motion to correct the low blood glucose may overshoot the mark and result in rebound hyperglycemia (Somogyi effect). Unrecognized hypoglycemia during sleep may lead to hyperglycemia which prompts the physician or the patient to increase an already overly high insulin dose and thereby compound the problem.[53]

Signs and Symptoms. Common symptoms of an insulin reaction include sweating, tremor, faintness, hunger, headache, numbness or tingling of the tongue or lips, rapid heart action, double or blurred vision, and unsteady gait. During more severe episodes, the patient may become unconscious and may also have convulsions. In those receiving regular insulin, such reactions appear most commonly 3 or 4 hours after a meal before which insulin has been taken, but they may also occur in the interval between the administration of the insulin and the taking of food if that period is unduly prolonged. Usually reactions occur about 8 to 10 hours after lente or NPH insulin has been given, and 12 to 24 hours after ultralente or protamine zinc insulin. Lack of adequate food, particularly carbohydrate, either in the diet or as a reserve stored in the body, favors hypoglycemia. The same is true if for some reason food remains overly long in the stomach or is lost by vomiting. Consequently, emaciated patients eating a meager diet are susceptible to insulin reactions. Likewise, unusual or strenuous exercise, by its demand on sources of energy, may precipitate hypoglycemia.

The signs and symptoms of an insulin reaction are by no means always the classical ones just mentioned. Indeed, when an insulin-treated diabetic child becomes quiet, lacks interest, and is unnaturally good, or, conversely, when the child is unusually fretful; when an adult diabetic acts ambitionless, depressed, and morose; or when an elderly man or woman becomes weak and faint, one should suspect a low blood glucose. If such changes occur some hours after a meal, particularly if the patient took the usual dose of insulin and in haste ate less than usual or engaged in unusual exercise, it can reasonably be assumed that hypoglycemia is present. Diabetics in such a condition may respond to questions automatically or, quite the reverse, may become emotionally unstable.

The symptoms of an insulin reaction are said to develop at times when the blood glucose is falling but is still above normal. It is probably true that a rapid decrease from high to considerably lower levels may give rise to symptoms. Such is usually not the case unless the blood glucose has fallen to 100 mg/dl or lower. Patients often attribute symptoms such as nervousness and sweating to an insulin reaction when they are actually due to intercurrent

disease or emotional upsets. Whenever practicable, the physician should secure blood for the later determination of its glucose content (or immediately by Chemstrips or Dextrostix) before administering carbohydrate for a suspected reaction. Apart from swift decreases, hypoglycemic signs and symptoms usually do not appear until the blood glucose falls to 50 mg/dl or lower.

Patients are puzzled when they experience symptoms characteristic of hypoglycemia but find that the urine contains sugar. They should be taught that the sugar may have been excreted by the kidneys minutes or hours previously and then retained in the urine in the bladder. In a true reaction, a second, freshly passed specimen of urine will be found to be sugar-free or nearly so provided the bladder was thoroughly emptied at the previous micturition. At such times the genuineness of the reaction is confirmed by prompt recovery following the administration of 5 to 15 g of carbohydrate.

Insulin Reactions Without Warning. The severity of symptoms of an insulin reaction does not parallel directly the degree of hypoglycemia. Blood glucose levels may be as low as 40 mg/dl without recognizable symptoms, particularly in children. At night, natural sleep may pass unnoticed into the stupor of hypoglycemia which, especially in patients with a low seizure threshold, may lead to convulsions.

Frequently reactions occur without warning, especially in a patient who has been taking insulin for 10 or more years. Such events emphasize the fact that warning signs, such as sweating, tremor, and tachycardia, commonly thought of as due to compensatory hyperactivity of the sympathetic nervous system and regarded as unpleasant by the patient, are actually a "blessing in disguise." Without them, the unattended patient having an insulin reaction may develop diminished cerebral function and confusion, poor coordination, unusual behavior such as negativism and belligerency, and finally coma, with or without convulsions.

The reason for the lack of warning of hypoglycemia, present or impending, is not entirely clear. Possibilities are: (a) in some patients, neuropathy may be responsible; (b) cerebral function may be compromised by neuroglucopenia and confusion result, thereby clouding appreciation of events; (c) certain end-organs may in time lose some degree of responsiveness to regulatory hormones; (d) lack of sympathetic (catecholamine) response provides an adequate basis for absence of warning signs, but the reason for such remains obscure.[54]

Course and Sequelae. If hypoglycemic episodes are of short duration, no recognizable permanent damage need be anticipated. After repeated episodes of severe insulin reactions, some degree of mental deterioration over the years would not be surprising. However, interpretation of such changes is difficult because of the influence of other factors such as complicating diseases and the passage of time with development of cerebral arteriosclerosis.

Certain clinical observations made during the course of severe hypoglycemic attacks are worthy of mention: (1) Stupor persisting for several hours despite restoration of a normal blood glucose level need not indicate a poor prognosis. Particularly in young and otherwise healthy patients, full recovery usually takes place within a few or several hours. This is often true despite such alarming signs as bilaterally positive Babinski responses, localized weakness, and hemiparesis. For further comment, see the following section on treatment. (2) The differential diagnosis between convulsions due to hypoglycemia and those due to epilepsy may indeed be difficult. Careful documentation by means of blood glucose determinations is essential. At times, in individuals who have basically a low seizure threshold, convulsions may be precipitated by hypoglycemia. Treatment may include administration of an anticonvulsant as well as measures to avoid hypoglycemia. (3) A single dose of regular insulin rarely has serious consequences even though the patient is alone. Almost invariably, if the person is in a warm, protected place and *no more insulin is given,* recovery will take place in time.

Treatment. The treatment of most insulin reactions is simple. Symptoms usually disappear in a few minutes after taking 5 to 15 g of carbohydrate in the form of sugar, candy, orange juice, ginger ale, cola drink, etc., requiring little or no digestion and which will be quickly absorbed.

In patients who cannot or will not swallow, the giving of glucagon subcutaneously or intramuscularly (0.5 to 1.0 mg in children and 1.0 mg in adults) often serves to restore a cooperative state in which carbohydrate may be given safely by mouth. Carbohydrate ingestion is important lest the blood glucose level fall again after the transient rise produced by glucagon. Every patient with a tendency to hypoglycemic episodes should keep in the refrigerator a glucagon kit for use by a knowledgeable family member. In place of glucagon, epinephrine (0.5 to 1.0 ml of 1:1000 solution) may be given subcutaneously but it is definitely less effective.

In treating at home a stuporous patient with clenched jaws, *tiny* amounts of a thick liquid as undiluted corn syrup, may be introduced carefully at intervals with a small spoon or straw in the space between the cheek and the gums. A preparation such as Instant Glucose, Reactose or Glutose may

be used similarly. These substances will slide down the esophagus (as do secretions of the mouth and nasopharynx) without the danger of getting into the trachea as posed by a thin liquid.[55]

If the unconscious patient is in the hospital, infirmary, or physician's office, quick relief may be secured by the injection of 20 ml or more of a 50% solution of glucose intravenously. Often the response is so prompt that before 10 ml of the solution are introduced, return to consciousness has occurred. Indeed, how so little carbohydrate could accomplish so prompt and startling an effect seems miraculous! In general, the greater the dose of insulin which is responsible for the reaction, and the longer the duration of the reaction (especially the unconsciousness), the more carbohydrate is required for sustained recovery. In patients in whom hypoglycemic coma has been present for several hours, glucose is given initially as a 50% solution in order to restore a normal blood glucose level quickly. In addition, in order to maintain a satisfactory level, it is usually necessary to follow this with a constant slow intravenous infusion of 5% solution of glucose in water (or in part in saline solution, if indicated).

MacCuish, Munro, and Duncan[56] state that if, despite the giving of glucose in severe reactions, unconsciousness continues beyond 30 minutes after the restoration and maintenance of normoglycemia (blood glucose, 90 to 180 mg/dl), cortisone given intravenously as a 100 mg bolus is often effective in restoring consciousness. If this fails to produce results in 30 to 60 minutes, they regard it advisable to proceed directly to the treatment of presumed cerebral edema with large doses of dexamethasone (10 mg intravenously) and/or 40 g mannitol given intravenously as a 20% solution over 20 minutes.

Prevention. The following measures are helpful in the prevention of hypoglycemic reactions due to insulin: (1) reasonable uniformity of diet, insulin, and exercise from day to day; (2) careful adjustment of the insulin program so that the type or types of insulin, dose, and time or times of administration are suited to the individual patient; (3) small between-meal and bedtime snacks consisting of food requiring digestion to provide slow absorption over an extended period of time; (4) regular testing of the urine and periodic testing of the blood, so as to foresee changing insulin requirements; (5) routine carrying of sugar, candy, or other readily absorbable carbohydrate which may be taken at the first warning of an oncoming reaction; (6) availability in the home of glucagon for prompt administration by another member of the family should hypoglycemic stupor occur; (7) in patients subject to reactions without warning, there must be re-education to recognize more subtle signs and symptoms of hypoglycemia such as lassitude, lethargy, hunger, inability to concentrate or think clearly; and paradoxically, at times, euphoria; and (8) all diabetics should carry an identification card in their pocket or wallet and, in addition, wear an identification bracelet or necklace.

Identification tags to be used in bracelets or necklaces may be obtained on application to Medic Alert Foundation, Turlock, California 95380. A tag and life registration are provided by payment of a fee (currently $15). Information regarding the patient is kept on file in the Central Office of the Medic Alert Foundation and is available for emergency use on a 24-hour a day basis by telephoning collect from any point in the world (the Medic Alert telephone number appears on the tag).

Effects Produced by Overly Large Doses of Insulin

The widespread use of insulin shock treatment of schizophrenia, introduced by Sakel in 1928 and in vogue for many years, afforded much opportunity for study of the changes which take place in the body following the administration of large doses of insulin. Data from such studies as well as those in animals are to be found in the literature of 35 to 40 years ago.[57] Then as now, attention was focused on the central nervous system. Functioning of the brain requires a constant supply of glucose and oxygen from the blood stream. Under normal (and hypoglycemic) conditions, the brain cannot utilize fatty acids or other substrates as do skeletal and cardiac muscle. (There is evidence that under special conditions the brain may obtain energy from ketone bodies.[58]) Overall rates of glucose consumption are maintained with decreasing plasma glucose levels until concentrations of about 35 to 40 mg/dl (2 mmol/L) are reached, at which point signs of neuroglucopenia become evident.

The brain normally uses glucose and oxygen at rates which, relative to other tissues, are high. Intracellular glycogen is also rapidly used and disappears quickly during ischemia but only after cerebral glucose has been depleted. It is stated that during severe hypoglycemia, oxygen use and the metabolic rate are decreased somewhat. Despite this, with sustained glucopenia, changes take place in the brain which may be irreversible. If death does not occur, higher (cerebral) centers are so damaged that a virtually decerebrate state is created and the patient becomes a ''vegetable.''

Himwich[59] divided the events occurring in marked hypoglycemia into five groups whose order of appearance can be explained on the basis of the metabolic rate of each region of the brain. According to him, first to suffer from glucose deprivation are, phylogenetically speaking, the newest portions of the brain, the cerebral hemispheres (especially the neocortex) and parts of the cerebellum, which metabolize at the highest rate. Each succeeding lower portion of the brain becomes involved in its turn. The medulla oblongata, the oldest part and the one with the lowest metabolic rate, functions long after the higher centers are able to do so. The five phases described by Himwich are: (1) cortical, (2) subcorticodiencephalic, (3) mesencephalic, (4) premyelencephalic, and (5) myelencephalic. Naturally the fifth stage is the most dangerous and is recognized by deep coma and the predominance of parasympathetic signs. The patient's respiration is shallow, the heart rate is slow, the skin is pale, and the pupils are contracted and no longer react to light. Perspiration is noted and the temperature is subnormal. The muscles are relaxed, the tendon jerks depressed, and the corneal reflex is entirely lost.

In studies carried out in primates, Meldrum and co-workers[60] found that the earliest brain abnormalities due to uncomplicated hypoglycemia are microvacuolation of cells after survival for a half-hour followed then by typical ischemic cell changes. Commonly there is diffuse involvement of the neocortex with changes in the occipital and parietal regions. The abnormality is at times focal but usually laminar, especially in the posterior half of the brain. Diffuse demyelination may accompany cortical changes. The hippocampi are almost always affected in a typical hypoxic necrosis. A third area involved is the corpus striatum.

Deaths Due to Insulin-Induced Hypoglycemia

Fortunately deaths due to insulin reactions are rare. Among 33,330 known deaths of Joslin Clinic patients from 1922 to 1979, only 85 (0.26%) were reported on death certificates to be caused by hypoglycemia due to insulin (See Table 13–16). However, and particularly in the more distant past, diagnoses often may have been made on circumstantial evidence rather than on blood glucose determinations, e.g., in unattended patients found dead. At any rate, many of these deaths occurred in patients at home or in widely scattered hospitals.

Among 2792 autopsies performed on diabetic patients at the New England Deaconess Hospital during the years, 1924–1980, in 19 cases (0.7%) death was ascribed to insulin-induced hypoglycemia (See Table 14–2). At the moment, information is not at hand to indicate how many of the 19 patients developed hypoglycemic coma elsewhere, were admitted to the hospital comatose, and never regained consciousness.

It is obvious that insulin hypoglycemia if not diagnosed and treated promptly, may result in serious brain damage and death. In the treatment of patients, particularly if one strives for normal or nearly normal blood glucose values, one must walk a thin line between hypoglycemia and hyperglycemia. Frequent and/or severe hypoglycemic episodes must be avoided. This is particularly true in the patient who has "reactions without warning" and those patients under treatment with pumps.

Apart from hypoglycemia due to insulin in the treatment of diabetes, there are, of course, other conditions in which this may occur and which are described in Chapter 40. Not to be forgotten is the fact that large doses of insulin have been used by both diabetic and non-diabetic persons with suicidal or alleged homocidal intent. At times the latter situation has been the subject of court action.

For further discussion of (1) hypoglycemia in relation to operating an automobile, particularly public service vehicles, and (2) hypoglycemia in general as a cause of death, see Chapter 45 and reference 61.

REFERENCES

1. Best, C.H.: The first clinical use of insulin. Diabetes 5:65, 1956.
2. Burrows, G.N., Hazlett, B.E., Phillips, M.J.: A case of diabetes mellitus. N. Engl. J. Med. 306:340, 1982. See also Marliss, E.B.: Insulin: sixty years of use. Ibid. p. 362.
3. Rizza, R.A., Gerich, J.E., Haymond, M.W., et al.: Control of blood sugar in insulin-dependent diabetes: comparison of an artificial endocrine pancreas, continuous subcutaneous insulin infusion, and intensified conventional insulin therapy. N. Engl. J. Med. 303:1313, 1980.
3a.Nathan, D.M., Lou, P., Avruch, J.: Intensive conventional and insulin pump therapies in adult Type I diabetics. Ann. Intern Med. 97:31, 1982.
3b.Buysschaert, M., Marchand, E., Ketelslegers, J.M., Lambert, A.E.: Comparison of plasma glucose and plasma free insulin during CSII and intensified conventional insulin therapy. Diabetes Care 6:1, 1983.
3c.Schiffrin, A., Belmonte, M.M.: Comparison between continuous subcutaneous insulin infusion and multiple injections of insulin. A one-year prospective study. Diabetes 31:255, 1982.
4. Chaskar, R., Chou, M.C.Y., Field, J.B.: Time-action characterics of regular and NPH insulin in insulin-treated diabetics. J. Clin. Endocrinol. Metab. 50:475, 1980.
5. Galloway, J.A., Bressler, R.: Insulin treatment in diabetes. Med. Clin. N. Am. 62:663, 1978.
6. Schlichtkrull, J., Brange, Aa.H., Christiansen, O., et al.: Monocomponent insulin and its clinical implications. In: Radioimmunoassay methodology and applications in physiology and clinical studies. Horm. Metab. Res. (Suppl.) 5:134, 1974.
6a.Meienhofer, J., Schnabel, E., Bremer, H., et al.: Synthese der Insulinketten und ihre Kombination zu insulaktiven Präparaten. Z. Naturforsch (B) 18:1120, 1963.
6b.Kung, Y.T., Da, Y.C., Huang, W.T., et al.: Total synthesis of crystalline insulin. Sci. Sinica (Peking) 15:544, 1966.
6c.Katsoyannis, P.G., Tometsko, A., Zalut, C.: Insulin peptides. XII. Human insulin generation by combination of synthetic A and B chains. J. Am. Chem. Soc. 88:166, 1966.
6d.Owens, D.R., Jones, M.K., Haynes, T.M., et al.: Human

insulin: study of safety and efficacy in man. Br. Med. J. 282:1264, 1981.
7. Goeddel, D.V., Kleid, D.G., Bolivar, F., et al.: Expression in Escherichia coli of chemically synthesized genes for human insulin. Proc. Natl. Acad. Sci. (USA) 76:106, 1979.
8. Skyler, J.S., Raptis, S. (Eds.: 32 papers): Symposium on Biosynthetic Human Insulin. Diabetes Care 4:139–264, 1981.
9. J.S. Skyler (Ed.): Symposium on Human Insulin of Recombinant DNA Origin (37 papers). Diabetes Care 5 (Suppl. 2):1–186, 1982.
10. Chance, R.E., Kroeff, E.P., Hoffman, J.A., Frank, B.H.: Chemical, physical and biologic properties of biosynthetic human insulin. Diabetes Care 4:147, 1981.
10a.Fineberg, S.E., Galloway, J.A., Fineberg, N.S., et al.: Safety, efficacy, and immunogenicity of human insulin of recombinant DNA origin. Diabetes. (In press).
10b.Fineberg, S.E., Galloway, J.A., Fineberg, N.S., Rathbun, M.J.: Immunologic improvement resulting from the transfer of animal-insulin-treated diabetic subjects to human insulin (recombinant DNA). Diabetes Care 5 (Suppl. 2):107, 1982.
11. Pirart, J., Lauvaux, J.P.: Remission in diabetes. In: E.F. Pfeiffer (Ed.): Handbook of Diabetes Mellitus. Munich, Lehmanns, 1971, pp. 443–502.
12. Jackson, R.L.: Remission phase of juvenile diabetes. (Letter). Diabetes Care 2:62, 1979.
12a.Lukens, F.D.W.: The rediscovery of regular insulin. N. Engl. J. Med. 272:130, 1965.
13. White, P., Marble, A., Bogan, I.K., Smith, R.M.: Enlargement of the liver in diabetic children. II. Effect of raw pancreas, betaine hydrochloride and protamine insulin. Arch. Intern. Med. 62:751, 1938.
14. Schmidt, M.I., Hadji-Georgopoulos, A., Rendell, M., et al.: Fasting hyperglycemia and associated free insulin and cortisol changes in "Somogyi-like" patients. Diabetes Care 2:457, 1979.
14a.Schmidt, M.I., Hadji-Georgopoulos, A., Rendell, M., et al.: The Dawn Phenomenon, an early morning glucose rise: implications for diabetic intraday blood glucose variation. Diabetes Care 4:579, 1981.
14b.Bolli, G.B., Gerich, J.E.: The "Dawn Phenomenon"—a common occurrence in both non-insulin-dependent and insulin-dependent diabetes mellitus. N. Engl. J. Med. 310:746, 1984.
14c.Schmidt, M.I., Lin, Q.X., Gwynne, J.T., Jacobs, S.: Fasting early morning rise in peripheral insulin: evidence of the Dawn Phenomenon in nondiabetes. Diabetes Care 7:32, 1984.
15. Hodge, R.H., Krongaard, L., Sande, M.A., Kaiser, D.L.: Multiple use of disposable syringe-needle units. J.A.M.A. 244:266, 1980.
15a.Koivisto, V.A., Felig, P.: Effect of leg exercise on insulin absorption in diabetic patients. N. Engl. J. Med. 298:79, 1978.
15b.Kemmer, F.W., Berchtold, P., Berger, M., et al.: Exercise-induced fall of blood glucose in insulin-treated diabetics unrelated to alteration of insulin mobilization. Diabetes 28:1131, 1979.
16. Perkin, F.S., Todd, G.M., Brown, T.M., Abbott, H.L.: Jet injection of insulin in treatment of diabetes mellitus. Proc. Am. Diab. Assoc. 10:185, 1930. See also Perkin, F.S.: Jet hypodermic injectors for use in diabetes. J.A.M.A. 195:844, 1966).
17. Danowski, T.S., Sunder, J.H.: Jet injection of insulin during self-monitoring of blood glucose. Diabetes Care 1:27, 1978.
18. Yamasaki, Y., Shichiri, M., Kawamori, R., et al.: The effectiveness of rectal administration of insulin suppository

on normal and diabetic subjects. Diabetes Care 4:454, 1981.

19. Moses, A.C., Gordon, G.S., Cary, M.D., Flier, J.S.: Effective nasal absorption of insulin from insulin-bile aerosols in normal and diabetic subjects. (Abstr.) Diabetes 32 (Suppl. 1):70, 1983.

20. Heuber, W., de Jongh, S.E., Laqueur, E.: Über Inhalation von Insulin. Klin. Wchnschr. 3:2342, 1924.

21. Gänssler, M.: Über Inhalation von Insulin. Klin. Wchnschr. 4:71, 1925.

22. Jensen, H.F.: Insulin: Its Chemistry and Physiology. New York, The Commonwealth Fund, 1938, pp. 92–97.

23. Goetz, F.C.: Early experiments in human pancreas transplantation. Diabetes 29 (Suppl. 1):1, 1980.

24. Soeldner, J.S., Chang, K.W., Aisenberg, S., et al.: Progress report—artificial implantable beta cell. In: Proceedings of the 1973 International Conference on Cybernetics and Society, November 5–7, 1973, Institute of Electrical and Electronics Engineers, Inc. New York, 1973, pp. 184–189.

25. Soeldner, J.S.: Treatment of diabetes mellitus by devices. Am. J. Med. 70:183, 1981.

26. Bessman, S.P., Hellyer, J.M., Layne, E.C., et al.: The total implantation of an artificial β-cell in a dog: Progress report. In: J.S. Bajaj (Ed.): Diabetes. International Congress Series No. 413. Amsterdam, Excerpta Medica, 1977, pp. 496–501.

27. Guyton, J.R., Soeldner, J.S., Giner, J., et al.: The development of an implantable electrochemical glucose sensor: response to glucose in bovine serum ultrafiltrate. In: Contributions to Workshop Schloss Reisenburg, 1978. Feedback-Controlled and Preprogrammed Insulin Infusion in Diabetes Mellitus. New York, Georg Thieme Verlag, 1979, pp. 25–26.

28. Pickup, J.C., Keen, H., Parsons, J.A., Alberti, K.G.M.M.: The use of continuous subcutaneous insulin infusion to achieve normoglycemia in diabetic patients. (Abstr.) Diabetologia 13:425, 1977. See also Br. Med. J. 1:204, 1978.

29. Pickup, J.C., Keen, H., Viberti, M.C., et al.: Continuous subcutaneous insulin infusion in the treatment of diabetes mellitus. Diabetes Care 3:290, 1980.

30. Tamborlane, W.V., Sherwin, R.S., Genel, M., Felig, P.: Reduction to normal of plasma glucose in juvenile diabetes by subcutaneous administration of insulin with a portable infusion pump. N. Engl. J. Med. 300:573, 1979.

31. Tamborlane, W.V., Sherwin, R.S., Genel, M., Felig, P.: Restoration of normal lipid and amino acid metabolism in diabetic patients treated with a portable insulin infusion pump. Lancet 1:1258, 1979.

32. Kroc Foundation Symposium on Insulin Delivery Devices (21 articles). Diabetes Care 3:253–370, 1980.

33. Bending, J.J., Pickup, J.C., Keen, H., et al.: Meeting the problems of first-generation insulin infusion pumps: clinical trial of a new miniature infuser. Diabetes Care 6:452, 1983.

34. Tamborlane, W.V., Sherwin, R.S., Koivisto, V., et al.: Normalization of the growth hormone and catecholamine response to exercise in juvenile-onset diabetic subjects treated with a portable insulin infusion pump. Diabetes 28:785, 1979.

35. Raskin, P., Pietri, A., Unger, R.H.: Changes in glucagon levels after four to five weeks of glucoregulation by portable insulin infusion pumps. Diabetes 28:1033, 1979.

36. Fredholm, N., Vignati, L., Brown, S.: Patient acceptance of open loop insulin therapy. Diabetes 32 (Suppl. 1):168A, 1983.

37. Vignati, L., Arastu, M., Ryan, P., MIller, D.: Assessment of glycemic control in IDDM with and without diabetic complications. Diabetes 30 (Suppl. 1):38A, 1981.

38. Vignati, L., Hare, J.W., Phillippe, M., et al.: Open loop

insulin infusion systems (OLIIS) during the first trimester of pregnancy. Diabetes 31 (Suppl. 2):173A, 1982.

39. Centers for Disease Control, Atlanta, Ga.: Deaths among patients using continuous subcutaneous insulin infusion pumps—United States. Morbid. Mortal. Weekly Report 31:80, 1982.

39a.Teutsch, S.M., Herman, W.H., Dwyer, D.M., Lane, J.M.: Mortality among diabetic patients using continuous subcutaneous insulin-infusion pumps. N. Engl. J. Med. 310:361, 1984.

39b.Goldstein, D.E.: Is glycosylated hemoglobin clinically useful? (Editorial). N. Engl. J. Med. 310:384, 1984.

40. Pietri, A., Dunn, F.L., Raskin, P.: The effect of improved diabetic control on plasma lipid and lipoprotein levels: a comparison of conventional therapy and continuous subcutaneous insulin infusion. Diabetes 29:1001, 1980.

41. Viberti, G.C., Pickup, J.C., Jarrett, R.J., Keen, H.: Effect of control of blood glucose on urinary excretion of albumin and B2 microglobulin in insulin-dependent diabetes. N. Engl. J. Med. 300:638, 1979.

42. Pietri, A., Ehle, A.L., Raskin, P.: Changes in nerve conduction velocity after six weeks of glucoregulation with portable insulin infusion pumps. Diabetes 29:668, 1980.

42a.Salans, L.B.: Proposed protocol for the clinical trial to assess the relationship between metabolic control and the early vascular complications of Type I (insulin-dependent) diabetes. (Letter). Diabetologia 24:216, 1983.

42b.Tchobroutsky, G., Job, D., Slama, G., Eschwege, E.: Therapeutic trials in Type I (insulin-dependent) diabetic patients on insulin: goals and tools (Letter). Diabetologia 24:217, 1983.

43. Paulsen, E.P.: An insulin degrading enzyme in a diabetic girl causing massive destruction of subcutaneous insulin (Abstr.). Diabetes 25 (Suppl. 1):334, 1976.

44. Berger, M., Cüppers, H.J., Halban, P.A., Offord, R.E.: The effect of aprotinin on the absorption of subcutaneously injected regular insulin in normal subjects. Diabetes 29:81, 1980.

45. Freidenberg, G.R., White, N., Cataland, S., et al.: Diabetes responsive to intravenous but not subcutaneous insulin: effectiveness of aprotinin. N. Engl. J. Med. 305:363, 1981.

46. Galloway, J.A., Spradlin, C.T., Nelson, R.L., et al.: Factors influencing the absorption, serum insulin concentration, and blood glucose responses after injections of regular insulin and various insulin mixtures. Diabetes Care 4:366, 1981.

47. Berson, S.A., Yalow, R.S.: Insulin antagonists, insulin antibodies and insulin resistance. Am. J. Med. 25:155, 1958.

48. Saudek, C.D., Boulter, P.R., Knopp, R.H., Arky, R.A.: Sodium retention accompanying insulin treatment of diabetes mellitus. Diabetes 23:240, 1974.

49. Antoniades, H.N., Gundersen, K., Beigelman, P.M., et al.: Studies on the state, transport and regulation of insulin in human blood. Diabetes 11:261, 1962.

50. Olefsky, J.M., Ciaraldi, T.P.: The insulin receptor: basic characteristics and its role in insulin resistant states. In: M. Brownlee (Ed.): Diabetes Mellitus. Islet Cell Function/ Insulin Action, Vol. II. New York, Garland STPM Press, 1981, pp. 73–116.

51. Davidson, J.K., DeBra, D.W.: Immunologic insulin resistance. Diabetes 27:307, 1978.

52. Davidson, J.K.: Personal communication.

53. Gale, E.A.M., Tattersall, R.B.: Unrecognized nocturnal hypoglycemia in insulin-treated diabetics. Lancet 1:1049, 1979.

54. Sussman, K.E., Crout, J.R., Marble, A.: Failure of warn-

ing in insulin-induced hypoglycemic reactions. Diabetes *12*:38, 1963.

55. Rosenbaum, H.M., Genuth, S.M., Kent, T., et al. (Letter). Garber, A.J. (Reply): Efficacy of instant glucose. J.A.M.A. *241*:1890, 1979.

56. MacCuish, A.C., Munro, J.F., Duncan, L.P.J.: Treatment of hypoglycemic coma with glucagon, intravenous dextrose and mannitol infusion in a hundred diabetics. Lancet *2*:946, 1970.

57. Sahs, A.L., Alexander, L.: Fatal hypoglycemia; clinico-pathologic study. Arch. Neurol. Psychiatr. *42*:286, 1959.

58. Owen, O.E., Morgan, A.O., Kemp, H.G., et al.: Brain metabolism during fasting. J. Clin. Invest. *46*:1589, 1967.

59. Himwich, H.D.: Brain Metabolism and Cerebral Disorders. Baltimore, Williams & Wilkins Co., 1951.

60. Meldrum, B.S., Horton, R.W., Brierly, J.B.: Insulin-induced hypoglycemia in the primate: relationship between physiological changes and neuropathology. In: J.B. Brierly and B.S. Meldrum (Eds.): Brain Hypoxia. Clinics in Developmental Medicine 39/40. London, Spastics Internat. Med. Publ., 1971, p. 207.

61. Marks, V., Rose, F.C.: Hypoglycaemia. 2nd ed. Oxford, Blackwell Scientific Publications, 1981, pp. 103–105.

20 Transplantation of the Pancreas and Islet Tissue

Stephen Podolsky and Alexander Marble

Although relatively few patients with insulin-dependent diabetes have obtained more than modest short-term help from pancreatic transplants, countless patients may, in the years ahead, benefit from experience gained during the past two decades. During this time, many important advances have been made in the techniques of surgery and immunosuppression as acquired both in humans and animals. It is now possible to isolate and transplant islet tissue and cells into diabetic animals and, in many instances, restore normal plasma levels of glucose and insulin.[1-6] For a wealth of detailed information and extensive bibliographies, the reader is referred to Sutherland's reviews of both experimental studies and clinical trials.[7-8b] These have been drawn upon freely in the preparation of this chapter.

The concept of treating diabetes by transplantation of the pancreas goes back many years prior to the discovery of insulin. In 1892, 3 years after his discovery with von Mering that removal of the pancreas caused diabetes in experimental animals,[9] Minkowski[10] attempted pedicle transplants of a pancreatic lobe into the abdominal wall. In the same year, Hedon[11] reported that transplantation of the remaining portion of a partially resected pancreas prevented the development of diabetes as long as the transplant remained in healthy condition. In a remarkable prediction made 2 decades before the discovery of insulin, Ssobolew[12,13] suggested pancreatic transplantation as a treatment for diabetes mellitus. However, it was not until December 16, 1966 that a pancreas transplant (a segmental graft) was performed in a human being. Done at the University of Minnesota, this failed in a few weeks because of technical problems and rejection.[14]

ISLET AND PANCREAS TRANSPLANTATION IN ANIMALS

It has been amply shown that the transfer of isolated islet tissue between rats from inbred strains can reverse streptozotocin diabetes and can ameliorate nephropathy which has developed in such diabetic animals.[3,4] This has led to a search for ways in which islet tissue or cultured beta cells might be effectively and safely implanted in human diabetic patients. A possible step in this direction was made with the findings of Lacy and coworkers[15] who, by maintaining islet allografts in culture for 7 days at 24°C, prolonged their survival more than 12-fold in diabetic rats who had received one injection of ALS (rabbit antiserum to rat lymphocytes).

Attempts in animals to secure viable and functional grafts of islet tissue have taken various forms: (1) transplantation of islets (after digestion of pancreatic tissue by collagenase) to various sites, including the peritoneal cavity and spleen. Fetal or neonatal islets are preferable due to the greater ratio of endocrine to exocrine tissue, thereby providing a larger yield of islets; (2) transfer of fetal pancreases as free, whole organ grafts; (3) embolization by injection of pre-treated islets into the portal vein (quite successful); (4) grafting into highly vascular organs such as the spleen of "purified" islet tissue or beta cells grown in tissue culture; or (5) placing in the blood stream of diabetic animals islet tissue or beta cells cultured in artificial capillary units or chambers[1,17] that protect them from lymphocytes or antibodies whose larger molecular weight prevents their passage through membranes permeable to insulin and glucose.

A few of these ingenious attempts have yielded initial success but none has demonstrated long-term viability and effectiveness in insulin production. The use of inbred strains of animals is helpful, but otherwise the problems encountered are similar to those found in human transplantation efforts, i.e., rejection and infection in an immunosuppressed recipient.

The first experimental pancreatic allotransplantations by direct vascular suture techniques were performed in animals by Delezenne and co-workers[18] and by Gayet and Guillaumie[19] in 1927 and by Houssay[20] in 1929. Interest waned until 1962 when, in dogs, heterotopic allotransplantation of the pancreas to the femoral vessels was carried out with cannulation of the attached duodenum for external drainage of digestive enzymes.[21] Both endocrine and exocrine functions of the donor pancreas were preserved, but only short-term survival ensued. Over the years a variety of surgical techniques were developed and applied, occasionally resulting in functioning transplants, documented by radioimmunoassay of insulin released by the grafted pancreatic or islet tissue.

EXPERIENCE IN HUMAN DIABETIC PATIENTS

As stated earlier, the first pancreas transplant performed in a human was done in 1966 but it was not until 12 years later that worldwide, more than 9 transplants were done in a single year.

Organ Transplant Registry

From December 16, 1966 until it was closed on June 30, 1977, the Organ Transplant Registry of the American College of Surgeons/National Institutes of Health, recorded 57 pancreas transplants in 55 patients with diabetes.[22] Only two of the patients were able to be maintained without insulin injections for longer than 1 year. One was a patient of Lillehei et al.[14] who received a pancreaticoduodenal graft, and the other, a patient of Gliedman et al.[23] who had a segmental pancreatic graft. Both patients died with functioning grafts at 12[14] and 49[23] months, respectively, after transplantation.

A new International Human Pancreas and Islet Transplant Registry was formed in 1979[24] under the auspices of the Scientific Studies Committee of the American Society of Transplant Surgeons. In Figure 20-1 is shown the distribution of the first 337 pancreas transplants in 316 patients performed in 46 medical centers through June 30, 1983 (including those reported to the earlier registry).[8a]

Ten groups performed more than 10 transplants; the total number was 248. Although nearly half of the 57 transplants reported to the original Organ Transplant Registry were pancreaticoduodenal, 256 of the 280 transplants carried out from July 1977 to June 30, 1983 were segmental.[8a]

Of the 337 transplants carried out at 15 different institutions between December 1966 and December 1982, 31 were functioning as of December 1983 for durations up to and including 12 months. The breakdown as regards length of reported functioning was as follows: 13–24 months, 14 transplants; 25–36 months, 12 transplants; 37–48 months, 1 transplant; 49–60 months, 3 transplants; 61 months and over, 1 transplant (65 months).[8a]

Types of Transplants

Each of the two main types of transplants, pancreaticoduodenal and segmental, has its advantages and disadvantages.

Pancreaticoduodenal Transplantation. With this procedure, the pancreas, duodenum, an aortic patch encompassing the coeliac axis and superior mesenteric artery, and the portal vein are removed as a single piece from the donor, and vascular anastomoses are made to the iliac vessels of the recipient.[8] Lillehei and colleagues[27] originally brought the duodenum out as a duodenostomy, and the pancreatic juices were collected from the duodenal stoma. In later patients the duodenum was connected directly to the patient's small intestine via a Roux-en-Y loop at the time of the transplantation.

About half of the pancreaticoduodenal grafts were technically satisfactory and functioned until rejection or death.[8] Complications such as vascular thromboses or infections occurred in other patients. Because of the technical difficulties and complications, this procedure has been largely abandoned in favor of segmental pancreas transplantation.

Segmental Pancreas Transplantation. Gliedman et al. at the Montefiore Hospital in New York, did the first large series (11 patients) of segmental grafts beginning in 1970.[23] The first (1966) pancreas transplant at the University of Minnesota, which has been the most active medical center in this field, was a segmental transplant[28] and almost all groups currently performing pancreas transplants use this procedure. The body and tail of the pancreas (approximately 50% of the organ) are removed, and the coeliac axis (or splenic artery) and portal vein (or splenic vein) are used for anastomoses to the iliac vessels of the diabetic recipient.[8] The segmental pancreas transplant allows the use of living related donors, since more than half of the pancreas can be removed from a normal individual without serious consequences, and the spleen will survive with blood from the short gastric vessels.[8] Figure 20–2 illustrates a technique of segmental pancreas transplantation.

Sutherland[26] states that in August, 1982, of 154 recipients of transplants since July 1, 1977, 106 or 69% were alive. There were 37 grafts which had functioned for 2 to 49 months. In the period named, of 163 transplants, 158 were of the segmental type.

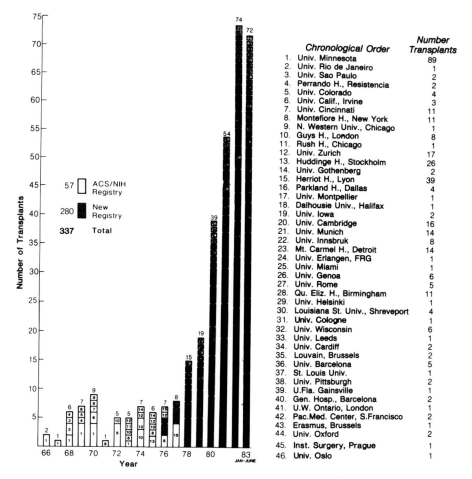

Chronological Order	Number Transplants
1. Univ. Minnesota	89
2. Univ. Rio de Janeiro	1
3. Univ. Sao Paulo	2
4. Perrando H., Resistencia	2
5. Univ. Colorado	4
6. Univ. Calif., Irvine	3
7. Univ. Cincinnati	11
8. Montefiore H., New York	11
9. N. Western Univ., Chicago	1
10. Guys H., London	8
11. Rush H., Chicago	1
12. Univ. Zurich	17
13. Huddinge H., Stockholm	26
14. Univ. Gothenberg	2
15. Herriot H., Lyon	39
16. Parkland H., Dallas	4
17. Univ. Montpellier	1
18. Dalhousie Univ., Halifax	1
19. Univ. Iowa	2
20. Univ. Cambridge	16
21. Univ. Munich	14
22. Univ. Innsbruk	8
23. Mt. Carmel H., Detroit	14
24. Univ. Erlangen, FRG	1
25. Univ. Miami	1
26. Univ. Genoa	6
27. Univ. Rome	5
28. Qu. Eliz. H., Birmingham	11
29. Univ. Helsinki	1
30. Louisiana St. Univ., Shreveport	4
31. Univ. Cologne	1
32. Univ. Wisconsin	6
33. Univ. Leeds	1
34. Univ. Cardiff	2
35. Louvain, Brussels	2
36. Univ. Barcelona	5
37. St. Louis Univ.	1
38. Univ. Pittsburgh	2
39. U.Fla. Gainsville	1
40. Gen. Hosp., Barcelona	2
41. U.W. Ontario, London	1
42. Pac.Med. Center, S.Francisco	2
43. Erasmus, Brussels	1
44. Univ. Oxford	2
45. Inst. Surgery, Prague	1
46. Univ. Oslo	1

Fig. 20–1. Number of pancreas transplants performed in the world by year and institution between December 1966 and June 30, 1983. Each institution is assigned a number according to the chronological order by which they did their first transplant. From Sutherland[8a] with permission of author and publishers.

SELECTION OF PATIENTS AND PROBLEMS IN TRANSPLANTATION

Patient Selection and Prevention of Graft Rejection

Most transplants have been done in patients with end-stage diabetic glomerulopathy and prior renal transplantation. There has been controversy over whether the kidney or the pancreas should be transplanted first, or whether the two organs should be grafted simultaneously. Since immunosuppressive therapy is obligatory for diabetic patients who have had or will require a renal transplant, it is likely that pancreas transplantation will continue to be performed primarily in these end-stage patients with a renal transplant. There is reason to suspect that if safe and adequate immunosuppressive therapy becomes available, transplantation of the pancreas into nonuremic diabetics may result in prevention or amelioration of characteristic complications of Type I diabetes.

It seems likely that cyclosporine A, available in recent years, may reduce the rejection rate of cadaver organ transplants. Although in adequate dosage it is a powerful immunosuppressive agent, its use as a single drug is limited by its toxic effects on the liver and kidney.[28a] Consequently, it has often been used in combination with more conventional therapy which includes azothioprine and prednisone.[29] The Canadian Multicentre Transplant Study Group concluded that cyclosporine is preferable to azothioprine in preventing renal transplant rejection.[30]

Management of Pancreatic Secretions

A variety of methods have been used to handle the secretions of segmental pancreas transplants by drainage or suppression. As summarized by Sutherland[8] these include: (a) deliberate cutaneous fistula; (b) duct ligation; (c) ductoureterostomy; (d) free peritoneal drainage; (e) pancreatojejunostomy; and (f) pancreatic duct occlusion by synthetic pol-

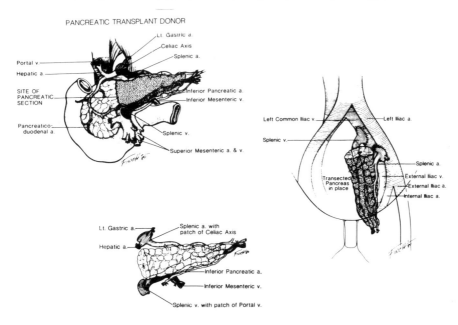

PANCREATIC TRANSPLANT DONOR

Fig. 20–2. Technique of segmental pancreas transplantation. Body and tail are transplanted with anastomoses of splenic vessels of donor pancreas to iliac vessels of recipient. From Sutherland[8] with permission of author and publishers.

ymers such as neoprene and prolamine. For technical details regarding these methods, the interested reader may consult the article by Sutherland.[8] At present, duct occlusion is the most favored, being used more often than any other technique. However, there has been concern that in the long run, fibrosis about the ducts may take place and cause damage to the endocrine tissue.

Returning to the transplant method of pancreatico-enteric anastomosis, there appears to be a consensus that, in contrast to segmental grafts, this more physiologic approach would better handle exocrine secretions if such could be accomplished without a significant risk of pancreatic fistulas and sepsis. This was taken up anew by workers at the Karolinska Institute in Stockholm who made various modifications of technical procedures. In a preliminary communication, they reported success with pancreatico-jejunal anastomosis in 3 consecutive patients with end-stage renal disease due to diabetic nephropathy who underwent combined renal and pancreatic transplantations.[31]

TRANSPLANTATION OF ISLET TISSUE

The promising results of transplantation of islet tissue in animals has naturally prompted trials in human patients. In his review, Sutherland[8a] states that 73 such operations were reported to the Registry as done prior to June 30, 1980, and 86 following that date for a total of 159 transplants performed up to June 30, 1983. The techniques were varied. fetal or adult islet tissue was used; sites of transplant included the portal vein, spleen and mus-

cle. In none of these cases has the recipient achieved independence from injected insulin. Sutherland concludes that a satisfactory method of allotransplantation of islet tissue is not as yet available for human use.

According to Sutherland's tabulations, 79 instances of islet autotransplantation were known to the Registry as of 1983. These were done in the attempt not to precipitate diabetes after extensive resection of the pancreas for malignancy or pancreatitis. Apparently about half of the recipients remained insulin independent.[8a]

MINNESOTA EXPERIENCE

In a separate report, Sutherland et al.[8b] have summarized the experience at the Hospitals of the University of Minnesota between July 1978 and December 1983. During this period, 75 patients with insulin-dependent diabetes received 85 grafts, 67 of which were segmental and 18 whole organ. At the time of the report, 23 (31%) of the recipients had functioning grafts, the longest duration of which was 65 months. Of the total, 50 transplants were from cadaver donors (32 segmental and 18 whole organ) and 35 were segmental from living related donors. Along with antilymphocyte globulin and prednisone, cyclosporine-A was used more than azathioprine as an immunosuppressive agent, although these workers apparently rated the two about the same in efficacy and found no significant difference in the survival of pancreas grafts.

Of the 23 patients who were not receiving exogenous insulin at the time of the report, 12 had normal or nearly normal glucose tolerance test results. Findings among the other patients varied from normal tolerance tests and normal 24-hour blood glucose profiles to grossly abnormal results by both means of evaluation. Results in this regard are in general in agreement with those of Pozza et al.[32]

The Minnesota group regards open biopsy of the pancreas graft as the best method to distinguish rejection from other possible causes of hyperglycemia in recipients of pancreas transplants. They find that vasculitis is the only certain criterion of rejection either of a pancreas or kidney transplant, although it does not necessarily indicate such.

Initially, pancreas transplantation was done by the Minnesota group (as by others) only in patients who had previously received kidney transplants. However, beginning in 1980, these workers have accepted non-uremic, non-renal-transplant patients whose complications of diabetes seemed more severe than the potential side effects of immunosuppression. They state that now such patients make up the majority of recipients (17 of 23 transplants in 1983). Since 1979, 32 (40%) of transplants have been segmental from living related donors (for a later report see Sutherland[33]).

The general consensus at present is that the progress made in the field of islet tissue and whole pancreas transplantation is encouraging. However, better solutions are needed for the problems of rejection and infection, and more information is required as to the length of life of the beta cell after successful transfer from one body to another.

FINAL COMMENT

An all-important question still to be answered is whether pancreas transplantation will provide prevention and/or amelioration of the vascular complications of diabetes. On the basis of experience in animals, mentioned earlier, there is a satisfying basis for hope that this may be the case. However, until truly long-term functioning of islet tissue or pancreatic transplants in human patients becomes a reality, it is not possible to assess benefits with certainty, aside from the expected freeing of the patient from daily insulin injections and other restrictions of present-day treatment. Nevertheless, in view of progress to date, one may justifiably look forward to continued advances.

REFERENCES

1. Leonard, R.J., Lazarow, A., Hegre, O.D.: Pancreatic islet transplantation in the rat. Diabetes 22:413, 1973.
2. Kemp, C.B., Knight, M.J., Scharp, D.W., et al.: Effect of transplantation site on the results of pancreatic islet isografts in diabetic rats. Diabetologia 9:486, 1973.
3. Mauer, S.M., Sutherland, D.E.R., Steffes, M.W., et al.: Pancreatic islet transplantation: effects on the glomerular lesions of experimental diabetes in the rat. Diabetes 23:748, 1974.
4. Mauer, S.M., Steffes, M.W., Sutherland, D.E.R., et al.: Studies of the rate of regression of the glomerular lesions of diabetic rats treated with pancreatic islet transplantation. Diabetes 24:280, 1975.
5. Matas, A.J., Payne, W.D., Grotting, J.C., et al.: Portal versus systemic transplantation of dispersed neonatal pancreas. Transplantation 24:333, 1977.
6. Pipeleers, D.G., Pipeleers-Marichal, M.A., Karl, J.E., Kipnis, D.M.: Secretory capability of islets transplanted intraportally in the diabetic rat. Diabetes 27:817, 1978.
7. Sutherland, D.E.R.: Pancreas and islet transplantation: I. Experimental studies. Diabetologia 20:161, 1981.
8. Sutherland, D.E.R.: Pancreas and islet transplantation: II. Clinical trials. Diabetologia 20:435, 1981.
8a. Sutherland, D.E.R.: Pancreas and islet transplant registry data. World J. Surg. 8:270, 1984.
8b. Sutherland, D.E.R., Chinn, P.L., Goetz, F.C., et al.: Minnesota experience with 85 pancreas transplants between 1978 and 1983. World J. Surg. 8:244, 1984.
8c. Benedetti, M.M., Hansen, B., Federlin, K., et al.: Report of the second workshop of the EASD Study Group on artificial insulin delivery systems, pancreas and islet transplantation (AIDSPIT). Diabetologia 26:169, 1984.
9. Von Mering, J., Minkowski, O.: Diabetes mellitus nach Pankreasextirpation. Arch. Exper. Path. Pharmakol. 26:371, 1889.
10. Minkowski, O.: Weitere Mitteilung über den diabetes mellitus nach Extirpation des Pankreas. Berlin Klin. Wochenschr. 29:90, 1892.
11. Hédon, E.: Fistule pancreatique. Compt. Rend. Soc. Biol. 44:678, 1892.
12. Ssobolew, L.W.: Zur normalen und pathologischen Morphologie der innern Secretion der Bauchspeicheldrüse. Virchows Arch. Path. Anat. 168:91, 1902.
13. Ssobolew, L.W.: Quoted by A.O. Whipple. A historical sketch of the pancreas. In: J.M. Howard and G.L. Jordan, Jr. (Eds.): Surgical Diseases of the Pancreas. Philadelphia, J.B. Lippincott Co., 1960, p. 2.
14. Lillehei, R.C., Ruiz, J.O., Acquino, C., Goetz, F.C.: Transplantation of the pancreas. Acta Endocrinol. (Kbh.) 83 (Suppl. 205):303, 1976.
15. Lacy, P.E., Davis, J.M., Finke, E.M.: Prolongation of islet allograft survival following in vitro culture (24 degrees C) and a single injection of A.L.S. Science 204:312, 1979.
16. Chick, W.L., Perna, J.J., Lauris, V., et al.: Artificial pancreas using living beta cells. Effect on glucose homeostasis in diabetic rats. Science 197:780, 1977.
17. Tze, J., Wong, F.C., Chen, L.M., O'Young, S.: Implantable endocrine pancreas unit used to restore normoglycemia in the diabetic rat. Nature 264:466, 1976.
18. Delezenne, C., Hallion, L., Gayet, R.: Sur le mecanisme de la secretion pancréatique. Mise en derivation d'une anse intestinale et d'un pancreas sur la circulation carotidojugulaire. Ann. Physiol. Physicochim. (Paris) 3:508, 1927.
19. Gayet, R., Guillaumie, M.: La regulation de la secretion interne pancréatique par un processus humorale, démontrée par des transplantations du pancreas. Experiences sur des animaux normaux. Compt. Rend. Soc. Biol. 97:1613, 1927.
20. Houssay, B.A.: Technique de la greffe pancreatico-duodenale au coul. Compt. Rend. Soc. Biol. 100:138, 1929.
21. DeJode, L.R., Howard, J.M.: Studies in pancreaticoduodenal homotransplantation. Surg. Gynec. Obstet. 114:553, 1962.
22. Gerrish, E.W.: Final newsletter, American College of Sur-

geons/National Institutes of Health Organ Transplant Registry, 1977.

23. Gliedman, M.L., Tellis, V.A., Soberman, R., et al.: Long-term effects of pancreatic transplant function in patients with advanced juvenile-onset diabetes. Diabetes Care *1*:1, 1978.

24. Sutherland, D.E.R.: International Human Pancreas and Islet Transplant Registry. Transplant Proc. *12* (Supp. 2):229, 1980.

25. Sutherland, D.E.R.: Report of International Human Pancreas and Islet Transplant Registry cases through 1981. Diabetes *31* (Suppl. 4):112, 1982.

26. Sutherland, D.E.R.: Current status of pancreas transplantation: Registry statistics and an overview. Transplant Proc. *15*:1303, 1983.

27. Lillehei, R.C., Idezuki, Y., Feemster, J.A., et al.: Transplantation of stomach, intestine, and pancreas: Experimental and clinical observations. Surgery *62*:721, 1967.

28. Kelly, W.D., Lillehei, R.C., Merkel, F.K., et al.: Allotransplantation of the pancreas and duodenum along with the kidney in diabetic nephropathy. Surgery *61*:827, 1967.

28a. Strom, T.B., Loertscher, R.: Cyclosporine-induced nephrotoxicity? Inevitable and intractable? (Editorial). N. Engl. J. Med. *311*:728, 1984.

29. Squifflet, J.-P., Sutherland, D.E.R., Rynasiewicz, J.J., et al.: Combined immunosuppressive therapy with cyclosporin A and azathioprine. A synergistic effect in three of four experimental models. Transplantation *34*:315, 1982.

30. The Canadian Multicenter Transplant Study Group: A randomized clinical trial of cyclosporine in cadaveric renal transplantation. N. Engl. J. Med. *309*:809, 1983.

31. Groth, C.G., Lundgren, G., Collste, H., et al.: Successful outcome of segmental human pancreatic transplantation with enteric exocrine diversion after modifications in technique. Lancet *2*:522, 1982.

32. Pozza, G., Traeger, J., Dubernard, J.M., et al.: Endocrine responses of Type I (insulin-dependent) diabetic patients following successful pancreas transplantation. Diabetologia *24*:244, 1983.

33. Sutherland, D.E.R., Goetz, F.C., Najarian, J.S.: Recent experience with 89 pancreas transplants at a single institution. Diabetologia *27* (Suppl.):149, 1984.

21 Oral Hypoglycemic Agents

Leo P. Krall

It is both presumptuous and counter-productive 60 years after the introduction of what ultimately became the biguanides[1] and 40 years after the start of the sulfonylurea[2-4] era, to re-invent the wheel by discussing extensively what is already documented and accepted. Most publications concerning diabetes in the past 20 years have often covered the same material, with entire books written about individual oral agents. One of these[5] has 625 pages with 1706 references. This chapter in the 11th edition had 247 references. Suffice it to say, it is more useful to start with a baseline of accepted information with the simple, all-encompassing quotation from the WHO (World Health Organization) Expert Committee on Diabetes Mellitus[6] that states succinctly: "Used selectively, oral agents occupy a place in diabetes therapy."

UPDATE

In spite of often sailing through tempestuous academic seas, the widespread therapeutic use of the oral agents continues. In the United States in 1980[7] the market for these products was $118,000,000 as compared to $104,000,000 spent on insulin. The cost of these agents constitutes a large part of the estimated 12 billion dollars spent annually on diabetes-oriented materials and services.

The number of patients using oral agents in the United States in 1980 was estimated as 1.8 million, and somewhat more than the estimate of 1.3 million taking insulin. In Europe and Japan the users of oral hypoglycemic agents greatly outnumber those treated with insulin. Moreover, given the generally poor effectiveness of the dietary prescription, many of the estimated 2,200,000 possibly under treatment with diet alone will eventually have oral agents or insulin added to the protocol.

The major changes in the universe of oral hypoglycemic agents during the past decade are these: (1) continuing, discordant notes pro and con the University Group Diabetes Program (UGDP); (2) the demise of phenformin in the United States and some fall from grace in certain other parts of the world; (3) further delineation of the extrapancreatic action of the sulfonylurea agents and their mechanism of action; and (4) the advent of the "second generation" of sulfonylurea compounds, as well as other oral blood glucose-lowering agents in various stages of planning or research.

EARLIER OBSERVATIONS

Early observations of substances effective in lowering the blood glucose level demonstrate that there is nothing completely new under the sun and that numerous compounds available in nature, though frequently toxic, are capable of accomplishing this.

Botanical and Sundry Natural and Ethnic Remedies

Plants have been sources of medication since antiquity and many ethnic groups have favorite remedies, real or imaginary, for diabetes. Scarcely any physician interested in diabetes worldwide has not had a patient bring him from some unknown source a packet of dried leaves that were said to lower blood glucose. Myrtillin[8] from blueberry leaves (whortleberry) has been investigated for many decades. Ivanka Frajevic[9] found that the extract, when purified, contained quercetin and s-methyl-methionine which had a definite if inconsistent hypoglycemic effect on alloxanized diabetic rats.

The extract of roots of the devil's club *(Fatsia horrida);* extract of raw cabbage; Cundeamor, made from *Momordica charantia;* Amellin, from *Scoperia dulcis;* sumach *(Rhustyphina);* Pterocarpus marsupium; Eugenia jambolana; Aspergillus niger; Fungi imperfecti* from avocado leaves; and others have been thought to have hypoglycemic properties.[10,11] A major drug of this type is hypoglycin, an extract of *ackee,* a native fruit of the West Indies. The list continues to grow. Other reported substances in this field, *Sarandi bianco* bark and *Skelly-F* both lowered the blood glucose in rats but required doses that were extremely high (as much as 500 to 1000 mg/kg).[12] Dr. S.S Ajgaonkar,

the leader of present-day studies of diabetes in India, has compiled a list of many exotic native remedies for diabetes, many of which apparently do decrease glycosuria.[13]

To demonstrate that hypoglycemic effect may be found in mundane things, Tjokroprawiro et al. of the School of Medicine, Airlangga University, Surbaya, Indonesia,[14,14a] in a prospective crossover study, observed that a diet of green beans and onions was accompanied by a reduction of blood glucose levels.

Guanidine Derivatives

The use of guanidine derivatives started with Watanabe[1] in 1918, and Frank and co-workers.[15-17] These homologues of guanidine, deca-methylene-diguanide (Synthalin A), were in use for a number of years by many physicians of that era. These substances eventually proved toxic with apparent liver damage.[4,18,19] In spite of this, Synthalin, a forerunner of the later biguanides, might not have disappeared so rapidly were it not for the development of insulin.

Early Sulfonylurea Compounds

Carbutamide (BZ-55) was the first modern clinically effective sulfonylurea.[20] The possible usefulness of sulfonamides in lowering blood glucose had been considered much earlier. Among the early workers were Ruiz et al.,[21] followed by the classic observations of Janbon,[2] as summarized by Loubatieres.[22]

Houssay[23] also described hypoglycemic effects in experimental animals but there was no widespread clinical application of these data until 1955 when Franke and Fuchs,[4] using carbutamide, observed hypoglycemic symptoms accompanied by low blood glucose levels. Soon many sulfonlyurea compounds were developed. These included tolbutamide, chlorpropamide, metahexamide, acetohexamide, tolazamide and many others. Two of the above (carbutamide and metahexamide) were

Table 21–1. Criteria for Degrees of Glycemic Control in Gauging Effectiveness of Treatment with Diet Alone or with Oral Hypoglycemic Agents. Values Listed are for Glucose (mg/dl) in Whole Venous Blood and in Serum (or Plasma)*

	Good		Fair		Poor
Relation to food	Whole blood	Serum or plasma	Whole blood	Serum or plasma	
Fasting	110	125	130	150	
1 hr. p.c.	150	170	180	200	All
2 hr. p.c.	130	150	150	170	other
3 hr. p.c.	110	125	130	150	values

*For the purpose of classification as to degree of control, 70% or more of the values must conform with the standards listed in the table. These standard values are the highest acceptable; one strives for values closer to normal if considered safe for the individual.

Table 21–2. World-Wide Available Oral Hypoglycemic Compounds by Generic and Trade Names*

1. ACETOHEXAMIDE
Antrepar, Dimelin, Dimelor, Dymelor, Gamadiabet, Hipoglicil, Metaglucina, Ordimel

2. AZEPENAMIDE
Betagon, Hexamyl, Perinase

3. BENZYLSULFONAMIDE
Gludinase, Glycodiazin, Gondofo, Oisen

4. BUFORMIN (Butyl Biguanide)
Bumel, Diabrin, Diabetos B., Diabetun S., Gliporal Lentocaps, P. 51084, Munel TM, Silubin, Retard, Silubin, Sindatil, Tidemol Ret, Probucal

5. CARBUTAMIDE
Alentin, Antidiabeticum, Butylsulfina, Carbutamidum, Carbutil, Dia Tablinen, Diabetamide, Glucidoral, Invenol, Midisol, Nadisan, Norboral Simplex, Norboral Vit., Orank, Retarden, Sulfadiabet, Yosulan

6. CHLORPROPAMIDE
Agnophenol, Apo-Chlorpropam, Bioglumin, Catanil, Chlopamide, Chloromide, Chloronase, Chlorpropamida MK, Chlorpropamide, Clordiabet, Clordiasan, Copamide, Dabinese, Diabamide, Diabet Pages, Diabetas, Diabetasi, Diabetex, Diabetics, Diabetil, Diabetoral, Diabikyn, Diabinese, Diabitex, Dianese, Galiron, Glucopless, Glucosulfina, Glynese, Melitase, Mellinese, Mellitos-C, Melormin, Nogluc, Nogral, Norboral, Novopropamide, Orabet, Oradian, P-604, Pamidin, Promide, Propamid, Shuabate, Stabinol, Sucrase, Toyomelin

18. GLYIBUZOL
Gluciase

19. GLYMIDINE
Redul

20. METAHEXAMIDE
Isodiane

21. METFORMIN (Methyl Biguanide)
Diabetosan, Diabex, Diabfor, Diformin -Ret., Glaformil, Gleofago, Glucinan, Glucofago, Glucophage, Glucophage -Ret., Glucophage Forte, Glucofagos, Gluformin, Glyciphage, Glycoran, Isotin, Melbin, Mellitin, Metformin, Metforminum, Metiguanide, Risidon, Rythmes, Stagid, Toulibor, Tolubol

22. PHENFORMIN (Phenethyl Biguanide)
Asipol, Azucaps, Biguanida Ret., Cronoformin, DB Retard, DBI Ret. T.D., Debei, Debeina, Debeone, Debynil, Diabetal, Diabiguan, Diabis Ret., Diaperos, Dibein, Dibein Retard, Dibotin, Dipar Retard, Fegunide, Glupostin, Glucopostin, Glucopostin Ret., Informin, Insogen, Insoral, Lentobetic, Meltrol, Normoglucina, Oradiabeta, Osmoform, Phenformin

23. TOLBUTAMIDE
Apo-Tolbutamide, Arcosal, Artosin, Artosina, Butamide, Debetos 500, Diaben, Diabuton, Diasulfon, Diabetos, Dolipol, Mellitos D, Mobinol, Neo Norboral, Neo Norboral Vit., Neobellin, Novobutamide, Oralin, Oramide, Ordiabet, Orinase, Osdiabet, Sinabetes, Tolbet, Tolbumid, Tolbutamid, Tolbutamid 500, Tolbutamid Tabline, Tolbutamid Ratio, Tolbutamida, Tolbutamide, Tolbutin, Tolbutone

7. GLIBORNURIDE — Glinor, Glitrim, Gluborid, Glutrid, Glutril, Glutrim
8. GLICLAZIDE — Diamicron
9. GLIPENTIDE — Staticum
10. GLIPIZIDE — Glibenese, Glucotrol, Micronese, Mindiab, Minidiab, Minodiab, Minodial
11. GLIQUIDONE — Glurenor, Glurenorm
12. GLISOXEPIDE — Bay 4321, Glucoben, Pro-Diaban
13. GLYBURIDE (Glibenclamide) — Adiab, Armoniol, Benclamide, Betanase, Clamid, Daonil, DiaBeta, Diaboral, Dimel, Euglucan, Euglucon-5, Euglyben, Euglykon, Gilamal, Gliben, Glibenclamida MK, Glibenclamidum, Glidiabet, Glinor, Glucolon, Glucoven, Glybenclamidum, Hemi-Daonil, Lisaglucon, Maninil, Micronese, Miglucan, Pira, Semi Daonil, Semi Euglucon
14. GLYBUTAMIDE — Clucidoral
15. GLYCODIAZINE — Glyconormal, Gondafon-28, Lycanol, Redul-28
16. GLYCLOPYRAMIDE — Deamelin-S
17. GLYCYCLAMIDE — Agliral, Diaboral

24. TOLAZAMIDE — Diabewas, Diabutos, Norglycin, Tolanase, Tolinas, Tolinase, Tolisan, Edudine, Guabeta N, Mellitol, Pramidex, Rastinon, Riboral, Tolgybuzamide, Tolnin, Tolurasi, Tolvit, Varoxina, Yosulan T
25. CARBUTAMIDE AND PHENFORMIN — Glucifrene
26. CHLORPROPAMIDE AND METFORMIN — Diabiformin, Diabiphage, Mellitron, Obinese
27. CHLORPROPAMIDE AND PHENFORMIN — Bidiabe, Biodiabes, Chlorformin, Combinacin, Diabetoplex, Diabis Compositum, Diabitol, Endiabin, Insogen Plus, Insone, Reobron, Trane, Zacharol
28. GLYBURIDE AND PHENFORMIN — Bi-Euglucon, Daopar, Gli-Norboral Cpto, Gliben F, Gliformin, Norglicem, Suguan
29. GLYCYCLAMIDE AND METFORMIN — Agliral Compuesto, Diabomet
30. GLYSOXEPIDE AND BUFORMIN — Sindiatil, Diabone
31. TOLBUTAMIDE AND METFORMIN — Glucosulfa
32. TOLBUTAMIDE AND PHENFORMIN — Melus, Oraleo, Tolbusan, Ultra-Norboral, 500
33. PHENFORMIN AND OXYPRODIOPHEN — DB Comb., Prodiaben

*All are sulfonylurea derivatives unless otherwise designated.

discontinued in the United States because of related cholangiostatic jaundice in patients.

Since "many are called but few are chosen," of the numerous sulfonylurea compounds studied, many have been found to be effective and potentially useful, but costs of research and marketing as well as the absence of any unique properties, caused their abandonment.

Other Blood-Glucose-Lowering Substances

Other agents, not specifically prepared for diabetics, have shown hypoglycemic properties. Decades ago, Blotner and Murphy[24] noted that, upon injection, preparations made from the liver of calves, lowered the blood glucose. Salicylates when used in the treatment of rheumatic fever in nondiabetic children, may cause lowering of the blood glucose.[25] Likewise, some antihistamines have this effect[26] as does imipramine.[27] The list of such substances is endless, including therapeutic compounds in common use, as propoxyphene (Darvon)[28] and the anti-arrhythmic drug, disopyramide (Norpace).[29,30] Thus, one should be aware of the many substances which produce hypoglycemic activity but which are not appropriate in the treatment of diabetes.

CRITERIA FOR EVALUATION OF ORAL HYPOGLYCEMIC AGENTS

It must be presumed that the oral hypoglycemic agents are intended as a means to help "control" the diabetes. Since most physicians are perfectionists by inclination and training, it is difficult to understand why in the past they have made extraordinary attempts to maintain all physiologic and chemical parameters at normal levels, and yet many have regarded normoglycemia as unimportant. Since the consequences of poorly controlled diabetes may take many years to develop, physicians are more likely to be concerned with what appear to be acute conditions with higher priority. While there is no complete, final proof of the value of tight regulation, increasingly "soft" evidence has pointed strongly in this direction, as summarized by Cahill et al.[31] Even those less enthusiastic about the virtues of tight control[32] suggest that "no one would disagree that it would be desirable to maintain the blood glucose of diabetic patients at normal levels if it were possible to do so safely." Deckert et al.[33] have demonstrated the beneficial effect on survival among various populations of insulin-dependent diabetics with an improved degree of diabetes control.

Too often reports of effectiveness of therapeutic methods have given no standard for evaluation. The words "control" and "regulation" mean little without such criteria. At the Joslin clinic, the effect of oral hypoglycemic compounds has been measured by the criteria cited in Table 21–1. While these may seem strict to some, they are considerably above the normal blood glucose levels in the nondiabetic, and are an attempt at practicality with avoidance of hypoglycemic reactions.

The diagnostic criteria suggested by the National Diabetes Data Group (NDDG) (see Table 15–2) present a dilemma because a fasting plasma glucose of 140 mg/dl (= about 120 mg/dl for whole blood) or an elevated plasma glucose greater than 200 mg/dl (= about 175 mg/dl for whole blood) at two hours is required for the diagnosis of diabetes. These values are obviously higher than those used by many clinical centers (See Tables 15–5 and 15–6). This brings up an interesting philosophic point. Are the NDDG criteria too lax? Or are the standards of Conn and Fajans, Joslin, et al. too rigid? If they are too rigid, then most patients treated with oral agents could be considered adequately controlled, making them almost 100% effective—which is not true.

In the treatment of diabetes, the choice to be made is the means of ensuring that there is adequate insulin action at the cellular level. A patient who does well with dietary restriction alone uses his own endogenous insulin, and this is also the case with effective oral agent therapy. Other patients require exogenous insulin given by injections. In any case, insulin is the only treatment available.

PRESENTLY AVAILABLE COMPOUNDS

Until May 1984, when glipizide and glyburide (glibenclamide) received F.D.A. approval for marketing in the United States, no new oral hypoglycemic compounds had become available for more than 20 years. Tabulation included only tolbutamide (Orinase), chlorpropamide (Diabinese), acetohexamide (Dymelor), and tolazamide (Tolinase). The removal of phenformin (DBI and Meltrol) from the market in 1977 by Federal fiat is discussed later in this chapter. However, these and many other compounds are used worldwide, and because the jet age has made travel commoner, Table 21–2 lists most available oral hypoglycemic compounds by both generic and trade names. The "second generation" compounds are discussed later.

In general, the present-day sulfonylurea agents are so well-known and documented that repetition is unnecessary. The first four compounds long available in the United States have a similar mechanism of action. The structural relationships are shown in Figure 21–1. The basic functional parts of the compounds are a benzene ring + a sulfonyl group + a urea. With tolbutamide (Orinase), a methyl group is added to the para-position of the

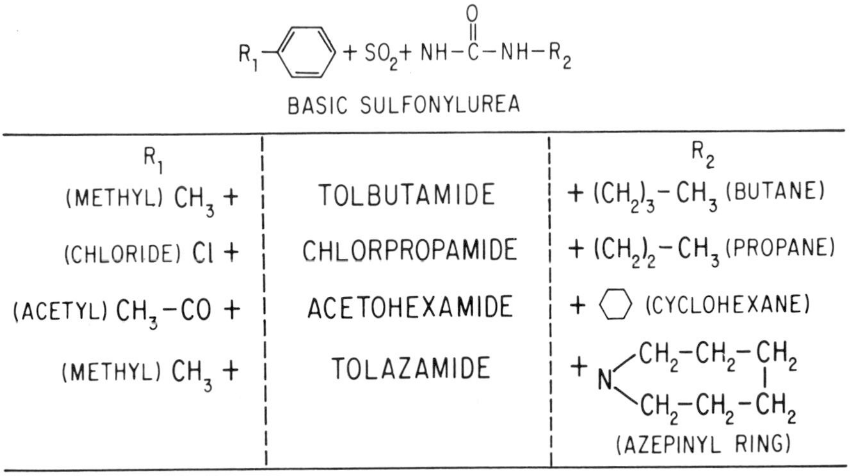

$$R_1 - \langle \text{benzene ring} \rangle + SO_2 + NH - \overset{\overset{O}{\parallel}}{C} - NH - R_2$$

BASIC SULFONYLUREA

R₁		R₂
(METHYL) CH_3 +	TOLBUTAMIDE	+ $(CH_2)_3 - CH_3$ (BUTANE)
(CHLORIDE) Cl +	CHLORPROPAMIDE	+ $(CH_2)_2 - CH_3$ (PROPANE)
(ACETYL) $CH_3 - CO$ +	ACETOHEXAMIDE	+ ⬡ (CYCLOHEXANE)
(METHYL) CH_3 +	TOLAZAMIDE	+ $N\begin{smallmatrix} CH_2-CH_2-CH_2 \\ \\ CH_2-CH_2-CH_2 \end{smallmatrix}$ (AZEPINYL RING)

Fig. 21–1. Formulas of the "first generation" sulfonylurea oral hypoglycemic compounds, and their relation to each other.

benzene ring and a butane to the urea group. For chlorpropamide (Diabinese), chloride is attached in the para-position of the benzene ring and a propane group added to the urea. For acetohexamide (Dymelor), an acetyl group is placed at the para-position of the benzene ring and a cyclohexane radical added to the urea. For tolazamide (Tolinase), methyl is at the para-position as in tolbutamide but, instead of a butane, a hexhydroazepinyl group is added to the urea group. Thus, the main basic structure with minor changes, prevails for all of these. This might be analogous to the fact that all automobiles are basic boxes with wheels, the differences being in performance, design and, of course, price. While sulfonylureas are much the same, slight differences in chemical structure and in metabolic fate when ingested, result in functional differences between these agents, which affect their potency and duration of action (See Table 21–3 and Figure 21–1).

Differences in Metabolism and Excretion. Since the beta cell stimulatory factor is similarly available in sulfonylureas, the fate of these compounds after ingestion is of basic importance.

It is difficult to be precise about duration of action of oral agents. Much data are based on "half-life" studies, which are averages. Repeated half-life studies of a pharmaceutical compound in the same person may give varying results, depending on liver and kidney function and other factors at a given time. Thus, while tolbutamide is the hypoglycemic agent of shortest duration and usually two or more doses are needed daily, Lozano-Castaneda and co-workers[34] showed that significant numbers of patients were adequately regulated with single doses of tolbutamide daily, proving again that each patient must be observed and treated as an individual (Table 21–4).

Tolbutamide (Orinase). This is the oldest and until recently most widely used oral compound in the United States. It was introduced in 1956, almost simultaneously with carbutamide, which was short-lived. Its characteristics are shown in Table 21–3. Wide use made it a subject for the University Group Diabetes Program discussed later. Tolbutamide is

Table 21–3. Fate and Approximate Duration of Action of the Sulfonylurea Oral Hypoglycemic Compounds Available in the United States before May 1984

Compound	Metabolized	Urinary Excretion in 24 Hours	Hypoglycemic Activity of Metabolites	Approximate Effectiveness in Hours
Tolbutamide	Rapidly	Nearly all	Inactive	6–10 (short)
Tolazamide	Rapidly	85%	+ †	12–18 (intermediate)
Acetohexamide	Rapidly	60%	+ + + ‡	12–20 (intermediate)
Chlorpropamide	Less than 1%	60%	Inactive	20–60 (long)

*It must be understood that "half-life" figures are only approximate, vary from patient to patient, and sometimes in the same individual. Listed in the last column above are estimated total durations of effect.
†Actually six major metabolites are formed; only three are hypoglycemic and only mildly so.
‡Although the metabolite is more hypoglycemic than the original, only minute amounts remain as metabolites.

Table 21–4.   Dosage of Presently Available Sulfonylurea Oral Hypoglycemic Compounds

Compound	Available Tablet	Starting Dose	Daily Dose Range (Grams)	Maximal Daily Dose (Grams)	Frequency
TOLBUTAMIDE (Orinase)	250 mg 0.5 g	0.5 g	0.5–3.0	2.0–3.0	Usually divided doses, 1–3 times daily
TOLAZAMIDE (Tolinase)	100 mg 250 mg 500 mg	100 mg	0.1–1.0	1.0	Single or divided doses
ACETOHEXAMIDE (Dymelor)	250 mg 500 mg	250 mg	0.25–1.5	1.5	Single or divided doses
CHLORPROPAMIDE (Diabinese)	100 mg 250 mg	100–250 mg	0.1–0.5	0.5	Single dose

carboxylated in the liver, rapidly metabolized, and almost entirely excreted in the urine as carboxytolbutamide. The derivative product is metabolically inert and the duration of action is usually about 6 to 10 hours. Its short active life and complete metabolization make it a useful choice for patients with diminished excretory functions, and less prone to cause severe or prolonged hypoglycemic reactions.

Chlorpropamide (Diabinese). Chlorpropamide is probably the most active hypoglycemically, longest in duration, and most widely used oral agent in the United States. It has been available since 1957. In contrast to the other oral agents, it has an anti-diuretic effect, discussed later. It is rapidly absorbed from the gut, and, following a single dose of 250 mg, has a peak plasma concentration of 20 to 30 mg/ml in about 4 to 6 hours, taking several days to eliminate the drug completely. The duration of chlorpropamide activity may be as long as 40 to 60 hours, although this would be rare, and the level of activity decreases as time progresses.

It has been widely accepted that chlorpropamide is not metabolized to any significant extent, being bound quite inexorably to protein. This has been questioned by Campbell et al.,[35] who quoted a representative of the manufacturer as stating that chlorpropamide has a variable hepatic metabolism, a renal excretion of unchanged drug between 6 and 60%, and a biological half-life of about 36 hours. Within 96 hours, 80 to 90% of a dose has been excreted in the urine. Early reports indicated that less than 1% of the drug is metabolized. However, later studies using sophisticated analytical techniques indicate that as much as 80% may be metabolized in diabetic patients, and 2 hours after chlorpropamide administration, the unchanged drug accounted for 95% of the total, but some metabolites had shorter elimination half-lives and the activity of these metabolites is unknown. In other words, results of this study suggested that chlorpropamide *is* metabolized in some patients

which, if true, may account for some of its strange interactions.

Chlorpropamide is considered to be an effective oral hypoglycemic agent. However, some precaution should be taken in its use, particularly with patients with decreased renal output, lest hypoglycemia occur.

Tolazamide (Tolinase). Structurally, tolazamide is similar to tolbutamide with a few significant changes. While readily absorbed from the gastrointestinal tract, this absorption takes place more slowly than with tolbutamide or chlorpropamide. The onset of hypoglycemic effect in fed diabetic patients occurs at 4 to 6 hours following ingestion, with duration of maximal hypoglycemic effect of about 10 hours. A rise in blood glucose becomes evident at 14 to 16 hours after the medication has been taken. About 85% of tolazamide is excreted in the urine within 24 hours. It has six metabolite products, three of which are only weakly hypoglycemic. Relatively few severe hypoglycemic reactions have been reported with tolazamide, and while it is said to be 5 to 9 times more potent than tolbutamide in laboratory animals,[36] a difference of this degree has not been observed in clinical practice. Although it has a more prolonged hypoglycemic effect than tolbutamide, it has been generally a safe and effective compound.

Acetohexamide (Dymelor). This is another compound of intermediate duration similar in effect to the other sulfonylurea compounds. It has been available since 1963 and is considered to be more active than tolbutamide. It is reduced rapidly in the liver to L-hydroxyhexamide and 60% is excreted in 24 hours, but the metabolite has considerable hypoglycemic activity, more than twice that of the original compound. Hence the duration of action is about 12 to 20 hours with a possible continued hypoglycemic activity for a longer period due to a residual hypoglycemic metabolite. Acetohexamide is also excreted by the kidneys and must be used carefully in patients with renal impairment. The dosage frequency is much like that of tolazamide.

When effective in lesser amounts, it may be used once daily, but if the dose requirement is greater than 1.0 g daily, it may be used in split doses. Although acetohexamide and tolbutamide have nearly the same biological half-life, the active metabolite keeps acetohexamide active longer. It also has a moderate but definite uricosuric property.[37]

DIFFERENCES IN THE FIRST GENERATION ORAL AGENTS

Since all the first generation oral hypoglycemic agents are effective in the same type of patients with Type II diabetes (NIDDM), how does the physician decide which to prescribe? Tests used formerly to determine patients most likely to succeed with oral therapy (e.g., the sulfonylurea response test described by Marble[10a]), while sometimes useful, were not infallible. Mahler[38] studied 12 obese and 8 lean diabetic patients by means of a tolbutamide response test in which levels of plasma glucose, C-peptide, and insulin were determined following the intravenous administration of 1 g of tolbutamide. A positive response was defined as a fall in glucose greater than 15% after 60 minutes. The patients were non-ketotic, maturity-onset diabetics who had been on insulin treatment until 1 day prior to the study. Of the 12 obese patients, 7 proved to be responders whereas of the 8 lean patients, only 2 responded positively. A fall in the blood glucose in the obese patients was accompanied by a rise in immunoreactive insulin and C-peptide levels. On the other hand, in the 2 lean patients who were responsive to tolbutamide, the drop in blood glucose was not correlated with either a rise in IRI or C-peptide levels. This difference in response of the obese and lean patients suggested to Mahler that there might be other mechanisms by which tolbutamide given intravenously lowers the blood glucose in such patients. He concluded that the intravenous tolbutamide test might be a valid indicator of those maturity-onset diabetic patients who would be responsive to treatment with diet and oral agents.

In practice, however, most clinicians use a trial-and-error method in prescribing oral agents, since even the most experienced clinician cannot always determine outcome in advance. Their choice of drug is often influenced by recollection of the therapeutic compound used during their training or by opinions expressed in medical literature.

The intensity of hypoglycemic effect is one means of making a selection. On this basis, tolbutamide is clearly mildest and chlorpropamide, most effective. On the other hand, the most potent agents are more likely to produce side effects as well as other undesirable responses. Duration of action is also a relevant matter. With patient compliance as a goal, this is more easily achieved with a single daily dose of a longer-acting medication (90% ± of compliance by patients) than with multiple doses of shorter-acting agents (30 to 50% of compliance.) Vinik[39] has documented that even with the least active type of oral agent, effective duration may be as long as 20 hours, and indicated, as did Lozano-Casteneda,[34] that in certain instances a single daily dose of tolbutamide may be as effective as divided doses, although this has not been the usual clinical experience. Clearly all of these oral agents are effective to some degree, but individual responses must be taken into account. One must consider side effects, potential toxicity, number of doses daily, and even patient idiosyncracies in making the initial choice of agent.

PRIMARY MECHANISM OF ACTION OF SULFONYLUREA AGENTS

It is believed that the primary action of the sulfonylurea agents is to stimulate insulin release, because functioning pancreatic islets are needed for the effectiveness of these compounds. Although there has been disagreement as to whether the insulin output is actually increased,[39a] the release is at least triggered.[40-43] It is accepted that after sulfonylurea use, there is a degranulation of the beta cells,[44,45] and some agreement as to how regranulation results from long-term sulfonylurea use.[46,47] There is also general consensus[41] concerning the inhibition of glucose formation from liver glycogen.[48,49] There is some disagreement about the details of sulfonylurea activity, since these agents appear also to increase the insulin stimulatory effect of glucose.[50,51] Also, there appears to be direct interaction with the membrane of the beta cell itself with changes in intracellular calcium,[52,53] during the process of insulin release.

Another phenomenon is that with continued administration of sulfonylureas, there appears to be improved glucose tolerance in the face of unaltered plasma insulin levels.[54-57] Lebovitz et al.[58] also showed that with chronic use of a second generation sulfonylurea, glipizide, the rate of insulin-mediated glucose disappearance became more efficient after a time. Blumenthal[59] demonstrated that chlorpropamide potentiated the ability of endogenous insulin to inhibit gluconeogenesis. Grodsky[60] found that one effect of chlorpropamide on beta cells was to stimulate insulin release in the early part of the reaction area. The so-called betacytotropic action resulting in insulin release is most active during the degranulation period.[61] With first generation drugs, there is a refractory period during which the beta cells no longer react despite stimulation.[61] It is claimed that this does not occur with second generation agents.[62]

Another topic of ongoing debate is whether or not chronic administration of sulfonylureas causes a deficit in circulating glucagon.[63] While some workers have found evidence of this,[64] it is now believed[65] that there is no glucagon decrease.

The most exciting recent development concerning the value of oral agents is the evidence of their effect on the insulin receptors. These are the glycoproteins which are on or in the cell membranes. Their function is to recognize insulin when it reaches this membrane and to bind it. The combination is thought then to generate a soluble second messenger which initiates cellular events. For insulin to work, every event in the series must work.[66] The receptor effect has been most pronounced with the second generation agents, but there is evidence of this even in the presently available oral agents. In obese persons, there are reduced numbers of insulin receptors, but weight loss and exercise can increase them. There is evidence that the oral agents increase the receptor sites in membranes of human monocytes[67] and also cause a significant increase in insulin receptor sites in hepatic cell membranes of mice. Prince and Olefsky[68] showed increased insulin receptors on human fibroblasts in vitro. Vigneri and co-workers,[68a] however, comparing in-vitro, insulin-binding effects of biguanides and sulfonylureas, were unable to reproduce these data and, indeed, found that while biguanides enhanced insulin binding, sulfonylureas of both generations failed to have any major direct effect. Archer[69] has also made notable contributions in the investigation of the effects of sulfonylurea agents on erythrocytes. Eaton et al.[70] described patients with insulin resistance and decreased erythrocyte insulin receptor binding, whose erythrocyte receptor bindings were restored to normal with the aid of tolbutamide. This effect has been reported to be more effective with second generation agents.[71] Holle et al.,[72] using a biguanide, metformin, showed increased specific binding of insulin as well as an increase in the actual number of receptors. The effectiveness of the oral agents on the receptor system is well described by Skillman and Feldman.[51] These observations added to previously accepted mechanisms of action encourage the use of oral hypoglycemic agents in appropriate patients.

In *summary,* the most direct effects of the sulfonylureas are related to the release of some insulin from viable beta cells, although just how much, is debatable. This occurs in many ways, probably affecting the beta cells themselves, increasing the rate of ionic changes in calcium, potassium and sodium. Insulin secretion is enhanced in response to blood glucose. However, more than these actions occur as suggested by Shenfield et al.,[73] Barnes et

al.,[74] and Dunbar and Foa.[75] Along with inhibiting gluconeogenesis, possible effects on glucagon, inhibition of prostaglandin secretion, the effects on the sensitivity and actual increased number of insulin receptor binding sites make the explanation of sulfonylurea effectiveness much more plausible than the earlier observations of 10 to 20 years ago.

SECONDARY OR EXTRAPANCREATIC ACTIONS

In addition to the already discussed effects of sulfonylureas on endogenous insulin, these agents also have effects on many body organs as indicated by Feldman and Lebovitz[76] in their classic review of the extrapancreatic actions of the sulfonylureas. Many of these actions have been demonstrated in vitro with concentrations far in excess of those ordinarily attained in clinical use. This makes it difficult to determine effects that might occur with clinical doses in man. As Roth[77] has pointed out, many of the sulfonylurea actions are caused by as yet undefined mechanisms and they have multiple effects in various tissues.

Blood

Since the blood stream is the internal transport system, this is a logical place to start, although some of the effects have been discussed under "receptors." Most instructive are the findings that blood elements and functions may be altered in uncontrolled diabetes (see Chapter 37). These malfunctions are often reversed by improved treatment with sulfonylurea agents.[78–84]

Insulinase

In 1955, Mirsky[86–87] described the insulinase system, showing insulinase to be in high concentration in the liver. He noted that diabetics had a greater insulinase activity than did nondiabetics, leading him to believe that insulin was destroyed more rapidly in the former. Tolbutamide was shown to be a non-competitive inhibitor of this system, suggesting that it could prolong the half-life of insulin.[87]

Effect on Lipids

Szücs and Csapo[88] studied 918 patients and found hyperlipemia in 8% of the insulin-treated group and in 26% of those treated with carbutamide, an early sulfonylurea agent. They suggested that the latter group had an increased number of chylomicrons at the expense of the alpha fraction of lipoproteins. However, reports of the effects of sulfonylureas on blood fat fractions are in conflict. Belknap and his group[89] evaluated the effect of tolbutamide on triglyceride levels of patients with mild glucose intolerance, and found that tolbutamide had little effect on either blood triglycerides or glucose tolerance. In another study,[90] they concluded that a year of therapy improved glucose tolerance without any apparent effect on triglycerides.

Stone[91] reported that tolbutamide exerts an antilipolytic effect on adipose tissue.

Effect on Thyroid

Reports of sulfonylurea effects on the thyroid are also confusing.[92,93] These effects are reported as goitrogenic with an implied unduly high incidence of hypothyroidism in patients treated with these drugs. Hunton and associates[94] stated unequivocally that hypothyroidism develops in approximately 20% of diabetics treated with sulfonylureas for five or more years. This was later documented by both Brown[95] and Seegers.[96] In another study, Burke and co-workers[97] disagreed with the previous findings and denied any antithyroid effects from sulfonylurea therapy. A review of long-term studies fails to show any significant referral to hypothyroidism and although possibilities of this should be considered, the Joslin clinic experience suggests that this does not constitute a problem of any magnitude.

Effect on the Heart

Since the crux of the University Group Diabetes Program (UGDP) criticism focused on the alleged effect on the human heart by sulfonylureas, this must be considered. Here, again, the evidence is sometimes conflicting. Studies have been done under different circumstances and dosages; some have been done in animals and some in humans, with no firm conclusion. However, if any medication modestly effective in lowering blood glucose levels, shows risk of heart damage, the use of that agent must be reconsidered. The UGDP discussion is presented later in this chapter, but some of the questions arose with an early report by Bloodworth,[98] who demonstrated the presence of microgranulomata in the heart muscle of sulfonylurea-treated patients. Palmer et al.[99] reported an increased demand for oxygen in isolated heart muscle treated with tolbutamide. While it had been shown that tolbutamide had a minimal effect on the papillary muscle in a cat, no such effect was seen in that muscle in a human.[77]

From the results of their studies on isolated animal hearts, Linden and Brooker[100] concluded that the slight inotropic action of sulfonylureas is not mediated by cyclic AMP, but may result from an effect upon myocardial calcium metabolism. Hildner et al.[101] evaluated nondiabetic subjects during cardiac catheterization with the injection of tolbutamide intravenously, and demonstrated an inotropic effect at 5 to 15 mintues with a return to normal values at 30 minutes. They noted that while the effects on the human heart were minimal, they could not be completely discounted in the heart of a diabetic with atherosclerosis. Curtis et al.,[102] on the other hand, firmly concluded that tolbutamide had no deleterious effect on the heart. Sykes et al.[103] were convinced that patients with uncontrolled diabetes are subject to an increased adrenergic stimulus to the cardiovascular system, which stimulus disappears with therapy. They stated unequivocally that there is no evidence of positive inotropic action of sulfonylureas. Crockett et al.[104] concluded that acute intravenous tolbutamide has no significant inotropic effect in intact human heart muscle, and stated that a positive inotropic effect is found in animal and human hearts in vitro, although not in vivo.[105] Brown and Brown agreed with this opinion and concluded that tolbutamide does not potentiate the effect of catecholamines on cardiac cyclic AMP concentration.[106] One hundred and one Joslin Clinic patients who had taken tolbutamide for 8–10 years continuously were examined by Balodimos and Marble[107] for diabetic angiopathy. Findings were compared with those in 87 patients who had never received oral agents and who had been treated either with diet alone or with small doses of insulin. Vascular disease—cerebral, cardiac, and peripheral—had occurred with equal frequecy in the two groups. In a later study,[108] these workers compared postmortem findings in 55 patients who had received sulfonylurea therapy for an average of almost 4 years with those of control subjects who had been treated with insulin or diet alone. Pathologic evidence of myocardial infarction, diabetic nephropathy, and cerebrovascular disease was found with equal frequency in the two groups.

This evidence against inotropic effects of sulfonylureas is also sustained in the second generation compounds. Crouchman[109] stated that neither tolbutamide nor glurenorm (a second generation agent) produced any positive inotropic effect that could be associated with cardiovascular problems. Deineka et al.,[110] in Kiev, discussing glibenclamide, reported that it did not change arterial pressure or inhibit cardiac activity. Barjot,[111] noting that while more than 50% of diabetics die from myocardial infarction, glibenclamide, a second-generation sulfonylurea, has no inotropic effect on an already known ischemic heart nor does it have antidiuretic hormone (ADH)-like effect. Nevertheless, he urged caution in choosing oral agents.[112] While it is difficult to reconcile divergent views from reputable investigators, careful evaluation results in the conclusion that while there may be deleterious inotropic effects on damaged hearts in some animals and in human muscle in in vitro experiments, there is probably no evidence of any danger to intact human hearts in vivo.

Effect on the Kidneys

The kidneys are one area where the sulfonylureas, particularly chlorpropamide, may have a love-hate relationship because, as Fine and Shedrovilzky[113] pointed out, in susceptible persons with a large water intake, chlorpropamide could have an ADH-like action. Their patient developed water retention, hyponatremia, and symptoms of water intoxication. Andreani et al.[114] and Blotner[115] advocated the use of chlorpropamide in the treatment of certain patients with diabetes insipidus. Moses[116] referred to the earlier work of Arduino et al.[117] who stated in their 1966 report that the useful antidiuretic action of chlorpropamide in patients with diabetes insipidus was proportionate to the patient's ability to liberate ADH and to concentrate urine in response to dehydration. Marcondes and Gental[118] remarked that the state of hydration modulated the action of chlorpropamide somewhat independently of the antidiuretic hormone. In other words, the antidiuretic effect of chlorpropamide, like that of vasopressin, reduces the excretion of water in the absence of changes in the rates of glomerular filtration. Chlorpropamide also appears to potentiate the effect of vasopressin and increase water permeability of the distal nephrons.[119] In another study, Moses and Miller[120] concluded that for chlorpropamide to produce antidiuresis, some low level of endogenous ADH must be present. Liberman et al.,[121] in attempting to explain the mechanism of the antidiuretic effect of chlorpropamide, found measurements that suggested that the presence of endogenous ADH is required for the effect, although their study did not answer the critical question as to whether chlorpropamide *causes* the release of ADH as well as *augmenting* the peripheral action of the hormone. Hagen emphasized that dilutional hyponatremia from tolbutamide treatment has also been reported in diabetes,[122] but in contrast to chlorpropamide, tolbutamide in the amounts used in treating patients with diabetes does not usually interfere with water excretion, although on rare occasions minimal water retention is possible. Tolazamide has no antidiuretic action but, in fact, has mild diuretic activity in the proximal tubules.

The dimensions of this continuing discussion have increased through the years. A drug-induced syndrome with inappropriate secretion of ADH has long been known. The finding of this effect with clofibrate, carbamazepine and other drugs provides evidence that this response is common. Indeed,

Miller and Moses[123] show that, to some degree, many compounds have this tendency, including ADH analogs, nicotine, some narcotics, biguanides, and even antineoplastic agents.

Effect on the Liver

It is known that sulfonylureas promote inhibition of gluconeogenesis, but this role may be more sophisticated than that of a passive partner during metabolism. One example is hypoglycemia despite no continued increased insulin release due to the antilipolytic effect that inhibits gluconeogenesis.[124] Blumenthal[59] described hepatic gluconeogenesis suppression during sulfonylurea administration. Colwell[125] found that while oral tolbutamide administration per se produced only a modest reduction in blood glucose, there was a much greater decrease in blood glucose if the sulfonylurea was given intraportally. He attributed this to direct action on the liver by tolbutamide. Marshall,[126] citing other studies, suggested that the sustained action of the sulfonylureas may be due partly to reduced hepatic uptake of endogenously secreted insulin. Both Breidahl et al.[127] and Feldman and Lebovitz[76] have reviewed these particular extrapancreatic influences.

Other actions on the liver include the inhibition of triglyceride lipase[130] and, most importantly, the potentiation of insulin action on the liver. Feinglos and Lebovitz[67] extensively studied this function because of its clinical relevance and in this excellent report discussed the possibilities, concluding that the ability of chronic sulfonylurea treatment to potentiate insulin action ameliorated a major abnormality in IDDM. They suggested that this activity was associated with an increase in insulin receptors available in plasma membranes.

Other Extrapancreatic Effects

Of the general potpourri of secondary and sometimes tertiary effects of sulfonylurea use,[128] probably the most valid are the effects on cell receptors just discussed[129] as well as generally improved hormone-receptor interaction.[130] Obviously, these effects on receptor sites have markedly changed the concept of sulfonylurea action as previously reported.[131]

There are other extrapancreatic effects, although some are not of major importance. However, the report that glyburide stimulates the release of gut factors (duodenal insulin releasing activity [DIRA]) in humans[132] is significant in the understanding of these agents. A report by Couturier et al.[133] indicated that the results of ionophore-mediated calcium counter-transport studies supported the view that insulinotrophic action of sulfonamides depends on the ionophore capacity. Following this line of reasoning, they gained the impression that patients with well-controlled diabetes treated with sulfonylurea therapy, have normal intermediary metabolite concentrations in comparison to those in patients with poor control. Greenfield et al.[134] reported that the hypoglycemic effect of glipizide, for example, appeared to correlate with the decrease in insulin resistance. Pope and co-workers[134a] found that in 3T3-L1 adipocytes glyburide treatment either potentiates or mimics the actions of insulin. Another factor influencing the hypoglycemic effect was the action of sulfonylurea on the dynamics of insulin release. Hecht et al.[135] demonstrated that in diabetes, initial insulin release is delayed even though subsequent release may be normal. Early release has a marked influence on glucose tolerance, and their study demonstrated that chronic treatment with these agents may not be related to acute treatment, since while glucose tolerance improved, insulin levels are not necessarily increased in spite of the hypoglycemic effect. While reviewing whether or not tolbutamide and glucose activate the metabolic pathway or the receptors in the beta cell, Ganda et al.[136] found that tolbutamide appears to cause peak insulin response earlier than glucose, while Koncz et al.,[137] using glucose or tolbutamide intravenously, in two consecutive pulses 30 and 60 minutes apart, demonstrated that insulin secretory response was altered during subsequent stimulations. This is an apparent characteristic of the first-generation compounds.

In *summary*, the simple act of insulin release from the beta cells, while vital, no longer suffices as an explanation of the activity of the sulfonylurea agents. While there is no insulin-release stimulation as well as response to rising blood glucose levels, there is also an effect on the beta cell membrane receptors, in addition to possible decrease of uncertain degree, in glucagon secretion. In addition to the increased insulin-receptor binding sites, there is enhancement of insulin hormonal release by the gastrointestinal stimulus along with decreased gluconeogenesis. Other suggested influences are calcium, sodium and potassium, as well as possible inhibition of prostaglandin. These increased roles of sulfonylurea activity, while helping explain their effects, are of some concern, since few effective therapeutic agents act in isolated focus on only their target areas, but may overflow into other systems as well.

ORAL HYPOGLYCEMIC AGENTS IN NONDIABETIC CONDITIONS

Other uses not related to diabetes have been reported, but interest in these is limited, and few have found any degree of clinical acceptance. One, already mentioned, that has been considered worth-wile is chlorpropamide in the treatment of milder forms of diabetes insipidus. The use of tolbutamide in treating cystic fibrosis of the pancreas was reported by Rosan and associates.[138] Tolbutamide has also been used in attempted treatment of Parkinsonsim, with generally indifferent results. Still another study suggested the helpful effect of treatment of young patients suffering from achondroplasia.[139]

These adaptations often reflect the ingenuity and desperation of physicians in their attempts to solve medical problems for which there is so far no specific treatment.

INDICATIONS FOR THE USE OF ORAL HYPOGLYCEMIC AGENTS

These have changed little since the previous edition of this book.[106] In fact, the defining of Type I (IDDM) and Type 2 (NIDDM) diabetes draws the line sharply for use or non-use. Even the best classifications, however, are not air-tight compartments. For example, there are rare youngsters who at an early age develop adult type diabetes and who may, at least for a time, respond to oral agent therapy. On the other hand, some older patients, theoretically the ideal choice for treatment with oral agents, may be insulin-dependent. This is an area where medical judgment is a prime requisite.

A laudable by-product of the UGDP controversy is the unanimous emphasis on diet for treatment of all diabetics. This applies as well when oral agents are used. Rough guidelines for choosing those who might be treated adequately with oral agents are: (a) those with onset of diabetes after the age of 40; (b) those with duration of diabetes of 10 years or less; (c) those using a daily dose of insulin of 20 to 30 units or less. No clinician with vast experience in diabetes would have any difficulty recalling numerous exceptions to these rules. There are patients who fit all the "suitable for oral agents" criteria, but still do not respond well. Skillman and co-workers[140] have shown that advancing age is not a sinecure for successful sulfonylurea use because older patients may have long-term diabetes.

The Joslin Clinic experience shows that the best chance for therapeutic success is in the group from the 5th to the 7th decade of life.[141] "*Good*" or "*Fair*" control as classified in Table 21–1, can be anticipated in about 70% of carefully selected patients, at least for a time, with primary (initial) failure in the rest. Occasionally there is the insulin-resistant patient who may be responsive to the use of these agents for a period of time.[142]

What about the patient with persisting significant hyperglycemia but without the classical triad of polyuria, polydipsia, and polyphagia? If one aims for a goal of normoglycemia as a possible deterrent to further deterioration as well as amelioration of complications, then after treatment with appropriate diet alone has been tried without success, it would seem feasible to try oral agents. Certainly no one espouses persisting hyperglycemia as a therapeutic goal. Some symptoms of a non-specific nature may be associated with diabetes. These might include unexplained weight loss, fatigue, frequent infections, etc.

Sometimes oral agents are unwisely prescribed during the initial treatment of diabetes. If a patient presents with diabetes which has been grossly out of control for many months, with greatly elevated blood glucose levels, weight loss, acetone in the urine, and excessive physical fatigue, it is unlikely that such a patient will respond to an oral hypoglycemic agent. Instead, initial treatment in this case should consist of diet and insulin. Once metabolic balance has been restored and there is evidence of beta cell viability, it is possible that treatment with a sulfonylurea compound may be effective.

There is also a debatable but intriguing suggestion that early use of oral agents in subjects with impaired glucose tolerance might prevent frank diabetes later. One such report by Sartor and colleagues[143] is based on surveys in Sweden where early, recently detected diabetics were treated with diet and these compounds. The results suggested that improvement in glucose tolerance was substantial. Paasikivi and Wahlberg[144] indicated that the progress of arterial disease, possibly fueled by impaired carbohydrate metabolism, might be retarded by early and vigorous tolbutamide therapy. A thought-provoking note provided by Kosaka et al.[145] indicated that good treatment of overt diabetes increases the insulin response regardless of what form the treatment takes, and this results in eventual better insulin output, improved receptor mechanisms and decreased insulin resistance.

Another controversial and provocative consideration is the possible use of oral agents in the moderately obese patient with hyperglycemia who does not respond to diet therapy. In the past, biguanides were thought to be preferable to sulfonylureas because the latter provoke insulin release, compounding the weight problem. However, glucose is a potent stimulus for insulin release. If the oral agents can decrease the blood glucose level and also improve the cell receptor system, might this not be a logical approach, especially if barely adequate doses of sulfonylurea were used?

CLINICAL USAGE

Onset of Treatment

Before starting treatment with any oral agent, it is imperative that a trial of treatment with diet alone

be carried out for a period of at least two to three weeks. If this fails, one starts patients with oral hypoglycemic therapy in a low starting dose, which is increased in small increments at intervals of 2 or 3 days, until both fasting and 2-hour postprandial levels of blood glucose are acceptable. In starting, tolbutamide could be begun safely with 0.5 g twice daily, and tolazamide or acetohexamide with an initial dose of 250 mg once or twice daily. Chlorpropamide should be started cautiously with a single 250 mg dose in the morning. Starting, usual, and maximal dosages are shown in Table 21–4.

There is disagreement about the hazards of changing over from insulin to oral agents. Actually, except for the longer duration compounds, sulfonylureas pose no threat of hypoglycemia if the dose is increased slowly as the insulin is gradually decreased. One must be aware of the longer effect of intermediate or longer-acting (ultralente or protamine zinc) insulins when initiating oral compounds in persons treated with insulin. The patient and physician must be in close communication during the transition from insulin to an oral agent. The patient should report to the physician in person or by telephone every few days. If there is obvious primary oral agent failure, the drug should be discontinued immediately and the patient returned to insulin. Equally close communication should be maintained during initiation of oral hypoglycemic therapy, following treatment with diet alone.

Combination Therapy

At times a successful treatment method is the concomitant use of biguanide and sulfonylurea agents. Because the sulfonylureas initiate insulin release, this provides a basis for the effectiveness of biguanides. Both apparently have an effect on receptor sensitivity; thus the use of both agents is often found to be complementary. The combination is effective in many patients when neither of the agents individually controls the blood glucose adequately.[146–150] With this combined effectiveness, the use of oral agents is prolonged sometimes for a number of years in some persons who might otherwise have required treatment with insulin. In countries in which biguanide compounds are still available, combinations with metformin and bu-

Table 21–5. Use of Oral Agents and Insulin by Age Groups As Reported by the National Health Interview Survey (1976)

Age group years	Patients using	
	Oral agents %	Insulin %
20–39	14.7	30.5
40–59	36.1	21.8
60 and older	50.1	16.9

formin are widely used. In the Joslin Clinic experience, longer than 20 years, prior to the discontinuance of biguanides, the most effective dosage was tolbutamide, 2.0 g, chlorpropamide 0.5 g, acetohexamide 1.5 g, or tolazamide 1.0 g along with a 50-mg phenformin capsule twice daily. Natrass et al.[153] reported that certain metabolic abnormalities found in patients treated with phenformin alone (increased blood lactate, alanine, ketones,etc.) were also present with combined therapy and that these were accentuated in the presence of microangiopathy.

Oral Compounds and Insulin. Treatment with a biguanide and insulin has occasionally been suggested but rarely justified. Earlier papers[152] proposed that this combination might stabilize juvenile-onset (Type I) diabetes, but while the short-term effects seemed promising, longer follow-up showed that the real effect was probably due to the remission of this type of diabetes. This combination was not widely used and appeared to be effective only in selected cases.[153,154] Another early hope was that adding biguanide to insulin might result in a reduction in insulin requirement, but while some in the study group averred that they had greater freedom from hypoglycemic reactions, the results were generally inconclusive,[155] although Molnar and colleagues[156] documented a series in which phenformin was used successfully to reduce the insulin requirement in certain insulin-resistant patients.

Early reports also suggested that sulfonylureas and insulin would provide an effective combination.[157,160] With the new knowledge of effects on receptors, the theoretical possibility is intriguing, but experience with this combination has not been impressive. Camerini-Davalos et al.[161] in a juvenile camp study, found that the addition of sulfonylurea to insulin made no real difference. In general, it would appear that the addition of oral hypoglycemic agents to insulin therapy is a useless exercise.

Other Combinations. In the literature are recorded the effects of other possible combinations. These often involve compounds that appear to enhance the oral agent. One of these is the antilipemic agent, halofenate. Kudzma and Friedberg[162] reviewed the experience of Jain et al.,[163] reporting that this compound when added to the sulfonylureas, potentiated their effect and increased blood tolbutamide levels, although there was no effect on persons treated wtih diet alone.

In *summary,* the judicious combining of a sulfonylurea with a biguanide (where available) may salvage some instances of therapeutic failure with one oral agent alone. Some patients might profit from other possible oral agent combinations or by

treatment with an oral agent and insulin therapy. However, treatment with more than one modality confuses many patients and, in general, the simpler the regimen, the greater the chance of success.

Contraindications

If the indications for the use of oral agents are observed, the contraindications are almost automatic. The sulfonylureas have no place in the treatment of insulin-dependent diabetes. The presence of parenchymal disease of the liver or kidney, pregnancy, lactation, or periods of major stress should also preclude the use of sulfonylureas. Since these agents are especially effective in older patients with viable beta cell function and short-duration diabetes, without undue stress, the candidates least likely to succeed can largely be avoided. The National Health Interview Survey in 1976 reported the use of oral agents and insulin by age group (Table 21–5).

Drug Failure

Primary Failure. Primary failure with oral hypoglycemic compounds poses no problem since if they are immediately ineffective, they are promptly discontinued. The term "primary" failure is defined arbitrarily as failure to respond to treatment within 1 month. As a clinical rule of thumb, of any 10 seemingly ideal candidates for oral agent therapy, about 5 will demonstrate early effectiveness, another three will be borderline, while the remaining 2 will fail for reasons unknown. The measure of a physician's astuteness is his judgment not only in prescribing, but also in knowing when to discontinue oral agents and substitute insulin.

Secondary Failure. Secondary failure, as defined here, indicates a good initial response to the oral agents (for at least 1 month) with decreasing effectiveness and eventual failure. There is copious literature on this subject. Stowers et al.[164] state that the failure rate with use of sulfonylureas depends on strictness of the selection criteria, and that most of the poorly selected patients fail in the first year of treatment; thereafter, the failure rate is about 5% per year. It was once thought that all orally treated patients would eventually be secondary failures if treated thus long enough, but this is not true, since some patients have been successfully treated with oral agents for 20 years or longer.

It is impossible to get solid data concerning the true percentage of secondary failures, and even less specific are the reasons for failure. Published rates of secondary failure range from 0.3%[165] to about 30%,[166,167] but the latter authors indicated that their data were skewed since when early failures were deleted, the longer term failure rate dropped to

6.5%. Camerini-Davalos and Marble[168] reported that of 1965 patients treated with sulfonylureas during a 5-year period, treatment was discontinued in 22% because of secondary failure. In the first year of treatment, the failure rate was 4.1%; in the second year, 9.4%; in the third year, 11.6%; in the fourth year, 9.0%; and in the fifth year, 7.5%. They concluded that poor initial selection of patients, disregard of diet, inadequate doses and/or temporary metabolic stress were the reasons for failure. They also reported that true secondary failure (agent failure) occurred in only 16 of 432 patients or 3.7% of the entire series of 1965 patients.

Ztrauzenberg et al.[169] concluded that the highest failure rate occurs 3 to 4 years after beginning treatment, and that in later years the incidence of failure does not increase further. Some reports[170] indicate that the greater potency of chlorpropamide results in fewer secondary failures. The National Health Interview Survey found that while 67.5% of diabetic patients were treated with oral agents at one time, when the survey was conducted in 1976, only 40.1% had continued with this form of treatment.

What happens to the patient after discontinuing oral therapy due to secondary failure? Are unusually large doses of insulin required because of beta cell exhaustion? This has seemed not to be the case in the experience of Joslin Clinic nor in the study carried out by Ross and Borthwick.[171]

In *summary,* while there is a substantial incidence of secondary failure with the present oral hypoglycemic agents, this may be the result of poor patient selection, lack of diet adherence, increased stress, or simply the inability of the beta cells to respond to oral therapy as the diabetes increases in duration. However, since it is now understood that the activity of sulfonylureas is not limited to the release of insulin, it must be assumed that other factors, such as increased insulin resistance, may lead to secondary failures.

Side Effects and Toxicity

Side Effects. Side effects usually result from abnormal physiologic responses to a particular medication, without altered organ structure. They may be annoying or worrisome, but generally are harmless if the offending substance is discontinued.

Any active medication may produce side effects, whether these compounds be aspirin, morphine or any agent in between. With the oral agents in current use, side effects have not been a major problem, except for those resulting from biguanides. Minor side effects include gastrointestinal distress, anorexia, vomiting, malaise, fever, skin eruptions, muscular weakness, lethargy and dizziness. Considering the vast number of persons treated with

sulfonylurea compounds, the frequency of these problems is strikingly low. Shen and Bressler[172,173] estimated the rate for all side effects as 3.2% for tolbutamide and 6.0% for chlorpropamide, but there are lower (.05%)[174] as well as higher estimates.[175–177] Kilo[177] has stated categorically that except for occasional mild hypoglycemia, he has seen no serious side effects after 20 years of prescribing oral agents. Observing 2500 patients, Marble and Camerini[178] reported a frequency of 0.9% of side effects, with most of these being attributed to allergic dermatitis or mild gastrointestinal disturbances. These were several cases of purpura and a case of jaundice in a patient with previously known hepatic disease. This correlates with O'Donovan's report of 0.5%.[174] Knowles[179] agrees that minor dermatitis and gastrointestinal upsets cause most side effects. Reactivation of peptic ulcers after the use of a sulfonylurea drug has been reported,[180] but this is rare. Pruritus is often the first symptom of allergic hypersensitivity. Only rarely has exfoliative dermatitis been reported.

The biguanides, on the other hand, have a much higher incidence of side effects, almost all in the gastrointestinal tract. These are readily reversible with discontinuance of the compound.

Disulfiram-Like Reactions. Over the course of time, emphasis has varied on pertinent aspects of a therapeutic agent. A paragraph from the 11th edition described the annoying non-dangerous acute flushing of the skin surface and other vascular phenomena in patients who used alcohol while under treatment with sulfonylurea agents, most often chlorpropamide.[10c] This phenomenon continues to occur and generally starts within 10 minutes after drinking alcohol. The flushing and facial warmth are often embarrassing and sometimes distressing. Some patients suffer severe pounding headaches, breathlessness, nausea and tachycardia.[181–183] It has been estimated that as many as 10 to 30% of those using oral hypoglycemic agents have at least mild symptoms after alcohol intake. Recently this phenomenon has assumed new importance. The original disulfiram (Antabuse) affected the intermediate metabolism of alcohol after ethanol was converted to acetaldehyde. This was used to discourage alcoholics.[184] Recently, in patients treated with chlorpropamide, this flushing was thought to be due to increased sensitivity to the peptide enkephalin, which can be blocked by the opiate antagonist, naloxone.

Pyke and associates[185] have related the chlorpropamide alcohol flushing (CPAF) to genetic predisposition to diabetes, and believe that this is an autosomal trait and a good genetic marker for Type II diabetes. They indicated that this syndrome, present in about 20% of patients with Type II diabetes mellitus, can be detected with a single challenge CPAF test before the onset of glucose intolerance. They further suggested there was less diabetic retinopathy among those with NIDDM who reacted positively to the CPAF challenge and that blindness from retinopathy was mainly confined to CPAF-negative cases.[186] They also reported that blocking CPAF by indomethacin (Indocin) suggested an association between prostaglandins and diabetic vascular complications.[187] Needless to say, while interesting and possibly significant, this view is not yet completely accepted since DeSilva et al.,[188] in their series, did not confirm the high estimates of the incidence of the CPAF phenomenon in NIDDM. Because this was considered as a possible genetic marker for one type of NIDDM, a workshop was held (1980) under the auspices of the National Institutes of Health and the International Diabetes Epidemiology Group.[189] It was concluded that while the CPAF findings to date are suggestive of an inherited trait, (a) its relationship to diabetes is still unclear; (b) it is not a consistent phenomenon; and (c) it is present in 30 to 40% of persons with NIDDM and 10% of insulin-dependent diabetics used as controls.

Toxicity. Toxicity is defined here as structural or functional change that can be measured objectively. The documented toxicity of the sulfonylurea compounds has been low indeed considering the wide use of these agents. If toxicity appears, the drug must be discontinued immediately and, when indicated, supportive measures must be instituted as well.

Hepatic Damage. Because it is an organ of detoxification, the liver is a target for toxic reactions. The range of damage can vary from impaired liver function to severe jaundice due to cholestatic obstruction. Bradley and associates[190] demonstrated the frequent occurrence of changes in liver function as part of the usual diabetic syndrome while Camerini-Davalos and co-workers[191] found a significant rise in alkaline phosphatase levels during the first few months of therapy with tolbutamide. Obviously the more potent an agent, the greater likelihood of liver impairment. Toxicity of this type was responsible for the withdrawal of the oral agents, carbutamide and metahexamide years ago in the United States, although they are still used abroad. This jaundice of cholestatic origin often involves mixed hepatocellular elements as well.[192,193] Marble and Camerini-Davalos[178] showed that after long-term use of carbutamide, there was impaired liver function with both bromsulphalein retention and increased alkaline phosphatase levels. Earlier, chlorpropamide was implicated in liver function abnormalities.[194] Brown

and co-workers compared the bile stasis to the type of jaundice resulting from thorazine hydrochloride or methyl testosterone therapy.[195]

Questions remain. How often is liver damage found? Is it serious or preventible? The numbers are actually small. Stowers and Bewsher[196] reviewed 333 cases, finding jaundice in 0.4% of chlorpropamide-treated and none in tolbutamide-treated patients. Skillman[140] found no liver changes during 916 patient-months with chlorpropamide treatment and 815 patient-months of tolbutamide. Haunz and Cornatzer[197] noted that there had been little or no jaundice reported since 1960. The relative disappearance of alleged chlorpropamide-induced jaundice coincides with the recommended limitation of a 500 mg daily dose. This was further documented by Fineberg[198] and Hamff et al.[199] who stated that any intracanalicular biliary stasis results from daily chlorpropamide doses greater than 500 mg daily. In their series, some patients returned to the same agent with a reduced dose of 250 mg daily without any recurrence of jaundice. In the Joslin Clinic series, Cervantes-Amezcua[200] studied 479 patients treated with chlorpropamide and noted only 1 case of jaundice; this occurred after 3 weeks of therapy. This patient suffered malaise, anorexia, nausea, pruritus and hepatomegaly. Liver function tests revealed a bromsulphalein retention of 19%, alkaline phosphatase of 49.2 Bodansky units, and a transaminase value of 324 units. Liver biopsy showed canalicular bile stasis but no hepatocellular damage. The patient improved with conservative therapy, and all liver function returned to normal after 2 months.

From these data, it is evident that the number of patients with hepatotoxic manifestations from sulfonylurea therapy are few.

Hematologic Toxicity. Of all possible toxic reactions in oral agent-treated patients, hematologic dyscrasias are the most threatening. They are infrequent but may be serious when they do occur. The number of reported cases has declined, suggesting better use of the oral agents or greater alertness by physicians. All of the first-generation agents have been implicated at one time or another. Agranulocytosis had previously been reported in patients treated with chlorpropamide.[201,202] This blood dyscrasia can have fatal results,[203] although with greater alertness and specific treatment, recent studies report remission and recovery.[204] An even more troublesome group, although fortunately fewer, are those who develop bone marrow aplasia resulting in pancytopenia.[201,205] In one case, however, the patient had also been treated with methyldopa for a year prior to oral agent therapy. Borish[206] reported a recent patient who recovered rapidly when medication was discontinued. Red blood cell aplasia has been rarely reported.[207,208] Logue[209] described a chlorpropamide-induced immune hemolytic anemia. Thrombocytopenia has been documented on rare occasions.[210,211] In a report by Cunliffe et al.,[212] the presence of an immunologic mechanism was shown to cause thrombocytopenia. Tolbutamide has been associated with pancytopenia[201,213,214] and myeloblastic anemia.[215] These have been rare instances of tolbutamide-induced hemolytic anemia.[216]

Another nonspecific problem reported was gastrointestinal bleeding following sulfonylurea therapy; this problem abated when the agent was discontinued.[217] Geary[218] reviewed sulfonylurea agents and other medications potentially indicted as causes of hematologic disturbances. While these complications are infrequent, one can neither ignore such problems nor dismiss them as unimportant.

Severe Dermatologic Toxicities. Although dermatologic manifestations were mentioned as "side effects," there is a rare but occasional toxic skin reaction. Tullet[219] reported a case of toxic erythema, while generalized exfoliative dermatitis was described by Rothfeld and associates.[220]

Other Manifestations. There are other isolated reports of suspected sulfonylurea toxicity, but many are difficult to prove. An important precaution in the use of any medication is recognition of the possibility of toxicity resulting from impaired renal function. In a comprehensive review, Bennett et al.[221] listed the hypoglycemic agents among the common medications that might produce prolonged hypoglycemia in the presence of azotemia. Gonzalez[222] also noted an enhanced response to tolbutamide in uremia although responses among uremic subjects are inconsistent. There have been no major differences in this respect between the sulfonylurea and control groups. The data of Balodimos and co-workerss[223,224] also indicated that post-mortem findings in both groups were similar.

SPECIAL PROBLEMS

Hypoglycemia

Inasmuch as lowering blood glucose is a goal of treatment, it would seem specious to list this as either side effect or toxicity, since a therapeutic agent should not be faulted for being too effective. Since any substance lowering blood glucose can cause hypoglycemia, it should come as no surprise that this can occur with oral hypoglycemic agents. This, however, is probably a manifestation of overdosage, relative or actual, as well as inadequate food intake. It must be constantly borne in mind that combining oral agents with other medications is a possible cause, as is any substance which either prolongs duration of action or slows elimination.

Minor reactions such as dizziness, weakness, extreme hunger or anxiety may occur as with insulin. This should be considered particularly when treating older patients who are often susceptible to cerebral glucose insufficiency.[224a] There should be particular caution in treating patients with these agents for nondiabetic reasons.[225,226] For example, Conn and coworkers[227] reported prolonged hypoglycemia after using tolbutamide in a person suffering from cirrhosis and malnutrition. Hypoglycemia caused by these agents, has been reported extensively in the literature.[228,229] The report of Spurny[230] is of particular significance because in a protracted tolbutamide-induced hypoglycemia, the half-life of the drug was estimated to be almost 70 hours in contrast to the usual 4 hours. These, of course, are rare episodes.

As might be anticipated, chlorpropamide, with longer duration of action and delayed excretion, is more often implicated in severe hypoglycemic reactions than is tolbutamide,[231] although these episodes are often due to misuse of the agent. For example, Dahl et al.[232] reported 5 patients with profound hypoglycemia allegedly caused by chlorpropamide. Three of these were diabetic; one took the agent by error and the fifth attempted suicide. The authors observed the inordinately slow response to intravenous glucose therapy and stated that the usual hypoglycemic warning symptoms did not seem to appear. They were concerned about the possibility of mistaking hypoglycemia in elderly persons for a cerebrovascular accident. Greenberg et al.[233] reported a rise in blood insulin levels and hypoglycemic symptoms persisting for 4 days in a 3½-year-old child who had ingested chlorpropamide tablets.

Acetohexamide has been reported as a cause of prolonged hypoglycemic reactions.[234,235] The deep hypoglycemia may not respond rapidly to the release of glucose from glycogen in the liver or even to glucose given intravenously, thereby resulting in prolonged coma. Stowers[164] admonishes that: "It is not sufficient merely to restore consciousness by intravenous glucose or an injection of glucagon; it is necessary to guard against the return of hypoglycemia."

Seltzer[236] points out in a classic review that a long-acting oral agent should be used warily in older patients, particularly in those who are not under close observation by friends or family. He states that every unconscious diabetic patient should be considered hypoglycemic until proven otherwise. Active measures may be needed, and these might include 10% glucose by vein, for as long as a day or two, and adding treatment with hydrocortisone and glucagon if needed until persisting hyperglycemia signals an end to the condition. Kaplinsky and Frankl[237] claim that chlorpropamide-induced hypoglycemia is often misdiagnosed because patients may arrive at the hospital with a normal serum glucose level; they noted that correction of a low glucose level in the cerebrospinal fluid occurs hours after improvement in the plasma glucose level. A high index of suspicion should also exist in the presence of any atypical encephalopathy. Here, cerebrospinal fluid examination may be useful.

Sometimes hypoglycemia may result from an inadvertent large dose of sulfonylureas. Miller et al.[238] reported a bizarre case in which a healthy nondiabetic 15-year-old male athlete took 3 tablets (presumably 500 mg each) of tolbutamide. They were labeled "Upjohn" and he assumed that they were a variety of stimulant or "uppers." He was admitted unconscious to the hospital and recovered. Here, a combination of inadequate food intake, exercise and alcohol added to tolbutamide, nearly culminated in tragedy.

Frerichs et al.[239] reviewing the subject, found that in most instances, hypoglycemic reactions are the result of the cumulative effect of the oral agents plus the potentiating effects of other concurrent medications.

Pregnancy

There is little in world medical literature concerning use of these compounds during pregnancy. One reason the oral agents have not been widely used in treatment of pregnant diabetics is that most of these patients are in the younger age group in whom these agents are usually not effective. Another reason is awareness by physicians of the potential teratogenic effect of medications, since it is known that many common and widely used drugs have induced malformation in animal fetuses when given in large doses. Jackson and associates[240] described perinatal mortality in a series of young diabetics treated with sulfonylureas. In the control group treated with insulin and diet, the fetal mortality was a high 20%. In the 42 patients treated wtih sulfonylureas, the offspring of women treated with tolbutamide had a mortality of 23% as compared with 65% for those threated with chlorpropamide. Previously, Campbell[241] described multiple congenital abnormalities in the fetus of a patient well controlled throughout pregnancy with tolbutamide, but did not necessarily implicate the compound. On the other hand, years ago White[242] observed that both tolbutamide and phenformin had been used without any untoward results in some of her pregnant patients, although in this series, the use of oral agents was limited to about 1%.

Dolger and co-workers[243] reported several series of pregnant patients who were treated with oral agents and had no resulting problems. Others have observed that there is already such a high degree of congenital malformation in the offspring of diabetics, that it is difficult to attribute these to the use of oral agents. Douglas and Richards[244] studied 128 pregnancies, and concluded that while there is evidence of teratogenic effect in animals if given large enough doses of sulfonylureas, the incidence of abnormality in the infants of their group was well below the general average for the offspring of diabetic mothers. Moss and associates,[245] reviewing the literature, stated that while safety and efficiency in pregnancy have not been established, there is also little evidence of any deleterious effect related to their use. However, Miller and co-workers[246] warned that because tolbutamide crosses the placental barrier freely, it might be a basis for problems. Brown and Gabert,[247] early adherents of tight control during diabetic pregnancies, state that since adequate control in pregnancy gives the best chance for success, oral agents might be helpful in obtaining such control.

On the other hand, Stowers[164] reports danger in using therapeutic agents in diabetic women of childbearing age. During the early developmental state of the fetus, sulfonylurea might be given to a mother who may not be aware of her pregnancy. A recent study by Watson et al.[248] reported in vivo cytogenic activity of the sulfonylurea drugs in humans, and warned against their use in pregnancy, but Sutherland[249] noted that chlorpropamide in doses of 100 mg daily had not shown any adverse effect on perinatal mortality, but rather that this amount might reverse chemical diabetes in women. Another possible danger is hypoglycemia in a newborn infant whose mother had been treated with oral agents during pregnancy.[250]

In conclusion, despite the fact that some physicians have successfully treated pregnant women judiciously with oral hypoglycemic agents, it is safest for most physicians to be aware that safety and usefulness of these drugs during pregnancy have not been established from the standpoint of the mother or the fetus. Therefore, they are not recommended for the management of diabetes during pregnancy.[251]

Surgery and Other Stresses

Whether or not a patient continues treatment with oral agents during surgery depends on (1) the severity of diabetes and (2) the extent and duration of the surgery. In general, it is wisest to substitute insulin for oral agents prior to and during any major surgery. In a patient using a long-duration agent, there should be several days of insulin therapy with no oral compound prior to surgery. This precaution may not be necessary for minor surgery under local anesthesia, especially if postoperatively the patient can eat a normal diet. It should be remembered that surgery and general anesthesia are stress factors. When the postoperative course has stabilized, treatment with oral hypoglycemic agents may often be resumed, if they were truly effective prior to the operation.

The Aging Patient

Since diabetes is a disease of aging, especially in the developed portions of the world, treatment of older persons with diabetes is an increasing problem. Oral agents are used widely in this age group. As a rule, although not always, diabetes with late onset is of the NIDDM type. There has been much debate as to how vigorous therapy should be in elderly patients. The goal should be to keep the patient functioning, avoiding extremes of very high or low blood glucose levels, ketoacidosis, hyperosmolar and lactic acidoses, and infections. Also the elderly patient living alone and often with poor vision, may find it difficult to use insulin, or will simply refuse. Shagan,[252] in reviewing the problems of treating older diabetics, stresses that habit, other medical problems, financial problems, lack of home resources, comprehension or acceptance, play a part in the treatment of these patients. In older persons, there is often a high renal threshold for sugar, making it difficult to evaluate the degree of control on the basis of urine tests. The older person also may not want or cannot afford to have frequent blood glucose determinations. This may account for the increased frequency of hyperosmolar acidosis in this group.[253] Elderly patients are most likely to be affected by severe prolonged hypoglycemia. In such patients, the shorter-acting oral agents would seem more appropriate.

Older persons living alone should develop a "buddy system" with friends, whereby they contact one another daily by telephone or in person when possible. While the attention required by older diabetics may be minimal, it is an irreducible minimum that is most vital. See also Chapter 25, "Diabetes in the Elderly."

Combination of Oral Agents with Other Medications

Much new information has recently become available in this regard. The effects of any medication will never be better known until it is marketed.[254,255] Combinations of medications, while possibly altering the action of one another, may not be harmful, although dosage adjustment may be necessary. Some substances not used for therapeutic purposes can also affect medications, e.g., alcohol, which is considered to be hypoglycemic because it hinders gluconeogenesis and release of glucose. Prolonged intake of ethanol decreases the half-life of tolbutamide,[255,257] possibly due to an effect on hepatic enzymes. The effect is not quite as strong with acetohexamide, but ethanol combined with phenformin can contribute to lactic acidosis.[257,258] From experience it would appear that hypoglycemia is the most common effect of alcohol on diabetes.[259]

There are many medications in common use that affect blood glucose in either direction. These, of course, would have an effect on the use of oral hypoglycemic agents either directly or indirectly. Some of these, described by Kimble,[260] include medications that tend to increase blood glucose levels such as asparaginase; birth control compounds (causing diminished glucose tolerance possibly related to estrogen); corticosteroids (which promote gluconeogenesis, antagonizing the effects of insulin); diuretics (which decrease glucose tolerance); diphenylhydantoin (which impairs insulin release); dextrothyroxin, nicotinic acid and a whole series of sympathomimetic agents (which stimulate the breakdown of glycogen to glucose). They include also the anabolic steroids; monoamine oxidase (MAO) inhibitors (which block homeostatic response to hypoglycemia); pentamidine; propranolol (which blocks liver glycogenolysis occurring in response to lowered blood glucose levels as well as masking symptoms of hypoglycemia); salicylates (although these require daily doses of 5 g or more); and theophylline. Not all the mechanisms of action are known. These may be due to inhibition of metabolism, protein displacement, or decreased excretion. Other drugs in this category are sulfisoxazole and phenylbutazone. There is also wide variation of the effects of drug metabolism on individual diabetics.[261] Likewise, the diabetes per se does not seem to change the drug metabolizing capacity of the liver. There is variance of effect among the interactions of the individual oral agents with other compounds. Brown[262] observed that agreement between experimental data and the calculated competitive binding equation is poor, but stated that glyburide, a new oral hypoglycemic agent, is less susceptible to displacement by acidic drugs than are tolbutamide and chlorpropamide. This is discussed later. Summaries of drug interactions are readily available and comprehensive. Some noteworthy publications on the subject are those by the American Pharmaceutical Association;[263] that of Griffin and d'Arcy,[264] and that by Hansten,[265] as well as the summaries in the Medical Letter.[266]

While some of the previously mentioned drug

combination actions are of interest, others have more clinical importance. This is true of widely used anticoagulants such as bishydroxycoumarin (Dicumarol), in which the mechanism is inhibition of the enzymes responsible for the metabolism of oral agents.[267] Thus, tolbutamide levels rise to 2 to 4 times the control values, and the disappearance of tolbutamide sometimes slows from a half-life of about 5 ato 17 hours.[268] Tolbutamide, however, is not influenced by the metabolism of warfarin[269] or phenindione.[270] These anticoagulant-oral agent interactions have also been shown with chlorpropamide[271] and presumably with other oral agents as well. A study by Poucher and Vecchio[269] disagreed with some reports, blaming them on laboratory variations as well as differences in vitamin K intake, and claiming that the few instances of apparent effect of tolbutamide on anticoagulant therapy were due to chance variation. However, it appears that some anticoagulants have a greater margin of safety than others in patients treated with oral agents.

Propranolol, a commonly used beta-adrenergic blocking agent, is used cautiously in patients with diabetes because it not only prevents rapid release of glucose from the liver but can mask the effects of hypoglycemic reactions. Newer agents of this type that are more beta-specific and without membrane-stabilizing activity, are safer in diabetics at risk from reactions.[272] Podolsky and Pattavina[273] reported that sulfonylurea-stimulated insulin release in patients with NIDDM can be abolished by administration of propranolol.

While many drugs exercise an adverse effect on one or another hypoglycemic agent, the actual dangers are quite small. Table 21–6 lists many drugs reported to affect sulfonylurea agents. However, in the Joslin Clinic, by practicing cautious and meticulous follow-up in prescribing thiazides, salicylates, and corticosteroids, these have been used without significant difficulty. Sound clinical judgment and astute observation are most important in a clinician using any therapeutic agent, and the oral hypoglycemic agents are no exception.

RISE AND FALL OF THE BIGUANIDES

When the Secretary of Health, Education and Welfare banned the use of phenformin in July of 1977 as an "imminent hazard to the public health,"[274] he removed from use in the United States an agent that had a controversial as well as an often useful existence. It was first described in the literature in 1957 by Pomeranze and associates[275] and Krall and Camerini-Davalos.[276] Phenformin (DBI, Meltrol) with the chemical name of N^1-phenethylbiguanide HCl, was one of a number of biguanide preparations that had clinical trials

at the Joslin Clinic. These included the amyl-, methylbenzyl-, butyl-, and isoamyl- biguanides. Of these, the phenethyl form was most potent, although with the greatest frequency of side effects.

Phenformin is no longer available except to physicians filing an IND (Investigational New Drug) application with the Food and Drug Administration (FDA), but it may be obtained free of charge by physicians who qualify, although they must file reports with the FDA on all patients. When the IND ruling was established, it was done because it was decided that a small population existed for whom the benefits might outweigh the risks. At present, the number of users in the U.S. continues to decline, the active number at present is about 1,200, and the cumulative total is about 4,000 patients. When phenformin was removed from the market, there were an estimated 350,000 persons using the compound.[277] Ordinarily, a drug so removed merits little discussion, except that the biguanides, like the legendary phoenix, keep rising from their own ashes. While some countries have banned or limited their use, they are still available in much of the world, either in their original form or as analogs (metformin and buformin). The biguanides were derived from an earlier guanidine-related compound, decemethylene diguanidine, known as Synthalin A.[278]

No single mechanism of action ever completely explains the mode of action of the biguanides. Among the documented mechanisms are: increased glucose utilization by anaerobic glycolysis (Williams[279]), and promotion of intracellular Embden-Meyerhoff glycolysis (Steiner and Williams[280]). Wick and Stewart[281] concluded that the lactic acid produced was utilized by peripheral tissues. Others suggested decreased gluconeogenesis (Meyer et al.[282] and Searle and Gulli[282a]); increased insulin uptake and insulin clearance (Butterfield and Whichelow[283]); overcoming beta cell inertia (Grodsky and co-workers[284]); and inhibition of transport through the intestinal wall (Kruger et al.[285] and Caspary and Creutzfeldt[286,287]). Cohen and co-workers[288] demonstrated involvement of phenformin in increasing insulin binding, thus enhancing tissue sensitivity to insulin. In short, these evaluations often used different standards with different research models and with varying dose concentrations, causing the scientific literature to be much like the traditional blind men around the elephant, each feeling a different portion of the anatomy, and each with a different impression of the overall structure.

These agents, active only in the presence of endogenous insulin, but having no effect on the beta cells, are often misused. For example, their use with insulin in an attempt to control unstable dia-

Table 21–6. Compounds and Medications that may Influence the Effectiveness of Oral Hypoglycemic Compounds*

A. *Interactions that may worsen diabetes.*
1. *Glucocorticosteroids* such as hydrocortisone and derivatives, especially in large doses, aggravate both subclinical and overt diabetes by increasing glucose output from liver.
2. *Oral contraceptives* may impair glucose tolerance in nondiabetics and worsen latent diabetes, presumably due to increased peripheral insulin resistance.
3. *Oral diuretics*, especially thiazides, cause both extra- and intra-cellular potassium depletion, and probably decreased insulin secretion. Chlorthalidone is the most potassium wasting.
4. *Diazoxide*, a salt-retaining thiazide as well as a potent insulin secretion blocker, has therapeutic limitations.
5. *Sympathomimetic agents* in addition to epinephrine and norepinephrine, amphetamines, ephedrine, phenylephrine and phenylpropranolamine, stimulate glucose output from liver and block insulin secretion.
6. *Nicotinic acid*, often used to treat hypercholesterolemia, may aggravate diabetes by causing liver cell damage.

B. *Interactions that may cause hypoglycemia.*
1. *Alcohol* blocks glucose output by liver. Insulin-plus-alcohol hypoglycemia is worsened by failure of liver to release stored glucose when needed.
2. *Bishydroxycourmarin* prolongs activity of tolbutamide. Avoid this effect by using warfarin instead for anticoagulation therapy with sulfonylurea-treated persons.
3. *Phenylbutazone* replaces sulfonylureas from protein-binding sites, prolonging hypoglycemia. Indomethacin is drug of choice over phenylbutazone as an anti-inflammatory agent.
4. *Salicylates* in large doses (i.e. 4 or more g daily) have a primary hypoglycemic effect.
5. *Sulfonamides* such as sulfisoxazole, sulfaphenazole, and sulfadimidine prolong metabolic activity of sulfonylureas by displacing them from protein binding sites.
6. *Propranolol* and other beta-adrenergic blocking agents prevent rapid release of glucose from liver.

*Adapted from Refs. 273a and 273b.

betes, is occasionally useful in a few isolated cases. However, this combination has shown no impressive results in any large series of patients over any duration. Biguanide was sometimes prescribed for obese patients[289,290] in preference to sulfonylurea because of the alleged lipogenicity of sulfonylureas as compared to biguanides. Czyzyk and co-workers[291] attributed the absence of weight increase to malabsorption of glucose in both humans and dogs when phenformin or butyl-biguanide (buformin) was used. The use of a biguanide in combination with a sulfonylurea is well recognized as effective. The insulin availability, initiated by the sulfonylureas, coupled with the effect of biguanides to increase this insulin effectiveness, made these quite complementary. Recent data indicating increased cell binding sensitivity make these reasons for effectiveness more plausible. Mehnert and Seitz[146] and Beaser[147] were among the first to use this combination therapy, although the Joslin Clinic series started in 1959.[148]

A daily dosage of 2.0 g of tolbutamide, 0.5 g of chlorpropamide, or 1.0 g of acetohexamide or tolazamide in addition to 50 or 100 mg of phenformin were effective in regulating the blood glucose in many patients. In one series (Table 21–7) in which only 9% of 217 patients were adequately regulated with single-dose chlorpropamide therapy, the rate of improvement rose to 60% when the biguanide was added. Mehnert and Standl[292] as well as Czyzyk[293] are cautious enthusiasts for this combination therapy. The discontinuance of phenformin in the United States, without an available alternate biguanide, adversely affected the "con-

trol" of certain patients in whom treatment with sulfonylureas alone was inadequate, and who could not or would not use insulin.[294,295]

The problems leading to the decline of the use of phenformin were numerous. The biguanides became available almost simultaneously with the sulfonylureas that were both effective and less difficult to use. In the Untied States in the last decade, a climate of introspection and cynicism regarding medication made it easy to denigrate unreasonably a therapeutic agent, especially when others, simpler to use, were available. Willy Gepts[296] summed it up well: "In the controversy on the subject of the value of oral therapy in diabetes, many objections expressed in opposition have undeniable theoretic value, but these do not always stem from factual observation."

Lactic Acidosis

What were some of the problems which ultimately led to the demise of phenethyl biguanide availability in the United States? There were annoying side effects, to be sure, largely restricted to the gastrointestinal tract and apparently not related to blood glucose levels.[276] Distressing flatulence, anorexia, nausea, vomiting and diarrhea were estimated as high as 30%.[10d] While better patient selection and use of the long-acting spansule decreased the frequency of these side effects, they were always a threat.[297,298] However, an estimated 400,000 persons in the United States were under treatment daily with this agent, alone or in combination with sulfonylureas. In spite of side effects, there was little or no reported toxicity and

Table 21–7. Results of Combined Oral (Phenformin + Chlorpropamide) Therapy in a Group of 217 Patients Whose Control Was Inadequate with One Type of Oral Compound Alone

Previous Control with Single Oral Agent (205 Chlorpropamide-Treated and 12 Phenformin-Treated Patients)		Control with Chlorpropamide + Phenformin	
Good	2% }	Good	37% }
Fair	7% } 9% satisfactory	Fair	23% } 60% satisfactory
Poor	91%	Poor	40%

no evidence of hypoglycemia caused by biguanide alone, nor were there reports of kidney or liver damage attributable to their use. In the Joslin Clinic series of more than 3000 patients, there was only one known incident of blood platelet sensitivity to phenformin.[10d]

However, in 1959, Walker[299] described excessive rise of blood lactate after exercise in young diabetic patients treated with phenformin, concluding that ketonuria had been present in most of these. Tranquada and co-workers[300] described a syndrome of severe metabolic acidosis that was usually fatal. Huckabee[301] demonstrated that accumulation of lactic acid in the blood sufficient to decrease the sodium bicarbonate and pH, occurs if tissue anoxia appears. Daughaday,[302] emphasized that lactic acidosis occurs in both nondiabetics and diabetics when hypoxia is present, including diabetics under poor control, especially when there is circulatory collapse. The condition of excessive lactate and its relationship to phenformin have been thoroughly described and phenformin-induced lactic acidosis and its treatment are discussed in Chapter 26. Originally thought to be a limited phenomenon, more critical later reports disclosed that lactic acidosis was prevalent enough to warrant due caution in the use of phenformin.

Other biguanides, notably metformin and buformin (methylbiguanide and butylbiguanide) not only had fewer reported side effects but also much less reported lactic acidosis.[303] Czyzyk[293] agrees, but notes that although lactic acidosis is rare, it is still an important consideration, since the mortality rate may be as high as 50%.[304,305] Dembo,[306] however, concluded that the problem of lactic acidosis, although related to phenformin, was caused in large part by poor use of this agent. Often the implicating facts were discovered post hoc. Obviously, poor patient choice was an important factor. However, while lactic acidosis occurred most frequently in older persons with kidney, heart or liver failure, there was probably a much greater incidence than had been reported, since the condition was not suspected until relatively recently. Conlay and Lowenstein[307] concluded that most of their lactic acidosis patients had been treated with phenformin,

and that this condition could be phenformin-induced without other precipitating factors. Wicklmayr et al.[308] found that the enhancing of muscle glucose uptake with lactate release could be of clinical importance since an 8-fold increase of muscle lactate and pyruvate release was found in one of their fatal cases. There have been numerous summaries.[309,310] For example, Alberti and Nattrass[311] described lactic acidosis as "not uncommon," concluding that lactic acidosis "is often not diagnosed, or diagnosed too late." Nattrass et al.[312] compared blood lactate concentrations in biguanide-treated patients. They found truly elevated levels occurring with phenformin, moderately elevated levels with metformin, and normal levels with glibenclamide (glyburide). However, Assan and co-workers[313] reported that lactic acidosis could result from any biguanide, citing five such cases secondary to acute renal failure while the sixth took a massive dose of metformin in a suicide attempt.

Gale and Tattersall[314] despaired that phenformin-induced lactic acidosis was ever preventable, concluding that while many medications had serious side effects, they continue in use because of some unique benefit that outweighs the risk, but such was not the case with phenformin which, at best, is a weak hypoglycemic agent. They opted for metformin as a much safer drug, a view echoed by Nattrass and Alberti[315] who pointed out that metformin produces lactic acidosis uncommonly. They concluded that "biguanides may still have a role in the treatment of hyperglycemia," but espoused metformin as the biguanide of choice, alerting physicians that those who use biguanides must understand that while treating diabetes, they may be creating further abnormalities by the mechanisms of action of these compounds.

In *summary*, it is questionable whether phenformin itself was solely responsible for lactic acidosis or whether this was due to the misuse of the agent. It seems strange that a medication used for more than 20 years with about 10 million patient years (20 × 500,000 patients per year in the United States alone), and which was possibly connected with 400 deaths often due to misuse, should have been removed by administrative fiat. The Food and

Drug Administration admittedly has responsibility for the safety of therapeutic agents and this presumably also covers opportunity for misuse. With the long history, reports of side effects, and in the highly charged medico-political milieu of the late 70s, it is easy to see how phenformin became such easy prey. In the world view, buformin and particularly metformin are considered superior to and safer than phenformin.[316–319] There is even a report by Coetzee and Jackson[320] of the use of metformin in pregnant diabetics. Taton[321] blames the phenformin results on the fact that the side chain length of phenformin *increases the force of binding.* Other forms of biguanide continue in extensive use world-wide, but phenformin still has an occasional supporter.[322]

THE UNIVERSITY GROUP DIABETES PROGRAM (UGDP)

Observers of the University Group Diabetes Program (UGDP) from its inception in 1961, the UGDP report at the Annual Meeting of the American Diabetes Association (ADA) in 1970 and in the years since, are either completely bored by the topic or so ideologically polarized that little can be said to change their opinions. The topic has been adequately covered in reports of diverse origin, often bent according to prejudices of the authors. However, since a whole new generation of physicians has started to practice medicine, the topic is briefly summarized, with the hope that the dilemma may be resolved before this chapter is in print.

In *summary,* the UGDP reports concerned 823 patients with allegedly recent adult-onset diabetes, studied in 12 centers nationwide. These were divided about equally into four treatment groups; *placebo, tolbutamide* (fixed dose, 1.5 g daily), *insulin standard* (fixed dose, 10 to 16 units of lente insulin daily, according to estimated body surface), and *insulin variable* (dose of insulin varied to achieve "satisfactory control" as in conventional treatment). Eventually there were 89 deaths, of which 61 were said to be of cardiovascular causes. The cardiovascular deaths occurred in 4.9% of patients receiving the placebo, in 12.7 of those receiving tolbutamide, in 6.2% of those treated with a fixed dose of insulin, and in 5.9% of those treated with a variable dose of insulin. The upward trend in deaths from cardiovascular disease appeared to take place after about 3½ years of the study.[323–326] These findings were challenged by many, including Keen et al.,[327] Paasikivi,[328] and a long-term retrospective study.[329] The last-named report concerned a cohort study involving 2167 patients first seen at the Joslin Clinic within 1 year of onset of diabetes and who had been treated for at least 90% of the time by one of 3 programs: diet alone, tolbutamide, or insulin.[329] These patients, all 40 years or over at the time of entry into the study, were followed to death or up to 10 years. By the end of the study, 40.8% of the patients had died. There was no significant difference in the percentage of those dying of cardiovascular-renal disease among the insulin and tolbutamide groups. Among the female patients there was no difference between these 2 groups with regard to percentage of deaths ascribed to coronary artery disease. Among male patients there was a significantly greater percentage of coronary artery disease reported in those on tolbutamide as compared to those on insulin. However, when risk factors were taken into account and relative survival rates determined, the difference was no longer important.

Criticisms, charges, counter-charges, and analyses of these and other studies continued for the last 2 decades, so it is not surprising that the practicing physicians of the world are confused.

A basic criticism of the UGDP study was the method of patient choice. Patients had to remain free of ketosis and other acute symptoms of diabetes during a 1-month observation period, were treated with a prescribed diet alone, and then were assigned randomly to 1 of the 4 patient groups. The criteria included the selection of patients free of life-endangering disease so they could have a minimal life expectancy of at least 5 years. Otherwise, there were no restrictions regarding age, sex, previous history, smoking, elevated blood lipids, overweight, or indeed any of the cardiovascular risk factors that are commonly accepted. Tolbutamide was the only oral agent used, although phenformin was added to the study 18 months after the other groups were started. This phenformin group consisted of 204 patients at six of the centers. Although phenformin differs radically from the sulfonylurea agents both in formula and action, the reported results indicated that the death rate from cardiovascular disease was 12.7% (26 out of 204 patients) in the phenformin group as compared to 3.1% (2 out of 64 patients) in the placebo group. It is strange that the cardiovascular death rates for the two insulin groups were higher than the placebo group although lower than that of phenformin, which understandably added to the confusion of interpreting these data.

Feinstein[330] criticized the variances in choice of doses, particularly standard insulin doses in an unchanging pattern, and indicated major inconsistencies in the inclusions and exclusions of patients for the study.

While admitting flaws in the UGDP, Simmons[331] of the Food and Drug Administration stated the study was the best available to date, adding, "It is the privilege of every physician to accept, to reject or to reserve judgment of the UGDP findings." In 1970, an ad hoc committee of the American Diabetes Association (ADA) tentatively accepted the possible hazard of tolbutamide and advised that, in general, it and other oral hypoglycemic agents not be used. The committee recommended restriction of their use to "diabetes of mild or moderate severity in a patient who proves to be poorly controlled with diet and who is unable or unwilling to take insulin."[331a] In a report published in 1979,[331b] the ADA liberalized its stand as indicated in the following statement:

> "Physicians continue to emphasize dietotherapy as the prime form of treatment for maturity-onset diabetes with appropriate use of an oral sulfonylurea or insulin only after diet therapy alone has clearly failed to achieve desired therapeutic goals. The choice of a sulfonylurea or insulin will be left to the judgment of the physician after discussion with the patient."

This is the core of the arguments. In due time, the Committee for the Assessment of Biometric Aspects of Controlled Trials of Hypoglycemic Agents[332] somewhat supported the UGDP data, stating that the UGDP was entitled to draw these conclusions from the material which they had used, archly suggesting that a study is no better than the data which go into it. This declaration likewise did little to settle the debate since the UGDP group staunchly defended their data.[333] Even the statistical performance was attacked by Feinstein[334,335] and O'Sullivan.[336] Meanwhile, the Food and Drug Administration (FDA) accepted the UGDP suggestion that tolbutamide could be unsafe but when they announced intent of warning inserts in the sulfonylurea packaging, a significant group of diabetologists formed the Committee on the Care of the Diabetic (CCD). They voiced disagreement with the threat to the freedom of medical practice and objected to medical decisions made by governmental bureaus. They contested the FDA action, filing suit against the Secretary of Health, Education, and Welfare (HEW) and the Commissioner of FDA, and named some members of the pharmaceutical industry as co-defendants in attempting to prevent biased prescribing regulations and package inserts.

Meanwhile, arguments continued. Davidson[337] was strong in his belief that rigid diet control could more safely replace oral agents. The arguments ranged from highly literate[338] to modestly acrimonious,[339] and continued.[340,341] Eventually, Medical Letter[342] recommended caution in use until "more studies" were performed. The Chairman of the CCD and co-workers[343] cited 20 reports against and 11 for UGDP conclusions. Among the former

were those of Leibel,[344] Seltzer,[345] Keen et al.,[346] and Marble.[347] Seltzer[347a] later expressed his opinion that the UGDP conclusions were becoming increasingly untenable and that, properly used, sulfonylureas are both effective and safe.

Tzagournis and Reynertson[348] in referring to the UGDP-indicted phenformin, cited their own study which showed no difference in survival between patients treated with phenformin and those treated with diet alone. This was reinforced by Chakrabarti and Fearnley[349] who reported that a combination of phenformin and ethylestrenol had a sustained favorable effect on blood fibrinolytic activity and plasma-fibrinogen levels over a 36-month period in survivors of myocardial infarction.

While some criticisms of the UGDP study are obviously picayune, a natural result of a study which some believe was directed against a popular, widely used therapeutic method, certain of the UGDP results are curious. Since the bulk of the alleged cardiovascular deaths occurred in three institutions, one wonders why only those three, and what were the circumstances? Moss[350] questioned the choice of patients studied. Table 21–8 suggests that in the UGDP selection process, the risk factors were greater in the tolbutamide than in the placebo group. The most devastating counter-UGDP charges, however, came from Kilo,[351] one of the original UGDP investigators who later disagreed with the published conclusions. One disillusionment with the study was the fact that no one outside the UGDP, not even the FDA, has ever seen the raw data on which the conclusions were based. In breaking with the UGDP, Kilo offered evidence following a case-by-case audit of computer records of the original patients of the UGDP program, stating that the data were flawed, the patients improp-

Table 21–8. Significant Cardiovascular Risk Factors in the Placebo and Tolbutamide Group Selection Prior to the Study* (University Group Diabetes Program)

	Frequency (%)	
	Placebo Group	Tolbutamide Group
Age over 55	41.5	48.0
Treated with digitalis	4.5	7.6
History of angina	5.0	7.0
Abnormal EKG findings	3.0	4.0
Elevated cholesterol (over 300)	8.6	15.1
Mean fasting blood glucose over 110 mg/dl	63.5	72.1
Decreased visual acuity (over 20/200)	4.5	7.5
Significant arterial calcification	14.3	19.7

There were no significant differences between the groups regarding sex, race, or creatinine greater than 1.5 mg/dl.
*Adapted from Moss.[350]

erly selected, and the study population largely composed of allegedly traditionally unreliable patients. He further claimed insufficient follow-up, poorly managed diabetes, hypertension and other risk factors, and also that many patients changed from the originally assigned medication to another. He also stated that a disproportionate number of subjects in the insulin-variable group, at an increased risk for cardiovascular disease at the time of entry into the study, were eliminated, and that in the remaining subjects, cardiovascular deaths in the placebo group were 4 times more frequent than in the insulin-variable group. He urged the FDA to reconsider the UGDP conclusions regarding tolbutamide toxicity based on inconclusive evidence,[352] which suggestion the FDA ignored. Kilo et al.[353] found cardiovascular deaths in 11 of 80 patients in the placebo group followed over the ensuing years, increasing the cardiovascular death rate from 4.9 to 13.8% between 1969 and 1974 in these former placebo patients, as compared to patients in the insulin standard (7.8%) and in the insulin variable group (9.6%) during those years. The group[354] also attacked "inappropriate data analysis." A Williamson and Kilo[355] study concerning all cardiovascular deaths listed by fasting blood glucose control, showed that the greatest number of deaths (20.4%) occurred in the tolbutamide group with an *average* fasting blood glucose level greater than 200 mg/dl compared with 10.0% of those with fasting blood glucose under 200 mg/dl. (See Table 21–9). However, when subjects dropped out of the study, changed medication, or were otherwise excluded for appropriate reasons, the results were further enhanced because in the group with fasting blood glucose below 200 mg/dl, the rate was 9.4% while in those with fasting levels above 200 mg/dl, the death rate was 25.0%. Certainly, fasting blood glucose levels of 200 mg/dl or above cannot in any way be considered as "regulated," much less, "controlled."

The controversy and agonizing over sulfonylurea use is largely a U.S.A. problem since many governments, including those of West Germany, Canada, Great Britain, Sweden, East Germany, and others reviewed the UGDP data and took no comparable action.[356,357] Dr. Charles Edwards, FDA Commissioner at the time of the original UGDP report, states now that he does not agree with the findings of the study, and that the original error was to accept statistical data without looking deeply into them.[356] An incisive statement was that of Leibel,[358] "The Biometric Committee buried the UGDP Study when they stated that the co-variables in the baseline may have been responsible for the mortality outcome and that randomization. . . . would not solve this problem."

In *summary,* the physicians in the original UGDP study were unquestionably well intentioned participants, attempting to determine in a scientific fashion the effect or lack of effect of widely used oral agents with diabetic patients. They would probably organize the study differently at this time. The results which apparently surprised even them, had probably statistical flaws based on questionable patient selection, and certainly not the same type of follow-up intensity common in the patient-physician relationship in private practice. These results were obtained in out-patient clinic populations who possibly had less motivation in control measures.

One cannot completely ignore the UGDP data since death is a definitive end-point in any study. The general, although not universal, reaction to the UGDP report is that the study organization and later conclusions drawn from data were somehow flawed. However, the lesson should not be dismissed completely. It is difficult to accept the thesis that insulin is no better than oral agents, which are no better than placebo; and if one assumes that the oral agents were poorly used, then possibly this was also true of the other therapeutic modalities. Clearly, the UGDP results point to the need for using the oral agents more circumspectly. The Joslin Clinic along with many others, has always tried to use oral agents only in selected patients, but possibly there are even tighter patient choices and more discrimination than before the UGDP report. Likewise, patients treated with oral agents who consistently have normal blood glucose levels, should have the dosage titrated downward or be treated with diet alone. There is no more virtue in poor control with oral agents than with inappropriate use of insulin. If euglycemia is a standard, one must assume that many of the UGDP patients were poorly regulated. With recent emphasis on blood glucose levels as close to normal as possible as a goal in therapy, the UGDP inference may be valid that much treatment of diabetes as practiced now, is not adequate. Oral agents have been too widely and too readily used in patients who may

Table 21–9. Percentage of Deaths in Each Study Group Related to the Mean Fasting Blood Glucose Level (University Group Diabetes Program)

	Mean Fasting Blood Glucose	
	Below 200 mg/dl	Above 200 mg/dl
	Percent	Percent
Placebo	5.2	4.7
Tolbutamide	9.6	18.0
Insulin, Constant	10.1	14.0
Insulin, Variable	5.1	5.6

either not have needed them or in whom they were not effective. The very simplicity of their use makes misuse possible. The "diabetes pills" became a magic shibboleth to many who thought that the use of the agents would protect them from their self-destructive dietary habits.

Apparently the controversy is drawing to a conclusion. Efforts by the Committee on the Care of the Diabetic served to document the disagreement with the interpretation of the UGDP findings. On May 1, 1938 the Food and Drug Administration (FDA) approved the release for sale of second generation oral agents. In the Federal Register,[358a] the FDA summarizes almost a decade of debate in relatively evenhanded fashion. While insisting that the UGDP findings be printed in labeling, after discussion pro and con the UGDP report ends with Solomonic equanimity that on the one hand,[385b] "The UGDP study provides adequate evidence to support a warning of risk of increasing CV mortality," and on the other, "The agency does not believe, however, that the UGDP study alone provides conclusive evidence of such risk, nor does the information from all studies taken together provide such evidence." In releasing these drugs for sale, the FDA required that package inserts inform physicians that the primary form of treatment for non-insulin-dependent diabetics should be diet, exercise, and weight reduction (where applicable), and that "glucose lowering drugs are indicated only when such a program has clearly failed to reduce symptoms and/or blood glucose levels."[358c]

The FDA[358c] strongly recommends that patients be informed by their physicians of the possible advantages and risks of using these drugs, and told of alternate methods of therapy.

While neither the most zealous physician, pro- or anti-UGDP, will be completely satisfied by these regulations, they do represent progress toward permitting the physician to use judgment in prescribing appropriate therapy, including the second-generation oral agents widely used throughout the world. These regulations, of course, also apply now to all available agents. If there is a lesson to be drawn from this odious drama, it is that medical differences and arguments should be settled in scientific forums and not in either politically charged governmental agencies or courts of law.

THE SECOND GENERATION ORAL AGENTS

It is easy to agree with Klimt[359] when he states that if glucose control could be shown to be effective in avoiding the major complications of diabetes, ". . . it might be argued that a drug which regulated blood sugar levels equally strictly, but more conveniently, and did not cause serious side effects, would be a useful supplement to insulin

and diet therapy. This would be particularly true in view of the difficulty of determining the right diet and then getting the patient to maintain it." Likewise, there is acute nonavailability of insulin in much of the world due chiefly to its cost which is excessive for patients in economically deprived countries. It is in this light that information regarding the second generation hypoglycemic agents widely used in the world, will be summarized to see if these drugs may close some of the gap between what is now available for treatment and the unassailable goal expressed in the quotation above.

By definition, the second generation sulfonylurea agents are those recently developed, about 25 years after the original compounds. These have the same general mode of action as the earlier sulfonylurea agents. However, the newer substances are said to be more efficient and effective in smaller doses and are presumably more precise in their targeted action. While there are about a dozen agents in this category, discussion here is limited to those most recently made available in the U.S.A., viz., glyburide (glibenclamide) and glipizide. A third, gliclazide, is mentioned because of reports of some unusual properties. Characteristics of the second generation agents are shown in Table 21–10.

Glyburide, available here since May 1984, is sold as Diabeta (Hoechst-Roussel Pharmaceuticals) or Micronase (Upjohn Company). It is the most widely used oral hypoglycemic agent in the world, outside the western hemisphere. The other compound, glipizide, is marketed as Glucotrol (Roerig Div., Pfizer Labs). Figure 21–2 shows the formulas of the second generation compounds, their relationship to each other, and (by comparison with Fig. 21–1) to the first generation agents. The other new agent, also extensively used world-wide, is gliclazide, marketed as Diamicron (Servier). Most mechanisms of action of the present sulfonylureas also apply to these. Because of their possible eventual availability, it is important to ask, "Are these really different from the first generation drugs?"

Glyburide (Glibenclamide). This drug, known in early research literature as HB-419, became available in Europe after a symposium in Rottach-Egern, Germany in 1969.[360] This agent requires viable islet cells for successful use but has a high potency whereby a few (5 to 10) mg are as effective as 1000 or more of tolbutamide. There is allegedly less secondary failure because of its potency. On the other hand, this feature increases the risk of hypoglycemic episodes. It is not quite correct to state that it is 100 to 500 times more potent than existing agents because it is used in fractional doses compared to present compounds. It is more accu-

Table 21–10. Characteristics and Dosage of "Second-Generation" Oral Hypoglycemic Agents*

Compound Generic	Trade Name (Manufacturer)	Daily Dose	Starting Dose	Duration of Action	Dose Frequency
Glyburide (Glibenclamide)	Diabeta (Hoechst-Roussel) Micronase (Upjohn)	2.5 to 20 mg	2.5–5.0	12–24 hrs.	Single or Divided
Glipizide	Glucatrol (Roerig)	5–40 mg.	5–20 mg.	10–16 hrs.	Usually Divided
Gliclazide	Diamicron (Servier)	80–320 mg.	80–160 mg.	10–20 hrs.	Single or Divided
compared to: Tolbutamide	Orinase (Upjohn)	500–3000 mg.	500–1000 mg.	6–10 hrs.	Divided

*Tablet sizes available are as follows: Glibenclamide (glyburide)—Hoechst (DiaBeta) and Upjohn (Micronase), 1.25 mg, 2.5 mg, 5.0 mg; Glipizide—Roerig (Glucatrol), 5.0 mg.

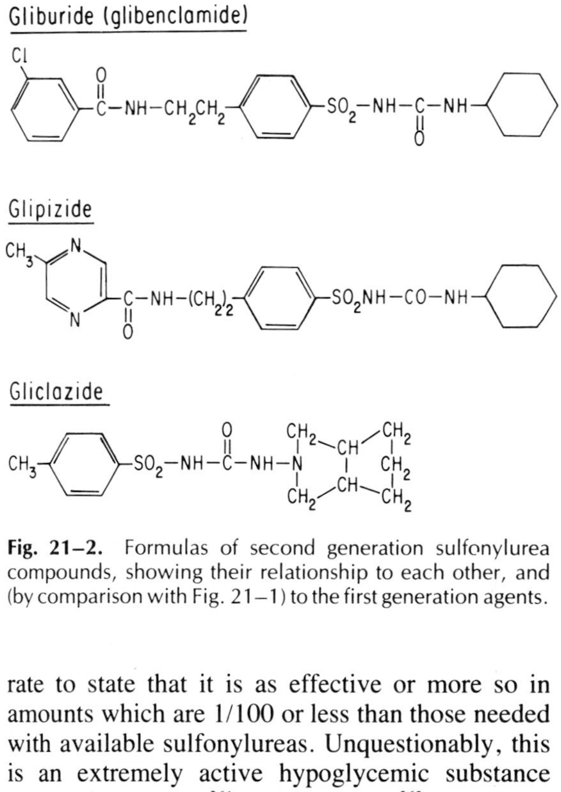

Gliburide (glibenclamide)

Glipizide

Gliclazide

Fig. 21–2. Formulas of second generation sulfonylurea compounds, showing their relationship to each other, and (by comparison with Fig. 21–1) to the first generation agents.

rate to state that it is as effective or more so in amounts which are 1/100 or less than those needed with available sulfonylureas. Unquestionably, this is an extremely active hypoglycemic substance (Loubatieres et al.[361]). Ritien et al.[362] found that with glyburide, 17 of 40 secondary failures with older sulfonylureas were adequately treated for long periods. Krall[363] cautiously noted the effectiveness of glyburide, especially with patients with borderline regulation or failure when treated with older compounds. A review by Müller et al.[364] summarizes the results of 5053 patients treated with a therapeutic dose range of 1.25 to 20 mg daily, stating that 80% of all patients were adequately treated with 10 mg a day. There was no evidence of toxicity although hypoglycemia leading to discontinuance was observed in 1.7%. A later fol-

lowup (Krall et al.[365]) noted that glyburide was probably a most effective sulfonylurea agent because patients who had secondary failures with first generation compounds could often be regulated for a period by adding a biguanide agent, whereas if a patient failed with glyburide, the addition of biguanides made no difference at all. The secondary failure rate was remarkably low, with adequate effective control of about 75% of selected patients. Ahuja,[366] O'Sullivan,[367] Luntz,[368] and Beyer and Schöffling[369] reported good clinical results with glibenclamide, and Breidahl[370] considered it potent enough to salvage patients with secondary failure with other agents. Longer term studies were impressive.[371] It is reported that 80% of patients in a worldwide study were able to achieve good results with a single dose daily,[372] although the criteria for the results were not given. The half-life of glyburide is shorter (under 3 hours) than that of the other sulfonylureas, but the duration of a compound's half-life and effective action do not always coincide. Also, the metabolites of glyburide have no hypoglycemic activity.[373] This compound, as with tolazamide and acetohexamide, has little or no antidiuretic action.[374] There has been no evidence of disulfiram-like effects following alcohol ingestion.[367,375]

Interaction with Other Therapeutic Agents. Like earlier sulfonylureas, this agent may interact with other drugs[265] with certain exceptions, e.g., phenylbutazone. The first generation drugs carry a strong negative charge by which they bind to albumin and when used with another negatively charged drug, the oral agent may be dislodged from the albumin, freeing it to increase hypoglycemic potential. Glyburide carries a much smaller charge and binds to albumin non-ionically, and therefore is less likely to be dislodged. This reduces the potential for hypoglycemia when used in combination with such other compounds as aspirin and other therapeutic agents.[376]

Hypoglycemic Reactions. In the early years of use of glibenclamide in Germany (1969 to 1972), reports emanated from that country[239] concerning numerous deaths from hypoglycemia brought about by this potent drug. These reports of severe hypoglycemia were misinterpreted. At a FDA committee hearing (1974),[377] it was determined that only a few cases could be even remotely associated with severe hypoglycemia due to glyburide. Although during those years, 1,633,000 patients were treated with glyburide, the total deaths in the fourth year were only 2.17 per 100,000 per year.[378] Even the 22 cases cited were due to attempted suicide, to neglect in supervising nursing home patients, or to some other negligence in use of the compound. A hearing determined that there was no unusual hypoglycemic risk from the use of this agent. However, as always, patient selection is of paramount importance and use of this drug should be approached cautiously and intelligently in elderly patients with compromised hepatic or renal function as well as in debilitated patients with irregular or inadequate food intake. Care must be taken also with those patients treated with multiple therapeutic agents that may affect the response to the oral hypoglycemic agent.

Comparisons with Other Oral Hypoglycemic Agents. It is difficult to compare medications tested in different studies under different circumstances and with different patients. If these agents have short half-lives, why the relatively long-term activity? Owens et al.[379] indicated that glibenclamide produced an early, profound blood glucose decrease and this remained constant through the day. The resorption is retarded because of poor solubility, but effective therapeutic levels are reached rapidly since only a minimal therapeutic plasma level is required. However, effective plasma levels have sometimes been found for more than 20 hours.[380] Another reason for prolonged effectiveness of glibenclamide is that while the trigger-releasing effect is of short duration, there is also reported a release of a gastrointestinal factor which amplifies the initial effect.[381] This was also emphasized by Zermatten[132] who reported that glibenclamide enhanced DIRA (duodenal insulin releasing activity) in humans. Repeated intravenous doses of first generation drugs indicated a lag phase with decreased output of insulin from the beta cells, whereas repeated intravenous injections of glibenclamide bring a response as strong as the initial impact, as long as endogenous insulin is available. It appears that glibenclamide has a "hit and run" effect, triggering insulin release although remaining only briefly in the body.

In comparing the effects of diet alone to those of diet and glibenclamide in Type II diabetics, after 10 days of treatment, the group of patients treated by diet alone had a 37% increase in insulin sensitivity with a 36% rise in receptor binding affinity. After 10 days, the group treated with diet and 10 mg daily of glibenclamide evidenced an 83% increase in insulin sensitivity, while insulin binding had increased by 80% as a result of increase in the number of receptors. Others have also shown that glibenclamide appears to stimulate insulin sensitivity due to an increase in the acutal number of insulin receptors.[71,382]

The most dramatic demonstrations of the rapid dispersal by the body of glibenclamide are the radiograms taken in mice. These compared several sulfonylureas for distribution and accumulation in certain cells, with readings at 5 minutes, 1 hour, and 8 hours after infusion of the oral agents. As shown in Fig. 21–3,[383,384] glibenclamide, while present in the liver, gut mucosa, kidney, pancreas and heart after 5 minutes, is found only in the liver and gut in 1 hour, with small amounts in the liver and a residual only in the gut at 8 hours. On the other hand, chlorpropamide with its longer duration of action, shows large amounts in most viscera at the end of 1 hour and even at 8 hours, a sizeable residue. Tolbutamide (not shown) is present in large amounts at one hour with a small residue only in the cecum in 8 hours.

In *summary,* this second generation agent is more potent than the first generation group, and while its mode of action is somewhat the same, it has the unique feature of long action despite a short half-life, and short duration in the body. Side effects are minimal and toxic reactions have not been shown. Hypoglycemic episodes, however, are always a threat, particularly in the older or malnourished patient. The metabolite is inert, excreted in both urine and feces, giving an alternate route of excretion. It has no antidiuretic effect, no disulfiram-like effect, and no known untoward effect on the heart. Pfeiffer[385] stated that glibenclamide is a greater potentiator than the older sulfonylureas. Also, it has extra-beta cell actions, particularly the stimulation of somatostatin and the inhibition of glucagon as well as its effect on receptor cells.[385a] It must be observed, however, that there is a great variance in the effect on insulin receptors.[385b]

While glyburide offers a fresh approach in a generally tired field, it is not a "Wunderkind" and there are some dissenting opinions concerning its superiority over chlorpropamide when both are effective. Chlorpropamide has a longer duration of action in the body. Glyburide, with its extra-pancreatic effects and effectiveness despite short duration in the body, may produce a more satisfactory

Chlorpropamide

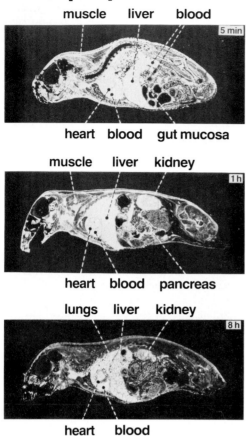

Glibenclamide

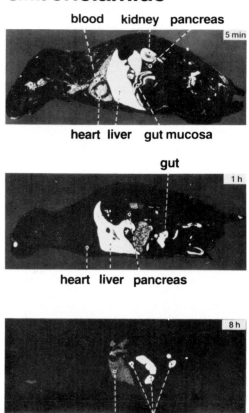

Fig. 21–3. Autoradiograms taken in mice at 5 minutes, 1 hour, and 8 hours after injection of tagged chlorpropamide and glibenclamide.

result. Although one would not discontinue use of an already successful agent in favor of glyburide, its use should be considered when available for patients with marginal results or secondary failure with other agents. As with other sulfonylureas, glyburide will not stimulate the release of insulin where no viable beta cells are present. In summary, this agent, glyburide, is considered to be the most effective oral hypoglycemic agent available to date.

Glipizide (Glucotrol). Another second generation oral agent, glipizide,shares some of the characteristics of glibenclamide. It is almost completely absorbed after oral administration and when compared with glibenclamide, plasma concentrations are about twice as great. It is eliminated by metabolic biotransformation and excretion of the metabolites in the urine. The metabolites have no hypoglycemic activity. The half-life is about 3 to 4 hours. Only about 6% of the administered drug is excreted in the urine, and bile is essentially unchanged in 24 hours. It is also more potent per dose

than tolbutamide. Its duration of action is shorter than that of glyburide (Brogden et al.[386]). The pattern of insulin release is much like that of other oral agents. There has been no evidence of effect on heart rate, blood pressure or electrocardiogram in heart studies,[387] and it appears to have no antidiuretic effect.[388] The compound is well tolerated by most patients except for the few temporary side effects common to all sulfonylureas. The daily dose is larger than that of glyburide, being in the range of 15 to 20 mg daily with a maximum recommended daily dose of 40 mg, usually in divided doses. Brogden et al.[386] summarized the results of numerous studies, concluding that under double-blind conditions, glipizide was superior to placebo or diet alone, somewhat comparable to glibenclamide and chlorpropamide, and superior to tolbutamide. No significant hematologic or gastrointestinal side effects or toxicity have been reported. Johannessen and Fagerberg[389] believe that glipizide achieved a better control of the post-prandial glucose load than that possible with presently available oral agents. Some interesting data from Allen and associates[389a] suggest that improved plasma glucose regulation can be achieved in some patients with insulin-requiring Type II diabetes by combining glipizide with insulin therapy. DeLeeuw et al.[390] stated that the frequency of primary failures with glipizide was slightly more than with glyburide and chlorpropamide. In vivo studies with glipizide suggest that it too increases the number of insulin receptors on the target membrane, thereby enhancing insulin sensitivity. In another trial, Fineberg and Schneider[391] demonstrated increased insulin sensitivity and stated that in comparison with tolbutamide, both had efficacy and safety, but only glipizide had chronic effects upon insulin secretion. Feinglos and Lebovitz[391a] likewise reported that unlike other sulfonylureas, glipizide caused a sustained, long-term increase in glucose-stimulated insulin secretion. Camerini-Davalos et al.[392] in a 3-year study measuring muscle capillary basement membrane thickness in chemical diabetics treated with glipizide compared to those given placebo, have found the membrane to be significantly thicker in the placebo group. In addition,[393] while studying the effect of glipizide on capillary basement membrane width, they found that glucosyltransferase activity (GTA), a collagen synthesizing membrane, was decreased in the treated group as compared to the placebo.

In *summary,* this is another second generation agent, widely used in Europe, which has recently become available in the United States. It does not appear to be quite as potent as glyburide. Ferguson,[394] in his series, indicated that several doses daily would probably be necessary. However, glipizide clearly has advantages over some first generation compounds, and will be useful in Type II diabetes.

Gliclazide (Diamicron-Servier). Gliclazide is also a sulfonylurea which stimulates insulin release and has an extrapancreatic action as well. In many respects, it is much like other second generation agents,[395] with complete absorption by the digestive tract, reaching a peak of plasma concentration in 2 to 6 hours. It has a half-life of 10 hours, with a longer action than other second generation agents, and is used widely abroad.[396] Campbell and associates,[396a] measuring plasma concentrations of gliclazide in health volunteers and diabetic patients, found significant differences in the rates of absorption and elimination, although once a threshold drug concentration was attained, there was little relation between these levels and clinical activity. It is eliminated mostly through the urine and partly in the feces. Up to this point it would appear to be another effective second generation agent with an

unusually wide range of dosage needed for effectiveness (80 to 240 mg daily). Asmal et al.[397] found no essential difference in the type of control between gliclazide and chlorpropamide, nor any evidence of short-term toxicity. While its action is thought by some to be a bit weaker than that of glibenclamide, Fagerberg[398] demonstrated that for identical diabetic control, plasma insulin levels are lower with gliclazide. It has been reported frequently that gliclazide has an action on fibrinolysis and platelet adhesiveness and, indeed, it has been suggested that it may be useful in the prevention or treatment of diabetic microangiopathy. If this proves to be true, the compound could be an important addition to diabetic treatment in preventing complications. Desnoyers and Saint-Dizier[399] reported that blood platelets in diabetics have increased adhesive, aggregative, and also pro-coagulant factor release functions. The authors demonstrated in both animals and humans that gliclazide has an anti-aggregation property, increases the release of plasminogen activator from the vessel wall, and inhibits activity at different stages of thrombus formation. Tsuboi et al.[400] have shown an inhibitory effect of gliclazide on prostaglandin and thromboxane synthesis in guinea-pig platelets. This effect gives an inhibition of arachidonate release from platelets leading to the blockage of the first step of the platelet plug formation. Ponsei et al.[401] observed a marked, progressive and persistent effect of gliclazide on different tests of platelet function during the 12-month treatment.

In his study, Almer[402] first used chlorpropamide for more than 5 years, noting abnormal fibrinolytic activity in vascular walls in 40% (a higher proportion than the 23% in unselected diabetics and 5% in controls). Half of those patients with the changes were then treated with gliclazide for 6 months, after which the endothelial activator was normalized. These early reports suggest that this oral antidiabetic agent may have a protective effect in regard to early diabetic angiopathy. For example, Duhault and co-workers[403] postulated that many of the difficulties with thrombotic phenomena are due to an increase of the release of platelet factors, and showed that gliclazide pre-treatment in experimental animals prevented the formation of aggregates and prevented obstruction in the retinal microcirculation in animals. Regnault[404] reported on a controlled study of diabetic patients, randomly allocated to two treatment groups: Group I with gliclazide alone or combined with another agent, and Group II with another sulfonylurea alone or similarly combined. The patient characteristics were identical for both groups at baseline and after 3 years, the metabolic states of both groups appeared to be identical, but the evolution of retinopathy differed remarkably with the percentage of deterioration being 34% in Group I and 71% in Group II. Although the studies are relatively short-term, they bear watching. There are those who, while hopeful, are seeking more conclusive evidence.

If confirmed, the possibilities are noteworthy. If indeed, as reported, this is a hypoglycemic agent that also regulates platelet function, decreases adhesiveness, reduces platelet aggregation, slows development of non-proliferative retinopathy, and delays new lesions, it merits at least serious investigation and observation.

OTHER POSSIBLE HYPOGLYCEMIC AGENTS UNDER STUDY

Other compounds are reported to have varying degrees of hypoglycemic effect. Some, neither sulfonylureas nor biguanides, are undergoing clinical trials. Chang et al.[405] have published results with ciglitazone (5-[4-(1-methylcyclohexylmethoxyl) benzyl]-thiazolidine-2,4-dione), which exerts a hypoglycemic effect in hyperglycemic animal models (obob and dbdb mice, diabetic Chinese hamsters, and streptozotocin diabetic rats). Another apparently effective oral agent, methyl-2-tetradecylglycidate (McN-3716), with relatively limited study as a hypoglycemic agent, seems to act by inhibiting fatty acid oxidation.[406] Several years ago in a flurry of reports, an isoxazolypyridinium salt compound was said to lower blood glucose levels in certain animals.[407] More recently, reports have demonstrated the anti-hyperglycemic effect of fenfluramide (Pondimin[408]). This anorectic agent resembles amphetamine in structure, but does not stimulate the central nervous system, and has had some limited use in the treatment of obesity. While it apparently increases glucose uptake by muscle, it has had limited usefulness in diabetes. A few studies have attempted to assess the effect of sodium oxaloacetate on diabetes with inconclusive results.[409]

In addition to these, reports in the literature describe exotic combinations with known oral agents. These usually involve non-diabetes-oriented compounds which might enhance effectiveness of known hypoglycemic agents. These include the alpha-glucosidase inhibitors such as Acarbose, the alpha-glucosidase inhibitor BAY g 5421,[410] one of a group of new complex oligosaccharides of microbial origin that inhibit gastrointestinal absorption of carbohydrates.[411] Although there appears to be a hypoglycemic effect, flatulence, a limiting side effect, has been reported.[412,413] This group has recently become popularized as "starch-blockers" claimed to be useful in preventing starch (carbohydrate) absorption, resulting in lower blood glucose with the ultimate goal of weight loss. Although they have found some use in parts of Europe, results of investigations are so sparse as to have occasioned a recent recommendation by the FDA against their use. These, while interesting, have no use in the practice of medicine at this time. There are also other possibly useful compounds,[414,415] but the history of blood glucose-lowering agents shows that very few of those which seem promising ever reach the market.

SUMMARY

After reviewing the enormous literature concerning the oral hypoglycemic era extending for more than 2 decades, it is easy to be neither wildly enthusiastic for, nor adamantly against their use. Clearly they are another step in the evolving therapy of diabetes. They are far from perfect, and the early hope that they were "oral insulin" has long since disappeared. On the positive side, anything that makes the treatment of a complicated condition like diabetes simpler for masses of people is, by definition, an advance in public health. It is specious to argue that they "only lower blood sugar levels" because if they release insulin, decrease resistance to insulin, and also sensitize the receptors while utilizing the patient's endogenous insulin, they have achieved some goals of treatment. Patients so treated must be constantly monitored. Considering their world-wide use, they are among the safest therapeutic agents known. The physician must always consider the potential exotic as well as mundane complications, because of rare but possible incidents such as the encephalopathy reported by Turkington.[416] Jordan and co-workers[417] summarized a group of cases of sulfonylurea-induced factitious hypoglycemia in patients suspected of having insulin-secreting tumors. The diagnoses were made by determining blood sulfonylurea levels.

The emergence of the second generation oral agents is a hopeful development. While not significantly more potent than the first generation agents, unquestionably they are at least effective in smaller doses. Some may cause greater release of insulin and have continued effectiveness in spite of their short half-life. They seem to have significant action on receptors, with decreasing resistance to such insulin as is available.

The lessons of the UGDP are obvious in that poor control is not meritorious under any circumstances and in understanding that while helpful, the oral agents are not miracle drugs. The greatest danger with oral agents is their misuse. Recently a patient admitted to a hospital ward was completely debilitated, having lost 30 kg of weight. His muscles were so atrophied that he could scarcely walk without assistance. Ketoacidosis finally precipitated his hospitalization. He had been treated with double the recommended dose of an ineffective sulfonylurea for this entire period, but responded rapidly to insulin therapy. The poor use of these compounds is a greater threat to the oral agents than are the results of a statistical survey. Future oral agents will probably be more effective by increasing sensitivity and numbers of receptors rather than simply stimulating insulin release. The most accurate statement regarding their effective use is that which opened this chapter, "Used selectively, oral drugs occupy a place in diabetes therapy."

Greek mythology told of the 7 daughters of Atlas who were metamorphosed into stars. These were known as the Pleiades, described now in astronomy as a cluster of stars quite visible to the unaided eye. In literature, the Pleiades were used to designate those ideas that measure the differences between success and failure. For successful use of oral hypolgycemic agents, the advice of the "Pleiades" is: (1) Do not treat with oral agents the patient whose pancreas cannot respond. (2) Make certain that the patient fits the selective criteria, although there may be exceptions. (3) Always keep in mind that diet therapy is basic and vital. (4) Continue to monitor the patient's blood and urine glucose and the glycosylated hemoglobin levels. (5) Do not accept fasting urine test results for monitoring control. (6) Anticipate that stresses such as infection make control less likely and affect control negatively. (7) Know when to change to a stronger oral agent or when to discontinue this treatment and start insulin.

REFERENCES

1. Watanabe, C.K.: Studies in the metabolic changes induced by administration of guanidine bases. I. Influence of injected guanidine hydrochloride upon blood sugar content. J. Biol. Chem. 33:253, 1918.
2. Janbon, M., Chaptal, J., Vedel, A., Schaap, J.: Accidents hypoglycemiques graves par un sulfamidothiazol. Montpelier Med. 21–22:441, 1942.
3. Loubatieres, A.: The hypoglycemic sulfonamides: history and development of the problem from 1942 to 1955. Ann. N.Y. Acad. Sci. 71:4, 1957.
4. Franke, H., Fuchs, J.: Eine neues antidiabetisches Prinzip. Ergebnisse klinischer Untersuchungen. Dtsch. med. Wochenschr. 80:144, 1955.
5. Tucker, H.A.: Oral Antidiabetic Therapy 1956–1965 with Particular Reference to Tolbutamide (Orinase). Springfield, Charles C Thomas, 1965.
6. WHO Expert Committee on Diabetes Mellitus, Second Report. Technical Report Series 640. Geneva, WHO, 1980, p. 31.
7. King, S.R.: Industry Review. Prospects in Diabetes Therapy. New York, F. Eberstadt & Co., Inc. Oct. 3, 1980.
8. Allen, F.M.: Blueberry leaf extract; physiologic and clinical properties in relation to carbohydrate metabolism J.A.M.A. 89:1577, 1927.
9. Franjevic, I.: The antidiabetic action of myrtillin from whortleberry. Med. Sci. Thesis, Univ. of Zagreb, 1980.
10. Krall, L.P.: The oral hypoglycemic agents. In: A. Marble, P. White, R.F. Bradley, L.P. Krall (Eds.): Joslin's Diabetes Mellitus, 11th Ed. Philadelphia, Lea & Febiger, 1971. pp. 302–338.
10a. Ibid. p. 310.
10b. Ibid. p. 309.
10c. Ibid. p 308–309.
10d. Ibid. p. 319.
11. Mahler, R.J.: Personal communication.
12. Galloway, J.A.: Personal communication.
13. Ajgaonkar, S.S.: Herbal drugs in the treatment of diabetes. A review. IDF Bulletin 24:October, 1979, p. 10.
14. Pikir, B.S., Tjokroprawiro, A., Pranawa, et al.: The effect of onion on blood sugar and blood lipid levels of patients with diabetes mellitus. (Abstract). In: H. Hornbostel, G. Strohmeyer, E. Schmidt (Eds.): XVth International Congress of Internal Medicine. Hamburg, 18th/22nd August, 1980. Amsterdam, Excerpta Medica, 1980. p. 50.
14a. Tjokroprawiro, A., Budhiarta, Wibowo, J.A., et al.: The effect of green bean (phaseolus vulgaris, L) on blood sugar levels of patients with diabetes mellitus. (Abstract). In: Ibid. p. 50.
15. Frank, E., Stern, R., Nothmann, M.: Die Guanidin- und Dimethylguanidin-Toxikose des Säugetiers und ihre physio-pathologische Bedeutung. Z. ges. exp. Med. 24:341, 1921.
16. Frank, E., Nothmann, M., Wagner, A.: Über synthetisch dargestellte Körper mit insulinartiger Wirkung auf den normalen und diabetischen Organismus. Klin. Wochenschr. 5:2100, 1926.
17. Frank, E., Nothmann, M., Wagner, A.: Die Synthalin Behandlung des Diabetes mellitus. Dtsch. med. Wochenschr. 52:2067, 1926.
18. Bertram, F.: Zum Wirkungsmechanismus des Synthalins. Dtsch. Arch. f klin. Med. 158:76, 1927.
19. Bertram, F.: Die Behandlung des Diabetes mellitus mit kleinen Dosen von Guanidinderivaten. Med. Klin. 24:1229, 1928.
20. Bertram, F., Benfeldt, E., Otto, H.: Über ein wirksames perorales Antidiabeticum (BZ-55) Dtsch. med. Wochenschr. 80:1455, 1955.
21. Ruiz, C.L., Silva, L.L., Libenson, L.: Contribucion al estudio sobre la composicion quimica de al insulina. Estudio de algunos cuerpos sinteticos sulfurados con accion hipoglucemiante. Rev. Soc. Argent. Biol. 6:134, 1930.
22. Loubatieres, A.: I. Analysis of the betacytotropic action of the hypoglycemic sulfonamides. Basis for its use in the treatment of diabetes. Presse Méd. 68:1421, 1960.
23. Houssay, B.A.: Action of sulphur compounds on carbohydrate metabolism and on diabetes. Am. J. Med. Sci. 219:353, 1950.
24. Blotner, H., Murphy, W.P.: Effect of certain liver extracts on the blood sugar of diabetic patients. J.A.M.A. 94:1811, 1930.
25. Reid, J., MacDougall, A.I., Andrews, M.M.: Aspirin and diabetes mellitus. Br. Med. J. 2:1071, 1957.
26. Graf, W., Nilzen, A.: Histamine, antigen and blood sugar. Acta Dermatovener (Stockholm) 28:7, 1948.
27. Kaplan, S.M., Mass, J.W., Pixley, J.M., Ross, W.D.: Use of imipramine in diabetes. J.A.M.A. 174:511, 1960.
28. Wiederholt, I.C., Genco, M., Foley, J.M.: Recurrent episodes of hypoglycemia induced by propoxyphene. Neurology 17:703, 1967.
29. Quevedo, S.F., Krauss, D.S., Chazan, J.A., et al.: Fasting hypoglycemia secondary to disopyramide therapy. J.A.M.A. 245:2424, 1981.
30. Douglas, R.G., Jr., Betts, R.F.: Influenza virus. In: G.L. Mandell, R.G. Douglas, Jr., J.E. Bennett (Eds.): Prin-

ciples and Practice of Infectious Diseases. New York, John Wiley & Sons, Inc., 1979, pp. 1135–1167.

31. Cahill, G.F., Jr., Etzwiler, D.D., Freinkel, N.: "Control" and diabetes. N. Engl. J. Med. 294:1004, 1976.

32. Siperstein, M.D., Foster, D.W., Knowles, H.C., Jr., et al.: Control of blood glucose and diabetic vascular disease. N. Engl. J. Med. 296:1060, 1977.

33. Deckert, T., Poulsen, J.E., Larsen, M.: Prognosis of diabetics with diabetes before the age of thirty-one. II. Factors influencing the prognosis. Diabetologia 14:371, 1978.

34. Lozano-Castaneda, O., Villasenor, H., Gonzalez-Millan, H., Rull, J.A.: Treatment of diabetes with a single dose of tolbutamide. In: W.J.H. Butterfield, W. Van Westering (Eds.): Tolbutamide After Ten Years. Proceedings of the Brook Lodge Symposium, Augusta, Michigan. March 6–7, 1967. New York, Excerpta Medica Foundation 1967, p. 298.

35. Campbell, R.K., Hansten, P.D.: Metabolism of chlorpropamide. Diabetes Care 4:332, 1981.

36. Tolinase. Animal Studies. In: Physicians' Desk Reference. Oradell, N.J. Medical Economics Co., 1984, p. 2050.

37. Yu, T-F., Berger, L., Gutman, A.B.: Hypoglycemic and uricosuric properties of acetohexamide and hydroxyhexamide. The Upjohn Company, 1968, p. 23.

38. Mahler, R.J.: Personal communication.

39. Vinik, A.I., Jackson, W.P.U., Keller, P., Marine, N.: Metabolic studies in diabetics on tolbutamide. Comparison of a single dose with a divided dose regimen. Diabetologia 4:203, 1968.

39a. Elkeles, R.S., Heding, L.G., Paisey, R.B.: The long-term effects of chlorpropamide on insulin, C-peptide, and proinsulin secretion. Diabetes Care 5:427, 1982.

40. Conference on the effects of the sulfonylureas and related compounds in experimental and clinical diabetes. Ann. N.Y. Acad. Sci. 71:1, 1957.

41. Renold, A.E., Winegrad, A.I., Froesch, E.R., Thorn, G.W.: Sulfonylurea Symposium: Studies on the site of action of the arylsulfonylureas in man. Metabolism 5:757, 1956.

42. Loubatieres, A.: The mechanism of action of hypoglycemic sulfonamides. A concept based on investigations in animals and in man. Diabetes 6:408, 1957.

43. Bänder, A.: The mode of hypoglycemic action of the sulfonylureas D 860 and BZ 55. German Med. Monthly 4:373, 379, 1959. (Translated from Dtsch. med. Wochenschr. 84:996, 1959.)

44. Gepts, W., Christophe, J., Belleno, R.: Étude experimentale de l'action du BZ 55 sur le rat normal ou alloxanise. Ann. Endocrinol. 17:278, 1956.

45. Volk, B.W., Goldner, M.G., Weisenfeld, S., Lazarus, S.S.: Functional and histological studies concerning the action of sulfonylureas. Ann. N.Y. Acad. Sci. 71:141, 1957.

46. Creutzfeldt, W., Deterling, L., Welte, O.: Das B-Zellensystem von normalen und hypophysektomierten Ratten sowie von Kaninchem unter D 860 und diabetogenen Hormonen. Dtsch. med. Wochenschr. 82:1564, 1957.

47. Davidson, J.K., Haist, R.E.: Islet weight studies in rats treated with tolbutamide. Diabetes 11 (Suppl.):115, 1962.

48. Bänder, A., et al.: Über die orale Behandlung des Diabetes mellitus mit N-(4-methylbenzolsulfonyl)-N′=butyl-harnstoff (D860). Dtsch. med. Wochenschr. 81:823, 887, 1956.

49. Bertram, F., Kuntze, J.: Aktuelle Diabetesfragen. Stuttgart, Georg Thieme, 1957.

50. Cerasi, E., Luft, R., Efendic, S.: Decreased sensitivity of the pancreatic beta cells to glucose in prediabetic and diabetic subjects. A glucose dose-response study. Diabetes 21:224, 1972.

51. Skillman, T.A., Feldman, J.M.: The pharmacology of sulfonylureas. Am. J. Med. 70:361, 1981.

52. Grodsky, G.M., Epstein, G.H., Fanska, R., Karam, J.H.: Pancreatic action of sulfonylureas. Fed. Proc. 36:2714, 1977.

53. Klöppel, G., Schäfer, H-J.: Effects of sulfonylureas on histochemical and ultracytochemical calicum distribution in B-cells of mice. Diabetologia 12:227, 1976.

54. Malaisse, W.J., Mahy, M., Brisson, G.R., et al.: The stimulus-secretion coupling of glucose-induced insulin release. VIII. Combined effects of glucose and sulfonylureas. Eur. J. Clin. Invest. 2:85, 1972.

55. Duran Garcia, S., Jarrousse, E., Rosselin, G.: Biosynthesis of proinsulin in newborn rat pancreas. J. Clin. Invest. 57:230, 1976.

56. Boyden, T.W.: The proper place of oral hypoglycemics in diabetes management. Drug Therapy 66:March, 1978.

57. Tsalikian, E., Dunphy, T.W., Bohannon, N.V., et al.: The effect of chronic oral antidiabetic therapy on insulin and glucagon responses to a meal. Diabetes 26:314, 1977.

58. Lebovitz, H.E., Feinglos, M.N., Bucholtz, H.K., Lebovitz, F.L.: Potentiation of insulin action: a probable mechanism for the antidiabetic action of sulfonylurea drugs. J. Clin. Endocrinol. Metab. 45:601, 1977.

59. Blumenthal, S.A.: Potentiation of the hepatic action of insulin by chlorpropamide. Diabetes 26:485, 1977.

60. Grodsky, G., Landahl, H., Curry, D., et al.: A two-compartment model for insulin secretion. Adv. Metab. Disord. 1:45, 1970.

61a. Hellman, B., Täljedal, I-B.: Effects of sulfonylurea derivatives on pancreatic beta cells. In: A. Hasselblatt, F.V. Bruchhausen (Eds.): Insulin. Pt. 2. Berlin, Springer, 1975, pp. 175–194.

62. Samols, E., Tyler, J.N., Miahle, P.: Suppression of pancreatic glucagon release by the hypoglycemic sulfonylureas. Lancet 1:174, 1969.

63. Podolsky, S., Lawrence, A.M.: Control of hyperglycemia in maturity onset diabetes mellitus. Lack of change in insulin and glucagon levels with long term sulfonylurea therapy. In: R.A. Camerini-Davalos, B. Hanover (Eds.): Treatment of Early Diabetes. New York, Plenum, 1979, pp. 381–385.

64. Marco, J., Valverde, I.: Unaltered glucagon secretion after seven days of sulfonylurea administration in normal subjects. Diabetologia 9 (Suppl.):317, 1973.

65. Pek, S., Fajans, S.S., Floyd, J.C., Jr., et al.: Failure of sulfonylureas to suppress plasma glucagon in man. Diabetes 21:216, 1972.

66. Olefsky, J.M., Reaven, G.M.: Effects of sulfonylurea therapy on insulin binding to mononuclear leukocytes of diabetic patients. Am. J. Med. 60:89, 1976.

67. Feinglos, M.N., Lebovitz, H.E.: Sulfonylureas increase the number of insulin receptors. Nature 276:184, 1978.

68. Prince. M.J., Olefsky, J.M.: Direct in vitro effect of a sulfonylurea to increase human fibroblast insulin receptors. J. Clin. Invest. 66:608, 1980.

68a. Vigneri, R., Pezzino, V., Wong, K.Y., Goldfine, I.D.: Comparison of the in vitro effect of biguanides and sulfonylureas on insulin binding to its receptors in target cells. J. Clin. Endocrinol. Metab. 54:95, 1982.

69. Archer, J.A.: Insulin receptors on erythrocytes: influence of oral antidiabetic agents. Upjohn Monograph #8875. Oct. 1979.

70. Eaton, R.P., Galagan, R., Kaufman, E., et al.: Receptor depletion in diabetes mellitus: correction with therapy. Diabetes Care 4:299, 1981.

71. Beck-Nielsen, H., Pedersen, O., Lindskov, H.O.: Increased insulin sensitivity and cellular insulin binding in obese diabetics following treatment with glibenclamide. Acta Endocrinol. 90:451, 1979.

72. Holle, A., Mangels, W., Dreyer, M., et al.: Biguanide treatment increases the number of insulin-receptor sites on human erythrocytes. N. Engl. J. Med. 305:563, 1981.

73. Shenfield, G.M., Logan, A., Shirling, D., Baird, J.: Plasma insulin and glucose levels in maturity onset diabetics treated with chlorpropamide. Diabetologia 13:367, 1977.

74. Barnes, A.J., Crowley, M.F., Garbien, K.J.T., Bloom, A.: Effect of short and long term chlorpropamide treatment on insulin release and blood glucose. Lancet 1:69, 1974.

75. Dunbar, J.C., Foa, P.P.: An inhibitory effect of tolbutamide and glibenclamide (Glyburide) on the pancreatic islets of normal animals. Diabetologia 10:27, 1974.

76. Feldman, J.M., Lebovitz, H.E.: Appraisal of the extrapancreatic actions of sulfonylureas. Arch. Intern. Med. 123:314, 1969.

77. Roth, J.: NIH Conference. Sulfonylureas: effects in vivo and in vitro. Ann. Intern. Med. 75:607, 1971.

78. Bagdade, J.D., Stewart, M., Walters, E.: Impaired granulocyte adherence. A reversible defect in host defense in patients with poorly controlled diabetes. Diabetes 27:677, 1978.

79. Bagdade, Nielson, K.L., Bulger, R.: Reversible abnormalities in phagocytic function in poorly controlled diabetic patients. Am. J. Med. Sci. 263:451, 1972.

80. Bagdade, J.D., Root, R.K., Bulger, R.J.: Impaired leukocyte function in patients with poorly controlled diabetes. Diabetes 23:9, 1974.

81. Nolan, C.M., Beaty, H.N., Bagdade, J.D.: Further characterization of the impaired bactericidal function of granulocytes in patients with poorly controlled diabetes. Diabetes 27:889, 1978.

82. Bagdade, J.D., Walters, E.: Impaired granulocyte adherence in mildly diabetic patients. Effects of tolazamide treatment. Diabetes 29:309, 1980.

83. Wolff, F., Grant, A.: Effect of tolbutamide on blood pressure. N. Engl. J. Med. 284:915, 1971.

84. Levey, G.S.: The effects of sulfonylureas. A peripheral metabolic process. Fed. Proc. 36:2720, 1977.

85. Mirsky, I.A., Perisutti, G., Dixon, F.J.: The destruction of I131 labelled insulin by rat liver extracts. J. Biol. Chem. 214:397, 1955.

86. Mirsky, I.A.: The role of insulinase and insulinase inhibitors. Metabolism 5:138, 1956.

87. Mirsky, I.A., Diengott, D.: The hypoglycemic response to insulin in man after sulfonylurea by mouth. J. Clin. Endocrinol. 17:603, 1957.

88. Szücs, S., Csapo, G.: Serum total lipid and lipoprotein fractions in diabetic patients treated with insulin or carbutamide. Am. J. Med. Sci. 246:710, 1963.

89. Belknap, B.H., Amaral, J.A.P., Bierman, E.L.: Plasma lipids and mild glucose intolerance. I. The response of plasma triglycerides to high carbohydrate feeding and the effect of tolbutamide therapy. In: Ref. 34. p. 159.

90. Belknap, B.H., Amaral, J.A.P., Bierman, E.L.: Plasma lipids and mild glucose intolerance. II. A double blind study of the effect of tolbutamide and placebo in mild adult diabetic outpatients. Ibid., p. 171.

91. Stone, D.B., Brown, J.D., Cox, C.P.: Effect of tolbutamide and phenformin on lipolysis in adipose tissue in vitro. Am. J. Physiol. 210:26, 1966.

92. Achelis, J.O., Hardebeck, K.: Über eine neue blutzuckersenkende Substanz. Dtsch. med. Wochenschr. 80:1452, 1955.

93. Brown, J., Solomon, D.H.: Mechanism of anti-thyroid effects of a sulfonylurea in the rat. Endocrinol. 63:473, 1958.

94. Hunton, R.B., Wells, M.V., Skipper, E.W.: Hypothyroidism in diabetics treated with sulfonylurea. Lancet 2:449 1965.

95. Brown, J., Solomon, D.H.: Effects of tolbutamide and carbutamide on thyroid function. Metabolism 5:813, 1956.

96. Seegers, W., McGavack, T.H., Haar, H.O., et al.: Influence of arylsulfonylureas on thyroid function in older diabetic men and women. J. Am. Geriatr. Soc. 5:739, 1957.

97. Burke, G., Silverstein, G.E., Sorkin, A.: Effect of longterm sulfonylurea therapy on thyroid function in man. Metabolism 16:651, 1967.

98. Bloodworth, J.M.B., Jr.: Morphologic changes associated with sulfonylurea therapy. Metabolism, 12:287, 1963.

99. Palmer, R.F., Lasseter, K.C., McCarthy, J.: Tolbutamide: an inotropic effect on rabbit atria. Lancet 1:604, 1967.

100. Linden, J., Brooker, G.: The positive inotropic action of sulfonylureas. A mechanism independent of cyclic adenosine 3',5' monophosphate. Diabetes 27:694, 1978.

101. Hildner, F.J., Yeh, B.K., Javier, R.P., et al.: Inotropic action of tolbutamide on human myocardium. Cathet. Cardiovasc. Diagn. 1:47, 1975.

102. Curtis, G.P., Setchfield, J., Lucchesi, B.R.: the cardiac pharmacology of tolbutamide. J. Pharm. Exp. Therap. 194:264, 1975.

103. Sykes, C.A., Wright, A.D., Malins, J.M., Pentecost, B.L.: Changes in systolic time intervals during treatment in diabetes mellitus. Br. Heart J. 39:255, 1977.

104. Crockett, S.E., Marsh, D., Lewis, R.P., Tzagournis, M.: Lack of cardiac inotropic effect of tolbutamide in intact man. Metabolism 23:763, 1974.

105. Crockett, S.E., Marsh, D., Lewis, R., Tzagournis, M.: Inotropic effects of tolbutamide in intact man. Diabetes 22:293, 1973.

106. Brown, J.D., Brown, M.E.: The effect of tolbutamide on contractility and cyclic adenosine 3':5'-monophosphate concentration in the intact beating rat heart. J. Pharm. Exp. Therap. 200:166, 1977.

107. Balodimos, M.C., Marble, A.: Diabetic angiopathy and sulfonylurea therapy. Minn. Med. 51:1341, 1968.

108. Balodimos, M.C., Marble, A., Rippey, J.H., et al.: Pathological findings after long-term sulfonylurea therapy. Diabetes 17:503, 1968.

109. Crouchman, M., Woodward, G., Greenberg, M., Keen, H.: Inotropic effects of tolbutamide and glurenorm compared with isoprenaline in diabetic patients and controls. Therapiewoche 26:50, 1976.

110. Deineka, G.K., et al.: Effect of glybenclamide on some values of the cardiovascular system and carbohydrate balance. Farm. ZH (Kiev) 31:48, 1976.

111. Barjot, B.: Les antidiabétiques oraux et le coeur: l'interêt du glibenclamide. In: Flammarion (Ed.): Journées Annuèlles de Diabétologie de l'Hotel-Dieu. Paris, Medecine-Sciences. 1977, p. 358.

112. Barjot, B.: Données actuelles sur le mode d'action du glibenclamide. In: Flammarion et Cie (Eds.): Extrait des Journees Annuèlles de Diabétologie. Hotel-Dieu 1978. Paris. Soulisse et Cassegrain, 1978, pp. 325–331.

113. Fine, D., Shedrovilzky, H.: Hyponatremia due to chlorpropamide. A syndrome resembling inappropriate secretion of antidiuretic hormone. Ann. Intern. Med. 72:83, 1970.

114. Andreani, D., Cinotti, G.A., Stirati, G.: Chlorpropamide

in idiopathic diabetes insipidus. Metabolism *18*:874, 1969.

115. Blotner, H.: The use of chlorpropamide in the treatment of diabetes insipidus. J. Maine Med. Assn. *61*:59, 1970.

116. Moses, A.M.: Effects of sulfonylurea drugs on water metabolism. In: H. Rifkin (Ed.): Proceedings of the Brook Lodge Symposium, Augusta, Michigan, Nov. 25–27, 1974, Amsterdam, Excerpta Medica, 1975: pp. 105–119.

117. Arduino, F.F., Feraz, P.J., Rodrigues, J.: Antidiuretic action of chlorpropamide in idiopathic diabetes insipidus. J. Clin. Endocrinol. Metab. *26*:1325, 1966.

118. Marcondes, M., Genta, E.N.: Antidiuretic action of chlorpropamide in diabetes insipidus patients and in normal subjects. Am. J. Med. Sci. *273*:185, 1977.

119. Earley, L.E.: Editorial: Chlorpropamide antidiuresis. N. Engl. J. Med. *284*:103, 1971.

120. Miller, M., Moses, A.M.: Mechanism of chlorpropamide action in diabetes insipidus. J. Clin. Endocrinol. Metab. *30*:488, 1970.

121. Liberman, B., Borges, R., Wajchenberg, B.L.: Evidence for a role of antidiuretic hormone (ADH) in the antidiuretic action of chlorpropamide. J. Clin. Endocrinol. Metab. *36*:894, 1970.

122. Hagen, G.A., Frawley, T.F.: Hyponatremia due to sulfonylurea compounds. J. Clin. Endocrinol. Metab. *31*:570, 1970.

123. Miller, M., Moses, A.M.: Drug-induced states of impaired water excretion. Kidney Int. *10*:96, 1976.

124. Debeer, L.J., Thomas, J., Mannaerts, G., DeSchepper, P.J.: Effect of sulfonylurea on triglyceride metabolism in the rat liver. J. Clin. Invest. *59*:185, 1977.

125. Colwell, A.R.: Potentiation of insulin action on the liver by tolbutamide. Metabolism *13*:1310, 1964.

126. Marshall, A., Gingerich, R.L., Wright, P.H.: Hepatic effect of sulfonylureas. Metabolism *19*:1046, 1970.

127. Breidahl, H.D., Ennis, G.C., Martin, F.I.R., et al.: Insulin and orl hypoglycemic agents. I. Physiological and clinical pharmacological aspects. Drugs *3*:79, 1972.

128. Davidoff, F.: Hepatic effects of oral hypoglycemic drugs. Fed.Proc. *36*:2724, 1977.

129. Lebovitz, H.E., Feinglos, M.N.: Sulfonylurea drugs; mechanism of antidiabetic action and therapeutic usefulness. Diabetes Care *1*:189, 1978.

130. Flier, J.S., Kahn, C.R., Roth, J.: Receptors, antireceptor antibodies, and mechanisms of insulin resistance. N. Engl. J. Med. *300*:413, 1979.

131. Kahn, C.R.: Role of insulin receptors in insulin-resistant states. Metabolism *29*:455, 1980.

132. Zermatten, A., Heptner, W., Delaloye, B., et al.: Extrapancreatic effect of glibenclamide: stimulation of duodenal insulin-releasing activity (DIRA) in man. Diabetologia *13*:85, 1977.

133. Couturier, E., Anjaneyulu, R., Anjaneyulu, K., et al.: Effects of gliclazide and diazoxide upon ionophore-mediated calcium countertransport. (Abstr.) Diabetologia *19*:266, 1980.

134. Greenfield, M.S., Doberne, L., Rosenthal, M.: The mechanism of sulfonylurea action in man. (Abstr.). Diabetes *30* (Suppl. 1):50A, 1981.

134a. Pope, S.R., Burns, D.M., Miljus, R.A., Miller, R.E.: Glyburide increases glucose transport and glycerol-3-P dehydrogenase activity in cultured 3T3-L1 adipocytes. Diabetes *32* (Suppl. 1):24a, 1983.

135. Hecht, A., Gershberg, H., Hulse, M.: Effect of chlorpropamide treatment on insulin secretion in diabetics: its relationship to the hypoglycemic effect. Metabolism *22*:723, 1973.

136. Ganda, O.P., Kahn, C.B., Soeldner, J.S., Gleason, R.E.: Dynamics of tolbutamide, glucose, and insulin interre-

lationships following varying doses of intravenous tolbutamide in normal subjects. Diabetes *24*:354, 1975.

137. Koncz, L., Soeldner, J.S., Smith, O.T.M., Gleason, R.E.: Insulin secretory dynamics after two consecutive intravenous stimulations with glucose and/or tolbutamide. Metabolism *28*:1183, 1979.

138. Rosan, R.C., Kayne, H.L., Nieland, M.L., Schwachman, H.: Some metabolic responses to intravenous tolbutamide in patients with cystic fibrosis of the pancreas. Metabolism, *13*:480, 1964.

139. Collipp, P.J., et al.: Tolbutamide aids youths with achondroplasia. J.A.M.A. (Medical News) *226*:617, 1973.

140. Skillman, T.A., Hamwi, G.J., Driskill, H., Penrose, M.H.: Oral hypoglycemic therapy: long-term results in older diabetic patients. Geriatrics *16*:209, 1961.

141. Sugar, S.J.: Clinical experience with more than 100 patients treated with Orinase. Med. Ann. D.C. *26*:293, 1959.

142. Rendell, M., Slevin, D., Meltz, G., et al.: A case of maturity-onset diabetes mellitus resistant to insulin but responsive to tolbutamide. Ann. Intern. Med. *90*:195, 1979.

143. Sartor, G., Scherstén, B., Cartström, S., et al.: Ten-year follow-up of subjects with impaired glucose tolerance. Prevention of diabetes by tolbutamide and diet regulation. Diabetes *29*:41, 1980.

144. Paasikivi, J., Wahlberg, F.: Preventive tolbutamide treatment and arterial disease in mild hyperglycaemia. Diabetologia *7*:323, 1971.

145. Kosaka, K., Kuzuya, T., Akanuma, Y., Hagura, R.: Increase in insulin response after treatment of overt maturity-onset diabetes is independent of the mode of treatment. Diabetologia *18*:23, 1980.

146. Mehnert, H., Seitz, W.: Weitere Ergebnisse der Diabetesbehandlung mit blutzuckersenkenden Biguaniden. München. med. Wochenschr. *100*:1849, 1958.

147. Beaser, S.B.: Therapy of diabetes mellitus with combinations of drugs given orally. N. Engl. J. Med. *259*:1207, 1958.

148. Krall, L.P., Balodimos, M.C.: Combined sulfonylurea-biguanide therapy of diabetes mellitus. In: Ref. 34, p. 303.

149. Goodman, J.I.: Role of phenformin (DBI) as an adjuvant in oral antidiabetic therapy. Metabolism, *14*:1153, 1965.

150. Unger, R.H., Madison, L.L., Carter, N.W.: The proper choice of oral antihyperglycemic therapy in diabetes mellitus. Postgrad Med. *29*:40, 1961.

151. Nattrass, M., Todd, P.G., Turnell, D., Alberti, K.G.M.M.: Metabolic abnormalities during combined sulphonylurea and phenformin therapy in maturity-onset diabetics. Diabetologia *14*:389, 1978.

152. Krall, L.P., White, P., Bradley, R.F.: Clinical use of the biguanides and their role in stabilizing juvenile-type diabetes. Diabetes *7*:468, 1958.

153. Faludi, G.: Oral therapy of diabetes in the elderly. Geriatrics *18*:452, 1963.

154. Goldner, M.G., Weisenfeld, S.: Oral hypoglycemic agents. In: M. Ellenberg, R. Rifkin (Eds.): Clinical Diabetes Mellitus. New York, McGraw-Hill Book Co., 1962, p. 229.

155. Jakobson, T., Kahanpaa, A., Berglund, B.: Experience with phenethylbiguanide (DBI) tablets and time-disintegration capsules (DBI-TD) administered as an adjunct to insulin or sulfonylurea drugs in previously treated diabetic patients. Ann. Med. Intern. Fenn. *54*:109, 1965.

156. Molnar, G.D., Striebel, J.L., Goetz, F.C., McGuckin, W.F.: On the use of phenformin to reduce high insulin requirements in diabetes mellitus. Proc. Mayo Clin. *37*:455, 1962.

157. Lazarus, S.S., Volk, B.W.: Physiological basis of the effectiveness of combined insulin-tolbutamide therapy in stable diabetes. Ann. N.Y. Acad. Sci. 82:590, 1959.

158. Fabrykant, M., Ashe, B.I.: Combined insulin-tolbutamide therapy in the management of insulin-dependent diabetes. Metabolism 7:213, 1958.

159. Otto, H., Otto-Benfeldt, E.: Use of combined treatment with insulin and sulphonylurea compounds in diabetes mellitus. Indian J. Med. Sci. 21:221, 1967.

160. Unger, R.H.: Therapy: insulin with oral hypoglycemic agents. In: T.S. Danowski (Ed.): Diabetes Mellitus: Diagnosis and Treatment. New York, American Diabetes Association, Inc., 1964, p. 99.

161. Camerini-Davalos, R., Marble, A., White, P., et al.: Effect of sulfonylurea compounds in diabetic children. N. Engl. J. Med. 256:818, 1957.

162. Kudzma, D.J., Friedberg, S.J.: Potentiation of hypoglycemic effect of chlorpropamide and phenformin by halofenate. Diabetes 26:291, 1977.

163. Jain, A.K., Ryan, J.R., McMahon, F.G.: Potentiation of hypoglycemia effect of sulfonylureas by halofenate. N. Engl. J. Med. 293:1283, 1975.

164. Stowers, J.M., Borthwick, L.J.: Oral hypoglycaemic drugs: clinical pharmacology and therapeutic use. Drugs 14:41, 1977.

165. Stötter, F.S., Seidler, I., Dorfmüller, M.F., et al.: Report on experiences in one and one half years of oral treatment of diabetes with tolbutamide. Ann. N.Y. Acad. Sci. 71:280, 1957.

166. DeLawter, D.E., Moss, J.M., Tyroler, S., Canary, J.J.: Secondary failure of response to tolbutamide treatment. J.A.M.A. 171:1786, 1959.

167. Krall, L.P., Bradley, R.F: "Secondary failures" in the treatment of diabetes mellitus with tolbutamide and with phenformin. Diabetes 11 (Suppl.):88, 1962.

168. Camerini-Davalos, R., Marble, A.: Incidence and causes of secondary failure in treatment with tolbutamide. Experience with 2,500 patients treated up to five years. J.A.M.A. 181:1, 1962.

169. Ztrauzenberg, S.E., Haller, H., Meyer, H.: Problem of late failure in oral diabetes therapy with sulfonylurea preparations. Schweiz Med. Wochenschr. 95:628, 1962.

170. Evans, J.R., Evans, B.K., Evans, G.R.: Improved quality of maintenance with Diabinese (chlorpropamide) reduces the likelihood of secondary failure. J. Amer. Geriat. Soc. 12:195, 1964.

171. Ross, I.S., Borthwick. L.J.: Tablet failure—Does insulin improve control? (Abstr.) Diabetologia 21:321, 1981.

172. Shen, S.W., Bressler, R.: Clinical pharmacology of oral antidiabetic agents. Part 1. N. Engl. J. Med. 296:493, 1977.

173. Shen, S.W., Bressler, R.: Clinical pharmacology of oral antidiabetic agents. Part 2. N. Engl. J. Med. 296:787, 1977.

174. O'Donovan, C.J.: Analysis of long-term experience with tolbutamide (Orinase) in the management of diabetes. Curr. Ther. Res. 1:880, 1959.

175. Mehnert, H., Camerini-Davalos, R., Marble, A.: Results of long-term use of tolbutamide (Orinase) in diabetes mellitus. J.A.M.A. 167:818, 1958.

176. Schöffling, K., Pfeiffer, E.F., Steigerwald, H., et al.: Die Nebenwirkungen der langfristigen D 860-Behandlung. Dtsch. med. Wochenschr. 82:1537, 1957.

177. Kilo, C.: Personal communication.

178. Marble, A., Camerini-Davalos, R.: Clinical experience with sulfonylurea compounds in diabetes. Ann. N.Y. Acad. Sci. 71:239, 1957.

179. Knowles, H.C., Jr.: Toxic effects of sulfonylurea and biguanides when used in treatment of diabetes mellitus. C.M.D. 33:1196, 1966.

180. Tolbutamide and gastric secretion. (Editorial). J.A.M.A. 179:221, 1962.

181. Signorelli, S.: Tolerance for alcohol in patients on chlorpropamide. Ann. N.Y. Acad. Sci. 74:900, 1959.

182. Fitzgerald, M.G., Gaddie, R., Malins, J.M., O'Sullivan, D.J.: Alcohol sensitivity in diabetics receiving chlorpropamide. Diabetes 11:40, 1962.

183. Alcohol sensitivity to sulphonylureas. (Leading article). Br. Med. J. 2:586, 1964.

184. Disulfiram (Antabuse). Med. Letter 22:No. 1, Jan. 11, 1980.

185. Pyke, D.A., Leslie, R.D.G.: Chlorpropamide-alcohol flushing: a definition of its relation to non-insulin-dependent diabetes. Br. Med. J. 2:1521, 1978.

186. Leslie, R.D.G., Barnett, A.H., Pyke, D.A.: Chlorpropamide alcohol flushing and diabetic retinopathy. Lancet 1:997, 1979.

187. Barnett, A.H., Spiliopoulos, A.J., Pyke, D.A.: Blockade of chlorpropamide-alcohol flushing by indomethacin suggests an association between prostaglandins and diabetic vascular complications. Lancet 2:164, 1980.

188. DeSilva, N.E., Tunbridge, W.M.G., Alberti, K.G.M.M.: Low incidence of chlorpropamide-alcohol flushing in diet-treated, non-insulin-dependent diabetes. Lancet 1:128, 1981.

189. Workshop sponsored by the International Diabetes Epidemiology Group and National Institutes of Health, Washington, D.C., June 13–14, 1980.

190. Bradley, R.F., Sagild, U., Schertenleib, F.E.: Diabetes mellitus and liver function. N. Engl. J. Med. 253:454, 1955.

191. Camerini-Davalos, R., Lozano-Castaneda, O., Marble, A.: Five years' experience with tolbutamide. Diabetes 11 (Suppl):74, 1962.

192. Zimmerman, H.J.: Drugs and the liver. D.M. May, 1963, p. 1.

193. Baird, R.W., Hull, J.C.: Cholestatic jaundice from tolbutamide. Ann. Intern. Med. 53:194, 1960.

194. Warner, R. Personal communication.

195. Brown, G., Zoidis, J., Spring, M.: Hepatic damage during chlorpropamide therapy. J.A.M.A. 170:2085, 1959.

196. Stowers, J.M., Bewsher, P.S.: The long-term use of sulfonylureas in diabetes mellitus. Lancet 1:122, 1962.

197. Haunz, E.A., Cornatzer, W.E., Luper, M.: Liver function in chlorpropamide therapy. Five year clinical study of 181 patients. J.A.M.A. 188:237, 1964.

198. Fineberg, S.K.: Clinical experience with chlorpropamide and comparative evaluation with tolbutamide. J. Am. Geriat. Soc. 8:441, 1960.

199. Hamff, H., et al.: The effects of tolbutamide and chlorpropamide on patients exhibiting jaundice as result of previous chlorpropamide therapy. Ann. N.Y. Acad. Sci. 74:820, 1959.

200. Cervantes-Amezcua, A., Naldjian, S., Camerini-Davalos, R., Marble, A.: Long-term use of chlorpropamide in diabetes. J.A.M.A. 193:759, 1965.

201. White, L.L.R.: Fatal marrow aplasia during chlorpropamide therapy. Br. Med. J. 1:691, 1962.

202. Stein, J.H., Hamilton, H.E., Sheets, R.F.: Agranulocytosis caused by chlorpropamide. A case report with confirmation by leukoagglutination studies. Arch. Intern. Med. 113:186, 1964.

203. Karlin, H.: Fatal agranulocytosis following chlorpropamide treatment of diabetes. N. Engl. J. Med. 262:1076, 1960.

204. Tucker, S.C., Lynch, J.P., Ansell, B.F., Jr.: Chlorpro-

pamide-induced agranulocytosis. J.A.M.A. *238*:422, 1977.

205. McMurdoch, J., Speirs, C.F., Mace, M.: Fatal marrow aplasia after chlorpropamide and methyldopa. (Letter to the Editor). Lancet *1*:207, 1968.

206. Borish, L.C.: Personal communication.

207. Recker, R.R., Hynes, H.E.: Pure red blood cell aplasia associated with chlorpropamide therapy. Patient summary and review of the literature. Arch. Intern. Med. *123*:445, 1969.

208. Teoh, P.C., Tan, D.K.S., Da Costa, J.L., Chew, B.K.: Acquired pure red-cell aplasia in adults. Med. J. Aust. *2*:373, 1973.

209. Logue, G.L., Boyd, A.E., III, Rosse, W.F.: Chlorpropamide-induced immune hemolytic anemia. N. Engl. J. Med. *283*:900, 1970.

210. Grace, W.J.: Thrombocytopenia in a patient taking chlorpropamide. N. Engl. J. Med. *260*:711, 1959.

211. Morley, A., Hirsh, J.: A case of thrombocytopenia associated with chlorpropamide therapy. Med. J. Aust. *2*:988, 1964.

212. Cunliffe, D.J., Gorst, D.W., Palmer, H.M.: Chlorpropamide-induced thromboyctopenia. Postgrad. Med. J. *53*:87, 1977.

213. Jost, F.: Blood dyscrasias associated with tolbutamide therapy. J.A.M.A. *169*:1468, 1959.

214. Chapman, I., Cheung, W.H.: Pancytopenia associated with tolbutamide therapy. J.A.M.A. *186*:595, 1963.

215. Janbon, M., Lazerges, P., Metropolitanski, J.M.: Étude du métabolisme du sulfa-isopropylthiodiazol (VK 57 ou 2254 RP) chez le sujet sain et en cours de traitement. Comportement de la glycémie. Montpellier Méd. *21-22*:489, 1942.

216. Malacarne, P., Castaldi, G., Bertusi, M., Zavagli, G.: tolbutamide-induced hemolytic anemia. Diabetes *26*:156, 1977.

217. Gelfand, M.L.: Gastrointestinal bleeding during tolbutamide therapy. J.A.M.A. *171*:258, 1959.

218. Geary, C.G.: Blood and neoplastic diseases. Acquired aplastic anemia. Br. Med. J. *1*:432, 1974.

219. Tullet, G.L.: Fatal case of toxic erythema after chlorpropamide (Diabinese). Br Med. J. *1*:148, 1966.

220. Rothfeld, E.L., Goldman, J., Goldberg, H.H., Einhorn, S.: Severe chlorpropamide toxicity. J.A.M.A. *172*:54, 1960.

221. Bennett, W.M., Singer, I., Coggins, C.H.: Guide to drug usage in adult patients with impaired renal function. J.A.M.A. *223*:991, 1973.

222. Sinclair, C., Danowski, T.S.: Enhanced response to tolbutamide in uremia. Acta Diabet. Lat. *9*:373, 1972.

223. Balodimos, M.C., Rippey, J.H., Marble, A.: Causes of death and pathological findings in diabetic patients treated with sulfonylurea compounds. In: 7th International Congress of Gerontology. Vienna, Austria, June 26–July 2, 1966, p. 1.

224. Balodimos, M.C., Marble, A., Rippey, J.H., et al.: Pathological findings after long-term sulfonylurea therapy. Diabetes *17*:503, 1968.

224a. Nowak, S.M., McCaleb, M.L., Lockwood, D.H.: Extrapancreatic action of sulfonylureas: hypoglycemic effects are not dependent on altered insulin binding or inhibition of transglutaminase. Metabolism *32*:398, 1983.

225. Yonet, H.M., Ballard, H.S.: Prolonged severe hypoglycemia following tolbutamide therapy for paralysis agitans. N.Y. J. Med. *61*:1939, 1961.

226. Schwartz, J.F.: Tolbutamide-induced hypoglycemia in Parkinson's disease: a case report. J.A.M.A. *176*:106, 1961.

227. Conn, H.J., Perlmutter, M., Silverstein, J.N., Numeroff,

M.: Prolonged hypoglycemia in response to intravenous tolbutamide in a patient with Laennec's cirrhosis and severe malnutrition. J. Clin. Endocrinol. *24*:28, 1964.

228. Kindschi, L.G.: Hypoglycemic coma in a diabetic patient treated with tolbutamide. Wisc. Med. J. *65*:120, 1966.

229. Brown, J.D., Stone, B.: Tolbutamide-induced hypoglycemia. Am. J. Clin. Nutr. *15*:144, 1964.

230. Spurny, O.M., Wolf, J.W., Devins, G.S.: Protracted tolbutamide-induced hypoglycemia. Arch. Intern. Med. *115*:53, 1965.

231. Karon, E.H., Kremer, J.L.: Severe, recurrent hypoglycemia due to chlorpropamide therapy. Minn. Med. *48*:1017, 1965.

232. Dall, J.L.C., Conway, H., McAlpine, S.G.: Hypoglycaemia due to chlorpropamide. Scot. Med. J. *12*:403, 1967.

233. Greenberg, B., Weihl, C., Hug, G.: Chlorpropamide poisoning. Pediatr. *41*:146, 1968.

234. Dougherty, J.: Hypoglycemic stupor caused by acetohexamide. N. Engl. J. Med. *274*:1256, 1966.

235. Alexander, R.W.: Prolonged hypoglycemia following acetohexamide administration. Report of two cases with impaired renal function. Diabetes *15*:362, 1966.

236. Seltzer, H.S.: Drug-induced hypoglycemia. A review based on 473 cases. Diabetes *21*:955, 1972.

237. Kaplinsky, N., Frankl, O.: The significance of the cerebrospinal fluid examination in the management of chlorpropamide-induced hypoglycemia. Diabetes Care *3*:248, 1980.

238. Miller, D.R., Orson, J., Watson, D.: Letter to the Editor: Up John, down glucose. N. Engl. J. Med. *297*:339, 1977.

239. Frerichs, H., Deuticke, U., Creutzfeldt, W.: A side effect of oral antidiabetics: hypoglycemia. Med. Klin. *68*:363, 1973.

240. Jackson, W.P.U., Campbell, G.D., Notelovitz, M., Blumsohn, D.: Tolbutamide and chlorpropamide during pregnancy in human diabetes. Diabetes *11* (Suppl.):98, 1962.

241. Campbell, G.D.: Possible teratogenic effect of tolbutamide in pregnancy. (Letter to the Editor). Lancet *1*:891, 1961.

242. White, P.: Pregnancy and diabetes, medical aspects. Med. Clin. North Am. *49*:1015, 1965.

243. Dolger, H., Bookman, J.J., Nechemias, C.: The diagnostic and therapeutic value of tolbutamide in pregnant diabetics. Diabetes *11* (Suppl.):97, 1962.

244. Douglas, C.P., Richards, R.: Use of chlorpropamide in the treatment of diabetes in pregnancy. Diabetes *16*:60, 1967.

245. Moss, J.M., DeLawter, D.E., Gallagher, E.J.: Oral hypoglycemic drugs; comparative evaluation of tolbutamide, chlorpropamide and phenformin. Med. Times *92*:645, 1964.

246. Miller, D.I., Wishinsky, H., Thompson, G.: Transfer of tolbutamide across the human placenta. Diabetes *11* (Suppl.):93, 1962.

247. Brown, G.D., Gabert, H.: Long-term experience with DBI (phenformin). Appl. Ther. *4*:451, 1962.

248. Watson, W.A.F., Petrie, J.C., Galloway, D.B., et al.: *In vivo* cytogenic action of sulphonylurea drugs in man. Mutation Res. *38*:71, 1976.

249. Sutherland, H.W., Stowers, J.M., Cormack, J.D., Bewsher, P.D.: Evaluation of chlorpropamide in chemical diabetes diagnosed during pregnancy. Br. Med. J. *2*:9, 1973.

250. Zucker, P., Simon, G.: Prolonged symptomatic neonatal hypoglycemia associated with maternal chlorpropamide therapy. Pediatrics *42*:824, 1968.

251. Physician's Desk Reference, 38th Edn. p. 2041, 1984.

252. Shagan, B.P.: Diabetes in the elderly patient. Med. Clin. N. Am. *60*:1191, 1976.

253. Podolsky, S.: Hyperosmolar nonketotic coma in the elderly diabetic. Med. Clin. N. Am. *62*:815, 1978.

254. Melmon, K.L., Neirenberg, D.W.: Editorial. Drug interactions and the prepared observer. N. Engl. J. Med. *304*:723, 1981.

255. Greenblatt, D.J., Sellers, E.M., Shader, R.I.: Drug disposition in old age. N. Engl. J. Med. *306*:1081, 1982.

256. Kater, R.M.H., et al.: Increased rate of tolbutamide metabolism in alcoholic patients. J.A.M.A. *207*:363, 1969.

257. Carulli, N., et al.: Alcohol-drugs interaction in man: alcohol and tolbutamide. Eur. J. Clin. Invest. *1*:421, 1971.

258. Johnson, H.K., Waterhouse, C.: Relationship of alcohol and hyperlactatemia in diabetic subjects treated with phenformin. Am. J. Med. *45*:98, 1968.

259. Editorial: Alcohol and hypoglycemic coma. J.A.M.A. *206*:639, 1968.

260. Kimble, M.A.: Diabetes. J. Am. Pharmaceut. Assoc. *NS14*:80, 1974.

261. Salmela, P.I., Sotaniemi, E.A., Pelkonen, R.O.: The evaluation of the drug-metabolizing capacity in patients with diabetes mellitus. Diabetes *29*:788, 1980.

262. Brown, K.F., Crooks, M.J.: Displacement of tolbutamide, glibenclamide and chlorpropamide from serum albumin by anionic drugs. Biochem. Pharmacol. *25*:1175, 1976.

263. Amer. Pharmaceut. Assoc.: Evaluations of Drug Interactions. Washington, Amer. Pharmaceut. Assoc. 1977, pp. 35–42.

264. Griffin, J.P., D'Arcy, P.F.: A Manual of Adverse Drug Interactions. Bristol, John Wright & Sons Ltd., 1975, pp. 160–170.

265. Hansten, P.D.: Drug interactions. In: Clinical Significance of Drug-Drug Interactions and Drug Effects on Clinical Laboratory Results. Philadelphia, Lea & Febiger, 1976, pp. 56–69.

266. Adverse interactions of drugs. The Med. Letter *23*:(Issue 578), 1981.

267. Ebert, R.V.: (Editorial). Oral anticoagulants and drug interactions. Arch. Intern. Med. *121*:373, 1968.

268. Sise, H.S. (Editorial note). Potentiation of tolbutamide by dicumarol. Ann. Intern. Med. *67*:460, 1967.

269. Poucher, R.L., Vecchio, T.J.: Absence of tolbutamide effect on anticoagulant therapy. J.A.M.A. *197*:121, 1966.

270. Kristensen, M., Hansen, J.M.: Potentiation of the tolbutamide effect by dicumerol. Diabetes *16*:211, 1967.

271. Hansen, J.M., Christensen, L.K.: Drug interactions with oral sulphonylurea hypoglycaemic drugs. Drugs *13*:24, 1977.

272. Deacon, S.P., Karunanayake, A., Barnett, D.: Acebutolol, atenolol, and propranolol and metabolic responses to acute hypoglycaemia in diabetics. Br. Med. J. *2*:1255, 1977.

273. Podolsky, S., Pattavina, C.G.: Hyperosmolar nonketotic diabetic coma: a complication of propranolol therapy. Metabolism *22*:685, 1973.

273a. Seltzer, H.S.: Medications and drugs that affect diabetes. In: L.P. Krall, K.G.M.M. Alberti (Eds.): World Book of Diabetes in Practice. Amsterdam, Excerpta Medica, 1982, pp. 148–150.

273b. Avery, G.S.: Drug interactions that really matter: a guide to the major importance of drug interactions. Drugs *14*:132, 1977.

274. Food and Drug Administration: Phenformin: removal from general market. FDA Drug Bulletin *7*:14, 1977.

275. Pomeranze, J., Fujiy, H., Mouratoff, G.T.: Clinical report of a new hypoglycemic agent. Proc. Soc. Exp. Biol. Med. *95*:193, 1957.

276. Krall, L.P., Camerini-Davalos, R.: Early clinical evaluation of a new oral non-sulfonylurea hypoglycemic agent. Proc. Soc. Exp. Biol. Med. *95*:345, 1957.

277. Food and Drug Administration: Report of the Endocrinologic and Metabolic Drugs Advisory Committee, Vol. I. Department of Health and Human Services, FDA, Oct. 15, 1981.

278. Staub, H.: Über Synthalin. Schweiz. Med. Wochenschr. *57*:1141, 1927.

279. Williams, R.H., Tanner, D.C., Odell, W.D.: Hypoglycemic actions of phenethyl-, amyl-, and isoamyl-diguanide. Diabetes *7*:87, 1958.

280. Steiner, D.F., Williams, R.H.: Actions of phenethylbiguanide and related compounds. Diabetes *8*:154, 1959.

281. Wick, A.N., Stewart, C.J.: Tissue distribution of administered DBI and its relationship to DBI action (Abstract). Clin. Res. *7*:111, 1959.

282. Meyer, F., Ipaktchi, M., Clauser, H.: Specific inhibition of gluconeogenesis by biguanides. Nature *213*:203, 1967.

282a. Searle, G.L., Gulli, R.: The mechanism of the acute hypoglycemic action of phenformin (DBI). Metabolism *29*:630, 1980.

283. Butterfield, W.J.H., Whichelow, M.J.: The hypoglycemic action of phenformin. Effect of phenformin on glucose metabolism in peripheral tissues. Diabetes *11*:281, 1962.

284. Grodsky, G.M., Karam, J.H., Pavlatos, F.C., Forsham, P.H.: Reduction by phenformin of excessive insulin levels after glucose loading in obese and diabetic subjects. Metabolism, *12*:278, 1963.

285. Kruger, F.A., Altschuld, R.A., Hollobaugh, S.L., Jewett, B.: Studies on the site and mechanism of action of phenformin. II. Phenformin inhibition of glucose transport by rat intestine. Diabetes *19*:50, 1970.

286. Caspary, W.F., Creutzfeldt, W.: Analysis of the inhibitory effect of biguanides on glucose absorption: inhibition of active sugar transport. Diabetologia *7*:379, 1971.

287. Caspary, W.F., Creutzfeldt, W.: Inhibition of intestinal amino acid transport by blood sugar lowering biguanides. Diabetologia *9*:6, 1973.

288. Cohen, D., Pezzino, V., Vigneri, A., et al.: Phenformin increases insulin binding to human cultured breast cancer cells. Diabetes *29*:329, 1980.

289. Danowski, T.S.: Diabetes mellitus and obesity. Phenformin hydrochloride as a research tool. Diabetes *16*:600, 1967.

290. Stowers, J.M., Bewsher, P.D.: Studies on the mechanism of weight reduction by phenformin. Postgrad Med. J. *45*:13, 1969.

291. Czyzyk, A., Tawecki, J., Sadowski, J., et al.: Effect of biguanides on intestinal absorption of glucose. Diabetes *17*:492, 1968.

292. Mehnert, H., Standl, E.: Biguanides—an unfinished story. In: W.K. Waldhausl (Ed.): Diabetes 1979. Proceedings of the 10th Congress of the International Diabetes Federation, Vienna, Austria, Sept. 9–14, 1979. Amsterdam, Excerpta Medica, 1980. p. 615.

293. Czyzyk, A.: The use of biguanide derivatives in the treatment of diabetes. In: J.S. Bajaj (Ed.): Diabetes. Proceedings of the 9th Congress of the International Diabetes Federation, New Delhi, India, Oct. 31–Nov. 5, 1976. Amsterdam, Excerpta Medica, 1977, pp. 442–450.

294. Dolger, H.: Personal communication.

295. Siitonen, O., Aro, A., Huttunen, J.K., et al.: Effect of discontinuation of biguanide therapy on metabolic control in maturity-onset diabetics. Lancet *1*:217, 1980.

296. Gepts, W.: Histopathology of the islets of Langerhans after oral treatment of diabetes. Le Diabète *6*:215, 1958.

297. Krall, L.P., Bradley, R.F.: Long-term phenformin therapy for diabetes, with emphasis on the older patient. Geriatrics *17*:337, 1962.

298. Krall, L.P.: Ten years' experience with biguanides in the treatment of diabetes mellitus. In K. Oberdisse, H. Daweke, G. Michael (Eds.): 2nd International Biguanid Symposium am 5 und 6 Mai, 1967. Düsseldorf, Stuttgart, Georg Thieme Verlag, 1968, p. 161.

299. Walker, R.S.: Preliminary observations on phenethyldiguanide. Br. Med. J. 2:405, 1959.

300. Tranquada, R.E., Bernstein, S., Martin, H.E.: Irreversible lactic acidosis associated with phenformin therapy. Report of three cases. J.A.M.A. *184*:159, 1963.

301. Huckabee, W.E.: Abnormal resting blood lactate. II. Lactic acidosis. Am. J. Med. *30*:840, 1961.

302. Daughaday, W.H., Lipicky, R.J., Rasinski, D.C.: Lactic acidosis as a cause of nonketotic acidosis in diabetic patients. N. Engl. J. Med. *267*:1010, 1962.

303. Bachman, W., Mehnert, H.: Oral hypoglycemic agents. In: Progress in the Topics of Diagnosis, Pathophysiology and Therapy of Diabetes. Proceedings of the IV Mediterranean Symposium of Diabetology. Corfu, Greece, May 1, 1979. Milan, Elli & Pagani, 1980, pp. 147–155.

304. Luft, D., Schmülling, Eggstein, M.: Lactic acidosis in biguanide-treated diabetics: a review of 330 cases. Diabetologia *14*:75, 1978.

305. Mizrahi, A.: Workshop discussion: Metabolic effects of biguanides. USV International, Paris, May, 1975.

306. Dembo, A.J., Marliss, E.B., Halperin, M.L.: Insulin therapy in phenformin-associated lactic acidosis. A case report, biochemical considerations and review of the literature. Diabetes *24*:28, 1975.

307. Conlay, L.A., Loewenstein, J.E.: Phenformin and lactic acidosis. J.A.M.A. *235*:1575, 1976.

308. Wicklmayr, M., Dietze, G., Mehnert, H.: Effect of phenformin on substrate metabolism of working muscle in maturity onset diabetics. Diabetologia *15*:99, 1978.

309. Kreisberg, R.A.: Lactate homeostasis and lactic acidosis. Ann. Intern. Med. *92*:227, 1980.

310. Misbin, R.I.: Phenformin-associated lactic acidosis: pathogenesis and treatment. Ann. Intern. Med. *87*:591, 1977.

311. Alberti, K.G.M.M., Nattrass, M.: Lactic acidosis. Lancet 2:25, 1977.

312. Nattrass, M., Todd, P.G., Hinks, L., et al.: Comparative effects of phenformin, metformin and glibenclamide on metabolic rhythms in maturity-onset diabetics. Diabetologia *13*:145, 1977.

313. Assan, R., Heuclin, Ch., Ganeval, D., et al.: Metformin-induced lactic acidosis in the presence of acute renal failure. Diabetologia *13*:211, 1977.

314. Gale, E.A.M., Tattersall, R.B.: Can phenformin-induced lactic acidosis be prevented? Br. Med. J. 2:972, 1976.

315. Nattrass, M., Alberti, K.G.M.M.: Biguanides. (Editorial). Diabetologia *14*:71, 1978.

316. Pirart, J., Rutman, S.: Un nouvel antidiabetique per os: le NN dimethylbiguanide. Essais therapeutiques alternes avec un placebo et un sulfamide. Acta Clinica Belgica, T. *XVI*:575, 1961.

317. Björntorp, P., Carlström, S., Fafferberg, S.E., et al.: Influence of phenformin and metformin on exercise induced lactataemia in patients with diabetes mellitus. Diabetologia *15*:95, 1978.

318. Bergman, U., Bowman, G., Wiholm, B-E.: Epidemiology of adverse drug reactions to phenformin and metformin. Br. Med. J. 2:464, 1978.

319. Bruns, W., Bibergeil, H.: The therapy with oral antidiabetic drugs. In: H. Bibergeil (Ed.): Diabetes mellitus. Ein Nachschlagewerk für die diabetologische Praxis. Jena, Fischer-Verlag, 1978, pp. 251–270.

320. Coetzee, E.J., Jackson, W.P.U.: Metformin in management of pregnant insulin-dependent diabetics. Diabetologia *16*:241, 1979.

321. Taton, J.: Personal communication.

322. Valenta, L.J.: Letter to the Editor. Phenformin in diabetes mellitus. Ann. Intern. Med. *85*:126, 1976.

323. Klimt, C.R., Knatterud, G.L., Meinert, C.L., Prout, T.E.: The University Group Diabetes Program: A study of the effects of hypoglycemic agents on vascular complications in patients with adult-onset diabetes. Part I. Design, methods, and baseline characteristics. Diabetes *19* (Suppl. 2):747, 1970.

324. Klimt, C.R., Knatterud, G.L., Meinert, C.L., Prout, T.E.: The University Group Diabetes Program: A study of the effects of hypoglycemic agents on vascular complications in patients with adult-onset diabetes. Part II. Mortality results. Diabetes *19* (Suppl. 2):789, 1970.

325. Goldner, M.G., Knatterud, G.L., Prout, T.E.: Effects of hypoglycemic agents on vascular complications in patients with adult-onset diabetes. Part III. Clinical implications of UGDP results. J.A.M.A. *218*:1400, 1971.

326. Knatterud, G.L., Meinert, C.L., Klimt, C.R., et al.: Effects of hypoglycemic agents on vascular complications in patients with adult-onset diabetes. Part IV. A preliminary report on phenformin results. J.A.M.A. *217*:777, 1971.

327. Keen, H., Jarrett, R.J., Chlouverakis, C., Boyns, D.R.: The effect of treatment of moderate hyperglycemia on the incidence of arterial disease. Postgrad. Med. J. 44 (Suppl.):960, 1968.

328. Paasikivi, J.: Long-term tolbutamide treatment after myocardial infarction. A clinical and biochemical study of 178 patients without overt diabetes. Acta Med. Scand. Suppl. *507*:1, 1970.

329. Marble, A.: Letter to the Editor. J.A.M.A. *232*:808, 1975.

330. Feinstein, A.R.: A critique of the UGDP study. In: Summaries of Presentations at AMA Convention, June 24, 1971. Ardsley, Geigy Pharmaceuticals, 1971, p. 5.

331. Simmons, H.E.: FDA viewpoint. In: Ibid. ref. 330.

331a. Ricketts, H.T.: The University Group Diabetes Program. A study of the effects of hypoglycemic agents on vascular complications in patients with adult-onset diabetes (editorial statement). Diabetes *19* (Suppl. 2):iii, 1970.

331b. American Diabetes Association: Policy Statement. The UGDP controversy. Diabetes Care 2:1, 1979.

332. Special Contribution. Report of the Committee for the Assessment of Biometric Aspects of Controlled Trials of Hypoglycemic Agents. J.A.M.A. *231*:583, 1975.

333. Cornfield, J.: The University Group Diabetes Program. A further statistical anaylsis of the mortality findings. J.A.M.A. *217*:1676, 1971.

334. Feinstein, A.R.: Clinical biostatistics. VIII. An analytical appraisal of the University Group Diabetes Program (UGDP) study. Clin. Pharmacol. Ther. *12*:167, 1971.

335. Feinstein, A.R.: Clinical biostatistics. XXXVI. The persistent biometric problems of the UGDP study. Clin. Pharmacol. Ther. *19*:572, 1976.

336. O'Sullivan, J.B., D'Agostino, R.B.: Decisive factors in the tolbutamide controversy. J.A.M.A. *232*:825, 1975.

337. Davidson, J.K.: The FDA and hypoglycemic drugs. J.A.M.A. *232*:853, 1975.

338. Schwartz, T.B.: The tolbutamide controversy: a personal perspective. Ann. Intern. Med. *75*:303, 1971.

339. Moser, R.H.: Editorial. Let's stop the Donnybrook. A perspective on the UGDP-Biometric Society study. J.A.M.A. *231*:1274, 1975.

340. Skyler, J.S.: The UGDP and insulin therapy. Editorial. Diabetes Care *1*:328, 1978.

341. Knatterud, G.L., Klimt, C.R., Levin, M.E., et al.: Letter

to the Editor. The UGDP and insulin therapy: a reply. Diabetes Care 2:247, 1979.

342. Phenformin and vascular complications of diabetes. The Medical Letter *14*:Issue 339, p. 1, 1972.

343. Bradley, R.F., Dolger, H., Forsham, P.H., et al.: Settling the UGDP controversy? J.A.M.A. *232*:813, 1975.

344. Leibel, B.: An analysis of the University Group Diabetes Program: Data results and conclusions. Can. Med. Assoc. J. *105*:292, 1971.

345. Seltzer, H.S.: A summary of criticisms of the findings and conclusions of the University Group Diabetes Program (UGDP). Diabetes *21*:976, 1972.

346. Keen, H., Jarrett, R.J., Fuller, J.H.: Tolbutamide and arterial disease in borderline diabetics. In: W.J. Malaisse, J. Pirart (Eds.): Diabetes. Amsterdam. Excerpta Medica, 1974. pp. 588–601.

347. Marble, A.: Oral hypoglycaemics: A balanced view. In: J.S. Bajaj (Ed.): Diabetes. Amsterdam. Excerpta Medica, 1977. pp. 451–455.

347a.Seltzer, H.S.: Efficacy and safety of oral hypoglycemic agents. Ann. Rev. Med. *31*:261, 1980.

348. Tzagournis, M., Reynertson, R.: Mortality from coronary heart disease during phenformin therapy. Ann. Intern. Med. *76*:587, 1972.

349. Chakrabarti, R., Fearnley, G.R.: Phenformin plus ethyloestrenol in survivors of myocardial infarction. Three-year pilot study. Lancet *2*:556, 1972.

350. Moss, J.M.: Oral hypoglycemics and the UGDP. Current Prescribing *12*:13, 1979.

351. Kilo, C.: Controlling diabetes: should you believe the UGDP? Modern Medicine, Sept. 15–30, 1978, p. 49.

352. Kilo, C.: The use of oral hypoglycemic agents. Hospital Practice. March, 1979, p. 103.

353. Kilo, C., Williamson, J.R., Choi, S.C., MIller, J.P.: Refuting the UGDP conclusion that insulin treatment does not prevent vascular complications in diabetics: In: R.A. Camerini-Davalos, B. Hanover (Eds.): Treatment of Early Diabetes. New York, Plenum, 1979, pp. 307–312.

354. Kilo, C., Miller, J.P., Williamson, J.R.: The crux of the UGDP: spurious results and biologically inappropriate data analysis. Diabetologia *18*:179, 1980.

355. Kilo, C., Miller, J.P., Williamson, J.R.: The Achilles heel of the University Group Diabetes Program. J.A.M.A. *243*:450, 1980.

356. Kolata, G.B.: Controversy over study of diabetes drugs continues for nearly a decade. Science *203*:986, 1979.

357. Schliack, V., Bibergeil, H., Haller, H.: Comment of the "Zentraler Gutachterausschluss für Arzneimittelverkehr, Sektion Humanmedizin" of the GDR to "The Question of an Elevated Cardiovascular Risk upon Long Term Application of Oral Antidiabetic Drugs." Medicamentum *17*:115, 1976.

358. Leibel, B.S. Personal communication.

358a.Rules and Regulations. Wednesday, April 11, 1984. Federal Register *49*:No. 71, pp. 14303–14330.

358b.Ibid., p. 14328.

358c.Ibid., p. 14327.

359. Klimt, C.R.: Oral hypoglycaemics after the UGDP. In: J.S. Bajaj (Ed.): Diabetes. Amsterdam, Excerpta Medica, 1977. pp. 416–425.

360. Levine, R., Pfeiffer, E.F. (Eds.): HB 419: A new oral antidiabetic drug. (Papers presented at the Tegernsee Conference, in Rottach-Egern, Germany, January 27–29, 1969.) Horm. Metab. Res. *1* (Suppl. 1):1–92, 1969.

361. Chapal, J.: Pharmacological study of a new particularly active hypoglycemic sulfonamide: Glibenclamide (HB 419). In: Ibid. Ref. 360. pp. 18–24.

362. Retiene, K., Petzoldt, R., Althoff-Zucker, C., et al.: Clin-

ical studies on Glibenclamide (HB 419). In: Ibid. Ref. 360. pp. 55–60.

363. Krall, L.P.: A critical appraisal of the new sulfonylurea HB 419 (Glibenclamide). In: Ibid. Ref. 360. pp. 85–87.

364. Müller, R., Bauer, G., Schröder, R., Saito, S.: Summary report of clinical investigation of the oral antidiabetic drug HB 419 (Glibenclamide). In: Ibid. Ref. 360. pp. 88–92.

365. Krall, L.P., Sinha, S., Goldstein, H.H.: Glibenclamide (HB 419, Daonil) in the clinical practice of diabetes. Aust. NZ J. Med. *1* (Suppl. 2):57, 1971.

366. Ahuja, M.M.S., Gupta, S.P., Sehgel, V.K.: Efficacy of glibenclamide in maturity-onset diabetics as maintenance therapy. Horm. Metab. Res. *5*:160, 1973.

367. O'Sullivan, D.J., Cashman, W.F.: Blood glucose variations and clinical experience with glibenclamide in diabetes mellitus. Br. Med. J. *2*:572, 1970.

368. Luntz, G.R.W.N.: Clinical use of glibenclamide in diabetes mellitus. Postgrad. Med. J. (Dec. Suppl.):84, 1970.

369. Beyer, J., Schöffling, K.: Clinical experience with glibenclamide in 300 diabetics. Postgrad. Med. J. (Dec. Suppl):78, 1970.

370. Breidahl, H.D.: Clinical experience with glibenclamide—Daonil. Aust. NZ J. Med. *1* (Suppl. 2):63, 1971.

371. Davidson, M., Lewis, A.A.G., de Mowbray, R.R.: Clinical experience with glibenclamide in 129 unselected diabetic patients. Postgrad. Med. J. (Dec. Suppl.):70, 1970.

372. Rupp, W., Christ, O., Fullberth, W.: Studies on the bioavailability of glibenclamide. Arzneim-Forsch *22*:471, 1972.

373. Heptner, W., et al.: Metabolization of HB 419 in animals. Arzneim-Forsch *19*:1400, 1969.

374. Rado, J.P., et al.: Investigation of the diuretic effect of glibenclamide in healthy subjects and in patients with pituitary and nephrogenic diabetes insipidus. Horm. Metab. Res. *6*:289, 1974.

375. Anderson, J., et al.: Clinical and metabolic study in diabetic patients treated with glibenclamide. Br. Med. J. *2*:568, 1970.

376. Skillman, T.G., Feldman, J.M.: The pharmacology of sulfonylrueas. Am. J. Med. *70*:361, 1981.

377. Committee of the Food and Drug Administration. Vol. I. 1974.

378. Medical Research Dept., Hoechst AG: Information on HB 419. (Glibenclamide; Glyburide). Position Paper on German and U.S. Experience Relative to Glyburide-Associated Deaths due to Hypoglycemia. Frankfurt FRG, 1974.

379. Owens. D.R., Biggs, P.I., Shetty, K., Wragg, K.G.: The effect of glibenclamide on the glucose and insulin profile in maturity onset diabetics following both acute and long term treatment. Diabete Metabol. *6*:219, 1980.

380. Müller, R.: Personal communication. March 18, 1969.

381. Heptner, W., Zermatten, A., Kellner, H-M., et al.: Extrapancreatic and pancreatic actions of glibenclamide in rats. Diabetologia *13*:339, 1977.

382. Sorenson, N.S., Pedersen, O., Lindskov, H.O.: A stimulatory effect of diet and glibenclamide on insulin sensitivity and insulin binding. (Abstract). Dibetologia *15*:271, 1978.

383. Hellmann, B., Idahl, L.A., Tjälve, H., et al.: Beobachtungen zum Wirkungsmechanismus des hypoglykämisch wirsamen Sulfonylharnstoff-Präparates HB 419. Arzneim. Forsch. *19*:1472, 1969.

384. Kellner, H.M., Heptner, W.: Personal communication. 1977.

385. Pfeiffer, E.F.: Personal communication.

385a.Olefsky, J.M., Kolterman, O.G.: Mechanisms of insulin resistance in Type II diabetes mellitus and the effects of sulfonylurea treatment. In: Mngola, E.N. (Ed.): Diabetes

1982. Proceedings of the 11th Congress of the International Diabetes Federation, Nairobi, Kenya, Nov. 10–17, 1982. Amsterdam, Excerpta Medica, 1983, pp. 177–187.

385b. Fleig, W.E., Nother-Fleig, G., Fussganger, R., Ditschuneit, H.: Glyburide affects insulin action but not insulin binding in cultured hepatocytes. Diabetes 32 (Suppl. 1):60a, 1983.

386. Brogden, R.N., Heel, R.C., Pakes, G.E., et al.: Glipizide: a review of its pharmacological properties and therapeutic use. Drugs 18:329, 1979.

387. Kojima, M., Shintomi, K., Ochiai, T., et al.: Pharmacological studies on glipizide. I. General pharmacological effects of glipizide. Pharmacometrics (Japan) 7:1197, 1973.

388. Fernandez, P., Singer, I.: Enhancement of ADH-induced water flow in isolated toad urinary bladders by two new sulfonylureas. (Meeting abstract). Clin. Res. 23:219A, 1975.

389. Johannessen, A., Fagerberg, S.E.: Glipizide, a new oral antidiabetic agent. (Report of a controlled clinical study in Sweden). Diabetologia 9 (Suppl.):339, 1973.

389a. Allen, B.T., Feinglos, M.N., Lebovitz, H.: Combined insulin, glipizide treatment of non-insulin dependent diabetes mellitus. Diabetes 32 (Suppl. 1):35a, 1983.

390. DeLeeuw, I., DeBaere, H., Decraene, P., et al.: An open comparative study of the efficacy and tolerance of a new antidiabetic agent: glipizide. Diabetologia 9 (Suppl.):364, 1973.

391. Fineberg, S.E., Schneider, S.H.: Glipizide versus tolbutamide, an open trial. Effects on insulin secretory patterns and glucose concentrations. Diabetologia 18:49, 1980.

391a. Feinglos, M.N., Lebovitz, H.E.: Sulfonylurea treatment of insulin-independent diabetes mellitus. Metabolism 29:488, 1980.

392. Camerini-Davalos, R.A., Velasco, C., Glasser, M., Bloodworth, J.M.B., Jr.: Drug-induced reversal of early microangiopathy. N. Engl. J. Med. 309:1551, 1983.

393. Camerini-Davalos, R.A.: Personal communication.

394. Ferguson, B.D.: Personal communication.

395. Malaisse, W.J., Couturier, E., Valverde, I.: The insulinotropic action of gliclazide: possible mode of action. In: H. Keen, A.D.S. Caldwell, M. Murphy, C. Bowker (Eds.): Gliclazide and the Treatment of Diabetes. London, Royal Society of Medicine International Congress and Symposium Series No. 20, 1980, pp. 37–42.

396. H. Keen, A.D.S. Caldwell, M. Murphy, C. Bowker (Eds.): Gliclazide and the Treatment of Diabetes. London, Royal Society of Medicine International Congress and Symposium Series No. 20, 1980.

396a. Campbell, D.B., Adriaenssens, P., Hopkins, Y.W., et al.: Pharmacokinetics and metabolism of gliclazide: a review. In: Keen, H., Caldwell, A.D.S., Murphy, M., Bowker, C. (Eds.): Gliclazide and the Treatment of Diabetes. London, Royal Society of Medicine, 1980, pp. 71–82.

397. Asmal, A.C., Leary, W.P., Thandroyen, F., et al.: An evaluation of the efficacy and safety of gliclazide compared to chlorpropamide. In: Ibid. ref. 396.

398. Fagerberg, S.E., Gamstedt, A.: Paired observations between different sulfonylureas in antidiabetic treatment. In: Ibid. Ref. 396. pp. 143–150.

399. Desnoyers, P., Saint-Dizier, D.: Gliclazide: haemobiological properties. A synopsis with emphasis on inhibition of platelet coagulant factors. In: Ibid. Ref. 396. pp. 19–27.

400. Tsuboi, T., Fujitani, J., Maeda, K., et al.: Effects of gliclazide on prostaglandin and thromboxane synthesis in guinea pig platelets. Thrombosis Res. 21:103, 1981.

401. Ponari, O., Civardi, E., Megha, S., et al.: Anti-platelet effects of long-term treatment with gliclazide in diabetic patients. Thromb. Res. 16:191, 1979.

402. Almer, L.: The effects of gliclazide on the fibrinolytic system. In: Ibid. Ref. 396. pp. 201–205.

403. Duhault, J., Regnault, F., Boulanger, M., Tisserand, F.: Prevention of experimental obstructions in the retinal microcirculation. Arterial fluorescein studies. Ophthalmologica (Basel) 170:345, 1975.

404. Regnault, A.F.: Prognosis of non-proliferative diabetic retinopathy during treatment with gliclazide. In: Ibid. Ref. 396. pp. 249–257.

405. Chang, A.Y., Wyse, B.M., Gilchrist, B.J.: Ciglitazone, a new hypoglycemic agent. 1. Studies in ob/ob and db/db mice, diabetic Chinese hamsters, and normal and streptozotocin-diabetic rats. Diabetes 32:830, 1983.

406. Tutwiler, G.F., Kirsch, T., Mohrbacher, R.J., Ho, W.: Pharmacologic profile of methyl 2-tetradecylglycidate (McN-3716). An orally effective hypoglycemic agent. Metabolism 27:1539, 1978.

407. Riggi, S.J., Blickens, D.A., Boshart, C.R.: A new oral hypoglycemic agent: 1-methyl-4-(3-methyl-5-isoxazolyl) pyridinium chloride. Diabetes 17:646, 1968.

408. Turtle, J.R., Burgess, J.A.: Hypoglycemic action of fenfluramine in diabetes mellitus. Diabetes 22:858, 1973.

409. Yoshikawa, K.: Studies on anti-diabetic effect of sodium oxaloacetate. Tohoku J. Exp. Med. 96:127, 1968.

410. Vierhapper, H., Bratusch-Marrain, P., Waldhäusl, W.: Long-term treatment of sulphonylurea-treated diabetics with the a-glucosidase inhibitor Bay g 5421 (Acarbose). (Letter to the Editor). Diabetologia 20:586, 1981.

411. Schmidt, D.D., Frommer, W., Junge, B., et al.: alpha-glucosidase inhibitors. New complex oligosaccharides of microbial origin. Naturwissenschaften 64:535, 1977.

412. Walton, R.J., Sherif, I.T., Noy, G.A., Alberti, K.G.G.M.: Improved metabolic profiles in insulin-treated diabetic patients given an alpha-glucosidehydrolase inhibitor. Br. Med. J. 1:220, 1979.

413. Sachse, G., Willms, B.: Effect of the a-glucosidase inhibitor Bay g 5421 on blood glucose control of sulphonylurea-treated diabetics and insulin-treated diabetics. Diabetologia 17:287, 1979.

414. Gerich, J.E., Lorenzi, M., Bier, D.M., et al.: Effects of physiologic levels of glucagon and growth hormone on human carbohydrate and lipid metabolism. Studies involving administration of exogenous hormone during suppression of endogenous hormone secretion with somatostatin. J. Clin. Invest. 57:875, 1976.

415. Brown, M., Rivier, J., Vale, W.: Somatostatin: Analogs with selected biological activities. Science 196:1467, 1977.

416. Turkington, R.W.: Encephalopathy induced by oral hypoglycemic drugs. Arch. Intern. Med. 137:1082, 1977.

417. Jordan, R.M., Krammer, H., Riddle, M.R.: Sulfonylurea-induced factitious hypoglycemia. A growing problem. Arch. Intern. Med. 137:390, 1977.

22 Exercise and Diabetes

Louis Vignati and Lee N. Cunningham

The triad of insulin, diet and exercise has been the basis for treatment of diabetes for the past 60 years. Each of these therapeutic modalities can have an impact on the health of the diabetic and each, individually or in combination with the others, has a place in the treatment regimen. Exercise programs in conjunction with diet, insulin or oral hypoglycemic agents can affect glycemic control, weight, cardiovascular risk factors and the mental health status of the patient.

The physiology of exercise is well understood in the normal nondiabetic in whom the changes caused by physical work are proportional to the duration and intensity of physical activity as well as the physical fitness level of the person exercising. The physiologic changes that occur during exercise in the diabetic are not as clear since changes in metabolism with exercise in the diabetic are de-pendent also on the plasma insulin level and the degree of metabolic or glycemic control prior to physical work. However, some parallels can be drawn between the nondiabetic and the diabetic.

This discussion will contrast the metabolic changes occurring in nondiabetic persons and in those with Types I and II diabetes. The discussion will also serve to suggest a method of prescribing exercise programs.

BENEFITS OF EXERCISE

Although there is no firm evidence that physical fitness prevents complications of diabetes, it is well known that in nondiabetic persons, a regular program of endurance exercises can reduce risk factors associated with macrovascular disease. Sustained endurance exercise decreases blood lipids,[1-3] reduces blood pressure, increases collateral circulation (particularly in those patients with peripheral vascular disease), decreases resting and exercise heart rate,[4] increases oxygen transport by increasing 2,3-diphosphoglycerate and decreasing blood viscosity, and improves glucose tolerance in normal individuals. It is reasonable to assume that some of the same benefits to the cardiovascular system would accrue as well to the diabetic under a proper exercise regimen. Indeed, diabetics exhibit changes in blood lipids that parallel those of nondiabetics during endurance training.[1] The effects which occur within the metabolic system during training include an increased insulin sensitivity,[5,6] improved fuel oxidation rates,[7] increased oxidative enzymes,[8] increased storage of muscle glycogen,[9] increased amino acid uptake, and increased maximal oxygen consumption.[8] However, some recent evidence suggests that exercise training may not improve glycemic control. Wallberg-Henriksson et al.[9a] reported no significant improvement in glycosylated hemoglobin, 24-hour urinary glucose excretion, and home-monitored urine tests despite increases in maximal oxygen consumption and muscle oxidative capacity following a 16-week aerobic training program.

Weight reduction is often an important goal in the treatment of maturity-onset diabetes. Here again, a regular program of physical activity is beneficial in part because there is an increased insulin responsiveness when there is a change of body composition toward a greater percentage of lean body mass.[10,11] Often the obese patient notes a change in clothes size and improvement in glucose control before changes in scale weight. The psychologic benefit derived from activity is apparent, both for the insulin-dependent and noninsulin-dependent diabetic. Table 22–1 lists the possible benefits of endurance exercise to the diabetic.

PHYSIOLOGY OF EXERCISE IN THE NONDIABETIC INDIVIDUAL

Metabolic Fuel Utilization and Production

Muscle is capable of oxidizing two metabolic fuels—glucose and free fatty acids—in order to generate the cyclic nucleotides necessary for muscular contraction. The availability of these two fuels is dependent on the circulating concentrations of regulatory hormones. Insulin is the preeminent controlling hormone. During exercise, however, glucagon, catecholamines, and cortisol also contribute to regulating the availability of metabolic fuel. The intensity and duration of the physical activity determines the contributory role of each hormone. The oxidation of fuels is dependent also on the relative plasma concentrations of glucose or free fatty acid, with muscle utilizing that fuel which is in greater abundance.

In the post-absorptive state, 90% of muscle energy at rest is generated by the oxidation of free fatty acids as reflected by respiratory quotients of 0.7. As work is performed, glucose oxidation increases at a proportionally greater rate than the increased oxidation of free fatty acids. The available glucose comes from plasma glucose, muscle

Table 22–1. Benefits of Regular Endurance Exercise for the Diabetic Patient

Metabolic Effects
Increased insulin sensitivity (decreased insulin requirements)
Normalization of fuel oxidation rates
Increased oxidative enzymes
Increased storage of glycogen
Increased amino acid uptake
Increased maximal oxygen uptake

Cardiovascular Effects
Decreased hemoglobin A_{1c}
Decreased triglycerides
Increased HDL-cholesterol
Lower resting blood pressure
Improved peripheral circulatory characteristics
Increased oxygen transport (2,3 DPG, viscosity)*
Increased cardiac dynamics (stroke value and cardiac output).

*Increased red cell 2–3 diphosphoglycerate; decreased blood viscosity.

or hepatic glycogen, and hepatic gluconeogenesis. Muscle glycogenolysis accounts for glucose availability during short bursts of physical activity. As muscular activity is prolonged, hepatic glycogenolysis is the source of increased availability of glucose. After about 15 minutes of moderate exercise, hepatic gluconeogenesis begins to have a major role in providing glucose for muscle cells. Hepatic gluconeogenesis is enhanced by increased flux from muscle of the major gluconeogenic substrate, alanine. Alanine is derived from carbon "skeletons" generated by glycolysis and by oxidation of branched chain amino acids within the muscle.

During the initial phase of muscle activity, the utilization of both glucose and free fatty acids increases, the glucose at this point more rapidly than the free fatty acids. When exercise is prolonged more than 30 minutes, free fatty acids, generated by adipocyte lipolysis, account for a major portion of muscle fuel requirements, and in more prolonged exercise gradually supplant the utilization of glucose.[12,12a]

Production of both glucose and free fatty acids for utilization by muscle is facilitated by production and release of the regulatory hormones, catecholamines, glucagon and growth hormone. The amount of these hormones released is modified by the state of physical fitness of the patient.[13,14]

The post-exercise recovery phase is characterized by restoration of muscle and hepatic glycogen stores, provided that sufficient insulin is available.[15–18a] Lactate produced during aerobic exercise is recycled to glucose via the Cori cycle, with the major portion oxidized by mitochondria.[18b] Accelerated glycogenic activity continues for 12 to 24 hours following prolonged exercise, and is insulin-dependent. This recovery phase may contribute to the post-exercise hypoglycemia seen in young diabetics after strenuous prolonged exercise.

PHYSIOLOGY OF EXERCISE IN THE DIABETIC INDIVIDUAL

Glucose and Fatty Acid Metabolism

The adaptation to exercise by diabetic muscle is dependent on the metabolic status of the patient. This in turn is determined not only by the immediate insulin availability, but also by the prior metabolic control as reflected in plasma glucose, ketoacid levels and the state of hydration.[18c] The noninsulin-dependent diabetic responds normally to the exercise stimulus. The metabolic response to exercise in insulin-dependent diabetics in good control does not differ from the normal individual, although endurance may be less.[18] Several theories related to oxygen delivery have been proposed to account for this.[19–21]

In diabetics under only fair glycemic control, the adaptation to muscle work parallels the normal person. However, the conversion from resting to working metabolism occurs more rapidly in the diabetic as a result of higher basal circulating levels of free fatty acids[22] and circulating gluconeogenic substrates. At rest, alanine flux from muscle is 2 times greater in the diabetic with fair control than in the nondiabetic.

Clinically it is recognized that exercise in poorly controlled diabetics can lead to increased blood glucose and ketoacids,[23] even precipitating diabetic coma in some cases.[24,25] Wahren and colleagues reported that short-term exercise in hyperglycemic patients (i.e., blood glucose greater than 350 mg/dl) may have an intensifying rather than an ameliorating effect upon the diabetic state.[26] Moxness et al. observed no rise in ketones in normal and pancreatectomized dogs after moderately severe exercise when the initial blood glucose levels were below 400 mg/dl,[27] but hyperglycemia resulted when the resting glucose levels were above 400 mg/dl.[28-32] Others have found a small rise in glucose in diabetics with only fair control whose blood glucose levels at rest averaged 332 mg/dl. This was accompanied by increased plasma glucagon and cortisol levels and an exacerbation of ketosis. In the untreated diabetic, the liver is already metabolically prepared for gluconeogenesis. Thus, plasma glucose can increase in early exercise as the result of hepatic gluconeogenic capability, coupled with decreased assimilation and inhibition of glycolysis by intracellular acidosis,[33] as well as lactate oxidation by acetoacetate[34] and by free fatty acids.

In the untreated insulin-dependent diabetic, the metabolic adaptation to exercise is exaggerated; there is an overproduction of free fatty acids from adipocyte lipolysis that is not seen in the noninsulin-dependent diabetic[35] or in the diabetic adequately treated with insulin.[36] The overproduction of ketoacids with strenuous exercise in poorly controlled diabetes may also be related to excess catecholamine release.[37] In contrast, exercise in the well-controlled patient can result in decreased ketone production.[38]

CHANGES IN INSULIN AND COUNTERREGULATORY HORMONES IN NORMAL INDIVIDUALS AND DIABETICS

Deviation from the desired steady state with respect to glucose, results not from response of diabetic muscle to exercise, but from deviations from the norm of counterregulatory hormones. All organisms strive to maintain blood glucose in a narrow physiologic range. During exercise, when glucose utilization is increased, hormonal adjustments occur which enhance glucose production. These changes maintain the balance between glucose utilization and production, despite alterations in energy expenditure. Insulin, catecholamines, glucagon, growth hormone and cortisol affect glucose homeostasis in response to exercise.

Insulin

Insulin appears to be the predominant hormone influencing the regulation of metabolic fuel availability in man. Working muscle is more sensitive to insulin action than is muscle at rest, resulting in a greater assimilation of glucose per unit of insulin during exercise.[39] This increased sensitivity of muscle to insulin occurs even with mild exercise[40-42] and the effect lasts beyond the active exercise period.[43]

Numerous factors have been postulated[44] to explain the responsiveness of muscle to insulin during exercise. By increasing blood flow, muscular work may increase the size of the perfused capillary bed and the available number of insulin receptors.[45] Noninsulin hormonal factors in blood and lymph, which increase glucose utilization, have been proposed.[46,47] Other nonhormonal factors have also been suggested as active at the cellular level.[48]

Counterbalancing this increased sensitivity to insulin or insulin-like factors is a concomitant decrease in the production of pancreatic insulin in both normal and noninsulin-dependent diabetic persons during exercise.[43,49-51] Following exercise programs which lead to increased endurance fitness, there is a decreased response of insulin production to carbohydrate loads[52-55] in normal subjects. The resultant decline of plasma insulin levels facilitates glucose homeostasis during exercise because low insulin levels promote glycogenolysis,[55] gluconeogenesis and lipolysis.[56,57] In the insulin-dependent diabetic, plasma insulin levels do not decrease during exercise and on occasion may increase, depending on absorption from depot sites.

Catecholamines

Release of catecholamines is a normal response to stress. Strenuous exercise (75% of VO_2 max*) results in increased levels of circulating catecholamines,[58] particularly norepinephrine. Secretion of norepinephrine or epinephrine is proportional to the amount of work performed. Mild exercise of less than 50% VO_2 max. does not cause an increase of norepinephrine or epinephrine, whereas working at 98% VO_2 max. doubles norepinephrine levels and

---

*VO_2 max is the maximal level of oxygen consumption above normal and is directly related to the quantity of work done.

has a slight effect on epinephrine levels.[13,14,37] The potential effect of rising norepinephrine levels on maintenance of metabolic fuel supply is significant because norepinephrine inhibits insulin secretion,[59] while at the same time it stimulates glucagon[60,61] and growth hormone secretion.[62,63] In addition, norepinephrine enhances lipolysis and glycogenolysis.

Catecholamine secretion in diabetics is variable in response to muscular work, depending on the degree of metabolic control of diabetes and possibly on the presence of microangiopathy or autonomic neuropathy. Insulin-dependent diabetics who are well controlled have a normal increment of catecholamine release when exercised.[64] In uncontrolled ketotic diabetics, however, norepinephrine release can increase dramatically. Eight-hundredfold increases have been reported.[64] The abnormal increases of systolic pressure[65] and heart rate seen in some diabetics may be explained in part by this superphysiologic response. The abnormally elevated catechol secretion is modified in diabetics under certain conditions. The presence of clinical microangiopathy is associated with a blunted response of catechol secretion to exercise.[66] Physical training also modifies norepinephrine release in response to exercise.

Glucagon

In normal individuals, pancreatic glucagon secretion increases minimally during moderate exercise,[67-69] but increases significantly during strenuous exercise. Diabetics exhibit a similar pattern of glucagon release.[70]

Growth Hormone

Changes in circulating growth hormone with muscular work is a well recognized phenomenon,[13,71,72] which can be blunted by the infusion of glucose during the exercise period.[62] In both the insulin-dependent and noninsulin-dependent diabetic, there is a higher than normal growth hormone secretion with exercise,[63,73-75] which can be reduced by adequate insulin therapy.[76] Growth hormone release during strenuous exercise may also be modulated by catecholamines, with the effect of further enhancing the availability of free fatty acids for muscle metabolism.

Cortisol, Thyroxine, Testosterone

Plasma cortisol levels increase minimally with strenuous exercise in both normal individuals and diabetic patients under treatment. However, poor control of diabetes results in an increased cortisol response with exercise.[13,28] No changes take place in the thyroid hormones, triiodothyronine, reverse triiodothyronine and thyroxine,[28] when exercise is undertaken. In the diabetic, a higher than normal secretion of testosterone occurs after exercise,[28] although the significance of this is unknown.

EFFECT OF PHYSICAL FITNESS ON GLUCOSE TOLERANCE

Physical activity or inactivity has a profound effect on the body's ability to handle a carbohydrate load. Nondiabetic patients, when placed at bed rest, have impaired glucose tolerance[77] which is unrelated to changes of body weight, although it may reflect changes in the ratio of body fat to lean body mass. Contrariwise, endurance training can exert a positive influence on the disposal of a glucose load. In well-trained, middle-aged, nondiabetic men[78] and in maturity-onset diabetics following endurance training, a lower blood glucose value at all points during an oral glucose tolerance test was found as compared to controls.

In the person with noninsulin-dependent diabetes, the utilization of glucose by peripheral tissues is enhanced if exercise is taken after 50 g of glucose orally.[79] Although a few reports have indicated a worsening of glucose tolerance with exercise,[80-82] this effect is observed only after acute short-term exercise, as opposed to regular progams of physical activity that result in an increased physical fitness of the patient. Benefit can be gained from mild exercise (30 to 40% VO_2 max),[83,84] and glucose tolerance uniformly improves with moderate physical activity (greater than 50% VO_2 max).[85]

Glucose intolerance related to obesity, has been shown to diminish with exercise, regardless of whether or not changes in total body weight occur.[10,11] The obese diabetic patient has an excess of circulating insulin,[86,87] but demonstrates resistance to the insulin by peripheral tissues. Regular physical activity reduces the insulin resistance and results in lower levels of circulating insulin.[43] Bjorntorp et al.[54] showed that after an 8-week period of training, insulin levels during an oral glucose tolerance test were lower in obese subjects by about one-half. Leon and co-workers[52] reported that following a 16-week vigorous walking program, decreased insulin:glucose ratios were observed in obese young men at 2 hours after a glucose load. These data suggest that physical training increases sensitivity to insulin, and that regular exercise would help delay or prevent the emergence of maturity-onset diabetes, or correct glucose intolerance in obese patients.

A mechanism that influences both glucose uptake and insulin sensitivity at the cell surface has been suggested. It has been reported that after a 6-week period of bicycle training, insulin binding to monocyte receptor sites was increased, thereby allowing greater insulin-mediated glucose uptake which in turn promoted oxidation of glucose and its glycolytic products.[88] Costill and co-workers[8] have shown that in insulin-dependent diabetics and in normal controls, the activity of several skeletal muscle enzymes, commonly considered markers of carbohydrate and lipid oxidation, was elevated at the conclusion of a 10-week exercise program. In addition, the phenomenon of increased glycogen and utilization storage,[23] during and after physical activity, influences glucose metabolism so that there is enhanced glucose uptake associated with endurance exercise.[27] Taken together, these data clearly suggest that endurance exercise has the potential of influencing fuel utilization in both the juvenile and maturity-onset diabetic in conjunction with insulin or diet therapy.

THE EXERCISE PROGRAM

Introduction to Exercise Prescription

Endurance exercise can be prescribed for the diabetic patient in the same manner as diet and insulin. It is possible to quantify the amount of exercise that a patient is capable of handling, and then to suggest a plan to reach the individual's optimal fitness level. To quantify endurance exercise, 4 important factors must be considered.[105] These are (1) the type or mode of activity, (2) the duration of each training session, (3) the frequency of the training sessions, and (4) the intensity of the training during each workout.

The human body adapts to two types of training: (1) endurance and (2) strength.[90] *Endurance training* is characterized by exercise that requires great expenditures of energy. It stimulates the cardiorespiratory system by utilizing a large portion of the skeletal muscle mass for at least 15 minutes per exercise session. Certain physical activities, which have the potential to use large amounts of energy, are shown in Table 22–2. *Strength training,* on the

other hand, is characterized by exercise such as weight-lifting, which applies heavy resistance to specific muscle groups. It is important to note that most physicians and physiologists regard endurance exercise as the more appropriate type of activity for adults because of the stress that is placed upon the cardiovascular and metabolic systems. Consequently, because of the frequency of cardiovascular disease in diabetes[95,99,100] and the necessity to control hyperglycemia and to assure normal lipid metabolism,[101,102] it is logical that endurance exercise constitutes the major portion of any training program for a diabetic. However, attention should be given also to exercises that promote muscular strength, endurance, and flexibility and enhance musculoskeletal development.

The Evaluation of Patients for Entry into an Endurance Fitness Program

Prior to embarking upon any exercise program, the patient must undergo a thorough physical examination. This is important at any age. The medical assessment should include a personal medical history, urine and blood studies, resting electrocardiogram (ECG), and eye and nerve evaluation. As shown in Table 22–3, the patient may then be classified as asymptomatic or symptomatic (e.g., as having uncontrolled diabetes, significant retinopathy, neuropathy, nephropathy, ischemic heart disease, or peripheral vascular disease, etc.) The symptomatic patient must be evaluated further prior to the exercise prescription. If the disease condition is related to the complications of long-term diabetes, the physician must decide whether that patient should start an exercise program or wait until the abnormality is corrected. An exercise ECG must be included in the battery of additional tests[103,104] if the decision is made to start the exercise program. In fact, any patient with complications of diabetes must be closely evaluated and monitored during the exercise training sessions by taking pulse, blood pressure, and ECG recordings.

Table 22–2. Physical Activities Beneficial to Patients with Diabetes

Individual Activities		Team Sports
Walking	Badminton	Soccer
Running—jogging	Golf	Basketball
Bicycling (incl. stationary)	Wrestling	Volleyball
Swimming	Fencing	Hockey (ice and field)
Dancing	Stair climbing	Lacrosse
Rope skipping	Calisthenics	
Skiing (downhill and	Tennis	
cross-country)	Handball	
Rowing	Squash	
Skating	Racquetball	

Any of the physical activities listed above can be used in an exercise program which will be beneficial to the diabetic. These activities have been selected because they place a high energy demand upon the body. How hard these activities are played should be regulated by the appropriate percent of the maximal heart rate for a given fitness level. The heart rate should be monitored periodically.

Table 22–3.   Evaluation for Entry into an Endurance Fitness Program

Resting screening: medical history, physical examination, evaluation of control of diabetes (DM), relevant urine and blood studies, clinical evaluation of function of heart, kidneys, eyes, nervous system, and peripheral circulation

Cardiovascular status	Age	Duration of DM	Exercise ECG needed
Asymptomatic	< 30 yrs	< 20 yrs	No
	20–30 yrs	> 20 yrs	Advisable
	31–45 yrs	Any duration	Advisable
	> 45 yrs	Any duration	Recommended
Symptomatic	All ages	Any duration	Yes

The safest approach is to assign those patients with vascular complications to a cardiac rehabilitation program. Many hospitals, YMCAs, and universities conduct such programs under the supervision of trained medical personnel.

If the initial evaluation at rest reveals no metabolic or cardiovascular problems, and if the patient is under 30 years of age with fewer than 15 years of diabetes, the physician may allow the patient to start immediately with the endurance program without an exercise stress test. Recent exercise stress testing with ECG monitoring was carried out at the Joslin Research Laboratory of 60 healthy insulin-dependent diabetic patients between the ages of 18 and 30 years, with fewer than 20 years of diabetes. These studies showed no significant S-T segment depressions (an indicator of cardiac ischemia) or unusual arrthythmias which could contraindicate participation in a moderate endurance exercise program (unpublished data). However, for patients from 20 to 30 years of age with 20 years or more of diabetes, and for patients between 31 and 45 years of age, an exercise stress test is highly advisable prior to writing the exercise prescription. For any patient over 45 years of age, the exercise stress test should be mandatory before the exercise prescription is written, regardless of the duration of diabetes.

In addition to the medical screening, the physician should make an assessment of the patient's endurance fitness capacity if the exercise prescription is to be individualized. The best single index of endurance fitness capacity is the measurement of maximal oxygen uptake[89,93,97] which reflects the effectiveness of the transport of oxygen and its utilization at the tissue level[94] (See Table 22–4). Although the laboratory measurement of maximal oxygen uptake is the most precise, some field methods that are less demanding in terms of time, equipment, and personnel can easily evaluate large groups of healthy diabetics with good precision. These techniques include the use of a stationary bicycle ergometer,[106,107] treadmill,[104] or performance tests such as swimming, bicycling, or running.[108] The estimation of maximal oxygen consumption may be determined during the exercise

Table 22–4.   Criteria for Establishing Endurance Fitness Levels Based upon Maximal Oxygen Consumption

Endurance Fitness Level	VO_2 max (ml/kg/min)
Very low	< 30
Low	30–36
Moderate	36–42
High	42–50
Athlete	> 50

stress test, either directly in laboratories with oxygen and carbon dioxide gas analyzers, or indirectly by using the well-known relationship between heart rate and oxygen consumption.[106]

A less precise method, but in many ways the most appropriate, is simply to have the patient exercise moderately with the activity that will be used for training. For example, if the patient should select walking as the training mode, then a comfortable walk would be undertaken, and a notation made of the time and distance. The strategy then is for the patient to increase gradually the speed and/or distance throughout the training period.

The Quantification of Endurance Exercise

Mode of Training. The mode of training is important and must include only high-energy-cost activities. These activities should require at least 5 to 7 times more energy than the resting energy expenditure to have beneficial effects in terms of diabetes control.[67] The high-energy-cost physical activities listed in Table 22–2 have the potential to increase energy expenditure to proper levels. Although not included, some work activities may be used as substitutes for those listed. Wood cutting and splitting, digging, lawn mowing, and farming if done at the proper intensity and continued for an appropriate duration, may be added to the list of high-energy-cost exercise.

Because of weather variations, several different fitness training activities may be necessary in a northern climate. The mode of training during the winter months may be outdoor activities such as cross-country skiing, downhill skiing, and indoor sports like racquetball, handball, basketball, or swimming, and exercise such as rope-skipping or pedaling a stationary ergometer. During warmer weather, jogging, hiking, tennis, or golf played without use of a cart, may be used as the training activity.

Duration and Frequency. The duration and frequency of the activity sessions are dependent upon the patient's age, time availability, and level of endurance fitness. A young athlete can handle safely 2 hours of hard training, 6 to 7 days per week. Most adults, however, have time constraints; consequently, the physician should suggest a more realistic time commitment.

Several exercise training studies have reported significant gains in aerobic capacity with training sessions of 15 to 30 minutes, 3 times per week, at an intensity of 60 to 90% of the maximal age-adjusted heart rate.[89] Training sessions of 45 minutes, 5 times per week, were associated with muscle and joint soreness, as well as a large dropout rate. It has been suggested[91] that a workout time of 15 to 30 minutes 3 times per week is the minimal commitment to endurance exercise training in order to produce health and fitness benefits. Persons with poor fitness levels should increase exercise to 5 to 7 days per week, but the duration of the training sessions must be reduced to 5 to 10 minutes at the start.

Intensity. The intensity of the exercise should be controlled by monitoring the heart and other signs of stress (Table 22–5). There is a well-known relationship between heart rate and oxygen consumption because, to improve endurance fitness, the patient must work at a specific percentage of the maximal oxygen uptake. The patient should use the pulse at the carotid artery or at the temple, or simply place his hand on his chest. To obtain a fairly accurate exercise heart rate, a 10-second count is taken starting within 5 seconds from the time the activity has ended.[105] Multiplying this find-

ing by 6 will yield the minute rate. This technique for monitoring heart rate is invalid in persons with cardiac neuropathy or patients who are on adrenergic blocking agents with a low maximal heart rate. In addition, during endurance exercise the heart rate of diabetic subjects was found to be 15 to 30 beats/minute higher at the same percentage of the maximal oxygen consumption when compared to nondiabetic subjects.[64,109] It has been suggested that this is related to the extraordinary rise in catecholamines, which has been noted in diabetic patients both at rest and during exercise.[64] The overestimation of heart rate would reduce the exercise intensity resulting in safer exercise, particularly for the less fit, poorly controlled diabetic.

Aside from heart rate, the patient, exercise leader, or exercise partner should watch for the usual signs of overstress such as labored breathing, facial pallor, and/or light-headedness. Exercise should be enjoyable and performed at a comfortable rate well within the patient's tolerance. An exercise intensity as low as 60% of the age-adjusted maximum heart rate can result in beneficial effects for the diabetic patient. This would give a heart rate of approximately 110 beats/minute for a 35-year-old.

Table 22–5 suggests a percentage of the age-adjusted maximum heart rate for training according to fitness category. For example, a 40-year-old in the low endurance fitness category may exercise at 60 to 70% of the maximum heart rate. The rate of fitness improvement must be carefully controlled based on the patient's age, health, starting level of fitness, adaptability to exercise stress, and the impact upon diabetic control. Consequently the 40-year-old mentioned above may be able to increase the intensity of exercise progressively to 70 to 80% of the maximal age-adjusted heart rate (127 to 146 beats per minute). There is little need for the adult exerciser to increase the intensity of the training

Table 22–5. Exercise Heart Rate by Age

Age	Predicted Maximal Heart Rate	90% max	85% max	80% max	75% max	70% max	65% max	60% max
15	193	174	164	154	145	135	125	116
20	191	172	162	153	143	134	124	115
25	189	170	161	151	142	133	123	113
30	186	167	158	149	140	130	121	111
35	184	166	156	147	138	129	120	110
40	182	164	155	146	137	127	118	109
45	180	162	153	144	135	126	117	108
50	178	160	151	142	134	125	116	107
55	175	158	149	140	131	123	114	105
60	173	156	147	138	130	121	112	104
65	171	154	145	137	128	120	111	103

Age-adjusted heart rates and the percentage of the maximal rates are shown above. For example, a 50-year-old Type II diabetic with low levels of endurance fitness should train at 60–70% of the maximal age-adjusted heart rate, 107–125 beats per minute.

beyond this level. Training at 90% of the maximal heart rate must be reserved for athletes.

In terms of intensity, it is important to "train, but not to strain." Patients should be counseled to "listen" to their bodies. They should reduce the exercise rate when the training becomes uncomfortable.

In summary, the development and maintenance of cardiovascular fitness require a frequency of training of 3 to 5 days per week of 15 to 60 minutes of continuous high energy expenditure activity per training session, at an intensity of 60 to 90% of the age-adjusted maximum heart rate.

The Exercise Prescription. Patients who are just starting an endurance training program need precise exercise goals, such as how long, how frequent, and how intense an exercise session should be. To provide that kind of guidance, Tables 22–2, 5, and 6 together illustrate a suggested program that is distributed to patients who attend an optional lecture given weekly at the Joslin Diabetes Center. The plan is essentially adopted from the American College of Sports Medicine position statement for prescribing exercise in healthy adults.[91] We suggest any of the activities shown in Table 22–1 as the mode of exercise with a great emphasis upon walking, for a number of reasons. First, walking is an efficient activity that involves little cost or equipment. Second, walking is basically a safe activity in terms of intensity in healthy adults. Table 22–6 suggests the number of sessions per week, the duration of each activity session, and the total minutes of exercise per week. The prescription is based on time of exercise. Only exercise that is of a proper intensity is included within the total time per day or per week. Patients may shift into a higher fitness level when they comfortably achieve the required total time per week for a given fitness category. We suggest that the moderate fitness level is a realistic goal for most diabetic patients without vascular disease. The program requires about 3 hours per week of endurance exercise at the appropriate intensity.

When choosing a specific exercise activity for the diabetic, considerations must be given to concomitant diabetic complications. Patients with peripheral vascular disease associated with thin, easily abraded skin, or those with prior amputation secondary to vascular disease, should not undertake activities which traumatize the feet such as vigorous walking, jogging or tennis.

An open lesion of the foot would be a contraindication to any walking program. Caution must also be used in activities which could result in trauma to the feet in patients with peripheral neuropathy or a history of neuropathic ulcers. In addition, foot abnormalities such as corns, calluses, ingrown toenails, digital deformities (hammer toes, bunions) should be treated by a competent podiatrist prior to engaging in a walking program. In some cases, special footwear will be required.

The existence of background retinopathy should not prevent participation in a routine endurance training program. However, in the presence of proliferative retinopathy, or for 3 weeks following laser therapy, strenuous physical activities should be avoided, particularly those involving increased intra-abdominal pressure or Valsalva-like maneuvers,[110] such as weight-lifting or sprinting. During the immediate period following laser therapy, these patients should be restricted from activities such as lifting objects weighing more than 5 pounds and contact sports.

ADJUSTMENT OF TREATMENT REGIMEN WITH EXERCISE

The Maturity-Onset Diabetic

It has been suggested that endurance training may provide the greatest potential benefits to maturity-onset diabetics and obese patients, because exercise decreases insulin resistance and glucose intolerance.[7,102] In some patients, the dose of oral agents must be reduced or the diet adjusted when an exercise program is undertaken. It should always be kept in mind that oral hypoglycemic agents can produce clinical hypoglycemia under certain conditions.

The Insulin-Dependent Diabetic

Insulin dependency should never be considered a contraindication to involvement in physical ac-

Table 22–6. The Exercise Prescription

Fitness level	Time/Week (Minutes)†	Frequency (Sessions/Week)	Duration (Min./Session)	Intensity* (% Max HR)
Very low	40–80	4–6	10–20	60
Low	90–120	4–6	15–30	60–70
Moderate	120–180	3–5	30–45	70–80
High	180–300	3–5	30–60	70–80
Athlete	300–840	5–7	60–120	70–90

*See the Exercise Intensity Table (Table 5).
†Exercise time should include only those periods when the body is in motion at the required intensity.

tivities. Exercise in the insulin-dependent diabetic improves overall control of blood glucose, minimizes blood glucose excursions and leads to higher self-esteem. Diabetic children have been shown to do less well in motor performance parameters such as speed, agility, and power, than their nondiabetic counterparts.[111,112] Although equal work capacity has been demonstrated in other studies,[113] poor performance on physical fitness tests may be the result of lack of participation in sports because of overprotective parents. At the Joslin Clinic, and at summer and holiday camps for diabetics, children are encouraged to participate in any sport up to the level of their ability.

The importance of educating the patient and the family cannot be overemphasized because no single diet formula and insulin dose can be applied. In order to avoid hypoglycemic reactions, the diabetic must make adjustments to diet and insulin according to the patient's own response to physical exertion. The increased utilization of glucose in response to exercise is balanced by increased production of glucose, which is induced by changes in the regulatory hormones. Hypoglycemia occurs when glucose production fails to keep pace with glucose utilization and is not compensated for by ingestion of carbohydrate.

For patients near or at ideal body weight, no change in insulin dose will be needed for sporadic, moderate exercise of short duration (i.e., less than 30 minutes) once the initial adjustments to exercise training are made. However, for exercise of this intensity and duration, the diabetic may need a 25–30 g carbohydrate snack. This should be in the form of readily assimilated carbohydrate, such as fruit or a bread exchange.

For exercise of one to two hours' duration, such as hiking, bicycling, or skiing, added snacks before and during exercise are indicated at periodic (60 minute) intervals. It is recommended that these snacks contain both carbohydrate and protein. An additional 25 to 50 g carbohydrate snack is occasionally necessary after vigorous exercise to prevent hypoglycemia.

Prolonged exercise, as might be encountered while hiking or skiing all day, requires an increase in the number and quantity of meals, and a decrease in insulin dose. Backpacking, for example, requires an estimated intake of 5,000–6,000 calories per day.[114] In this situation the patient should decrease insulin initially by 25% of the usual dose. On prolonged wilderness expeditions, diabetic boys decreased their insulin requirement by 50%.[115]

A program of graded physical exercise leading to increased physical fitness necessitates a gradual adjustment of insulin, usually within the first 2 weeks. In a study of 100 diabetics, ages 17 to 62,

who were active runners and joggers, the average decrease in the daily insulin dose was 17 units.[116]

The overweight diabetic who participates in a physical exercise program for purposes of weight reduction will need to decrease the insulin dose on days of increased activity in order to avoid an added caloric intake, which would be counterproductive.

The site of insulin injection may also be an important factor in precipitation of hypoglycemia during exercise. During moderate (50% VO_2 max.) exercise in the insulin-dependent diabetic, no change in blood glucose occurs if insulin is given by intravenous infusion.[117] However, if insulin is given subcutaneously into an exercising limb, its absorption will be increased as compared to that when given into a relatively inactive area. This can result in suppression of hepatic glycogenolysis and gluconeogenesis[87,118–122] leading to hypoglycemia. Juvenile diabetics prone to insulin reactions should take insulin over the abdomen or flanks while exercising.

SUMMARY

Because the diabetic is more inclined to vascular complications, a careful screening procedure prior to the exercise program is critical. The organization of exercise training for the adult diabetic should include two distinct programs: (1) the adult fitness program for the diabetic *without* vascular complications, and (2) a cardiac rehabilitation program for diabetics *with* vascular complications. Important considerations for the insulin-dependent diabetic, prior to and during exercise, include the time of day, the injection site used, the feeding schedule, and the state of metabolic control. An endurance training program may be a valuable adjunct to the therapy regimen for the noninsulin-dependent diabetic since only a minor modification of the metabolism is required for normalization. Several disturbances of the cardiovascular system are noted with diabetes such as an elevated heart rate, decreased oxygen transport, reduced peripheral blood flow, and a reduced potential for achieving maximal oxygen consumption. The exercise program for the healthy diabetic is planned in the same manner as for any healthy adult. When taken together, hopefully the benefits of regular endurance exercise would include cost-effectiveness in terms of fewer sick days and fewer long-term vascular complications.

REFERENCES

1. Larsson, Y., Sterky, G., Persson, B., Thoren, C.: Effect of exercise on blood lipids in juvenile diabetes. Lancet *1*:350, 1964.
2. Wertz, S.H., Eagleson, H.M.: The effect of exercise therapy on blood sugar and cholesterol levels. J. Assoc. Phys. Ment. Rehab. *20*:46, 1966.

3. Wood, P.D., Haskell, W.L., Stern, W.P., et al.: Plasma lipoprotein distributions in male and female runners. Ann. N.Y. Acad. Sci. 30:748, 1977.

4. Wallin, C.C., Schendel, J.: Physiological changes in middle-aged men following a ten-week jogging program. Res. Q. Am. Assoc. Health Phys. Educ. 40:600, 1969.

5. LeBlanc, J., Nadeau, A., Boulay, M., Rousseau-Migneron, S.: Effects of physical training and adiposity on glucose metabolism and ^{125}I-insulin binding. J. Appl. Physiol. 46:235, 1979.

6. Koivisto, V.A., Soman, V., Conrad, P., et al.: Insulin binding to monocytes in trained athletes: changes in the resting state and after exercise. J. Clin. Invest. 64:1011, 1979.

7. Saltin, B., Lindgärde, F., Houston, M., et al.: Physical training and glucose tolerance in middle-aged men with chemical diabetes. Diabetes 28 (Suppl):30, 1979.

8. Costill, D.L., Cleary, P., Fink, W.J., Foster, C., et al.: Training adaptations in skeletal muscle of juvenile diabetics. Diabetes 28:818, 1979.

9. Maehlum, S., Høstmark, A.T., Hermansen, L.: Synthesis of muscle glycogen during recovery after prolonged severe exercise in diabetic subjects. Effect of insulin deprivation. Scand. J. Clin. Invest. 38:35, 1978.

9a. Wallberg-Henriksson, H., Gunnarsson, R., Henriksson, J., et al.: Increased peripheral insulin sensitivity and muscle mitochondrial enzymes but unchanged blood glucose control in Type I diabetics after physical training. Diabetes 31:1044, 1982.

10. Holm, G., Björntorp, P., Jagenburg, R.: Carbohydrate, lipid and amino acid metabolism following physical exercise in man. J. Appl. Physiol. 45:128, 1978.

11. Holm, G., Sullivan, L., Jagenburg, R., Björntorp, P.: Effects of physical training and lean body mass on plasma amino acids in man. J. Appl. Physiol. 45:177, 1978.

12. Costill, D.L., Coyle, E., Dalsky, G., et al.: Effects of elevated plasma FFA and insulin on muscle glycogen usage during exercise. J. Appl. Physiol. 43:695, 1977.

12a. Newsholme, E.A.: The control of fuel utilization by muscle during exercise and starvation. Diabetes 28(Suppl. 1):1, 1979.

13. Hartley, L.H., Mason, J.W., Hogan, R.P., et al.: Multiple hormonal responses to prolonged exercise in relation to physical training. J. Appl. Physiol. 33:607, 1972.

14. Hartley, L.H., Mason, J.W., Hogan, R.P., et al.: Multiple hormonal responses to graded exercise in relation to physical training. J. Appl. Physiol. 33:602, 1972.

15. Maehlum, S.: Muscle glycogen synthesis after a glucose infusion during post-exercise recovery in diabetic and non-diabetic subjects. Scand. J. Clin. Lab. Invest. 38:349, 1978.

16. Maehlum, S., Høstmark, A.T., Hermansen, L.: Synthesis of muscle glycogen during recovery after prolonged severe exercise in diabetic and non-diabetic subjects. Scand. J. Clin. Lab. Invest. 37:309, 1977.

17. Maehlum, S., Felig, P., Wahren, J.: Splanchnic glucose and muscle glycogen metabolism after glucose feeding during postexercise recovery. Am. J. Physiol. 235:E255, 1978.

18. Pruett, E.D.R., Maehlum, S.: Muscular exercise and metabolism in male juvenile diabetics. I. Energy metabolism during exercise. Scand. J. Clin. Lab. Invest. 32:139, 1973.

18a. Calles, J., Cunningham, J.I., Nelson, L., et al.: Glucose turnover during recovery from intensive exercise. Diabetes 32:734, 1983.

18b. Gaesser, G.A., Brooks, G.A.: Metabolic basis of excess post-exercise oxygen consumption: a review. Med. Sci. Sports Exerc. 16:29, 1984.

18c. Krzentowski, G., Pirnay, F., Pallikarakis, N., et al.: Glucose utilization during exercise in normal and diabetic subjects: the role of insulin. Diabetes 30:983, 1981.

19. Helmreich, E., Cori, C.F.: Studies of tissue permeability. II. The distribution of pentoses between plasma and muscle. J. Biol. Chem. 224:663, 1957.

20. Bergman, H., Björntorp, P., Conradson, T-B., et al.: Enzymatic and circulatory adjustments to physical training in middle-aged men. Eur. J. Clin. Invest. 3:414, 1973.

21. Roch-Norlund, A.E.: Muscle glycogen synthetase in patients with diabetes mellitus. Basal values, effect of glycogen depletion by exercise, and effect of treatment. Scand. J. Clin. Lab. Invest. 29:237, 1972.

22. Arvidson, G., Carlstrom, S.: Studies on fatty acid metabolism in diabetics during exercise. 3. Individual plasma-free fatty acids in newly diagnosed juvenile diabetics during exercise. Acta. Med. Scand. 181:631, 1967.

23. Marble, A., Smith, R.M.: Exercise in diabetes mellitus. Arch. Int. Med. 58:577, 1936.

24. Barringer, T.B.: The effect of exercise upon the carbohydrate tolerance in diabetes. Am. J. Med. Sci. 151:181, 1916.

25. Lawrence, R.D.: The effect of exercise on insulin action in diabetes. Br. Med. J. 1:648, 1926.

26. Wahren, J.: Glucose turnover during exercise in healthy man and in patients with diabetes mellitus. Diabetes 28 (Suppl. 1):82, 1979.

27. Moxness, K.E., Molnar, G.D., McGuckin, W.F.: Exercise and blood glucose concentration in intact and pancreatectomized dogs. Diabetes 13:37, 1964.

28. Berchtold, P., Berger, M., Cüppers, H.J., et al.: Non-glucoregulatory hormones (T_4, T_3, rT_3, TSH, testosterone) during physical exercise in juvenile type diabetics. Horm. Metab. Res. 10:269, 1978.

29. Berger, M., Berchtold, P., Cüppers, H.J., et al.: Metabolic and hormonal effects of muscular exercise in juvenile type diabetics. Diabetologia 13:355, 1977.

30. Berger, M., Hagg, S., Ruderman, N.B.: Glucose metabolism in perfused skeletal muscle: Interaction of insulin and exercise on glucose uptake. Biochem. J. 146:231, 1975.

31. Richardson, R.: Factors determining the effect of exercise on blood sugar in the diabetic. J. Clin. Invest. 13:949, 1934.

32. Standl, E., Janka, H.-U., Dexel, T., Kolb, H.J.: Muscle metabolism during rest and exercise: Influence on the oxygen transport system in normal and diabetic subjects. Diabetes 25:914, 1976.

33. Vignati, L., Cahill, G.F.: Biochemical abnormalities produced by acid base disturbances. In: E.D. Robin (Ed.): The Extra-Pulmonary Manifestations of Respiratory Disease. New York, Marcel Dekker, 1978, pp. 345–361.

34. Berger, M., Hagg, S.A., Goodman, M.N., Ruderman, N.B.: Glucose metabolism in perfused skeletal muscle. Effects of starvation, diabetes, fatty acids, aceto-acetate, insulin and exercise on glucose uptake and disposition. Biochem. J. 158:191, 1976.

35. Carlstrom, S.: Studies on fatty acid metabolism in diabetics during exercise. V. Plasma concentration of free fatty acids and glycerol in newly-diagnosed adult diabetics during exercise. Acta. Med. Scand. 182:363, 1967.

36. Carlstrom, S., Studies on fatty acid metabolism in diabetics during exercise. VII. Plasma glycerol concentrations in juvenile diabetics during exercise before and after adequate insulin treatment. Acta. Med. Scand. 186:429, 1969.

37. Chin, A.K., Evonuk, E.: Changes in plasma catechol-

amine and corticosterone levels after muscular exercise. J. Appl. Physiol. *30*:205, 1971.

38. Sestoft, L., Trap-Jensen, J., Lyngsooe, J., et al.: Regulation of gluconeogenesis and ketogenesis during rest and exercise in diabetic subjects and normal men. Clin. Sci. Mol. Med. *53*:411, 1977.

39. Wahren, J., Felig, P., Ahlborg, G.A.: Glucose metabolism during leg exercise in man. J. Clin. Invest. *50*:2715, 1971.

40. Dorchy, H., Ego, F., Baran, D., Loeb, H.: Effect of exercise on glucose uptake in diabetic adolescents. Acta. Paediatr. Belg. *29*:83, 1976.

41. Dorchy, H., Nisct, G., Ooms, II., et al.: Study of the coefficient of glucose assimilation during muscular exercise in diabetic adolescents deprived of insulin. Diabete Metab. *3*:31, 1977.

42. Hunter, W.M., Sukkar, M.Y.: Changes in plasma insulin levels during muscular exercise. J. Physiol. *196*:110P, 1968.

43. Fahlen, M., Sternberg, J., Björntorp, P.: Insulin secretion in obesity after exercise. Diabetologia *8*:141, 1972.

44. Kalant, N., Leibovici, T., Rohan, I., McNeill, K.: Effect of exercise on glucose and insulin utilization in the forearm. Metabolism *27*:333, 1978.

45. Garratt, C.J., Butterfield, W.J.H., Abrams, M.E., et al.: Effect of exercise on peripheral uptake of I[131] iodo insulin and glucose in nondiabetics. Metabolism *21*:36, 1972.

46. Goldstein, M.S.: Humoral nature of hypoglycemia in muscular exercise. Am. J. Physiol. *20*:67, 1961. Diabetes *10*:232, 1961.

47. Cochran, B., Jr., Marbach, E.P., Poucher, R., et al.: Effect of acute muscular exercise on serum immunoreactive insulin concentration. Diabetes *15*:838, 1966.

48. Dulin, W.E., Clarke, J.J.: Studies concerning a possible humoral factor produced by working muscles. Its influence on glucose utilization. Diabetes *10*:289, 1961.

49. Björntorp, P., DeJounge, K., Sjöström, L., Sullivan, L.: The effect of physical training on insulin production in obesity. Metabolism *19*:631, 1970.

50. Vranic, M., Kawamori, R., Peks, S., et al.: The essentiality of insulin and the role of glucagon in regulating glucose utilization and production during strenuous exercise in dogs. J. Clin. Invest. *57*:245, 1976.

51. Nikkila, E.A., Taskinen, M.R., Miettinen, T.A., et al.: Effect of muscular exercise on insulin secretion. Diabetes *17*:209, 1968.

52. Leon, A.S., Conrad, J., Hunninghake, D.B., Serfass, R.: Effect of a vigorous walking program on body composition and carbohydrate and lipid metabolism of obese young men. Am. J. Clin. Nutr. *32*:1776, 1979.

53. Krotkiewski, M., Mandroukas, K., Sjöström, L., Sullivan, L., et al.: Effects of long-term physical training on body fat, metabolism and blood pressure in obesity. Metabolism *28*:650, 1979.

54. Björntörp, P., DeJounge, K., Sjöström, L., Sullivan, L.: The effect of physical training on insulin production in obesity. Metabolism, *19*:631, 1970.

55. Lohmann, D., Liebold, F., Heilmann, W., et al.: Diminished insulin response in highly trained athletes. Metabolism *27*:521, 1978.

56. Koivisto, V.A., Akerblom, H.K., Kiviluoto, M.K.: Metabolic and hormonal effects of exercise in the severely streptozotocin-diabetic rat. Diabetologia *10*:329, 1974.

57. Ahlborg, G., Felig, P., Hagenfeldt, L., et al.: Substrate turnover during prolonged exercise in man. Splanchnic and leg metabolism of glucose, free fatty acids, and amino acids. J. Clin. Invest. *53*:1080, 1974.

58. Kozlowski, S., Nazar, K., Taton, J., et al.: Plasma catecholamines during sustained isometric exercise in healthy subjects and patients with essential hypertension and diabetes mellitus. In: E. Usdin, R. Kvetnansky, I.J. Kopin (Eds.): Catechols and Stress. Oxford, Pergamon Press, 1976, pp. 531–37.

59. Wright, P.H., Malaisse, W.J.: Effects of epinephrine, stress and exercise on insulin secretion in the rat. Am. J. Physiol. *214*:1031, 1968.

60. Luyckx, A.S., Lefebvre, P.J.: Mechanism involved in the exercise-induced increase in glucagon secretion in rats. Diabetes *23*:81, 1974.

61. Harvey, W.D., Faloona, G.R., Unger, R.H.: The effect of adrenergic blockade on exercise-induced hyperglucagonemia. Endocrinology *94*:1254, 1974.

62. Hansen, A.P.: The effect of intravenous glucose infusion on the exercise-induced serum growth hormone rise in normals and juvenile diabetics. Scand. J. Clin. Lab. Invest. *28*:195, 1971.

63. Hansen, A.P.: The effect of adrenergic receptor blockade on exercise-induced serum growth hormone rise in normals and juvenile diabetics. J. Clin. Endocrinol. Metab. *33*:807, 1971.

64. Christensen, N.J.: Abnormally high plasma catecholamines at rest and during exercise in ketotic juvenile diabetics. Scand. J. Clin. Lab. Invest. *26*:343, 1970.

65. Langer, L., Bergentz, B.E., Bjure, J., Fagerberg, S.E.: The effect of exercise on hematocrit, plasma volume and viscosity in diabetes mellitus. Diabetologia *7*:29, 1971.

66. Nazar, K., Taton, J., Chwalbinska-Moneta, J., Brzezinska, A.: Adrenergic responses to sustained handgrip in patients with juvenile-onset-type diabetes mellitus. Clin. Sci. Mol. Med. *49*:39, 1975.

67. Vranic, M., Kawamori, R., Wrenshall, G.A.: The role of insulin and glucagon in regulating glucose turnover in dogs during exercise. Med. Sci. Sports *7*:27, 1975.

68. Bottger, I., Schlein, E.M., Faloona, G.R., et al.: The effect of exercise on glucagon secretion. J. Clin. Endocrinol. Metab. *35*:117, 1972.

69. Felig, P., Wahren, T., Hendler, R., Ahlborg, G.: Plasma glucagon levels in exercising man. N. Engl. J. Med. *287*:184, 1972.

70. Garlaschi, G., di Natale, B., del Guercio, M.J., et al.: Effect of physical exercise on secretion of growth hormone, glucagon and cortisol in obese and diabetic children. Diabetes *24*:758, 1975.

71. Federspil, G., Udeschini, G., DePalo, C., Sicolo, N.: Role of growth hormone in lipid mobilization stimulated by prolonged muscular exercise in the rat. Horm. Metab. Res. *7*:484, 1975.

72. Schalch, D.S.: The influence of physical stress and exercise on growth hormone and insulin secretion in man. J. Lab. Clin. Med. *69*:256, 1967.

73. Passa, A., Gauville, C., Canivet, J.: Influence of muscular exercise on plasma level of growth hormone in diabetics with and without retinopathy. Lancet *2*:72, 1974.

74. Hansen, A.P.: Abnormal serum growth hormone response to exercise in maturity-onset diabetics. Diabetes *22*:619, 1973.

75. Hansen, A.P.: Abnormal serum growth hormone response to exercise in juvenile diabetics. J. Clin. Invest. *49*:1467, 1970.

76. Tchobroutsky, G., Lenormand, M-E., Michel, G., Assan, R.: Lack of post prandial exercise-induced growth hormone secretion in normoglycemic, insulin-treated diabetic men. Horm. Metab. Res. *6*:184, 1974.

77. Lipman, R.L., Raskin, P., Love, T., et al.: Glucose intolerance during decreased physical activity in man. Diabetes *21*:101, 1972.

78. Björntorp, P., Fahlén, M., Grimby, G., et al.: Carbo-

hydrate and lipid metabolism in middle-aged, physically well-trained men. Metabolism 21:1037, 1972.

79. Whichelow, M.J., Butterfield, W.J.H., Abrams, M.E., et al.: The effect of mild exercise on glucose uptake in human forearm tissues in the fasting state and after oral glucose administration. Metabolism 17:84, 1968.

80. Davidson, P.C., Shane, S.R., Albrink, M.K.: Decreased glucose tolerance following a physical conditioning program. Circulation 34:Suppl. III-7, 1966.

81. Dieterle, P., Bachl, I., Bachl, G., et al.: Muscle metabolism during exercise in diabetics and in obese during starvation. Horm. Metab. Res. 10:263, 1978.

82. Montoye, H.J., Block, W.D., Metzner, H., Keller, J.B.: Habitual physical activity and glucose tolerance. Males age 16–64 in a total community. Diabetes 26:172, 1976.

83. Klachko, D.M., Lie, T.H., Cunningham, E.J., et al.: Blood glucose levels during walking in normal and diabetic subjects. Diabetes 21:89, 1972.

84. Zinman, B., Murray, F.T., Vranic, M., et al.: Glucoregulation during moderate exercise in insulin-treated diabetics. J. Clin. Endocrinol. Metab. 45:641, 1977.

85. Maehlum, S., Pruett, E.D.: Muscular exercise and metabolism in male juvenile diabetics. II. Glucose tolerance after exercise. Scand. J. Clin. Lab. Invest. 32:149, 1973.

86. Kreisberg, R.A., Boshell, B.R., Di Placido, J., Roddam, R.F.: Insulin secretion in obesity. N. Engl. J. Med. 276:314, 1967.

87. Perley, M.J., Kipnis, D.M.: Plasma insulin responses to oral and intravenous glucose: studies in normal and diabetic subjects. J. Clin. Invest. 46:1954, 1967.

88. Soman, V.R., Koivisto, V.A., Deibert, D., et al.: Increased insulin sensitivity and insulin binding to monocytes after physical training. N. Engl. J. Med. 301:1200, 1979.

89. Pollock, M.L.: The quantification of endurance training programs. In: J.H. Wilmore (Ed.): Exercise and Sport Sciences Review. Vol. 1. New York, Academic Press, 1973, p. 155.

90. Edington, D.W., Edgerton, V.R.: The Biology of Physical Activity. Boston, Houghton Mifflin Co., 1976.

91. American College of Sports Medicine, Position Statement. The recommended quantity and quality of exercise for developing and maintaining fitness in healthy adults. Med. Sci. Sports 10:vii, 1978.

92. Barnard, R.J.: Long-term effects of exercise on cardiac function. In: J.H. Wilmore, J.F. Keough (Eds.): Science and Medicine in Sports. Vol. 3. New York, Academic Press, 1975, p. 113.

93. Clausen, J.P.: Effect of physical training on cardiovascular adjustments to exercise in man. Physiol. Rev. 57:779, 1977.

94. Holloszy, J.O.: Adaptation of skeletal muscle to endurance exercise. Med. Sci. Sports. 7:155, 1975.

95. McMillan, D.E.: Exercise and diabetic microangiopathy. Diabetes 28 (Suppl.):103, 1979.

96. Morganroth, J., Maron, B.J.: The athlete's heart syndrome: a new perspective. Ann. N.Y. Acad. Sci. 301:931, 1977.

97. Rowell, L.B.: Circulation. Med. Sci. Sports. 1:15, 1969.

98. Wahren, J., Felig, P., Hagenfeldt, L.: Physical exercise and fuel homeostasis in diabetes mellitus. Diabetologia 14:213, 1978.

99. Brownlee, M., Cahill, G.F., Jr.: Diabetic control and vascular complications. In: R. Paoletti and A.M. Gotto, Jr. (Eds.): Atherosclerosis Reviews. Vol. 4. New York, Raven Press, 1979, pp. 29–70.

100. Colwell, J.A., Halushka, P.V., Sarji, K.E., et al.: Vascular disease in diabetes. Arch. Intern. Med. 139:225, 1979.

101. Bennion, L.J., Grundy, S.M.: Effects of diabetes mellitus on cholesterol metabolism in man. N. Engl. J. Med. 296:1365, 1977.

102. Ruderman, N.B., Ganda, O.P., and Johansen, K.: The effect of physical training on glucose tolerance and plasma lipids in maturity-onset diabetes. Diabetes 28 (Suppl. 1):89, 1979.

103. Levitas, I.M., Kristal, J.J.: Exercise test valuable in spotting coronary disease in young diabetics. Medical Tribune. Jan. 26, 1972, p. 20.

104. Levitas, I.M., Kristal, J.J.: Stress exercise testing of the young diabetic for the detection of unknown coronary artery disease. Isr. J. Med. Sci. 8:845, 1972.

105. Pollack, M.L., Broida, J., Kendrick, Z.: Validity of the palpation technique of heart rate determination and its estimation of training heart rate. Res. Quart. 43:77, 1972.

106. Astrand, P.O.: Aerobic work capacity in men and women with special reference to age. Acta Physiol. Scand. 49 (Suppl. 169):1, 1960.

107. Edgren, B., Marklund, G., Nordesjo, L.O., Borg, G.: The validity of four bicycle ergometer tests. Med. Sci. Sports 8:179, 1976.

108. Cooper, K.H.: The Aerobics Way. New York, M. Evans & Co., 1977.

109. Wahren, J., Hagenfeldt, L., and Felig, P.: Splanchnic and leg exchange of glucose, amino acids and free fatty acids during exercise in diabetes mellitus. J. Clin. Invest. 55:1303, 1975.

110. Franken, S.: The history of patients with diabetic retinopathy. Ophthalmologica 175:49, 1977.

111. Etkind, E.L., Cunningham, L.N.: Physical abilities of diabetic boys. Presented at International Symposium Commemorating 50th Ann. of Insulin, Israel, Oct. 1971. Isr. J. Med. Sci. 8:848, 1972.

112. Hebbelinck, M., et al.: Physical development and performance capacity in a group of diabetic children and adolescents. Acta Paediatr. Belg. 28 (Suppl.):151, 1974.

113. Olavi, E., Hirvonen, L., Peltonen, T., Välimäki, I.: Physical working capacity of normal and diabetic children. Ann. Pediat. Fenn. 11:25, 1965.

114. Labrenz, J.B.: Planning meals for the backpacker with diabetes—nutritional values of freeze-dried foods. J. Am. Diet. Assoc. 61:42, 1972.

115. Etzwiler, D.D.: When the diabetic wants to be an athlete. The Physician & Sport Medicine 2:45, 1974.

116. Flood, T.M.: Who's running? Diabetes Forecast 32:20, 1979.

117. Murray, F.T., Zinman, B., McClean, P.A., et al.: The metabolic response to moderate exercise in diabetic man receiving intravenous and subcutaneous insulin. J. Clin. Endocrinol. Metab. 44:708, 1977.

118. Koivisto, V.A., Felig, P.: Effects of leg exercise on insulin absorption in diabetic patients. N. Engl. J. Med. 298:79, 1978.

119. Kawamori, R., Vranic, M.: Mechanism of exercise-induced hypoglycemia in depancreatized dogs maintained on long-acting insulin. J. Clin. Invest. 59:331, 1977.

120. Rennie, M.J., Park, D.M., Sulaiman, W.R.: Uptake and release of hormones and metabolites by tissues of exercising leg in man. Am. J. Physiol. 231:967, 1976.

121. Vranic, M., Kawamori, R., Wrenshall, G.A.: Mechanisms of exercise-induced hypoglycemia in depancreatized insulin-treated dogs. Diabetes 23 (Suppl.):353, 1974.

122. Zinman, B.: Exercise and diabetic control. Primary Care 4:637, 1977.

Color Plates

Plate I

PANCREAS: NORMAL AND DIABETIC

A. Normal human islet of Langerhans. Gomori's aldehyde fuchsin counterstained with Gomori's trichrome method. The blue-purple granules fill β cells ×250, (#72-A-181).

B. Normal human islet of Langerhans stained with the immunoperoxidase method, labeling insulin. The brown granules in the β cells identify insulin ×250 (#76-S-42).

C. "Hyalinized" islet of Langerhans with residual well-granulated β cells. The pale amyloid centrally replaces part of the islet tissue. Gomori's aldehyde fuchsin counterstained with Gomori's trichrome ×250 (X72-A-183).

D. Poorly granulated islet of Langerhans. Blue-purple granules of β cells are nearly completely absent in the central islet. The patient was a 74-year-old woman with a 6-year history of diabetes mellitus treated with diet and sulfonylurea. Gomori's aldehyde fuchsin and trichrome ×250 (#253410).

E. Juvenile onset, insulin-dependent diabetes mellitus. The central islet is small, shrunken with pyknotic cells and non-granulated. By immunocytochemical techniques, such islets appear to be formed largely of PP cells. The 33-year-old man with diabetes of 22 years' duration died because of diabetic nephropathy and had severe diabetic retinopathy. Pancreas weighed 80 g. Gomori's aldehyde fuchsin and trichrome ×250 (#239932).

F. Inverse ratio of islet cells with the blue-gray β cells in the minority. Fifty-seven-year-old man with diabetes of 2 years' duration that had been controlled on diet alone. Patient died of myocardial infarct. Chrome-alum hematoxylin and phloxine stain ×250 (#213515).

PLATE I

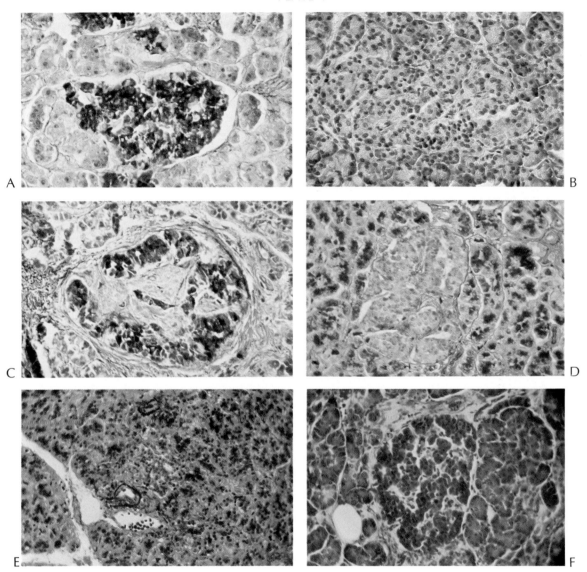

Plate II

KIDNEY AND RETINA

A. Advanced diabetic nephropathy causing the death of the patient. The glomerulus illustrates severe diffuse mesangial change, arteriolosclerosis and capsular drops. The patient was a 65-year-old woman with diabetes mellitus for 17 years. Periodic acid-Schiff and hematoxylin ×250 (#72-A-200).

B. Nodular glomerulosclerosis, the Kimmelsteil-Wilson lesion of diabetic nephropathy, the cause of death of the patient. Fifty-four-year-old woman with diabetes for 3 years. Periodic acid-Schiff and hematoxylin ×400 (#176147).

C. Glycogen infiltration of renal tubules, the Armanni-Ebstein lesion. The bright red droplets are glycogen. An 8-year-old boy who died in ketoacidosis with a 7-year history of diabetes. Periodic acid-Schiff and hematoxylin ×250 (#238575).

D. Retinal microaneurysm of diabetic retinopathy. Note the thickened capillary walls. Layer of rods and cones at bottom of picture. Patient was a 71-year-old woman with diabetes for 11 years and cataracts. Periodic acid-Schiff and hematoxylin stain ×250 (#218005).

E. Diabetic retinopathy with disruption of granular layers, edema and exudates. The patient was a 67-year-old woman who had diabetes for 21 months and also had diabetic nephropathy. Layer of rods and cones at bottom of picture. Periodic acid-Schiff and hematoxylin ×100 (#236904).

F. End-stage retinitis proliferans with complete destruction of the retina. Sixty-eight-year-old woman with diabetes mellitus for 41 years H & E ×100 (#280250).

PLATE II

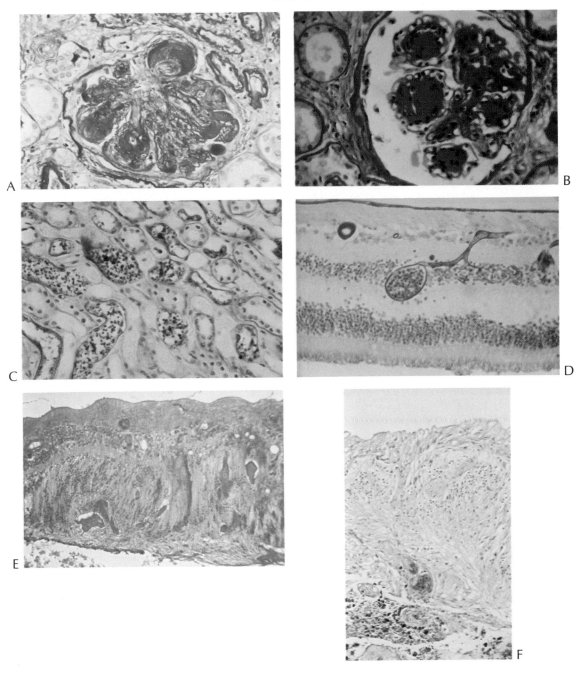

Plate III

DIABETIC RETINOPATHY

Thirty-one-year-old patient with diabetes of 11 years' duration with poor control of diabetes.

A. Optic disc edema with associated superficial hemorrhages adjacent to disc. No new vessels.
B. Six months later after coming under excellent control of diabetes. Complete remission of the optic disc edema without progression to neovascularization. (See Fig. 29–3.)

Forty-two-year-old patient with diabetes of 10 years' duration with diabetic maculopathy.

C. Ring of hard exudate adjacent to center of fovea. See fluorescein angiogram (Fig. 29–6).
D. Laser treatment marks noted in area of leakage as seen on fluorescein angiogram (Fig. 29–6).
E. Macular edema and hard exudates completely cleared; old laser burns seen as pigmented clumps. See fluorescein angiogram (Fig. 29–6).

Thirty-year-old patient with diabetes of 11 years' duration with diabetic macular edema and New Vessels Elsewhere (NVE).

F. Thickening in region of center of macula with hemorrhages and microaneurysms near center of macula. NVE also noted nasal to center of macula.
G. More New Vessels Elsewhere (NVE) seen nasal to disc. See Figure 29–7 for fluorescein angiography.

PLATE III

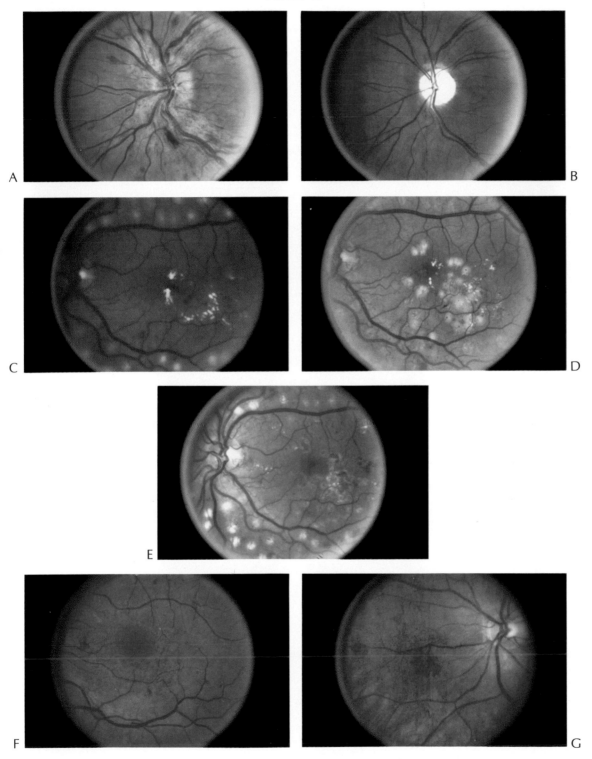

Plate IV

DIABETIC RETINOPATHY

Twenty-five-year-old patient with diabetes of 15 years' duration.

A. New Vessels Elsewhere with pre-retinal hemorrhage represent high risk characteristics. (See Fig. 29–8.)
B. Laser lesions photographed immediately after treatment. Note white round laser burns scattered more densely through the areas of new vessels.

Twenty-three-year-old patient with diabetes of 13 years' duration.

C. New vessels on Optic Nerve Head (NVD) and New Vessels Elsewhere near the disc (NVE). Photographed prior to treatment.
D. Pigmented laser lesions noted throughout the area around the disc (optic nerve head) with regression of all new vessels and remaining persistent small patch of fibrosis (FPD) on disc. (See Fig 29–9.)

Twenty-two-year-old patient with diabetes of 16 years' duration.

E. New vessels and pre-retinal hemorrhage temporal to macular area representing high risk characteristics (HRC).
F. New vessels elsewhere with soft exudates and intraretinal microvascular abnormalities (IRMA's).
G. One year later with extensive vitreous hemorrhage and active fibroproliferative tissue with traction elevation of retina as seen on ultrasound. (See Fig. 29–10).
H. After successful vitrectomy, visual recovery to 20/50. Remaining fibrosis is inactive with all traction relieved.

PLATE IV

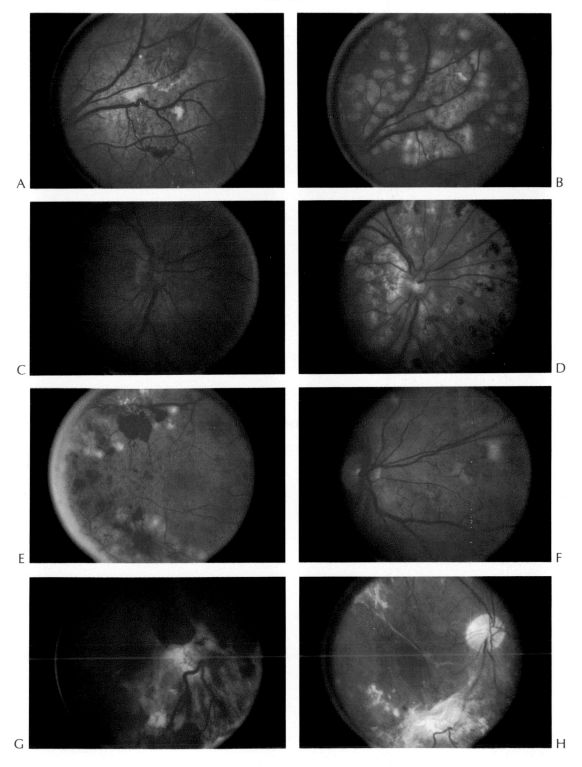

Plate V

SKIN LESIONS

A. This severe *burn* on the plantar surface of the foot resulted from injudicious use of a hot water bottle by a person with neuropathy and decreased circulation.
B. *Necrobiosis Lipoidica Diabeticorum* is almost always associated with diabetes. This is an early lesion which is difficult to diagnose at this stage. Often bilateral and in the pretibial areas, it is not limited to this site.
C. More advanced *Necrobiosis Lipoidica*. The danger is trauma which may result in infection. This has already advanced to ulceration on one side. See footnote beneath legends for Plate VI.
D. Severe *Necrobiosis Lipoidica* with ulceration and infection. Because of the poor circulation at sites of lesions, these stubbornly resist treatment.
E. Extreme case of *lipoatrophy* related to insulin injections.
F. Severe *lipoatrophy* at the site of insulin injections in the deltoid area. The outline of the underlying muscle can be seen through the skin. Lipoatrophy occurred frequently prior to the introduciton of purified insulins.

PLATE V

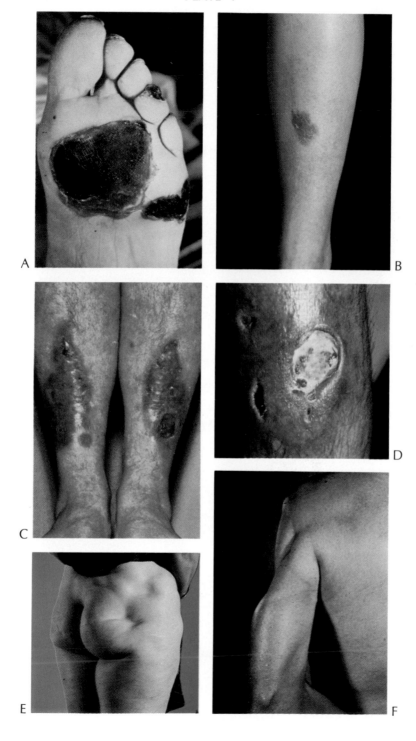

Plate VI

SKIN INFECTIONS AND XANTHOMATA

A. A classic *carbuncle*, at one time the nemesis of the diabetic, occurs infrequently since the development of antibiotic therapy. However, any skin infection must be watched carefully, especially since these lesions are susceptible to autoinoculation.

B. Common *epidermophytosis* (''athlete's foot'') which, if unnoticed and untreated, can cause serious problems in feet with poor circulation.

C. *Candida mycosis* is found in sweaty areas of the body that lend themselves to mycotic infections of this type. The axilla is a common site.

D. Classic *Xanthomata*. These yellow-orange lesions can appear rapidly and may be found anywhere on the body, but most often around the forearms and elbows.

E. A group of discrete *Xanthomata* in a fairly typical site.

Plates V C and VI A and C are used with the permission of Prof. med. G. Brehm of the Dermatological Clinic, Mainz, F.R.G. (Director: Prof. Dr. med. G. W. Korting), reproduced from ''Diabetes in Pictures,'' Farbwerke Hoechst, A. G., Frankfurt (Main).

PLATE VI

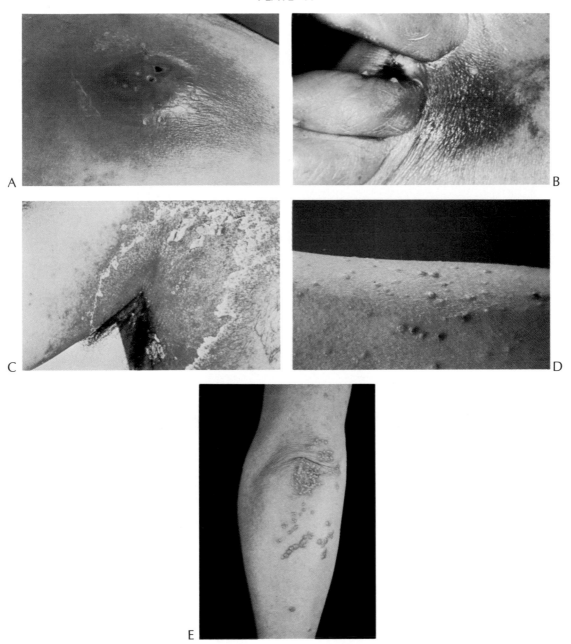

23 Education: A Treatment For Diabetes*

Leo P. Krall

> THIS BUILDING
> GIVEN BY
> THOUSANDS OF PATIENTS
> AND THEIR FRIENDS
> PROVIDES AN OPPORTUNITY
> FOR MANY
> TO CONTROL THEIR DIABETES
> BY METHODS OF TEACHING
> HITHERTO AVAILABLE TO
> THE PRIVILEGED FEW

This message, carved in stone on the face of the Diabetes Treatment Unit in 1955, demonstrates the dedication of the Joslin Diabetes Center to the education of the diabetic patient. This active concern with educating patients started some 70 years ago when Dr. Elliott P. Joslin realized the importance of educating both persons with diabetes and their families in order to sustain life. This was long before education became an accepted part of treatment. It was once considered a luxury. Dr. Joslin's attitude was "The diabetic who knows the most lives the longest." More recently the World Health Organization has stated that "Education is a cornerstone of diabetic therapy and vital to the integration of the diabetic into society."[1]

In spite of general agreement concerning its necessity, the adoption of education as a part of treatment for diabetes has been agonizingly slow and ineffective. In fact, until recent years medical texts often ignored the topic.

*The cooperation of Sylvia J. Brown, Ph.D., Northeastern University, Boston, Massachusetts, in the preparation of this chapter is gratefully acknowledged.

465

THE IMPORTANCE OF EDUCATION

With some conditions it is not critical that the patient understand the disease as long as appropriate medical instructions are followed. Diabetes is different. Assuming the diabetic is in close rapport with a knowledgeable and interested physician and is seen several times yearly, there are still most days when independent decisions must be made, and the ability to cope depends on appropriate responses. While patients cannot be their own physicians, they should at least be able assistants to skilled physicians because the success of therapy depends on their joint knowledge and cooperation.

Moreover, in recent years, education has come out of narrow, institutional walls and as a treatment has become a national and international concern. The American Hospital Association Bill of Rights states that "it is also the legal responsibility of the medical profession to the health care consumer to provide patient education as part of the total health care given."[2] Education is a preventive measure as well as a means of rehabilitation. Assal and Martin[3] state that management of diabetes includes prevention of poor control, and this goal can be reached only by careful education. About 80 years ago, Jose Marti, a Cuban patriot, stated succinctly: "It is better to build a fence around the edge of a mountain cliff than to build a hospital under the cliff."

The objective of this chapter is to discuss *why* diabetics should be taught, *who* should teach them, *what* they should be taught, and *how* this teaching should be made effective with appropriate evaluation at pertinent steps along the way. Also an analysis of international educational issues will be presented at the end of the chapter.

WHY EDUCATE THE PERSON WITH DIABETES?

In the simplest terms, the best reason for educating the person with diabetes concerning the life-long problems of his or her condition, is survival. Beyond this, the purposes of instruction of the patient may be stated in detail as listed below. Certain of these items will be discussed at length.

1. To live longer and happily. Quantity of life is important but so is quality.
2. To help the patient manage the diabetes so as to have fewer complications and fewer days of illness.
3. To function and cope with the problems of modern living.
4. To live more productive and useful lives.
5. To be less costly economically to self, family, community, and to the health system under which the patient lives.

6. In this modern litigious age, the legal focus increasingly implies that the inadequately informed patient may be a potential plaintiff.

To Insure a Longer Life for the Diabetic

The life span of the diabetic has been consistently lengthening since the use of insulin and other treatment measures, from pre-insulin days to the present. For example, even those with onset under age 10, who in pre-insulin days averaged a further duration of life of only 2½ years, by 1968 averaged nearly 30 additional years. Since 1968 this has increased significantly, but survival over this longer period requires more basic knowledge as well as familiarity with the many intricacies of diabetes management. Among the factors in the survival of patients with insulin-requiring diabetes for 50 years or longer, as reported by Cochran et al.,[4] is careful management of diabetes. It is clear that this is made possible only by considerable knowledge of the disease. Deckert and associates[5] reach similar conclusions, reporting that longevity with diabetes requires frequent medical contact to get good metabolic control and that even the act of giving insulin accurately requires knowledge and education. Williams[6] points out that, barring major illness, the physician or other health professionals will probably not have direct contact with the average diabetic for more than 6 to 12 of the patient's 5800 waking hours per year. This clearly emphasizes the need to educate patients so they can better manage their diabetes.

To Improve the Quality of Life

As people live longer, they seek to improve their life style, a phenomenon not limited to diabetes. A patient who is not knowledgeable about diabetes and cannot carry out instructions, is more likely to require medical or even hospital attention due to frequent hypoglycemic reactions, recurring bouts of ketoacidosis or complications of the cardiovascular system, eyes, nerves, kidneys, and feet. Persons poorly educated regarding diabetes may also be subject to more psychological concerns about diabetes so that they are unable to work efficiently or enjoy normal lives.

To Decrease the Cost of Diabetes Care

While it is generally agreed that education can be a major factor in decreasing costs of hospitalization, not until this fact can be proved conclusively regarding diabetic patients will ample money be made available for the needed education.

While "hard" evidence regarding economic benefits of education is incomplete, ample "soft" evidence suggests that the training of health personnel in keeping patients informed and in contact with trained helpers may indeed pay economic dividends. Two classic and widely quoted efforts in this direction are those by Miller and Goldstein[7] and Runyan.[8,9] The first of these studies involved two new programs, a telephone answering service and the screening of all candidates for hospitalization by either a nurse practitioner or a resident in the diabetes service. While these measures were not strictly "education," the educational process was part of the system in that people were trained to cope with patients. Emergency Room visits were remarkably reduced and the admissions for diabetic coma, for example, were reduced by two-thirds. The authors claimed a potential saving of between $1,700,000 and $3,500,000 for the diabetes service. In other studies, decentralized care using simple but rigid protocols without direct physician supervision was instituted. In 1972, more than 8500 patients made 35,000 visits to the clinics involved. In these reports, although chronic diseases other than diabetes were mentioned, this, along with hypertension and cardiac problems, accounted for 95% of admissions. For diabetes, there was a 49% reduction in total hospital days. In commenting on these, Williams,[10] in a superb review, pointed out that this research (which took place in California and Tennessee) showed effectiveness of geographic accessibility for patients as well as the significant role of specially trained clinicians. The Los Angeles clinic did cut health care delivery costs under those circumstances, but while the telephone answering service and intervention by persons with less expensive training than physicians were noteworthy, there was little to suggest that education per se (except of the concerned health team members) had achieved this difference in cost.

On the other hand, regarding education per se, Geller and Butler[11] made a specific study of educational deficits as a cause of hospital admissions for diabetes in a community hospital. They found that 27% of the patients had a specific education deficit which was responsible for their hospitalization, while another 20% had both educational and psycho-socio-economic problems. Davidson and co-workers[12] have established a program at the Emory University School of Medicine teaching hospital, providing care for 8000 diabetic patients, including a significant number of previously undiagnosed diabetics. The program includes facilities and the training of personnel for appropriate patient education and early detection. With these patients, about 75% of whom had less than 9th grade education and often could neither read nor write, Davidson et al. found, as a result of their efforts, that they had notably fewer hospital admissions, effecting a sizeable savings. For example, they made significant inroads in preventive foot care as well as ketoacidosis, which in 1969 had cost the hospital over $1,500,000. In evaluating cost effectiveness, the authors suggest the hospital had saved about $3,700,000 over a period of 8 years (1971 to 1978). This is a striking instance of effective health and education planning on a grand scale.

Kilo and his group, in a report by Dudley[13] concerning the diabetes educator's role in patient teaching, claimed that following survival education which enabled their patients to become independent by using self-report and daily feedback tools, there was consistent improvement in patient blood glucose levels, with glycosylated hemoglobin levels of 5.5 to 8.5 in 60% of 70 patients and levels of 8.6 to 10.5 in another 25%. They were also able to reduce the hospitalizations of insulin-dependent diabetics, since in a 2½-year period, 49% of the patients had no hospitalizations and 21% had only one. In diabetes data compiled in 1977 by the U.S. Department of Health, Education and Welfare, 37% of all diabetic admissions in the United States from 1967 to 1973 in patients aged 10 to 38 years were for ketoacidosis, and the average length of stay was from 7.18 to 9.44 days. This was in marked contrast to the data of Kilo et al. which showed no patients hospitalized for that condition.

The Joslin Clinic experience in educating patients, while extensive and perhaps episodic, has furnished some evidence of being able to relate patient education to lowered costs.[14] In 1969, for example, there were about 4500 admissions of diabetic patients to the New England Deaconess Hospital. Of these, 417 were admitted for foot complications (Table 23–1). They were hospitalized for 10,742 patient days. During the same period (Table 23–2), the total N.E.D.H. admissions, including those with diabetes, numbered 10,321, and they utilized 119,870 admission days. At that time, the average cost per hospital day was $101.08, not including medical or surgical fees. Therefore, the annual hospital cost for patients with severe foot

Table 23–1. Admissions of Diabetics with Foot Lesions, New England Deaconess Hospital, Boston, MA, USA—January 1–December 31, 1969

Condition	No. Cases	Patient Days
Gangrene	142	4,719
Infection	32	724
Ulcer	159	3,391
Charcot joint	6	64
Abscesses, cellulitis	33	580
Osteomyelitis	45	1,264
	417	10,742

Table 23–2.   New England Deaconess Hospital Admissions—January 1–December 31, 1969

	Admissions	Patient Hospital Days	Hospital Days Per Patient
TOTAL hospital admissions *including* diabetics	10,321	119,870	11.61
TOTAL diabetic patients for foot problems only	417	10,742	25.76

In 1969—hospital costs average $101.08 daily *not* including medical or surgical fees. Total cost $1,085,801 or $2,604 per diabetic foot patient.

In 1981—average cost of hospitalization per day (USA) $285.*

*U.S. News and World Report, March 8, 1982, page 62.

lesions and complications in this one hospital alone, was over $1 million. These costs have risen markedly since, due to various causes including inflation.

In attempting to determine how many of these admissions might have been prevented, 100 consecutive hospitalized foot patients were interviewed, their charts examined, and their cases discussed with their surgeons. An attempt was made to determine if these foot complications might have been prevented by earlier discovery of the lesions or better initial treatment on the part of either patient or primary physician. Of the 100 interviewed, probably 34 admissions could have been prevented, while 41 others might have been prevented. If half of the "possibles" were preventable, then about 54% of these complications might have been avoided. In attempting to pursue the reasons for the hospital admissions, patients were interviewed to determine their previous exposure to educational information. Choosing only those known to have diabetes at least five years, Table 23–3 shows that of the 100 queried, only 38 had ever been exposed to what might be termed adequate information. Furthermore, exposure to information does not in any way assure that the patient has learned or can apply that information.

A similar questionnaire was used with 100 con-

Table 23–3.   Interviews with 100 consecutive outpatients known to have had diabetes 5 or more years

Classification of Amount of Diabetes Education to Which They Had Been Exposed	Number
1. GOOD: Attendance at organized course at least 5 days in last year	13
2. ADEQUATE: Same as above but within last 5 years	25
3. FAIR: Outpatient teaching but not in organized consecutive days	36
4. POOR: Were told "something about diabetes" but no organized course	16
5. NONE: No particular access to information	10
Total	100

secutive outpatients, whatever the reason for their visit. In attempting evaluation, a tally of acute complications in the previous 12 months was loosely related to their degree of exposure to information (Table 23–4). Even in this unscientific patient sampling, it was possible to discern some relationship between the number and degree of complications and the degree of exposure to information.

Increasingly, third party insurance carriers are becoming aware of the possible dollar value of patient education and some have already agreed to pay charges for organized patient educational activities. At the national level, the former Department of Health, Education and Welfare Health Insurance Benefits Advisory Council strongly urged private carriers to pay for the costs of patient education. The state of California has enacted a law (S.B. 1187, January, 1982), which gives approval to group insurance coverage for out-patient diabetes education. Such coverage, however, does not include Medicaid or Medicare.[15] Nordberg and King[16] noted that while the value of patient education is unquestioned, it takes both ingenuity and persistence to ferret out those who could be induced to pay for educational programs, as was achieved at a Takoma Park, Maryland Hospital.[17] Furthermore, a Medicare directive (1976),[18] while apparently not widely implemented, indicates under the heading of Patient Education Programs that although "the law does not specifically identify patient education programs as covered services, reimbursement may be made under Medicare for such programs furnished by providers of services such as hospitals. . . . to the extent that the programs are appropriate, integral parts. . . . necessary to the treatment of individuals' illness or injury—for example, educational activities carried out by nurses teaching patients to give themselves necessary injections, etc."

So, the issue is still not clear-cut. Education is still too often considered as something "desirable" but not really necessary.

Potential Malpractice Problems

In this day of sensitivity to potential lawsuits for alleged malpractice or negligence in patient treat-

Table 23–4. Total of Acute Complications During the Previous 12 Months Among 100 Consecutive Diabetic Outpatients Related to the Amount of Diabetes Education*

Degree of Education	Group 1 "Good"	Group 2 "Adequate"	Group 3 "Fair"	Group 4 "Poor"	Group 5 "None"
Number in Each Group	13	25	36	16	10
Severe insulin reaction	3	10	75	30	30
Ketoacidosis	0	1	2	2	1
Infection—urinary tract	1	0	3	0	4
Infection—skin	0	2	2	3	2
Illness requiring help in insulin adjustment	1	2	1	4	3
Telephone or other help needed	3	8	8	10	15

*Using criteria for exposure to education defined in Table 18–4—not to be confused with evaluation of education.

ment, there is a danger of lawsuits stemming from presumed inadequate information or education. A $525,000 lawsuit was settled out of court in Sacramento, California, one of three recent medicolegal developments relating to the alleged liability of a physician in diabetes.[19] While this case per se did not directly relate to education, it is possible to envision situations fraught with medico-legal peril. For example, injuries resulting from automobile accidents said to be due to insulin-caused hypoglycemia, might be claimed to have resulted from inadequate instruction in preventing such incidents.

The end of this section is a good time to muse about possible dramatic monetary savings by improved education of patients. For example, if patient education efforts could cut the average daily dose of insulin used by an estimated 2,000,000 persons with diabetes, at current prices the savings could amount to at least $30 million annually in the United States alone. The question is not whether we can afford education, but how can we afford to do without it?

WHO SHOULD BE TAUGHT?

The person most in need of instruction is obviously the patient. However, in order to reach the patient effectively, education must be directed first to the teachers, whoever they may be, for unless the teachers are taught, they cannot teach. Ideally, the teaching of educators is a simple pyramid (Fig. 23–1) where each level is an immediate contact with the next level, with education broadly expanding to the patient. Often, realistically, this does not take place.

Layers of Educators: Physicians

To achieve appropriate diabetes educational levels, there must be certain layers. Unquestionably, education in diabetes must start with the physician. Unfortunately, some are not well informed in the

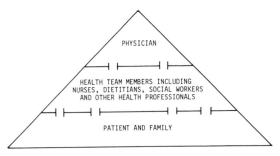

Fig. 23–1. Theoretical ideal teaching scheme for information to diabetics.

modern treatment of diabetes, perhaps because they have a greater interest in other phases of medicine. In 1977, a sample physician survey was conducted for the American Diabetes Association[20] to ascertain the degree of interest in diabetes. Among a representative sampling of 100 physicians to whom questionnaires were sent, 58% replied. The results indicated that while diabetes is commonly seen in the practices of general and family physicians and internists (an average of 10 patients per week), only about 40% of the general physicians thought that members of their specialty were very well informed on the subject, although this percentage rose to 70% among internists. Those surveyed were largely interested in learning more about the areas of "drug therapy" or "diet and nutrition," but only 26% had interest in the psychological problems of diabetics.

The very volume of new information in the field of diabetes causes delay in reaching physicians. For example, Kessner[21] noted that 2 years after the findings of the well-designed clinical trial of photocoagulation in diabetic retinopathy were reported, only 33% of primary care physicians were even aware of the study. Howver, those who were informed of the study results changed their practice habits and referred more diabetic patients to ophthalmologists at an earlier stage of retinopathy. This lack of awareness of the modern benefits of early eye referral becomes crucial since it has been shown[22] that potentially serious mistakes in diagnosis are often made by physicians.

The attempt to keep physicians up to date via continuing education is enormous. Accredited A.M.A. courses have jumped from 5,200 to more than 22,000 in a 6-year period and the registrations of physicians increased from about 300,000 to about 1,470,000 in that time.[23] However, Kessner's data suggest that other and stronger efforts must be made to keep physicians informed regarding current methods of treatment and diagnosis.[23a] Thus, an important part of the educational effort in the field of diabetes must include education of physicians.

Another concern is that of Czyzyk[24] who finds that physicians are not always the best teachers. Indeed, a serious criticism of medical education is that not enough is done to encourage medical students and residents to teach and reach the patient. Yet, the family oriented physician must play a central role in diabetes education throughout the world. This places a tremendous responsibility on the physician not only as an educator but as one attuned to family problems.[25] There is evidence that the modern physician is interested in responding to this challenge.[26]

Layers of Educators: The Health Team Concept

Due to increased technical aspects of health care and education and increased medical intervention into medical situations once deemed hopeless, the responsibility for sharing the burdens of instructing and educating, especially in long-term chronic illness, now includes health professions from various disciplines, i.e., a health team approach. Members of the allied health professions, such as nurses and dietitians, often have great understanding and acceptance of patients, and are readily related to by patients. Jackson noted at the Diabetes Update session of the I.D.F. Congress in New Delhi (1976): "For many newly diagnosed diabetics, the doctor is a remote deity whose pronouncements have a scriptural value and are voiced in a confusing new language which, to them, is often incomprehensible." The non-physician professionals have made a great impact on health education in the last decade.[27]

At one time, the health "educator" was an occasional nurse who had acquired special knowledge about diabetes in a hospital setting and taught patients about their disorder. At present, patients are taught by various members of a health care team, including: (1) the nurse, whose practical knowledge of insulin injection technique, care of equipment and general health is augmented by (2) the dietitian with a practical knowledge of nutrition as well as awareness of local dietary habits and availbility of foods; (3) the social worker who understands patients' psychosocial background and can help them to cope with diabetes; (4) the pharmacist who not only knows the differences in action of medications and testing materials, but often must serve as a primary health education resource; (5) the podiatrist who advises about foot care; and (6) the physiotherapist who may need to develop exercise activities suited to the patient's needs and abilities. There is scarcely a discipline or resource which may not be involved in diabetes education.

A summary in Lancet[28] states that while it is not a new concept to include the nurse in the team managing diabetes, the modern trend allows the nurse to assume a rightful place on the team beside the physician, "equal in importance but different in emphasis." There are numerous data in recent literature calling attention to the fact that the nurse educator has become a necessary cost-effective addition to the health care team[29] and increasingly, this means greater competence in applying modern methodology to teaching.[30]

Primary diabetes knowledge is also a responsibility for the occupational health professional.[31] The passage of the Occupational Safety and Health Act of 1970 brought new attention to the needs of industrial employees. Modern industry with complicated techniques and expensive machinery necessitates the knowledge of an employee's diabetes and potential hazards, e.g., preventable hypoglycemic reactions.

The role of the pharmacist is not to be underestimated.[32] From time immemorial, the pharmacist in the corner drugstore was a source of emergency information, often known as "Doc" by persons who came to obtain necessary medications. Patients in one survey were shown to have visited their pharmacists 5.2 times more often than they saw their physicians. The pharmacist's role has now expanded, involving not only community pharmacists but also highly skilled hospital-based pharmacists. Why should not pharmacists know at least as much about diabetes as a well educated patient?

While this increasing focus on higher levels of education for the diabetes educator is important, with increased specialization, the educational process certainly becomes much more expensive, possibly more effective, and sometimes less available. While no one denies the need for increased training for all professionals, there is the obvious danger of providing superb training for a smaller group of patients, whereas the crucial need is for basic survival information for all patients. While the team concept is valid, it is often available only in large (often university group) centers.

The development of improved information techniques must also take into account the smaller hospitals and clinics scattered at distances from large centers. Their needs must not be forgotten. Where larger teams are not available, a dedicated, well-informed, sympathetic nurse or other health professional can perform wonders. The education of patients should become a continuing process because a patient once taught, does not necessarily remain at that level without continuous replenishment of knowledge.

The Patient and Associates

"For want of a nail a shoe is lost, For want of a shoe the horse is lost, For want of a horse, the rider is lost."

George Herbert, *Jacula Prudenuum,* 1641

This aptly describes the problem of the person with diabetes. Education is probably the most vital part of treatment, and if this is not achieved, all may be lost. Without education of the patient to understand what is being done with and for him, the whole therapeutic system unravels.[33]

It has long been known that many efforts to teach patients may achieve results that are far from ideal.[34] A study of 162 diabetic patients from 3 clinics and 22 private physicians showed that 58% made errors in insulin dosage; of this total, 35% of the errors were potentially serious (measured dose differed from that prescribed by 15% or more). In another study,[35] a 7-day record kept by 17 patients showed not only inadequate and inaccurate food intake but omission of regular meals during 40% of the patient days. Gozzi and co-workers showed marked communication gaps between patients and physicians during a study involving 8.2 patient visits.[36] Part of the communications block came about because either the physician allegedly interrupted the patient's comments or both physician and patient talked at the same time in 63% of the situations. Also reported were vague and inappropriate comments by the physician, or simply "not listening to what the patient was trying to say." Obviously, physicians must make a conscious effort to understand what the patients need and want to know, and whether subsequent teaching has actually been successful.

Although the patient with diabetes is the primary target of the educational goal, others beside the patient must be involved. This is especially true of youngsters whose parents need to be gracefully immersed in information aiding the survival of their offspring. Also, as Jackson[37] asserted, the example given by parents is the basic model that children use in developing health practices as well as their

future life style. Education may pay off significantly in this group: Guthrie and Guthrie[38] reported, as a result of an intensive education and follow-up system, only 1.5% of a population of 300 Midwestern children with diabetes were re-hospitalized for any reason during a 6-year period of time (0.25% admissions per year).

Others who should learn about diabetes[39] include close family members, relatives, close neighbors and business associates of the patient, who should all be aware of potential diabetes problems. Persons who are frequently with the patient include employers, employees, fellow workers, friends, teachers, clergy, and possibly pharmacists. People who might occasionally come in contact with diabetic persons include hospital and clinical support personnel, police, firemen, service personnel, airline and other transportation employees. Increasingly, transport workers are faced with problems of diabetic passengers, and can be very helpful if they are aware of symptoms of a hypoglycemic episode. Police likewise can be helpful if they recognize a hypoglycemic reaction and provide a sweet drink rather than assume that the diabetic patient is drunk.

WHAT SHOULD BE TAUGHT?

Minimal Survival Information

The American Diabetes Association suggests that the first level of education include the guidelines for initial diabetes management. The following basic information should be given at the time of diagnosis or immediately afterward:

A definition of diabetes and its relationship to blood and urine glucose.

Diet: Not only general information but a specific meal plan.

Urine testing.

Action of insulin or oral agents.

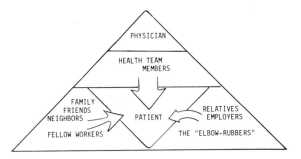

Fig. 23–2. The ideal teaching scheme for diabetes. From: Krall, L.P.: The direct and indirect members of the diabetic's universe. In: G. Steiner and P.A. Lawrence (Eds.): Educating Diabetic Patients. New York, Springer Publishing Company, Inc. 1981. p. 253. Used by permission.

Techniques of insulin injection.

Care of insulin and syringes.

Symptoms and treatment of uncontrolled diabetes.

Meaning of acetonuria.

Symptoms and treatment of hypoglycemia.

What to do in case of acute complications related and unrelated to diabetes.

Sick day rules.

Care of the feet.

In teaching the patient, it is important to avoid either supplying insufficient information or inundating the patient with too much. The former "worst case" situation is typified by a patient who is told that tests indicate diabetes, gets 15 minutes of hurried instruction in injecting insulin, is given a diet, and arrives home, confused, depressed, bitter at his/her fate, and with a sackful of insulin, syringes and needles, cotton balls, alcohol, and possibly a not very personalized mimeographed diet sheet. At the other extreme, too much information too soon to a new diabetic may overwhelm the learning system.

Primary: Early Instruction

This information should essentially be "survival information." For a patient who presents with newly diagnosed diabetes, reassurance is vital and it is hardly necessary to discuss long-term complications. Information should be offered to the patient in small increments as he is capable of accepting it. Otherwise, it is like plugging a huge electrical appliance into a small capacity electric outlet. As to diet, patients should be able to demonstrate the exchange system by actually choosing food from a hospital or restaurant, selecting the food they like, and know the reason for eating meals and snacks on time.

Secondary: Important and Useful Information

This information enables the patient to travel and to be comfortable with a wide variety of diets, such as at parties and picnics, thereby adding pleasure to necessity. More complex preventive measures as well as adjustment of diet and insulin should be taught in order to meet changes in activities. Patients at this level are not only capable of preventing ketoacidosis and severe hypoglycemic reactions, but must also know when to seek aid.

Tertiary: More Sophisticated Aids to a Better Life Style

This type of information answers questions such as: Can a diabetic have a successful pregnancy? Will offspring of diabetic parents have diabetes? It deals with employment choices and the ability to

solve the problem of living with diabetes. While the learning of these items is not important early, it is vital for a better life. People with diabetes must accept certain changes in life patterns, not needed for nondiabetics. The sooner they adapt to these, the closer to normal can be their life style. They must, however, be convinced that this is a good exchange.

OBJECTIVES: WHAT EDUCATIONAL GOALS ARE DESIRED?

Of all the educational goals desired for the diabetic, the first objective is an *increase in a patient's knowledge*. Without knowledge, there is no basis for a change in attitude or life style. The second of these is *attitudinal change* because without motivation, the knowledge gained will not be put to use. The ultimate result is an appropriate *change in behavior and compliance* in self-care. The final result should be improved quality of life.

Knowledge

The knowledge requirement for diabetics is formidable. The authors of a recent book concerning the education of diabetics[40] cover 106 pages of topics deemed important for the diabetic patient as minimal information. Entire manuals[41] have told the diabetic what he should know, and no one has yet complained that a patient knew too much. In transferring knowledge, it is important to avoid discouragement for patients who feel hopeless because they seem unable to absorb the mass of data. This often results in escape and laxness with the regimen. The burden of diabetes learning must not be placed entirely on the patient but should be shared with family members as well.

To pour information into people without explaining its importance is counterproductive.[42] The person who knows *why* he is supposed not to exceed the speed limit—because (a) there is a penalty for doing so; (b) it is a hazard to his own safety as well as that of others—is more likely to comply than one who knows only that it is against the law.

Attitude and Motivation

Many diabetes programs founder on the reefs of insufficient motivation and poor attitude. Without these, compliance will never take place. Wysocki and co-workers[43] surveyed health behavior and its determinants among insulin-dependent diabetics in Warsaw. They found an appalling lack of compliance and noted that the greatest deterrent was the lack of understanding of the condition and of what was expected of the patient. As one might expect, given these factors, the study also uncovered a lack of adequate motivation. Basic to all of this is the fact that patient responses are strongly influenced by the attitude and teaching process of the physicians or other teachers. The interest of the physician in a given disease condition is vital and the study cited previously[20] indicated that when a physician saw only few patients with a given problem, not only did he know less about it, but often was less interested as well. If motivation and interest do not stem from the fountainhead, what can one expect from the patient? A famous cartoon depicted an obese physician with a cigar in his hand, telling a patient to change his life style, i.e., follow a diet, lose weight, and discontinue smoking, a point that may have been lost by the lack of example. Czyzyk and co-workers[44] reiterate that diabetes cannot be treated without motivation, and point out that the periods in which motivation are most important are: (a) the immediate post-diagnosis period when attempts should be made to reduce fear, anxiety, and even anger of the patient and to stabilize the emotional response; (b) the period of basic education, to take place within a few weeks after the initial diagnosis, with planning for future training with the help of psychological evaluation; (c) continually thereafter, as the state of "being diabetic" requires constant reinforcement and re-education. Many patients in the early phase of their diabetes take care of themselves, but later, with the absence of stimuli, become bored with the subject. Motivation must be constant. Attitudes also depend on understanding.

Compliance

Compliance is neither automatic nor accidental. There are occasional patients who strive to improve and attain perfection in the care of their diabetes, but these people are self-motivated and often are attracted to clinics known for zealous diabetes care. But how can other patients (certainly the majority) achieve the necessary change of behavior? Morreau[45] stated: "The client must want to change existing behaviors that impede his progress;" but before this is achieved, it is important to assess the degree of patient motivation to determine future progress. The person involved first must be convinced that the effort toward change in life style is worthwhile. For example, if a diet given to a patient has marked ethnic differences from the foods to which the patient is accustomed, he is less likely to follow that diet. To achieve patient compliance, the diet must be planned around foods which the patient likes.[46] Likewise, it must be understood that both patient and teacher must put effort into the educational process. A useful method is something known as a health care "contract."[47] It means that the patient and the teacher share responsibility for achieving mutually agreed upon goals. In its sim-

plest form, a "contract" is a written agreement between patient and physician. The contract includes a description of what is to be achieved, what the patient must do, and what steps must be taken to reach that goal. It must be understood that parties of *both* parts are accessories to this agreement. Then, like a contract, it can be signed. This reinforces the patient's sense of active participation in his or her own diabetic care.

As Alivisatos[48] stated, patient compliance is the outcome of the interaction of a number of factors between the physician, the disease state, the treatment regimen, and the therapeutic milieu. West et al.[49] measured outpatient compliance in insulin-dependent diabetic patients and found that errors, such as improper insulin doses, occurred when the patient did not understand diet or other phases of instruction by the physician. Communication is most vital[50] and patients had a significantly better response in understanding and recall if they were given written instructions by their physicians.[51] Other types of communication were those used at the Mayo Clinic, where dismissal interviews between patients and their physicians were recorded on cassettes, and patients were given the cassettes to take home. A later questionnaire to the patients indicated that 91% felt they better understood the physician's instructions, 75% found it helpful to have relatives listen to the tapes, and 62% preferred the recording to a follow-up letter.[52]

Improved Quality of Life

The motivation for patient compliance is the anticipation of improved quality of life. This tenet is the sine qua non of modern diabetes therapy. While it is not fully understood just how many complications may be prevented or ameliorated, without a doubt there are rewards. It is clearly known, for example, that severe hypoglycemic reactions, ketoacidosis, serious infections, and even limb loss, may be prevented. Perhaps as important in daily living, the person who constantly vacillates between insulin reactions and hyperglycemia simply does not enjoy a good life style.

METHODS OF TEACHING

How does one teach? What materials and equipment are necessary? What is the best way to teach?

The fact that there is no one "right" answer to these questions may confuse and even discourage institutions from trying to develop sound educational programs. Ajgaonkar[53] differentiated between education programs that use a more personal approach, as in diabetes clinics, health centers, physicians' offices, camps and other community locations, as opposed to those emanating from more impersonal mass informational media such as magazines, books and newspaper articles as well as lectures, radio, television, and more recently, videotape. Where does one begin? The choice of method depends on the goal of one's educational program (i.e., what one hopes that patients will learn) as well as the type of persons to be taught, their motivation, their willingness to learn, and what aids to teaching are available. Modern equipment can be useful, but no discovery has yet been made that will replace the motivated and enthusiastic teacher and a willing student.

Education is an ongoing process. Sims[54] maintains that the person with diabetes cannot possibly absorb all that should be learned in several days in an acute care setting. Patients need to know where to seek continuing support and further information when needed. Large clinical groups may have an advantage since it may cost less to teach patients in classes than individually. The Grady Memorial Hospital Counseling Program in Atlanta[55] is outstanding in this respect. However, teaching should not be limited to hospitalized patients; these facilities may be used efficiently for educating outpatients as well. For example, Heller et al.[56] organized a series of 1-day symposia for patients at risk, and being treated, for diabetes-related kidney disease. Many nationally sponsored diabetes control projects, administered by various states, have developed a model for ongoing outpatient educational programs which are then carried out at various locations throughout the area. Innovative thinking can convert any institution with facilities and imagination into a teaching center.

For example, for adult patients with multiple health problems who have limited mobility, income and/or education, the use of home health aides as patient educators has been found successful.

Videotapes are frequently used in teaching today. Patients appear to learn as well from videotape as from trained nurses.[57] The easily made tapes are the natural sequelae to the teaching machines of the recent past. In the future, videotapes will be widely used at home as well as in institutions.

For much of the world in the foreseeable future, the lecture method will probably continue to be widely used. With an experienced teacher presenting material in an orderly fashion, using simple teaching aids, and stimulating general discussion by posing questions, the results may be excellent. If this method is used ideally, the listener not only may acquire information, but may learn from questions raised by peers, and experience the benefits of being with a group of people who have similar problems and concerns.

One obstacle with the lecture method is the difficulty in holding the attention of listeners beyond about 20 minutes, unless the speaker is excep-

tional. One must accept the fact that within a few weeks many tend to forget about 75% of what they have heard.[58] Consequently, repetition is necessary. However, while change of attitudes can often be better accomplished by role playing, group discussions, field experiences and other methods, the lecture is likely to remain a favored means of group communication.[59]

Probably the primary method of teaching patients will continue to be one-on-one teaching, i.e., physician with patient, nurse with patient, etc. This method builds on the typical patient relationship and is one with which both parties are likely to be comfortable. Further, questions of special interest to an individual are more easily answered in this setting. Also, follow-up and monitoring (two critical aspects of ongoing education) are facilitated.

Whenever possible the use of accompanying written materials is recommended to supplement the in-hospital or office education. Patients can then review important information at home. Such materials may be obtained from many sources such as diabetes associations, clinical centers, pharmaceutical education programs, and health education publishing companies. Annotated bibliographies of a wide variety of teaching tools, e.g., foot care, diet and recipes, diabetes in youth and the elderly, may be obtained at no cost from the National Diabetes Information Clearinghouse, sponsored by the National Institutes of Health.

In summary, to do the best possible job, each institution or group must analyze its needs, goals, audience and resources, and use whatever help is obtainable from persons knowledgeable in the art of teaching. The new devotion and intensity regarding the art and science of diabetes education is best summarized by the comprehensive monograph on that subject by Assal et al.[59a]

EDUCATIONAL APPROACHES

Assessing Needs

Planning of objectives for patient education is important, but this cannot be accomplished until the patient and his or her needs are identified. Assessing needs determines what the patient already knows about diabetes, as well as the general level of education, physical status, home situation, emotional readiness, etc.[60] This information can be obtained by the following techniques: interview, questionnaire, paper and pencil test, observation, simulation, and/or examination of the medical record.

Planning and Setting Goals

Hess[61] indicated that a common mistake is to state objectives that are neither clearly specified nor properly sequenced, noting that sequenced objectives facilitate communication, provide proper order, and make it possible to begin with what the patient already knows and fill in the gaps where needed. The planning process may be broken down into (1) stating the ultimate goals of the program; (2) providing specific educational objectives; (3) selecting or devising education programs to enable the patient to achieve these goals; and finally (4) helping the patient accept them in accordance with his own behavioral pattern and life style. Again, the objectives must not be impossible. There must also be a good balance between the organization of program and material content, since an unbalanced program is no program.

Program Settings

Out-Patient Facilities. Many physicians have an assistant and/or a part-time nurse but no real access to diet service. Diabetics may become lost in the large volume of patient visits. To provide effective out-patient education in these limited facilities, some physicians invite their patients and their families to the office one evening a week for a discussion of diabetes followed by a question-and-answer session. Another approach is to schedule appointments for all diabetic patients on one day, and have a teaching nurse available to instruct patients. Also, a group of cooperating physicians in an area may organize such classes jointly, supporting an educator for this purpose. The present influx of teaching devices, videotape teaching systems, publications, etc., can be an enriching factor of any of these teaching programs. Referral of patients to diabetes teaching centers and/or to dietitians may also be necessary for some patients.

In those situations where out-patient offices are in conjunction with a larger institution, such as the Joslin Clinic out-patient service and its relationship to the Diabetes Treatment Unit of the New England Deaconess Hospital, this is not a great problem. Another example is the diabetic day care center at the Maricopa County General Hospital (California), consisting of two rooms for blood testing and individual instruction regarding insulin usage. A conference room for classes was provided by the hospital.[62] Obviously this has filled a need since 3021 patient visits to the diabetic day care center were registered in a one-year period, with instruction in English and Spanish.

In-Patient and Hospital-Based Settings. These provide excellent opportunities for teaching because they often have more room, more resources, and more staff as well as the possibility of diverting staff from one function to another.

Because of its size and the long tradition of education, which has in various forms been available for the last three-quarters of a century, the diabetes education program at the Joslin Clinic is quite comprehensive.[63,64] This started at the turn of the century when Dr. Elliott P. Joslin practiced out of his own home. Later, in 1928 he hired and trained the first teaching nurse to assist as his "wandering nurse" who accompanied newly diagnosed diabetic patients, usually children, to their homes during their period of adjustment. Later, Dr. Joslin adapted a small boarding house across the street from the Deaconess Hospital to house ambulatory patients who needed treatment and instruction but not detailed nursing care. The George F. Baker Clinic building at the New England Deaconess Hospital, occupied first in 1934, was a pioneer diabetes center, including quite remarkably for that time, space for teaching, research, adult and juvenile admissions, a delivery room and eye unit, and even a small gymnasium for exercise and recreation.

The present in-patient ambulatory Diabetes Treatment Unit, administered by the Deaconess Hospital, has 70 beds which cost less than those in the main hospital, due to minimal staffing and the ability of patients to help take care of themselves, under supervision. Formal classes are given every day of the year by physicians, nurses and dietitians. Patients also have frequent contact with each other. This facility has special programs for young diabetics. Severely ill patients requiring bed care are treated in the main part of the Deaconess Hospital. Institutions of this type are being developed in many areas.

To determine whether an individual educational program is successful, the patient's progress should be monitored continually. Assuming that the prescribed diet and insulin dose are optimal, it is possible to assess the degree of patient success in understanding educational material by comparing the original learning goals with the evaluation results. By this means it is possible to modify the teaching program to a level which may be grasped by the patient. Interviewing patients in person or by telephone or requesting that they keep records for later review, may help the instructor to make an assessment of the extent of the patient's achievement of goals, However, it is important to consider that any method may yield biased results since experience shows that data kept and reported by the patient may be unreliable. Monitoring and follow-up should take place both during and after an educational program to be sure desired learning and behavioral changes are maintained.[65]

Simulation techniques are also useful in adjusting programs and may be particularly effective in diet instruction.[66] For instance, the proper use of food models permits assessment of patients' knowledge and behavior regarding food choices. Further instruction to help the patient avoid any mistakes in the future can then be based on a realistic view of the exact nature of the patient's problems.

Education for Special Groups

The Young Patient. Young patients present a major challenge because they live the longest and are potentially subject to the complications which may arise from diabetes of long duration. They also develop diabetes at a time when they are working at developmental tasks such as the need for autonomy, a sense of adequacy, and a feeling of normalcy and independence. During this period of psychological growth and change, it is particularly difficult to incorporate into their lives the regimentation required by diabetes care. Despite these difficulties, it is important to give youngsters a good start in learning to care for their diabetes toward the goal of increasing their longevity with a minimum of morbidity.

Education is a vital part of treatment for young people with diabetes. Done well, it can make a significant difference. A special clinic at Oxford, England, directed especially at young people, showed a marked decrease in hospital admissions for this group over a 7-year period[67] not only because of better medical care but also due to improvement in patient education. In a study conducted in a clinic in Israel, Laron[68] found the degree of control so superior after the use of a special multidisciplinary team, that there were fewer complications and almost no need for hospitalization. Laron emphasized that instruction of members of the family of the affected youngster is important since the child cannot shoulder all of the responsibility of care, particularly at an early age.[69] In another special pilot program of service and education for inner city children with diabetes in Detroit, a similar significant reduction in hospital admissions was recorded.[70]

The teaching of young patients requires all of the ingenuity and resources available. Not only do the capacities of youth to understand the nature of diabetes differ at various ages, but so do their abilities to engage in various kinds of self-care procedures. Age level also affects what is relevant for youth to learn. Some of the knowledge and skills required by adolescents to care for their diabetes within the context of their day-to-day activities are irrelevant to the pre-schooler. It is essential, therefore, that age-appropriate educational materials and activities be utilized. Admittedly, the education of this age group is complex, but the rewards, when successful, are great. (See Chapter 24)

The Older Patient. The elderly diabetic also presents difficulties. One must consider how much

one desires to or can change the life style of an elderly person. Kratzer[71] asks "Is it possible to change the life style of a forgetful 73-year-old widower who lives alone and who has recently been diagnosed as having diabetes mellitus?" Since about 20% of all diabetics are diagnosed after age 65, many older persons are asymptomatic but still require care. On the other hand, there are older persons who are insulin-dependent with "juvenile-type" diabetes. A significant number of these persons become ketoacidotic, and the proportion of loss of limbs is highest in this group. Hypoglycemia may also pose a particular threat to older patients.

Grobin[72] stresses the fact that health professionals need remotivation concerning care of elderly patients because there is a tendency to take their diabetes and other problems lightly. Senior citizens require special assistance in coping with general problems such as limited funds, which result in inability to afford a nutritious diet, or adequate dental care; and loneliness which could decrease motivation to care for one's diabetes. While their diabetes education may be less detailed than that for the young, a program for them[73] must be sympathetic, their life style and ethnic food preferences must be considered, and they must be permitted to make decisions about required changes. This is important for their independence and self-esteem. The British Diabetic Association has organized holidays for elderly persons with diabetes at a resort in Bournemouth, Dorset,[74] and a program of diabetes education was inaugurated in this holiday environment, away from the tense hurried city atmosphere.

Illiterate or Low Educational Levels. The illiterate or low educational level diabetic presents another challenge to teachers. It has been believed that many at this level suffer more problems, as emphasized by a unique Warsaw study[75] in which some 4,300 diabetics aged 18 to 68 were followed for 5 years. The age-standardized mortality rates for diabetics with high levels of education did not exceed the expected rates for the Warsaw general population, while the rates for diabetics in the lower education groups significantly exceeded the expected values. The protecting effect of higher education levels may be due to better health education and regular health behavior patterns. One reason the uneducated are harder to reach is because of the inability of many educators to understand that persons with different educational levels have different responses and levels of motivation.[76] Most popular publications aim at high school or higher reading levels, perhaps because authors feel these are the people who buy books and read them, and it is easier to be a clever author for a high-level readership.

H.E.W.'s "Right to Read Office" claims that 23 million Americans are functionally illiterate.[77] While many can speak articulately, they neatly conceal the fact that they did not learn to read adequately during that "narrow window in time—usually between the first and fourth grades."

Indigent patients in out-patient clinics are inadequately taught because traditional treatment programs are often planned for the more affluent patients who may be more highly motivated.[78] Even the diets include generous amounts of expensive protein foods and three regularly scheduled meals a day, which may be a novelty to a surprising number of Americans as well as to persons elsewhere in the world. Furthermore, in certain cultures, a hospital is regarded as simply a place to die and not a place to go for preventive care. The attitude is the same toward visits to a physician.

Other Factors Interfering with Educational Programs. There are other reasons for less than ideal educational results. These may include inadequate cooperation within a team of educators, inability to afford educational services, language barriers, ethnic considerations, inadequate materials, prejudice, superstition, and others to be overcome by the educator at whatever level. Assal[79] noted that failures may begin with the physician's lack of recognition that teaching is a real aspect of therapy and a subconscious feeling that education decreases the physician's medical identity and authority, as well as failure to appreciate that the role of the doctor must be shared with others.

Difficulties presented by language barriers and ethnic groupings are readily understood, Many people who live within ethnic enclaves do not feel comfortable, are distrustful, and regard anything outside of their own ethnic sphere as alien. This is particularly true of first generation immigrants, although this prejudice may subconsciously carry over into the next generation. It is necessary for an educational center to find translators within the patient's family, particularly the younger members or, lacking such, other patients, hospital staff members, or anyone understanding the patient's language. It may be awkward, time-consuming or expensive, but patient care itself is hopeless without a means to communicate with the patient. No medical institution in the United States can now consider itself to be an educational or treatment center without available persons proficient in Spanish. It is estimated that about 15 million persons in the country are more comfortable with that language.

Another reason for education failure is inadequate materials. There is no longer any excuse for outdated, uninteresting, and poorly conceived materials since improved versions are increasingly available from major clinics, the American Diabetes Association, the American Association for Diabetes Educators, and Juvenile Diabetes Foundation as well as various pharmaceutical companies.

Another barrier is that of medical orders. Studies have shown that the greater the number of medications and complexity of regimen, the greater the number of errors and indifference on the part of the patient.[80] Another reason for breakdown in understanding is too many conflicting new ideas too early and too often as well as the use of technical jargon in talking down to patients.

Costs of education are a barrier. It has been realized[81] that many who have lost their jobs because of insulin reactions or have lost time from employment because of illness, are unable to spend time or money on educational programs. Thus the most needy are often not helped by effective programs. Some progress has been made in classifying diabetes instruction programs as an educational work adjustment service, enabling more people to benefit by providing some form of tuition reimbursement.

EVALUATION OF EDUCATION

In a world of diminishing available resources for many necessities, funding for patient education as well as for disease prevention is being increasingly questioned. For some years after the discovery of insulin, the simple transmission of information was considered to be sufficient "education." More recently, there has been a shift from simply imparting information to an attempt to influence and change the very life style of those with diabetes through long-term behavioral changes. In addition, there has been an increased interest in evaluating whether diabetes instruction programs make any difference in patient behavior and ultimately in blood glucose levels and long-term complications. If evaluation is able to prove effectiveness of education, it may strengthen the case for obtaining more funding for educational efforts.

Martin[82] urges that "evaluation" not be a "frightening" word since we continually evaluate every service in life. He also discusses the difficulties evaluators encounter in trying to determine the effectiveness or usefulness of education in diabetes, e.g.: (a) objectives not clearly stated; (b) lack of reliable indices to measure the impact of a program; (c) personal and organizational dislike of being evaluated; and (d) shortage of sophisticated evaluation consultants.

The questioning of effectiveness of education applies not only to patient teaching but to the efficiency of continuing and postgraduate medical education programs. Even the recently accepted concept of continuing education programs for physicians is now questioned with the recent observation[83] that millions of dollars are expended for this but few have succeeded in determining whether it is effective.

Because the rapid growth of patient education has been recent, little thought has been given to evaluation until the last few years. The criticism has been made that "the educator tends to place more emphasis on imparting knowledge and less on evaluating what the learner has assimilated and applied to his daily life style."[84] Even the discipline of evaluation becomes questioned, because in determining need, educational objectives, attitudinal and behavioral objectives, the process of evaluation itself may come into conflict with those who would prefer to spend available funds directly on services. It is evident that while the process of evaluation is neither an exact nor completely developed science, remarkable improvements and refinements are being made.

Diabetes educational programs set up with built-in evaluation processes[86] may be ideal, but given the disparity of the needs of individuals as well as the limited resources, one must determine the priorities while not discouraging application of any evaluative process that is practicable, useful and affordable. One cannot wait for the evaluative process to be perfected any more than for any other discipline that, like education or, indeed, medicine, is in a constant state of evolution.

In an oversimplistic sense, a sign near a frozen pond stating, "Danger, Thin Ice, Keep Off!" may save lives. Is this simply "informative" or "educational?" Studies could be made to determine the numbers who died falling through ice, the onset of freezing weather in the area, etc. The educational evaluation process would, however, concern itself with why people persist in skating on thin ice despite warning signs and why people ignore the signs. Is there a better way of warning the skaters? While information, per se, is a vital first step in saving lives, it may not be sufficient to change behavior, which is one of the goals of education for improving diabetes care.

While this may appear to be ridiculous analogy, in much of the world there is little or no information available to diabetics. Many do not know the differences in insulin, for example, nor its proper use, action and how to prevent or treat hypoglycemic reactions. It seems important to teach with whatever resources are available, meanwhile inserting systems of evaluation in order to continually improve educational processes.

GLOBAL PROBLEMS AND THE INFLUENCE OF EDUCATION

The Developed Nations

Much of what has been discussed, except for basic principles of education, may be useful in only a portion of the developed world. One cannot ignore the great bulk of the world's population in discussing education, since there is still opportunity to greatly impact world diabetes. The "developed" nations (those in most of Europe, North America, Australia, New Zealand, Japan, etc.) have the ability and resources to help themselves educationally if they should choose to do so and if the priorities are established. What about the rest of the world's estimated population of 4,321,000,000 persons with its increasing number of diabetics? For example, the ASEAN* nations of Thailand, Singapore, Indonesia, Malaysia and the Philippines encompass 265,000,000 persons in addition to about one billion Chinese and three-quarters of a billion inhabitants in India who have enormous health problems especially with chronic conditions. Yet somehow this tremendous mass of suffering humanity escapes the attention of the rest of the world except on the rare occasions when a television spectacle brings this briefly into our homes.

The Developing Nations

How does one define "Developing Nations"? There are numerous definitions measured by different standards and the terms are confusing because "developing nations," "non-aligned nations," and "Third World," etc., are sometimes incorrectly used interchangeably because the non-aligned designation is political rather than economic. For example, the Institute for Developing Countries in Zagreb lists 114 developing nation members and these are further divided into United Nations members, OPEC members, least developed countries, sea-less countries, and island countries, etc.[87] The World Bank[88] divides the developing countries on the basis of the 1975 gross national product (GNP) per capita into low-income countries with per capita incomes of $300 (U.S.) and below and middle-income countries with per capita incomes of above $300 (U.S.). They are further divided into those countries which are oil exporters, the industrialized nations, the centrally planned economies (CPE), and other divisions based on GNP and financial status. In general, economists tend to group countries according to their realized national income per capita as developed, medium developed, and less developed

*ASEAN = Association of South East Asian Nations.

countries. Other means of classification as developing nations include the literacy rate and also access to raw materials.[89] Unfortunately, the great
bulk of the world's population that continues to
burgeon is, by any standard, the poorest portion
of the world. The World Development Report for
1981 estimated that about 750,000,000 people live
in absolute poverty and that the total will increase
by the end of the century. Of the so-called 30 poorest nations on earth, 20 are in Africa and the others
are scattered around the world from Yemen to
Haiti. These have 207,000,000 people with a des-
perate future.[90]

There are differences which also divide many of
the "developing nations" into poor, poorer, poorest. For example, the life expectancy in years is
age 45 in the least developed countries; age 60 in
others; and age 72 in the developed nations. The
public health expenditure is $1.70 (U.S.) per capita
in the poorest, $6.50 in the more developed and
$244 in developed countries.[91] These problems
have an obvious influence on public health problems, communicable diseases, malnutrition and increases in population which overwhelm the limited
resources, particularly since the available medical
services often are concentrated in urban areas.[92]
Meanwhile, the population of the world grows,
with a possible 5.3 billion in 1990 and an estimated
6 billion by the year 2000. It is apparent that while
it is important for most of the world, diabetes is
not the *most* important problem at this time. However, diabetes is being used as a model by the
World Health and other organizations because it is
one of the more identifiable chronic illnesses, is
worldwide, and moreover is a disease for which
education may give the most aid per dollar outlay
in alleviating these problems.

Diabetes in Developing Nations

Diabetes is not only a disease of the affluent
because as rapidly as adequate food and increased
living standards occur, diabetes reaches into all
nations. The global overview of epidemiology dealt
with in Chapter 2 shows an over-all prevalence rate
of diabetes in the age group of 15 years and above,
at about 2%. This increases to 4 to 7% if the population is restricted to 40 years and older.[93]

Bajaj notes that not all of these persons have
classical diabetes. For example, calcific pancreatic
diabetes, common in many developing nations,
may be due to intake of tapioca (cassava) tuberous
root.[93] It is also possible that a deficiency of dietary
fiber may lead to a noninsulin-dependent diabetes.[94] Furthermore, over-nutrition and obesity
can influence a population where heredity and genetic predisposition provide a background. For example, those Indians who have migrated to other

parts of the world and enjoy modern urban facilities
have an increased prevalence of diabetes mellitus.[93]
The projected prevalence of diabetes in the developing countries during the next two decades is
likely to show a disproportionate increase. However, the problems of improved health go beyond
diabetes since diabetes is only one marker of decreased health opportunities for the developing
world. The World Health Organization (WHO) has
set as its goal, endorsed by 150 member nations,
"Health for all by the year 2000." Some people
feel that this is a cruel hoax that cannot be
achieved,[95] citing that "the cost of a massive and
concerted World Health diabetes program would
be between $12 and $20 billion over a period of
20 years. This is roughly what is now spent on
defense in less than 2 weeks." Even the cost of
safe water and sanitation is almost beyond comprehension because this requires an investment in
the range of $150 to $650 per capita in areas where
the average per capita income is less than a total
of $200.[96]

However, for developing as well as for developed nations, diabetes care will not improve until
a state of better general health is achieved. The
first World Conference on Primary Health Care
which took place in Alma-Ata (USSR) in 1978[97]
under the joint auspices of WHO and UNICEF,
agreed that developing countries must improve
their primary health care systems in a realistic general national plan, because there is no way to insure
proper diabetes care without generally improved
health. For example, the diabetes death rate is
higher in Chile than in the United States, and also
the rate of tuberculosis in that country is as it was
in the United States some decades ago. Many of
these problems relate to malnutrition. In Ecuador
(population 8 million persons, est. 1978), the Ministry of Public Health states that more than 750,000
children suffer from some degree of malnutrition
as do many adults.[98] There is then a link between
poverty, malnutrition, infections such as tuberculosis, and eventually diabetes.

Role of Organizations in Education

While the fight against diabetes must continue
in many ways, one of the most productive is education. The more people know about diabetes, the
better they will be able to fight it. Information and
education at all levels can therefore help to promote
both early detection and proper care. It is also true
that those areas with a great lack of resources need
organizational help. Calderon[99] warns that in modern diabetes care, "the use of increasingly sophisticated and expensive machinery is imposing a
heavy burden on the very limited health budgets
for diabetes throughout Latin America." Any prog-

ress in the fight against diabetes requires government help in those places where often less than 15% of the rural population and other underprivileged groups have access to adequate health services. In diabetes care in those countries, education must be part of the general health structure. Knowledge is particularly needed in some of the developing countries where the physician/population ratio is about 1 per 10,000. For example, the ratio is about 1 physician per 14,500 population in Indonesia and about 1 per 15,415 in Tanzania. Efforts in education are complicated by varying degrees of illiteracy. The adult literacy rate is as low as 10% in Ethiopia, 26% in Bangladesh, and 30% in Kenya. Educational efforts, therefore, must be bold and imaginative to make any impact. Recommendations of the WHO Expert Committee on Diabetes Mellitus[100] call attention to the need for the establishment of special centers in developing countries to encourage learning. These activities must be aimed at the patient and especially at health care personnel, particularly where physicians are and will be in short supply. Indeed, WHO is attempting to organize these activities because diabetes with its global distribution and long-term complications becomes increasingly important now that acute infectious diseases are gradually coming under control.[101] A liaison with the International Diabetes Federation (IDF), which started under the presidency of Rolf Luft and continued under that of Albert Renold,[102] emphasized the training of health personnel (Joint Postgraduate Course in Diabetes, Nairobi, Kenya, December, 1978). In addition, symposia were conducted on health education and diabetes (Geneva, 1979), and programs in Health Care Delivery in Developing Countries, at Dubrovnik in 1979, and at Opatija (Yugoslavia) in 1982.

Because of the importance of this effort, the World Bank decided to lend money for health projects that are in accordance with WHO policies. Luft[103] emphasized that education is as essential in diabetes as drugs, diet and exercise, since the latter measures will be useless unless the patient has received adequate understandable instruction. He ended his plenary lecture at the New Delhi IDF Congress in 1976 with the challenge that "National associations must work now in conjunction with governmental departments, trusts and foundations; with leaders of clinical and basic sciences; and with and for the diabetic community to insure that facilities for training are made available so that the quality of life of the patient is consequently improved."

Possible Solutions

Since even developed nations have difficulty in facing the problems of education costs and allocation of resources, it is important that developing nations solve their problems with ingenuity and boldness in addition to seeking all the possible help that can be obtained. Lambo[104] states that "We in WHO have come to the conclusion that science and technology per se are not magic wands and that a judicious selection (of health and economic measures) can produce amazing results if properly applied." Technology per se is no longer the only solution.

A first step must be increased communication and interchange of medical and educational literature between the different countries, especially those with similar cultural roots. One problem has been the fact that education in diabetes matters has been funneled in many countries through small numbers of physicians, with the effect of developing a corps of "elite" physicians who are well informed in matters of diabetes at a world level. This is called the "funnel effect" because much information goes into the top of the funnel with little coming out the narrow bottom. The "funnel" must be inverted in order to broadcast needed information to the largest number of health care personnel. Calderon[90] has pointed out that the majority of physicians in many Latin American countries must rely on information they received at medical schools, even though these physicians must care for the great bulk of patients with diabetes.

In response to this need, the Joslin Diabetes Center, using Joslin and Harvard Medical School faculty, organized by Dr. Sebastian Rodriguez of Miami, and generously funded previously by U.S.V. Pharmaceutical and more recently by Pfizer-Latin America, organized programs on "Diabetes in Relation to General Medicine" for practicing clinicians of Latin America. The first of these was in connection with the University of Buenos Aires in 1971. Since then, the program has expanded to most of Latin America during the past 14 years. Visiting Joslin-Harvard staff were catalysts and most of the faculty were clinicians and researchers from each country. An international course of this type (*Phase 1*) is useful since it focuses on diabetes and raises the consciousness level of diabetes education. There have been 13 Latin American and a total of 20 such world-wide courses. These have stimulated a significant exchange at all levels between Latin American and North American institutions.

To decentralize diabetes education from the capital city and make it available for physicians of the regional medical schools, Drs. Joseph Garcia-Reyes and Oscar Lozano-Casteneda organized *Phase 2* in Leon, Mexico at the University of Guadalajara. This resulted in the development of Spanish language videotape sessions to update diabetes education in areas far from the main centers. *Phase 3* of this educational effort will extend diabetes education further into distant rural areas with small teams of physicians, who will make rounds in hospitals, meet the staffs, and close the educational gap between the university and sparsely settled regions, hoping to improve diabetes care in even the smallest hamlets.

There must be increased use of "traditional doctors" who can be given further training in countries where there is a paucity of modern medical facilities. WHO monitors claims concerning the efficacy of certain traditional systems of medicine and medications, and is considering ways to train existing health workers to a level at which they can provide acceptable care. Given the meager financial resources of developing nations, apparently unorthodox solutions will have to be used if the goal of improved health for most or all of the world by the year 2000 is to be approached.

Another possibility would be for contiguous developed nations to "adopt" or "couple" with developing nations to share resources and information, and certainly developing nations must as far as possible cope with their own needs. In Yugoslavia, Prof. Zdenko Skrabalo and associates are developing a model program not only to educate and treat the diabetics in that country of 22 million, but also to foster medical education and technological advances among developing nations.

It is in the developing countries that education can have its greatest impact in teaching preventive medicine and early care. They may have the opportunity to slow down and divert the plague of diabetes before it greedily consumes the resources of these nations. Prevention is always less costly than rehabilitation.

But important as is money to fund education, imagination and new ideas have found a home in some of the less affluent countries that have developed ingenuity in coping with their education problems. Jackson[105] cited some of the excellent methods developed in some of these countries. He noted excellent 3-minute films for teaching in Cuba, after which nurses and dietitians answered questions. In Egypt, displays of plastic foods gave guidance about meals. In the Dominican Republic, small groups of patients cluster around nurse educators and receive a remarkable amount of information without much visual aid material. In Bogota, Colombia, a dedicated group of volunteers not only provide teaching to groups of patients, but also look after particular districts of the city, and persons of means are encouraged to "adopt" a juvenile-onset (Type I) diabetic, providing insulin for this patient whose very life depends on it. Singapore has done an outstanding job in communi-cations since its journal "Disbet" is produced in English, Chinese, Malay as well as another dialect, Tamil. In the Netherlands, Pelser and Groen organize small groups of diabetics who educate each other. Certainly there is no one ideal educational method. While the Diabetes Treatment Unit at the Joslin Diabetes Center may be a good model for some countries, in many areas the educational forms must be designed to meet greater needs and sparser resources. Nonetheless, even the simplest education forms can save lives.

The necessary steps are: (1) to raise the index of suspicion and diabetes awareness for detection and early care; (2) early and immediate education of health personnel; (3) education of all diabetics with at least survival information. This can succeed only if these countries have access to basics such as testing materials, insulin, etc., While there will not be enough physicians in the near or intermediate future for many of these countries, an infrastructure of health educators, nurses, dietitians or, as in Kenya, well-trained nonprofessional health associates, can teach and handle many needs. As important as is education for the highly developed, industrialized areas of the world, it can be more effective and less costly in the developing countries.

SUMMARY

Everyone admits that education is vital, important and useful in diabetes. Yet, while agreeing with its importance, there is a relatively small expenditure of available funds in this area. Former United States President Carter[106] stated "It is time for us to get back to the basics. The basis of any health care system is to care about people and prevent disease or injury. In recent years we (U.S.A.) have spent 40¢ out of every dollar on hospitalization. . . yet we have spent only 3¢ on disease control and prevention, less than one-half cent on health education, and one-quarter of a cent on environmental health research." Education, therefore, must depend on support from groups who understand its value and necessity. Of course, the educators also have a responsibility to prove unequivocally that health education is a good financial investment as well as a moral obligation to help others. Fragments of evidence suggest this is true but until there is better evidence that investment in this course does indeed ultimately save considerable money and suffering, the difficulties of supporting the health education system will continue.

It must also be clearly understood that "education" does not mean the same thing to everyone. There is no one system that will suffice for even the United States, to say nothing of the whole world. However, since the evidence of the absolute necessity for the education of the diabetic is so impelling, there can be no excuse for neglecting this essential part of treatment of diabetes, utilizing whatever resources are available. At stake is the very survival of the patient.

How much education? Dr. Elliott P. Joslin was fond of quoting Isadore, Archbishop of Seville (c. 570–636): "Learn as if you were to live forever. Live as if you were to die tomorrow."

REFERENCES

1. Education. In: WHO Expert Committee on Diabetes Mellitus. Second Report. Technical Report Series 646. Geneva, World Health Organization, 1980, p. 58.
2. American Hospital Association: A patient's bill of rights. 840 North Shore Drive, Chicago, Ill. 1975.
3. Assal, J.P., Martin, D.B.: Management of juvenile diabetes mellitus. In: J.G. Cull, R.E. Hardy (Eds.): Counseling and Rehabilitating the Diabetic. Springfield, Charles C Thomas, 1974, p. 40.
4. Cochran, H.A., Jr., Marble, A., Galloway, J.A.: Factors in the survival of patients with insulin-requiring diabetes for 50 years. Diabetes Care 2:363, 1979.
5. Deckert, T., Poulsen, J.E., Larsen, M.: Prognosis of diabetics with diabetes onset before the age of thirty-one. II. Factors influencing the prognosis. Diabetologia 14:371, 1978.
6. Williams, T.F.: The need for diabetes education. In: G. Steiner, P.A. Lawrence (Eds.): Educating Diabetic Patients. New York, Springer Publishing Co. 1981, pp. 3–11.
7. Miller, L.V., Goldstein, J.: More efficient care of diabetic patients in a county-hospital setting. N. Engl. J. Med. 286:1388, 1972.
8. Runyan, J.W., Jr.: Decentralized medical care of chronic disease. Trans. Assoc. Am. Phys. 86:237, 1973.
9. Runyan, J.W., Jr.: The Memphis Chronic Disease Program: comparisons in outcome and the nurse's extended role. J.A.M.A. 231:264, 1975.
10. Williams, T.F.: Health services research and diabetes. Diabetes Care 2:237, 1979.
11. Geller, J., Butler, K.: Study of educational deficits as the cause of hospital admission for diabetes mellitus in a community hospital. Diabetes Care 4:487, 1981.
12. Davidson, J.K., Alogna, M., Goldsmith, M., Borden, J.: Assessment of program effectiveness at Grady Memorial Hospital—Atlanta. In: G. Steiner, P.A. Lawrence (Eds.): Educating Diabetic Patients. New York, Springer Publishing Co., 1981, pp. 329–348.
13. Kilo, C., Dudley, J.D.: Kilo Diabetes Research Foundation, St. Louis, Mo.: Personal communication. Dec. 14, 1981.
14. Krall, L.P.: Pourquoi éduquer les diabétiques? In: M. Rathery (Ed.): Journées Annuelles de Diabetologie de L'Hotel-Dieu 1976. Paris, Flammarion Medicine-Sciences, 1976, pp. 71–78.
15. Insurance for outpatient education. Diabetes Dateline 3:2, March/April, 1982.
16. Nordberg, B., King, L.: Third-party payment for patient education. Am. J. Nurs. 76:1269, 1976.
17. Nordberg, T.: Qualifying for third party reimbursement: two case histories. Diabetes Educator. 21, 1977.
18. Patient education programs. In: Medicare Regulations Regarding Patient Education. #27.201 and #27.202, March, 1976, pp. 9025–9026.
19. Thomas vs. Hutchinson, California, Superior Court, Sacramento Co., Docket No. 221636, 1974. (malpractice suit)
20. Analytical Research Service Co.: Physicians' Interest/Activity in Diabetes. Prepared for: American Diabetes Association. Oct. 1977.
21. Kessner, D.M.: Diffusion of new medical information. Editorial. Am. J. Publ. Health 71:367, 1981.
22. Sussman, E., Tsiaras, W., Soper, K.: Physician diagnosis of diabetic eye disease. Diabetes 30(Suppl. 1):33A, 1981.
23. Current status of continuing medical education. In: Report of the Council on Medical Education: C (I-80). Chicago, Illinois, American Medical Association.
23a. Kessner, D.M.: Diffusion of new medical information. Am. J. Public Health 71:367, 1981.
24. Czyzyk, A.: Diabetic problems in East European countries. I.D.F. Bulletin 27:14 Jan. 1982.
25. Hunt, J.A.: Diabetes and the family physician. I.D.F. Bulletin 26:3 June, 1981.
26. Bryan, T., Huffman, B.L., Kahn, G., et al.: Is patient education alive and well? Patient Care Feb. 15, 1982, pp. 227–243.
27. A.R. Van Son (Ed.): Diabetes and Patient Education: A Daily Nursing Challenge. New York, Appleton-Century-Crofts, 1982.
28. Editorial: The place of nurses in management of diabetes. Lancet 1:145, 1982.
29. Dudley, J.D.: The diabetes educator's role in teaching the diabetic patient. Diabetes Care 3:127, 1982.
30. Simonds, S.K.: Competency-based training for the diabetes educator. The Diabetes Educator, 5, Spring, 1978.
31. Felton, J.S.: Health education—A responsibility of the occupational health professional. J. Occup. Med. 19:344, 1977.
32. Krall, L.P.: The pharmacist's role in treating the diabetic. The Apothecary 92:21, Jan. 1981.
33. Serantes, N.A.: Education del diabetico. INDEN 6:26, 1981.
34. Watkins, J.D., Roberts, D.E., Williams, T.F., et al.: Observation of medication errors made by diabetic patients in the home. Diabetes 16:882, 1967.
35. Williams, T.F., Anderson, E., Watkins, J.D., Coyle, V.: Dietary errors made at home by patients with diabetes. J. Am. Dietetic Assoc. 51:19, 1967.
36. Gozzi, K., Morris, M.J., Korsch, B.: Gaps in doctor-patient communication; implications. Am. J. Nurs. 69:529, 1969.
37. Jackson, R.L.: Education of the parents of a child with diabetes. Nutrition Today, May/June, 1980, p. 30.
38. Guthrie, D.W., Guthrie, R.A.: The parents and education. The Diabetes Educator, March, 1975, p. 13.
39. Krall, L.P.: The direct and indirect members of the diabetic's universe. In: G. Steiner, P.A. Lawrence (Eds.): Educating Diabetic Patients. New York, Springer Publishing Co., 1981, pp. 252–259.
40. Steiner, G.: The nature of diabetes: etiology, pathophysiology, and clinical implications. In: Ibid., pp. 25–29.
41. L.P. Krall (Ed.): Joslin Diabetes Manual, 11th Ed. Philadelphia, Lea & Febiger, 1978.
42. Sims, D.: Please don't tell me what to do unless you tell me why: a diabetic speaks out. The Diabetes Educator, Winter 1977–78, p. 13.
43. Wysocki, M., Czyzyk, A., Slonska, Z., et al.: Health behaviour and its determinants among insulin-dependent diabetics. Results of the Diabetes Warsaw Study. Diabete Metab. (Paris), 4:117, 1978.
44. Czyzyk, A., Wysocki, M.: Education and motivation of the diabetic patient. IDF Bulletin 26:10, Oct. 1981.
45. Morreau, L.E.: Assessing and modifying patient motivation. In: G. Steiner, P.A. Lawrence (Eds.): Educating

Diabetic Patients. New York, Springer Publishing Co., 1981, pp. 133–145.

46. Premack, D.: Toward empirical behavioral laws: I. Positive reinforcement. Psych. Rev. 66:219, 1959.

47. Morreau, L.E.: Motivating patients toward self-management. In: D.D. Etzwiler, K. Hess, A. Hirsch, L. Morreau (Eds.): Education and Management of the Patient with Diabetes Mellitus, 2nd Ed. Elkhart, Ind., Ames Company Div. Miles Laboratories, Inc. 1978, pp. 18–26.

48. Alivisatos, J.G.: Personal communication.

49. West, T.E.T., Read, P., Camps, B., et al.: An out-patient study of compliance in insulin treated diabetic patients. (Abstract). Diabetologia 15:280, 1978.

50. Ley, P.: Toward better doctor-patient communications. In: A.E. Bennett (Ed.): Communications Between Doctors and Patients. Oxford, The Nuffield Provincial Hospitals Trust. Oxford University Press, 1976, p. 77.

51. Ellis, D.A., Hopkin, J.M., Leitch, A.G., Crofton, J.: "Doctor's orders": controlled trial of supplementary, written information for patients. Br. Med. J. 1:456, 1979.

52. Butt, H.R.: A method for better physician-patient communications. Ann. Intern. Med. 86:478, 1977.

53. Ajgaonkar, S.S.: Personal communication.

54. Sims, D.F.: The suggestions of a cooperative client. In: G. Steiner, P.A. Lawrence (Eds.): Educating Diabetic Patients. New York, Springer Publishing Co., 1981, pp. 12–20.

55. Davidson, J.K.: Grady Memorial Hospital counseling program for patients with diabetes mellitus. Patient Counseling and Health Education 1:38, 1978.

56. Heller, D.R., Unger, K., Malarick, C., et al.: Living with diabetes and kidney disease: a one-day patient symposium. The Diabetes Educator. Summer, 1981, p. 21.

57. Reith, S., Fraser, K.J., McEwan, C.: Education of diabetic patients and professional staff by videotape. The impact of television and an evaluation of its efficacy. (Abst.). Diabetologia 20:674, 1981

58. Werner, C., Dickinson, G.: The lecture in analysis and review of research. Adult Education. Winter, 1967, p. 86.

59. Barzansky, B., Foley, R.: Effective lecturing. When and how. Physician East. December, 1980. p. 22.

59a.J.-Ph. Assal, M. Berger, N. Gay, J. Canivet (Eds.): Diabetes Education. How to Improve Patient Education. International Congress Series No. 624. Amsterdam. Excerpta Medica, 1983.

60. Redman, B.: The Process of Patient Teaching in Nursing, 3rd Ed. St. Louis, C.V. Mosby, 1976.

61. Hess, R.M.: Setting goals for patient education. In: D.D. Etzwiler, K. Hess, A. Hirsch, K. Morreau (Eds.): Education and Management of the Patient with Diabetes Mellitus. Elkhart, Inc. Ames Company, 1978, pp. 13–17.

62. Verso, M.A.: This is how wo do it at. . . Diabetes Day Care: A method for diabetic education and control. The Diabetes Educator, Spring, 1978, p. 16.

63. Stevens, A.D.: Diabetes education program—Joslin Clinic, Boston. In: S. Steiner, P.A. Lawrence (Eds.): Educating Diabetic Patients. New York, Springer Publishing Co., 1981, pp. 263–271.

64. Stevens, A.D., Bradley, R.F.: The team approach to patient education and management. In. H. Rifkin, P. Raskin (Eds.): Diabetes Mellitus Vol. V. Bowie, Maryland, Robert J. Brady Co., 1981, pp. 145–152.

65. Cammarata, D.: Group interaction as a teaching method. The Diabetes Educator, Fall, 1976, p. 9.

66. Porter, S.F.: Simulation techniques applied to diet instruction. The Diabetes Educator, Spring, 1978, p. 11.

67. Hardie, J., McPherson, K., Baum, J.D.: Hospital admission rates of diabetic children. Diabetologia 16:225, 1979.

68. Laron, Z.: More on diabetic control. J. Pediatr. 92:340, 1977.

69. Laron, Z.: The role of education in the treatment of diabetic children. I.D.F. Bulletin, 26:20, June, 1981.

70. Hoffman, W.H., O'Neill, P., Khoury, C., Bernstein, S.S.: Service and education for the insulin-dependent child. Diabetes Care 1:285, 1978.

71. Kratzer, J.B.: The elderly diabetic: an educator's challenge. The Diabetes Educator, Fall, 1979, p. 11.

72. Grobin, W.: Role of the health professionals in managing diabetes in the aged. The Diabetes Educator, Fall, 1977, p. 5.

73. Bernstein, R.: Diabetes teaching program for senior citizens. The Diabetes Educator, June, 1975, p. 24.

74. Diment, P.E.: Education of the elderly diabetic in a holiday situation. I.D.F. Bulletin 26:7, October, 1981.

75. Krolewski, A., Czyzyk, A.: Factors influencing mortality and social status of diabetics. In: Abstracts of 28th Scientific Conference of Diabetologic Section of Polish Association of Internal Medicine, Lodz, 1979.

76. Redman, B.K.: Planning and evaluation of patient education. The Diabetes Educator, June, 1975, p. 11.

77. Doak, L.G., Doak, C.C.: Diabetes education for adults with low literacy skills. The Diabetes Educator, Winter, 1978–79, p. 9.

78. Anderson, R.S.: Teaching and management problems with indigent diabetic patients. Medical Tribune, November 1, 1963.

79. Assal, J-Ph.: Overall educational problems encountered by physicians and paramedical personnel. Presented at a symposium sponsored by the Swiss Diabetes Association and the International Diabetes Federation, Geneva, Switzerland Sept. 27, 1977. Symposium entitled: Patient Education Methods and Teaching Aids in Diabetes Mellitus.

80. Hulka, B.S., Cassel, J.C., Kupper, L.L., Burdette, J.A.: Communication, compliance, and concordance between physicians and patients with prescribed medication. Am. J. Pub. Health 66:847, 1976.

81. Schluneger, R.: Creative growth makes a difference. The Diabetes Educator, Summer, 1980, p. 31.

82. Martin, D.L.: Evaluation of health programs. In: G. Steiner, P.A. Lawrence (Eds.): Educating Diabetic Patients. New York, Springer Publishing Co., 1981, pp. 189–198.

83. Sibley, J.C., Sacket, D.L., Neufeld, V., et al.: A randomized trial of continuing medical education. N. Engl. J. Med. 306:511, 1982.

84. Chisholm, S.: Evaluation of the diabetic learner. The Diabetes Educator, Summer, 1978, p. 18.

85. Boutaugh, M.L., Hull, A.L., Davis, W.K.: An examination of diabetes educational assessment forms. The Diabetes Educator, Winter, 1982, p. 29.

86. Laugharne, E., Steiner, G.: Tri-hospital diabetes education centre: a cost effective, cooperative venture. The Canadian Nurse, Sept. 1977, p. 14.

87. Skrabalo, Z., and Komar, S.: Personal communication.

88. International Bank for Reconstruction and Development World Bank: World Development Report, 1979. Oxford, Oxford University Press, 1979.

89. Prof. J. Bajaj, India: Personal communication.

90. French, D.: Poorest of the poor. Forbes, July 20, 1981. p. 37.

91. Dark times for the young and vulnerable. The Economist, Dec. 26, 1981, p. 80.

92. Agarwal, B.L.: Rheumatic heart disease unabated in developing countries. Lancet 2:910, 1981.

93. Bajaj, J.S.: Delivery of health care for diabetics in developing countries. (Zagreb). June 1, 1980, p. 1.

See also:
Bajaj, J.S.: Epidemiology of diabetes in developed and developing countries. Diabetologia Croatica (Zagreb) *9* (Suppl. 1):33, 1980.

94. Anderson, J.W., Midgley, W.R., Wedman, B.: Fiber and diabetes. Diabetes Care *2*:369, 1979.
95. Taylor, C.E.: Health for all-most. Harvard Medical Alumni Bulletin, Summer, 1981, p. 36.
96. Hoet, J.: Health care in South America. I.D.F. Bulletin *27*:33, Jan. 1982.
97. Primary health care: International Conference on Primary Health Care, Alma-Ata, U.S.S.R., September, 1978, Geneva, World Health Organization, 1978.
98. Mendoza, M.: Desnutricion afecta a mas de 750 mil ninos ecuatorianos. El Comercio, Quito, Ecuador, Oct. 4, 1981, p. 1.
99. Calderon, R.: The special needs of Latin America in the field of diabetes. I.D.F. Bulletin *26*:15, October, 1981.

100. Recommendations. In: WHO Expert Committee on Diabetes Mellitus. Second Report. Series 646. Geneva, World Health Organization, 1980, p. 65.
101. Alberti, K.G.M.M.: The WHO Expert Committee on Diabetes Mellitus: a call for action (Editorial). I.D.F. Bulletin *25*:3, June, 1980.
102. Renold, A.E.: Report from the President: Closer collaboration of I.D.F. with the World Health Organization. I.D.F. Bulletin *26*:3, February, 1981.
103. Luft, R.: Extract from the Plenary Lecture: Diabetes an International Disease. I.D.F. Bulletin *22*:10, Jan. 1977.
104. Lambo, T.A.: A new world in the making. Delivery of Health Care for Diabetics in Developing Countries. 2:2, June 1, 1981.
105. Jackson, J.G.L.: Personal communication.
106. Quotation from former President James E. Carter. Medical World News, November 29, 1976.

24 Diabetes in Youth

Donna Younger, Stuart J. Brink, Donald M. Barnett,
Samuel M. Wentworth, Joan Leibovich, and Paul B. Madden

Children with diabetes participate in one of the most dramatic achievements of modern medicine. There are people alive today who developed insulin-dependent diabetes more than 60 years ago at a time when the prognosis was for 6 to 24 months of progressive wasting until coma and death.

Prior to the development of antimicrobial agents, the discovery of insulin prolonged the mean duration of life for the child with diabetes to 5 or 6 years. The use of sulfonamides and antibiotics re-

duced the threat from overwhelming infection markedly, improving the life expectancy of the youngster with diabetes to several decades.[1] Since these dramatic turning points in medical history, however, progress has been painfully slow. Although insulin is now used more effectively, the outlook is still unpredictable even with the best of current practices. Although examples of fulfilled adulthood offer encouragement to both physicians and patients, all too often the blight of diabetes strikes during the prime of life with an unrelenting series of increasing disabilities leading to death. Faced with the present statistics on the morbidity and mortality of Type I (insulin-dependent diabetes (IDDM), the challenge to medical science is clear: to devise means for prevention or early cure. In the indefinite interim until these urgently hoped-for goals have been reached, the corresponding challenge to medical practice is to meet the needs of the patient and family, encouraging the most effective use of current methods of treatment even though cumbersome and woefully imperfect.

This chapter begins with a discussion of the disease—its prevalence, etiology, diagnosis, association with other conditions, and clinical course—and then turns to present management practices. Throughout, there is emphasis on the special physical and emotional factors that operate when diabetes affects the young.

PREVALENCE

Diabetes mellitus is the most common endocrine disorder of childhood and adolescence. In 1973, 13 children per 10,000 under the age of 17 in the United States had known diabetes.[2] One may estimate, therefore, that approximately 86,000 of the 66 million children under age 17 in the United States have diagnosed diabetes.[3] This is about 2% of patients of all ages with known diabetes, assuming conservatively that about 2% of the population has known overt diabetes. On the basis of a survey of children of school age in Minnesota in 1975, the prevalence of diabetes mellitus was found to be 1 per 529 students (1.89 per 1,000), 95% of whom were receiving insulin.[4]

Epidemiologic studies concerning diabetes in the young in the United States and Canada have shown an annual incidence that ranges from 6 to 12.1 cases per 100,000 per year, with an average of 8.8.[5,6] Admittedly, some of these are flawed by the variety and inadequacy of reporting systems. The highest incidences are reported in Scandinavian countries where there is a formalized method of reporting health statistics.

Type I diabetes occurs almost equally in males and females. An unpublished study of 1246 patients with onset before the age of 18, seen by one of us (S.J.B.) at the Joslin Clinic between 1978 and 1982, revealed 614 males and 632 females (1:1.03) (Fig. 24–1). A multi-centered study which summarized experiences at the Pittsburgh Children's Hospital, the University of Texas Hospital in Galveston, the University of Florida Hospital in Gainesville, and the Melbourne (Australia) Children's Hospital, reported a male:female ratio of 1.2:1 among Type I diabetics.[7]

There is a higher incidence of diabetes in more industrialized societies.[8] The increased availability of medical care and biochemical testing services have been suggested as contributing to the frequency of known diabetes.

ETIOLOGY

Despite its prevalence among children, many facts about insulin-dependent diabetes remain un-

clear. Perhaps most elusive is its etiology. A great deal of investigaton centers on this point, resulting in a nearly constant flow of new information.

Several factors influence the risk for development of diabetes. A Montreal study found the risk for diabetes in siblings of diabetic children to be approximately 15 times higher than in a control population. If the child had a Type I diabetic sibling and parent, the risk factor was reported as about 45 times higher.[9] Interestingly, there is some increased risk to a child who has a Type I diabetic sibling and a Type II diabetic parent.[10] Studying the empirical risks in relatives of children with diabetes, Simpson hypothesized polygenic susceptibility to the phenotypic expression of insulin-dependent diabetes.[11,11a,11b] Priscilla White's survey of 1072 Joslin Clinic patients with 20 or more years' duration of Type I diabetes with onset under age 15, revealed that 18% had a diabetic grandparent, 14% had a diabetic parent, and 1% had a diabetic child.[12] One of the most significant studies in the epidemiology of diabetes is the twin study by Pyke et al.[13] which revealed only a 50% concordance in identical twins when the first twin developed diabetes before the age of 40 (in contrast to almost 100% concordance when the index twin developed diabetes after age 40). When diabetes developed in the second twin, it was usually diagnosed within 3 years of the first. A Joslin Clinic review of 15 families with multiple non-twin siblings with diabetes revealed an average time span

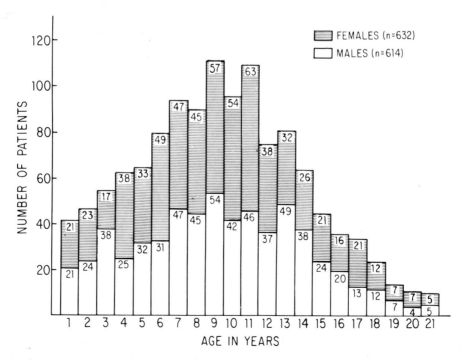

Fig. 24–1.   Age at first visit to the Joslin Clinic, of 1246 patients (614 males and 632 females), with onset of diabetes before age 18 (experience of S.J. Brink).

Table 24–1. Empiric Risk for Development of Type I Diabetes When First Degree Relative Has Known Diabetes*

Relative(s) with Diabetes	Approximate Risk for Development of Diabetes (percent)
A parent	2–3
A parent and one sibling	11–13
One sibling	2–6
More than one sibling	6–7
A child	1–3
None known	0.1

*Adapted from Wagener[10]

of 87 months between the diagnosis of the first child and the second.[13a]

Studies of the histocompatibility locus on the sixth chromosome have provided some help in understanding the patterns observed. Several studies have outlined the genetic and clinical heterogeneity of diabetes in children[14–16] (see also Chapter 4). The role of histocompatibility antigens (HLA), specifically B-8 and B-15, was first suggested by Nerup.[17] The chance of developing diabetes is increased 2.5 fold if one of these two loci is present.[18] It was quickly discovered that there was a genetic heterogeneity even within the HLA system, with the conclusion that B8 and B15 were not directly responsible for insulin-dependent diabetes but that there is a linkage disequilibrium with other genes at the HLA loci. The D, Dr, and Dw loci are also involved. D3, D4, Dr3, and Dr4 are found with increased frequency in the diabetic population, with Dr4 present in 56.3% of affected individuals.

Although different loci are associated with diabetes in different population groups, Sakurami et al. state that increased frequencies of Dr4 in diabetic patients are similar in Caucasians, American Blacks, and Japanese.[19] B8 has been associated with increased frequency of high islet cell antibody levels, lack of antibody response to exogenous insulin, potentially increased risk of microvascular

disease,[18] and coexisting coeliac disease.[20] On the other hand, B15 has been linked with increased insulin antibodies and earlier age at onset.[18] The exact HLA combination that results in the code necessary for Type I diabetes in childhood remains an area of active research. The differences in presentation, course, and potential involvement of non-genetic factors continue to cloud the picture.

Islet Cell Antibodies

In an effort to evaluate the role of HLA loci in the pathogenesis of diabetes, there has been a search for indicators of the involved immunopathology. Studies by Bottazzo,[21] Irvine,[22] Bright,[23] and Neufeld[24] confirm a high frequency of islet cell antibodies in newly diagnosed children with Type I diabetes. Neufeld reported 74% incidence of antibodies in the first three months of the diagnosis in Caucasians.[24] The incidence of antibodies at onset in Blacks is significantly lower (33%) according to this study. IDDM is less common and milder in African Blacks than in Caucasians. The incidence of antibodies in 33% of American Blacks with diabetes may reflect the racial mixture found.[24] The frequency of positive antibody tests declines with duration of diabetes to 5.5% after 10 years.[23] If duration and race are not taken into account, about 33% of all diabetic patients have positive islet cell antibody titers.[23,24]

Recent studies at the E.P. Joslin Research Laboratory were concerned with islet cell antibodies and beta cell function in an unusual set of monozygotic triplets and a set of twins initially discordant for insulin-dependent diabetes.[24a] The subjects were participants in an on-going prospective study of "genetic pre-diabetes" carried out since 1966 under the direction of J.S. Soeldner. One of the two nondiabetic triplets and the nondiabetic twin developed insulin-dependent diabetes after 8 and 36 years of discordance, respectively. Islet cell antibodies were detected in the triplet and in the twin 8 and 5 years respectively before the onset of

Table 24–2. Increased Risk of Diagnosed Diabetes (Any Type) by Age 19 or Less When a Living Relative (Proband) Has Known Diabetes*

Age of Proband at Onset (Years)	Relationship	Increased Risk of Diabetes for Relative Compared to Controls
0–19	Parent	X5
	Sibling	X15
	Children†	X22
≥20	Parent	No data
	Sibling	X7
	Children†	X5

*Adapted from Simpson[11b]
†Children with one diabetic parent (onset at any age). The risk is increased an additional 3-fold if both parents have diagnosed diabetes.

Table 24–3. Prevalence of Islet Cell Antibodies in Patients With Insulin Dependent Diabetes

	Percent
IDDM at onset	60–85
2 months after onset	50
1 year after onset	50
3 years after onset	20
IDDM; 1st-degree relatives	10
NIDDM	3
Controls	0.5–1.7
Other autoimmune endocrinopathies	about 8

*Adapted from Nerup[17]

overt diabetes. No islet cell antibodies were detected in the serum of the third triplet who remained healthy with as yet no evidence of diabetes 17 years after its development in the index triplet. These results suggested that there is a latent period for the development of overt diabetes during which islet cell antibodies are present, and suggest that antibodies may be useful as an early marker of beta cell destruction. Obviously, further studies are needed to establish definitely such predictive value. However, the results of this study are compatible with those of other workers.[24b]

In their studies of autoimmunity in the pathogenesis of Type I diabetes, Kaldany et al.[24c] of the Joslin Clinic Research Laboratory found that reinjected labeled, autologous lymphocytes were first distributed in the patients' lungs, liver, and spleen. In 72 hours they could not be found in the lungs and liver but were still in the spleen and also in the pancreas of two of three acute-onset patients. The authors suggest that this mononuclear cell infiltration may be a marker of insulitis and aid in the selection of those patients who might benefit from immunosuppressive treatment.

Further evidence of autoimmune aspects of the etiology of diabetes in children is found in the increased levels of antibodies to other endocrine tissues. The most common is thyroid, but elevated gastric parietal cell and adrenocortical antibodies are found as well. The majority of patients with elevated thyroid antibody titers remain euthyroid. In patients studied by Riley, 55% were euthyroid, 7% were hyperthyroid, and 38% hypothyroid.[25]

Seasonal Variation in Onset

A seasonal variation in onset of Type I diabetes in children was first reported by Adams in 1926.[26] Several studies since that time have confirmed the observation that the diagnosis of diabetes in children is more commonly made during the winter than the summer.[27] This observation was one of the factors which prompted speculation that there may be environmental influences that precipitate dia-

betes in children. The seasonal variation in onset has led to the epidemiologic search for an association between infections and the onset of diabetes in children[28–33] (Table 24–4). Strang first reported 1864 cases of diabetes developing in the wake of clinical mumps (epidemic parotitis). Mumps continues to be considered as a possible etiologic agent.[29] The onset of diabetes has also been linked to congenital rubella,[34] infectious hepatitis,[35] and Coxsackie viruses.[36,37] Studies of viral involvement in the pathogenesis of diabetes have included the use of Coxsackie,[38] encephalomyocarditis,[39] and Venezuelan encephalitis[40] viruses in animal models. Interest in the relationship between viral infections and the pathogenesis of human diabetes remains high because of the obvious potential for prevention or early intervention.

Gleason et al.[33] examined the seasonal distribution of onset of insulin-dependent diabetes in 1142 Joslin Clinic patients (598 males and 544 females) who were less than 21 years of age at onset and had developed diabetes between January 1, 1964 and December 31, 1973. Significant peaks were noted during the first 5 months of the year with maximum in either January or February. The most pronounced seasonal variation was found in a subgroup of 129 diabetics less than 15 years of age with onset less than 2 months prior to diagnosis and with no family history of diabetes. Considerable variation in incidence from year to year did not correlate with fluctuations in the reported incidence in Massachusetts of aseptic meningitis, rubella, rubeola, or mumps. Preliminary analysis of results in a later study of 154 patients suggests no greater frequency of elevated antibody titers against Coxsackie B1-6, mumps, or cytomegalic virus than in a matched control group of siblings and close friends of the patients.

Effect of Other Variables on Onset of Diabetes

Several studies have correlated the onset of diabetes with periods of rapid growth (Fig. 24–3). Most reports describe the ages of peak incidence as just prior to the rapid growth at puberty. A smaller peak has been found around the age of 5 which corresponds to a less dramatic but definite period of rapid growth. Attempts to correlate the onset with changes in growth hormone secretion have not been successful. There is some theoretical speculation that the determining factor may be somatostatin rather than growth hormone.

A recent review by one of us (S.W.) of the records of Type I patients seen in the Joslin Clinic and others seen earlier in Indiana, showed a much less dramatic increase in onset at the ages shown in Figure 24–3. It is not clear whether this repre-

Table 24–4. Comparison of Incidence of Diabetes, Seasonal Peaks, and Ages at Onset in Six Populations

Study	West et al.[28]	Sultz et al.[29]	Bloom et al.[30]	Cristau et al.[31]	Wentworth et al.[32]	Gleason et al.[33]
Population	Montreal	New York	England Ireland	Copenhagen	Indiana	Massachusetts
Age Range of Patients Studied	<17 years	<18 years	<16 years	<30 years	<16 years	<21 years
Years Studied	1971–77	1948–72	1972–74	1970–74	1959–72	1964–73
Mean Annual Incidence	8.8	6.1–11.0	7.67	13.2		
Seasonal Peaks of Onset	November January		October	October January	November February	January March
Peak Age at Onset:						
Male	12 years	9–12 years	11–12 years	14 years	5 & 11 years	12 years
Female	11 years	9–12 years	10 years	12 years	10–11 years	10–13 years

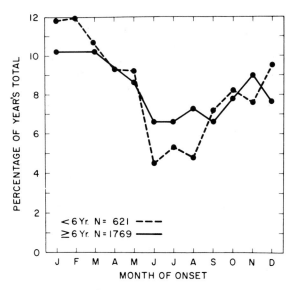

Fig. 24–2. Seasonal onset of IDDM in 2390 children in 3 U.S. cities (Pittsburgh, Gainesville and Galveston). (Fleegler et al.[7]) (Used by permission of the authors and publisher.)

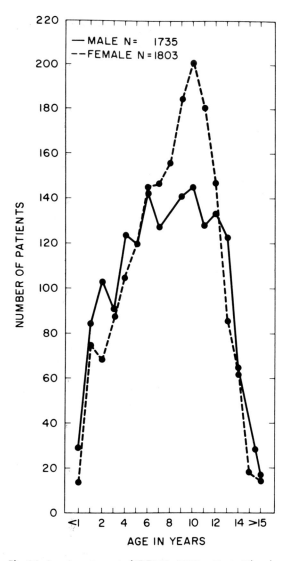

Fig. 24–3. Age at onset of IDDM in 3538 patients (Fleegler et al.[7]). Note that the peak coincides with prepubertal growth spurts. (Used by permission of the authors and publisher.)

sents an actual change in the pattern of onset or difference in the referral base of the younger patients.

A study of 624 youth-onset Type I patients at the Joslin Diabetes Center revealed that the incidence of diabetes increases in children of older mothers. This was particularly noticeable in families of large sibships. For example, in 69% of large families the diabetic child was fifth or sixth. The occurrence of diabetes corresponded more to maternal age than birth order.[41]

Even food additives have been suggested as a cause of ketosis-prone diabetes.[42] Offhand, this seems unlikely but is cited here because of its uniqueness and the intensity with which the study was carried out in Iceland.

These multiple associations suggest factors possibly involved in the onset of Type I diabetes in childhood. Although this does not negate the influence of genetic predisposition, it does complicate the search for non-genetic factors which may precipitate the onset of diabetes or protect an individual from it. Physical trauma, dietary history, or emotional stress have not been recognized as factors which precipitate the onset of diabetes in children.

In summary, the etiology of classical insulin-dependent diabetes in children may involve one or a combination of several of the following factors: (a) hereditary influences which result in malfunction of the beta cells; (b) viral insult to susceptible beta cells; (c) autoimmune reactions; (d) environmental factors such as growth, puberty or toxic

substances. Other factors that have been suggested include abnormalities of end organ receptor sites, and/or production of abnormal insulin.[43]

CLASSIFICATION

None of the terms that have been used in classifying diabetes has been entirely satisfactory. Even when limited to the diabetes that occurs during childhood years, there is a wide spectrum of severity. A joint effort of the National Diabetes Data Group (NDDG)[44] and the Lawson Wilkins Pediatric Endocrine Society[45] produced the following classification of diabetes in children and adolescents. Type I or insulin-dependent diabetes; Type II or non-insulin-dependent diabetes; impaired glucose tolerance; reactive hypoglycemia of early diabetes; diabetes neonatorum; and secondary disorders of glucose metabolism. The focus of this chapter will be primarily on Type I diabetes. For a more complete presentation of this classification, see Chapter 15.

Type I or Insulin-Dependent Diabetes Mellitus (IDDM)

This type of diabetes, previously called juvenile, juvenile-onset, ketosis-prone, and unstable ("brittle") diabetes, may begin with intermittent hyperglycemia but usually progresses quite rapidly to being markedly symptomatic until the course is modified by specific therapy. The severity of associated signs and symptoms generally relates to the extent of hyperglycemia and insulinopenia and their duration. Priscilla White's studies of juvenile diabetes at the Joslin Clinic included patients with onset under the age of 15. Other studies referred to in this chapter include those with onset up to age 20.

Type II or Non-Insulin-Dependent Diabetes Mellitus (NIDDM)

This type is occasionally seen in young people (Maturity Onset Diabetes in Youth; MODY). In contrast to typical juvenile-onset type diabetes, such patients generally are overweight, in their teens or older, and are members of a family with multiple cases of diabetes in a pattern consistent with autosomal dominant inheritance. Tattersall and Fajans[46] reported that of the young patients they studied with MODY, 85% had a parent with diabetes; direct vertical transmission of diabetes through three generations was present in 46% of their families; chemical diabetes was diagnosed by standard glucose tolerance testing in 53% of tested siblings; and even though they were young, most of the patients could be treated satisfactorily with diet or diet and oral hypoglycemic compounds. This has been noted particularly in those patients who are relatively hyperinsulinemic in proportion to the blood glucose levels.[47]

The youngsters with NIDDM initially vary in clinical course and pattern of inheritance. Progression to insulin-requiring diabetes occurs more often in those with delayed and subnormal serum insulin levels in response to a glucose challenge. Patients with "high" serum insulin response curves have only rarely progressed to insulin-requiring diabetes.[15]

Impaired Glucose Tolerance (IGT) (Chemical Diabetes, Asymptomatic Hyperglycemia)

This disorder is being recognized in young people with increasing frequency because of the following factors: (1) urinalyses and screening serum profiles, increasingly performed for pre-school and pre-camp yearly examinations, and as standard hospital admission evaluations; (2) increased sophistication and knowledge of diabetes by the general public; and (3) heightened awareness of potential diabetes in families with known diabetes.

Diabetes Neonatorum

The syndrome of transient diabetes mellitus of the newborn (congenital neonatal pseudodiabetes or paradiabetes mellitus infantum) first described in 1842 by Kitselle in his own son[48] is found in infants who are small for gestational age (SGA) and who develop an unusual pallor and an aged appearance. In spite of severe dehydration, such children remain remarkably alert and open-eyed.[49] Ramsey[50] was the first to document that hyperglycemia and glycosuria were part of this condition. These SGA infants characteristically develop polyuria which is followed by sudden weight loss, and yet only 30% have acetonuria.[49] Symptoms may develop as early as 1 day of age or as late as 6 weeks. Blood glucose levels at the time of diagnosis range between 250 and 2000 mg/dl. There is a family history of diabetes in only 35% of these infants; however, it has been reported that there may be an unusually flat line in the results of the glucose tolerance test of the mother during pregnancy.[51] A single case of macroglossia associated with transient diabetes has been reported.[52]

During the acute phase of diabetes neonatorum, insulin levels are either undetectable or are remarkably low in relation to the existing blood glucose level. Administration of tolbutamide and theophyllin do not result in an increase in insulin release.[53] Hypothalamic imbalance, adrenocortical imbalance, infection, insulin resistance and hypoinsulinism have been suggested as the causes of insulin lack. Based on several studies, it appears that the syndrome is due to delay in maturation of the beta cell and/or its adenyl cyclase-cyclic adenosine monophosphate system.[54] Since insulin has been identified as an intra-uterine growth factor,[55] the association between this syndrome and SGA might be expected. More recent work has suggested the growth retardation may actually be related to both insulin lack and decrease in the amount of somatomedin-C/insulin-like growth factor #1.[56] An unpublished report of a patient cared for by one of us (S.W.) follows.

A full-term male infant was born with an uncomplicated gestational history. There was no family history of diabetes and the mother (para 1, gravida 2) had no elevation of her blood glucose during the pregnancy. Although the child was noted to be small for gestational age at the time of birth, his initial neonatal course was uneventful. After 5 days in the hospital, the mother and child returned to their rural home. On the eighth day the mother began to be concerned that he was not thriving, having noticeably lost weight. Since the child was being breast-fed, the exact intake was not known, thereby tempering some of the initial concern about the lack of weight gain. Rather suddenly during the evening of the ninth day, the child became noticeably dry and lethargic. The parents took him to a neighboring city where a pediatrician discovered that the blood glucose level was 990 mg/dl.

The infant was admitted to a hospital and cared for in an Intensive Care Unit. He had arrived comatose, moderately acidotic, and was estimated to be 15% dehydrated. Intravenous infusion of insulin was started after an initial insulin bolus of 0.2 µ/kg had been given. The infusate was calculated to administer 0.05 µ/kg/hr. For the next 48 hours the child's blood glucose continued to improve as did his hydration and clinical condition. On the third day the child was able to return to oral feedings. On the fourth day, he was started on a dosage of regular insulin every 6 hours. This was later changed to two small doses of NPH insulin a day. Over a period of the next 15 months, the insulin dose was gradually decreased while his blood glucose control was carefully monitored at home with the use of a glucose meter. At 15 months of age, insulin was discontinued. For the next three months, periodic blood glucose tests were done at home. When values remained normal pre- and post-prandially, monitoring was discontinued.

Although the child was dramatically ill at the time of diagnosis, the response to insulin administration indicated remarkable insulin sensitivity. Treatment of hyperglycemia in such patients consists of multiple doses of regular insulin given subcutaneously or by constant intravenous infusion of insulin with appropriate fluids to correct dehydration. Characteristic of the syndrome is the temporary nature of the glucose intolerance. The need for insulin may be as short as 14 days or as long as 18 months.[49] As the dysmature beta cells complete their maturation, glucose tolerance improves progressively. The child passes through a period of delayed serum insulin response to a glucose challenge. During this phase the increasing growth hormone secretion would appear to be paradoxical to the progressive normalization of glucose tolerance. Follow-up of individuals with this syndrome over periods ranging from 3 to 25 years has revealed no patients who have developed diabetes.[49]

Separation between classical insulin-dependent diabetes (IDDM) of childhood and transient diabetes neonatorum is made by observing the clinical course. The diagnosis of IDDM is rare under the age of 6 months and the child is usually significantly acidotic at the time of diagnosis. The presence of hyperglycemia and dehydration with only mild to moderate ketonuria in a child under 6 months of age directs consideration to the syndrome of transient diabetes of the newborn.

Secondary Disorders of Glucose Metabolism

Some common and other uncommon clinical situations that should be considered before making the diagnosis of primary diabetes mellitus are listed below.

Acute Gastroenteritis and Hypernatremic Dehydration with Hyperglycemia.[57] Hyperglycemia occurs in as many as 50% of infants with acute vomiting and diarrhea associated with hypernatremia. Usually the serum sodium concentration is greater than 150 mEq/L and is accompanied by a moderately severe disturbance in acid-base status. The hyperglycemia varies widely in degree (from 130 to 180 mg/dl to 600 to 1200 mg/dl). Too rapid reduction of glucose levels by insulin may increase the already high risk of cerebral edema by causing rapid shifts in osmolality. Initially, therapy should be directed toward correcting the electrolyte and water deficits present in such infants. The hyperglycemia often is only a temporary metabolic phenomenon. If insulin is necessary usually only small doses are needed. The blood glucose should be monitored frequently.

Cystic Fibrosis. This is initially seen in childhood and may be complicated by secondary diabetes. Fibrosis develops around the islets and is associated with progressive carbohydrate intolerance which may require insulin therapy. Severe diabetes is an uncommon component of the syndrome and, even when insulin is needed, the diabetes in these patients is usually of the nonketotic type. With improved methods of treatment, children with cystic fibrosis now live well into the third decade, thus contributing to an increase in the incidence of diabetes. Close collaboration with the nutritionist is crucial for optimal control of the metabolic disturbances created primarily by the characteristic malabsorption.[58,59]

Nondiabetic Glycosuria. Renal glycosuria[60] is an asymptomatic euglycemic condition which should be distinguished from the nonspecific melituria associated with the Fanconi syndrome. It is a benign condition with no associated abnormality in glucose metabolism or insulin secretion. The diagnosis is usually made in the second decade of life.

During pregnancy or with starvation, there can be excessive ketosis and dehydration which, when superimposed upon renal glycosuria,[60] leads to diagnostic problems. See Chapter 15 for a more complete discussion of the nondiabetic meliturias.

ASSOCIATION OF CHILDHOOD DIABETES WITH OTHER CONDITIONS

Impaired glucose tolerance of variable severity is associated with certain other syndromes or conditions usually diagnosed in the childhood years. Neither the syndromes nor the diabetes associated with them are particularly common. Some of these conditions are listed below.

Diabetes Mellitus with Optic Atrophy with or without Deafness. Although this complex has been recognized for over a century, less than 50 cases have been reported in the literature.[61] The average age at onset of diabetes is 7.5 yr (range, 3 to 15), and that of optic atrophy, 10.8 yr (range 4 to 24). Deafness, if present, generally occurs subsequently. Variants of this syndrome include *diabetes insipidus with or without optic atrophy* (Wolfram's syndrome or DIDMOAD).[62]

Friedreich's Ataxia with Progressive Cerebellar and Spinal Cord Dysfunction. Diabetes may be present in as many as 20% of patients with this condition.[63] The mean age at onset of diabetes is 11.9 yr (range 8 to 14); the diabetes is typically of the insulin-dependent ketosis-prone type.

Refsum's Syndrome. This is another rare form of hereditary ataxia with onset late in childhood or adolescence. The clinical presentation is that of progressive cerebellar ataxia, distal weakness, sensory loss, retinitis pigmentosa, deafness, and ichthyosis with or without hypogonadism. Diabetes reportedly appears first.

Alstrom's Syndrome. This syndrome is characterized by infantile obesity, retinal degeneration, deafness, and slowly progressive chronic nephropathy, plus diabetes with insulin resistance. There may be associated acanthosis nigricans and scoliosis.

Laurence-Moon-Biedl Syndrome. This syndrome has a variable phenotype and includes obesity, mental deficiency, retinitis pigmentosa, polydactyly, and hypogonadotrophic hypogonadism, with or without diabetes.

Prader-Willi Syndrome. A complex of hypotonia ("floppy infant"), hypogonadism, hypomentia, and obesity (HHHO), this syndrome is associated with hyperphagia and small stature. Diabetes typically occurs in adolescence and closely resembles the stable non-insulin dependent, Type II variety. Allowing for the inherent problem of weight reduction in such patients, diet therapy may be all that is necessary to control hyperglycemia. Insulin may be needed if caloric reduction cannot be enforced.

Werner's Syndrome. This syndrome is a phenomenon of extremely premature aging with baldness, premature atherosclerosis and its associated complications, cataracts, short stature, hypogonadism (both sexes), along with a mild relatively insulin-resistant diabetic state in 50% of all such patients.

The Siep-Lawrence (Bernardinelli) Syndrome.[64] This condition, with its congenital total lipodystrophy, should be distinguished from the non-inherited partial and total lipoatrophies. At birth or soon thereafter, such children have many endocrine and metabolic abnormalities, including accelerated growth, lack of adipose tissue, muscle hypertrophy, hypertriglyceridemia, polycystic ovaries, and acanthosis nigricans, in addition to insulin-resistant, non-ketotic diabetes. Patients may be retarded and generally have hepatomegaly with progressive hepatic insufficiency leading to an early death. Partial lipodystrophy is a different complex seen in females with onset of diabetes between 5 and 15 years of age, with hepatomegaly and a high frequency of glomerulonephritis and hydronephrosis.

Klinefelter's[65,66] Turner's,[67] and Down's[68] Syndromes. These syndromes have been associated with an increased frequency of chemical and overt diabetes as well as a higher likelihood of positive thyroid antibodies and clinical thyroid disease, including goiter and hypo- and hyper-thyroidism.[69] These three entities and their variants suggest a genetic link with chromosomes other than the sixth and its histocompatibility locus. They also provide some insight into the factor(s) governing the immune process. Diabetes may occur in as many as 8% of those with Klinefelter's. As many as 20% of patients with Turner's syndrome may have abnormal carbohydrate tolerance and 50% may have positive thyroid antibodies. Data associating diabetes and/or impaired glucose tolerance with Down's syndrome are currently considered conflicting and incomplete. They may have more to do with maternal age as reported from studies at the Joslin Clinic.[41]

Drugs. Diabetes may also be seen as a result of the treatment of the child for some other condition. Two of the drugs which may precipitate diabetes in the child are corticosteroids[70] and L-asparaginase.[71] Since these are frequently used together in the treatment of leukemia, there is a high risk in this group[72] for the development of a diabetes-like state. Less frequently, other drugs may cause abnormalities of glucose tolerance which are usually less severe. These include the thiazides, diazoxide, estrogens, oral contraceptives, glucagon, epinephrine and cogeners, thyroid hormones, chlorpromazine, diphenyhydantoin, ethacrynic acid, indomethacin, isoniazid, lysergide (LSD), marijuana, nalidixic acid, nicotinic acid, and pentamidine.

DIAGNOSIS

Oral glucose tolerance tests (OGTT) are rarely needed to diagnose Type I diabetes in children because of characteristic symptoms, glycosuria with or without acetonuria, or random blood glucose levels greater than 200 mg/dl. However, a glucose tolerance test (GTT) may be helpful to delineate the status of a youngster with other forms of glucose intolerance. In carrying out an OGTT, care must be taken to prepare the patient properly and to follow the standardized protocol for the test (see Chapter 15). Prior to giving the loading dose of glucose (1.75 g/kg of ideal body weight up to a maximum of 75 g), the fasting blood glucose should be determined. If it is 140 mg/dl or greater (serum or plasma value), a complete GTT may be unnecessary and, in fact, may be contraindicated. In selected patients, it may be helpful to obtain plasma insulin levels as well as those for glucose during a GTT.

Glycosylated hemoglobin (HbA$_1$) (discussed in Chapters 10 and 15) may provide a valuable, easy means to screen for glucose intolerance. Through its use along with a fasting and post-prandial blood glucose, significant hyperglycemia may be documented without subjecting the child to an entire GTT. If the results are equivocal, a complete GTT may be obtained. O'Sullivan has stated that it is possible to predict from the results of an OGTT during pregnancy which mothers at risk for diabetes are likely to progress to overt diabetes over the long term. [73] Most investigators believe, however, that with children, neither the OGTT nor the HbA$_1$ in borderline situations provides an accurate method for estimating risk of future development of diabetes in the child.

Early in the course of juvenile-onset diabetes mellitus (JODM) and over a period of years in maturity-onset diabetes in the young (MODY), the impairment of glucose tolerance may be characterized by waxing and waning, showing spontaneous improvement or deterioration of metabolic integrity. This does not happen later in the course of JODM, a fact that professionals sometimes forget when bright pre- to early adolescents decide to demonstrate that they have achieved a late and total remission. Because of the variable prognosis for patients with impaired glucose tolerance or early diabetes progressing to overt diabetes, therapeutic programs designed to forestall total insulin deficiency are difficult to assess. Hemoglobin A$_1$ or A$_{1c}$ determinations may allow better assessment of hyperglycemia during the weeks preceding diagnosis.

CLINICAL COURSE

Priscilla White has characterized five distinct phases of diabetes in the child. They include (1) the acute onset; (2) remission or lessening; (3) intensification; (4) total diabetes; and (5) total diabetes compounded. [12,74]

Acute Onset

The onset of diabetes in children is usually symptomatic. Commonly, it is reported to the physician that symptoms have been present for only a few days or weeks, although in some cases, for many months. Parents and children can often name the day or week of the onset of symptoms. Polydipsia is extreme and may lead to enuresis. The appetite becomes insatiable, mainly noticeable at night. When diabetes becomes decompensated, loss of appetite, nausea and vomiting occur. Abdominal pain and cramps in the legs are common complaints. Fatigue is conspicuous. Failure in school may replace satisfactory achievement. Vision may become blurred. The child may be irritable. The physical signs observed most frequently are those of weight loss and dehydration. The level of blood glucose at the time of diagnosis is generally markedly elevated, although increasing public awareness and routine biochemical health screening have led recently to diagnosis before the blood glucose levels are strikingly abnormal. The early course may be so rapid that ketosis, or even severe ketoacidosis with coma, may occur before the diagnosis is established. Ketosis with depression of the serum bicarbonate to less than 9 mEq/L was present in 15% of children at the Joslin Clinic at initial presentation.[74a] Despite the degree of chemical disturbance and acutely ill appearance, most children are alert and functioning at a fairly satisfactory level. Because of the potential for dangerously rapid deterioration within a day or two if appropriate treatment is not given, a child needs prompt medical attention at the first indication of glycosuria and/or hyperglycemia.

Remission of Diabetes

Within days, weeks or months after initiating therapy, from one-third to one-half of all children with newly diagnosed diabetes experience a marked lessening in the clinical and biochemical expression of the condition. Rarely, glucose tolerance may return to normal, indicating a complete remission. If total remission occurs, blood glucose levels remain normal on dietary therapy. In a majority of children there is a partial remission wherein responsiveness to sulfonylureas and biguanides has been noted. However, low-dose insulin therapy is usually continued. During this lessening phase, patients tend to have random blood glucose values within the normal range because of the appropriately variable secretion of endogenous insulin (which may be determined indirectly through the measurement of C-peptide levels).

A review of the records of 334 juvenile patients seen at the Joslin Clinic between 1953 and 1958 disclosed a remission in 100 of these. More boys than girls experienced a remission. The children least likely to have a remission were infants and prepubescent girls. Of the youngsters who experienced a remission, 42% were overweight, 30% were of standard weight, and 20% were underweight.[1] Brush reported similar statistics.[75] Vigorous initial treatment of the diabetes seems more likely to induce a remission than does a less aggressive approach. The termination of remission followed a growth spurt in 46% of the children, infections in 40%, poor control in 8%, puberty in 5%, and hypoglycemia in 3%. It may be that maintenance of normoglycemia during a remission prolongs somewhat its duration which usually varies from a few weeks to several months.[75a] The occurrence or absence of a detectable remission period seems of no prognostic value. This period is a single event within the first year after diagnosis, and does not recur. Apparent remissions later in the course require careful evaluation. Endocrine failure, such as hypothyroidism should be considered, but the most common cause of apparent late remissions relates to surreptitious manipulation of the insulin dose or inappropriate recording of the home monitoring tests. For a further discussion of remission, see Chapter 19.

Intensification and Total Diabetes

During the first several years of childhood diabetes, the clinical and biochemical evidence is consistent with the progressive loss of residual insulin production. A few youngsters, especially those whose diabetes started in infancy or early childhood, seem to have total diabetes (i.e., a total dependence on exogenous insulin to sustain life) from the beginning. Although clinically it would appear that within 1 to 5 years after onset of diabetes, most children show little or no evidence of endogenous insulin production, determinations of serum C-peptide following glucagon stimulation indicate residual beta cell activity, albeit slight, for a good many years. For example, Madsbad et al.[75b] reported that among 267 patients with onset of insulin-dependent diabetes prior to age 20, 56 or 21% had residual beta cell function. This was true in 25 or 65.8% of those with duration of diabetes up to 5 years, but in only 9 or 15.3% of those with duration of 5 to 9.9 years. Ludvigsson and Heding[75c] suggest that preservation of residual beta

cell function depends on early diagnosis of diabetes and prompt intensive treatment. See also the review article by Hoekstra, et al.[75d]

Clinically, the total diabetic state is characterized by rapid onset of ketosis should insulin be omitted for even a single day. There may be increasing episodes of night-time to early morning hypoglycemia in a patient who previously had satisfactory 24-hour control on a single dose of intermediate-acting insulin given before breakfast. Whether treated with a single daily injection or a split dose (two or more injections daily) from diagnosis, the insulin requirement per kilogram of body weight increases as does the variability of blood and urine tests for sugar, usually over a period of several years. Historically, this transition was documented in acute testing by loss of response to sulfonylureas[76] in most children with diabetes of one or more years' duration.

Total Diabetes Compounded

This is the term Priscilla White used to characterize the tendency of many juvenile patients with diabetes of relatively long duration to have fluctuations in blood glucose while being treated with what seems to be an optimal dosage of insulin and an appropriate diet. Increasing post-prandial hyperglycemia may occur although dietary habits are not changed. At the same time there is a greater tendency to unanticipated hypoglycemia, unexplained by variations in meals and/or exercise. Frequently there is increasing difficulty in recognizing early warning symptoms of hypoglycemia with resultant management problems, despite careful precautions taken by the patient. In other words, unstable diabetes becomes even more unstable. Some of these problems may be related to irregular insulin absorption and/or disposition. Variability in endogenous contra-insulin hormones may play a role.[76a]

TREATMENT

As indicated in earlier chapters, there is increasing evidence suggesting that long-term complications of diabetes may be minimized or postponed by successful management of hyperglycemia. As for any diabetic patient, insulin, diet, exercise, and general health maintenance measures must be integrated within the treatment program. There are, however, special considerations in planning diabetes treatment for the child. The diabetes care should be adjusted to the child's development and ever-changing level of responsibility. Proper attention must be given to the particular educational, psychologic, and emotional needs of the entire family, beginning as soon as diabetes is diagnosed. For treatment to succeed, the continuing cooperation of the parents and the child is essential. Current medical practices will be discussed first.

In many cases, because of the abrupt onset and acutely progressive nature of diabetes, it seems imperative to admit the child promptly to the hospital. However, if the family is considered able, the patient with minimal symptoms can be treated initially as an outpatient. This allows for adjustment of the treatment of diabetes without placing the child and family in the foreign, stressful environment of the hospital. Usually the family is instructed in urine and blood testing and given basic information about diabetes at the initial visit. Frequent subsequent visits are used to assess and expand skills and knowledge, to make necessary changes in insulin dosage, and to provide needed psychologic support to the entire family. The schedule of return visits varies from family to family but most are seen on a daily basis during this period of initial adjustment. If distance precludes this, hospital admission is usually advisable, preferably to an ambulatory in-patient unit that emphasizes education as intrinsic to optimal therapy. The frequency of visits is decreased once initial material is mastered and the family no longer requires such intensive support.

After the period of introduction to the details of diabetes and its treatment, the child may be admitted to a Diabetes Treatment Unit (DTU) (see Chapter 16), if such is available, for more intensive education and supportive milieu therapy. In this setting, the dose of insulin may be adjusted every 4 to 12 hours. Such alterations are made on the basis of capillary blood glucose levels before breakfast, lunch, and the mid-afternoon snack. If needed, additional tests may be made before the evening meal, before the bedtime snack, and during the middle of the night (to detect asymptomatic hypoglycemia). The careful monitoring of blood glucose facilitates the determination of the insulin doses, and expedites the individualization of an optimum treatment plan. It has been our experience that many children have better blood glucose patterns with two doses of insulin daily, within a short period of time after initiation of therapy. If results later indicate that insulin twice daily is no longer necessary, the second injection may be discontinued. However, many physicians find that continuing a twice daily insulin schedule facilitates optimal treatment later in the course of diabetes.

With children under 8 years of age it is extraordinarily helpful if a parent is admitted to the DTU as a guest. This allows for intensive instruction of the parent as well as avoidance of the trauma of separation for the child.

Diet

A Structured Nutritional Program. Good nutrition is certainly an important item in the treatment of the growing young person with diabetes. Any meal plan developed for children should be appropriate for age in types and amounts of foods and times of eating. This is particularly true when dealing with teenagers.

Quantitative vs Free Diet Approach. The limitations of the inflexible dosages of exogenous insulin currently prescribed for replacing variable amounts of endogenous insulin have resulted in decades of argument: whether one should prescribe diet with a quantitative approach in order to achieve a relatively stable eating pattern around which the doses of insulin can be planned; or allow the general eating habits for the family and the patient's appetite to determine the calories consumed daily. There are many other factors that determine the blood glucose concentration at any particular time, including the level of physical activity and all of the counterregulatory hormones. As a result, some physicians have concluded that the best approach is to allow youngsters to eat whatever others in the family are eating (except for sugar, sweets and pastries), taking frequent snacks throughout the waking hours to avoid hypoglycemia, and covering with insulin as needed.[77]

Unfortunately, the complex and subtle systems that balance hunger and satiety for the multiplicity of nutrients make it difficult for a patient to maintain a steady balance in the disordered metabolism of diabetes. It is our belief that in most young patients, a quantitative approach to nutrition promotes more stable blood glucose levels. One must, however, go beyond fixed dietary schedules such as those widely available on a printed single sheet of paper or in brief booklets. A thorough understanding of the nutritional content of foods and the ability to use this knowledge to adjust the food intake in relation to variable and unpredictable levels of physical activity, are achievements that can be accomplished only by continuing educational programs over a period of years. This does not obviate making treatment initially as simple as possible. To go from rules of grammar and memorizing vocabulary to fluency in a new language takes time. Similarly, using nutritional information effectively requires time and intense, ongoing education.

Modification of Traditional, Quantitative Formula. In prescribing diets, the traditional formula of 40% of the calories as carbohydrate, 20% as protein, and 40% as fat is modified to accommodate problems of individual patients. Furthermore, in the present day, in the hope of minimizing atherogenesis, the prescription is more apt to provide 45 to 50% of calories as carbohydrate, 20% as protein, and 30 to 35% as fat. One-fifth of each of these components is given for breakfast and a mid-morning snack, two-fifths are used for the mid-day meal and afternoon snack, and the remaining two-fifths for the evening meal and bedtime snack.

A study done at camps for children with diabetes, supervised medically by Joslin Clinic physicians, indicated that serum cholesterol and triglyceride levels could be reduced by emphasizing polyunsaturated fats within the diet prescription.[78] It is important to adapt the caloric prescription to the young patient's need for growth and weight gain. Initially a dietary program may be started with 1000 kcal for age one, plus 100 kcal for each additional year of age. The meal plan must be modified frequently for changes in the level of activity such as participation in athletics. There must often be two or more diets prescribed: one for the most active days of sports, another for less active school days, and others as needed for particular activity patterns. Nutritional programs must be monitored several times a year to adjust the caloric level for age, weight, height and level of activity and to maintain the patient's growth pattern along with normal isodromes.

Food is often a major problem for youngsters with diabetes.[79] Probably those who most commonly over-eat are adolescents. Over-eating begins with a tremendous calorie requirement for the active teenager with or without diabetes. Males do not seem to become obese while this readily occurs in teenage girls. In addition, some teens feel a need to prove to their peers that there is "nothing wrong" with them. Consumption of large amounts of food, particularly concentrated carbohydrates, is used to prove this point.

Counselling and open discussion of ways to reduce to an appropriate meal plan are integral parts of any dietary prescription in teenagers. A third factor in over-eating may be a fear of hypoglycemia, a complication which is dreaded by most adolescents. Holidays are difficult times for most children and adolescents with diabetes. Birthdays, Thanksgiving, etc., are common times of overeating in most households. Since this inability to take part in the celebration is often resented by young people with diabetes, we have found it desirable to permit planned over-eating on a few special occasions. Planning ahead for such times permits increasing the insulin dose prior to the increased eating, and scheduling an active period afterward. A holiday program which has seemed to work well with our patient population is to schedule the morning insulin and breakfast late (8:30 or so) and then eat a double or triple snack at about

11:30 AM, with the large meal at about 2:00 to 3:00 PM. Prior to the meal, a dose of regular insulin is given in an amount equal to 10 to 20% of the child's 24-hour insulin requirement. A well balanced meal is given with no restriction on quantities, and tastes of a small amount of concentrated carbohydrates are permitted. The evening dose of insulin, if used, is given at about 7:00 PM, followed by a double snack. This method permits the child to participate in the celebration of the holiday but prevents extreme swings in the blood glucose.

Insulin

Insulin Dosage. Because in newly diagnosed diabetes there may be considerable sensitivity to insulin, one should begin treatment on the day of diagnosis with small doses, preferably of regular insulin, increasing the amount as necessary. This cautious approach can avoid initial overtreatment. Even relatively mild symptoms of hypoglycemia early in the course of treatment can be frightening to the patient and family and consequently interfere with the most effective use of insulin for years and even decades thereafter.

In general, treatment begins with 0.25 unit of insulin per kg of body weight. If there is chronic ketosis, the dose may be up to 0.5 U/kg initially. (The treatment of decompensated diabetic ketoacidosis in children is discussed later in the chapter). The practice at the Joslin Clinic is to start intermediate acting insulin (lente or NPH) either immediately or the morning after initial treatment rather than trying to "cover the urine tests" with multiple doses of regular insulin beyond the first day of treatment. Being cautious during the first few days does not negate the goal of rapidly achieving blood glucose levels close to normal during the "onset phase" in hope of inducing a remission.[75a]

After the first day, the majority of children are treated with a mixture of regular and intermediate (lente or NPH) insulin. In instituting insulin treatment, we have found it necessary as a rule to increase the dose daily up to a plateau at about day 5 to 7, and then to decrease the dose gradually from about day 7 to 14. A decreasing requirement for exogenous insulin marks the beginning of a remission phase, but only rarely is the dose reduced to zero.

At the Joslin Clinic, treatment with insulin is usually continued during remission, even if only a token dose such as two units daily can be tolerated. Discontinuance of insulin at the time of remission and later necessary resumption when this phase subsides, seems to be associated with psychologic confusion for the patient and the family. In addition, it is thought that the incidence of increased insulin antibodies and overt insulin allergy may be related to a break in the continuity of insulin therapy. Children continue to be monitored with daily urine tests and occasional home blood glucose determinations during this period.

Treatment During "Total Diabetes." As the remission wanes, there is a decrease in the endogenous insulin supply as indicated by declining C-peptide levels and increased hemoglobin A_1 or A_{1c}. When this occurs, there is a gradual increase in insulin need. As the intensification to "total diabetes" occurs, insulin requirements increase to a level of 0.7 to 1.0 U/kg per day. This increase is usually gradual although it may be abrupt. During the intensification phase, many patients who have been successfully controlled with a single mixed dose or even a single injection of one type of insulin, will need an evening dose of insulin as well. This consists of regular or combined regular and intermediate insulins before supper, or only intermediate insulin before supper or at bedtime. In general, regular insulin is to be avoided at bedtime because of possible hypoglycemic episodes during the night. Diabetes management must be planned individually in order to achieve optimal results. The goal is to obtain blood glucose levels as close as possible to physiologic concentrations without significant hypoglycemia. Except in general terms, there seems to be no single ideal or "right" program for every patient or for any one juvenile patient over a long period of time. Rather, in each case one must carefully evaluate the degree of success obtained when the child is on a single or split dose schedule, using one (or usually two) types of insulin.[80] Using a mixture of intermediate- and short-acting insulins both morning and evening, approximately two-thirds of the total dose is given in the morning and one-third in the evening. These general rules must be modified to suit individual needs as determined by the blood glucose indices. Trends nationally and internationally appear to be toward this method of management.[81–83] Lente and NPH have been used essentially without preference as intermediate insulins at the Joslin Clinic.

Because of its very slow absorption from the injection site, ultralente insulin, combined with multiple doses of regular insulin, has been suggested in the treatment of children in order to provide more stable blood glucose patterns. The goal is, specifically, better blood glucose levels at night. However, the children we have evaluated on this type of program usually have not achieved the desired results, possibly because of (a) problems in making appropriate alterations of insulin dosages based on home monitoring of blood glucose levels; (b) variations in the duration of effect of ultralente insulin with differing injection sites; or (c) continued dietary noncompliance.

The timing of insulin doses must be adjusted to mealtimes and vice versa.[83a] Insulin should be given about 30 to 45 minutes before breakfast if regular insulin is being used. If the dose is delayed, an increase in the blood glucose during the first hours after arising may take place even if fasting is maintained.

After the young person is fully grown, the dose requirement may decrease somewhat. If the diet is not decreased as growth is completed, adolescent girls often become overweight or frankly obese. This contingency must be anticipated so that diet and insulin prescriptions may be tailored simultaneously to prevent the problem rather than correct it after excess weight has been gained. Boys, on the other hand, often need to continue increasing their daily caloric intake and insulin dose until 18 to 20 years of age before a similar reduction is indicated. After the fourth decade of juvenile-onset diabetes, there may be a significant drop in the daily insulin requirement, even in the absence of overt renal disease, hypoendocrine function, significant weight change, or decrease in food intake.[84] In teaching patients and their families to use insulin effectively, it is important to continue to emphasize the need for balancing the insulin doses to an appropriate meal plan of high nutritional value, to be taken daily at regularly scheduled times.

Use of Devices in the Administration of Insulin. Although the current insulin infusion pumps will probably be viewed soon as primitive devices, there is at present a great deal of interest in their use.[85] Patients are now requesting treatment with the pump because they hope that with its use, more satisfactory management is possible. Often there is limited knowledge of the chores involved in effective pump usage. Some possible current indications for using an insulin pump in management of Type I diabetes include "brittle" diabetes, growth failure, earlier-than-usual complications, insulin resistance, pregnancy, and a highly motivated patient who is well informed about the pump and its use. All patients should be screened and fully informed about the operation of the pump prior to making a final decision about its use. Although a growing number of Joslin Clinic patients are using insulin pumps, the indications for their use are limited.[85a] Because of the danger of hypoglycemia, *pumps should not be used by patients who are subject to insulin reactions without warning.* (See also Chapter 19.)

Exercise

Exercise is an important part of the treatment of the child with diabetes.[85b] Most children are naturally active so that it is not necessary to provide a formal exercise prescription. They ordinarily engage in bursts of extreme exercise erratically alternating with periods of decreased activity. It is essential that the patient and family understand the effects of exercise on the blood glucose so that appropriate anticipatory adjustments of diet and/or insulin may prevent hypoglycemia and assure as safe a blood glucose level as possible. Because of the erratic nature of exercise in most children, the use of supplemental calories rather than reduction of insulin dosage usually provides more satisfactory results. Participation in regular programs of exercise is of benefit and makes management of diabetes easier. Exercise is discussed in detail in Chapter 22.

COMPLICATIONS OF INSULIN THERAPY

Hypoglycemia

Among the complications of the treatment of diabetes, hypoglycemia is one of the most dreaded by young patients. Teenagers are particularly apprehensive primarily because of potential embarrassment if witnessed by peers. It is not uncommon for teenagers to eat excessively to over-insure against such episodes. For younger children, an illustrated reminder card indicating symptoms and treatment is helpful for teachers, scout leaders, and others temporarily caring for youngsters (Fig. 24–4).

Of great concern to patients and parents is the possibility of chronic neurologic dysfunction resulting from hypoglycemic episodes. This fear comes not only from concerns expressed by health care personnel, but also from the experience of seeing the acute symptoms during severe insulin reactions (e.g. seizures and even paralysis). Seizures or other neurologic signs may be seen with hypoglycemia in up to 38% of patients.[86] Electroencephalographic (EEG) abnormalities have been reported in 25% of children with diabetes compared with 10 to 15% of a control population.[87] The highest frequency of abnormalities occurred in children who had had five or more episodes of hypoglycemia with loss of consciousness and/or convulsions. Others have described persistent EEG abnormalities in a small series of patients in approximately the same frequency following hyperosmolarity associated with ketosis.[88] This would suggest that the finding of abnormal EEGs in children with insulin-dependent diabetes should not be presumed related to hypoglycemia.

No special studies have been carried out recently, but it has been our clinical impression that in young patients, hypoglycemic episodes, some severe, have not had a residual adverse effect on cerebral function. Of possible relevance in this regard was the observation of Priscilla White that of 478 patients studied after more than 30 years of juvenile-onset, insulin-dependent diabetes, 40% had attended college, 9% graduate school, and 34% had entered professions. The scholastic levels attained compared favorably to those of members of the general population and the number who had entered professions was truly remarkable.[74]

In all insulin programs—single or split dose—care must be taken to avoid nocturnal hypoglycemia. The use of a single daily dose does not necessarily protect the patient from this problem, and the use of two doses does not necessarily create it. Eighteen percent of children in a population which would not be considered "tightly controlled" were found to have asymptomatic nocturnal hypoglycemia. In the series reported by Winter, the blood glucose fell at a rate of 20 to 25 mg/dl per hour during episodes of nocturnal hypoglycemia with an average low point of 50 mg/dl.[89] The physiologic response to this process is release of glucose stores resulting in morning hyperglycemia. Although the child may sleep through the periods of hypoglycemia, he or she upon arising may complain of a variety of symptoms including headache, bad dreams, night sweats, abdominal pain, and malaise. The recurring nature of this rebound (Somogyi) phenomenon may be mistaken for a school avoidance problem. Urine tests in the morning may be positive for sugar and/or ketones. After breakfast, the symptoms generally resolve slowly so that by noon, the child usually feels well. After identifying this pattern, reduction in the insulin dose results in improvement of the symptoms. It is often the morning dose of intermediate insulin that needs to be decreased (see Chapter 19).[89a]

Local and Systemic Problems

A more extensive discussion of these complications resulting from insulin therapy, is presented in Chapters 19 and 38. Since 1973 when further purification of insulin was achieved, there has been a recognizable decrease in such complications. Now that biosynthetic human insulin is available, patients who receive this product solely from the start of their insulin treatment, will be followed carefully to determine the frequency of untoward responses, especially of immunologic nature.

Lipoatrophy. Lipoatrophy at the site of or within the dermatome of an injection site was formerly the most common local complication of insulin therapy. Although the exact cause is not certain, it is believed to be an expression of local allergy. It is physically harmless, but cosmetically a source of significant concern. Insulin lipoatrophy may involve some sites only, or virtually all injection sites. In most patients, the condition is im-

Diabetes and Me

My name is _____

I have diabetes and take insulin daily.

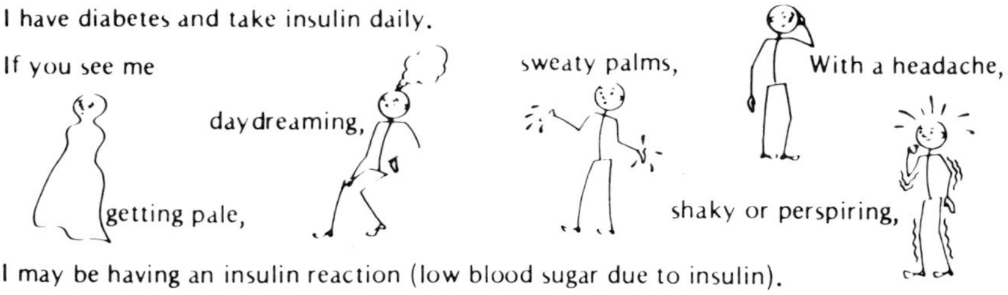

If you see me   daydreaming,   sweaty palms,   With a headache,

getting pale,   shaky or perspiring,

I may be having an insulin reaction (low blood sugar due to insulin).

Please give me: sugar   coke   gingerale   candy   fruit juice

Keep a watchful eye!

In case of need, call Dr. _____ (Telephone) _____

Parent's Signature _____ (over)

A Few Facts About Diabetes

Diabetes Mellitus is an hereditary disease in which the pancreas fails to supply enough effective insulin. The body is therefore unable to use food properly. Common initial symptoms are excessive urination, thirst, hunger, loss of weight and weakness.

Careful attention to diet, exercise and medication make it possible for a person with diabetes to live a life which is close to normal.

An "insulin reaction" may occur if the dose of insulin has been excessive, if there has been unusual physical activity, or if the prescribed amount of food has not been taken. The symptoms of an insulin reaction vary. Most young diabetics are aware when they need extra carbohydrate.

For further information you may contact the

Youth Committee
Joslin Diabetes Foundation
One Joslin Place
Boston, Massachusetts 02215
(617) 732-2400

JC 158 2/78

Fig. 24–4. Card (front and back) prepared for distribution to school teachers and other supervisors regarding diabetes and hypoglycemic episodes.

proved by the injection of highly purified insulin, usually of pork origin, directly into the affected area or at its margins if direct injection is too painful. Since the use of insulin to which the patient is not allergic may result in hypertrophy of subcutaneous fat, the end result may be, hopefully, a more normal contour. Of 310 patients with local lipoatrophy treated in this fashion, 99% showed improvement.[90] It is essential to return to the usual pattern with deliberately wide scattering of the sites within the rotational areas once a normal contour is achieved, to prevent the continuing development of hypertrophy. Returning to the area of previous atrophy periodically is essential; otherwise the "controlled hypertrophy" may begin to disappear with reappearance of the atrophy. If lipoatrophy does recur, it is much more difficult to treat successfully a second time.

Hypertrophy. Hypertrophic lipodystrophy can be induced in animal models with repeated injections of insulin into the same area.[90] The degree to which subcutaneous areas become firm and enlarged probably depends on the proportion of fibrous and fatty tissue present at the site. Although this problem is also chiefly cosmetic, there may also be "trapping" of insulin in the area, resulting in significant hypoglycemia at unusual times, when this insulin is released. A study of 58 patients showed equivocal results when purified insulin was used to treat this condition.[90]

Local Cutaneous Allergy. This condition is characterized by burning, itching, rash or hives at the site of injection. Poor injection technique, use of cold insulin or alcohol allergy should be ruled out. In a study of 153 patients with local allergy, a majority had other allergies, many had coexisting subcutaneous lipoatrophy and 24% had a history of interruption of insulin therapy. Eighty percent improved with change to purified pork insulin and 15% showed improvement with the use of purified beef insulin. The remaining 5% required desensitization.[90]

MONITORING THE CLINICAL COURSE AND EFFECTIVENESS OF TREATMENT

Continued Monitoring and Management. After a child leaves the hospital environment, many aspects of diabetes management change, not the least of which is the ease of monitoring. In the hospital, tests are taken by professionals whenever required. Tests on double-voided ("second") urine specimens and tests of 4- or 24-hour collections of urine are done routinely. Clinical observations and data thereby accumulated in a controlled environment by experienced personnel facilitate decisions concerning adjustments in treatment. At home, the child and the family cannot continue this high level of generation of data and still maintain a normal life style. Home monitoring, like other home care programs, must be tailored to the family's life style. Frequency of monitoring, dietary constancy, and regular schedules become modified by what the patient and family are able and/or willing to do. This should not prevent continued striving for the best care possible.

Urine Testing. Urine testing by home monitoring remains the classical standard of control. The degree of correlation between results of tests of urine and of blood glucose remains a topic of debate, but admittedly is often poor.[90a] Correlation is difficult because of the rate of glucose clearance, wide range of blood glucose covered by each percentage of urine test, and variable "renal thresholds" for children. "Double voided" urine specimens (i.e. not the first one after food) have traditionally been used in an effort to improve the correlation. Young children find double voiding difficult. Care must be taken to avoid what Krauser has referred to as "iatrogenic urinary retention,"[91] i.e., stressing the use of a second voided urine specimen so strongly that the child partially voids each time to satisfy the request for a second specimen.

A frequently employed method of testing the urine of children uses a Clinitest tablet with 2 drops of urine and 10 drops of water (2-drop method). This permits measurement of up to 5% sugar concentration in the urine. Methods measuring only up to 2% concentration have a range too narrow for the daily variations in most children. Falsely positive results may be obtained because of other substances which reduce alkaline copper reagents (see Chapter 15).

Methods specific for glucose involve the use of strips impregnated with glucose oxidase. Those in common use are TesTape, Diastix, and Chemstrip uG. The use of test strips provides obvious convenience, particularly away from home. Problems with these methods include difficulty in matching colors, inhibition of glucose color change by ketone reagents, need for exact timing and loss of glucose oxidase activity (if the test strip has been inadvertently exposed to humidity). These difficulties were studied in detail by Feldman and Lebovitz.[92] Some methods include a section on the same strip for the testing of ketones. Such strips cost more and this is often a needless expense. If a test for ketones is desired, Acetest, Ketostix, or Chemstrip uK may be used.

Twenty-four Hour Urine and Block Collections. An additional method of monitoring diabetes at home is through the use of 24-hour urine collections. The complete 24-hour collection or the four 6-hour fractions or blocks, provide additional information about the total quantity of sugar lost in the urine over the entire 24 hours and specific portions thereof. The results can be compared to the carbohydrate intake for that day. Under ideal conditions, a 24-hour urine sample should contain no sugar. An acceptable goal is 5 to 10% of 24-hour carbohydrate intake. Fractional or block urine tests can provide useful information about the time period (morning, afternoon, evening, or night) during which the largest amount of sugar is lost.

Blood Glucose. One of the major changes in diabetes management in recent years has been the introduction of home glucose monitoring by means of test strips with or without a reflectance meter providing a digital read-out. This allows maintenance of blood glucose levels below the so-called renal threshold, as well as the capability of confirming suspected hypoglycemia in an incipient or asymptomatic phase.

Monitoring programs used by patients vary widely. Some patients do four or more blood glucose tests a day. Others do one a day, staggering the time so that all times are covered in the course of a week. The most commonly used schedule is to do four blood glucose tests a day for 2 or 3 days a month, and otherwise to rely on urine testing alone.

In addition to home monitoring, blood glucose determinations are routinely done at each visit to the Joslin Clinic. A capillary blood specimen from a finger pad or an ear lobe is used for children, most of whom express strong preference for this method. It is extremely helpful to discuss the current blood glucose result with the patient and family at the time of the visit since it can serve as a springboard for discussion of management problems.

Like the urine tests, results of the tests for blood glucose levels should not be classified as either "good" or "bad," but seen merely as an index for the ongoing modification of treatment.

Glycosylated Hemoglobin (HbA₁). In spite of the introduction of home blood glucose monitoring, use of periodic 24-hour urine tests for glucose, and/or individual random urine tests, the total data input remains, at best, episodic. Although these tests provide valuable information for recognition of daily, weekly, and week-end patterns, they do not integrate the effect of treatment over time. Fortunately, now generally available are facilities for determining the glycosylated hemoglobin (HbA₁), the percentage of which appears to be a direct indication of the general level of the blood glucose over the preceding few weeks.[93] Hemoglobin A₁ in association with plasma insulin or C-peptide assays may provide indices of endogenous insulin production.

The nondiabetic value for total HbA₁ varies by method and laboratory but is approximately 5.5 to 7.5%. Values in children with IDDM even during periods of excellent treatment are at least 1 to 3 points higher than normal. The values are proportionately higher when treatment results are less than successful, with extremes up to about 20%. False elevations in children may be caused by the presence of renal failure or hemoglobin F or, on the other hand, falsely low values are seen when hemoglobins S, C, or D are present.[94] There is an inverse correlation with metabolic control and a direct correlation with the age of the child but not duration of diabetes.[95] Glycosylated hemoglobin is discussed further in Chapters 10, 15, and 19.

Determinations of HbA₁ at intervals provide for the young patient, family and clinical team an index as to whether management strategies are achieving improving or deteriorating results. Comparison of sequential reports avoids the confusion caused by transient fluctuations in blood and urine tests for glucose. It does not, however, obviate the need for conventional tests of urine and blood to detect metabolic patterns.

Blood Lipids. Morrison et al.[96] presented useful guidelines for assessing blood lipids in children. Using values above the 90th percentile for age as abnormal (184 mg/dl for total cholesterol and 104 mg/dl for triglycerides, through age 19), 50% of the boys and 32% of the girls with diabetes were found to have elevated lipid values. Abnormal lipid levels were present in 40% of the children and teenagers at some time during a year's monitoring at the Joslin Clinic.[97] Similar results were reported by Chase.[98] The significance of such findings is not yet clear, but the implications for future vascular compromise are a matter of concern. It should be possible to alter such abnormalities with a diet low in cholesterol and saturated fats, supplemented by a sustained exercise program, as well as improved degrees of blood glucose control. Triglycerides are affected most by impairment in glucose metabolism, but cholesterol levels may also be affected by long-standing hyperglycemia. Improved diabetes management can reduce blood lipids in adults, but this relationship is not as well documented for youngsters with diabetes.

Growth. Growth is an important clinical indication of overall general health and well-being in children and adolescents, at least for the short term of 20 years or so. Changes in weight and height reflect the net metabolic balance of total body homeostasis: energy intake, utilization and expenditure. If the insulin-deficient state is corrected sufficiently, the youngster with insulin-dependent diabetes should grow in a fashion comparable to nondiabetic peers, consistent with genetic potential. Height and weight should be measured at each out-patient visit and *plotted on standard growth grids*. The 1976 National Center for Health Statistics curves[99] provide such standards for boys and girls. Initial baseline data on the patient should include heights and weights of immediate family members (grandparents, parents, aunts, uncles, and siblings) to allow a rough estimation of growth potential. Past growth data are almost always available from other physicians, clinic visits or school records, and should be charted on the growth grid. If a child has fallen behind in height or weight at the time of diagnosis of diabetes, the initiation of prompt and appropriate treatment should quickly return the child to the former percentile and pattern of growth. The obese youngster should be encouraged to achieve a more appropriate percentile of weight gradually over a period of months, rather than abruptly, so that the linear growth expectation may be met.

Growth Retardation Associated with Poor Diabetes Control. In the 1930s, prior to the advent of long and intermediate acting insulins, severe growth failure, with deficits of 4 or more inches, were noted in 25% of the boys and 10% of the girls with diabetes followed at the Joslin Clinic. Short stature was usually found in a child who had had diabetes for more than 5 years, and was most frequent in those children who had developed diabetes before they were 10 years of age.[100,101]

Growth Failure. The extreme of diabetes-related growth disorders is known as the Mauriac syndrome, characterized by short stature, hepatomegaly, and protuberant abdomen. For further discussion, see Chapter 19.

Today, such severe growth failure is much less common.[102] Research has produced contradictory conclusions in the analysis of growth patterns in diabetic populations. Genetic,[103-105] nutritional,[106,107] and psychologic[108] factors have been implicated, but the strongest case has been made for the over-all metabolic impairment of the diabetic state.[109,110]

From March, 1978 to March, 1982, 65 children (6% of 616 boys and 4% of 669 girls) seen at the Joslin Clinic had a significant decrease in linear growth velocity which was attributed to unsuccessful diabetes management. Clinically, the impairment of growth correlated with excessive hyperglycemia and extensive caloric loss (glycosuria) for months prior to evaluation. With improved diabetes treatment, growth resumed at a more normal rate but usually at a lower percentile line; in a few, "catch-up" growth occurred.[107a] Of these 65 children, 17 (1% of total sample) also had hepatomegaly. Values for serum glutamic oxaloacetic transaminase (SGOT) were sometimes significantly elevated, but plasma bilirubin levels were usually normal. All 17 children with hepatomegaly subsequently improved in an ambulatory in-patient hospital setting (Diabetes Treatment Unit) with insulin given twice daily. Symptoms related to uncontrolled diabetes (polyuria, weakness, nocturia, enuresis) abated and glycosuria decreased from 100 to 220 g to 15 to 30 g per 24 hours (10 to 20% of the carbohydrate intake). Hepatomegaly and serum enzyme values reflecting abnormal liver function resolved within 1 to 4 weeks. The psychosocial milieu of these children often was less than optimal and there was a tendency for recurrent bouts of ketoacidosis, over-insulinization, lack of compliance with dietary plans, and neglect of home monitoring.

A chart in Figure 24-5 illustrates growth failure in a youngster with diabetes. The curve demonstrates what is probably an "over-insulinization growth spurt" phenomenon between onset of diabetes at ages 4 and 9 years. Subsequent fall-off in velocity of height increase can be seen between ages 9 to 14. At age 15 years and 8 months, this patient was at the average height for a 13-year-old boy, i.e., 8 inches shorter than the 50th percentile for age. During the next 2 years, growth was appropriate, but the deficit was not overcome. Bone age was 1 year behind his chronologic age which is not considered a significant deficit. Delayed epiphyseal closure may allow a partial "closing of the gap" by extending the growth years (Fig. 24-5).

A comparison of height and weight gain of identical twin sisters, one with diabetes and one without, illustrates the problem (Fig. 24-6) which may not be evident until later unless careful charting is done. Any falling away from the normal growth percentile for a particular child demands careful re-

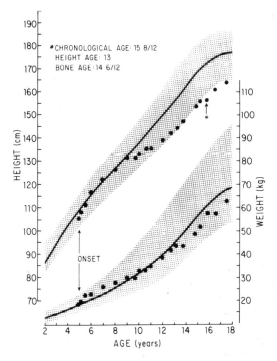

Fig. 24-5. Failure in linear growth beginning at about age 9 at a period of poor control of diabetes (see text).

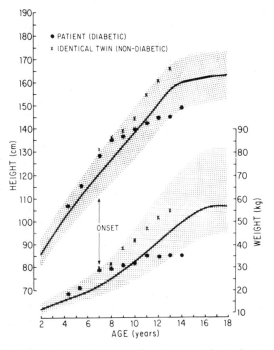

Fig. 24-6. Contrasting growth patterns in identical twins non-concordant for diabetes. Note that impaired growth in the diabetic appeared 3 to 4 years after onset (see text).

evaluation of the diabetes treatment program as well as other factors that may affect growth.

Pubertal Development. As part of the evaluation of pubertal development, careful Tanner staging[111] should be recorded in pre-adolescents and adolescents from onset to completion of puberty. The pubertal process in any child almost invariably takes 4 years from onset to full adult sexual reproductive capacity. Girls in whom the onset of diabetes was pre-pubertal may experience some delay in menarche. Extreme delay may occur in those youngsters with the longest duration of diabetes, the earliest ages at onset, and the most erratic patterns of glycemic excursions. Similar delayed adolescence is seen in males although details are more difficult to document. Tattersall and Pyke support these clinical impressions with their comparison data from twins.[112] They conclude that difficulty in the management of diabetes is the most likely reason for growth impairment and pubertal delay. If diabetes goes out of control for a significant period of time, previously regular menses may cease or become irregular; with improved treatment, regular menstruation should resume.

Not to be forgotten is the need for instruction of patients in this age group regarding sexual development, pregnancy, and contraception. In some instances, this will reinforce information obtained at home or in school; in others, this will introduce such education. At the Joslin Clinic, such instruction is accomplished both individually and in classes.

The effect of menses upon fluctuations of glucose levels is highly variable throughout the monthly cycle. Generally, each individual has a fairly characteristic pattern. This usually consists of increased glycosuria for a few days premenstrually with an increased insulin requirement that subsequently returns to base-line one to several days after the onset of menses. Recognition of a particular pattern for the individual is important in order to make appropriate anticipatory adjustments of the daily treatment schedule. Severe dysmenorrhea does not seem to be more frequent among diabetic young women, but if anorexia or nausea occurs, changes in caloric and fluid intake will require appropriate insulin adjustments.

Other Aspects of Regular Follow-up. Children with Type I diabetes have traditionally been seen by a physician every 2 or 3 months. These visits offer an opportunity to evaluate the patient not only physically, but also chemically through the use of blood glucose, hemoglobin A_1 or A_{1c}, and review of home monitoring records. Equally important is provision of time to answer questions, discuss problems, provide support, and continue education.

The physical examination should place special emphasis on systems that are affected by diabetes. As previously mentioned, growth rate and weight gain should be reviewed at each visit. Since weight problems commonly plague the teen-age girl with diabetes, a program aimed at preventing obesity should be considered in the early months of puberty. Teenage girls will often accept the concept of caloric (and insulin) reduction more readily when it is recommended in the context of avoiding obesity rather than in relation to diabetes treatment. By the time obvious obesity has occurred, treatment is difficult. Over-insulinization may be the real culprit in such young women, leading them to take excessive food to treat impending or actual hypoglycemia.

Fluctuations in weight of 2 to 5 kg (4 to 11 lb) over a few days are experienced by some adolescent girls. These most often occur with difficulties in diabetes management which may or may not be in relation to one or another phase of the menstrual cycle. Significant edema may occur when a child who has been chronically in poor control is brought under satisfactory control. This "insulin edema" occurs within a few days of improved control and lasts for a week to a month or more. Salt restriction is sometimes helpful and diuretics may be transiently needed, but may be over-used by patients for weight control.

School performance is generally normal for most youngsters with diabetes. Nevertheless, it is important that each aspect of the child's participation in school be examined carefully in terms of management. All people involved in any part of the youngster's day, teachers and substitute teachers, transportation, and cafeteria workers, coaches, scout leaders, extracurricular activity leaders, guidance personnel, nursing personnel, etc., need to be taught about the nature of diabetes and its treatment. Special attention should be given to the symptoms and signs of possible hypoglycemia. Along with the necessary medical knowledge, these adults must learn how to avoid causing inappropriate anxiety and/or embarrassment.

COMPLICATIONS

In the past, many physicians caring for children with diabetes have thought that their patients during childhood and adolescence would be spared from the vascular and neurologic complications of diabetes. However, as attention has been directed toward early detection of such, most of these have been found in the pediatric age group. Although neuropathy, proteinuria, necrobiosis, retinopathy, nephropathy, and hypertension occur in less than 15% of this population, the impact of early diagnosis and treatment makes screening of great importance in children (Table 24–5).

Periodic evaluation of *incipient retinal or renal problems* should be made. Detection may bring more family support for intensive diabetes treatment. Routine checks should be made for protein in the urine.[112a] As discussed elsewhere, hypertension is of significant prognostic importance. Through the use of blood pressure grids with values adjusted appropriately for age, early identification and treatment of hypertension may decrease long-term cardiovascular morbidity.[113] Since atherosclerosis is commonly associated with diabetes, periodic evaluation of fasting lipids should be carried out. The diet recommended by the American Heart Association can be integrated into the diabetes meal plan to lower the intake of saturated fat and thereby lower cholesterol levels. Limiting the use of dietary fat and adding fiber to meals for the entire family will increase nutrition awareness and create a positive atmosphere regarding the specific dietary requirements for the entire treatment of diabetes.

Thyroid Dysfunction is not rare in children with diabetes, and elevated antithyroid antibody titers are quite common. The latter may be helpful in deciding which children need periodic tests of thyroid function.

Smith and colleagues[114] present evidence for a 10-fold increased prevalence of IgA deficiency and suggested that a more aggressive course of diabetes takes place in such patients.

Necrobiosis Lipoidica Diabeticorum may occur early in diabetes, even before any clinical manifestations of diabetes are evident. It has occasionally been described in young patients even prior to the diagnosis of diabetes. It can be significantly disfiguring for young women. See Chapters 38 and 42 for further discussions.

Limited Joint Mobility (LJM) of the hands of patients with IDDM was studied at the Joslin Clinic in a group of 103 subjects 3 to 22 years of age. LJM, found in 32 patients, was independent of age and sex but increased with duration of diabetes, with peak occurrence in those with IDDM for more

Table 24–5. Frequency of Clinical Findings in 1246 Joslin Clinic Patients, Age 1–21 Years Experience of S.J. Brink, 1978–82 (unpublished data)

	Girls	Boys	Total
	n = 669 (100%)	n = 616 (100%)	n = 1285 (100%)
Psychosocial Dysfunction including School Problems	194 (29%)	175 (28%)	369 (29%)
Recurrent Ketoacidosis	47 (7%)	18 (3%)	65 (5%)
Convulsions	40 (6%)	41 (7%)	81 (6%)
Impaired Growth Pattern	28 (4%)	37 (6%)	65 (5%)
Insulin Allergy, Local	13 (2%)	7 (1%)	20 (1%)
Systemic	1 (<1%)	1 (<1%)	2 (<1%)
Hepatomegaly	10 (1.5%)	7 (1%)	17 (1%)
Obesity (>120% Ideal Weight for Height)	115 (11%)	28 (5%)	143 (11%)
Enuresis 1° and 2°	38 (6%)	61 (10%)	99 (8%)
Urinary Tract Infection	23 (3%)	5 (1%)	28 (2%)
Hypertension (> 120/90)	14 (2%)	11 (2%)	25 (2%)
Edema	25 (4%)	1 (<1%)	26 (2%)
Goiter*	74 (11%)	28 (5%)	102 (8%)
Hypothyroidism†	60 (9%)	31 (5%)	91 (7%)
Clinical	28 (4%)	12 (2%)	40 (3%)
Compensated‡	32 (5%)	19 (3%)	51 (4%)
Addison's Disease	1 (<1%)	2 (<1%)	3 (<1%)
Vitiligo	7 (1%)	5 (1%)	12 (1%)
Primary Amenorrhea/Delayed Puberty	23 (3%)	4 (<1%)	27 (2%)
Diabetic Retinopathy	39 (6%)	18 (3%)	57 (4%)
Diabetic Nephropathy	18 (3%)	11 (2%)	29 (2%)
Diabetic Neuropathy	32 (5%)	20 (3%)	52 (4%)
Cataracts	7 (1%)	4 (<1%)	11 (1%)
Gastrointestinal Dysfunction	36 (5%)	15 (2%)	51 (4%)
Limited Joint Mobility	29 (7%)	68 (17%)	97 (12%)
Klinefelter's Syndrome	—	4 (<1%)	4 (<1%)
DIDMOAD§	3 (1%) (sisters)	0	3 (<1%)
Prader-Willi Syndrome	0	1 (<1%)	1 (<1%)

*Goiter with or without thyroid dysfunction
†Hypothyroidism with or without goiter
‡Elevation of serum thyroid stimulating hormone with otherwise normal thyroid function tests
§Diabetes insipidus and diabetes mellitus with optic atrophy and deafness

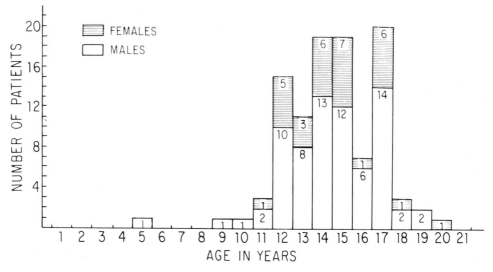

Fig. 24–7. Age of patients at time of recognition of contractures of fingers (limited joint mobility).

than 5 years.[115] In a subsequent study[116] of 819 children and teenagers with IDDM, LJM was found in 68 males and 29 females, 17 and 7% respectively of the 398 males and 421 females. The earliest age of discovery of LJM was in a child 5 years old; the peak onset was between 12 and 17 years. LJM has also been found at the time of diagnosis of IDDM. The risk for complications of IDDM in patients with LJM was noted to be 4:1 for retinopathy, hypertension or neuropathy and 6:1 for nephropathy (see Figs. 24–7, 24–8, and 42–4).

Ketoacidosis. In Chapter 26 the causes, consequences, and management of diabetic ketoacidosis are discussed in detail. In young people, ketoacidosis severe enough to require hospitalization is generally preventable. The underlying difficulties almost always include one or more of the following problems: (1) failure to take all or part of the prescribed insulin dose; (2) failure to adjust the dose of insulin for growth and level of physical activity; (3) failure to take extra insulin, salt and fluids for intercurrent illness (especially if febrile); (4) failure to adjust the insulin dose because urine or blood tests were omitted or results reported incorrectly; (5) chronic overdosage of insulin resulting in hypoglycemia followed by rebound hyperglycemia and ketonemia; (6) severe physical or emotional stress which stimulates counterregulatory hormones such as epinephrine, norepinephrine, glucagon and glucocorticoids which alter liver metabolism with resulting marked hyperglycemia and sometimes ketosis. A few children with recurrent stress-related episodes have been successfully treated in part with the use of beta adrenergic blockade.[117]

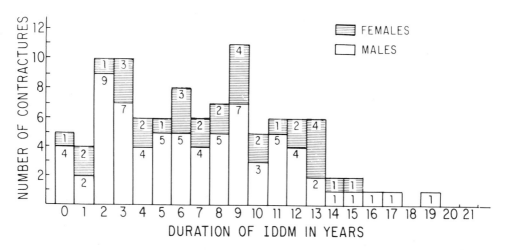

Fig. 24–8. Duration of diabetes at time of recognition of limited joint mobility.

Guidelines for home management of diabetes during acute illness to prevent ketoacidosis include the following: (1) continue usual insulin dose; (2) test blood preferably, or urine for glucose, and urine for acetone every 2–4 hours; (3) contact the physician or clinic and arrange for frequent communication; (4) replenish fluids with broth, soup, juice, and other beverages to maintain pre-illness weight; (5) give supplementary regular insulin subcutaneously every 4 to 6 hours in doses equivalent to about 10 to 20% of the usual total daily insulin requirement; (7) double the supplementary dose or increase its frequency to every 2 hours if there is not evidence of progressive improvement in the tests and in the way the child looks and feels.[118]

The problem of recurrent hospitalization for diabetic ketoacidosis frequently involves unrecognized, deliberate attempts by the young patient to deal with diabetes inappropriately. By partial or complete omission of treatment, the youngster may be testing a personal hypothesis that the diagnosis was a mistake. The use of denial permits avoidance of the painful envy and impaired self-image that healthy peers evoke. Sometimes it is peer ridicule that leads to avoidance tactics. A certain amount of experimentation is normally a part of early adolescence. However, if the child's manipulations of diet and insulin are ignored or are met with inappropriate responses, ketoacidosis may ensue. The medical emergency may produce secondary gains such as expressions of love and concern, and thereby lead to repetition of the behavior-induced sequence.

The monitoring of fluid and electrolyte balance must be frequent and precise in children as in adults since parameters change rapidly in both. Frequent neurologic evaluation is needed to identify incipient cerebral edema since this complication may be a threat to children more often than to adults. The early signs are usually subtle, but clearly identifiable, such as changes in sensorium often evident as quieting in a previously combative or thrashing child. Corticosteroids and/or mannitol have been used in treatment, but with questionable results.

Treatment of ketoacidosis is usually uneventful and rapid in children if constant infusion insulin therapy is used (Table 24–8). For further details of the treatment of ketoacidosis, see Chapter 26.

PSYCHOSOCIAL ASPECTS OF TREATMENT

Physicians and parents must work together in encouraging progressive emotional growth as well as providing physical care for the chronically ill child. The primary focus must be on the development of the child, not on the illness.

Onset. The manner in which the child and family experience the onset of juvenile diabetes depends

Table 24–6. Management of Diabetic Ketoacidosis in a Young Person

A. Emergency recognition of presenting problems
  Circulatory status: is patient in shock?
  Respiratory difficulties: need for airway?
B. Initial clinical assessment
  Estimate degree of dehydration: extreme dryness of skin and mucosae; soft and sunken eyeballs.
  Is Kussmaul's respiration present? Acetone breath?
  Check pulse, respiratory rate, blood pressure.
  Measure height and weight; estimate body surface.
C. Initial evaluation at bedside.
  Urine for sugar and acetone.
  Rapid blood glucose estimate with glucose oxidase strips.
  Serum acetone by test strips or tablets.
D. Prompt and adequate initial treatment: see text, Table 24–8, and Chapter 26.
  Regular insulin: continuous IV infusion (or IM or SC).
  Fluid and electrolyte replacement.
  Establish and maintain flow chart.
E. Laboratory studies: blood glucose, pH, BUN, creatinine, electrolytes, complete blood count, urine analysis, Ecg (if indicated).
F. Further assessment: more detailed history and complete P.E.
  Search for causes and complications of DKA. Institute treatment.
  Aspirate stomach (carefully), esp. if patient is unconscious.
G. Re-evaluate therapy hourly at first and later q 2–4 h.
H. Respond to psychologic needs of patient and family.
I. Initiate or review education to prevent recurrence.

upon their personalities and capacity to cope with stress, previous experience with psychologically similar events, and the child's age-related developmental stage. However, one can expect manifestations of the commonly felt grief at the time of the initial diagnosis regardless of the family's particular psychologic style and personal history. The emotional sequelae are parallel to those of the bereaved: shock, disbelief, denial, anger, and depression.

Once treatment begins and the external signs of illness recede, parents often find it difficult to believe their child is ill. They still must face the overwhelming facts, however, and need time to express a whole range of emotional responses. Most parents do move beyond denying diabetes and become concerned with their role in "causing" the disease.

The onset of juvenile diabetes usually brings intensive medical attention involving procedures which are unfamiliar to the family and which often occur in a hospital setting. It is during this turmoil that the seeds for preventing future difficulties can be sown. One critical task for the medical team is their understanding and handling of the painful feelings experienced by the family and child. With the recognition and acceptance by the staff that a

Table 24–7. Estimated Water and Electrolytes Needed (for Maintenance plus Losses) During the First 24 Hours of Treatment of Young Persons with Moderate to Severe Diabetic Ketoacidosis Assuming 10% ± Dehydration

	Maintenance (kg/24 hr)		Replacement (per kg)	2 yr (12 kg) 0.6 m² ±	5 yr (20 kg) 0.8 m² ±	10 yr (30 kg) 1.0 m² ±	16 yr (60 kg) 1.6 m² ±
H_2O	50–100 ml		75–150 ml	2400 ml	3600 ml	4700 ml	8000 ml
Na^+	3 mEq	+	5–8 mEq	115–120 mEq	180–200 mEq	270–290 mEq	530–560 mEq
K^+*	1–2 mEq	+	3–6 mEq	90–95 mEq	145–150 mEq	210–220 mEq	410–425 mEq
Cl^-	1–2 mEq	+	3–5 mEq	80–95 mEq	125–150 mEq	180–210 mEq	350–395 mEq
PO_4			1 mEq	12 mEq	20 mEq	30 mEq	60 mEq
Mg^{++}			0.5 mEq	6 mEq	10 mEq	15 mEq	30 mEq

*Any infusion containing potassium in concentration greater than 40 mEq/L requires electrocardiographic monitoring.

Body surface area may be calculated by using a special formula or nomogram to be found in metabolism or pediatrics texts or in manuals such as that of the Children's Hospital Medical Center in Boston: J.W. Graef, T.E. Cone, Jr. (Eds.): Manual of Pediatric Therapeutics, 2nd Ed. Boston, Little, Brown and Company, 1980.

In practice, the amounts noted in the table above must be adjusted to recognize the needs of the individual patient both initially and as treatment progresses. When the patient is able to ingest and retain fluid and then soft solids, one must slowly provide such and let Nature assist in the replacement of losses. If this proves successful, one may discontinue the intravenous infusion containing insulin, having given an appropriate dose of regular and lente (or NPH) insulin subcutaneously 15–20 minutes before.

Magnesium levels may be elevated at the beginning of treatment and then with hydration fall rapidly as often potassium does. Only rarely has any clinical expression of this shift been recognized (see pp. 536 and 852). Ordinarily, magnesium is not included in the perfusion fluid.

The extent to which bicarbonate should be administered has long been controversial. In any case, it is good to be conservative, restricting its use to situations in which the blood pH is 7.10 or below and the total serum CO_2 is less than 5 mEq/L.

Table 24–8. Continuous Insulin Infusion in Diabetic Ketoacidosis

1. Loading Dose: 0.1–0.2 U/kg IV push, after flushing tubing with regular insulin (no albumin used)
2. 0.1 U/kg IV per hour regular insulin
3. Monitor blood glucose response at 1 hour; double dose if no decrease or switch to an alternate insulin treatment plan
4. Expect blood glucose to decline 50–100 mg/dl per hour
5. Give 5% dextrose IV infusion at about 100 ml/kg/hour when blood glucose is approximately 250–300 mg/dl
6. When blood glucose is 250 mg/dl or less, give a mixture of equal doses of regular and intermediate insulin subcutaneously for a total of 0.25 U/kg and discontinue insulin infusion after 15–20 min
7. Evaluate water, sodium, potassium, phosphate and bicarbonate therapy frequently *and* independently of insulin treatment

range of emotions is normal and should be expressed, most parents will respond with relief.

Initial teaching of the family must emphasize the most immediate and straightforward necessities of the treatment: (1) giving insulin, (2) testing urine or blood, (3) recognizing and treating hypoglycemia, and (4) maintaining contact with the medical team. Families may feel overwhelmed by the large body of knowledge that will become useful in time but which they find remote or irrelevant initially and much of which they will consider themselves inadequate to grasp. Over a period of months, parents and children will increasingly be able to absorb more complex information about the course of diabetes.

It is tempting to reassure the family that the child can resume a "normal" life. But such encouraging statements, directed at parents who are eager for such reassurance, will in fact create a climate of denial and distrust in the family's relationship with health professionals. The existence of diabetes does necessitate alterations in the lives of the child and family. A more appropriate goal is the striving for the most nearly normal childhood and adulthood possible, given the inherent nature of the condition and the demands of its management.

Remission. When a period of remission follows shortly after onset, there are additional factors which will influence the acceptance of diabetes. Since remission typically occurs when the adjustment to the disease is relatively incomplete, this period is often experienced as a release from the disease; there is a hope that the diagnosis was in error or that the illness has magically vanished. It is essential to continue professional involvement and treatment during the remission phase in order to prepare the family for the inevitable re-emergence of more unstable diabetic symptoms.

Insulin Reactions. Possibly the most anxiety-producing aspect of diabetes in children is the fear of insulin reactions. Parents and children alike associate reactions with not only loss of control, danger of head and other injuries, convulsions, and coma, but also almost universally with death. The child's own anxieties about insulin reactions create tension about potential embarrassment in the presence of peers, both in school and in play activities. This may sometimes hinder a confident approach to scholastic achievement as well as social relationships.

Stages of Development

The impact of diabetes on the view that children have of themselves affects their understanding and handling of the situation according to the phase of development the child is in and the nature of the parents' involvement in it (Table 24–9).

First Year of Life. An infant establishes confidence in the environment primarily through relationship with parents and their responses to the child's needs. The more comfortable these parents become about their competence in handling their infant's diabetic care, the more relaxed they will be in responding to their baby's needs.

Most toddlers fear insulin injections and blood tests. Injection sites that they can watch are important to some children; sites they cannot see readily are important to others. Capillary blood tests which minimize pain, and consequently fear, are usually preferred to venipuncture.

Pre-School Children (3 to 5 Years). The pre-school youngster normally has intense concerns about body strength and intactness and fears their being damaged. The adults in the child's world should be sensitive to these concerns and offer reassurance and support.

School Age Children (6 to 11 Years). One of the major steps a child of school age takes is the gradual shifting of emotional attachment from the immediate family to contemporaries. The child may feel "different," and, therefore, somehow inadequate, compared to peers and may try to hide the "differentness" by keeping the illness a secret. The child's sensitivity to others' learning of the diabetic condition must be considered. Informing teachers and others privately rather than in the presence of other children assures the youngster's welfare while permitting the choice to inform others personally.

The impact on the personality created by the diagnosis of diabetes in pre-adolescent years is often greater than in an adult due to the fact that personality is still evolving an ego identity and self-esteem. The adolescent needs to be accepted by peers; unfortunately, many teenagers feel that the diagnosis and treatment of diabetes separates them

Table 24–9.　Psychological Aspects of Caring for Children and Youth With IDDM*

	Impact of Diagnosis		Major Development Issues	Management Implications	
	Parents	Child		Parents	Professionals
Infants	Shock, disbelief, denial, anger, guilt, depression. Affects capacity to learn regimen.	Responds to added tension and discomfort.	Trusting relationship: interaction with parents about food.	Difficulties in differentiating hypoglycemic reactions from "normal" distress. Monitoring of diabetes felt as "overwhelming" and "lonely."	Constant availability of medical team.
Toddlers	"	Regression: motor, speech development, toilet training.	Early steps toward autonomy: balkiness, stubbornness. Exploration of environment without judgment.	Temper tantrums in child interfere with distinguishing insulin reactions, giving injections, and blood tests.	Select least painful sites for injections and blood tests.
Pre-school	"	Regression in social behavior and skills. May "cling" more.	Intense concerns about body strength and "intactness." May view diabetes management as "punishment." Fears injections and blood testing as bodily injury.	Normal moodiness easily confused with hypoglycemic reactions.	"
School Age	"	Depression, regression; withdrawal from social, athletic activities; school work may be affected. Aware of genetic factors.	Curiosity, development of motor, intellectual, social skills. Attachment shifts gradually from family to peers: sensitive to feeling "adequate."	Encourage self-monitoring: recognize hypoglycemic reactions; participate in diet planning; help in blood testing; draw up and occasionally inject insulin. All activities to be supervised.	Begin seeing child alone during office visits.
Adolescence	"	Similar to adult grieving; recognizes implication of diabetes, potential complications. Aware of genetic factors.	Identity formation, intense body awareness, sexual identity. Dependence-independence struggle with parents and authorities: defiance. Measures self against peers; diabetes may make feel less adequate.	Experimentation: omitting insulin and blood testing, not following diet; in extreme situations DKA and recurrent DKA indicates need for psychiatric intervention. Discretion needed in physical contact: information about sexuality and diabetes beneficial. Capable of some self-management, still needing overall adult supervision and involvement.	As "neutral" adult assure confidentiality and privacy at visits.
Young Adults	"	"	Emotional ties to family lessen; career development; interpersonal commitment. Concerns about possible diabetes complications and effect on future goals.	Young adult responsible for diabetes management; shares information with others.	Continuing relationship beneficial to prepare for possible future physical complications.

*Prepared by J.B. Leibovich, ACSW, LICSW, Joslin Clinic.

from their peers. No treatment program, lax or strict, seems to be totally exempt from this impact. Since teenagers with diabetes, particularly boys, have been noted to develop lower ego and self-esteem than their peers,[119] the lack of caring about one's self may result in poorer metabolic control,[120] particularly if the family does not provide adequate support.[121]

Typically, much of the energy of children between the ages of 6 and 11 is channeled into learning academic, social, and physical skills, discovering how things work and cause-effect relations. In the search for reasons for the diabetes, the child may assume personal blame (e.g., for eating too much candy) or blame parents (e.g., for somehow not providing protection). This distortion of cause and effect reasoning is typical of the young child and will flourish unless the youngster is encouraged to ask questions and express feelings and fears openly. Diabetes is particularly mysterious because its course involves hidden internal bodily functions.

Children at this age often become inquisitive about the diabetic regimen and even choose to take an active part in it. Permitting the youngster to help test blood and/or urine, draw up and occasionally give insulin injections, and play a part in planning the diet, will promote a sense of mastery. Self-confidence will be enhanced and satisfaction achieved as the child gains approval for the successful execution of these tasks. It is hazardous, however, for parents to relinquish their close supervision of each aspect of the diabetic regimen. The school-age child is not sufficiently mature to take on this responsibility which involves life-and-death issues.

In the pre- and early adolescent age group, regardless of the specific individual overall adjustment, there is typically a manipulation of tests and/or test reports. Even if previously cooperative in handling home testing efficiently, the child 10 or 12 years of age and older may refuse outright to cooperate with testing or may dilute the urine specimens to create acceptable results. The testing may not seem of immediate importance to the child or in any way related to the possibility of feeling ill. By trying to produce satisfactory test results without the necessary self-discipline, the child seeks approval while at the same time denying the existence of diabetes. Parents and physicians should attempt to counter this kind of manipulation by balancing close supervision of the child's participation in treatment with encouragement for that participation. If at all possible, they should avoid direct and punitive confrontations, with their potential for the child's loss of face and increased feelings of anger and inadequacy.

Adolescence (12 to 17 Years). The course of adolescence is normally tumultuous: the teenager increasingly strives to establish an individual identity. In the process, the youngster must gradually give up the satisfaction of childhood and look ahead with anxiety and excitement to a time of being self-sufficient. Most adolescents feel that both the diagnosis and the treatment of diabetes separate them from their peers. During this period of life when the body usually undergoes dramatic changes, there is intense focus upon the physical being. This preoccupation with bodily functions and their adequacy increases when the juvenile with diabetes must concentrate more attention on somatic events. Many adolescents with diabetes are especially vulnerable to feelings of defectiveness or weakness especially in comparison to nondiabetic contemporaries. Joining friends in drinking alcohol or taking drugs may prove tempting as a way of gaining social acceptance and demonstrating similarity to peers. A change in regimen may be perceived as a worsening of the diabetes and therefore an increased threat to health rather than as the usual clinical course of the condition. It is essential that the physician make clear that an increased or split dose of insulin is prescribed for greater balance and a somewhat closer match to normal physiology.

Early in adolescence, youngsters normally tend to react not only with pleasure but also with guilt and confusion about their increased sexual interest. The task of easing these anxieties and diminishing the distortion in the adolescent's fantasies about the relation of diabetes and sexuality is not an easy one. Teenagers are typically guarded in revealing their sexual thoughts to others, especially adults. A willingness to discuss and help correct information acquired from other children and the adolescent's own imaginings is important. Furthermore, the professional must anticipate the need to repeat facts about sexuality, as the adolescent often "forgets" in an unconscious effort to deny anxiety-producing knowledge.

Another aspect of the increased sexuality of adolescents is reflected in modesty about parents' observing them in the bathroom or while dressing. The direct involvement of the parents with the child's body, e.g., in obtaining urine samples or in giving insulin injections, must be treated with great discretion to minimize physical contact, "exposure," and the embarrassment and other uncomfortable feelings they are likely to generate.

A teenager's striving toward self-identity pivots around the issue of dependence on family. Teenagers may be tempted to experience for themselves the limits of the dangers of their condition in order to confront personally the reality of diabetes. Frequently, the diabetic regimen itself is associated with the teenager's perceptions of the world of parents and authority. By defying their guidelines for diabetes management, the child tries to become detached from their values and find a personal identity. Even the formerly cooperative child who has mastered the techniques of diabetes care may experiment with the regimen some time and to some degree during adolescence (e.g., by occasionally omitting insulin or ignoring the prescribed diet). The ramifications of this experimentation create a difficult situation for parents and others overseeing diabetic management. When the resulting lapses bring repeated episodes of ketoacidosis or other serious clinical problems, the adults in charge are compelled to assume a closer supervision of the teenager's management. This is best achieved with understanding and realistic limit-setting without critical or devaluing responses toward the adolescent. By virtue of being outside of the parent-child struggle, the physician can often play a crucial role in defusing the intensity of the parent-child confrontation. The adolescent may perceive guidelines drawn by professionals as less threatening to becoming self-sufficient than those that come from parents. If the physician can be seen as a friendly, non-critical, accessible and flexible individual, the teenager may feel safe to air any worries and be more likely to follow the physician's advice.

The promise of confidentiality between the adolescent and the medical staff is essential to developing a trusting relationship. Thus, the adolescent should be seen alone for at least a portion of each visit and rarely, if ever, excluded from discussion with parents. It may be helpful to suggest, prior to adolescence, that youngsters have some time alone with the physician during their visits. This will establish a pattern for contact during a period when a teenager's reticence may prevent expression of a wish for such privacy.

The physician who has been consistently involved with the teenager and family can determine when the diabetic fluctuations are within the limits of a normal "testing out" period or when they should be viewed as a form of self-destructive behavior, such as repeated episodes of ketoacidosis. Psychiatric intervention may be necessary for both child and parents to prevent serious medical complications that may arise from such behavior. (See Chapter 44.)

Late Adolescence (18 to 20 Years). The young adult living away from home must make provision for medical emergencies. This often involves having a trusting relationship with a friend or roommate who has been taught methods for treating insulin reactions. Young women contemplating pregnancy must include diabetes in this planning. Early pregnancies (by the late 20s) are usually rec-

ommended, and this fact may put pressure on both the young woman and her partner. Possible physical complications of long-term diabetes create additional pressures on intimate relationships as well.

Although the onset of diabetes rarely occurs in late adolescence, the emergence of complications often does. The young adult will benefit from an ongoing relationship with the physician in beginning to deal with physical complications, the emotional issues accompanying them, or even the recognition of potential for future complications. All of these will have a marked effect on immediate future plans for education and life style.

Coping with Difficulties in Child Rearing

Working with families who have children with juvenile-onset diabetes has revealed issues which present the most crucial difficulties these parents face in child rearing: dependence-independence conflict, discipline, responses of siblings, and facing fears of death and acute and long-term complications.[121a]

Dependence-Independence. The presence of diabetes often affects the balance between dependence and independence which varies according to the changes in the development of the child. The medical team can assist parents in transferring some responsibility to others by educating school personnel, camp directors, athletic coaches, and others in the handling of possible emergencies. In overcoming their reluctance to trust others to protect and care for their children, parents and youngsters will benefit from the reassurance that they can indeed survive alone for periods of time and rely on others to share the burden.

Discipline. Another area of special difficulty for the families of children with diabetes is discipline, which is too often equated with punishment. Parents often find it troublesome to set limits for their diabetic youngsters, feeling that to do so would place yet another pressure on them. Children often re-enforce this tendency by using diabetes as an excuse for what would otherwise be unacceptable behavior. Parents can be helped to view their limit setting as an important part of teaching their children various forms of self-control and acceptable behavior. Failure to provide firm guidelines actually constitutes a disservice to any youngster, with or without diabetes, who will one day live and work by standards of the world outside the childhood home.

Siblings. Siblings of children with diabetes are also greatly influenced by the daily routine of the condition and by the family's emotional involvement in it. They need to be a part of the education and open discussions, both within the family and at times with health personnel, as they too may harbor concerns about their diabetic sister or brother and the illness. Jealousy and resentment are sometimes felt by the healthy sibling as special attention in time, energy, and emotion is given to the diabetic child. Physicians can heighten parents' awareness of this need. How the total family incorporates the facts and requirements of diabetes into their life varies greatly but non-diabetic siblings play a vital role in this process.

Team Approach. Ideally, a physician's appropriate medical treatment for the fluctuating pattern of diabetes in a growing child should be supplemented by the contributions of a team of other professionals, i.e., nurses, social workers, and dietitians, each of whom supplies education, treatment and support for the family over a long period of years. Their knowledge and understanding of the family enables them to be most effective at critical phases in the course of the illness.

At the Joslin Clinic, the Youth Division was established to meet the needs of children with diabetes and their families. Staffed by specialized teaching nurses and pediatric endocrinologists, in consultation with psychiatric social workers and youth counselors, the aim is to provide therapeutic, educational, supportive, and counselling services to families in situations in which: (1) juvenile diabetes is newly diagnosed; (2) medical problems arise which result from difficulties in management and/or from the natural course of the illness (e.g., during adolescence or in a child with "brittle" diabetes); (3) interpersonal or social difficulties arise, attributable at least in part to diabetes or the family's response to it (e.g., frequent school absences or children lacking in self-confidence); (4) parents are tense, confused, or uncertain about handling their child's care (e.g., parents of children under 5 years or of adolescents).

Groups and Other Programs. The Clinic's programs promote overall self-esteem and a sense of mastery in the child and his family through various activities. One method proven successful in assisting families at the Joslin Clinic has been holding parent discussion groups led by a psychiatric social worker. Such groups provide an opportunity for lessening the isolation experienced by many families. In an atmosphere of mutual support and sharing, participants are encouraged to air their feelings of self-blame and resentment along with the fears of death and future complications. As parents recognize that some difficulties are inevitable, they gain increased confidence about their own ability to cope effectively. Expressing and confronting their own sad and frightening feelings—sometimes for the first time—parents are better able to encourage the same process in their

diabetic children and siblings, thereby easing tensions within the family.

Groups for diabetic children organized by age levels and led by trained professionals are similarly beneficial. Activity-oriented group sessions for young children and "rap sessions" for older ones allow feelings of being alone and different to be expressed through an interchange of similar worries, questions, and experiences.

When the physician does not have readily available the resources of a specialized juvenile diabetes treatment team, the patient may be referred to a medical center or local diabetes association. Such settings, in which diabetes is the specific focus, give families the comfortable feeling that their special needs are provided for. Families can also increase their sense of proficiency and self-confidence through contacts with other families who share similar concerns or through working themselves to establish special programs for juvenile diabetes.

One example of a volunteer program, supervised by professionals, matches the family of a newly diagnosed juvenile diabetic with a family of similar background who have already achieved a positive adjustment to the illness. Through frequent informal meetings about similar problems, the recipient's family gains not only a source of support, but also a model for positive identification. For the more experienced family there is the opportunity to build further confidence and mastery by demonstrating their success and channeling their energies in a productive direction.

Diabetes in Young Adulthood. The incidence of new diabetes in individuals between the ages of 15 to 20 years is less than at ages 10 to 12. Whether the young person has recently diagnosed diabetes or has been living with it since early childhood, the primary issue at this age is concern about the actual or potential manifestation of physical damage related to the chronic syndrome. Some patients are overwhelmed by the fear of physical impairment whereas others actively suppress these concerns. Often patients obtain information from inappropriate sources, and tend to confuse their own prognosis with inadequately understood statistics and bits of information designed to dramatize the disabilities associated with diabetes in behalf of fund-raising. The primary tasks of late adolescence and young adulthood are those of separation from parents, usually by seeking education, a career, or a job away from home, finding a partner with whom to share one's life, and ultimately making decisions about having a family. Concerns about the presence of a chronic illness may inhibit this progression. Some young people make decisions based on incomplete information, which change the course of their lives. Some avoid marriage or permanent relationships, seek sterilization, or fail to commit themselves to endeavors that take long periods of time.

From time to time, it is necessary to discuss with care and understanding the prognosis for quality and duration of life with young adult patients, and to review the known facts about the long-term outcome of youth-onset diabetes. The great difficulty in predicting prognosis stems from major deficiencies of available information. No large prospective longitudinal cohort study has been completed. Retrospective analyses of patients whose diabetes started some years or decades ago do not represent the improved outlook for those starting therapy in more recent times. It is not definitely known whether the clustering of clinical problems as seen in young adults with long-term diabetes represents the results of treatment or is an expression of the heterogeneity of youth-onset diabetes, or both. An active approach to the management of diabetes as well as general health issues are usually associated with less depression than a passive nihilistic attitude toward the disease.

As the duration of diabetes lengthens in patients who escape the microvascular manifestations of diabetes in eyes and kidneys, it can be increasingly reassuring that the long-term prognosis is good (see Chapter 12). Those with diabetes of more than 25 years' duration face predominantly macrovascular disease, more often involving the heart than the lower extremities. This may be more reassuring than the physician might anticipate. Heart attacks and strokes in later life are considered "normal" and it is generally known that many survive such acute episodes and do well. Gangrene and major amputations are disfiguring, disabling, and irreparable and almost uniquely associated with diabetes. Good preventive foot care can go a long way to avoiding such problems. (For further details, see Chapter 35.)

There is now increasing evidence that successful long-term management of diabetes can postpone major complications of the disorder (see Chapters 1, 10 and 19). This evidence includes indications of possible reversibility or, at least, delay in progression, of which patients should be made aware.

Even under the best circumstances, disciplined regulation of food and especially of carbohydrate intake in teenagers is a large task. By age 20, most young adults with diabetes should be independent of their parents. Their concern for other young people with diabetes, as well as their own health, can impel them to move on with treatment of their condition. Peer support becomes helpful as they join with each other in efforts to promote research toward better treatment of diabetes. Even chroni-

cally depressed and angry young people, resentful of the effect of diabetes on their lives, may achieve a sense of satisfaction by monitoring urine and blood glucose and adjusting treatment, thus gaining a sense of control of the diabetes.

Optimism for the Future. The use of home glucose monitoring makes the correction of blood glucose levels more possible. Interest in newer technical aspects of care such as the "open loop" pump is high in young adults. These methods, coupled with intensive monitoring, can demonstrate to the patient the ability to master a serious chemical fault. This new-found strength also enhances other aspects of the individual's self-esteem. Increased responsibility for all phases of life can be helped by this ability to deal effectively with one's medical problems. The reality of improved insulin delivery systems in the 1980s gives increased hope of minimizing the long-term complications of diabetes. The physician must continue to be optimistic about ongoing advances in medical science that may prevent or ameliorate the complications of diabetes.

CAMPS FOR DIABETIC CHILDREN

Since their inception in the 1920s, camping programs for young people with diabetes have been recognized as beneficial both emotionally and educationally. In about 1925 or 1926, the first summer camp for diabetic children was established by Dr. Leonard F.C. Wendt[122] of Detroit, but was later discontinued. The first one to have continuous operation (except for war years) is Camp Ho-Mita-Koda, founded in 1929 by Dr. Henry John of Cleveland. The Joslin Clinic program had its origin in 1925 when a Deaconess Hospital nurse took one child to her home in Ogunquit, Maine, for the summer. The result was so impressive that the following summer, 5 children were sent and by 1931, 28 children. In 1932, the Clara Barton Birthplace Camp for Girls was established in North Oxford, Massachusetts, by the Universalist Alliance[123] and continues today under the sponsorship of the Unitarian Universalist Women's Federation. The Elliott P. Joslin Camp for Boys was established in 1948 at Charlton, Massachusetts, three miles away, and has been in continuous operation since.

In the early years, camps were often considered "hospitals in the woods." They were geared to health care delivery and education with exercise relegated to a secondary role. Slowly, exercise became a more important focus of the camp programs. Camps such as the Clara Barton and Joslin have integrated sports into their programs. Dr. Mary Olney pioneered the concept of wilderness camping for children with diabetes at Camp Bearskin Meadow in California, and Dr. Donnell Etzwiler introduced wilderness canoe experiences at Camp Needlepoint in Minnesota.

During the summer of 1940, there were in the United States approximately 18 summer camps[124] specifically for children with diabetes. The number of camps has grown steadily with 48 operating in 1973[125] and 69 in 1983,[126] plus 13 in Canada. In a study done by the International Diabetes Federation in 1979, it was learned that 20 of the 24 nations surveyed reported the presence of organized camping programs for people with insulin-dependent diabetes.[127]

In addition to the more traditional residential summer camping, other programs have developed to help meet diverse needs. In the summer of 1982 several day camps were inaugurated for children with diabetes and members of their families. Such programs include wilderness camping, bicycling camps, family camps, and winter camping programs. Success in these efforts has led to camps for senior citizens with diabetes. One of the first such was developed in 1970 by Drs. Joseph C. Shipp and Addison Scoville in Florida.[128] Smaller programs for adolescents such as winter camps and wilderness programs differ from the traditional summer camp program by giving the teenagers virtually all of the responsibility for their diabetes management under the supervision of medical and counseling staffs. Similar programs including week-end retreats are being developed by diabetes groups throughout the country for young people and their families.

During the first 50 years of diabetes camping, the professionals involved have had informal communication with each other. In 1974, Dr. Etzwiler established the first International Diabetes and Camping Workshop,[129] which provided an official forum in which health care professionals and administrators of diabetes camps could work together. Since that time, there have been eight such workshops permitting camp personnel from all over the world to meet, share resources and experiences, promote new camp programs, improve those presently available, and to develop guidelines for diabetes camping programs internationally. The ninth such conference was held May 19–22, 1984 at the Elliott P. Joslin Camp for Boys, Charlton, Massachusetts. It was sponsored by the American Diabetes Association and hosted by the Joslin Camp and the nearby Clara Barton Birthplace Camp for Girls.

The Committee on Camps of the American Diabetes Association has developed minimum standards of health and safety for camps which accept children with insulin-dependent diabetes. In March, 1982, the American Camping Association accepted these standards to be used for accreditation of all camps which accept children with diabetes, an important step toward insuring that camping experiences for children with diabetes are healthful and safe.

At the first International Workshop on Diabetes and Camping, it was decided that camps specializing in diabetes should be referred to as "Camps for Children with Diabetes" thus recognizing that the primary purpose of these camps is the recreational experience of the youngsters. Planning focuses on providing maximum stimulation and enjoyment for the child, commensurate with good treatment of diabetes. Camping is defined by the American Camping Association as a "sustained experience which provides a creative, recreational and educational opportunity in group living out-of-doors. It utilizes trained leadership and resources of natural surroundings to contribute to each camper's mental, physical, social and spiritual growth."[130] It is the goal of the diabetes camp professionals to help campers learn to live with their diabetes so that the disease no longer inhibits their lives inappropriately.

Professionals at such camps have the challenge of treating the diabetes optimally while helping the child to participate fully in a total camp experience. The American Diabetes Association's Committee on Camps in 1976 suggested a list of objectives for camps for children with diabetes,[131] the first of which is to provide an enjoyable recreational camping experience for children with diabetes mellitus.

Diabetes education remains an important part of the total program, and must be carried out in the context of the camp environment so that learning is enjoyed more and retained better. Diabetes specialty camps strive to provide freedom, understanding, and nurturing of the ego.[132] Freedom from discrimination, guilt, and overprotectiveness of parents is promoted, thereby engendering in the children a feeling of independence based on competence. The camp leaders strive to promote better comprehension of self as well as of diabetes management, providing the young person with increasing perspective about making good decisions, based on awareness of options. Nurturing the ego enhances self-esteem and self-confidence. The camp environment provides a unique opportunity for young people to associate in a peer group in which all are learning to deal with similar issues about managing diabetes successfully. Here also there are positive role models a few years older who have mastered some of the problems with diabetes management each young person must face. It was noted in a study by McCraw and Travis[133] that the boys and girls who attended their diabetes camp showed a significant increase in self-esteem. It is the belief of many who work with young people with diabetes that this helps a young person manage the diabetes effectively. Camping programs provide a most significant impact on many young people with diabetes, often creating the central core of support for them as they are growing up.

The technical aspects of the treatment programs that have been described here are in a state of evolution and flux. Patients, families and physicians must remain diligent, open-minded and optimistic in their striving to promote the best of health for young people who live with the daily challenge of diabetes.

REFERENCES

1. White, P., Graham, C.A.: The child with diabetes. In: A. Marble, P. White, R.F. Bradley, L.P. Krall (Eds.): Joslin's Diabetes Mellitus, 11th Ed. Philadelphia, Lea & Febiger, 1971. pp. 348, 354.
2. Gorwitz, K., Howen, G., Thompson, T.: Prevalence of diabetes in Michigan school-aged children. Diabetes 25:122, 1975.
3. U.S. Department of Health, Education and Welfare Service: Diabetes Data Compiled 1977, DHEW Publication No. (NIH) 78–1468, U.S. Government Printing Office, 1978.
4. Kyllo, C.J., Nuttall, F.Q.: Prevalence of diabetes mellitus in school-age children in Minnesota. Diabetes 27:57, 1978.
5. LaPorte, R.E., Fishbein, H.A., Drash, A.L., et al.: The Pittsburgh Insulin-dependent Diabetes Mellitus Registry. Diabetes 30:279, 1981.
6. Ehrlich, R.M., Walsh, L.J., Falk, J.H., et al.: The incidence of Type I (insulin-dependent) diabetes in Toronto. Diabetologia 22:289, 1982.
7. Fleegler, F.M., Rogers, K.D., Drash, A.L., et al.: Age, sex, and season of onset of juvenile diabetes in different geographic areas. Pediatr. 63:376, 1979.
8. North, A.F., Gorwitz, K., Sulfa, H.A.: A secular increase in the incidence of juvenile diabetes mellitus. J. Pediatr. 91:706, 1977.
9. West, R., Belmonte, M.M., Colle, E., et al.: Epidemiologic survey of juvenile-onset diabetes in Montreal. Diabetes 28:690, 1979.
10. Wagener, D.K., Sacks, J.M., LaPorte, R.E., MacGregor, J.M.: The Pittsburgh Study of Insulin-dependent Diabetes Mellitus. Diabetes 31:136, 1982.
11. Simpson, N.E.: The genetics of diabetes: a study of 233 families of juvenile diabetics. Ann. Hum. Genet. 26:1, 1962.
11a. Simpson, N.E.: Diabetes in the families of diabetics. Canad. Med. Assn. J. 98:427, 1968.
11b. Simpson, N.E.: The genetics of diabetes mellitus—a review of family data. In: W. Creutzfeld, J. Köbberling, J.V. Neel (Eds.): The Genetics of Diabetes Mellitus. Heidelberg, Springer Verlag, 1976, pp. 12–20.
12. White, P.: Natural course and progress of juvenile diabetes. Diabetes 5:445, 1956.
13. Pyke, D.A., Nelson, P.G.: Diabetes mellitus in identical twins. In: W. Creutzfeld, J. Köbberling, J.V. Neel (Eds.): The Genetics of Diabetes Mellitus. Heidelberg, Springer Verlag, 1976. pp. 194–202.
13a. Wentworth, S.M.: Unpublished data.
14. Rotter, J.I., Rimoin, D.L.: Heterogeneity in diabetes mellitus. Update, 1978. Diabetes 27:599, 1978.
15. Fajans, S., Floyd, J.C., Jr., Taylor, C.I., Peck, S.: Heterogeneity of insulin responses in latent diabetes. Trans. Assoc. Am. Physicians 87:83, 1974.
16. S. Fajans (Ed.): Diabetes Mellitus. Fogarty International Center Series, 1976. DHEW Publication No. (NIH) 76, 854.
17. Nerup, J., Andersen, O., Christy, M., et al.: HLA autoimmunity, virus, and the pathogenesis of juvenile diabetes mellitus. Acta Endocrinol. 83 (Suppl. 205) 167, 1976.
18. Rotter, J.I., Rimoin, D.L.: The search for genetic markers. Diabetes Care 2:215, 1979.
19. Sakurami, T., Ueno, Y., Nagoka, K., et al.: HLA-DR specifications in Japanese with juvenile-onset insulin-dependent diabetes mellitus. Diabetes 31:105, 1981.
20. Koivisto, V.A., Kuitunen, P., Tillikainen, A., et al.: HLA antigens in patients with juvenile diabetes mellitus, coeliac disease and both of the diseases. Diabete Metab. 3:49, 1977.
21. Bottazzo, G.R., Doniach, D., Pouplard, A.: Humoral autoimmunity in diabetes mellitus. Acta Endocrinol. 83 (Suppl. 205):55, 1976.
22. Irvine, W.J., Barnes, E.W.: Addison's disease, ovarian failure, and hypothyroidism. Clin. Endocrinol. Metab. 4:379, 1975.
23. Bright, G.M., Blizzard, R.M., Kaiser, D.L., et al.: Organ specific antibodies in children with common endocrine diseases. J. Pediatr. 100:8, 1982.
24. Neufeld, M., Maclaren, N.K., Riley, W.J., et al.: Islet cell and other specific antibodies in U.S. Caucasians and Blacks with insulin-dependent diabetes mellitus. Diabetes 29:589, 1980.
24a. Srikanta, S., Ganda, O.P., Eisenbarth, G.S., Soeldner, J.S.: Islet-cell antibodies and beta-cell function in monozygotic triplets and twins initially discordant for Type I diabetes mellitus. N. Engl. J. Med. 308:322, 1983.
24b. Gorsuch, A.N., Spencer, K.M., Lister, J., et al.: Evidence for a long prediabetic period in Type I (insulin-dependent) diabetes mellitus. Lancet 2:1363, 1981.
24c. Kaldany, A., Hill, T., Wentworth, S., et al.: Trapping of peripheral blood lymphocytes in the pancreas of patients with acute-onset insulin-dependent diabetes mellitus. Diabetes 31:463, 1982.
25. Riley, W.J., Maclaren, N.K., Lezotte, D.C., et al.: Thyroid autoimmunity in insulin-dependent diabetes mellitus. The case for routine screening. J. Pediatr. 99:350, 1981.
26. Adams, S.F.: The seasonal variation in the onset of acute diabetes. Arch. Intern. Med. 37:861, 1926.
27. Maclaren, N.K.: Viral and immunological basis of beta cell failure in insulin-dependent diabetes. Am. J. Dis. Child. 131:1149, 1977.
28. West, R., Colle, E., Belmonte, M.M., et al.: Prospective study of insulin-dependent diabetes mellitus. Diabetes 30:584, 1981.
29. Sultz, H.A., Hart, B.A., Zielezny, M., Schlesinger, E.R.: Is mumps virus an etiological factor in juvenile diabetes mellitus? J. Pediatr. 86:654, 1975.
30. Bloom, A., Hayes, T.M., Gamble, D.R.: Register of newly diagnosed diabetic children. Br. Med. J. 3:580, 1975.
31. Christau, B., Kromann, H., Andersen, O., et al.: Incidence, seasonal and geographic patterns of juvenile-onset insulin-dependent diabetes in Denmark. Diabetologia 13:281, 1977.
32. Wentworth, S.M., Gregory, R.I.: Indiana's camp for diabetic children. A 16-year follow-up. J. Ind. State Med. Assn. 65:316, 1972.
33. Gleason, R.E., Kahn, C.B., Funk, I.B., Craighead, J.E.: Seasonal incidence of insulin-dependent diabetes (IDDM)

in Massachausetts, 1964–1973. Int. J. Epidemiol. *11*.39, 1982.

34. Menser, M.A., Forrest, J.M., Bransby, R.D.: Rubella infection and diabetes mellitus. Lancet *1*:57, 1978.
35. Adi, F.C.: Diabetes mellitus associated with epidemic of infectious hepatitis in Nigeria. Br. Med. J. *1*:183, 1974.
36. Champsaur, H.F., Bottazzo, G.F., Bertrams, J., et al.: Virologic, immunologic and genetic factors in insulin-dependent diabetes mellitus. J. Pediatr. *100*:15, 1982.
37. Cudworth, A.G., Gamble, R.R., White, G.B.B.: Etiology of diabetes: a prospective study. Lancet *1*:1880, 1975.
38. Coleman, T.J., Taylor, K.W., Gamble, D.R.: The development of diabetes following Coxsackie B virus infection in mice. Diabetologia *10*:755, 1974.
39. Yoon, J.W., Notkins, A.L.: Virus-induced diabetes mellitus. J. Exp. Med. *143*:1170, 1976.
40. Rayfield, E.J., Gorelkin, L., Curnow, R.T., Jahrling, P.B.: Virus-induced pancreatic disease by Venezuelan encephalitis virus. Alterations in glucose tolerance and insulin release. Diabetes *25*:623, 1971.
41. Flood, T.M., Brink, S.J., Gleason, R.E.: Increased incidence of Type I diabetes in children of older mothers. Diabetes Care *5*:571, 1982.
42. Helgason, T., Jonasson, M.R.: Evidence for a food additive as a cause of ketosis-prone diabetes. Lancet *2*:716, 1981.
43. Sanders, H.J.: Diabetes: rapid advances, lingering mysteries. Chemical and Engineering News. March, 1981, pp. 30–46.
44. National Diabetes Data Group: Classification and diagnosis of diabetes mellitus and other categories of glucose intolerance. Diabetes *28*:1039, 1979.
45. Rosenbloom, A.L., Kohrman, A., Sperling, M.: Classification and diagnosis of diabetes mellitus in children and adolescents. J. Pediatr. *98*:320, 1981.
46. Tattersall, R.B., Fajans, S.S.: A difference between the inheritance of classical juvenile-onset and maturity-onset type diabetes in young people. Diabetes *24*.44, 1975.
47. Rosenbloom, A.L.: Insulin responses of children with chemical diabetes mellitus. Am. J. Dis. Child. *282*:1228, 1970.
48. Kitselle, J.F.: Ein Fall von Diabetes bei einem Kinde. Kinderheilk *18*:313, 1842.
49. Cornblath, M., Schwartz, R.: Disorders of Carbohydrate Metabolism. Philadelphia, W.B. Saunders Co., 1976. pp. 218–227.
50. Ramsey, W.R.: Glycosuria in the newborn. Treatment with insulin. Trans. Am. Pediatr. Soc. *38*:100, 1926.
51. Gerrard, J.W., Chin, W.: The syndrome of transient diabetes. J. Pediatr. *61*:89, 1962.
52. DaCou-Voutatakis, C., Anagnostakis, D., Xanthou, M.: Macroglossia, transient neonatal diabetes mellitus and intrauterine growth failure: a new distinct entity? Pediatrics *55*:127, 1975.
53. Sodoyez-Goffaux, F., Sodoyez, J.C.: Transient diabetes mellitus in a neonate. Evaluation of insulin, glucagon, and growth hormone secretion and management with a continuous low-dose insulin infusion. J. Pediatr. *91*:395, 1977.
54. Pagleara, A.S., Earl, E.K., Kipnis, D.M.: Transient neonatal diabetes; delayed maturation of the pancreatic B-cell. J. Pediatr. *82*:97, 1973.
55. Thorsson, A.V., Hintz, R.L.: Insulin receptors in the newborn. N. Engl. J. Med. *297*:908, 1977.
56. Blethen, S.I., White, N.H., Santiago, J.V., Daughaday, W.H.: Plasma somatomedins, endogenous insulin secretion, and growth in transient neonatal diabetes mellitus. J. Clin. Endocrinol. Metab. *32*:144, 1981.

57. Finberg, L.: Hypernatremic (hypertonic) dehydration in infants. N. Engl. J. Med. *289*:196, 1973.
58. Rosen, R.C., Schwachman, H., Kulcycki, L.L.: Progressive impairment of insulin production for release in diabetes mellitus and cystic fibrosis of the pancreas. Laboratory and clinical observations. Am. J. Dis. Child. *104*:652, 1962.
59. Handwerger, S., Roth, J., Gorden, P., et al.: Glucose intolerance in cystic fibrosis. N. Engl. J. Med. *281*:451, 1969.
60. Krane, S.M.: Renal glycosuria. In: J.B. Stanbury, J.B. Wyngaarden, D.S. Fredrickson (Eds.): The Metabolic Basis of Inherited Disease, 4th Ed. New York, McGraw-Hill Book Co., 1977, pp. 1607–1617. (See also 5th Ed., 1983, pp. 1806–1807, in which appears an adaptation of the summary from the former edition.)
61. Rose, R.C., Fraser, G.R., Friedman, A.I., Kohner, E.M.: The association of juvenile diabetes mellitus and optic atrophy: clinical and genetical aspects. Quart. J. Med. *35*:385, 1966.
62. Raiti, S., Plotkin, S., Newns, G.H.: Diabetes mellitus and insipidus in two sisters. Br. Med. J. *2*:1625, 1963.
63. Thoren, C.: Diabetes mellitus in Friedreich's ataxia. Acta Pediatr. (Upps) *51* (Suppl. 135):239, 1962.
64. Smith, D.W.: Recognizable Patterns of Human Malformation, 2nd Ed. Philadelphia, W.B. Saunders Co., 1976. p. 357.
65. Zuppinger, K., Engel, E., Forbes, A.P., et al.: Klinefelter's syndrome. A clinical and cytogenic study in 24 cases. Acta Endocrinol. *54* (Suppl.):113, 1967.
66. Valloson, M.B., Forbes, A.P.: Autoimmunity in gonadal dysgenesis and Klinefelter's syndrome. Lancet *1*:648, 1967.
67. Engel, E., Forbes, A.P.: Cytogenic and clinical findings in 48 with congenitally defective or absent ovaries. Medicine (Balt.) *44*:135, 1965.
68. Mellon, J.P., Day, B.Y., Green, D.M.: Mongolism and thyroid autoantibodies. J. Ment. Defic. Res. *7*:31, 1963.
69. Schöffling, K., Schade, Ch.: Diabetes mellitus and impaired glucose tolerance in diseases with chromosomal aberrations. In: W. Creutzfeld, J. Köbberling, J.V. Neel (Eds.): The Genetics of Diabetes Mellitus. Heidelberg, Springer Verlag, 1976, pp. 125–137.
70. Perlman, K., Ehrlich, R.M.: Steroid diabetes in childhood. Am. J. Dis. Child. *136*:64, 1982.
71. Whitecare, J.P., Bodey, G.P., Hill, C.S., Samaan, N.A.: Effect of L-asparaginase on carbohydrate metabolism. Metabolism *19*:581, 1970.
72. Pui, C.H., Burghen, G.A., Bowman, P.W., Aur, R.J.A.: Risk factors for hyperglycemia in children with leukemia receiving L-asparaginase and prednisone. J. Pediatr. *99*:46, 1981.
73. O'Sullivan, J.B.: Gestational diabetes and its significance. In: R.A. Camerini-Davalos, H.S. Cole (Eds.): Advances in Metabolic Disorders, Suppl. 1, New York, Academic Press, 1970, pp. 339–346.
74. White, P.: Childhood diabetes. Its course and influence on the second and third generations. Diabetes *9*:345, 1960.
74a. Reference 1. p. 340.
75. Brush, J.M.: Initial stabilization of the diabetic child. Am. J. Dis. Child. *67*:429, 1944.
75a. Ludvigsson, J., Heding, L.G., Larsson, Y., Leander, E.: C-peptide in juvenile diabetics beyond the postinitial remission phase. Acta Paediatr. Scand. *66*:177, 1977.
75b. Madsbad, S. Faber, O.K., Binder, C., et al.: Prevalence of residual beta-cell function in insulin-dependent diabetics in relation to age at onset and duration of diabetes. Diabetes *27* (Suppl. 1):262, 1978.

75c. Ludvigsson, J., Heding, L.G.: Beta-cell function in children with diabetes. Diabetes 27 (Suppl. 1):230, 1978.

75d. Hoekstra, J.B.L., van Rijn, H.J.M., Erkelens, D.W., Thijssen, J.H.H.: C-peptide. Diabetes Care 5:438, 1982.

76. Camerini-Davalos, R.A., Marble, A., White, P., et al.: Effect of sulfonylurea compounds in diabetic children. N. Engl. J. Med. 256:817, 1957.

76a. White, N.H., Skor, D.A., Cryer, P.E., et al.: Identification of Type I diabetic patients at increased risk for hypoglycemia during intensive therapy., N. Engl. J. Med. 308:485, 1983.

77. Knowles, H.C., Guest, G.M., Lampe, J., et al.: The course of juvenile diabetes treated with unmeasured diet. Diabetes 14:239, 1965.

78. Kaufmann, R.L., Assal, J.P., Soeldner, J.S., et al.: Plasma lipid levels in diabetic children. Effect of diet restricted in cholesterol and saturated fats. Diabetes 24:672, 1975.

79. Belmonte, M.M., Gunn, T., Gonthier, M.: The problem of "cheating" in the diabetic child and adolescent. Diabetes Care 4:116, 1981.

80. Langdon, D.R., James, F.D., Sperling, M.A.: Comparison of single and split-dose insulin regimens with 24-hour monitoring. J. Pediatr. 99:854, 1981.

81. Jackson, R.L., Guthrie, R.A.: The Child with Diabetes Mellitus. (Kalamazoo, Mich.—The Upjohn Company) 1975.

82. Wentworth, S.M., Alles, B., Russell, B.: Care of children with diabetes in Indiana. J. Indiana State Med. Assoc. 75:120, 1982.

83. Ward, G.M., Simpson, R.W., Ward, W.A., Turner, R.C.: Comparison of two twice daily insulin regimens. Diabetologia 21:383, 1981.

83a. Dimitriadis, G.D., Gerich, J.E.: Importance of timing of preprandial subcutaneous insulin administration in the management of diabetes mellitus. Diabetes Care 6:374, 1983.

84. Paz-Guevara, A.T., Hus, T.H., White, P.: Juvenile diabetes mellitus after forty years. Diabetes 24:559, 1975.

85. Soeldner, J.S.: Treatment of diabetes mellitus by devices. Am. J. Med. 70:183, 1981.

85a. Stewart, C., Brink, S.J., Wentworth, S.: Insulin pump treatment (CS11) failure in children and adolescents. (Abstr.) Pediatr. Res. April, 1983.

85b. Campaigne, B.N., Gilliam, T.B., Spencer, M.I., et al.: Effects of physical activity program on metabolic control and cardiovascular fitness in children with insulin-dependent diabetes mellitus. Diabetes Care 7:57, 1984.

86. Eeg-Olofsson, O.: Hypoglycemia and neurologic disturbances in children with diabetes mellitus. Acta Paediatr. Scand. (Suppl) 270:91, 1977.

87. Haumont, D., Corchy, H., Pelc, S.: EEG abnormalities in diabetic children. Clin. Pediatr. 18:750, 1979.

88. Tsalikian, E., Becker, D.J., Crumrine, K., et al.: Electroencephalographic changes in diabetic ketosis in children with newly and previously diagnosed diabetes mellitus. Pediatrics 99:355, 1981.

89. Winter, R.J.: Profiles of metabolic control in diabetic children. Frequency of asymptomatic nocturnal hypoglycemia. Metabolism 30:66, 1981.

89a. Bolli, G.B., Gerich, J.E.: The "Dawn Phenomenon"—a common occurrence in both non-insulin-dependent and insulin-dependent diabetes mellitus. N. Engl. J. Med. 310:746, 1984.

90. Wentworth, S.M., Galloway, J.A., Davidson, J.A., et al.: The use of the purified insulins in the treatment of patients with insulin lipoatrophy. Presented at the International Diabetes Federation Meeting. Vienna, Austria, September 13, 1979.

90a. Hayford, J.T., Weydert, J.A., Thompson, R.G.: Validity of urine glucose measurements for estimating plasma glucose concentration. Diabetes Care 6:40, 1983.

91. Krauser, K.: Correlation between blood values and double voided urines. Masters thesis. Indiana University, 1981.

92. Feldman, J.M., Lebovitz, F.L.: Tests of glycosuria. Diabetes 22:115, 1973.

93. Dunn, P.J., Cole, R.A., Soeldner, J.S., et al.: Temporal relationships of glycosylated hemoglobin concentrations and glucose control in diabetes. Diabetologia 17:213, 1979.

94. Wentworth, S.M., Russell, B., Alles, B.: Clinical use of glycosylated hemoglobin. J. Indiana State Med. Assoc. 74:574, 1981.

95. Daneman, D., Wolfson, D.H., Becker, D.J., Drash, A.L.: Factors affecting glycosylated hemoglobin values in children with insulin-dependent diabetes. J. Pediatr. 99:84, 1981.

96. Morrison, J.A., deGroot, I., Edwards, B.K., et al.: Lipids and lipoproteins in 1926 school children age 6 to 17 years. Pediatr. 62:990, 1978.

97. Brink, S.J.: Blood lipids in Type I juvenile diabetes mellitus (Abstr.) Pediatr. Res. 14:568, 1980.

98. Chase, H.P.: Juvenile diabetes mellitus and serum lipids and lipoprotein levels. Am. J. Dis. Child. 130:1113, 1976.

99. National Center for Health Statistics Growth Charts, 1976. Monthly Vital Statistics Report #25. No. 3, Suppl. (HRA) 76–1120. Health Resources Administration, Rockville, Maryland, June, 1976.

100. Joslin, E.P., Root, H.F., White, P.: The growth, development and prognosis of diabetic children. J.A.M.A. 85:420, 1925.

101. Wagner, R., White, P., Bogan, I.K.: Diabetic dwarfism. Am. J. Dis. Child. 63:667, 1942.

102. Lee, R.G.L., Bode, H.H.: Stunted growth and hepatomegaly in diabetes mellitus. J. Pediatr. 91:82, 1977.

103. Doud, H.: Some aspects of growth in diabetic children. Postgrad Med. (Suppl.) 46:616, 1976.

104. Fisher, A.C., Machler, H.S., Marks, H.H.: Long-term growth of diabetic children. Am. J. Dis. Child. 64:413, 1942.

105. Boyd, J.D., Kantrow, A.D.: Retardation of growth in diabetic children. Am. J. Dis. Child. 55:460, 1938.

106. Jackson, R.L., Kelly, H.G.: Growth of children with diabetes mellitus in relationship to level of control of the disease. J. Pediatr. 29:316, 1946.

107. Jackson, R.L., Holland, E., Chatman, I.D., et al.: Growth and maturation of children with insulin-dependent diabetes mellitus. Diabetes Care 1:96, 1978.

107a. Rudolf, M.C.J., Sherwin, R.S., Markowitz, R., et al.: Effects of intensive insulin treatment on linear growth in the young diabetic patient. J. Pediatr. 101:333, 1982.

108. Laron, Z.: Treatment of diabetes in children revisited. Pediatr. Annals 3:63, 1974.

109. Sivan, S.K., Kayner, I.H.: Does control influence the growth of diabetic children? Arch. Dis. Child. 48:109, 1973.

110. Sterky, G.: Growth pattern in juvenile diabetes. Acta Med. Scand. Suppl. 177:82, 1967.

111. Craig, J.O.: Growth as a measure of control in the management of diabetic children. Postgraduate Med. 46 (Suppl.):607, 1970.

112. Tattersall, R.B., Pyke, D.A.: Growth in diabetic children. Lancet 2:1105, 1973.

112a. Ellis, D., Becker, D.J., Daneman, D., et al.: Proteinuria in children with insulin-dependent diabetes: Relationship to duration of disease, metabolic control, and retinal changes. J. Pediatr. 102:673, 1983.

113. The National Heart, Lung, and Blood Institutes Task Force on Blood Pressure Control in Children: Report of Task Force on Blood Pressure Control in Children. Pediatrics. Supplement 59 (5):797–820, May, 1977.

114. Smith, W.I., Jr., Rabin, B.S., Huellmantel, A., et al.: Immunopathology of juvenile-onset diabetes mellitus. I. IgA deficiency and juvenile diabetes. Diabetes 27:1092, 1978.

115. Starkman, H., Brink, S.: Limited joint mobility of the hand in Type I diabetes mellitus. Diabetes Care 5:534, 1982.

116. Brink, S.: Limited joint mobility (LJM) as a risk factor for complications in youngsters with IDDM. (Abstr.) Diabetes 32 (Suppl. 1):16a, 1983.

117. Baker, L., Barcai, A., Kaye, R., Haque, N.: Beta adrenergic blockade and juvenile diabetes: acute studies and long-term therapeutic trial. Evidence for the role of catecholamines in mediating diabetic decompensation following emotional arousal. J. Pediatr. 75:19, 1969.

118. Kogut, M.D.: Pathogenesis, diagnosis and treatment of diabetic ketoacidosis. Curr. Probl. Pediatr. 6: (4) 1, 1976.

119. Hauser, S.T., Pollets, D., Turner, B.L., et al.:Ego development and self-esteem in diabetic adolescents. Diabetes Care 2:465, 1979.

120. Simonds, J., Goldstein, D., Walker, B., Rawlings, S.: The relationship between psychological factors and blood glucose regulation in insulin-dependent diabetic adolescents. Diabetes Care 4:610, 1981.

121. Anderson, B.J., Miller, J.P., Auslander, W.F., Santiago, J.V.: Family characteristics of diabetic adolescents: relationship to metabolic control. Diabetes Care 4:586, 1981.

121a.Banion, C.R., Miles, M.S., Carter, M.C.: Problems of mothers in management of children with diabetes. Diabetes Care 6:548, 1983.

122. Stephens, J.W., Marble, A.: Place and value of summer camps in management of juvenile diabetes. Amer. J. Dis. Child. 82:259, 1951.

123. White, P.: Diabetes in Childhood and Adolescence. Philadelphia, Lea & Febiger, 1932, pp. 222–224.

124. Shanahan, M.: Camping Provisions for Diabetic Children in the United States. Thesis. Deposited in the University Library of the University of California, July 23, 1947.

125. American Diabetes Association, Inc.: 1973 List of Summer Camps for Children with Diabetes. New York, American Diabetes Association, Inc.

126. American Diabetes Association, Inc.: 1983 List of Summer Camps for Children with Diabetes. New York, American Diabetes Association, Inc.

127. Etzwiler, D.D.: International study on juvenile diabetes. IDF Bulletin 24:Feb. 1979, pp. 18–19.

128. Shipp, J.C.: Adults away. Diabetes Forecast 34:March/April, 1981, p. 39.

129. Etzwiler, D.D., Robb, J.R.: First International Workshop on Diabetes and Camping. May 8, 9, 10, 1974. Camp Needlepoint, Hudson, Wisconsin.

130. American Camping Association: Standards with Interpretation for the Accreditation of Organized Camps. 1980.

131. Skyler, J.S., and Camps Committee Members: Recommended Standards for Camps for Children with Diabetes. Committee on Camps, New York, American Diabetes Association, Inc., 1976.

132. Skyler, J.: Camping for Youth with Diabetes Mellitus. First International Workshop on Diabetes and Camping. May 8, 1974. Camp Needlepoint, Hudson, Wisconsin.

133. McCraw, R.K., Travis, L.B.: Psychological effects of a special summer camp on juvenile diabetics. Diabetes 22:275, 1973.

25 Diabetes in the Elderly

Alexander Marble

The average duration of life in the United States has increased steadily from 47 years in 1900 to an estimated 74 years in 1980.[1] In the latter year, people aged 65 years and over numbered 25.5 million or 11.3% of the total population of approximately 222 million.[2] These increases in the older segment reflect great progress in the prevention of perinatal and infant mortality as well as the extraordinary advances in the prevention and treatment of disease in general. Persons with diabetes have shared in all of this and in addition, have benefited dramatically and uniquely from the discovery of insulin in 1921.

It has been estimated that 5% of the population has some degree of glucose intolerance, ranging all the way from a slight, asymptomatic and often undiagnosed state to overt diabetes of the insulin-dependent variety (Type I). Large though the estimate of 5% seems, the actual percentage is much greater in persons over the age of 50. Studies, such as those of Tokuhata[3] in Pennsylvania, suggest that in the elderly, the prevalence of diabetes and impaired glucose tolerance may be 20% or more. This is based on the fact that known diabetes is often not even mentioned on death certificates of persons with known diabetes who die of atherosclerotic cardiovascular disease or other conditions which have a much greater morbidity and mortality in diabetic than in nondiabetic individuals.

National recognition of the growing elderly population with its unique problems came in 1974 with the creation of the National Institutes on Aging, an important function of which is to stimulate geriatric research. In October, 1976, Congress established the National Diabetes Advisory Board to advise Congress and the Secretary of Health, Education and Welfare on the implementation of a "Long-Range Plan to Combat Diabetes" (P.L. 94–562). This was designed to expand and coordinate the national effort both in research and in diabetes control, health care and education.

Since May, 1970, the Joslin Diabetes Center has been privileged to award a 50-Year Medal and Certificate to over 700 patients who, with one rare exception,[4] have had well-documented, insulin-dependent diabetes (IDDM) for 50 years or more. One of these (JC 2808)[4a] had had extremely unstable diabetes for over 64 years when in May, 1983 he died at 87 of acute myocardial infarction. There is good basis for believing that in the world today there are sizeable, although untabulated, numbers of persons who have had IDDM for a half-century or more.

In the past decade or two, interest has run high in the diabetes of young people, especially those with IDDM who comprise perhaps 95% of those with onset under age 20, and the majority of those with onset under age 40. This upsurge of interest and accelerated research are most gratifying and hopefully intensive work will continue. However, one needs to keep prominently in mind that the vast bulk of diabetic patients are over the age of 40 to 50 years, and for the most part have non-insulin-dependent diabetes (NIDDM; Type II) and impaired glucose tolerance (IGT; formerly called "chemical" diabetes). Taken as a whole, this is a heterogenous group, composed both of persons with idiopathic and those with secondary glucose intolerance. Much more attention should be paid also to this vast group both in the laboratory and clinic. Study and treatment should be more aggressive than it currently is, especially for those in the three decades between 40 and 70, in the hope of preventing or reducing morbidity and mortality arising from macro- and micro-vascular diseases as well as neuropathy.

Elsewhere in this book, many topics have been presented that apply to the elderly diabetic. However, in view of the growing number of older persons with diabetes and the special problems that they have, it has seemed wise and appropriate to prepare this chapter for a more specific discussion. To avoid duplication, reference will be made frequently to other chapters.

DIAGNOSIS

Methods and standards of diagnosis and classification of diabetes, including those recently proposed,[5] are outlined and assessed in Chapter 15 and therefore will not be repeated here. However, it is worth pointing out that when specific values for circulating glucose are given, one must be sure whether reference is made to plasma, whole venous, or capillary blood and whether to fasting or postprandial samples (and, if the latter, how long after food).

Among those interested in diabetes there has long been a nagging question as to whether the same diagnostic standards should be applied to older persons as to young people. Some have proposed, and many others have accepted, the dictum that beginning at, say, 50 years of age, blood glucose values required for diagnosis during an oral tolerance test be increased either arbitrarily by 10 mg/dl per decade or by use of an age-adjusted nomogram.[6] This is based on the results of most surveys indicating that in the majority of persons in the general population, glucose tolerance deteriorates progressively as age advances. However, the degree to which this occurs varies considerably from 4 to 14 mg/dl (mean, 9 mg/dl) per decade.[7] Values obtained in the fasting state show only minor (1 to 2 mg/dl) progression by decade. From his studies, DeFronzo[7] concluded that the impairment in glucose tolerance is due largely to decreased sensitivity of tissues to insulin caused by the aging process. He assigned a secondary role to decreased physical activity, reduction in lean body mass and obesity.

In evaluating the published results of surveys designed to determine the frequency of diabetes in the general population, one should keep in mind that the subjects should have been in good general health, physically active, and nonobese. They should have had a food intake of at least 150 to 250 g of carbohydrate for at least 3 days prior to the test. Otherwise, one runs the risk of overestimating the prevalence of impaired glucose tolerance (IGT) in the nonobese healthy population. In this connection, in ordinary clinical practice, if fasting and random postprandial blood glucose values are within a normal range, no formal glucose tolerance test is necessary.

The level of glycosylated hemoglobin (HbA₁) has been reported to increase with age and to correlate with the fasting blood glucose.[8] However, definite standards in this regard remain to be worked out.

TYPE OF DIABETES

One ordinarily thinks of older persons with diabetes as having the non-insulin-dependent type (Type II). This is true in perhaps 70 to 80% of those who are 50 years of age or older. However, with increases in longevity, persons of older ages now include (a) large numbers of those with onset of Type I diabetes before the age of 30 to 40 years. An impressive number of these have hard-to-manage, unstable ("brittle") diabetes which poses difficult problems for both patient and physician. Another sizeable number have (b) Type I diabetes with onset after age 40 or later. Finally, there are (c) those persons who, although not truly insulin-dependent (i.e., do not need it for survival), benefit from endogenous insulin in order to provide optimal treatment. In keeping with the thesis presented earlier, it is likely that many more patients with Type II diabetes should be treated with insulin.

TREATMENT

In planning treatment for older persons, one keeps in mind that "health in the elderly is best measured in terms of function."[9] Restoration of functional activity not only allows the patient to preserve independence which is prized by all, but reduces the need for costly care in a nursing home and the amount of services required from the community. Common sense dictates that individuals must be evaluated not only according to the chronologic age but also by (a) the biologic age, namely the degree of integrity of vital organs and their functions and (b) the psychologic age which reflects the patient's temperament, disposition and zest for living.

Principles of Management

Continuity and Adequacy of Treatment. The older diabetic patient should be seen at regular intervals, varying in length according to individual needs, and preferably by a single physician who, in the present day, may well become the "primary" physician. Older patients appreciate greatly having "my doctor" who knows them well and to whom they may turn for advice and help both during and between visits. It is important that the physician not have rigid and pre-conceived standards that preclude excellent treatment of older persons with Type II diabetes.

Time at Visits. Elderly patients are apt to have many problems, some physical, some emotional, and some social, to which the physician must be prepared to deal with true concern and desire to help. "I like my doctor but he is always too busy to talk to me" is a comment heard much more frequently than it should be.

Approach to the Patient. As with all patients, the elderly individual should be treated as a whole person and not simply from the standpoint of diabetes. At each visit, unless these are quite frequent, an interval history and a relevant physical examination should be done to discover new complications if present and to call the attention of the patient and family to items of preventive care. Social conditions including economic status, place and mode of living, family composition, and habits of eating must be taken into account, particularly in caring for the older person.

Diet

Unless the elderly patient has ketoacidosis or symptoms of diabetes or an accompanying disease, the first approach in treatment should be solely that of an individually planned diet, particularly if the patient is overweight as is often the case. Under the physician's supervision, written instructions regarding the type and quantity of food should be given to the patient by a dietitian or teaching nurse. For best success, an accompanying family member should also be present so as to secure understanding and hopefully compliance. The diet plan must be outlined in simple terms for easy reference at home (to be posted in the kitchen and not filed in some drawer!). Such instruction must be amplified and questions answered at subsequent visits.

Over many years, elderly men and women have established certain habits of living and eating so that in planning the diet, their likes and dislikes should be taken into account as much as possible. Similarly, economic status, ethnic background, literacy, and similar factors must be kept in mind. Special attention should be given to instances in which the dietary history indicates an inadequacy of certain items, especially protein, vitamins, minerals and calories which are essential for maintenance of satisfactory (not excessive) weight, strength, and general health.

The greatest problem often arises with those of limited means who live alone in cramped quarters. Understandably, these persons are apt to dislike planning a meal, preparing vegetables, cooking the food, and then sitting down to eat alone. The result is that, from a nutritional standpoint, often the selection of food is considerably less than ideal. For such people, programs such as meals for Senior Citizens, provided by a city or town in schools or other public buildings, have the added great social advantage of permitting people to be with others

and to enjoy their company. Loneliness is often the greatest "disease" of the elderly person.

In planning the diet, other issues of special importance to the elderly arise from the digestive tract. Many lack teeth or have ill-fitting dentures so that the proper chewing of food is difficult, and the use of soft food necessary. Many are troubled with gastric and intestinal gas. This may at times be due to aerophagia but more commonly to the type of food and altered bowel function (malabsorption and decrease in specific enzymes). In prescribing diets for diabetic patients in general, it is customary to include liberal amounts of leafy green vegetables for vitamin and mineral content, satiety value and fiber content. However, in many people, foods which are high in fiber are also gas-forming and may cause considerable abdominal distress, so that the physician or dietitian must alter the diet plan accordingly. An important source of excess production of gas is deficiency to a variable degree of the enzyme, lactase. This deficiency increases with age and should be suspected particularly in older people who appear to be troubled unduly, especially after consuming milk and milk products.

Insulin and Oral Hypoglycemic Agents

For full discussion of these agents, see Chapters 19 and 21, respectively. However, a few general comments are indicated here. Since the majority of older diabetic persons have NIDDM, treatment with diet alone may suffice to restore the blood glucose to a normal or near-normal level. This is true especially if the patient is overweight and if restriction of calories is successful in lowering weight. However, in nonobese patients and in those in whom a reasonable food intake fails to control the blood glucose, the use of insulin or sulfonylurea compounds may be necessary. Obese, asymptomatic older patients should be allowed to give caloric restriction ample opportunity to bring about loss of weight and glycemic control (See Chapters 17 and 18). However, there should be no hesitancy whatever in treating with insulin those elderly patients who are underweight and have persistent hyperglycemia that does not respond to a sulfonylurea compound.

It is axiomatic that in the attempt to secure satisfactory blood glucose levels, care must be taken not to produce frequent or severe episodes of hypoglycemia. This is admittedly difficult in patients with unstable diabetes treated aggressively with insulin. However, almost always a reasonable compromise may be obtained. In this connection, it is well to keep in mind that in older diabetic patients, there may be adequate endogenous insulin which is not available to body tissues as in obese individuals with reduced insulin receptor sites. Reduction in body weight often corrects this difficulty.

Emphasis on serious attempts to lower body weight assumes added importance because of the finding that atherosclerotic states are often associated with elevated plasma insulin levels and exaggerated response of insulin to glucose given orally.[10] This is true particularly in patients with Type II diabetes who are obese and inactive physically.

Although the use of phenformin was banned in the United States in 1977 because of the possibility of lactic acidosis, it and other biguanides are still available in many other countries. Metformin and buformin are effective drugs and apparently their use has been linked with lactic acidosis to a smaller extent than phenformin.[11] Nevertheless, it must be emphasized that regardless of which biguanide is used, it must not be prescribed for patients with significant cardiac, hepatic or renal insufficiency or other conditions which in themselves might render the patient more likely to develop lactic acidosis.

Exercise

Like their younger counterparts, patients who are in their 60's or older benefit greatly by regular physical activity. The fortunate can swim, play golf, or even tennis. Others may dance, bowl, or engage in other forms of less strenuous activity. Except for those who are truly incapacitated, almost everyone, even if confined indoors, can find some form of exercise for arm and leg muscles. The best exercise for many is simply walking as briskly as permissible in view of heart, lung or joint problems. Such brisk walking is best done out-of-doors, and for those with ample time, walking two or more times a day is desirable unless the weather is inclement (See Chapter 22).

Hospitalization

In the United States, persons 65 years of age or older are admitted to hospitals much more frequently than are younger people. Those with diabetes spend twice as many days in the hospital as do nondiabetic individuals.[12] The causes for admissions are the same as for nondiabetics plus a larger proportion of conditions due to micro- and macro-vascular disease, or to other conditions such as infections, neuropathy, etc. All of these causes for admission are in addition to those for the management of diabetes itself and treatment of acute complications including ketoacidotic and hyperosmolar coma. The total cost of hospitalization is tremendous—whether paid by the patient, insurance, or welfare agencies—and this creates a challenging area for preventive medicine and cost containment. The hospice concept—relatively new in the United States—deserves more attention. Its use might well lower costs for the care of terminally ill patients but, more importantly, it would provide a more pleasant and comfortable environment during final days or weeks.

COMPLICATIONS

Acute

That hyperosmolar, nonketotic coma occurs more frequently in older than in younger patients is well known (see Chapter 26), but not so well appreciated is the occurrence of ketoacidotic coma and pre-coma in a significant number. Some years ago during a 15-year period, among 401 cases of ketoacidotic coma admitted to the Joslin Clinic service of the New England Deaconess Hospital, 51 or 12.7% were in patients aged 60 or over. Six of the 51 patients died; four of them had an accompanying acute myocardial infarction, probably a precipitating event of the ketoacidosis.[13]

Other acute complications to which the older diabetic is prone include infections and hypoglycemia. The latter may appear more insidiously in the old than in the young or at least, less well perceived. Of special note is hypoglycemia due to chlorpropamide which may occur particularly in thin, elderly patients who live alone, eat little and irregularly, and may even forget to eat. Usually it is easy to restore consciousness with glucose given intravenously but hypoglycemia is apt to recur due to the long-sustained action of this sulfonylurea agent. Consequently, the patient should be kept under observation for some hours as in an Emergency Ward overnight. It must also be kept in mind that severe hypoglycemia may occur in elderly persons who use alcohol to excess and who do not have an adequate food intake. Worth mentioning is the fact that in some patients taking beta-blocking drugs such as propranolol, the symptoms of hypoglycemia may be masked.

Chronic

The chronic complications are well known, especially coronary, cerebral, and peripheral vascular disease, retinopathy, nephropathy, and neuropathy of various types. They may appear to occur earlier in the course of Type II than Type I diabetes but the insidious start and early asymptomatic course often make it difficult to establish a probable date of onset. Special mention is due retinopathy, both background and proliferative, by no means uncommon in older patients (see Chapter 29); infection and gangrene of the feet (Chapters 34 and 35); chronically painful peripheral neuropathy; and diabetic amyotrophy, affecting especially older men (see Chapter 31).

For almost all chronic complications, treatment at present consists chiefly of palliative and "stop-gap" measures. Although these may provide great benefit, it is obvious that prevention is the necessary and desirable answer to the difficult problems presented.

HYPERGLYCEMIA: DISEASE OR NATURAL CONSEQUENCE OF AGING?

The elderly diabetic person is by no means immune from microvascular disease. However, the following discussion will concentrate on the related atherosclerosis which by its characteristic of arterial occlusion, contributes greatly to the high morbidity and mortality among older diabetic patients as expressed in cerebral, coronary and peripheral vascular disease. As factors for the development of atherosclerosis, various items have been suggested and investigated. Among these are hyperlipidemia, hypercholesterolemia, obesity, cigarette smoking, and the aging process. In the patient with diabetes or impaired glucose tolerance (IGT), the unique risk factor is hyperglycemia of varying degree, depending upon the severity of the metabolic disorder and the type and intensity of treatment employed. For a detailed discussion regarding macrovascular disease and diabetes, see Chapter 11. In the comments that follow here, the emphasis will be on the possibility of reducing the frequency of atherosclerotic complications and the question as to whether one should consider hyperglycemia as part of a specific disease process or a natural consequence of aging.

It is obvious that here one enters the broad and ill-defined area of what constitutes disease. Are progressive increases in the blood glucose during the last decades of life to be regarded as simply part of the process of growing old, for which serious treatment is not indicated? Or, should they be considered in the same light as other conditions which are related to the passing years such as elevated blood pressure or cardiac and cerebral vascular difficulties which are regarded as diseases worthy of prevention and treatment?

Evidence is mounting to indicate that reduction is possible in the degree of hypertension and the vascular complications just mentioned. In recent years, there has been a gratifying decline in coronary and cerebral vascular mortality in the general population of the United States.[14] This has occurred coincident with warnings from the Surgeon General regarding the dangers of cigarette smoking (heeded by large numbers of adults), and from the American Heart Association and others as to the risk of obesity, hypertension, and the excessive use of saturated fats, oils, and foods with high sodium and cholesterol content. A corresponding decrease in deaths from heart attacks and stroke has taken place in the diabetic population (see Chapter 13).

Hyperglycemia in the person with untreated diabetes varies from being constant and severe in overt diabetes to being slight and asymptomatic in the state now proposed to be called not diabetes but instead, "impaired glucose tolerance." In the last several years, Type I diabetes has been treated with much greater zeal and vigor. However, there is real basis for concern that persons in the category of Type II diabetes and IGT will in this regard be neglected or forgotten. There are some data indicating that persons with IGT, if untreated, will experience further deterioration in glucose tolerance.[15] Furthermore, there is evidence that those persons whose intolerance is not quite enough to classify as Type II diabetes, may develop over the years the same vascular and neurologic complications as their counterparts with overt diabetes, although not to the same degree.[16]

Ideally, one should try to obtain conclusive data from long-term, controlled, longitudinal studies to compare over a period of years the extent of atherosclerosis and its complications in a sizeable group of persons treated carefully with another group treated in present-day conventional fashion. In the first group, one would attempt to approach euglycemia as nearly as possible (with care not to produce frequent or severe hypoglycemic episodes in those using insulin). Obviously, such studies are extremely difficult to carry out and if one were planned on a large scale, the first and preliminary step would be to determine the feasibility of securing and maintaining excellent glycemic control in a study group over many years. To be expected are problems administering such a project including: (1) human frailty shown by the patient in failure to follow a prescribed diet, to avoid weight gain, to take insulin 2 or more times daily, and to monitor the blood glucose frequently; (2) difficulty in maintaining the interest and enthusiasm of clinical investigators in a long-term project; (3) attrition of subjects due to disinterest, change of residence, long continued illness, and death; (4) great cost which would need to be funded in the same manner as other projects of clinical investigation.

Studies along the general lines noted above have been carried out in Bedford,[17] England and Tecumseh,[18] Michigan and the prospective Whitehall study[19] of male British civil servants. The projects were of different type and design, but all three showed a definite, and in some instances a striking, influence of control of diabetes on vascular disease and deaths therefrom.

In summary, although the data at hand are not as conclusive as one demands with an experiment in the laboratory, there is evidence to indicate that among the items to be considered in the pathogenesis of atherosclerosis, hyperglycemia must be considered a risk factor of great importance.[20-22] Furthermore, indication is strong that if the blood glucose could be maintained at a level approaching euglycemia, the morbidity and mortality from vascular disease in diabetic patients would be significantly lowered. Allowing for the fact that one must take care in the elderly to avoid hypoglycemic episodes in those under treatment with insulin, there is still much room between that point and the average random blood glucose values commonly obtained and accepted. Improved treatment and more satisfactory control of diabetes in older patients may be expected to lead to improved health, higher quality of life in general, and economic benefits to the community at large.

REFERENCES

1. U.S. Public Health Service. National Center for Health Statistics, 1980.
2. Metropolitan Life Foundation: Continued increase in the elderly population. Statistical Bulletin 63:6 (July-Sept.) 1982.
3. Tokuhata, G.K., Miller, W., Digon, E., Hartman, T.: Diabetes mellitus: an underestimated health problem. J. Chron. Dis. 28:23, 1975.
4. Armitage, M., Frier, B.M., Duncan, J.P.: A misplaced medal? 50 years of unnecessary insulin treatment. Br. Med. J. 286: 844, 1983.
4a. Beckner, E.R.: Sixty-two years with diabetes. Keeping the lion caged. IDF (International Diabetes Federation) Bulletin 25:11, (Oct.) 1980.
5. National Diabetes Data Group: Classification and diagnosis of diabetes mellitus and other categories of glucose intolerance. Diabetes 28:1039, 1979.
6. Andres, R.: Aging and diabetes. Med. Clin. North Am. 55:835, 1971.
7. DeFronzo, R.A.: Glucose tolerance and aging. Diabetes Care 4:493, 1981.
8. Graf, R.J., Halter, J.B., Porte, D., Jr.: Glycosylated hemoglobin in normal subjects and subjects with maturity-onset diabetes. Evidence for a saturable system in man. Diabetes 27:834, 1978.
9. The Public Health Aspects of the Aging of the Population. Copenhagen, World Health Organization, 1959. Cited by Kennie, D.C.: Good health care for the aged. J.A.M.A. 249:770, 1983.
10. Stout, R.W.: The role of insulin in atherosclerosis in diabetics and nondiabetics. A review. Diabetes 30 (Suppl. 2): 54, 1981.
11. Cohen, R.D., Woods, H.F.: Lactic acidosis revisited. (Review article). Diabetes 32:181, 1983.
12. Kane, R., Solomon, D., Beck, J., et al: The future need for geriatric manpower in the United States. N. Engl. J. Med. 302:1327, 1980.
13. Barnett, D.M., Wilcox, D.S., Marble, A.: Diabetic coma in persons over 60. Geriatrics 17:327, 1962.
14. Walker, W.J.: Changing life style and declining vascular mortality—a retrospective. (Editorial). N. Engl. J. Med. 308:649, 1983.
15. Sartor, G., Schersten, B., Carlström, S., et al: Ten-year follow-up of subjects with impaired glucose tolerance. Prevention of diabetes by tolbutamide and diet regulation. Diabetes 29:41, 1980.
16. Keen, H., Jarrett, R.J., Fuller, J.H., McCartney, P.: Hyperglycemia and arterial disease. Diabetes 30(Suppl. 2):49, 1981.
17. Keen, H., Rose, G.A., Pyke, D.A., et al: Blood sugar and arterial disease. Lancet 2:505, 1965.
18. Ostrander, L.D., Jr., Francis, T., Jr., et al: The relation of cardiovascular disease to hyperglycemia. Ann. Intern. Med. 62:1188, 1965.
19. Fuller, J.H., Shipley, M.J., Rose, G.A., et al: Coronary heart disease risk and impaired glucose tolerance. The Whitehall Study. Lancet 1:1373, 1980.
20. Bell, E.T.: Arteriosclerotic gangrene of the lower extremities in diabetic and nondiabetic persons. Am. J. Clin. Pathol. 28:27, 1957.
21. Keen, H., Jarrett, R.J., Fuller, J.H., McCartney, P.: Hyperglycemia and arterial disease. Diabetes 30 (Suppl. 2):49, 1981.
22. Colwell, J.A., Lopes-Virella, M., Halushka, P.V.: Pathogenesis of atherosclerosis in diabetes mellitus. Diabetes Care 4:121, 1981.

26 Coma in Diabetes

Louis Vignati, A. Cader Asmal, William L. Black, Stuart J. Brink, and John W. Hare

Coma in a diabetic patient may be the end result of one of several conditions which may occur in both diabetic and nondiabetic persons, or it may represent a specific complication of the diabetes itself. In the latter category are included diabetic ketoacidosis (DKA), nonketotic hyperosmolar coma, hypoglycemia, lactic acidosis and possibly end-stage renal failure. Of these, the most important by far is DKA. The features, pathogenesis, and management of DKA and of some of the other diabetes-specific comas will be reviewed in this chapter.

DIABETIC KETOACIDOSIS

The terms DKA, precoma, and coma are used somewhat interchangeably to describe differing degrees of acute decompensation of diabetes of which clinically the cardinal features are dehydration and alterations in the sensorium. The biochemical hallmarks of the disorder are hyperglycemia (blood glucose levels usually greater than 350 mg/dl), ketonemia (plasma ketone levels usually greater than 5 mmol/L) and acidosis (plasma bicarbonate levels usually less than 9 mEq/L). Despite the imprecise terminology, a common denominator of the acute metabolic decompensation is the urgent need for insulin and replacement of fluid and electrolytes lost during the development of this unique complication.

Pathogenesis

Diabetic ketoacidosis develops in a milieu of severe insulin deficiency and excess levels of counterregulatory hormones. While the respective contribution of these factors is the subject of controversy, insulin deficiency per se is an essential condition for the development of ketoacidosis, although insulin antagonism may accelerate its progress or compound its severity. In order to place the pathogenesis of ketoacidosis into perspective, a brief account of the physiology of insulin and the contra-insulin hormones will be reviewed here. For further details the reader is referred to Chapters 3, 6, 8 and 9.

Insulin

The importance of insulin deficiency in precipitating ketoacidosis is underscored by the integral role that insulin subserves in the metabolic homeostasis of the body. Insulin is the pre-eminent hormone of anabolism and this function is most clearly observed in muscle, adipose tissue, and liver. At these sites, insulin interacts with its specific receptor[1,1a,2] and triggers a number of biochemical events,[3] culminating in the well-recognized biologic effects of the hormone. The identity of the second messenger of insulin action, represented by alterations in the intracytoplasmic concentrations of adenosine monophosphate cyclic nucleotide (cAMP), cellular ion flux, polarization of cell membrane, etc., has thus far escaped elucidation.[3]

Effects of Insulin on Muscle. The insulin receptor interaction on the muscle cell membrane promotes the intracellular transport of glucose,[4] potassium,[5] amino acids,[6] phosphorus and ketones;[7] stimulates glycolysis, glycogenesis, and protein synthesis;[8] and suppresses protein catabolism and amino acid release[5] (Fig. 26–1).

Effects of Insulin on Adipose Tissue.[9] The insulin receptor interaction on the adipocyte membrane triggers a series of important reactions culminating in the inhibition of lipolysis and stimulation of lipogenesis. The increase of glucose uptake which accompanies insulin action has the effect of augmenting glucose utilization via both the glycolytic and the hexose phosphate shunt pathways. Enhanced activity of the former yields increased amounts of α-glycerophosphate and acetyl-CoA, and of the latter, increased cellular levels of reduced nucleotide adenine dinucleotide phosphate (NADPH). The accumulation of these substrates favors lipogenesis. On the other hand, insulin, by mechanisms probably related to alterations in the levels of cAMP, lowers the activity of adipocyte hormone-sensitive lipase activity (also known as triglyceride lipase). This results in an inhibition of triglyceride hydrolysis. Conversely, insulin stimulates adipose tissue lipoprotein lipase activity thereby promoting the peripheral dismantling of triglycerides and uptake of fatty acids by the adipocyte (Fig. 26–2).

Effects of Insulin on the Liver (Fig. 26–3). The insulin receptor interaction on the hepatocyte membrane initiates several intracytoplasmic enzymatic reactions but has no direct influence on the cellular influx of glucose. Glucose metabolism

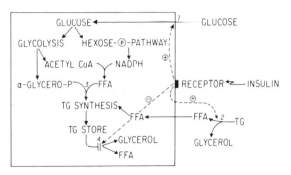

1. Glucose uptake stimulated
2. Lipoprotein lipase synthesis increased
3. Lipogenesis increased
4. Lipolysis inhibited

Fig. 26–2. The actions of insulin on adipocytes. Insulin promotes glucose and fatty acid uptake, favors lipogenesis, and inhibits lipolysis.

by the liver is modulated by a specific glucokinase which differs from other hexokinases by its higher Km (10 mmol/L) for glucose,[10] and its regulation by the prevailing glucose and insulin concentrations.[11] This ensures that hepatic glucose uptake is stimulated only when the blood glucose concentration is significantly elevated. Under these circumstances the glucose that is taken up is channeled through the pathway of glycogenesis, an event favored by the simultaneous insulin-mediated activation of glycogen synthetase activity[12] (Fig. 26–3).

Insulin favors the induction of several key glycolytic enzymes (phosphofructokinase, pyruvate kinase, and pyruvate dehydrogenase), and the suppression of important gluconeogenic enzymes (pyruvate carboxylase, phosphoenol pyruvate carboxykinase, fructose-1-6-diphosphatase, and glucose-6-phosphatase).[13,14] The blockade of hepatic amino acid uptake by insulin[15] reduces the supply of important gluconeogenic precursors. Inhibition of liver phosphorylase activity[11] by insulin ensures that glucose is not released into the circulation in the presence of hyperglycemia.

Insulin activates enzymes of the hexose phosphate shunt pathway, as well as two key lipogenic enzymes (acetyl-CoA carboxylase and fatty acid synthetase) in the liver.[16] These alterations promote hepatic lipogenesis and at the same time present an environment that is unfavorable for ketogenesis.[17]

Biochemical Consequences of Insulin Deficiency. Lack of insulin is invariably accompanied by an excess of counterregulatory hormone, such as glucagon, cortisol, catecholamines, or growth hormone, and the clinical picture seen is a composite one reflecting both events (Figs. 26–4 and 26–5). This consideration, as well as the differ-

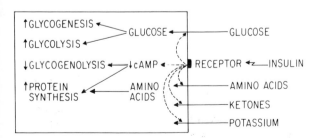

Fig. 26–1. The actions of insulin on muscle. Insulin stimulates the uptake of substrates across the muscle membrane, and independently promotes protein synthesis.

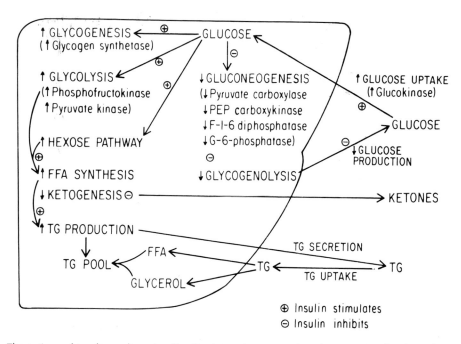

Fig. 26–3. The actions of insulin on liver. Insulin stimulates glucose uptake, glycogenesis, glycolysis, fatty acid synthesis and triglyceride production, and inhibits glycogenolysis, gluconeogenesis, and ketogenesis. PEP = phosphoenolpyruvate; FFA = free fatty acid; TG = triglyceride; F = fructose; G = glucose.

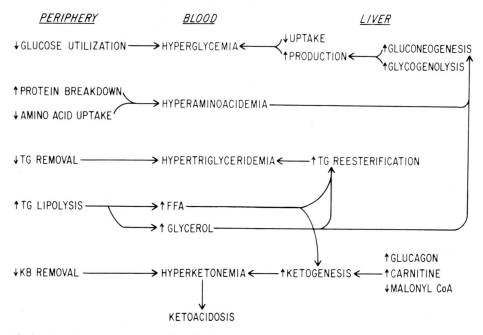

Fig. 26–4. The biochemical consequences of insulin lack.

ential sensitivities of tissues to the effects of insulin (such as lipolysis in adipose tissue or glucose uptake in muscle) account for the varying rates of appearance of the metabolic abnormalities in the course of DKA.

Hyperglycemia is a result of both increased hepatic gluconeogenesis and glycogenolysis, and de-

creased peripheral glucose utilization. Glucose production by the liver is stimulated by the heightened activity of gluconeogenic and glycogenolytic enzymes and by the accelerated influx of gluconeogenic precursors to the liver.

The increased plasma concentrations of the branched-chain amino acids (leucine, isoleucine,

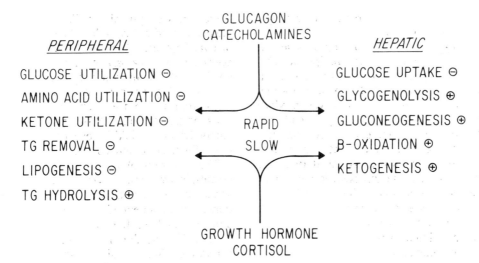

Fig. 26–5. The role of counterregulatory hormones in amplifying the consequences of insulin deficiency through a rapid (glucagon and catecholamines), or a slow (cortisol or growth hormone) action. The four hormones may not necessarily demonstrate all the effects on the liver and periphery.

and valine) and also α-aminobutyrate, reflect increased protein breakdown or reduced peripheral amino acid uptake.[15] On the other hand, the concentration of gluconeogenic amino acids such as glycine, alanine, threonine and serine is diminished because of augmented hepatic removal.[15]

Hypertriglyceridemia is the result both of defective removal of and overproduction of triglyceride. The former is brought about by a lipoprotein lipase deficiency as a result of insulin lack which is also responsible for the latter, caused by the enhanced hepatic reesterification of free fatty acids (FFA) released in the periphery.

Ketosis occurs when there is simultaneous hepatic hyperketogenesis and diminished peripheral ketone utilization.

Counterregulatory Hormones

Controversy pervades the issue of the relative importance of insulin deficiency as opposed to an excess of counterregulatory hormones in the pathogenesis of DKA.[19–30] This is engendered in part by the design of experimental studies that have sought to place the physiologic role of the anti-insulin factors into perspective. A major drawback of these investigations is that in attempting to dissect out the role of insulin and its antagonists, few if any have directly examined the influence of three parameters that may exercise a significant influence on insulin action, viz. residual β-cell function, the degree of insulin binding to antibody, and the status of the insulin receptors and post-receptor pathways. Until this is known, attempts to assign a primary role to insulin deficiency or to an excess of counterregulatory hormones in the pathogenesis of DKA are not very meaningful. In the present state of

knowledge it is perhaps prudent to accept that, while insulin deficiency is an essential condition for the occurrence of DKA, an excess of anti-insulin factors is necessary for the development of the whole picture.[30]

Glucagon. By virtue of its many diabetogenic actions,[19] glucagon occupies a pre-eminent position as a counterregulatory hormone. Glucagon has a potent hepatic glycogenolytic,[12] and gluconeogenic effect.[31] It increases adipocyte lipolysis,[19] accelerates hepatic ketogenesis independently of the lypolytic action,[32] and also possibly limits peripheral ketone utilization.[33] Glucagon is devoid of a direct effect on peripheral glucose utilization[19] and does not increase amino acid flux across the forearm.[34]

In patients with poorly controlled diabetes, basal glucagon levels are elevated[35] and dynamic responses altered. There is a failure of suppression of glucagon levels by a glucose load,[36] and an exaggerated glucagon rise in response to protein administration.[37] In DKA, plasma glucagon concentrations are markedly elevated[20,21] and considered by some to exert the dominant influence in bringing about the severe metabolic decompensation.[20]

The results of several studies designed to delineate the role of hyperglucagonemia in the evolution of ketoacidosis have been contradictory. Several workers have established evidence in support of a prominent role for glucagon,[22,23] whereas others have failed to confirm this in the absence of insulin lack.[24–27] Studies in pancreatectomized patients have yielded equally inconclusive results.[28–29]

On the basis of the available data, it would appear that glucagon is one of several contra-insulin factors that contribute to the metabolic derangements of uncontrolled diabetes.[27]

Growth Hormone. Pharmacologic doses of growth hormone (GH) depress peripheral glucose,[38] and possibly ketone utilization[39] and stimulate adipocyte lipolysis[40] and hepatic ketogenesis.[41] Physiologic doses of GH, however, produce less pronounced changes, especially in carbohydrate metabolism.[22] One explanation for this may be the slowness of onset of GH activity because of de novo protein synthesis.[30] A corollary of this is that once the activity is expressed, it may persist beyond the period of normalization of the GH levels. If this is the case, the absence of significant GH elevation in plasma would not exclude significant GH modulation of metabolic activity, a view that may be of relevance to the observation that GH levels are not universally elevated in ketoacidotic patients.

Cortisol. The counterregulatory effects of cortisol are typified by protein breakdown, gluconeogenesis, glycogen synthesis,[42] lipolysis,[43] ketogenesis, suppression of peripheral glucose,[44] and ketone[39] utilization. Cortisol infusion in diabetics provokes a delayed but significant hyperglycemic and ketonemic response.[30] Plasma cortisol secretion rates in DKA have been reported to be increased.[45-47] Thus, while excessive elevation of cortisol levels clearly contributes to the development of DKA, there is no direct evidence that it initiates the metabolic derangement.

Catecholamines. An increase in plasma catecholamine levels (or increased sympathetic activity) is accompanied by enhanced lipolysis,[48] glycogenolysis,[49] ketogenesis,[50] augmented glucagon,[51] and growth hormone[52] secretion, attenuated insulin release[53] and peripheral glucose[39] and ketone utilization.[39] The relevance of these metabolic effects of catecholamines is underscored by the potential role of stress in precipitating DKA[30] and in increasing plasma catecholamine concentration.[54] The available data demonstrating an elevation of catecholamine levels in DKA are, however, limited,[54,55] and more direct evidence is needed to uphold the concept that such elevations are indeed the triggering mechanism in the pathogenesis of DKA.

Ketogenesis

Ketogenesis occurs within the mitochondria of liver cells. Accelerated ketogenesis, as in uncontrolled diabetes, is due to two factors: (1) an augmented supply of FFA, the predominant precursor of ketone synthesis, to the liver; and (2) an alteration of the hepatic metabolism away from FFA synthesis to FFA oxidation.[56,57]

Insulin deficiency is the primary stimulus for adipose tissue lipolysis, while glucagon excess is the primary stimulus for hepatic ketogenesis.[11] The plasma FFA elevation mediated by peripheral lipolysis promotes a parallel increase in hepatic FFA uptake. Fatty acids within the liver follow one of two main disposal pathways: esterification within the cytoplasm to triglycerides, cholesterol, and phospholipid esters; or β-oxidation within the mitochondrium to yield ketone bodies, or CO_2 and H_2O (Figs. 26–6 and 26–7).

The direction of fatty acid flux is determined essentially by the rate at which they are translocated across the mitochondrial membrane. Fatty acid translocation is dependent on activation and transport. Long-chain fatty acids initially react with CoA, ATP, and thiokinase, forming an acyl-CoA derivative. This combines with carnitine and carnitine acyl-transferase-I which translocates the residue across the inner mitochondrial membrane. Carnitine acyl-transferase-II releases acyl-CoA into the mitochondrial matrix.[56,57]

Diminished activity of carnitine acyl-transferase-I reduces translocation of FFA, and increased activity promotes fatty acid oxidation and ketogenesis. Acyl-transferase activity is stimulated by raised carnitine concentrations,[58] as well as by depressed carbohydrate metabolism in general,[17] and reduced malonyl-CoA levels[59] in particular. Malonyl-CoA appears to be a pivotal substrate in fatty acid metabolism. Its synthesis is favored by a milieu conducive to lipogenesis. Inhibition of its production has the effect of terminating fatty acid synthesis on the one hand, and of stimulating fatty acid oxidation on the other. In DKA, serum carnitine levels have been shown to be reduced, whereas those of acyl-carnitine are raised.[60]

Mitochondrial β-oxidation of acyl-CoA residues yields acetyl CoA. Its further disposition is dependent on the intramitochondrial ratio of acetyl-CoA to CoA.[61] If the ratio is high, the formation of acetoacetyl-CoA is favored; if the ratio is low, citrate is formed. The rate of acetoacetyl-CoA formation is thus the most important determinant of ketone body synthesis, a process that is almost wholly dependent on the mitochondrial translocation of acyl-CoA by carnitine acyl-transferase. Once formed, acetoacetyl-CoA is the immediate precursor of the three ketones synthesized in the liver: acetoacetate, betahydroxybutyrate, and acetone. The hepatic biosynthesis of ketones provides an important alternative fuel source for muscle and, in states of starvation, for the brain.[62] In uncontrolled diabetes, the rate of ketone generation is excessive and unmatched by the capacity of peripheral tissues to utilize ketones under the influence of the prevailing insulin[63-65] and glucose concentrations.

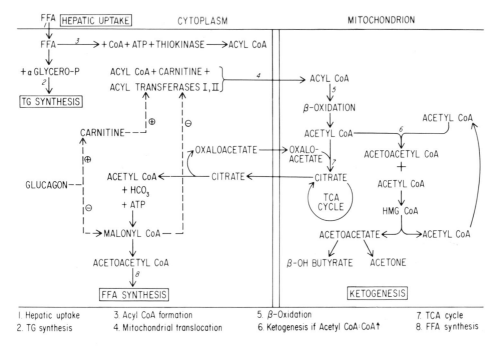

Fig. 26–6. Normal ketogenesis in the liver. The fate of the hepatic fatty acid taken up is determined by the level of hepatic de novo fatty acid synthesis, which modulates hepatic ketogenesis. CoA = coenzyme A; TCA = tricarboxylic acid cycle; HMG-CoA = β-hydroxy-β-methyl glutaryl-CoA.

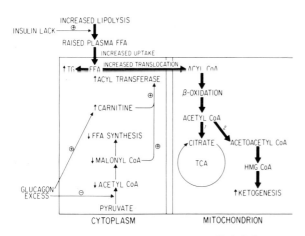

Fig. 26–7. Hyperketogenesis in uncontrolled diabetes is brought about both by insulin lack which increases substrate availability of fatty acid to the liver, and by glucagon excess which raises carnitine and lowers malonyl CoA levels, thereby augmenting mitochondrial fatty acid translocation.

Figure 26–8 illustrates the physiologic and clinical consequences of insulin lack.

Clinical Presentation

Cause of Ketoacidosis. While deliberate or misguided omission or reduction of insulin dosage is perhaps the commonest cause of decompensation in a previously well-stabilized patient, incidental and apparently minor factors, such as a common cold, urinary tract infection, or gastric upset, may well play an important contributory role. Clearly, any major stress, such as that of an acute infection, myocardial infarction, surgery, or cerebral vascular accident, may easily precipitate DKA. In some cases no cause is readily identifiable. The ingestion of concentrated glucose-containing food is not a predisposing factor, unless there is concomitant and well-advanced insulin deficiency. The rate of development of the ketoacidosis is variable and dependent on factors such as the presence and nature of acute precipitating circumstances and the inherent instability of the disease. If DKA is the presenting feature of new-onset diabetes, its evolution tends to be more gradual than if the decompensation arises in a patient with preexisting diabetes. In the latter, especially if control has been indifferent over the preceding period, DKA may develop within hours after omission of insulin.

Symptoms and Signs. Usual symptoms at presentation are those of progressive polydipsia, polyuria, weakness, malaise, nausea, vomiting and abdominal pain. Symptoms of the precipitating illness may overshadow those of the diabetes; conversely, the precipitating event may remain unobtrusive unless specifically sought out as in the case of a silent myocardial infarct. Physical examination may reveal evidence of varying degrees of dehydration ranging from mild tachycardia without orthostatic hypotension to severe hypovolemia and shock. In

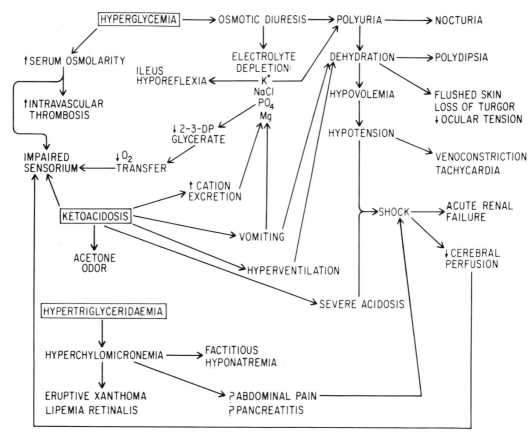

Fig. 26–8. The clinical features secondary to the physiologic consequences of insulin lack and counterregulatory hormone excess.

the severely acidotic patient, Kussmaul "air hunger" respiration may be evident, and the odor of acetone may be detected in the breath. The mental status may be completely clear, variably clouded, or the patient may be deeply comatose. About 10% of the patients described by Alberti and Hockaday in 1977[66] fell into the last-named category whereas a much smaller percentage of the patients seen now at the Joslin Clinic present in such a critical state. Hopefully, this is due to improved education of patient and family. The presence of abdominal distention and tenderness, the pathogenesis of which remain obscure, may direct attention to the possibility of an acute underlying surgical problem. Generally, correction of the ketoacidosis controls the vomiting and the abdominal pain. Physical examination may bring to light the precipitating factors of the DKA, such as pneumonia, meningitis, or a cerebral vascular accident.

Diagnosis. The diagnosis of DKA is based on the combination of a compatible clinical history, physical examination, and the presence of significant glycosuria and ketonuria. Blood studies help to confirm the diagnosis, provide an index of the

severity of the decompensation, and permit rationalization of therapy. The level of blood glucose is generally in excess of 350 mg/dl and that of ketones greater than 5 mmol/L. A clinical assessment of the severity of the ketosis can be made at the bedside using crushed Acetest tablets. Acetest measures the amount of acetoacetate in solution and becomes positive at a concentration of 0.1 mmol/L. As the ratio of the acetoacetate to betahydroxybutyrate is about 1:3, the serum dilution at which Acetest shows a trace of ketones is multiplied by a correction factor of 0.4. Thus, if the dilution is 1:32, the total ketone concentration is 12.8 mmol/L (32 × 0.4). On occasion the ratio of acetoacetate to betahydroxybutyrate may exceed 1:3, in which case the Acetest would underestimate the severity of the ketoacidosis. During treatment of DKA, betahydroxybutyrate concentrations fall because of conversion to acetoacetate. Thus, the Acetest may continue to be positive at the original or even higher dilutions during the initial stages of treatment.

The serum electrolytes depict no characteristic pattern in DKA. The serum sodium may be raised, lowered, or normal. Hypernatremia reflects a severe water loss whereas hyponatremia may be factitious due to marked hyperglycemia or hyperlipidemia. More importantly, although there is always a significant total body potassium depletion, the intial serum potassium level may be normal or even elevated due to dehydration and this has important implications for the therapeutic management of the patient in DKA. A metabolic acidosis as demonstrated by a fall in pH and serum bicarbonate concentration is an integral component of the decompensation. Plasma phosphate and magnesium levels may also be depressed. In contrast, plasma lipids may be markedly elevated with the lipemia causing a factitious hyponatremia. The white cell count is often elevated to 20,000 or more with a shift to the left. Serum amylase and creatinine kinase levels may also be raised, contributing to confusion in diagnosing such disease states as pancreatitis and coronary insufficiency.

Treatment of Diabetic Ketoacidosis

The successful treatment of the patient with diabetic ketoacidosis is one of the most rewarding experiences in clinical medicine. The success of the outcome is based on the recognition that DKA is a medical emergency. Early recovery and minimal mortality require prompt diagnosis and initiation of intensive therapy. In Table 26–1, the necessary steps are summarized in outline form. The problems listed below should be identified specifically and dealt with appropriately.

(1) *Unconsciousness,* when present in a diabetic ketoacidotic patient demands no less an intense approach to its management than when it occurs in a nondiabetic, i.e., close observation of vital signs and, if indicated, the establishment of an airway with administration of oxygen.

(2) *Dehydration,* with its attendant hypovolemia and hypotension require immediate correction with intravenous infusions of fluids.

(3) *Hyperglycemia* and *Ketoacidosis,* both of which respond dramatically to adequate insulin therapy.

(4) *Precipitating Factors* should be sought assiduously and dealt with definitively.

(5) *Special Measures.* A rapid evaluation should be made for the possible need of the following measures in the management of the patient:

(a) A central venous pressure line (usually not necessary).

(b) Urinary catheterization (to be avoided if possible).

(c) Electrocardiographic monitoring.

(d) Gastric lavage.

(e) Intubation, rarely necessary.

Because DKA is a metabolic state in flux and is dramatically influenced by medical intervention, it is essential that as management progresses according to plan, all relevant clinical, biochemical, and therapeutic changes be accurately recorded on a flow sheet. The vigilance of physicians and nurses needs constant focus on the following:

(1) the development of complications of DKA;

(2) the hazards of precipitating complications through mismanagement (Table 26–2).

There is no substitute for constant surveillance by the physician of the ever-changing scene. This responsibility cannot be delegated.

Insulin and Fluids. The placement of the following discussion of fluid and electrolyte replacement before that of insulin should not be interpreted as downgrading the all-important role of insulin in treatment. It should be given at once after diagnosis, usually at the same time that the administration of fluids is begun.

Fluid Replacement

The partial correction of dehydration within the first few hours of treatment will in itself bring about a substantial reduction in hyperglycemia and ketonemia. While there is no disagreement that saline solution is the initial fluid of choice in the replacement of lost water and electrolytes, there is no consensus as to whether 0.9 or 0.45% saline solution should be the fluid used initially and as to whether potassium or bicarbonate should be infused from the very beginning.[66a] When used alone as the initial replacement fluid, 0.9% saline solution has several advantages over alternative approaches. It is ideal for the correction of extracellular fluid depletion with attendant hypovolemia and hypotension. It can be infused as rapidly as the dehydration dictates. Since it is distributed to the intravascular and extravascular spaces, it is less likely to precipitate cerebral edema, a real possibility with hypotonic fluids. Its initial use without additives such as potassium and bicarbonate does not place a restraint on the speed of its administration, which is vital to its role in correcting the depletion of extracellular fluid. Moreover, its rate of infusion need not be based on prior knowledge of the existing electrolyte status.

Disadvantages of 0.9% saline solution include the precipitation of congestive heart failure, especially in the elderly or in those with preexisting heart disease when the fluid is infused too rapidly. Much less commonly, the development of hypernatremia or of hyperchloremic acidosis, if the saline solution is infused over a prolonged period, may be a possible hazard associated with its use. Some studies have indicated that this develops due to renal wasting of bicarbonate in preference to chloride.[66b] Still others believe that hyperchloremic

Table 26–1.   Schematic Outline for Treatment of Diabetic Ketoacidosis (DKA)

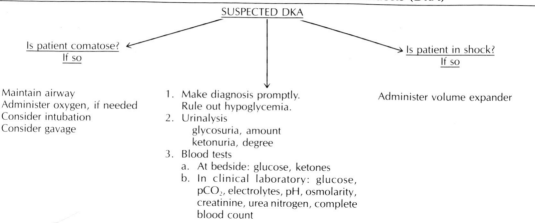

SUSPECTED DKA

Is patient comatose?
If so

Is patient in shock?
If so

Maintain airway
Administer oxygen, if needed
Consider intubation
Consider gavage

1. Make diagnosis promptly.
   Rule out hypoglycemia.
2. Urinalysis
   glycosuria, amount
   ketonuria, degree
3. Blood tests
   a. At bedside: glucose, ketones
   b. In clinical laboratory: glucose,
   pCO_2, electrolytes, pH, osmolarity,
   creatinine, urea nitrogen, complete
   blood count

Administer volume expander

4. If bedside tests confirm clinical impression of diabetic ketoacidosis, start treatment immediately with insulin and fluids.
5. Begin therapy with regular insulin by (a) "low dose" continuous intravenous, (b) intramuscular, or (c) "high dose" subcutaneous routes. See text and Tables 24–4 and 24–5 for details.
6. Commence intravenous infusion of 0.9% saline. Rate and amount to be determined by severity of dehydration.
7. Maintain timed flow sheet: treatment measures, vital signs, fluids, electrolytes, etc.
8. Identify and treat precipitating factors, e.g., infection, myocardial infarct, trauma, etc.
9. Identify need for special procedures, e.g., central venous pressure line, urinary catheter, electrocardiograph, etc.
10. At appropriate time commence potassium replacement: "piggy-back" potassium supplement or saline infusion.
11. Check blood glucose every 1–2 hours and electrolytes every 2–4 hours initially.
12. Consider need for bicarbonate replacement.
13. Consider possible benefit from phosphate supplementation.
14. Continue above regimen until blood glucose drops to range of 250 mg/dl. Then shift infusion to 5% dextrose in water and follow potassium response with increased vigilance.

Table 26–2.   Diabetic Ketoacidosis: Frequent Errors and Problems

1. Delay in diagnosis.
2. Delay in starting treatment.
3. Inadequate physician supervision throughout treatment until recovery. May occur at times of change of treatment personnel.
4. Aspiration of stomach contents due to failure to consider lavage (done carefully!).
5. Insulin dosage: (a) too little delays recovery; (b) overzealous use may cause hypoglycemia and hypokalemia.
6. Fluid replacement: (a) if tardy, may lead to shock; (b) if excessive, may precipitate cardiac failure and pulmonary edema.
7. Potassium replacement: if timing and amount are not appropriate, potentially lethal hypo- or hyperkalemia may result.
8. Bicarbonate replacement: (a) if none used, severe acidosis may persist in some patients, leading to shock; (b) if too much is given, metabolic acidosis may be induced.
9. Unrecognized cerebral edema.
10. Failure to monitor urine output hourly and be guided by results (should be at least 30–60 ml/hr). Progressive decrease is an ominous sign.
11. Recurrent ketoacidosis due to failure to give insulin subcutaneously 20–30 min. prior to stopping insulin infusion.
12. Too great reliance on electrocardiogram as index of serum potassium level.

DEATH DUE TO UNCOMPLICATED DIABETIC KETOACIDOSIS SHOULD NOT OCCUR!

acidosis may be a presenting metabolic pattern independent of treatment modality.[66c]

An exception to the use of 0.9% saline solution initially would be the existence of severe shock at presentation, in which circumstance a plasma volume expander, such as human serum albumin or low molecular weight dextran would be the preferred fluid if available *without delay*.

The rate of fluid replacement is determined by the severity of the extracellular fluid dehydration,

the age of the patient and the presence or absence of underlying heart disease. Accurate assessment of dehydration and the volume of replacement fluid is difficult and is at best estimated by clinical judgment. A physiologic approach to fluid replacement takes into account (a) maintenance needs, (b) replacement requirement, and (c) ongoing losses. A pediatrician, if available, may be consulted to evaluate the fluid and electrolyte requirements of young children. Weight loss, if known, may serve as a useful index of the extent of dehydration and thus the body weight may be employed to calculate replacement volume. The body surface area permits an estimation of the maintenance fluid requirement. Table 26–3 illustrates the fluid and electrolytes deficits which may be incurred during the development of DKA.[67]

In general, sodium depletion may be of the magnitude of 500 to 600 mEq and water loss in the order of 6 to 8 liters. A minimal detectable level of dehydration represents approximately 5% loss of body weight. The maximal acute body weight loss compatible with life, is estimated to be approximately 20%, a state that is invariably accompanied by shock. Thus, the initial approach to the correction of the problem of extracellular fluid depletion is the administration of 0.9% saline solution. In adults with *severe* dehydration, 1 liter of 0.9% saline solution may be infused over a 15 to 20 minute period and up to 3 liters in the first 2 hours. In elderly patients with less severe dehydration and the possibility of preexisting heart disease, the first liter may be given over a period of two hours. The clinical evaluation of the changes in pulse, respiration and blood pressure and the assessment of tissue turgor with or without the usage of central venous pressure measurement, help to guide the rate of replacement. Thus, the clinical response of the patient as well as the estimated fluid and electrolytes deficits illustrated in Table 26–3 provides some sort of measure of the volume of saline solution replacement required. In general, the fluid replacement which is initiated with 0.9% saline solution, is continued until such time as the blood glucose drops to a value in the range of 250 mg/dl or less. At this point, usually between 4 and 6 hours after the initiation of therapy, significant dehydration should have been corrected and the infusion fluid can be replaced by 5% dextrose in water or saline. Assessment of plasma electrolytes done at this time will afford a guide to further potassium therapy.

The shift to 5% dextrose in water serves two purposes. First, it represents a vehicle for the replenishment of free water, the loss of which is greater than that of sodium and which can never be restored with the use of 0.9% saline solution

alone. Second, 5% dextrose in water introduces additional carbohydrate at a time when the blood glucose level tends to fall more rapidly but ketogenesis has not been completely reversed. The 5% dextrose in water will prevent the development of hypoglycemia but more importantly the glucose substrate may serve to suppress lipolysis and ketogenesis and possibly enhance ketone utilization. Inadequate carbohydrate administration at this stage of management delays the reversal of ketosis, which may persist for several days and increase the difficulty of stabilization of the diabetes. Depending on the urine output, the 5% dextrose in water is infused at a rate of between 150 and 200 ml of fluid per hour in adults and at appropriately lower rates in children. The dextrose in water is continued for as long as the patient is considered to require intravenous fluid administration; i.e., when there is no further nausea and vomiting and the patient is able to tolerate fluids by mouth.

Electrolyte Replacement

Potassium. In the development of DKA there is a total body potassium loss of approximately 500 mEq in adults. However, this loss may not be reflected in the serum potassium concentration which initially may be raised, normal, or low. If the serum concentration is raised and potassium is infused with the very first liter of saline replacement, the consequence could be disastrous unless the rate of infusion were so drastically reduced as to defeat the primary object of intravenous fluid replacement; i.e., the restitution of the extracellular fluid volume to normal. If the initial serum potassium concentration is low, and no potassium is given, the effects could be equally deleterious to the heart, especially as saline infusion will cause further hemodilution and promote diuresis, and the insulin will promote the transfer of potassium into the cells concomitant with glucose uptake. On the other hand, even if the serum potassium level is low, and notwithstanding the total body potassium depletion, too rapid an infusion of the potassium itself is hazardous as a sudden hyperkalemia can also induce cardiac arrest. Thus, the replacement of the potassium is fraught with hazard if not appropriately carried out.

A rational and pragmatic approach to potassium administration is to infuse saline at a rate dictated by the patient's dehydration, and to attach to it in "piggyback" fashion another bottle containing between 20 and 40 mEq/L of potassium chloride. This could be administered at a variable rate depending upon the urinary output and the level of the serum potassium. Provided that this kind of precaution is undertaken, potassium replacement could be initiated with the first liter of saline infusion, espe-

Table 26–3. Average Losses of Water and Electrolytes in Severe Diabetic Ketoacidosis

Constituent	Per kg body weight
Water	75–100 ml
Sodium	8 mEq
Chloride	5 mEq
Potassium	6 mEq
Phosphorus	1 mEq
Magnesium	0.5 mEq

cially as early therapy has been reported to decrease morbidity and mortality.[68] The potassium replacement rate should be increased under the following circumstances: (a) when the serum concentration drops below 3 mEq/L; (b) if there is a simultaneous infusion of bicarbonate; or (c) when insulin is administered with 5% dextrose in water.[69-71] In the last-named circumstance, the administration of potassium is mandatory as the serum potassium may fall to dangerously low levels at this stage of management. Potassium replacement should be controlled by serial serum potassium estimations and selectively by electrocardiographic monitoring.[72]

Bicarbonate. Over the past 10 years the use of bicarbonate in the management of DKA has undergone a dramatic change. The previous practice of some clinicians was to administer fairly large doses of bicarbonate based on the arbitrary calculation of apparent bicarbonate deficits. The injudicious use of large amounts of bicarbonate over a short space of time resulted in a reversal of the severe metabolic acidosis to one of an acute metabolic alkalosis with the precipitation of severe hypokalemia.[73,74] At the same time the correction of the systemic acidosis frequently led to a paradoxical acidosis within the central nervous system with a sudden and unexpected worsening of the patient's mental status.[74] With the recognition that overzealous replacement with bicarbonate could precipitate serious adverse effects on acid-base balance, the tendency now is to use bicarbonate with greater circumspection. In general, its usage is avoided during the initial phases of management of DKA and is considered only when the metabolic acidosis is severe, e.g., when the arterial pH is less than 7 or the bicarbonate value less than 5 mEq/L, particularly when prior rehydration and treatment with insulin has failed to correct the acidosis. Under such circumstances up to 200 mEq of bicarbonate may be infused slowly over 2 to 4 hours. This slow rate of administration of bicarbonate, while promoting the restoration of the acid-base disturbance towards normal, avoids the acute hazards associated with the rapid administration of large amounts. This is true also with children in whom much smaller amounts suffice (40–80 mEq/m^2 infused over 2 hours).

Phosphate. Severe hypophosphatemia, especially if chronic, may be accompanied by several clinical consequences including dizziness, dysarthria, irritability, confusion and coma,[75] and biochemically by a deficiency of red cell 2–3 diphosphoglycerate (2, 3-DPG). As early as 1948 Franks[76] reported the occurrence of severe hypophosphatemia (plasma phosphate concentrations less than 0.6 mEq/L) during the therapy of DKA. It has since been documented that despite elevation of initial plasma phospate levels, a significant fall may occur within 30 minutes of commencing therapy because of intracellular glycogen deposition.[77-79] However, it has yet to be shown that the falls in plasma phosphate levels occurring during the course of management of DKA are associated in any way with the development of clinical manifestations.[80,80a] On the other hand, the reduction of 2,3-DPG concentration[81-84] that accompanies phosphate depletion has been theorized to limit the delivery of oxygen to peripheral tissues in ketoacidosis by shifting the oxygen dissociation curve to the left.[85] Acidosis itself, however, causes a decrease in hemoglobin affinity with oxygen through the Bohr effect and thus compensates for the effect of the fall in 2,3-DPG level.

Thus, the opposing actions of reduced levels of 2,3-DPG and acidosis on hemoglobin affinity for oxygen result in no net effect on this function in DKA.[85] Quite possibly, the rapid administration of bicarbonate may reverse the protective effect of acidosis on hemoglobin affinity and cause a decreased tissue release of oxygen and consequent hypoxia. On the basis of such considerations, Ditzel and associates[86] have recommended the usage in adults of 65 mEq of phosphate over the first 24 hours of DKA and have demonstrated that this restores the 2,3-DPG levels to normal within hours.[83] This intervention, however, has not been shown to influence the recovery rate, morbidity, or mortality from DKA. Phosphate replacement is not part of the standard regimen of treatment of DKA in the Joslin protocol.

Trace Mineral Deficit Therapy. While deficits of trace elements such as zinc, selenium, and chromium may occur during the course of DKA, no recognizable clinical correlates have been shown to accompany such changes, and at present there is no indication for any specific replacement.[77,78] Magnesium depletion may accompany the development of DKA (see Table 26–3), and predispose to cardiac arrythmias.[78a] That this requires correction in the acute stage of management remains to be shown.

Treatment with Insulin

The traditional approach to the treatment of DKA based on the administration of large doses of insulin, subcutaneously or intravenously, has been largely supplanted in recent times by the use of low dose insulin either as continuous intravenous infusions or as intermittent intramuscular injections. However, controlled trials in the hands of experienced clinicians have not shown any significant decrease in mortality.

Intravenous Infusion. Studies since 1974 in both children and adults have repeatedly documented the safety and efficacy of low dose intravenous infusions of insulin in the correction of DKA.[87-98] Despite the existence of insulin resistance,[98a] low-dose infusion regimens provide plasma insulin levels that exert a maximal hypoglycemic effect. The generally employed infusion dose is 0.1 unit of insulin per hour per kg of body weight, which may be preceded by a single loading dose of 0.2 U/kg body weight. The infusion is administered either by the use of special pumps such as the Harvard, Imed, or Evac types or with the use of a pediatric infusion set. The dose of insulin infused is adjusted to maintain plasma concentrations of insulin between 60 and 100 μU/ml of insulin.[94,98,99] These levels effectively inhibit glycogenolysis and lipolysis and serve to suppress the elevated concentrations of counterregulatory hormones.[100] Blood glucose levels should fall predictably—at approximately 10% per hour. The acidosis is corrected more slowly than with the use of larger doses of insulin, thus reducing the likelihood of precipitating severe hypokalemia. The use of an insulin infusion pump permits the possibility of titrating insulin doses quite rapidly in responses to changes in blood glucose concentration (Table 26–4).

Notwithstanding these benefits of intravenous infusion, several disadvantages have also to be considered. Inadvertent discontinuation of the infusion is a major hazard and constant surveillance of the infusion system has to be maintained by the responsible physician and nursing staff. A not uncommon error is the failure to administer a dose of regular insulin (with or without lente or NPH insulin) subcutaneously 20 to 30 minutes prior to discontinuance of the intravenous infusion. This is necessary because of the very short half-life of insulin given intravenously.

A theoretical problem of intravenous insulin administration is that of the adsorption of the hormone to the plastic syringe or tubing.[101,102] It has been suggested that the addition of albumin to the intravenous solution could circumvent this difficulty. In practice, however, it has been found that once the infusion system has been initially flushed[103] with the insulin solution, there is no significant further adsorption to the tubing. The delivery to the tissues appears to be adequate and poses no major problem in the clinical management. It has also been argued that the low dose insulin infusion may not be as effective as the previously employed intermittent high doses because of possible insulin resistance in states of DKA. Insulin receptor activity has been shown to be markedly depressed when the blood pH is less than 7.0.[104] In practice, however, insulin resistance has not been found to be of significant clinical concern in the vast majority of patients treated.[105,106] If an adequate blood glucose response fails to occur within the first few hours of commencing insulin therapy, doubling the infusion rate invariably overcomes the apparent resistance and permits correction of the ketoacidosis.

Intramuscular Insulin Injection. Based on the knowledge that insulin given intramuscularly is more rapidly absorbed than when administered subcutaneously[107,108] and that a relatively constant serum insulin concentration can be attained by repeated injections of insulin at 1- to 2 hour intervals,[109] a treatment program was devised[110] for the management of acute DKA in adults using between 5 to 10 units of insulin intramuscularly hourly. The efficacy of this approach has been extensively investigated and verified in a large number of studies in both adults and children.[87,88,110–113] In children an initial loading dose of 0.25 U/kg of body weight

Table 26–4. Continuous Insulin Infusion Guidelines

1. Place 1 ml of U100 regular insulin in 100 ml of normal saline (can be 50 units insulin in 50-ml syringe if Harvard pump is to be used) for a concentration of 1 unit per ml.
2. Attach intravenous tubing and pre-flush to allow adherence of insulin to plastic. Not necessary to use albumin.
3. Set up piggyback system into existing intravenous line. Use Harvard, IVAC, or IMED pump (or even pediatric drip set).
4. Give 0.2 units per kg of actual body weight as intravenous bolus.
5. Give 0.1 unit per kg of actual body weight per hour intravenous as continuous drip.
6. Expect initial drop in blood glucose from rehydration and then approximately 10% drop from original blood glucose level each hour (e.g., 50–70 mg/dl per hour).
7. Monitor blood glucose at 1 hour and then every 2–4 hours to make sure blood glucose is falling. Urine should be checked for glucose every 2–4 hours. Plasma electrolytes should be checked every 2–6 hours until stable.
8. Double rate of infusion or shift to alternative protocol if blood glucose does not fall in 2 hours.
9. Calculate estimated time when blood glucose will reach 250–300 mg/dl range.
10. Stop insulin infusion when blood glucose reaches 250± mg/dl and change intravenous solution to contain 5% dextrose.
11. Because of short half-life of intravenous insulin, insulin (regular or regular plus lente or NPH) must be given 20–30 minutes before discontinuing insulin infusion. Dosage adjusted according to duration of diabetes, degree of ketoacidosis, age of patient, body size, known sensitivity to insulin, amount of insulin given so far in treatment, or other factors affecting amount of insulin needed (pregnancy, renal failure, ongoing infection, etc.).

followed by a dose of 0.1 U/kg/hr has been shown to achieve a satisfactory reversal of DKA.

This intramuscular route is a satisfactory alternative for low-dose intravenous infusion and for the formerly popular high-dose subcutaneous route. It has been shown to share many of the advantages of the low dose intravenous insulin infusion system. Its major additional advantage over the infusion system is its inherent simplicity that obviates the need for an infusion pump with its attendant risk of failure to operate.

A chief shortcoming of the intramuscular route is the inability to deliver an adequate amount to a severely dehydrated patient in whom insulin absorption from the site of injection may be defective until the tissue perfusion has been corrected. In this sort of situation, a small dose of insulin may be administered intravenously at the same time as the first dose of insulin is given intramuscularly.

Subcutaneous Administration of Insulin. This route, used for many years is still a valid choice for the physician if the following principles of treatment are observed: (1) prompt diagnosis and initiation of therapy; (2) continuous close supervision by the physician with adjustment of treatment as indicated by the condition of the patient and the results of laboratory studies; (3) immediate giving of insulin and starting of fluids intravenously; (4) initial insulin dose of 20 to 100 units subcutaneously (SC) plus a similar dose intravenously (IV) in adults, or 5 to 20 units (SC) plus 5 to 20 units (IV) in children with actual amounts adjusted according to the age of the patient and severity of ketoacidosis; (5) determination of blood glucose after 2 hours, and on the basis of the results, then and at intervals of 2 to 4 hours, giving insulin in doses in the range of those just quoted; (6) if in periodic tests, expected improvement in blood values does not occur, increase in the size of doses of insulin (see Table 26–5).

One of the most common criticisms of this method is the danger of hypoglycemia. Experience has shown that this is rarely a problem if the amounts of insulin given in the first few hours approach the expected total dose. Overly large doses should be avoided later in treatment, particularly if the blood glucose is falling satisfactorily. When the blood glucose has fallen to the range of 250 mg/dl, the fluid given intravenously should be shifted to 5% dextrose solution.

More detailed discussions of the "high-dose" method may be found in the 11th edition of this book and other texts.

While both recent innovations, i.e., the use of low doses of insulin either intravenously or intramuscularly, have helped to rationalize the management of DKA, the importance of meticulous attention of the physician to this and other details of treatment cannot be overemphasized. Apart from adequate amounts of insulin, foremost is the need for the vigorous restoration of the depleted extracellular fluid volume to normal. Also of great importance is scrutiny for any precipitating factors. The risks for the development of complications either from the ketoacidosis or from injudicious therapy are always present. In the management of DKA there is no room for complacency.

The Complications and Mortality of DKA

The complications of DKA may be iatrogenic or reflect the severity of the underlying metabolic abnormality. In any case their development increases the morbidity and mortality of the ketoacidotic episode. The most serious inherent complications are the development of severe shock and the persistence of coma. Both may lead to death. Shock can be prevented by effective early rehydration and correction of acidosis. The presence of full coma in DKA has a significant impact on the mortality rate. Unconsciousness, especially if present for 8 or more hours before treatment, carries a poor prognosis, as do serum pH values of 7.0 or below. Insofar as the role of iatrogenic factors is concerned, delay in diagnosis and tardy or inadequate insulinization may aggravate any preexisting coma and dehydration, and inappropriate fluid replacement may precipitate shock with tubular necrosis. On the other hand, overzealous administration of insulin may cause hypoglycemia, and overhydration with inappropriate fluids may lead to hypernatremia, hyperchloremic acidosis, or cerebral edema.

Cerebral Edema. Discussions of brain edema occurring in the course of treatment of DKA are filled with contradictions. Its frequency is not clear: published estimates range from "rare" to "not uncommon." Death is not common as judged by reported instances. However, it is likely that some cases may remain undiagnosed, and it is entirely possible that nonfatal cerebral edema may be more common than ordinarily thought. Fein and colleagues[114] found that the serial echoencephalograms of 9 of 11 patients showed significant decreases in lateral ventricle width during treatment, and in 7 of the 11 patients there were "hash" marks characteristic of cerebral edema. However, as recognized clinically, the condition is so uncommon that in a large series of patients with DKA, no case may be seen or, at least, recognized.

As to the cause of cerebral edema, there is no common agreement. Many have thought that it may be caused by too rapid a correction of serum osmolarity, body fluid loss, and hyperglycemia, with overly zealous giving of fluids (especially hypo-

Table 26–5. Guide to Initial (First Hour) Insulin Dosage in Treatment of Diabetic Coma by High Dose Method (Units of Regular Insulin)

Type of Patient	Immediate	At 1 hr when blood glucose is known and if bicarbonate is 9 mEq/L or less*			
		Blood glucose level mg/dl			
		B.G. <300	> 300	> 600	> 1000
Adult or mature adolescent	20–50 I.V. + 20–50 S.C.	0	20–50 I.V. + 20–50 S.C.	100–150 I.V. + 100–150 S.C.	150–200 I.V. + 150–200 S.C.
Adult or mature adolescent. No insulin for many hours or unconscious	50–100 I.V. + 50–100 S.C.	0	50–100 I.V. + 50–100 S.C.	150–200 I.V. + 150–200 S.C.	200–300 I.V. + 200–300 S.C.
Children age 10 or more and not fully grown	10–20 I.V. + 10–20 S.C.	0	10–20 I.V. + 10–20 S.C.	50–70 I.V. + 50–70 S.C.	80–100 I.V. + 80–100 S.C.
Children under age 10 or diagnosis in coma	5–10 I.V. + 5–10 S.C.	0	5–10 I.V. + 5–10 S.C.	30–40 I.V. + 30–40 S.C.	40–50 I.V. + 40–50 S.C.

*If 10 to 15 mEq/L and clinical condition warrants, give the lower number of units of insulin indicated.

Table 26–6. Causes of Death During or Following Coma in 94 Patients

Causes of Death	Jan. 1, 1923 to Jan. 1, 1957	Jan. 1, 1957 to Jan. 1, 1967	1974 to 1980
Uncomplicated coma	24	5	0
Sepsis and metastatic infection	19		1
Pneumonia	12		1
Pancreatitis	3	1	
Cardiac	3	3	3
Pulmonary embolism	1		
Pulmonary infarct with empyema	1		
Hemorrhage from duodenal ulcer	2		
Cerebral hemorrhage or infarct	2	2	1
Alkalosis	1		
Infected burn	1		
Nephropathy (with anuria)	3	1	1
Acute edema of lungs	1		
Encephalopathy	1		
Pseudomembranous duodenojejunitis		1	
TOTAL	74	13	7

tonic solutions) and insulin. However, Carroll and Matz[115] state that in their patients no instance of cerebral edema "occurred with the rapid infusion of large volumes of hypotonic solutions."

Despite these differing ideas and experiences,[116] it can be assumed that, in general, brain edema is more likely to occur if hypotonic fluids are used *too early* in treatment[117-122] and if the blood glucose falls too rapidly to a level below 250± mg/dl. Although the replacement of lost body fluid is an extremely important part of the treatment of DKA, this must be done with forethought and with careful observation of the patient as therapy progresses. It must be kept in mind that in the replacement of fluids as well as that of electrolytes, all calculated deficits need not be made up completely. Instead, treatment should be flexible, working toward a stage of recovery in which the patient may take

and retain fluids by mouth. In addition, Nature should be allowed to help complete the process of full recovery.

Cerebral edema should be thought of in patients whose sensorium continues to be depressed despite satisfactory improvement in the results of chemical tests. Headache and increasing lethargy, although nonspecific, should raise the possibility of cerebral edema. Increasing intraocular pressure, unequal or dilated pupils, and diminished response of the pupils to light are among the changes that may be observed. Fever, not present at the initiation of treatment, and increase in blood pressure may be noted. If suspicion grows, special procedures such as lumbar puncture (cautiously done!) should be considered to determine cerebrospinal pressure. The electroencephalogram may be of value.

Treatment is unsatisfactory when the patient

Table 26–7. Reported Experiences in Treatment of Diabetic Ketoacidosis

	No. Cases Diabetic Ketoacidosis	Mortality (%)	Sex M	Sex F	Mean Age Range	Duration of Diabetes (Yrs.)	No. in Coma on Admission	No. of Coma Patients Dying	Diabetes Recently Diagnosed (%)	Mean Blood Sugar on Admission	Mean CO₂ Range* vol. %	Total Insulin 1st 24 hrs
Dillon & Dyer[123] 1931–1936	268	43.7	81	187	38	—	79	64 (81%)	37	Not Given†	6–29 vol. %	Not Stated
Brøchner-Mortensen[124] 1930–1945	106	25.4	51	55	—	—	28	17 (61%)	13	—	—	—
Zieve & Hill[125] 1930–1948	124	29.0	55	69	36.6 (11–77)	5.4	33	—	17	533 (188–1165)	9.2 (3.6–20.7)	220
Martin, Smith, Wilson[67] (26 pts.)	29	24.0	16	10	14–73	—	—	—	—	—	Bl. Ket. 89–225 mg%	>200
Harwood[126] 1944–1950	67	1.5	33	34	(36–75)	—	1	0	23	597 (156–1280)	7.2 (3.7–12.3)	1280
Pease & Cooke[127] 1932–1941	63	61.9	—	—	—	—	} 74	} 57 (77%)	—	—	—	—
1941–1950	122	22.1	—	—	—	—			—	—	—	—
Brakier & Brull[128] 1951–1954	64	20.3 <age 50–6.2 >age 50–37.5	20	44	<50–32 >50–32	—	—	—	—	>500	10–40 vol. %	200–300 1st 3 hr.
Greenaway & Read[129] 1950–1955 (58 pts.)	69	16.0	20	38	38.3	6–10 median	14	43 (6%)	17 (mortality 43%)	400–600 median	<10	320–720
Cohen et al.[130] 1952–1955 severe k.d.	73	5.5	34	39	36.6 (3–80)	10.2	} 8 2	} 1 (13%) 1 (50%)	29	388 (200–599) 358 (191–532)	5.0 (0–10) 12.5 (10.1–15)	751 433
(6) moderate k.d.												

Study												
Skillman et al.[131]												
1947–1951	140	31.4	—	—	40.2 (13–72)	—	—	—	—	556 (133–1390)	8.1 (2.7–14)	392 } 1st
1952–1956	172	14.5	—	—	42.4 (15–84)	—	—	—	—	507 (197–1180)	8.9 (3.5–14)	456 } 6 hr.
Derot & Tchobroutsky[132]												
(117 pts.)	133	12.0	51	66	14–81	1–20	50 (37%)	11 (22%)	18	200–1000	10–15 (20%)	Not Given
No. *not* comatose							83 (63%)	5 (6%)			<10 (80%)	
Pines[133]												
1940–1952	110	13.0	—	—	—	—	—	—	—	—	—	—
1952–1961	131	4.0	—	—	—	—	—	—	—	—	—	—
Schneider & Winckler[134]												
1949–1961	135	15.4	62	73	(1–78)	—	62	23 (37%)	43	777	—	—
(23)					—							
FitzGerald, O'Sullivan & Malins[135]												
1955–1959	160	12.0	60	100	39.6	—	—	—	—	—	—	—
Asfeldt[136]												
1943–1963	119	6.7	40	79	36 (0.7–79)	7.1	25	26 (24%)	16	>479 (214–1424)	8.6 (0–18)	189
Joslin Clinic[136a]												
1965–1966	43	4.6	—	—	28.1	9.2	—	—	—	587	7	223
Beigelman[136b]												
1965–1968	482	9	153	187	38 (14–84)	—	—	32	—	705	—	540
Joslin[‡]												
1979–	42	4.7	17	25	36 (6–86)	—	—	—	—	—	—	—

*Expressed in mEq/L unless otherwise specified.

†Mortality for patients with initial blood glucose 700 mg or more = 57.7%; for those with initial blood glucose 400 mg or less = 29.1%.

‡Unpublished

reaches an advanced stage. In addition to general measures, low molecular weight dextran, mannitol, and large doses of corticosteroids have been suggested.

The dangers of *hypokalemia* are well known. This event may be an early feature of the DKA or may be precipitated by inadequate potassium replacement particularly in the face of bicarbonate usage or when glucose and insulin are infused. *Hyperkalemia* may be equally hazardous to the patient if an attempt is made to correct the potassium deficit too aggressively, especially if there is underlying renal failure. While the dangers of severe metabolic acidosis in leading to a state of irreversible shock are unquestioned and potentially lethal, equally dangerous is the injudicious use of excessive amounts of *bicarbonate*. All of these problems in the management of DKA are compounded in patients who have concomitant complications of diabetes such as severe sepsis, cerebral vascular accident, and myocardial infarction. The recognition of the ease with which such dangerous complications may develop emphasizes once more the need for a constant surveillance of diabetic patients in coma by all personnel involved in management.

Table 26–6 shows the *causes of death* in patients admitted in diabetic coma at the Joslin Clinic between 1923 and 1980. In the preinsulin era mortality in diabetic coma ranged between 40 and 70%. Since the advent of insulin, there has been a steady decline in the mortality from DKA. Concomitant aggressive treatment of infections and cardiovascular catastrophes has reduced the mortality even further. Infections and/or cardiovascular complications associated with DKA, however, remain the major causes of death during episodes of DKA.

Among patients treated by Joslin Clinic physicians at the New England Deaconess Hospital during 1956 through 1966, the *mortality from DKA* was 1.1% whereas during the period from 1970 to 1980, the mortality was less than 0.5%. Between the years 1977 and 1980, there were no deaths in patients admitted with uncomplicated DKA; the total mortality was less than 5% including those with complications which in themselves were potentially fatal, e.g., acute myocardial infarction. Reported results in the treatment of patients with DKA are summarized in Table 26–7. Although imprecise terminology and definition of DKA and coma make comparison of results between centers of dubious value, nonetheless the table does provide some insight into the progressive improvement in the mortality in diabetic ketoacidosis over the last 50 years. Two caveats emerge from the combined experience of management of diabetic ketoacidosis in various centers: (1) the prompt recognition of DKA and initiation of treatment are imperative and (2) decrease in mortality is clearly related to a maximal effort to provide optimal insulin, fluid, and electrolyte therapy especially during the earlier stages of DKA.

Prevention of Diabetic Ketoacidosis

The prevention of ketoacidosis should be the main objective in the management of diabetes. This is particularly important in patients with long-duration diabetes and underlying vascular disease. DKA, especially if repetitive, can also precipitate neuropathy and accelerate microangiopathy.

The availability of adequate medical advice has been shown to reduce the incidence of emergency room visits for diabetics. Nonetheless, the thrust of the preventive measures should be directed toward better education of patients, their families, and associates of the early warning signs of acidosis and of emergency measures that can be undertaken to prevent further progression. Patients and relatives should be taught that the deterioration of urine and blood tests for glucose and ketones, accompanied by the constellation of symptoms that characterize uncontrolled diabetes, namely thirst, polyuria, nausea, vomiting, enuresis, and malaise, especially in the presence of infection, should indicate the urgent need for greater attention to the diabetes. While the development of ketoacidosis is not a sudden event, the omission of insulin under such circumstances may cause the full-blown picture to develop with alarming rapidity.

The sick-day rules taught patients at the Joslin Clinic summarize the salient features in the prophylaxis of DKA (Table 26–8). They are taught that, as soon as they feel ill or find that the control of diabetes is not satisfactory, they are to increase the frequency of urine testing both for glucose and ketones. In addition, they are instructed to carry out frequent blood glucose tests at home using Chemstrips or Dextrostix with or without glucose meters. Many Joslin Clinic patients with insulin-dependent (and some with noninsulin-dependent) diabetes have been trained in home blood glucose monitoring.

With impending ketoacidosis, patients are encouraged to consume as much fluid as they can. In particular, they are encouraged to take additional amounts of salt with their fluids in order to replace salt lost in the urine. When anorexia, nausea and vomiting occur, beverages containing sugar may be tried in small amounts frequently in an attempt to decrease the contribution of starvation ketosis to the ketonemia. Fruit juices and most commercially available ginger ale and soft drinks contain approximately 10% sugar with a reasonable sodium content. When complemented by broth and chicken soup, this is usually sufficient to compensate for

Table 26–8. Sick Day Guidelines as Taught to the Patient

1. Always take your daily dose of insulin. *Never omit it, even if you are unable to eat.*
2. Test urine or blood glucose every 2 to 4 hours. A minimum of four times a day (before each meal and at bedtime) is absolutely essential. Use freshly voided urine. For blood glucose tests use Dextrostix or Chemstrip bG with or without a glucose meter. If you are feeling too sick to test, ask someone to do it for you or call your physician.
3. If urine glucose is 1% or more, or blood glucose is higher than about 200 mg/dl, test also for urine ketones. *Do this when ill from any cause.* If ketones are present along with high glucose levels, you *always* need extra insulin. Regular (short acting) insulin should be used. Guidelines for how much Regular insulin should be used and how often to take it appear below. Do not use extra insulin if only ketones are present or if tests for glucose indicate less than 1%.
4. Take liquids every hour. Refer to the food suggestions for sick days which appear below. If unable to take liquids because of nausea or vomiting, contact your physician, who may prescribe medication to stop the nausea or vomiting.
5. Rest and keep warm. Do not exercise. Have someone take care of you.
6. If you are vomiting or are in pain, contact your physician at once.
7. Food. If you are too ill to follow your usual diet plan, eat or drink whatever you can tolerate and retain. Drink at least 6 to 8 glasses of fluid a day, taking some each hour. Use water, fruit juices, regular soft drinks, tea, consomme, and broth (made from bouillon cubes). With improvement, gradually return to a soft solid diet and then to regular meal plan.
8. Extra insulin. If tests indicate need for extra insulin over and above your regular dose, every 3 or 4 hours take 20% (1/5) of your usual dose when well. Thus, if your usual total daily dose is 40 units, take 8 units of regular insulin every 3 or 4 hours, depending on the outcome of blood and urine tests. Keep a record of all doses of insulin taken each day (together with time of day when taken).

the extra losses induced by the osmotic diuresis. Foods containing potassium such as bananas and juices can be helpful if they are tolerated. Body weight should be determined, if possible, every 6 to 12 hours as a guide to the adequacy of fluid replacement particularly in small infants and children. In the absence of vomiting, most patients can maintain body weight despite ongoing losses due to increased urination. Increasing anorexia with reduced fluid and caloric intake presages a more serious deterioration in control. Unless combated with increased insulin therapy, this situation will lead to imminent DKA. Therefore, of equal importance to the advice to increase the frequency of monitoring, liberalizing fluid, electrolytes, and, possibly, sugar intake, is the injunction to supplement the daily insulin dose.

A major factor working against the patient's ability to adequately handle metabolic decompensation at home is the failure of the patient and family to understand that despite the anorexia and nausea the presence of hyperglycemia and ketosis increase rather than reduce the need for insulin replacement. A rule of thumb prescribed to patients is that, if necessary, an additional 20% of the total daily insulin dose should be taken as regular insulin every 4–6 hours, guided by determinations of glucose in blood and urine. Superimposed acute illness as a stress leading to the threat of decompensated ketoacidosis is often self-limited. Appropriate vigilance is the key factor to successful early therapeutic intervention and cannot be over-emphasized. Repeated acute episodes of vomiting, persistent weight loss, and abdominal pain associated with worsening of symptoms warrant emergency out-patient care or hospitalization.

Instruction of patient and family, as well as psychosocial assessment and support, are often of great value in the prevention of repetitive bouts of DKA.

HYPERGLYCEMIC HYPEROSMOLAR NONKETOTIC COMA

Hyperglycemic hyperosmolar nonketotic coma is a frequently lethal complication of diabetes characterized by marked hyperglycemia, plasma hyperosmolarity, profound dehydration, absence of severe ketoacidosis, and variable mental status.

Pathogenesis

In Figure 26–9 are shown those factors thought to play an important role in the evolution of hyperosmolar coma. Hyperglycemia produces an osmotic diuresis which in turn causes dehydration and loss of electrolytes. Dehydration is known to increase the secretion of counter-regulatory hormones glucagon, cortisol and epinephrine. Hypokalemia impairs insulin secretion. These two effects worsen hyperglycemia, perpetuating the cycle.

Half of the patients with hyperosmolar coma have a precipitating illness, most frequently infection. Gram negative pneumonia is particularly common.[137] Infection (especially of the urinary tract), myocardial infarction, cerebral vascular accident, and other acute illnesses initiate the cycle by increasing secretion of stress hormones. About half the patients have previously undiagnosed (and therefore untreated) diabetes. In these as well as patients taking phenytoin or diazoxide (both of which impair insulin secretion), inadequate insulin

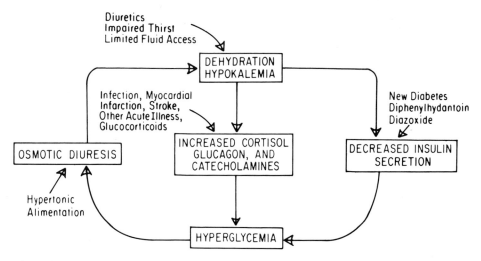

Fig. 26–9. The cycle of events culminating in hyperosmolar hyperglycemic nonketotic coma.

triggers the coma. Patients taking thiazides or loop diuretics, those with impaired thirst, or bedridden patients unable to communicate their thirst, enter the cycle as a result of dehydration. Hypertonic alimentation acts by directly producing an osmotic diuresis. Propranolol, cimetidine, chlorpromazine, and various cytotoxic agents contribute to the syndrome by unknown mechanisms.

The explanation for the absence of significant ketogenesis is unknown. Some patients with diabetic ketoacidosis have higher serum osmolarities and insulin levels than some patients with hyperosmolar coma. There exist patients who at one time or another have had both types of coma.

Impairment of mental status correlates with the degree of hyperosmolarity, a direct reflection of intracellular dehydration.[138] Many patients have focal symptoms such as hemiparesis or seizures.

Clinical Presentation

A typical patient is elderly (average age, 60 years) and in about half the time a known diabetic, usually Type II. One series of hyperosmolar patients included 18% who were under age 50 years[115] and the syndrome has been seen in infants. There is a history of several days (3 days to 3 weeks) of polyuria and the patient is brought to the emergency room because of increasing obtundation, seizures, or symptoms of a stroke.

Physical examination shows evidence of dehydration, the most reliable signs being orthostatic hypotension and failure of the jugular veins to fill while supine. Many patients are in frank shock. There may be evidence of an underlying precipitating illness.

The plasma glucose is at least 600 (average =

1000) mg/dl. The osmolarity, calculated as shown below, is at least 350 (average = 380) in mOsm/L.

$$mOsm/L = 2 \ (Na + K \ mEq/L) \ +$$

$$\frac{(glucose \ mg/dl)}{18} + \frac{(BUN \ mg/dl)}{2.8}$$

Example (normal):

$$2 \ (140 + 4) + \frac{90}{18} + \frac{20}{2.8} = 300 \ mOsm/L$$

The plasma acetoacetate as estimated by the nitroprusside reaction is negative if the serum is diluted beyond 2:1. The serum sodium may be high or low, the former signifying severe dehydration. This is because the initial effect of hyperglycemia is to increase extracellular osmolarity, drawing water from inside the cells and thereby diluting the serum sodium. Table 26–9 shows a computational example illustrating this effect. As diuresis proceeds, the initially low serum sodium tends to increase, since the urine produced approximates half-normal saline solution, i.e., more water is lost than sodium.

The serum potassium may also be low, normal, or, less frequently, high. Hyperkalemia is common on presentation of ketoacidosis and is generally attributed to the acidosis which is rarely a significant factor in hyperosmolar coma. However, there are some data suggesting that hyperosmolarity itself may lead to expulsion of potassium from cells. Insulin drives potassium into cells, so its absence probably contributes to hyperkalemia. Regardless of the serum potassium, the total body loss is sub-

Table 26–9. How Hyperglycemia Shifts Fluid, Lowering Plasma Sodium

Blood glucose level	Volume (liters)		Plasma Sodium (mEq/L)	Plasma Glucose (mg/dl)	Plasma Osmolarity (mOsm/L)
	Intra-cellular	Extra-cellular			
Normoglycemia	26	14	135	90	275
Hyperglycemia	25	15	126	612	286

The first row shows typical values for a normoglycemic patient. Urea crosses membranes so fluid shifts do not affect its contribution to osmolarity, which has therefore been ignored. Entries in the second row were calculated by assuming that glucose rises enough to attract one liter from the intracellular fluid, raising the extracellular volume an equal amount. Since the total number of sodium atoms does not change, the new plasma sodium is 14/15 of the old. Since total intracellular osmols do not change, the new osmolarity is 26/25 of the old. From these two numbers, the new glucose is computed. Note:

(1) Sodium fell by 1.7 mEq/L for each 100 mg/dl rise in glucose.
(2) A glucose rise of about 500 mg/dl shifts a liter of fluid from intracellular to extracellular space.

stantial with estimates ranging from 400 to 1000 mEq.

Serum bicarbonate generally exceeds 12 mEq/L (average 17) and the pH usually exceeds 7.2 (average 7.26). The anion gap is calculated as follows:

$$Anion\ gap = (Na + K) - (Cl + HCO_3)$$

Example:

$$(140 + 4) - (100 + 28) = 16\ mEq/L.$$

In hyperosmolar coma the anion gap is elevated, averaging 34 mEq/L which is somewhat surprising since levels of acetoacetate or lactate are not high enough to account for the unmeasured anion(s). Serum blood urea nitrogen is invariably high (average about 90 mg/dl).

Treatment

Published algorithms for treating hyperosmolar coma differ in detail. Reversal of precipitating factors, compulsive attention to the rapidly changing metabolic state of the patient, and individualization of therapy are more important than the differences between the various acceptable therapeutic stratagems.

Fluid Replacement. Aggressive fluid replacement is crucial in the treatment of hyperosmolar coma. Dehydration is profound, approximating a quarter of total body water, or an eighth of normal total body weight. Although severe, the degree of water loss is often not apparent because hyperglycemia attracts water into the extracellular space supporting the circulation, and acts as a diuretic, maintaining urination. The presence or absence of skin tenting, soft eyeballs, and axillary sweat are not of much help in guiding fluid replacement in these elderly patients. Neither are hemoconcentration, hyperproteinemia, or azotemia. A premorbid weight, if available, can allow a quantitative estimate of the fluid deficit.

Rehydration is the mainstay of therapy. Several patients have been treated successfully without insulin, using only fluid and electrolyte replacement. With rehydration alone, glucose may fall at about 20 mg/dl per hour.[139,140]

There is agreement that most of the fluid loss should be replaced with half normal saline solution, except that if the patient is hypotensive, normal saline or even colloid solutions should be used.

We believe that in all cases the first liter or two should be normal (0.9%) saline, following which half-normal saline solution may be given. Rapid expansion of the intravascular space is the first priority since death may result from myocardial infarction, stroke, pulmonary emboli, and renal shutdown—all associated with the impaired circulatory state. Even if the patient is initially normotensive, shock may develop after insulin is given, when decreasing hyperglycemia permits water to return to the intracellular space, depleting the vascular system.[141,142]

Another point of view is that in the absence of frank hypotension, half-normal saline should be used exclusively. It has been claimed that one can expand the intravascular space as rapidly by giving half-normal saline solution at twice the rate and at the same time produce a rapid fall in the hyperosmolarity. Although unproven, it is reasonable to suppose that decreasing the duration of hyperosmolarity would be beneficial. Brain swelling due to rapid infusion of hypotonic fluid has not been a problem and animal data suggest that rapid falls in osmolarity will do no harm provided treatment is slowed when the blood glucose reaches 250 mg/dl.[143] This is in striking contrast to ketoacidosis in which symptomatic cerebral edema is not uncommon.

Elderly patients may have a history of heart disease and are often oliguric. Nonetheless they require rapid administration of large volumes of fluid. Although general guidelines are given below, there is no substitute for assessment of the patient every 1 to 2 hours and appropriate adjustment of subsequent fluid administration. A reasonable target is to give 6 liters in the first 12 hours and another 5 over the next 24 hours. It is convenient to write fluid orders for 2-hour intervals since this simplifies keeping records of administered volume, sodium, and potassium. One may give 2 liters over the first 2 hours, a liter every 2 hours for the next 6 hours, and then 500 ml every 2 hours until repletion is complete. This totals 6 liters in the first 12 hours and another 6 in the next 24 hours. As mentioned, the first liter or two should be normal saline, followed by half-normal saline solution.

Arousable patients do not require a central venous line since one can check postural signs, follow neck veins, listen to lungs, and watch the urine output. When patients are obtunded, a central venous line is helpful. Normal saline can then be infused at a liter per hour until the central venous pressure exceeds zero.

Although the giving of plasma or whole blood are often recommended when patients are hypotensive, these products would probably increase the already high incidence of thromboembolic events.

Potassium. Potassium replacement must be guided by serum levels. The total body potassium loss is profound (400 to 1000 mEq), and after receiving insulin, the patient's potassium will plummet abruptly, an effect exaggerated by the struggle of the kidneys to retain sodium because of volume depletion. The resulting hypokalemia can produce ileus, respiratory paralysis, or even ventricular fibrillation.

Serum potassium should be monitored every 2 hours so long as it is between 3 and 5 mEq/L, otherwise hourly. The electrocardiogram may be helpful during the first few hours of treatment when electrolytes are rapidly changing. An arbitrary but reasonable approach to potassium replacement is to give nothing, 10, 20, or 30 mEq per hour, respectively, depending on whether the serum potassium exceeds 5, lies between 4 and 5, between 3 and 4, or is less than 3 mEq/L. If the serum potassium is less than 5 mEq/L, repletion should begin even if the patient is not yet urinating. After 36 hours one can expect to have given about 300 mEq of potassium of which perhaps half will have been excreted in the urine. Since only a small portion of the potassium will be replaced by the time acute therapy is over, the patient will generally need oral supplements for approximately a week.

Insulin. Insulin should be given in small amounts, either intravenously or intramuscularly.[144,145] A reasonable plan is to give a bolus of 10 units of regular insulin intravenously, followed by an infusion of 0.1 unit/kg/hr until the blood glucose is down to 250 mg/dl. At this point the intravenous insulin infusion may simply be stopped, in contrast to ketoacidosis, in which the absence of a subcutaneous depot of insulin may lead to the immediate redevelopment of hyperglycemia and ketosis. If insulin is stopped, there is no need to add glucose to the intravenous fluids in order to prevent hypoglycemia. Many patients will need no further insulin. Those that do may be given regular insulin every 6 hours until lente or NPH insulin can be started daily before breakfast.

Occasionally, as in the case of patients with ketoacidosis, one may encounter insulin resistance. If so, one should double the infusion rate of insulin if there has been no fall of glucose in the first hour. With certain patients it may be necessary to repeat the doubling several times.

Insulin may be given intramuscularly if the facilities for intravenous infusion are not available. The efficiency of intramuscular insulin is well documented for ketoacidosis, but less well for hyperosmolar coma. Doses are identical with those for DKA except that the initial loading dose should be doubled, half given as an intravenous bolus, and the other half intramuscularly. Subsequent injections may be given hourly. Rehydration is especially crucial if one is relying on intramuscular absorption.

Hypophosphatemia occurs in hyperosmolar coma just as it does in DKA. One should give no more than 40 mEq/L of potassium as the phosphate salt. Even this amount contains a gram of elemental phosphorus which can lower serum calcium significantly in normal persons. Patients with hyperosmolar coma have lost calcium and magnesium and are presumably prone to significant hypophosphatemia. Further phosphorus repletion can be done over the following week.

In some patients, hyperosmolar coma is triggered by an acute event such as myocardial infarction or cerebrovascular accident and will therefore not recur if the patient survives. In others (up to one-half) no precipitant will be found. Common reversible factors include neglected diabetes; limited fluid access due to dementia, inanition, or paralysis; and infection (all patients should have appropriate cultures of blood, body surfaces and excreta).

Differential Diagnosis. Patients with uncontrolled diabetes and renal failure with anuria may be deceptively similar to those with hyperosmolar coma at presentation. Both groups present with extremely high blood glucose levels as well as elevated urea nitrogen and creatinine concentrations. The former, however, tend to be anemic (not hemoconcentrated), hyponatremic, hyperkalemic, and with extracellular volume overload, often presenting with congestive heart failure. The distinction is of some importance since large volumes of fluid are dangerous in the aneuric patient. Here therapy should consist of insulin alone. By shifting water intracellularly, insulin will also decrease the heart failure. Of course, dialysis will ultimately be required. A substantial number of patients with hyperosmolar coma will subsequently be found to have at least mild renal impairment.

Prognosis

In one older series,[141] the mortality was 40%. Half the deaths were due to underlying illness and the remainder were attributed to the effects of dehydration. Of this latter group, half died within 24 hours in intractable shock. The other half died of thromboembolic complications such as pulmonary embolus. When treatment is delayed, the number of deaths thought to be directly attributable to hyperosmolarity increases. In a 1983 publication, Carroll and Matz[115] reported that there were 9 deaths among 89 patients of all ages with hyperosmolar, nonketotic coma; all deaths occurred in the group of 64 patients over the age of 50 years.

The survivors of hyperosmolar coma often turn out to have relatively mild diabetes which can be managed with appropriate diet and/or oral hypoglycemic agents. Repeat episodes are common. The patient and his family should be instructed to obtain medical consultation rapidly for every acute medical illness, to follow the diet and take the appropriate hypoglycemic agents faithfully, and to test for glycosuria frequently.

LACTIC ACIDOSIS

Lactic acidosis is a metabolic acidosis in which the blood pH is lowered because of the accumulation of lactic acid. It results from a variety of conditions that prevent the utilization of pyruvate and thus lactate, allowing lactic acid to contribute its hydrogen ions, thereby lowering the pH. When buffering capacities are exceeded, the pH falls and lactic acidosis ensues. The most common etiology is hypoperfusion of tissue which results in anaerobic glycolysis, accumulation of pyruvate, and an altered redox situation so that pyruvate is converted to lactate.

Kreisberg[146] has listed 30 items in a classification of causes of lactic acidosis. In addition to 8 conditions with impaired tissue perfusion and oxygenation, he cites 22 others in which there is no obvious impairment of tissue perfusion and oxygenation. These include 6 associated disorders (e.g., diabetes, liver disease, renal failure, etc.), 11 drugs, and 5 hereditary expressions of enzyme deficiency.

Lactic acidosis deserves discussion here not only because the clinical state must be differentiated from that of diabetic ketoacidosis but also because it may occur in certain diabetic patients treated with biguanides.[147] The latter situation, in which there were some deaths, led in 1977 to the sudden withdrawal of phenformin (DBI) from the market in the United States by the Food and Drug Administration (see Chapter 21). However, phenformin is still used in some countries. Furthermore, related biguanides, such as metformin and buformin (especially metformin), are also used outside the U.S.A.

In a literature review covering the period of 1959 to 1977, Luft, Schmülling and Eggstein[148] found reports of 330 diabetic patients who developed lactic acidosis during treatment with a biguanide. Of these, 166 or 50.3% had died. They quote both the French and Swiss experience as indicating considerably less lactic acidosis in patients treated with metformin than those who had received phenformin or buformin. In contrast to phenformin, metformin is not metabolized by the liver, but in patients with satisfactory renal function, is rapidly excreted by the kidney. It seems clear that if biguanides are prescribed, they should not be used in patients with impaired hepatic or renal function.[149] (See also Chapter 21.)

Under normal conditions, lactate and pyruvate co-exist in the blood plasma in a ratio of about 10:1 with lactate concentration in the range of 0.6 to 1.0 mmol/L and that of pyruvate, about 0.1 mmol/L. An increase in lactate may follow physical exercise but the situation is benign due to a corresponding increase in pyruvate. In lactic acidosis the plasma lactate is 2 to 5 mmol/L or more and usually substantially greater. Lactate and pyruvate may be measured directly but facilities are usually not available readily enough for clinical purposes. When the physician suspects that lactic acidosis may be present, a determination of electrolytes will often yield helpful results. The "anion gap" or difference between the sum of the plasma sodium and potassium minus the sum of chloride and the bicarbonate is usually less than 16 mmol/L. The anion gap of 16 mmol/L includes protein and a wide variety of organic acids which normally circulate. When the anion gap is greater than this, it suggests that an additional organic acid is present. If the patient's history does not suggest other causes of metabolic acidosis, lactic acidosis may be presumed to be present.

Lactic acidosis occurs with increased frequency in patients with diabetes, hepatic or renal disease. It is invariably present to some degree in patients in shock. Since hypoperfusion is a common complication of ketoacidosis or hyperosmolar coma, some lactate accumulation is also frequently present in these conditions. Therefore, a seriously ill patient with ketoacidosis or hyperosmolar coma may likely also have some element of lactic acidosis. It should also be noted that a seriously ill patient with hyperosmolar coma may have a metabolic acidosis because of hypoperfusion and lactate accumulation, but no significant ketoacidosis.

Lactate and pyruvate exist in the cytosol whereas beta-hydroxybutyrate (β-HOB) and acetoacetate (AcAc) are in the mitochondria. Both are redox couples and indicate the relative acid-base status of their respective compartments. However, there are mechanisms for the transfer of hydrogen ions back and forth between the cytosol and mitochondria. This is clinically important because in a patient with ketoacidosis in whom hydrogen ion is released by β-HOB, and in whom some hypoperfusion is present, the formation of lactate may be favored. Moreover, as lactate accumulates and hydrogen ion is released from it, it may further increase the β-HOB:AcAc ratio. In this event, a severe mixed acidosis may be present, but the contribution of the ketoacidosis may be underestimated because most of the circulating ketoacids will be β-HOB which is not detected by the nitroprusside reaction.

The treatment of lactic acidosis includes the following: (1) discontinuance or correction of any probable incitant; (b) overcoming of shock by measures designed to maintain acceptable blood pressure and adequate cardiac output; (c); neutralization of acidosis by means of a base, usually sixth molar sodium bicarbonate, intravenously; and (d) correction of diabetic ketoacidosis, if present, by appropriate amounts of insulin, fluids, and electrolytes.

Since the amount of bicarbonate required differs widely from patient to patient, there should be frequent monitoring of acid-base indices and the clinical response to treatment. It must be emphasized that, although in some patients aggressive treatment may be definitely indicated, rapid and complete correction of the acidosis is not necessary or even desirable lest volume overload with low blood potassium and calcium result. Kassirer[150] has suggested one plan, namely to raise the level of plasma bicarbonate by 4 to 6 mEq/L initially and then to 14 to 16 mEq/L in 24 hours.

ALCOHOLIC KETOACIDOSIS

Alcoholic ketoacidosis is encountered in both nondiabetic and diabetic persons of both sexes. It is usually seen in heavy users of alcohol and often in those who have recently stopped or suddenly decreased alcohol consumption because of prolonged abdominal discomfort and vomiting with consequent starvation.[151]

Ethanol is primarily metabolized to acetalde-

hyde, which is further altered to acetate. Both of these steps generate hydrogen ions which favor the formation of betahydroxybutyrate or, for that matter, lactic acid. Ethanol has an inhibitory effect on fatty acid oxidation but as blood levels fall, and in association with lipolysis, ketoacid may be formed. If diabetes is present, the stage is set for an even more prompt development of ketoacidosis. Alcohol has several other metabolic effects and in particular, inhibits gluconeogenesis. Thus, patients with alcoholic ketoacidosis may have a low, normal, or high glucose level. In some patients with diabetes, the ingestion of alcohol is a substantial contributor to the development of diabetic ketoacidosis.

In patients without significant complications, treatment with 5% dextrose in water (or saline initially) and minimal amounts of sodium bicarbonate intravenously, usually results in a favorable outcome. Insulin may or may not be indicated, depending upon the nature of the diabetes.

MIXED SYNDROMES

From the foregoing, it is evident that a patient with diabetes may have several coexisting and overlapping syndromes. Diabetic ketoacidosis (DKA) and hyperglycemic hyperosmolar nonketotic coma are obviously closely related, both having insulin lack as a common feature. In hyperosmolar coma, the insulin lack may be less severe whereas dehydration and hyperosmolarity are more severe than in ketoacidosis. Alcohol may be a substantial contributor to the development of DKA or may cause alcoholic ketoacidosis with modest hyperglycemia which may be mistaken for the more serious syndrome of DKA. Lactate may accumulate in any of the three conditions resulting in a mixed acidosis in DKA and alcoholic ketoacidosis and a more seriously ill patient with hyperosmolar coma.

Treatment of the individual patient is directed by the physician's impression as to which condition is the dominant one, keeping in mind that these syndromes may coexist. Once this decision is made, treatment should be directed primarily at the one considered to be the most important in the illness at hand.

REFERENCES

1. Kahn, C.R.: Role of insulin receptors in insulin resistant states. Metabolism 29:455, 1980.
1a. Kahn, C.R.: The insulin receptor and insulin: the lock and key to diabetes. Clin. Res. 31:326, 1983.
2. Gorden, Ph., Carpentier, J-L., Freychet, P., Orci, L.: Internalization of polypeptide hormone. Mechanism, intracellular localization and significance. Diabetologia 18:263, 1980.
3. Baxter, J.D., MacLeod, K.M.: Chapter 4. Molecular basis of hormone action. In: P.K. Bondy and L.E. Ro-

senberg (Eds.): Metabolic Control and Disease. Philadelphia, W.B. Saunders Co., 1980, pp. 104-160.

4. Levine, R., Goldstein, M.S.: On the mechanism of action of insulin. Rec. Prog. Horm. Res. *11*:343,1955.

5. Felig, P.: Chapter 6. Disorders of carbohydrate metabolism. In: P.K. Bondy and L.E. Rosenberg (Eds.): Metabolic Control and Disease. Philadelphia, W.B. Saunders Co., 1980, pp. 276-392.

6. Manchester, K.L.: Insulin and protein synthesis. In: G. Litwack (Ed.): Biochemical Action of Hormones, Vol. I. New York, Academic Press, 1970, pp.267-320.

7. Sherwin, R.S., Hendler, R.G., Felig, P.: Effect of diabetes mellitus and insulin on the turnover and metabolic response to ketones in man. Diabetes *25*:776, 1976.

8. Jefferson, L.S.: Role of insulin in the regulation of protein synthesis. Diabetes *29*:487, 1980.

9. Khoo, J.C., Steinberg, D., Thompson, B., Mayer, S.E.: Hormonal regulation of adipocyte enzymes. The effects of epinephrine and insulin on the control of lipase, phosphorylase kinase, phosphorylase, and glycogen synthase. J. Biol. Chem. *248*:3823, 1973.

10. Shrago, E., Lockhart-Ewart, R.B.: Chapter 2. Carbohydrate metabolism and its implications. In: H.W. Katzen and R.J. Mahler (Eds.): Advances in Modern Nutrition. Vol. 2. Diabetes, Obesity and Vascular Disease: Metabolic and Molecular Interrelationships. Part I. New York, John Wiley & Sons, 1978, pp. 7–36.

11. Liljenquist, J.E., Keller, U., Chiasson, J-L., Cherrington, A.D.: Insulin and glucagon actions and consequences of derangements in secretion. In: L.J. DeGroot (Ed.): Endocrinology, Vol. 2. New York, Grune & Stratton, 1979, p. 981.

12. Hers, H.G.: The control of glycogen metabolism in the liver. Ann. Rev. Biochem. *45*:167,1976.

13. Weber, G.: Integrative action of insulin at the molecular level. In: E. Shafrir (Ed.): Impact of Insulin on Metabolic Pathways. New York, Academic Press, 1972, pp. 151–161.

14. Mayes, P.A.: Regulation of carbohydrate and lipid metabolism. In: H.A. Harper, V.W. Rodwell, P.A. Mayes (Eds.): Review of Physiological Chemistry. 16th Ed. Los Altos, Lange Medical Publication, 1977, pp. 321–336.

15. Felig, P., Marliss, E., Ohman, J.L., Cahill, G.F.: Plasma amino acid levels in diabetic ketoacidosis. Diabetes *19*:727, 1970.

16. Volpe, J.J.: Lipid metabolism: fatty acid and cholesterol biosynthesis. In: H.M. Katzen, R.J. Mahler (Eds.): Advances in Modern Nutrition, Vol. 2. Diabetes, Obesity and Vascular Disease: Metabolic and Molecular Interrelationships. Part I. New York, John Wiley & Sons, 1978, pp. 37–125.

17. Woodside, W.F., Heimberg, M.: Effects of anti-insulin serum, insulin, and glucose on output of triglycerides and on ketogenesis by the perfused rat liver. J. Biol. Chem. *251*:13, 1976.

18. Schade, D.S., Eaton, R.P.: Dose response to insulin in man: differential effects on glucose and ketone body regulation. J. Clin. Endocrinol. Metab. *44*:1038, 1977.

19. LeFebvre, P.J., Luyckx, A.S.: Glucagon and diabetes: a reappraisal. Diabetologia *16*:347, 1979.

20. Müller, W.A., Faloona, G.R., Unger, R.H.: Hyperglucagonemia in diabetic ketoacidosis. Its prevalance and significance. Am. J. Med. *54*:52, 1973.

21. Unger, R.H., Orci, L.: Role of glucagon in diabetes. Arch. Intern. Med. *137*:482, 1977.

22. Gerich, J.E., Schneider, V.S., Lorenzi, M., et al. Role of glucagon in human diabetic ketoacidosis: studies using somatostatin. Clin. Endocrinol. *5*(Suppl.):299, 1976.

23. Raskin, P., Unger, R.H.: Hyperglucagonemia and its suppression. N. Engl. J. Med. *299*:433, 1978.

24. Felig, P., Wahren, J., Sherwin, R., Hendler, R.: Insulin, glucagon, and somatostatin in normal physiology and diabetes mellitus. Diabetes *25*:1091, 1976.

25. Clarke, W.L., Santiago, J.V., Kipnis, D.M.: The effect of hyperglucagonemia on blood glucose concentrations and on insulin requirements in insulin-requiring diabetes mellitus. Diabetes *27*:649, 1978.

26. Perry-Keene, D.A., Alford, F.P., Chisolm, D.J., et al.: Glucagon and diabetes. I. The failure of hyperglucagonaemia to influence the response of established diabetic ketoacidosis to therapy. Clin. Endocrinol. (Oxf.) *6*:417, 1977.

27. Barnes, A.J., Kohner, E.M., Bloom, S.R., et al.: Importance of pituitary hormones on aetiology of diabetic ketoacidosis. Lancet *1*:1171, 1978.

28. Winegrad, A.I., Morrison, A.D.: Diabetic ketoacidosis, nonketotic hyperosmolar coma and lactic acidosis. In: L.J. DeGroot (Ed.): Endocrinology. Vol. 2. New York, Grune & Stratton, 1979, pp. 1025–1042.

29. Alberti, K.G.M.M., Nattrass, M.: Severe diabetic ketoacidosis. Med. Clin. North Am. *62*:799, 1978.

30. Schade, D.S., Eaton, R.P.: Pathogenesis of diabetic ketoacidosis. A reappraisal. Diabetes Care *2:296,* 1979.

31. Chiasson, J-L., Liljenquist, J.E., Sinclair-Smith, B.C., Lacy, W.W.: Gluconeogenesis from alanine in normal postabsorptive man. Intrahepatic stimulatory effect of glucagon. Diabetes *24*:574, 1975.

32. Park, C.R., Exton, J.H.: Glucagon and the metabolism of glucose. In: D.J. Lefebvre, R.H. Unger (Eds.): Glucagon. Molecular Physiology, Clinical and Therapeutic Implications. Oxford, Pergamon Press, 1972, pp. 77–108.

33. Schneider, H., Fineberg, S.E., Blackburn, G.: The effects of physiologic variations in glucagon concentrations upon human forearm tissues. Diabetes *25* (Suppl. 1): 341, 1976.

34. Pozefsky, T., Tancredi, R.G., Moxley, R.T, et al : Metabolism of forearm tissues in man. Diabetes *25*:128, 1976.

35. Gerich, J.: On the causes and consequences of abnormal glucagon secretion in human diabetes. In: P.P. Foa, J.S. Bajaj, N.L. Foa (Eds.): Glucagon: Its Role in Physiology and Clinical Medicine. New York, Springer, 1977, pp. 617–641.

36. Müller, W.A., Faloona, G.R., Aguilar-Parada, E., Unger, R.H.: Abnormal alpha-cell function in diabetes. N. Engl. J. Med. *283*:109, 1970.

37. Wise, J.K., Hendler, R., Felig, P.: Evaluation of alpha-cell function by infusion of alanines in normal, diabetic and obese subjects. N. Engl. J. Med. *288*:487, 1973.

38. Fineberg, S.E., Merimee, T.J.: Acute metabolic effects of human growth hormone. Diabetes *23*:499, 1974.

39. Eaton, R.P., Schade, D.S.: Modulation and implications of the counter-regulatory hormones: glucagon, catecholamines, cortisol, and growth hormone. In: H.W. Katzen, R.J. Mahler (Eds.): Advances in Modern Nutrition, Vol. 2. Diabetes, Obesity, and Vascular Disease. Metabolic and Molecular Interrelationships. Part 1. New York, John Wiley & Sons, 1978, pp. 341–372.

40. Raben, M.S., Hollenberg, C.H.: Effect of growth hormone on plasma fatty acids. J. Clin. Invest. *38*:484, 1959.

41. Felig, P., Marliss, E.B., Cahill, G.F.: Metabolic response to human growth hormone during prolonged starvation. J. Clin. Invest. *50*:411, 1971.

42. Exton, J.H., Miller, T.B., Harper, S.C., Park, C.R.: Carbohydrate metabolism in perfused livers of adrenalectomized and steroid-replaced rats. Am. J. Physiol. *230:*163, 1976.

43. Fain, J.N., Scow, R.O., Chernick, S.S.: Effect of glu-cocorticoids in metabolism of adipose tissue *in vitro*. J. Biol. Chem. *238*:54, 1963.

44. Olefsky, J.M.: Effect of dexamethasone on insulin bind-ing, glucose transport and glucose oxidation of isolated rat adipocytes. J. Clin. Invest. *56*:1499, 1975.

45. Gerich, J.E., Martin, M.M., Recant, L.: Clinical and metabolic characteristics of hyperosmolar nonketotic coma. Diabetes *20*:228, 1971.

46. Sperling, M.A., Bacon, G., Kenny, F.M., Drash, A.: Cortisol secretion in acidotic and non-acidotic diabetes mellitus. Am. J. Dis. Child. *124*:690, 1972.

47. Jacobs, H.S., Nabarro, J.D.N.: Plasma 11-hydroxycor-ticosteroid and growth hormone levels in acute medical illnesses. Br. Med. J. *2*:595, 1969.

48. Vaughan, M., Steinberg, D.: Glyceride biosynthesis, glyceride breakdown, and glycogen breakdown in adipose tissue: mechanisms and regulations. In: A.E. Renold, G.F. Cahill (Eds.): Handbook of Physiology, Section 5: Adipose Tissue. Am. Physiol. Soc., Washington, D.C., 1965, pp. 239–252.

49. Sherline, P., Lynch, A., Glinsmann, W. H.: Cyclic AMP and adrenergic receptor control of rat liver glycogen me-tabolism. Endocrinology *91*:680, 1972.

50. Exton, J.H., Park, C.R.: Interaction of insulin and glu-cagon in the control of liver metabolism. In: R.O. Greep, E.B. Astwood, D.F. Steiner, N. Freinkel (Eds.): Hand-book of Physiology, Section 7: Endocrinology. Vol. 1. Am. Physiol. Soc., Washington, D.C., 1972, pp. 437–455.

51. Gerich, J.E., Karam, J.H., Forsham, P.H.: Reciprocal adrenergic control of pancreatic alpha and beta cell func-tion in man. Diabetes *21*(Suppl. 1):332, 1972.

52. Blackard, W.G., Heidingsfelder, S.A.: Adrenergic re-ceptor control mechanism for growth hormone secretion. J. Clin. Invest. *47*:1407, 1968.

53. Porte, D.: Sympathetic regulation of insulin secretion. Its relation to diabetes mellitus. Arch. Intern. Med. *123*:252, 1969.

54. Christensen, N.J.: Catecholamines and diabetes mellitus. Diabetologia *16*:211, 1979.

55. Bolli, G., Compagnucci, P., Cartechini, M.G., et al: Urinary excretion and plasma levels of norepinephrine and epinephrine during diabetic ketoacidosis. Arch. Diabetol. Lat. *16*:157, 1979.

56. McGarry, J.D., Foster, D.W.: Regulation of hepatic ke-togenesis. In: L.J. DeGroot (Ed.): Endocrinology,Vol. 2. New York, Grune & Stratton, 1979, pp. 997-1006.

57. McGarry, J.D., Foster, D.W.: Ketogenesis and its reg-ulation. Am. J. Med. *61*:9, 1976.

58. McGarry, J.D.: New perspectives in the regulation of ketogenesis. Diabetes *28*:517, 1979.

59. McGarry, J.D., Mannaerts, G.P., Foster, D.W.: A pos-sible role for malonyl-CoA in the regulation of hepatic fatty acid oxidation and ketogenesis. J. Clin. Invest. *60*:265, 1977.

60. Genuth, S.M., Hoppel, C.L.: Plasma and urine carnitine in diabetic ketosis. Diabetes *28*:1083, 1979.

61. Sauer, F., Erfle, J.D.: On the mechanism of acetoacetate synthesis by guinea pig liver fractions. J. Biol. Chem. *241*:30, 1966.

62. Cahill, G.F., Herrera, M.G., Morgan, A.P., et al. Hor-mone-fuel interrelationships during fasting. J. Clin. In-vest. *45*:1751, 1966.

63. Ruderman, N.B., Goodman, M.N.: Inhibition of muscle acetoacetate utilization during diabetic ketoacidosis. Am. J. Physiol. *226*:136, 1974.

64. Owen, O.E., Block, B., Patel, M., et al. Human splanch-nic metabolism during diabetic ketoacidosis. Metabolism *26*:381, 1977.

65. Balasse, E.O., Havel, R.J.: Evidence for an effect of insulin on the peripheral utilization of ketone bodies in dogs. J. Clin. Invest. *50*:801, 1971.

66. Alberti, K.G.M.M., Hockaday, T.D.R.: Diabetic coma: a reappraisal after 5 years. Clin. Endocrinol. Metab. *6*:421, 1977.

66a.Lever, E., Jaspan, J.B.: Sodium bicarbonate therapy in severe diabetic ketoacidosis. Am. J. Med. *75*:263, 1983.

66b.Oh, M.S., Banerjii, M.A., Carroll, H.J.: The mechanism of hyperchloremic acidosis during recovery phase of dia-betic ketoacidosis. Diabetes *30*:310, 1981.

66c.Adroque, H.J., Wilson, H., Boyd, A.E., et al.: Plasma acid-base patterns in diabetic ketoacidosis. N. Engl. J. Med. *307*:1603, 1982.

67. Martin, H.E., Smith, K., Wilson, M.L.: The fluid and electrolyte therapy of severe diabetic acidosis and ketosis. A study of twenty-nine episodes (twenty-six patients). Am. J. Med. *24*:376, 1958.

68. Kogut, M.D.: Pathogenesis, diagnosis and treatment of diabetic ketoacidosis. Curr. Prob. Pediat. *VI*:3, 1976.

69. Andres, R., Baltzan, M.A., Cader, G., Zierler, K.L.: Effect of insulin on carbohydrate metabolism and on po-tassium in the forearm of man. J. Clin. Invest. *41*:108, 1962.

70. Kamminga, C.E., Willebrands, A.F., Groen, J., Blick-man, J.R.: Effect of insulin on potassium and inorganic phosphate content of medium in experiments with isolated rat diaphragms. Science *111*:30, 1950.

71. Rebar, B., Omachi, A., Rebar, J., Jr.: Effects of glucose infusion on dog myocardial metabolism. Circ. Res. *7*:977, 1959.

72. Soler, N.G., Bennett, M.A., Fitzgerald, M.G., Malins, J.M.: Electrocardiogram as a guide to potassium replace-ment in diabetic ketoacidosis. Diabetes *23*:610, 1974.

73. Assal, J.P., Aoki, T.T., Manzano, F.M., Kozak, G.P.: Metabolic effects of sodium bicarbonate in the manage-ment of diabetic ketoacidosis. Diabetes *23*:405, 1974.

74. Ohman, J.L., Jr., Marliss, E.B., Aoki, T.T., et al.: The cerebrospinal fluid in diabetic ketoacidosis. N. Engl. J. Med. *284*:283, 1971.

75. Alberti, K.G.M.M., Knochel, J.P.: The pathophysiology and clinical characteristics of severe hypophosphatemia. Arch. Intern. Med. *137*:203, 1977.

76. Franks, M., Berris, R.F., Kaplan, N.O., Myers, G.B.: Metabolic studies in diabetic acidosis; effect of admin-istration of sodium phosphate. Arch. Intern. Med. *81*:42, 1948.

77. Butler, A.M., Talbot, N.B., Burnett, C.H., et al. Meta-bolic studies in diabetic coma. Trans. Assoc. Am. Phy-sicians *60*:102, 1947.

78. Nabarro, J.D.N., Spencer, A.G., Stowers, J.M.: Meta-bolic studies in severe diabetic ketosis. Quart. J. Med. *21*:225, 1952.

78a.McMullen, J.K.: Asystole and hypomagnesaemia during recovery from diabetic ketoacidosis. Br. Med. J. *1*:690, 1977.

79. Riley, M.S., Schade, D.S., Eaton, R.P.: Effects of insulin infusion on plasma phosphate in diabetic patients. Me-tabolism *28*:191, 1979.

80. Zipf, W.B., Bacon, G.E., Spencer, M.L., et al.: Hypo-calcemia, hypomagnesemia, and transient hypoparathy-roidism during therapy with potassium phosphate in dia-betic ketoacidosis. Diabetes Care *2*:265, 1979.

80a.Fisher, J.N., Kitabchi, A.E.: Randomized study of phos-phate therapy in the treatment of diabetic ketoacidosis. J. Clin. Endocrinol. Metabol. *57*:177, 1983.

81. Guest, G.M., Rappaport, S.: Role of acid-soluble phos-

phorus compounds in red blood cells in experimental rickets, renal insufficiency, pyloric obstruction, gastroenteritis, ammonium chloride acidosis and diabetic acidosis. Am. J. Dis. Child. 58:1072, 1939.

82. Alberti, K.G.M.M., Emerson, P.M., Darley, J.H., Hockaday, T.D.R.: 2,3-diphosphoglycerate and tissue oxygenation in uncontrolled diabetes mellitus. Lancet 2:391, 1972.

83. Andersen, H., Ditzel, J.: Importance of plasma inorganic phosphate in the treatment of diabetic ketoacidosis. Diabetes 22(Suppl.):293, 1973.

84. Gerson, J., Bessman, A.N.: Nucleotide phosphate, 2,3-DPG and inorganic phosphate flux in diabetic ketoacidosis. Clin. Res. 22:191A, 1974.

85. Bellingham, A.J., Detter, J.C., Lenfant, C.: The role of hemoglobin affinity for oxygen and red-cell 2,3-diphosphoglycerate in the management of diabetic ketoacidosis. Trans. Assoc. Am. Physicians 83:113, 1970.

86. Ditzel, J.: Improved erythrocytic oxygen release following a dietary supplement of calcium diphosphate to diabetic and healthy children. Diabetologia 10:363, 1974.

87. Soler, N.G., Wright, A.D., Fitzgerald, M.G., Malins, J.M.: Comparative study of different insulin regimens in the management of diabetic ketoacidosis. Lancet 2:1221, 1975.

88. Fisher, J.N., Shahshahani, M.N., Kitabchi, A.E.: Diabetic ketoacidosis low-dose insulin therapy by various routes. N. Engl. J. Med. 297:238, 1977.

89. Alberti, K.G.M.M.: Low dose insulin in the treatment of diabetic ketoacidosis. Arch. Intern. Med. 137:1367, 1977.

90. Völlm, V.K.R.: On the preservation of insulin in a physiological sodium carbonate solution; on the problem of therapy of the diabetic coma with a continuous intravenous drip infusion of insulin. Schweiz. Med. Wochenschr. 90:1080, 1960.

91. Page, M.M., Alberti, K.G.M.M., Greenwood, R., et al: Treatment of diabetic coma with continuous low-dose infusion of insulin. Br. Med. J. 2:687, 1974.

92. Kidson, W., Casey, J., Kraegen, E., et al.: Treatment of severe diabetes mellitus by insulin infusion. Br. Med. J. 2:691, 1974.

93. Semple, P.F., White, C., Mandersen, W.G.: Continuous intravenous infusion of small doses of insulin in treatment of diabetic ketoacidosis. Br. Med. J. 2:694, 1974.

94. Sönksen, P.H., Srivastava, M.C., Tompkins, C.V., Nabarro, J.D.N.: Growth-hormone and cortisol responses to insulin infusion in patients with diabetes mellitus. Lancet 2:155, 1972.

95. Weber, M.E., Abbassi, V.: Continuous intravenous therapy in severe diabetic ketoacidosis: variations in dosage requirement. J. Pediatr. 91:755, 1977.

96. Lightner, E.S., Kappy, M.S., Revsin, B.: Low-dose intravenous insulin infusion in patients with diabetic ketoacidosis: biochemical effects in children. Pediatrics 60:681, 1977.

97. Kaufman, I.A., Keller, M.A., Nyhan, W.L.: Editorial: Diabetic ketosis and acidosis: The continuous infusion of low doses of insulin. J. Pediatr. 87:846, 1975.

98. Martin, M.M., Martin, A.A.: Continuous low-dose infusion of insulin in the treatment of diabetic ketoacidosis in children. J. Pediatr. 89:560, 1976.

98a. Barrett, E.J., DeFronzo, R.A., Bevilacqua, S., et al.: Insulin resistance in diabetic ketoacidosis. Diabetes 31:923, 1982.

99. Genuth, S.M.: Metabolic clearance of insulin in man. Diabetes 21:1003, 1972.

100. Heber, D., Molitch, M.E., Sperling, M.A.: Low-dose continuous insulin therapy for diabetic ketoacidosis. Arch. Intern. Med. 137:1377, 1977.

101. Weisenfield, S., Podolsky, S., Goldsmith, L., Ziff, L.: Adsorption of insulin to infusion bottles and tubing. Diabetes 17:766, 1968.

102. Semple, P., Ratcliffe, J.C., Manderson, W.G.: Letter: Carrier solutions for low-level intravenous insulin infusion. Br. Med. J. 4:228, 1975.

103. Peterson, L., Caldwell, J., Hoffman, J.: Insulin adsorbance to polyvinylchloride surfaces with implications for constant-infusion therapy. Diabetes 25:72, 1976.

104. Roth, J., Muggeo, M.: Insulin receptors and hyperglycemia. In: H. Rifkin, and P. Raskin (Eds.): Diabetes Mellitus, Volume V. Rowie, Md., R.J. Brady Co., 1981, pp. 63–77.

105. Madison, L.L.: Low-dose insulin: A plea for caution. N. Engl. J. Med. 294:393, 1976.

106. Balasse, E.O.: Acido-cetose diabetique: Aspects physiopathologiques et therapeutiques recents. Diabete Metab. 2:87, 1976.

107. Katsch, G.: Insulinbehandlung des diabetischen Komas. Dtsch. Gesundheits 1:651, 1946.

108. Guerra, S.M.O., Kitabchi, A.E.: Comparison of the effectiveness of various routes of insulin injection: insulin levels and glucose response in normal subjects. J. Clin. Endocrinol. Metab. 42:869, 1976.

109. Binder, C.: Absorption of injected insulin. A clinical-pharmacological study. Acta Pharmacol (Kbh.) (Suppl.) 2:1, 1969.

110. Alberti, K.G.M.M., Hockaday, T.D.R., Turner, R.C.: Small doses of intramuscular insulin in the treatment of diabetic "coma". Lancet 2:515, 1973.

111. Moseley, J.: Diabetic crises in children treated with small doses of intramuscular insulin. Br. Med. J. 1:59–61, 1975.

112. Kitabchi, A.E., Ayyagari, V., Guerra, S.M.O.: The efficacy of low dose versus conventional therapy of insulin for treatment of diabetic ketoacidosis. Ann. Intern. Med. 84:633, 1976.

113. Menzel, R., Zander, E., Jutzi, E.: Treatment of diabetic coma with low-dose injections of insulin. Endokrinologie 67:230, 1976.

114. Fein, I.A., Rockow, E.C., Sprung, C.L., Grodman, R.: Relation of colloid osmotic pressure to arterial hypoxemia and cerebral edema during crystalloid volume loading of patients with diabetic ketoacidosis. Ann. Intern. Med. 96:570, 1982.

115. Carroll, P., Matz, R.: Uncontrolled diabetes mellitus in adults: exercises in treating diabetic ketoacidosis and hyperosmolar nonketotic coma with low-dose insulin and a uniform treatment regimen. Diabetes Care 6:579, 1983.

116. Foster, D.W., McGarry, J.D.: The metabolic derangements and treatment of diabetic ketoacidosis. N. Engl. J. Med. 309:159, 1983.

117. Alberti, K.G.M.M., Hockaday, T.D.R.: Diabetic coma: a reappraisal after five years. Clin. Endocrinol. Metab. 6:421, 1977.

118. McGarry, J.D., Foster, D.W.: Regulation of ketogenesis and clinical aspects of the ketotic state. Metabolism 21:471, 1972.

119. Kitabchi, A.E., Young, R., Sacks, H., Morris, L.: Diabetic ketoacidosis: reappraisal of therapeutic approach. Ann. Rev. Med. 30:339, 1979.

120. Kreisberg, R.A.: Diabetic ketoacidosis: new concepts and trends in pathogenesis and treatment. Ann. Intern. Med. 88:681, 1978.

121. Levine, S.N., Loewenstein, J.E.: Treatment of diabetic ketoacidosis. Arch. Intern. Med. 141:713, 1981.

122. Clements, R.S., Jr., Prockop, L.D., Winegrad, A.I.: A

mechanism to explain acute cerebral edema during the treatment of diabetic acidosis. Diabetes *17*(Suppl. 1):299, 1968.

123. Dillon, E.S., Dyer, W.W.: Factors influencing the prognosis in diabetic coma. Ann. Intern. Med. *11*: 602, 1937.

124. Brøchner-Mortensen, K.: Om prognosen for coma diabeticum. Ugeskr. Laeg. *108*:607, 1946.

125. Zieve, L., Hill, E.: Descriptive characteristics of patients with moderate or severe diabetic acidosis; relation to recovery or death. Arch. Intern. Med. *92*:51, 1953.

126. Harwood, R.: Diabetic acidosis; results of treatment in 67 consecutive cases. N. Engl. J. Med. *245*:1, 1951.

127. Pease, J.C., Cooke, A.M.: The family doctor and diabetic coma. Br. Med. J. 2:336, 1951.

128. Brakier, T., Brull, L.: Acidose diabétique. Le Diabéte 7:146, 1955.

129. Greenaway, J.M., Read, J.: Diabetic coma: a review of 69 cases. Aust. Ann. Med. 7:151, 1958.

130. Cohen, A.S., Vance, V.K., Runyan, J.W., Jr., Hurwitz, D.: Diabetic acidosis: an evaluation of the cause, course and therapy of 73 cases. Ann. Intern. Med. *52*:55, 1960.

131. Skillman, T.G., Wilson, R., Knowles, H.C., Jr.: Mortality of patients with diabetic acidosis in a large city hospital. Diabetes 7:109,1958.

132. Derot, M., Tchobroutsky, G.: L'acidocétose diabétique. Facteurs déclenchants, évolution et mortalité dans 133 observations consécutives. Presse Med. *71*:2017, 1963.

133. Pines, K.L.: Diabetic acidosis. In: M. Ellenberg and H. Rifkin (Eds.): Clinical Diabetes Mellitus. New York, McGraw-Hill Book Co., 1963, p. 340.

134. Schneider, K.W., Winckler, H.: Diabetic coma--still a problem. German Med. Monthly 8:244, 1963.

135. Fitzgerald, M.G., O'Sullivan, D.J., Malins, J.M.: Fatal diabetic ketosis. Br. Med. J. *1*:247, 1961.

136. Asfeldt, V.H.: Ketoacidosis diabetica. A prognostic and therapeutic study of 119 consecutive cases. Danish Med. Bull. *12*:103, 1965.

136a.Bradley, R.F.: Diabetic ketoacidosis and coma. Table 14–1. In: A. Marble, P. White, R.F. Bradley, L.P. Krall (Eds.): Joslin's Diabetes Mellitus, 11th ed. Philadelphia, Lea & Febiger, 1971, p. 363.

136b.Beigelman, P.M.: Severe diabetic ketoacidosis (diabetic "coma"). 482 episodes in 257 patients; experience of three years. Diabetes *20*:490, 1971.

137. Arieff, A.I., Carroll, H.J.: Nonketotic hyperosmolar coma with hyperglycemia: clinical features, pathophys-

iology, renal function, acid-base balance, plasm. cerebrospinal fluid equilibria and the effects of therapy in 37 cases. Medicine *51*:73, 1972.

138. Arieff, A.I., Kleeman, C.R.: Cerebral edema in diabetic comas. II. Effects of hyperosmolality, hyperglycemia and insulin in diabetic rabbits. J. Clin. Endocrinol. Metab. *38*:1057, 1974.

139. Przasnyski, E.J., Fariss, B.L.: Hyperosmolar hyperglycemic nonketotic syndrome treated without insulin: case reports. Milit. Med. *143*:556, 1978.

140. Waldhäusl, W., Kleinberger, G., Korn, A., et al.: Severe hyperglycemia: effects of rehydration on endocrine derangements and blood glucose concentration. Diabetes *28*:577, 1979.

141. McCurdy, D.K.: Hyperosmolar hyperglycemic nonketotic diabetic coma. Med. Clin. North Am. *54*:683, 1970.

142. Brown, R.H., Rossini, A.A., Callaway, C.W., Cahill, G.F., Jr.: Caveat on fluid replacement in hyperglycemic, hyperosmolar, nonketotic coma. Diabetes Care *1*:305, 1978.

143. Arieff, A.I., Carroll, H.J.: Cerebral edema and depression of sensorium in nonketotic hyperosmolar coma. Diabetes *23*:525, 1974.

144. Bendezu, R., Wieland, R.G., Furst, B., et al: Experience with low-dose insulin infusion in diabetic ketoacidosis and diabetic hyperosmolarity. Arch. Intern. Med. *138*:60, 1978.

145. Boehme, W., Rossetto, B., Davis, J., et al.: Low-dose insulin for diabetic nonketotic hyperosmolar coma. J.A.M.A. *242*:1260, 1979.

146. Kreisberg, R.A.: Lactate homeostasis and lactic acidosis. In: H. Rifkin and P. Raskin (Eds.): Diabetes Mellitus, Volume V. Bowie, Maryland. R.J. Brady Co., 1981, pp. 203–211.

147. Misbin, R.I.: Phenformin-associated lactic acidosis: pathogenesis and treatment. Ann. Intern. Med. *87*:591, 1977.

148. Luft, D., Schmülling, R.M., Eggstein, M.: Lactic acidosis in biguanide-treated diabetics. Diabetologia *14*:75,1978.

149. Assan, R., Heuclin, Ch., Ganeval, D., et al.: Metformin-induced lactic acidosis in the presence of acute renal failure. Diabetologia *13*:211, 1977.

150. Kassirer, J.P.: Current concepts: serious acid-base disorder. N. Engl. J. Med. *291*:773, 1974.

151. Kreisberg, R.A.: Diabetic ketoacidosis: New concepts and trends in pathogenesis and treatment. Ann. Intern. Med. *88*:681, 1978.

27 Heart Disease and Diabetes Mellitus

O. Stevens Leland and Peter C. Maki

Heart disease occurs eventually in a majority of patients with diabetes mellitus and continues to be the outstanding factor in overall diabetic morbidity and mortality rates. Atherosclerotic coronary vascular disease is by far the most frequent type of cardiac involvement and, for reasons that are as yet unclear, is more common in diabetics than in the nondiabetic population.[1] However, diabetics in some less affluent societies have fewer cardiovascular complications than either diabetics or nondiabetics in this country.[2–4] This raises the important possibility that macrovascular disease is not a necessary component of diabetes and that other factors are operative. Among these, environmental influences, diet, body weight, physical activity, and age at onset, are suspect.

Other etiologic forms of heart disease may also be encountered relatively frequently. Diabetics have an increased risk of congestive heart failure.[5] A cardiomyopathy specific to diabetes has recently been described. The prevalence of this complication and the magnitude of its contribution to diabetic morbidity and mortality remain uncertain. Hypertensive heart disease is frequent in the setting of diabetes. Hemochromatosis may involve the heart and should not be overlooked in the diabetic with myocardial disease of uncertain etiology and with less than expected response to treatment. Cardiac considerations may play a paramount role in the diabetic undergoing pregnancy, surgery, or in the setting of renal failure or vascular disease elsewhere. Although as many other forms of heart disease occur in those with diabetes as in the nondiabetic, this chapter will emphasize selected features of cardiac problems which the diabetic most often encounters.

BIOCHEMICAL CHANGES IN THE DIABETIC HEART

It has not yet been possible to establish a direct link between the metabolic derangements characterizing diabetes and any form of cardiac disease encountered clinically in the diabetic. In fact, in the well-controlled diabetic, the generation of energy for myocardial contraction and active transport mechanisms proceeds normally.[6]

The heart consists of aerobic tissue and the adenosine triphosphate (ATP) required for fuel is generated largely by oxidative phosphorylation. Quantitatively the most important substrates utilized to manufacture ATP are the fatty acids which generally account for 60 to 70% of oxidative phosphorylation, but under some conditions may account for as much as 100%.[7] Fatty acids reach the heart attached to proteins, are transported into the myocardium, and enter the mitochondria via the carnitine-dependent system. They are used directly for ATP synthesis, being broken down two carbons at a time to acetyl coenzyme A which enters the tricarboxylic acid cycle.

During oxidative metabolism, electrons from the hydrogens of intermediary products are transported by cytochrome enzymes, regenerating large amounts of ATP. All enzymes required in the tricarboxylic acid cycle, and the cytochrome enzymes involved in the reduction of oxygen, are located in the mitochondria, which makes up 35% of the total myocardial volume, and in which the processes of oxidative phosphorylation take place.[7]

The glycolytic pathways serve as back-up systems for the restoration of ATP, and can function both aerobically and anaerobically. Both glucose and its storage polymer, glycogen, require ATP during initial metabolic steps. However, ATP is then produced in excess during further breakdown. If the oxygen available to the heart does not allow restoration of ATP by normal oxidative processes, anaerobic glycolysis provides a short-term alternative for energy production. Enzymatic systems for anaerobic glycolysis are found in the sarcoplasm or attached to the sarcoplasmic reticulum. Amino acids liberated by protein breakdown can also participate in the citric acid cycle after transamination, but are not a major source of muscle energy except in starvation.

Myocardial metabolism in the poorly-controlled diabetic or fasting animal is characterized by almost exclusive oxidation of fatty acids and ketone bodies, and a low rate of glucose utilization.[8] Myocardial uptake of free fatty acids (FFA) is dependent on the level of circulating FFA and the metabolic state of the myocardium. Low insulin levels and increased FFA and ketone bodies further inhibit glucose transport. Concurrent inhibition of phosphofructokinase and increased levels of glucose-6-phosphate result in elevated myocardial glycogen stores. Associated with the enhanced oxidation of FFA and ketone bodies are an increased level of intracellular triglycerides and a faster rate of lipolysis, which appear to reduce the sensitivity to insulin of myocardial tissue.[8]

PATHOLOGIC CHANGES IN THE DIABETIC HEART

The cardiac changes which have been related to diabetes involve both the vascular system and the myocardial interstitium. The former includes the microvasculature, the small and medium sized intramural vessels, and the larger chiefly epicardial vessels. These are affected under differing circumstances and to varying degrees. However, recent theories suggest that initial events in both the microvasculature and the macrovasculature may involve similar pathways of endothelial damage followed by platelet adherence and aggregation.[9,10]

Changes are often not uniform throughout the vascular tree, but rather predominantly involve either larger or smaller vessels. Atherosclerosis in the larger vessels is most frequent. Occasionally microvascular disease is seen in the absence of large vessel disease, although the reverse is more common.

Microangiopathy may encompass a sequence of changes beginning with functional abnormalities and proceeding to endothelial damage, basement membrane thickening, and hematologic disturbances such as increased plasma viscosity, red cell and platelet aggregation and microthrombi.[10] Thickening and duplication of the pericapillary basement membrane is a generalized phenomenon in diabetes and has been seen in patients with impaired glucose tolerance, as well as long-standing, insulin-dependent diabetes.[11] It has been described in many organs, including the heart. Quantitative studies suggest the average thickness of basal laminae around the myocardial capillaries may be less than that reported in skeletal muscle.[12] An increase in permeability of cellular elements of the capillary wall or of the basement membrane, with consequent passage and deposition of glycoprotein material resulting in gradual additions to the laminar width may underlie these changes.[13] This process is not unique to diabetes mellitus and its functional significance to the myocardium is unknown.

Capillary microaneurysms involving the retina are considered a hallmark of diabetes mellitus. In properly injected and cleared specimens of myocardial tissue, Factor et al.[14] found saccular microaneurysms in 3 of 6 long-term diabetics (2 of whom did not have retinopathy or nephropathy) and in none of 8 nondiabetic controls. Microaneurysms were not localized to any given depth or area of myocardium, nor were they closely associated with the extensive fibrosis also often encountered.

Changes in the small and medium sized vessels (50 to 500 micra), which are predominantly intramural, rarely are due to atherosclerosis. Blumenthal and associates[15] examined intramural coronary artery branches in 116 diabetic patients and 105 nondiabetics. All patients had severe atherosclerosis of the epicardial vessels, but in only one instance were substantial lipid-filled atheromata noted beyond the point of entry into the muscular wall of the heart. Diabetics frequently had lesions in the intramural small vessels. Two-thirds of the diabetics had lesions classified by the authors as proliferative, a prevalence 2½ times that found in nondiabetics. These lesions consisted of endothelial proliferation and swelling of subendothelial histiocytes to form mounds, capillary projections, bridges, and eccentric masses of cells occasionally progressing to marked narrowing or complete obliteration of small arteries and venules. These small vessels may be involved in other diseases, such as hypertension,[16] and by a variety of pathologic processes including thickening by deposits of PAS staining material, and occlusion by platelet aggregates or atheromatous debris after rupture of an atheroma in a larger vessel upstream. The functional significance of such lesions in the diabetic is under investigation, particularly with respect to the increased incidence of congestive heart failure and the possible existence of a specific diabetic cardiomyopathy described in subsequent sections. The suggestion that changes in the vasa vasorum accelerate atherosclerosis is not supported by the frequent dissociation between extensive microvascular and macrovascular disease.[17]

Atherosclerosis of epicardial vessels in diabetics is indistinguishable from that in nondiabetics except for increased severity, as noted in the following sections. Early suggestions that the lesions are chemically different have not been confirmed.

Alterations in cardiac myofibrils occur as the result of these vascular changes, but the myocardial interstitium may be separately involved with deposition of PAS-staining material (probably glycoprotein) and extensive fibrosis. None of the alterations is specific to diabetes. Rather, the diabetic heart is characterized by the unusual severity of these abnormalities. The hearts of diabetic patients dying with severe myocardial failure, but with no large vessel atherosclerotic disease, have frequently shown extensive interstitial deposits of PAS-staining material and fibrosis.[18,19] The precise relation between these changes in the failing heart and the metabolic alterations produced by diabetes is unclear. Changes in myocardial compliance appear closely associated with these interstitial abnormalities.

CORONARY ARTERY DISEASE—GENERAL CONSIDERATIONS

The frequency and severity of atherosclerotic vascular disease involving the heart continues to present the diabetologist with a formidable challenge, despite the national trend toward decreasing cardiovascular mortality.[20] Atherosclerosis, neither specific for diabetes nor its inevitable consequence, remains the single most important cause of heart disease and death in the diabetic (Table 27–1).

Occurrence. The occurrence of coronary atherosclerotic heart disease in the diabetic and in the nondiabetic may be contrasted as follows: (1) the overall frequency is much increased; (2) this increase is particularly striking among women; (3) clinically encountered disease is often more advanced than in the nondiabetic; (4) even younger

Table 27–1. Joslin Clinic: Total Deaths and Deaths Due to Atherosclerotic Cardiac Disease (By Decade)

Period	Total No.	Deaths Due to Atherosclerotic Cardiac Disease	
		No.	%
1950–1959	9851	4985	50.6
1960–1968	5009	2690	53.7
1969–1979	6533	3560	54.5

patients are frequently affected. These aspects will be discussed in turn.

Frequency. Autopsy studies have long documented the increased frequency and severity of coronary disease among diabetics. Root et al. in 1939 found coronary artery disease in 51% of 349 diabetics and 18% of 3,400 nondiabetics at the New England Deaconess and Massachusetts General Hospital, a ratio of 2.8:1.[21] In a subsequent study using careful injection techniques for studying the coronary arteries, Stearns et al.[22] noted significant disease in 74% of diabetics compared to only 37% of nondiabetics. In Bell's series of 1,559 autopsies performed on diabetic persons between 1910 and 1951, vascular disease "chiefly gangrene, coronary disease, and renal arteriosclerosis" was causative or a major factor contributing to death in 49.3% of cases in contrast to 24.5% for the nondiabetic.[23] Many other autopsy studies have documented similar findings with a frequency in the diabetic about 2½ times the control group.[24–26] Several others however, could not confirm these findings.[27,28] In the necropsy study by Waller, the average number of 3 main vessels narrowed by 75% was identical in diabetics whose onset occurred after age 30 and controls. However, left main coronary disease was significantly greater in diabetic patients.[28a] In 1968 the International Atherosclerosis Project assessed 34,000 autopsies from 13 national centers. In this study diabetics had more fatty streaks in the coronary arteries and more raised lesions, fibrous plaques, calcification and coronary stenosis than nondiabetic controls.[29] A similar increase in coronary atherosclerosis was noted by Vigorita, who found no correlation between the presence or severity of coronary disease and the duration of adult onset diabetes.[29a] Further detailed pathologic findings are discussed in Chapter 14.

Mortality statistics reported from diabetic clinic populations have highlighted the consequences to be expected from these autopsy findings. Excess mortality is primarily the result of excess atherosclerotic heart disease.[30–32] Kessler reported a retrospective 26-year follow-up study of 21,447 diabetic patients seen at the Joslin Clinic between January, 1930 and July, 1956.[30] A significant excess risk of death from coronary atherosclerotic heart disease was observed compared to expected sex and age specific rates for the general population of Massachusetts over the same time. Similarly, Krolewski assembled statistics from 4 large diabetic clinics in Warsaw which confirmed a 2 times higher mortality for cardiovascular disease in diabetics compared with the general population of Warsaw.[31] The mortality statistics reported by Hayward from the Birmingham, England diabetic clinic also showed an excess of deaths compared to the population of West Midlands.[32]

Selective population studies have confirmed the excess risk of heart disease. Data from the Framingham Study have given us important insights into the incidence of coronary disease in an adult population followed for 20 years.[33] Six percent of the women and 8% of the men in this population of 1,529 subjects were diagnosed as diabetic. Overall the incidence of cardiovascular disease among diabetic men was roughly twice that among nondiabetic men. Among diabetic women the incidence of cardiovascular disease was almost 3 times that among nondiabetic women. In the Tecumseh Study the known diabetics were found to have at every age level 2 to 3 times more vascular disease than would have been expected from the population as a whole.[34]

Other approaches to obtaining data on cardiovascular morbidity include surveys of hospitalized or outpatient diabetic population and follow-up data.[35–40] These studies all reflect the high prevalence of both symptomatic and asymptomatic (Class I) coronary disease in selective diabetic populations.[40a]

Atherosclerotic cardiac disease continues to account for a majority of deaths in the Joslin Clinic population (Table 27–1). During the past decade cardiac disease accounted for 54.5% of all deaths. The persistence of this problem over the past 30 years is also shown. In contrast is the recent decline in heart disease mortality experienced nationwide. In the 1950s coronary heart disease mortality was still increasing, having been the leading cause of death in the United States for many years. By 1960 arteriosclerotic heart disease accounted for 29% of the total deaths.[41] In the early 1960s it began to plateau, and since 1968 there has been a greater than 20% decline in coronary heart disease mortality.[20] The explanation for this remains obscure, although modification of risk factors as well as improvements in medical care presumably contribute.[42]

In populations with a low overall prevalence of atherosclerosis, coronary artery disease in diabetics

is also reduced.[2,3] In Japan death was attributed to coronary heart disease in only 6% of a large series of post-mortem examination of diabetics.[43] The experience in Nigeria[44] and Central America[45] is similar. These reports strongly suggest the thesis that atherosclerotic disease in the diabetic is subject to the same environmental conditions as that in the nondiabetic and allow the conjecture that the high frequency of such disease in diabetics in certain countries is not an inevitable consequence of hyperglycemia.[46] Rather the diabetic appears to be particularly susceptible to the atherogenic factors operating in a population.

Sex. Relative freedom from significant coronary heart disease is well established in the nondiabetic female during the premenopausal years. Morphologic data are available from the large autopsy series of Clawson showing a male to female ratio of 8:1 among patients without hypertension.[47] Age matched data for the general population are even more striking. Oliver reports a male to female ratio of 16:1 under age 40, 7:1 between ages 40 and 49, falling with each decade to a ratio of 1:1 at age 70 or over.[48]

This decrease in risk enjoyed by younger women in the general population is lost in the diabetic patient. Clawson and Bell studied data obtained at autopsy in 50,000 subjects and found fatal coronary heart disease to be 3 times as frequent among diabetic as among nondiabetic males.[49] The excess of coronary deaths in diabetic women was particularly striking in the Framingham study.[50] Data confirming the reversal of the expected male/female ratio in the Joslin Clinic experience and elsewhere have been summarized.[51,52] In the large series of diabetic patients with acute myocardial infarction reported by Partamian and Bradley representing the Joslin Clinic experience, young premenopausal females as well as older women were affected more frequently than diabetic men.[52]

Severity. In addition to the autopsy studies reviewed above which have documented the increased severity of atherosclerotic coronary disease in diabetics seen at autopsy, there is now evidence that the diabetic patient seen for symptomatic coronary disease must already be considered a sicker patient than an otherwise similar nondiabetic individual. Dortimer compared 37 diabetic patients with 79 control subjects matched for sex, age, hypertension, hyperlipidemia, and smoking.[53] Diabetics had more diseased vessels, greater severity of disease in the involved segments of those vessels, and a higher incidence of multivessel disease. Similar findings were presented by Hamby[54] who found increased disease in persons with "chemical" as well as clinical diabetes, compared to the nondiabetic population. In that study, the extent of disease could not be related to the duration of symptoms. Whether such findings reflect a more aggressive disease pattern or a relative lack of early warning symptoms in the diabetic or both is a matter for speculation. In a study of the hearts of 316 diabetic residents of Rochester, Minnesota who died between 1945 and 1970, Waller, Palumbo, and Connolly[54a] found that the diabetic patients had a much greater extent of CAD than the 219 nondiabetic patients matched as to age, sex, and duration of heart disease. These workers emphasized that the diagnosis and treatment of CAD in patients with diabetes should be approached aggressively.

Age. Ischemic heart disease in the diabetic may be seen to involve both older patients with Type II, noninsulin-dependent diabetes in whom coronary atherosclerosis has been accelerated, and younger patients with Type I, insulin-dependent diabetes who have aggressive premature macrovascular, as well as microvascular complications. Increasing age is a recognized risk factor in both the diabetic and nondiabetic, and atherosclerotic heart disease complicates the course of adult onset diabetes with increasing frequency in the older age groups. Too often symptomatic coronary disease becomes the prominent clinical feature in the Type II diabetic diagnosed in the 6th to 7th decade of life. In such patients the date of onset of the diabetes is often uncertain, and "chemical" diabetes may have been present for years. This makes difficult a correlation between the duration of diabetes and the severity of atherosclerosis. Vigorita noted that although on the average diabetic patients had more coronary disease, including both more diffuse disease and more myocardial infarcts, progression of the atherosclerotic disease was unrelated to the duration or severity of known diabetes.[29a]

In contrast, the diabetic who becomes insulin dependent during his first few decades of life may pursue a course which after 20 or more years is dominated by the microvascular complications of diabetes leading to retinopathy, nephropathy, or neuropathy. Symptomatic coronary disease often develops in the 4th or even 3rd decade and frequently pursues a relentless course.

There is hope but no firm evidence that with excellent and continuous control of diabetes, sequelae in severe form may be postponed or prevented, although presently many such patients do not live beyond their mid-forties.

At the New England Deaconess Hospital where 20% of autopsies are on diabetic subjects, 11 of 12 subjects 35 years or less dying with acute myocardial infarction were diabetic.[55] Kessler noted excess deaths from coronary disease in each sex and nearly all groups age 35 and over. Neither cross-sectional analysis nor cohort analysis gave evidence of a substantial variation of risk with age.[30]

Data are not available regarding the prevalence of severe coronary disease in young diabetics without symptoms of cardiac or other vascular disease. However, silent high-grade coronary obstructive disease was found in more than one-third of a group of juvenile-onset diabetics with severe diabetic nephropathy (average age, 34 years and duration of diabetes, 21 years).[56] The likely occurrence of coronary heart disease among younger diabetic patients (age 20 to 40), female or male, with or without hypertension and/or hyperlipidemia, cannot be emphasized too strongly.

Risk Factors. Hypertension, hyperlipidemia, obesity, and smoking are among the widely accepted factors which increase the risk of atherosclerosis.[33,57–59] These factors are often operative in diabetics, particularly those with Type II diabetes, many of whom are overweight, hypertensive, and have elevated levels of serum cholesterol and triglycerides.[60] The generally higher mortality rate from coronary disease in diabetics can in part be explained by the increased interplay of multiple risk factors,[61,62] although diabetics appear to cope about as well with these risk factors as do nondiabetics.[33] Moreover, even after these risk factors are taken into account, there seems to be an unknown "diabetic factor" which is responsible for much of the higher incidence of cardiovascular complications.[63,64] This is especially true in women for whom diabetes is a much greater relative risk than in males.[33,52,64] The anatomic and clinical counterparts of this epidemiologic observation have not been clearly identified.

Hypertension. Hypertension is common in diabetics. Among diabetic employees of the Dupont Company, Pell and D'Alonzo reported a 54% higher prevalence of hypertension compared to age, sex, and employment matched nondiabetic controls.[61] Moreover the prevalence in diabetic women was higher than in men. In the Framingham Study the blood pressure of diabetics was significantly higher than in matched nondiabetics.[64] Similarly, in the Tecumseh Study, Epstein analyzed subgroups of the population by blood pressure levels and noted an increasing prevalence of diabetes in the quartiles with higher blood pressures.[60] Others have not been able to confirm this association of diabetes and hypertension.[46,62,65]

Elevated systolic blood pressure levels have been noted in diabetic children.[66] Fifty-four percent of juvenile diabetics at the Joslin Clinic who survived 35 years had hypertension associated with diabetic nephropathy.[67] Hypertension in adult onset Type II diabetes is seen under a variety of clinical circumstances including essential hypertension, atherosclerosis, renal artery disease, parenchymal renal disease or alterations of the renin angiotensin system. These aspects are discussed in detail in Chapter 28. The importance of even mild hypertension in contributing to coronary disease mortality has recently been documented in a randomized study of 10,940 hypertensives with diastolic blood pressures between 90 and 104 mm Hg.

Those receiving intensive medical treatment to bring the diastolic pressure to 90 mm Hg or less had a 17% lower mortality and a 26% reduction in coronary artery disease compared to controls.[68]

Lipids. A close link between glucose intolerance and blood triglyceride levels has long been observed.[69,70] Gross hyperlipidemia, mainly hypertriglyceridemia, frequently accompanies uncontrolled insulin-dependent diabetes. Lack of insulin is associated with underactivity of the enzyme lipoprotein lipase.[71] This enzyme is responsible for the hydrolysis of circulating triglycerides.

Diabetics of both sexes in the Framingham population had substantial and significant elevations of very low density lipoprotein (VLDL), the lipoprotein carrying primarily triglyceride.[72] Many investigators have reported elevated levels of triglyceride, cholesterol, or both in diabetics with atherosclerosis.[73–76] The higher incidence of myocardial infarction and mortality in patients with severe forms of diabetes has been related to high levels of both of these lipids.[77] However, a causal determination of the serum cholesterol reflects the risk of coronary disease as well as any of the blood lipid fractions.[78]

Risk of cardiovascular disease in the older age groups has been best related to high density lipoprotein (HDL), with which it relates inversely.[72,79–81] HDL may act to interfere with cellular uptake of cholesterol[82] and act as a "scavenger" lipoprotein, transporting cholesterol from blood vessels to the liver. Particularly in women, the association of diabetes and a low HDL cholesterol level is associated with an elevated risk.[83] However, HDL cholesterol has actually been higher in some middle age diabetic populations than in age and sex matched nondiabetic controls.[84]

Obesity. Many studies have associated Type II diabetes with obesity.[85] In turn, marked obesity may contribute as a major risk factor in the development of coronary artery disease. Keen et al. noted an excess of new complaints of angina in the most overweight in a population otherwise similar in respect to hypertension, smoking, and history of vascular disease.[86] Others have attributed excess risk in the obese to its association with hypertension[87] and elevated cholesterol[88], and generally obesity has not appeared as a separate special risk factor when epidemiologic data are assessed by multivariate analysis.[89]

In the diabetic population a similar lack of interaction between relative weight and cardiovascular risk has been found.[33,58] Diabetic women may be an exception.[83] However, even among women, the more important variables are diabetes and a low HDL cholesterol.[83]

Cigarettes. In 1964 the report of the Advisory Committee to the Surgeon General advised that smoking was a health hazard.[90] Despite the suggestion that the connection between coronary disease and smoking is an example of guilt by association,[91] current estimates suggest there are a quarter of a million smoking-related coronary deaths yearly.[92] Heavy smoking almost doubles the cardiovascular mortality under age 65 and the proportion of deaths that are sudden increases progressively. The National Pooling Project combined the prospective information from the Framingham, Albany, Chicago, and Western Collaborative studies and reported data on about 7,000 men.[93] Among those with hypertension and elevated cholesterol, cigarette smoking increased the risk of death 4-fold.

Oral Contraceptives. Oral contraceptives are associated with excess cardiovascular risk primarily from myocardial infarctions and cerebrovascular accidents in women over 35 years.[94] Dalen has recently reviewed the cardiovascular risk which, although small, is increased 4-fold as compared to that in women not taking such drugs.[95] Excess risk is seen primarily in older women and in the presence of other risk factors for premature coronary atherosclerosis, including diabetes.[96]

In addition, interaction may occur with other risk factors which are found in the diabetic. In a large prospective study, hypertension appeared in 4% of users of oral contraceptives compared to 1.5% of nonusers, a 2.7–fold increase.[97] Even nonhypertensives may experience progressive rises in blood pressure over a 4-year period, averaging 14.2 mm Hg systolic and 8.5 mm Hg diastolic compared to nonusers.[98] Lipid disturbances have also been attributed to the estrogenic component of the pill.[99] In Framingham, oral contraceptive users had a small increase in cholesterol (2.9%) but a substantial increase in triglyceride (37%), and VLDL.[100] Despite the possibility that oral contraceptives may act to increase atherosclerosis, the observation that excess risk disappears when oral contraceptives are discontinued suggest they may act primarily to precipitate symptomatic disease in patients with underlying atherosclerosis.[101] Use of alternate means of contraception seems preferable for the juvenile onset diabetic, particularly as she enters her 4th decade and if hypertension or lipid abnormalities are present.

Clinical Features of Coronary Artery Disease

Coronary artery disease both in diabetics and nondiabetics becomes clinically manifest as angina pectoris, myocardial infarction, congestive failure, arrhythmia, or sudden death. In others it may be asymptomatic and go undetected. Selected aspects pertinent to the diabetic are discussed below. The likelihood of a particular clinical manifestation may vary with the sex of the patient and possibly with the severity and control of the diabetes. The risk of cardiovascular disease is about the same for diabetic men and women, being essentially double that of the nondiabetic population.[1] However, the relative risk of congestive failure is twice as high for diabetic women as diabetic men, a risk nearly 4-fold that of the general population. Furthermore diabetic women are twice as likely as diabetic men to experience death from cardiovascular disease.[1]

Clinical recognition of coronary disease begins with an awareness of the marked frequency of this complication. Even young diabetics in their late 20s or 30s who have had diabetes for 20 years or more may develop symptomatic coronary atherosclerotic disease. Moreover the symptoms are often atypical. The clinician who is not constantly alert for the more subtle manifestations of ischemic disease or who excludes the possibility because of the patient's youthfulness, lack of other risk factors, or sex may unwittingly contribute to a critical delay in proper diagnosis and treatment.

When a patient gives a history of typical angina pectoris, anatomically severe coronary atherosclerotic disease will be confirmed in more than 90% of instances.[102] The diabetic may also present with vague and atypical chest, neck or upper extremity pain, or epigastric discomfort. A wide variety of symptoms may be "anginal equivalents." Fatigue, particularly when produced abruptly by exercise and relieved promptly with rest, may signal ischemic heart disease. Unexplained nausea, vomiting, hyperglycemia, or stroke may precede unstable coronary disease or myocardial infarction. In our experience, when angina pectoris occurs in the young patient with juvenile-onset diabetes, it is particularly likely to have atypical features.

Case Report. JZ, Case #51539, a 32-year-old housewife with diabetes of 20 years' duration, controlled on 34 units of NPH insulin, was hospitalized for pneumonia and responded to treatment with tetracycline. One week later she developed paroxysmal tachycardia for which she was digitalized intravenously. Subsequent changing T waves were attributed to digitalis. She remained tired and noted episodes of dull, mild, mid-chest pressure responding to rest only after about

20 minutes. Repeated electrocardiograms with patient off digoxin showed ST-T abnormalities in the inferolateral leads. The possibility of viral myocarditis was raised. Atypical unpredictable chest discomfort persisted and eventually coronary angiography documented severe diffuse coronary artery disease involving all three coronary systems, and a dilated hypokinetic left ventricle. Coronary bypass surgery was not advised because of severe distal coronary artery involvement. During the next 5 years she continued to have angina pectoris and required hospitalization twice for unstable symptoms. Otherwise she remained able to do light housework and take care of her children. Her angina occasionally was exertional, but frequently was not, and mild discomfort often persisted for several days. Variation in location, quality and intensity were recorded. Occasionally episodes of sudden and profound exertional fatigue overwhelmed her. More recently, she has developed progressive microvascular retinal disease and symptoms of autonomic gastropathy; however, the atypical anginal symptoms have diminished. Present medications include digitalis, nitrates, beta blocking agents and quinidine.

Comment. The diagnosis of coronary disease was not initially considered in this young premenopausal normotensive woman. Initial EKG changes were attributed to digoxin given for an arrhythmia. Her anginal syndrome included many atypical features and was associated with severe widespread coronary vascular obstruction documented angiographically (Fig. 27–1).

Conversely, atypical chest symptoms in a young Type I diabetic may not necessarily indicate obstructive coronary disease. Normal vessels in a 24-year-old juvenile onset diabetic (Fig. 27–2) contrast markedly with the diffuse lesions noted in Figure 27–1.

Myocardial Infarction. Patients with acute myocardial infarction may present with atypical features.[52,103] These include not only atypical pain, but nausea, vomiting, or congestive failure. Frequently changes in diabetic control provide an important warning, and the wise clinician will regard otherwise minor symptoms more closely when accompanied by increasing glycosuria or other evidence of hyperglycemia.

Pain. Bradley and Schonfeld[104] noted that 42% of diabetics compared with 6% of nondiabetics had no history of chest pain during acute infarction. However, the myocardial infarction was rarely truly "silent." Only 5% of the diabetics and none of the nondiabetics were entirely asymptomatic. Similarly during 18 years of medical follow-up of the Framingham population, 23% of electrocardiographically documented myocardial infarctions were discovered only by routine electrocardiogram.[105] Thirty-nine percent of the infarctions

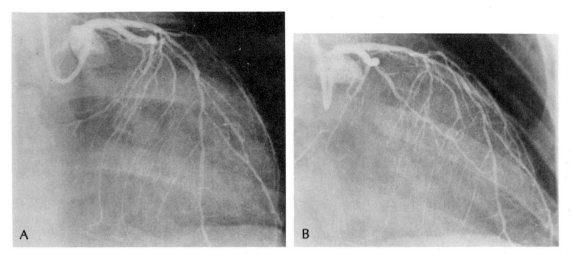

Fig. 27–1. A. Left Anterior Oblique (LAO) and B. Right Anterior Oblique (RAO) views of the left coronary system of 32-year-old female with juvenile-onset diabetes mellitus. Narrowing of major vessels is diffuse, and widespread narrowing of first and second order branches is present. Extensive collateral vasculature is seen.

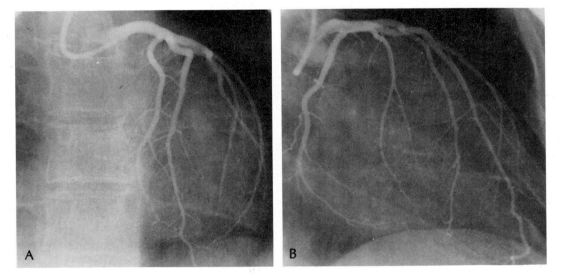

Fig. 27–2. A. Left Anterior Oblique (LAO) and B. Right Anterior Oblique (RAO) views of normal vessels in a 24-year-old juvenile diabetic.

were unrecognized clinically among the diabetic population compared with 22% in the nondiabetic population. Only half of these infarctions were judged truly silent and only 17% reported no interim illnesses or symptoms of any sort. The apparent increase of unrecognized infarcts among diabetics did not reach clinical significance, however.[105] These estimates of asymptomatic infarctions agree closely with those made in other studies.[106,107]

The presence or absence of chest pain may be an index of pain sensitivity. Patients with unrecognized myocardial infarction in the Framingham population had a strikingly low prevalence of angina before discovery of the infarct and a decreased

incidence of angina even after discovery of the infarct.[105] The mechanism of diminished pain may be related to diabetic autonomic neuropathy. Pathologic changes in nerve fibers consisting of beaded or spindle-shaped thickenings as well as fragmentation and diminution of fibers have been found in diabetics with painless infarcts but not in a control group.[108] Alternatively, the diffuse changes in small intramural myocardial blood vessels seen in some diabetic hearts may play a role.[109] It has also been reported that, despite their diabetes, subjects with painless infarcts visit their physicians less frequently for routine care.[105] This suggests that denial of illness may be a factor.

Regardless of its mechanism, the absence of typical chest pain in the patient with diabetes mellitus may result in a delay in treatment during the early crucial phases of myocardial infarction. Delay in recognizing an acute infarction may contribute to excess mortality before hospitalization or delay proper triage after the hospital is reached. Soler et al.[103] reported higher early mortality among patients with infarction who had no pain and were sent to the general medical floors rather than the Coronary Care Unit (CCU).

Metabolic Response to Myocardial Infarction. The myocardial metabolic response during acute myocardial infarction is the consequence of a non-uniform process, with areas of anoxic myocardium interspersed with adjacent islands of hypoxic or normally aerobic tissue. Opie has reviewed studies of myocardial glucose and fatty acid metabolism during myocardial infarction.[110] During anoxia, free fatty acids cannot be utilized for energy. Glycolysis is accelerated and lactate is produced instead of pyruvate. However, anaerobic energy production is not sufficient to provide for the needs of working muscle. Once cardiac glycogen has been consumed, total reliance for energy must depend on the provision of glucose in the extracellular fluid. Opie calculates that the maximum rates of glycolysis which could be achieved in infarcting myocardium by glucose and insulin administration could contribute significantly to energy needs.[110] Anoxia itself accelerates glycolysis even in the severely diabetic heart in the absence of added insulin.[110a]

During anoxia, free fatty acid uptake by the myocardium falls markedly and intracellular accumulation occurs.[111] Free fatty acid may be toxic to the myocardium, causing both arrhythmias and depressed contractility,[112] although such findings have not been confirmed by all observers.[113]

The systemic metabolic response to myocardial infarction is determined mainly by the plasma catecholamine concentration in response to stress.[114] Norepinephrine released from post-ganglionic nerve endings and tissue stores, and epinephrine released from the adrenal medulla are present in high concentrations in plasma during the first 24 hours; the levels are related to the severity of the infarct.[115,116] Norepinephrine activates the adenyl cyclase system in adipose tissue, leading to hydrolysis of stored triglycerides and release of free fatty acids and glycerol into the circulation.[117] Epinephrine stimulates glycogenolysis in liver and muscle, raising blood glucose levels. It also suppresses beta cell activity in the pancreas.[118] Reduction of insulin secretion has been documented after myocardial infarction both after intravenous glucose loading[119] and by an intravenous tolbutamide test.[120] Patients with shock may have virtually absent insulin secretion. These changes may result in marked hyperglycemia. Hypoinsulinemia cannot always be implicated in hyperglycemic patients, however, since elevated immunoreactive insulin levels may be found.[121] Nevertheless, insulin responses may be blunted and inappropriately low for the degree of hyperglycemia present.[122] Cortisol secretion,[123] glucagon levels,[124,125] and plasma growth hormone levels[126] are also increased and may contribute to elevations of blood glucose. These responses are similar to those occurring with surgical stress[127] and a variety of clinical situations combining starvation and stress.[127a]

Blood Glucose and Myocardial Infarction. Glucose intolerance has been noted in a high percentage of those with angiographically documented coronary artery disease in the absence of acute infarction.[128] Hyperglycemia is also a striking early feature of response to stress, as noted in the previous section. Pearson compared patients with recent myocardial infarction to those with recent trauma producing bone injury and found abnormal intravenous glucose tolerance tests in 75.5% of cardiac patients and 68% of bone trauma patients in the first few days.[129] Abnormal carbohydrate metabolism is magnified after the stress of acute infarction and has been reported in the majority of instances.[130,131] The often complex interrelationships responsible for hyperglycemia during the acute phase of myocardial infarction have been discussed by Prakash and Chhablani.[121] Hyperglycemia not related to acute stress has also been encountered in the setting of noncoronary heart disease with a low cardiac output and an abnormally low insulin response.[132,133] Some cardiac patients may also show evidence of increased insulin resistance which additionally contributes to hyperglycemia.[134]

Carbohydrate intolerance often persists well beyond 3 days when catecholamine levels have returned to normal; and when cortisol, glucagon, and growth hormone are no longer elevated. Ravid, Berkowicz and Sohar reported the persistence of carbohydrate abnormalities in 169 nondiabetic patients studied during the first 72 hours after acute infarction. Elevated fasting blood glucose levels were found in 48% and abnormal oral glucose tolerance tests in 73%. At 6 years, 80% of the 30 survivors with an initially elevated fasting blood glucose had either latent or overt diabetes. Of those with only an initially abnormal 2-hour blood glucose, 37% continued to show abnormal values.[135] Measurement of Hb_{A1} may help to separate hyperglycemia due to stress from that due to diabetes mellitus.[135a,135b]

Mortality after Myocardial Infarction. The increased risk faced by the diabetic of death from myocardial infarction is a combination both of the greater prevalence of coronary artery disease and for an increased case fatality rate. Nearly all investigators have reported a higher hospital mortality (Table 27–2). Several recent reports have indicated a fatality twice that of age- and sex-matched nondiabetic controls,[103,136–138] although an increase in mortality has not been found by all.[139]

Excess risk is present for both sexes and all ages, although the greatest excess appears among younger patients[52,136] and among women, whose mortality exceeds that of diabetic men.[51,103,138] More than two-thirds of diabetics less than 40 years old with acute myocardial infarction reported in the study of Partamian and Bradley, died.[52] Often such young juvenile-onset diabetic patients have extensive coronary macrovascular disease, as well as severe microvascular disease with nephropathy. Angiographically, their vessels may take on a "cobweb" appearance reflecting the marked diffuse reduction in vascular lumen (Fig. 27–1). It seems probable that the aggressive nature of the vascular disease which resulted in its premature appearance is also responsible for its often fatal consequence. Among older Type II diabetic patients, anatomic coronary disease is also more severe than among controls[53,54] and presumably contributes to the less favorable outcome. Tansey et al. have pointed out that the high mortality among such diabetics is largely accounted for by obese women whose mortality (43%) was twice that of other diabetics and 3 times that of nondiabetics (14%).[138] These patients had a higher incidence of congestive failure; as would be expected, patients with evidence of more profound myocardial damage were those with the highest mortality. In the Swedish Cooperative CCU study of 2,008 patients with acute myocardial infarction, 41% of the diabetics had a history of congestive failure, significantly higher than nondiabetics.[137] The diabetic with anterior infarction may be at particularly high risk.[137a] Other consequences of profound myocar-

Table 27–2. Acute Myocardial Infarction—Hospital Mortality

Author (Year)	Ref. (#)	Number of Patients	Mortality %	
			Diabetic	Nondiabetic
Bradley (1965)	(52)	258	38	
Soler (1975)	(103)	285	39.7	18
Harrower (1976)	(141)	94	24	19
Lichstein (1976)	(142)	265	24	
Czyzyk (1980)	(136)	154	36	18

dial damage including shock, myocardial rupture, and a history of multiple myocardial infarctions are also more common.[52] Not all studies agree that left ventricular tree wall rupture, reported in as many as 9% of diabetics, is increased.[28a] Excess hypertension and possibly more renal and widespread vascular disease may contribute.

Poor diabetic control is also associated with a high mortality. Bradley and Bryfogle reported 85% mortality in myocardial infarction complicated by ketoacidosis.[51] Soler et al. similarly noted 87% mortality in those with blood glucose values greater than 400 mg/dl on admission.[103] Hyperglycemia marked to this degree partly reflects the severity of the infarction.

Diabetics well controlled by medication and those on diet alone have a hospital mortality comparable to nondiabetics.[140,141] Soler et al. suggested that diabetics on oral agents have a higher mortality than those on insulin.[140] This observation could not be confirmed by Harrower and Clarke[141] or Lichstein et al.[142] who found no significant difference in mortality. Czyzyk et al. reported increased risk, particularly among those on insulin.[136]

Several reports suggest that primary ventricular fibrillation (ventricular fibrillation not precipitated by profound myocardial impairment) may be increased in the diabetic (Table 27–3). Soler et al. reported that primary ventricular fibrillation occurred in 12% of his patients on oral agents versus 3 and 7% on insulin or diet alone.[140] In a combined study from 3 hospitals of 265 patients with diabetes mellitus and acute myocardial infarction, this potentially lethal arrhythmia was twice as frequent in those on oral drugs as in those on diet alone.[142] Ten of 151 patients on oral agents developed ventricular fibrillation, whereas only 2 of 54 on insulin did so; the numbers were too small to achieve statistical significance.

Whether there is a subpopulation of diabetics who are unusually likely to develop primary ventricular fibrillation during the hospital phase of their acute myocardial infarct is unclear. However, the possibility that ventricular fibrillation may develop late, after transfer from the Coronary Care Unit, is deserving of comment (Table 27–3). In the above studies more than one-third of all primary ventricular fibrillation occurred after transfer from the CCU and was almost universally fatal. This group contributes significantly to the late mortality as well as the overall mortality, and represents a failure of hospital care for a potentially highly salvageable population. In contrast, survivors of infarction evaluated by 24-hour EKG monitor prior to discharge from the hospital were found to have a similar prevalence of ventricular ectopy, including

Table 27–3. Incidence of Primary Ventricular Fibrillation in Diabetics with Acute Myocardial Infarction: Percent of Episodes Occurring After Day Four (and Outcome)

Author	Ref. (#)	Patients No.	Total VF No.	Total VF %	Late VT (% of total)	Mortality of Late VF	Mortality of (%)
Harrower	(141)	94	10	(9.4)	5 (50)	5	(100)
Soler	(140)	184	15	(8.2)	5 (33)	5	(100)
Lichstein	(142)	265	14	(5.3)	11 (79)	10	(91)

ventricular tachycardia, when compared to non-diabetics.[142a]

Other arrhythmias and conduction disturbances are also more common in the diabetic in the setting of acute myocardial infarction and are associated with the increased incidence of congestive failure. In the Swedish Cooperative Study, both atrial fibrillation and left bundle branch block were more common.[137] Czyzyk et al. reported that the prognosis for diabetics with arrhythmias or disorders of conduction were 3 times worse than for the non-diabetic group irrespective of hemodynamic complications.[136]

A consecutive series of Joslin Clinic diabetic patients hospitalized at the New England Deaconess Hospital during 1979–1980 with acute myocardial infarction emphasizes the particularly adverse experience of diabetic women (Table 27–4). Female mortality was 37%, 3-fold that of diabetic males. In part, this could be attributed to a somewhat older female population (67.6 years) compared to the male group (58.4 years). Women also had more congestive heart failure. More than one-half of all women had congestive heart failure compared to 29% of the men, despite the apparent similarity of the infarct location and type, and of the years of diabetes. Ten of the 16 women who developed congestive heart failure died and 6 of these were in cardiogenic shock.

The overall mortality (23%) did not vary with either the location or type (transmural vs subendocardial) of infarct. Of those who died 87% had CHF (Killip, Class III or IV) compared to 27% of the survivors. Left bundle branch block was associated with CHF and shock. Of those with left bundle branch block 4 of 6 died, whereas only 1 of 7 with right bundle branch block died.

This experience and those of others suggest that significant further reduction in Coronary Care Unit mortality is likely only when efforts to preserve and improve myocardial function are successful. Further studies are needed to provide confirmation of excess ventricular dysfunction in women with long-standing diabetes in the setting of acute myocardial infarction.

Hospital Treatment. Management of the acute and chronic phases of myocardial infarction is in most respects identical to that in the nondiabetic. Detailed discussion is beyond the scope of this chapter. Diabetic control is worth emphasizing. Most diabetics should be placed on insulin during the early stages for prompt control of the blood sugar in the range of 150 to 200 mg/dl, since the energy requirement of anaerobic tissue is supplied by circulating glucose when myocardial glycogen is depleted. Severe hyperglycemia is to be avoided and may be associated with hemodynamic instability. Adverse hemodynamic changes may also accompany insulin administration. Hypotension and tachycardia have occurred, particularly in association with autonomic neuropathy.[143,144] Insulin infusion can be used for effective control, with careful monitoring of serum potassium as well as glucose.[144a] Conversely, hypoglycemia not only deprives the ischemic cell of required substrate but also may provoke further sympathoadrenal discharge, increasing myocardial damage and provoking arrhythmias.[145,146] Experimental evidence which suggests that an infusion of glucose-insulin-potassium may have a protective effect against my-

Table 27–4. Acute Myocardial Infarction After Prolonged Diabetes Mellitus, Male vs. Female. (Joslin Clinic Experience at the New England Deaconess Hospital, 1979–1980).

	No.	(%)	Age	Diabetes (Yrs.)	Type T	Type SE	Location A	Location P	CHF	(%)	Mortality	(%)
Male	34	(53)	58.4	20.1	27	7	15	13	10	(29)	4	(12)
Female	30	(47)	67.6	17.8	20	10	16	5	16	(53)	11	(37)
Total	64	(100)	62.1	19.1	47	17	31	18	26	(41)	15	(23)

T = transmural
SE = subendocardial
A = anterior, anteroseptal, anterolateral
P = posterior, inferior
CHF = Killip Class III or IV.

ocardial ischemia[147] has not yet led to routine clinical application. In fact, clinical verification of the efficacy of the many varied exciting research approaches to limiting infarct size by metabolic or pharmacological interventions still lies ahead. Recent efforts acutely to restore coronary blood flow, using intracoronary or intravenous streptokinase, often with mechanical recanalization within a few hours of infarction, have increased the possibility that myocardium can be salvaged.

Pending additional confirmation of the unusual frequency of ventricular fibrillation and late death, particular attention to antiarrhythmic control seems warranted. Prophylactic use of lidocaine is generally indicated initially. The duration of monitoring for warning arrhythmias will need to be individually determined. It is our practice to continue ambulatory monitoring in a "stepdown unit" after discharge from the CCU. It should be recalled that high-grade, dangerous yet asymptomatic, ventricular arrhythmias may occur at the time of hospital discharge in patients whose ectopy initially seemed well controlled[148]. Congestive failure, left bundle branch block and atrial fibrillation may all indicate particularly high risk patients who require precise control of their hemodynamic status and whose recovery phase may be prolonged.

For many diabetics whose myocardial infarctions are complicated by severe pump failure, optimal cardiac care may require central hemodynamic monitoring. Occasionally other interventions such as intraaortic balloon pumping, pacemakers or treatment of respiratory, renal, or nutritional failure or infection may further complicate management. In these instances, adjustment of parenteral medication including vasodilators, vasopressors, diuretics, antiarrhythmics, and opiates is required to optimize left ventricular performance. By adjusting the left ventricular pressure and cardiac index, coronary flow and tissue perfusion are maintained.

In view of frequent re-infarction, high subsequent mortality during recurrence, and the all too frequent complication of sudden death,[50,64,103] careful evaluation is particularly important prior to discharge for residual highly jeopardized areas of myocardium and for potentially lethal arrhythmias.

Recent large scale clinical trials of beta blocking agents appear to confirm the benefit of long-term beta blockade in reducing mortality in post-infarct patients.[149a,149c] Specific information relating to the subgroup of diabetic patients is not yet available. Acute-phase trials of beta-blocking agents given during the initial hours of acute myocardial infarction are presently being conducted.[149b] Results of several studies suggest a reduction of mortality and morbidity in selected patients.[149c,149d]

Selected Aspects of Angina Management

Diabetes Control. Many diabetics will need to confront a previously cavalier attitude toward their frequently uncontrolled hyperglycemia and excess caloric intake. Metabolic instability is all too often partner to a pattern of increasing angina. Conversely, an improvement in angina is often associated with better diabetes control. Proper cardiac treatment includes a wide range of general and pharmacologic interventions including treatment of the metabolic disturbance; and benefit may be difficult to attribute specifically to carbohydrate restriction, glucose-lowering agents, or changes in life style or activity. The occasional patient with a normal vascular tree after many years of well controlled diabetes hints that the possibilities of prevention may lie partially with optimal metabolic control.

The report that oral agent therapy may increase cardiovascular mortality has stimulated considerable controversy. The University Group Diabetes Study found an increased cardiovascular mortality in diabetic patients on oral antidiabetic agents.[150a,150b] This study prompted the Food and Drug Administration to issue warnings regarding these agents.[151] However, its conclusions have not been universally accepted.[152,153,153a] For further discussion, see Chapter 21.

Risk Factor Management. Epidemiologic evidence continues to give strong support to risk factor intervention to combat atherosclerosis, a strategy which appears particularly appropriate in the diabetic.[41a,154] Aspects of hypertension, lipid abnormalities, obesity, and diet and their management are discussed in Chapters 28, 11, 18, and 17. Alternatives to oral contraception should be sought, particularly for diabetics in their mid or late 30s or those with hypertension, lipid disturbance or clinical heart disease. Cigarette smoking increases an already high risk. The diabetic male with hypertension and lipid disturbances who insists on smoking is flirting with disaster. The risk of cardiovascular disease increases by elevenfold in the presence of hypertension, an elevated serum cholesterol, and cigarette use compared to risk in the absence of these factors.[154a] In general, the physician managing a diabetic patient should keep in mind the strong possibility of eventual coronary disease, and begin risk factor intervention even in the absence of clinical symptoms. Alertness to these aspects ensures that the diabetic patient broadens his knowledge beyond immediate diabetic care and includes the variety of interventions which may help to reduce future atherogenic complications.

Pharmacologic Agents. The rationale, dose and

response to medication given for the control of angina pectoris are similar in the diabetic and non-diabetic. Nitroglycerin, generally accompanied by a beta blocking agent and/or a calcium blocking agent, remains central to most treatment plans whether or not other agents are added. Brief comments follow on particular features to consider in diabetic patients.

Nitrate Therapy. Nitrates remain the cornerstone of angina therapy in the diabetic, as in the nondiabetic. Angina is the result of imbalance between myocardial oxygen supply and demand, and nitrates produce hemodynamic changes which result in reduction of myocardial oxygen consumption. Nitrates relax vascular smooth muscle.[155] This action is particularly marked in the venous capacitance bed and results in peripheral venous pooling. The cardiac consequences are a decrease in preload and a consequent reduction in cardiac output. The arteriolar resistance bed is also dilated, augmenting a fall in blood pressure and resultant reflex tachycardia.

The induced hypotension may be of special concern to diabetics whose cardiovascular reflexes are impaired through the development of autonomic neuropathy.[156] The clinical consequences may be an increase in coronary ischemia or a reduction in cerebral blood flow leading to cerebrovascular symptoms and syncope. Orthostatic instability should be a warning that cardiovascular reflexes are impaired. However, postural hypotension often is not present in those who have autonomic impairment and cannot be relied upon as a predictor of potential nitrate hypotension. Therefore, nitrate should be started under close supervision, although it will usually be well tolerated in full dosage.

Beta Blocking Agents. Beta blocking agents have assumed an important role in angina control and despite potential problems in diabetics, serious problems usually can be circumvented. Beta blockers reduce myocardial oxygen consumption by reducing all its major determinants: rate, contractility and blood pressure (a major component of wall tension).[157] Potentially detrimental effects including an increase in intracardiac volume,[158] increased coronary resistance,[159] and decreased coronary blood flow[160] do not outweigh this effect. Perfusion of the subendocardium is maintained or increased[161] and clinically important decreases in cardiac performance are generally avoided. Beta blocking agents also reduce platelet aggregation.[162,162a] Platelet function is abnormal in diabetes (see Chapters 10 and 37). The role of platelet aggregates in diabetic small vessel disease of the heart and in coronary atherosclerosis is under study.

Recommended doses are determined primarily by the symptomatic response. Inhibition of exercise tachycardia may be a helpful guide, with reductions of 15 to 30% being achievable.[162b] Reduction in resting rate, particularly in the diabetic with autonomic neuropathy, may be unreliable in the author's experience. The magnitude of dose effect depends importantly on the prevalent sympathetic tone,[163] an important consideration particularly in instances of myocardial failure associated with myocardial catecholamine depletion. There is a widespread individual variation in plasma levels from equal oral doses.[163]

At least two groups of beta-adrenoreceptor sites have been identified: B1 receptors which can be blocked by cardioselective beta-blocking agents, and B2 receptors, which cannot.[163a] B1 receptors generally mediate the effect of the neuronally released transmitter, norepinephrine, whereas B2 receptors generally respond to the hormone, epinephrine. B1 receptors affect cardiac stimulation, renin release, and lipolysis; B2 receptors affect vasodilation, glycogenolysis, and bronchodilation. Cardioselective beta-blocking agents have therefore been regarded as vascular-sparing, energy-sparing, and bronchosparing. However, no clinical studies suggest that any one of the many beta-blocking agents has major advantages over the others in treating angina. In the diabetic, cardioselectivity may reduce certain side effects.

Propranolol, the prototype non-selective beta-blocker, can be associated with hypoglycemia, particularly in the insulin-dependent diabetic.[157,163] Propranolol interferes with the sympathetic stimulation of glycogenolysis and the release of glucose from liver and muscle stores. Ordinarily this effect does not change the hypoglycemic response of insulin but hypoglycemia has been prolonged when mobilization of liver glycogen is inhibited by ketoacidosis, alpha blockade, starvation or other factors.[156,163]

Hypoglycemia may also provide a stimulus to unopposed alpha vasoconstriction during beta blockade. This can result in increases in diastolic and mean arterial blood pressure, and hypertensive crisis has been reported in a patient newly treated with propranolol, in conjunction with hypoglycemia.[164]

Of special concern has been the impaired recognition of hypoglycemia when it does occur. Beta blockade interferes with sympathetically mediated symptoms related to hypoglycemia. However, sweating and hunger sensations are not impaired and most diabetics continue to be able to recognize symptoms of impending hypoglycemia.

Propranolol may also inhibit insulin release. The possibility of further reducing insulin reserve in the Type II diabetic must be considered.[165] However, Hedstrand reported that there was no change in insulin secretion to a glucose challenge after 1 year on propranolol.[166]

In theory a selective beta 1 blocking agent would have advantages over nonselective beta blockage in the diabetic patient. In an insulin-dependent (Type I) diabetic who may be prone to hypoglycemic episodes, a beta 1 blocking agent may cause less inhibition of glycogen mobilization than the nonselective agent. In addition, the non-insulin-dependent (Type II) diabetic should secrete more endogenous insulin when given a selective beta 1 blocking agent since insulin secretion is under the control of beta 2 receptors and secretion is reduced with beta 2 blockade.

Other complications must be considered. Congestive failure can usually be managed with standard therapy, and a beta blocker continued at a lower dose. Atrioventricular block, possibly more common among diabetics, may also be aggravated. Claudication due to severe peripheral vascular disease may increase, and rarely non-selective beta blockade is associated with gangrene. Hyperosmolar nonketotic coma has been described in a patient on propranolol.[167] Respiratory, gastrointestinal, and neurologic complications are similar in the diabetic and in the nondiabetic. The abrupt discontinuation of beta blocking agents in patients with severe angina may precipitate increased angina or infarction.[159,168]

Despite the clinical evidence described, significant adverse effects are infrequently reported in diabetics taking propranolol. We continue to use a nonselective beta blocker in the insulin-resistant diabetic who has no severe peripheral vascular disease and in whom possible adverse effects are carefully sought. The drug appears to be more hazardous in the insulin-dependent diabetic with extensive atherosclerosis. Such individuals may be best treated with a beta 1 selective blocker, although even then, in clinical use, the caveats noted remain applicable.

Calcium Channel Blocking Agents. The calcium channel blocking agents are potent dilators of coronary and peripheral arteries. Their clinical efficacy in angina relates to their ability to decrease afterload, myocardial contractility, and heart rate and increase coronary blood flow. The individual blockers have different relative potencies on various cardiovascular functions, although all have negative chronotropic, ionotropic and dromotropic properties.[168a] The presently used agents, nifedipine, verapamil, and diltiazem are effective both in classic and variant angina.[168a] Nifedipine appears to increase fasting glucose concentrations and delay insulin response in normal individuals[168b] and in diabetics.[168c] Verapamil has been reported to have hyperglycemic effects unrelated to insulin and may

affect hepatic handling of glucose.[168d] These alterations have not prevented clinical use in diabetic patients.

Unstable Angina. Unstable angina is a particular challenge in the diabetic. The cardiac problem demands immediate concern and is often associated with severe vascular lesions elsewhere. Cerebrovascular, renal, and peripheral vascular disease as well as the metabolic disorder may at times require modification of the therapeutic regimen.

Approximately three-quarters of patients hospitalized with unstable angina will respond to standard measures.[169,170,171] Rest, sedation and the quiet of a supportive hospital environment as well as adjustments in short and longer acting nitrates together with a beta and/or a calcium channel blocking agent are helpful in most. Some may benefit from adjustment in hemodynamic status,[172] and treatment of arrhythmia, thyrotoxicosis or other contributory factors. The role of anticoagulation continues to be uncertain.

The more severely unstable group, particularly those with refractory hypertension or congestive failure, may respond to intravenous vasodilating drugs (especially nitroglycerin) aimed at systemic arteriolar and/or venodilation, although caution is required.[173] Similar effects may be approached mechanically via the intra-aortic balloon pump,[174] although the latter generally conveys only short-term benefits and cannot be used in patients with severe peripheral vascular disease. When effective, each of these measures has by differing mechanisms reduced the oxygen demands of the myocardium. Vasodilators may also augment coronary flow.

Approaches to improving blood supply have been based on attempts to reduce coronary spasm, to dissolve clots, to dilate constricted segments, and to bypass the narrowed or occluded segment.[175] Arterial spasm, of central importance in variant or Prinzmetal angina, may also play a role in atherosclerotic coronary disease.[176] However, the precise role of spasm in the pathogenesis of unstable angina remains unclear.

Recent studies have suggested the possibility of using fibrinolytic agents to dissolve clots forming in the coronary tree of those with impending infarction.[177] Early studies have documented dissolution of clot after infusing streptokinase directly into the coronary vessel. A direct approach by catheter to the coronary tree is also used in balloon angioplasty.[178] A highly select group of angina patients may be found to have focal subtotal occlusions with soft atheromata which can be compressed by balloon dilatation of the vessel resulting in restoration of blood flow. Although the indications and limitations of this procedure have not been fully defined, it is clear that many individuals with complete occlusions or with distal disease will not be candidates. Surgical bypass procedures are advised for an increasing number of patients but generally do not need to be performed on an urgent basis.[179]

Coronary Angiography

Coronary angiography is indicated in all individuals for whom these direct techniques of augmenting coronary flow are contemplated.[180] Diabetes is not considered a contraindication to coronary surgery and even after many years of insulin-dependent diabetes, some patients may still be anatomically excellent candidates for surgery. One Joslin patient who has required insulin for diabetes of 43 years' duration had suitable anatomy for bypass grafting and the grafts were widely patent when restudied 3 years later.[181]

Angiography is also occasionally required to establish a diagnosis, particularly when symptoms are atypical and other laboratory tests equivocal. The association of many years of diabetes and suggestive, though atypical, chest pain does not automatically imply coronary disease. One of our teaching films of normal coronary anatomy was obtained from a woman who has been a diabetic for 41 years.

Coronary angiography is generally well tolerated by the diabetic patient, and cardiovascular risks and complications are those found in nondiabetics with similar disease.[182] Insulin requirements must be adjusted on the day of angiography, generally by giving half the usual dose prior to the study and the remainder thereafter. The presence of peripheral vascular disease may dictate the route employed for catheterization. The hazard of iodinated contrast media in the presence of renal failure is well known,[183] and when the creatinine clearance is reduced, the volume of contrast media must be strictly limited, hypotension avoided, and hydration and urinary output maintained. Patients with severe chronic renal failure should be dialyzed as soon as possible after the angiographic procedure is completed, and their insulin dose reduced to avoid hypoglycemia.[184]

Angiographic criteria for operability have been arbitrarily defined as (1) greater than 70% reduction in lumen diameter of a major proximal coronary artery; (2) a patent coronary artery distal to the obstruction with a diameter greater than 1.5 mm; and (3) acceptable left ventricular performance (ejection fraction greater than 30%, left ventricular end diastolic volume less than 125 ml/m²).[185]

Coronary angiography is generally performed during hospitalization in the 15 to 20% of patients with refractory symptoms in the anticipation that surgery will be required for relief, and with the knowledge that the 1-year mortality in such patients on medical treatment may approach 43%.[170] In the majority who respond to therapy, as well as for other patients with chronic coronary disease, angiography provides an important basis for therapeutic and prognostic evaluation.

Understandably, prognosis appears to depend on the amount of jeopardized myocardial tissue, as well as the remaining ventricular function, reflecting the amount of damage already done.[186] Left main coronary artery obstruction has been found in 4 to 20% of individuals and has an extremely poor prognosis. Bypass surgery improves survival in this subgroup.[187] There is increasing evidence that bypass surgery performed by the most experienced groups improves the prognosis of patients with severe three-vessel disease and with certain types of two-vessel disease.[188] Such claims remain controversial and many such patients are offered surgery only if intractable symptoms are not effectively managed by alternative methods.[189] A variety of factors in addition to the anatomic findings dictate the course of action, including the wishes of the patient, the philosophy of the clinician, other laboratory evidence of myocardial ischemia and functional deficit, and the experience and results of the surgical team.

Approximately 10% of patients are found to have no fixed obstructive lesions. They can be reassured that their long-term prognosis is excellent.[190] In addition, 10 to 20% of patients are inoperable because of diffuse distal vessel disease or diffuse myocardial scar. In our experience the subgroup of juvenile-onset diabetics who present with symptomatic coronary disease in their early 30s or 40s after 20 or more years of diabetes are more likely to have inoperable disease than these figures imply. A surgical approach has been possible in less than 50% of outpatients in this category.

Surgical Management

Restoration of blood flow to ischemic myocardium is now possible in most patients. Over 90% of initially satisfactory grafts remain patent at 1 year, and the operative morbidity, particularly that from intraoperative myocardial infarction, is reported in recent studies to be approximately 6% or less. The operative mortality has been reduced to 1% or less for all but the most unstable and poorest risk category of patients.[188] These overall figures do not distinguish between diabetics and nondiabetics.

When total revascularization is possible and all narrowed vessels are bypassed with widely patent grafts, no residual laboratory evidence of ischemia is present postoperatively and ischemic pain disappears. Even in patients with residual ischemic damage and incomplete revascularization, substantial symptomatic benefit is the rule. A marked decrease or absence of angina is recorded in 70 to 90% of patients postoperatively.[189]

We now offer surgery to patients with unstable angina who remain symptomatic despite appropriate hospital management. For the majority who initially respond to medical therapy, for those who have chronic stable angina, and for those whose coronary disease has resulted in myocardial infarction without angina pectoris, consideration for surgery is individualized. Many patients with angina will eventually develop intolerable symptoms. Thirty percent of those randomly selected for medical therapy in a recent prospective trial of unstable angina eventually elected surgical treatment.[191] Anatomic considerations including the localization and severity of coronary lesions, and the amount of jeopardized myocardium may provide sufficient reason for operation in other patients whose prognosis can thereby be improved. Survival for large groups of patients treated surgically now approaches that of the general population.

Follow-up studies show that 60% or more of patients are still markedly improved after 5 years.[192] Disease may be expected to progess in the native circulation[193] and further attrition in graft patency is to be expected. Until an understanding of ways to prevent atherosclerosis is achieved, surgery will continue to be palliative rather than curative. Long-term follow-up of selected populations may be expected to show that palliation for those with the most aggressive varieties of atherosclerosis, such as Type I juvenile onset diabetics, may be of shorter duration.

Most Joslin Clinic patients undergoing bypass surgery are adult onset diabetics. Coronary surgery has also been effective in the smaller group of cardiac patients whose diabetes started in the second decade of life and was present 20 or 30 years later with severe ravages of microvascular disease. Thirteen Joslin Clinic patients with juvenile onset diabetes for an average of 30 years when they came to coronary artery bypass grafting at an average age of 44.[193a] Twelve had class IV angina despite maximal nitrate and beta blocking therapy. Retinopathy was present in 85%, neuropathy in 69%, peripheral vascular disease in 38%, and nephropathy in 15%. Surgery was possible despite the prolonged duration of diabetes and the severe microvascular complications. There was no operative mortality and at an average 6 year follow-up, 11 of 13 continued to have marked symptomatic improvement. One died of myocardial infarction, although at autopsy the graft remained patent.

Coronary disease, particularly persistent angina pectoris, contributes importantly to maternal mortality in the diabetic (see Chapter 33).

As shown in the case report below, a successful coronary artery bypass graft may enable a patient to undergo pregnancy successfully.

Case Report: CR, Case #44599, a 28-year-old social worker with diabetes of 22 years' duration on 8 units of clear and 34 units of NPH insulin, was hospitalized in 1972 after 1 week of severe classical angina pectoris and dyspnea. She was not obese and blood pressure was 112/76. There were no cardiac abnormalites on examination. She did have microaneurysms in the right fundus, but no proteinuria or neuropathy. Cholesterol, triglyceride, and resting electrocardiogram were all normal. Subsequent coronary angiography showed marked diffuse narrowing in the proximal one-third of the left anterior descending coronary artery. The left ventriculogram was normal. Symptoms persisted, progressing despite medical therapy, and 3 weeks later she underwent surgical interposition of a vein graft from the proximal aorta to the left anterior descending coronary artery by Dr. Wilford B. Neptune. Seven months later she became pregnant. She had no cardiac complications, and delivered a full-term normal boy 16 months after surgery. Two years later repeat angiography showed a patent graft, although disease had progressed in the mid and distal portions of the left anterior descending coronary artery, and the vessel was totally obstructed proximal to the graft insertion. Minimal nonobstructive irregularities were also noted in the right coronary artery. She experienced several episodes of transient exertional chest pain and underwent abortion of a 10-week fetus and tubal ligation. During the subsequent 8 years despite documented progression of disease in coronary circulation, she has been free of angina, is presently active as a housewife and mother of a first grade child, and enjoys political activities and social work.

We apply the same considerations toward evaluating the diabetic patient for coronary bypass surgery as we do for the nondiabetic patient. In general diabetic patients have a slightly higher risk for coronary artery bypass surgery than nondiabetic patients, probably because of increased coronary disease as well as vascular disease elsewhere.[194] Salomon et al. reported a 12-year experience with 3707 patients, including 162 diabetics treated with insulin and 250 diabetics on diet only or oral agents. Diabetics had more hypertension, ventricular hypertrophy, diffuse disease, and grafts per patient. Perioperative mortality was 5.1% for non-insulin-dependent diabetics and 4.5% for insulin-dependent diabetics compared to 2.5% in nondiabetics. Total hospital days were greater and ten-year survival less.[194a] Johnson noted a similar increase in mortality.[194b]

Several days of preoperative preparation are required to be certain of appropriate metabolic control and proper insulin treatment. Generally half the usual dose of long-acting insulin is given pre-operatively on the day of surgery and the remainder given in the recovery room. Supplemental increments of regular insulin are given subcutaneously in order to keep the blood glucose below 250 mg/dl on the night of surgery. Alternatively insulin can be delivered throughout surgery and for the first 24 hour postoperative period by insulin pump, with close monitoring for maintenance of blood glucose levels. Insulin infusion rates may range from 2 to 30 units/hour. Blood glucose is monitored every 2–4 hours or more during rewarming, transfusion, and ionotropic therapy.[194c] At least 150 g/day of glucose is given intravenously to suppress starvation ketosis.

CONGESTIVE HEART FAILURE

Epidemiologic studies suggest a marked increase in the incidence of congestive failure in diabetics. Diabetic males aged 45 to 74 who were followed over 18 years in the Framingham Study were twice as likely to develop congestive failure as their non-diabetic cohorts.[195] Even more remarkable was a 5-fold increase in congestive failure among diabetic women. The increased risk was limited to the 40% of all diabetics who required insulin and was not attributed either to known coronary disease or to the risk factors of blood pressure, cholesterol, or relative weight. This striking epidemiologic observation suggests that the clinician might expect to see large numbers of diabetic women presenting with, and dying of, congestive heart failure of uncertain etiology. However, it is more usual for an etiologic diagnosis to be established. These observations do indicate that the female diabetic may pay a disproportionate price in myocardial dysfunction no matter what the underlying diagnosis.

Many patients with coronary artery disease eventually develop congestive failure. Severe myocardial dysfunction may be the first evidence of underlying coronary disease even in patients who have never had chest pain or EKG evidence of ischemia.[196,197] The designation "ischemic cardiomyopathy" has been applied to such patients. However, this term inappropriately suggests a primary myopathic origin. Alternatively, myocardial disease due to diabetes has been suggested as underlying some of the congestive failure. This is discussed in a later section. Cardiomyopathy and coronary disease may coexist but their relative contributions to congestive symptoms in an individual patient are difficult to assess.[198]

Because diabetes is common, diabetics encounter many other forms of heart failure. Hypertensive heart disease with congestive heart failure is seen especially in the setting of obesity and renal disease. Valvular heart disease, although not ob-

viously increased in frequency in the diabetic, occurs often enough to consider this cause in any person with heart failure of obscure etiology. Less common causes to be excluded include alcoholic and hypertrophic cardiomyopathy, congenital heart disease, thyroid disorders, pericardial disease, hemochromatosis, a host of infiltrative disorders, and the myocarditides.

The bedside diagnosis of cardiac decompensaion in the diabetic may be difficult under several circumstances. Myocardial failure may be missed, particularly when due to transient ischemia. Acute ischemia is associated with poor diastolic compliance; and marked increases in end diastolic pressure may occur abruptly, resulting in pulmonary edema in the absence of any cardiac dilatation. Type I diabetics with severe diffuse macrovascular coronary disease may maintain a normal heart size by chest x-ray in the presence of acute severe congestive failure. Occasionally the proper diagnosis of congestive failure due to coronary disease may not be recognized because of the nearly normal heart size. This "small stiff heart syndrome" may be particularly common in diabetics.[199,200] With therapy, echocardiographic evidence of left ventricular dysfunction may entirely disappear in such instances, raising additional doubt about the proper diagnosis of ischemic cardiac failure.

Myocardial failure may be prematurely diagnosed in diabetics with chronic renal failure who are hypertensive. Such patients may have a marked left ventricular impulse, gallop sounds, x-ray findings of marked cardiomegaly and pulmonary congestion, and laboratory evidence of anemia. The clinical appearance may resemble well advanced congestive failure, but may instead reflect a markedly elevated cardiac output and a hyperdynamic circulation relating to volume overload and anemia.[201]

In a study of myocardial function in azotemic diabetics, we noted normal rest and exercise left ventricular end diastolic pressures, normal left ventricular end diastolic volumes, and normal or elevated ejection fractions in 7 patients. The mean cardiac index was 6 liters/min./m^2. Despite this normal ventricular function, 5 of the 7 had an S$_3$ gallop and these had cardiomegaly on physical examination. Two had x-ray evidence of congestive failure. The coexistence of chronic volume overload and severe anemia was associated with a hyperdynamic circulation and elevated cardiac output in these patients, who were all initially suspected to have important myocardial dysfuntion (Table 27–5).

Proper control of diabetes is important in the management of congestive failure. It has been pointed out that high blood sugars contribute to

Table 27–5. Clinical Findings Suggesting Myocardial Disease in Azotemic Patients With Normal Ventricular Function*

Clinical Findings	No.
Left ventricular impulse	5
Cardiomegaly	3
S₃/S₄	3/6
Xray CHF	2

Hemodynamic Data	
Left ventricular end diastolic pressure (mm/Hg)	
Rest	10
Exercise	12
Left ventricular end diastolic volume (ml/m²)	85
Stroke volume (ml/beat)	111
Cardiac index (liters/min/m²)	6
Ejection fraction (%)	83

CHF = Congestive heart failure.
S_3/S_4 = Ventricular and atrial gallops.
*Modified from D'Elia et al.[201]

osmotic gradients in tissues and pulmonary edema can result.[202] Control of the blood glucose may coincide with clearing of the edema. Metabolic acidosis may further impair myocardial function and contribute both to hyperkalemia and lethal arrhythmias. Serum potassium must be watched closely. The insulin-deficient diabetic has lost a homeostatic defense against hyperkalemia, and particular care is necessary when using aldosterone antagonists or other potassium-retaining diuretics, with or without potassium supplementation.[203] Conversely, hypokalemia impairs insulin secretion.[203a]

ARRHYTHMIAS AND SUDDEN DEATH

Some aspects of cardiac arrhythmias in the diabetic with acute myocardial infarction have been reviewed. Arrhythmias also may be a prominent manifestation of chronic coronary artery disease, but the influence of diabetes in such instances is unknown. Since sudden death is a particular risk for the diabetic (see below), an increased likelihood of dangerous arrhythmias in the diabetic is suggested.

Sinoatrial dysfunction may be more common in diabetics. Phillips noted diabetes in 68% of 31 patients with chaotic atrial mechanism.[204] However, the relationship is not clear.[205] Bradycardia arrhythmias and third degree AV block may also be more common.[206,206a,206b] Both coronary disease and primary degeneration and fibrosis of the conducting system are common underlying etiologies. Degenerative changes of the fibrous cardiac skeleton as seen in mitral annular calcification is also more common among diabetics.[207]

Sudden death is a frequent complication of coronary artery disease and is the fate of about 20%

of individuals with acute myocardial infarction. Conversely, severe coronary disease is found in about 75% of those resuscitated after sudden death.[208] Sudden death is also high in populations without known coronary disease but with antecedent coronary risk factors such as diabetes.[209] This complication and its prevention is therefore of particular concern to the diabetic who has an increased frequency of coronary disease, myocardial infarction and cardiovascular mortality. In the Framingham population diabetics had an excess risk of sudden death.[210] Strategies applicable to the important problem of sudden death have been reviewed.[211]

NONCORONARY HEART DISEASE

Autonomic Neuropathy

Autonomic neuropathy frequently involves the heart of the diabetic.[212] Physiologic rate control is altered[213,214] and severe forms may be associated with impairment of the myocardial adaptation to stress.[215] Neuropathy may also reduce appreciation of ischemic pain[108] and may change responses to some pharmacologic agents. Early autonomic neuropathy may also underlie certain laboratory abnormalities encountered in asymptomatic diabetics.

The pathogenesis of autonomic neuropathy is controversial and is discussed in detail in Chapter 31. One theory implicates the sorbitol pathway—an alternate pathway for glucose metabolism in which glucose is converted to sorbitol and then to fructose. Sorbitol and fructose accumulate in Schwann cells, causing changes in osmotic gradients and in intracellular electrolytes which result in cell damage.[216]

Cardiac autonomic neuropathy may involve both sympathetic fibers and the vagus nerve.[217] Degenerative changes are seen in cells of the sympathetic ganglia, rami communicantes, and Schwann cells. Structural changes in the vagus nerve are not seen, but functional impairment is noted frequently and may affect the esophagus and stomach, as well as the heart (Chapter 40).

Normally, reflex heart rate changes are determined by variations in parasympathetic tone.[218] Beta-adrenergic activity affects basal heart rate but plays little role in baroreceptor reflex heart rate control. Impairment in vagal control of heart rate in diabetics is frequent and leads to diminished spontaneous variation of heart rate at rest or with deep inspiration.[213,214,217,219] Sympathetic impairment is more difficult to assess, but may also be common.[217] Decreased sympathetic outflow to the heart and resistance vessels accompanies a decrease in systemic pressure. Exercise capacity and maximum exercise heart rate may be reduced.[219a]

A variety of maneuvers designed to test the afferents to the heart may show impairment. These include tilting, the Valsalva maneuver, carotid sinus pressure, handgrip, and responses to amyl nitrate.[217,220] Vibratory sense is always impaired.[219a]

The transplanted heart is a model of the total cardiac denervation which can be approached in severe cases of diabetic autonomic dysfunction. With the removal of autonomic tone the intrinsic rate of the sinus node increases and beat-to-beat variability in heart rhythm disappears.[221] The early response to a demand for an increased cardiac output during stress is not met by rate change. Rather, modification of myocardial performance after denervation depends on changes in venous filling and the response to circulatory catecholamines.[222] This inability initially to increase cardiac output by appropriate rate adjustment may contribute to postural hypotension and to reduced exercise response.[223] Hypersensitivity of the denervated heart to norepinephrine has been demonstrated in dogs[224] but not in man.[225] It is of potential concern, however, and cardiac arrest has been related to diabetic autonomic neuropathy.[226]

Acute myocardial infarction has been reported as a complication of diabetic neuropathy.[227] It has been suggested that autonomic neuropathy may also prevent adequate slowing of heart rate in response to beta blockade, leading to a therapeutic drug failure.[217] Depletion of norepinephrine stores in the cardiovascular system of diabetic patients has been reported and may possibly contribute to higher cardiac mortality.[215] Ewing et al. noted a 56% 5-year mortality rate in patients with autonomic symptoms and abnormal function tests. Half of these deaths were considered possibly attributable to autonomic neuropathy.[227a]

One may speculate that the diabetic with autonomic neuropathy leading to myocardial catecholamine depletion is much more vulnerable to insult from the wide spectrum of possible myocardial diseases. Those insults which otherwise might be associated with borderline myocardial function produce frank congestive heart failure when autonomic neuropathy has resulted in catecholamine depletion.

Diabetic Cardiomyopathy

Coronary angiography has made it possible to identify during life patients with myocardial dysfunction without significant coronary obstruction. Because the presence of nonobstructed coronaries does not always exclude dysfunction on an ischemic basis from coronary spasm, embolus, or occlusion with recanalization, the term "diabetic cardiomyopathy" has been proposed.[228,229]

Reviewers of cardiomyopathy in the 1960s observed that populations of patients with primary myocardial disease contained an excess of diabetics.[230,231] In 1974 a series of diabetic patients was reported with normal coronary arteries by angiography and clinical or hemodynamic evidence of cardiovascular dysfunction.[229] This association has since been extended to diabetics with hypertension[19] and chronic renal disease.[201,228] History and physical examination revealed findings indistinguishable from congestive heart failure due to other causes. Hemodynamic studies demonstrated a spectrum of abnormalities from simple elevation of the left ventricular end diastolic pressure to severely depressed ejection fraction.[201,232] In patients examined postmortem, multiple histologic abnormalities were observed including the deposition of PAS positive material in the interstitium and small vessels, microvascular endothelial proliferation, interstitial and perivascular fibrosis, and patchy myocytolysis.[19,229]

Regan et al. reported the post-mortem examination of 13 diabetics.[233] Nine had no significant coronary disease, although 6 had been in clinical heart failure at death. Mild thickening of intramyocardial vessels was noted; however, the existence of narrowing was equivocal. Marked accumulation of PAS positive material was seen in the myocardial interstitium, a finding rarely present in normal individuals. Variable degrees of patchy fibrosis without inflammatory cells were present. Electron microscopy revealed the accumulation of collagen and amorphous material, presumably the PAS positive material observed, as well as lipid bodies. Muscle samples showed increased triglyceride levels in comparison to nondiabetic normal controls.

The same group reported that dogs made diabetic by alloxan developed hemodynamic changes 1 year later which could not be attributed to a direct effect of alloxan on the myocardium.[234] A decrease was seen in left ventricular distensibility characterized by increased left ventricular end diastolic pressure and abnormal responses to saline infusion and pressor agents. Histology showed PAS positive material similar to that noted earlier in humans, and accumulation of triglycerides was also suggested.

The same methods were applied to the study of 12 insulin-resistant diabetics without significant coronary occlusions by angiography. Eight had no prior heart failure by history. Abnormal left ventricular pressure volume curves were present, although the ejection fractions were within normal limits. The response to angiotensin paralleled that in experimental animals: the left ventricular end diastolic pressure rose abnormally, but stroke volume failed to increase normally. These data were felt compatible with an early cardiomyopathy.

Case report. AM, Case #88610, a 61-year-old diabetic male taking 38 units of NPH insulin, was hospitalized for evaluation of severe diabetic amyotrophy and incidentally found to have rapid atrial flutter. There was no past history of chest pain, hypertension, pulmonary or liver disease, recent febrile illness, or excess alcohol intake. Blood pressure was 140/80, left ventricular apex in sixth interspace at the anterior axillary line, scattered rales at lung bases, hemoglobin 15.8, creatinine 1.1, bilirubin 0.6, T3 and folic acid normal. The arrhythmias persisted despite quinidine, digoxin, and furosemide and reappeared 4 days after electrical reversion. During the next 9 months he remained in atrial fibrillation free of overt congestive failure. His amyotrophy and neuropathy subsequently became much improved; he no longer had severe burning discomfort in his legs or required a wheelchair. Accompanying this response his cardiac status improved and he returned to normal sinus rhythm for the first time. However, during the next 4 years progressive and increasingly refractory cardiac decompensation appeared with a return of atrial flutter and fibrillation, progressive retinopathy, neuropathy, and nephropathy. His death was attributed to congestive failure.

At postmortem examination, his heart was markedly enlarged, weighing 860 g. There was mild atherosclerosis involving only the right posterior descending coronary artery. Microscopically there was marked interstitial and subendocardial fibrosis. Many muscle fibers were hypertrophied; some showed myocytolysis. No infarcts were seen. The small intramyocardial blood vessels showed moderate to marked thickening of their walls with narrowing of the lumen (Fig. 27–3 to 27–5). In summary, the myocardial changes were consistent with those seen in cardiomyopathy of diabetes mellitus.

Comment. This diabetic died with marked cardiomegaly after a course characterized by progressive cardiac failure. The findings were consistent with cardiomyopathy perhaps partly aggravated by minor coronary disease. An unusual feature was the apparent clinical association between regression and progression of his cardiac disease along with similar changes in his peripheral muscle and neuropathic symptoms.

The etiology of the functional myocardial abnormality is uncertain. Cardiomyopathy often coexists with microangiopathy.[228,229] In addition, a positive correlation has been made between the severity of microvascular disease in other tissues and cardiac abnormalities found during noninvasive testing.[235,236] Vascular injection techniques have shown the presence of capillary microaneurysms in the heart analogous to the structure seen in eye and kidney.[11] Other microcirculatory abnormalities in diabetics may coexist, including platelet defects (both increased aggregation and adhesiveness[10]), increased plasma viscosity,[237] de-

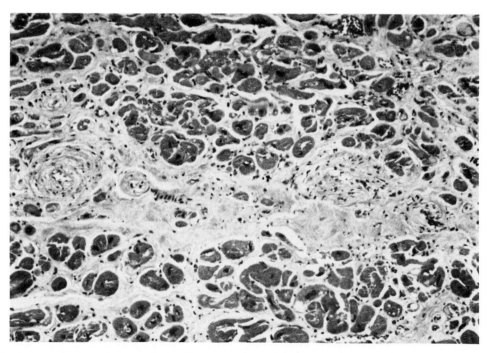

Fig. 27–3. Low power view of myocardium with considerable diffuse fibrosis. A small artery with marked narrowing of lumen is seen near left upper corner.

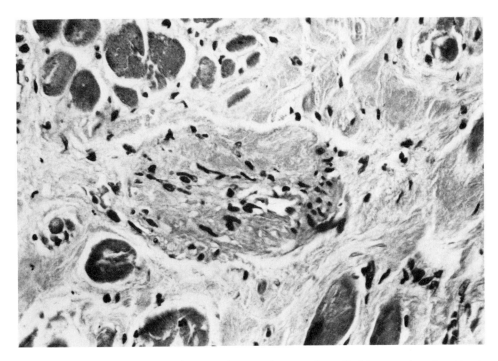

Fig. 27–4. A small intramyocardial artery with severe changes. The muscular wall of the artery is replaced by dense fibrous tissue and the lumen is markedly narrowed. Notice the dense homogenous fibrous tissue in the adventitia and adjacent myocardium, separating individual muscle fibers.

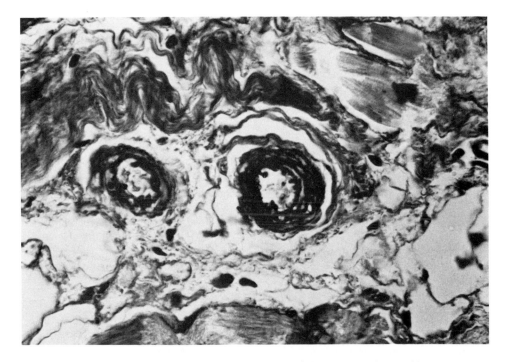

Fig. 27–5. Small intramyocardial arterioles with thickened media with fraying and splitting of layers. PAS reaction.

creased red cell deformability,[237] reduced oxygen carrying capacity,[238] and primary capillary basement membrane thickening.[239] However, these findings may reflect the increased incidence of independent complications in patients with diabetes of long duration.

The significance of small vessel disease is also disputed and whether such changes might contribute to myocardial ischemia, remains uncertain.[15,240,241] Small vessel disease was noted in 72% of diabetic hearts and 28% of nondiabetic hearts by Zoneraich. However, atrial pacing has failed to demonstrate ischemia in at least one study of diabetics with cardiomyopathy.[233]

The presence of PAS positive material in histologic specimens of diabetics with cardiomyopathy, a finding not seen in normal or diabetic patients without cardiomyopathy,[228,229,233,242,243] raises the possibility that glycoprotein deposits may accumulate in myocardial cells and lead to functional abnormalities. This process would be analogous to the combination of glucose with hemoglobin in the red cell.[244] The interstitial tissue of heart muscle is the primary site determining compliance. In addition to glycoprotein, alterations may include deposition of collagen and fibrosis,[19] and lipid accumulation in the form of triglyceride.[244a]

One implication of such a mechanism would be the possibility of favorably altering the metabolic balance away from tissue deposition. From an empiric standpoint the goal of minimizing hyperglycemia should be attempted. Vigorous treatment of associated hypertension must be emphasized in the patient developing clinical myocardial dysfunction, and exposure to potential toxins such as alcohol prevented. Renal failure may also be associated with a spectrum of contributing abnormalities.[201,228]

Preclinical Heart Disease

Laboratory tests in asymptomatic diabetics show a surprisingly high prevalence of cardiac abnormalities both among younger individuals with juvenile onset diabetes and older subjects with longstanding diabetes. The significance of such findings is obscure because of the lack of specificity of any of these tests and the ignorance of underlying mechanisms responsible for the abnormality.

Electrocardiography. Zoneraich reported electrocardiographic abnormalities in 51%, and vectorcardiographic abnormalities in 75% of a group of ambulatory asymptomatic diabetics between ages 15 to 81.[245,246] Evidence of myocardial infarction was present in 14%, whereas 41% had distortions of the QRS vector loop, twice the prevalence of age and sex matched controls. In addi-

tion, 25% of the diabetics showed intra-atrial conduction disturbances.[246]

Systolic Time Intervals. The duration of electromechanical systole can be subdivided into preejection and ejection periods. Temporal alterations of electromechanical ventricular systoles are characteristic of early myocardial dysfunction. The preejection period reflects the rate of rise of left ventricular pressure and generally becomes prolonged with disease.[247] The left ventricular ejection time shortens with either decreased stroke volume or more rapid ejection.[248] The ratio between these variables is customarily employed as a single measure of left ventricular performance. In asymptomatic diabetes this ratio has been increased, although generally within the normal range.[249,250] Several authors have noted that the degree of such abnormalities was directly related to the severity of microvascular disease as manifested by neuropathy, retinopathy, and nephropathy.[235,236] Abnormalities may become more marked under the influence of alcohol, utilized as a further metabolic depressant.[251] Although these findings may represent preclinical diabetic cardiomyopathy, they are subject to a number of other considerations. Changes in blood sugar affect systolic time intervals,[252] as do changes in systemic venous return,[249] cardiac autonomic neuropathy,[248] or even inapparent coronary disease.[253]

Echocardiography and Stress Testing. Echocardiograms in young diabetics may show abnormalities of systolic or diastolic function.[254,255] In fact, Lababidi et al. reported a high prevalence of abnormalities determined by M-mode echocardiography in 107 Type I diabetics with an average age of 13.8 years. These included increased chamber dimensions, reduced intraventricular septal excursion, and occasional septal hypertrophy.[255a] Exercise testing in similar patients suggests that some diabetics may achieve a slightly low maximum oxygen consumption and heart rate. Abenavoli reported treadmill or scintigraphic abnormalities in 7 of 12 asymptomatic diabetic males undergoing exercise testing. Five had focal perfusion defects on myocardial scintigraphy suggesting that subclinical coronary disease was responsible.[255]

The Joslin Clinic is presently studying cohorts of asymptomatic juvenile diabetics to determine the incidence of functional disturbances and evaluate their progression and clinical significance during medical follow-up.

OTHER FORMS OF MYOCARDIAL DISEASE WITH DIABETES

When considering the less common diseases in which myocardial dysfunction and diabetes mellitus are associated, one must recall that a variety of pathologic processes can cause glucose intolerance. Hemochromatosis is an example. The abnormal deposition of iron in the tissues results in impaired function of both heart and endocrine pancreas. Although hepatic failure is the most common presenting problem, both congestive heart failure and diabetes mellitus each occasionally develop as initial manifestations. Because evidence suggests that early phlebotomy or other treatment may ameliorate myocardial failure, early diagnosis is essential.[256]

A variety of endocrine abnormalities which result in glucose intolerance may also display prominent cardiac manifestations. Hyperthyroidism, especially in older patients, can develop with cardiac failure and atrial arrhythmias in the setting of a hyperdynamic circulation. Similarly, an autopsy series of patients with pheochromocytoma demonstrated active myocarditis, presumably from the toxic effects of excess circulating catecholamines.[257] A majority of these patients showed signs of congestive failure. Although patients with Cushing's syndrome rarely display edema, sodium retention and edema formation is a reported adverse effect of corticosteroid administration.[258] Acromegaly is frequently associated with diabetes mellitus and a variety of cardiovascular disorders, including hypertension, cardiomyopathy, premature coronary atherosclerosis, and arrhythmias.[259] Finally, several chronic inflammatory illnesses, among them infectious endocarditis, can produce glucose intolerance and congestive heart failure in the susceptible individual.

Among the diseases which appear to be linked statistically to diabetes mellitus, the endocrine deficiency disease of hypothyroidism is a well known cause of cardiac enlargement and pericardial effusion, and may display findings suggestive of congestive heart failure. Myotonic dystrophy displays a variety of unusual clinical features including cardiomyopathy and atrial arrhythmias, as well as an increased incidence of diabetes mellitus.[260]

An unrelated syndrome worthy of mention is the recently identified cardiomyopathy of newborns born of diabetic mothers. This entity can appear both in congestive and hypertrophic forms and is generally transient in nature.[261,262]

Although these conditions are rare in comparison to the seemingly ubiquitous associations of coronary artery disease, hypertension and diabetes, early diagnosis will depend on an appreciation of their possible occurrence, especially when atypical features are present.

REFERENCES

1. Kannel, W.B., McGee, D.L.: Diabetes and cardiovascular disease: The Framingham study. J.A.M.A. *241*:2035, 1979.

2. Gordon, T., Garcia-Palmieri, M.R., Kagan, A., et al.: Differences in coronary heart disease in Framingham, Honolulu and Puerto Rico. J. Chronic Dis. *27*:329, 1974.

3. West, K.M.: Diabetes in American Indians and other native populations of the New World. Diabetes *23*:841, 1974.

4. Prosnitz, L.R., Mandell, G.L.: Diabetes mellitus among Navajo and Hopi Indians: The lack of vascular complications. Am. J. Med. Sci. *253*:700, 1967.

5. Kannel, W.B., Hjortland, M., Castelli, W.P.: Role of diabetes in congestive heart failure: the Framingham study. Am. J. Cardiol. *34*:29, 1974.

6. Most, A.S., Brachfeld, N., Gorlin, R. et al.: Free fatty acid metabolism of the human heart at rest. J. Clin. Invest. *48*:1177, 1969.

7. Davies, R.E.: Biochemical processes in cardiac function. In: E. Braunwald (Ed.): The Myocardium: Failure and Infarction. New York, H.P. Publishing Co., 1974. pp. 29–35.

8. Neely, J.R., Rovetto, M.J., Oram, J.F.: Myocardial utilization of carbohydrate and lipids. Prog. Cardiovasc. Dis. *15*:289, 1972.

9. Ross, R., Glomset, J.A.: The pathogenesis of atherosclerosis. N. Engl. J. Med. *295*:420, 1976.

10. Colwell, J.A.: Pathogenesis of diabetic vascular disease: New concepts. In: S. Podolsky (Ed.): Clinical Diabetes: Modern Management. New York, Appleton-Century-Crofts, 1980, pp. 363–372.

11. Siperstein, M.D., Unger, R.H., Madison, L.L.: Studies of capillary basement membranes in normal subjects, diabetic, and prediabetic patients. J. Clin. Invest. *47*:1973, 1968.

12. Fischer, V.W., Barnes, H.G., Leskier, L.: Capillary basement thickness in diabetic human myocardium. Diabetes *28*:713, 1979.

13. Williamson, J.R., Kilo, C.: Basement-membrane thickening and diabetic microangiopathy. Diabetes *25*(Suppl. 2): 925, 1976.

14. Factor, S.M., Okun, E.M., Minase, T.: Capillary microaneurysms in the human diabetic heart. N. Engl. J. Med. *302*:384, 1980.

15. Blumenthal, H.T., Morris, A., Goldenberg, S.S.: A study of lesions of the intramural coronary artery branches in diabetes mellitus. A.M.A. Arch. Path. *70*:13, 1960.

16. James, T.N.: Pathology of small coronary arteries. Am. J. Cardiol. *20*:679, 1967.

17. Yodaiken, R.E.: The relationship between diabetic capillaropathy and myocardial infarction. Diabetes *25* (Suppl. 2) 928, 1976.

18. Regan, T.J., Lyons, M.M., Ahmed, S.S., et al.: Evidence for cardiomyopathy in familial diabetes mellitus. J. Clin. Invest. *60*:885, 1977.

19. Factor, S.M., Minase, T., Sonnenblick, E.H.: Clinical and morphological features of human hypertensive-diabetic cardiomyopathy. Am. Heart J. *99*:446, 1980.

20. R. J. Havlik, M. Feinleib (Eds.): Proceedings of the Conference on the Decline in Coronary Heart Disease Mortality. United States Department of Health, Education & Welfare. Public Health Service, National Institutes of Health. NIH Publication No. 79–1610, 1979.

21. Root, H.F., Bland, E.F., Gordon, W.H., White, P.D.: Coronary atherosclerosis in diabetes mellitus: A postmortem study. J.A.M.A. *113*:27, 1939.

22. Stearns, S., Schlesinger, M.J., Rudy, A.: Incidence and clinical significance of coronary artery disease in diabetes mellitus. Arch. Intern. Med. *80*:463, 1947.

23. Bell, E.T. A postmortem study of vascular disease in diabetics. A.M.A. Arch. Pathol. *53*:444, 1952.

24. Feldman, M., Feldman, M., Jr.: The association of cor-

onary occlusion and infarction with diabetes mellitus. A necropsy study. Am. J. Med. Sci. 228:53, 1954.

25. Goldenberg, S., Alex, M., Blumenthal, H.T.: Sequelae of arteriosclerosis of the aorta and coronary arteries. A statistical study in diabetes mellitus. Diabetes 7:98, 1958.

26. Goodale, F., Daoud, A.S., Florentin, R., et al.: Chemico-anatomic studies of arteriosclerosis and thrombosis in diabetics. I. Coronary arterial wall thickness, thrombosis, and myocardial infarcts in autopsied North Americans. Exper. Mol. Pathol. 1:353, 1962.

27. Vikhert, A.M., Zhdanov, V.S., Matova, E.E.: Atherosclerosis of the aorta and coronary vessels of the heart in cases of various diseases. Atheroscl. Res. 9:179, 1969.

28. Ledet, T.: Histological and histochemical changes in the coronary arteries of old diabetic patients. Diabetologia 4:268, 1968.

28a. Waller, B.F., Palumbo, P.J., Roberts, W.C.: Status of the coronary arteries at necropsy in diabetes mellitus with onset after age 30 years. Analysis of 229 diabetic patients with and without clinical evidence of coronary heart disease and comparison to 183 control subjects. Am. J. Med. 69:498, 1980.

29. Robertson, W.B., Strong, J.P.: Atherosclerosis in persons with hypertension and diabetes mellitus. In: H.C. McGill, Jr. (Ed.): Geographical Pathology of Atherosclerosis. Baltimore, Williams & Wilkins, 1968.

29a. Vigorita, V.J., Moore, G.W., Hutchins, G.M.: Absence of correlation between coronary arterial atherosclerosis and severity or duration of diabetes mellitus of adult onset. Am. J. Cardiol., 46:535, 1980.

30. Kessler, I.I.: Mortality experience of diabetic patients. A twenty-six-year follow-up study. Am. J. Med. 51:715, 1971.

31. Królewski, A.S., Czyzyk, A., Janeczko, D., Kopczyński, J.: Mortality from cardiovascular diseases among diabetics. Diabetologia 13:345, 1977.

32. Hayward, R.E., Lucena, B.C.: An investigation into the mortality of diabetics. J. Institute of Actuaries 91:286, 1965.

33. Kannel, W.B., McGee, D.L.: Diabetics and cardiovascular risk factors: the Framingham study. Circulation 59:8, 1979.

34. Ostrander, L.D., Jr., Francis, T., Jr., Hayner, N.S. et al.: The relationship of cardiovascular disease to hyperglycemia. Ann. Intern. Med. 62:1188, 1965.

35. Keen, H., Rose, G., Pyke, D.A., et al.: Blood-sugar and arterial disease. Lancet 2:505, 1965.

36. Bryfogle, J.W., Bradley, R.F.: The vascular complications of diabetes mellitus. A clinical study. Diabetes 6:159, 1957.

37. Liebow, I.M., Hellerstein, H.K., Miller, M.: Arteriosclerotic heart disease in diabetes mellitus. A clinical study of 383 patients. Am. J. Med. 18:438, 1955.

38. Anderson, R.S., Ellington, A., Gunter, L.M.: The incidence of arteriosclerotic heart disease in Negro diabetic patients. Diabetes 10:114, 1961.

39. Lundbaek, K.: Late developments in long-term diabetic vascular disease. In: K. Oberdisse, K. Jahnke (Eds.): Diabetes Mellitus, Third Congress of the International Diabetes Federation, Dusseldorf, 21–25 July, 1958. Stuttgart, George Thieme Verlag, 1959, pp. 141–150.

40. Schlesinger, F.G., Franken, S., van Lange, L. Th. P., Schwarz, F.: Incidence and progression of retinal and vascular lesions in long-term diabetes. A follow-up of a group of patients over 7 years. Acta Med. Scand. 168:483, 1960.

40a. Keen, H., Jarrett, R.J., Fuller, J.H., McCartney, P.: Hyperglycemia and arterial disease. Diabetes 30 (Suppl. 2):49, 1981.

41. Rosenberg, H.M., Klebba, A.J.: Trends in cardiovascular mortality with a focus on ischemic heart disease: United States 1950–1976. In: R. J. Havlik, M. Feinleib (Eds.): Proceedings of the Conference on the Decline in Coronary Heart Disease Mortality. United States Department of Health, Education & Welfare. Public Health Service, National Institutes of Health. NIH Publication No. 79–1610, 1979, pp. 11–16.

42. Eleventh Bethesda Conference: Prevention of coronary heart disease. Am. J. Cardiol. 47:713, 1981.

43. Goto, Y., Fukuhara, N.: Cause of death in 933 diabetic autopsy cases. J. Japanese Diabetic Soc. 11:197, 1968.

44. Greenwood, B.M., Taylor, J.R.: The complications of diabetes in Nigerians. Tropical and Geographical Medicine 20:1, 1968.

45. West, K.M., Kalbfleisch, J.M.: Diabetes in Central America. Diabetes 19:656, 1970.

46. Jarrett, R.J., Keen, H.: Diabetes and atherosclerosis. In: H. Keen and R.J. Jarrett (Eds.): Complications of Diabetes. London, E. Arnold, 1975. pp. 179–203.

47. Clawson, B.J.: Incidence of types of heart disease among 30,265 autopsies, with special reference to age and sex. Am. Heart J. 22:607, 1941.

48. Oliver, M.F.: Sex differences. In: L. MacDonald (Ed.): The Proceedings of a Conference in London at the Royal College of Physicians of London: Pathogenesis and Treatment of Occlusive Arterial Disease. London, Pitman Medical Publishing Co. Ltd., 1960, pp. 124–132.

49. Clawson, B.J., Bell, E.T.: Incidence of fatal coronary disease in nondiabetic and in diabetic persons. A.M.A. Arch. Pathol. 48:105, 1949.

50. Garcia, M., McNamara, P., Gordon, T., et al.: Cardiovascular complications in diabetics. In: R.A. Camerini-Davalos, H.S. Cole (Eds.): Vascular and Neurological Changes in Early Diabetes. New York, Academic Press, 1973, pp. 493–499.

51. Bradley, R.F., Bryfogle, J.W.: Survival of diabetic patients after myocardial infarction. Am. J. Med. 20:207, 1956.

52. Partamian, J.O., Bradley, R.F.: Acute myocardial infarction in 258 cases of diabetes. Immediate mortality and five-year survival. N. Engl. J. Med. 273:455, 1965.

53. Dortimer, A.C., Shenoy, P.N., Shiroff, R.A., et al.: Diffuse coronary artery disease in diabetic patients: fact or fiction? Circulation 57:133, 1978.

54. Hamby, R.I., Sherman, L., Mehta, J., Aintablian, A.: Reappraisal of the role of the diabetic state in coronary artery disease. Chest 70:251, 1976.

54a. Waller, B.F., Palumbo, P.J., Connolly, D.C.: Distribution of coronary artery disease in diabetic and nondiabetic hearts. Diabetes 25 (Suppl. 1):346, 1976.

55. Meissner, W.A., Legg, M.A.: The pathology of diabetes. In: A. Marble, P. White, R.F. Bradley, L. Krall (Eds.): Joslin's Diabetes Mellitus, 11th Ed. Philadelphia, Lea & Febiger, 1971, p. 174.

56. Weinrauch, L.A., D'Elia, J.A., Healy, R.W., et al.: Asymptomatic coronary artery disease: angiographic assessment of diabetics evaluated for renal transplantation. Circulation 58:1184, 1978.

57. Stamler, J.: Atherosclerotic coronary heart disease. In: K.E. Sussman, R.J.S. Metz (Eds.): Diabetes Mellitus, 4th Ed. New York, Am. Diabetes Assoc., 1975, pp. 229–241.

58. Goodkin, G.: Mortality factors in diabetes. A 20-year mortality study. J. Occup. Med. 17:716, 1975.

59. Kannel, W.B.: Some lessons in cardiovascular epidemiology from Framingham. Am. J. Cardiol. 37:269, 1976.

60. Epstein, F.H.: Hyperglycemia. A risk factor in coronary artery disease. Circulation 36:609, 1967.

61. Pell, S., D'Alonzo, C.A.: Some aspects of hypertension in diabetes mellitus. J.A.M.A. 202:104, 1967.

62. Freedman, P., Moulton, R., Spencer, A.G.: Hypertension and diabetes mellitus. Q. J. Med. 27:293, 1958.

63. Pell, S., D'Alonzo, C.A.: Factors associated with long-term survival of diabetics. J.A.M.A. 214:1833, 1970.

64. Garcia, M.J., McNamara, P.M., Gordon, T., Kannel, W.B.: Morbidity and mortality in diabetics in the Framingham population. Sixteen year follow-up study. Diabetes 23:105, 1074.

65. Pyke, D.A.: Arterial disease and diabetes. In: W.G. Oakley, D.A. Pyke, K.W. Taylor (Eds.): Clinical Diabetes and its Biochemical Basis. Oxford, Blackwell, 1968, pp. 506–541.

66. Moss, A.J.: Blood pressure in children with diabetes mellitus. Pediatrics 30:932, 1962.

67. White, P.: Natural course and prognosis of juvenile diabetes. Diabetes 5:445, 1956.

68. Hypertension Detection and Follow-Up Program Cooperative Group: Five-year findings of the hypertension detection and follow-up program. J.A.M.A. 242:2572, 1979.

69. Levy, R.I., Glueck, C.J.: Hypertriglyceridemia, diabetes mellitus and coronary vessel disease. Arch. Intern. Med. (Chicago) 123:220, 1969.

70. Kyner, J.L., Levy, R.I., Soeldner, J.S., et al.: Lipid, glucose, and insulin interrelationships in normal, prediabetic, and chemical diabetic subjects. J. Lab. Clin. Med. 88:345, 1976.

71. Olefsky, J.M., Farquhar, J.W., Reaven, G.M.: Reappraisal of the role of insulin in hypertriglyceridemia. Am. J. Med. 57:551, 1974.

72. Gordon, T., Castelli, W.P., Hjortland, M.L., et al.: High density lipoprotein as a protective factor against coronary heart disease. The Framingham Study. Am. J. Med. 62:702, 1977.

73. Albrink, M.J., Lavietes, P.H., Man, E.B.: Vascular disease and serum lipids in diabetes mellitus. Observations over thirty years (1931-1961). Ann. Intern. Med. 58:305, 1963.

74. Santen, R.J., Willis, P.W., 3rd., Fajans, S.S.: Atherosclerosis in diabetes mellitus. Correlations with serum lipid levels, adiposity, and serum insulin levels. Arch. Intern. Med. 130:833, 1972.

75. Wardle, E.N., Piercy, D.A., Anderson, J.: Some chemical indices of diabetic vascular disease. Postgrad. Med. J. 49:1, 1973.

76. Kissebah, A.H., Siddiq, Y.K., Kohner, E.M., et al.: Plasma-lipids and glucose insulin relationship in noninsulin-requiring diabetics with and without retinopathy. Lancet 1:1104, 1975.

77. Keys, A., Taylor, H.L., Blackburn, H., et al.: Coronary heart disease among Minnesota business and professional men followed fifteen years. Circulation 28:381, 1963.

78. Kannel, W.B.: Lipid profile and the potential coronary victim. Am. J. Clin. Nutrition 24:1074, 1971.

79. Barr, D.P., Russ, E.M., Eder, H.A.: Protein-lipid relationships in human plasma. II. In atherosclerosis and related conditions. Am. J. Med. 11:480, 1951.

80. Gofman, J.W., Young, W. Tandy, R.: Ischemic heart disease, atherosclerosis and longevity. Circulation 34:679, 1966.

81. Castelli, W.P., Doyle, J.T., Gordon, T., et al: HDL cholesterol and other lipids in coronary heart disease. The cooperative lipoprotein phenotyping study. Circulation 55:767, 1977.

82. Miller, G.J., Miller, N.E.: Plasma-high-density-lipoprotein concentration and development of ischemic heart disease. Lancet 1:16, 1975.

83. Gordon, T., Castelli, W.P., Hjortland, M.C., et al.: Diabetes, blood lipids, and the role of obesity in coronary heart disease risk for women. Ann. Intern. Med. 87:393, 1977.

84. Nikkilä, E.A., Hormila, P.: Serum lipids and lipoproteins in insulin-treated diabetes. Demonstration of increased high density lipoprotein concentrations. Diabetes 27:1078, 1978.

85. West, K.M., Kalbfleisch, J.M.: Influence of nutritional factors on prevalance of diabetes. Diabetes 20:99, 1971.

86. Keen, H., Jarrett, R.J., Fuller, J.H.: Tolbutamide and arterial disease in borderline diabetics. In: W.J. Malaisse, J. Pirart (Eds.): Diabetes. Proceedings of the 8th Congress of the International Diabetes Federation, Brussels, July 15–20, 1973. International Congress Series No. 312. Amsterdam, Excerpta Medica, 1974, pp. 588–601.

87. VanBuchem, F.: Coronary heart disease in seven countries. VIII. Zutphen, a town in the Netherlands. Circulation 41(Suppl. 1) & 42: I–76–I–87, 1970.

88. Chapman, J.M., Massey, F.J., Jr.: The interrelationship of serum cholesterol, hypertension, body weight, and risk of coronary disease. Results of the first ten years' follow-up in the Los Angeles heart study. J. Chronic Dis. 17:933, 1964.

89. Keys, A., Aravanis, C., Blackburn, H., et al.: Coronary heart disease: overweight and obesity as risk factors. Ann. Intern. Med. 77:15, 1972.

90. Smoking and Health Report of the Advisory Committee to the Surgeon General of the Public Health Service, U.S. Dept. of Health, Education, and Welfare, Public Health Service Publication No. 1103. Washington, D.C., U.S. Govt. Printing Office, 1964.

91. Seltzer, C.C.: Smoking and coronary heart disease: what are we to believe? Am. Heart J. 100:275, 1980.

92. Kannel, W.B.: Update on the role of cigarette smoking in coronary artery disease. Am. Heart J. 101:319, 1981.

93. McGee, D., Gordon, T.: The results of the Framingham Study applied to four other United States based epidemiologic studies of cardiovascular disease. In: W.B. Kannel, T. Gordon (Eds.): The Framingham Study, Section 31. Department of Health, Education, and Welfare Publication No. (NIH) 76–1083, 1976.

94. Royal College of General Practitioners' Oral Contraception Study: Mortality among oral-contraceptive users. Lancet 2:727, 1977.

95. Dalen, J.E., Hickler, R.B.: Oral contraceptives and cardiovascular disease. Am. Heart J. 101: 626, 1981.

96. Mann, J.I., Doll, R., Thorogood, M., et al.: Risk factors for myocardial infarction in young women. Br. J. Prev. Soc. Med. 30:94, 1976.

97. Fisch, I.R., Frank, J.: Oral contraceptives and blood pressure. J.A.M.A. 237:2499, 1977.

98. Weir, R. J., Briggs, E., Mack, A., et al.: Blood pressure in women taking oral contraceptives. Br. Med. J. 1:533, 1974.

99. Hazzard, W.R., Spiger, M.J., Bagdade, J.D., Bierman, E.L.: Studies on the mechanism of increased plasma triglyceride levels induced by oral contraceptives. N. Engl. J. Med. 280:471, 1969.

100. Kannel, W.B.: Oral contraceptives, hypertension, and thromboembolism. Int. J. Gynaecol. Obstet. 16: 466, 1978–1979.

101. Rosenberg, L., Hennekens, C.H., Rosner, B., et al.: Oral contraceptive use in relation to nonfatal myocardial infarction. Am. J. Epidemiol. 111:59, 1980.

102. Diamond, G.A., Forrester, J.S.: Analysis of probability

as an aid in the clinical diagnosis of coronary-artery disease. N. Engl. J. Med. *300*:1350, 1979.

103. Soler, N.G., Bennett, M.A., Pentecost, B.L., et al.: Myocardial infarction in diabetes. Q. J. Med. *44*:125, 1975.

104. Bradley, R.F., Schonfeld, A.: Diminished pain in diabetic patients with acute myocardial infarction. Geriatrics *17*:322, 1962.

105. Margolis, J.R., Kannel, W.S., Feinleib, M., et al: Clinical features of unrecognized myocardial infarction—silent and asymptomatic. Eighteen-year follow-up: the Framingham study. Am. J. Cardiol. *32*:1, 1973.

106. Roseman, M.D.: Painless myocardial infarction: A review of the literature and analysis of 220 cases. Ann. Intern. Med. *41*:1, 1954.

107. Lindberg, H.A., Berkson, D.M., Stamler, J., Poindexter, A.: Totally asymptomatic myocardial infarction: an estimate of its incidence in the living population. Arch. Intern. Med. *106*:628, 1960.

108. Faerman, I., Faccio, E., Milei, J., et al.: Autonomic neuropathy and painless myocardial infarction in diabetic patients. Histological evidence of their relationship. Diabetes *26*:1147, 1977.

109. Friedberg, C.K.: Pathogenesis of the pain of myocardial infarction. In: Diseases of the Heart. Philadelphia, W.B. Saunders Co., 1966, p. 799.

110. Opie, L.H.: Metabolic response during impending myocardial infarction. I. Relevance of studies of glucose and fatty acid metabolism in animals. Circulation *45*:483, 1972.

110a. Morgan, H.E., Cadenas, E., Regen, D.M., Park, C.R.: Regulation of glucose uptake in muscle: II. Rate-limiting steps and effects of insulin and anoxia in heart muscle from diabetic rats. J. Biol. Chem. *236*:262, 1961.

111. Evans, J.R.: Cellular transport of long chain fatty acids. Can. J. Biochem. *42*:955, 1964.

112. Kurien,V.A., Yates, P.A., Oliver, M.F.: The role of free fatty acids in the production of ventricular arrhythmias after acute coronary artery occlusion. Eur. J. Clin. Invest. *1*:225, 1971.

113. Regan, T.J., Markov, A., Oldewurtel, H.A., Burke, W.M.: Myocardial metabolism and function during ischaemia: response to L-noradrenalin. Cardiovasc. Res. *4*:334, 1970.

114. Oliver, M.F.: Metabolic response during impending myocardial infarction. II. Clinical implications. Circulation *45*:491, 1972.

115. Gazes, P.C., Richardson, J.A., Woods, E.F.: Plasma catecholamine concentrations in myocardial infarction and angina pectoris. Circulation *19*:657, 1959.

116. Lukomsky, P.E., Oganov, R.G.: Blood plasma catecholamines and their urinary excretion in patients with acute myocardial infarction. Am. Heart J. *83*:182, 1972.

117. Gupta, D.K., Young, R., Jewitt, D.E., Hartog, M.: Increased plasma-free-fatty-acid concentrations and their significance in patients with acute myocardial infarction. Lancet *2*:1209, 1969.

118. Porte, D., Jr., Graber, A.L., Kuzuya, T., Williams, R.H.: The effect of epinephrine on immunoreactive insulin levels in man. J. Clin. Invest. *45*:228, 1966.

119. Allison, S.P., Hinton, P., Chamberlain, M.J.: Intravenous glucose tolerance, insulin, and free fatty acid levels after myocardial infarction. Br. Med. J. *4*:776, 1969.

120. Taylor, S.H., Saxton, C., Majid, P.A., et al: Insulin secretion following myocardial infarction. With special respect to the pathogenesis of cardiogenic shock. Lancet *2*:1373, 1969.

121. Prakash, R., Chhablani, R.: Immunoreactive serum insulin and growth hormone response in patients with prein-

farction angina and acute myocardial infarction. Chest *65*:408, 1974.

122. Kurt, T.L., Genton, E., Chidsey, C., 3rd, et al.: Carbohydrate metabolism and acute myocardial infarction: circulating glucose, insulin, cortisol and growth hormone responses and excretion of catecholamines. Chest *64*:21, 1973.

123. Logan, R.W., Murdoch, W.R.: Blood levels of hydrocortisone transaminases and cholesterol after myocardial infarction. Lancet *2*:521, 1966.

124. Laniado, S., Segal, P., Esrig, B.: Secretion of endogenous immunoreactive glucagon following acute myocardial infarction in man: its role in the pathogenesis of post-infarction hyperglycemia. Am. J. Cardiol. *31*:144, 1973.

125. Willerson, J.T., Hutcheson, D.R., Leshin, S.J., et al.: Serum glucagon and insulin levels and their relationship to blood glucose values in patients with acute myocardial infarction and acute coronary insufficiency. Am. J. Med. *57*:747, 1974.

126. Lebovitz, H.E., Schultz, K.T., Matthews, M.E., Scheele, R.: Acute metabolic responses to myocardial infarction. Changes in glucose utilization and secretion of insulin and growth hormone. Circulation *39*:171, 1969.

127. Ross, H., Johnston, I.D.A., Welborn, T.A., et al.: Effect of abdominal operation on glucose tolerance and serum levels of insulin, growth hormone, hydrocortisone. Lancet *2*:563, 1966.

127a. Meguid, M.M., Collier, M.D., Howard, L.J.: Uncomplicated and stressed starvation. Surg. Clin. North Am. *61*:529,1981.

128. Heinle, R.A., Levy, R.I., Fredrickson, D.S., Gorlin, R.: Lipid and carbohydrate abnormalities in patients with angiographically documented coronary artery disease. Am. J. Cardiol. *24*:178, 1969.

129. Pearson, D.: Intravenous glucose tolerance in myocardial infarction. Postgrad. Med. J. *47*:648, 1971.

130. Boden, G.: Incidence and cause of glucose intolerance (GI) after acute myocardial infarction (AMI) in man. Diabetes *19* (Suppl. 1): 378, 1970.

131. Datey, K.K., Nanda, N.C.: Hyperglycemia after acute myocardial infarction. N. Engl. J. Med. *276*:262, 1967.

132. Aronow, W.S., Kent, J.R.: Plasma insulin response to an oral glucose load in noncoronary heart disease. Chest *59*:184, 1971.

133. Ettinger, P.O., Oldewurtel, H.A., Dzindzio, B., et al.: Glucose intolerance in nonischemic cardiac disease. Role of cardiac output and adrenergic function. Circulation *43*:809, 1971.

134. Vallence-Owen, J., Ashton, W.L.: Cardiac infarction and insulin antagonism. Lancet *1*:1226, 1963.

135. Ravid, M., Berkowicz, M., Sohar, E.: Hyperglycemia during acute myocardial infarction. A six-year follow-up study. J.A.M.A. *233*:807, 1975.

135a. Soler, H.G., Frank, S.: Value of glycosylated hemoglobin measurements after acute myocardial infarction. J.A.M.A. *246*:1690, 1981.

135b. Husband, D.J., Alberti, K.G.M.M., Julian, D.G.: "Stress" hyperglycaemia during acute myocardial infarction: an indicator of pre-existing diabetes? Lancet *2*:179, 1983.

136. Czyzyk, A., Królewski, A.S., Szabowska, S., et al.: Clinical course of myocardial infarction among diabetic patients. Diabetes Care *3*:526, 1980.

137. Henning, R., Lundman, T.: Swedish Cooperative CCU Study: A study of 2008 patients with acute myocardial infarction from twelve Swedish hospitals with coronary care unit. Part I: A description of the early stage. Part II: The short-term prognosis. Acta Med. Scand. *198* (Suppl. 586): 1–64, 1–35, 1975.

137a.Weitzman, S., Wagner, G.S., Heiss, G., et al.: Myocardial infarction site and mortality in diabetes. Diabetes Care 5:31, 1982.

138. Tansey, M.J.B., Opie, L.H., Kennelly, B.M.: High mortality in obese women diabetics with acute myocardial infarction. Br. Med. J. 1:1624, 1977.

139. Kvetny, J.: Diabetes mellitus and acute myocardial infarction. Acta Med. Scand. 200:151, 1976.

140. Soler, N.G., Bennett, M.A., Lamb, P., Pentecost, B.L., Fitzgerald, M.G., Malins, J.M.: Coronary care for myocardial infarction in diabetics. Lancet 1:475, 1974.

141. Harrower, A.D., Clarke, B.F.: Experience of coronary care in diabetes. Br. Med. J. 1:126, 1976.

142. Lichstein, E., Kuhn, L.A., Goldberg, E. et al.: Diabetic treatment and primary ventricular fibrillation in acute myocardial infarction. Am. J. Cardiol. 38:100, 1976.

142a.Smith, J.W., Buckels, L.J., Carlson, K., Marcus, F.I.: Clinical characteristics and results of noninvasive tests in 60 diabetic patients after acute myocardial infarction. Am. J. Med. 75:217, 1983.

143. Page, M.M., Smith, R.B., Watkins, P.J.: Cardiovascular effects of insulin. Br. Med. J. 1:430, 1976.

144. Alexander, W.D., Oake, R.J.: The effect of insulin on vascular reactivity to norepinephrine. Diabetes 26:611, 1977.

144a.Gwilt, D.J., Nattrass, M., Pentecost, B.L.: Use of low-dose insulin infusions in diabetics after myocardial infarction. Br. Med. J. 285:1402, 1982.

145. Parsonnet, A.E., Hyman, A.S.: Insulin angina. Ann. Intern. Med. 4:1247, 1931.

146. Libby, P., Maroko, P.R., Braunwald, E.: The effect of hypoglycemia on myocardial ischemic injury during acute experimental coronary artery occlusion. Circulation 51:621, 1975.

147. Maroko, P.R., Libby, P., Sobel, B.E. et al.: Effect of glucose-insulin-potassium infusion on myocardial infarction following experimental coronary artery occlusion. Circulation 45:1160, 1972.

148. Vismara, L.A., Amsterdam, E.A., Mason, D.T.: Relation of ventricular arrhythmias in the late hospital phase of acute myocardial infarction to sudden death after hospital discharge. Am. J. Med. 59:6, 1975.

149. Taylor, G.J., Humphries, J.O., Mellits, E.D., Pitt, B., Schulze, R.A., Griffith, L.S., Achuff, S.C.: Predictors of clinical course, coronary anatomy and left ventricular function after recovery from acute myocardial infarction. Circulation 62:960, 1980.

149a.May, G.S.: A review of long-term beta-blocker trials in survival of myocardial infarction. Circulation 67 (Suppl.) I-46, 1983.

149b.Braunwald, E., Muller, J.E., Kloner, R., Maroko, P.R.: Role of beta-adrenergic blockade in the therapy of patients with myocardial infarction. Am. J. Med. 74:113, 1983.

149c.Hjälmarson, A., Herlitz, J., Holmberg, S., et al.: The Göteborg metoprolol trial. Effects on mortality and morbidity in acute infarction. Circulation 67(Suppl.):I–26, 1983.

149d.Yusuf, S., Sleight, P., Rossi, P., et al.: Reduction in infarct size, arrhythmias, and chest pain by early intravenous beta blockade in suspected acute myocardial infarction. Circulation 67 (Suppl.):I-32, 1983.

149e.Gundersen, T., Kjekshus, J.: Timolol treatment after myocardial infarction in diabetic patients. Diabetes Care 6:285, 1983.

150. The University Group Diabetes Program: A study of the effects of hypoglycemic agents on vascular complications in patients with adult-onset diabetes. I. Design, methods, and baseline results. Diabetes 19: (Suppl. 2): 747, 1970.

150a.University Group Diabetes Program: Effects of hypo-glycemic agents on vascular complications in patients with adult-onset diabetes. VII. Mortality and selected nonfatal events with insulin treatment. J.A.M.A. 240:37, 1978.

150b.University Group Diabetes Program: Effects of hypoglycemic agents on vascular complications in patients with adult-onset diabetes. VIII. Evaluation of insulin therapy: final report. Diabetes 31 (Suppl. 5):1, 1982.

151. Federal Register 42(88), Friday, May 6, 1977. Food & Drug Admin. pp. 23170–74.

152. Bradley, R.F.: UGDP Study and the treatment of diabetes mellitus. Drug Therapy, 54, June, 1971.

153. Kilo, C., Miller, J. Ph., Williamson, J.R.: The crux of the UGDP. Spurious results and biologically inappropriate data analysis. Diabetologia 18:179, 1980.

153a.Skyler, J.S.: Complications of diabetes mellitus: relationship to metabolic dysfunction. Diabetes Care 2:499, 1979.

154. Kannel, W.B.: Some lessons in cardiovascular epidemiology from Framingham. Am. J. Cardiol. 37:269, 1976.

154a.Kannel, W.B., Schatzkin, A.: Risk factor analysis. Prog. Cardiovasc. Dis. 26:309, 1984.

155. Parratt, J.R.: Pharmacological approaches to the therapy of angina. Adv. Drug. Res. 9:103, 1974.

156. Vaisrub, S.: Diabetes and the heart: the autonomic connection. In: S. Zoneraich (Ed.): Diabetes and The Heart. Springfield, Charles C Thomas, 1978, pp.161–174.

157. Sostman, H.D., Langou, R.A.: Contemporary medical management of stable angina pectoris. Am. Heart J. 95:775, 1978.

158. Gibson, D.G.: Pharmacodynamic properties of beta adrenergic receptor blocking drugs in man. Drugs 7:8, 1974.

159. Wolfson, S., Heinle, R.A., Herman, M., Kemp, H.G., Sullivan, J.M., Gorlin, R.: Propranolol and angina pectoris. Am. J. Cardiol. 18:345, 1966.

160. Wiener, L., Dwyer, E.M., Jr., Cox, J.W.: Hemodynamic effects of nitroglycerin, propranolol, and their combination in coronary heart disease. Circulation 39:623, 1969.

161. Winbury, M.M., Weiss, H.R., Howe, B.D.: Effects of beta-adrenoreceptor blockade and nitroglycerin on myocardial oxygenation. Eur. J. Pharmacol. 16:271, 1971.

162. Frishman, W.H., Weksler, B., Christodoulou, J.P. et al.: Reversal of abnormal platelet aggregability and change in exercise tolerance in patients with angina pectoris following oral propranolol. Circulation 50:887, 1974.

162a.Weksler, B.B., Gillick, M., Pink, J.: Effect of propranolol on platelet function. Blood 49:185, 1977.

162b.Alderman, E.L., Davies, R.O., Crowley, J.J., et al.: Dose response effectiveness of propranolol for the treatment of angina pectoris. Circulation 51: 964, 1975.

163. Shand, D.G.: Propranolol. N. Engl. J. Med. 293:280, 1975.

163a.Lands, A.M., Arnold, A., McAuliff, J.P., et al.: Differentiation of receptor systems activated by sympathomimetic amines. Nature 214:597, 1967.

164. McMurtry, R.J.: Propranolol, hyperglycemia, and hypertensive crisis. (Letter). Ann. Intern. Med. 80:669, 1974.

165. Cerasi, E., Luft, R., Efendic, S.: Effect of adrenergic blocking agents on insulin response to glucose infusion in man. Acta Endocrinol (Kbh.) 69:335, 1972.

166. Hedstrand, H., Aberg, H.: Insulin response to intravenous glucose during long-term treatment with propranolol. Acta Med. Scand. 196:39, 1974.

167. Podolsky, S., Pattavina, C.G.: Hyperosmolar nonketotic diabetic coma: a complication of propranolol therapy. Metabolism 22:685, 1973.

168. Allan, R., Genovese, B.: Propranolol withdrawal. (Letter). Ann. Intern. Med. 82:431, 1975.

168a.Stone, P.H., Antman, E.M., Muller, J.E., Braunwald,

E.: Calcium channel blocking agents in the treatment of cardiovascular disorders. Part II. Hemodynamic effects and clinical applications. Ann. Intern. Med. 93:886, 1980.

168b.Charles, S., Ketelslegers, J.-M., Buysschaert, M., Lambert, A.E.: Hyperglycaemic effect of nifedipine. Br. Med. J. 283:19, 1981.

168c.Giugliano, D., Torella, R., Cacciapuoti, F., et al.: Impairment of insulin secretion in man by nifedipine. Eur. J. Clin. Pharmacol. 18:395, 1980.

168d.Röjdmark, S., Andersson, D.E.H., Hed, R., Sunblad, L.: Effect of verapamil on glucose response to intravenous injection of glucagon and insulin in healthy subjects. Horm. Metab. Res. 12:285, 1980.

169. Fischl, S.J., Herman, M.V., Gorlin, R.: The intermediate coronary syndrome: Clinical, angiographic, and therapeutic aspects. N. Engl. J. Med. 288:1193, 1973.

170. Stoner, J., Harrison, D.C.: Medical and surgical approach to unstable angina. In: R.S. Eliot (Ed.): Contemporary Problems in Cardiology, Vol. 3: Cardiac Emergencies. New York, Futura Publishing Co. Inc. 1977, pp. 337–355.

171. Hugenholtz, P.G., Michels, H.R., Serruys, P.W., Brower, R.W.: Nifedipine in the treatment of unstable angina, coronary spasm, and myocardial ischemia. Am. J. Cardiol. 47:163, 1981.

172. Crawford, M.H., LeWinter, M.M., O'Rourke, R.A., Karliner, J.S., Ross, J.: Combined propranolol and digoxin therapy in angina pectoris. Ann. Intern. Med. 83:449, 1975.

173. Parker, M., Meller, J., Medina, N. et al.: Provocation of myocardial ischemic events during initiation of vasodilator therapy for severe chronic heart failure. Am. J. Cardiol. 48:939, 1981.

174. Weintraub, R.M.,Voukydis, P.C., Aroesty, J.M., et al.: Treatment of preinfarction angina with intra-aortic balloon counterpulsation and surgery. Am. J. Cardiol. 34:809, 1974.

175. Muller, J.E., Gunther, S.J.: Nifedipine therapy for Prinzmetal's angina. Circulation 57:137, 1978.

176. Maseri, A., Pesola, A., Mimmo, R., et al.: Pathogenetic mechanisms of angina at rest. Circulation (Suppl) 52:89, 1975.

177. Rentrop, P., Blanke, H., Karsch, K.R.: Selective intracoronary thrombolysis in acute myocardial infarction and unstable angina pectoris. Circulation 63:307,. 1981.

178. Gruntzig, A.R., Senning, A., Siegenthaler, W.E.: Nonoperative dilatation of coronary-artery stenosis: Percutaneous transluminal coronary angioplasty. N. Engl. J. Med. 301:61, 1979.

179. Mundth, E.D., Austen, W.G.: Surgical measures for coronary heart disease. N. Engl. J. Med. 293:75, 1975.

180. King, S.B., Douglas, J.S.: Coronary arteriography and left ventriculography: Indications. In: J.S. Hurst (Ed.): The Heart, New York, McGraw-Hill Book Co., 1978, pp. 398–400.

181. Leland, O.S., Jr.: Diabetes and the heart. In: G.P. Kozak (Ed.): Clinical Diabetes Mellitus. Philadelphia, W.B. Saunders, Co., 1981, pp. 302–316.

182. Abrams, H.L., Adams, D.F.: The complications of coronary arteriography. Circulation 52 (Suppl. II): 11, 1975.

183. Weinrauch, L.A., Healy, R.W., Leland, O.S., Jr., et al.: Coronary angiography and acute renal failure in diabetic azotemic nephropathy. Ann. Intern. Med. 86:56, 1977.

184. Weinrauch, L.A., Healy, R.W., Leland, O.S., Jr., et al.: Decreased insulin requirement in acute renal failure in diabetic nephropathy. Arch Intern. Med. 138:399, 1978.

185. National Cooperative Study: Unstable angina pectoris: National Cooperative Study Group to Compare Medical

and Surgical Therapy: I. Report of protocol and patient population. Am. J. Cardiol. 37:896, 1976.

186. Plotnick, G.D., Conti, C.R.: Unstable angina: angiography, short- and long-term morbidity, mortality and symptomatic status of medically treated patients. Am. J. Med. 63:870, 1977.

187. Takardot, Hultgren, H.N., Lipton, M.J., et al.: The VA cooperative randomized study of surgery for coronary arterial occlusive disease. II. Subgroup with significant left main lesions. Circulation 54:(Suppl. III): 107, 1976.

188. Hurst, J.W., King, S.B., 3rd, Logue, R.B., et al.: Value of coronary bypass surgery. Controversies in cardiology: Part I. Am. J. Cardiol. 42:308, 1978.

189. McIntosh, H.D., Garcia, J.A.: The first decade of aorto-coronary bypass grafting 1967–1977. A review. Circulation 57:405, 1978.

190. Proudfit, W.L., Bruschke, V.G., Sones, F.M., Jr.: Clinical course of patients with normal or slightly or moderately abnormal coronary arteriograms: 10-year followup of 521 patients. Circulation 62:712, 1980.

191. National Cooperative Study: Unstable angina pectoris: National Cooperative Study Group to Compare Surgical and Medical Therapy. II. In-hospital experience and initial follow-up results in patients with one, two, and three vessel disease. Am. J. Cardiol. 42:839, 1978.

192. Anderson, R.P., Rahimtoola, S.H., Bonchek, L.A., et al.: The prognosis of patients with coronary artery disease after coronary bypass operations. Time-related progress of 532 patients with disabling angina pectoris. Circulation 50:274, 1974.

193. Kramer, J.R., Matsuda, Y., Mulligan, J.C., et al.: Progression of coronary atherosclerosis. Circulation 63:519, 1981.

193a.Batist, G., Blaker, M., Kosinski, E., et al.: Coronary bypass surgery in juvenile onset diabetes. Am. Heart J. 106:51, 1983.

194. Draskoczy, S.P., Leland, O.S., Bradley, R.F.: Aorto-coronary bypass in the diabetic patient. Kidney Int. 6(Supp. I):37, 1974.

194a.Salomon, N.W., Page, U.S., Okies, J.E., et al.: Diabetes mellitus and coronary artery bypass. Short-term risk and long-term prognosis. J. Thorac. Cardiovasc. Surg. 85:264, 1983.

194b.Johnson, W.D., Pedraza, P.M., Kayser, K.L.: Coronary artery surgery in diabetics. 261 consecutive patients followed four to seven years. Am. Heart J. 104:823, 1982.

194c.Elliott, M.J., Gill, G.V., Home, P.D., et al.: A comparison of two regimens for the management of diabetes during open-heart surgery. Anesthesiology 60:364, 1984.

195. Kannel, W.B., Hjortland, M., Castelli, W.P.: Role of diabetes in congestive heart failure: The Framingham study. Am. J. Cardiol. 34:29, 1974.

196. Burch, G.E., Giles, T.D., Colcolough, H.L.: Ischemic cardiomyopathy. Am. Heart J. 79:291, 1970.

197. Dash, H., Johnson, R.A., Dinsmore, R.E., et al.: Cardiomyopathic syndrome due to coronary artery disease. I. Relation to angiographic extent of coronary disease and to remote myocardial infarction. Br. Heart J. 39:733, 1977.

198. Dash, H., Johnson, R.A., Dinsmore, R.E., et al.: Syndromes of coronary artery disease in diabetics and non-diabetics. Circulation 49–50 (Suppl. III): 109, 1974.

199. Dodek, A., Kassebaum, D.G., Bristow, J.D.: Pulmonary edema in coronary-artery disease without cardiomegaly. Paradox of the stiff heart. N. Engl. J. Med. 286:1347, 1972.

200. Zoneraich, S., Zoneraich, O., Gupta, M.P.: Severe coronary artery disease masquerading as cardiomyopathy. Angiology 25:583, 1974.

201. D'Elia, J.A., Weinrauch, L.A., Healy, R.W., et al. Myocardial dysfunction without coronary artery disease in diabetic renal failure. Am. J. Cardiol. 43:193, 1979.
202. Axelrod, L.: Response of congestive heart failure to correction of hyperglycemia in the presence of diabetic nephropathy. N. Engl. J. Med. 293:1243, 1975.
203. Cox, M., Sterns, R.H., Singer, I.: The defense against hyperkalemia: the roles of insulin and aldosterone. N. Engl. J. Med. 299:525, 1978.
203a.Grunfeld, C., Chappell, D.A.: Hypokalemia and diabetes mellitus. Am. J. Med. 75:553, 1983.
204. Phillips, J., Spano, J., Burch, G.: Chaotic atrial mechanism. Am. Heart J. 78:179, 1969.
205. Kones, R.J., Phillips, J.H., Hersh, J.: Mechanism and management of chaotic atrial mechanism. Cardiology 59:92, 1974.
206. Gadboys, H.L., Wisoff, B.G., Litwak, R.S.: Surgical treatment of complete heartblock. J.A.M.A. 189:97, 1964.
206a.Johansson, B.W.: Adams-Stokes syndrome. A review and follow-up study of forty-two cases. Am. J. Cardiol. 8:76, 1961.
206b.Hasslacher, C., Wahl, P.: Diabetes prevalence in patients with bradycardia arrhythmias. Acta Diabetol. Lat. 14:229, 1977.
207. Korn, D., DeSanctis, R.W., Sell, S.: Massive calcification of the mitral annulus. A clinicopathological study of fourteen cases. N. Engl. J. Med. 267:900, 1962.
208. Perper, J.A., Kuller, L.H., Cooper, M.: Arteriosclerosis of coronary arteries in sudden unexpected deaths. Circulation 52 (Suppl. 3): 27, 1975.
209. Clinical predictors and characteristics of sudden coronary death syndrome. In: Proceedings of First U.S./USSR Symposium on Sudden Death. United States Health, Education and Welfare, United States Public Health Service, National Institutes of Health Publication No. (NIH) 78-1470, pp. 99-116, 1978.
210. Doyle, J.T., Kannel, W.B., McNamara, P.M., et al.: Factors related to suddenness of death from coronary disease—combined Albany & Framingham studies. Am. J. Cardiol. 37:1073, 1976.
211. Lown, B.: Cardiovascular collapse and sudden cardiac death. In: E. Braunwald (Ed.): Heart Disease. A Textbook of Cardiovascular Medicine. Philadelphia, W.B. Saunders, Co. 1980, pp. 778-817.
212. Bennett, T., Hosking, D.J., Hampton, J.R.: Cardiovascular control in diabetes mellitus. Br. Med. J. 2:585, 1975.
213. Bennett, T., Fenton, P.H., Fitton, D., et al.: Assessment of vagal control of the heart in diabetes. Measures of R-R interval variation under different conditions. Br. Heart J. 39:25, 1977.
214. Wheeler, T., Watkins, P.J.: Cardiac denervation in diabetes. Br. Med. J. 4:584, 1973.
215. Neubauer, B., Christensen, N.J.: Norepinephrine, epinephrine and dopamine contents of the cardiovascular system in long-term diabetics. Diabetes 25:6, 1976.
216. Gabbay, K.G.: The sorbitol pathway and the complications of diabetes. N. Engl. J. Med. 288:831, 1973.
217. Lloyd-Mostyn, R.H., Watkins, P.J.: Defective innervation of heart in diabetic autonomic neuropathy. Br. Med. J. 3:15, 1975.
218. Leon, D.F., Shaver, J.A., Leonard, J.J.: Reflex heart rate control in man. Am. Heart J. 80:729, 1970.
219. Fraser, D.M., Campbell, I.W., Ewing, D.J., et al.: Peripheral and autonomic nerve function in newly diagnosed diabetes mellitus. Diabetes 26:546, 1977.
219a.Hilsted, J.: Pathophysiology in diabetic autonomic neuropathy: cardiovascular, hormonal, and metabolic studies. Diabetes 31:730, 1982.
220. Bennett, T., Farquhar, I.K., Hosking, D.J., Hampton, J.R.: Assessment of methods for estimating autonomic nervous control of the heart in patients with diabetes mellitus. Diabetes 27:1167, 1978.
221. Cannom, D.S., Graham, A.F., Harrison, D.C.: Electrophysiological studies in the denervated transplanted human heart. Response to atrial pacing and atropine. Circ. Res. 32:268, 1973.
222. Carleton, R., Heller, S.J., Najafi, H., Clark, J.G.: Hemodynamic performance of a transplanted human heart. Circulation 40:447, 1969.
223. Friedman, S.A., Freiberg, P., Colton, J.: Vasomotor tone in diabetic neuropathy. Ann. Intern. Med. 77:353, 1972.
224. Cooper, T., Willman, V.L., Potter, L.T., Hanlon, C.R.: Pharmacologic responses of the denervated heart. In: A.N. Brest: Heart Substitutes: Mechanical and Transplant. Springfield, Charles C Thomas, 1966, pp. 247-253.
225. Cannom, D.S., Rider, A.K., Stinson, E.B., et al.: Electrophysiologic studies in the denervated transplanted human heart. Am. J. Cardiol. 36:859, 1975.
226. Garcia-Búnuel, L.: Cardiorespiratory arrest in diabetic autonomic neuropathy. (Letter.) Lancet 1:935, 1978.
227. Almog, C., Pik, A.: Acute myocardial infarction as a complication of diabetic neuropathy. J.A.M.A. 239:2782, 1978.
227a.Ewing, D.J., Campbell, I.W., Clarke, B.F.: Assessment of cardiovascular effects in diabetic autonomic neuropathy and prognostic implications. Ann. Intern. Med. 92:308, 1980.
228. Rubler, S., Dlugash, J., Yuceoglu, Y.Z., et al.: New type of cardiomyopathy associated with diabetic glomerulosclerosis. Am. J. Cardiol. 30:595, 1972.
229. Hamby, R.I., Zoneraich, S., Sherman, L.: Diabetic cardiomyopathy. JAMA 229:1749, 1974.
230. Hamby, R.I.: Primary myocardial disease. A prospective clinical and hemodynamic evaluation of 100 patients. Medicine 49:55, 1970.
231. Varnauskas, E., Ivemark, B., Paulin, S., Ryden, B.: Obscure cardiomyopathies with coronary artery changes. Am. J. Cardiol. 19:531, 1967.
232. Regan, T.J., Haider, B., Lyons, M.M.: Altered ventricular function and metabolism in diabetes mellitus. In: S. Zoneraich (Ed.): Diabetes and The Heart. Springfield, Charles C Thomas, 1978, pp. 123-136.
233. Regan, T.J., Lyons, M.M., Ahmed, S.S., et al.: Evidence for cardiomyopathy in family diabetes mellitus. J. Clin. Invest. 60:884, 1977.
234. Regan, T.J., Ettinger, P.O., Khan, M.I., et al: Altered myocardial function and metabolism in chronic diabetes mellitus without ischemia in dogs. Cir. Res. 35:222, 1974.
235. Seneviratne, B.I.: Diabetic cardiomyopathy: the preclinical phase. Br. Med. J. 1:1444, 1977.
236. Shapiro, L.M., Leatherdale, B.A., Mackinnon, J., Fletcher, R.F.: Left ventricular function in diabetes mellitus. II. Relation between clinical features and left ventricular function. Br. Heart J. 45:129, 1981.
237. McMillan, D.E.: Plasma protein changes, blood viscosity, and diabetic microangiopathy. Diabetes 25 (Suppl. 2):858, 1976.
238. Ditzel, J.: Oxygen transport impairment in diabetes. Diabetes 25 (Suppl. 2): 832, 1976.
239. Williamson, J.R., Kilo, C.: Current status of capillary basement-membrane disease in diabetes mellitus. Diabetes 26:65, 1977.
240. Pearce, M.B., Bulloch, R.T., Kizziar, J.C.: Myocardial small vessel disease in patients with diabetes mellitus. Circulation 48: (Suppl.): IV-6, 1973.
241. Zoneraich, S., Silverman, G.: Myocardial small vessel

disease in diabetic patients. In: S. Zoneraich (Ed): Diabetes and the Heart. Springfield, Charles C Thomas, 1978, pp. 3–18.

242. Ledet, T.: Histological and histochemical changes in the coronary arteries of old diabetic patients. Diabetologia 4:268, 1968.

243. Crall, F.V., Jr., Roberts, W.C.: The extramural and intramural coronary arteries in juvenile diabetes mellitus: analysis of nine necropsy patients aged 19 to 38 years with onset of diabetes before age 15 years. Am. J. Med. 64:221, 1978.

244. Bunn, H.F., Gabbay, K.H., Gallop, P.M.: The glycosylation of hemoglobin: relevance to diabetes mellitus. Science 200:21, 1978.

244a. Regan, T.J., Haider, B., Lyons, M.M.: Altered ventricular function and metabolism in diabetes mellitus. In: S. Zoneraich (Ed.): Diabetes and the Heart. Springfield, Charles C Thomas, 1978, p. 127.

244b. Shapiro, L.M., Howat, A.P., Calter, M.M.: Left ventricular function in diabetes mellitus. I. Methodology and prevalence and spectrum of abnormalities. Br. Heart J. 45:122, 1981.

245. Zoneraich, S., Zoneraich, O., Rhee, J.J.: The electrocardiogram in diabetic patients without clinically apparent heart disease: echocardiographic correlations. In: S. Zoneraich (Ed.): Diabetes and the Heart. Springfield, Charles C Thomas, 1978, pp. 57–65.

246. Zoneraich, O., Zoneraich, S.: A vectorcardiographic study of spatial P, QRS, and T-loops in diabetic patients without clinically apparent heart disease. In: S. Zoneraich (Ed.): Diabetes and the Heart. Springfield, Charles C Thomas, 1978, pp. 66–77.

247. Metzger, C.C., Chough, C.B., Kroetz, F.W., et al.: True isovolumic contraction time. Its correlation with two external indices of ventricular performance. Am. J. Cardiol. 25:434, 1970.

248. Lewis, R.P., Boudoulas, H., Welch, T.G., et al.: Usefulness of systolic time intervals in coronary artery disease. Am. J. Cardiol. 37:787, 1976.

249. Ahmed, S.S., Jaferi, G.A., Narang, R.M., et al.: Preclinical abnormality of left ventricular function in diabetes mellitus. Am. Heart J. 89:153, 1975.

250. Rynkiewicz, A., Semetkowska-Jurkiewicz, E., Wyrzy-kowski, B.: Systolic and diastolic time intervals in young diabetics. Br. Heart J. 44:280, 1980.

251. Rubler, S., Sajadi, R.M., Araoye, M.A., Holford, F.D.: Noninvasive estimation of myocardial performance in patients with diabetes. Effect of alcohol administration. Diabetes 27:127, 1978.

252. Sykes, C.A., Wright, A.D., Malins, J.M., et al.: Changes in systolic time intervals during treatment of diabetes mellitus. Br. Heart J. 39:255, 1977.

253. Shapiro, L.M., Leatherdale, B.A., Coyne, M.E., et al.: Prospective study of heart disease in untreated maturity onset diabetics. Br. Heart J. 44:342, 1980.

254. Sanderson, J.E., Brown, D.J., Rivellese, A., Kohner, E.: Diabetic cardiomyopathy? An echocardiographic study of young diabetics. Br. Med. J. 1:404, 1978.

255. Abenavoli, T., Rubler, S., Fisher, V.J., et al.: Exercise testing with myocardial scintigraphy in asymptomatic diabetic males. Circulation 63:54, 1981.

255a. Lababidi, Z.A., Goldstein, D.E.: High prevalence of echocardiographic abnormalities in diabetic youths. Diabetes Care 6:18, 1983.

256. Powell, L.W., Isselbacher, K.J.: Hemachromatosis. In: K.J. Isselbacher, R.D. Adams, E. Braunwald, et al. (Eds.): Harrison's Principles of Internal Medicine, 9th Ed. New York, McGraw-Hill Book Co., 1980, pp. 488–491.

257. Radtke, W.E., Kazmier, F.J., Rutherford, B.D., Sheps, S.G.: Cardiovascular complications of pheochromocytoma crisis. Am. J. Cardiol. 35:701, 1975.

258. Melby, J.C.: Systemic corticosteroid therapy: pharmacology and endocrinologic considerations. Ann. Intern. Med. 81:505, 1974.

259. McGuffin, W.L., Sherman, B.M., Roth, J., et al.: Acromegaly and cardiovascular disorders. A prospective study. Ann. Intern. Med. 81:11, 1974.

260. Adams, R.D., Bradley, W.G., Rebeiz, J.J.: Progressive muscular dystrophy. In: K.J. Isselbacher, R.D. Adams, E. Braunwald, et al. (Eds.): Harrison's Principles of Internal Medicine, Ninth Ed. New York, McGraw-Hill Book Company, 1980, p. 2062.

261. Wolfe, R.R., Way, G.L.: Cardiomyopathies in infants of diabetic mothers. Johns Hopkins Med. J. 140:177, 1977.

262. Gutsegell, H.P., Speer, M.E., Rosenberg, H.S.: Characterization of the cardiomyopathy in infants of diabetic mothers. Circulation 61:441, 1980.

28 Hypertension in the Diabetic Patient

A. Richard Christlieb

Of the currently recognized risk factors for cardiovascular disease, hypertension and diabetes mellitus appear to be the best indicators in predicting cardiovascular morbidity and mortality. Their coexistence in the same patient compounds the risk for cardiovascular events as clearly demonstrated by the results of the Framingham Study.[1-3] The processes leading to coronary heart disease, stroke, peripheral vascular disease, and congestive heart failure are all accelerated in the hypertensive compared with the normotensive diabetic. This adverse effect of hypertension in the diabetic is not limited to the major arteries. Both nephropathy and retinopathy may also be accelerated when hypertension is present.

Recently, we reported a longitudinal assessment of a homogeneous population of insulin dependent diabetic patients with the onset of diabetes under age 21 who were first seen at the Joslin Clinic in 1939 within 1 year of the onset of diabetes.[4] These patients were followed until death or through 1980. Ninety percent survived to 20 years of diabetes, 77% to 30 years, and 46% to 40 years. These survival rates exceed those generally recorded from cross-sectional data. Coronary heart disease deaths accounted for 48% of the mortality and renal deaths for 31%, but most of these patients had both coronary and renal disease. Cardiac deaths were spread over the complete age spectrum, whereas renal deaths occurred between the ages of 30 and 45 years. Hypertension was present in all patients dying a renal death and in all but 3 patients dying a coronary heart disease death. Hypertension was rarely observed in the survivors, a significant difference from both the cardiac and renal death groups. In these patients, neither smoking nor blood lipid abnormalities appeared to add significantly to the risk, presumably because of the overwhelming impact of the hypertension.

From the data currently available, it is estimated that hypertension is approximately twice as common in the diabetic as in the nondiabetic population.[5] This estimate is derived from population surveys, many of which have inherent deficiencies. Generally, blood pressure measurements were not well standardized, control data were infrequently used, and the diabetic population was incompletely sampled. Further, diastolic hypertension was generally not differentiated from systolic hypertension.

To further evaluate the prevalence of hypertension in the diabetic population, approximately 1000 Joslin Clinic patients were studied under standardized conditions.[4] So that comparison could be made with data from the general population as recorded in the Framingham population[6] and in the United States Survey of Hypertension,[7] hypertension was defined as a blood pressure of greater than 160/95 mm Hg, a conservative definition by current standards. In all age groups with diabetes from 0 to 10 years or from 15 to 25 years' duration, the prevalence of hypertension was significantly higher and in females and older males was generally twice that of the comparative populations. Such studies leave little question that hypertension is more prevalent in the diabetic than in the nondiabetic population.

One must therefore question what etiologic factors are instrumental in increasing the prevalence of hypertension in the diabetic. Some surgically curable forms of hypertension are associated with impaired glucose tolerance and could be expected to be found frequently in diabetics. This does not occur. Cushing's disease, primary aldosteronism and pheochromocytoma are not found with any greater frequency in the diabetic than in the non-diabetic population. Acceleration of the athero-sclerotic process results in a high incidence of an-atomic stenosis in the renal arteries of diabetics.[8] Despite this, hypertension due to physiologically significant renal artery stenosis may be no more common in diabetics than in nondiabetics.[9] There-fore, it must be postulated either that the multiple mechanisms responsible for hypertension in the nondiabetic occur with greater frequency in dia-betics or that additional mechanisms are involved in the hypertensive process in diabetes. Further, diastolic hypertension must be differentiated from systolic hypertension and the mechanisms involved in each process discussed separately.

The level of blood pressure is governed by the cardiac output and the degree of peripheral vascular resistance. Cardiac output is affected by many fac-tors including stroke volume, heart rate, myocar-dial contractility, blood volume, and the degree of venous tone which regulates venous return to the right side of the heart. Factors affecting peripheral vascular resistance include anatomic changes in the microvasculature and the numerous vasoactive sub-stances which are known as the vasopressor and vasodepressor hormones. Although much knowl-edge has been accumulated concerning these fac-tors in normotension and in hypertension, the pre-cise abnormalities involved in the hypertensive process remain largely undefined. An increase in cardiac output with peripheral vascular resistance remaining unchanged will result in elevated blood pressure. Similarly, increased peripheral vascular resistance with no change in blood volume or car-diac output will also result in increased pressure. There are some data suggesting that an imbalance between vasopressor mechanisms such as the renin-angiotensin-aldosterone system and catechol-amines, and the vasodepressor factors such as cer-tain prostaglandins and the kallikrein system may result in diastolic hypertension through alterations in peripheral vascular resistance. To date, most research in this area in the hypertensive diabetic population has involved the renin-angiotensin-al-dosterone system and catecholamines. These hor-mones appear to be normally responsive in patients with uncomplicated diabetes but are often abnor-mally decreased when the diabetes is complicated by hypertension and nephropathy or neuropathy.

Systolic hypertension, so frequently observed especially in the elderly diabetic population, is etiologically related to the accelerated rate of ath-erosclerosis. As will be discussed, systolic hyper-tension may be of three different types. Orthostatic

hypotension, associated with either normal or el-evated supine blood pressures, occurs when most or all of the factors involved in the maintenance of upright blood pressure fail.

In this chapter, the current state of the art con-cerning the pathophysiology involved in each of the types of hypertension encountered in the dia-betic population will be discussed (Table 28–1). Using this knowledge of pathophysiology, a ra-tional approach to therapy based upon the mech-anisms of action of various antihypertensive agents will be presented.

PATHOPHYSIOLOGY

Diastolic Hypertension

Diastolic hypertension occurs when the periph-eral vascular resistance is disproportionately ele-vated in relation to the cardiac output and the blood volume. Generally, the systolic pressure is elevated proportionately, thus maintaining the pulse pres-sure near normal. Of the vasoactive hormones reg-ulating peripheral vascular resistance, only the renin-angiotensin system and catecholamines have been studied in patients with diabetes mellitus. Understanding the alterations in these systems which are observed in diabetics with diastolic el-evations of the blood pressure is important in a rational approach to antihypertensive therapy. Prior to reviewing these alterations, it seems appropriate to review the function of the renin-angiotensin-aldosterone system in normal physiology.

The maintenance of normal fluid and electrolyte balance and blood pressure at precise levels is de-pendent in part upon alterations in the activity of the renin-angiotensin-aldosterone system. Renin it-self is an enzyme which is produced in the juxta-glomerular cells of the kidney. Upon release from these cells, this enzyme cleaves a polypeptide from a large protein called renin substrate which is made in the liver. The resultant decapeptide, known as angiotensin I, is essentially inactive and remains in the circulation only transiently. Angiotensin I is converted to the octapeptide, angiotensin II, by an

Table 28–1.   Hypertension in Diabetes Mellitus

Diabetes without nephropathy
1) "Essential" hypertension
2) Systolic hypertension
    a) Isolated
    b) Inappropriately elevated diastolic pressure
    c) Elevated diastolic pressure
Diabetes with nephropathy
    Renal ("diabetic") hypertension
Diabetes with neuropathy
    Supine hypertension with orthostatic hypotension

enzyme which is found in abundance in the pulmonary circulation. Angiotensin II is the active peptide which increases peripheral vascular resistance through vasoconstriction and stimulates the secretion of aldosterone from the adrenal cortex. The potent mineralocorticoid effect of aldosterone promotes sodium retention and potassium excretion at the level of the distal renal tubule. Normally, sodium retention is accompanied by water retention. Therefore an increase in aldosterone produces extracellular fluid expansion including expansion of the plasma volume. By contrast, a deficiency of aldosterone will result in natriuresis, decreased plasma volume, and potassium retention.

The mechanisms responsible for the release of renin are multiple and their order of dominance is incompletely defined. A few such mechanisms include changes in blood volume, blood pressure, posture, sympathetic vasomotor activity, renal tubular sodium concentration, and total body sodium balance. Probably all are interrelated in effecting changes in the release of renin, but blood volume is a major factor. Simply stated, an increase in volume suppresses and a decrease in volume stimulates the activity of this system. This concept is helpful in understanding the alterations in the function of this system in diabetics with associated hypertension.

Hypertension without Renal Disease

In diabetics with hypertension but no renal disease, plasma renin activity generally is normal. As discussed, volume depletion will usually result in stimulation of renin activity. Despite such stimulating maneuvers as sodium depletion and upright posture, a small sub-group of these patients have low renin activity[10,11] (Fig. 28–1). Low plasma renin activity under similar conditions has been observed repeatedly in from 20 to 30% of persons with essential hypertension. Elevated renin activity is uncommon in both groups. These similarities in renin activity between nondiabetic patients with essential hypertension and hypertensive diabetic patients without clinical evidence of renal disease, suggest either one of two possibilities. First, the hypertension in this group of diabetics may be essential hypertension, i.e. the result of alterations of blood pressure homeostatic mechanisms which are similar to those in the nondiabetic hypertensive population. Second, factors associated with the altered glucose metabolism in the diabetic may initiate the hypertensive process and subsequently decrease renin activity.

The first hypothesis is supported by observations that the prevalence of hypertension increases between the ages of 30 and 50 years in the diabetic just as in the nondiabetic population. Additionally,

hypertension is especially prevalent in patients with noninsulin-dependent diabetes. Frequently the hypertension precedes the diagnosis of diabetes mellitus. In other patients, hypertension is diagnosed soon after the diabetes is discovered. Such proximity of the two diagnoses renders it unlikely that altered glucose metabolism is responsible for initiating the hypertension. These observations together with those concerning plasma renin activity suggest that the hypertension may be of the essential type and therefore do not explain the increased prevalence in diabetics.

The second hypothesis relates to factors associated with abnormal glucose metabolism which may cause the hypertension. It is clear that in many nondiabetic patients with hypertension, an expanded blood volume with increased cardiac output is the initiating factor. Later, vasoconstriction sustains the chronic phase of hypertension. Blood volume expansion could explain the genesis of hypertension in diabetics, especially in those whose onset of hypertension occurs several years following the diagnosis of diabetes. Studies have shown that hyperglycemia is associated with hypervolemia in diabetic rats[12] and very likely in humans with poorly controlled but non-ketotic diabetes.[13] Further, such patients have an increased total body sodium.[11] These observations can readily be explained. The osmotic effect of elevated glucose in the extracellular fluid compartment results in expansion of this space at the expense of intracellular dehydration. Blood volume expansion therefore occurs with hyperglycemia as long as the fluid intake remains adequate to compensate for the fluid losses in the urine. Another possible cause for blood volume expansion is hyperinsulinemia itself, which enhances renal tubular sodium absorption.[13a] This volume expansion over a prolonged period could result in increased cardiac output and hypertension, especially in those whose diabetes is chronically under poor control. Both the increased prevalence of hypertension and the suppression of renin activity in a certain subsegment of this hypertensive diabetic population can be explained by this hypothesis.

Using either hypothesis, it appears that in the hypertensive diabetic population without clinically significant renal disease, the hypertension may be the result of altered blood pressure homeostatic mechanisms similar to those initiating hypertension in the nondiabetic population. This then would be "essential hypertension." Treatment of these patients therefore would be similar to that proposed for the treatment of nondiabetic persons with essential hypertension. In practice, this group clearly responds to antihypertensive regimens similar to

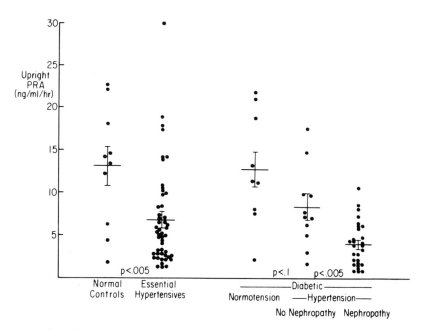

Fig. 28–1. Comparison of upright plasma renin activity (PRA) in non-diabetic and diabetic subjects. Mean PRA is normal in normotensive subjects and is decreased in non-diabetics with essential hypertension and in diabetics with hypertension but no nephropathy. Hypertensive diabetics with nephropathy all have low or low normal PRA. (Used with permission of the author and publisher.[10])

those used for essential hypertension in nondiabetic individuals.

Hypertension with Nephropathy

Diabetic glomerulosclerosis with the clinical syndrome known as diabetic nephropathy occurs eventually in virtually all persons with onset of diabetes early in life. Diabetic nephropathy remains a major problem even in diabetics with the onset of their disease following the age of 40. Hypertension almost universally accompanies diabetic nephropathy and clearly is etiologically related to the renal disease and therefore is a true "diabetic hypertension."

The histologic, histochemical, and histoimmunologic characteristics of diabetic nephropathy are discussed in Chapter 30. Diffuse glomerulosclerosis is the histologic lesion most frequently found in the clinical syndrome of diabetic nephropathy and therefore is the lesion that correlates best with the associated hypertension.[14] Associated arteriolar hyalinization involving the afferent arteriole results in a decreased diameter of the arteriolar lumen, thus increasing peripheral vascular resistance. This pathologic process may be the major event that initiates the hypertension in diabetics with nephropathy.

Diffuse glomerulosclerosis and narrowing of the lumen of the afferent arterioles are not the only abnormalities involved in hypertension associated with nephropathy. Alterations have also been noted in the function of the renin-angiotensin-aldosterone system. In diabetic patients with clinical nephropathy defined as greater than 2 g of protein in the urine daily, both plasma renin activity[10] and plasma aldosterone[15] are significantly decreased (Figs. 28–1 and 28–2). Several mechanisms have been studied which may be involved in decreasing the renin activity in such patients. (1). Progression of the nephropathy decreases free water clearance, resulting in elevated blood volume. Hyperglycemia if inadequately treated results in hyperosmolality and further elevates the blood volume. This increased volume is sensed by the kidney and results in a suppression of renin release. (2). The hyalinization in the afferent arteriole accounts for decreased renin activity. This hyalinization can produce a barrier between the juxtaglomerular cells and the arteriolar lumen, preventing the release of renin into the circulation,[16] or can destroy the juxtaglomerular cells.[5] (3). Diabetics with nephropathy may have defective synthesis of renin. In these patients, much of the renin is a relatively inactive, high molecular weight substance which has been termed "big renin" or "pro-renin."[17,18] Large amounts of pro-renin are frequently present with either low or normal levels of circulating renin activity. (4). Both circulating and locally released catecholamines may be decreased. In diabetics with neuropathy, plasma levels of catecholamines are

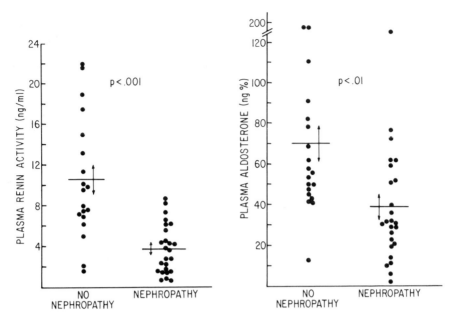

Fig. 28–2. Plasma renin activity (left panel) and plasma aldosterone (right panel) in diabetic patients with and without nephropathy. (Used with permission of the author and publisher.[15a])

distinctly low.[11,19] Additionally, increased vascular reactivity to exogenous norepinephrine has been observed in patients with diabetic retinopathy.[20] Such an observation suggests that there may be at least partial autonomic denervation. These defects will result in decreased catecholamine stimulation of renin release.

The amount of sodium reaching the renal tubule at the level of the macula densa also plays a role in regulating renin release. In the diabetic with a glucose osmotic diuresis, changes in the renal tubular sodium could be expected to result in a decrease in renin release and renin activity. This hypothesis was tested comparing alloxan-treated diabetic rats with phlorhizin-treated renal glycosuric rats.[21] Although the two groups of animals had similar glucose osmotic diureses, the diabetic rats had decreased renin activity, whereas the phlorhizin treated rats had elevated renin activity. These results sugsest that a glucose osmotic diuresis does not decrease renin activity.

It is clear that hypertension associated with diabetic nephropathy is a "low renin hypertension" with several mechanisms acting to decrease the renin. What then are the mechanisms causing the increased blood pressure? Both cardiac output and peripheral vascular resistance are elevated. Cardiac output is elevated secondary to increased blood volume due to decreased free water clearance and the accelerated heart rate resulting from the anemia of renal failure. Peripheral vascular resistance is increased secondary to the renal arteriolar hyalin-ization which decreases the diameter of the arteriolar lumen.

With a progressive increase in both cardiac output and peripheral vascular resistance, a rapid acceleration of the blood pressure could be expected. Frequently the hypertension does become severe but an occasional patient will remain normotensive, suggesting that compensatory mechanisms are operative. The low renin activity and aldosterone provide such a mechanism (Fig. 28–3). Low renin activity is generally associated with low circulating levels of angiotensen II. Such a deficiency together with low circulating catecholamines would therefore decrease peripheral vascular resistance. The low angiotensin II would also decrease aldosterone release. If sensed by the distal renal tubule of the diseased kidney, this hypoaldosteronism would provide natriuresis followed by a decrease in plasma volume.

Therefore, through deficiencies of these hormones, hypotensive mechanisms are present to compensate for those processes which elevate the blood pressure.[22] Maintenance of normal blood pressure will be sustained as long as the hypotensive mechanisms can balance the hypertensive ones. With progressive deterioration of renal function, however, free water clearance will continue to decrease, thus increasing blood volume, and cardiac output and peripheral vascular resistance will continue to increase. Hypertension then is the result of these mechanisms exceeding those of an antihypertensive nature.

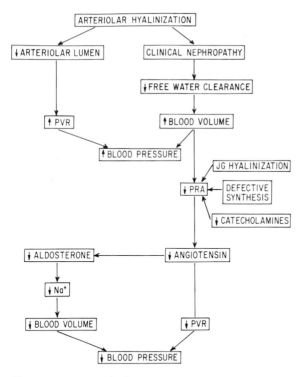

Fig. 28–3. Proposed schema depicting the factors tending to increase the blood pressure (upper section) and those tending to decrease the blood pressure (lower section) in patients with diabetic nephropathy. When the antihypertensive factors can no longer compensate for those increasing the blood pressure, hypertension results. PVR = peripheral vascular resistance. JG = juxtaglomerular. PRA = plasma renin activity. (Used with permission of the author and publisher.[22])

Classical malignant hypertension is distinctly rare in patients with diabetic nephropathy. This can be explained by the low renin activity and angiotensin II which usually are markedly elevated in malignant hypertension. However, accelerated hypertension including hypertensive encephalopathy may be observed.

Although the low renin activity and low aldosterone may serve as compensatory mechanisms minimizing the hypertension in patients with diabetic nephropathy, the hypoaldosteronism has the potential for producing life-threatening hyperkalemia. The two major factors controlling potassium homeostasis in normal physiology are (1) mineralocorticoids and (2) glucose and insulin. A severe deficiency of aldosterone can result in hyperkalemia in patients without renal disease and this is exaggerated if renal disease is present. The presence of diabetes further complicates the situation. When both aldosterone and insulin deficiency are present, acute infusions of glucose will result in hyperkalemia.[23] With the prior administration of desoxycorticosterone acetate and adequate replace-

ment of insulin, the hyperkalemic response is abolished. Further, poor control of the diabetes in such patients will frequently result in hyperkalemia which is reversed with adequate diabetic control.[15] Such studies emphasize both the independent and the combined effects of insulin and aldosterone in regulating serum potassium and stress the necessity of adequate insulin therapy in patients with hypertension associated with diabetic nephropathy and hypoaldosteronism. It is of interest that despite hypoaldosteronism, the serum sodium is frequently normal or only mildly decreased.

Systolic Hypertension

Elevated systolic pressure can be present in several nondiabetic conditions including the hyperkinetic heart syndrome and in hypermetabolic states such as anemia, hyperthyroidism, and in Paget's disease where arteriovenous shunting occurs. When such conditions are eliminated as diagnostic possibilities, systolic hypertension in the diabetic may be of three types: (1). Isolated systolic hypertension in which there is an elevation in the systolic pressure with either a low or low normal diastolic pressure. This produces a widening of the pulse pressure with the mean blood pressure maintained at normal or near-normal levels. (2). Elevation in systolic pressure associated with a normal diastolic pressure. Here both the pulse pressure and the mean blood pressure are elevated, suggesting that the diastolic pressure is disproportionately elevated. (3). Systolic hypertension accompanied by an elevated diastolic pressure with the mean pressure significantly elevated.

Regardless of the type of systolic hypertension encountered, the etiology of the elevated systolic pressure is the same, a loss of major arterial elasticity associated with the atherosclerotic process. It is this elastic property of major vessels (compliance) that allows for sudden changes in volume occurring during the phases of the cardiac cycle. The large arteries will normally expand during systole in order to accommodate the abrupt increase in intra-arterial volume resulting from ejection of blood from the heart. This expansion limits the degree to which systolic pressure will be elevated. The vessels then contract as blood passes through the arteriolar system thus maintaining intra-arterial volume and pressure. With progressive atherosclerosis in the diabetic, the large arteries lose their elasticity and gradually become rigid. Any given volume of blood ejected from the left ventricle will enter an arterial system which, to a greater or less degree, is incapable of expanding. The systolic pressure will thus be increased.

The diastolic pressure is determined by the degree of resistance in the arteriolar system. Vasoconstriction of these resistance vessels will increase and vasodilatation will decrease the diastolic pressure. The mean blood pressure is determined by both the systolic and the diastolic pressures. Therefore, in order for the mean blood pressure to remain normal in the presence of an elevated systolic pressure, peripheral vascular resistance must decrease, thus lowering the diastolic pressure. In isolated systolic hypertension, this condition prevails. Should both the cardiac output and the peripheral resistance remain constant in the presence of an elevated systolic pressure, the mean blood pressure increases. In this situation, although the diastolic pressure may be within acceptable limits of normal, the peripheral vascular resistance is inappropriately elevated. A disproportionately high systolic pressure together with an elevated diastolic pressure implies a definite increase in peripheral vascular resistance. Cardiac output must then increase, resulting in a further increase in systolic pressure in order to maintain flow through the arteriolar bed to the capillaries.

Orthostatic Hypotension

This is common in patients with diabetes both with or without supine hypertension. Sometimes it is observed in patients with diabetic nephropathy, especially in its early stages. More frequently, it is encountered in those with neuropathy involving both the peripheral and autonomic nervous systems.

Maintenance of the erect blood pressure involves the integrity of multiple blood pressure homeostatic mechanisms. Among these are the baroceptor reflexes, various vasoactive hormones, cardiac output, and blood volume. Because these mechanisms compensate for one another, it is unlikely that a compromise in the function of any one will result in orthostatic hypotension. However, should several of the mechanisms be compromised simultaneously as may occur in the diabetic population, an inability to maintain the erect posture will ensue. Baroceptor reflexes are frequently blunted in patients with neuropathy.[24] Circulating catecholamines generally are low.[19,25] Some diabetic patients with orthostatic hypotension, however, may have normal or elevated circulating catecholamines but vascular resistance to these vasopressors limits their effectiveness.[25] The renin-angiotensin-aldosterone system is low and cannot be normally stimulated.[11,26] In patients with neuropathy, hypoalbuminemia secondary to urinary protein losses may occur prior to any clinically significant compromise in renal function. A contracted plasma volume ensues. Severe coronary heart disease or diabetic cardiomyopathy may result in decreased myocardial contractility and a decrease in cardiac output.

Therefore, in the diabetic population, each of these mechanisms responsible for the maintenance of upright blood pressure may be compromised. The combined deficiency in these mechanisms in any given individual will result in orthostatic hypotension.

THERAPY

Few studies are available to evaluate the effect of antihypertensive therapy on cardiovascular morbidity and mortality in the diabetic population. In assessing the effect of such therapy, it is necessary therefore to extrapolate from the results of studies in the general hypertensive population. Although this is not a scientific approach, it is reasonable considering the increased rate of development of vascular disease in diabetics which is further increased when hypertension is present.

The results of both animal and human studies attest to the fact that hypertension accelerates both macrovascular and microvascular disease. In animals treated with diets containing varying amounts of cholesterol, the atherosclerosis process is further increased with higher dietary cholesterol content and a further increase occurs when hypertension is present.[27] Microvascular disease is accelerated in diabetic rats in the presence of hypertension. This was demonstrated by creating Goldblatt hypertension.[28] Compared with kidneys of normotensive diabetic rats, the protected kidneys showed decreased diabetic glomerular changes, whereas the unprotected kidneys demonstrated accelerated changes. More recently, Mogensen has reported that appropriate antihypertensive therapy can delay the progression of renal failure,[28a] a finding confirmed by Parving et al.[28b]

The Framingham Study,[29] in which approximately 5,000 men and women were involved, documented the detrimental effect of hypertension on morbidity and mortality. Cardiovascular events were clearly dependent on the level of blood pressure. Surprisingly, the systolic blood pressure was found to be as reliable as the diastolic or mean blood pressure in predicting these events which included heart failure, myocardial infarction, stroke and peripheral vascular disease. The risk was incremental, increasing with increasing levels of blood pressure. Further analysis of the data demonstrated that in patients with diabetes, these morbid events were increased in the presence of hypertension.[3]

As previously discussed, systolic hypertension results from major arterial atherosclerosis. The Framingham results suggest that the hypertension itself has the potential to accelerate the atherosclerotic process. Such will result in further decreases in arterial compliance and further increases in the systolic blood pressure. In addition to the adverse effects of systolic hypertension on the coronary arteries, the overall cardiac effect must be considered. The greatest amount of work performed by the heart occurs during cardiac systole. With elevations of the systolic pressure, myocardial energy requirements are exaggerated and result in increased oxygen demands and utilization. When continued for a prolonged period of time, myocardial failure is often the end result.

Results of studies in the nondiabetic hypertensive population suggest that anti-hypertensive therapy is beneficial in decreasing the incidence of cardiovascular morbidity and mortality in certain segments of this population. Probably the Veterans Administration Cooperative Study is the best known in this field.[30] Patients with moderately severe hypertension (diastolic blood pressure 115 to 130 mm Hg) were followed for 3 years. Severe complicating events occurred in 43% of placebo-treated patients but in only 3% of those receiving antihypertensive therapy. Obviously, this was a high risk population initially. The results, however, document the benefit of lowering the blood pressure pharmacologically.

Although the Veterans Administration data are not conclusive for patients with diastolic pressures between 90 and 104 mm Hg,[31] antihypertensive therapy did provide significant protection against cardiovascular events in patients over the age of 60 years.[32] Recently, however, the 5-year results of the Hypertension Detection and Follow-up Program have been reported and clearly demonstrate the value of antihypertensive therapy for patients with diastolic blood pressures between 90 and 104 mm Hg.[33] Of the almost 8000 patients with this level of blood pressure, one half were assigned to a "stepped care" systematic antihypertensive program. The goal of therapy was a reduction in diastolic blood pressure to less than 90 mm Hg in those with a diastolic blood pressure of more than 100 or a 10 mm Hg decrease for those with a diastolic blood pressure between 90 and 100 mm Hg. The other half were referred to their usual physicians for standard antihypertensive treatment. In the stepped care group, there were 45% fewer deaths attributed to cerebrovascular disease and 46% fewer deaths from acute myocardial infarction. For all cardiovascular diseases, there were 26% fewer deaths in the stepped care compared with the referred care group. One can anticipate that larger differences would have resulted had the patients receiving stepped care been compared with a placebo-treated group.

To date, there are no reports of the results of studies to assess the effect of antihypertensive therapy in patients with isolated systolic hypertension or in those with systolic hypertension associated with a normal (inappropriately elevated) diastolic pressure.

Hypertension is a chronic disease. The effects on the vascular system are not evident until hypertension has been present for many years. Considering the accelerated vascular disease, hypertension must be treated early and aggressively, especially when superimposed upon diabetes.

Treatment of the diabetic patient with hypertension is complex and involves more than the routine use of antihypertensive drugs. Familiarity with the underlying pathophysiology in each of the types of hypertension is necessary in prescribing a rational therapeutic program. It is also essential to be familiar with the treatment of diabetes and its many complications. Complications such as diabetic cardiomyopathy, coronary heart disease, cerebral vascular disease, nephropathy, neuropathy with orthostatic hypotension and impotence all may present specific problems with antihypertensive drugs.

Mechanism of Action and Complications of Antihypertensive Drugs in the Diabetic

Before assuming the responsibility for antihypertensive therapy in patients with diabetes mellitus, it is important that the physician have an understanding of the mechanisms decreasing blood pressure and of the various adverse effects of antihypertensive drugs as they relate to diabetics. Certainly these drugs can aggravate hyperglycemia and hypoglycemia, electrolyte imbalance, heart and cerebrovascular disease, and neuropathic symptoms. A brief overview of these complications is presented in Table 28–2.

Diuretic Drugs

Although the mechanism of antihypertensive action of these drugs is not clear, acutely they cause a decrease in plasma volume. Chronically, because of intra-arteriolar sodium depletion, vascular responsiveness to endogenous vasopressors is blunted.

One well-recognized complication of both the thiazide and the "loop" (furosemide and ethacrynic acid) diuretic drugs is hypokalemia which may at times suppress insulin release.[34,35] Therefore, in diabetics who are not dependent on exogenous insulin and whose diabetes is controlled with either diet alone or with diet and oral glucose-lowering agents, treatment with these diuretics may decrease glucose tolerance and result in hyperglycemia. This complication should not be observed in patients with total insulin dependence. Should hyperglycemia be associated with diuretic-induced

Table 28–2.   Antihypertensive Drug Complications in Diabetic Patients*

Drug	Possible Complications
Diuretics	
A. potassium losing	
1. thiazides	Hypercholesterolemia
2. furosemide	Hyperglycemia in insulin-dependent diabetes
3. ethacrynic acid	
B. potassium sparing	
1. spironolactone	Hyperkalemia with cardiac arrhythmias
2. triamterene	
3. amiloride	
Alpha adrenergic inhibitors	
A. prazosin	Orthostatic hypotension
Beta adrenergic blocking drugs	
A. propranolol	Heart failure
B. metoprolol	Prolongation of recovery from hypoglycemia
C. nadolol	Obscuring of symptoms of hypoglycemia
D. atenolol	Hypertension during hypoglycemia
E. timolol	Hyperosmolar coma (one report)
F. pindolol	Aggravation of peripheral vascular disease
Sympathetic inhibitors	
A. methyldopa	Orthostatic hypotension
B. clonidine	Impotence
C. reserpine	
D. guanethidine	
Vasodilators	
A. hydralazine	Aggravation of coronary heart disease
B. minoxidil	Excessive hair growth
Converting Enzyme Inhibitor	
A. captopril	Proteinuria
	Renal failure

*See appropriate texts or Physician's Desk Reference for complete information regarding drug complications.

hypokalemia, potassium supplementation or the addition of a potassium-sparing diuretic such as spironolactone or triamterene will generally reverse the abnormality. There is, however, some evidence that the thiazides may cause a decrease in glucose tolerance independent of a hypokalemic action.[36] Further studies are necessary before this concept can be accepted.

Thiazide diuretics have been reported to elevate serum cholesterol.[37] Whether this elevation is sufficient to accelerate further the atherosclerotic process remains to be determined. These drugs are generally an integral part of any antihypertensive program and this potential complication should not preclude their use.

The potassium-sparing diuretics, spironolactone, triamterene, and amiloride should not be used in patients with nephropathy accompanied by azotemia. Furthermore, they should not be used in the occasional patient with hypoaldosteronism. When used in either group of patients, they may precipitate severe hyperkalemia with associated cardiac arrhythmias.

Alpha-Adrenergic Blocking Drugs

Prazosin has been used in the United States for antihypertensive therapy since 1976. Original studies suggested that it, like hydralazine, acted as a direct vasodilator. Subsequent studies, however, show that its action in reducing peripheral vascular resistance is through blockade of vascular alpha adrenergic mechanisms.[38] Because its antihypertensive effect is striking when compared with another alpha adrenergic blocker, phentolamine, it is probable that prazosin acts through other mechanisms also. In addition to decreasing peripheral vascular resistance, it affects the capacitance side of the circulation, causing venous dilatation and decreased return of blood to the right heart. Because of this, little change in cardiac output occurs. This is a distinct advantage over the direct vasodilator, hydralazine, in many patients. Generally, prazosin should be used in conjunction with a diuretic and often with a beta adrenergic blocking agent. Severe orthostatic hypotension may occur, especially following the first dose of this drug or when the dosage has been increased. It is important to initiate treatment with the smaller dose and to warn patients of this potential side effect. It is advisable for the patient to remain supine for 5 to 6 hours following the first dose.

Beta-Adrenergic Blocking Drugs

There are two types of beta adrenergic blocking drugs. The nonselective beta blockers, such as propranolol, timolol, pindolol, and nadolol, will block the beta 1 and the beta 2 adrenergic receptors. Cardioselective beta blockers, such as metoprolol and atenolol, when used in low dosages, will block selectively the beta 1 receptors. With high doses, however, selectivity may be lost and the beta 2 receptors may also be blocked.

There are several antihypertensive mechanisms that account for the effectiveness of these drugs. First, they decrease cardiac output by decreasing myocardial contractility through competitive antagonism of catecholamines on the adrenergic receptor sites. Second, they decrease plasma renin activity, thereby decreasing angiotensin II, thus lowering peripheral vascular resistance and decreasing the stimulus for aldosterone secretion. Third, sympathetic outflow to peripheral nerves is reduced through a central nervous system effect.

These drugs must be used cautiously in patients with diabetes.[39,40] Cardiac failure due to coronary heart disease, hypertensive heart disease, and cardiomyopathy is frequent in the diabetic population. Overt heart failure can be precipitated in patients with a borderline myocardial reserve with any further depression of myocardial contractility. Frequent monitoring for symptoms and signs of heart failure is essential, even in adequately digitalized patients.

Catecholamine stimulation of pancreatic beta receptors will cause insulin to be released. Therefore, beta blockade can inhibit insulin release, and hyperglycemia ensues. In one patient, non-ketotic hyperglycemic coma was associated with propranolol therapy.[41]

Glucagon can be released via catecholamine stimulation of beta 2 receptors. Therefore, nonselective beta blockade can be expected to inhibit glucagon release, thus impeding glycogenolysis and gluconeogenesis and thereby aggravating hypoglycemia. The results of studies to evaluate such effects have shown that the nadir of blood glucose during insulin-induced hypoglycemia is not altered by beta adrenergic blockade.[42,43] The recovery phase from hypoglycemia, however, is delayed with propranolol but not with small doses of cardioselective drugs.

Catecholamine release associated with hypoglycemia accounts for some of the symptoms of hypoglycemia. Because of this, there has been some resistance to using beta adrenergic blockers in diabetic patients for fear that hypoglycemic symptoms may be masked. Only the symptoms produced by the sympathoadrenal response such as palpitation, anxiety, tremor, and sweating could be expected to be blunted. Hypoglycemic symptoms are multiple and vary among patients. Palpitation secondary to tachycardia is relatively uncommon. Sweat-

ing, a complex response, is actually increased after beta blockade. Although some hypoglycemic symptoms may be blunted in the occasional patient following beta blockade, this rarely produces a problem. However, patients to be treated with these drugs must be warned that symptoms of hypoglycemia may be diminished.

Normal catecholamine-induced cardiovascular responses to hypoglycemia include an increase in heart rate and an elevation of systolic pressure with a reduction in diastolic pressure, thus maintaining a normal mean pressure. Resistance vessels are constricted through catecholamine stimulation of alpha receptors and dilated by stimulation of the beta 2 receptors. This stimulation of beta 2 receptors accounts for the reduction in diastolic blood pressure during hypoglycemia. Nonselective beta blockade leaves the vasoconstrictive alpha receptors unopposed with a resultant increase in both the systolic and diastolic pressure. By contrast, cardioselective blockers produce a relatively normal blood pressure response to hypoglycemia.[43] That these effects may be important in the choice of beta adrenergic blockers in the diabetic patient is emphasized by the report of a patient who developed a hypertensive crisis in response to hypoglycemia soon after the initiation of propranolol therapy.[44] As previously mentioned, with large doses of cardioselective blockers, both beta 1 and beta 2 blockade may occur. This loss of selectivity is believed responsible for severe hypertension developing in a patient treated with metoprolol.[45]

A further caution for the use of beta blockers in the diabetic patient is the potential for aggravating peripheral vascular disease. This can occur through blockade of the beta 2 mediated vasodilatory responses.

Although beta adrenergic blocking agents have the potential to produce several adverse effects in diabetic patients, in practical experience, these drugs have rarely caused difficulty. The differences between nonselective and cardioselective beta blockers should be considered when these drugs are used to treat the diabetic population.

Sympathetic Inhibitors

This group of drugs includes methyldopa, clonidine, guanabenz, reserpine, and guanethidine. In general, they act by inhibiting sympathetic responses, either at the periphery or through stimulation of central alpha adrenergic receptors, thus decreasing peripheral vascular resistance. The standing blood pressure frequently may be lowered to a degree greater than the supine blood pressure. As discussed earlier, orthostatic hypotension is often present when diabetes is complicated by autonomic neuropathy. Therefore, when prescribed to a patient with pre-existing orthostatic hypotension, these drugs may result in an intolerable decrease in the upright blood pressure with subsequent fainting or decreased blood flow to vital organs. This could precipitate transient ischemic episodes, angina, or compromised renal function as manifested by a rise in blood urea nitrogen or creatinine. It is essential to follow the therapeutic response with both supine and standing blood pressure determinations, using the standing blood pressure as a guide to the therapeutic result. Should symptoms of compromised flow to vital organs occur, drug dosage must be decreased and possibly the drug must be discontinued. Elevation of the head of the bed during the night can be helpful in reducing supine blood pressure and minimizing the orthostatic drop which is most prominent in the morning.

Impotence is another adverse effect of this group of drugs. It is most frequently encountered with guanethidine and is uncommon with clonidine. As diabetic neuropathy is often associated with impotence, the use of these drugs in patients with partial impotence may produce complete cessation of sexual function. This side effect may be intolerable and limit patient compliance with an antihypertensive drug program. Should it occur, other antihypertensive agents should be substituted.

Vasodilator Drugs

Hydralazine and minoxidil are the two vasodilators available in the United States for the long-continued oral treatment of hypertension. Minoxidil should be reserved for resistant hypertension. Both drugs should be used with appropriate diuretics. These drugs act by directly decreasing peripheral vascular resistance. They have no effect on the venous side of the circulation and, therefore, venous return to the right heart is not impaired and cardiac output is increased. This increased cardiac work can precipitate angina pectoris, aggravate pre-existing angina, or, theoretically, even cause myocardial infarction in a patient with severe coronary atherosclerosis. Their use in any patient with active coronary disease must be weighed, recognizing that hypertension itself adversely affects myocardial function. By lowering the blood pressure, an overall improvement in myocardial reserve usually results. Combining vasodilators with a beta adrenergic blocking agent in patients without congestive heart failure will minimize the increase in cardiac output and have an additive effect in lowering the blood pressure.

Converting Enzyme Inhibitors

Captopril is the only drug of this class currently available, and its use should be restricted to moderate to severe hypertensives. Its efficacy in diabetics has yet to be shown. Because its action is due largely to inhibition of the conversion of angiotensin I to angiotensin II, it is of limited value in the presence of diabetic nephropathy where renin is low. Further, this drug can cause proteinuria and renal failure.

SPECIFIC ANTIHYPERTENSIVE PROGRAMS

In this section, specific antihypertensive programs for each type of hypertension in the diabetic will be outlined. These programs are based upon the basic pathophysiology and the mechanisms of antihypertensive drug action that have been discussed. Initial and maximum daily dosage of the major antihypertensive drugs are listed in Table 28–3. For prescribing information and a complete discussion of the adverse effects of these drugs, the reader should consult standard pharmacology texts, the package insert, or the Physicians' Desk Reference.

Essential Hypertension in the Diabetic (Table 28–4)

Because hypertension in the diabetic without clinically evident renal disease may be secondary to mechanisms similar to those involved in essential hypertension, the guidelines proposed for antihypertensive therapy by the Joint National Commission on Detection, Evaluation, and Treatment of High Blood Pressure can be followed.[46] However, hypertension in the diabetic should be treated earlier and more aggressively than as proposed by this Committee. This aggressive approach is justified because the additional adverse vascular effects of hypertension superimposed upon diabetes may lead to early morbidity and mortality. Diabetics with diastolic pressures over 90 mm Hg should be treated with the goal of reducing the standard blood pressure to as close to 120/80 mm Hg as possible. Frequently it is advisable to have the blood pressure recorded at home by the patient's family. Antihypertensive drug therapy must be individualized because of the various complications of diabetes which may be compounded with the use of these drugs.

In the mild to moderate hypertensive diabetic patient with a diastolic blood pressure of 90 to 114 mm Hg, treatment can be initiated with mild sodium restriction (no added salt diet) and either a thiazide diuretic given daily in the morning or a beta adrenergic blocking agent given in small doses. Propranolol 20 mg twice daily, metoprolol 50 mg twice daily or small doses of another beta blocker (see Table 28–3) will generally start the program without adverse drug effects. Gradually increasing dosages of these drugs may be necessary

Table 28–3. Initial and Maximum Dosage of Antihypertensive Drugs

	Mild to Moderate Hypertension (Diastolic 90–114 mm Hg)		Severe Hypertension (Diastolic 115–129 mm Hg)	
	Initial dose (mg/day)	Maximum dose (mg/day)	Initial dose (mg/day)	Maximum dose (mg/day)
Diuretics*				
Alpha adrenergic blocking agents				
prazosin	2	15	2	20
Beta adrenergic blocking agents				
propranolol	40	320	160	480
metoprolol	100	400	100	450
nadolol	40	160	160	320
atenolol	50	100	50	100
timolol	20	40	20	60
pindolol	20	40	20	60
Sympathetic Inhibitors				
methyldopa	500	2000	750	2500
clonidine	0.1	1.0	0.1	2.4
reserpine	0.1	0.25	Probably not effective	
guanethidine	10	100	25	300
Vasodilators				
hydralazine	50	300	100	300
minoxidil	Not indicated		5	(40–100)
Converting enzyme inhibitor	Not indicated			
captopril			75	300

*See appropriate texts or Physician's Desk Reference for complete prescribing information regarding individual drugs.
Diuretics, reserpine, minoxidil, nadolol, atenolol and guanethidine generally can be prescribed once daily.
Other drugs should be given in divided doses 2 to 4 times daily.

Table 28–4. Proposed Progressive Antihypertensive Therapy without Nephropathy (see text)

Diastolic pressure	Initial drugs		Add if blood pressure reduction not optimal	
90–114 mm Hg	thiazide diuretic	+ →	beta adrenergic blocker or reserpine or methyldopa or clonidine or prazosin	+ → hydralazine
	beta adrenergic blocker	+ →	thiazide diuretic	+ → prazosin or hydralazine
115–129 mm Hg	thiazide + beta adrenergic blocker or methyldopa or reserpine or clonidine or prazosin	+ →	hydralazine or minoxidil	+ → guanethidine

(see Table 28–3). Propranolol may be increased to 80 mg, and metoprolol to 100 mg, 3 or 4 times daily. If the desired reduction in blood pressure is not achieved with either a diuretic or beta adrenergic blocking agent alone, then combining the two drugs will often achieve a satisfactory antihypertensive response.

Alternatively in the patient not achieving the desired response on a diuretic alone after 1 month, methyldopa 250 mg twice daily, (increasing if necessary up to 2 g daily in divided doses), reserpine 0.25 mg daily, clonidine 0.1 mg daily (increasing up to 1 mg daily in divided doses), or prazosin 1 mg twice daily (increasing to 15 mg daily in divided doses), or guanabenz 4 mg twice daily (increasing to 16 mg twice daily), may be added. Virtually all patients with mild hypertension will be controlled on such a program. Should the blood pressure remain elevated following 2 months of increasing doses of this combined therapy, hydralazine (25 mg twice daily up to 300 mg daily in divided doses) or prazosin (1 mg twice daily up to 15 mg daily in divided doses) can be added. Hydralazine in doses greater than 300 mg daily should be avoided as this drug may be associated with a lupus erythematosus-like syndrome.

Until the blood pressure has been adequately controlled, patients should be seen every 2 to 4 weeks. Following control, office visits at intervals of 3 to 6 months are usually adequate.

With more severe hypertension in which diastolic blood pressures are 115 mm Hg or greater, antihypertensive therapy should be initiated with a concomitant use of two drugs and, with higher pressures, occasionally treatment should be initiated with three drugs, especially if there is evidence of end organ damage. A diuretic, together with a beta adrenergic blocking drug and a vasodilator, is a rational program. As an alternative, a diuretic can be started concomitantly with methyldopa, clonidine, prazosin or guanabenz and a vasodilator. Almost invariably, the desired antihypertensive effect can be achieved with increasing doses of these drugs. If the blood pressure is not adequately controlled, minoxidil can be substituted for hydralazine, initiating therapy with 5 mg daily and increasing the dose by 5 mg every 1 to 2 days up to a maximum of 40 mg. Occasionally, higher doses may be needed. Patients must be aware that excessive generalized hair growth usually occurs, a side effect which is especially distressing to women. Rarely is it necessary to add guanethidine. However, should it be needed, the starting dose is 25 mg daily with gradual increases to as high as 300 mg daily in divided doses. Often, other antihypertensive agents can be deleted as the dose of guanethidine is increased. Such patients should be

seen weekly until the desired reduction in blood pressure has been achieved. Following that, they may be seen at 2- to 4-month intervals.

"Diabetic Hypertension"

This type of hypertension in patients with diabetic nephropathy is a low renin hypertension associated with elevated blood volume, increased cardiac output, and increased peripheral vascular resistance. Therefore, antihypertensive therapy should be directed toward reversing each of these abnormalities (Table 28–5).

Adequate diuretic therapy is essential. Thiazide diuretics are often effective before the onset of azotemia and in the early azotemic phase of nephropathy. Should hypokalemia occur, it can be treated with potassium supplementation or with the concomitant use of one of the potassium sparing diuretics, spironolactone or triamterene. Extreme caution must be observed with frequent monitoring of the serum potassium and creatinine since the use of these drugs in azotemic patients or in patients with hypoaldosteronism can result in severe hyperkalemia. With progression of the renal disease, the thiazide diuretics are generally ineffective and "loop" diuretics should be started. Because of their prompt onset and short duration of action, they should be given in divided dosage. An initial dosage of 20 to 40 mg of furosemide twice daily can be increased to 160 mg twice daily depending on the clinical response. Excessive diuresis will result in volume depletion and a further decrease in the glomerular filtration rate. Therefore, in the treatment of the edematous patient, it is generally advisable to maintain trace edema.

When the hypertension is not adequately controlled with this diuretic program alone, other antihypertensive medications must be added. Because of the increase in peripheral vascular resistance, a vasodilating agent appears to be the best second choice. Coronary heart disease or diabetic cardiomyopathy is present in many of these patients. Further, cardiac output is usually increased secondary to the anemia. Therefore, prazosin which does not increase cardiac output appears to have advantages over hydralazine. Initial doses of 1 mg twice daily can be increased to 20 mg daily in divided doses. One of the beta adrenergic blocking agents can then be added if needed. As alternatives to the beta adrenergic blocking agents, methyldopa in divided doses of 500 mg to 2.5 g daily or clonidine in divided doses of 0.2 to 2.4 mg daily may be used. The antihypertensive response to reserpine in these patients has generally been poor, possibly because of the pre-existing catecholamine depletion. With the above combinations of antihyper-

Table 28–5.   Proposed Progressive Antihypertensive Therapy in Diabetics with Nephropathy (see text)

	Initial drug	Add if desired blood pressure reduction not achieved		
No azotemia	thiazide		propranolol or	
		prazosin or hydralazine $+$ $\longrightarrow$	metoprolol or methyldopa or $+$ $\longrightarrow$	minoxidil or guanethidine
Azotemia	furosemide		clonidine	

tensive agents, minoxidil or guanethidine is rarely needed.

With progression of the renal disease, the hypertension becomes more difficult to control. Consideration should be given to ultrafiltration dialysis and/or renal transplantation when the serum creatinine approaches 5 mg/dl. Once on hemodialysis, the hypertension generally can be controlled by the removal of excess fluid which decreases the plasma volume. Diuretics at this stage are of little value. Should the hypertension persist, nondiuretic antihypertensive agents can be used. It is not uncommon for a patient to require decreased dosages of these drugs on days of dialysis.

Systolic Hypertension

At the present time, there are no conclusive data concerning the effectiveness of antihypertensive treatment in patients with isolated systolic hypertension or with systolic hypertension associated with normal diastolic blood pressure (inappropriately elevated diastolic pressure). Therefore, one can neither recommend that such patients receive antihypertensive therapy nor outline a specific antihypertensive program for them. The individual physician must decide whether or not to treat and which drug to use if treatment is undertaken. Justification for treatment can be obtained from the accumulated evidence associating isolated systolic hypertension with an increase in cardiovascular morbidity and mortality. Additionally, cardiac work and the chance of myocardial failure will be decreased by lowering the systolic pressure. However, isolated systolic hypertension may be nothing more than a manifestation of diffuse vascular atherosclerosis which by itself will lead to increased cardiovascular morbidity and mortality. The adverse effects of antihypertensive drugs themselves cannot be overlooked. Until evidence that lowering this systolic hypertension will result in a decrease in cardiovascular morbidity and mortality, a physician who elects not to treat cannot be criticized.

When the systolic blood pressure is disproportionately elevated with regard to an elevated diastolic pressure, antihypertensive therapy should be initiated. Because the cardiac output is a major factor in increasing the systolic blood pressure, it would seem reasonable to use drugs that would decrease cardiac output and also decrease the elevated peripheral vascular resistance. Both methyldopa and the beta adrenergic blocking drugs used alone or with diuretics represent the most rational approach to therapy. In choosing a drug which results primarily in vasodilatation, prazosin is preferable to hydralazine since it does not increase the cardiac output.

When initiating antihypertensive therapy for systolic hypertension, therapy should be started with small doses of these drugs and increased gradually and cautiously. Not only must the standing blood pressure be monitored closely but also the patient should be observed for any signs of compromise in function of the cerebral, cardiac, or renal circulations.

Orthostatic Hypotension

Probably the most difficult hypertensive problem to treat in the diabetic patient is supine hypertension with orthostatic hypotension. Occasionally, the orthostatic hypotension can be so severe as to prevent the patient from assuming the upright posture. With lesser degrees, antihypertensive medications to control the supine pressure may result in intolerable orthostatic hypotension. If associated with hypoaldosteronism, renal sodium losses can result in sodium depletion. Blunted vascular responsiveness to endogenous vasopressor hormones and some degree of volume depletion will ensue. To treat the hypoaldosteronism, mineralocorticoid replacement with 9-alpha fluorohydrocortisone in doses of 0.05 to 0.2 mg daily may be necessary. Although initially it may appear paradoxical to add a mineralocorticoid to the program for a patient with any form of hypertension, it must be remembered that this is merely replacing a hormone which is deficient in such patients. Restoring normal mineralocorticoid activity will increase vascular reactivity and plasma volume and in some will decrease the degree of orthostatic hypotension. Elastic support stockings during the day and 8 to 10-inch blocks under the head of the bed at night may minimize the morning orthostatic drop in blood pressure and lower the nocturnal supine hypertension. To decrease the blood pressure further during the night, hydralazine may be given in a single dose shortly before retiring. To increase the blood pressure during the day, ephedrine 25 mg 4 times daily is beneficial in some patients.

It must be recognized that despite these maneuvers and pharmacologic manipulations, supine hypertension with orthostatic hypotension may be benefited only minimally. As with many of the other neuropathic problems in the diabetic, orthostatic hypotension generally improves with time. Frequently this occurs with the onset and progression of diabetic nephropathy.

Hypertensive Emergencies

These are life-threatening disorders characterized by severe elevations of the blood pressure, arteriolar spasms, necrotizing arteriolitis, and end organ damage. Emergencies such as malignant hypertension, hypertensive encephalopathy, rapidly progressive renal failure, and left ventricular failure, may occur in the course of hypertension in the diabetic. Malignant hypertension, however, is distinctly rare in the hypertensive diabetic with nephropathy probably because of the marked suppression of the renin-angiotensin system. Such emergencies require immediate hospitalization and treatment. Diagnostic evaluation for surgically curable forms of hypertension should be delayed until the blood pressure is adequately controlled.

Principles of treatment of hypertensive emergencies in the diabetic are similar to those in the nondiabetic. Parenteral antihypertensive drugs should be started as soon as possible with oral antihypertensive drugs instituted when permitted by the patient's condition.

Of the many parenterally administered drugs, the 5 most useful are listed in Table 28–6. Reserpine

has not been included because of its marked sedative effect which may mask symptoms of central nervous system deterioration and because agents more recently introduced are more uniformly effective in lowering the blood pressure rapidly.

Sodium nitroprusside has a potent, predictable, and immediate antihypertensive effect. Constant monitoring, preferably in an intensive care facility, is essential. Because it affects both the resistance and the capacitance side of the circulation, cardiac output is not increased. Additionally, arterial pressure can be maintained at any level with adjustment of the infusion rate. These advantages render it useful in virtually any hypertensive emergency including active cerebral vascular disease where rapid and precipitous reduction in the blood pressure may be detrimental.

Trimethaphan, a ganglionic blocking agent, also has an immediate onset of action. Arterial pressure must be regulated by adjusting the infusion rate and as with nitroprusside, constant monitoring is mandatory. The tachyphylaxis which generally occurs in 12 to 24 hours, can be minimized by elevation of the head of the bed. Each of the side effects of ganglionic blockade including urinary retention, can occur with this drug. This is especially important in the diabetic population in whom bladder neuropathy is often present.

Diazoxide must be administered in an intravenous bolus to achieve its antihypertensive effect. Generally the blood pressure will become normal immediately. The drug may be repeated at 3- to 10-hour intervals as needed. Occasionally, hypotension will be produced. Because of this rare complication and the rapid lowering of blood pressure which accompanies the use of diazoxide, it should not be given to patients with acute coronary insufficiency or with active cerebral vascular disease. Since diazoxide may cause hyperglycemia, the blood glucose must be monitored closely, espe-

Table 28–6.   Parenterally Administered Drugs for Hypertensive Emergencies*

	Mechanism of Action	Cardiac Output	Dosage	Onset of Action	Duration of Action
Nitroprusside	Dilatation of arteries and veins	↓	0.03–0.5 mg/min IV Infusion	immediate	3–5 min
Trimethaphan	Ganglionic blocker	↓	1–15 mg/min IV Infusion	immediate	10 min
Diazoxide	Dilatation of arteries	↑	4 mg/kg IV Bolus	immediate	4–12 hrs
Hydralazine	Dilatation of arteries	↑	10–50 mg IM or IV	10–20 min	3–8 hrs
Methyldopa	Sympathetic inhibitor	—	500–1000 mg IV	2–3 hrs	6–12 hrs

*Consult package insert or appropriate texts for full prescribing information.
IV = Intravenous
IM = Intramuscular

cially in the diabetic. Because of its sodium retaining properties, it is necessary to accompany its use with diuretics (preferably furosemide given intravenously) in the acute situation.

Hydralazine may be administered by either the intravenous or intramuscular route. Arterial pressure will usually be reduced in 15 minutes. Repeated doses at 2- to 3-hour intervals are frequently necessary. It has limited antihypertensive effectiveness when used alone because the increased cardiac output it produces minimizes its vasodilatory effect. Further, in patients with severe coronary heart disease, this increase in cardiac output can be detrimental. Concomitant use of propranolol intravenously in doses of 1 to 2 mg is frequently helpful to decrease further the arterial pressure and to lower the cardiac output.

Methyldopa has a slow onset of action, making it a poor choice when immediate reduction of the blood pressure is essential. Further, its action is variable with little or no reduction in blood pressure achieved in some patients. It can be used, however, in malignant hypertension or as adjunctive therapy to other drugs such as hydralazine. Although its sedative effect may be useful in agitated patients, it may mask important central nervous system symptoms.

Use of these drugs in hypertensive emergencies will produce sodium retention and plasma volume expansion. Therefore a loop diuretic should be given intravenously at the onset of therapy. Antihypertensive medications should be started orally as soon as permissible clinically. As these become effective, the parenteral medications can be tapered gradually and finally discontinued.

CONCLUSIONS

Hypertension in the diabetic patient is of several types, each with different mechanisms producing the elevation in arterial pressure. Understanding these mechanisms and the mode of action of the various antihypertensive drugs will provide the physician with the necessary knowledge to approach antihypertensive therapy rationally. Adverse effects of these drugs which are peculiar to the patient with diabetes, necessitate special precautions in their use.

REFERENCES

1. Kannel, W.B., Wolf, P.A., Verter, J., McNamara, P.M.: Epidemiologic assessment of the role of blood pressure in stroke: The Framingham Study. J.A.M.A. 214:301, 1970.
2. Kannel, W.B., Hjortland, M., and Castelli, W.P.: Role of diabetes in congestive heart failure. The Framingham Study. Am. J. Cardiol. 34:29, 1974.
3. Kannel, W.B.: Diabetes and cardiovascular disease: The Framingham Study: 18-year follow-up. Cardiol. Digest 5:11, 1976.
4. Christlieb, A.R., Warram, J.H., Królewski, A.S., et al.: Hypertension: the major risk factor in juvenile onset insulin dependent diabetics. Diabetes 30 (Suppl.2):90, 1981.
5. Christlieb, A.R.: Diabetes and hypertensive vascular disease. Am. J. Cardiol. 32:592, 1973.
6. Gordon, T., Shurtleff, D.: Means at each examination and interexamination variation of specified characteristics: Framingham Study Exam 1 to Exam 10. Section 29, The Framingham Study, NIH Publication No. 74:478, 1974.
7. Gordon, T., Devine, B.: Hypertension and hypertensive heart disease in adults: United States 1960–62. National Center for Health Statistics Series 11, No. 13, 1966.
8. Shapiro, A.P., Perez-Stable, E., Moutsos, S.E.: Coexistence of renal arterial hypertension and diabetes mellitus. J.A.M.A. 192:813, 1965.
9. Munichoodappa, C., D'Elia, J.A., Libertino, J.A., et al.: Renal artery stenosis in hypertensive diabetics. J. Urol. 121:555, 1979.
10. Christlieb, A.R., Kaldany, A., D'Elia, J.A.: Plasma renin activity and hypertension in diabetes mellitus. Diabetes 25:969, 1976.
11. de Chatel, R., Weidmann, P., Flammer, J., et al.: Sodium, renin, aldosterone, catecholamines, and blood pressure in diabetes mellitus. Kidney Int. 12:412, 1977.
12. Christlieb, A.R.: Renin, angiotensin, and norepinephrine in alloxan diabetes. Diabetes 23:962, 1974.
13. Christlieb, A.R., Assal, J.P., Katsilambros, N., et al.: Plasma renin activity and blood volume in uncontrolled diabetes: ketoacidosis, a state of secondary aldosteronism. Diabetes 24:190, 1975.
13a. DeFronzo, R.A.: The effect of insulin on renal sodium metabolism. Diabetologia 21:165, 1981.
14. Gellman, D.D., Pirani, C.L., Soothill, J.F., et al.: Diabetic nephropathy: a clinical and pathologic study based on renal biopsies. Medicine (Balt.) 38:321, 1959.
15. Christlieb, A.R., Kaldany, A., D'Elia, J.A., Williams, G.H.: Aldosterone responsiveness in patients with diabetes mellitus. Diabetes 27:732, 1978.
15a. Christlieb, A.R.: Nephropathy, the renin system, and hypertensive vascular disease in diabetes mellitus. Cardiovascular Med. 3:417, 1978.
16. Schindler, A.M., Sommers, S.C.: Diabetic sclerosis of the renal juxtaglomerular apparatus. Lab. Invest. 15:877, 1966.
17. Day, R.P., Luetscher, J.A., Gonzales, C.M.: Occurrence of big renin in human plasma, amniotic fluid and kidney extracts. J. Clin. Endocrinol. Metab. 40:1078, 1975.
18. deLeiva, A., Christlieb, A.R., Melby, J.C., et al.: Big renin and biosynthetic defect of aldosterone in diabetes mellitus. N. Engl. J. Med. 295:639, 1976.
19. Christensen, N.J.: Plasma catecholamines in long-term diabetics with and without neuropathy and in hypophysectomized subjects. J. Clin. Invest. 51:779, 1972.
20. Christlieb, A., Janka, H-U., Kraus, B., et al.: Vascular reactivity to angiotensin II and to norepinephrine in diabetic subjects. Diabetes 25:268, 1976.
21. Christlieb, A.R., Long, R.: Renin-angiotensin system in phlorhizin compared with alloxan diabetes in the rat. Diabetes 28:106, 1979.
22. Christlieb, A.R.: Renin-angiotensin-aldosterone system in diabetes mellitus. Diabetes 25 (Suppl. 2):820, 1976.
23. Goldfarb, S., Cox, M., Singer, I., Goldberg, M.: Acute hyperkalemia induced by hyperglycemia: hormonal mechanisms. Ann. Intern. Med. 84:426, 1976.
24. Lloyd-Mostyn, R.H., Watkins, P.J.: Total cardiac denervation in diabetic autonomic neuropathy. Diabetes 25:748, 1976.
25. Cryer, P.E., Silverberg, A.B., Santiago, J.V., Shah, S.D.: Plasma catecholamines in diabetes. The syndromes of hy-

poadrenergic and hyperadrenergic postural hypotension. Am. J. Med. *64*:407, 1978.

26. Christlieb, A.R., Munichoodappa, C., Braaten, J.T.: Decreased response of plasma renin activity to orthostasis in diabetic patients with orthostatic hypotension. Diabetes *23*:835, 1974.

27. Freis, E.D.: Hypertension and atherosclerosis. Am. J. Med. *46*:735, 1969.

28. Mauer, S.M., Steffes, M.W., Azar, S., et al.: The effects of Goldblatt hypertension on development of the glomerular lesions of diabetes mellitus in the rat. Diabetes *27*:738, 1978.

28a.Mogensen, C.E.: Antihypertensive treatment of inhibiting the progression of diabetic nephropathy. In: J. Ditzel (Ed.): Diabetes and Diabetes Treatment, III. Proceedings of 3rd Nordic Symposium on Diabetes. Aalborg, Denmark, Nordisk Insulin Laboratories, 1979, pp. 103–108.

28b.Parving, H.H., Anderson, A.R., Smidt, U.M., Svendsen, P.A.: Early aggressive anti-hypertensive treatment reduces rate of decline in kidney function in diabetic nephropathy. Lancet *1*:1175, 1983.

29. Kannel, W.B., Gordon, T., Schwartz, M.J.: Systolic versus diastolic blood pressure and risk of coronary heart disease. Am. J. Cardiol. *27*:335, 1971.

30. Veterans Administration Cooperative Study Group: Effects of treatment on morbidity in hypertension: results in patients with diastolic blood pressure averaging 115 through 129 mm Hg. J.A.M.A. *202*:1028, 1967.

31. Veterans Administration Cooperative Study Group on Antihypertensive Agents: Effects of treatment on morbidity in hypertension: II. Results in patients with diastolic blood pressures averaging 90 through 114 mm Hg. J.A.M.A. *213*:1143, 1970.

32. Veterans Administration Cooperative Study Group on Antihypertensive Agents: Effects of treatment on morbidity in hypertension: III. Influence of age, diastolic pressure, and prior cardiovascular disease, further analysis of side effects. Circulation *45*:991, 1972.

33. Hypertension Detection and Follow-Up Program Cooperative Group: Five-year findings of the Hypertension Detection and Follow-Up Program. I. Reduction in mortality of persons with high blood pressure, including mild hypertension. J.A.M.A. *242*:2562, 1979.

34. Conn, J.W.: Hypertension, the potassium ion and impaired carbohydrate tolerance. N. Engl. J. Med. *273*:1135, 1965.

35. Sagild, U., Andersen, V., Andreasen, P.B.: Glucose tolerance and insulin responsiveness in experimental potassium depletion. Acta Med. Scand. *169*:243, 1961.

36. Lewis, P.J., Petrie, A., Kohner, E.M., Dollery, C.T.: Deterioration of glucose tolerance in hypertensive patients on prolonged diuretic treatment. Lancet *1*:564, 1976.

37. Grimm, R.H., Leon, A., Hunninghake, D., et al.: Increased lipids and lipoproteins in diuretic-treated mild hypertensives. Am. J. Cardiol. *43*:419, 1979 (Abstract).

38. Graham, R.M., Pettinger, W.A.: Prazosin. N. Engl. J. Med. *300*:232, 1979.

39. Christlieb, A.R., Maki, P.C.: The effect of beta-blocker therapy on glucose and lipid metabolism. Primary Cardiology *Suppl. 1*:47, 1980.

40. Waal-Manning, H.J.: Can β-blockers be used in diabetic patients? Drugs *17*:157, 1979.

41. Podolsky, S., Pattavina, C.G.: Hyperosmolar nonketotic diabetic coma: a complication of propranolol therapy. Metabolism *22*:685, 1973.

42. Deacon, S.P., Karunanayake, A., Barnett, D.: Acebutolol, atenolol, and propranolol and metabolic responses to acute hypoglycaemia in diabetics. Br. Med. J. *2*:1255, 1977.

43. Lager, I., Blohmé, G., Smith, U.: Effect of cardioselective and nonselective β-blockade on the hypoglycemic response in insulin-dependent diabetics. Lancet *1*:458, 1979.

44. McMurty, R.J.: Propranolol, hypoglycemia, and hypertensive crisis. Ann. Intern. Med. *80*:669, 1974.

45. Shepherd, A.M.M., Lin, M-S., Keeton, T.K.: Hypoglycemia-induced hypertension in a diabetic patient on metoprolol. Ann. Intern. Med. *94*:357, 1981.

46. The 1980 Report of the Joint National Committee on Detection, Evaluation, and Treatment of High Blood Pressure. Arch. Intern. Med. *140*:1280, 1980.

29 The Eyes and Diabetes

Lloyd M. Aiello, Lawrence I. Rand, John G. Sebestyen, Jeffrey N. Weiss, Michael J. Bradbury, M. Zafer Wafai, and Jose C. Briones

Although the ocular complications of diabetes continue to pose a significant threat to the vision of patients, new methods of treatment are now available for some of the more severe stages of diabetic retinopathy which make the visual prog- nosis for the diabetic patient much more encour- aging. The primary purpose of this chapter is to present major new findings in such a way as to provide useful guidelines for those caring for the diabetic patient and thereby encourage timely treat- ment. The diabetic who first visits an ophthalmol- ogist with severe loss of vision and vitreous hem- orrhage should become a thing of the past. Participants in a Diabetes Screening Workshop held in Atlanta in May, 1978 recommended that the screening of diabetic populations for retinop- athy should be "an integral and routine part of the clinical care of diabetic patients."[1]

At the Joslin Clinic there is a strong working relationship between internists, pediatricians, ne- phrologists, and ophthalmologists. At medical vis- its to the Clinic, the patient is questioned concern- ing blurring or loss of vision and the occurrence of symptoms of flashes of light or floaters. The eyes are examined by direct ophthalmoscopy, pay- ing particular attention to new vessels on the optic nerve head (NVD), macular edema and exudates, venous beading, and any changes in the degree of hemorrhages and microaneurysms. Patients in whom the above lesions or other significant ophthalmoscopic changes are noted are referred to the William P. Beetham Eye Research and Treat- ment Unit. Baseline (screening) ophthalmologic examinations are recommended in juvenile-onset, insulin-dependent diabetes (IDDM) after 5 years of diabetes or earlier if symptoms or other com- plications including joint contractures[2] develop.

Patients with adult-onset diabetes should be seen by an ophthalmologist soon after onset. Though in most instances these screening examinations yield normal or near-normal findings, they serve to in- troduce the diabetic to what will probably be a lifetime of ocular surveillance, and detect those few unsuspected cases of advanced retinopathy with short duration of diabetes.

DEFINING THE PROBLEM

It has been estimated that 300,000 people are at risk of blindness from diabetic retinopathy in the

United States today.[3] While this figure may be overly generous, it is clear that diabetic retinopathy and other diabetic eye changes represent an important public health problem. Recognition of this is indicated by the fact that the only three large-scale clinical trials initiated in the last 12 years by the National Eye Institute have concerned themselves with diabetic retinopathy.

Because it is not mandatory to report to government health agencies data regarding blindness, loss of vision, or diabetic retinopathy, precise statistics concerning the incidence and prevalence of retinopathy and consequent loss of vision are not readily available. Data from the U.S. Model Reporting Area (MRA)[4] suggest that diabetic retinopathy may be responsible for about 10% of new blindness at all ages and for about 20% of new blindness between the ages of 45 and 74. In addition, 8.5 persons per 100,000 population are registered as legally blind from diabetic retinopathy. These figures do not include those individuals blinded by cataract or glaucoma related to diabetes or others with lesser levels of visual impairment. It has been estimated that loss of income and public welfare expense due to diabetic retinopathy are about $75 million annually.[5]

How common is retinopathy in the diabetic population? Numerous studies in the past have yielded varying results, depending on who was doing the examination, how it was performed, and how retinopathy was defined. In analyzing the available data, the sex of the patient, age at onset and duration of diabetes, and age of the patient at the time of examination need to be taken into consideration. Because of the non-standard conditions existing in various studies reporting prevalence, it is probably not useful to discuss the results of these early surveys.

Several recent studies using more strict criteria to determine the prevalence of retinopathy in the diabetic population stratified by duration of diabetes, have shown that retinopathy is more common within the first 10 years of diabetes than was previously thought. Davis et al.[6] defined retinopathy as the presence of one or more definite microaneurysms or any other more severe lesion of retinopathy found in any of 7 stereoscopic fundus photographic fields. He reported a prevalence of about 69% after 6 years of insulin-dependent diabetes; the patients were drawn from general diabetes practices in Wisconsin. This figure approached 100% after 14 years of diabetes and reached 100% at 18 years. In stratifying Davis' data in those patients less than 20 years of age with diabetes for 5 to 10 years, 63% had retinopathy by evaluation of stereo fundus photographs. Malone and co-workers,[7] using color photographs of a more

limited area of the fundus, found that 10% of patients less than 18 years of age with less than 10 years of diabetes had retinopathy, but 71% of this same group had evidence of retinopathy on fluorescein angiography. A remarkable finding was that 67% of 30 patients less than 18 years of age with diabetes of less than 1 year had evidence of retinopathy by fluorescein angiography. This has not been found by others using this procedure. Frank[8] studied a juvenile-onset population from a general diabetes clinic with both photography and angiography. He found no evidence of retinopathy by angiography in 60 children with diabetes of less than 5 years' duration and only 27% had retinopathy after 5 to 9 years of diabetes. Palmberg and associates[9] also studied a juvenile-onset population with fundus photography and angiography. He, too, failed to find the large number of patients with retinopathy after 1 year of diabetes; only 26% had evidence of such by 5 years. After 5 years there was a rapid increase in the prevalence of retinopathy with 60% having some evidence after 7 years. By 17 years of diabetes, all of the patients had some evidence of retinopathy.

Though there still appears to be some difference in findings, it is generally agreed that retinopathy frequently makes an appearance after 5 years of diabetes and that half of the patients have some evidence in less than 10 years. Despite the fact that angiography is theoretically more sensitive, the groups of Davis and Palmberg found an equally high prevalence without the use of this more invasive technique. Though all of the studies mentioned have been made in ophthalmologically unselected populations, the numbers of patients have been relatively small (120 to 420), and in many cases the duration of retinopathy before examination is unknown. Rand[10] tried to develop cumulative incidence data from prevalence data in an attempt to determine sample sizes for clinical studies. Klein, in a population-based study in Wisconsin, has found similar prevalence rates.[10a] Surprisingly, however, he also found that about 50% of patients with over 15 years of diabetes had evidence of proliferative diabetic retinopathy. In a Joslin cohort study there was found a 60% cumulative incidence of proliferative retinopathy by 40 years' duration of diabetes.[10b]

While most investigators agree that duration of diabetes is an important determinant of retinopathy, other factors are not so clear-cut. Most have found that retinopathy develops sooner after diagnosis of maturity-onset diabetes than after diagnosis of the juvenile-onset type.[11,12] Some patients are first diagnosed as diabetic by ophthalmologists because of retinopathy. Clearly, the possibility of long asymptomatic periods prior to diagnosis make difficult the dating of onset and duration, especially in noninsulin-dependent diabetes. Study of the Pima Indians,[13] a group with prevalence of diabetes greater than 40% (diabetes mostly of noninsulin-dependent type) showed no relationship between age at diagnosis and frequency of retinopathy. A retrospective study of Joslin Clinic patients[14] showed the prevalence of retinopathy to be related to age only if diabetes had been present for less than 10 years. The duration of diabetes had a much greater influence than age on the prevalence of retinopathy. Comparing patients 60 years old with similar duration of diabetes, virtually no difference was found in the prevalence of retinopathy, whereas 5 additional years of diabetes (up to 15 total) doubled the prevalence.

Formerly it was thought that the status of the eyes in a person with diabetes was a good index of systemic prognosis. Recent evidence developed by Davis and associates[15] strongly suggests that this is indeed true and to some degree confirms work previously done by Caird and co-workers.[16] The results of a study of 709 diabetics, some drawn from general diabetes practices and others from a retinopathy specialty clinic, showed that the survival rate in patients with no retinopathy or only microaneurysms was little different from that in the general population (0.99 vs 1.00). The relative survival rate in those patients with non-proliferative retinopathy characterized by hemorrhages and/or exudates but without new vessels or vitreous hemorrhage, was less (0.81) and that for patients with proliferative retinopathy, even less (0.56). Impairment of visual acuity was also shown to be inversely related to survival. After adjustment for sex, age at diagnosis and duration of diabetes, these differences remained significant. The results of this study strengthen the role of the development of progression of diabetic retinopathy as an endpoint in diabetes intervention studies. It also makes suspect the use of microaneurysm counts as a meaningful way of quantifying retinopathy. Joslin Clinic cohort data and unpublished data from the Diabetic Retinopathy Study show that mortality in patients with proliferative retinopathy is strongly related to kidney status. Almost all deaths among retinopathy patients occurred among those who already had persistent proteinuria and an elevated creatinine level at the time of or shortly following diagnosis of proliferative retinopathy.

THE EFFECT OF DIABETES ON OCULAR FUNCTION AND STRUCTURE

Each part of the visual system (Fig. 29–1) is susceptible to the harmful effects of diabetes which range from changing refractive errors to progressive disease of the eye itself, including cornea, iris,

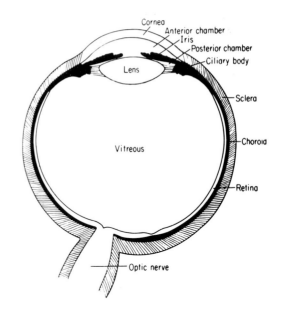

Fig. 29–1. Diagram of the eye. Diabetes affects all portions of the eye except perhaps the choroid and sclera.

lens, retina, optic nerve, extraocular muscles, and orbit. Even the periocular structures such as the extraocular muscles, orbit, and sinuses can be affected. The severity of these complications extends from a simple change in eyeglass prescription to irreversible total blindness. Orbital complications can be life-threatening and severe eye disease often is associated with serious systemic complications which can lead to death.

Even a small reduction in vision can have important effects on the patient's life style. Reduction in vision to less than 20/40 in the better eye will prohibit the patient from obtaining a driver's license in most states. A further reduction in visual acuity will make it difficult to measure and administer insulin. Low vision aids and large print reading material may be necessary in order to function. "Legal blindness" is defined as a best corrected visual acuity of 20/200 or worse in the patient's better eye, or a reduction in visual field to less than 20 degrees in both eyes. Although the patient can still be ambulatory with this vision, it will be difficult or impossible to perform most types of work. If the vision is reduced to counting fingers, hand motions, or light perception, the patient is dependent on a white cane or guide dog to get around in unfamiliar surroundings. The person with no light perception whatsoever is handicapped still further by not being able to tell whether it is night or day, and only then is considered totally blind.

The cornea (Fig. 29–1) of the diabetic patient can be affected in several ways. A classic sign is the presence of corneal striae (sometimes called

Beetham's lines), secondary to severe ocular hypotony. Formerly, this was seen most often in patients with frequent episodes of ketoacidosis and dehydration. It is rarely seen today because of the early and effective treatment available for ketoacidosis. Another condition encountered in diabetics is recurrent corneal erosion. The corneal epithelium of diabetic eyes is susceptible to corneal abrasion which does not heal rapidly as it would in the nondiabetic patient. The defect is in the basement membrane of the epithelium with resultant poor adherence to the overlying epithelial surface of the cornea. When these abrasions do heal, the patient may often have recurrent breakdown in those areas, with the reappearance of the symptoms of corneal abrasion. These include pain, foreign body sensation, photophobia, and decreased vision. Some of these are difficult to treat and can lead to more serious corneal complications such as corneal ulcers and decreased visual acuity from corneal scarring.

If there is faulty healing of the corneal epithelium in the diabetic, infections can be more serious than in the nondiabetic patient. While a corneal ulcer is an ophthalmic emergency in any patient, the diabetic patient may be at even greater risk. In the diabetic, prompt diagnosis and treatment of any red and painful eye are indicated.

Those diabetic patients who wear hard contact lenses must be especially careful to avoid corneal abrasion from wearing the lenses longer than recommended. Over-wearing of contact lenses is a problem in any patient, but with a poorly healing epithelium in a diabetic patient, it can create long-term difficulties. Soft contact lenses have a lower risk of producing a corneal abrasion, but must be cared for meticulously to avoid the possibility of contamination and subsequent infection.

The corneal epithelium is sometimes removed during vitrectomy surgery for the complications of diabetic retinopathy. This is in effect an iatrogenic corneal abrasion and is sometimes difficult to heal with recurrent epithelial breakdown and decreased vision. It should be kept in mind as a cause of pain in the eye of a patient who has had a vitrectomy.

THE IRIS, ANTERIOR CHAMBER, AND CILIARY BODY

The *iris* (Fig. 29–1) is the anterior portion of the uveal tract which consists of the iris, ciliary body, and choroid. It is a circular moving diaphragm with a central opening, the pupil, and forms a border between the anterior and posterior chambers of the eye. The sphincter muscle of the iris, located within a connective tissue framework, is capable of constricting the pupil. The blood vessels of the iris have a slightly corkscrew shape which allows them to vary their length during dilation and contraction of the iris.

Diabetes uniformly affects the iris. The presence of diabetes in life can be inferred by the finding of glycogen deposition in pigment epithelium of the iris in post-mortem specimens. The pupils of diabetic patients may not dilate as readily to mydriatic drops.[17]

The *anterior chamber* (Fig. 29–1) is the space bounded anteriorly by the corneal endothelium and posteriorly by the anterior surface of the iris and lens. Where the surface of the iris and the posterior surface of the cornea meet is known as the angle of the eye. This is an important structure as the outflow of aqueous fluid and the maintenance of intraocular pressure are dependent on structures in this angle. In the angle is the trabecular meshwork which lies internal to Schlemm's canal. It is through this structure that aqueous fluid drains from the eye.

The *ciliary body* (Fig. 29–1) is part of the uveal tract and is commonly divided into two parts, the pars plana and the pars plicata. The pars plana is approximately 4 mm long and extends from the posterior edge of the ciliary processes to the beginning of the retina. The pars plicata consists of 70 to 80 prominent folds or ciliary processes which are oriented in an anterior-posterior direction and are responsible for the production of aqueous fluid. Lying within the stroma of the ciliary body are the ciliary muscles which control accommodation by effecting a change in the shape of the lens.

The most important disease state arising from affection of the anterior chamber and ciliary body is *glaucoma* which is more common in diabetics than in the population at large.

GLAUCOMA AND DIABETES

The frequency of glaucoma is 5% in the diabetic population as compared to 2% in the population at large. There are many different types of glaucoma. Perhaps the broadest definition is that glaucoma is a condition in which the intraocular pressure is sufficient (usually greater than 22 mm Hg) to cause damage to the optic nerve (cupping) and thereby changes in the visual field. Central vision often remains normal until late in the disease. There are three main types of glaucoma in relation to the diabetic as well as general population: (a) chronic open angle, (b) narrow angle, and (c) neovascular.

Chronic open angle glaucoma appears to be more common in diabetics than nondiabetics. The outflow channel of the eye, in the angle formed by the posterior cornea and the anterior iris surface, appears normal on examination. The defect is thought to be in the microscopic outflow channels located within this angle. Treatment is designed to lower the intraocular pressure and prevent damage to the optic nerve head. This is accomplished by topical miotic and epinephrine compound drops and/or a beta blocking agent such as timolol (Timoptic), also administered topically. Carbonic anhydrase inhibitors as acetazolamide (Diamox) are also used to decrease aqueous production and lower the intraocular pressure. In some cases in which the pressures cannot be controlled medically, filtering surgery can be performed to create a new outflow channel and thus lower the intraocular pressure. Laser trabeculoplasty is now usually performed first, thereby reducing the need for surgery.

Narrow angle glaucoma is a rare but clinically impressive type which sometimes includes a hereditary component. In this acute glaucoma, the normal angle outflow channels are closed because of apposition of the iris to the posterior corneal surface. The intraocular pressure rises rapidly to high levels with resultant pain, decreased vision, halo around lights, and often nausea and vomiting. This is not more common in the diabetic than in the general population. One should keep in mind the possibility of glaucoma in the differential diagnosis of nausea and vomiting in the diabetic. The treatment is to break the attack medically, and perform a peripheral iridectomy by surgery or laser iridotomy, thus restoring the normal aqueous flow in the eye. This is an emergency and if the diagnosis is suspected, immediate ophthalmic consultation should be obtained. Since this type of glaucoma can be caused by dilation of the pupil, mydriatic eye drops should be used with caution if a narrow angle is suspected.

Neovascular glaucoma is most frequently thought of as associated with diabetes and results from the formation of new blood vessels on the surface of the iris and in the angle of the eye (rubeosis iridis). This is usually seen in association with significant proliferative retinopathy.

Diabetes is probably the most common cause of neovascular glaucoma. Central retinal vein occlusion, the second most common cause, is quite often associated with diabetes and hypertension in persons over 40 years of age. The earliest signs of *rubeosis iridis* are seen in angiograms showing leakage of fluorescein from blood vessels around the pupillary margin of the iris (Fig. 29–1). Slit-lamp examination is required to see the new vessels at the second stage when they appear as tiny tufts of dilated capillaries at the pupillary margin. The angle of the eye (site of the aqueous outflow) is usually not involved unless new vessels are first seen around the pupillary margin. Typically, these new vessels are initially thin walled. With time, fibrovascular membranes develop, causing radial contraction with the result that the pupil is distorted

and the posterior iris pigment epithelium pulled through the pupil onto the anterior surface of the iris (ectopic uveae). As these new vessels extend into the angle, they, along with the fibrous membrane which accompanies them, start to occlude the aqueous outflow channel, resulting in an increase in intraocular pressure. The end stage is a "zipped up" angle secondary to the fibrovascular growth in the filtration angle with the pulling of the iris over the angle to the cornea occluding the angle. The resulting high intraocular pressure leads to pathologic cupping and atrophy of the optic nerve. Extensive neovascularization of the angle may occur within days after rubeosis iridis is noted or may progress slowly over a period of years. The vessels present around the pupillary margin may disappear from slit-lamp view and suddenly recur with rapid progression over a period of time as short as 1 week.

This iris neovascularization responsible for neovascular glaucoma appears to be directly related to posterior segment pathology. One histopathologic study of diabetic eyes[17] reported a 90% incidence of retinal neovascularization in patients with rubeosis iridis. This condition appears directly related to the duration of diabetes, being infrequent in adult-onset diabetes of less than 15 years' duration. In fact, 76% of rubeosis iridis occurs in patients with duration of 15 years or more. However, the average age of patients with neovascular glaucoma due to diabetes is approximately 45 years, as compared to an average age of 57 years in patients with neovascular glaucoma due to central retinal vein occlusion. The time interval between extensive retinal disease and the development of rubeosis iridis is much more prolonged than is the interval for development of this condition in patients with central retinal vein occlusion. This may be related to the gradual progression of the retinal disease as opposed to the acuteness of vein occlusion.

Due to the unpredictable course of rubeosis iridis and subsequent neovascular glaucoma, prophylactic treatment is difficult. It is known that the development of neovascular glaucoma in one eye is positively correlated with the development of this condition in the opposite eye.

Therapy for Neovascular Glaucoma. The prognosis for the treatment of neovascular glaucoma remains guarded although new breakthroughs in surgical management offer rays of hope. The major goal is the prevention of the elevation in intraocular pressure by treatment of angle neovascularization before closure of the filtration angle. Goniophotocoagulation of the filtration angle frequently results in the successful occlusion and regression of these new vessels. This procedure often requires multiple sessions. Goniophotocoagulation is often used in conjunction with panretinal photocoagulation to permit time for the latter to be effective. Panretinal photocoagulation may have its effect by reducing the presumed release of "angiogenesis factor" and thus removing the stimulus for neovascularization. Obviously, this can be done only in the presence of clear ocular media. Panretinal photocoagulation alone is often effective in obtaining regression of iris and angle neovascularization.

If angle neovascularization is extensive or fibrovascular membranes have formed, resulting in an angle closure with subsequent elevation of the intraocular pressure, then a combination of medical and surgical therapy is indicated. Beta adrenergic blocking agents and carbonic anhydrase inhibitors will depress aqueous formation, thus lowering the intraocular pressure. However, one should not allow a false sense of security to prevail since the intraocular pressure may normalize and yet the angle continue to close. Cycloplegic agents such as atropine may often relieve the pain associated with neovascular glaucoma and when combined with topical steroids make the eye feel more comfortable and quiet the associated inflammation prior to surgical intervention. The present operation of choice is trabeculectomy which creates an outflow channel from the anterior chamber of the eye through the sclera and under the conjunctiva, forming a "filtering bleb." Unfortunately, because of the active neovascularization tendencies these eyes exhibit, this filtration bleb may frequently become scarred from fibrovascular overgrowth. Topical steroids must be continued after surgery to help prevent this complication. New techniques involving the implantation of valves or drainage tubes within the eye are presently under investigation. In eyes that have little chance for visual rehabilitation, cyclocryotherapy has been used to reduce the intraocular pressure and associated pain. This procedure carries a high risk of phthisis bulbi resulting from the total suppression of aqueous production. In addition, it is accompanied by severe hyperemia and transient increases in intraocular pressure, and may have to be repeated for future control of intraocular tension. However, as a last resort, cyclocryotherapy is useful so that retrobulbar alcohol injections and enucleation may be reserved for more severe cases.

In summary, at the earliest signs of rubeosis iridis, panretinal photocoagulation should be performed in an effort to prevent the progression of neovascularization into the angle. If angle involvement by new vessels has occurred, panretinal photocoagulation may frequently be sufficient to result in regression of the new vessels and avoid neovascular glaucoma. However, if these new vessels are extensive, goniophotocoagulation is performed along with panretinal photocoagulation. When the media are opaque and iris neovascularization has occurred, pan-retinal cryotherapy or a more heroic measure—cataract extraction and vitrectomy may be performed in conjunction with intraoperative endopanretinal photocoagulation; or panretinal photocoagulation may be tried in the immediate postoperative period.

When the patient has actual neovascular glaucoma, medical therapy is indicated to quiet the eye; panretinal photocoagulation is performed if the media are clear, and a definitive filtering procedure is planned. If cataract or vitreous hemorrhage prevent panretinal photocoagulation, medical therapy is instituted and the combined cataract extraction/vitrectomy panretinal endo-photocoagulation and filtering procedure or subsequent panretinal photocoagulation may be considered. This procedure is extensive and the prognosis is poor.

In the eye blind from neovascular glaucoma, atropine and steroids topically are often necessary to control pain. Cyclocryotherapy may be used and should this fail, alcohol injection or enucleation may be necessary.

Although the prognosis for iris neovascularization is guarded, definitive advances have been made. Hopefully, further studies into the etiology of diabetic retinopathy and rubeosis iridis will result in a more direct approach to the prevention of this disastrous ocular complication of diabetes.

THE LENS

The lens (Fig. 29–1) is an elliptical-shaped avascular transparent structure with two convex surfaces which is located behind the iris and pupil and anterior to the vitreous. It is held in place by zonules which are tiny fibers attaching at the equator of the lens and to the ciliary body. A change in tension of these zonules affects the shape of the lens. It receives nourishment from the aqueous humor produced by the ciliary processes. The capsule is elastic and allows the lens to change shape easily and thereby alter refraction of light.

Refractive Changes[17]

Diabetic patients have the same range of refractive errors as nondiabetics but there is some evidence that they become presbyopic at a younger age than persons in the general population. Quite often the presenting sign of diabetes is myopia induced by hyperglycemia. Patients who formerly could see clearly at a distance, rather suddenly find that they are nearsighted. Patients who had required reading glasses or bifocals find that they can read without such aid. Although distance vision has decreased, patients often interpret the increase in near vision as an improvement in sight. Refractive errors change along with blood glucose; diabetic patients often state that vision is less clear at certain times of the day. Eyeglasses should not be prescribed unless the blood glucose is controlled and in approximately the same range that it will be when the eyeglasses will be used. For this reason, the diabetic should always inform the ophthalmologist or optometrist who is prescribing eyeglasses that he or she has diabetes and that the blood glucose is under control and at its usual level. Upper respiratory infections and other illnesses can affect the blood glucose and therefore, glasses should not be prescribed during an acute illness. Indeed, up to a 10 diopter shift in refractive error is possible.[17] In children who are first treated for diabetes, early hypoglycemia may induce several diopters of hyperopia (farsightedness). This often requires several weeks to stabilize. Incidentally, there may be an uncorrectable blurring of vision associated with rapidly decreasing or increasing blood glucose on an acute basis. Under these situations, the vision cannot be corrected to its best possible acuity.

Diabetics often complain of visual disturbances in association with hypoglycemic episodes. These are not refractive errors but are commonly due to central nervous system effects of hypoglycemia. Commonly, patients experience a typical pattern preceding such episodes, including phenomena such as aura, visual darkening or narrowing. These become useful warning signs of hypoglycemia to the patient and family.

Cataracts

While cataracts as a whole[16-18] may not be more frequent in diabetic patients than in the general population, they are 4 to 6 times more likely to develop at a younger age and to progress more rapidly. In the U.S. there are more than 200,000 people (primarily diabetics) between the ages of 14 and 44 with cataracts. A cataract is defined as an opacity in the crystalline lens which interferes with vision. There are many different types of cataracts, classified as to severity and location in the lens.

Classically, the ''diabetic'' or floccular cataract consists of showers of small granular opacities (''Christmas tree'' pattern). These appear as ''snowflake'' dots directly under both the anterior and posterior lens capsules. It was noted particularly in the pre-insulin and early insulin eras, associated with episodes of acute, severe ketoacidosis, but occurs rarely today. Clinical observation suggests that it may be related to the degree of sustained hyperglycemia. As seen formerly, this type of cataract occurs especially in insulin-dependent adolescents and young adults. It progresses

rapidly in a matter of a few to several weeks. Van Heyningen[19] has sought the pathogenesis of this metabolic cataract and postulates that increased concentrations of glucose enter the lens and activate the enzyme aldose reductase which favors the conversion of glucose to sorbitol. Sorbitol is not promptly metabolized, but through osmotic effect, draws water into the lens, bringing with it sodium which damages the lens fibers and results in cataract formation.[20]

More common are cortical spokes of the lens which are best appreciated with the pupil well dilated. Fortunately, this type of lens opacity does not usually interfere with vision.

The most common kinds of cataracts in both the diabetic and nondiabetic populations are the nuclear sclerotic and posterior subcapsular types. In nuclear sclerotic cataracts, the nucleus of the lens becomes more dense, turning a brownish-yellow color and preventing light from passing through. Early in the course of development of these cataracts, the lens loses its ability to change shape easily and nearsightedness results. Since most of these patients are at an age where they need bifocals or reading glasses, this newly acquired tendency to myopia with the ability to read without eyeglasses is often interpreted as an increase in visual acuity. In reality, distance vision has decreased.

The second major kind of cataract, the posterior subcapsular type, is an opacity on the back surface of the lens, just beneath the lens capsule. This is particularly devastating to vision because under situations in which the pupil is miotic, the light must pass directly through the center of the lens and is blocked by the opacity at its back surface. These patients have poor vision in bright sunlight or when trying to read, since the pupil is smaller under these conditions. Patients get along fairly well under conditions of dimmer lighting when the pupil is larger and allows more light to pass around the opacity and be focused on the retina. The pupil of the diabetic is often smaller than that of the nondiabetic; it dilates poorly, making a posterior subcapsular cataract a real problem.

One last type of cataract which should be mentioned is the mature cataract which consists of a totally white lens, all parts of which are now opaque. This usually appears as a white pupil and vision is reduced to light perception.

Surgical extraction is the only treatment for cataracts. This is indicated when the patient is unable to get along with decreased vision due to the cataract. After cataract extraction, the eye no longer has its focusing power and this must be corrected by means of aphakic eyeglasses or contact lenses. In addition, it is now possible to implant an intraocular lens directly into the eye. This newer procedure is not recommended routinely in the diabetic patient, especially in the presence of significant diabetic retinopathy, primarily because of the possibility of developing rapidly progressive diabetic retinopathy, requiring frequent examination and treatment. It is often difficult to examine and treat the fundus of an eye with an intraocular lens in place. Older patients ($>$ 60 years) with minimal or no retinopathy may, however, be reasonable candidates for intraocular lens implantation.

In eyes with both cataracts and proliferative diabetic retinopathy, there is a danger of neovascular glaucoma if the cataract is removed before adequate panretinal photocoagulation has been performed. These are complicated cases and should be managed by an ophthalmologist experienced in such problems. From the point of view of the internist or generalist, it is essential that the diabetes be in good control at the time of surgery. Severe hypoglycemic episodes are especially dangerous to a recently operated eye because of the possibility of wound rupture.

Effect of Cataract Surgery on Neovascularization. In addition to the accepted complications of cataract surgery in the total population, cataract extraction in the patient with diabetes carries an increased risk of rubeosis iridis, neovascular glaucoma, acceleration of proliferative diabetic retinopathy (PDR) with or without vitreous hemorrhage, and difficulty in corneal wound and epithelial healing. A retrospective evaluation of 154 patients, in whom intracapsular cataract extraction of one eye was performed with no surgery on the other eye for at least 1 year later, was made with particular attention to known preoperative retinal status and postoperative complications (Table 29–1). If an ocular complication had occurred within 6 weeks after cataract extraction, it was considered a result of surgery. Complications occurred in two categories: (a) vitreous hemorrhage and (b) rubeosis iridis with neovascular glaucoma. Diagnoses of rubeosis iridis and neovascular glaucoma were made on accepted clinical criteria. Iris fluorescein angiography was not available. No patient had rubeosis iridis preoperatively. The preoperative retinopathy status was divided into three categories: (a) no proliferative (PDR) or nonproliferative diabetic retinopathy (NPDR); (b) quiescent PDR (in remission); (c) active PDR with or without vitreous hemorrhage.

Looking at the total of 154 patients without regard to preoperative status of the retina, 12 of the 154 operated eyes and 6 of the 154 unoperated eyes developed postoperative vitreous hemorrhage; the difference was not statistically significant (NS). Twelve of 154 operated eyes and 1 of the 154 unoperated eyes developed postoperative rubeosis iridis with subsequent neovascular glaucoma within the 6-week postoperative period; this was highly significant (p = $<$ .005). In those patients who had no diabetic retinopathy or mild or moderate NPDR preoperatively, 7 of the 108 operated eyes and none of the 103 unoperated eyes developed postoperative vitreous hemorrhage (NS). In the same group of patients, 3 of the 108 operated eyes and none of the 103 unoperated eyes developed postoperative rubeosis iridis with subsequent neovascular glaucoma (NS). In patients with quiescent PDR preoperatively, 2 of 31 operated eyes and 3 of 20 unoperated eyes developed postoperative rubeosis iridis with subsequent neovascular glaucoma (NS). In patients with active PDR preoperatively, 3 of 15 operated eyes and 2 of 31 unoperated eyes developed postoperative vitreous hemorrhage (NS). In the same group of patients, 6 of 15 operated eyes and none of 31 unoperated eyes developed postoperative rubeosis iridis with subsequent neovascular glaucoma within the 6 week postoperative period (p = $<$ .001).

In conclusion, corneal healing did not present a significant problem in the postoperative phase. Exacerbation or acceleration of the PDR and vitreous hemorrhage may occur following cataract extraction in patients with diabetes. However, a leading risk factor was the presence of active PDR producing the major complication of rubeosis iridis with subsequent neovascular glaucoma within 6 to 8 weeks following surgery.

We recommend, therefore, that diabetic patients be examined early, the retinal status be evaluated as the cataracts develop, and laser photocoagulation performed as soon as indicated by the high risk characteristics of the Diabetic Retinopathy Study.[21] If progression of the cataract may prevent such treatment later, earlier laser photocoagulation should be considered. In addition, laser photocoagulation in the immediate postoperative 6 week period should be performed if active PDR is known to be present preoperatively or is found to be present immediately postoperatively.

THE VITREOUS, OPTIC NERVE AND RETINA

The *vitreous* (Fig. 29–1) is a transparent gel which occupies about ⅔ of the volume of the eye. It is about 4 ml in volume and consists of water, collagen, and hyaluronic acid. It is located behind the lens and anterior to the retina. It is attached firmly to the vitreous base at the ora serrata where the retina ends and the pars plana begins. It is also attached less firmly to the optic nerve head posteriorly and to the macula. With aging, the vitreous tends to liquefy. The posterior surface of the vitreous (posterior hyaloid) may pull away from the retina as liquefaction progresses, causing the struc-

Table 29–1. Summary of Findings on 154 Patients Within 6 Weeks After Intracapsular Cataract Extraction in One Eye

	Operated Eyes (Number)	Unoperated Eyes (Number)	Statistical Significance
Examining patient without regard to pre-operative status of retina			
Number of eyes involved	154	154	
Postoperative vitreous hemorrhage	12	6	N.S.
Postoperative rubeosis iridis with subsequent neovascular glaucoma	12	1	<.005
Patients with no DR* or mild or moderate nonproliferative DR preoperatively			
Number of eyes involved	108	103	
Postoperative vitreous hemorrhage	7	0	N.S.
Postoperative rubeosis iridis with subsequent neovascular glaucoma	3	0	N.S.
Patients with quiescent proliferative DR preoperatively			
Number of eyes involved	31	20	
Postoperative vitreous hemorrhage	2	3	N.S.
Postoperative rubeosis iridis with subsequent neovascular glaucoma	3	1	N.S.
Patients with active proliferative DR preoperatively			
Number of eyes involved	15	31	
Postoperative vitreous hemorrhage	3	2	N.S.
Postoperative rubeosis iridis with subsequent neovascular glaucoma	6	0	<.001

*DR = Diabetic retinopathy.

ture of the vitreous body to collapse. The posterior vitreous face provides the scaffold for growth of new blood vessels on and above the retinal surface. Liquefaction and contraction of the vitreous play an important role in the evolution of proliferative diabetic retinopathy.

The *optic nerve* (Figs. 29–1 and 29–2) consists of nerve fibers, neuroglia, and microglia. Its blood supply is from a periaxial system derived from the pia mater and an axial system with vessels derived from the central artery of the nerve which enters the optic nerve approximately 10 mm behind the globe. It runs into the eye and divides on the nerve head into the retinal arteries and is accompanied by a vein which becomes the central retinal vein.

The optic nerve itself is not directly affected by diabetes. Optic atrophy, however, may be seen in diabetic patients after long-standing proliferative retinopathy has gone into remission. In this condition, the disc is usually pale and the retinal blood vessels narrowed and atrophic. Swelling of the optic nerve head (Plate III, A, B) may be seen along with dilated nerve head capillaries in young patients with juvenile-onset, insulin-dependent diabetes. It is not a well-defined clinical entity and may in some cases be a manifestation of early disc neovascularization. This disc swelling is usually not accompanied by visual loss or systemic complications of diabetes. There is usually little as-

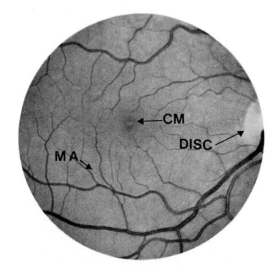

Fig. 29–2. Almost normal posterior pole of retina in diabetic patient. Temporal portion of optic nerve head (DISC) noted. Center of macula (CM) is normal showing retinal capillaries ending at 300–500 microns from center of macula (CM). Rare microaneurysms are seen. Note normal arterial and venous systems.

sociated retinopathy and the edema may resolve in a short time.[22]

However, swelling of the optic nerve head, in association with considerable diabetic changes (Fig. 29–3, Plate III, A, B) should be considered preproliferative diabetic retinopathy until proven otherwise. Patients with this condition should be followed carefully and photocoagulation strongly considered if PDR develops. Finally, any swollen optic nerve head should be studied to rule out papilledema since a diabetic patient may have any of the usual causes of this condition. This is particularly true when the disc edema is bilateral and is seen in the presence of little or no retinopathy.

Embryologically, the *retina* (Figs. 29–1 and 29–2) is derived from a single continuous sheet of neural ectoderm. The optic vesicle invaginates, forming the optic cup which is lined by the neural ectoderm and which then differentiates into the sensory retina and the retinal pigment epithelium.

The retina is a transparent sheath of neural tissue which lines the inside of the eye and lies behind the vitreous and on Bruch's membrane over the choroid. It extends from the optic disc posteriorly to the ora serrata anteriorly; the latter is the dividing line between retina and pars plana of the ciliary body. An important landmark on the retina is the *macula lutea* (center of macula) (Fig. 29–2), an area of slightly yellowish pigmentation measuring 1.5 mm (or the size of the optic nerve head) and lying 2.5 mm temporal to the center of the optic nerve. The fovea is the area in the center of the macula and yields a bright light reflex on direct ophthalmoscopy. Only the fovea is capable of 20/20 vision; all other areas see less clearly. Damage to the fovea alone may result in poor visual acuity, whereas with the fovea intact, 20/20 vision may be present despite extensive damage to the remaining retina. The retinal blood vessels form vascular arcades which, on the temporal side, enclose the macular area. The vortex veins of the choroid, seen through the retina as branching darker structures, are useful as points of reference for other lesions in the retina.

The retina consists of 10 layers which are distinguishable on light microscopy. These layers are, from the vitreous side to the scleral side: (1) the internal limiting membrane; (2) the nerve fibers; (3) ganglion cell; (4) inner plexiform; (5) inner nuclear; (6) outer plexiform; (7) outer nuclear layers; (8) the external limiting membrane; (9) the rods and cones; and (10) the retinal pigment epithelium. Light energy must normally pass through the transparent anterior retinal layers to reach the retinal pigment epithelium and photoreceptors. There the light energy is converted chemically into a nerve impulse which is transmitted through the neural elements to the nerve fiber layer close to the vitreous and hence to the optic nerve and then back to the brain. The vascular supply of the retina consists of the retinal blood vessels which supply the inner half of the retina and the choroidal vasculature which serves the outer half. The thickness of the retina varies from 0.5 mm near the optic disc to 0.2 mm at the equator and 0.1 mm at the ora serrata.

DIABETIC RETINOPATHY

The primary effect of diabetes on the retina appears to be on its capillaries. Exactly what aspect of diabetes causes these changes remains unclear. The elevated blood glucose still seems a likely cause although the basic insulin lack (relative or absolute) and altered levels of other substrates and hormones may also play an important role. Whatever the cause, the diabetic capillaries become functionally less competent.

Functional changes in the retinal circulation have been reported to precede structural changes. These include alterations in retinal blood flow,[23] and breakdown in the blood-retinal barrier resulting in abnormal leakage from retinal blood vessels as measured by vitreous fluorophotometry.[24] At present we believe that neither retinal blood flow measurements nor vitreous fluorophotometry are of value in the ophthalmic care of the diabetic patient. We have had extensive personal experience with both of these techniques and find them to be exciting research tools which may in the future help identify those patients who are most at risk to de-

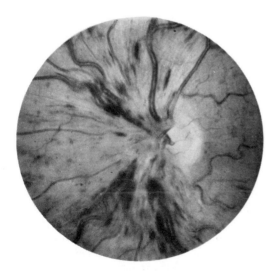

Fig. 29–3. Optic disc edema in 31-year-old patient with diabetes of 11 years' duration. Edema of the disc is associated with many superficial hemorrhages adjacent to the disc which do not extend into the mid-periphery. With the institution of excellent control of diabetes, spontaneous remission often occurs. (See Plate III, A and B.)

velop severe retinovascular disease. However, much more basic and clinical work must be done first. Differences in retinal circulation between diabetic and nondiabetic persons remain to be found.

Vitreous fluorophotometry, despite all the publicity, is really in its infancy. Although many of the previously reported findings of differences between diabetics and normals may be correct, much additional work is needed on the determinants of the phenomena in order to standardize measurements and make them more nearly reproducible. It was originally thought that leakage came from retinal vessels. Other investigators[24a] have pointed out the possible contributions of leakage from the choroid through the pigment epithelium. It may be several years before vitreous fluorophotometry has evolved to the point of being a valuable clinical adjunct. The details of the pathologic and clinical aspects of diabetic retinopathy will be presented in sections that follow.

Natural Course of Diabetic Retinopathy

There are 5 basic clinical pathologic processes that may be recognized in diabetic retinopathy: (Figs. 29–4–9) (a) formation of microaneurysms (outpouchings of the capillary wall); (b) closure of retinal capillaries and arterioles; (c) increased vascular permeability of retinal capillaries and arterioles; (d) proliferation of new vessels and fibrous glial tissue; (e) contraction of vitreous and fibrous glial proliferation with subsequent retinal detachments due to traction. These processes are manifested in four clinical disease stages: background (BDR), preproliferative (PPDR), proliferative (PDR), and quiescent diabetic retinopathy (QDR). (See Figs. 29–4–9 and Plates III, IV.)

Background retinopathy may be further divided into a true benign background stage consisting of a few microaneurysms or small hemorrhages and a transitional stage, indicating the first occurrence of lesions such as soft exudates, venous beading, and intraretinal microvascular abnormalities, which, when present to a greater degree, make an eye pre-proliferative.

As mentioned above, the microaneurysm is ophthalmoscopically the earliest definitive sign of diabetic retinopathy (Fig. 29–2). Other techniques, however, such as angiography and vitreous fluorophotometry, may detect earlier abnormalities such as capillary leakage (Fig. 29–7).

Retinal capillary occlusion (''dropout'') is ophthalmoscopically seen adjacent to areas of capillary dilatation. The latter areas are often described as having intraretinal microvascular abnormalities (IRMA) (Figs. 29–4 and 29–7). This term has been used because in some respects, these vessels resemble neovascularization and they may, indeed, represent intraretinal proliferation. Other workers, however, believe that these are pre-existing capillaries which have dilated due to the increased hydrostatic pressure associated with the adjacent capillary dropout. If fluorescein angiography is done, no perfusion is seen in the areas of retinal capillary occlusion. Adjacent dilated capillaries frequently show leakage of the fluorescein dye. If the parafoveal capillary bed is occluded and nonperfused, then central visual acuity will be lost and changes of diffuse macular edema (Figs. 29–6 and 29–7) or thickening of the retina will be seen. It is thought that these diffuse areas of macular edema may be a stimulus to neovascularization. Pre-capillary retinal arteriolar obstruction occurs in the medium to large arterioles and may also result in capillary dropout in the distribution of the obstructed arterioles.

Other frequent ophthalmoscopic findings are ''cotton-wool'' spots or soft exudates (Figs. 29–4, 5, 8, 9). These are microinfarcts in the nerve fiber layer and may be associated with large flame-shaped hemorrhages. Venous beading (VCAB) (Figs. 29–4, 5, 8, 9), characterized by a regular dilatation and narrowing of the venules with associated white threadlike arterioles, may be observed particularly peripheral to the area of these microinfarcts. Fluorescein angiography clearly indicates that these areas of focal non-perfusion are considerably larger than that area visualized by the ophthalmoscope. Arterioles, adjacent to or passing through the areas of non-perfusion, show stumps

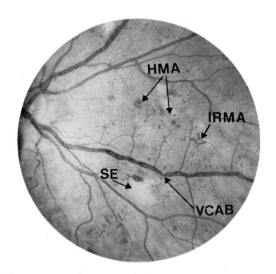

Fig. 29–4. Diabetic retinopathy entering the pre-proliferative stages. Moderate amount of hemorrhages and microaneurysms (HMA), soft exudates (SE), venous caliber abnormalities (VCAB), and intraretinal microvascular abnormalities (IRMA) suggest that this eye will progress to neovascularization (proliferating diabetic retinopathy [PDR]).

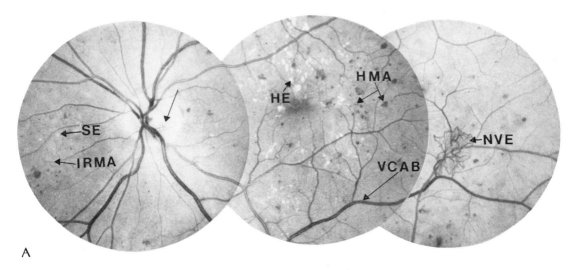

A

Fig. 29–5A. Proliferative diabetic retinopathy (PDR) without high risk characteristics (HRC). Red-free photographs. 5A. PDR without HRC characterized in this figure by New Vessels Elsewhere (NVE) in association with PPDR characteristics including SE, IRMA, HMA, and VCAB. Also macular edema characterized by hard exudates (HE). Combination of PPDR with PDR suggest more rapid progression may occur to HRC.

of occluded arterioles near MA (Fig. 29–6) in addition to venous beading with staining of the venule walls by the fluorescein dye (Fig. 29–8C). This is indicative of increased permeability of the vessel. If this process occurs in the macular area with obstruction of macular arterioles, the resultant visual acuity loss may be considerably more significant than that seen with retinal capillary occlusion as described above. With large areas of peripheral arteriolar occlusion (Figs. 29–8B, 8C), abnormalities may be observed on testing of visual fields. These areas may also represent a stimulus for neovascularization and, as such, are photocoagulated in order to reduce this effect.

The mechanism for retinal capillary and/or arteriolar occlusion is certainly not clear. Many theories have been put forth. Pericyte dropout has been implicated as leading to microaneurysm formation with endothelial cell proliferation and increased amounts of basement membrane. A defect in vascular autoregulation may result in mechanical obstruction of the vessels. Defective platelets and erythrocytes in the diabetic patient may result in blockage of capillaries or arterioles. Sorbitol accumulation with hyperosmotic swelling in the vascular endothelium may also be a factor. The ultimate clinically important outcome of this vascular occlusion is retinal neovascularization (Figs. 29–5, 8, and 9).

Retinal vessel neovascularization may be divided into a growth phase and a contraction phase. The active stage of fibrovascular tissue growth is apparently stimulated by retinal ischemia, especially by the large areas of retinal arteriolar occlusion as described above. New vessels without visible fibrous tissue initially undergo rapid growth which then gradually slows and eventually regresses. These new vessels may regress without fibrous proliferation, but in most cases, this does not occur. The new vessels alone, or those associated with the fibrous growth, (Fig. 29–5B) often adhere to the cortical vitreous, especially if the vitreous has not spontaneously detached from the retina. With the neovascular tissue in place, should the vitreous detach from the retina, hemorrhage will result. (Figs. 29–5B, 8; Plate IV A, B, E, F, G, H.) If the fibrous and vascular tissue grows tangentially across the retina, the macula may be mechanically distorted or obstructed (Plate IV G). This may result in surface wrinkling of the retina with a resultant decrease in central vision. Fibrovascular contraction may result in elevation of the new vessels, detachment of the vitreous from the retina, hemorrhage into or behind the vitreous, and traction between the vitreous and the retina resulting in a traction retinal detachment (Plate IV G).

Background Retinopathy

Microaneurysms (Fig. 29–2). The hallmark of diabetic retinopathy is the capillary microaneurysm, an out-pouching of a capillary wall which, when filled with blood, is seen as a small red dot with discrete borders. This is regarded by many as the first clinical sign of retinal involvement with diabetes. Others with experience in looking at the diabetic fundus may rightly argue that capillary dilation and increased venous tortuosity and engorgement (Fig. 29–4) often precede microaneurysms, but these are subtler and less reproducible findings. The findings in previously presented stud-

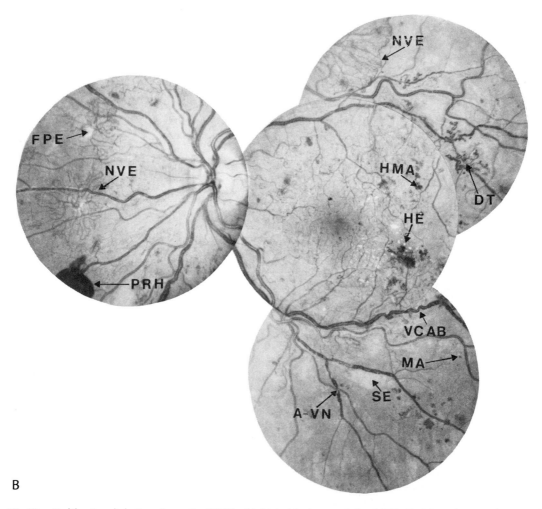

Fig. 29–5B. Proliferative diabetic retinopathy (PDR) with high risk characteristics (HRC). Red-free photographs. 5B. All of the above characteristics are present, that is PPDR and PDR along with pre-retinal hemorrhage, making this patient fall into the High Risk Characteristic (HRC) group. Note also that there is a tendency to develop fibrous tissue (FPE) within the NVE. Arterial venous nicking (A-VN) is also present. In summary, this eye has all the characteristics: macular edema (ME), pre-proliferative diabetic retinopathy (HMA, VCAB, SE), as well as proliferating diabetic retinopathy (NVE, FPE, PRH).

ies indicate that if one looks closely enough, one will probably find at least one microaneurysm in either eye of over 50% of juvenile-onset, insulin-dependent patients (IDDM) who have had diabetes for 5 to 10 years. The cause of the development of microaneurysms is unknown. In the past there has been speculation as to the role of weakening of the capillary wall and loss of vascular tone due to loss of pericytes or mural cells on the development of microaneurysms, but no clear cause and effect relationship has been proven. Using retinal trypsin digest techniques[25] and more recently fluorescein angiography (Fig. 29–7), it can be seen that microaneurysms occur most commonly in areas of abnormal or even partially occluded capillaries. It is thought that they are more common on the venous side of the capillary bed in the inner plexiform and inner nuclear layers of the retina. A particularly common place to look for microaneurysms is in the area temporal to the center of the macula (Figs. 29–6, 7) which is the watershed between the superior and inferior temporal vasculature. A patient with only microaneurysms indicating diabetic retinopathy is, for the most part, at limited risk of visual loss from diabetes unless there is marked progression or an unusually large number of these lesions in the macular region (Figs. 29–6, 7). Should microaneurysms leak fluid causing macular edema, central vision can be impaired (Figs. 29–6, 7). This is the most common cause of visual impairment in diabetics, particularly those in the older age groups.

Hemorrhages and Exudates. Along with microaneurysms, intraretinal hemorrhages (Figs. 29–5–7) and hard or waxy exudates (Fig. 29–6, Plate III C, D, E) make up what is called back-

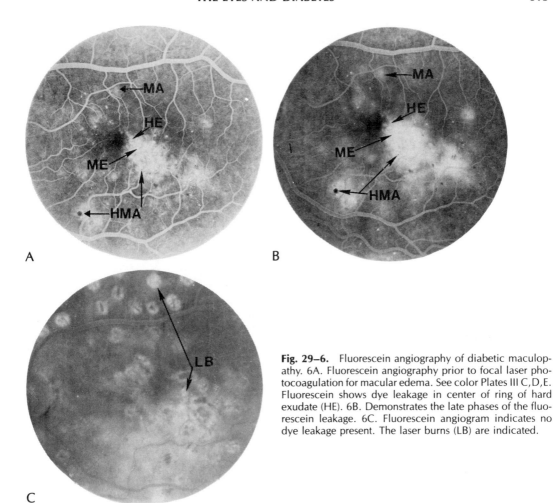

A

B

C

Fig. 29–6. Fluorescein angiography of diabetic maculopathy. 6A. Fluorescein angiography prior to focal laser photocoagulation for macular edema. See color Plates III C,D,E. Fluorescein shows dye leakage in center of ring of hard exudate (HE). 6B. Demonstrates the late phases of the fluorescein leakage. 6C. Fluorescein angiogram indicates no dye leakage present. The laser burns (LB) are indicated.

ground or simple diabetic retinopathy. Both of these lesions may result from either leakage of red blood cells or other blood components from microaneurysms or other weakened vasculature. They are by no means specific for diabetes and may be seen in many other forms of retinovascular disease, particularly that associated with hypertension. Hemorrhages from diabetic retinopathy are typically "dot and blotch" in shape and are deep in the retina (Figs. 29–4, 5). Superficial flame-shaped hemorrhages in the nerve fiber layer, typical of hypertension, also are frequently seen in diabetes (Figs. 29–3, 4). Small dot hemorrhages are difficult to distinguish from microaneurysms. Large numbers of blotch hemorrhages may be a sign that the disease is entering an active phase. Preliminary reports of data in the Diabetic Retinopathy Study[26] show extensive intraretinal hemorrhages to be a risk factor for the development of severe visual loss in the presence of proliferative retinopathy.

Hard or Waxy Exudates (Fig. 29–6; Plate III C, D, E). These highly refractile, yellow-white,

discrete deposits seen in the retina, and particularly in the macula, are a sign of a leaky capillary bed. These exudates which lie deep in the outer plexiform layer of the retina are usually associated with edema of the retina. The term "diabetic maculopathy" refers to the exudates, edema, and leaky microaneurysms seen frequently in the macular region in diabetic patients. There are three basic shapes of exudates: discrete dots, rings, and plaques. Most discrete dots if followed long enough, will disappear as others develop and if sequentially traced, will form rings. Exudates usually are deposited at the junction of healthy and unhealthy retina where fluid is absorbed. Leaking microaneurysms are usually found in the center of the rings (Fig. 29–6). For the past 14 years, edema and exudates which threaten or involve the macula, have been treated with photocoagulation. Though many clinicians have achieved satisfactory results with this technique, others find it less uniformly successful. This issue will be discussed further in the section on clinical trials. Many previously pub-

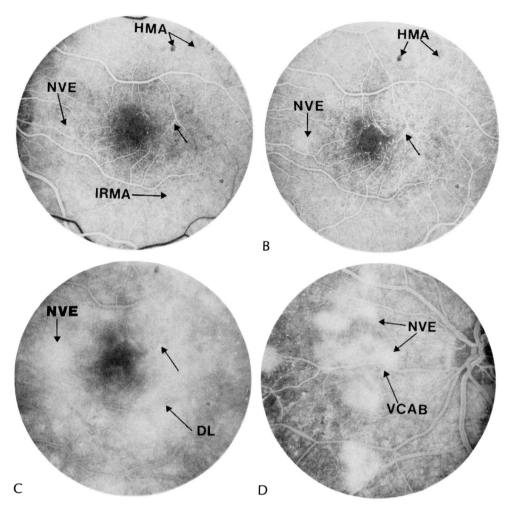

Fig. 29–7. Fluorescein angiogram of diabetic maculopathy and New Vessels Elsewhere in a 30-year-old patient with diabetes of 11 years' duration. (See Plate III F and G.) 7A. Early phase of fluorescein angiograms showing arterial phase with microaneurysmal dilatations along the capillary (see unmarked arrows), IRMA, and NVE. 7B. Reveals these changes in more detail with early and moderate leakage of dye. 7C. Shows diffuse leakage (DL) from the microaneurysms and IRMA's and NVE. 7D. Shows leakage from the new vessels in the nasal retina (see Plate III G) and staining of venous walls (at sites of VCAB).

lished studies evaluated diets and clofibrate (Atromid-S) for the treatment of exudative retinopathy.[27–30] In general, it can be said that once vision is decreased due to exudates, it does not recover regardless of therapy. Edema may, however, cause widely fluctuating vision and may improve considerably. The influence of therapy is unclear. At the present time, we are no longer routinely recommending the use of clofibrate in exudative diabetic retinopathy.

The presence of macular edema has classically been thought of as a manifestation of retinopathy in noninsulin-dependent diabetes (NIDDM). We have observed that the presence of macular edema in an insulin-dependent diabetic (IDDM), particularly a young person, may be an ominous sign of rapidly progressing disease that often is refractory

to treatment. In that sense, macular edema in a young patient fits in with the next group of pre-proliferative lesions. Macular and generalized retinal edema in an insulin-dependent diabetic may also be a sign of impending renal disease; the serum creatinine should be determined whenever this is found.

Table 29–2 summarizes the progression of diabetic retinopathy as seen clinically. Following the occurrence of disc neovascularization with or without vitreous hemorrhage (Fig. 29–9; Plate IV C, D), or New Vessels Elsewhere (NVE) with vitreous hemorrhage (Fig. 29–8; Plate IV A, B), the eye is at high risk to go on to severe visual loss from fibrous proliferation and traction detachment or neovascular glaucoma. Laser panretinal photocoagulation will induce remission and reduce severe visual loss by 50 to 60% (Tables 29–3 and 4).

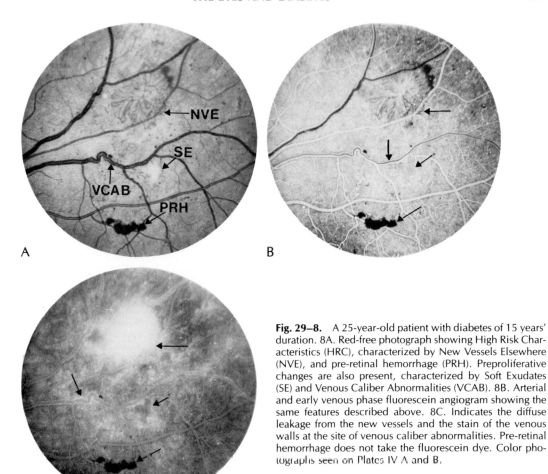

Fig. 29–8. A 25-year-old patient with diabetes of 15 years' duration. 8A. Red-free photograph showing High Risk Characteristics (HRC), characterized by New Vessels Elsewhere (NVE), and pre-retinal hemorrhage (PRH). Preproliferative changes are also present, characterized by Soft Exudates (SE) and Venous Caliber Abnormalities (VCAB). 8B. Arterial and early venous phase fluorescein angiogram showing the same features described above. 8C. Indicates the diffuse leakage from the new vessels and the stain of the venous walls at the site of venous caliber abnormalities. Pre-retinal hemorrhage does not take the fluorescein dye. Color photographs seen on Plates IV A and B.

OCULAR RISK FACTORS FOR THE DEVELOPMENT OF SEVERE VISUAL LOSS

The Diabetic Retinopathy Study (DRS) Research Group[31] has examined fundus photographs to determine risk factors for the development of severe visual loss of PDR. Stereo fundus photographs were obtained of seven standard fields in each eye of the 1,742 participating patients as a baseline, and then annually during the course of the study. Using methods for quantifying fundus photographic lesions, a multivariate linear regression model was used to evaluate the influence of lesions in the untreated eyes as compared to the end point visual acuity. Forty-seven photographically graded lesions were added to the regression equation in order to select those lesions most closely associated with an endpoint visual acuity of less than 5/200. It became apparent that new vessels on the disc (NVD) (Fig. 29–9) clearly have the strongest influence on the development of the endpoint. This is especially important because these may be detected with direct ophthalmoscopy. Other important lesions (Fig. 29–5, 8; Plates III F, G, IV A, B,

C, D) were hemorrhages and microaneurysms, neovascularization at areas other than the disc, vitreous hemorrhages, arteriolar abnormalities, venous caliber abnormalities, and perivenous exudates. Lesions in the opposite photocoagulated eye were also predictive of the endpoint in the untreated eye but to a lesser extent. The presence of disc neovascularization, venous caliber abnormalities, hemorrhages and microaneurysms, vitreous hemorrhages and preretinal hemorrhages appear to be the most significant findings in the opposite photocoagulated eye.

The Early Treatment Diabetic Retinopathy Study (ETDRS)[32] should provide further insight into the findings, as seen photographically, that contribute to the development and progression of diabetic retinopathy.

NON-OCULAR CLINICAL FACTORS INFLUENCING THE DEVELOPMENT AND RATE OF PROGRESSION OF DIABETIC RETINOPATHY

The onset and progression of diabetic retinopathy may be influenced by clinical factors other than

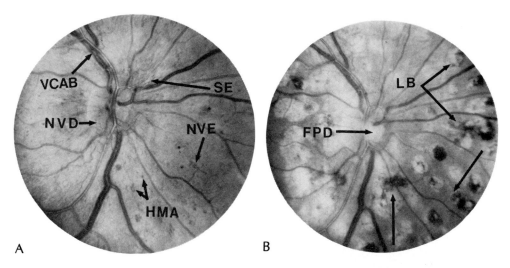

Fig. 29–9. A 20-year-old patient with diabetes of 10 years' duration. 9A. Prior to laser treatment; New Vessels on the Optic Nerve (NVD) and New Vessels Elsewhere (NVE) associated with other active changes as hemorrhages and micro-aneurysms (HMA), Soft Exudate (SE), and Venous Caliber Abnormalities (VCAB). 9B. Results of laser photocoagulation treatment: New Vessels on Disc (NVD) have cleared and left small fibrous membrane (FPD); New Vessels Elsewhere (NVE) have completely cleared. (See unmarked arrows.) Laser burns noted surrounding the disc 360 degrees (LB). See Plate IV C and D. This case represents high risk characteristics with excellent response to laser treatment.

Table 29–2. Types of Diabetic Retinopathy

A. Background or non-proliferative diabetic retinopathy (BDR) (NPDR).
  1. Microaneurysms with or without associated small blotch hemorrhages.
  2. Hard exudates.
  3. Minor venous abnormalities, characterized by irregularities in the width of the vein.
  4. Arteriolar narrowing.
  5. Arteriolar venular nicking.
  6. Retinal edema.

B. Preproliferative diabetic retinopathy (PPDR).
  1. Cotton-wool spots (soft exudates).
  2. Venous abnormalities characterized by beading and duplication.
  3. Intraretinal microvascular abnormalities (IRMA).
  4. Areas of non-perfusion or capillary closure.
  5. Macular edema in a young patient.

C. Proliferative diabetic retinopathy (PDR).
  1. Vasoproliferation
    a. New vessels on the disc (NVD).
    b. New vessels elsewhere (NVE).
    c. Fibrous tissue membrane associated with the new vessels.
  2. Fibrous growth stage with contraction.
    a. Retinal hemorrhage.
    b. Vitreous hemorrhage.
    c. Traction retinal detachment.

ocular. Most important of these are age of the patient at onset of diabetes, duration of diabetes, degree of control of hyperglycemia, blood pressure, pregnancy, and renal disease.

During the 5-month period between March 1 and July 31, 1980, 568 Eye Unit patients had photographs taken for diabetic retinopathy.[10] The information collected at the time of photography included the age at onset of diabetes, duration of known diabetes, sex, visual acuity, and retinopathy status based on clinical examination. Seven standard stereo photographic fields were taken of both eyes in each patient. Sets of photographs (both eyes) of 343 patients were graded by a trained worker using a modified version of the classification scheme used in the Diabetic Retinopathy Study.[31] Retinopathy status was coded by that in the worse eye. The findings may be summarized as follows:

1. Patients who develop diabetes at 40 years or older differ from patients with classic juvenile-onset diabetes mellitus both demographically and in retinopathy status. Patients who develop diabetes between 20 and 39 share characteristics of both groups (Table 29–5). These older-onset patients make up a significant proportion (22.1%) of those patients with PDR in the Joslin Clinic Eye Unit population.

2. There appears to be an excess of females over males in the older-onset group; however, among those with PDR, males equal females (Table 29–6).

3. The development of PDR within the first 10 years of known diabetes occurs most frequently in

Table 29–3. Cumulative 2-Year Rates of Severe Visual Loss* Eye with High Risk Characteristics**

	Untreated	Treated	Z Value***
Moderate or severe New Vessels Elsewhere (NVE); no New Vessels on the Disc (NVD); with Hemorrhage	29.7	7.2	3.0
Mild NVD; NVE; with Hemorrhage	25.6	4.3	2.9
Moderate or Severe NVD; NVE; no Hemorrhage	26.2	8.5	4.7
Moderate or Severe NVD; NVE; with Hemorrhage	36.9	20.1	3.1

*Visual acuity of ≤5/200 at two or more consecutively completed follow-up visits.
**High-risk characteristics defined at time of 1976 protocol changes are:
    (1) Moderate or severe NVE with vitreous or preretinal hemorrhage, or both.
    (2) Mild NVD with vitreous or preretinal hemorrhage or both.
    (3) Moderate or severe NVD without vitreous or preperipheral hemorrhage.
    (4) Moderate or severe NVD with vitreous or preretinal hemorrhage or both.
***Z value: Observed difference between the cumulated 2-year rates observed in the untreated and treated groups divided by the standard error of the difference.[63]

Table 29–4. Cumulative 2-Year Rate of Severe Visual Loss* Eyes Without High Risk Characteristics**

	Untreated	Treated	Z Value***
No New Vessels; no Hemorrhage	3.6	3.0	0.4
Mild NVE; no NVD; no Hemorrhage	6.8	2.0	1.8
Moderate or severe NVE; no NVD; no Hemorrhage	6.9	4.3	1.0
Mild NVD; NVE; no Hemorrhage	10.5	3.1	2.4

*Visual acuity of ≤5/200 at two or more consecutively completed follow-up visits.
**High-risk characteristics defined at time of 1976 protocol changes are:
    (1) Moderate or severe NVE with vitreous or preretinal hemorrhage, or both.
    (2) Mild NVD with vitreous or preretinal hemorrhage or both.
    (3) Moderate or severe NVD without vitreous or preperipheral hemorrhage.
    (4) Moderate or severe NVD with vitreous or preretinal hemorrhage or both.
***Z value: Observed difference between the cumulated 2-year rates observed in the untreated and treated groups divided by the standard error of the difference.[63]

Table 29–5. Percentage Distribution by Clinical Examination of Retinopathy Status (Worse Eye) According to Age at Onset of Diabetes*

Age at Onset of Diabetes	NDR	BDR	PPDR	PDR	Total
0–19	41.9	45.7	36.8	52.9	47.2
20–39	19.4	23.7	21.1	25.0	23.4
≥40	38.7	30.6	42.1	22.1	29.4
	100.0	100.0	100.0	100.0	100.0
N	62	186	76	244	568

NDR: No diabetic retinopathy.
BDR: Background diabetic retinopathy.
PPDR: Preproliferative diabetic retinopathy.
PDR: Proliferative diabetic retinopathy.

*From Aiello et al.[11]

this older onset group (Table 29–7). Most patients in this group who develop PDR will do so within 10 years after onset of diabetes.

5. Visual disability was more common in older-onset patients. As in other onset groups, it is most common if proliferative disease is present; but, on the other hand, over 40% of visual disability in the older onset group occurred in patients without PDR (Table 29–8).

6. PDR occurs in non-insulin-taking diabetics commonly with duration of diabetes of 10 years or less. These patients are at significant risk of visual disability.

7. Macular edema (Figs. 29–6, 7; Plate III C, D, E) is more common in the older onset group and occurs equally at all stages of retinopathy, i.e., in association with background diabetic retinopathy (BDR), pre-proliferative diabetic retinopathy (PPDR), and PDR. In younger onset groups, macular edema occurs primarily in association with pre-proliferative or proliferative disease (Table 29–9).

8. Macular edema in patients less than 50 years of age is usually associated with PDR regardless of the age at onset of diabetes.

9. We cannot estimate from our data what proportion of the general adult-onset diabetic population develop serious eye problems. Klein and co-workers have found that approximately 20% of

Table 29–6. Sex Distribution by Age at Onset and Retinopathy Status

Age at Onset	Retinopathy Status										
	NDR*		BDR**		PPDR***		PDR****		All	
	M	F	M	F	M	F	M	F	M	F
<20	9	16	42	43	15	13	57	72	123	144
20–39	5	7	21	23	12	4	38	22	76	56
≥40	7	17	17	40†	11	21	25	28	60	106†

*No diabetic retinopathy
**Background diabetic retinopathy
***Pre-proliferative diabetic retinopathy
****Proliferative diabetic retinopathy
†95% confidence interval for male-female distribution does not include 50%.

From Aiello et al.[11]

Table 29–7. Percentage Distribution of Patients with PDR* According to Duration and Age at Onset of Diabetes
(Numbers of patients in parentheses)

Age at Onset	Duration					
	10	11–15	16–20	21–25	25	Total
<20	3.1 (4)	14.7(19)	31.8(41)	19.4(25)	31.0(40)	100.0(129)
20–39	6.6 (4)	13.1 (8)	23.0(14)	19.7(12)	37.7(23)	100.0 (61)
≥40	38.9(21)	24.1(13)	29.6(16)	7.4 (4)	0.0 (0)	100.0 (54)

*PDR: proliferative diabetic retinopathy.

From Aiello et al.[11]

Table 29–8. Distribution of Visually Disabled Patients (20/40 in Better Eye) According to Age at Onset of Diabetes and Retinopathy Status
(Percentage of patients in parentheses)

Status of Retinopathy	Age at Onset of Diabetes			
	<20	20–39	≥40	Total
NDR*	1	0	3	5
BDR**	0	0	6	5
PPDR***	1	1	3	5
PDR****	18(90.0)	12(92.3)	16(57.1)	46
Total disabled	29(7.5)	13(9.8)	28(16.8)	61(10.7)
Total Patients	268	133	167	568

*No diabetic retinopathy.
**Background diabetic retinopathy.
***Preproliferative diabetic retinopathy.
***Proliferative diabetic retinopathy.

From Aiello et al.[11]

insulin-taking and 10% of noninsulin-taking diabetics who developed diabetes over age 30 had PDR.[33] However, the fact that these patients, whether taking insulin or not, can develop the full spectrum of diabetic eye disease, and if they do, are more likely to do it quickly and more frequently with visual disability, should cause physicians to be unusually watchful in following them. We suggest that adult-onset diabetics be seen by an ophthalmologist shortly after diabetes is discovered, and at least yearly thereafter, unless problems develop after which more frequent follow-up is indicated. In most cases, the classic juvenile IDDM

patients in the absence of symptoms do not need to be seen by an ophthalmologist until diabetes has been present for about 5 years. After 5 years, IDDM patients should have an ophthalmologic examination yearly. Patients with severe non-proliferative retinopathy should be followed at 4- to 6-month intervals to watch for the development of new vessels.

This suggestion of careful screening and follow-up could generate a large patient population in which a majority of examinations may reveal no retinopathy. Cooperation between the ophthalmologist and internist/diabetologist/family practitioner

Table 29–9. Distribution of Macular Edema (Either Eye) by Age at Onset of Diabetes and Retinopathy Status Based on Grading of Stereo Photographs

Age at Onset	NDR*	BDR**	PPDR***	PDR****	All Retinopathy Groups	
0–19	(8)	2(39)	3(12)	14(51)	19(110)	17.3%
20–39	(10)	8(35)	8(16)	22(47)	38(108)	35.2%
40	(18)	14(43)	20(25)	20(39)	54(125)	44.8%
Total	None(36)	24(117)	31(53)	56(137)	111(343)	32.4%
%	——	20.5	58.5	40.9	32.4	

*No diabetic retinopathy.
**Background diabetic retinopathy.
***Preproliferative diabetic retinopathy.
***Proliferative diabetic retinopathy.

Figures within parentheses are those with retinopathy and those outside are those who also had macular edema.

From Aiello et al.[11]

with training of non-ophthalmic physicians to identify diabetic retinopathy accurately, would do much to distribute the responsibility of interim screening of these patients and increase the yield of treatable disease seen by the ophthalmologist.

Hyperglycemic Control

The issue of whether control of hyperglycemia influences the development or progression of retinopathy is beyond the scope of this brief section. Suffice it to say that a large body of evidence has been accumulated, most of which favors the hypothesis that control makes a difference, at least in the earlier stages of retinopathy.[34–38] Records of 360 Joslin Clinic juvenile diabetics[36] who had been followed from 20 to 40 years were reviewed, defining stages of control of diabetes and retinopathy. Of the patients with *good* control, 7% were found to have marked or extreme retinopathy. Of the patients with *fair* control, 19% had marked or extreme retinopathy. Of the patients with poor control, 43% had marked retinopathy.

Though most studies appear to show that better control is associated with less retinopathy, no previous study has been able to demonstrate adequately that differences in control achieved did not reflect "lesser" degrees of diabetes, and therefore less resultant retinopathy. Only a randomized study can definitively answer this question, and this is the basic clinical question in all studies of complications in diabetic patients.

The randomized study of Job and colleagues[34] showed less progression in microaneurysm counts in a group of diabetic patients assigned to multiple daily injections of insulin (+ 1.8 Ma/yr) than in a group assigned to single daily insulin injections (+ 7.2 Ma/yr). However, the results of this study have not been well accepted. This may be due to the relatively small differences in glycemic control achieved between the two treatment groups, the 20% (10/52) drop-out rate during the first year, and

the 9 additional patients who did not receive the assigned therapy.

The studies of Engerman[38] also supported the beneficial effect of diabetes control in an animal model of diabetes. Alloxan diabetic dogs allowed to have poorly controlled diabetes, routinely developed background retinopathy after 3 to 5 years. Intensive control of diabetes with insulin resulted in freedom from retinopathy in many animals or in much lower microaneurysm counts after similar durations of diabetes. The recent findings of diabetes-like retinopathy in galactose-fed animals is exciting, and is evidence in favor of a direct role for hyperglycemia in the development of diabetic retinopathy.[38a] With the advent of newer techniques (e.g., the insulin pump), the need for a controlled clinical trial to anwer this question is more imperative and realistic. Indeed, a multicenter clinical trial sponsored by the National Institute of Arthritis, Diabetes, Digestive and Kidney Diseases has recently been designed to answer this question. This study (Diabetes Control and Complications Trial) (DCCT) will test insulin-dependent diabetics between the ages of 10 to 28 years. Patients will be randomized to two forms of therapy: those tightly controlled by insulin infusion pumps, multiple injections of daily insulin, etc., as available, and those controlled by conventional means. Separate groups of patients without retinopathy and with minimal retinopathy may be studied. If this is done properly, it may well provide the definitive answer to this question.

Blood Pressure

Although diabetic patients with hypertension may be at higher risk for developing severe diabetic retinopathy than comparable patients without hypertension, the relationship found in cross-sectional studies is not striking. Klein et al. in such a study of diabetic retinopathy and its association with risk variables, found a positive relationship with proliferating disease (PDR) and elevated diastolic blood pressure.[10a,33]

The Pima Indian Study[39] is one of the few longitudinal studies which have examined the relationship between blood pressure and diabetic retinopathy. Over a 5-year interval, the incidence of "exudates" in those diabetic individuals with systolic blood pressure of 145 mm Hg or higher was more than twice those with pressures of less than 125 mm Hg. These data must be interpreted with caution; of 284 eyes in nondiabetic individuals, 12% were found to have similar "exudates," suggesting that drüsen and diabetic hard exudates were not distinguished. This study also failed to find similar association between blood pressure and hemorrhages. In a case-control study comparing long-term diabetic patients with PDR with duration-matched patients with minimal or no retinopathy, there is a marked excess of hypertensive patients in the PDR group.[40] Further analysis of those data shows that after controlling for the effects of renal disease the importance of hypertension is greatly diminished but not entirely eliminated.

The importance of hypertension as a risk factor for diabetic retinopathy requires further study. Since the prevalence of hypertension is higher in diabetic patients than in nondiabetics,[41] and since hypertension is an additional known cardiovascular risk factor in patients already at high risk,[42] we suggest that blood pressure control is an important part of overall diabetes care. Referral to internists for treatment of those patients found to have hypertension is consistent with optimal ophthalmologic care.

Pregnancy

Since no control studies have been done, we are unable to state definitely whether pregnancy is a risk factor for the progression of retinopathy. In a review of the literature, Rodman et al.[43] found 201 cases of pregnant diabetic patients either without retinopathy or with only the non-proliferative type at the onset of pregnancy (17 patients—18%). This retinopathy progressed during pregnancy and 4 of these 17 patients developed PDR at the onset of pregnancy; 32 (15.9%) experienced progression during pregnancy.

In a retrospective study[44] at the Beetham Eye Unit of the Joslin Clinic, the effects of pregnancy on diabetic retinopathy with and without laser treatment were evaluated. Records and photographs of 64 patients whose eyes were examined through a successful pregnancy by one of us (LMA) during 1975 to 1977 were reviewed by the same examiner to document changes in status regarding retinopathy. Of these 64 patients, 43 had background angiopathy or early neovascularization and were not treated by laser; they showed progression of retinopathy to a more severe stage during the pregnancy, peaking in the third trimester, and then regressing to a less severe stage in 3 to 6 months postpartum. Ten patients had successful laser treatment prior to onset of pregnancy and during pregnancy no progression occurred. Five patients were in spontaneous remission of retinopathy at onset of pregnancy and remained stable during pregnancy. In these groups, no change in visual acuity occurred during or after pregnancy. However, 6 eyes of patients with neovascularization on the disc present in the first trimester, experienced rapid progression in the second and third trimesters. Four of these responded to laser treatment but the two with advanced disc neovascularization did not, and went on to blindness.

A more recent study of our patients summarized findings in 80 pregnant diabetics seen during the period April 1980 to April 1981.[45] These patients were examined weekly for pre-natal care and diabetes control at the Pregnancy Clinic of the Joslin Clinic. At intervals during pregnancy and postpartum, eye examinations were performed. The best correctable vision, an anterior segment examination with slit-lamp, applanation tonometry, and a dilated ophthalmoscopic examination were done at each eye visit, followed by stereo color photographs of seven standard fields of the retina in each eye as defined by the Diabetic Retinopathy Study (DRS).[31] The photographs at each visit were graded independently, using a modification of the DRS grading scheme. The results are shown in Table 29–10 in which it is evident that the average age for each retinopathy status is similar and clustered around the 25th to 27th year. Of greater significance is the duration of diabetes compared with the retinopathy status. As can be noted, the severity of the retinopathy seemed to be directly proportional to the duration of diabetes. Patients with no retinopathy showed the shortest duration of diabetes, compared to those with background and pre-proliferative retinopathy. Only 2 patients had proliferative retinopathy, numbers too small for evaluation.

Of the 80 patients, only 36 were seen at least twice during the course of the pregnancy with an average follow-up of 15.5 weeks. Initially, 6 of these had no retinopathy in either eye and did not develop such during the course of pregnancy. The remaining 26 had background retinopathy initially; during the course of pregnancy, 24 showed no progression and 2 developed pre-proliferative disease. Three had pre-proliferative changes; at first examination of these, 2 remained at the same stage whereas 1 developed proliferative changes and eventually required laser treatment. One patient on

Table 29–10. Retinopathy Status of 80 Pregnant Diabetics, According to Age and Duration of Diabetes

Status of Retinopathy	Patients No.	Age	(S.E.)	Duration	(S.E.)
No retinopathy	18	25.9	(1.74)	6.6	(1.0)
Background*	48	27.3	(0.66)	13.7	(0.95)
Pre-Proliferative**	12	26.2	(0.95)	17.7	(1.18)
Proliferative***	2	27.5	(5.5)	15.5	(4.5)
	80				

*Background retinopathy consists of microaneurysms and hemorrhages without the preproliferative characteristics defined by the ETDRS Manual of Operations.[36]
**Pre-proliferative retinopathy includes groupings of the following lesions: moderate to severe hemorrhages and microaneurysms, soft exudates, venous beading, and intraretinal microvascular abnormalities.[36]
***Proliferative retinopathy indicates the presence of definite neovascularization.

entry into the study had proliferative changes that also required additional laser treatment.

Considering eyes only, 17 eyes of the 80 patients had no diabetic retinopathy (NDR) and none of these developed retinopathy during the course of pregnancy. Forty-six eyes had background retinopathy (BDR) with 4 eyes developing pre-proliferative changes (PPDR). Of 6 eyes with pre-proliferative retinopathy upon entry into the study, 1 developed proliferative retinopathy (PDR) requiring laser during pregnancy. Two eyes had proliferative retinopathy requiring additional laser treatment.

Individual lesions were graded on the color photographs. In the majority of eyes, the hemorrhages and microaneurysms in Field 2 (the macular area), and the hemorrhages and microaneurysms in Fields 3 to 7 (the peripheral areas), stayed the same or became worse during the course of pregnancy (Table 29–11). There was also a tendency for a

Table 29–11. Course of Hemorrhages and Microaneurysms in Fields 2 and 3–7 During Pregnancy (49 Eyes)

	Field 2 (Macular area)	Fields 3–7 (Peripheral area)
Worse	22	25
Better	4	2
Same	23	22
	49	49

Table 29–12. Course of Individual Eye Lesions During Pregnancy

	Soft Exudates	VCAB*	IRMA**
Worse	13	13	12
Better	4	0	2
Same	11	4	13
	28	17	27

*Venous Caliber Abnormalities
**Intra Retinal Microvascular Abnormalities.

worsening or increase in soft exudates and venous caliber abnormalities (Table 29–12). Intraretinal microvascular abnormalities also, in general, did not improve and at best remained the same. Only 3 of 36 patients showed any changes in visual acuity with one patient with proliferative disease changing from 20/15 in each eye to 20/40 right eye and 20/30 in the left eye. Two patients with background retinopathy changed from 20/20 to 20/30 in each eye.

Summary of Pregnancy Data. 1. Most patients examined during pregnancy had some evidence of retinopathy. Also, since only 43% of the pregnant women were referred for examination, it is likely that the proportion of the patients with retinopathy in the group not seen was lower. Consequently, an accurate estimate of the prevalence of retinopathy in this group of pregnant diabetic women is not available.

2. In our study, most patients did not show a marked acceleration of retinopathy during pregnancy.

3. Patients with no retinopathy had significantly shorter duration of diabetes than those with retinopathy.

4. Patients with no retinopathy when first seen did not tend to develop such during the course of pregnancy.

5. Individual lesions tended to progress during pregnancy but this was sufficient to change the overall retinopathy grouping in only 5 of 71 eyes examined.

6. Visual acuity changes were uncommon.

7. Without a control group of non-pregnant women of comparable age, duration of diabetes, and retinopathy status, it is difficult to conclude whether or not pregnancy had any impact on retinopathy.

Recommendation. At the present time we recommend that all diabetics be seen by an ophthalmologist during the first month of pregnancy. If only minimal or no retinopathy is found, an additional visit is probably not necessary during pregnancy unless symptoms develop or retinal changes are noted during pregnancy at periodic examinations by the physician managing the diabetes. However, if more advanced retinopathy is found, additional visits during the pregnancy, even in the absence of symptoms, are reasonable and are recommended. Patients with pre-proliferative or proliferative disease should be seen every 1 to 2 months starting early in pregnancy. Patients with more than 15 years of diabetes should probably be seen more than once during the pregnancy regardless of retinopathy status. It is these patients that show the rare progression from minimal to significant retinopathy during pregnancy. Finally, we favor laser photocoagulation in pregnant patients when definite proliferative changes develop and in some patients with extremely active pre-proliferative retinopathy. This, in general, is earlier than we apply treatment in non-pregnant diabetic patients.

Renal Disease

With the advent of dialysis and renal transplantation for end-stage diabetic renal disease, ocular complications of kidney disease are seen more frequently by both internists and ophthalmologists. Two-year survival for dialysis patients is now 60% and the current survival rate for diabetics under 30 receiving a transplant, is 80%. Retinopathy has been reported to occur in 97% of uremic diabetics and to account for impaired sight in 50%.[46] Funduscopic changes in "renal retinopathy" consist of a hypertensive component and a renal component. The hypertensive changes are superficial retinal hemorrhage, cotton-wool spots, and narrowing and irregularity of the arterial tree. The renal component consists of a diffuse retinal and disc edema which has a characteristic opaque or translucent quality. Acute exacerbation of renal failure may be associated with the development of macular edema as a part of renal retinopathy in the diabetic patient. Treatment of the renal failure including diuretics may be accompanied by reduction of the general retinal and macular edema. Laser photocoagulation, in our hands, has not been effective in altering renal retinopathy. Renal retinopathy superimposed upon diabetic retinopathy predisposes the patient to neovascular glaucoma, makes laser photocoagulation much more difficult, and the beneficial results of treatment less likely to occur. Therefore, in the early stages of renal failure, consideration of laser photocoagulation is recommended prior to the appearance of the hypertensive renal component, as early as pre-proliferative or early stages of proliferative diabetic retinopathy.

Treatment for renal failure has also produced its own ocular problems. Transient rises in intraocular pressure have been noted during hemodialysis, particularly in eyes in which vitrectomy has been done. Therefore, glaucoma patients and others undergoing dialysis may require careful monitoring. An apparent increased risk of vitreous hemorrhage during hemodialysis may exist but has not been confirmed. Although heparinization may be implicated as causing hemorrhage, the occurrence of vitreous hemorrhage during hemodialysis is more likely to be related to rapid metabolic and blood pressure shifts. The frequency seems to have lessened in our experience with more sophisticated monitoring and reduced fluid load accumulation between dialysis treatments.

Summary. The management of the patient with, or at risk for, diabetic eye disease, especially diabetic retinopathy, requires knowledge of clinical nonocular risk factors which may influence the rate of progression of diabetic retinopathy. Prospective controlled randomized clinical trials are not available to substantiate the hazards discussed in this section. Nevertheless, in our opinion, the duration and age at onset of diabetes, degree of hyperglycemia, blood pressure, pregnancy, and renal disease are important clinical risk factors to be considered appropriately in the management of diabetic retinopathy.

TREATMENT OF DIABETIC RETINOPATHY

Bilateral adrenalectomy, anabolic steroids, vitamin P factors, antilipemics, hypophysectomy, radiotherapy, calcium dobesilate, calcium phosphate, fructose, vitamins C, E, and K, salicylates, cyclandelate (Cyclospasmol), and photocoagulation are among those therapies which have been proposed to prevent or treat diabetic retinopathy.

At the present time no medical therapy (aside perhaps from insulin) has been shown to alter the course of diabetic retinopathy beneficially. Aspirin is being studied in the ETDRS, and aspirin/dipyridamole (Persantine) is being studied in a French/English collaborative study.[47] Calcium dobesilate (Doxium) had no beneficial effect in a recently reported double-blind cross-over study[48] although some workers have regarded it as effective.[49,50] Clofibrate is still being used by some for exudative retinopathy but much less frequently than in previous years. This is partially due to reports of possible adverse systemic effects,[51] as well as lack of real evidence that it is effective.[29] Some believe that the drug still has not been adequately tested. However, due to lack of effectiveness, its use for retinopathy has been abandoned at the Joslin Clinic.

Pituitary Ablation for Proliferative Diabetic Retinopathy

Pituitary ablation has been a controversial means of treatment for PDR ever since it was first introduced by Luft in 1952.[52] Further impetus resulted from Poulsen's report in 1953[53] that one of his patients gained considerable angiopathic improvement of diabetic retinopathy following the development of acute pituitary insufficiency after delivering her child (Sheehan's syndrome).

Due to the fact that photocoagulation was not extensively used for proliferative diabetic retinopathy until 1962, several methods and techniques of pituitary ablation were developed. These included surgical hypophysectomy, stalk section, transphenoidal hypophysectomy, Yttrium-90 implantation, X-radiation, proton beam irradiation, and stereotactic hypophysectomy using radiofrequency coagulation.

Growth hormone was thought to be the retinopathic factor after Lundbaek[54] showed that its concentration in blood of juvenile diabetics was 3 times that in the normal control group. Wright[55] postulated also that improvement of the retinopathy was greatest in patients with low growth hormone concentration (in 36 diabetic patients with yttrium 90). The most acceptable theories to explain the retinopathic mechanisms of growth hormone are: (a) It increases sorbitol synthesis resulting in retinal damage by an osmotic mechanism.[56] (b) It increases clotting properties of blood and platelets and could predispose the patient to vascular occlusion as seen on fluorescein angiography.[57] On the other hand, retinopathy is unknown in nondiabetic acromegalics who may have high levels of growth hormone, and retinopathy is not necessarily worse in diabetic acromegalics than in non-acromegalic diabetics. In addition, retinopathy may even progress in diabetic patients following well-performed pituitary ablation.[58]

Pituitary ablation may be effective and useful in a limited group of patients; only one Joslin Clinic patient has been considered in the past 5 years. Patients with severe PDR but with visual acuity of 20/100 or better in the remaining eye may benefit from pituitary ablation after all else fails provided no severe systemic disease (particularly cardiovascular or renal) exists and provided the patient is mature enough to maintain a lifelong program of judicious hormone replacement.

The ocular finding that may indicate consideration of pituitary ablation is florid diabetic retinopathy in which large networks of new vessels are present over the disc, especially if they are elevated and have fibrotic tissue interspersed among them. Large areas of capillary occlusion might contraindicate pituitary ablation for it often accompanies poor retinal function postoperatively. A pre-operative electroretinogram (ERG) may have prognostic importance.[59]

Kohner in 1976 compared the responses of PDR to laser and to pituitary ablation and concluded "It is suggested that for this rare form of retinopathy (florid), pituitary ablation remains the treatment of choice if vision is to be maintained."[60] McMeel and Field,[61] reporting the results in 57 patients who underwent transphenoidal radiofrequency pituitary ablation, observed the following: (a) a clearing of nonhemorrhagic vitreous turbidity; (b) lessening of intravitreous hemorrhages and retinal edema; (c) decreasing caliber of abnormally dilated capillaries and new vessels; (d) lessening engorgement and segmentation of the large retinal veins; and (e) decreasing fluorescein leakage as noted by angiography. They observed that intraretinal hemorrhages were most responsive to pituitary ablation. However, hard exudates cleared less dramatically. Of their patients, 74% maintained or improved their preoperative visual acuity.

Valone and McMeel[62] reported in 1978 on 10 eyes of diabetics with severe adolescent-onset proliferative retinopathy who underwent pituitary ablation. Eight of these 10 eyes maintained visual acuity of better than 20/200, compared to a control group of 12 eyes in which 11 became blind due to severe PDR and traction retinal detachment.

The number of patients considered for pituitary ablation at the Joslin Clinic is limited as laser photocoagulation has been effective and the risk:benefit ratio of the photocoagulation—vitrectomy alternative is considered more favorable. At last report, there were no major diabetes centers routinely using pituitary ablation.

Photocoagulation

Only photocoagulation has been proven effective for the treatment of diabetic retinopathy (DR). With the report issued in April 1976, The Diabetic Retinopathy Study (DRS) under the leadership of Matthew Davis demonstrated beyond a doubt, that photocoagulation reduced the rate of severe visual loss (SVL) (VA 5/200 at two consecutive follow-up visits) in eyes with proliferative diabetic retinopathy (PDR).[63] Subsequent reports of this and other studies have confirmed these findings.[63,64] Photocoagulation in this study consisted of a "scatter" panretinal treatment, placing burns in a grid pattern around the eye, avoiding the macula and other vital structures (Figs. 29–6C and 9B). Focal treatment of new vessels was done in addition to scatter. Both argon laser and xenon arc photocoagulation were used. In this randomized trial, the 4-year rate of SVL in eyes assigned to the no treatment group was 28.5%. This was reduced to 12% in eyes assigned to treatment. In addition, certain characteristics were identified which place the eye at particularly high risk of SVL. The most important of these appears to be new vessels on the optic disc (NVD), (Fig. 29–9; Plate IV C, D) as well as the presence of vitreous or preretinal hemorrhage (Table 29–3) (Figs. 29–5, 8; Plate IV A, B, E, F, G, H). The details of these high risk characteristics are outlined elsewhere,[21,65–69] but if present in an eye, the 2-year risk of SVL is 25% or greater. The DRS also found some adverse effects of photocoagulation, particularly in the xenon-treated eyes. These included small losses in central visual acuity, and constriction in peripheral visual fields. Because of these adverse effects, the DRS fell short of recommending photocoagulation for all eyes of the types included in the study (Table 29–13).

The 2-year risk of SVL was found low in eyes with severe non-proliferative (3%) (Fig. 29–4), and in some groups of eyes with proliferative retinopathy (Figs. 29–5A, 7C, 7D; Plate III G) in which only 10% or less of eyes show NVD and/ or vitreous or pre-retinal hemorrhage. Consequently, the study could not conclude that immediate photocoagulation of these eyes was preferable to careful follow-up with treatment applied when progression to a more severe stage occurred. A new study, the Early Treatment Diabetic Retinopathy Study (ETDRS), sponsored by the NEI, is presently underway at 24 medical centers to answer this question. In addition, the ETDRS will address the question of the effectiveness of argon laser photocoagulation in treating macular edema which is perhaps the most common cause of lesser degrees of visual impairment in the diabetic (Figs. 29–6, 7; Plate III C, D, E). All patients enrolled in the ETDRS will receive either 650 mg of aspirin or placebo to evaluate the influence of this platelet anti-aggregant on the progression of retinopathy. If the increased aggregability of diabetic platelets[70,71] contributes to the development of cap-

illary closure in the diabetic retina, reversal of the process may slow the progression of the disease.

Though impressive evidence exists that photocoagulation is effective both in preventing severe visual loss and in slowing progression of retinopathy,[69] its mechanism of action remains unclear. The two most promising hypotheses are:

1. Photocoagulation destroys hypoxic retina which is producing a diffusable vasoproliferative substance necessary for new blood vessel growth, the removal of which leads to regression of new blood vessels.

2. Photocoagulation alters the metabolic relationship betwen the retina and underlying choroid, allowing the choroid to supply a greater proportion of retinal metabolic requirements (which are now decreased due to destruction of large areas of retina, particularly high metabolically active rod outer segments) and resulting in decreased stimulus for vasoproliferation via a specific diffusable substance or otherwise.

We personally favor some form of latter hypothesis though the evidence for either is not overwhelming. The effectiveness of photocoagulation may not be via reversal of processes that cause retinopathy to develop or progress. An understanding of how photocoagulation works should provide insight into the pathophysiology of retinopathy.

Progress of Early Treatment Diabetic Retinopathy Study

The ETDRS has been recruiting patients since December, 1979. Over 4000 have completed evaluations for study entry, and over 3000 have been treated in that time. We have enrolled several new clinics in the study to speed up patient recruitment. It is anticipated that recruitment will continue through 1984. Data are reviewed at 3- to 6-month intervals. To date, there have been no recommendations from the Data Monitoring Committee to alter study treatments. This would imply that unacceptable levels of adverse effects from one or another treatment have not been identified, and also that additional data are necessary to answer conclusively the questions for which the study was designed. We anticipate that that data will be available by the time the study is concluded, and the ETDRS will provide useful clinical guidelines concerning treatment of pre-proliferative and early proliferative stages of diabetic retinopathy as well as macular edema.

Vitrectomy

Counting laser photocoagulation as the first, a second major advance in the treatment of diabetic retinopathy has been the development of vitreous

Table 29–13. Estimated Percentages of Eyes with Harmful Effects Attributable to DRS Treatment

	Argon	Xenon
Decrease in Visual Acuity		
1 line	11	19
>2 lines	3	11
Constriction of Visual Field (Goldman IVe4) to an average of		
≤45°, >30° per meridian	5	25
≤30° per meridian	0	25

From Diabetic Retinopathy Study Research Group.[69a]

surgery. Though many people have made major contributions, Machemer et al.[72-75] developed the first clinically useful vitreous suction/cutting instrument. Since then, several workers have developed instruments for performing pars plana vitrectomy. He is responsible for popularizing this technique which is capable of restoring useful vision in eyes previously blind from vitreous hemorrhage.[72] Removal of the blood-filled vitreous (vitrectomy) is done through a small incision(s) using small pen-like instruments capable of cutting vitreous and membranes, extracting them from the eye by suction, and maintaining the integrity of the eye by infusion of fluids and gases.[72] In addition to removing opacities, vitrectomy can release traction on the retina which may have been causing or threatening retinal detachment. Though not the rule, visually impaired eyes can be restored to useful vision. Vitrectomy is undoubtedly a medical miracle in selected cases, able to do things unheard of only 15 years ago. It does, however, remain a risky procedure which should not be offered to a patient lightly. Data gathered by the Diabetic Retinopathy Vitrectomy Study (DRVS) during its design phase, showed that approximately 25% of eyes undergoing vitrectomy in diabetic patients lost vision from a complication of surgery.[76]

The modern era of vitreous surgery began with Kasner[77,78] who developed the technique of subtotal excision of formed vitreous. First, he showed that the eye can withstand extensive removal of the vitreous and its replacement with saline solution. Second, he demonstrated that this approach is suitable for a number of disease states, including diabetic vitreous hemorrhage, which have cloudy or opaque vitreous as a common feature, and which would be inoperable by any other means. Third, his initial success stimulated the development of new instrumentation and techniques to explore the full potential of vitrectomy.

The development of modern surgical microscopes and of suitable miniaturized instrumentation which made surgery possible from a small entry wound (pars plana approach) while maintaining the configuration of the globe and near-normal intraocular pressure, broadened considerably the scope of vitreous surgery.[73-75,79-81] It opened the way to the treatment of several opacifying and proliferative vitreous diseases which previously were considered beyond help; also it afforded a more promising treatment modality for several kinds of complicated retinal detachments.

The various instruments differ from each other in size, weight, and cutting action (rotating, oscillating, guillotine), and speed, and in the mode by which suction is applied (manual via syringe, or motor-driven vacuum pump). The improved instrumentation brought with it the need for improved illumination. Both the coaxial light of the operating microscope and the slit illumination give rise to disturbing light reflexes when the surgery proceeds to the mid- or posterior vitreous. However, using an intraocular fiberoptic light source, the light reflexes are completely eliminated and maximum illumination is provided in the vitreous cavity.[82,83]

Indications for Vitrectomy (Plate IV E, F, G, H). The present indications for trans-pars plana vitrectomy in diabetic patients consist of non-absorbing (after 6–12 months) vitreous hemorrhage, opaque vitreous or epiretinal membranes, and traction retinal detachment involving or imminently threatening the macula.

(1) Non-absorbing Vitreous Hemorrhage. Vitreous hemorrhages originate from retinal neovascularization which is either in the plane of the retina or, more often, already proliferating into the vitreous cavity. A small hemorrhage may clear spontaneously in the course of a few weeks or several months. While it is present it prevents light from reaching the retina, thereby causing various degrees of visual impairment. If a vitreous hemorrhage fails to absorb, it may remain in the vitreous cavity as liquid or semi-liquid blood, whitish gray degenerated blood, or may wholly or partially organize, forming "white blood" in the vitreous. The long-standing presence of blood in the vitreous cavity may also have some toxic effect on the retina because of the liberation of hemosiderin from the red blood cells; however, this toxic effect remains in question. To intervene surgically and remove the blood from the vitreous cavity may serve a triple purpose: (a) it creates clear optical media; (b) it removes substances which are possibly retinotoxic; and (c) it removes the matrix upon which fibrous proliferation could grow. One has to weigh these possible advantages of early surgery against the fact that hemorrhages signify activity of PDR. Operating in the presence of active retinopathy may expose the patient to yet another hemorrhage.

A large scale nationwide survey is being conducted by the Diabetic Retinopathy Vitrectomy Study (DRVS), mentioned earlier, to investigate the possible benefit of early vitrectomy in cases of fresh vitreous hemorrhage. Another phase of the DRVS is designed to investigate the effect of vitrectomy on eyes that have clear media (no significant vitreous hemorrhage) but show progressive retinal detachment due to traction, secondary to active fibrovascular PDR. This results from the clinical impression that pathologic neovascularization may recede after the scaffolding upon which it grows has been removed by vitrectomy.

The pre-operative evaluation of retinal function is of paramount importance. Pupillary response, light projection, entopic phenomena, and two-point light discrimination have been found to be fairly dependable tests in the presence of opaque media. Electrophysiologic testing (electroretinography, electrooculography, visually evoked response) has not been particularly useful for clinical purposes even though it is valuable as a research tool. Ultrasonographic evaluation is an absolute necessity if the retina cannot be visualized satisfactorily. The posterior hyaloid cone, the relation of major fibrous bands to the retina, and the presence or absence of retinal detachment can be demonstrated by this technique.

During vitrectomy the lens must be removed in certain instances. The indications for removal are: (a) the lens already has opacities and following vitrectomy, these opacities often increase, necessitating cataract operation at a later date; (b) during surgery, clouding of the posterior lens capsule often occurs which makes manipulation near or on the surface of the retina hazardous; (c) should any hemorrhage occur during surgery, the blood has free access to the outflow channels and can clear spontaneously more easily if the lens has already been removed; and (d) the diabetic patient is more prone to cataract development and progression than a nondiabetic. Some surgeons formerly removed the lens routinely during diabetic vitrectomy because of these four reasons. However, recent evidence[84] indicates that the postoperative occurrence of neovascular glaucoma is significantly lower if the integrity of the lens is preserved during vitrectomy.

(2) Vitreous or epiretinal membranes, a second indication for vitrectomy, are direct results of non-absorbing hemorrhages. Most often, partial or complete posterior vitreous detachment co-exists with hemorrhages. The posterior hyaloid forms a cone which anteriorly, at its broader part, is adherent to the vitreous base while posteriorly, at its apex, is connected to the optic nerve head. This cone serves as a matrix upon which neovascularization and fibrous proliferation can grow. While contracting, it exerts traction on the retina at locations where abnormal vitreo-retinal adhesions exist. As a result, it can cause new hemorrhages by rupturing neovascular fronds which originate from the retinal vessels and invade the vitreous body. In the presence of hemorrhage, the posterior hyaloid may opacify, taking the color and shape of a yellow-ochre conical membrane which prevents useful vision. Behind it there is usually either red or partially degenerated blood which has not been absorbed.

Epiretinal membranes sometimes form on the surface of the retina. They may cause retinal wrinkling and, if present on the posterior pole, distortion of the retinal image.

(3) Traction Retinal Detachments (Plate IV G). Posterior vitreous detachment and fibro-proliferative growth are the two components of this condition. Pre-retinal fibrous tissue growing onto the posterior hyaloid surface may eventually contract, resulting in a tractional retinal detachment. This typically occurs along the superior and inferior vascular arcades, although it may be observed at other retinal locations as well. The progression of a traction retinal detachment is usually quite slow and may arrest spontaneously at any stage. For this reason, the mere presence of a traction retinal detachment does not constitute an indication for vitrectomy unless the macular area is involved or acutely threatened.

Pre-Existing Ocular Risk Factors. There are three pre-existing ocular risk factors which have an influence on the visual results after vitrectomy: (1) rubeosis iridis; (2) traction retinal detachment; and (3) occluded retinal vasculature.

(1) *Rubeosis iridis* when present pre-operatively, may have two manifestations. One is the appearance of tightly looped blood vessels forming clusters around the pupillary border without peripheral extensions, and the other consists of arborizing blood vessels invading the filtration angle of the anterior chamber and causing neovascular glaucoma.

(2) *Traction retinal detachment* is usually recognized pre-operatively. The extent of the retinal detachment and the location of the traction bands and abnormal vitreo-retinal connections may be assessed visually if the media are clear. Should the presence of a cataract or hemorrhage obscure the view of the fundus, one must rely on an ultrasound examination (Fig. 29–10). Although ultrasonography has made great advances, interpretation may in some cases be difficult.

The presence of traction retinal detachment makes vitrectomy more difficult technically. The first step in a successful vitrectomy is the release of any antero-posterior traction. This is achieved by making an equatorial circular cut in the hyaloid cone (circumcision of the cone). The second step, equally important, is the release of tangential traction on the retina. This is accomplished by fragmenting and/or delaminating the epiretinal membranes. During the circumcision of the posterior vitreous cone, and particularly during the delamination of epiretinal membranes, the detached retina may come dangerously close to the posterior hyaloid and during the separation of the two structures, iatrogenic breaks may result.

If the vitrectomy is anatomically successful, the functional result will depend on how much macular

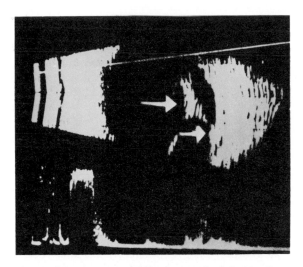

Fig. 29–10. A 22-year-old patient with diabetes of 16 years' duration whose proliferative diabetic retinopathy went on to vitreous hemorrhage and fibrous proliferation requiring vitrectomy. Ultrasound examination reveals fibrous membranes from back of vitreous with traction on retina (see arrows). See Plates 6, 6A–6H.

damage exists in the form of exudates, hemorrhages or impaired circulation (Plate 6, 6D).

(3) *Occluded retinal vasculature* cannot be recognized in the presence of opaque refractive media. This determination can only be made after the vitreous cavity has been sufficiently cleared to permit visual assessment of the status of the retina.

Intraoperative Complications. Complications during surgery may involve practically all the ocular structures: cornea, iris, lens, and retina. The cornea may develop epithelial or stromal edema, folds in Descemet's membrane, and endothelial damage. The iris may be accidentally cut or torn, causing intraocular bleeding or permanent deformity of the pupil. Touching the lens with an instrument will cause cataract formation. Posterior subcapsular lens opacities may also develop during a prolonged operation, making the visualization of deeper structures extremely difficult. Retinal complications include intraocular hemorrhage from the cutting of vascularized fibrous tissue and the creation of iatrogenic retinal breaks. Each of these complications must be treated individually if success is to be achieved. Corneal epithelial edema seriously impairs ocular visualization. Removal of the edematous epithelium restores the clarity of vision for the surgeon. Stromal edema and folds in Descemet's membrane are usually the result of a prolonged procedure or of profound ocular hypotony. Choosing the right kind of infusion solution and maintaining near-normal intraocular pressure during surgery usually obviates this problem.

If the lens opacifies to such an extent that it interferes with visualization, the surgeon has no choice but to remove it. This can be done through the same entry wound which had already been made for the vitrectomy. Either the vitreous suction-cutter or a lens fragmentation instrument may be used for this maneuver.

Intraocular hemorrhage may be treated in two ways. The intraocular pressure can be raised above the retinal vascular pressure, causing collapse of the bleeding vessel, or the site of the hemorrhage may be directly treated by either bipolar cautery or underwater diathermy.

Retinal breaks, whether pre-existing or iatrogenic, must be treated at the time of surgery. The surgeon has his choice of using conventional scleral buckling procedures or cryopexy in combination with complete intraocular fluid-gas exchange.

Postoperative Complications. All ocular structures may become involved in the postoperative course. Corneal complications are quite frequent; the most troublesome among them is the delayed healing of the corneal epithelium. Lubrication of the eye, pressure bandage, and therapeutic soft contact lens are the modes of treatment. It may take several weeks or sometimes months before the epithelium adheres firmly to Bowman's membrane. Stromal edema is usually the result of the decompensation of the corneal endothelium. It may require penetrating keratoplasty if vision is seriously affected despite medical therapy.

Rubeosis iridis may be seen after any type of intraocular surgery in the diabetic patient. It occurs particularly in 4 to 8 weeks postoperatively following vitrectomy in combination with lensectomy. For this reason, if a cataract is present and removal of the lens is necessary, we believe that it is safer to do it first and follow with the vitrectomy 1 to 2 months later. If the eye survives the cataract extraction without the development of rubeosis iridis, it can be predicted more safely that this complication will not occur after vitrectomy. The exceptions are those eyes which are known to harbor traction retinal detachment in addition to the cataract since the removal of a cataract allows the vitreous body to move forward. If the retina is attached to the posterior hyaloid, the forward shifting of the vitreous body tends to increase the extent of the retinal detachment. Also, it has been observed that rubeosis iridis following intraocular surgery occurs more frequently in those eyes which have a retinal detachment that fails to reattach.

Rubeosis iridis and neovascular glaucoma are frequently seen as complications of vitrectomy. A frequency of from 12 to 36% has been reported in patients who underwent lensectomy at the time of vitrectomy. If lensectomy is not performed at this time, the complication rate is reported to be 5.5%

to 8%. It is apparent that cataract extraction appears to be directly related to the post-operative development of rubeosis and neovascular glaucoma in vitrectomy patients. It is reported that if rubeosis iridis is present prior to vitrectomy, neovascular glaucoma will occur in 33% of the patients within 6 months as compared to a frequency of 17% if the condition is not present.

The pathogenesis for the development of rubeosis iridis is not known. If retinal tissue does liberate an angiogenesis factor, then the removal of the lens will allow the substance to bathe the iris with the resulting new rubeotic response.

In our experience, approximately 60% of the eyes that develop rubeosis iridis can be salvaged with vigorous use of strong topical corticosteroids, panretinal photocoagulation, and gonio-photocoagulation. Usually at least two of the three treatment modalities are used concurrently.

Repeated intraocular hemorrhages after vitrectomy tend to clear more rapidly than they do in eyes that have not undergone such surgery. This is true particularly in eyes in which the lens was removed, probably because the normal outflow channels are more easily accessible to the intraocular blood. Vitreous washout is indicated if the hemorrhage does not clear within a reasonable time. No definite time limits can be established, but we believe that a minimum of 2 to 3 months should be allowed before another surgical intervention is contemplated.

Retinal breaks and retinal detachments must be treated as if vitreous surgery had not preceded them. Some vitreous surgeons routinely employ an encircling silicone band on the equator of the globe, claiming that it diminishes the incidence of post-operative aphakic retinal detachment.[84]

Fibrinoid syndrome[85] is an infrequent but extremely severe postoperative complication. It can occur between 2 days and 2 weeks after vitrectomy. The corneal surface becomes irregular and, concurrently, white criss-cross strands appear in the vitreous cavity. They attach to each other and to the retina, and unless the fibrinous reaction can be controlled, the contraction of the fibrinous strands causes retinal detachment. The cause of this complication is unknown. It was found that multiple surgical procedures performed during the same operation (lens surgery, vitrectomy, and retinal detachment procedure) significantly increase its frequency. It is assumed that extensive surgery may cause a change in vascular permeability, resulting in the appearance of the fibrin-like material in the vitreous cavity. Therefore, it seems important to do as simple a procedure as possible which will accomplish the objective of the operation and refrain from unnecessary manipulation.

Therapy is purely symptomatic and is aimed at reducing the fibrinous reaction. Large doses of steroids given systemically (as much as 100 mg of prednisone a day) offer the only hope, but the prognosis is guarded. We had 16 eyes that developed this complication and only 9 could be saved.

Glial regrowth may occur, especially in those cases where extensive epiretinal membrane peeling was performed. The reforming of membranes may cover large areas of the retina, and, through shrinkage, cause retinal detachment.

Results of Vitrectomy in Joslin Clinic Patients. Between January, 1976 and June 30, 1981, 359 eyes of 326 diabetic patients of the W. P. Beetham Eye Unit of the Joslin Clinic underwent simple vitrectomy or vitrectomy combined with one or more other procedures. The courses of 112 of those who consecutively had the operation were analyzed. One patient died in renal failure 1 year after the operation; death due to myocardial infarction occurred in 1 patient in 2 years, and in 2 others, in 3 years after surgery. The remaining 108 patients had a minimum of a 4-year follow-up after surgery. All but one of the patients were insulin-dependent. The sex distribution and the age spread within the two sexes were approximately equal. All patients were hospitalized at least 48 hours before the planned surgery and underwent a thorough medical evaluation. Particular attention was paid to the control of diabetes, to normalization of high blood pressure, to correction of renal failure insofar as possible, and to cardiac supportive measures when needed.

For the purpose of this analysis, patients with diastolic blood pressure of 90 mm Hg and above were regarded as hypertensive. Blood urea nitrogen (BUN) levels of 20 mg/dl and serum creatinine of 1.2 mg/dl were regarded as the upper limits of normal in determining impaired renal function. Three patients had had kidney transplants and three patients were on chronic hemodialysis at the time of surgery.

When analyzing the results of the operation, one has to differentiate between anatomic and functional success. An operation is considered anatomically successful when, in the case of non-absorbing hemorrhages and/or opaque membranes, the blood or membranes are removed from the vitreous cavity, thus allowing light to reach the retina. In the case of traction retinal detachment, anatomical success means the release of traction bands and reattachment of the retina. Functional success involves a degree of visual improvement which can occur only after anatomic improvement has taken place. In this group of patients the number of hypertensive and normotensive individuals were approximately equal. The number of patients with impaired, and of those with normal, renal function were also close, with the differences statistically not significant. Therefore, it appeared that the presence of hypertension and of impaired renal function had no influence on the success of these vitrectomies in diabetic patients. Examination of the visual results revealed that 44 of 112 patients (39.3%) achieved vision of 20/200 or better and 28 had "traveling" vision (20/300 to finger counting). Thirteen patients (16.0%) could see hand movements or had light perception only, while 27 patients (20.5%) lost even light perception. Three of the 27 eyes that had lost light perception had to be enucleated due to intractably painful glaucoma (Table 29–14).

The causes of loss of light perception are neovascular glaucoma, occluded retinal vasculature, and traction retinal detachment that was not successfully re-attached or had been of such long duration that the retina could not recover after re-attachment. It is known from retinal detachment surgery that good macular function cannot be expected if the macula had been detached for more than 2 weeks. If the retinal vasculature is occluded, one cannot expect good central visual acuity. In our 112 patients, 57 had traction retinal detachment of various durations, some for as long as several years. The incidence of neovascular glaucoma is definitely higher in those patients who had a traction retinal detachment pre-operatively than in those who did not have this risk factor. Occluded retinal vasculature and the above mentioned two conditions are responsible for the cases that had poor visual results.

It is noteworthy that only two of the 112 patients developed retinal detachment postoperatively. One of them became inoperable and the other one was successfully re-attached but the post-operative vision was only light perception.

The visual improvement usually reaches its final level between 3 and 4 months postoperatively. There were some patients, however, who showed a slow, gradual visual improvement for up to 1 year after the operation.

Longer Term Follow-up. An analysis of results was carried out in a subset of 66 patients followed for 60 to 78 months after vitrectomy. In this group, 80 eyes had undergone surgery. At the time of the extended follow-up, 6 of the females and 6 of the males had died. The visual results in the 80 operated eyes are shown in Table 29–15. "Economically useful vision" (20/20 to 20/100) was attained in 28 eyes and "traveling" or "get-around" vision in 38 eyes (20/200 to finger counting and perception of hand movements or simply of light). Fourteen eyes had no light perception.

The renal status of the patients (32 females and 34 males) prior to vitrectomy is shown in Table 29–16. In 51.5%, blood urea nitrogen (BUN) was above the value of 20 mg/dl; in 43.9%, the serum creatinine was above 1.2 mg/dl; and in 42.4% proteinuria was present.

Vitrectomy in Diabetic Renal Failure Patients. Twenty-three of the previously mentioned 326 vitrectomy patients followed in the W. P. Beetham Eye Unit were known to have chronic renal failure and were undergoing hemodialysis or had had a kidney transplant. In these 23 patients, 36 eyes were operated upon. Two eyes were disqualified from this study because of lack of follow-up,

Table 29–14. Diabetic Vitrectomies
Visual results, 112 cases

Age at surgery		20/20-20/50	20/60-20/200	20/300-CF	HM-LP	NLP
20–39	F	1	5	4	1	9
	M	3	6	1	0	2
40–54	F	1	2	1	1	4
	M	0	2	2	3	3
55–69	F	3	9	8	3	3
	M	1	7	6	1	6
70+	F	2	0	3	2	0
	M	0	2	3	2	0
Total		11	33	28	13	27

Economically useful — 44

Traveling vision

Table 29–15. Vitrectomy in Diabetic Patients
Follow-Up from 60 to 78 Months
Visual Results

Visual function	Visual limitations	Number of eyes
Economically useful vision	20/20-20/40	7
	20/50-20/100	21
Traveling vision*	20/200-CF	31
	HM-LP	7
No light perception		14

*CF = counts fingers
HM = sees hand movements
LP = light perception

leaving the number included in the special study at 34.

There were 13 males and 10 females with only 1 female having undergone kidney transplant. The patients' ages ranged between 23 and 61 years, with an average of 40.2 years. It is noteworthy that the average age of the dialysis patients was 41.9 years, whereas that of the transplant patients was 36 years. The duration of diabetes ranged between 9 and 35 years with an average of 20.6 years. The average duration of diabetes for the dialysis patients was 19.5 years and, for the transplant patients, 24 years. All patients but one were insulin-dependent.

The indications for vitrectomy were either dense, non-absorbing vitreous hemorrhage (in 31 eyes) or traction retinal detachment involving or threatening the macula (in 3 eyes) or a combination of both. Pre-operative evaluation included determination of best corrected visual acuity, intraocular pressure with applanation tonometry, biomicroscopy, a fundus drawing, and vitreous study. Ultrasound was performed when indicated.

The pre-operative visual acuity of the patients varied from 20/200 to light perception. The intraocular pressure ranged between 11 and 21 mm Hg. Three eyes had rubeosis iridis before surgery and all of them progressed rapidly to neovascularization and hemorrhagic glaucoma which resulted in total blindness.

Most of the operations were done using the O'Malley ocutome, with a few exceptions where the Duvas roto-extractor or the Tolentino-Banko nibbler were used. The operation was usually carried out under general anesthesia (unless contraindicated). The Zeiss microscope with coaxial light and intraocular illumination was used in all cases. The distribution of procedures in these 34 eyes is shown in Table 29–17.

Six patients had already had kidney transplants. At the time of surgery, the renal function of 4 of these was within normal limits, while 2 patients had rejected their implants and were back on hemodialysis. Seventeen patients were undergoing hemodialysis, usually 3 times a week, with normal blood urea nitrogen and creatinine values at the time of surgery.

The follow-up ranged between 3 and 62 months with an average of 23 months. Thirteen of 34 eyes (38%) lost light perception from rubeosis iridis which evolved into neovascular and/or hemorrhagic glaucoma and subsequent pthisis bulbi. This figure is higher but not statistically different from the overall figures for neovascular glaucoma following vitrectomy reported in the literature to date (25 to 30% in some series). Subdividing by surgical procedure, simple pars plana vitrectomy had a 21.4% risk of total visual loss which is closer to the previously reported figures. However, if a secondary procedure such as lensectomy, intracapsular cataract extraction, scleral buckling, or cryopexy was added, the risk of neovascular glaucoma and blindness was high (50%). Whether this increased risk is due to the surgery itself or to the conditions that made additional surgery necessary, is unclear from our data.

Further studies are in progress to determine the significance of these findings in relation to diabetics without renal failure, the extent of vitreous hemorrhage and/or retinitis proliferans pre-operatively, duration and extent of renal disease prior to surgery, duration of diabetes, and other possible factors that could influence the outcome.

OPHTHALMOPLEGIA

Diabetes can be the cause of extraocular muscle palsies involving the 3rd (oculomotor), 4th (troch-

Table 29–16. Vitrectomy in Diabetic Patients
Follow-Up from 60 to 78 Months
Renal Status Before Surgery

	Blood Urea Nitrogen		Serum Creatinine		Proteinuria	
	High	Normal	High	Normal	Present	Absent
Females	14	18	10	22	9	23
Males	20	14	19	15	19	15
Total	34	32	29	37	28	38
Total Percent	51.5%	48.5%	43.9%	56.1%	42.4%	57.6%

Table 29–17. Vitrectomy in Diabetic Patients with Renal Failure

Type of surgery	Eyes operated on	TVL* percent
Vitrectomy (simple)	14	21.4%
Vitrectomy and lensectomy	4	
Vitrectomy and intracapsular cataract extraction	8	50%
Vitrectomy and 360 degree scleral buckle	3	
Vitrectomy, lensectomy, cryopexy, and 360 degree scleral buckle	5	
Total	34	

*TVL = Total visual loss

lear), and 6th (abducens) cranial nerves. Diplopia may be the presenting sign of previously undiagnosed diabetes, especially in the adult. In the case of 3rd nerve palsy, the eye is directed down and out with ptosis of the eyelid on that side. There may be pain associated with or preceding the palsy. The pupil is generally normal and reacts in the usual manner; indeed, the fact that the pupil is spared is a major differentiating point between the diabetic 3rd nerve palsy and that due to intracranial aneurysm or tumor. Aneurysm is a life-threatening condition and must be ruled out in any patient with a 3rd nerve palsy.

The diabetic patient with a 6th nerve palsy also complains of a sudden onset of double vision. The affected eye is turned inward toward the nose since the 6th nerve innervates the lateral rectus muscle which turns the eye outward. There are multiple causes of 6th nerve palsy because of its long intracranial course. When the 4th cranial nerve, which innervates the superior oblique muscle, is affected, there is usually a vertical diplopia with tilting of the visual images.

The hallmark of diabetic nerve palsies is that they usually resolve with recovery or beginning of recovery in a few weeks to 4 to 6 months. Any nerve palsy which does not show signs of recovery in 6 months may well not be of diabetic origin. Causes of nerve palsy other than diabetes should be considered initially and further evaluation carried out in case of lack of recovery after a reasonable interval. Whereas the 3rd, 4th, and 6th nerve palsies constitute external ophthalmoplegia, diabetic patients may also develop internal ophthalmoplegia, i.e., abnormalities of the pupil and accommodative mechanisms of the eye. The pupil may become sluggishly reactive in diabetics and this is thought to be due to a neuropathy of the nerves supplying the iris. The pupil is usually smaller in patients with long-standing diabetes. Rubeosis iridis can also affect the pupil and restrict its movement or sometimes may give the appear-

ance of a dilated pupil because of ectropion uveae (the turning outward of the iris pigment epithelium at the pupillary border). In eyes that have been photocoagulated heavily, there is often a poorly reactive dilated pupil. This is thought to be due to the effects of photocoagulation on the ciliary nerves which supply the iris sphincter muscles and travel in the choroid behind the retina under the area photocoagulated. Photocoagulation directed to the iris itself causes a somewhat dilated and poorly reactive pupil.

ORBITAL COMPLICATIONS

The bony orbit of the skull serves as a protective socket for the eye. Infections can occur in the orbit and are usually due to external puncture wounds or to spread from adjacent sinus cavities. Orbital cellulitis is a dangerous condition and if it spreads posteriorly to the cavernous sinus, can be fatal. It is characterized by massive swelling of the orbital and periorbital tissues and eyelids, along with pain, decreased vision and immobility of the eye. Since patients with poorly-controlled diabetes do not handle infection well, prompt treatment is imperative.

A classic infection of the orbit in the diabetic is mucormycosis, a fungal infection which usually spreads from adjacent sinuses. The typical presentation is in a patient whose diabetes is grossly out of control and who often is in ketoacidosis. Careful examination of the nose or soft palate frequently reveals the underlying eschar characteristic of this disease. The signs and symptoms of this potentially fatal orbital infection include ptosis, chemosis, extraocular muscle palsy, internal ophthalmoplegia, reduced vision and pain. The diagnosis is confirmed by biopsy. Intravenous amphotericin B and orbital exenteration are the treatments of choice.

ROLE OF NON-OPHTHALMIC PHYSICIANS IN MANAGING DIABETIC EYE DISEASE

Now that photocoagulation has proven effective in reducing the rate of severe visual loss from PDR, it is particularly important that patients with treatable stages of retinopathy be detected and referred to an ophthalmologist for appropriate treatment. Physicians can increase the likelihood of early treatment by:

1. Developing an understanding of the natural history of diabetic retinopathy and the current indications for photocoagulation as developed by the Diabetic Retinopathy Study (DRS).

Untreated eyes whose risk of severe visual loss (SVL) is greater than 25% over a 2-year follow-up period are called "high risk" and prompt photocoagulation of these eyes has been recommended. In Table 29–3 are shown the degrees of high risk as suggested by the DRS (Figs. 29–5B, 8, 9; Plate IV C, D, E, F, G, H).

Because 8 to 20% of photocoagulated eyes (depending on the treatment modality used) have an early persistent decrease in visual acuity of one or more lines on the visual acuity chart in excess of what might be expected from the natural course of the disease process, and also because constriction of the visual field has been noted following treatment (Table 29–14), photocoagulation has not been routinely recommended for eyes at lesser risk of severe visual losses (Table 29–4). It may be preferable to observe lesser risk patients for signs of progression before photocoagulation is initiated so those eyes that never progress would be spared the risk of treatment. The appropriate time to initiate photocoagulation is being investigated by a new clinical trial, the Early Treatment Diabetic Retinopathy Study (ETDRS).

2. Developing a regular pattern of referral with an ophthalmologist(s) knowledgeable in diabetic eye disease for baseline (pre-symptomatic) evaluation.

    a. Juvenile onset patients after 5 years of diabetes.

    b. Adult onset patients at time of onset of diabetes or soon thereafter.

3. Questioning the patient at regular intervals about ocular symptoms: persistent blurry vision, floaters, dots, or flashes of light.

4. Examining the retina (dilated pupil encouraged) at regular intervals with particular attention to certain key lesions including new vessels on the optic disc (NVD) (Fig. 29–9; Plate IV C, D); new vessels elsewhere (NVE) (Figs. 29–5, 7, 8; Plates III F, G, IV A, B); pre-retinal hemorrhage (Figs. 29–5B, 8; Plate IV A, B, E, F, G, H); vitreous hemorrhage (Plate IV E, F, G, H); venous beading (Figs. 29–5, 8); arteriolar white threads; exudates in the macular region (Figs. 29–6, 7; Plate III C, D, E); cotton-wool spots (Figs. 29–4, 5A and 5B); and intraretinal microvascular abnormalities (IRMA's) (Figs. 29–4, 5A).

The combination of a baseline ophthalmologic examination with interval evaluation and questioning by a knowledgeable non-ophthalmic physician should reduce the number of patients who develop severe hemorrhage and blindness without ever having had the opportunity to receive photocoagulation therapy.

REFERENCES

1. Herron, C.A.: Screening in diabetes mellitus: report of the Atlantic Workshop. Diabetes Care 2:357, 1979.
2. Brink, S.: Limited joint mobility (LJM) as a risk factor for complications in youngsters with IDDM. (Abstr.) Diabetes 32 (Suppl. 1):16a, 1983.
3. National Advisory Eye Council: Vision Research: a National Plan: 1978–1982. 1977. DHEW Publ. (NIH) 78–1258.
4. Kahn, H.A., Moorehead, H.B.: Statistics on Blindness in the Model Reporting Area 1969–1970. DHEW Publ. (NIH) 73–427.
5. Westat Inc: Summary and Critique of Available Data on the Prevalence and Economic and Social Cost of Visual Disorders and Disabilities. NIH, Feb. 16, 1976.
6. Davis, M.D., MacCormick, A.J.A., Harris, W.A.C., Haug, G.A.: Diabetic Retinopathy Prevalence and Importance. XXII. Concilium Ophthalmologicum Paris 1974. ACTA Vol. I, Paris, Masson, 1976, pp. 165–173.
7. Malone, J.I., Van Cader, T.C., Edwards, W.C.: Diabetic vascular changes in children. Diabetes 26:673, 1977.
8. Frank, R.N., Hoffman, W.H., Podgor, M.J., et al.: Retinopathy in juvenile-onset diabetes of short duration. Ophthalmol. (Rochester, MN) 87:1, 1980.
9. Palmberg, P., Smith, M., Waltman, S., et al.: The natural history of retinopathy in insulin-dependent juvenile-onset diabetes. Ophthalmol. (Rochester, MN) 88:613, 1981.
10. Rand, L.I.: Recent advances in diabetic retinopathy. Am. J. Med. 70:595, 1981.
10a. Klein, R., Klein, B.E., Moss, S.E., et al.: The Wisconsin Epidemiologic Study of Diabetic Retinopathy. II. Prevalence and risk of diabetic retinopathy when age at diagnosis is less than 30 years. Arch. Ophthalmol. 102:520, 1984.
10b. Krolewski, A.S., Rand, L.I., Warram, J.H., Christlieb, A.R.: Development of proliferative retinopathy in juvenile onset IDDM—40 years follow-up study (Abstract). Invest. Ophthalmol. Vis. Sci. (Suppl.):128, 1984.
11. Aiello, L.M., Rand, L.I., Briones, J.C., et al.: Diabetic retinopathy in Joslin Clinic patients with adult-onset diabetes. Ophthalmol. (Rochester, MN) 88:619, 1981.
12. Caird, F.I., Garrett, C.J.: Prognosis for vision in diabetic retinopathy. Diabetes 12:389, 1963.
13. Dorf, A., Ballantine, E.J., Bennett, P.H., Miller, M.: Retinopathy in Pima Indians. Relationships to glucose level, duration of diabetes, and age at examination in a population with a high prevalence of diabetes mellitus. Diabetes 25:554, 1976.
14. Kahn, H.A., Bradley, R.F.: Prevalence of diabetic retinopathy. Age, sex, and duration of diabetes. Br. J. Ophthalmol. 59:345, 1975.
15. Davis, M.D., Hiller, R., Magli, Y.L., et al.: Prognosis for life in patients with diabetes: Relation to severity of retinopathy. Trans. Am. Ophthalmol. Soc. 77:144, 1979.
16. Caird, F.I., Pirie, A., Ramsell, T.C.: Diabetes and the Eye. Oxford, Blackwell Publications, 1969, p. 69.
17. Waite, J.H., Beetham, W.P.: The visual mechanism in diabetes mellitus; comparative study of 2002 diabetics and 457 non-diabetics for control. N. Engl. J. Med. 212:367, 1935 and 212:429, 1935.
18. Olson, L.: Anatomy and embryology of the lens. In: T.D. Duane (Ed.): Clinical Ophthalmology. Hagerstown, MD. Harper & Row, 1979, Vol. I. pp. 1–8.
19. Van Heyningen, R.: Experimental studies on cataracts. Invest. Ophthalmol. 15:685, 1976.
20. Chumblay, L.C.: Ophthalmology in Internal Medicine. Philadelphia, W.B. Saunders Co., 1981, p. 38.
21. The Diabetic Retinopathy Study Research Group. The third report: Four risk factors for severe visual loss in diabetic retinopathy. Arch. Ophthalmol. 97:654, 1979.
22. Pavan, P.R., Aiello, L.M., Wafai, M.Z., Briones, J.C.: Optic disc edema in juvenile-onset diabetes. Arch. Ophthalmol. 98:2193, 1980.
23. Kohner, E.M., Hamilton, A.M., Saunders, S.J., et al.: The retinal blood flow in diabetes. Diabetologia 11:27, 1975.

24. Waltman, S.R., Oestrich, C., Krupin, T., et al.: Quantitative vitreous fluorophotometry. A sensitive technique for measuring early breakdown of the blood-retinal barrier in young diabetic patients. Diabetes 27:85, 1978.

24a. Kirber, W.M., Nichols, C.W., Laties, A.M.: Fluorescein studies on the RPE in streptozotocin diabetes. Invest. Ophthalmol. Vis. Sci. 17 (ARVO suppl.):225, 1978.

25. Yanoff, M., Fine, B.S.: Ocular Pathology; a Text and Atlas. Chapter 15. Hagerstown, MD. Harper & Row, 1975, pp. 566–585.

26. Rand, L.I., The Diabetic Retinopathy Study Research Group: Fundus photographic risk factors for development of severe visual loss in proliferative diabetic retinopathy (Abstr.) Invest. Ophthalmol. Vis. Sci. 19:198, 1980.

27. Duncan, L.J.P., Cullen, J.F., Ireland, J.T., et al.: A three-year trial of Atromid therapy in exudative diabetic retinopathy. Diabetes 17:458, 1968.

28. Van Eck, W.F.: The effect of a low fat diet on the serum lipids in diabetes and its significance in diabetic retinopathy. Am. J. Med. 27:196, 1959.

29. Cullen, J.F., Town, S.M., Campbell, C.J.: Double-blind trial of Atromid-S in exudative diabetic retinopathy. Trans. Ophthalmol. Soc. UK 94:554, 1974.

30. King, R.C., Dobree, J.H.: Exudative diabetic retinopathy. Br. J. Ophthalmol. 47:666, 1963.

31. The Diabetic Retinopathy Study Research Group: Report 7: A modification of the Airlie House Classification of Diabetic Retinopathy. Invest. Ophthalmol. Vis. Sci. 21, part 2:210, 1981.

32. Rand, L.I.: The Early Treatment Diabetic Retinopathy Study. In: E.A. Friedman, A. L'Esperance, Jr. (Eds.): Diabetes Renal-Retinal Syndrome Prevention and Management. New York, Grune & Stratton, 1982, pp. 155–170.

33. Klein, R., Klein, B.E., Moss, S., et al.: The Wisconsin Epidemiologic Study of Diabetic Retinopathy. III. Prevalence and risk of diabetic retinopathy when age at diagnosis is 30 or more years. Arch. Ophthalmol. 102:527, 1984.

34. Job, D., Eschwege, E., Buyot-Argenton, C., et al.: Effect of multiple daily insulin injections on the course of diabetic retinopathy. Diabetes 25:463, 1976.

35. Knowles, H.: The control of diabetes mellitus and the progression of retinopathy. Summary of papers. In: M.F. Goldberg, S.L. Fine (Eds.): Symposium on the Treatment of Diabetic Retinopathy. PHS Publication #1890, 1968, pp. 115–117 and 129–131.

36. Bradley, R.F., Ramos, E.: The eyes and diabetes. In: A. Marble, P. White, R.F. Bradley, L.P. Krall (Eds.): Joslin's Diabetes Mellitus, 11th Ed. Philadelphia, Lea & Febiger, 1971, pp. 485–486.

37. White, N.H., Waltman, S.R., Krupin, T., Santiago, J.V.: Reversal of abnormalities in ocular fluorophotometry in insulin-dependent diabetes after five to nine months of improved metabolic control. Diabetes 31:80, 1982.

38. Engerman, R., Bloodworth, J.M.B., Jr., Nelson, S.: Relationship of microvascular disease in diabetes to metabolic control. Diabetes 26:760, 1977.

38a. Engerman, R.L., Kern, T.S.: Experimental galactosemia produces diabetic-like retinopathy. Diabetes 33:97, 1984.

39. Knowler, W.C., Bennett, P.H., Ballintine, E.: Increased incidence of retinopathy in diabetes with elevated blood pressure. A six-year follow-up study in Pima Indians. N. Engl. J. Med. 302:645, 1980.

40. Rand, L.I.: Hypertension, smoking and other risk factors for diabetic retinopathy. In P. Henkind (Ed.): Acta XXIV. International Congress of Ophthalmology. Vol. 2. Philadelphia, J.B. Lippincott Company, 1982, p. 715.

41. Janka, H.U., Sandl, E., Bloss, G., et al.: Zur Epidemiologie der Hypertonie bei Diabetikern. Dtsch. Med. Wochenschr. 103:1540, 1978.

42. Christlieb, A.R., Warram, J.H., Krolewski, A.S., et al.: Hypertension: The major risk factor in juvenile-onset diabetics. Diabetes 30 (Suppl. 2):90, 1981.

43. Rodman, H.M., Singerman, L.J., Aiello, L.M., et al.: Diabetic retinopathy and its relationship to pregnancy. In: T.R. Merkaty, P.A.J. Adams (Eds.): The Diabetic Pregnancy, a Perinatal Perspective. New York, Grune & Stratton, 1979, pp. 73–91.

44. Aiello, L.M.: Pregnancy and diabetic retinopathy. Laser therapy. Presented at the Diabetes 1979 Proceedings of the 10th Congress of the International Diabetes Federation. Vienna, Austria, Sept. 9–14, 1979.

45. Briones, J.C., Rand, L.I., Aiello, L.M., et al.: Diabetic retinopathy in pregnancy. Presented at the New England Ophthalmological Society, May, 1981.

46. Friedman, E.A., L'Esperance, F.A., Jr.: Diabetes renal-retinal syndrome: the prognosis improves. (Editorial) Arch. Intern. Med. 140:1149, 1980.

47. DAMAD Study Group: Controlled clinical trial of the effect of aspirin and aspirin + dipyridamole on the development of diabetic retinopathy. I. General protocol. Diabete Metab. 8:91, 1982. (Eng. abstract).

48. Stamper, R.L., Smith, M.E., Aronson, S.B., et al.: The effect of calcium dobesilate on non-proliferative diabetic retinopathy. A controlled study. Ophthalmol. (Rochester, MN) 85:594, 1978.

49. Freyler, H.: Microvascular protection with calcium dobesilate (Doxium) in diabetic retinopathy. Ophthalmologica (Basel) 168:400, 1974.

50. Larsen, H.-W., Sander, E., Hoppe, R.: The value of calcium dobesilate in the treatment of diabetic retinopathy. A controlled clinical trial. Diabetologia 13:105, 1977.

51. Committee of Principal Investigators: A cooperative trial in the primary prevention of ischemic heart disease using clofibrate. Br. Heart J. 40:1069, 1978.

52. Luft, R., Olivecrona, H., Sjögren, E.: Hypophysectomy in man. Nord. Med. 47:351, 1952.

53. Poulsen, J.E.: The Houssay phenomenon in man: recovery from retinopathy in a case of diabetes with Simmonds' disease. Diabetes 2:7, 1953.

54. Lundbaek, K., Malmros, R., Andersen, H.C., et al.: Hypophysectomy for diabetic angiopathy. A preliminary report. Diabetes 11:474, 1962.

55. Wright, A.D., Kohner, E.M., Oakley, N.W., et al.: Serum growth hormone levels and the response of diabetic retinopathy to pituitary ablation. Br. Med. J. 2:346, 1969.

56. Beaumont, P., Schofield, P.J., Hollows, F.C., et al.: Growth hormone, sorbitol, and diabetic capillary disease. Lancet 1:579, 1971.

57. Kohner, E.M.: Diabetic retinopathy. Clin. Endocrinol. Metab. 6:345, 1977.

58. Kelly, W.F., Anapliotou, N., Joplin, G.F.: Pituitary ablation and its effect on diabetic retinopathy. Int. Ophthalmol. Clin. 18:165, 1978.

59. Wafai, M.Z., Hirose, R., McMeel, J.W.: Unpublished data.

60. Kohner, E.M., Hamilton, A.M., Joplin, G.F., Fraser, T.R.: Florid diabetic retinopathy and its reponse to treatment by photocoagulation or pituitary ablation. Diabetes 25:104, 1976.

61. McMeel, J.W., Field, R.A.: Pituitary ablation: treatment for diabetic retinopathy. In R.J. Brockhurst, S.A. Boruchoff, B.T. Hutchinson, et al. (Eds.): Controversy in Ophthalmology. Philadelphia, W.B. Saunders Co., 1977, pp. 686–693.

62. Valone, J.A., McMeel, J.W.: Severe adolescent-onset proliferative diabetic retinopathy, the effect of pituitary ablation. Arch. Ophthalmol. 96:1349, 1978.

63. The Diabetic Retinopathy Study Research Group: Prelim-

inary report on effects of photocoagulation therapy. Am. J. Ophthalmol. *81*:383, 1976.

64. Ederer, F., Hiller, R.: Clinical trials, diabetic retinopathy and photocoagulation. A re-analysis of five studies. Surv. Ophthalmol. *19*:267, 1975.

65. Ederer, F.: Randomized controlled clinical trial. National Eye Institute Workshop for Ophthalmologists. Why do we need controls? Why do we need to randomize? Am. J. Ophthalmol. *79*:758, 1975.

66. Rand, L.I., Kupfer, C.: Clinical trials in diabetic retinopathy. Ophthalmol. Clin. Diabetic Retinopathy *18*:17, 1978.

67. Davis, M.D.: Randomized controlled clinical trial. National Eye Institute Workshop for Ophthalmologists. Application of the principles of clinical trials. Am. J. Ophthalmol. *79*:779, 1975.

68. The Diabetic Retinopathy Study Research Group: Photocoagulation treatment of proliferative diabetic retinopathy. The second report of diabetic retinopathy study findings. Trans. Am. Acad. Ophthalmol. Otolaryngol. *85*:82, 1978.

69. The Diabetic Retinopathy Study Research Group: Photocoagulation treatment of proliferative diabetic retinopathy. A short report of long range results. Diabetic Retinopathy Study (DRS) Report Number Four. In: Proceedings of the 10th Congress of the International Diabetes Federation. Amsterdam, Excerpta Medica, 1980, pp. 789–794.

69a. The Diabetic Retinopathy Study Research Group: Photocoagulation treatment of proliferative diabetic retinopathy. Clinical application of Diabetic Retinopathy Study (DRS) findings, DRS Report Number 8. Ophthalmol. *88*:583, 1981.

70. Sagel, J., Colwell, J.A., Crook, L., Laimins, M.: Increased platelet aggregation in early diabetes mellitus. Ann. Intern. Med. *82*:733, 1975.

71. Dobbie, J.G., Kwaan, H.C., Colwell, J.A.: Suwanwela, N.: The role of platelets in pathogenesis of diabetic retinopathy. Trans. Am. Acad. Ophthalmol. Otolaryngol. *77*:43, 1973.

72. Machemer, R., Aaberg, T.M.: Vitrectomy, 2nd ed. New York, Grune & Stratton, 1979.

73. Machemer, R., Parel, J.-M., Buettner, H.: A new concept for vitreous surgery. I. Instrumentation. Am. J. Ophthalmol. *73*:1, 1972.

74. Machemer, R.: A new concept for vitreous surgery. II. Surgical technique and complications. Am. J. Ophthalmol. *74*:1022, 1972.

75. Machemer, R., Norton, E.W.D.: A new concept for vitreous surgery. III. Indications and results. Am. J. Ophthalmol. *74*:1032, 1972.

76. The Diabetic Retinopathy Vitrectomy Study Group: The Diabetic Retinopathy Vitrectomy Study: an explanation for patients. Group H. National Eye Institute (NEI), Bethesda, MD. National Institutes of Health, 1976.

77. Kasner, D.: Vitrectomy, a new approach to the management of vitreous. Highlts. Ophthalmol. *11*:304, 1968.

78. Kasner, D.: The technique of radical anterior vitrectomy in vitreous loss. In A. Balding, J. Welsh, R.C. Welsh (Eds.): The New Report on Cataract Surgery. Proceedings of the First Cataract Surgery Congress, 1969, Miami Beach. Miami, Miami Educational Press, 1969, pp. 1–4.

79. Douvas, N.: The cataract roto-extractor. (A preliminary report). Trans. Am. Acad. Ophthalmol. Otolaryngol. *77*:792, 1973.

80. Peyman, G.A., Dodich, N.A.: Experimental vitrectomy: instrumentation and surgical technique. Arch. Ophthalmol. *86*:548, 1971.

81. O'Malley, C., Heintz, R.M.: Creation of vitrectomy instruments, ideals, and practicalities. In A.R. Irvine, C. O'Malley (Eds.): Advances in Vitreous Surgery. Springfield, Charles C Thomas, 1976, pp. 319–327.

82. Thorpe, H.: Ocular endoscope. Trans. Am. Acad. Ophthalmol. Otolaryngol. *38*:442, 1929.

83. Leydhecker, F.K.: Zur Entfernung nichtmagnetischer-Fremdkörper aus dem Augeninnern. Klin. Augenheilk. *141*:665, 1940.

84. Blankenship, G.W.: The lens influence on diabetic vitrectomy results. Report of a prospective randomized study. Arch. Ophthalmol. *98*:2196, 1980.

85. Sebestyen, J.G.: Fibrinoid syndrome, vitrectomy surgery, and diabetes. Ann. Ophthalmol. *14*:853, 1982.

30 Diabetic Nephropathy

John A. D'Elia, Antoine Kaldany, Donald G. Miller, Nicolas N. Abourizk, and Larry A. Weinrauch

Much effort has been devoted to understanding diabetic microvascular disease and its impact on renal complications since the classic report by Kimmelstiel and Wilson.[1] However, in spite of impressive progress in certain areas, much confusion and disagreement remain. We shall review the main facts, summarizing clinical, pathologic and experimental data, and analyze their impact on the clinical management of the diabetic patients, particularly as seen at the Joslin Clinic.

PATHOPHYSIOLOGY

Renal Abnormalities Associated with Onset of Diabetes

In early studies of renal size in persons with newly diagnosed diabetes, Mogensen and Anderson[2] found a 20 to 25% increase in calculated kidney weight compared to normal subjects. The increase in renal mass involved the glomeruli, tubules, and glomerular capillaries[3-5] and while the total number of cells remained unchanged, isolated cells were larger.[3,5] Similar results were obtained in rats made diabetic with streptozotocin, namely, increase in renal weight with parallel increase in protein synthesis and cellular hypertrophy.[6,7] Kidney weight returned to normal following insulin therapy and adequate control of blood glucose levels.[7,8] The glomerular basement membrane may well increase in volume with the overall renal hypertrophy, but it is not thickened at this early stage.[7-9]

A number of functional abnormalities are present in the kidney in early diabetes, especially if poorly regulated. Renal "hyperfunction" at this stage is characterized by a 20 to 30% increase in the glomerular filtration rate (GFR) without a proportional rise in renal plasma flow.[10] The filtration fraction is increased as well.[11,12] The tubular maximum resorption rate for glucose (TmG) increases proportionately to the rise in GFR, indicating that the renal threshold remains constant and that the tub-ulo-glomerular balance is intact.[10,12,13] The in-creased GFR may be seen with proteinuria (up to 2 g/day); both are reversible with insulin therapy, resulting in the so-called "intermittent protein-uria."[10] The strong correlation between abnormal renal function and renal size in persons with early diabetes,[2] and reversal toward normal with insulin therapy,[14] was confirmed in animal studies where kidney weight and blood glucose correlated closely.[15]

The glomerulus is not permanently altered by the stress of the abrupt onset of diabetes. Tests of the glomerular sieving function show the expected inverse relationship between molecular weight and clearance. This can be tested by various sizes of dextrans[12] or by analysis of the clearance ratio of IgG to transferrin.[16] The transcapillary escape rate for albumin is only transiently elevated during pe-riods of poorly controlled diabetes.[17]

Renal Involvement in Long-Term Diabetes

In long-term diabetes, the most striking altera-tions are found in the glomeruli and the blood ves-sels. Light microscopic study of glomeruli show various abnormalities: a nodular lesion, a diffuse lesion (nodular and diffuse forms of intercapillary glomerulosclerosis), an exudative or fibrin-cap le-sion and the capsular-drop lesion. The nodular le-sion, described by Kimmelstiel and Wilson in 1936,[1] is thought to be pathognomonic of diabetes mellitus.[18] The diffuse form of intercapillary glom-erulosclerosis is characterized by the presence of increased amounts of eosinophilic, PAS-positive material within the mesangium. In most cases, ad-vanced changes of diffuse glomerulosclerosis co-exist with small or large localized nodules. It is unusual to observe advanced nodular changes in the absence of some evidence of the diffuse le-sion.[18] Mesangial cell proliferation may be seen in the diffuse form of intercapillary glomerulo-sclerosis, with subsequent difficulties in distin-guishing this lesion from a generalized and diffuse proliferative glomerulonephritis. Although no con-sistent relationship can be found between the se-verity of the clinical features (such as proteinuria, hypertension, and azotemia) and the histopathol-ogy, Gellman et al.[19] noted that the closest corre-lation occurs in the diffuse form of intercapillary glomerulosclerosis. The capsular drop lesion and the fibrin cap are not specific for diabetes since they can be found in arteriosclerosis and in some cases of glomerulonephritis.[18]

Electron microscopy has allowed a better appre-ciation of the nature of glomerular lesions in dia-betic nephropathy. It is now recognized that no-dular glomerulosclerosis results from an increase in the mesangial matrix.[20–22] Early mesangial cell proliferation[23] is gradually replaced by increase in mesangial matrix, and eventually the mesangial cells atrophy completely as a fully developed nod-ule takes shape.[20–23]

Glomerular size may present a striking degree of heterogeneity in diabetic glomerulosclerosis. From a Danish morphometric study,[5] it was con-cluded that enlarged glomeruli are due to compen-satory hypertrophy rather than to excessive depo-sition of basement membrane material. Although sclerosis of glomeruli progresses slowly and is seen in advanced stages only after 10 to 20 years of diabetes,[18,24] the rate of glomerular dysfunction ap-pears to proceed irrevocably along a straight line when the reciprocal of serum creatinine is plotted on one axis versus time on the other.[5,18] This proc-ess may well play a role in the rapid progression of the clinical syndrome once established.[5]

PATHOGENESIS OF DIABETIC GLOMERULAR DISEASE

The glomerular involvement in persons with in-sulin-dependent diabetes represents the local expression of generalized diabetic microangiopa-thy. Patients with Kimmelstiel-Wilson disease often have retinal, neurologic, and cardiac abnor-malities. Two major hypotheses have been ad-vanced over the years to explain the pathogenesis of diabetes mellitus and diabetic microangiopathy.

1. The *"genetic defect hypothesis"* envisions the disease as a primary genetic, somatic cell defect that is largely independent of the absence of ade-quate insulin effect,[25] resulting in accelerated rate of cell death and cell regeneration. In support of their hypothesis, Vracko and Benditt[25,26] suggest that the presence of several layers of basement membrane material, as seen in electron micro-scopic studies of diabetic capillaries, may indicate successive cell generation.[25] Cell debris can often be identified between the individual lamina.[25,26] Siperstein et al.[27,28] reported the presence of sig-nificant thickening of the basement membrane of capillaries taken from the quadriceps muscle of diabetic patients and nondiabetic offspring of dia-betic patients, thus suggesting that the alteration occurs independent of carbohydrate intolerance. Finally, Goldstein et al. reported a decreased rate of growth of fibroblasts obtained from prediabet-ics,[29] which would be consistent with the presence of primary mesenchymal disturbance.

2. The *"metabolic hypothesis"* ascribes the vascular and basement membrane alterations to pri-mary disturbances in lipid, glycoprotein, protein and carbohydrate metabolism resulting from a de-ficiency in insulin effect. This hypothesis seems to us to be the more tenable of the two because of

the evidence outlined below. In recent years it has won increasing support from clinicians and investigators alike.

a. Clinical and histologic studies involving quantitative electron microscopy show normal vascular structure at the moment of acute onset of diabetes.

b. Microvascular disease is found in persons with apparently non-genetic diabetes secondary to pancreatic or endocrine diseases,[30-32] but only after many years of diabetes.

c. Many large studies have indicated the beneficial effect of good glycemic control. In animal models, thickening of glomerular basement membranes could be slowed, or even prevented, with good control of diabetes.[8,33]

d. Diabetic vascular lesions can be seen within 5 years in biopsies of normal kidneys transplanted into diabetic patients.[34]

The concept of diabetic angiopathy as a secondary phenomenon implies that if diabetics are studied at the time of onset of diabetes, there should be no demonstrable basement membrane abnormalities. Also, progressive increase and worsening of microvascular lesions should be demonstrable. In Østerby's analysis of sequential renal biopsies, the progressive nature of glomerular basement membrane thickening in juvenile diabetics is clearly documented.[9] In another prospective study from Japan, progressive hyaline sclerosis of afferent and efferent renal arterioles was demonstrated as well.[35] Further, the progressive nature of these lesions was confirmed by analysis of biopsies obtained from kidneys transplanted in insulin-dependent diabetics.[34] Finally, it is extremely unusual to find changes of advanced glomerulosclerosis in children.[18]

Spiro[36] has reported an increase of a basement membrane glucosyltransferase in the renal cortex of diabetic rats. This increased enzymatic activity is partially reversible with insulin therapy if instituted early.

The pathway of glucose to glycoprotein is independent of insulin.[37] Hence, an excess of glucose with concomitant lack of insulin would divert greater amounts of glucose to the synthesis of glycoproteins.[38] Thus, a correlation exists between long-standing poor control of diabetes and the increased frequency and severity of vascular disease.

Biochemical analysis of glomerular basement membrane in diabetic patients revealed an increase in hydroxyproline[39] and decrease in proline.[40] The increase in glomerular size and mass may well be consequent to the increase in basement membrane collagen.[41]

Whether or not growth hormone is involved in the development of diabetic nephrosclerosis remains to be proven. It is noteworthy that in selected cases, stabilization of diabetic retinopathy may be achieved by pituitary ablation. Furthermore, growth-hormone-deficient dwarfs with diabetes show little angiopathy.[42] The effects of increased growth hormone and hyperglycemia have been combined in the glucose-growth hormone hypothesis, according to which "growth hormone increases the synthesis of the peptide chain and perhaps enhances hydroxylase activity while glucose increases the activity of the specific glycosyl-transferases."[43]

CLINICAL MANIFESTATIONS AND CLINICAL COURSE

Until recently, diabetic nephropathy inevitably led to death. Now, with the development of dialysis and renal transplantation, renal failure in the diabetic is treatable. This has focused more attention from clinicians on the renal complications of diabetes.

Glomerulosclerosis and the Nephrotic Syndrome

Only a minority of diabetics develop overt clinical renal disease. The earliest change is the development of an increased GFR which is reversible with better control of the blood glucose. This is followed by intermittent proteinuria which, after a variable period of time, becomes persistent. It is unusual to see persistent proteinuria in people with diabetes with duration of less than 10 years. However, by 15 years of diabetes, up to 33% of diabetics may have persistent proteinuria and occasionally the person with adult onset diabetes may manifest proteinuria earlier. In some cases, this may be due to a period of unrecognized diabetes prior to diagnosis.

The proteinuria is selective and its severity is variable. In many diabetics, proteinuria is mild and of no clinical significance. However, a minority of diabetics have heavy proteinuria (> 3 g/day) and develop the nephrotic syndrome with hypoalbuminemia, edema, and hyperlipidemia. In these patients, synthesis of albumin is inadequate to replace albumin lost through the kidney (Table 30–1). This leads to hypoalbuminemia with resultant decreased plasma oncotic pressure. Transudation of water into the extracellular space decreases plasma volume and causes the edema. Hypovolemia causes the kidney to retain sodium and water, thus making the edema even worse. Hypertriglyceridemia and hypercholesterolemia may arise from increased triglyceride and cholesterol synthesis coupled with increased lipoprotein synthesis.

Table 30–1.   Mechanism of Edema Formation in the Nephrotic Diabetic

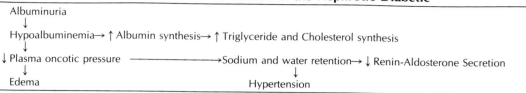

Albuminuria
↓
Hypoalbuminemia→ ↑ Albumin synthesis→ ↑ Triglyceride and Cholesterol synthesis
↓
↓ Plasma oncotic pressure ———————————→Sodium and water retention→ ↓ Renin-Aldosterone Secretion
↓   ↓
Edema   Hypertension

Therapy for the nephrotic syndrome in the diabetic is symptomatic only. The diabetic should be placed on moderate sodium restriction (1 to 2 g daily) plus diuretics if necessary to control edema. In addition, the patient should receive a protein diet of high biologic value in order to encourage maximum albumin synthesis. However, with the development of renal insufficiency and azotemia, the protein intake must be restricted. This is unfortunate because diabetes is one of the few causes of nephrotic syndrome in which the urinary albumin loss does not always decrease as renal function deteriorates.

Renal Insufficiency

Not all diabetics with proteinuria go on to develop renal insufficiency and then renal failure. The rate of deterioration is variable, but tends to be constant for any given diabetic.[44] Overall, an average of 4 to 6 years elapses from the onset of proteinuria until the development of renal failure.[45–47] During this time the diabetic develops the problems seen in any person with renal insufficiency: anemia, renal osteodystrophy, neuropathy, hypertension, and eventually uremic symptoms. In addition, diabetics may develop hyporeninemic hypo-aldosteronism and insulin sensitivity. Anemia often first develops when renal function has declined to 20 to 25% of normal. It is due mainly to inhibition of erythropoietic effect on bone marrow function by retained nitrogenous wastes with resultant decrease in red blood cell production. In addition, patients develop deficient blood clotting due to an excess of guanine that inhibits platelet aggregation and an excess of blood vessel prostacycline and a deficiency of thromboxane. This may lead to blood loss, especially from oozing through the gastrointestinal tract. In most cases the hematocrit stabilizes between 20 to 30%, although in rare cases it may be as low as 15%. If the hematocrit is under 18 to 20%, other causes of anemia should be excluded before assuming the person is anemic only because of renal disease. There is no specific therapy for anemia, unless deficiencies of iron, folate, vitamin B_{12} or pyridoxine can be demonstrated. Red blood cell transfusions may be necessary should the patient be symptomatic or the hematocrit dangerously low (< 17%). Large transfusion requirements may occur in patients with myelofibrosis associated with prolonged secondary hyperparathyroidism.

Renal Osteodystrophy

Bone change may represent a serious complication of renal disease. It is usually manifested as osteomalacia and/or osteitis fibrosa cystica. The causes are a deficiency of 1,25 $(OH)_2$ vitamin D and secondary hyperparathyroidism. The kidney is responsible for the conversion of 24 OH vitamin D to 1,25 $(OH)_2$ vitamin D. Less 1,25 $(OH)_2$ vitamin D is produced as GFR progressively falls below 20 to 25 ml/min. This results in less calcium absorption from the gastrointestinal tract, hypocalcemia, and osteomalacia. Renal excretion of phosphorus is impaired as renal insufficiency develops. This is partly compensated by an increase in phosphorus excretion per nephron, caused by an increase in parathormone. However, this compensation fails as the nephron population decreases and the patient eventually becomes hyperphosphatemic. Thus the diabetic with renal insufficiency suffers from a deficiency in vitamin D and from secondary hyperparathyroidism, with resultant hypocalcemia, hyperphosphatemia and bone disease. It has been shown that measures which normalize the serum calcium and phosphorus may retard the development of renal osteodystrophy. Therefore, the serum calcium and phosphorus should be checked periodically when the serum creatinine rises above 2.5 mg/dl. If the serum phosphorus is elevated, foods rich in phosphorus such as milk and milk products should be restricted and if necessary, a phosphate binder such as sucralfate (Carafate) should be given with meals. If a patient is hypocalcemic (and not hyperphosphatemic), he should be given supplemental calcium 1 to 2 g daily and, if necessary, vitamin D or vitamin D analogs (dihydrotachysterol or 1,25 (OH_2), vitamin D).

Neuropathy

People with severe renal insufficiency (GFR < 10 ml/min) may develop a combined sensory-motor peripheral neuropathy. As diabetics may already have peripheral neuropathy, it can be difficult to distinguish the diabetic from the uremic neuropathy. At times it may not be until after dialysis or transplantation that the two forms can be differentiated, since uremic neuropathy will be arrested or ameliorated with improvement in the uremia. In addition, the diabetic with autonomic neuropathy may suffer from nausea, vomiting, diarrhea, and light-headedness at a lesser degree of uremia than the uremic nondiabetic.

Finally, as renal function deteriorates (GFR of 5 to 10 ml/min), the diabetic may develop all of the symptoms of uremia: lethargy, anorexia, nausea, vomiting, pruritus, shortness of breath (from acidosis or congestive heart failure), edema, and even seizures and coma. Uremic pericarditis may develop.

SPECIAL ASPECTS OF RENAL INSUFFICIENCY IN THE DIABETIC

Although hyporenin-hypoaldosteronism is seen in the nondiabetic, it has most often been described in the diabetic with mild renal insufficiency.[48-50] These patients have hyperkalemia disproportionate to their degree of renal insufficiency, associated with an impaired ability to secrete potassium. Decreased levels of serum aldosterone and often plasma renin have been found. Postulated causes include fibrosis of the renin-producing interstitial cells, renal denervation, decreased catecholamine, and chronic expansion of the plasma volume. Therapy includes potassium restriction, potassium exchange resins, and at times mineralocorticoid replacement. Mineralocorticoid replacement itself, however, does not completely reverse the syndrome.

The development of renal insufficiency appears to make many diabetics more sensitive to insulin.[51] Therefore, they may develop repeated bouts of hypoglycemia if their insulin dose is not reduced. The cause of this increased insulin sensitivity is probably decreased renal degradation of insulin as the kidney fails. Diabetic control is also made more difficult because the urinary glucose threshold may change, and therefore urine glucose may not accurately reflect blood glucose. In this case, the patient may have to monitor the blood glucose at home to guide the regulation of the insulin dose. We have seen several patients with severe diabetic retinopathy and nephropathy who no longer require exogenous insulin.[51a]

Not all renal insufficiency in diabetics is caused by the diabetes.[52,52a] A nondiabetic cause of renal failure should be suspected if the kidneys are small, if there is no or minimal proteinuria, or if there is an abrupt deterioration in renal function. In particular, the physician should look for volume depletion, renal papillary necrosis, and a urinary tract infection. Contrast studies may induce renal failure more commonly in Type I diabetics than Type II

diabetics or nondiabetics.[53-56a] The renal failure is usually transient, but may at times be permanent. Therefore, contrast studies should be done only when absolutely necessary. The diabetic should be well hydrated, a minimal dose of dye used, and urine volume and creatinine should be carefully followed after the study.

Maintaining a high index of suspicion for nondiabetic etiologies in renal insufficiency patients is of practical as well as academic interest.[52] In collaboration with Drs. Scott Robertson and Ann Crosson of the New England Deaconess Hospital, we have already identified 23 patients with renal disease that was out of proportion to retinal involvement and who on biopsy were shown to have a variety of nondiabetic diagnoses.[52a] Obtaining a correct diagnosis allowed successful therapeutic intervention in 3 cases (2 cases involved medical therapy, 1 surgical). In the remainder, therapy was not directly altered, but a more firm prognosis was possible. Table 30-2 lists the diagnostic categories derived.

Case 108984 illustrates this point. This 34-year-old white male came to the Joslin Clinic with a history of diabetes for 7 years, requiring 24 units of insulin in split doses. On this regimen his blood glucose levels had been reasonably well controlled and he had had few complaints. His physicians, however, had been noting proteinuria for several years, which they assumed was caused by diabetes. He had no hypertension and no edema, but he did have an elevated serum cholesterol for which he had been placed on a diet restricted in cholesterol and saturated fats.

On admission to the New England Deaconess Hospital, physical examination was unremarkable, vital signs and fundi were normal, and there was no edema. However, the results of laboratory studies revealed a serum creatinine of 2.0 mg/dl and a urea nitrogen (BUN) of 30 mg/dl. The urinary sediment contained 6 rbd/phpf, protein was present in the urine to the extent of 15 g/24 h, and the creatinine clearance was 77 ml/min., serum albumin was 2.5 g/dl and cholesterol, 432 mg/dl. Intravenous pyelograms were normal.

Because of the discrepancy between the renal disease and the absence of apparent disease in the retina, fluorescein angiograms were performed which revealed the presence of two retinal holes but essentially no evidence of diabetic retinopathy. The origin of the renal lesion was thus pursued with a biopsy which revealed typical changes of membranoproliferative glomerulonephritis.

Treatment with prednisone was begun empirically when the serum creatinine rose to 2.7 mg/dl after initial reduction in proteinuria and stabilization of creatinine and blood urea nitrogen (BUN). He was continued on prednisone for 8 months with stabilization of the renal status, although he showed no further improvement. One year after stopping steroids, the creatinine and BUN remained stable at 2.0 and 30 mg/dl, respectively.

Thus, 10 years after the onset of proteinuria, the patient's renal function remains remarkably good. Though

Table 30–2.   Nondiabetic Renal Diseases in a Diabetic Population

A.	Glomerular Disorders.	
	1. Acute glomerulonephritis	3
	2. Unspecified glomerulopathy with subendothelial dense deposits	3
	3. Lupus nephritis	3
	4. Scleroderma nephritis	2
	5. Membranous glomerulopathy	2
	6. Membranoproliferative glomerulonephritis	1
	7. Minimal change disease	1
	8. Focal sclerosis	1
	9. Renal vein thrombosis	1
	10. Wegener's granulomatosis with rapidly progressive glomerulonephritis	1
B.	Tubular Disorders.	
	1. Acute tubular necrosis	>100*
	2. Polycystic kidney disease	2
	3. Reflux nephropathy	1
	4. Nephrolithiasis, papillary necrosis	1
	5. Amyloid obstruction of ureters	1

*In addition to the 23 patients mentioned in the text, more than 100 instances of acute tubular necrosis were noted.

the value of therapy cannot be definitely documented, the patient's course reflects the disservice that might have resulted had he been advised 10 years ago of the prognosis on the basis of renal disease due to diabetes.

The Role of Hypertension

Hypertension is found in the majority of diabetics with renal insufficiency. This is a serious problem, since increased blood pressure adds to the increased risk of atherosclerosis already present in the diabetic. In addition, the adverse effect of severe hypertension on renal function has been well documented.

Therapy must be individualized. There are many therapeutic approaches, but in our opinion sodium restriction and diuretics are the mainstays of therapy. Patients should be limited to less than 2 g of sodium daily. If the patient is still hypertensive, a thiazide diuretic should be added. If the patient has a GFR of < 20 ml/min, the thiazides may be ineffective and metolazone, furosemide or ethacrynic acid should be used. Diuretics act to reduce blood pressure initially by decreasing blood volume and later, via unknown mechanisms, by reducing peripheral vascular resistance. Hypokalemia is an uncommon problem with diuretics and can be managed by the judicious use of potassium supplements. Potassium-sparing agents (triamterene, spironolactone, or amiloride) may cause fatal hyperkalemia in the diabetic with renal insufficiency.

If the blood pressure is not controlled with the above measures, the addition of another antihypertensive drug (e.g. propranolol, prazosin, methyldopa, clonidine, reserpine, or minoxidil) is indicated. Propranolol is highly effective, but its β-adrenergic blockade may mask the symptoms of insulin-induced hypoglycemia in which the diabetic may become comatose. Prazosin, a vasodilator, may have an advantage over hydralazine in that it does not induce reflex tachycardia. Minoxidil is the most potent vasodilator known and may be effective even if prazosin or hydralazine are not. Diabetics with postural hypotension due to autonomic neuropathy may still be hypertensive when supine, making blood pressure control difficult.

Once proteinuria develops in a diabetic, there is low plasma renin activity as hypertension is recorded. Causes of decreased renin secretion in the presence of hypertension in diabetic neuropathy include items in Table 20–2.

Indications for Dialysis and Transplantation

The indications for dialysis or transplantation are the same in the diabetic as in the nondiabetic. These include development of uremic symptomatology, uremic pericarditis, progressive neuropathy, fluid overload, uncorrectable acidosis, and hyperkalemia. In our experience, the diabetic may suffer uremic symptoms, including neuropathy, sooner than the nondiabetic. In particular, nausea and vomiting from uremic exacerbated diabetic autonomic neuropathy may lead to volume depletion and further renal deterioration. Retinopathy may appear to progress more rapidly. Therefore, the diabetic is often started on dialysis or given a renal transplant before the nondiabetic.

Fluid Overload. While fluid overload is no more common in diabetics with proteinuria than in patients with other nephrotic states (amyloidosis, membranous nephropathy, lupus membranous nephropathy, membranoproliferative glomerulonephropathy), pathologic complications associated with diabetes may magnify the loss of volume regulation that occurs as glomerular and tubular function diminish (Table 30–3).

Although increases in total body water secondary to renal insufficiency are distributed across all fluid

Table 30–2a. Mechanisms of Decreased Renin and Aldosterone Secretion in Diabetic Nephropathy (Low Renin Hypertension)

A. Hyperosmolar volume expansion
B. Hyperkalemia*
C. Decreased conversion of (inactive) "big" renin†
D. Decreased catechol stimulation of juxtaglomerular apparatus (neuropathy)†
E. Hyaline sclerosis of afferent arterioles to juxtaglomerular apparatus†
F. Adrenal cortical enzyme deficiency (18-hydroxylase)‡

*Causes increased aldosterone.
†Aldosterone decrease secondary to decreased renin.
‡Renin unchanged or increased secondary to decreased aldosterone.

Table 30–3. Factors Which Alter the Volume of Fluid Compartments in Patients with Diabetic Nephropathy

		Increase	Decrease
A.	Total Body Water	Renal insufficiency	Diabetic diarrhea Deficiency of antidiuretic hormone

B.	Intravascular Volume	Hyperosmolarity
		  Sodium
		  Glucose
			Hypoproteinemia

C.	Intracellular Volume	Insulin	Hyperosmolarity
D.	Interstitial Volume	Hypoproteinemia Excess insulin, fluorocortisol Vasodilating antihypertensives	Diuretic

compartments, the physician is most concerned with the consequences of increased intravascular volume. Even in the presence of dehydration, mild to moderate renal insufficiency may be responsible for congestive heart failure when increased blood glucose leads to hyperosmolar nonketotic coma. Renal tubular transport of glucose and sodium reflect the state of volume depletion or expansion in parallel.[57] Thus, even in the presence of hyperglycemia, dehydration may enhance glucose reabsorption and worsen hyperosmolarity.

Axelrod[58] has described reversal of pulmonary edema by insulin therapy in a diabetic man whose urine output had been markedly curtailed by renal insufficiency. The process of normalizing an elevated blood glucose of 932 mg/dl was calculated to shift 1.2 liters of fluid into the intracellular space. Repetition of this experience provided convincing evidence that urinary or gastrointestinal fluid losses were not primarily responsible for the reversal of his clinical fluid overload state. Since Axelrod's observation, we have been able to confirm this entity of hyperosmolar pulmonary interstitial edema reversible with insulin therapy on eight separate occasions in four individuals who were functionally anephric hemodialysis patients. This reversal of pulmonary edema was achieved without change in body weight because of an average shift of 30 mOsm/L that could be almost entirely accounted for by a diminution in blood glucose from a mean of 870 to 150 mg/dl. The correction of

hyperglycemia ameliorates congestive heart failure by shifting glucose with water from the extracellular (intravascular) compartment to the intracellular compartment. In our patients, a mean fluid shift of 1.3 liters was accomplished without complications such as hypotension, hypoglycemia, hypokalemia, or manifestation of cerebral edema.[58a]

An increase in palpable interstitial peripheral edema occurs as serum albumin concentration falls during early and middle stages of diabetic nephropathy. In this situation, vasodilating antihypertensive drugs (hydralazine, prazosin, minoxidil, nifedipine) have been found to aggravate the formation of ankle edema. Sodium retention with the large doses of insulin used to treat ketoacidosis may be associated with sufficient accumulation of extracellular fluid to become palpable as edema.

A decrease in total body water may follow the repeated bouts of watery diarrhea associated with diabetic enteropathy (Table 30–3). A specific subgroup of diabetics with congenital deficiency of antidiuretic hormone and optic edema has been described.[59] In our experience, they span a spectrum of partial to complete deficiency of vasopressin.

Postural hypotension in patients with peripheral neuropathy and watery diarrhea may be minimized by use of fludrocortisone. When this drug is used in pharmacologic doses (0.3 to 1.0 mg/day), it may eventually produce fixed hypertension.[60]

Coronary Artery Disease. In diabetic patients with symptoms of dyspnea and interstitial pulmonary edema in the context of chronic renal failure, it is often quite difficult to determine whether the etiology is cardiac or renal. It is not surprising to find that large vessel coronary artery disease will be the major determinant of survival in these individuals, regardless of the mode of therapy for chronic renal failure.[61,62] While estimates of risk for the development of symptomatic coronary disease may vary based on the criterion of hyperglycemia used for the diagnosis of diabetes mellitus, in our experience 40 to 50% of diabetic patients under evaluation for severe renal insufficiency have significant coronary artery disease without definite symptoms, an observation confirmed by the Cleveland Clinic Group.[63,63a] The risk factors are many, including hypertension, hypertriglyceridemia, diminution of high-density lipoprotein cholesterol, hyperuricemia, and perhaps secondary hyperparathyroidism.[64]

Large vessel coronary artery disease is usually implicated when typical anginal chest pain occurs with or precedes interstitial pulmonary edema. However, even the addition of electrocardiographic changes to this clinical syndrome will not assure demonstrable obstructive lesions on coronary angiography. Electrocardiographic changes suggestive of an acute myocardial process may be mimicked by an exacerbation of hypertension (left ventricular diastolic overload), by hypotension secondary to depletion of blood volume, or by arrhythmias with aberrant conduction. Particularly confusing situations may arise when severe hyperkalemia occurs acutely, since the peaked T wave also occurs with a hyperacute ischemic process. Diabetics with renal failure are more susceptible to rapid swings in blood potassium which parallel rises and falls in blood glucose caused by deficiencies in both insulin and aldosterone. When acute hyperkalemia and acute interstitial pulmonary edema accompany hyperglycemia, treatment of all three problems may sometimes be accomplished with insulin alone as in the case originally described above by Axelrod.[58,58a]

In view of the difficulty in determining whether or not obstructive coronary atherosclerosis is present, *coronary angiography* may be indicated, but not before the multiple risks associated with this procedure have been considered. Some of these include arterial trauma with ischemic damage to a limb or loss of potential arteriovenous fistula hemodialysis access site. Radiographic contrast material is now widely recognized as a potential nephrotoxin in patients with underlying renal disease. Most instances of acute renal damage secondary to infusion of radiographic contrast material are reversible unless the baseline creatinine clearance is less than 25 ml/min or the serum creatinine greater

than 3.0 to 4.0 mg/dl. In these instances, availability of chronic dialytic therapy must be guaranteed before proceeding with the potentially nephrotoxic procedure.

The need for *noninvasive cardiac tests* is compelling. However, the existing technology does not satisfy the requirement for unequivocal results. For example, exercise testing in patients with proliferative retinopathy may exacerbate visual difficulties. Also, a combination of peripheral vascular disease plus metabolic neuropathy may make use of the treadmill quite difficult; bicycle ergometry is a potential alternative. Resting thallium scintigraphy may be relatively insensitive to the presence of ischemic coronary disease. Enhanced sensitivity may be achieved with exercise, atrial pacing, and vasodilating drugs. Because of the invasive nature of atrial pacing and intravenous vasodilators, these procedures are generally used only on an experimental basis. While specificity is high with regional abnormalities in blood flow, even adequate exercise testing may not delineate local defects in diffuse three-vessel obstructive disease. Echocardiography is routinely useful in detecting cardiac valve motion abnormalities, pericardial thickening or effusion, chamber dilatation, myocardial hypertrophy, and end-diastolic pressure elevation, but its usefulness in detecting coronary artery disease is negligible. An indirect method of evaluating coronary artery disease, study of ventricular wall motion by radioisotope blood pool scanning, holds considerable promise, as does nuclear magnetic resonance. The presence of segmental myocardial dysfunction on any of the above tests may enable the cardiologist to avoid coronary angiography in selected instances. When coronary angiography is required, it can often be delayed until the natural progression of diabetic nephropathy results in a requirement for dialysis.

Although premature or accelerated atherosclerosis is well-known in patients with diabetic nephropathy, coronary disease appears to be no different anatomically from that seen in the nondiabetic population. Thus, there is no convincing evidence for a specific entity sometimes referred to as "diabetic coronaries." As prognosis in these patients appers to be related to the presence or absence of significant coronary disease regardless of the means of treatment for renal insufficiency, the delineation of a high-risk group might be useful in decision-making.

Table 30–4 shows cardiac catheterization data from two groups of patients with diabetic nephropathy who were similar with regard to degree of azotemia, anemia, and hypertension as well as presence or absence of a surgically created arteriovenous fistula. Despite depressed left ventricular

Table 30–4. Cardiac Catheterization Data in Diabetic Nephropathy

	Patients number	Creatinine mg/dl	HGB g/dl	Mean BP mm Hg	LVEDP mm Hg	CO L/min	EF %
A. No Significant Coronary Disease							
1. With AV Fistula	7	7.3	7.5	107	11	10.5	77
2. Without AV Fistula	3	7.9	9.8	95	17	9.0	82
Mean	10	7.5	8.2	103	13	10.0	79*
B. Significant Coronary Disease							
1. With AV Fistula	7	8.2	9.0	109	20	9.7	64
2. Without AV Fistula	2	9.7	8.9	106	20	5.8	—
Mean	9	8.5	8.9	108	20	9.3	64*

HGB = Hemoglobin
LVEDP = Left Ventricular End-diastolic Pressure
CO = Cardiac Output
EF = Ejection Fraction
*$p < 0.05$ by unpaired t-test.

function in the group with obstructive coronary disease, groups were not definable by chest x-ray, cardiac output, clinical instances of fluid overload, or response to potent diuretics. Subsequent longitudinal follow-up, however, served to emphasize the predictive value of cardiac catheterization by demonstrating significant differences in survival within 2 years.[62,63] Patients with normal arteriograms had a 4-fold greater survival than those with significant coronary artery disease.

Myocardial Dysfunction. Numerous studies have presented both clinical and laboratory evidence of myocardial dysfunction in diabetic patients.[65–70] Segmental myocardial dysfunction can almost always be ascribed to localized coronary artery obstruction. Global myocardial dysfunction may relate to diffuse severe coronary artery disease or to a primary disease of the myocardium in the absence of coronary artery obstruction. Various hemodynamic stresses may result from hypertension,[71] deficiency of high-energy phosphates[72] or thiamine,[73] anemia[74] or iron overload,[75] surgical arteriovenous fistulas[76] with shunt greater than 10% of cardiac output, and perhaps uremic toxins[77,78] in these patients before or after dialysis has begun. Other nutritional (protein/calorie) deficiencies may contribute further to atrophy of the heart.[79] These factors, individually or in sum, may promote ventricular dilatation with diminished contractility at any given level of end-diastolic pressure or volume. However, higher pressure-volume settings may produce more easily those contraction abnormalities that characterize clinical cardiomyopathy as depicted by ventriculography or by diminution of the ejection fraction. It is, therefore, not surprising that in our experience most diabetic patients with cardiomyopathy have rather marked fluid overload hypertension secondary to nephrotic syndrome.

Depending upon the criteria used to define myocardiopathy, it is possible to estimate the prevalence of this entity at various stages of renal insufficiency. Within a small group of diabetic patients with hypertension and azotemia who are shown to have nearly normal coronary anatomy, there appears to be a subset with normal heart size, but abnormal pressure-volume relationships (Table 30–5). Such patients maintain normal cardiac output with a slight decrease in ejection fraction. Patients with clinical myocardiopathy demonstrate cardiomegaly with a diffusely abnormal ventriculogram, characterized by diminished contractility. The hemodynamic data of this subset of patients include a marked increase in left ventricular end-diastolic pressure and volume, as well as a slight decrease in cardiac output coupled with a significant diminished ejection fraction.[80]

Persons with nondiabetic cardiomyopathies appear to have a survival of about 5 years independent of etiology. In the context of potentially reversible disease (anemia, malnutrition, uremia), however, the prognosis may be better. Our experience thus far would suggest that myocardial dysfunction alone does not contraindicate renal transplantation since no cardiac deaths have occurred during 3 follow-up years. Some improvement in clinical myocardial function may be confirmed by cardiac echogram within the first year following successful renal transplantation.

A uremic cardiomyopathy has been described in the nondiabetic population.[78] This entity, attributed to direct uremic toxicity, may be reversed with dialysis. The patient may have hypotension, cardiomegaly, pericarditis, and increased sensitivity to digitalis. It is difficult to determine whether the primary mechanism is direct uremic toxicity or fluid overload with increased ventricular wall tension and displacement of the Starling curve. Regardless of which cause is primary, efforts to restore renal function would be the most logical form of therapy.

Finally, it should be mentioned that in our ex-

Table 30–5. Cardiac Catheterization Data from Diabetic Patients with Azotemic Nephropathy Found to Have No Significant Obstructive Coronary Artery Disease

	Patients Number	MAP mm Hg	LVEDP mm Hg	LEVDV ml/m	CO L/min	EF %
Normal Myocardial Function	7	100	10	85	10	83
Pressure Volume Abnormalities	4	113	20	90	10	70
Myocardiopathy*	4	105	24	105	7	47

MAP = Mean Aortic Pressure
LVEDP = Left Ventricular End-Diastolic Pressure
LVEDV = Left Ventricular End-Diastolic Volume
CO = Cardiac Output
EF = Ejection Fraction
*Defined by diffusely abnormal ventriculogram

perience diabetic cardiomyopathy has been encountered in juvenile diabetics with azotemic nephropathy.[80] This includes clinical signs of congestive heart failure and abnormal left ventricular pressure-volume kinetics in the absence of angiographically demonstrable coronary artery disease. Although this could be due to cardiac microangiopathy as reported recently,[80a] it seems that such a cardiac dysfunction is ameliorated after renal transplantation.

Pericardial Disease. Aseptic fibrinous pericarditis may be a cause of death in severe renal insufficiency, usually because of tamponade leading to restrictive heart failure. Occasionally acute intrapericardial hemorrhage may occur following the use of heparin for hemodialysis. It has been suggested that diabetics with renal failure have a higher incidence of pericarditis than patients with other types of kidney disease, but to date no studies support an infectious etiology. The presence of hypotension, cardiomegaly, and right heart failure in a patient with pericardial pain and a three-component friction rub remains an ominous sign that may not be relieved by dialysis alone. Direct surgical intervention on the pericardium may be required.

Hypertension. Special problems may be expected in the treatment of the hypertensive patient who suffers from both renal failure and diabetes mellitus. This is naturally so because even potent loop diuretics may be ineffective as creatinine clearance falls below 10 to 15 ml/min in a hyperosmolar state. Also, combined diabetic-uremic neuropathy promotes the antihypertensive effect of methyldopa, clonidine, and prazosin so as to limit their usefulness in certain individuals who find postural hypotension intolerable (Table 30–6). Another problem associated with clonidine and prazosin is fluid retention, which is tolerable or intolerable depending upon the response to diuretics. Vasodilators, particularly hydralazine, may also increase myocardial oxygen consumption leading to angina, palpitations, and a worsening of

Table 30–6. Side Effects of Drugs Used to Control Hypertension in the Azotemic Diabetic

Postural hypotension: methyldopa, clonidine, prazosin
Impotence: methyldopa, guanethidine
Angina pectoris or palpitation: hydralazine, prazosin
Congestive heart failure: propranolol, nifedipine
Impaired response to hypoglycemia: propranolol
Tachyphylaxis: prazosin
Increased hair growth: minoxidil

congestive heart failure. Such problems as diminished diuretic responsiveness, increased myocardial oxygen consumption, and fluid retention may combine to dictate the need for earlier institution of dialysis than might have been necessary for a similar level of creatinine clearance in a normotensive patient.

Although nondiuretic drug therapy for increased blood pressure may continue to be required after a stable dialysis schedule has been established, the dosage levels generally can be reduced. This follows directly from the elimination of excess total body salt and water, but indirectly from the need to avoid sudden hypotension during ultrafiltration hemodialysis. Angina pectoris, atrial or ventricular arrhythmias, and pulmonary edema may complicate hemodialysis when an anemic patient becomes suddenly hypotensive during ultrafiltration, resulting in an attempt to correct for fluid deficit by the rapid infusion of several hundred milliliters of normal saline solution. One guideline involves withholding the vasodilator antihypertensive drug for several hours just prior to each hemodialysis treatment. Nevertheless, individuals with combined diabetic-uremic neuropathy may experience uncomfortable hypotensive symptoms during hemodialysis even if antihypertensive therapy is withdrawn entirely.

The severity of autonomic neuropathy (including emesis of undigested food; frequent, watery diarrhea) parallels the degree of azotemia. Addition of sympathoplegic drugs, such as guanethidine may, in this situation, be contraindicated. Clinical hypoglycemic reactions may be blunted in the difficult-to-control diabetic when beta-adrenergic blockers (propranolol, metopralol) are used.

Despite the multitude of side effects potentially involved in the use of potent antihypertensive drugs in diabetics with renal failure, we believe it is crucial to limit deterioration of retinal and glomerular circulations by application of the principles outlined in Chapter 28 on hypertension. Further major arterial deterioration involving cerebral, coronary, and peripheral vessels probably occurs in much the same way as is seen in nondiabetic patients with renal insufficiency.

Malnutrition. Several nutritional problems occur occasionally in hospitalized diabetics with chronic renal failure. Despite dietary therapy, the uremic patient is often left with borderline nutrition. Diets low in protein and electrolytes can be difficult to maintain, and anorexia due to uremic toxins and emotional depression further diminish food intake. Loss of blood from frequent phlebotomy and gastrointestinal bleeding, and loss of protein and amino acids in peritoneal and hemodialysis, further deplete the patient's nutritional status.

If the patient then encounters severe complications (e.g., severe infection, pernicious vomiting, or diabetic gastroparesis) leading to increased protein breakdown and/or decreased capacity to eat, another route of nutrient delivery is necessary. Work in collaboration with Dr. Gerald Batist and Dr. Bruce Bistrian of the New England Deaconess Hospital has shown that such a patient can now be "fed" via a catheter placed in a large central vein. One can use a solution consisting of 4.5 to 6.5% crystallized amino acids and 25 to 40% dextrose, with the addition of regular insulin and various electrolytes in accordance with serum levels. Lipid emulsions can also be added. Approximately 50 kcal/kg/day are supplied. Parameters indicative of malnutrition include anthropometric measurements of body weight, muscle mass, and body fat stores. Plasma levels of total protein, albumin, and transferrin show significant depletion.[81]

By monitoring carefully the above described parameters of nutritional status with a close eye to electrolytes and glucose, patients can be fed successfully for short courses of up to 6 weeks. Data show improved levels of body weight, serum protein, and transferrin in 7 such patients.[82]

The breakdown of the amino acids given intravenously, as well as the breakdown of endogenous protein as seen in conditions of stress, may result in elevation of blood urea nitrogen (BUN), which may require additional dialysis to prevent uremic symptoms. However, positive nitrogen balance can be maintained by this means. Concomitantly, with new cell production, electrolytes such as potassium and phosphorus are shunted extracellularly. This may result in diminished serum levels of these salts, and care must be taken not to lower them dangerously during dialysis. Measurements of the overall balance of protein nitrogen absorbed versus nitrogen excreted as waste products in blood (BUN) and urine show definite movement in favor of intake. Diabetes is controlled with regular insulin in the solution given intravenously and additional insulin is given in accordance with frequent blood glucose measurements. During this period of total parenteral nutrition, attention is directed to relieving the acute event leading to this increased nutritional requirement. Patients generally feel better and appetites improve, so that physical therapy may be initiated to mobilize the patient.

THE DIABETIC RENAL-RETINAL SYNDROME

Patients with diabetic nephropathy may suffer simultaneously from a progressive retinopathy with visual failure. This diabetic renal-retinal syndrome results from long-standing progressive microangiopathy. Its pathogenesis involves a series of microcirculatory changes including basement membrane thickening, mural cell dysfunction, permeability disorders and small vessel occlusion.[83–85] Consequently, hypoxic cell damage and/or deposition of biochemically abnormal basement membrane glycoproteins ensues. Although these changes seem to be generalized throughout the body,[80a,86] they are clinically serious and devastating disorders of eye and kidney.

The need to cope with the ocular complications, which calls for a collaborative approach, is becoming recognized in uremic diabetics. Using current methods of treatment, prolongation of useful life has become possible in diabetics with advanced microvascular complications.

Microcirculatory Disease in the Eye and the Kidney

The pericyte of the retinal capillary and the mesangial cell of the renal glomerulus are parallel elements in the pathogenesis of diabetic microcirculatory disease. Early in this syndrome, there is a conspicuous, but enigmatic, selective loss of the retinal capillary pericyte, a cell which normally is present in a ratio of 1:1 with ordinary endothelial cells.[87] Mesangial cell dysfunction, on the other hand, involves two basic abnormalities. First, the mesangium, in diabetes, exhibits a marked increase in contractile actomyosin-like proteins,[88] the importance of which in physiologic control of glomerular filtration and blood flow is under active study.[89] Second, in alloxan-diabetic rats, there is an advanced mesangial insufficiency in clearing accumulating basement membrane macromolecular proteins and peptide derivatives; the insufficiency appears to be reversible with improved control of the insulin-deficient state.[90]

Another aspect of the process of capillary damage involves metabolic and cellular changes that lead to stasis in the microcirculation. An increase in red cell[91] and platelet aggregation,[92,93] together with a decrease in red cell deformability and fibrinolysis,[91] may cause mechanical reduction of local blood flow in retinal and glomerular capillaries. The situation may be further aggravated by a hyperviscosity state, associated with either an increased concentration or glycosylation of plasma proteins.[82,94] Microvascular stasis may play a central role in inducing regional ischemia, a basic process underlying retinal and renal complications.[91,95]

Permeability and structural disorders of endothelial basement membrane contribute to the pathogenesis of the microcirculatory disease. The integrity of the basement membrane may possibly be altered by excess glycosylation of polypeptide constituents resulting in the breakdown of blood-retinal barriers. Subsequent increases in permeability may lead to intra-retinal edema and to deposition of globin and/or albumin in the glomerulus as well as to proteinuria.[40,91,96] The unique patterns of glomerular hyalinization in diabetes are generally understood to be a part of a basement membrane disorder in which enzymatic synthesis of a basement-membrane-like material is enhanced. Moreover, this material is glycosylated and, hence, rendered less susceptible to proteolytic degradation.[97]

There is increasing evidence that hyperglycemia and relative insulin deficiency are responsible for the sequence of abnormalities outlined above.[91] A genetic susceptibility cannot be completely ruled out. Advent of better modes of delivery of insulin, including open- and closed-loop systems, may eventually clarify the role of the genetic component.[98]

Natural Course: Clinical Parallels in Renal and Ocular Failure

The clinical relationship between diabetic nephropathy and diabetic retinopathy is revealed through their parallel natural courses and the interdependence of their various treatment modalities. Strong evidence supports the belief that duration of diabetes and degree of glycemic control influence the natural course of diabetic retinopathy, exerting a profound effect upon its time of onset and severity.[99] Generally, background retinopathy precedes proteinuria, which is an early clinical sign

of diabetic nephropathy. Retinopathy may coincide with the onset of biochemical or histologic glomerular basement membrane changes, which may occur several years prior to proteinuria.[100] In advanced diabetic nephropathy, fixed proteinuria parallels in degree the severity of the retinopathy.[100] While diabetic retinopathy is invariably a concomitant finding in clinically detectable Kimmelstiel-Wilson nephropathy, the reverse is not necessarily true.

Observations of a higher incidence of hypertension in diabetic patients raise the question of its relation to the pathogenesis of microangiopathic renal-retinal diabetic disease.[101-104] There have been attempts to define an entity of "diabetic hypertension" whose etiology is probably renal, whose mechanism might involve a state of hyporeninemia, and whose incidence parallels closely that of proteinuria in juvenile-onset diabetes.[105] These mechanisms might coexist with an essential and/or systolic atherosclerotic type of hypertension. Despite a prominent association of retinopathy with raised systolic blood pressure[106] and the corollary that hypertension may hasten its course, there is as yet no proven role of hypertension in diabetic retinopathy.[99,107]

Methods of treatment for diabetic nephropathy include long-term hemodialysis, peritoneal dialysis, and renal transplantation. Despite improvement in the survival rate of patients treated with long-term hemodialysis, there continues to be concern that hemodialysis may be associated with potential acceleration of progression of retinopathy to proliferation and to hemorrhage.[108] Of less concern are those alterations in visual acuity associated with marked glycemic fluctuations.

The reasons for retinopathic deterioration during chronic hemodialysis are not clear, but factors such as systemic heparinization, marked glycemic (and hence osmolal) fluctuations, and undulating blood pressure levels play an exacerbating role. Superimposed upon these factors is the variation in intraocular pressure during hemodialysis. Experimental hypovolemia (dehydration in uremic dogs) or hyperosmolality (addition of solute to hemodialysis bath solution) may induce a significant decrease in intraocular pressure in uremic animals.[109] Conversely, a small but significant rise in intraocular pressure has been demonstrated during euvolemic hemodialysis in patients with no evidence of ocular disease. This rise in intraocular pressure can be blocked with acetazolamide.

Since patients with sequelae of proliferative retinopathy (vitreous hemorrhage with fibrosis, retinal detachment, rubeosis iridis) may suffer hazardous changes in intraocular pressure during hemodialysis, the dialysis team must minimize the degree of these fluctuations by removing excess body water slowly. Considering the potential for increased ocular morbidity with functional visual disability that is associated with chronic hemodialysis, attempts to use long-term peritoneal dialysis are quite reasonable, and, in at least one center, have revealed a marked diminution in visual complications with no progress in retinopathic sequelae.[108] Peritoneal and hemodialysis, nevertheless, lead to good survival rates for uremic diabetics whose prognosis would have been dim a few years ago. Promising results are also obtained from renal transplantation where even better survival rates and rehabilitation are to be expected.[110,111]

Blindness and traction retinal detachment are now amenable to vitrectomy.[112,113] Since an increasing number of patients with diabetic nephropathy are being kept alive by maintenance hemodialysis, their proliferative retinopathy will require surgical intervention in some cases, despite reluctance to operate in the presence of intermittent anticoagulation. Recent preliminary data with short-term follow-up show that major eye surgery (mainly vitrectomies and cataract extractions) can be performed safely on insulin-dependent diabetic patients being treated for their advanced nephropathies.[114] The relative safety is reassuring to patients treated medically with chronic hemodialysis or with renal transplantation, considering the high-risk nature of such categories of patients. However, one of the observed complications of vitrectomies is devastating in that 10 to 20% of diabetic post-vitrectomy patients may develop rubeosis iridis with hemorrhagic glaucoma and blindness.[112] It may be that hemodialysis precipitates this complication in diabetic post-vitrectomy patients, probably by causing anticoagulation on one hand, and variation in intraocular pressure (accompanying hydration and glycemic osmolal changes) on the other. It is not uncommon to encounter acute severe unilateral glaucomatous eyes in patients with post-vitrectomy rubeosis iridis during hemodialysis.

It is generally agreed that by the time nephropathy results, virtually all diabetics will have some grade of retinopathy.[115] Despite reports of disparity in onset or course,[116] patients with advanced diabetic microangiopathy in general have coexistent renal and retinal disease—the diabetic renal-retinal syndrome. Joint efforts by the nephrologist, transplant surgeon, ophthalmologist, and diabetologist can positively alter the prognosis of diabetics suffering from this syndrome.[117]

MANAGEMENT OF PATIENTS

The Renal Unit Team

In the management of patients with chronic renal disease, it has been found helpful, and indeed imperative, to have a team of both physician and nonphysician members in order to provide a smooth course for the patient and family, particularly as the need for dialysis approaches.

Renal Unit Nurse. A specially trained nurse is essential in the day-to-day practice of internal medicine among diabetic patients with renal insufficiency. These patients may be in a state of disbelief, denial, anger, and resentment following the diagnosis. The Renal Unit Nurse can help provide much needed emotional support as well as perform certain medical services. At the direction and under the supervision of the physician, the nurse may assist in the adjustment of drugs for hypertension, in the interpretation of dietary prescriptions for uremia, in the management of altered insulin requirements during hemo- or peritoneal dialysis, and in the early detection of such critical complications of renal transplantation as iatrogenic Cushing's syndrome, sub-acute allograft rejection, opportunistic infection, and toxic bone marrow suppression. At the Joslin Clinic, the Renal Unit Nurse has developed teaching materials including a teaching guide for dialysis, a booklet of basic information for prospective kidney donors, and a programmed case review quiz for home study by prospective kidney transplant recipients and their families (See Table 30-7).

The Renal Unit Nurse may assist in directing patient follow-up after discharge from the hospital. This service, under the direction of the physician, includes the regulation of drugs for hypertension based upon multiple determinations of the blood pressure by the patient or family at home; detection of asymptomatic urinary tract infections following renal transplantation; and review of the patient's technique in the rapid determination of the blood glucose by use of capillary glucose measuring strips. Helpful in assisting the Renal Unit Nurse are volunteers who are willing to invest time and energy in the continuing education of the individual patient. Group activities for patients, such as those sponsored by the Juvenile Diabetes Foundation or the National Kidney Foundation, are often conceived and organized by such well-motivated volunteers. Our family workshops have been greatly helped by the contributions of nurses and physicians who regularly perform dialysis at home.

The Renal Unit Nurse may be of great help in the clinical research program by monitoring the accurate recording of data in legible form. The basic work in this regard is usually the responsibility of the patient.

Renal Unit Dietitian. The specialized knowledge and skill of the dietitian in nutritional assessment and treatment is essential to patient care, since dietary modification plays a major role in the long-

Table 30-7. Renal Failure and Diabetes - Nursing Inservice Guidelines

	Dialysis/Transplant in Diabetics		
	Hemodialysis	Peritoneal Dialysis	Renal Transplant
Preparation	Creation of a vascular access (surgical procedure) AV fistula (internal) requires 4–6 weeks maturation. External shunt can be used immediately.	Requires access to peritoneum: temporary catheter inserted at bedside. Permanent (Tenckhoff) inserted in O.R. Both immediately usable.	Needs blood/tissue typing and recipient evaluation. Related donor must be screened for diabetes.
Hospitalization	Required for access. Dialysis can be done as outpatient or at home (4–8 weeks training period) with partner.	Required for catheter placement. Dialysis can be done as outpatient or at home (2–4 weeks training period) if vision is adequate or an assistant available.	Varies from 3–8 weeks for recipient, 10–14 days for donor (major surgery).
Follow-up	Dialysis need usually permanent. Follow-up with physician as needed; average 15 hrs/week.	Again dialysis permanent (unless transplant occurs). Need periodic cultures of peritoneal drainage. Average 30 hours/week.	Need regular (weekly, monthly, yearly, etc.) visits to physician after discharge.
Diet	Usually: Na⁺, K⁺, protein and fluid restriction.	Na⁺, K⁺, fluid restriction	Possible Na⁺ restriction.
Insulin/DM	Dose may decrease on dialysis days. Use glucose oxidase impregnated paper.	May increase on dialysis days. Use glucose oxidase impregnated paper.	May increase while on large doses of steroids. Can use urine testing.
Medications	Vitamins, iron, folic acid, PO₄ binders, antihypertensives.	Same	Immunosuppressives (prednisone/azothiaprine), diuretics, antihypertensives.
Problems/Complications	Hypoglycemia on dialysis. Cardiac ischemia and peripheral vascular steal syndromes.	Hyperglycemia. Catheter obstruction problems. Infection (peritonitis) requires intraperitoneal instillation of antibiotics. Constipation may be associated with decreased clearance of uremic toxins.	Rejection. Increased risk of infection and other side effects of steroids. Nephropathy can affect transplant kidney if diabetes is poorly controlled for years. Azothiaprine causes bone marrow suppression (neutropenia).
Nursing	Monitor blood pressures, inter-dialytic weight gains. Reinforce diet, meds, insulin, fistula care (medic alert care). Need much support through 3 phases of adjustment, euphoria, depression, long-term adjustment.	Monitor blood pressures, weight gains, etc. Teach infection control, and assess technique to do dressing changes. (May need VNA support). Emotional support: body image varies greatly among individuals.	Patient to learn to monitor blood pressures, temps, weights, I/O's. Should recognize signs/symptoms of rejection episodes, early infection. Need good physical (oral) hygiene and follow-up (ophthalmology, dental, GYN, etc.). Nephropathy can affect transplant kidney.

term management of both diabetes and chronic renal insufficiency. Initial contact of the patient with the Renal Unit Dietitian occurs during hospitalization in the pre-dialysis stages of renal failure. The dietitian uses pertinent data from the medical record and subjective information from the patient interview to evaluate nutritional status and to plan appropriate intervention in collaboration with the physician. The prescribed meal plan must meet the patient's metabolic and psychologic needs with consideration of the various restrictions imposed by renal disease. Recognizing the importance of involving patients in their own treatment, the dietitian works closely with each individual in setting nutritional goals and provides periodic feedback to the physician regarding progress. Frequent patient visitation cultivates the trust and rapport necessary for effective nutrition counseling.

Before discharge from the hospital, the patient and/or family members must have sufficient knowledge to select and prepare meals properly in accordance with dietary restrictions which are often complex. Unless thoroughly informed and repeatedly encouraged, the patient who in the past has had difficulty in adapting to restrictions imposed by diabetes alone, may be overwhelmed by the added restrictions imposed by renal failure.

Renal Unit Chaplain. Hospital chaplains are important members of the team in providing spiritual and emotional support to patients and/or families who have been struggling to cope with an unrelenting series of setbacks. The patient's relationship with the chaplain permits exploration of such issues as hope, anger, and the fear of death which often play an important role in coping with and recovering from serious illness. As an attentive listener to the patient's concerns, the chaplain may often function in much the same way as a professional counselor.[118]

Renal Unit Social Worker. End-stage renal disease (ESRD) has an enormous impact on patients, affecting nearly every aspect of their lives. Patients must contend not only with concerns about health and physical functioning, but also with such matters as employability, social roles, finances, and emotional health. These issues may be even more pressing for the patient with diabetes who has suffered, or is threatened with, further complications of this primary disease. The Renal Unit Social Worker is uniquely qualified to intervene in those areas that cannot be treated by dialysis, medication, or transplantation.[119]

As physicians, surgeons, nurses, and dietitians work to improve the physical condition of the patient, and as the chaplain attempts to provide emotional and spiritual support, the Social Worker helps the patient adjust to ESRD by arranging such services as giving information concerning and referral to community agencies and other support appropriate to the needs of the individual patient. Just as each patient with ESRD presents a special medical situation that falls within the broad spectrum of end-stage renal disease, he/she also presents a unique psychosocial picture that lies within the broad spectrum of human behavior under stress. The Renal Unit Social Worker makes an assessment of each patient and an individual plan to suit the physical, emotional, and social needs.

It is valuable to encourage an informal self-help network among patients. Patients with diabetes often feel singled out and alone in their struggle against deteriorating health. They may think that no one can understand how they feel without having the same experiences. Encouraging these patients to talk to one another has been helpful in decreasing their sense of isolation and helping them face the reality of their situation.

ACUTE RENAL IMPAIRMENT SUPERIMPOSED ON CHRONIC RENAL FAILURE

The presence of concomitant vascular disease or exacerbation of pre-existing renal insufficiency in the azotemic patient may require that radiographic studies be performed utilizing contrast agents that are excreted by the kidney. It had been reported since the early 1960s that intravenous infusion pyelography with iodinated contrast material is a relatively safe procedure, even in patients with depressed renal function.[120–124] However, several papers have subsequently described acute renal failure in azotemic diabetics after excretory urography, emphasizing the potential risk in the presence of dehydration and cautioning against the use of these procedures without a specific indication.[53,55,125–149] A large study from the Mayo Clinic indicated that diabetics with normal renal function rarely developed acute oliguric renal failure following excretory urography.[54] Other prospective studies suggest that both diabetic and nondiabetic patients with chronic renal insufficiency may have a 50% (10 to 90%) incidence of superimposed acute renal impairment following the infusion of iodinated contrast. Among patients with severe renal insufficiency at baseline, up to 50% may develop irreversible renal failure in this setting.[53,56a,128,148] Table 30–8 summarizes the literature. Table 30–9 summarizes factors apparently related to the likelihood of developing varying degrees of acute renal failure following the use of contrast dye.

Fortunately renal function returns to the levels observed prior to the use of contrast dye, or nearly so, in most instances within a period of 5 to 10

Table 30–8. Review of Acute Renal Failure in Azotemic Diabetics Induced by Iodinated Contrast Media

Author	Baseline serum creatinine, mg/100 ml	Number of Patients	Study
Bergman et al. 1968[125]	4.5	1	Intravenous pyelography (IVP)
Pillay et al. 1970[126]	4.2 (1.9–9.6)	4	IVP
Barshay et al. 1973[127]	3.4 (2.1–5.0)	5	IVP
Feldman et al. 1974[149a]	5.0	1	IVP and coronary angiography
Diaz-Buxo et al. 1975[54]	4.3	8	IVP
Weinrauch et al. 1977[128]	6.8	12	IVP and coronary angiography
Weinrauch et al. 1977[56]	1.6	1	Cerebral angiography
Weinrauch et al. 1978[55]	2.8	1	Cerebral angiography
Harkonen & Kjellstrand 1977[53]	2.0	22	IVP
Shafi et al. 1978[148]	3.7	11	Infusion IVP (300 ml dye)
Krumlovsky et al. 1978[138]	2.37	3	Hydrated before IVP, cholecystogram, and coronary angiography
Ansari & Baldwin 1976[129]	2.0–3.6	4	IVP, renal angiography
	0.8–2.6	7	Oral cholecystogram
Carvallo et al. 1978[135]	1.3–5.0	4	Infusion IVP
Swartz et al. 1978[134]	1.0–7.8	8	IVP, cholecystogram, other angiography

Table 30–9. Acute Renal Failure Following Intravenous Pyelogram: Proposed Pathophysiologic Mechanisms and Risk Factors

1. Decreased renal perfusion
   A. Hyperosmolarity of injected dye
   B. Dehydration
   C. Low cardiac output states
   D. Hypotension
   E. Severe vascular disease
   F. Catheter trauma
   G. Decreased renal blood flow and glomerular filtration. Vasoconstriction of the renal vascular bed. Crenation of erythrocytes and increased blood viscosity.
2. Pre-existing renal disease
3. Diabetes mellitus
4. Severe liver disease and/or hemorrhage
5. Concomitant use of nephrotoxic drugs
6. Repeat contrast dye injection
7. Multiple myeloma
8. Tamm-Horsfall protein precipitation
9. Hypersensitivity reaction to contrast material
10. Circulating immune complexes
11. Hyperuricemia and increased uric acid secretion
12. Dosage of injected dye

days. However, as emphasized in the results from two dialysis and transplant centers dealing with large diabetic populations,[53,128] apparently irreversible deterioration to the temporary or permanent need for dialysis occurred in one-half or more of patients whose initial serum creatinine was 5.0 mg/dl or more. The likelihood of sustained renal damage is considerably less in those whose observed creatinine levels, prior to the use of contrast dye, were nearer to the normal range (fewer than 20% among patients with serum creatinine levels of less than 4.0 mg/dl).

Clearly the indications for using contrast material, particularly that to be given intravascularly, must be carefully assessed in patients with increased susceptibility to acute renal failure. The possible diagnostic benefit of alternative procedures (such as ultrasound) should be considered, and potentially susceptible patients should be monitored for renal function before and after the administration of dye. Facilities that administer contrast dye to patients at risk should be prepared to provide adequate back-up dialysis.

HEMODIALYSIS

Effect on Symptoms

The current era of experience with chronic hemodialysis for diabetic patients began with Kolff's challenge entitled "The Sad Truth about Hemodialysis in Diabetic Nephropathy."[150] Nevertheless, experience with several surgical vascular access procedures (particularly the Brescia-Cimino internal arteriovenous (AV) fistula), and aggressive use of antibiotics for AV fistula superficial cellulitis, as reported by Barcenas and co-workers,[151] have allowed more and more diabetics to achieve consistent therapy for uremic complications including fluid overload, uremic neuropathy, and malnutrition associated with vomiting. Hyperkalemia is most easily controlled with dietary manipulation and hemodialysis against a low bath potassium concentration, although on occasion fluorohydrocortisone is required for those individuals with severe inhibition of the renin-aldosterone secretory response.[152]

Fluid overload states, both intra- and extra-vascular, as well as volume-overload hypertension (low renin, low aldosterone), are usually well managed by ultrafiltration hemodialysis, as in the non-diabetic patient. However, marked hyperglycemia may impede smooth ultrafiltration because of the added osmolar load. A confusing array of symptoms may occur during the course of hemodialysis with either hypotension or hypoglycemia, so that careful documentation of blood pressure and blood glucose must precede volume replacement with colloid-saline versus a hyperosmolar glucose infusion. Rapid estimation of blood glucose from the dialyzer is possible utilizing capillary glucose measuring strips. Hypotension in the diabetic patient may also be due to the presence of symptomatic or asymptomatic coronary artery disease or myocardial dysfunction, both of which have an increased prevalence in diabetics. Rapid volume changes producing hypotension must be scrupulously avoided because of the concomitant presence of cerebral, coronary, and peripheral vascular disease which may thereby be aggravated. Hemodialyzed diabetic patients with neuropathy of the autonomic nervous system may lack the usual baroreceptor responses needed to counteract shock due to volume-contraction. This observation by Alancot and co-workers[153] applies also to hypertensive patients treated with beta-adrenergic blocking agents.

Neuropathy involving sympathetics may hinder those catecholamine-mediated cardiovascular reflexes that support blood pressure during ultrafiltration hemodialysis.[153] Therefore, patients with diabetic neuropathy may experience refractory hypotension requiring colloid and/or saline infusions, thereby reversing volume control initiated by ultrafiltration. Many studies suggest that hypertension in diabetic nephropathy is volume-dependent, associated with low renin, as well as low aldosterone secretory responses. When these factors are taken into consideration, a measure of the adequacy of hemodialysis therapy among diabetics is the control of hypotension as well as hypertension. Bicarbonate dialysate has replaced acetate in those diabetics who suffer recurrent vomiting, cramps, headache, and hypotension during hemodialysis. If management along these lines is not adequate, then peritoneal dialysis may well be indicated.

Diabetics respond as well as other individuals with chronic renal failure to hemodialysis for treatment of metabolic acidosis with hyperphosphatemia. It is our impression that diabetics more often than nondiabetics demonstrate a pericardial friction rub that is usually, but not always, responsive to increased dialysis time or increased dialyzer surface area. We have noted only two instances of cardiac tamponade among several hundred diabetic patients with renal failure. This hemodynamic emergency may be promptly relieved by creation

of a pericardial window. Among nondiabetics, the low incidence (3%) of this complication and the efficacy of surgical therapy have been reported by Ghavamian[154] and by Silverberg.[155]

We find no increased susceptibility to hemodialysis-associated hepatitis among diabetics as compared to nondiabetics: the incidence at the Joslin Clinic is similar to that reported by Garibaldi[156] from an extensive survey conducted by the Center for Disease Control (i.e., abnormal liver function tests in about 3 cases per 100 at risk, with icterus in only 1 case per 100).

Other complications of hemodialysis, such as ascites,[157] spontaneous retroperitoneal bleeding,[158] and subdural hematoma[159] have been documented as less than 1% in our experience with diabetic renal failure patients. We have seen two instances of fatal dialysis encephalopathy.[160] Vertebral osteomyelitis was studied in our general group of hospitalized patients; surprisingly, there were no instances of this complication among diabetics with arteriovenous vascular access.[161] This was unlike the experience of Leonard et al.[162] who reported several instances of osteomyelitis involving both diabetics and nondiabetics on an active dialysis service.

As renal failure progresses to the point where dialysis is required, individuals with quiescent gastric stasis associated with diabetic gastropathy may experience a discomforting sense of fullness, with intermittent vomiting and associated loss of appetite. Apparently, the autonomic neuropathy associated with diabetic gastropathy does not entirely impair gastric acid secretion. Therefore, cimetidine in small doses may be quite useful in controlling gastric acid hypersecretion of uremic diabetics. (Warning: accumulation of cimetidine and diazepam may result in prolonged stupor in the dialysis patient.) A subset of uremic diabetics have as their predominant clinical problem a pernicious vomiting, with or without upper gastrointestinal bleeding leading to severe malnutrition. Although no sequential studies have yet been reported of gastrointestinal motility following institution of dialysis therapy, it would appear that improvement occurs as uremia is corrected with hemodialysis. The effect of metaclopramide on gastric motility in diabetic gastroenteropathy, with the added problem of severe renal insufficiency, also has not yet been reported. Although we would expect the drug to be without significant effect in the face of untreated uremia, it may be of some value in stable dialysis patients with diabetic gastropathy, either orally or intravenously for those who cannot tolerate the oral route.

Accumulation of this dopamine antagonist in the dialysis patient may result in fleeting, awkward, extrapyramidal movements or even persistent dystonia with fever and seizures. This neuroleptic malignant syndrome requires a dopamine agonist such as bromocriptine.

In several instances, intravenous hyperalimentation has been necessary when even nasogastric tube feedings were not tolerated. Since the safety margin for pulmonary edema may be quite narrow in patients on maintenance hemodialysis, the fluid-volume intake required for nasogastric tube feedings or intravenous hyperalimentation must be carefully monitored.

In parallel with diabetic gastroenteropathy (which probably has a neuropathic component), certain classic forms of diabetic neuropathy may be exacerbated by uremia. Peripheral sensory and motor-nerve deficiencies that are reversible with prompt institution of vigorous hemodialysis would be considered due to uremia. However, accelerated vascular disease of the vasa nervora may be induced by hyperlipidemia associated with either poorly controlled diabetes or inadequately dialyzed uremia, thereby leading to identical degrees of segmental demyelination. Thus, one-third of hemodialyzed diabetics may experience an increase in peripheral neuropathy, one-third may show no change, and one-third may actually improve within several months of hemodialysis. Other components of the diabetic neuropathy syndrome, such as amyotrophy and the Charcot-joint deformity, generally do not improve in concert with successful removal of middle-molecule uremic toxins (molecular weight 500 to 10,000 daltons).[163]

As renal failure worsens, the precarious course of retinopathy in a longstanding diabetic is not always predictable. If high blood pressure and fluid overload are aggressively controlled by dialysis or transplantation, the malignant procession of retinal edema, vitreous hemorrhage with scarring, macular or optic nerve head neoproliferation, and retinal-scleral separation/detachment may be halted, stabilized, or even reversed. For the group at risk, roughly one-third will be blind before dialysis is required. Our observations of uremic diabetic patients with partially or completely intact vision prior to institution of hemodialysis suggest that, if each patient is used as his or her own control, the incidence of retinal hemorrhage may not be altered significantly after hemodialysis has been started.[164] We believe that patients should be enrolled in a prospective study of early intervention with either peritoneal or hemodialysis or, conceivably, even transplantation, since loss of vision and its consequences (e.g., restricted social life and dwindling self-respect) may lead later to refusal of dialysis.

When cataract or vitrectomy surgery has been required among patients with diabetic nephropathy,

the best results have been noted either early in azotemia or following successful transplantation. Nevertheless, diabetic patients on maintenance hemodialysis may have sufficient cardiovascular stability, adequate hemostasis, and an intact resistance to infection so as to withstand general anesthesia, followed by several weeks of healing. As of July, 1980, 50 diabetic nephropathy patients from our practice had undergone major eye surgery at either the Massachusetts Eye and Ear Infirmary or the New England Deaconess Hospital.[114] Of these, 30 had not yet required chronic hemodialysis, 15 were receiving maintenance hemodialysis, and 5 had previously undergone renal transplantation. Two dialysis-dependent patients died postoperatively of uremic complications. Since 1980 approximately 100 such procedures have been performed on Joslin Clinic patients with a single postoperative death due to a cerebrovascular accident.

Drug management of diabetic retinopathy in maintenance dialysis patients requires special considerations. Acetazolamide, used to lower intraocular pressure in hemorrhagic glaucoma, produces profound metabolic acidosis in patients with chronic renal failure when used in full doses (250 mg 2 to 4 times per day). After chronic dialysis has been started, full doses may be required again, since hemodialysis may cause a modest increase in intraocular pressure, even in individuals without eye disease.[165] Extra doses of acetazolamide, intravenously or by mouth, may be required prior to or during hemodialysis treatments associated with eye pain and increased intraocular pressure. A rare patient with eye pain during hemodialysis may be found to have a chronic elevation of intraocular pressure complicated by an acute rise during ultrafiltration hemodialysis.

Doses of clofibrate, used to control waxy exudates on the macula, should be reduced from 500 mg 4 times per day to 500 mg per day in chronic renal failure, because of renal and muscle toxicity. However, since this drug is not dialyzable, its dosage cannot be liberalized after maintenance hemodialysis has been instituted. Using clofibrate in the uremic diabetic with progressive neuromuscular dysfunction obviously is contraindicated.[166] Despite increased cardiovascular morbidity among patients on hemodialysis, the myopathic effects of clofibrate contraindicate its use unless on a protocol basis.

Adequate blood glucose control is difficult to achieve in the chronic hemodialysis diabetic patient.[167] In order to minimize wide fluctuations in blood glucose concentration, we have usually split the morning insulin dose before and after a morning hemodialysis, emphasizing that breakfast must be eaten with the first insulin dose. Since food and drink are forbidden in our hemodialysis unit (in an attempt to limit dissemination of hepatitis virus via salivary droplets), insulin hypoglycemic reactions occurring during the course of hemodialysis treatment are reversed with intravenous infusions of hyperosmolar glucose (50 g per 100 ml) so as to limit the volume of fluid intake. Blood glucose concentration may subsequently rise abruptly from less than 50 mg/dl to more than 250 mg/dl. Capillary glucose measuring strips may be useful for rapid determinations using blood removed from the arterial line. We have also treated hypoglycemia in chronic dialysis patients by intramuscular injections of small doses of glucagon (0.1 to 0.5 mg) in an attempt to avoid precipitating nausea and vomiting, which may accompany injections of a full vial (1.0 mg).

Among insulin-dependent diabetics with chronic renal failure, an abrupt decrease in renal function will result in a sudden decrease in insulin requirement. Several proposed mechanisms include decreased renal binding and degradation of insulin,[51] decreased substrate availability from gluconeogenic amino acids,[168] decreased hepatic glycogenolysis,[169] and increased insulin sensitivity.[170] We have also observed slowly progressive decreases in insulin requirement in severe long-standing hemodialysis patients, probably because of a progressive loss of lean body mass or perhaps related to a diminution of endogenous creatinine clearance from 5 to 1 ml/min, with subsequent loss of insulin binding and degradation. We have treated five blind diabetics whose insulin dependence of greater than 10 years' duration has been eliminated some time after starting chronic dialysis.[51a]

Non-insulin-dependent diabetics with severe renal dysfunction can be managed with tolbutamide, since this sulfonylurea drug is largely metabolized in the liver. However, use of some sulfonylurea drug such as chlorpropamide or acetohexamide in diabetic patients on maintenance dialysis is strictly contraindicated since their metabolism involves the kidney to a large extent. Treatment of profound and prolonged hypoglycemia in instances of sulfonylurea overdose among diabetics with severe renal impairment may include intravenous glucose, intramuscular glucagon, and either intravenous or intramuscular glucocorticoid over prolonged periods as required. Another drug contraindicated among diabetic patients on maintenance dialysis is phenformin, which is not dialyzable. A lack of renal function needed to metabolize phenformin allows accumulation of the drug, with production of excess lactic acid. The finding of an increased degree of anion gap in a diabetic hemodialysis patient should raise the question of low-grade lactic acidosis with impending beta hydroxybutyric acid ketoacidosis.

Effect on Longevity and Life-style

Survival of diabetic patients with chronic hemodialysis has improved sufficiently to make this treatment comparable to live-related-donor renal transplantation.[164] Dependence on the center performing dialysis, and its high cost, have promoted the development of home dialytic therapy, even for diabetics. It has been suggested that patients undergoing hemodialysis experience acceleration of existing vascular disease (already an early event in diabetics).[171] However, since the "natural progression" of atherosclerosis is not known, it may be presumptuous to assert at this time that we have accelerated or prevented atherogenesis with one or another therapy. Until prospective anatomic studies are available, or better markers for accelerated atherogenesis are produced, or long-term morbidity-mortality statistics are published, it is unlikely that questions regarding acceleration of vascular disease can be answered.

Perhaps the single most important factor in rehabilitation and/or continued employment is the preservation of eyesight. The experience of Shapiro et al.[172] appears representative with regard to the incidence of blindness among diabetics just prior to hemodialysis therapy; 22% of his patient group were totally blind and an additional 8% had unilateral blindness. When these patients were followed for 2 to 4 years of dialysis, one-third of the eyes at risk developed new blindness, mainly during the first 12 months of hemodialysis. Mitchell and colleagues have reviewed their extensive Mayo Clinic experience to compare the effect of treatment modality on visual acuity.[108] Thirty-six hemodialysis patients were compared with 11 peritoneal dialysis patients for a mean follow-up of about 6 months. None of the hemodialysis patients had improved visual acuity, 4 patients deteriorated, and 8 of 55 (15%) eyes at risk worsened to an acuity of 20/200. By contrast, 2 of the peritoneal dialysis patients achieved an improved acuity and none deteriorated, so that none of 14 eyes at risk were determined blind by the criterion of 20/200. This study had patient groups that were fairly comparable with regard to angina, hypertension, myocardial infarction, cerebrovascular accidents, and peripheral vascular disease. The only problem we have with accepting the conclusion that peritoneal dialysis spares useful vision is the short follow-up period in both groups. It is not clear that peritoneal dialysis will make any real difference to patients who remain on a chronic dialysis program rather than undergoing the rigors of transplantation. It is also unknown if these findings, already alluded to by Oreopolous,[173] will be reproduced in the majority of other centers that are now beginning to apply peritoneal dialysis techniques to diabetics.

The survival of useful arteriovenous access routes among diabetic patients with advanced renal failure is somewhat diminished when compared to equally azotemic nondiabetics.[174] This problem may cause an increased amount of work disability since there are increased hospitalizations for access revision. Because of increased clotting and infection problems with the Scribner external shunt, we have eliminated its use, depending instead on intermittent peritoneal dialysis or the Uldall subclavian catheter while awaiting maturation of a Brescia-Cimino arteriovenous fistula. Nevertheless, the de novo failure rate of arteriovenous fistulae prior to the needling process for hemodialysis therapy has been sufficiently high to require us to apply the bovine arteriovenous graft or the polytetrafluorethylene graft to about 100 patients under our care with excellent results. Surgeons working with renal failure in diabetic patients must skillfully avoid creating an excessively large arteriovenous fistula since both "steal" syndromes[175] and high-output heart failure[176] are more detrimental in this group.

PERITONEAL DIALYSIS

The development of continuous ambulatory peritoneal dialysis (CAPD) in 1978 by Popovich et al. has greatly enhanced the use of this procedure in the diabetic patient with renal failure.[177] CAPD is a method of prolonged in-dwelling peritoneal dialysis in which the patient undergoes 3 to 5 exchanges of 2 liters of dialysate fluid every 4 to 8 hours. This provides continuous removal of fluid and toxins. Studies to date by Oreopoulos suggest that survival in diabetics on CAPD is comparable to that of hemodialysis or cadaver transplantation.[173] Through continuous fluid removal, CAPD may permit liberalization of fluid and salt intake and thus be of particular benefit to the diabetic with associated heart failure.[178]

It has been suggested, though not proved, that blood pressure is better controlled in patients on CAPD as compared with hemodialysis. Early fears that orthostatic hypotension and peripheral vascular disease might be aggravated by CAPD in the diabetic patient have not been substantiated. There is reasonable evidence that patients on CAPD are less anemic than those on hemodialysis. This may be due to the absence of blood loss associated with the latter procedure. Non-diabetic patients on CAPD gain weight secondary to dextrose absorption from the dialysate and, in addition, may suffer from hypertriglyceridemia. Over time some patients also develop hernias. These problems appear

to be less significant in the diabetic patients, although the reasons for this are obscure.

Problems with CAPD include technical difficulties with catheters resulting in poor fluid inflow and outflow and catheter-associated peritonitis. At the present time, patients experience one episode of catheter-associated peritonitis approximately every 12 to 20 months. While usually controlled with antibiotics added to the dialysate, peritonitis can account for a substantial morbidity in the occasional patient.[177]

As might be expected, blood glucose elevation leading to dangerous hyperosmolarity has occasionally occurred with peritoneal dialysate glucose concentrations of 4.25 g/100 ml. Therefore, regular insulin administered subcutaneously every 6 hours may be required over and above the ordinary intermediate-acting insulin dose given as usual in the morning. For intensive care units treating diabetics with acute renal failure, a continuous subcutaneous insulin infusion may be the most convenient method of insulin management. For chronic peritoneal dialysis at home, supplemental insulin can be administered by adding it to the dialysate with each of the 3 to 5 exchanges performed daily. The estimated (regular) insulin requirement can be computed and divided equally among the number of dialysis treatments that are to be administered. Patients undergoing continuous ambulatory peritoneal dialysis come to a new steady-state of insulin requirement. Studies using home blood glucose monitoring and hemoglobin A_{1c} tests have shown that there is good control of blood glucose in these patients.[179]

Extrapolation from experience with chronic peritoneal dialysis among nondiabetic patients allows considerable optimism for management of uremic complications, including hyperkalemia, pericarditis, and fluid-overload. When biventricular failure is unresponsive to medical management in patients with moderate renal insufficiency, peritoneal dialysis is recommended to relieve the failing heart prior to the onset of uremic symptoms.[179a] The long-term effect of CAPD on diabetic complications—including proliferative retinopathy and various aspects of peripheral and sympathetic neuropathy such as gastroenteropathy, amyotrophy, and Charcot joint—must await further passage of time.

With the advent of CAPD, the use of *intermittent* peritoneal dialysis (IPD) in both the nondiabetic and diabetic patient has declined. However, there are still some diabetic patients who because of cardiac disease or difficulty with vascular access are poor candidates for hemodialysis, and yet are too disabled or not motivated to do CAPD at home. For these patients, either home or in-center IPD is of benefit.

RENAL TRANSPLANTATION

Live-Related-Donor Allograft

Initially, poor results were associated with renal transplantation in the diabetic patient, most likely because advanced deterioration of cardiac, peripheral nerve and nutritional status made it difficult for these patients to undergo the stress of general anesthesia with subsequent immunosuppression. Performance of a bilateral nephrectomy in addition to transplantation in early reports was associated with a 10 to 15% surgical mortality in the diabetic group. Currently, the survival of a diabetic patient undergoing live-related-donor renal allograft without bilateral nephrectomy approximates the 80 to 90% survival at 2 years seen among nondiabetics.[180] In the absence of coronary artery disease, the survival rate for cadaveric allograft recipients is also reassuringly high. However, when coronary artery disease and severe rejection reactions are combined, survival is quite a bit lower, i.e., 40% at 2 years. Nevertheless, we have been gratified to note the improvement in quality of life following both live-related and cadaveric renal transplantation for diabetics with known severe coronary artery disease.[181]

Transplantation in the diabetic patient is no longer experimental and tends to occur earlier than in the nondiabetic. After the onset of moderately severe renal failure (serum creatinine = 5 mg/dl), functional renal deterioration appears to progress at a more rapid rate in diabetic than in nondiabetic patients with renal transplantation advisable within 6 to 12 months. For this reason, prevailing practice favors elective live-related renal transplantation once the serum creatinine exceeds 5.0 mg/dl. This occurs prior to the time when symptoms are far advanced, certainly prior to the time when hypertension and volume overload result in gross deterioration of left ventricular function. Thus, in the ideal situation, the individual with chronic renal failure undergoes several weeks to months of hemodialysis or short-term peritoneal dialysis prior to transplantation to limit fluid overload and to allow for blood transfusions. If blood transfusions are not indicated for a particular live-related transplantation, this procedure can be performed without prior dialysis treatment.

Effect on Symptoms. When frequency and duration of episodes of rejection are few and short-lived, good blood volume control is achieved within several days of diuresis. Thereafter, the patient experiences a new freedom from dialysis dependency. Blood pressure control becomes easier as volume becomes more nearly normal. However, the high-dose glucocorticoids that are used in the first 6 weeks post-transplantation tend to expand volume because of salt retention. Blood pressure elevation may continue through this period until prednisone dosage has declined to less than 20 mg per day. Patients with pre-existent non-renal (essential) hypertension will continue to require antihypertensive therapy.

For individuals known to have normal coronary anatomy and normal cardiac function, the added stress of glucocorticoid therapy is well tolerated postoperatively. However, for those patients who do have regional myocardial dysfunction, slight increases in circulating blood volume may continue to hamper rehabilitation until about 6 months postoperatively, when prednisone doses have been tapered to maintenance levels ($\sim$12.5 mg/day). Where diffuse myocardial dysfunction has been associated with normal coronary arteries, long-term allograft survival has been associated with improvement in myocardial function. During the profound diuretic phase that may follow successful transplantation, borderline hypotension and hypovolemia may be responsible for thrombosis of previously established arteriovenous fistula access routes for hemodialysis.

Transfusions have now been shown independently by Opelz et al.[182] and Vincenti et al.[183] to be associated with an improved acceptance rate for both related and non-related renal allografts. Postulated mechanisms for this are enhancement of tolerance for exposure to foreign antigens versus elimination of hyperreactors from the pool of transplant recipients. Thus, it is common practice to give 5 to 15 units of blood during the months which precede surgery, while the patient is being maintained on either peritoneal or hemodialysis. For this reason, with large-scale diuresis following successful transplantation, it is unusual for transfusions to be required acutely. On chronic follow-up, one finds that uninhibited erythropoietin bone marrow stimulation from the functioning allograft returns hemoglobin levels to normal within 9 months of successful surgery. At this point, in female patients, the normal menstrual cycle may be re-established for the first time in several years. These cycles are ovulatory and pregnancy with a subsequent normal gestation leading to birth has been noted.

Several centers have reported that *erythrocytosis* may occur in the nondiabetic during the year following successful transplantation. The mechanism is not yet fully understood, although it is known to involve bone marrow stimulation by both erythropoietin from the allograft and glucocorticoid therapy. Perhaps the reactivation of bone marrow in some of these patients is enhanced by early chronic lung disease induced by cigarette smoking. In our own transplantation population, we see this more often in males than in females. Interestingly, the only women who have exhibited significant erythrocytosis (Hgb. > 16.0 g/dl) after successful transplantation have continued to have secondary amenorrhea or have initiated cigarette smoking. Postoperative bleeding induced by peptic ulcer, related to stress and/or exogenous corticosteroids, is seen in 1% of transplantation patients. One patient who had received large doses of glucocorticoids following prolonged rejection of a live-related allograft experienced a sudden massive gastrointestinal hemorrhage. Another patient who preoperatively had a history of peptic ulceration did not have any sign of gastrointestinal bleeding despite equally large doses of exogenous steroids.

As previously summarized, the mechanism for *hypertension* in diabetic nephropathy is related to an expanded blood volume associated with a low-renin, low-aldosterone response. We do not have sufficient data to delineate the mechanism of post-transplant hypertension in the diabetic. However, several studies suggest that, in the nondiabetic with this condition, a common mechanism involved is increased renin secretion without a high volume state.[184–186] Several instances of allograft renal-artery stenosis producing hypertension have now been documented with varying levels of plasma renin activity. Similarly, there are now good studies on alternate-day glucocorticoid therapy showing improved control of blood volume and blood pressure in the successfully transplanted nondiabetic; these parameters have yet to be adequately evaluated among diabetic allograft recipients. Insulin-dependent diabetics may experience difficulty in insulin adjustment with use of alternate-day steroids.

In our experience, *peripheral neuropathy,* extending from simple numbness to profound proximal lower extremity weakness, has improved following successful renal transplantation. The best results have been associated with live-related transplantation, in all likelihood because of the shorter, less severe rejection periods and resulting in lower total doses of glucocorticoid immunosuppression. Diabetic complications, such as Charcot joint deformity, may actually be exacerbated by an aggressive rehabilitation program that encourages greater use of neuropathic extremities, possibly hastening trauma to the plantar surface of the denervated foot. Since there is no way of predicting which patient may develop Charcot joint deformities, we have established frequent visits to our podiatric and physical therapy centers for those individuals who require foot braces to sustain a flaccid ankle joint. At the earliest indication of traumatic arthropathy, non-weight bearing is begun. Substantial improvement may occur in pe-

ripheral numbness and muscle weakness following live-related allograft transplantation.

In summary, the more profound the symptoms of neuropathy are at the time of transplantation, the less likely these symptoms are to be totally reversible. If overall rehabilitation of neuromuscular function has been rewarding with live-related transplantation, patients with profound *gastroenteropathy* have not usually undergone elective transplantation because of severe malnutrition with associated vascular complications. Fortunately, several of our chronic renal failure patients with gastric stasis at the time that dialysis was begun appear to have stabilized nicely with control of uremia by transplantation. In a striking instance of life-threatening maldigestion-malabsorption reversed by transplantation, pancreatitis, gastroparesis, and enteropathy were stabilized largely by means of intravenous hyperalimentation. The patient with latent gastric stasis may notice a recurrent tendency to postprandial fullness, which may eventually deteriorate into vomiting and malabsorption if renal function declines some time after successful transplantation.

Long-Term Follow-Up. Studies of nondiabetic patients who have been successfully transplanted have revealed persistent *hyperlipidemia* and no improvement in high-density lipoprotein cholesterol levels; these levels remained depressed during a period of hemodialysis and following successful renal transplantation.[187] The progression of cerebral and peripheral vascular disease following successful transplantation is disturbingly consistent among individuals whose atherosclerotic disease is markedly advanced at the time they undergo transplantation. Thus, among patients who remain hypertensive following successful transplantation, stroke ranks third behind myocardial infarction and infection as a factor producing severe morbidity. Additionally, amputation procedures are required in about 25% of successfully transplanted diabetic patients followed for greater than 2 years with normal renal function. These amputation procedures include digits of the upper extremities in vascular territories previously involved in arteriovenous access procedures (the minority), as well as lower extremity amputations following minor or major trauma. We have now seen several instances of amputations proximal to the digit level in our successfully transplanted patients. Below-knee amputations have been reported and should be expected with application of renal therapy to a wider range of susceptible patients. Thus, the progress of peripheral vascular disease in the diabetic patient on glucocorticoid immunosuppression following successful transplantation may not be significantly different from the progression in the diabetic patient with an equal degree of atherosclerosis without renal insufficiency.

While *cataracts* are perhaps more frequent in the diabetic than the nondiabetic patient on dialysis, both groups experience an increase in cataract formation with glucocorticoid treatment following transplantation. Several instances of cataract surgery have been recorded among our patients whose renal function approached normal after transplantation. Patients with successful transplantation have been characterized by such a marked diminution in recurrent retinal hemorrhage that hemorrhagic glaucoma is an unusual complication compared with the hemodialysis group. When increased intraocular pressure has occurred during hemodialysis or peritoneal dialysis prior to transplantation, acetazolamide therapy has been required in reduced doses which can subsequently be liberalized as renal function improves. Surgical ophthalmologic procedures performed when renal function has improved have been rewarded with good results. Several instances of cataract removal and of vitrectomy reconstruction without complication are recorded among our successfully transplanted patients.

As transplantation is extended to the older diabetic group, it is to be expected that retinal fatty deposits ("waxy exudates") will occur in the interval beyond follow-up. In those patients with near-normal renal function and rehabilitated neuromuscular ability, diminished doses of clofibrate may be indicated. Currently available data suggest that visual acuity may be stabilized in diabetics with near-normal renal function following allograft transplantation. However, these data are based on 2 to 4 years' follow-up. As patients are followed for longer periods, it is to be expected that those aspects of diabetic retinal microangiopathy which depend upon glucose dysmetabolism will continue to progress. In 2 patients with a mean follow-up of 6 years after live-related allograft transplantation, we have now seen progression of proliferative retinopathy and, in one of those patients, a rather marked deterioration of acuity has occurred. Thus, we plan to consider open-loop insulin pump therapy for well-motivated individuals willing to perform home capillary blood glucose monitoring, provided that experience with this form of insulin delivery has been thoroughly evaluated in diabetics with fewer complications. Contrary to the situation of patients on dialytic therapy, chronic stable doses of insulin can be established more easily for transplantation patients, once they are past the stage of acute rejection. However, in the 3 months that follow transplantation, varying blood glucose ranges have required frequent insulin adjustment as renal failure is reversed and appetite augmented by glu-

cocorticoids. Obviously, the use of steroids every other day presents a challenge for the diabetic transplant recipient hoping to control blood glucose with one simple insulin dose.

Given the trend toward earlier transplantation and shorter courses of immunosuppressives, the era of transplantation for diabetics has matched closely the era of decreased complications in parathyroid function and bone integrity as consequences of chronic renal failure. We have seen only two instances of necrosis of the femoral head or atraumatic fractures among several hundred diabetic patients treated with either dialysis or transplantation. However, following traumatic fracture, we have found two additional patients with poor bone healing. One of these has had a parathyroidectomy. Symptoms of tertiary hyperparathyroidism following successful transplantation have not been observed among our patients and have not been reported from other centers treating diabetics in this way.

Our longest surviving transplant patient developed a gastric adenocarcinoma in the ninth year following cadaveric allograft placement by Dr. Anthony Monaco at the Boston City Hospital. She subsequently succumbed to hepatic metastases. It is likely that we will experience more malignancies as the procedure becomes more widespread. We do not have any evidence at this time, however, of any significant difference between the diabetic and non-diabetic population in this regard. We have had no cases of steroid-induced pancreatitis.

Effect on Survival and Life-style. The survival of patients without significant coronary artery disease (symptomatic or asymptomatic) parallels that of the nondiabetic population. Renal live-related allograft transplantation has an 80 to 90% survival at 2 years, which is virtually the same as the survival rate in nondiabetics. In conjunction with Drs. John Libertino and Leonard Zinman of the Lahey Clinic, we are following several diabetic individuals who are back to work with normal renal function more than 5 years after a successful transplant.[180,181]

Causes of death following transplantation in diabetic patients without coronary disease are equally divided between stroke and infection. Surprisingly, opportunistic infection with unusual bacterial, fungal, parasitic, or viral organisms has not hampered the transplantation program in diabetic patients. We have had a single instance of asymptomatic fungal meningitis diagnosed fortuitously by the discovery of cryptococcal organisms in the urine following which a culture of cerebrospinal fluid revealed similar organisms. This patient was successfully treated with amphotericin B and 5-fluorocytosine.

Urinary tract infections occur in approximately 80% of our group and are related to Foley catheter drainage for about 2 weeks following surgery. This is probably not different from the incidence of urinary tract infections in nondiabetic transplant groups. We have applied to the diabetic transplant patient in our institution the practice current in some centers of utilizing prophylactic broad spectrum antibiotics in the post-transplant stage to limit the incidence of urinary tract and wound infections. However, given that wound infection superimposed upon chronic urinary tract infection is associated with a high incidence of transplant allograft rejection, careful monitoring of prothrombin and partial thromboplastin times is needed when decreased renal function allows antibiotic accumulation to sterilize the bowel. Vitamin K replacement may prevent major hemorrhage.[187a] Our experience with collections of lymph in the pelvic area would suggest that when intraperitoneal drainage becomes necessary because of allograft ureteral obstruction, this simple procedure is not complicated by superinfection.

Cadaveric Transplantation

It is generally accepted that allograft survival following non-related transplantation is less than that following related donation. However, in some centers, improved immune suppression has been so successful that non-related renal transplantation from cadavers may soon replace related allografts from parent to child.[188] At this time, however, no specific information is available with regard to diabetic patients at these centers. Many active transplantation centers refuse to perform cadaveric transplantation in the juvenile-onset diabetic because of increased risk of sepsis and shortened survival secondary to vascular disease. The use of sibling-to-sibling donation in diabetics involves the added problem of the possibility of ultimate development of diabetes in the donor.

Contrary to European statistics among nondiabetics, data for U.S. nondiabetics show little correlation between HLA histocompatibility-typing and allograft-survival for cadaveric transplantation. Since only small numbers of diabetics have been followed so far, it is not yet possible to ascertain whether HLA typing plays a major role in organ survival in either the European or U.S. cohorts.

Effect on Symptoms. For the 40% of diabetic renal failure patients achieving near-normal renal function following cadaveric transplantation, control of blood volume is no longer a problem. However, as with successful live-related transplants, blood pressure may remain elevated until prednisone doses have been decreased to less than 15 mg/day. Reports of improved blood pressure control with alternate-day steroids are of great interest for those cadaveric-allograft recipients who chronically require 15 to 25 mg of prednisone per day to maintain graft survival with adequate function.

Since maintenance glucocorticoid doses have averaged about twice those achieved among successful live-related allograft recipients, we have noted greater morbidity and mortality due to sepsis. Whereas no patients in our live-related transplantation group have died with sepsis, three of our recipients of cadaveric grafts had terminal pneumonia and two had fatal wound infections. Other steroid-related complications include the chronic depression of HDL cholesterol and the potential for accelerated cataract formation. Two diabetic complications—motor neuropathy and gastroenteropathy—which have been rather well stabilized following successful live-related transplantation, have not remitted with the usual level of renal function seen between rejections in the cadaveric recipients (creatinine > 2 mg/dl). Treatment of motor neuropathy requires optimal nutrition, minimal glucocorticoid dosage, and sufficient energy for daily physical therapy. Treatment of gastroenteropathy requires reduction to a minimum of azotemia (creatinine < 2 ml/dl) and prednisone dosage.

Immunosuppressives. Two new agents in immunotherapy, now well tested in diabetic renal recipients, are (1) the OKT_3 monoclonal antibody against thymus-derived helper cells and (2) cyclosporine. The OKT_3 monoclonal antibodies as a refinement of antithymocyte globulin (ATG) exert their major contribution during acute allograft rejection. This treatment thus is superimposed on prednisone and azathioprine. Unfortunately, these antibodies add to the bone marrow suppression induced by azathioprine, sometimes resulting in unwanted degrees of neutropenia and thrombocytopenia. Since these preparations may be irritating to blood vessels and may exert febrile reactions, they are delivered in the most dilute form via a central venous catheter which may be a source of transdermal infection.

Cyclosporine replaces azathioprine and diminishes required prednisone doses. In our experience, it is more effective than azathioprine with a lesser tendency to bone marrow suppression. Its drawbacks include a very significant nephrotoxicity which causes considerable confusion in the treatment of allograft rejection. The rule is "When in doubt, lower the dose of cyclosporine." Although blood levels of this drug are useful when too high, there is no guarantee at what point the nephrotoxic effect will be seen in a particular renal transplant patient. Since lymphomatous tumors appear with long-term use of cyclosporine, it is prudent to be prepared to shift to azathioprine at any time. These tumors often regress with elimination of cyclosporine. High cost also has encouraged a view toward limiting the use of cyclosporine to 1 year or less.

STRATEGY OF MANAGEMENT IN DIABETIC NEPHROPATHY

We have described a multidisciplinary approach for evaluating the diabetic patient with progressive deterioration in renal function. As is apparent from Table 30–10, most of these patients are managed by the primary internist throughout the major portion of their course. In the past, the onset of symptomatic uremia or fluid overload was the natural signal for consulting a renal specialist. However, numerous experiences have convinced us that renal function may deteriorate quickly without apparent cause. We therefore advise construction of an arteriovenous fistula for hemodialysis when the serum creatinine is greater than 3 to 4 mg/dl to allow sufficient time for maturation to occur (assuming a greater amount of peripheral vascular disease than occurs among nondiabetic patients with renal disease).

Despite obvious advantages of involving the renal team earlier, the patient usually prefers that the primary internist remain his or her central physician for as long as possible, and the wisdom of this preference should be acknowledged. During the time that it takes to have the arteriovenous fistula constructed and matured, family members require an education in the physical and emotional changes to be expected as renal function terminates. The family should be convened for tissue typing in preparation for live-related transplantation, without undue pressure from the physician. Economic and emotional problems that would otherwise surface at times of intense physical stress can be more dispassionately examined while the patient remains asymptomatic.

The appearance of volume-dependent hypertension, anemia, and metabolic bone diseases (osteitis fibrosa cystica, osteomalacia, osteosclerosis) coincides with progressive deterioration in renal function below a glomerular filtration rate of 25 ml/min and a serum creatinine of 4 mg/dl. Downward adjustment of insulin dose is necessary as metabolism of insulin by the kidney diminishes. Diabetic neuropathy is magnified by uremic neuropathy, resulting in diminished tolerance for methyldopa and prazosin or the requirement for fludrocortisone. Postural hypotension, sexual impotence, fatigue, and depression may accompany use of antihypertensive drugs, leading to non-compliance. Visual disturbances, more than any other clinical problem, will occupy the patient's attention. In our experience, severely increased blood pressure, associated with rapid deterioration in visual and renal function, may well be an indication for initiation of hemodialysis despite fears of retinal hemorrhage secondary to use of heparin anticoagulation.

Development of orthopnea and dyspnea in the edematous diabetic patient may herald the need for dialysis as diuretics in high doses become less effective. A decade ago, the diabetic in this situation was considered pre-terminal in many hospitals. Now, however, the transplantation and vascular surgical consultants have settled upon a series of options depending upon urinary bladder function,

Table 30–10.   Stages of Renal Failure

Serum Creatinine mg/dl	Symptoms	Signs	Physicians	Treatment
0.5 to 3.0	—	Proteinuria Hypertension (mild) Hypertriglyceridemia	Internist	Diuretics, thiazide Diabetes control
3.1 to 6.0	Orthostatic hypotension Hypoglycemia	Anemia Hyperphosphatemia Hypoproteinemia Neuropathy Hypertension (moderate) ↓ insulin need Edema	Internist + Nephrologist + Vascular Access Surgeon	Diuretics—loop diuretic Phosphate binders Other antihypertensives Beta adrenergic blockade Vasodilators False neurotransmitters Alpha adrenergic blockade Fludrocortisone
6.1 to 9.0	Vomiting Deteriorating vision Dyspnea, orthopnea	Hypertension (severe) Osteodystrophy Fluid overload Retinal edema and hemorrhages	Internist + Nephrologist + Transplant Surgeon	Protein restriction Potassium restriction Dialysis

left ventricular cardiac function, and integrity of the peripheral circulatory system. Individuals with urinary ureteral reflux are likely to have chronic active pyelonephritis or reflux nephropathy, neither of which will be improved by immunosuppression. Poor cardiac function due to coronary artery disease may be associated with some improvement as blood pressure is normalized along with renal function, but many transplant patients with severe coronary artery disease do not tolerate the postoperative stress. Obviously, chronic foot ulcers may become acutely worsened with immunosuppression and peripheral vascular insufficiency.

The Renal Dietitian plans menus for dietary phosphate and potassium restriction, while phosphate binders and fludrocortisone may help to control hyperphosphatemia and hyperkalemia, respectively. While protein restriction is rather rigorous at the initiation of dialytic therapy, experience may later show improved muscle strength with a more liberal diet plus slightly longer dialysis treatments. A treatment team composed of renal nurses and social workers may give sufficient support to help resolve complex problems arising out of so many setbacks. Unfortunately, the divorce rate for married couples in which one partner is diabetic with an elevated serum creatinine concentration is unquestionably even greater than the high figure for the general population. Family dissolution can seriously demoralize a patient and thereby impede treatment. The psychiatric and ministerial services find their functions limited to passive non-intervention when they have been consulted too late. When an unemployed dialysis or transplant patient finds a new way of earning a salary after a period of rehabilitation, this is ranked highly on the team's list of achievements.

Our group has found asymptomatic coronary artery disease to be the major organic determinant in rehabilitation of diabetics with chronic renal failure. Results of coronary angiography have been used as a rational insight into the natural history of these patients treated with dialysis or transplantation, particularly since non-invasive cardiac testing is notoriously unreliable as a predictor of coronary artery disease in asymptomatic patients. Since radiographic contrast material is nephrotoxic, coronary angiography is best postponed until total deterioration of renal function has occurred and the individual has adjusted to dialytic therapy. Whether the patient has severe coronary artery disease or not, a successful live-related renal transplant appears to offer better rehabilitation statistics than either cadaver-allograft renal transplantation, hemodialysis, or peritoneal dialysis. However, no prospective studies have been done to compare several groups of diabetic patients with the same distribution of coronary anatomic characteristics. Since survival statistics for dialysis procedures have shown improvement annually for the past decade, at this time the physician, patient and family must make some decisions without the benefit of proven guidelines.

REFERENCES

1. Kimmelstiel, P., Wilson, C.: Intercapillary lesions in glomeruli of kidney. Am. J. Pathol. *12*:83, 1936.
2. Morgensen, C.E., Andersen, M.J.F.: Increased kidney size and GFR in early juvenile diabetics. Diabetes *22*:706, 1973.
3. Østerby, R., Gundersen, H.J.G.: Glomerular size and structure in diabetes mellitus. I. Early abnormalities. Diabetologia *11*:225, 1975.
4. Kroustrup, J.P., Gundersen, H.J.G., Østerby, R.: Glomerular size and structure in diabetes mellitus. III. Early enlargement of the capillary surface. Diabetologia, *13*:207, 1977.
5. Gundersen, H.J.G., Østerby, R.: Glomerular size and structure in diabetes mellitus. II. Late abnormalities. Diabetologia, *13*:43, 1977.
6. Ross, J., Goldman, J.K.: Effect of streptozotocin-induced diabetes on kidney weight and compensatory hypertrophy in the rat. Endocrinology, *88*:1079, 1971.
7. Seyer-Hansen, K.: Renal hypertrophy in streptozotocin diabetic rats. Clin. Sci. Mol. Med. *51*:551, 1976.
8. Rasch, R.: The effect of diabetic control on kidney weight, glomerular volume and glomerular basement membrane thickness. (Abstract) Diabetologia *13*:426, 1977.
9. Østerby, R.: Early phases in the development of diabetic glomerulopathy. Acta Med. Scand. (Suppl.) *574*:3, 1975.
10. Mogensen, C.E.: Renal function changes in diabetes. Diabetes *25* (Suppl):872, 1976.
11. Ditzel, J., Junker, K.: Abnormal GFR, RPF and renal protein excretion in short-term diabetics. Br. Med. J. *2*:13, 1972.
12. Mogensen, C.E.: Kidney function and glomerular permeability to macromolecules in early juvenile diabetes. Scand. J. Clin. Lab. Invest. *28*:79, 1971.
13. Mogensen, C.E.: Maximum tubular reabsorption capacity for glucose and renal hemodynamics during rapid hypertonic glucose infusion in normal and diabetic subjects. Scand. J. Clin. Invest. *28*:101, 1971.
14. Mogensen, C.E., Andersen, M.J.F.: Increased kidney size and GFR in untreated juvenile diabetics. Normalization by insulin treatment. Diabetologia, *11*:221, 1975.
15. Seyer-Hansen, K.: Renal hypertrophy in experimental diabetes: relation to severity of diabetes. Diabetologia, *13*:141, 1977.
16. Jerums, G., Post, R., Miller, M., Barzellato, E.: Differential renal protein clearance in diabetes. Diabetes *22*:104, 1973.
17. Parving, H.: Increased microvascular permeability to plasma proteins in short- and long-term juvenile diabetics. Diabetes *25* (Suppl. 2):884, 1976.
18. Heptinstall, R.H.: Diabetes mellitus and gout. In: R.H. Heptinstall (Ed.): Pathology of the Kidney, 2nd Ed. Boston, Little Brown & Co., 1974, pp. 929–975.
19. Gellman, D.D., Pirani, C.L., Soothill, J.F., et al.: Diabetic nephropathy: a clinical and pathologic study based on renal biopsies. Medicine *38*:321, 1959.
20. Sabour, M.S., MacDonald, M.K., Robson, J.S.: An electron microscopic study of the human kidney in young diabetic patients with normal renal function. Diabetes *11*:291, 1962.

21. Suzuki, Y., Churg, J., Grishman, E., et al.: The mesangium of the renal glomerulus. Electron microscopic studies of pathologic alterations. Am. J. Path. *43*:555, 1963.

22. Fisher, E.R., Perez-Stable, E., Amidi, M., et al.: Ultrastructural renal changes in juvenile diabetics. J.A.M.A. *202*:291, 1967.

23. Kimmelstiel, P.: Diabetic nephropathy. In: F.K. Mostofi, D.E. Smith (Eds.): The Kidney. Baltimore, Williams & Wilkins, 1966, pp. 226–252.

24. Bell, E.T.: Renal vascular disease in diabetes mellitus. Diabetes *2*:376, 1953.

25. Vracko, R., Benditt, E.P.: Manifestations of diabetes mellitus—their possible relationships to an underlying cell defect. A review. Am. J. Path. *75*:204, 1074.

26. Vracko, R.: Basal lamina layering in diabetes mellitus: evidence for accelerated rate of cell death and cell regeneration. Diabetes *23*:94, 1974.

27. Siperstein, M., Raskin, P., Burns, H.: Electron microscopic quantification of diabetic microangiopathy. Diabetes *22*:514, 1973.

28. Williamson, J., Kilo, C.: A common sense approach resolves the basement controversy and the NIH Pima Indian study. Diabetologia *17*:129, 1979.

29. Goldstein, S., Littlefield, J.W., Soeldner, J.S.: Diabetes mellitus and aging: diminished plating efficiency of cultured human fibroblasts. Proc. Natl. Acad. Sci. (USA) *64*:155, 1969.

30. Burton, T.Y., Kearns, T.P., Rynearson, E.H.: Diabetic retinopathy following total pancreatectomy. Proc. Mayo Clin. *32*:735, 1957.

31. Ennis, G., Miller, M., Unger, F.M., Unger, L.: Intercapillary glomerulosclerosis in diabetes secondary to chronic relapsing pancreatitis. Diabetes *18*:333, 1969.

32. Becker, D., Miller, M.: Presence of diabetic glomerulosclerosis in patients with hemochromatosis. N. Engl. J. Med. *263*:367, 1960.

33. Ørskov, H., Olsen, T.S., Nielsen, K., et al.: Kidney lesions in rats with severe long-term alloxan diabetes. Diabetologia *1*:172, 1965.

34. Mauer, S.M., Barbosa, J., Vernier, R.L., et al.: Development of diabetic vascular lesions in normal kidney transplanted into patients with diabetes mellitus. N. Engl. J. Med. *295*:916, 1976.

35. Takazakura, E., Nakamoto, Y., Hayakawa, H.: Onset and progression of diabetic glomerulosclerosis; a progressive study based on serial renal biopsies. Diabetes *24*:1, 1975.

36. Spiro, R.G.: Biochemistry of the renal glomerular basement membrane and its alterations in diabetes mellitus. N. Engl. J. Med. *288*:1337, 1973.

37. Spiro, R.G.: Role of insulin in two pathways of glucose metabolism: *in vivo* glucosamine and glycogen synthesis. Ann. N.Y. Acad. Sci. *82*:366, 1959.

38. Spiro, R.G.: Glycoproteins and diabetes. Diabetes *12*:223, 1963.

39. Klein, L., Butcher, D.L., Sudilovsky, H., et al.: Quantification of collagen in renal glomeruli isolated from human non-diabetic and diabetic kidneys. Diabetes *24*:1057, 1975.

40. Westberg, N.G.: Biochemical alterations of the human glomerular basement membrane in diabetes. Diabetes *25* (Suppl 2):920, 1976.

41. Butcher, D., Kikkawa, R., Klein, L., Miller, M.: Size and weight of glomeruli isolated from human diabetic and non-diabetic kidneys. J. Lab. Clin. Med. *89*:544, 1977.

42. Merimee, T.J., Fineberg, S.E., Hollander, W.: Vascular disease in the chronic HGH-deficient state. Diabetes *22*:813, 1973.

43. Spiro, R.G.: Search for a biochemical basis of diabetic microangiopathy. Claude Bernard Lecture. Diabetologia *12*:1, 1976.

44. Jones, R.H., Mackay, J.D., Hayakawa, H., et al.: Progression of diabetic nephropathy. Lancet *1*:1105, 1979.

45. Andersen, A.R., Andersen, J.K., Christiansen, J.S., Deckert, T.: Prognosis for juvenile diabetics with nephropathy and failing renal function. Acta Med. Scand. *203*:131, 1978.

46. Kussman, M.J., Goldstein, H.H., Gleason, R.E.: The clinical course of diabetic nephropathy. J.A.M.A. *236*(16):1861, 1976.

47. Scribner, B.H.: Discussion: The problem of end-stage diabetic nephropathy. Kidney Int. *6* (Suppl.):S21, 1974.

48. Christlieb, A.R., Kaldany, A., D'Elia, J.A., Williams, G.H.: Aldosterone responsiveness in patients with diabetes mellitus. Diabetes *27* (7):732, 1978.

49. Perez, G.O., Lespier, L., Jacobi, J., et al.: Hyporeninemia and hypoaldosteronism in diabetes mellitus. Arch. Intern. Med. *137*:652, 1977.

50. Perez, G.O., Lespier, L., Knowles, R., et al.: Potassium homeostasis in chronic diabetes mellitus. Arch. Intern. Med. *137*:1018, 1977.

51. Weinrauch, L.A., Healy, R.W., Leland, O.S., et al.: Decreased insulin requirement in acute renal failure in diabetic nephropathy. Arch. Intern. Med. *138*:399, 1978.

51a. D'Elia, J.A., Kaldany, A., Miller, D.G., et al.: Elimination of requirement for exogenous insulin therapy in diabetic renal failure. Clin. Exp. Dial. Apheresis *6*:75, 1982.

52. Wass, J.A., Watkins, P.J., Dische, F.E., Parsons, V.: Renal failure, glomerular disease and diabetes mellitus. Nephron *21*:289–296, 1978.

52a. Robertson, W.R., Crosson, A., Wafai, Z., et al.: Nondiabetic renal disease in diabetic patients. Kidney International *14*:660, 1978.

53. Harkonen, S., Kjellstrand, C.M.: Exacerbation of diabetic renal failure following intravenous pyelography. Am. J. Med. *63*:939, 1977.

54. Diaz-Buxo, J.A., Wagoner, R.D, Hattery, R.R., Palumbo, P.J.: Acute renal failure after excretory urography in diabetic patients. Ann. Intern. Med. *83*:155, 1975.

55. Weinrauch, L.A., Robertson, W.S., and D'Elia, J.A.: Contrast media-induced acute renal failure. Use of creatinine clearance to determine risk in elderly diabetic patients. J.A.M.A. *239*:2018, 1978.

56. Weinrauch, L.A., Friedberg, S.R., D'Elia, J.A.: Acute renal failure after cerebral arteriography in a diabetic patient. Neuroradiology *12*:197, 1977.

56a. D'Elia, J.A., Gleason, R.E., Alday, M., et al.: Nephrotoxicity from angiographic contrast material. Am. J. Med. *72*:719, 1982.

57. Kurtzman, N., Pillary, V.: Renal reabsorption of glucose in health and disease. Arch. Intern. Med. *131*:901, 1973.

58. Axelrod, L.: Response of congestive heart failure to correction of hyperglycemia in the presence of diabetic nephropathy. N. Engl. J. Med. *293*:1243, 1975.

58a. Kaldany, A., Curt, G.A., Estes, N.M., et al.: Reversible acute pulmonary edema due to uncontrolled hyperglycemia in diabetics with renal failure. Diabetes Care *5*:506, 1982.

59. Rose, F., Fraser, G., Friedmann, A., and Kohner, E.: The association of juvenile diabetes mellitus and optic atrophy. Quart. J. Med. *35*:385, 1966.

60. Chobanian, A.V., Volicer, L., Tifft, C.P., et al.: Mineralocorticoid-induced hypertension in patients with orthostatic hypotension. N. Engl. J. Med. *301*:68, 1979.

61. Bennett, W., Kloster, F., Rosch, J., et al.: Natural history of asymptomatic coronary arteriographic lesions in dia-

betic patients with end-stage renal disease. Am. J. Med. 65:779, 1978.

62. Weinrauch, L., D'Elia, J., Healy, R., et al.: Asymptomatic coronary artery disease: angiography in diabetic patients before renal transplantation. Relation of findings to postoperative survival. Ann. Intern. Med. 88:346, 1978.

63. Weinrauch, L., D'Elia,: J., Healy, R., et al.: Asymptomatic coronary artery disease: angiographic assessment of diabetics evaluated for renal transplantation. Circulation 58:1184, 1978.

63a. Braun, W.E., Phillips, D., Vidt, D.G., et al.: Coronary arteriography and coronary artery disease in 99 diabetic and non-diabetic patients on chronic hemodialysis and transplantation programs. Trans. Proc. 13:128, 1981.

64. Kannel, W., Hjortland, M., Castelli, W.: Role of diabetes in congestive heart failure: the Framingham study. Am. J. Cardiol. 34:29, 1974.

65. Ahmed, S.S., Jaferi, G.A., Narang, R.M., Regan, T.J.: Preclinical abnormality of left ventricular function in diabetes mellitus. Am. Heart J. 89:153, 1975.

66. Seneviratne, B.I.: Diabetic cardiomyopathy: the preclinical phase. Br. Med. J. 1:1444, 1977.

67. Rubler, S., Sajadi, M.R.N., Araoyhe, M.A., Holford, F.D.: Noninvasive estimation of myocardial performance in patients with diabetes. Effect of alcohol administration. Diabetes 27:127, 1978.

68. Hamby, R.I., Zoneraich, S., Sherman, L.: Diabetic cardiomyopathy. J.A.M.A. 229:1749, 1974.

69. Regan, T.J., Lyons, M.M., Ahmed, S.S., et al.: Evidence for cardiomyopathy in familial diabetes mellitus. J. Clin. Invest. 60:884, 1977.

70. Regan, T.J., Ettinger, P.O., Khan, M.I., et al.: Altered myocardial function and metabolism in chronic diabetes mellitus without ischemia in dogs. Circ. Res. 35:222, 1974.

71. Kim, K., Onesti, G., Schwartz, A., et al.: Hemodynamics of hypertension in chronic end-stage renal disease. Circulation 46:456, 1972.

72. Ditzel, J., Anderson, H., Peters, N.D.: Oxygen affinity of haemoglobin and red cell 2,3-diphosphoglycerate in childhood diabetes. Acta Paedieatr. Scand. 64:355, 1971.

73. Weiss, S., Wilkins, R.: The nature of cardiovascular disturbances in nutritional deficiency states (beri-beri). Ann. Intern. Med. 11:104, 1937.

74. Del Greco, F., Simon, N., Roguska, J., and Walker, C.: Hemodynamic studies in chronic uremia. Circulation 40:87, 1969.

75. Engle, M.A., Erlandson, M., Smith, C.H.: Late cardiac complications of chronic, severe, refractory anemia with hemochromatosis. Circulation 30:698, 1964.

76. Johnson, G., Jr., Blythe, W.: Hemodynamic effects of arteriovenous shunts used for hemodialysis. Ann. Surg. 171:715, 1970.

77. Pund, E.E., Jr., Hawley, R.L., McGee, H.J., Blount, S.G., Jr.: Gouty heart. N. Engl. J. Med. 263:835, 1960.

78. Bailey, G.L., Hampers, C.L., Merrill, J.P.: Reversible cardiomyopathy in uremia. Trans. Am. Soc. Artif. Intern. Organs 13:263, 1967.

79. Smythe, P.M., Swanepoel, A., Campbell, J.A.H.: The heart in kwashiorkor. Br. Med. J. 5271, 1:67, 1962.

80. D'Elia, J., Weinrauch, L., Healy, R., et al.: Myocardial dysfunction without coronary artery disease in diabetic renal failure. Am. J. Cardiol., 43:193, 1979.

80a. Factor, S.M., Okun, E.M., Minase, T.: Capillary microaneurysms in the human diabetic heart. N. Engl. J. Med. 302:384, 1980.

81. Miller, D.G., Levine, S., Bistrian, B., D'Elia, J.A.: Diagnosis of protein calorie malnutrition in diabetic patients on hemodialysis and peritoneal dialysis. Nephron 33:127, 1983.

82. Batist, G., Bistrian, B., Kaldany, A., et al.: Use of intravenous total parenteral nutrition in diabetic renal failure. Nephron 7:21, 1981.

83. Neetens, A.: Microcirculation in the diabetic eye. Adv. Microcirc. 8:55, 1979.

84. McMillan, D.E.: Deterioration of the microcirculation in diabetes. Diabetes 24:944, 1975.

85. Ditzel, J.: Functional microangiopathy in diabetes mellitus. Diabetes 17:388, 1968.

86. Williamson, J.R., Kilo, E.: Vascular complications in diabetes mellitus. N. Engl. J. Med. 302:399, 1980.

87. Kohner, E.M.: Diabetic retinopathy. Clin. Endo. Metab. 6:345, 1977.

88. Scheinman, J.I., Fish, A.J., Michael, A.F.: The immunohistopathology of glomerular antigens. The glomerular basement membrane, collagen, and actomyosin antigens in normal and diseased kidneys. J. Clin. Invest. 54:1144, 1974.

89. Deen, W.M., Robertson, C.R., Brenner, B.M.: Glomerular ultrafiltration. Fed. Proc. 33:14, 1974.

90. Mauer, S.M., Steffes, M.W., Michael, A.F., Brown, D.M.: Studies of diabetic nephropathy in animals and man. Diabetes 25 (Suppl. 2):850, 1976.

91. Brownlee, M., Cahill, G.F., Jr.: Diabetic control and vascular complications. In: R. Paoletti and A.M. Gotto, Jr. (Eds.): Atherosclerosis Reviews, Vol. 4. New York, Raven Press. 1979, pp. 29–70.

92. Sagel, J., Colwell, J.A., Crook, L., Laimins, M.: Increased platelet aggregation in early diabetes mellitus. Ann. Intern. Med. 82:733, 1975.

93. Colwell, J.A., Halushka, P.V., Sarji, K., et al.: Altered platelet function in diabetes mellitus. Diabetes 25 (Suppl. 2):826, 1976.

94. McMillan, D.E.: Disturbance of serum viscosity in diabetes mellitus. J. Clin. Invest. 53:1071, 1974.

95. Kohner, E.M., Oakley, N.W.: Diabetic retinopathy. Metabolism 24:1085, 1975.

96. Beisswenger, P.J., Spiro, R.G.: Studies on the human glomerular basement membrane. Composition, nature of the carbohydrate units and chemical changes in diabetes mellitus. Diabetes 22:180, 1973.

97. Birkeland, A.J., Christensen, T.B.: Resistance of glycoproteins to proteolysis, ribonuclease-A and -B compared. J. Carbohydrates-Nucleosides-Nucleotides 2:83, 1975.

98. Hanna, A.K., Minuk, H.L., Albisser, A.M., et al.: A portable system for continuous intravenous insulin delivery: characteristics and results in diabetic patients. Diabetes Care 3:1, 1980.

99. Kohner, E.M., Dollery, C.T.: Diabetic retinopathy. In: H. Keen and J. Jarrett (Eds.): Complications of Diabetes. London, Edward Arnold Publications, 1975, pp. 7–98.

100. Cameron, J.S., Ireland, J.T., Watkins, P.J.: The kidney and renal tract. In: H. Keen and J. Jarrett (Eds.): Complications of Diabetes. London, Edward Arnold Publications, 1975.

101. Root, H.F., Sharkey, T.P.: Arteriosclerosis and hypertension in diabetes. Ann. Intern. Med., 9:873, 1936.

102. Pell, S., D'Alonzo, C.A.: Some aspects of hypertension in diabetes mellitus. J.A.M.A. 202:104, 1967.

103. Freedman, P., Moulton, R., Spencer, A.G.: Hypertension and diabetes mellitus. Quart. J. Med. 27:293, 1958.

104. Pell, S., D'Alonzo, C.A.: Factors associated with long-term survival of diabetics. J.A.M.A. 214:1833, 1970.

105. Christlieb, A.R.: Diabetes and hypertensive vascular disease. Mechanisms and treatment. Am. J. Cardiol. 32:592, 1973.

106. Knowler, W.C., Bennett, P.H., Ballintine, E.J.: Increased incidence of retinopathy in diabetics with elevated blood pressure. A six-year follow-up study in Pima Indians. N. Engl. J. Med. *302*:645, 1980.

107. Knowles, H.C.: Discussion: vascular and visual complications. Kidney Int. Suppl. *1*:41, 1974.

108. Mitchell, J.C., Frohnert, P.P., Kurtz, S.B., Anderson, C.F.: Chronic peritoneal dialysis in juvenile-onset diabetes. A comparison with hemodialysis. Mayo Clinic Proc. *53*:775, 1978.

109. Sitprija, V., Holmes, J.H., Ellis, P.P.: Changes in intraocular pressure during hemodialysis. Invest. Ophthalmol. *3*:273, 1964.

110. Rao, K.V., Sutherland, D., Kjellstrand, C.M., et al.: Comparative results between dialysis and transplantation in diabetic patients. Trans. Am. Soc. Artif. Intern. Organs *23*:427, 1967.

111. Ramsay, R.C., Knobloch, W.H., Barbosa, J.J., et al.: The visual status of diabetic patients after renal transplantation. Am. J. Opthalmol. *87*:305, 1979.

112. Machemer, R., Aaberg, T.M.: Selection of patients. In: Vitrectomy, Chap. 1, 2nd Ed. New York, Grune & Stratton, 1979.

113. McMeel, J.W.: The treatment of diabetic retinopathy. Perspectives in Ophthalmology *2*:275, 1978.

114. Abourizk, N., Arastu, M.I., Arora, T., et al.: Ocular surgery in patients with diabetic nephropathy. Diabetes Care *3*:530, 1980.

115. Balodimos, M.C.: Diabetic nephropathy. In: A. Marble, P. White, R.F. Bradley, and L.P. Krall (Eds.): Joslin's Diabetes Mellitus, 11th Ed. Philadelphia, Lea & Febiger, 1971, pp. 526–561.

116. Oakley, W.G., Pyke, D.A., Tattersall, R.B., Watkins, P.J.: Long-term diabetes. A clinical study of 92 patients after 40 years. Quart. J. Med. *43*:145, 1974.

117. Friedman, E.A., L'Esperance, F.A., Jr.: Diabetic renal-retinal syndrome. The prognosis improves. Arch. Intern. Med. *140*:1149, 1980.

118. Anderson, R.: The role of the chaplain as a member of the renal dialysis kidney transplant team. In: N. Levy (Ed.): Psychological Factors in Hemodialysis and Transplantation. New York, Plenum Publishing Company. 1980, pp. 61–70.

119. D'Elia, J.A., Piening, S., Kaldany, A., et al.: Psychosocial crisis in diabetic renal failure. Diabetes Care *4*:99, 1981.

120. Fulton, R.E., Witten, D.M., Wagoner, R.D.: Intravenous urography in renal insufficiency. Am. J. Roentgenology, Radium Therapy, Nuclear Med., *106*:623, 1969.

121. Schwartz, W.B., Hurwit, A., Ettinger, A.: Intravenous urography in the patient with renal insufficiency. N. Engl. J. Med. *269*:277, 1963.

122. Bosniak, M.A., Schweizer, R.D.: Urographic findings in patietns with renal failure. Radiol. Clin. North Am. *10*:433, 1972.

123. Talner, L.B.: Urographic contrast media in uremia. Physiology and pharmacology. Radiol. Clin. North Am. *10*:421, 1972.

124. Doust, B.D., Redman, H.C.: The myth of 1 ml/kg in angiography. A study to determine the relationship of contrast medium dosage to complications. Diagnostic Radiology *104*:557, 1972.

125. Bergman, L.A., Ellison, M.R., Dunea, G.: Acute renal failure after drip infusion pyelography. N. Engl. J. Med. *279*:1277, 1968.

126. Pillay, V.K., Robbins, P.C., Schwartz, F.D., Kark, R.M.: Acute renal failure following intravenous urography in patients with long-standing diabetes mellitus and azotemia. Radiology *95*:633, 1970.

127. Barshay, M.E., Kaye, J.H., Goldman, R., Coburn, J.W.: Acute renal failure in diabetic patients after intravenous infusion pyelography. Clin. Nephr. *1*:35, 1973.

128. Weinrauch, L.A., Healy, R.W., Leland, O.S., Jr., et al.: Coronary angiography and acute renal failure in diabetic azotemic nephropathy. Ann. Intern. Med. *86*:56, 1977.

129. Ansari, Z., Baldwin, D.S.: Acute renal failure due to radio-contrast agents. Nephron *17*:28, 1976.

130. Milman, N., Stage, P.: High dose urography in advanced renal failure. II. Influence on renal and hepatic function. Acta Radio *15*:104, 1974.

131. Agarwal, B.N., Cabebe, F., McCormick, C.: Letter: Renal effects of urography in diabetes mellitus. Ann. Intern. Med. *83*:902, 1975.

132. Matz, R., Camacho, F., Sable, R., Seinfeld, D.: Renal effects of urography in diabetes mellitus. Ann. Intern. Med. *83*:902, 1975.

133. Alexander, R.D., Berkes, S.L., Abuelo, G.: Contrast media-induced oliguric renal failure. Arch. Intern. Med. *138*:381, 1978.

134. Swartz, R.D., Rubin, J.E., Leeming, B.W., Silva, P.: Renal failure following major angiography. Am. J. Med. *65*:31, 1978.

135. Carvallo, A., Rakowski, T.A., Argy, W.P., Jr., Schreiner, G.E.: Acute renal failure following drip infusion pyelography. Am. J. Med. *65*:38, 1978.

136. Hanaway, J., Black, J.: Renal failure following contrast injection for computerized tomography. J.A.M.A. *238*:2056, 1977.

137. Appell, R.A., Lytton, B.: Reversible renal failure following intravascular contrast radiography. J.A.M.A. *238*:1947, 1977.

138. Krumlovsky, F.A., Simon, N., Santhanam, S., et al.: Acute renal failure. Association with administration of radiographic contrast material J.A.M.A. *239*:125, 1978.

139. Teal, J.S., Rumbaugh, C.L., Segall, H.D., et al.: Acute renal failure following spinal angiography with methylglucamine iothalamate. Case report. Radiology *104*:561, 1972.

140. Port, F.K., Wagoner, R.D., Fulton, R.E.: Acute renal failure after angiography. Am. J. Roentgenol. Radium Ther. Nucl. Med. *121*:544, 1974.

141. Light, J.A., Hill, G.S.: Acute tubular necrosis in a renal transplant recipient: complication from drip-infusion excretory urography. J.A.M.A. *232*:1267, 1975.

142. Dudzinski, P.J., Petrone, A.F., Persoff, M., Callaghan, E.E.: Acute renal failure following high dose excretory urography in dehydrated patients. J. Urol. *106*:619, 1971.

143. D'Elia, J., Alday, M., Gleason, R., et al.: Acute renal failure following angiography. Prospective study of 150 patients, preliminary results. Proceedings of a Clinical Dialysis and Transplantation Forum (National Kidney Foundation) *8*:123, 1978.

144. D'Elia, J.D., Curt, G.A., Trey, C., et al.: Risk of acute renal failure following angiography in the elderly: a case report. Angiography, *30*:205, 1979.

145. Reiss, M.D., Bookstein,: J.J., Bleifer, K.H.: Radiology aspects of renovascular hypertension. Part 4. Arteriographic complications. J.A.M.A. *221*:375, 1972.

146. Brewster, D.C., Retana, A., Waltman, A.C., Darling, R.C.: Angiography in the management of aneurysms of the abdominal aorta. Its value and safety. N. Engl. J. Med. *292*:822, 1975.

147. Older, R.A., Miller, J.P., Jackson, D.C., et al.: Angiographically induced renal failure and its radiographic detection. Am. J. Roentgenol. *126*:1039, 1976.

148. Shafi, T., Chou, S.Y., Porush, J.G., Shapiro, W.: Infusion intravenous pyelography and renal function. Effects

in patients with chronic renal insufficiency. Arch. Intern. Med. *138*:1218, 1978.

149. VanZee, B.E., Hoy, W.E., Talley, T.E., Jaenike, J.R.: Renal injury associated with intravenous pyelography in non-diabetic and diabetic patients. Ann. Intern. Med. *89*:51, 1978.

149a.Feldman, H.A., Goldfarb, S., McCurdy, D.K.: Recurrent radiographic dye-induced acute renal failure. J.A.M.A. *229*:72, 1974.

150. Ghavamian, M., Gutch, C., Knopp, K., Kolff, W.: The sad truth about hemodialysis in diabetic nephropathy. J.A.M.A. *222*:1386, 1972.

151. Barcenas, C., Fuller, T., Elms, J., et al.: Staphylococcal sepsis in patients on chronic hemodialysis regimens: intravenous treatment with vancomycin given once weekly. Arch. Int. Med. *136*:1131, 1976.

152. Christlieb, A., Kaldany, A., D'Elia, J.: Plasma renin activity and hypertension in diabetes mellitus. Diabetes *25*:969, 1976.

153. Alancot, I., DeGoulet, P., Juillet, Y., et al.: Hemodynamic evaluation of hypotension during chronic hemodialysis. Clin. Nephrol. *8*:312, 1977.

154. Ghavamian, M., Gutch, C., Hughes, R., et al.: Pericardial tamponade in chronic-hemodialysis patients; treatment by pericardectomy. Arch. Intern. Med. *131*:249, 1973.

155. Silverberg, S., Oreopoulos, D., Wise, D., et al.: Pericarditis in patients undergoing long-term hemodialysis and peritoneal dialysis. Incidence, complications and management. Am. J. Med. *63*:874, 1977.

156. Garibaldi, R., Forrest, J., Bryan, J., et al.: Hemodialysis-associated hepatitis. J.A.M.A. *225*:384, 1973.

157. Gotloib, L., Servadio, C.: Ascites in patients undergoing maintenance hemodialysis. Report of six cases and physiopathologic approach. Am. J. Med. *61*:465, 1976.

158. Milutinovich, J., Follette, W., Scribner, B.: Spontaneous retroperitoneal bleeding in patients on chronic hemodialysis. Ann. Intern. Med. *86*:189, 1977.

159. Leonard, A., Shapiro, F.: Subdural hematoma in regularly hemodialyzed patients. Ann. Intern. Med. *82*:650, 1975.

160. Mahurkar, S., Dhar, S., Salta, R., et al.: Dialysis dementia. Lancet *1*:1412, 1973.

161. Cooppan, R., Schoenbaum, S., Younger, M., et al.: Vertebral osteomyelitis in insulin dependent diabetics. S. Afr. Med. J. *50*:1993, 1976.

162. Leonard, A., Comty, C., Shapiro, F., et al.: Osteomyelitis in hemodialysis patients. Ann. Intern. Med. *78*:651, 1973.

163. Babb, A., Popovich, R., Christopher, T., Scribner, B.: The genesis of the square meter-hour hypothesis. Trans. Am. Soc. Artif. Intern. Organs *17*:81, 1971.

164. Totten, M., Izenstein, B., Gleason, R., et al.: Chronic renal failure in diabetes: survival with hemodialysis versus transplantation. J. Dialysis *2*:17, 1978.

165. Sitprija, V., Holmes, J., Ellis, P.: Changes in intraocular pressure during hemodialysis. Invest. Ophthalmol. *3*:273, 1964.

166. Langer, T., Levy, R.: Acute muscular syndrome associated with administration of clofibrate. N. Engl. J. Med. *279*:856, 1968.

167. Miller, D.G., Hampton, L., Vlachokosta, F., et al.: The use of an open-loop insulin pump in Type I diabetics with renal insufficiency. Diabetic Nephropathy *3*:19, 1984.

168. Garber, A., Bier, D., Cryer, P., Pagliara, A.: Hypoglycemia in compensated chronic renal insufficiency. Substrate limitation of gluconeogenesis. Diabetes *23*:982, 1974.

169. Rutsky, E., McDaniel, H., Tharpe, D., et al.: Sponta-neous hypoglycemia in chronic renal failure. Arch. Intern. Med. *138*:1364, 1978.

170. Field, J.: Angiography, acute renal failure and decreased insulin requirements in diabetes mellitus. Editorial. Arch. Intern. Med. *138*:354, 1978.

171. Lindner, A., Charra, B., Sherrard, D., Scribner, B.: Accelerated atherosclerosis in prolonged maintenance hemodialysis. N. Engl. J. Med. *290*:697, 1974.

172. Shapiro, F.L., Leonard, A., Compty, C.M.: Mortality morbidity and rehabilitation results in regularly dialyzed patients with diabetes mellitus. Kidney Inter. *6*: (Suppl. 1):S8, 1974.

173. Oreopoulos, D.: Maintenance peritoneal dialysis. In: E. Friedman (Ed.): Strategy in Renal Failure. New York, Wiley Medical Publications, 1978, pp. 393–414.

174. Buselmeir, R., Najarian, J., Simmons, R., et al.: A-V fistulas and the diabetic: ischemia and gangrene may result in amputation. Trans. Am. Soc. Artif. Intern. Organs *19*:49, 1973.

175. Bussell, J., Abbot, J., Lim, R.: A radial steal syndrome with arteriovenous fistula for hemodialysis: studies in seven patients. Ann. Intern. Med. *75*:387, 1971.

176. Ahearn, D., Maher, J.: Heart failure as a complication of hemodialysis arteriovenous fistula. Ann. Intern. Med. *77*:201, 1972.

177. Popovich, R.P., Moncrief, J.W., Nolph, K.D., et al.: Continuous ambulatory peritoneal dialysis. Ann. Intern. Med. *88*:449, 1978.

178. Shapira, J., Lang, R., Jutrin, I., et al.: Peritoneal dialysis in refractory congestive heart failure. Part 1. Intermittent peritoneal dialysis. Peritoneal Dialysis Bulletin *3*:130, 1983.

179. Amair, P., Khanna, R., Leibel, B., et al.: Continuous ambulatory peritoneal dialysis in diabetics with end-stage renal disease. N. Engl. J. Med. *306*:625, 1982.

179a.Weinrauch, L.A., Belok, S., Healy, R.W., et al.: Peritoneal dialysis in refractory biventricular failure. Clin. Exp. Dial. Apheresis (accepted for publication).

180. Libertino, J., Zinman, L., Salerno, A., et al.: Diabetic renal transplantation. J. Urol. *124*:593, 1980.

181. D'Elia, J.A., Weinrauch, L.A., Kaldany, A., et al.: Improving survival after renal transplantation for diabetic patients with severe coronary artery disease. Diabetes Care *4*:380, 1981.

182. Opelz, G., Terasaki, P.: Improvement of kidney-graft survival with increased numbers of blood transfusions. N. Engl. J. Med. *299*:799, 1978.

183. Vincenti, F., Duca, R., Amend, W., et al.: Immunologic factors determining survival of cadaver-kidney transplants. N. Engl. J. Med. *299*:793, 1978.

184. Linas, S., Miller, P., McDonald, K., et al.: :Role of the renin-angiotensin system in post-transplantation hypertension in patients with multiple kidneys. N. Engl. J. Med., *298*:1440, 1978.

185. Rao, T., Gupta, S., Butt, K., et al.: Relationship of renal transplantation to hypertension in end-stage renal failure. Arch. Intern. Med. *138*:1236, 1978.

186. Whelton, P., Russell, R., Harrington, D., et al.: Hypertension following renal transplantation: causative factors and therapeutic implications. J.A.M.A. *241*:1128, 1979.

187. Bagdade, J., Albers, J.: Plasma high-density lipoprotein concentrations in chronic hemodialysis and renal-transplant patients. N. Engl. J. Med. *296*:1436, 1977.

187a.Clark, J., Hochman, R., Rolla, A.R., et al.: Coagulopathy associated with the use of cephalosporin or moxalactum antibiotics in acute and chronic renal failure. Clin. Exp. Dial. Apheresis *7*:177, 1983.

188. Ascher, N., Simmons, R., Fryd, D., Najarian, J.: Superior results of well matched cadveric grafts as compared to parental grafts. Proc. Clin. Dial. Transplant Forum *7*:11, 1977.

31 The Nervous System and Diabetes

Simeon Locke and Daniel Tarsy

Involvement of the nervous system in persons with diabetes has long been recognized. Rollo[1] is credited with having first recorded this association in 1798, and until the middle of the 19th century, diabetes itself was ascribed to a disorder of the central nervous system. Marchal de Calvi[2] in 1864 first suggested that diabetes might be the cause rather than the effect of neuropathy. Subsequent reports appeared with increased frequency and demonstrated the clinical acumen of the era. Pavy's[3] description in 1885 is noteworthy in its completeness:

"The usual account given by these patients of their condition is that they cannot feel properly in their legs, that their feet are numb, that their legs seem too heavy— as one patient expressed it, 'as if he had twenty pound weights on his legs, and a feeling as if his boots were a good deal too large for his feet'. Darting or 'lightning' pains are often complained of. Or there may be hyperesthesia, so that a mere pinching up of the skin gives rise to great pain; or, it might be, the patient is unable to bear the contact of the seam of a dress against the skin on account of the suffering it causes. Not infrequently there is deep-seated pain, located, as the patient describes it, in the marrow of the bones, which are tender on being grasped; and I have noticed that these pains are generally worse at night. With this there is the usual loss or impairment of the patellar tendon reflex."

Interest in the neurologic symptoms associated with diabetes has continued[4-8] and in fact, in recent years, has increased greatly as new techniques for study have become available. Disorders of the peripheral nervous system have attracted more attention than those of the central nervous system largely because the latter frequently represent manifestations of an associated illness rather than of diabetes itself.

PERIPHERAL NERVOUS SYSTEM

Complication or Concomitant?

Involvement of the peripheral nervous system by diabetes is referred to as diabetic neuropathy. This noncommittal term makes no implication about the nature or location of the pathologic process. Similarly, it takes no stand on whether involvement of the peripheral nervous system constitutes a complication or a concomitant of the metabolic disorder. Although an increasing bulk of evidence favors the concept that the neuropathy is due to diabetes, particularly if it is poorly controlled, it is clear that characteristic symptoms of neuropathy may occur without clinically manifest diabetes.[9] Furthermore, the not infrequent lack of relation between the duration or severity of abnormal glucose metabolism and the presence of neuropathy is consistent with the possibility that peripheral neuropathy may be a concomitant abnormality.[10] Increased blood glucose is frequently noted in patients with peripheral neurologic manifestations but ketosis does not appear to be a factor in the development of symptoms. Paradoxically, symptoms of peripheral nerve involvement may appear when the diabetes is first brought under control; fortunately such symptoms usually subside with maintenance of good metabolic control.[6]

Despite the suggestion that neuropathy is due to a *metabolic* defect in diabetes, proponents of a *vascular* etiology argue that the parallel with nephropathy and retinopathy suggests that microangiopathy may also be causative in the production of peripheral neurologic manifestations.[11] Perhaps both vascular and metabolic disorders are at work.[12] It is worth recalling the division of the mixed spinal nerve into A, B, and C fibers on the basis of conduction velocity. Characteristically, ischemic processes affect the large myelinated, rapidly conducting A fibers first.[13] The selective involvement of small fibers which conduct pain and autonomic impulses[14] is reminiscent of the effect of procaine and its derivatives and suggests a metabolic mode of action.

Types

Many classifications of diabetic neuropathy have been proposed. In 1936 Jordan,[15] following a study of patients with neuropathy at the Joslin Clinic, recognized three types: (1) a "hyperglycemic" type with symptoms but without signs and with prompt reversal by treatment of diabetes; (2) a circulatory-degenerative type; and (3) a neuritic type. Similarly, Treusch[16] wrote of (1) diabetes with pain in which the diabetes is out of control and symptoms improve with treatment; (2) ischemic neuropathy; (3) diabetic polyneuritis; and (4) visceral neuritis. The classification of Goodman and coworkers[17] includes (1) functional neuropathy with uncontrolled diabetes and no objective evidence of neurologic involvement ("hyperglycemic neuritis" of Jordan or Treusch's "diabetes with pain"); (2) organic neuropathy in which objective signs are present; and (3) post-treatment neuropathy. A division into symmetric sensory and an asymmetric motor neuropathy has been suggested.[18]

An anatomic rather than a clinical classification has also been proposed[19] (Fig. 31–1), using a typical spinal segment as the point of departure. When the lesion is of nerve root, the disorder is referred to as a *radiculopathy*. When a mixed spinal nerve is affected, it produces a *mononeuropathy*. If the affection is of the distal portions of many nerve fibers, it is classified as *polyneuropathy*.

Pathology

Woltman and Wilder in 1929[20] emphasized the location of disease in peripheral nerves and, based on studies of limbs amputated for arteriosclerotic gangrene, attributed the changes to occlusive disease of the vasa nervorum. The suggestion of a "generalized, specific, diabetic, vascular disease, not identical with" arteriosclerosis or atherosclerosis, was also made by Lundbaek in 1954.[21] With van Gieson's stain, vascular changes appear similar to those of hypertension, but with the periodic acid Schiff (PAS) reagent, a distinction between the two can be made.[22] Characteristically, intraneural vessels demonstrate stenosis, hyalinization, and subendothelial PAS-positive staining material.[23]

Although other investigators[24–27] were not impressed with the severity of vasa nervorum involvement and argued against a correlation between vascular lesions and extent of neuropathy, later electron microscopic studies have shown hyperplasia of capillary endothelial and pericyte basement membranes and thickening of the perivascular space to be more frequent in diabetic neuropathy than in other acquired neuropathies.[28–30] Similar basement membrane thickening has been observed in perineurial cells of sural nerves and dorsal root ganglia of diabetics when compared with similar tissues of nondiabetics matched for age and severity of neuropathy.[27] Whether such changes are etiologically important for diabetic neuropathy is uncertain. Related to suggestions concerning diabetic microangiopathy in renal and retinal capillaries,[31] are proposals that excessive capillary permeability may allow access to the endoneurial space by putative toxins which are normally excluded by the blood-nerve barrier.[32] Although such toxins have not been identified, the endoneurial vessels of alloxan-diabetic rats show increased permeability to protein which, by leakage into the endoneurial space, may produce edema, increased interstitial pressure, compromised capillary flow and filtration, and resultant nerve fiber injury.[33] Endoneurial edema and associated shrinkage of Schwann cells have also been demonstrated in the nerves of rats with streptozotocin diabetes.[34] However, in another study, blood-nerve barrier permeability has been found normal in alloxan and streptozotocin diabetic rats and a mutant diabetic mouse.[35,36] Increased platelet aggregation and microvascular occlusion by aggregates[37] or fibrin[38] have been reported in sural nerve biopsies from diabetics. The relevance of these findings for pathogenesis of diabetic neuropathy, remains to be determined[39] (Fig. 31–2).

In most diabetic patients, neuropathy appears to occur in a mixed pattern affecting large and small myelinated and unmyelinated nerve fibers,[30] although a few patients can be found on either end of the spectrum with predominantly small or large fiber dysfunction.[40,41] The pathologic changes in axons, myelin, and Schwann cells are qualitatively nonspecific with no features to distinguish diabetic polyneuropathy from other chronic axonal neuropathies.[30] There has been considerable debate concerning whether segmental demyelination or axonal degeneration is the primary abnormality in

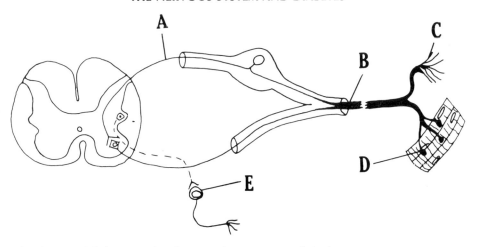

Fig. 31–1. Classification of diabetic peripheral neuropathy on an anatomic basis

	Structure	Disorder	Etiology	Signs and Symptoms
A	Nerve root	Radiculopathy	Probably vascular	Pain and sensory loss in distribution of a dermatome.
B	Mixed spinal or cranial nerve	Mononeuropathy	Probably vascular	Pain, weakness, reflex change, sensory loss in distribution of mixed spinal or cranial nerve.
C	Nerve terminals	Polyneuropathy	Metabolic?	Glove and stocking sensory loss; mild peripheral weakness, absent reflex.
D	Nerve terminal? Muscle?	Diabetic amyotrophy	Unknown	Anterior thigh pain, proximal weakness of legs.
E	Sympathetic ganglion	Autonomic neuropathy	Unknown	Postural hypotension, anhydrosis, impotence, gastropathy, vesical atony.

(Used with permission of author and publisher[19]).

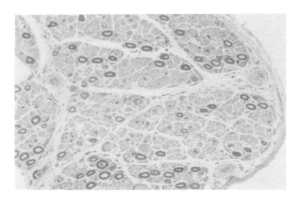

Fig. 31–2. Epon section of sural nerve in a case of diabetic neuropathy. Note the extensive demyelination and the thickening of vessel walls.

diabetic neuropathy. Some investigators have held that segmental demyelination, presumably due to a metabolic disturbance affecting Schwann cell function, is the primary abnormality.[27,42] Thomas and Lascelles,[26] from results with teased fiber preparations, emphasized segmental demyelination and remyelination as the main pathologic change of diabetic neuropathy, but also identified prominent

axonal degeneration in severe cases. They considered it unresolved as to whether axonal loss was secondary to demyelination or was an independent process. Behse et al.[29] found evidence of loss of large and small myelinated fibers and unmyelinated fibers; they believed that axonal degeneration and Schwann cell damage proceed independently of each other (Fig. 31–3).

More recently, electromyographic[29,43] and

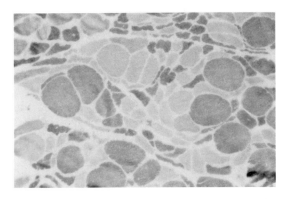

Fig. 31–3. Muscle biopsy from a patient with diabetic neuropathy. Small group atrophy is evident.

morphologic[29,40] evidence has shown that axonal degeneration appears early in the course of human diabetic neuropathy. Although experimental findings have not been uniform,[40] studies in several animal models of diabetes have indicated that axonal degeneration may actually be the primary event.[38,45,46] Segmental demyelination is known to occur as a secondary response to primary axonal disease in other peripheral neuropathies,[47,48] but the precise relationship of segmental demyelination to axonal degeneration in diabetic neuropathy remains an open question.[6,38,44]

Some investigators have suggested a primary neuronal degeneration with loss of axons in peripheral nerves and nerve roots, and loss of dorsal root ganglion cells and anterior horn cells with secondary degeneration of posterior columns of spinal cord and muscle.[25,49] Location of the disorder at the nerve cell body may result in initial manifestations appearing at the periphery due to a "dying back" from the nerve terminals.[50] Accordingly, the changes in neuromuscular endings in diabetic neuropathy studied by staining with intravital methylene blue are understandable.[51–53] Of great interest is the pathologic finding of end plate changes in patients with diabetes without overt signs of neuropathy.[53] Biopsy findings must, of course, be evaluated with caution since collateral regeneration[54] may complicate the interpretation. In cats made diabetic with alloxan, intravital stain showed degeneration of the end plate, atrophy of the subneural apparatus, presence of growth cones, and collateral branching of the terminal axon.[55]

The pathologic basis of diabetic *autonomic* neuropathy is incompletely understood. A number of investigators have identified abnormalities in paravertebral sympathetic ganglia including neurons distended by accumulations of lipid-rich material,[56–58] vacuolar degeneration of neurons produced by dilatation of endoplasmic reticulum,[23,58,59] and mononuclear cell infiltration of autonomic nerve bundles and ganglia.[58] Loss of myelinated nerve fibers has also been described in sympathetic communicating rami,[59,60] vagus nerve,[58,61] postganglionic sympathetic nerves,[14] and splanchnic nerves.[60] Neuronal vacuolation in the myenteric plexus of Auerbach, however, occurs no more frequently in diabetics with diarrhea than in nondiabetic controls.[62]

Based on the careful study of a small number of cases, the pathologic basis of diabetic *mononeuropathy* is believed to be ischemic infarction of nerve. Raff and colleagues[63] described a single patient found to have numerous microinfarcts in the proximal portions of obturator, femoral, sciatic, and tibial nerves. Occurrence of these infarcts has been emphasized in bridging interfascicular nerve

bundles, similar to the distribution of microinfarcts in other ischemic mononeuropathies.[30] Although fibrosis and hyalinization of small arterioles and capillaries were prominent, most infarcts did not relate to identifiable vascular occlusions. Three cases of diabetic oculomotor nerve palsy have also been studied pathologically.[64–66] All three demonstrated a localized zone of ischemic nerve injury. Both myelin and axonal degeneration occurred in 2 cases[64,66] and predominantly demyelination was present in the 3rd case.[65] In all 3 instances, an exhaustive search for a responsible occluded vessel was unrevealing.

Pathophysiology

The relationship between the diabetic neuropathies and the metabolic aspects of diabetes remains unknown. Observations that peripheral neuropathy may be the initial manifestation of diabetes and failure in many patients to produce improvement in neuropathy by aggressive management of hyperglycemia, have contributed to the concept that peripheral neuropathy may result from a pathophysiologic process independent of glucose and insulin metabolism. On the other hand, abundant evidence indicates that the frequency and severity of diabetic neuropathy does show an overall correlation with the duration of disease[67] and degree of diabetic control.[4,25,68,69] The observations that patients with newly diagnosed diabetes and laboratory animals with experimental diabetes both show slowing in nerve conduction velocity which is preventable in laboratory animals[70] and partially correctable in humans by insulin treatment,[71–73] support the concept of an early, reversible impairment in nerve function in diabetes due to biochemical changes that precede structural abnormalities of axons or myelin.

Since segmental demyelination was felt at one time to be the hallmark of diabetic neuropathy, early studies were directed toward identifying a metabolic defect affecting Schwann cells and myelin. A series of in vitro studies of lipid metabolism in nerve from animals with experimental diabetes have shown abnormalities in mechanisms of lipid synthesis and percentage composition of individual lipid constituents of myelin.[6,44,74–76] Unfortunately, the results of such studies have not been uniform and their relationship to actual nerve function is uncertain.[44]

It has been suggested that hyperglycemia may have an adverse effect on Schwann cell integrity by means of increased activity in the polyol pathway.[77] Since peripheral nerve does not require insulin for intracellular diffusion of glucose, the enzymatic conversion of glucose to sorbitol by aldose reductase and subsequent conversion of sorbitol to fructose are directly related to plasma glucose concentration.[77] The levels of nerve glucose, sorbitol, and fructose are all elevated in hyperglycemic diabetic animals, and decrease following insulin treatment.[78] The sorbitol and fructose content of sural nerve taken from diabetic patients is related to the median fasting blood glucose level but shows wider variability than for nondiabetic control nerves and does not appear to be related to the severity of neuropathy.[79] Since most polyol activity in peripheral nerve occurs in the Schwann cell,[77] it was predicted that the osmotic effect of sugar accumulation would result in edema and cell death. Contrary to this expectation, Schwann cell volume has been shown to decrease rather than increase in animals with experimental diabetes.[34] Earlier demonstrations that nerve edema does occur appear to be explained by increased endoneurial rather than intracellular edema.[44] Despite these findings, and since the implication of endoneurial edema for nerve function is unknown, there continues to be active interest in the possible benefits of blocking sorbitol synthesis by use of aldose reductase inhibitors in patients with diabetic neuropathy.[6,8,44]

More recently it has been suggested that abnormalities of axonal myoinositol metabolism may be important in the pathophysiology of diabetic neuropathy.[44,70] Myoinositol is a polyalcohol which is normally present in high concentrations in peripheral nerve and other tissues. Although its role in nerve function is unknown, the turnover of phospholipids containing myoinositol increases following nerve impulse and synaptic transmission.[44] In rats with relatively severe experimental diabetes, a decline in nerve myoinositol concentration and a decrease in nerve conduction velocity can be prevented by treatment of hyperglycemia with insulin.[70] Dietary manipulation of myoinositol has a major effect on plasma and nerve concentrations in both normal and diabetic rats. In diabetic rats given a myoinositol supplemented diet, nerve myoinositol concentrations were increased and nerve conduction velocity was significantly faster than in diabetic rats receiving a standard diet.[70] Since similar results have not been obtained with diets containing still higher concentrations of myoinositol[70] and myoinositol has not been found to be reduced in sural nerve from diabetic patients,[79] and since the findings have not been confirmed in other laboratories,[80] the precise relationship of myoinositol metabolism to diabetic neuropathy remains uncertain. Preliminary clinical trials of myoinositol in patients with diabetic neuropathy have shown increased sensory nerve conduction velocity[8] and amplitude[82] of evoked sensory nerve action potentials but no change in motor nerve conduction velocity or vibration perception thresholds.[81-83]

CLINICAL OBSERVATIONS

Diabetic Radiculopathy

Diabetic radiculopathy is an infrequent form of peripheral neurologic involvement. It is of uncertain cause but, similar to peripheral mononeuropathies, may arise from ischemic infarction of nerve roots. The disorder is characterized by either lancinating or more continuous deep-seated pain in the distribution area of one or several dermatomes. When thoracic roots are involved, abdominal pain and weight loss may be prominent and exhaustive investigations for abdominal malignancy are often undertaken.[84-86] The presence of paresthesia or subtle sensory findings in a dermatomal distribution and segmental electromyographic abnormalities in paraspinal muscles[84-86] are helpful in identifying this condition. Although patients are typically uncomfortable, the prognosis is excellent with recovery usually occurring within several months. When an arm or leg is involved, a root-like pattern of sensory deficit may be found and a compressive lesion such as herniated nucleus pulposus or spondylosis may be suspected. The diagnosis of diabetic pseudotabes may be made[87] when (a) multiple nerve roots are affected; (b) posterior column degeneration with loss of position sense attends the process; (c) lancinating pain and ataxia are prominent, and (d) these are associated with pupillary involvement and trophic ulcers.

Diabetic Mononeuropathy

Mononeuropathy is particularly common in diabetics and may occur on the basis of a vascular lesion, entrapment, or trauma to superficially placed nerves.[88] Any major nerve trunk may be affected. When several nerve trunks are involved simultaneously, the disorder is classified as mononeuropathy multiplex. The femoral mononeuropathy which appears acutely with pain, motor and sensory deficit, and loss of knee jerk, is likely to be on an ischemic basis and, because of extensive anastomoses of collateral circulation, carries a good prognosis for complete recovery.[89,90] An isolated sciatic mononeuropathy may also occur on a similar basis.[91]

Carpal tunnel syndrome due to median nerve entrapment in the wrist is common among diabetics and produces a clinical syndrome indistinguishable from that occurring in nondiabetics. Occasionally, however, a distal median mononeuropathy may occur in the absence of the usual pain and sensory symptoms of carpal tunnel syndrome. In such cases a distal ulnar neuropathy often coexists[92] and both may be due to a "dying back" polyneuropathy rather than entrapment at the wrist. The finding of prolonged distal latencies in multiple nerve trunks rather than just in median nerve, will usually distinguish this situation from entrapment.

Peroneal mononeuropathy typically produces a sudden foot drop usually without associated pain and, in addition to vascular factors, may be due to trauma because of the superficial location of the nerve. Ulnar mononeuropathy is probably also related to the vulnerable position of the nerve at the elbow. Unlike femoral or peroneal neuropathy, however, symptoms usually appear insidiously and may be due to chronic trauma rather than an acute insult to the nerve.

Cranial Neuropathies

Cranial neuropathies belong to the category of mononeuropathies. They probably arise from a specific angiopathy and may be recurrent. The majority of cranial neuropathies affect the 3rd and 6th cranial nerves[93-95] while the 4th nerve is rarely affected alone.[95] In cases of 3rd nerve involvement, the pupil is usually spared. Onset of diplopia is often associated with pain behind or above the affected eye.[96,97] Unlike the painful ophthalmoplegia sometimes associated with temporal arteritis, eye muscle weakness occurs in a nerve distribution rather than from random ischemic muscle involvement.[98] The suggestion that the pain may be due to simultaneous involvement of the 1st and 2nd divisions of the trigeminal nerve within the cavernous sinus is supported by the occasional finding of sensory impairment in the distribution of these branches.[95] Differentiation from a structural lesion of the sphenoidal fissure or cavernous sinus is obviously important. The vascular etiology of diabetic ophthalmoplegia was confirmed by 3 cases of diabetic 3rd nerve palsy studied pathologically.[64-66] In all 3, focal ischemic nerve infarction was found. The peripheral location of the pupillary fibers allows them to be nourished by the venous blood of the cavernous sinus, accounting for the pupillary function. Recovery is usually complete within several weeks or months, suggesting that demyelination without significant axonal destruction may be the responsible lesion in most cases.[65] The Argyll Robertson pupil, if it occurs in diabetes, is exceedingly rare.[1,99,100]

Other cranial nerves are infrequently affected. In one uncontrolled study, impaired olfaction was reported in 35 of 58 diabetic patients with no evidence of nasal mucosa abnormality.[101] The occurrence of acute optic neuritis or progressive optic atrophy in association with diabetes should not be construed as a causal relation. The 2 cases of optic neuritis reported by Jordan[15] as having "no obvious cause unless it was diabetes" are examples of the lack of proven causality. Careful studies have

shown the condition to occur infrequently in diabetes[102,103] except in special circumstances such as the syndrome of juvenile-onset diabetes and optic atrophy (vide infra).[104]

Optic disc edema, indistinguishable in appearance from papilledema, with associated nerve fiber layer hemorrhages and "cotton wool spots," has been described in patients with juvenile-onset diabetes. This is usually associated with mild or transient impairment of visual acuity, normal visual fields with the exception of an enlarged blind spot, and a favorable prognosis. This condition is of obscure etiology but is believed to be due to a vasculopathy of the most superficial capillary layer of the disc and adjacent retina.[105,106] Anterior ischemic optic neuropathy may occasionally appear in diabetes. This is an ischemic infarction of the anterior optic nerve which produces acute optic disc edema and visual loss with subsequent development of optic atrophy. Although local vascular causes, especially arteriosclerosis, are common, there is no proven specific association of this condition with diabetes.[107]

Facial paralysis due to a 7th nerve involvement occurs with some frequency in diabetes[94,108] and apparently has a less favorable prognosis for full recovery than in nondiabetics,[109] but its designation as a diabetic mononeuropathy remains doubtful. Eighth nerve palsies on a diabetic basis seem most unlikely despite the report of 2 cases of nerve deafness.[1] The lower cranial nerves are never the site of a diabetic mononeuropathy.

Diabetic Polyneuropathy

By far the most frequent form of diabetic neuropathy is the distal, bilateral, comparatively symmetric polyneuropathy. Although predominantly sensory, motor abnormality is not uncommon and sometimes may be quite severe. The sensory loss and motor weakness affect the distal portion of the longest nerves first and do not conform to distribution of a nerve root or peripheral nerve. Rather, they are in the territory of overlapping peripheral terminals of many nerves. Feet are affected before hands, with the upper level difficult to define as it grades into normal. It is this distribution which produces the "glove and stocking" loss of sensation characteristic of the disorder. In severe cases distal portions of thoracic intercostal nerves may be affected there by producing midline sensory loss in a teardrop distribution over the anterior thorax and abdomen.[110] By contrast with thoracic truncal radiculopathy[84-86] this is a painless although persistent form of neuropathy.

In most patients with polyneuropathy, symptoms are minimal. When reported, they are usually noted as absence of sensation in contrast with the pain of mononeuropathy and radiculopathy. Painful paresthesia, hyperesthesia, dysesthesia, and episodic, discretely localized jabbing pains may occur, however. Burning sensation in the feet may occur but should also alert the physician to a concomitant toxic or deprivational state. When large fibers are affected early, vibration sense is often preferentially depressed.[111] Pain loss, impaired touch perception and decreased position sense rapidly supervene. Motor weakness is less prominent than sensory impairment but is often present, particularly in extensors and flexors of the toes. Atrophy may occur but often is not apparent until long after the onset of clinical weakness. Loss of bulk of the intrinsic muscles of hand and foot is sometimes striking and may produce a deformity similar to the claw hand and pes cavus of Charcot-Marie-Tooth disease. However, the diabetic claw foot never has the tight plantar fascia or short Achilles tendon of a true cavus deformity.[112]

Electromyography

Nerve conduction studies show relatively mild degrees of slowing in asymptomatic or mild cases[67,113,114] but may become profound in patients with significant weakness and large fiber sensory deficits for vibration and proprioception.[115] Although motor nerve conduction velocity measurements are often mildly abnormal in newly diagnosed diabetics, the most sensitive index of early or subclinical peripheral neuropathy is reduction in amplitude and dispersion of the sensory nerve action potential.[115-117] Electromyography discloses typical changes of denervation such as fibrillation potentials at rest and reduced recruitment of motor unit potentials during voluntary muscle contraction.[118,119] The distal gradient of involvement has been explained as the result of a "dying back" process in which a disturbance of neuronal and axonal integrity may result in degeneration of terminals and distal segments of nerve because these are most removed from the origin of neuronal nutrient transport systems.[50,120] This theory gains support from those cases of diabetic polyneuropathy in which there is a much more marked prolongation of distal motor latency than the slowing of nerve conduction velocity in more proximal nerve segments. An alternative explanation for involvement of the longest fibers is that these are more likely to be affected by a disease process in which lesions are randomly scattered along the length of the axon.[121] Evidence for random distribution of nerve lesions has been obtained for several other peripheral neuropathies and may well exist also in diabetic neuropathy.[121]

AUTONOMIC NEUROPATHY

Gastrointestinal Tract

Particularly difficult diagnostic problems may occur in patients with visceral autonomic neuropathy, particularly when combined with abdominal pain due to an associated thoracic radiculopathy. Disorders of motility include diminished esophageal peristalsis,[122] gastroparesis with impaired gastric emptying, gastric hypotonicity[123-126] and achlorhydria,[127] gallbladder dysfunction,[127,128] nocturnal or postprandial diarrhea, steatorrhea, and constipation (see Chapter 40).

Genitourinary Tract

Hypotonic neurogenic bladder, retrograde ejaculation, and sexual (erectile) impotence are the commonest manifestations of genitourinary disturbance (See Chapter 32). Hypotonic bladder is particularly common and appears insidiously with increasing intervals between voiding, progressive micturitional difficulty, and increasing residual urinary volume with heightened susceptibility to infection.[129] Electrophysiologic[130] and neuropathologic[131] evidence suggests that diabetic bladder dysfunction is due to abnormalities of the intrinsic sensory innervation of the bladder rather than pudendal neuropathy.[4] Retrograde ejaculation occurs due to incompetence of the internal bladder sphincter. Erectile impotence occurs sooner or later in 50 to 60% of diabetic males[132] and correlates with clinical or laboratory evidence of bladder dysfunction.[133] Differentiation from psychologic impotence or that due to drugs or other influences is obviously essential. Impotence in diabetes is usually gradual rather than abrupt in onset and characterized by complete absence of nocturnal erections. Monitoring of nocturnal penile tumescence is helpful in making this distinction.[134] Ellenberg found no evidence for an adverse effect of diabetes on female sexual function.[132]

Cardiovascular System

Postural hypotension is the most common cardiovascular effect of diabetic autonomic neuropathy.[135] Symptoms include lightheadedness, visual disturbance, and syncope on standing, but many patients are remarkably asymptomatic despite large drops in blood pressure. The importance of differentiation from hypoglycemic reactions and cerebral vascular insufficiency is obvious. The responsible lesion is presumed to be in the efferent limb of the reflex arc due to abnormalities of sympathetic innervation of the splanchnic, muscular or cutaneous circulations. Decreased plasma renin and noradrenaline responses to standing have also been reported[8,135] and may be contributory. Lack of compensatory tachycardia to postural change is often present and may increase symptoms. A number of cardiovascular reflex abnormalities with effects on heart rate have been identified in diabetic autonomic neuropathy, and their possible but unproven relationship to sudden cardiac death has been discussed.[8,135] See Chapters 27 and 28.

Sweating Disturbances

Peripheral vasomotor and sweating disturbances are common in diabetes and may result from polyneuropathy of mixed nerves or result from specific disturbances in postganglionic sympathetic innervation of the skin circulation.[136] Sweating disturbances include anhidrosis in the lower part of the body[137] sometimes associated with hyperhidrosis over the face and upper trunk.[4,138] Gustatory sweating may cause profuse perspiration over the face upon eating.[139]

Charcot-type Arthropathy

Whether the development of Charcot-like joint changes, with or without perforating ulcers, is related to deprivation of autonomic innervation or whether it results from a circulatory disorder, is still unresolved. Usually Charcot joints are ascribed to diminution of the nocifensive reflex attendant upon sensory loss. The small fiber affection responsible for diminished pain sensation may similarly result in autonomic nervous system dysfunction, producing a predisposition to neurogenic arthropathy.[140,141] Recurrent trauma in the presence of intact motor function, impaired pain perception, and diminished or absent proprioception which normally inhibits hypermobility,[141] results in thickening of the tarsal region, external rotation and eversion of the foot, and destruction of tarsal and metatarsal bones. Joint spaces are obliterated, and tarsal and metatarsal bones are separated and fragmented. There is radiologic evidence of atrophy of the phalanges, destruction of the epiphyses, erosion of joint surfaces, and restorative periosteal regeneration.[7,8,142-144] Swelling occurs in the absence of inflammation with neither tenderness nor temperature change prominent. *Neuropathic ulcers* occur on the plantar surface of the foot and, similar to Charcot joints, result from weight bearing on a foot with reduced sensory innervation. The common association with Charcot joints arises from excessive mechanical pressures on areas of the foot which normally do not bear weight.

DIABETIC AMYOTROPHY

Originally described by Bruns[144] in 1890, this disorder was redescribed by Garland and

Taverner[145] under the name of "diabetic myelopathy." Because convincing clinical and pathologic evidence for spinal cord involvement was not forthcoming, this syndrome was subsequently designated diabetic amyotrophy,[146] a deliberately noncommittal term with regard to precise locus of the disease process. The clinical picture is one of subacute painful weakness and atrophy of the pelvic girdle and thigh musculature. Affected muscles nearly always include the psoas and quadriceps, compromising thigh flexion and stabilization of the knee and producing a superficial similarity to the more restricted femoral mononeuropathy.[89] However, weakness of the glutei, hamstrings, thigh adductors, and occasionally distal muscles such as tibialis and peroneal muscles, indicates the more widespread distribution of the disorder.[147-149] Sensory signs or symptoms often occur and may include paresthesia or dysesthesia in anterior thigh or anteromedial lower leg. Pain is severe, typically located in the hip, buttock, and anterior thigh, and is described as a deep ache rather than the shooting radicular pain often associated with lumbar root compression.

Diabetic amyotrophy is typically unilateral in onset but there may be eventual involvement of the contralateral side. The knee jerk is nearly always reduced or absent on the affected side, while ankle jerks may remain preserved unless compromised by distal polyneuropathy. Plantar responses are usually flexor but sometimes equivocal or weakly extensor. Pain, sensory abnormalities, and weakness in thoracic root distribution may also occur in an affected patient.[86] Shoulder girdle involvement, however, is relatively uncommon and, when present, usually occurs together with significant leg weakness.[146,147,150-152] Bulbar involvement does not occur and if present, should suggest an alternative neurologic disorder. Diabetic amyotrophy occurs with a peak incidence in the 6th decade, characteristically in adult onset diabetes often of relatively brief duration. Although many patients are only mildly diabetic at the time of diagnosis, a number of authors have emphasized poor diabetic control in such patients.[146,148,151] Similar to thoracic radiculopathy, weight loss is usually prominent and, in some cases, is sufficiently great to suggest an occult carcinoma.

Differential diagnosis includes lumbar nerve root compression, neoplastic infiltration of lumbosacral plexus, motor neuron disease, primary myopathy, polymyositis, and vasculitis. Laminectomies and laparotomies are not infrequently carried out in such patients in search of a structural etiology. The lack of mechanical signs or symptoms, frequent nocturnal exacerbation of pain with failure to respond to bed rest, and extreme muscular wasting usually serve to distinguish diabetic amyotrophy from mechanical nerve root compression.

There has been considerable debate concerning the etiology and proper classification of diabetic amyotrophy.[153,154] The syndrome has variously been called asymmetric proximal motor neuropathy,[17] subacute proximal diabetic neuropathy,[152] proximal mononeuropathy multiplex,[63] or diabetic proximal amyotrophy.[154] The findings that conduction velocities of femoral or distal motor nerves are slow[115,149,155,156] and that nerve biopsies show features of demyelination in such patients,[26] prompted the early view that diabetic amyotrophy is a form of diabetic neuropathy with a predilection for proximal motor nerves rather than a disorder of anterior horn cells or muscle. A vascular etiology has been proposed for the more acute cases.[17,63,153] In one· pathologic study, numerous small vessel infarcts were found in the lumbosacral plexus and proximal nerve trunks of a patient who exhibited a rapid appearance of painful proximal neuropathy.[63] On the basis of these findings, the patient was believed to have ischemic mononeuropathy multiplex. Although acute cases of asymmetric proximal neuropathy associated with sensory involvement may be explained on this basis, the gradual clinical course, prominent weight loss, weakness in a distribution of more than one or two peripheral nerves, and the usual sparing of distal muscles, seem more suggestive of a metabolic rather than an ischemic disorder[149,152,153] (Fig. 31–4).

It has been suggested that the major abnormality in diabetic amyotrophy may lie in the intramuscular motor terminals of proximal nerves.[147,149] On muscle biopsy, the most characteristic pattern is single fiber atrophy in which the distribution does not conform to a pattern of motor unit atrophy or ischemic changes.[147,149,150–152] Grouped fiber atrophy suggesting a neurogenic process has also been demonstrated,[149,152] while histochemical staining of muscle has shown a mixture of type I and type II muscle fiber atrophy.[149,152] Single fiber atrophy with reduction of fiber size, preservation of cross striations, and condensation of sarcolemmal nuclei, may represent a form of early motor unit atrophy[157] in which the mechanism of denervation relates to changes at the motor end plate resulting in individual muscle fiber atrophy. Indeed, motor point biopsy studies of the motor end plate have demonstrated ballooned subneural elements, beaded and thickened terminal axons, and spherical axonal swellings with evidence of collateral reinnervation.[149] Electromyography discloses features of denervation without features of either anterior horn cell disease or primary myopathy.[149,152] Rare reports of myopathy[115] have been based largely on the finding of short duration, polyphasic potentials which may also occur on the basis of motor terminal disease rather than myopathy.[158] If in fact the locus of disease lies in terminal intramuscular branches of proximal nerves, the sparing of distal muscles and lack of significant sensory impairment which characterizes most cases, would be explained.[147,149]

SPINAL SYNDROMES

Although diabetic amyotrophy was initially referred to as diabetic myelopathy,[145] spinal cord disease is uncommon in diabetes despite early reports.[159–161] So-called spinal signs as well as pathologic evidence of spinal degeneration, particularly in posterior columns, may result from retrograde changes secondary to peripheral neuropathy or affection of dorsal root ganglia. Retrograde degeneration of cell[162,163] and tract[164,165] results from lesions of roots and nerves. Diabetics with peripheral neuropathy have, in fact, been reported to display slowing of conduction velocities in the dorsal column of the spinal cord as measured by somatosensory evoked potential techniques.[166,167] Specific examination of the spinal cord in several cases[168–170] failed to reveal unequivocal change.

Anterior spinal artery thrombosis is the common spinal vascular lesion to which patients with diabetes are subject.[171] Infarction of the anterior two thirds of the spinal cord may evolve subacutely and be preceded by pain. Motor loss associated with impaired perception of pain below the level of the lesion occurs in conjunction with comparative preservation of touch and position sense. Like syphilis, collagen disease, and dissecting aneurysm of the aorta, diabetes affects the appropriate order of vessels to produce the syndrome. Usually the level of involvement is related to one of the major radicular arteries. When cervical spondylosis occurs in diabetics, it may be particularly disabling because as-

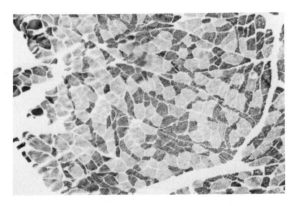

Fig. 31–4. Single fiber atrophy in a muscle biopsy obtained from a patient with diabetic amyotrophy.

sociated vascular involvement produces increased liability to ischemia from the compression.

INSULIN AND HYPOGLYCEMIA

Insulin treatment of diabetes may create problems of its own. Precipitation of symmetrical sensory neuropathy has been reported on numerous occasions[6,14,172–174] but has also been reported rarely after control with oral hypoglycemic agents and diet.[175]

Although no causal relationship has been demonstrated, neuropathy has appeared in nondiabetic patients with hyperinsulinism and profound hypoglycemia. In a patient with an islet cell adenoma, bilateral foot drop and atrophy of the small muscles of the hands occurred.[176] Paresthesias of the distal limbs, weakness, muscle atrophy, and fibrillation potentials have occurred in a hyperinsulin neuropathy, difficult to distinguish from the neuropathy of diabetes.[177] Hypoglycemic neuropathy may be exclusively motor, exclusively sensory, or sensorimotor. A syndrome indistinguishable from diabetic amyotrophy developed in conjunction with hypoglycemia.[178] The pathologic changes produced by hypoglycemia include vacuolation of the myelin sheath and damage to dorsal root ganglia, but nonmyelinated fibers appear more vulnerable than myelinated ones.[179]

Electrophysiologic studies in the acute stage have usually shown electromyographic evidence of denervation with normal nerve conduction velocities.[180,181] Taken together with pathologic evidence for anterior horn cell degeneration,[182] it has been suggested that hypoglycemic muscle wasting may be a neuronopathy of anterior horn cells rather than a peripheral neuropathy.[181]

All parts of the central nervous system may be affected including the spinal cord. Cellular changes are indistinguishable from those of severe anoxia (Fig. 31–5). Cell shadows, intracellular neurofibrillary clumping, damage to axis cylinders, and increase of glia have been noted in experimental animals.[183] The gradient of sensitivity of the central nervous system to hypoglycemia includes early depression of cortical and cerebellar activity, release of basal nuclear and hypothalamic function and appearance of mesencephalic and, ultimately, medullary levels of function.[184] There is, however, little correlation between the level of blood glucose and the symptoms of hypoglycemia.[185] Patients may complain early of hunger, nausea, and belching associated with bradycardia and hypotension. This phase of parasympathetic response is followed by decreased cerebral function which in turn is followed by sympathetic responses of tachycardia, anxiety, agitation and perspiration. Diplopia may be conspicuous, particularly if a heterophoria is

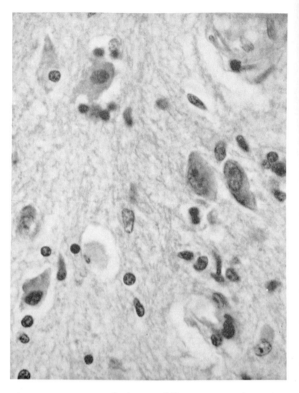

Fig. 31–5. Nerve cell changes following severe hypoglycemia. Contrast pyknotic cells with unaffected neurons. Section from hypothalamus.

present. Headache is often occipital. Stupor follows the sympathetic phase and ultimately gives way to coma. Patients may have no warning of an impending hypoglycemic reaction and manifest no sympathetic response.[186] A sympathetic response does not, of itself, imply a conscious warning. Hypothermia may be a clue to asymptomatic hypoglycemia.[187]

The early suppression of alpha activity and the ultimate appearance of delta waves during hypoglycemia, as revealed by the electroencephalogram, correlate with the decreased arteriovenous-oxygen difference. The low rate of cerebral oxygen consumption persists in the phase of posthypoglycemic coma when glucose administration does not reverse the clinical picture. In this stage, failure to utilize glucose occurs. The degree of altered function correlates directly with the blood glucose. Total stores of glycogen and glucose in the brain are estimated to be 2 g.[188] There is some evidence that the brain can utilize lipids as well as glucose.[189]

In highly susceptible persons, sulfonylurea compounds can produce histologic and physiologic lesions similar to those produced by insulin, through the mechanism of hypoglycemia. Patients complain of headache, drowsiness, confusion and paresthesia. Cranial nerve palsies, increased symptoms of paralysis agitans, and coma have been observed.[190] Hypoglycemic reactions due to sulfonylureas are particularly important to recognize since they have been reported to produce a slowly progressive hypoglycemic encephalopathy over a period of several months without the usual features of the more acute hypoglycemic reaction associated with insulin treatment.[191]

Convulsions may be a manifestation of an insulin reaction even without antecedent symptoms of hypoglycemia. There is nothing unique about the clinical characteristics of the seizures which differentiate them from a convulsive disorder of another cause. The question as to whether a patient with hypoglycemic seizures has epilepsy or whether the convulsion represents a manifestation of hypoglycemia is semantic. Seizures, after all, represent a paroxysmal discharge of cortical nerve cells resulting from any one of many possible initiating events. If hypoglycemia is the determinant, management of the convulsive disorder is best accomplished by skillful maintenance of blood glucose levels. Anticonvulsive medication has a role in the control of this disorder but cannot be relied on exclusively. Anticonvulsive medication probably can be continued with profit even in the absence of frank convulsions. In this way, a drug such as diphenylhydantoin may make the management of ''brittle'' diabetes somewhat easier.

When focal lesions of the brain, often well compensated and not discernible, are present, a diffuse metabolic disturbance such as hypoglycemia may initiate a seizure. The focal onset indicates the structural process as well as the metabolic derangement. Similarly, hypoglycemia may produce transient manifestations of focal vascular disease which are well compensated in the presence of a normal blood glucose. Clinical and experimental evidence indicates that, in the presence of an area of relative cerebral ischemia, hypoglycemia may produce a localized reversible paralysis of neuronal function. Localized impairment of oxygen can be demonstrated. Administration of glucose restores normal oxygen consumption and functional activity. If sufficiently prolonged, hypoglycemia in the presence of vascular insufficiency may produce irreversible focal necrosis.[192]

KETOACIDOSIS

The pathologic and physiologic effects of ketoacidosis are less easily delineated. This is partially due to the multiple associated abnormalities that are not strictly those of ketoacidosis. So-called ketoacidotic neuropathy undoubtedly represents pressure palsies of peripheral nerves sustained during loss of consciousness. Studies of the guinea pig[193] demonstrated unequivocal cytologic changes in nerve cells in experimentally induced ketoacidosis. Previously reported glial increase, damaged ganglion cells, and neuronophagia observed during acidosis in rabbits as well as in brains of patients with diabetic ketoacidosis, were attributed to agonal change. The clinical manifestations of ketoacidotic coma are no different from those of coma of any cause and may stimulate an acute neurosurgical emergency.[194] Only the knowledge of the underlying metabolic abnormality and the evidence of derangement of biochemical values allow conclusions as to etiologic background.

Posner and co-workers[195] have found that mental confusion and coma occur when the cerebrospinal fluid (CSF) pH falls below 7.15. Not only is the pH of CSF much more important than blood pH in the genesis of diabetic coma, but CSF pH lags behind blood pH improvement during treatment.[196] Posner and associates suggest that rapid and excessive administration of sodium bicarbonate may be related to the serious complication of cerebral edema that is sometimes seen in patients being treated for diabetic ketoacidosis. Presumably the use of alkali, especially by rapid direct intravenous injection, slows down the increase of CSF pH or, paradoxically, causes the CSF pH to fall further. The ensuing cerebral edema complicating the ketoacidosis may result in death, as has been reported by Young and Bradley.[197]

Cerebral intravascular coagulation with thrombosis in medium and smaller blood vessels has also been reported in association with fatal cases of diabetic ketoacidosis.[198] Continuous monitoring of cerebrospinal fluid pressure during the first 10 hours of treatment of 5 patients with diabetic ketoacidosis showed abnormally high cerebrospinal fluid pressure developing after therapy had produced a rapid fall in plasma glucose and osmolality.[199] Experiments on dogs made severely hyperglycemic suggest that acute cerebral edema during treatment of diabetic ketoacidosis comes from increased intracranial pressure after isotonic fluid therapy.[200] This may result in a rapid shift of water into cells when plasma glucose and osmolality are abruptly reduced.

The syndrome of nonketotic hyperglycemic coma occurs usually in elderly, noninsulin-dependent diabetics.[201,202] The most prominent accompaniments of this condition have been continuous focal epileptic seizures lasting several hours to days with transient postictal focal neurologic deficits. The seizures are nearly always poorly responsive to anticonvulsant medications but eventually respond to correction of the hyperosmolar state. It has been suggested that an underlying cerebral cortical ischemic infarction in conjunction with the abnormal osmotic state may be responsible for the focality of the seizures and neurologic signs.[202]

CENTRAL NERVOUS SYSTEM

Central neurons are not directly affected in diabetes mellitus. Their involvement reflects associated disease of large and small vessels or results from the metabolic derangements caused by prolonged hypoglycemia, anoxia, or ketoacidosis. The well-documented pathologic changes in patients with diabetes[203] have their clinical counterparts in insufficiency syndromes and cerebral infarction. Narrowing of large vessels, although common, rarely occurs singly; when major vessels are affected, usually more than one extracranial arterial trunk is involved. Common points of arteriosclerosis include the site of origin of the carotid artery at the aortic arch, the division of the innominate artery into subclavian and carotid, the ostia of the vertebral arteries, the parasellar region of the internal carotid artery, and 1.0 cm above the division of the common carotid artery. A single vessel may be involved at more than one site. Transient ischemic attacks herald an oncoming cerebral infarction. Symptoms indicate the area of insufficient blood supply and can be used in a general way to locate the site of vascular stenosis. Complex hemodynamic relations between affected vessels and collateral supply preclude absolute correlation between area of infarction and occluded vessel. Usually obstruction to a major artery causes infarction in the distribution of arterial terminals or the so-called border zone.[204]

General medical evaluation should be undertaken in all patients with cerebrovascular insufficiency. Repeated stereotyped transient ischemic attacks often imply the association of a structural stenosing lesion of a major vessel with a dynamic lesion which transiently reduces cerebral blood flow. Cardiac arrhythmia or embolization, loss of blood volume, anemia, and increased blood viscosity should be considered in evaluation of precipitating factors. Palpation of the carotid, superficial temporal, and the radial pulses, auscultation for bruits in head and neck, and evaluation of blood pressure in each arm provide useful inferential information about blood flow in the carotid bed. Of particular value are non-invasive carotid flow studies which, with present-day techniques, have a high degree of reliability, enabling the clinician to often avoid angiograms and their slight but definite risk. However, if the results of non-invasive studies are equivocal, angiography may need to be performed if intervention is seriously considered.[205] The choice of surgical method will vary with circumstance and surgeon. A careful functional evaluation should be undertaken prior to surgical reconstruction. Restoration of blood flow, no matter how successful, is ineffective once extensive cerebral infarction has occurred.

Cerebral infarction and focal encephalomalacia have been claimed to occur $1\frac{1}{2}$ times more frequently in diabetics than in nondiabetics.[206] This is related to the higher incidence of "hemodynamic disease of small intraparenchymal cerebral vessels," but the increase is of the same order of magnitude as increased frequency of hypertension in patients with diabetes. Whether diabetes is uniquely responsible for an increased risk of cerebrovascular disease distinct from the risk produced by frequently associated hypertension and lipid abnormalities, is uncertain. Prospective data from the Framingham Study, however, do indicate an increased risk of cerebral infarction in individuals with even slight glucose intolerance.[207] Proliferative lesions of small vessels occur $2\frac{1}{2}$ times more often in the diabetic than in the nondiabetic population. Clearly such a process enhances the liability to ischemic infarction related to impairment of circulation in the large vessels. Cerebral infarction in the patient with diabetes differs in no way from that in the nondiabetic patient. Major vessel syndromes, scattered subcortical infarcts, and lacunar states all occur, particularly in association with hypertension.[205] When diabetes is associated with hypertension, a lacunar state manifested by arteriosclerotic parkinsonism, pseudobulbar palsy, and dementia may occur. This is due to multiple small aneurysms of major vessels that usually relate to hypertension rather than to diabetes.

CONGENITAL AND INFECTIOUS DISEASES

Congenital Anomalies

Among the neurologic abnormalities associated with diabetes is the increased incidence of congenital anomalies in infants of diabetic mothers. Mental deficiency and cerebral diplegia have been specifically noted.[208] Periventricular leukomalacia attributed to anoxia in a "watershed" circulatory distribution in offspring of diabetic mothers is probably related to circulatory and respiratory disturbances in the infant rather than to maternal diabetes.[209]

An increased incidence of diabetes has been reported in association with several hereditary neurologic disorders including Friedreich's ataxia,[210] Refsum's syndrome,[211] spinocerebellar degeneration,[212] and myotonic muscular dystrophy.[213] A sporadic disorder of unknown cause in which juvenile diabetes is associated with optic atrophy, sensorineural hearing loss, cerebellar ataxia, and a number of other neurologic, ocular, and systemic abnormalities, has also been described.[104]

Mucormycosis

Although mucormycosis is a rare disease, a high percentage of those so afflicted are diabetic.[214] The fungus Rhizopus has broad, branching, nonseptate hyphae. Of the several forms of the disease, that with rapidly fatal vascular thrombosis is perhaps most characteristic. A cloudy antrum without fluid on x-ray study suggests infection following nasal entry. Extension upward produces orbital swelling, and from there the meninges and frontal lobes are often involved. The fungus invades the vessels to produce cavernous sinus thrombosis and carotid occlusion.[215] Usually the organism is not found in the spinal fluid.

CEREBROSPINAL FLUID

In all diabetics having neurologic disorders, spinal fluid alteration must be interpreted with caution. Clearly, increased pressure, dynamic block, and the presence of cellular elements or abnormal pigments have the same meaning in patients with diabetes that they do in nondiabetics. An increased protein content is difficult to interpret. Although it may represent alterations in the nervous system, neuropathy can occur without evident abnormality of the spinal fluid protein. The farther the process is from the subarachnoid space, the less likely there will be a reflection of that process in spinal fluid protein. Peripheral polyneuropathy occurring predominantly at nerve terminals need not be associated with abnormality of CSF protein. The increased vascular permeability associated with small vessel disease, however, may produce marked alteration in the spinal fluid protein, even in the absence of neuropathy.[216]

TREATMENT OF NEUROLOGIC DISORDERS

The treatment of neurologic disorders associated with diabetes must be directed toward both the diabetes and the neurologic process itself. The manifestations of disease of the central nervous system are treated in patients with diabetes just as in nondiabetics. The importance of diabetes control and the special hazards of hypoglycemia impose upon the clinician the need for special care and judgment.

Cerebrovascular Syndromes

Evaluation for those treatable causes of cerebrovascular insufficiency which have been discussed should be undertaken immediately. Medical management of the insufficiency syndromes has as its goal the support of cerebral circulation. In the case of transient ischemic attacks suggesting impending infarction or an evolving stroke, the patient should be placed at bed rest, the blood pressure should be maintained, and the patient adequately hydrated. Hypoglycemia must be avoided. If the patient is hypertensive and on medical treatment, only moderate reduction of the blood pressure should be attempted. The use of anticoagulants appears to be justified for specific indications such as recurrent cerebral emboli, increasingly frequent transient ischemic attacks, and rapidly evolving or fluctuating ischemic stroke (in which hemorrhage or tumor has been excluded by computed tomography of the brain). The potential risk of vitreous hemorrhage must be given special consideration in the diabetic population.

In the convalescence of patients with cerebrovascular insufficiency, ambulation should be undertaken gradually and cautiously, with frequent evaluation for postural hypotension. Return to normal activity should be permitted only when clinical evidence indicates establishment of adequate collateral circulation. Even then, hot baths, large meals, sudden alterations of posture, straining at stool with the attendant Valsalva maneuver, and other measures which acutely compromise blood flow, should be specifically interdicted.[205]

Diabetic Neuropathy

In a provocative (unsigned) editorial in *Lancet*, entitled, "Diabetic Neuropathy—Where are we now?", the author asks, "Can we do anything about neuropathy or do we just have to document it and commiserate with the patient?"[216a] Certainly, in view of currently inadequate knowledge, the treatment of diabetic neuropathy must be based largely on relief of symptoms.

Specific treatment directed at the presumed pathophysiologic basis of neuropathy with aldose reductase inhibitors (sorbinil) or myoinositol, is currently under investigation. The results to date with sorbinil have been encouraging but not positive enough to establish this substance as truly effective. For example, Judzewitsch et al. studied nerve conduction velocity in the peroneal motor, median motor, and median sensory nerves in 39 patients with stable diabetes. At the start of the study, these patients had abnormal nerve conduction velocities but no actual symptoms of neuropathy. The study consisted of a randomized, double-blind, cross-over trial with 9 weeks of treatment with sorbinil and 9 weeks with a placebo. At the end of the study, the nerve conduction velocity in all instances showed improvement in the sorbinil-treated group. The changes were small but significant.[216b] A double-blind study in patients with painful diabetic neuropathy has been reported to show improvement in pain, tendon reflexes, and sensory potential amplitude in the sural nerve.[216c] Certainly further long-term evaluation of sorbinil is indicated.

Although the precise relationship between poor diabetic control and peripheral neuropathy is uncertain, consensus favors maintenance of strict control of blood glucose levels in patients with or without diabetic neuropathy.[6] Service, et al. attempted to determine the relative effect of blood glucose levels on peripheral nerve function by comparing the results in a group of patients treated in a "rigorous" fashion with a similar group maintained on conventional treatment.[216d] In the former, an attempt was made to provide blood glucose values as nearly normal as possible. Starting with 33 insulin-treated patients whose durations of diabetes were only 2 years or less, Service and colleagues found a total of 20 patients suitable for comparison. After 3 years, no significant difference was observed between the two groups, and in neither group was there any significant improvement in peripheral nerve function. Both the authors and Windebank[216e] agreed that to bring out the advantage of strict glycemic control, future studies would need to have larger differences in the blood glucose levels of the strict control group and those patients treated by conventional standards. Furthermore, such a study would require an even longer duration, and the patients selected for the study would have to have a more advanced abnormality of peripheral nerve function than in the treatment trials just described.

More encouraging were the results of a study carried out by workers in England.[216f] Here, 74 patients with insulin-dependent diabetes and background retinopathy were randomized to continue with their usual care of diabetes or, in a second group, to be treated by a more intensive program, with a basal dose of ultralente insulin and regular insulin at mealtimes. Those in the first group attended the clinic more frequently, received closer supervision of their diet, and were taught to do home blood glucose monitoring. After 2 years, sensory nerve function was found to be significantly better preserved in the strictly controlled group than in the conventionally treated one. In addition, these workers report a significant improvement in the first group with regard to renal function, low density lipoprotein cholesterol values, and whole blood low-shear viscosity. The rate of progression of retinopathy was similar in the two groups.

Some patients with newly diagnosed diabetes may have a relatively mild distal polyneuropathy which is responsive to diabetes control. It should be kept in mind that some patients develop symptoms of neuropathy shortly after initiation of treatment which usually subside if the treatment is continued.[6] Care should be taken to avoid frequent or severe hypoglycemic reactions. Studies of the effect on nerve function of strict control of blood glucose by means of an "artificial pancreas" are beginning and will be watched with interest.[217] Unfortunately, vitamin therapy has not proved particularly helpful. There is no evidence to suggest thiamine deficiency. Serum pyruvate levels may be elevated in patients with diabetes, whether or not neuropathy is present.[218] Claims for improvement in vibration sense following treatment with vitamin B complex, niacinamide, and thiamine,[219] and the suggestion of good relief attendant upon treatment with vitamin B_{12} have not been substantiated.[16] Hypophysectomy produces no change in signs and symptoms of diabetic neuropathy[220] despite its known ameliorative effect on proliferative retinopathy.

In the management of the patient with diabetic neuropathy, it is extremely important to carry out appropriate studies to exclude the possibility that the neurologic symptoms are due to a disorder other than diabetes. This is true because to a large degree diabetic neuropathy is a diagnosis made by exclusion. Root lesions produced by herniated nucleus pulposus, arthritic spurs, and vasculitis, must be considered. Causes of mononeuropathy including compression, trauma, vascular lesions, and involvement of brachial or lumbar plexus by hemorrhage and neoplasm, should not be overlooked. Toxic causes of polyneuropathy including heavy metals, alcohol, nutritional deprivation, uremia and neurotoxic drugs, should be ruled out. Cauda equina tumor, neurofibroma, Paget's disease, and malignant or other disease of the vertebral body on occasion may give the erroneous impression of diabetic neuropathy.

The treatment of painful diabetic neuropathy is a major clinical problem. Pain and discomfort of several types may occur. Patients with distal sensory polyneuropathy usually describe tingling paresthesia of the feet, lower legs, and hands often associated with dysesthesia manifested by exaggerated sensitivity to light touch, clothing, or bed sheets. Patients with diabetic amyotrophy, acute radiculopathy, or acute femoral mononeuropathy usually describe deep, aching pain in the thigh, hip, or lower trunk, sometimes associated with superficial paresthesia or dysesthesia of the anterolateral thighs. Brief, lancinating pains of the extremities or trunk occasionally occur which presumably relate to disturbances in dorsal root ganglia or dorsal roots.

During the acute and painful phases of mononeuropathy and amyotrophy, relative rest is recommended. A cradle over the bed will protect the legs from the weight of the bed clothes. Passive and graduated active exercises are useful. Footdrop must be managed with appropriate supportive braces. Regular foot care is important for the patient with sensitive feet, and stringent measures must be taken to avoid trauma (See Chapter 35).

Since painful diabetic neuropathy may persist for months and occasionally years, continued use of narcotics should be avoided except as a last resort. When non-narcotic analgesics are effective, they should be taken on a carefully timed, regular basis throughout the day rather than allowing pain to increase repeatedly in crescendo fashion to unbearable proportions.

Anticonvulsants such as phenytoin, carbamazepine, and benzodiazepines have all been used to treat painful diabetic neuropathy. Despite initial reports of efficacy,[221] phenytoin (Dilantin) is usually ineffective in controlled studies and general clinical experience.[222] Carbamazepine (Tegretol) has been effective in one controlled study[223] and is more likely to be of benefit but, similar to phenytoin, may not be helpful.[6,224] Benzodiazepines such as diazepam (Valium) and clonazepam (Clonopin) are also ineffective.[225,226]

The use of phenothiazines, such as promazine (Sparine) or chlorpromazine (Thorazine) in painful neuropathy in general and diabetic neuropathy in particular, has been recommended and may be quite useful. These may be given alone or together with a non-narcotic analgesic. Combined use of a more potent phenothiazine such as fluphenazine (Prolixin, Permital) and a tricyclic antidepressant such as amitriptyline (Elavil) has recently been recommended.[227] The efficacy of this combination, as in other painful neuropathies or radiculopathies,[228,229] may relate to some poorly defined effect on central pain mechanisms.[230]

The pain of diabetic neuropathy not infrequently shows striking diurnal fluctuation, becoming more severe in the evening and at night. In this situation, a single daily dose of a sedative tricyclic such as amitriptyline or a phenothiazine such as promazine or chlorpromazine may be particularly effective in allowing sleep.

Emotional disturbances such as depression, anxiety, and insomnia are common accompaniments of chronic painful neuropathy.[225,231] Whether these occur as a result of the pain or are themselves predisposing factors in producing or enhancing the pain, is uncertain. In severe forms of diabetic neuropathy with anorexia and weight loss, pain usually precedes the appearance of depression.[231] It is important to note that, similar to other painful neuropathies such as postherpetic neuralgia or tic douloureux, the disappearance of pain is usually followed by remarkable resolution of depressive symptoms. In one study of painful diabetic neuropathy, a high incidence of psychologic and somatic symptoms usually associated with depression were identified.[225] Treatment with amitriptyline or imipramine produced remission of pain with concomitant relief of depression over a mean period of 10 weeks, a time course compatible with the antidepressant effect of these drugs. Regardless of whether depression is a primary or secondary process in painful diabetic neuropathy, its management frequently requires thoughtful emotional support and psychologic counselling in addition to pharmacologic treatment.

Management of *orthostatic hypotension* includes the use of 9-alpha-fluorohydrocortisone and avoidance of drugs which themselves may produce or potentiate the condition.[232] *Bladder dysfunction* may be benefited by use of cholinergic drugs such as urecholine or bethanecol, judicious use of transurethal surgery of the bladder neck, and the cautious use of intermittent catheter drainage.[223] *Male sexual (erectile) impotence* may be managed by use of a silicone penile prosthesis,[234] but first there should be avoidance of antihypertensive drugs which produce impotence, exploration of possible psychogenic causes, and in a very few selected cases, determination of the serum testosterone level (See Chapter 32). *Diabetic gastroparesis* has been benefited by treatment with metoclopramide (Reglan) which enhances gastric emptying.[235] *Diarrhea* may be managed with drugs which depress intestinal motility such as diphenoxylate (Lomotil), atropine, ambemonium or, for short-time use, codeine. When *steatorrhea* occurs due to reduced small bowel motility and stasis with bacterial overgrowth, antibacterial therapy may be helpful[236] (See Chapter 40). Non-weight-bearing is the most useful conservative treatment for Charcot-type arthropathy.[150] Lumbar sympathectomy has been discarded despite initial reports of success, while arthrodesis should be avoided in the early management of the unstable joint.[150] As for an ulcer in a neuropathic foot, bed rest with removal of any offending callus plus antibiotics will usually result in prompt healing provided the circulation is adequate (see Chapters 34 and 35).

In general, the outlook for the most frequent form of diabetic peripheral neuropathic involvement, symmetric polyneuropathy, is good. Although insensitivity or mild motor weakness may persist, functional impairment is uncommon. On the whole, recovery from a mononeuropathy is to be anticipated although when severe, as the result of a proximal vascular occlusion, collateral circulation may not be adequate. Ulnar neuropathy is perhaps the least reversible of the mononeuropathies. It is remarkable, however, how successful the patient may become in the use of the hands despite a significant ulnar neuropathy. Patients with diabetic amyotrophy universally recover clinical function despite the persistence of change as shown by biopsy. Although recovery usually requires 6 months to 2 years, as a rule, patients respond positively to the knowledge that this painful and disabling form of neuropathy at least carries a favorable prognosis.

In general, it can be said that the management of the neurologic complications of diabetes consists of good control of glucose metabolism, analgesia when needed, judicious use of braces in appropriate situations, care to avoid recurrent injury of nerve or joints, and continued encouragement.

REFERENCES

1. Rollo, cited by Martin, M.M.: Diabetic neuropathy. A clinical study of 150 cases. Brain 76:594, 1953.
2. Marchal de Calvi, C.J.: Recherches sur les accidents diabétiques. Paris, P. Asselin, 1864.
3. Pavy, F.W.: Introductory address to the discussion on the clinical aspect of glycosuria. Lancet 2: 1033, 1085, 1885.
4. Rundles, R.W.: Diabetic neuropathy: general review with report of 125 cases. Medicine 24: 111, 1945.
5. Eliasson, S.G.: Disorders of the nervous system in diabetes. Med. Clin. North Am., 55: 1001, 1971.
6. Thomas, P.K., Eliasson, S.G.: Diabetic neuropathy. In: P.J. Dyck, P.K. Thomas, E.H. Lambert (Eds.): Peripheral Neuropathy. Philadelphia, W.B. Saunders, 1975, Chapter 47.
7. Ellenberg, M.: Diabetic neuropathy: clinical aspects. Metabolism 25: 1627, 1976.
8. Spritz, N.S.: Nerve disease in diabetes mellitus. Med. Clin. North Am. 62:787, 1978.
9. Ellenberg, M.: Diabetic complications without manifest diabetes: complications as presenting clinical symptoms. J.A.M.A. 183:926, 1963.
10. Rudy, A.: Diabetic neuropathy. N. Engl. J. Med. 233:684, 1945.
11. Fagerberg, S.-E.: Diabetic neuropathy: a clinical and histological study on the significance of vascular affections. Acta Med. Scand. Suppl. 345:1, 1959.
12. Ellenberg, M.: Diabetic neuropathy. In: M. Ellenberg, H. Rifkin (Eds.): Diabetes Mellitus. Theory and Practice, 3rd ed. New Hyde Park, N.Y., Medical Examination Pub. Co., 1983, Chapter 35, pp. 777–801.
13. Stein, M.H., Wortis, H., Jolliffe, N.: Peripheral neuropathy: Evaluation of sensory findings. Arch. Neurol. Psychiatry 46: 464, 1941.
14. Martin, M.M.: Involvement of autonomic nerve fibers in diabetic neuropathy. Lancet 1: 560, 1953.
15. Jordan, W.R.: Neuritic manifestations in diabetes mellitus. Arch. Intern. Med. 57: 307, 1936.
16. Sprague, R.G., cited by Treusch, J.V.: Diabetic neuritis: a tentative working classification. Proc. Mayo Clin. 20:393, 1945.
17. Goodman, J.I., Baumoel, S., Frankel, L., et al.: The Diabetic Neuropathies. Springfield, Charles C Thomas, 1953.
18. Sullivan, J.F.: The neuropathies of diabetes. Neurology 8:243, 1958.
19. Locke, S.: The peripheral nervous system in diabetes mellitus. Diabetes 13:307, 1964.
20. Woltman, H.W., Wilder, R.M.: Diabetes mellitus. Pathologic changes in the spinal cord and peripheral ..erves. Arch. Intern. Med. 44:576, 1929.
21. Lundbaek, K.: Diabetic angiopathy: a specific vascular disease. Lancet 1:377, 1954.
22. Fagerberg, S.-E.: Neuropathie diabétique. World Neurol. 2:509, 1961.
23. Fagerberg, S.-E.: Studies on the etiology and pathophysiology of diabetic neuropathy. Proceedings: 4e Congès de la Fédération Internationale du Diabète: Ed. Médecine et Hygiène, Geneva, 1961, p. 449.
24. Dolman, C.L.: The morbid anatomy of diabetic neuropathy. Neurology 13:135, 1963.
25. Greenbaum, D., Richardson, P.C., Salmon, M.V., Urich, H.: Pathological observations on six cases of diabetic neuropathy. Brain 87:201, 1964.
26. Thomas, P.K., Lascelles, R.G.: The pathology of diabetic neuropathy. Quart. J. Med. 35:489, 1966.
27. Chopra, J.S., Hurwitz, L.J., Montgomery, D.A.D.: The pathogenesis of sural nerve changes in diabetes mellitus. Brain 92:391, 1969.
28. Vital, C., Le Blanc, M., Vallat, J.M., et al.: Étude ultrastructurale du nerf périphérique chez 16 diabétiques sans neuropathie clinique. Comparisons avec 16 neuropathies diabétiques et 16 neuropathies non diabétiques. Acta Neuropathol. (Berl.) 30:63, 1974.
29. Behse, F., Buchthal, F., Carlsen, F.: Nerve biospy and conduction studies in diabetic neuropathy. J. Neurol. Neurosurg. Psychiatry 40:1072, 1977.
30. Asbury, A.K., Johnson, P.C.: Pathology of Peripheral Nerve. Philadelphia, W.B. Saunders Co., 1978. Chapter 5.
31. Brownlee, M.: Alpha-2-macroglobulin and reduced basement-membrane degradation in diabetes. Lancet 1:779, 1976.
32. Johnson, P.C.: Fenestrated endothelium in the human peripheral nervous system. J. Neuropathol. Exp. Neurol. 36:607, 1977. (Abstract)
33. Seneviratne, K.N.: Permeability of blood-nerve barriers in the diabetic rat. J. Neurol. Neurosurg. Psychiatry 35:156, 1972.
34. Jakobsen, J.: Peripheral nerves in early experimental diabetes: expansion of the endoneurial space as a cause of increased water content. Diabetologia 14: 113, 1978.
35. Sima, A.A.F., Robertson, D.M.: The perineurial and blood-nerve barriers in experimental diabetes. Acta Neuropathol. (Berl) 41:189, 1978.
36. Sima, A.A.F., Robertson, D.M.: Peripheral neuropathy in the mutant diabetic mouse. Acta Neuropathol. (Berl.) 41:85, 1978.
37. O'Malley, B.C., Timperley, W.R., Ward, J.D., et al.: Platelet abnormalities in diabetic peripheral neuropathy. Lancet 2:1274, 1975.
38. Timperley, W.R., Ward, J.D., Preston, F.E., et al.: Clinical and histological studies in diabetic neuropathy. A reassessment of vascular factors in relation to intravascular coagulation. Diabetologia 12:237, 1976.
39. Bern, M.M.: Platelet functions in diabetes mellitus. Diabetes 27:342, 1978.
40. Bischoff, A.: Ultrastructural pathology of peripheral nervous system in early diabetes. Adv. Metab. Disord. 2 (Suppl.):441, 1973.
41. Brown, M.J., Martin, J.R., Asbury, A.K.: Painful diabetic neuropathy: a morphometric study. Arch. Neurol. 33:164, 1976.
42. Chopra, J.S., Sawhney, B.B., Chakravorty, R.N.: Pathology and time relationship of peripheral nerve changes in experimental diabetes. J. Neurol. Sci. 32:53, 1977.
43. Hansen, S., Ballantyne, J.P.: Axonal dysfunction in the neuropathology of diabetes mellitus: a quantitative elec-

trophysical study. J. Neurol. Neurosurg. Psychiatry *40*:555, 1977.

44. Clements, R.S., Jr.: Diabetic neuropathy—new concepts of its etiology. Diabetes *28*:604, 1979.
45. Schlaepfer, W.W., Gerritsen, G.C., Dulin, W.E.: Segmental demyelination in the distal peripheral nerves of chronically diabetic Chinese hamsters. Diabetologia *10*:541, 1974.
46. Powell, H., Knox, D., Lee, S., et al.: Alloxan diabetic neuropathy: electron microscopic studies. Neurology *27*:60, 1977.
47. Thomas, P.K.: The morphological basis for alterations in nerve conduction in peripheral neuropathy. Proc. R. Soc. Med. *64*:295, 1971.
48. Dyck, P.J., Johnson, W.J., Lambert, E.H., O'Brien, P.C.: Segmental demyelination secondary to axonal degeneration in uremic neuropathy. Mayo Clin. Proc. *46*:400, 1971.
49. Olsson, Y., Säve-Söderbergh, J., Sourander, P., Angervall, L.: A pathoanatomical study of the central and peripheral nervous system in diabetes of early onset and long duration. Path. Europ. *3*:62, 1968.
50. Coërs, C.: The Innervation of Muscle: A Biopsy Study. Springfield, Charles C Thomas, 1959.
51. Woolf, A.L., Malins, J.M.: Changes in the intramuscular nerve endings in diabetic neuropathy: a biopsy study. J. Path. Bact. *73*:316, 1957.
52. Harriman, D.: The diagnostic value of motor-point biopsy. In: H. Garland (Ed.): Scientific Aspects of Neurology. Baltimore, Williams & Wilkins, 1961, Chapter 3, pp. 37–45.
53. Coërs, C., Hildebrand, J.: Latent neuropathy in diabetes and alcoholism. Electromyographic and histological study. Neurology *15*:19, 1965.
54. Wohlfart, G.: Collateral regeneration in partially denervated muscles. Neurology *8*:175, 1958.
55. MacFadyen, D.J.: End plate morphology in neuropathies and myopathies. M. Sc. Thesis, University of Saskatchewan, 1961.
56. Appenzeller, O., Richardson, E.P., Jr.: The sympathetic chain in patients with diabetic and alcoholic polyneuropathy. Neurology *16*:1205, 1966.
57. Hensley, G.T., Soergel, K.H.: Neuropathologic findings in diabetic diarrhea. Arch. Pathol. *85*:587, 1968.
58. Duchen, L.W., Anjorin, A., Watkins, P.J., Mackay, J.D.: Pathology of autonomic neuropathy in diabetes mellitus. Ann. Intern. Med. *92* (Part 2):301, 1980.
59. Olsson, Y., Sourander, P.: Changes in the sympathetic nervous system in diabetes mellitus. A preliminary report. J. Neurovasc. Relat. *31*:86, 1968.
60. Low, P.A., Walsh, J.C., Huang, C.Y., McLeod, J.G.: The sympathetic nervous system in diabetic neuropathy: a clinical and pathological study. Brain *98*:341, 1975.
61. Kristensson, K., Nordborg, C., Olsson, Y., Sourander, P.: Brief reports. Changes in the vagus nerve in diabetes mellitus. Acta Path. Microbiol. Scand. (A) *79A*:684, 1971.
62. Berge, K.G., Sprague, R.G., Bennett, W.A.: The intestinal tract in diabetic diarrhea: a pathologic study. Diabetes *5*: 289, 1956.
63. Raff, M.C., Asbury, A.K.: Ischemic mononeuropathy and mononeuropathy multiplex in diabetes mellitus. N. Engl. J. Med. *279*:17, 1968.
64. Dreyfus, P.M., Hakim, S., Adams, R.D.: Diabetic ophthalmoplegia. Report of case, with postmortem study and comments on vascular supply of human oculomotor nerve. Arch. Neurol. Psychiatry *77*:337, 1957.
65. Asbury, A.K., Aldredge, H., Hershberg, R., Fisher,

C.M.: Oculomotor palsy in diabetes mellitus; a clinicopathological study. Brain *93*:555, 1970.
66. Weber, R.B., Daroff, R.B., Mackey, E.A.: Pathology of oculomotor nerve palsy in diabetics. Neurology *20*:835, 1970.
67. Mulder, D.W., Lambert, E.H., Bastron, J.A., Sprague, R.G.: The neuropathies associated with diabetes mellitus. A clinical and electromyographic study of 103 unselected diabetic patients. Neurology *11*:275, 1961.
68. Gregersen, G.: Diabetic neuropathy: influence of age, sex metabolic control, and duration of diabetes on motor conduction velocity. Neurology *17*:972, 1967.
69. Fraf, R.J., Halter, J.B., Halar, E., Porte, D.: Nerve conduction abnormalities in untreated maturity-onset diabetes: relation to levels of fasting plasma glucose and glycosylated hemoglobin. Ann. Intern. Med. *90*:298, 1979.
70. Winegrad, A.I., Greene, D.A.: Diabetic polyneuropathy: the importance of insulin deficiency, hyperglycemia and alterations in myoinositol metabolism in its pathogenesis. N. Engl. J. Med. *295*:1416, 1976.
71. Gregersen, G.: Variations in motor conduction velocity produced by acute changes of the metabolic state in diabetic patients. Diabetologia *4*:273, 1968.
72. Ward, J.D., Barnes, C.G., Fisher, D.J., et al.: Improvement in nerve conduction following treatment in newly diagnosed diabetics. Lancet *1*:428, 1971.
73. Fraser, D.M., Campbell, I.W., Ewing, D.J., et al.: Peripheral autonomic nerve function in newly diagnosed diabetes mellitus. Diabetes *26*:546, 1977.
74. Field, R.A., Adams, L.C.: Insulin response of peripheral nerve. II. Effects on lipid metabolism. Biochim. Biophys. Acta. *106*:474, 1965.
75. Eliasson, S.G., Samet, J.M.: Alloxan induced neuropathies: lipid changes in nerve and root fragments. Life Sci. *8*:493, 1969.
76. Brown, M.J., Iwamori, M., Kishimoto, Y., et al.: Nerve lipid abnormalities in human diabetic neuropathy: a correlative study. Ann. Neurol. *5*:245, 1979.
77. Gabbay, K.H.: The sorbitol pathway and the complications of diabetes. N. Engl. J. Med. *288*:831, 1973.
78. Ward, J.D., Baker, R.W.R., Davis, B.H.: Effect of blood sugar control on the accumulation of sorbitol and fructose in nervous tissues. Diabetes *21*:1173, 1972.
79. Dyck, P.J., Sherman, W.R., Hallcher, L.M., et al.: Human diabetic endoneurial sorbitol, fructose, and myoinositol related to sural nerve morphometry. Ann. Neurol. *8*:590, 1980.
80. Jefferys, J.G.R., Palmano, K.P., Sharma, A.K., Thomas, P.K.: Influence of dietary myoinositol on nerve conduction and inositol phospholipids in normal and diabetic rats. J. Neurol. Neurosurg. Psychiatry. *41*:333, 1978.
81. Clements, R.S., Jr., Vourganti, B., Kuba, T., et al.: Dietary myo-inositol intake and peripheral nerve function in diabetic neuropathy. Metabolism *28* (Suppl. 1):477, 1979.
82. Salway, J.G., Whitehead, L., Finnegan, J.A., et al.: Effect of myoinositol on peripheral-nerve function in diabetes. Lancet, *2*:1282, 1978.
83. Gregersen, G., Børsting, H., Theil, P., Servo, C.: Myoinositol and function of peripheral nerves in human diabetics. A controlled clinical trial. Acta Neurol. Scand. *58*:241, 1978.
84. Longstreth, G.F., Newcomer, A.D.: Abdominal pain caused by diabetic radiculopathy. Ann. Intern. Med. *86*:166, 1977.
85. Ellenberg, M.: Diabetic truncal mononeuropathy—a new clinical syndrome. Diabetes Care *1*:10, 1978.

86. Sun, S.F., Streib, E.W.: Diabetic thoracoabdominal neuropathy: Clinical and electrodiagnostic features. Ann. Neurol. 9:75, 1981.
87. Pryce, T.D.: On diabetic neuritis, with a clinical and pathological description of three cases of diabetic pseudotabes. Brain 16:416, 1893.
88. Fraser, D.M., Campbell, I.W., Ewing, D.J., Clarke, B.F.: Mononeuropathy in diabetes mellitus. Diabetes 28:96, 1979.
89. Calverley, J.R., Mulder, D.W.: Femoral neuropathy. Neurology 10:963, 1960.
90. Goodman, J.I.: Femoral neuropathy in relation to diabetes mellitus. Report of 17 cases. Diabetes 3:266, 1954.
91. Jacobs, E.M.: Diabetic sciatic neuropathy: report of a case. Diabetes 7:493, 1958.
92. Jung, Y., Homan, T.C., Gerneth, J.A., et al.: Diabetic hand syndrome. Metabolism 20:1008, 1971.
93. King, F.P.: Paralyses of the extraocular muscles in diabetes. Arch. Intern. Med. 104:318, 1959.
94. Ross, A.T.: Recurrent cranial nerve palsies in diabetes mellitus. Neurology 12:180, 1962.
95. Zorilla, E., Kozak, G.P.: Ophthalmoplegia in diabetes mellitus. Ann. Intern. Med. 67:968, 1967.
96. Jackson, W.P.U.: Ocular nerve palsy with severe headache in diabetics. Br. Med. J. 2:408, 1955.
97. Harris-Jones, J.N.: Ocular nerve palsies with headache in diabetes mellitus. Diabetes 5:128, 1956.
98. Barricks, M.E., Traviesa, D.B., Glaser, J.S., Levy, I.S.: Ophthalmoplegia in cranial arteritis. Brain 100:209, 1977.
99. Walsh, F.B.: Clinical Neuro-ophthalmology, 2nd ed. Baltimore, Williams & Wilkins, 1957.
100. White, P.: Juvenile diabetes. In: G.G. Duncan (Ed.): Diseases of Metabolism, 4th ed. Philadelphia, W.B. Saunders Co., 1959, Chapter 16, pp. 913–929.
101. Jørgensen, M.B., Buch, N.H.: Studies on the sense of smell and taste in diabetics. Acta. Otolaryng. 53:539, 1961.
102. Skillern, P.G., Lockhart, G., III: Optic neuritis and uncontrolled diabetes mellitus in 14 patients. Ann. Intern. Med. 51:468, 1959.
103. Tunbridge, R.E., Paley, R.G.: Primary optic atrophy in diabetes mellitus. Diabetes 5:29S, 1956.
104. Lessell, S., Rosman, N.P.: Juvenile diabetes mellitus and optic atrophy. Arch. Neurol. 34:759, 1977.
105. Pavan, P.R., Aiello, L.M., Wafai, M.F., et al.: Optic disc edema in juvenile-onset diabetes. Arch. Ophthalmol. 98:2193, 1980.
106. Lubow, M., Makley, T.A., Jr.: Pseudopapilledema of juvenile diabetes mellitus. Arch. Ophthalmol. 85:417, 1971.
107. Hayreh, S.S.: Anterior ischaemic optic neuropathy. I. Terminology and pathogenesis. Br. J. Ophthalmol. 58:955, 1974.
108. Korczyn, A.D.: Bell's palsy and diabetes mellitus. Lancet 1:108, 1971.
109. Adour, K.K., Wingerd, J.: Idiopathic facial paralysis (Bell's palsy): factors affecting severity and outcome in 446 patients. Neurology 24:1112, 1974.
110. Waxman, S.G., Sabin, T.D.: Diabetic truncal polyneuropathy. Arch. Neurol. 38:46, 1981.
111. Steiness, I.: Diabetic neuropathy. Vibration sense and abnormal tendon reflexes in diabetics. Acta. Med. Scand. Suppl. 394:1, 1963.
112. Simpson, J.: Chapter 8. In: D. Williams (Ed.): Modern Trends in Neurology, Series 3. London, Butterworth, 1962, p. 245.
113. Lawrence, D.G., Locke, S.: Motor nerve conduction velocity in diabetes. Arch. Neurol. 5:483, 1961.
114. Skillman, T.G., Johnson, E.W., Hamwi, G.J., Driskill, H.J.: Motor nerve conduction velocity in diabetes mellitus. Diabetes 10:46, 1961.
115. Lamontagne, A., Buchthal, F.: Electrophysiological studies in diabetic neuropathy. J. Neurol. Neurosurg. Psychiatry 33:442, 1970.
116. Downie, A.W., Newell, D.J.: Sensory nerve conduction in patients with diabetes mellitus and controls. Neurology 11:876, 1961.
117. Noël, P.: Sensory nerve conduction in the upper limbs at various stages of diabetic neuropathy. J. Neurol. Neurosurg. Psychiatry 36:786, 1973.
118. Fagerberg, S.-E., Petersen, I., Steg, G., Wilhelmsen, L.: Motor disturbances in diabetes mellitus. A clinical study using electromyography and nerve conduction velocity determination. Acta. Med. Scand. 174:711, 1963.
119. Thage, O., Trojaborg, W., Buchthal, F.: Electromyographic findings in polyneuropathy. Neurology 13:273, 1963.
120. Spencer, P.S., Schaumburg, H.H.: Central-peripheral distal axonopathy—the pathology of dying-back polyneuropathies. In: H.M. Zimmerman (Ed.): Progress in Neuropathology, Vol. 3. New York, Grune & Stratton, 1976. pp. 253–295.
121. Waxman, S.G.: Pathophysiology of nerve conduction: relation to diabetic neuropathy. Ann. Intern. Med. 92 (Part 2):297, 1980.
122. Mandelstam, P., Siegel, C.I., Leiber, A., Siegel, M.: The swallowing disorder in patients with diabetic neuropathy-gastroenteropathy. Gastroenterology 56:1, 1969.
123. Kassander, P.: Asymptomatic gastric retention in diabetics (gastroparesis diabeticorum). Ann. Intern. Med. 48:797, 1958.
124. Wooten, R.L., Meriwether, T.W.: Diabetic gastric atony: a clinical study. J.A.M.A. 176:1082, 1961.
125. Howland, W.J., Drinkard, R.U.: Acute diabetic gastric atony: gastroparesis diabeticorum. J.A.M.A. 185:214, 1977.
126. Campbell, I.W., Heading, R.C., Tothill, P., et al.: Gastric emptying in diabetic autonomic neuropathy. Gut 18:462, 1977.
127. Dotevall, G.: Gastric secretion of acid in diabetes mellitus during basal conditions and after maximal histamine stimulation. Acta. Med. Scand. 170:59, 1961.
128. Gitelson, S., Oppenheim, D., Schwartz, A.: Size of the gall bladder in patients with diabetes mellitus. Diabetes 18:493, 1969.
129. Ellenberg, M.: Development of urinary bladder dysfunction in diabetes mellitus. Ann. Intern. Med. 92 (Part 2):321, 1980.
130. Bradley, W.E.: Diagnosis of urinary bladder dysfunction in diabetes mellitus. Ann. Intern. Med. 92 (Part 2):323, 1980.
131. Mastri, A.R.: Neuropathology of diabetic neurogenic bladder. Ann. Intern. Med. 92 (Part 2):316, 1980.
132. Ellenberg, M.: Sexual function in diabetic patients. Ann. Intern. Med. 92 (Part 2):331, 1980.
133. Ellenberg, M.: Impotence in diabetes: the neurologic factor. Ann. Intern. Med. 75:213, 1971.
134. Karacan, I.: Diagnosis of erectile impotence in diabetes mellitus. Ann. Intern. Med. 92 (Part 2):334, 1980.
135. Ewing, D.J., Campbell, I.W., Clarke, B.F.: Assessment of cardiovascular effects in diabetic autonomic neuropathy and prognostic implications. Ann. Intern. Med. 92 (Part 2):308, 1980.
136. Barany, F.R., Cooper, E.H.: Pilomotor and sudomotor innervation in diabetes. Clin. Sci. 15:533, 1956.
137. Goodman, J.I.: Diabetic anhidrosis. Am. J.Med. 41:831, 1966.

138. Watkins, P.J.: Facial sweating after food: a new sign of diabetic autonomic neuropathy. Br. Med. J. *1*:583, 1973.

139. Foster, D.B., Bassett, R.C.: Neurogenic arthropathy (Charcot joint) associated with diabetic neuropathy. Report of two cases. Arch. Neurol. Psychiatry *57*:173, 1947.

140. Oakley, W., Catterall, R.C.F., Martin, M.M.: Aetiology and management of lesions of the feet in diabetes. Br. Med. J. 2:953, 1956.

141. Parsons, H., Norton, W.S.: The management of diabetic neuropathic joints. N. Engl. J. Med. *244*:935, 1951.

142. Naide, M., Schnall, C.: Bone changes in necrosis in diabetes mellitus. Differentiation of neuropathic from ischemic necrosis. Arch. Intern. Med. *107*:380, 1961.

143. Sinha, S., Munichoodappa, C.S., Kozak, G.P.: Neuroarthropathy (Charcot joints) in diabetes mellitus. (Clinical study of 101 cases). Medicine *51*:191, 1972.

144. Bruns, L.: Ueber neuritische Lähmungen beim Diabetes mellitus. Berl. Klin. Wochenschr. *27*:509, 1890.

145. Garland, H., Taverner, D.: Diabetic myelopathy. Br. Med. J. *1*:1405, 1953.

146. Garland, H.: Diabetic amyotrophy. Br. Med. J. *2*:1287, 1955.

147. Locke, S., Lawrence, D.G., Legg, M.A.: Diabetic amyotrophy. Am. J. Med. *34*:775, 1963.

148. Casey, E.B., Harrison, M.J.G.: Diabetic amyotrophy: a follow-up study. Br. Med. J. *1*:656, 1972.

149. Chokroverty, S., Reyes, M.G., Rubino, F.A., Tonaki, H.: The syndrome of diabetic amyotrophy. Ann. Neurol. 2:181, 1977.

150. Bischoff, V.A.: Zur diabetischen amyotrophie (neuromyopathie). Schweiz Med. Wochenschr. *89*:519, 1959.

151. Hamilton, C.R., Jr., Dobson, H.L., Marshall, J.: Diabetic amyotrophy: clinical and electronmicroscopic studies in six patients. Am. J. Med. Sci., *256*:81, 1968.

152. Williams, I.R., Mayer, R.F.: Subacute proximal diabetic neuropathy. Neurology *26*:108, 1976.

153. Asbury, A.K.: Proximal diabetic neuropathy, (Editorial). Ann. Neurol. 2.179, 1977.

154. Chokroverty, S.: Diabetic proximal amyotrophy. Muscle & Nerve *1*:507, 1978. (Abstract)

155. Gilliatt, R.W., Willison, R.G.: Peripheral nerve conduction in diabetic neuropathy. J. Neurol. Neurosurg. Psychiatry *25*:11, 1962.

156. Chopra, J.S., Hurwitz, L.J.: Femoral nerve conduction in diabetes and chronic occlusive vascular disease. J. Neurol. Neurosurg. Psychiatry *31*:28, 1968.

157. Locke, S.: Diabetic amyotrophy (Editorial). Diabetes *13*:541, 1964.

158. Engel, W.K.: Brief, small, abundant motor-unit action potentials. Neurology 25: 173, 1975.

159. Williamson, R.T.: Changes in the posterior columns of the spinal cord in diabetes mellitus. Br. Med. J. *1*:398, 1894.

160. Nonne, M.: Ueber Poliomyelitis anterior chronica als Ursache einer chronisch-progressiven atrophichen Lähmung bei Diabetes mellitus. Berl. Klin. Wochenschr. *33*:207, 1896.

161. Kraus, W.M.: Involvement of the peripheral neurons in diabetes mellitus. Arch. Neurol. Psychiatry *7*:202, 1922.

162. Logothetis, J., Baker, A.B.: Neurologic manifestations in diabetes mellitus. Med. Clin. N. Am. *47(6)*:1459, 1963.

163. Muri, J.: Diabetic arthropathy and intercapillary glomerulosclerosis. Report of case. Acta Med. Scand. *135*:391, 1949.

164. Bosanquet, F.D., Henson, R.A.: Sensory neuropathy in diabetes mellitus. Folia Psychiat. Neurol. Neurochir. Neerl. *60*:107, 1957.

165. Seitz, D.: Zur Klinik und Pathogenese der Polyneuritis diabetica. Deutsch Z. Nerveheilk. *175*:15, 1956.

166. Cracco, J., Castells, S., Mark, E.: Conduction velocity in peripheral nerve and spinal afferent pathways in juvenile diabetics. Neurology *30*:370, 1980.

167. Gupta, P.R., Dorfman, L.J.: Spinal somatosensory conduction in diabetes. Neurology *30*:414, 1980.

168. Skanse, B., Gydell, K.: A rare type of femoral-sciatic neuropathy in diabetes mellitus. Acta Med. Scand. *155*:463, 1956.

169. Matthews, W.B.: Discussion on some clinical, genetic and biochemical aspects of metabolic disorders of the nervous system. Proc. R. Soc. Med. *51*:859, 1958.

170. Garland, H.: Neurological complications of diabetes mellitus: clinical aspects. Proc. R. Soc. Med. *53*:137, 1960.

171. Stenvers, H.W.: Diabetic "myelopathy" with formation of aberrant nerve fibres in the spinal cord. In: A. Biemond (Ed.): Recent Neurological Research. Amsterdam, Elsevier, 1959, pp. 213–222.

172. Caravati, C.M.: Insulin neuritis: A case report. Va. Med. Mon. *59*:745, 1933.

173. Rudy, A., Hoffmann, R.: Skin disturbances in diabetes mellitus: their relation to vitamin deficiencies. N. Engl. J. Med. *227*:893, 1942.

174. Ebaugh, F.G., Holt, G.W.: Polyneuropathy and diabetes mellitus. Am. J. Med. Sci. *244*:110, 1962.

175. Ellenberg, M.: Diabetic neuropathy precipitating after institution of diabetic control. Am. J. Med. Sci. *236*:466, 1958.

176. Lidz, T., Miller, J.M., Padget, P., Stedem, A.F.A.: Muscular atrophy and pseudologia fantastica associated with islet cell adenoma of the pancreas. Arch. Neurol. Psychiatry *62*:304, 1949.

177. Mulder, D.W., Bastron, J.A., Lambert, E.H.: Hyperinsulin neuronopathy. Neurology *6*:627, 1956.

178. Williams, C.J., Amyotrophy due to hypoglycaemia. Br. Med. J. *1*:707, 1955.

179. Rosner, L., Elstad, R.: The neuropathy of hypoglycemia. Neurology *14*:1, 1964.

180. Danta, G.: Hypoglycemic peripheral neuropathy. Arch. Neurol. *21*:121, 1969.

181. Harrison, M.J.G.: Muscle wasting after prolonged hypoglycaemic coma: case report with electrophysiological data. J. Neurol. Neurosurg. Psychiatry *39*:465, 1976.

182. Tom, M.I., Richardson, J.C.: Hypoglycaemia from islet cell tumor of pancreas with amyotrophy and cerebrospinal nerve cell changes. J. Neuropath. Exp. Neurol. *10*:57, 1951.

183. Winkelman, N.W., Moore, M.T.: Neurohistopathologic changes with Metrazol and insulin shock therapy: an experimental study on the cat. Arch. Neurol. Psychiatry *43*:1108, 1940.

184. Himwich, E.W., Frostig, J.P., Fazekas, J.F., Hadidian, Z.: The mechanism of the symptoms of insulin hypoglycemia. Am. J. Psychiatry *96*:371, 1939.

185. Tschirgi, R.D.: Chemical environment of the central nervous system. In: J. Field (Ed.): Handbook of Physiology, Vol. III. Washington, D.C., American Physiological Society, 1960, Chapter 78, p. 1865.

186. Sussman, K.E., Crout, J.R., Marble, A.: Failure of warning in insulin-induced hypoglycemic reactions. Diabetes *12*:38, 1963.

187. Kedes, L.H., Field, J.B.: Hypothermia. A clue to hypoglycemia. N. Engl. J. Med. *271*:785, 1964.

188. Sokoloff, L.: Metabolism of the central nervous system in vivo. In: J. Field (Ed.): Handbook of Physiology, Vol. III. Washington, D.C., American Physiological Society, 1960, Chapter 77, p. 1843.

189. Abood, L.G.: Neuronal metabolism. In: J. Field (Ed.):

Handbook of Physiology, Vol. III. Washington, D.C., American Physiological Society, 1960, Chapter 75, p. 1815.

190. Bloodworth, J.M.B., Jr., Hamwi, G.J.: Histopathologic lesions associated with sulfonylurea administration. Diabetes *10*:90, 1961.

191. Turkington, R.W.: Encephalopathy induced by oral hypoglycemic drugs. Arch. Intern. Med. *137*:1082, 1977.

192. Meyer, J.S., Portnoy, H.D.: Localized cerebral hypoglycemia stimulating stroke. A clinical and experimental study. Neurology *8*:601, 1958.

193. Windle, W.F., Koenig, H., Jensen, A.: Histologic study of the brain in experimentally induced acidosis. Arch. Neurol. Psychiatry *56*:428, 1946.

194. Anderson, J.M.: Diabetic ketoacidosis presenting as neurosurgical emergencies. Br. Med. J. *3*:22, 1974.

195. Posner, J.B., Swanson, A.G., Plum, F.: Acid-base balance in cerebrospinal fluid. Arch. Neurol. *12*:479, 1965.

196. Posner, J.B., Plum, F.: Protection of CSF pH and of brain function during severe metabolic acidosis. Trans. Am. Neurol. Assoc. *91*:38, 1966.

197. Young, E., Bradley, R.F.: Cerebral edema with irreversible coma in severe diabetic ketoacidosis. N. Engl. J. Med. *276*:665, 1967.

198. Timperley, W.R., Preston, F.E., Ward, J.D.: Cerebral intravascular coagulation in diabetic ketoacidosis. Lancet *1*:952, 1974.

199. Clements, R.S., Blumenthal, S.A., Morrison, A.D., Winegrad, A.I.: Increased cerebrospinal-fluid pressure during treatment of diabetic ketosis. Lancet *2*:671, 1971.

200. Clements, R.S., Jr., Prockop, L.D., Winegrad, A.I.: A mechanism to explain acute cerebral edema during the treatment of diabetic acidosis. Diabetes *17* (Suppl. 1):299, 1968.

201. Maccario, M., Messis, C.P., Vastola, E.F.: Focal seizures as a manifestation of hyperglycemia without ketoacidosis. A report of seven cases with review of the literature. Neurology *15*:195, 1965.

202. Daniels, J.C., Chokroverty, S., Barron, K.D.: Anacidotic hyperglycemia and focal seizures. Arch. Intern. Med. *124*:701, 1969.

203. Grunnet, M.L.: Cerebrovascular disease: diabetes and cerebral atherosclerosis. Neurology *13*:486, 1963.

204. Romanul, F.C.A., Abramowicz, A.: Changes in brain and pial vessels in arterial border zones. A study of 13 cases. Arch. Neurol. *11*:40, 1964.

205. Locke, S.: Diabetes and the nervous system. Med. Clin. North Am. *49(4)*:1081, 1965.

206. Alex, M., Baron, E.K., Goldenberg, S., Blumenthal, H.T.: An autopsy study of cerebrovascular accident in diabetes mellitus. Circulation *25*:663, 1962.

207. Kannel, W.B.: Current status of the epidemiology of brain infarction associated with occlusive arterial disease. Stroke *2*:295, 1971.

208. Dekaban, A.S., Magee, K.R.: Occurrence of neurologic abnormalities in infants of diabetic mothers. Neurology *8*:193, 1958.

209. Driscoll, S.G.: The pathology of pregnancy complicated by diabetes mellitus. Med. Clin. North Am. *49(4)*:1053, 1965.

210. Podolsky, S., Sheremata, W.A.: Insulin-dependent diabetes mellitus and Friedreich's ataxia in siblings. Metabolism *19*:555, 1970.

211. Refsum, S.: Heredopathia atactica polyneuritiformis. A familial syndrome not hitherto described. A contribution to the clinical study of the hereditary diseases of the nervous system. Acta Psychiatr. Neurol. Suppl. 38, 1946.

212. Nakano, K.K., Dawson, D.M., Spence, A.: Machado disease: a hereditary ataxia in Portuguese emigrants to Massachusetts. Neurology *22*:49, 1972.

213. Huff, T.A., Horton, E.S., Lebovitz, H.E.: Abnormal insulin secretion in myotonic dystrophy. N. Engl. J. Med. *277*:837, 1967.

214. LeCompte, P.M., Meissner, W.A.: Mucormycosis of the central nervous system associated with hemochromatosis. Report of a case. Am. J. Pathol. *23*:673, 1947.

215. Baker, R.D.: Diabetes and mucormycosis. Diabetes *9*:143, 1960.

216. Kutt, H., Hurwitz, L.J., Ginsburg, S.M., McDowell, F.: Cerebrospinal fluid protein in diabetes mellitus. Arch. Neurol. *4*:31, 1961.

216a. Diabetic neuropathy—where are we now? (Editorial) Lancet *1*:1366, 1983.

216b. Judzewitsch, R.G., Jaspan, J.B., Polonsky, K.S., et al.: Aldose reductase inhibition improves nerve conduction velocity in diabetic patients. N. Engl. J. Med. *308*:119, 1983.

216c. Young, R.J., Ewing, D.J., Clarke, B.F.: A controlled trial of sorbinil, an aldose reductase inhibitor, in chronic painful diabetic neuropathy. Diabetes *32*:938, 1983.

216d. Service, F.J., Daube, J.R., O'Brien, P.C., et al.: Effect of blood glucose control on peripheral nerve function in diabetic patients. Mayo Clin. Proc. *58*:283, 1983.

216e. Windebank, A.J.: Diabetic control and peripheral neuropathy. Mayo Clin. Proc. *58*:344, 1983.

216f. Holman, R.R., Dornan, T.L., Mayon-White, V., et al.: Prevention of deterioration of renal and sensory-nerve function by more intensive management of insulin-dependent diabetic patients. A two-year randomized prospective study. Lancet *1*:204, 1983.

217. Daube, J.R., Service, F.J., Dyck, P.J.: Acute effects on nerve conduction of strict control of blood sugar with an artificial pancreas. Muscle & Nerve *3*:437, 1980. (Abstract).

218. Thompson, R.H.S., Butterfield, W.J.H., Fry, I.K.: Pyruvate metabolism in diabetic neuropathy. Proc. R. Soc. Med. *53*:143, 1960.

219. Collens, W.S., Rabiner, A.M., Zilinsky, J.D., et al.: The treatment of peripheral neuropathy in diabetes mellitus. Am. J. Med. Sci. *219*:482, 1950.

220. Lundbaek, K., Malmros, R., Andersen, H.C., et al.: Hypophysectomy for diabetic angiopathy. A preliminary report. Diabetes *11*:474, 1962.

221. Ellenberg, M.: Treatment of diabetic neuropathy with diphenylhydantoin. N.Y. State J. Med. *68*:2653, 1968.

222. Saudek, C.D., Werns, S., Reidenberg, M.M.: Phenytoin in the treatment of diabetic symmetrical polyneuropathy. Clin. Pharmacol. Ther. *22*:196, 1977.

223. Rull, J.A., Quibrera, R., González-Millán, H., Lozano Castañeda, O.: Symptomatic treatment of peripheral diabetic neuropathy with carbamazepine (Tegretol): double blind crossover trial. Diabetologia *5*:215, 1969.

224. Editorial. Painful diabetic neuropathy. Br. Med. J. *2*:349, 1977.

225. Turkington, R.W.: Depression masquerading as diabetic neuropathy. J.A.M.A. *243*:1147, 1980.

226. Gade, G.N., Hofeldt, F.D., Treece, G.L.: Diabetic neuropathic cachexia. Beneficial response to combination therapy with amitriptyline and fluphenazine. J.A.M.A. *243*:1160, 1980.

227. Davis, J.L., Lewis, S.B., Gerich, J.E., et al.: Peripheral diabetic neuropathy treated with amitriptyline and fluphenazine. J.A.M.A. *238*:2291, 1977.

228. Taub, A.: Relief of postherpetic neuralgia with psychotropic drugs. J. Neurosurg. *39*:235, 1973.

229. Dalessio, D.J.: Chronic pain syndromes and disordered

cortical inhibition: effects of tricyclic compounds. Dis. Nerv. System 28:325, 1967.

230. Basbaum, A.I., Fields, H.L.: Endogenous pain control mechanisms: review and hypothesis. Ann. Neurol. 4:451, 1978.

231. Ellenberg, M.: Diabetic neuropathic cachexia. Diabetes 23:418, 1974.

232. Schatz, I.J., Podolsky, S., Frame, B.: Idiopathic orthostatic hypotension: diagnosis and treatment. J.A.M.A. 186:537, 1963.

233. Frimodt-Møller, C., Mortensen, S.: Treatment of diabetic cystopathy. Ann. Intern. Med. 92 (Part 2):327, 1980.

234. Scott, F.B., Fishman, I.J., Light, J.K.: An inflatable penile prosthesis for treatment of diabetic impotence. Ann. Intern. Med. 92 (Part 2):340, 1980.

235. Longstreth, G.F., Malagelada, J.R., Kelly, K.A.: Metoclopramide stimulation of gastric motility and emptying in diabetic gastroparesis. Ann. Intern. Med. 86:195, 1977.

236. Green, P.A., Berge, K.G., Sprague, R.G.: Control of diabetic diarrhea with antibiotic therapy. Diabetes 17:385, 1968.

32 Sexual Dysfunction in Diabetes

Donald M. Barnett and Robert E. Desautels

Table 32–1. Types of Sexual Dysfunction

1. Loss of libido.
2. Orgasmic dysfunction.
3. Sexual inadequacy in the aging person.
4. Fertility disorders.

    In males:

5. Erectile impotence.
6. Retrograde ejaculation
7. Premature ejaculation.
8. Ejaculatory incompetence.

Poor sexual performance is of great concern to persons with diabetes mellitus. It follows fear of blindness and loss of limb in order of importance to many men with diabetes.

This chapter outlines ways whereby the physician can assess the sexual difficulties of which patients complain. In the past decade, male impotence has received greater attention than before due to clarification of frequency of this condition, improved diagnostic techniques and more treatment options. This topic will be emphasized and set in perspective with the generally improved quality of life that the person with diabetes has come to expect.

All men and women with diabetes should be helped to cope, when possible, with any obstruction to sexual expression in their daily lives.

CLASSIFICATION OF SEXUAL DYSFUNCTION

Since the work of Masters and Johnson in the 1960s, a number of clarifications of sexual problems have occurred.[1] The term "sexual dysfunction" covers a wide variety of problems that describe a whole range of conditions from diminished sexual desire to failure to experience orgasm or sexual pleasure.

Listed below are the problems that a physician may need to explore with a patient regarding a sexually related complaint. See Table 32–1.

1. Loss of Libido. This term, borrowed from the psychoanalytic literature, really describes decreased sexual desire. The urge to engage in sexual activity arises at mid-adolescence or late pubescence, coinciding with a rise in sex hormone levels and maturation. The libido of some persons increases as an outlet, it would seem, to unrelated life events, while others report a general decline in interest in sexual expression after 50 years of age. The level of sexual desire can vary due to medical conditions and medication changes as well. Therefore, this is the first type of sexual dysfunction about which to inquire. Decreased libido per se does not appear to be a special factor in the diabetic population. However, the physician needs to help the patient with discouragement or depression which may result from certain life events, leading to loss of sexual interest.

Certain medical conditions such as the hypoendocrinopathies, particularly hypoadrenalism and Klinefelter's syndrome, may cause a loss of sexual interest to be a prime complaint. Conditions of hyperendocrine functioning such as Cushing's syndrome and many chronic system failure disorders such as obstructive pulmonary disease and renal disease, also may cause loss of sexual drive.

2. Orgasmic Dysfunction refers to the inability to experience climactic sexual pleasure. This will be discussed in the section under sexual dysfunction in women where it has been almost exclusively described.

3. Sexual Inadequacy in the Aging Male or Female. This item relates particularly to sexual dysfunction in the aging male. Some confusion has existed for years over whether or not the male undergoes a menopause or "climacteric" similar to that of the female. From age 40 onward, males

may experience vascular instability with symptoms variously described as dizziness, sweating, paresthesias, and the like. Most often these are accompanied by problems with memory lapses, insomnia, irritability and in general, loss of psychologic stability. Some physicians have ascribed these problems to depression. For the diabetologist, it is important to rule out coronary artery disease or autonomic neuropathy.

These vasomotor symptoms need to be firmly dissociated from a sexual performance issue that all men seem to undergo as they reach middle age. Although, as shown clearly by Masters and Johnson, men in middle to advanced age never lose their facility for erection at any time, they do appear to become aroused, and to erect at a slower pace as age advances.[2] This physiologically slower sexual arousal pattern as well as decreased "ejaculatory demand" are often interpreted by the man and his partner as evidence of decreased sexual function. Following this slowing, discouragement usually develops and a pattern of loss of expectation ensues. Compounding difficulties of boredom with one's sexual partner, excessive alcohol ingestion, or the vasomotor male climacteric symptoms mentioned above, can all confuse the situation.

While the menopause and the passage of years do represent for many women a decreasing urgency for sexual relations, the prediction of this fact is not guaranteed. A minority of women complain of dyspareunia due to decreased vaginal lubrication, but most women with ongoing stable, intimate relationships seem to be little disturbed by diminution of this apparent estrogen-related trait.

It is important to realize that without appropriate study, one should not ascribe loss of sexual function to the age of any patient, diabetic or nondiabetic. There is abundant evidence that general information about sexual function and reassurance go a long way to improve this particular type of sexual dysfunction.

4. Fertility Disorders, secondary to errors of hormonal balance, while hinted at in earlier literature on "impotence," have not been noted in the Joslin Clinic experience. The problems of diabetic women are with the effects of pregnancy on the fetus, not on conception. The only direct problem with fertility relates to the male who experiences retrograde ejaculation which acts in most cases as built-in contraception, since in this condition, the sperm is propelled back into the bladder and becomes unavailable in a number adequate to initiate pregnancy.

5 and 6. Retrograde Ejaculation and Erectile Impotence, two entities more common in diabetic than in nondiabetic males, will be discussed later in this chapter.

7. Premature Ejaculation is the most common entity treated by sex therapists. It plagues younger males but may be corrected by behavior techniques amply illustrated by Masters and Johnson in their initial work on the subject.[3] This condition is no more common in diabetics than in nondiabetics.

8. Ejaculatory Incompetence, a problem opposite to premature ejaculation, i.e., failure to ejaculate despite adequate erectile function, is rare and has not been reported in men with diabetes. It is seen in older nondiabetic patients with emotional or "withholding" problems.

Identification of the entities that comprise sexual difficulties is necessary during the taking of the sexual history. One must keep in mind that many persons undergo periods when their sexual desire or sexual response seems to decline for brief periods (see later section under Sexual History). Assurance that this is expected and "normal" can be a tremendous help to many people of all ages.

NORMAL SEXUAL FUNCTION AND THE PERSON WITH DIABETES

Normal sexual function depends on an intact brain, spinal cord, and vascular supply. The peripheral nerve system, largely from the sacral plexus, also is needed to initiate and sustain sexual function.

Erection centers in the brain and spinal cord initiate activation of the autonomic system. Weiss has summarized what is known about the neurophysiologic response of erectile function.[4] The medical literature on the subject is largely the result of studies in paraplegic veterans and experimental animals. Three initiators of the sexual "reflex" appear to be: central (brain); tactile (external stimulation); and abdominal (internal stimulation). Any or all of these activators have been thought to play a part in the understanding of sexual function.

Figure 32–1 outlines what is needed to function normally. The absolute minimum is an intact lumbar spinal cord where sympathetic nerves exit, and the sacral cord where the nervi erigentes (parasympathetic nerves) leave (sacral 2–4). Additionally, the pudendal artery which derives from the internal iliac artery, needs to be patent in order to supply the genital tissue with an increased amount of blood during sexual arousal, excitation, and performance.

Activation of the autonomic nervous system takes two routes as implied in the above description of the spinal cord requirements for sexual performance. Vasodilation of the penis is sponsored by the parasympathetic outflow, while smooth and striated muscle contraction is inaugurated and sustained by sympathetic nervous supply of the autonomic plexus.

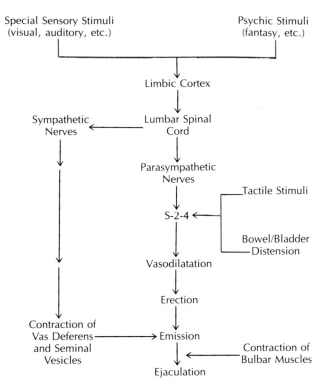

Fig. 32–1. Neurogenic and psychogenic mechanisms of penile erection and ejaculation. ("S" = sacral nerves.)

It has been postulated that valve-like structures, called "polsters" containing smooth muscle, are in the corpora cavernosa and under the control of the autonomic nervous system. Poor neural transmission presumably would disturb the steady state of increased inflow of blood into erectile tissue during sexual arousal. This site of a pathologic condition seems logical as an area for further consideration in the diabetic male, as reported in the work of Faerman et al.[5] who found histologic evidence of autonomic neuropathy in the neural fibers of the corpora cavernosa.

The musculature is involved in propelling sperm, prostatic fluid, and seminal vesicle contents forward in the ejaculatory phase of sexual functioning. Perineal nerves also are believed to be necessary to aid this expulsion of seminal fluid and require intact peripheral motor nerves to the perineal muscles. Contraction or maintenance of closure of the bladder neck by sympathetic stimulation is essential for normal ejaculation. Failure of this mechanism is the cause of retrograde ejaculation.

In the female, vasodilation and vaginal lubrication require a parasympathetic supply. Anticholinergic drugs such as belladonna preparations have been noted to decrease vaginal lubrication by the apparent blocking of this autonomic-parasympathetic function. By the same token, clitoral en-

gorgement ("female erection") could be blocked by similar agents.

The intact anatomic sequences necessary for normal sexual function can be greatly challenged by changes evoked in the course of the pathophysiologic development of diabetes. "Chronic diabetes syndrome" is the term given for the possible development of changes in structure and function of several major areas of the body. Table 32–2 (items 2 and 3) illustrates the possible effect of micro- and macro-angiopathy and disorders of the peripheral nervous system on sexual function in a person with diabetes. Problems of sexual function might be due to these disorders:

Table 32–2.   Causes of Impotence in Diabetic Men

1. Psychogenic factors.
2. Neuropathy.
   A. Autonomic neuropathy (sympathetic/parasympathetic)
   B. Motor neuropathy, i.e., perineal muscles
3. Macro- and micro-vascular abnormalities.
4. Hormone dysfunction.
5. Drugs and medications.
6. Local fibrous (collagen) tissue factors.
7. Mixed type - any of the above.

(a). neuropathy principally of the autonomic nerves, or

(b). large vessel narrowing in the aortic-iliac area. This site contributes to the Leriche syndrome and appears rarely in our clinical experience. More subtle forms of vascular inflow to the genital tissue are possible with narrowing or stenosis of the pudendal artery. Other possibilities are degenerative changes in the arteries to the shaft of the penis or in the capillary networks between the arterial inflow and venous outflow circulation, resulting in decreased shunting to these tissues. Still another possibility, that of venous incompetence, as a cause of impotence, has been suggested.

One problem observed by us in diabetic patients at surgery is fibrosis of the spongy tissue of the corpora cavernosa. It would seem likely that this change would have a significant effect upon the filling of the corpora with blood and the production of an erection. Insofar as we know, this cannot be corrected by any type of surgery available at this time.

A spectrum of the factors which could produce or promote physiologic impotence in diabetic males is illustrated in Table 32-2. The usual sequence might be that some decreased autonomic tone becomes coupled with some decreased vascular flow into denser than normal spongy tissue of the penile corpora.

IMPOTENCE IN MEN WITH DIABETES

Prevalence. The prevalence of erectile dysfunction or impotence in diabetic men is high. The results of major studies are summarized in Table 32-3 from which it is evident that about 40 to 50% of the men questioned reported trouble with penile erection.

In the Joslin Clinic studies reported in 1974[13] and in 1982,[14] the average age of the men involved was around 50 years.

In the 1974 study, the 175 subjects were selected and interviewed at random for their sexual history. Testosterone levels were determined on each subject and were found to be normal in all the men studied. The 48% who, by history, were impotent, included 8% in whom psychologic problems were prominent and 7% with grossly poor control of diabetes, leaving 33% in whom neither factor was evident. Of the total of 175 men, 52% denied sexual dysfunction. In both the 1974 and the 1982 studies, the percentages of men on insulin and on oral agents were about equal. Neuropathy seemed more prevalent than any other measured complication of diabetes, being present in 30% of the subjects in 1974 and 50% in the 1982 study. Nephropathy and retinopathy were about half as frequent as neuropathy.

Assessment of Impotence. With possibly a third of middle-aged diabetic men complaining of impotence, it is most important to assess correctly the problem. The first step is to obtain an accurate history. A good definition of impotence should include the following: inability to achieve and maintain an erection of sufficient rigidity for insertion and thrusting until completion of the sexual act.

Sexual History. Most men are deeply concerned with the change in their sexual performance, and welcome the chance to discuss their problem. Surprisingly, a number of men mention it first to a nurse who is attending them, and it is from this source that many physicians (who did not include the sexual inquiry in a review of systems) learn of the situation. Often it is wise to approach the matter of sexual function either at the time of the review of systems (under the heading of genitourinary system, for example) or just after completion of the genital or rectal examination.

It is important to question the man on his baseline performance level prior to the onset of the problem. It is remarkable to see the differences in what men call the "normal frequency" of sexual relations. Frequency of intercourse usually declines rapidly once performance becomes an issue. The power of suggestion in male sexual functioning works both ways in eliciting desire, and likewise in ways that discourage the man from sexual activity.

Table 32-3. Frequency of Erectile Impotence in Men with Diabetes*

Author	No. of Men	Age Range Years	Impotent Percent
Rundles, R.W. (1945)[7]	69	17–70+	27.5
Martin, M.M. (1953)[8]	70	20–70+	54.0
Rubin, A. et al. (1958)[9]	198	16–92	55.0
Montenero, P. et al. (1962)[10]	436	20–65	55.0
Schöffling, K. et al. (1963)[11]	314	16–65	53.0
Ellenberg, M. (1971)[12]	200	Not stated	59.0
Kolodny, R.C. et al. (1974)[13] (Joslin Clinic)	175	18–81	49.0
Faerman, I. et al. (1974)[5]	299	18–50	40.0

*Adapted from article by Schiavi and Hogan.[6]

In appropriate cases the sexual partner should be questioned. This is essential to substantiate many issues of frequency of intercourse, past and present, as well as other parts of the psychosocial history that may surround the sexual issue. Attitudes of the partners are of clinical importance. Many women unwittingly put demands on their husbands at the time of declining performance. They may imply that there are other partners that may be influencing their husband's performance. This should be elicited and delineated early in the assessment process.

Impotence is often described as becoming progressively worse in the diabetic male. Erections of only "50%" create above-average difficulty in completing the sexual act satisfactorily.

Additionally, the ability for the patient to experience erection during sleep, the ability to achieve full rigidity during solo or mutual masturbation, and even finding satisfaction in a full erection during oral intercourse, are additional pieces of information that may be offered by the patient if correctly questioned during the history taking. When one finds by history that sexual desire is diminished but erections during sleep and ability to masturbate are preserved, diabetes is an unlikely cause of the problem.

Impotence is "organic" or physical in etiology supposedly when it occurs in a more abrupt fashion, as after surgery. However, a blend of features characteristic of any etiology (psychologic, diabetic, or other organic dysfunction) can be seen with this type of history taking. As one learns more about the patient in question, the work situation and the family constellation, additional questioning will help clarify the problem.

Masters and Johnson[2] list several areas where impotence seems to occur as the male grows older. These can serve as the basis for pertinent questions as to the general quality and content of the patient's personal life. Is there:

(1) monotony with a repetitive sexual relationship?
(2) preoccupation with career areas of one's life?
(3) mental or physical fatigue?
(4) overindulgence in food and drink?
(5) physical or mental influence of the spouse?

The next step in the assessment of sexual dysfunction is to elicit all medications and alcohol consumption, past and present. These agents can alter sexual performance significantly at all levels. Also implied here is the fact that the physician should modify these medications when possible. Antihypertensives, sedatives, and alcohol are three major categories of drugs that should be carefully inventoried. The introduction of most antihypertensives in a treatment program can in many cases mark the time when sexual dysfunction or impotence started. Table 32–4 lists the drugs that have been reported most commonly to interrupt any or all of the three aspects of sexual function (i.e., libido, erection, and ejaculation). Ejaculation is linked to orgasmic function as they occur simultaneously and are apparently neurocerebrally related. Therefore, it is important to modify any drug plan where possible.

Physical Examination. The third part of the assessment and treatment process for impotence is to verify certain aspects of the genital system by a complete physical examination. The major emphasis should be on the vascular, neurologic, and rectal examinations. The Leriche syndrome or aortic iliac obstruction due to atherosclerosis is rare, but is denoted when femoral pulses are absent on physical examination or bruits are heard near bounding femoral pulses. Most middle-aged diabetic patients with peripheral vascular disease show absent foot pulses and often diminished or absent popliteal pulses, but usually have good femoral pulsations. Occasionally, arteriograms reveal a blocked pudendal artery that could account for diminished erectile function.

The basic neurologic examination will show that in a third to a half of patients, deep tendon reflexes are absent and peripheral sensation is diminished distally. However, a number of diabetic men with impotence have been found to have these functions intact. Absence or diminution of ankle reflexes, poor anal sphincter tone, and absent bulbocavernosus reflex are common occurrences in diabetic patients with impotence. Attention to these features leads one to believe that neuropathy is far more common than is reported.

The bulbocavernosus reflex is achieved by stimulating the glans penis by a sudden squeeze or pinch while the other index finger is in the anal canal. A sudden tightening of the anal sphincter can be felt about the examining finger in at least 85% of normal individuals. Absence of the reflex is suggestive, but not absolute evidence of neurologic impairment. The sacral latency test is a new electromyographic method of demonstrating the same effect with greater accuracy.[14a]

The determination of penile blood pressure provides a measure of the adequacy of penile blood flow. A 2.5-cm blood pressure cuff, placed at the base of the penis, and a Doppler apparatus to detect arterial pulsation are used for this determination. Blockage of penile arterial circulation is suspected when the penile systolic pressure is less than 75% of brachial artery systolic pressure.[15]

Laboratory Studies. Few laboratory tests are

Table 32–4. Drugs Reported to Have Caused Sexual Dysfunction*

Drug Drug Class Generic Name (Brand Name)	Adverse Effect		
	Ejaculation Difficulties	Erectile Problems	Decrease or Loss of Libido
Antihypertensives:			
Clonidine (Catapres)	+++	+++	−
Ganglionic blocking agents	+++	+++	−
Guanethidine (Ismelin)	++++	+++	+
Methyldopa (Aldomet)	+	++++	++++
Pargyline (Butonyl)	++++	++++	++
Phenoxybenzamine (Dibenzyline)	+++	−	−
Reserpine (various)	+	+++	++++
Diuretics:			
Chlorthalidone (Hygroton)	−	+	++
Spironolactone (Aldactone)	+	++	+
Anticholinergics:			
Atropine	−	++	+
Belladonna alkaloids (Donnatal and others)	−	++	+
Antidepressants:			
Amitriptyline (Elavil, Endep)	+++	+	++
Imipramine (Tofranil and others)	+	++	++
Doxepine (Sinequan)	−	+	+++
Antipsychotics:			
Phenothiazines:			
Chlorpromazine (Thorazine and others)	+	++	+
Thioridazine (Mellaril)	+++	+	++
Antiarrhythmics:			
Disopyramide (Norpace)	−	++	−
Anorexiants:			
Fenfluramine (Pondimin)	−	++	++
Alcohol	++	+++	+
Cannabis (Marijuana)	−	++	+
Other:			
Disulfiram (Antabuse)	−	++	−
17-alpha hydroxyprogesterone caproate (Delalutin)	−	++++	−

+ Adverse sexual side effect has been reported at least once.
++ Occurrence of sexual side effect is rarely experienced.
+++ Occurrence of sexual side effect is commonly experienced.
++++ Occurrence of sexual side effect is extremely common.
− Drug not usually associated with this sexual side effect.
*Adapted from O'Connor and Scavone.[16]

available than can aid in the diagnosis of impotence. The 1974 Joslin study showed no difference in testosterone levels between the men who complained of impotence and those in a matched control group. Therefore, this expensive test can be omitted except in unusual patients in whom androgen deficiency is suspected.

A profile of blood chemistry, sedimentation rate, and complete blood count are presumed to be part of the laboratory tests for any problem that could be related to debilitating situations. This would be of importance if loss of libido were postulated as the major problem in the differential diagnosis.

Most endocrinopathies that require screening involve issues primarily related to libido, but issues of erectile performance are often enmeshed in this complex problem. Evaluations for pituitary, thyroid, adrenal and prolactin function may be helpful in disorders where libido but not potency is the emphasis.

The degree of diabetes control plays a significant role in a minor group of patients. This can be assessed clinically by measuring glycosylated hemoglobin. Surprisingly high results can substantiate that grossly poor control has or will contribute to poor sexual function. Random blood glucose values should not be down-played as they too can help to confirm poor control. It is of interest to note that the urologic department of one of the largest diagnostic clinics in the country uses a glucose tolerance test as their only laboratory screening procedure for impotence. Often men have had the diagnosis of hitherto unsuspected diabetes made through investigation of the complaint of impotence. However, the sensitivity of the sexual reflex to even modest aberrations of glucose metabolism on the one hand, and the sparing of some of the most grossly uncontrolled or chronically ill patients on the other (e.g., people with uremia undergoing dialysis), remain a mystery.

Special laboratory testing can include the Nocturnal Penile Tumescence test (NPT). NPT was developed by Karacan[17] from his observations in the sleep laboratory. It has been noted that normal men from birth to old age uniformly erect in cycles that correspond to dream sleep (rapid eye movements [REM] during sleep). From a maximum of 32% or a total of 90 minutes of sleep spent with the penis in an engorged state to 20% or a total of 15 minutes in the same state by 70 years of age, is one observation from this work. The monitoring of this physiologic phenomenon has been incorporated into a measurement that helps differentiate the various disorders that result in impotence. Recent refinements in sleep laboratory techniques now distinguish between degrees of firmness of the penis and determinations of penile circumference in the tumescent state. However, it is possible to have an adequate NPT determination but still find a patient complaining of diminished penile rigidity.

The experience in Joslin Clinic patients with the NPT has been confined to those who are prospective candidates for the use of a penile prosthesis. It is hardly surprising, therefore, that we have found either absence or significant diminution in NPT routinely in the group of approximately 250 patients who have been evaluated in this way.

The NPT does not require the elaborate apparatus of the sleep laboratory but can be done at the patient's bedside or attached at home by use of a portable meter. A strain gauge 1-mm loop is placed around the penis near its base. As the loop stretches during erections, it is recorded on a tape similar to an electrocardiographic tracing (Fig. 32–2). The basic office screening process is summarized in Table 32–5. A simple apparatus has been devised for home use (Snap-Gauge made by Dacomed Corp., Minneapolis, MN 55420).[17a]

TREATMENT OPTIONS

The treatment options open to the patient with impotence as the main problem are outlined in Table 32–6. By no means is each type of treatment exclusive of the others.

Medical Treatment

The diabetologist/endocrinologist or general physician will need to emphasize better diabetes control, especially with tests such as glycosylated hemoglobin (HbA_1).

Medications to control hypertension are frequent offenders as the cause of impotence. Certain antihypertensives such as methyldopa (Aldomet) and clonidine (Catapres) should be avoided. A suggested program might include at first diuretics every other day with the addition of a peripheral vasodilator such as hydralazine. Beta blocker medications such as propranolol (Inderal) in small doses can be the third drug added cautiously. When treatment of hypertension is difficult, any appropriate combination of drugs must be used in such treatment, taking precedence over concern for sexual performance. If this sequence of events fails to provide satisfactory results, then a prosthesis should be considered. It is important that the physician combine basic sexual education with inquiry at every step of the assessment and treatment. It has been stated that there are 3 primary goals in treating impotence: (a) remove the man's fears regarding sexual performance; (b) reorient his in-

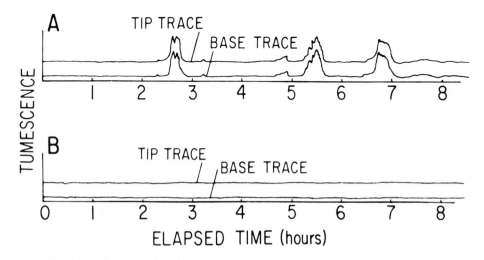

Fig. 32–2. Typical (condensed) nocturnal penile tumescence (NPT) patterns: *A.* This tracing indicates significant tumescence activity. Organic impotence can be ruled out. *B.* This tracing shows no tumescence activity, strongly indicating that the impotence is of organic nature. "Tip" and "base" refer to tracings taken respectively from the distal and proximal portions of the penis.

Table 32–5. Screening Tests for Impotence (History of unsatisfactory erections and normal libido)

Physical Examination and Laboratory Studies	Neuropathic Etiology Primarily	Vascular Etiology Primarily	Psychologic Etiology Primarily
Deep tendon reflexes	0 or decreased	Normal	Normal
Anal sphincter tone	Decreased	Normal	Normal
Bulbocavernosus reflex	0 or decreased	Normal	Normal
Penile blood pressure	Decreased or normal	Decreased	Normal
Nocturnal penile tumescence	0 or decreased	0 or decreased	Normal

Note: In the diabetic patient with organic impotence, the ability to achieve orgasm, usually with the production of ejaculate, is preserved.

Table 32–6. Treatment Options

1. Improved treatment of diabetes and other conditions.
2. Discontinuance or change of unnecessary medications and alcohol.
3. Sex education.
   A. Instruction in sexual information.
   B. Teaching sexual skills (maximizing intimacy, arousal).
   C. Marital or individual counseling.
4. Surgical options.
   A. Non-inflatable prosthesis (Carrion-Jonas type).
   B. Inflatable prosthesis (Scott type).
   C. Revascularization.

voluntary behavioral pattern so that he becomes an active participant rather than his usual one of a spectator (the most common problem found in relationship to impotence); and (c) relieve the fears of the woman regarding her partner's sexual performance.[18]

In a sense, these three primary goals are "sex therapy." However, this particular term has led to some misunderstanding about what is expected of the role of physician or therapist in guiding people to better sexual performance. Certainly crucial is a combination of skills including sound medical advice and correct referral to consultants who can assist the partners in better sexual expression. When appropriate, the patient and his partner should be referred to a surgeon who is knowledgeable and experienced in prosthetic correction of impotence.

The neat division between patients who have normal sexual drive and are free of psychosocial problems but have poor erection performance, on the one hand, and those with abrupt onset of impotence (usually a middle-aged male with only fair or even poor libido) that changes with psychosocial events on the other, is an oversimplification of the usual presentation of impotence. While the former will likely have minor psychologic overlay and the latter a major component of this factor, many patients appear to have a mixed clinical picture.

Within sex education are available a variety of options. While the individual physician may not feel comfortable with this type of assistance, sex therapists with these skills exist in large referral centers. It is particularly important when sexual performance is variable, marital strife obvious, and in situations largely not amenable to surgical correction, that this type of referral take place.

Information on sexual response and expectation is fundamental from this type of consultation, followed by discussion of ways sexual intimacy and arousal can be enhanced. Simultaneous counseling for patient and partner on issues unrelated to sexual performance is not uncommon since financial, job and past social difficulties all too often become indirectly focused on the sexual performance level of a couple's relationship.

Surgical Treatment

After medical problems have been corrected or treatment has been attempted for a period of time (1 to 3 months), lack of progress will necessitate a urologic consultation. When corrective measures fail, consideration of a prosthetic penile insertion is necessary.

Prosthetic Devices. Such devices are made of silicone elastomer and have been steadily developed since the 1950s. Presently, there are two basic models from which to choose. One is a non-inflatable prosthesis developed by Small and Carrion[19] and a modification by Jonas.[19a] The other is an inflatable prosthesis developed by Scott.[20] The non-inflatable silicone rod comes with or without a malleable core of wire. These paired silastic rods are implanted within the chamber of the corpora cavernosa. The use of twisted silver wire in the core of the rods has allowed more flexibility and greater concealment. Figure 32–3 illustrates these various models now available.

The inflatable prosthesis is a hydraulic system which employs a reservoir of fluid that can be pumped into two cylinders that inflate the tunica albuginea of the penis. The cylinders are located within the chambers of the corpora cavernosa. The pump which lies in the scrotum has a release valve

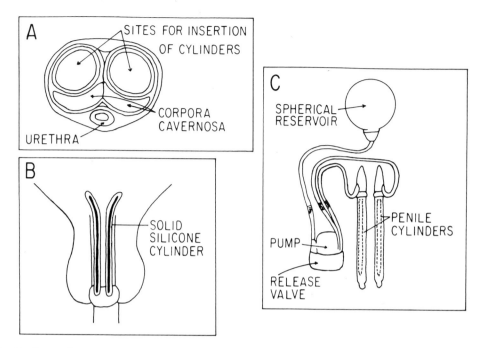

Fig. 32–3. Penile prostheses.
A. Cross section of penis showing location of sites for insertion of silicone cylinders, both solid and expandable. *B.* Solid, non-expandable cylinders in place (Small-Carrion or Jonas modification). *C.* Scott expandable cylinders, hydraulic pump (in scrotum) and reservoir for isotonic fluid (implanted beneath skin of abdominal wall). Adapted in part from Scott et al.[21]

on its side. A reservoir for fluid to fill the cylinders is placed in the superpubic area behind the abdominal wall.

Scott[21] reports only 1 of 50 cases where there was failure of the cylinder to "heal in." Six of 100 cylinders leaked when observed on an average of 16 months postoperatively. Replacement of cylinders and/or use of antibiotics corrected this problem.

Most series that have been reported in the literature show larger numbers of patients receiving a non-inflatable device, since these have been longer in use. Additionally, they are less involved from a surgical point of view, particularly related to mechanical problems. Both models have had virtually no rejection phenomenon or tissue mobility complications over a 5-year period.

The Joslin Clinic experience is summarized in Table 32–7. Final decision as to implantation of a prosthesis as well as the surgery itself was carried out by Dr. R. E. Desautels, urologist. The complication rate overall was less than 10% when all problems of major or minor infections, erosions or mechanical adjustment were considered.

Once the technical aspects of prosthetic implants are discussed with a couple, it is necessary to explain to them that a prosthesis is really an aid to help with the intromission of the penis into the vagina and not a device that will insure arousal of

the partners or guarantee orgasm for the female. The increased rigidity of the penis does not help with psychosocial problems that may have preceded or been attendant to the problem of impotence.

A follow-up of the penile prosthesis patients in the Joslin population reported by Beaser and associates,[14] showed that over 80% of patients were ultimately satisfied with the prosthetic devices (Table 32–8). It was instructive that even with the partner who for some reason was not consulted prior to the surgical procedure, satisfaction was about the same, in the 80 to 90% range, as in situations where partners were consulted.

Revascularization Procedures. Apart from removing discrete aorto-iliac blocks by endarterectomy to correct the Leriche syndrome which sometimes leads to impotence, newer approaches to smaller artery procedures have been explored recently. They have not been shown to be successful except in a few highly selected patients.[19b]

Retrograde Ejaculation. Retrograde ejaculation is seen more commonly in diabetics than in nondiabetics. However, in a random sampling of our patients, the prevalence is from 1 to 2%.[13] That retrograde ejaculation goes on to produce impotence has not been documented. Schiavi and Hogan[6] point out that retrograde ejaculation is "frequently unrecognized since the amount of ejaculate

Table 32–7. Experience with Penile Prostheses in Joslin Clinic Patients (R.E. Desautels, urologic surgeon)

Type of Prosthesis	Number Implanted	Type of Complications	Complications			
			Major		Minor	
			Number	Percent	Number	Percent
Small-Carrion	113	Loss of prosthesis:				
		Unilateral erosion	2	1.7		
		Bilateral erosion	1	.8		
		Bilateral infection	1	.8		
		Superficial infection			3	2.6
Jonas	71	Loss of prosthesis:				
		Unilateral erosion	1	1.4		
		Removal:				
		Psychologic. Not replaced			1	1.4
		Pain. (Replaced with Scott prosthesis)			2	2.8
		Adjustment:				
		Position change			1	1.4
		Shorten length			1	1.4
Scott	36	Failure:				
		2 adjusted. 1 replaced with Jonas prosthesis			3	8.4
		Loss of prosthesis:				
		Bilateral infection	1	2.8		
		Bilateral erosion	1	2.8		
		Adjustment:				
		Position change			2	5.6
TOTAL PROSTHESES	220	TOTAL COMPLICATIONS	7	3.1	13	5.9

Table 32–8. The Effect of Preoperative Consultations with Partners on Ultimate Patient/ Partner Satisfaction*

	Number of Patients	Ultimately Satisfied	
		Number	Percent
Patients:			
Consulted partners preoperatively	59	49	81
Did not consult partners preoperatively	23	19	83
	Number of Partners		
Partners:			
Were consulted by patients preoperatively	44	36	82
Were not consulted by patients preoperatively	9	8	89

*Number of respondents to these questions: Patients, 82; Partners, 53. No statistical difference was noted between satisfaction levels of the consulted versus the nonconsulted groups for both patients and partners.

Adapted from Beaser et al.[14]

may diminish progressively over an extended period of time without impairment of orgastic capacity. . . . Patients with retrograde ejaculation differ greatly in the quality and intensity of their orgastic experience with some indicating little change in orgastic satisfaction even with the total absence of ejaculate.''

There are a number of patients who appear to have retrograde ejaculation, but who do not have spermatozoa in the urine immediately after orgasm. It is presumed, therefore, that these individuals fail to ejaculate because of sympathetic nerve damage

producing absence of contraction of the vasa, seminal vesicles and prostate smooth muscle at the time of orgasm. The seminal fluid in this condition is thrust into the bladder rather than through the urethral canal at the time of orgasm. This is due apparently to a selective failure of the internal sphincter of the bladder to close properly during the sexual response. This event is often referred to by patients as a ''dry run.''

The spontaneous correction of this problem has also been reported. Medications have not been of help in bladder neck strengthening.

Case example: J.H., #09-90-20, a 35-year-old man with diabetes since age 10, married for 3 years, reported problems with lack of ejaculate in the previous year. Orgastic function was normal. He and his wife desired children and feared sterility. Several attempts at postcoital collection of seminal fluid proved unsatisfactory. A referral to a center over a 15 months' span proved successful with attainment of pregnancy after approximately 10 attempts at artificial insemination with cervical capping. This was done with concentrated specimens of seminal fluid from the husband's urine.

SEXUAL DYSFUNCTION IN WOMEN

Sexual dysfunction in women has not been well investigated. Two studies have confused the situation. Kolodny[22] found that in reviewing about 100 diabetic women and matched controls, 35% of them reported no orgastic response. On the other hand, Ellenberg[23] was unable to document sexual difficulties in a comparable group of women who had principally neuropathic dysfunction.

Diabetic women potentially have three basic sexual difficulties: arousal, painful intercourse, and a non-orgastic response. Diabetic and nondiabetic women are subject to problems related to lack of estrogen at the menopause, and some of these women experience decreased sexual desire or arousal, diminution of vaginal lubrication, and possibly less orgastic response than in the pre-menopausal period.

Diabetic women have an increased likelihood of some dyspareunia from vaginal infections. Monilial infections are more common in diabetic women. These infections are treated with vaginal inserts and creams applied to the vulvar tissue. Likewise, oral or vaginal estrogens should be prescribed when necessary.

The majority of impotent diabetic men are able to achieve orgasm. It would seem, therefore, unlikely that diabetes would significantly affect orgasm in women. Rather, problems might be related to lack of vasocongestion and clitoral engorgement. Methodologies for assessing vaginal and clitoral circulation have not been developed for the study of diabetic women.

The sexual response of women, of course, differs from that of men and appears to involve wider areas of psychologic response in order to achieve sexual satisfaction. With this in mind, the problems of arousal and orgasm might indicate depression in women with any of the chronic problems related to diabetes. However, this particular hypothesis needs further clarification.

It is possible that medications may block sexual function in women, although this has not been studied. Antihypertensives that often block the sympathetic part of the nervous system, theoretically may impede orgastic function. Therefore, when necessary, these medications should be eliminated. Anticholinergic medications block vaginal lubrication, and these may need to be changed or avoided for a time. Antidepressants work through an anticholinergic activity or response, and they may need to be changed if sexual dysfunction is evident. However, it is more likely that depression is the primary cause and should be treated in order to revive sexual function.

REFERENCES

1. Masters, W.H., Johnson, V.E.: Human Sexual Inadequacy. Boston, Little, Brown & Co., 1970.
2. Ibid, Chapter 12, p. 326.
3. Ibid, Chapter 3.
4. Weiss, H.D.: The physiology of human penile erection. Ann. Intern. Med. 76:793, 1972.
5. Faerman, I., Glocer, L., Fox, D., et al.: Impotence and diabetes. Histological studies of the autonomic nervous fibers of the corpora cavernosa in impotent diabetic males. Diabetes 23:971, 1974.
6. Schiavi, R.C., Hogan, B.: Sexual problems in diabetes mellitus: psychological aspects. Diabetes Care 2:9, 1979.
7. Rundles, R.W.: Diabetic neuropathy. Medicine 24:111, 1945.
8. Martin, M.M.: Diabetic neuropathy. A clinical study of 150 cases. Brain 76:594, 1953.
9. Rubin, A., Babbott, D.: Impotence and diabetes mellitus. J.A.M.A. 168:498, 1958.
10. Montenero, P., Donatone, E.: Diabete et activite sexuelle chez l'homme. Le Diabete 10:327, 1962.
11. Schöffling, K., Federlin, K., Ditschuneit, H., Pfeiffer, E.F.: Disorders of sexual function in male diabetics. Diabetes 12:519, 1963.
12. Ellenberg, M.: Impotence in diabetes: the neurologic factor. Ann. Intern. Med. 75:213, 1971.
13. Kolodny, R.C., Kahn, C.B., Goldstein, H.H., Barnett, D.M.: Sexual dysfunction in diabetic men. Diabetes 23:306, 1974.
14. Beaser, R.S., Van der Hoek, C., Jacobson, A.M., et al.: Experience with penile prostheses in the treatment of impotence in diabetic men. J.A.M.A. 248:943, 1982.
14a. Blaivas, J.G., O'Donnell, T.F., Jr., Gottlieb, P., et al.: Measurement of bulbocavernosus reflex latency time as part of a comprehensive evaluation of impotence. In A.W. Zorgniotti, G. Rossi (Eds.): Vasculogenic Impotence. Springfield, Ill., Charles C Thomas, 1980, p. 49.
15. Goldstein, I., Siroky, M.B., Nath, R.I., et al.: Vasculogenic impotence: role of the pelvic steal test. J. Urol. 128:300, 1982.
16. O'Connor, T.W., Scavone, J.M., Jr.: Drug-related sexual dysfunction. Apothecary 94:20, (Jan.) 1982.
17. Karacan, I.: Diagnosis of erectile impotence in diabetes mellitus: an objective and specific method. Ann. Intern. Med. 92:334, 1980.
17a. Ek, A., Bradley, W.E., Krane, R.L.: Snap-gauge band: new concept in measuring penile rigidity. Urology 21:63, 1983.
18. Masters, W.H., Johnson, V.E.: Ref. 1, p. 196.
19. Small, M.P., Carrion, H.M., Gordon, J.A.: Small-Carrion penile prosthesis: new implant for management of impotence. Urology 5:479, 1975.
19a. Krane, R.J., Freedberg, P.S., Siroky, M.B.: Jonas sili-

cone-silver penile prosthesis: initial experience in America. J. Urol. *126*:475, 1981.

19b.McDougal, W.S., Jeffery, R.F.: Microscopic penile revascularization. J. Urol. *129*:517, 1983.

20. Scott, F.B., Bradley, W.B., Timm, G.W.: Management of erectile impotence. Urology *2*:80, 1973.

21. Scott, F.B., Fishman, I.J., Light, J.C.: An inflatable penile prosthesis for treatment of diabetic impotence. Ann. Intern. Med. *92*:340, 1980.

22. Kolodny, R.C.: Sexual dysfunction in diabetic females. Diabetes *20*:557, 1971.

23. Ellenberg, M.: Sexual function in diabetic patients. Ann. Intern. Med. *92*:331, 1980.

33 Pregnancy and Diabetes

John W. Hare

In the pre-insulin era, a few pregnant women with diabetes were treated at the Joslin Clinic with modest success: two-thirds of the mothers and 40% of the infants survived.[1] After insulin became generally available in 1923, a dramatic improvement in maternal survival occurred and a steady improvement in fetal survival began (Table 33–1). In recent decades, maternal mortality has become virtually nonexistent and perinatal mortality now approaches that of normal pregnancies.

PERINATAL MORBIDITY AND MORTALITY

As with success in the treatment of any disease which still lacks a cure, new areas of concern become evident. Neonatal morbidity still afflicts half the infants; hypoglycemia, macrosomia, respiratory distress, hypocalcemia, and hyperbilirubinemia are all common. These complications present great challenges which deserve, and currently are receiving, much attention. Consequently, they will be dealt with at the start of this chapter.

Perinatal Complications

Hypoglycemia has occurred in nearly half of the infants delivered of Joslin Clinic patients and was more common in the more than one-third of the infants affected with macrosomia.[2] It is thought that *macrosomia* may occur because maternal hyperglycemia results in fetal hyperglycemia and stimulation of fetal hyperinsulinemia. Another possible mechanism is the transplacental passage of amino acids released from maternal protein stores[3] which stimulate the fetal islet. Since muscle tissue is quite sensitive to insulin, this offers a possible explanation for the fact that women with mild diabetes and modest hyperglycemia sometimes deliver macrosomic infants. However, precise correlations between maternal hyperglycemia and fetal macrosomia have been difficult to obtain. In the same series of infants,[2] hypocalcemia was present in 22% and hyperbilirubinemia in 19%.

For many years, special attention has been focused on the *respiratory distress syndrome,* a classic complication of infants born to diabetic mothers. Contributing to the prevalence of the syndrome has been premature delivery, induced to prevent intrauterine death in the last weeks of pregnancy. However, even when length of gestation and route of delivery are taken into account statistically, respiratory distress is almost 6 times as common in infants of diabetic as compared with nondiabetic mothers.[4] Thus, maternal diabetes per se predisposes the infant to respiratory complications. We have found the respiratory distress syndrome to occur in 8% and transient tachypnea of the neonate (a milder disorder) in 7% of infants delivered of Joslin Clinic patients; thus 1 of 6 infants is born with some respiratory disorder. This is a marked improvement over the 23.4% frequency of respiratory distress syndrome in Joslin Clinic infants delivered in the same hospital from 1958 to 1968.[4] Similar results have been reported by others for complications in the neonatal period.[5-7] Modern tools for assessment of intrauterine health and fetal lung maturity have allowed this improvement to occur and their use will be discussed below.

Now that most infants survive respiratory distress, a new concern has recently emerged; namely, the number that suffer from *congenital anomalies.* Pedersen comments that in his extensive experience, 40% of perinatal mortality now results from

Table 33–1. **Maternal and Fetal Mortality**

1898–1979
2505 Viable Pregnancies

Dates	Viable Pregnancies	Fetal Survival (%)	Maternal Survival (%)
1898–1910	10	40	67
1924–1938	128	54	}
1938–1958	900	86	} >99
1958–1974	1119	90	}
1975–1976	147	97	}
1977–1979	201	98	} 100

Perinatal Morbidity

1975–1976
147 Viable Pregnancies

Hypoglycemia (47%)	+ + + +
Poor Feeding (37%)	+ + +
Macrosomia (36%)	+ + +
Hypocalcemia (22%)	+ +
Hyperbilirubinemia (19%)	+ +
Respiratory Disease (17%)	+ +
Major Anomalies (9%)	+

congenital malformations.[8] Gabbe et al. note a comparable mortality from congenital malformations.[5] The Joslin Clinic has also experienced a substantial incidence of congenital anomalies, 9% major and 5% minor.[2] Of special note and concern are the relatively large numbers of neural tube and cardiac anomalies. For example, anencephaly and similar anomalies occur in 1 to 2% of all pregnancies treated at the Joslin Clinic.[9,2] The altered availability of substrate, especially glucose, may be operant in the genesis of malformations during early cell division.[10] More recent evidence indicates that ketone bodies, in combination with glucose, potentiate the teratogenic effect of the latter.[10a] For this reason, optimal glycemic control should be sought as soon after conception as possible,[11] or ideally before such.

Maternal Complications

Ketoacidosis, pyelonephritis, and toxemia may occur with increased frequency in diabetic pregnancies. Ketoacidosis often causes fetal demise, especially in the second trimester, and Pedersen has long considered pyelonephritis and toxemia additional threats to the fetus. Microvascular disease may progress during and because of pregnancy.[12] The coexistence of nephropathy with hypertension, proteinuria, and edema makes the diagnosis of preeclampsia difficult, if not impossible. The alterations in maternal metabolism and circulation cause increases in glycosuria and acetonuria so that urine testing requires special attention.

It is generally accepted that meticulous control of diabetes during pregnancy leads to the best outcome for the mother and fetus. After the discovery of pregnancy the mother should be seen weekly by a physician. If a woman seeks counseling prior to pregnancy, she should be encouraged and assisted to achieve the best possible control of diabetes from conception onward. As mentioned above, the fetus is of particular concern, and continued vigilance is required to protect both fetal and maternal health.

Normal fasting and postprandial blood glucose levels are evidence of optimal control. Karlsson and Kjellmer[13] found differences in perinatal mortality associated with the mean glucose level of the mother during the last weeks of pregnancy. In a group with a mean glucose level above 150 mg/dl, the mortality rate was 23.6%; from 100 to 150 mg/dl, the rate was 15.3%; and below 100 mg/dl, it was 3.8%. It should be pointed out that these data were obtained in women hospitalized from week 30 to 32 until delivery. Comparable control in active young out-patients with long-term insulin-dependent diabetes is difficult to achieve. It is desirable to minimize acetonuria, particularly in the third trimester, because this is reported to lower the child's intelligence when examined at age 4.[14] However, this has not been clearly proved.

PHYSIOLOGY OF NORMAL PREGNANCY

When normal pregnant women are fasted, hypoglycemia results, accompanied by brisk mobilization of fat and excretion of urinary ketones. The hypoglycemia is attended by a fall in circulating amino acids needed for gluconeogenesis. The blood glucose rises when alanine, the principal gluconeogenic amino acid, is adminstered.[15] The concept of "accelerated starvation" was first proposed by Freinkel.[16] Subsequent work in his laboratory further delineated the increase of lipid turnover[17] and the substrate deficiency syndrome of lowered amino acids in hypoglycemia.[18] Further investigations have shown that during gluconeogenesis, placental factors conserve nitrogen by decreasing the amount of urea nitrogen which can be reutilized.[19] Since placental lactogen also has a growth hormone-like effect which promotes muscle protein conservation and stimulates lipolysis, it seems that one function of the physiology of normal pregnancy is to promote maternal nitrogen conservation by diversion to fat as a fuel and away from protein. It should also be remembered that the conceptus is able to remove both glucose and amino acids from the maternal circulation. The placenta removes glucose by facilitated diffusion, and amino acids by active transport.[20] It makes teleologic sense for the mother to rely as little as possible on these compounds for substrate.

It is of key importance that extra insulin is needed to maintain proper metabolic balance during normal gravid physiology. The rapid fat turnover is exactly that–turnover–with rapid lipolysis as well as lipogenesis because of the availability of adequate insulin. If the supply of insulin is insufficient, rapid lipolysis and gluconeogenesis result in ketoacidosis. The liver is relatively resistant to insulin during pregnancy.[20] At that time, also, the maternal liver undergoes hypertrophy and hyperplasia and has a greatly enhanced potential for gluconeogenesis and accompanying ketogenesis[21] which must be restrained by adequate insulin.

The reason for increased insulin needs is not entirely known, although placental lactogen probably plays a role. It has been shown to be an insulin antagonist in normal humans.[22] In addition, steroids derived from placenta may alter insulin needs.[23] The placenta is also capable of binding and degrading insulin,[16] although this may not be quantitatively significant. Nonetheless, it is clear that the placenta has a central role in the alterations of metabolism in pregnancy.

Glucagon has been studied extensively in pregnancy because it has known contrainsulin and catabolic properties. It is not responsible for the diabetogenic nature of pregnancy in either gestationally diabetic[24,25] or juvenile diabetic women.[26] In fact, the elevated insulin levels characteristic of pregnancy result in increased insulin:glucagon ratios. It is of interest that following a glucose load, glucagon is more readily suppressed during pregnancy than afterward.[24] It has been suggested that this suppression permits accumulation of ingested fuels and is a feature of "facilitated anabolism" in pregnancy which counterbalances the "accelerated starvation" that occurs when food is withheld.[27] Thus, the mother is able to alternate between periods of enhanced catabolism and anabolism.

One additional normal alteration in the physiology of pregnancy has special relevance for the management of diabetes: cardiac output increases steadily until early in the third trimester. This results in a 30 to 50% increase in glomerular filtration rate. Since glycosuria occurs when the tubular maximum for glucose is exceeded, glucose is found in the urine at lower blood glucose levels than in the nongravid state.[28] Pregnant women with diabetes will find more sugar in the urine even with the same or better control of their disease. Ketones are also cleared readily by the kidney and appear more frequently in the urine for that reason as well as their increased production.

From the foregoing, several cardinal points about diabetic pregnancies emerge:

1. *Additonal insulin is required.* If insufficient beta cell reserve is present in a nondiabetic woman, gestational diabetes results. Women who already have insulin-dependent diabetes require substantially more exogenous insulin. The expected increase is from $1\frac{1}{2}$ to 3 times that of the nonpregnant requirement. Women with microvascular disease may not have a rise in insulin requirement because their placentas are smaller[12] and presumptively have smaller production of contrainsulin factors. It should be noted that placental lactogen cannot be the only factor causing a higher insulin requirement because its levels do not correlate with insulin dose needs.[29]

2. *More carbohydrate and protein must be provided* in the diet because of fetal needs and the ability of the placenta to remove glucose and amino acids from the mother.

3. Cardiorenal changes make glycosuria more prominent, and increased ketogenesis leads to more ketonuria. This makes urine testing more difficult to interpret. Women whose diabetes is well controlled still may have slight glycosuria and occasional ketonuria. Special care must be given to urine testing because physiologic mechanisms lead to an *increased danger of ketoacidosis* if insufficient insulin is present to restrain hepatic gluconeogenesis.

DIAGNOSIS OF THE DIABETIC PREGNANCY

Diabetes occurs in about 1% of pregnant women. Of these, only 1 in 10 will have been known to have had diabetes prior to pregnancy. Thus, the majority of patients with diabetes during pregnancy must have the diagnosis established while pregnant.

A variety of factors (Table 33–2) should alert the physician to the possibility of maternal diabetes. These include a family history of diabetes, obesity, age over 30, glycosuria, or a random plasma glucose level over 120 mg/dl. Perinatal features which should alert the physician to the possibility include a history of stillbirth or congenital anomalies, macrosomia, or polyhydramnios in this pregnancy or a prior one. If diabetes is suspected, a glucose tolerance test should be performed (Table 33–3). However, this is not necessary if fasting or random postprandial glucose levels clearly exceed the postglucose limits of normal shown in Table 33–3. As can be seen from the table, the fasting level is lower in pregnant than in nonpregnant diabetics for reasons discussed earlier. Thereafter, glucose disposal is slowed and the subsequent values are higher than in the nonpregnant diabetic.[30] Table 33–3 also gives plasma values for interpretation of results from laboratories which use this method.

White's Classification

Women who are known to have diabetes prior to pregnancy have been classified by Dr. Priscilla White into categories that are delineated by duration of diabetes and the presence of complications (Table 33–4). The classification has been more recently revised in order to separately consider gestational diabetes.[30a] Several points deserve comment. It is rare that insulin therapy is not required in a woman who is known to have diabetes before

pregnancy (i.e. not gestational). She is a Class A diabetic. When insulin is needed, she moves from Class A to B (or even Class C in the unusual circumstance of onset of diabetes under age 20). More typically, women with Class B or C diabetes have insulin-dependent diabetes, the age at onset or duration determining the class. The development of ketosis-prone insulin-dependent diabetes during, but not because of, pregnancy, results in assignment of class according to the patient's age. Longer term or younger onset diabetes is Class D. In addition, the presence of background retinopathy or hypertension places the patient in Class D, proliferative retinopathy or vitreous hemorrhage in Class R, significant proteinuria (greater than 500 mg/24 hrs) in Class F, and atherosclerotic heart disease in Class H. All of the categorizations based on complications are independent of the duration of diabetes or age at onset. The development during pregnancy of any of these complications changes the class.

Historically, the classification was used because of the higher likelihood of fetal morbidity and mortality with longer duration of diabetes or diabetes complicated by vascular disease. More recent experience has blurred fetal outcome as a distinguishing feature of the classes except for Class F.[31] Maternal outcome is affected only by Class H.[1] Class

Table 33–2. Risk Factors for Diabetes in Pregnancy

Maternal Features	Perinatal Features
Family history of diabetes	History of stillbirth
Obesity	History of congenital anomalies
Age over 30	Macrosomia before or presently
Glycosuria	
Random plasma glucose ≥120 mg/dl	Polyhydramnios before or presently

Table 33–3. Glucose Tolerance Test in Pregnancy*

	(Upper Limits of Normal)	
Time	Whole Blood (mg/dl)	Plasma (mg/dl)
Fasting	90	105
1 hr	165	190
2 hr	145	165
3 hr	125	145

*Taken in part from O'Sullivan and Mahan.[29a]

Table 33–4. Classification of Priscilla White

Gestational Diabetes	Abnormal GTT, but euglycemia maintained by diet alone
	Diet alone insufficient, insulin required
Class A	Diet alone, any duration or onset age
Class B	Onset age 20 or older and duration less than 10 years
Class C	Onset age 10–19 or duration 10–19 years
Class D	Onset age under 10 or duration over 20 years or background retinopathy or hypertension (not pre-eclampsia)
Class R	Proliferative retinopathy or vitreous hemorrhage
Class F	Nephropathy with over 500 mg/day proteinuria
Class RF	Criteria for both classes R and F coexist
Class H	Atherosclerotic heart disease clinically evident
Class T	Prior renal transplantation

All classes below A require insulin therapy. Note that Class D may be assigned even if onset/duration criteria are not met, e.g. background retinopathy. Classes R, F, RF, H and T have no onset/duration criteria but usually occur in long term diabetes.

E (calcification of pelvic vessels) has been dropped from the table because current practice proscribes pelvic x-rays during pregnancy. Class G (adverse obstetrical history) is no longer used. Class T has been added because of case reports of women bearing children after renal transplantation.[32,32a]

Gestational Diabetes

The White classification was intended for women whose insulin-dependent diabetes began prior to pregnancy. It is best to consider women with gestational diabetes apart from these. Gestational diabetes is a disorder arising because of the contrainsulin effects of pregnancy and would ordinarily not be insulin-dependent were it not for fetal considerations.[33] This condition may not become apparent until late in pregnancy because the diabetogenic effect is progressive from the end of the first until late in the third trimester. Most nondiabetic women have a 2-hour postprandial blood glucose value of less than 110 mg/dl during pregnancy and a fasting blood glucose of less than 90 mg/dl. If diabetes is suspected and a second trimester glucose tolerance test is normal, such a test should be repeated in the third. The discovery of gestational diabetes should prompt immediate dietary therapy. If this does not maintain postprandial blood glucose levels in the normal range, insulin therapy should be instituted.

In the strictest sense of the term, women with gestational diabetes should not require treatment after delivery, although a few may. Some of these women may have had latent diabetes which became manifest during pregnancy; others may have had mild diabetes, undiagnosed until pregnancy brought them under scrutiny. In the absence of data obtained when not pregnant, the diagnosis of gestational diabetes may be presumed but cannot be firmly established.

EFFECTS OF PREGNANCY ON THE INDIVIDUAL WITH DIABETES

Young diabetic women contemplating pregnancy, or who are already pregnant, are frequently concerned about the development of visual loss or renal failure.

Retinopathy

Neovascularization on the disc of the eye (proliferative retinopathy) may well progress to loss of vision.[34] If possible, pregnancy should be delayed when this condition is present. If such neovascularization is discovered early in pregnancy, interruption of the pregnancy may be considered. Previously photocoagulated proliferative retinopathy in a quiescent state has a good prognosis during pregnancy, often remaining quiescent. Neovascularization not on the disc, which antedates or occurs during the pregnancy, has far less serious visual prognosis than that on the disc. Nonproliferative (background) retinopathy has a low risk of progression to proliferative retinopathy and is not a cause for alarm. Background retinopathy often becomes more prominent during pregnancy and regresses post partum. Patients with any degree of retinopathy should be seen by an ophthalmologist for examination and fundus photography. They may be seen once or twice more during the pregnancy in routine follow-up, and much more frequently if necessary.

Nephropathy

If renal disease is not present prior to pregnancy, it will not develop.[12] Since retinopathy generally precedes nephropathy, the absence of retinal changes is particularly reassuring. The presence of significant proteinuria ($\geq$ 500 mg/24 hr) before or early in pregnancy is a cause for concern, even if the serum creatinine is normal. Dense proteinuria of 5 to 10 g per day may develop, often accompanied by hypertension and marked edema.[31] These women require weeks of bed rest at home or in the hospital from midpregnancy onward, which precludes employment or care of other children. When pregnancy counseling is sought and proteinuria is found, the patient should be forewarned. If proteinuria is discovered in a urine specimen early in pregnancy, a 24-hour urine test for protein and creatinine clearance should be obtained then and at monthly intervals thereafter. Worsening renal function evidenced by increased proteinuria, and particularly by declining creatinine clearance, requires a trial of modified bed rest at home. This can be done by minimizing activity and resting in bed for 2 hours morning and afternoon. Hypertension often accompanies nephropathy and can also be treated with bed rest. Diuretics are not ordinarily used in pregnancy because their volume constricting effect may worsen pre-eclampsia.[35] If stabilization of renal function or hypertension cannot be accomplished on an out-patient basis, then hospitalization of the patient becomes imperative, often for lengthy periods and sometimes throughout the remainder of the pregnancy.

If the serum creatinine is normal but the creatinine clearance is diminished, the above sequence is even more likely to develop. The clearance may not change or may even decline during pregnancy, instead of rising as it does in normal pregnant women. Pregnancy probably does not hasten the development of renal failure, but once renal failure is present, it proceeds inexorably. At this point, the natural history of renal failure is such that consideration of dialysis or renal transplantation is not far behind.[36] A serum creatinine level of 3.0 mg/dl is usually incompatible with fetal life.[37]

Neuropathy

Neuropathy may develop or progress during pregnancy but it is usually not a serious problem. Neuropathic ulceration of the feet is rare. Paresthesias are the most common neuropathic manifestation and usually require only reassurance. If necessary, analgesics may be given. Autonomic neuropathy manifested by gastropathy may worsen nausea. Frequent small meals often contribute to the patient's comfort and regulation of the diabetes.

Ketoacidosis

The metabolic alterations of pregnancy place the diabetic woman at particular risk for this hazard which often results in loss of the fetus. Careful attention to the regulation of diabetes is imperative, and in our patients has reduced the incidence of ketoacidosis to less than 5%.[2] Persistent glycosuria and ketonuria, especially if associated with nausea or polydipsia and polyuria, should be immediately brought to the physician's attention. Since ketoacidosis can develop in less than 24 hours during pregnancy, there should be no delay in seeking help.

EFFECTS OF DIABETES ON THE PREGNANCY

Several complications of pregnancy occur more commonly in diabetic women. The physician must be alert to their development.

Spontaneous Abortion. The rate of spontaneous abortion in women with diabetes is no greater than in the general population of pregnant women without diabetes. Fertility may be impaired if diabetes is so poorly controlled as to result in amenorrhea. However, once pregnant, no additional risk of early loss is imposed by the diabetes.

Urinary Tract Infection. The mechanical changes in renal drainage brought about by the enlarging uterus cause stasis and increased risk of pyelonephritis. Asymptomatic bacteriuria should be treated. Pyelonephritis may precipitate ketoacidosis and is itself considered by Pedersen[8] to be a prognostically bad sign. Urinary tract infections in nondiabetic women are known to adversely affect perinatal mortality, especially if maternal hypertension or acetonuria is present.[38] Obviously, these complications may also occur in diabetic women.

Headache. A few women develop severe headaches which require hospitalization and/or narcotic therapy. Complaints of headache should be promptly treated with potent analgesics if necessary to prevent progression to a degree of severity requiring hospitalization.

Preeclampsia. Preeclampsia has historically been a frequent complication of diabetic pregnancy[12] with poor prognosis for the fetus.[8] More recent experience has found the frequency of this complication to be only slightly higher than in the nondiabetic population.[5] Our Class F patients with nephropathy, edema, and hypertension are not generally considered to have preeclampsia. A program of modified bed rest at home is instituted if preeclampsia is suspected. Failure to normalize blood pressure necessitates hospitalization.

Polyhydramnios. Polyhydramnios occurs in a third of our patients. It is more common in diabetic women and not related to congenital anomalies. There is a suspicion that hyperglycemia is related to polyhydramnios and that better control of diabetes lessens the incidence. Since it is generally agreed that optimal control leads to the best outcome, no different approach is needed. Premature labor precipitated by polyhydramnios is the most serious complication.

Stillbirth. Death of the fetus in the last weeks of pregnancy is the classic obstetrical accident in the diabetic mother. It is not related to the severity or duration of diabetes because it occurs also in women with gestational diabetes treated with diet alone. It has indirectly been a cause of many fetal deaths because many women have been delivered prematurely to avoid a late loss of the infant. The cause remains an enigma. It appears to be metabolic since anatomic abnormalities of the fetus and placenta need not be present. Recent technical advances in assessing intrauterine health have reduced the incidence of stillbirth. Concomitantly, pregnancy is allowed to continue longer to avoid the respiratory complications of prematurity.

The Placenta. Placentas from diabetic mothers tend to be heavier than those from nondiabetic mothers with fetuses at the same gestational age and weight. In women with renal disease (Class F), the placenta is often smaller, not unlike those from women with nondiabetic renal disease. Placentas from diabetic mothers have large cellular congested villae. Chronic vascular thrombosis is common. Decidual vessels have arteriolar hyalinization in half the specimens and fibrinoid change and lipid deposition in the intima of larger vessels in one fifth.[39]

MANAGEMENT

Team Approach. A clear and steady improvement in outcome of diabetic pregnancies is reported by centers with skilled specialty consultants available. Ideal therapy requires a diabetologist, perinatologist, neonatologist, and obstetrician functioning as a team in close communication. If such help is not available, a team comprising an obstetrician, an internist, and a pediatrician should be constituted. An occasional solo success with diabetic pregnancy should not lead the practitioner to complacency. Even without a specialized team, loss rates are generally low, so that a perinatal mortality of 20% may escape notice when only a few patients a year are seen. In Table 33–5, the management of the pregnant diabetic woman is given in outline form from the first trimester through delivery and post partum.

First Trimester

Initial Examination. At the first visit, the internist should obtain a history of the duration and any complications of diabetes in the past. The physical examination should particularly seek evidence of complications of diabetes. Regardless of the findings on funduscopic examination, it is our practice to have an ophthalmologic examination done within a few weeks of the first visit. The obstetrical examination is important to confirm the dates of the pregnancy. Both physicians should be available to answer any questions that the patient may have.

Table 33–5. Management of Pregnancy in Diabetic Women

History and Physical (H&P)	Management Maneuvers	Laboratory
First Trimester		
Full H&P with special attention to diabetes and its complications. Refer to ophthalmologist if any retinopathy is present.	Calculation of and instruction in diet, instruction in home blood glucose monitoring, urine testing, and use of glucagon. Give iron and vitamins.	CBC, cholesterol, liver functions, uric acid, electrolytes, Rubella titer, blood group, antibodies, urine culture, 24-hour urine protein and creatinine clearance if proteinuria is present.
Weekly blood pressure, weight, funduscopic examination. Note edema if any.	Adjust insulin dose—often slightly less needed. Treat nausea. Emphasize need for regular home blood glucose testing. Review test results.	Weekly blood and urine glucose. Monthly Hb_{Alc}
Second Trimester		
Weekly blood pressure, weight, funduscopic examination. Note edema if any. Examination by ophthalmologist if retinopathy is present.	Anticipate rising insulin dose and change in complexity of insulin pattern—night dose and/or pre-meal regular may be needed. Review results of home blood glucose tests.	Weekly blood and urine glucose. Continue monthly Hb_{Alc}. Check for pyuria. Monthly 24-hr urine protein and creatinine clearance if proteinuria is present. Serum alpha fetoprotein. Ultrasound examination by week 20.
Third Trimester		
Weekly blood pressure, weight, funduscopic examination. Note edema if any. Examination by ophthalmologist if retinopathy is present.	Diabetes more stable. Continued rise in insulin dose until week 34–36; may then need decreased dose. Review results of home blood glucose tests.	Ultrasound examination. Weekly blood and urine glucose. Continue monthly Hb_{Alc}. Monthly 24-hr urine protein and creatinine clearance if proteinuria is present. Institute weekly NST* and E_3† at 32 weeks.
	Bed rest at home or hospital for edema, hypertension or declining renal function.	Weekly or twice weekly NST*, daily E_3 and urine glucose. Amniocentesis for L:S.‡ Several times daily blood glucose and urine.
	Hospitalize at 37–38 wks. Normal blood glucose preferred.	
Day of Delivery		
	One-third *pre-pregnancy* insulin dose in A.M. I.V. D5W§ at 125 ml/hr for labor or late cesarean section. Cautious use of insulin.	Blood glucose in A.M., in Recovery Room, and in P.M.
Postpartum		
Presence of anorexia or nausea, fever, or symptoms of infection.	Gradual increase of insulin dose and advancement of diet over 3–7 days if section done. If nursing, diet similar to pregnancy used.	Several times daily blood and urine glucose. Check for lactosuria. Urine culture if needed.
4–6 Weeks Postpartum		
Should have returned to full health and normal weight.	Adjust insulin dose. Continue iron if needed. Treat hypertension if present.	Blood and urine glucose. Follow-up of any earlier abnormalities in renal function.

*NST = Nonstress Test
†E_3 = Estriol
‡L:S ratio = Lecithin-sphyngomyelin ratio
§D5W = 5% Dextrose in water

Ideally, if the internist has followed the patient and knows of her desire to bear children, she should receive counseling in advance of conception.

Laboratory Studies. Tests done at the first visit should include an estimation of renal function, a urinalysis, and screening culture. If proteinuria is present, a 24-hour urine test for protein and creatinine clearance should be obtained. Significant bacteriuria should be treated with an appropriate antibiotic. Other determinations include hemoglobin or hematocrit, liver function tests, cholesterol, uric acid, electrolytes, rubella titer, and blood group antibody screening titers. Also needed is the institution of monthly determinations of hemoglobin A_{1c} to assist in evaluating metabolic control.

Patient Instruction. It is helpful to give the patient written information about her pregnancy, what to expect, what to be alert for, and whom to call if trouble arises. A printed sheet handed to pregnant patients at the Joslin Clinic, outlines maternal and fetal complications and lists pertinent telephone numbers for the hospitals, physicians, and obstetricians involved in her care. Some patients will require skilled psychologic and social service support to cope with the demands imposed by the pregnancy and its care.

At the first visit, the patient should receive instruction in diet, home glucose monitoring, urine testing, and use of glucagon if prescribed.

In the last few years *home glucose monitoring* has become the cornerstone of management. This may be done with a reflectance meter which utilizes glucose oxidase impregnated strips to measure capillary blood. A meter is not an absolute necessity, however, because sufficient accuracy can be obtained by the use of strips which are read by visual estimation.

Urine should be tested for glucose by the two-drop Clinitest method which permits determination of up to 5% glycosuria. Any specimen with more than 2% glycosuria should be tested for acetone. It is often helpful to test a morning specimen if aglycosuric, to see if overnight fasting has produced more than small amounts of acetone. If so, an additional carbohydrate snack at bedtime may help. If acetonuria is frequently present during the day, added carbohydrate and insulin may be given. Because many patients have great difficulty with insulin reactions, the use of glucagon may prove useful. Those women whose diabetes was quite stable before pregnancy usually do not need glucagon but those who have had unstable diabetes prior to pregnancy generally will. As a precautionary measure, another member of the household must be instructed in the indications for and actual use of glucagon.

Diet. By the end of pregnancy, a woman should have gained 10 to 15 kg, or about 25 pounds. The first trimester should result in a gain of 5 pounds or less, but a steady increase of about a pound a week should occur thereafter. The total caloric requirement is approximately 35 calories per kg of body weight, which can be met by the addition of about 300 calories per day to the diet prescribed prior to pregnancy.[40] Obese women need fewer calories, and the diet can be calculated on the basis of ideal body weight. Weight reduction should not be attempted during pregnancy. Because of first trimester nausea and third trimester uterine enlargement, some women will eat less at the beginning and end of pregnancy, but more in the middle. Since the fetus extracts glucose and amino acid, adequate carbohydrate and protein must be provided. Carbohydrate should make up 45–50% of the total calories needed. Most pregnant women require 200 or more grams of carbohydrate daily. The amount of protein should be 1.5 g/kg of body weight, and the remainder of calories should be fat. The expected calcium need of over a gram a day is best met with a quart of milk or its equivalent as cheese. If dairy products are not used, supplemental calcium may be given. Multivitamins, customarily containing folic acid, are usually prescribed. If considered necessary by the physician, folic acid, 0.5–1.0 mg daily, may be given as a supplement. Most women cannot meet their own and fetal needs for iron, so that supplements of this element are commonly used.

Insulin. The first trimester is often characterized by instability of the diabetes and frequent reactions. The insulin requirement may decline in the first trimester by 10%. Weekly blood and urine determinations of glucose and a record of insulin reactions and their time of occurrence, will assist in regulating the insulin dose.

The pattern of subcutaneous insulin administration may change during pregnancy, depending upon individual needs. Pattern I is a single dose of intermediate-acting insulin given daily before breakfast. Pattern II is a mixture of regular and intermediate insulins, also given before breakfast. Pattern III is a pre-breakfast mixture plus a dose of intermediate insulin given at supper or bedtime. Pattern IV is a mixture of regular and intermediate insulins given both pre-breakfast and pre-supper. Many women who require a Pattern I or II program before pregnancy will require a Pattern IV by the end of gestation. A gestational diabetic may be considered as beginning with a Pattern O. She will often progress to a Pattern II or III requirement. After the patient delivers, her insulin pattern usually reverts to its previous nonpregnant state.

The current standard of ideal control for pregnant

women with insulin-dependent diabetes requires daily fasting capillary values to be 100 mg/dl or less and postprandial capillary glucose levels to be 140 mg/dl or less. In addition, a monthly hemoglobin A_{1c} should be less than 7% (normal 4 to 6%). It is not possible to achieve this degree of excellent control in all women with Type I diabetes. In some, the disease is so unstable that an attempt at stringent management will result in incapacitating insulin reactions. Most patients, however, are able to do so if they and their physicians are well motivated.

We have had success with open loop *insulin infusion pumps* during all stages of pregnancy. They are safe and effective when used with home blood glucose monitoring. Considerable effort on the part of the patient is needed to operate the pump, follow the diet, and measure blood glucose. If a pump is not available or not desired, comparable effort with conventional insulin administration will probably give comparable results.

Sex Steroids. Female sex steroids have not been used at the Joslin Clinic since 1975. They were given to fill in a possible short supply of endogenous estrogen and progesterone being produced by a diseased placenta. Since the abortion rate is no higher in diabetic pregnancies than in nondiabetic, our present perinatal survival is comparable to that in other centers.[5,41] Because estrogen administration has been linked to vaginal carcinoma in female offspring of treated mothers, the use of these steroids no longer seems justified. However, we are thus far unaware of any case of vaginal carcinoma in the female progeny of our patients.

Second Trimester

The second trimester is a time of equanimity for the patient and physician. The risk of spontaneous abortion has passed, the diabetes becomes more stable, and troublesome nausea abates.

Weekly ophthalmologic examinations by the internist continue. If any question of significant change arises, the patient should be examined by the ophthalmologist who saw her in the first trimester. If necessary, photocoagulation with the laser can be safely performed at any time in pregnancy.

The urine should be re-examined, and if pyuria or bacteriuria is present, another urine culture should be done. If proteinuria was present before pregnancy, monthly monitoring of creatinine clearance and 24-hour protein should have been established.

Insulin. During the second trimester, although not always in the first weeks, as the unstable pattern of diabetes ameliorates, a progressive rise in the insulin requirement begins. The dose may not need to be increased each week, but by the end of the

trimester, a rise will have been noted. This change in physiology is probably related to the dominance of placental contrainsulin factors over fetal siphonage of substrate.[20] Because of the emergence of marked alterations in metabolism effected by the placenta, the risk of ketoacidosis increases. Continued vigilance and communication with the patient are necessary. By this time, regular urine testing should be a firmly established routine.

Special Tests. At the beginning of the second trimester, a serum alpha fetoprotein level should be determined. This is helpful but not unequivocal in excluding open neural tube defects. Early in the second trimester and before the 20th week, an ultrasonographic determination should be performed. It is important to date the pregnancy accurately, and this is an ideal time to do so. Furthermore, anencephaly, if present, is invariably detected as are occasionally more subtle but severe anomalies such as myomeningocele.

Third Trimester

Throughout the third trimester, regular monitoring of ophthalmologic and renal status and diabetes management should continue. If, during the progression of pregnancy hypertension, marked edema or proteinuria has developed, a program of modified bed rest at home may need to be instituted. As previously stated, 2 hours of lying on the left side, morning and afternoon, is helpful. Declining renal function may necessitate hospitalization and complete bed rest. With some women, this will have been necessary from late in the second trimester.

A second ultrasound test at the beginning of the third trimester documents fetal growth and confirms the dating obtained earlier. The best time for this is in the 28th to 30th week. A third ultrasound is done at 36 weeks to assess fetal size (macrosomia).

Insulin. The progressive rise in insulin requirement continues until about the 34th to 36th week. The diabetes becomes quite stable relative to its pre-pregnancy state. After delivery it will revert to its prior non-pregnant level of stability.[42] During this period, optimal control can be obtained because the likelihood of an insulin reaction is much less. The insulin dose can be increased to achieve near ideal postprandial glycemia. The patient's diabetes responds similarly to that of an obese person, with relative resistance to insulin and rare hypoglycemic reactions.

The requirement for insulin may decline substantially in the last weeks of pregnancy. Before present-day methods were available for assessing fetal health, and modest declines in insulin requirement were viewed with apprehension, a 50% fall in dose was considered an urgent sign of fetal distress. The physician should be reassured that a 25% decline in insulin requirement is not unusual today. The reason for this alteration is not known, but may represent the converse of the placental-fetal relationship mentioned earlier. Placental growth levels off late in pregnancy, but fetal growth does not, so that fetal removal of substrate increases relative to placental factors. Maternal early satiety (because of abdominal distension) may also contribute, particularly if polyhydramnios is present.

Antepartum Fetal Heart Rate Testing. Antepartum monitoring of the fetal heart rate has notably decreased the incidence of fetal mortality. One standard method has been the Oxytocin Challenge Test (OCT). A small amount of oxytocin, sufficient to cause uterine contractions, is infused into the mother. The resulting hypoxia is easily withstood by a healthy fetus; an unhealthy one decreases its heart rate after a contraction (late deceleration). This is a positive test and gives cause for urgent concern. A negative test provides a greater than 99% likelihood that no fetal demise will occur in the following week.[5,43] An equivocal test should be repeated.

More recently, the nonstress test (NST) has been devised. In this instance, no oxytocin is given. The fetal heart and movement are monitored. The presence of baseline variation in the heart rate and acceleration after movement, are termed a reactive test. This assurance of fetal well-being for the following week is nearly equivalent to that of a negative OCT.[44]

A weekly out-patient NST should be instituted at the 32nd week. Good results permit the mother to remain at home with safety, often for a longer period of time than was considered safe before the availability of these procedures. Once hospitalized, weekly tests are continued to assure the safety of waiting. Delivery may be elected when the lungs are mature, and needless premature delivery is avoided.

Estriol. The fetal adrenal gland produces a steroid precursor which is converted to estriol (E_3) in the placenta, conjugated in the maternal liver, and ultimately renally excreted. Substantial amounts of estriol are not found in nonpregnant women. The quantity may be measured in plasma or a 24-hour urine collection. Simultaneous measurement of the 24-hour urine creatinine permits the use of E_3: creatinine ratio to correct for variances in completeness of collection. A significant drop (usually 50% when compared to the mean level of the 3 previous days) indicates an acute failure in the system, presumably the fetal-placental unit. A fall in estriol may occur without fetal distress and the NST helps to decide if the decline was a false-positive one.

A non-reactive NST in conjunction with a falling estriol level virtually demands immediate delivery.

It is obvious from the foregoing that, to be of any value, estriol determinations must be done daily and results promptly reported. A report of a precipitous fall in estriol is of little help the day after fetal demise. If laboratory results cannot be secured in less than a day, it is pointless to order estriol determinations. Moreover, there is an increasing tendency to rely more on the NST and less on the measurement of estriol. Ultrasonographic assessment of specific fetal movements (Biophysical Profile) is gaining credence as an adjunct to the NST in some centers.

At the Joslin Clinic, weekly out-patient determinations are done from the 32nd week in 24-hour urine collections to establish each individual's excretion pattern, since there is considerable variation in normal values. Some women, particularly those with renal disease, are "chronic low excretors," and it is helpful to know this prior to hospitalization. Intrauterine growth retardation is also associated with low levels of urine excretion.

Gestational Diabetes in the Third Trimester. A particularly common problem encountered by physicians is the discovery of gestational diabetes well into the third trimester. The presence of the previously mentioned risk factors should prompt evaluation for diabetes, even if it had not been detected earlier, because the diabetogenic effect of pregnancy is maximal in the third trimester. Discovery of diabetes should call for immediate institution of dietary therapy. This may be done on an out- or in-patient basis. Plasma glucose should be controlled to levels below 105 mg/dl fasting and 120 mg/dl at 2 hours after a meal. If this degree of control is achieved, nothing more need be done until 40 weeks' gestation. At that time, if spontaneous labor has not occurred, the patient should be admitted and a fetal monitoring regimen instituted. If satisfactory control is not achieved with diet alone, insulin should be given. This may also be done on an out- or in-patient basis. After good control is achieved with insulin, the best course of management depends on the judgment and experience of the physician. It may be prudent to admit such patients at 38 weeks, although some physicians allow them to stay out of the hospital until 40 weeks has been reached.

Hospitalization. For many years a progressive risk to the fetus was noted with increasing duration or lower age at onset of diabetes. Because of this, the classification of Priscilla White was developed and subsequently widely adopted. In recent years, the relative risk between classes has become less distinct except for Class F (and probably H and T). The previous need for progressively earlier hospital admissions in categories B to D, is not now indicated. Most patients can be admitted safely between the 37th and 38th weeks and then often carried to the 38th or 39th week before delivery, if all indicators of fetal health are favorable. If the mother's diabetes is under ideal control, often admission can be delayed until week 38. If there is any question about maternal or fetal well-being, admission at 36 weeks is prudent.

Upon hospitalization, routine laboratory work should be done. The diabetes is managed with the benefit of several daily blood glucose and urine glucose determinations. Weekly or even biweekly NSTs should be continued and daily estriol determinations instituted.

Fetal Lung Maturity. Amniocentesis is performed soon after hospitalization. The fluid is analyzed for the lecithin-sphyngomyelin ratio (L:S ratio). When the lungs are mature and surfactant is present, lecithin is present in a concentration several-fold higher than sphyngomyelin. In most women, a ratio of 2:1 indicates that delivery may be carried out safely. However, in diabetic women, an added margin of safety is desired. Some infants will develop respiratory difficulty even though the L:S ratio indicates maturity. We have found a ratio of over 3.5:1 to be best.[2] There are variations in methodology and normal values in different laboratories. The L:S level considered safe in a particular laboratory for nondiabetic women, should be increased somewhat for diabetic women. An immature ratio is reason to wait several more days or a week to allow further lung development, provided that antepartum monitoring of the fetal heart and appropriate estriol levels allow the delay. Amniocentesis may be repeated one or more times if necessary, until lung maturity has been established.

The L:S ratio is currently in wide use. However, there are other substances present in amniotic fluid whose measurements may prove more reliable than the L:S ratio. As newer tests (e.g., saturated phosphatidyl choline) are validated and become generally available, they will probably supplant the L:S ratio.[45]

Management of Delivery

The decision as to timing and route of delivery is within the province of the obstetrician. If fetal health is good, the lungs are mature, and the cervix is favorable, induction is preferred. If induction cannot be accomplished, cesarean section must be performed. An elective cesarean section should be done in the morning to facilitate management of the diabetes. If proliferative retinopathy is present, cesarean section may be preferable to labor to avert the risk of vitreous hemorrhage which sometimes results from labor, and particularly from difficult

labor. The advice of an ophthalmologist may be necessary in this regard. If fetal distress supervenes, a cesarean section may be done even though the lungs are immature. The current level of neonatal care usually makes possible infant survival even if respiratory distress occurs.

Insulin. On the day of delivery, an exquisite sensitivity to insulin is present. The usual dose requirement on the day of delivery or first postpartum day is less than half the *pre-pregnancy* dose. In anticipation of delivery, a small amount of intermediate insulin should be given in the morning. An early morning cesarean section necessitates only normal saline as an intravenous fluid. If the operation is not to be performed until later in the day, dextrose should be infused intravenously at a rate of at least 5 g per hour. Other intravenous solutions are less desirable because they do not provide needed carbohydrate. Lactate is converted to glucose if gluconeogenesis is active, but Ringer's lactate solution provides less than optimal amounts of carbohydrate. A blood glucose determination should be obtained in the Recovery Room. Levels are often elevated because of the stress of delivery and additional intravenous fluids administered by the anesthesiologist. Modest doses of insulin may be given if the blood glucose is quite high, but levels tend to decline spontaneously several hours after delivery. Regular insulin requires particularly judicious use. If induction is attempted, the insulin dose should be reduced in anticipation of delivery. Even if induction fails, the mother may not require supplementary insulin because factors operative in active labor reduce the need for insulin. Some women will not return to their usual insulin requirement until the 2nd day after attempted induction.

An alternative method of management is to infuse intravenously the insulin as well as the glucose. The initial rate of insulin infusion is 1 to 2 units per hour and is adjusted based on hourly determinations of blood glucose. The infusion may be started early in the day and continued until the infant is delivered.

Postpartum Care

The Infant. At the time of delivery, the infant should be taken by the pediatrician and immediately placed in the Special Care nursery. Hypoglycemia is extremely common and is a consequence of fetal hyperinsulinemia.[46] It may occur in the 1st hour of life and must be actively sought because the infant may be lethargic rather than irritable as one might expect. A regimen of early feeding helps. After the 1st or 2nd day of life, it is unlikely to occur. As the risk of hypoglycemia abates, the pediatrician must be alert for tachypnea or respiratory distress, hypocalcemia, hyperbilirubinemia, and poor feeding. An examination for congenital anomalies should be done during the 1st day of life. If the infant is healthy and feeding well, it may be taken from the Special Care nursery after 1 or 2 days.

The Mother. Following a pelvic delivery, the mother may eat the same day. After a cesarean section, standard postoperative management with intravenous fluids is used. A progressive diet is instituted over the next several days. The initial content will necessarily be high in carbohydrate, because protein and fat are difficult to provide in liquid or soft diets. The low insulin requirement on the first day postpartum will slowly increase at a variable rate over the next few days. Because of the variable return to the pre-pregnancy requirement for insulin, frequent blood glucose determinations are needed. Urine should be checked with a glucose oxidase method as well as Clinitest to insure that significant lactosuria is not causing an overestimation of glycosuria. Most women will reach their pre-pregnancy insulin requirement by 1 week postpartum. Caution is necessary in the first 3 postpartum days to avoid hypoglycemia because of continued insulin sensitivity. Maternal growth hormone response is blunted in the immediate puerperium[47] and this is suggested as a cause for the insulin sensitivity. The abrupt withdrawal of placental hormones in the transition to the non-gravid state may induce other mechanisms. Whatever the precise cause, this clinical feature of parturition in the diabetic mother must be borne in mind. Since the 3rd trimester dose of insulin is quite high and the immediate postpartum requirement is only a fraction of the pre-pregnancy dose, the change in amount of insulin from the last day of pregnancy to the first nonpregnant day, is marked.

Nursing. If the mother is nursing, a diet similar to the pregnancy diet is needed to provide for the caloric needs of the growing infant. Although these demands are larger than those of a fetus, the diet need not be increased because the mother utilizes her physiologically acquired fat stores from the pregnancy.[40] Calcium should be supplemented in the form of a quart of milk daily. Iron supplementation is needed for 2 or 3 months, whether or not the mother is nursing. Because the infant is in a Special Care nursery, a breast pump is needed to maintain milk flow. There is no reason why diabetic mothers cannot nurse, although early delivery may make it difficult or impossible because milk formation is inadequate at that time.

When metabolic balance for the mother has been reached and recovery from delivery has occurred,

she may be discharged. This should occur by the 5th to 7th postpartum day.

At the postpartum check-up 4 to 6 weeks after delivery, the internist can ascertain the correctness of the insulin dose prescribed at discharge, and assess the status of any diabetic complications which may have been present. Renal function may need to be measured. Hypertension, if present, is treated in a standard fashion (i.e. diuretics may be used).

GENETIC COUNSELING

Parents may seek genetic counseling prior to a pregnancy or after delivery if an anomaly was present. The most commonly asked questions relate to the development of diabetes in the offspring. Many women with diabetes express reluctance to bear a child with a high likelihood of developing diabetes at an early age. Certainly, the presence of maternal diabetes increases the risk of its occurrence in the offspring. If the father or his immediate relatives have diabetes as well, the risk is even higher. However, it is not nearly as high as previously believed. If only maternal diabetes is present, the child has a less than 10% probability of developing diabetes. Even if both parents have diabetes, the likelihood of diabetes developing in the child is perhaps only 1 in 3. Although there is some tendency for the type of diabetes present in a parent to be passed to a child, many children in this group actually have a milder, insulin-independent type of diabetes. Also reassuring to prospective parents is the recognition that juvenile-onset diabetes is less genetically determined than is the maturity-onset type,[48] although the child's risk of development of diabetes is clearly higher than that of the population at large.

CONGENITAL ANOMALIES

The rate of development of congenital anomalies is more disturbing. With modern techniques in neonatology, congenital anomalies are emerging as the principal cause of death in diabetic pregnancy.[5,8] Those infants who do not have anomalies incompatible with life may face corrective surgery and life-long deformity. The incidence of serious anomalies in children of diabetic mothers, whether compatible or incompatible with life, demands that the mother be informed regarding this possibility at the outset of the pregnancy.

The occurrence of anomalies is more likely to be related to the metabolic milieu in early pregnancy than to genetic determinants. The crucial period of teratogenesis for the common anomalies in infants of diabetic mothers occurs within 9 weeks of the last menstrual period (within 7 weeks following conception[49]). For this reason, excellent control of diabetes is important in the earliest possible weeks of pregnancy, or preceding pregnancy if possible.

We have studied a group of insulin-dependent diabetic women in the 1st trimester, divided into a better controlled half and a more poorly controlled half, as determined by the hemoglobin A_{1c} level carried out before 14 weeks' gestation. The better controlled half had an anomaly rate of 3% (very near that of the general population). The more poorly controlled half had an anomaly rate of 22%, accounting for most of the malformations and all of the mortalities.[11]

Of particular concern is the frequency of neural tube defects.[50] Serum or amniotic fluid alpha fetoprotein level aids in discovering these defects early in pregnancy. Sensitive ultrasonographic technique often will identify a neural tube anomaly and is a helpful adjunct when the defect is closed and the alpha fetoprotein level is not elevated. If a mother has an infant with a neural tube defect, the likelihood of recurrence in a later pregnancy is increased but still low. The only exception is the autosomal recessive Meckel syndrome (occipital encephalocele, facial, genitourinary, and extremity anomalies). Rarely, chromosomal lesions will produce neural tube defects. If this has been the case, early amniocentesis for chromosomal studies is indicated in successive pregnancies.

Cardiac and renal anomalies are also common and frequently contribute to perinatal mortality.[51] They are not likely to recur in subsequent pregnancies if diabetes is the only contributory etiology. However, prior delivery of a malformed infant may increase the risk for malformation in a subsequent delivery. Although no woman is safe, there is less likelihood of congenital anomalies in patients with Class A or B diabetes.[8,2]

REFERENCES

1. Hare, J.W., White, P.: Pregnancy in diabetes complicated by vascular disease. Diabetes 26:953, 1977.
2. Kitzmiller, J.L., Cloherty, J.P., Younger, M.D., et al.: Diabetic pregnancy and perinatal morbidity. Am. J. Obstet. Gynecol. 131:560, 1978.
3. Metzger, B.E., Phelps, R.L., Freinkel, N.: Correlation of plasma amino acids with fetal macrosomia in gestational diabetes. Clin. Res. 24:502A, 1976. (Abstract)
4. Robert, M.F., Neff, R.K., Hubbell, J.P., et al.: Association between maternal diabetes and the respiratory-distress syndrome in the newborn. N. Engl. J. Med. 294:357,1976.
5. Gabbe, S.G., Mestman, J.H., Freeman, R.K., et al.: Management and outcome of pregnancy in diabetes mellitus, classes B to R. Am. J. Obstet. Gynecol. 129:723, 1977.
6. Ayromlooi, J., Mann, L.I., Weiss, R.R., et al.: Modern management of the diabetic pregnancy. Obstet. Gynecol. 49:137, 1977.
7. Pildes, R.S.: Infants of diabetic mothers. N. Eng. J. Med. 289:902, 1973.
8. Pedersen, J.: Goals and end-points in management of diabetic pregnancy. In: R.A. Camerini-Davalos, H.S. Cole (Eds.): Early Diabetes in Early Life. New York, Academic Press, 1975, pp. 381–391.
9. Hare, J.W.: Diabetes mellitus in pregnancy. Compr. Ther. 3:23, 1977.
10. Villee, D.B., Powers, M.L.: Effect of glucose and insulin on collagen secretion by human skin fibroblasts in vitro (letter). Nature 268:156, 1977.
10a.Lewis, N.J., Akazawa, S., Freinkel, N.: Teratogenesis from B-hydroxybutyrate during organogenesis in rat embryo organ culture and enhancement by subteratogenic glucose. Diabetes 32 (Suppl. 1):11a, 1983.
11. Miller, E., Hare, J.W., Cloherty, J.P., et al.: Elevated maternal hemoglobin A_{1c} in early pregnancy and major congenital anomalies in infants of diabetic mothers. N. Engl. J. Med. 304:1331, 1981.
12. White, P.: Pregnancy and diabetes. In: A. Marble, P. White, R.F. Bradley, L.P. Krall (Eds.): Joslin's Diabetes Mellitus. 11th Ed., Philadelphia, Lea & Febiger, 1971. pp. 581–598.
13. Karlsson, K., Kjellmer, I.: The outcome of diabetic pregnancies in relation to the mother's blood sugar level. Am. J. Obstet. Gynecol. 112:213, 1972.
14. Berendes, H.W.: Effect of maternal acetonuria on I.Q. of offspring. In: R.A. Carmerini-Davalos, H.S. Cole (Eds.): Early Diabetes in Early Life. New York, Academic Press. 1975, pp. 135–140.
15. Felig, P., Kim, Y.J., Lynch, V., Hendler, R.: Amino acid metabolism during starvation in human pregnancy. J. Clin. Invest. 51:1195, 1972.
16. Freinkel, N.: Effects of the conceptus on maternal metabolism during pregnancy. In: B.S. Leibel, G.A. Wrenshall (Eds.): On the Nature and Treatment of Diabetes. Amsterdam, Excerpta Medical Foundation, 1965, pp. 679–691.
17. Knopp, R.H., Herrera, E., Freinkel, N.: Carbohydrate metabolism in pregnancy. VIII. Metabolism of adipose tissue isolated from fed and fasted pregnant rats during late gestation. J. Clin. Invest. 49:1438, 1970.
18. Metzger, B.E., Hare, J.W., Freinkel, N.: Carbohydrate metabolism in pregnancy. IX. Plasma levels of gluconeogenic fuels during fasting in the rat. J. Clin. Endocrinol. Metab. 33:869, 1971.
19. Freinkel, N., Metzger, B.E., Nitzan, M., et al.: Accelerated starvation and mechanisms for the conservation of maternal nitrogen during pregnancy. Isr. J. Med. Sci. 8:426, 1972.
20. Felig, P.: Body fuel metabolism and diabetes mellitus in pregnancy. Med. Clin. N. Am. 61:43, 1977.
21. Metzger, B.E., Agnoli, F.S., Hare, J.W., Freinkel, N.: Carbohydrate metabolism in pregnancy. X. Metabolic disposition of alanine by the perfused liver of the fasting pregnant rat. Diabetes 22:601, 1973.
22. Beck, P., Daughaday, W.H.: Human placental lactogen: studies of its acute metabolic effects and disposition in normal man. J. Clin. Invest. 46:103, 1967.
23. Costrini, N.V., Kalkhoff, R.K.: Relative effects of pregnancy, estradiol, and progesterone on plasma insulin and pancreatic islet insulin secretion. J. Clin. Invest. 50:992, 1971.
24. Daniel, R.R., Metzger, B.E., Freinkel, N., et al.: Carbohydrate metabolism in pregnancy. XI. Response of plasma glucagon to overnight fast and oral glucose during normal pregnancy and in gestational diabetes. Diabetes 23:771, 1974.
25. Kuhl, C., Holst, J.J.: Plasma glucagon and the insulin: glucagon ratio in gestational diabetes. Diabetes 25:16, 1976.
26. Kitzmiller, J.L., Tanenberg, R.J. Aoki, T.T., et al.: Pancreatic alpha cell response to alanine during and after nor-

mal and diabetic pregnancies. Obstet. Gynecol. 56:440, 1980.

27. Freinkel, N., Metzger, B.E., Nitzan, M., et al: Facilitated anabolism in late pregnancy: Some novel maternal compensations for accelerated starvation. In: W.J. Malaisse, J. Pirart (Eds.): Diabetes. Proceedings of the 8th Congress of the International Diabetes Federation. Brussels, July 15–20, 1973. Amsterdam, Excerpta Medica, 1974, pp. 474–488.

28. Welsh, G.W., 3rd., Sims, E.A.H.: The mechanisms of renal glucosuria in pregnancy. Diabetes 9:363, 1960.

29. Spellacy, W.N., Cohn, J.E.: Human placental lactogen levels and daily insulin requirements in patients with diabetes mellitus complicating pregnancy. Obstet. Gynecol. 42:330, 1973.

29a.O'Sullivan, J.M., Mahan, C.M.: Criteria for the oral glucose tolerance test in pregnancy. Diabetes 13:278, 1964.

30. O'Sullivan, J.B., Mahan, C.M., Charles, D., Dandrow, R.V.: Medical treatment of the gestational diabetic. Obstet. Gynecol. 43:817, 1974.

30a.Hare, J.W., White, P.: Gestational diabetes and the White classification. Diabetes Care 3:394, 1980.

31. Kitzmiller, J.L., Brown, E.R., Phillippe, M., et al.: Diabetic nephropathy and perinatal outcome. Am. J. Obstet. Gynecol. 141:741, 1981.

32. Tagatz, G.E., Arnold, N.I., Goetz, F.C., et al.: Pregnancy in a juvenile diabetic after renal transplantation (Class T diabetes mellitus). Diabetes 24:497, 1975.

32a.Ogburn, P.L., Jr., Kitzmiller, J.L., Hare, J.W., et al.: Pregnancy following renal transplantation in diabetes mellitus. Diabetes 33(Suppl. 1):14a, 1984.

33. O'Sullivan, J.B., Gellis, S.S., Dandrow, R.V., Tenney, B.O.: The potential diabetic and her treatment in pregnancy. Obstet. Gynecol. 27:683, 1966.

34. Aiello, L.M.: Personal communication.

35. Redman, C.W.G.: Treatment of hypertension in pregnancy. Kidney Int. 18:267, 1980.

36. Kussman, M.J., Goldstein, H.H. Gleason, R.E.: The clinical course of diabetic nephropathy, J.A.M.A. 236:1861, 1976.

37. Katz, A.I., Davison, J.P., Hayslett, J.P.: Pregnancy in women with kidney disease. Kidney Int. 18:192, 1980.

38. Naeye, R.L. Causes of the excessive rates of perinatal mortality and prematurity in pregnancies complicated by maternal urinary-tract infections. N. Engl. J. Med. 300:819, 1979.

39. Driscoll, S.G.: The pathology of pregnancy complicated by diabetes mellitus. Med. Clin. N. Am. 49:1053, 1965.

40. Franz, M.: Nutritional management in diabetes and pregnancy. Diabetes Care 1:264, 1978.

41. Mintz, D.H., Skyler, J.S., Chez, R.A.: Diabetes mellitus and pregnancy. Diabetes Care 1:49, 1978.

42. Lev-Ran, A., Goldman, J.A.: Brittle diabetes in pregnancy. Diabetes 26:926, 1977.

43. Evertson, L.R., Gauthier, R.J., Collea, J.V.: Fetal demise following negative contraction stress tests. Obstet. Gynecol. 51:671, 1978.

44. Evertson, L.R., Paul, R.H.: Antepartum fetal heart rate testing: The non-stress test. Am. J. Obstet. Gynecol. 132:895, 1978.

45. Torday, J., Carson, L., Lawson, E.E.: Saturated phosphatidylcholine in amniotic fluid and prediction of the respiratory-distress syndrome. N. Engl. J. Med. 301:1013, 1979.

46. Phelps, R.L., Freinkel, N., Rubenstein, A.H., et al.: Carbohydrate metabolism in pregnancy. XV. Plasma C-peptide during intravenous glucose tolerance in neonates from normal and insulin-treated diabetic mothers. J. Clin. Endocrinol. Metab. 46:61, 1978.

47. Mintz, D.H., Stock, R., Finster, J.L., Taylor, A.L.: The effect of normal and diabetic pregnancies on growth hormone responses to hypoglycemia. Metabolism 17:54, 1968.

48. Ganda, O.P., Soeldner, J.S.: Genetic, acquired, and related factors in the etiology of diabetes mellitus. Arch. Intern. Med. 137:461, 1977.

49. Mills, J.L., Baker, L., Goldman, A.S.: Malformations in infants of diabetic mothers occur before the seventh gestational week. Implications for treatment. Diabetes 28:292, 1979.

50. Holmes, L.B., Driscoll, S.G., Atkins, L.: Etiologic heterogeneity of neural-tube defects. N. Engl. J. Med. 294:365, 1976.

51. Gabbe, S.G.: Congenital malformations in infants of diabetic mothers. Obstet. Gynecol. Surv. 32:125, 1977.

34 Surgery in Diabetes

Frank C. Wheelock, Jr., Gary W. Gibbons, and
Alexander Marble

Surgery in patients with diabetes presents all the problems of surgery in general, with additional ones peculiar to diabetes and its complications. Since surveys suggest that there are 6 to 10 million persons with diabetes in the United States at present, and since an estimated 25% of these will eventually need some type of surgery, the numbers involved are large. Great advances in the care of these patients have been made in recent decades so that the diabetic patient can usually be brought safely through the most complicated surgical procedures.

In this chapter we will discuss problems of pre-, intra-, and postoperative care and then will consider the management of some pathologic states peculiar to the diabetic.

PREOPERATIVE EVALUATION

In planning for surgery in the patient with diabetes, time should be allowed, if the surgical condition will permit, for careful study and treatment to insure that the patient is in as good general physical condition as possible. For patients under medical supervision prior to hospital admission, this period need not be lengthy, usually only 1 to 3 days, and rarely more than a week, unless additional time is necessary for study and treatment of the surgical condition such as a foot lesion. During this preparatory period, the following features should be kept in mind for evaluation and correction: (1) satisfactory control of the diabetic state; (2) support of the nutritional status by means of an intake thoroughly adequate in calories, protein, vitamins, and minerals; (3) treatment of anemia if present; (4) diagnosis, evaluation, and treatment of any complicating disease of a cardiac, pulmonary, renal or other origin; and (5) adequate hydration and correction of any electrolyte imbalance.

If cardiac disease is suggested by history, physical examination or electrocardiographic changes, stress testing, echocardiography and thalium scanning may be used in selected patients to determine the present level of cardiac function, extent of disease, and/or response to appropriate medication. In other patients, cardiac catheterization and coronary artery surgery might be indicated prior to elective general surgical procedures. More commonly, it is reasonable and safe to proceed with operation after suitable preparation, including the administration or adjustment of appropriate cardiac medication.

Renal disease is evaluated preoperatively by the more common tests of renal function, including blood urea nitrogen, serum creatinine, and urinalysis. A 24-hour urine collection for electrolytes, creatinine, urea nitrogen, and protein may be indicated as well as determination of the creatinine clearance. If renal disease is present, iodine-containing angiographic fluids should be used with care in small amounts. All patients undergoing angiography should be kept well hydrated, and monitoring of electrolytes and renal function before and after evaluation is essential. If possible, antibiotics which are potentially nephrotoxic should be avoided, especially combinations of drugs such as an aminoglycoside plus a cephalosporin. If potentially nephrotoxic antibiotics or other medications are necessary, careful daily monitoring of renal function and serum drug levels must be done, especially in patients with diminished renal function.

Evaluation of the cerebral circulation is indicated prior to major surgery especially in patients who have had diabetes for longer than 10 years. If neurologic symptoms are present which could be related to carotid stenosis or if a significant bruit is heard over the neck vessels in an asymptomatic patient, further studies should be carried out. (See section on Carotid Artery Surgery at the end of this chapter.)

Respiratory function is another important area to evaluate preoperatively. A simple test is to exercise the patient (if ambulatory) up and down a series of stairs to evaluate respiratory reserve. In addition, pulmonary function tests with arterial blood gases may be needed. Methods to improve respiratory function include the cessation of smoking. We have learned that if a chronic smoker stops for even a few days preoperatively, there is a decrease of respiratory complications postoperatively. Chest physiotherapy, breathing exercises including "spirocare," and ultrasonic nebulizers have been beneficial in specific instances. The use of intermittent positive pressure breathing (IPPB) is discouraged except as a means of delivering medications since its use has not been shown to be beneficial.

Of great importance is evaluation of the patient's nutritional status. Diabetic patients with poor control, diabetic gastroenteropathy or severe cardiovascular or renal disease are particularly prone to develop malnutrition[1] related mainly to a deficiency of protein reserves. A period of time spent in correcting this condition is well worthwhile prior to major surgical procedures.[2] Standard protocols of oral or intravenous hyperalimentation can be used in diabetic patients with careful monitoring of glucose[3,4] in blood and urine.

MANAGEMENT OF DIABETES

Many patients enter the hospital with diabetes under poor control. In some the diagnosis of diabetes may not have been made prior to admission or before the onset of the condition for which surgery is contemplated. In any case, the diet should be limited appropriately in carbohydrate, thoroughly adequate in protein, and at such a level of fat as is called for by the weight of the patient. With most adult patients, many of whom are elderly, the dietary prescription will range from 150 to 225 g of carbohydrate, 70 to 100 g of protein and 40 to 100 g of fat, furnishing from 1200 to 2200 calories per day. Although certain patients have diabetes which is well controlled by dietary restriction alone, the vast majority require insulin daily in dosage suited to the individual requirements. Most patients treated previously on oral hypoglycemic agents require insulin at least temporarily, during and following operation, and there should be no hesitancy in shifting such patients from oral compounds to insulin.

Of the various insulin programs which are possible, we have found most workable that in which a daily dose of isophane (NPH) or lente insulin, with or without an accompanying dose of regular insulin, is given before breakfast. In those patients with onset of diabetes prior to the age of 40 and in others with unstable, hard-to-manage diabetes, a smaller dose of NPH or lente insulin will be necessary at bedtime or before the evening meal, in which case it can be accompanied by a small dose of regular insulin. The regular and NPH or lente insulins are given in a single injection, drawing the regular insulin into the syringe first. For the principles used to guide adjustment of doses of insulin, see Chapter 19.

Treatment During and Following Operation

On the day of operation, hopefully scheduled for the early part of the forenoon, food is withheld and, in lieu thereof, fluid and dextrose are given intravenously. At the time that the intravenous infusion is started, insulin is administered in dosage of approximately one-half of that which has been found necessary previously. Thus, if the patient has been stabilized on a dose of 20 units of regular and 40 units of NPH insulin given daily before breakfast, on the day of the operation breakfast is omitted, an infusion of dextrose (usually 1000 ml of 5% in water) is started, and 8–10 units of regular plus 16–20 units of NPH insulin are given subcutaneously. Following surgery and on return to the recovery room, the same (or slightly smaller) amounts and types of insulin are given subcutaneously as were administered prior to the operation. Usually no more insulin will be necessary until the following morning. The intravenous infusion of dextrose (5% in water or saline solution) is continued to provide at least 100 to 150 g of carbohydrate on the day of surgery. One or more blood glucose determinations are made in the hours after the operation and the results reported promptly to alert the physician to any changes in treatment which may be necessary. A blood glucose level of 180 to 250 mg/dl is satisfactory when a glucose solution is being administered slowly.

The program outlined above, which includes the administration on the day of operation of an amount of insulin which approximates that found necessary on the days prior to surgery, has certain advantages over other programs commonly used: (1) The patient is adequately protected by insulin since the doses are decided upon and ordered in advance. (2) The physician is relieved of the necessity of obtaining urine specimens for analyses at intervals following surgery as required when regular insulin is given according to a sliding scale. Experience has shown that it is often difficult to obtain urine without catheterizing the patient, and this must be avoided in the diabetic patient unless absolutely necessary. (3) Hypoglycemia is less apt to occur than when regular insulin is given at intervals according to the outcome of urine tests. In a patient who is receiving glucose intravenously, the results of urine tests may be strongly positive and yet the blood glucose level not be exceptionally high. A large dose of insulin given solely because of a strongly positive urine test for sugar may produce hypoglycemia which in the fragile, elderly patient may be harmful.

Those not accustomed to the program discussed above may fear hypoglycemia because little or no food is taken orally on the day of operation to offset the effect of the insulin. However, the combination of dextrose given intravenously and the metabolic stress of surgery and anesthesia usually balance the effect of the insulin to a surprisingly close degree. As stated earlier, as an automatic "check and balance," one or more blood glucose determinations may be made in the middle or latter part of the afternoon of the day of the operation.

Further comment is necessary regarding two situations not covered above. The first has to do with conditions which demand prompt surgery. These may range all the way from emergencies requiring immediate action to conditions in which, although urgent, operation may be delayed for at least a few or several hours. In such cases the physician must adapt treatment to the situation presented. If symptomatic ketoacidosis is present, energetic treatment with insulin, fluids, and electrolytes (as and when indicated) may within a few or several hours bring a patient to a state acceptable for emergency surgery. The second situation concerns the time of day at which operation is done. Although the early forenoon is preferable, if this is not possible, the physician can adapt the orders and procedures to conform to the situation.

On the day following operation, the usual dose of insulin is given in the morning before breakfast or at the time of starting the first infusion of glucose and fluid. It is anticipated that no more insulin will be needed until the following morning. However, as guides, blood glucose determinations are made in the late forenoon and in the middle or latter part of the afternoon. Blood for these and other determinations mentioned earlier may be obtained by capillary samplings from the ear lobe or finger pad. Glucose tests may be made easily at the bedside with Chemstrip bG or Visidex II.

In those patients whose diabetes had been well controlled prior to operation by means of diet and oral hypoglycemic agents, oral medication usually can be resumed after a few days when the metabolic stress of the operation has diminished or disappeared.

INTRA-OPERATIVE MANAGEMENT

Anesthesia

In general the choice of anesthetic agent should be left to the anesthesiologist who may have certain preferences based on experience. It should not be forgotten that local anesthesia is excellent for many procedures including herniorrhaphy, carotid endarterectomy, dilatation and curettage, etc. However, local anesthesia should not be used for operations on the feet when ischemia is present. In many neuropathic cases, local amputations may be painlessly accomplished with no anesthesia.

Diabetic patients, especially those at considerable operative risk and undergoing major procedures, need constant intra-operative monitoring. Continuous electrocardiographic monitoring is standard now in all patients who have general or spinal anesthesia. A temperature probe, Foley catheter, radial artery line, central venous pressure catheter and even a Swan-Ganz catheter may be needed with the overall objective of maintaining body homeostasis and preventing complications. It is imperative that episodes of hypo- or hypertension be recognized and controlled immediately. For critically ill patients, especially those with hypertension or severe coronary artery disease, more commonly used medications such as lidocaine, dopamine, nitroprusside and propranolol should be readily available and in some instances already mixed in a continuous drip ready to run.

Fluid, Electrolyte and Acid-Base Balance

Transfusions are, of course, matched against blood loss. Balanced salt solutions are used to maintain intravascular volume and to replace physiologic losses which may be significant in lengthy and/or major intra-abdominal operations. Obviously dextrose must be included in the intravenous fluids or serious hypoglycemia may develop intra- or postoperatively. Careful monitoring of all intake and output is mandatory and should be periodically compared to the patient's vital signs and other hemodynamic measurements of the patient's overall general condition. Serum electrolytes, especially potassium, and arterial blood gases are measured as needed.

Sepsis

If an open lesion is present, or if the gastrointestinal or genitourinary tract is to be entered or manipulated, intravenous antibiotics are started preoperatively, in the hope that sudden bacteremia or wound infections can be avoided. Cephalosporins are the most commonly used antibiotics for prophylaxis. In many cases an isotonic antiseptic or antibiotic solution is also used locally to irrigate the incision prior to closure.

POSTOPERATIVE MANAGEMENT

Wound Healing. In patients whose diabetes is under good control, incisions heal at a normal rate except in areas where there is diminished blood supply. This coincides with Rosenthal's[5] experimental work in rats which found that those with controlled diabetes actually healed better than the normal animals. The rate of sepsis in clean incisions is in the range of 1 to 2%.

Cardiorespiratory Problems. After lengthy upper abdominal procedures, especially in patients with known respiratory disease, the patient may remain intubated on a volume respirator for hours or even days. Weaning and extubation are delayed until the patient is able to resume and maintain adequate respiratory function, and until measurements of arterial blood gases and acid-base balance yield acceptable results. Medications for pre- and postoperative pain and sedation must be kept at low dosage levels as many diabetic patients overreact to average doses.

The usual frequency of atelectasis is to be expected and is managed by standard techniques including early mobilization of the patient, coughing, and deep breathing exercises as well as incentive spirometry and chest physiotherapy. Fluid overload is of concern but can be avoided by judicious fluid and electrolyte replacement with careful monitoring of the patient's vital signs and hemodynamic status. Careful charting of all intake and output, daily weights, serial measurements of urine specific gravity, serum and urine osmolarity, and serum electrolytes can be extremely important in these patients.

Diabetic Concerns. We have seen more trouble from hypoglycemia than from hyperglycemia and therefore generally continue intravenous dextrose in one form or another until we are certain the patient is eating satisfactorily. The nursing staff is trained to report failure of the patient to eat adequately at any meal so that dextrose may be given intravenously if indicated.

Neuropathic Bladder. Paresis of the urinary bladder occurs with relative frequency in patients with long-term diabetes. If such bladders are left over-distended for significant periods, the muscles are stretched and subsequently are slow to regain tone. Frequent voiding in small amounts for a prolonged period should make the diagnosis of neuropathic bladder suspect. Bladder training and medications such as urecholine may be useful in restoring bladder tone.

INFECTIONS IN DIABETIC PATIENTS

There is no doubt that diabetes, especially if poorly controlled, affects the response to infection. The reason for this is not well understood but may be due to a reduced capacity of leukocytes to engulf and kill bacteria.[6] From a practical point of view, it is of the utmost importance that infection in diabetics be viewed with respect and treated carefully.[7] After obtaining appropriate cultures, one should administer antibiotics intravenously, put the affected part at rest, and institute adequate surgical drainage when indicated. It is difficult to persuade surgeons to drain infections adequately, particularly in the foot when the circulation may be diminished. The unalterable objective must be to obtain dependent drainage when the part is at rest. The incision must open fully all areas of infection and then taper proximally so that pus may run out unhampered; that is to say, the subcutaneous fat is cut further than the fascia and the skin further than the subcutaneous fat. Hot compresses or soaks are to be avoided at all times since they cause burns in a numb foot or increase metabolic demands in a foot deprived of arterial blood supply (see Chapter 36).

THE ACUTE ABDOMEN IN THE DIABETIC

An acute surgical abdomen may be well hidden in the diabetic, disguised by the lack of pain. This phenomenon is probably due to diabetic neuropathy but in any event presents a real danger as illustrated by the following case.

A 31-year-old diabetic woman was admitted with severe abdominal pain. She reported a week's history of mild discomfort and urine positive for glucose. She had continued working until 12 hours prior to admission when the severe pain appeared and she became dangerously ill. On admission her pulse was 140, blood pressure 95/50, temperature 104° F, and the white blood count was 24,000. Her abdomen was distended and rigid. At operation it was found that a large appendiceal abscess had ruptured flooding the abdomen with pus. Massive antibiotic therapy had been started on admission and continued. Postoperatively her temperature rose to 106.4° F and her pulse to 180. In the course of the next 10 weeks, the patient underwent an unbelievable series of 8 operations to drain abscesses, including an empyema and an operation to bypass a jejunal fistula. Eventually recovery was complete.

This case emphasizes the danger inherent in the paucity of symptoms which serious intra-abdominal disease may produce in the diabetic patient. It also illustrates the advantage and necessity of aggressive surgery in treating uncontrolled sepsis. None of the Attending Staff believed that this diabetic patient with undrained pus could survive without operation and yet the risk of surgery was considerable (absent systolic blood pressure during the initial part of the operation). Courage was drawn from the surgical principle that a patient, however ill, will usually tolerate an operation if it removes the disease process.

SURGERY OF THE BILIARY AND GASTROINTESTINAL TRACTS

Biliary Tract. It may be difficult to decide whether or not to remove a gallbladder containing stones and producing no symptoms. In general, we advise operation in good risk patients under the age of 70. This decision is based on the eventual likelihood of serious complications in the form of acute cholecystitis, common duct stones or cholangitis. Mundth[8] reported a 22% mortality for such acute problems in the diabetic as opposed to 0.7% in the nondiabetic. On the other hand, there is zero mortality for elective cholecystectomy in the diabetic.

Pancreas. Pancreatitis and carcinoma of the pancreas are more common in the diabetic than in the nondiabetic patient for reasons not well understood.[9,10] The management of these diseases is standard but in general relatively difficult with results less satisfactory than one might wish.

Stomach. The stomach presents one unique problem: that of gastric atony due to diabetic neuropathy. The symptoms are vague discomfort, weight loss, vomiting, and diarrhea. X-ray films (Fig. 34–1) show a large flaccid stomach which empties slowly through a normal or dilated pylorus or duodenum.[11] Gastrojejunostomy or gastrectomy have been disappointing, making medical management the preferred modality of treatment, including small meals, improving diabetic control and the like.[12] Newer medications such as metoclopramide

are being tried with some encouraging results, but further controlled clinical trials are needed.

Small and Large Intestine. Duodenal ulcer requiring surgery remains relatively rare in the diabetic population. If surgery is required, the type of operation is dictated by the clinical situation just as in the nondiabetic. Perforated ulcers may occur and produce little in the way of symptoms.

The most common problem in this area is carcinoma of the colon which is treated in the usual manner.

One should watch for the easily missed diagnosis of occlusion of the superior mesenteric artery. This diagnosis should be considered when there has been unexplained weight loss and abdominal pain after meals. Once outlined by aortogram, the obstruction lends itself well to surgical correction by artery grafting.

Constipation and episodic diarrhea secondary to diabetic gastroenteropathy are common. Severe constipation is not an infrequent complication of hospitalization, and attention to this should be part of all routine admission orders.

LOWER EXTREMITY PROBLEMS

It has been estimated that 25% of diabetic patients will develop foot or leg problems eventually, and in our experience these account for over half of all hospital admissions of diabetic patients (excluding those to in-patient units for ambulatory pa-

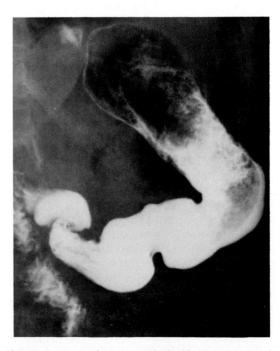

Fig. 34–1. X-ray showing residual of barium in stomach, and gastric and duodenal bulb atony and dilatation in a patient with diabetic neuropathy. (Ref. 11).

tients). There are three major pathologic entities which individually or in combination cause the problem: (1) purely infectious processes; (2) neuropathy; (3) situations developing as a result of arterial insufficiency.

Infections

The foot represents an area subjected to repeated minor trauma. Ingrown toenails, calluses, and blisters all can serve as portals of entry for bacteria. Seemingly benign, superficial, and localized ulcers can progress to those with extensive cellulitis, tissue destruction and systemic toxicity. This process may be governed by several factors including specific bacterial invasion, degree of control of diabetes, continued trauma, the severity of vascular disease and local care. It is imperative that the cardinal principles of treating infection be closely adhered to in the management of the infected diabetic extremity.

Prevalence and Types of Organisms. Previous publications have emphasized the importance of aerobic gram-positive and enteric gram-negative bacilli in diabetic foot ulcers. Louie, Bartlett and colleagues[13] reported a high frequency of anaerobes in 20 diabetic foot ulcers. Fierer, Daniel and Davis[14] made a similar observation in a review of 30 consecutive diabetics who required surgery for lower extremity infections and noted a large number of mixed infections which generally responded poorly to therapy.

We[15] studied 100 consecutive diabetic patients with foot lesions in an attempt to correlate particular pathogens with progression of the foot ulcer and to identify optimal antibiotic therapy. The patients were divided into three groups based on the severity of infection (Table 34–1). Patients with stable, uncomplicated ulcers (Group I) had an average of 2.9 isolates per ulcer (Table 34–1). The high frequency of gram-negative bacilli (35%) and anaerobes (53%) is surprising since none of the patients in this group required operations directly related to the septic complications of their ulcer. This suggests that treatment protocols including local care, rest to the injured part and broad spectrum antibiotics given orally may prevent deterioration of the ulcer and septic complications.

The majority of patients (83%) had moderately or severely infected foot ulcers. Although systemic toxicity was absent in some, the gravity of the problem was attested to by the fact that 85% of these patients required one or more operations. Fifty percent of the patients in the moderately infected group required a forefoot amputation (toe, toe plus metatarsal or transmetatarsal) and 20% required a major amputation (below or above knee). In 20% of these patients, arterial revascularization was performed which permitted a subsequent lesser amputation than would have been required otherwise.

Cultures of the moderately infected ulcers (Table 34–2) revealed an average of 2.9 isolates per patient. Aerobic gram-positive organisms were the most prevalent (85% of patients), while aerobic gram-negative bacilli were found in 58% of these patients. Only gram-negative bacilli were cultured from 5 patients. Of the aerobes isolated, a significant finding was the presence of Enterococcus and Proteus species (50% of patients). Anaerobic cultures were positive in 34% of the patients with Peptostreptococcus being the most frequently isolated anaerobe.

Patients comprising Group III (Table 34–1) had severely infected ulcers with marked tissue destruction and with lymphangitis, poorly-controlled diabetes, elevated temperature and malaise being the most frequent systemic manifestations. They averaged 3.2 bacterial isolates per ulcer, the highest of the three groups (Table 34–2). Gram-positive aerobic organisms were present in 93%, while aerobic gram-negative bacilli were isolated in 50% of these ulcers. Enterococcus and Proteus species were cultured in 64%. Anaerobes were present in 69% of the Group III ulcers and of note was a high frequency of Bacteroides species.

Only one of the 42 patients with severe infection avoided operation and multiple operations were required in 36% of this group. Sixty-seven percent of the patients underwent a forefoot amputation (toe, toe plus metatarsal or transmetatarsal), and over one-third of the patients required a major amputation. When a severe foot infection involved Enterococcus, Proteus species, Pseudomonas or anaerobic organisms and antibiotic therapy was not directed specifically against these organisms, the prognosis was especially poor.

Treatment. Because patients with uncontrolled diabetes tend to tolerate infection poorly, it is imperative that treatment for moderately and severely infected foot ulcers begin immediately after diagnosis. Ulcers with a fetid odor or the presence of crepitation due to subcutaneous gas should be particularly suspect for the presence of anaerobic organisms. Our experience with patients with moderately or severely infected ulcers indicates that a single antibiotic is seldom sufficient initially. Since aerobic gram-positive and gram-negative organisms and anaerobic bacteria are frequently isolated and since there is a major threat to limb survival, initial broad-spectrum intravenous antibiotic coverage for all of these bacteria is indicated on admission as soon as appropriate cultures are obtained. Reasonable combinations of intravenous antibiotics might be (1) an aminoglycoside plus

Table 34–1.   Characterization of 100 Consecutive Foot Ulcers

Groups and Characteristics of Ulcers	Organisms Found Percentage of Patients Affected		Initial Treatment
Group I (17 patients) Stable uncomplicated ulcers Superficial lesion No cellulitis No bone involvement No systemic toxicity No threatened limb loss	Average 2.9 isolates per patient Aerobes — Gram-pos. cocci (88%) Gram-neg. rods (35%) Anaerobes—(53%)		Rest of injured part Local care Broad spectrum oral antibiotic Special shoeing
Group II (41 patients) Moderately infected ulcers Up to 2 cm cellulitis Some deep soft tissue and/or bone destruction No systemic toxicity Threatened limb loss	Average 2.9 isolates per patient Aerobes — Gram-pos. cocci (85%) Gram-neg. rods (58%) Anaerobes—(34%)		Complete bed rest Local care Thorough debridement and dependent drainage Intravenous broad spectrum antibiotics covering aerobic and anaerobic microorganisms. Changed when specific sensitivities are available.
Group III (42 patients) Severely infected ulcers More than 2 cm cellulitis Extensive tissue and/or bone destruction Systemic toxicity Threatened limb loss	Average 3.2 isolates per patient Aerobes — Gram-pos. cocci (93%) Gram-neg. rods (50%) Anaerobes—(69%)		As for Group II

ampicillin plus clindamycin or (2) a cephalosporin plus choloramphenicol. Careful monitoring for signs of antibiotic toxicity is mandatory. As soon as bacterial sensitivity studies are available, appropriate changes should be made in these medications. Particular attention should be paid to a positive culture for Pseudomonas (present in 14% of our cases). We have found this organism to be responsible for continuing and extensive tissue destruction. The most effective treatment at this time appears to be a combination of an aminoglycoside plus carbenicillin, ticarcillin, or piperacillin. Similarly, ulcers from which Enterococcus plus Proteus species are isolated (50% of patients) demand aggressive antibiotic therapy as do ulcers yielding anaerobic organisms on culture. Newer antibiotics with specific antimicrobial spectrums may have promise for the future, but carefully designed clinical trials are needed before these become a standard part of treatment protocols for moderately and severely infected diabetic foot ulcers.

In addition to adequate antibiotic therapy, limb salvage is favored by management of diabetes, aggressive nutritional support, complete rest of the injured part, extensive debridement, adequate dependent drainage, appropriate arterial reconstruction and well chosen, conservative amputation. Warm or hot soaks or compresses should *never* be used as they may produce a burn, introduce more

bacteria, or cause more tissue destruction, especially in an already ischemic extremity. Similarly we do not think it appropriate to use whirl-pool baths when an open lesion is present.

Peripheral Neuropathy

The patient with long-standing diabetes, particularly if control of the disease has been poor, is prone to develop neuritis, usually involving first the lower legs and feet. The underlying pathologic and physiologic states are poorly understood, but the clinical picture is easily recognized. The sympathetic nerves or ganglia are also affected so that sweating and other signs of vasomotor activity are absent in the affected areas. Strangely, severe pain may occur at a time when sensation to vibration, light touch, or painful stimuli is reduced or lacking. Narcotics stronger than codeine must be avoided because of the obvious danger of addiction in this condition which may well last a long time.

The more common complication of the neuropathy results from loss of sensation in the foot.[16] In the normal foot, minor discomfort triggers a shift in stride or weight-bearing to protect an area under stress. In the neuropathic foot, there is little or no sensation to effect such a change. Consequently large calluses may form owing to constant relentless weight-bearing on one area. Such a callus becomes rock hard and just about as dangerous as a small stone inside a shoe would be. Eventually a

Table 34–2. Frequency of Isolation of Bacterial Species

	GROUP I (17 patients) Patients affected No.	GROUP II (41 patients) Patients affected No.	GROUP III (42 patients) Patients affected No.
Gram-pos. aerobes	15	35	39
Staph. aureus	9	23	22
Staph. epidermidis	6	14	12
Streptococcus	6	10	13
Enterococcus	4	12	16
Diphtheroids	5	7	7
Total no. isolates	30	66	70
Gram-neg. aerobes	6	24	21
E. Coli	2	3	7
Proteus	1	10	11
Klebsiella	1	4	4
Enterobacter	0	5	3
Serratia	1	1	0
Pseudomonas	1	10	3
Total no. isolates	6	33	38
Anaerobes	9	14	29
Clostridia	0	0	2
Bacteriodes	4	3	12
Peptococcus	9	13	21
Total no. isolates	13	16	35
Rare organisms			
Citrobacter	1	1	2
Herellea	0	0	1
Total no. isolates	50	116	136
Average number of isolates per patient	2.9	2.9	3.2

subcutaneous hemorrhage or blister and then an ulcer form underneath the callus with subsequent infection. Local pain is absent so that the destruction may be widespread before the problem is recognized.

Prevention of Neuropathic Ulceration. Neuropathic feet are prone to develop bone and joint abnormalities such as hallux rigidus, bunion, hammer toe, or deformed metatarsals. These put unusual stresses on the skin and cause ulcers. Proper podiatric appliances or orthopedic surgical correction of these conditions can prevent serious complications. In addition, all diabetics should be instructed to:

1. Avoid hot applications or soaks.
2. Avoid strong local medicines.
3. Give careful attention to toe nails.
4. Avoid walking barefoot.
5. Take the time and effort to see that shoes fit properly.
6. Inspect the feet daily or, if vision is poor, have someone else do so.

Treatment of Foot Ulcers

Small superficial ulcers in feet with good circulation will heal if calluses are trimmed, weight bearing is eliminated by bed rest or crutches, and appropriate dressings are used. In most cases we elect to use one-quarter strength povidone-iodine (Betadine) dispensed from a dropper bottle for convenience. Plain gauze without a cotton center is moistened with the solution and cut to fit the ulcer. A dry, sterile dressing is applied over this and changes are made from 1 to 3 times a day. It has been shown experimentally that this medication does not interfere with healing. If extensive necrosis is present, surgical debridement and diluted Dakin's solution are used for a time, switching to isotonic Betadine when pink granulation appears. When healing has occurred, a podiatric appliance is made to insure that the area has minimal pressure.

Recurrent ulcers constitute a special category since a great deal of fibrosis occurs in the involved area. Thick, hard, avascular scar tissue makes a poor bed for the thin healing epithelium and results in further recurrence. It then becomes necessary to remove the area including the underlying bony prominence, frequently by means of a single toe and metatarsal head amputation or an osteotomy if feasible.

Large, deep ulcers with or without surrounding

infection usually require definitive surgery. Most of these are secondary to calluses that in turn are caused by excess pressure from a bony prominence which, whether or not involved by osteomyelitis, must be removed. The only question is whether it is wise to carry out the procedure in one stage or to drain the soft tissue first and then remove the offending area at a second operation. In general, if x-ray or clinical examination shows involvement of the bone, a one-stage procedure is better. If there is widespread sepsis with intact bones and joints, occasionally two operations are preferable. In either event, all necrotic tissue must be removed, avoiding unnecessary sacrifice of viable skin. Dependent drainage must be established (assuming that the patient will lie supine while convalescing). If the infection is well localized, portions of the incision may be closed, leaving adequate dependent areas open for drainage. In other instances secondary closures of incisions after 4 or 5 days may be time-saving. This would be done only if all areas were clean and granulating well.

Thus far single toe and metatarsal head amputations have been discussed, but it is important to point out that at times a transmetatarsal amputation of all toes may give a better result. This procedure permits excision of some plantar skin in the form of a triangle around an ulcer beneath one or more metatarsal heads, or over the medial aspect of the first or lateral aspect of the 5th metatarsal head.

Extensive Sepsis of Foot. Occasionally extensive sepsis will develop in a neglected lesion on a neuropathic foot, requiring amputation of the foot. However, unless there is involvement of the ankle or tarsal joints, or there is associated ischemia, the foot is salvageable, at least in part. The effort of saving the foot may be time-consuming but is worthwhile if the patient is otherwise in reasonably good condition, and especially if there has already been a major amputation of the other extremity.

It is of great importance to keep in mind the cardinal principle of surgery in diabetic patients: *thoroughly adequate incision and drainage of any infected area must be accomplished.* In some patients with neglected neuropathic involvement, infection may extend above the ankle into the lower leg following the tendon sheaths. The remedy may lie in extending the incision from the foot along the tendon sheath in continuity almost to the knee if need be. Through-and-through drainage with a tunnel between two incisions is seldom advisable; rather, the whole area should be laid open. Areas of skin loss on the dorsum or plantar aspect of the foot or on the leg may eventually need split-thickness skin grafting.

Another important finding in such feet may be the presence of gas in the tissue, whether felt as crepitus or detected by x ray. This is due to facultative and obligate anaerobic bacteria either clostridial or non-clostridial. This infection is treated by adequate debridement and drainage (making sure no closed spaces remain) plus intravenous antibiotics.

Occasionally even the neuropathic foot with good circulation is not salvageable and a major amputation is necessary. The level of choice is, of course, below the knee to permit use of the knee joint with a prosthetic limb. At times the foot may be so infected that a guillotine amputation just above the ankle is needed to control infection, followed by a definitive reamputation below the knee when the patient's condition permits. It is not necessary or possible to perform the initial guillotine amputation above the level of cellulitis; the inflammation will clear with the aid of antibiotics once the source of the sepsis has been removed. The site of the guillotine amputation should be low so that it is not necessary to divide much muscle and that there is room to perform a definitive closed procedure a few inches more proximal at a later time.

Neuropathic Arthropathy (Charcot Joint)

In 1868, Charcot described neuropathic joint changes associated with tabes dorsalis. The same changes can occur in diabetic neuropathy, usually after 12 to 18 years of diabetes.[17] The foot usually has good circulation and always has poor sensation. Swelling, ulcers, increased temperature, and bone or joint deformity appear. Because of destruction of the sympathetic nerve fibers, the foot does not sweat. X-rays confirm the diagnosis. An extreme case is illustrated in Figure 34–2. Treatment consists of prolonged rest with absolutely no weight bearing. This is continued until the physical signs subside and x-rays show stabilization of the bone process—possibly a period of 6 to 12 weeks or even more. After this, the Podiatry Department is asked to make a suitable orthotic to accommodate the resulting deformity. It is possible to mistakenly diagnose this disease process as osteomyelitis. It should be kept in mind that the latter rarely occurs in a diabetic foot without an associated skin ulcer serving as a portal of entry for bacteria.

ARTERIAL INSUFFICIENCY

Arterial disease, particularly involving the lower extremity, is common among adult diabetic patients. The number of men and women so affected is about equal, in contrast to the nondiabetic population in which the frequency of arterial insufficiency is much greater among males.

Pathology

The cause of the diabetic's tendency to develop arterial occlusion is not known.[18] The smallest ar-

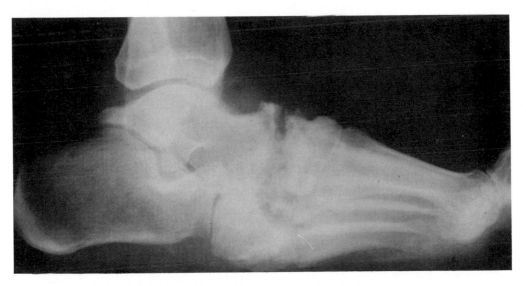

Fig. 34–2. Diabetic neuropathic foot (Charcot joint). The patient, a 31-year-old man, had had diabetes for 14 years. Note the dissolution of the outlines of the tarsal bones.

terioles are involved quite definitely in many diabetics. The larger vessels also are frequently occluded; the first and commonest vessels to be so involved are the tibial arteries in the lower leg. These are usually patent in nondiabetics, even when there may be diffuse arterial degeneration elsewhere. Forty percent of diabetic patients who have no pedal pulses and arterial insufficiency of the foot still have palpable popliteal pulses which indicate open aorta, iliac, and femoral arteries. This situation is almost never seen in the absence of diabetes. In addition to tibial artery disease, many diabetics have occlusions of the larger arteries such as the aorta, iliac, and femoral. If one or more of these vessels is occluded and tibial occlusions are also present, the resulting symptoms are magnified greatly. If, in addition to these two areas, there is extensive disease of vessels of microscopic size, then a most serious problem exists. An added problem is the fact that the diabetic has little ability to develop good collateral circulation.

The actual morphologic pathology of the large vessel wall is not much different from that in the nondiabetic with atherosclerosis. The intima is thickened by fatty deposits occurring in plaques which are most commonly located at bifurcations, on the posterior wall of arteries, or where the artery is naturally rather constricted by muscles and fascia as in the adductor canal. The fact that local blocks occur while the remaining arterial tree is patent is important when arterial reconstruction is considered. The diabetic artery does develop an unusual amount of medial calcification which does not in itself occlude the lumen.

The development of areas of necrosis (gangrene) is frequently related to minor trauma in a foot already inadequately supplied with blood. The injury may be due to pressure from a tight shoe or stocking, the application of heat or strong medication, an ingrown toenail or injury incurred while nails were being trimmed, an injury from a blow of some sort, or a number of other causes. The result may be either a thrombosis of small arterioles in or near the skin or the introduction of infection from a break in the epidermis. A vicious cycle is thus established: thrombosis of vessels leads to necrosis of tissue which in turn leads to infection and to further thrombosis.

Symptoms of Arterial Insufficiency

The earliest sign of inadequate arterial supply is the appearance of claudication. This may involve various muscle groups, depending on the location of the occlusion in the artery; the area possibly involved reaches from the buttock to the foot. Of interest is the fact that while pain is the symptom usually noted, some patients may describe only fatigue, weakness, or numbness.

The next more serious symptom consists of pain at rest, usually night pain. This may be relieved by sitting with the feet dependent, a position in which gravity may favor the entry of additional blood into the feet.

The third symptom is the development of skin necrosis, usually but not always caused by a minor injury. The amount of pain accompanying the appearance of necrosis (gangrene*) will vary greatly from patient to patient. Neuropathy may lessen or abolish pain in the diabetic, even though a gangrenous area is present. When pain is present, it can serve as a useful index of the effectiveness of treatment. This is so because, when the infection comes under control, or when collateral circulation builds up, the pain stimulus to the nerve ending is reduced. The disappearance of the pain while the patient is at rest may mean that maximum improvement has been attained by conservative means and that the patient is ready for any local surgery which may be indicated.

Signs of Arterial Insufficiency

1. Pulses. The aorta and common iliac pulses are palpable in most persons of average size if they can be encouraged to relax sufficiently. At times one or the other iliac pulse may be missing, which helps to localize the arterial blockage. The femoral pulses are easily felt and can be graded from 1 to 4 plus. The presence of a thrill or bruit should be noted, the latter by use of a stethoscope over the aortic, iliac, and femoral areas. A narrowing of 50% or more will usually produce a bruit. If the aorta or iliac artery is completely occluded and if a weak femoral pulse fed by collaterals is present, there will be no bruit. The popliteal pulse, often difficult to locate even though present, is best felt with the patient supine, just lateral to the sagittal section of the knee. If the examiner uses both hands, the fingertips of one overlapping those of the other, it is easy to obtain just the correct amount of pressure without losing an accurate sense of touch. Both posterior tibial and dorsalis pedis pulses are felt for carefully. If there is doubt as to whether one is feeling one's own pulse or the patient's, a check against the patient's radial pulse quickly settles the question.

2. Temperature. In testing temperature, comparisons between the two feet and legs are valuable. Also to be noted is the level of temperature change between a cool foot and the normal skin more proximal if such a line of demarcation exists.

3. Nutrition. The condition of the skin and subcutaneous tissues is informative. If the skin is thin-appearing and white, and if the subcutaneous tissues have wasted away, arterial circulation is poor and probably has been so for some time.

4. Hair and Nails. The absence of hair on the dorsum of the foot and the lack of normal nail growth and appearance may indicate chronic ischemia.

5. Sweating. The absence or presence of moisture on the skin may be of great value in determining whether or not a sympathectomy would be of value. A cool, moist foot may reflect vasospasm, suggesting functional sympathetic nerves.

6. Color. The skin color should be noted, particularly if sympathetic activity is indicated by changes from time to time under stress. Redness which blanches with pressure may indicate cellulitis or severe ischemia. A red tone to the skin which does not blanch with pressure is sometimes found with severe ischemia and is due to leakage of blood from fragile capillaries in or beneath the skin.

7. Venous Filling Time. If the patient's legs are elevated until the dorsal foot veins are empty and appear as valleys, and if the patient then sits with his legs dependent, it is possible to measure accurately the time it takes for the veins to fill. One should take as the end point the number of seconds needed for any segment of vein to fill enough to become even a small "hill" above the skin level. This number can be accurately obtained. If, in the absence of varicose veins, the time is less than 20 seconds, the collateral circulation to the foot is satisfactory.

8. Rubor on Dependency. A bright or dusky red color may develop on dependency if the circulation is quite poor. Presumably this is due to dilated capillaries beneath thin skin through which blood is flowing quite slowly owing to lack of arterial pressure.

9. Sensation. Lack of sensation may be due to neuropathy, but may also accompany sudden arterial occlusion. In the latter, it is a bad prognostic sign.

10. Motor Power. Foot drop or other paralysis may be due to either neuropathy or severe sudden arterial occlusion more proximally.

11. Oscillometry. Either with a standard aneroid manometer or with an oscillometer the amplitude of the pulse may be measured at various levels in the thigh, calf, and ankle. This supplements one's clinical evaluation of the pulse in the major arteries, but does not help with the evaluation of the collateral circulation when proximal major arterial blocks exist.

By training one's powers of observation, it is entirely possible to evaluate with reasonable accuracy the arterial circulation and thereby decide whether symptoms can be explained on a vascular basis, and whether enough circulation exists to heal a given lesion or to permit conservative amputation in the foot.

The Vascular Laboratory

By providing a simple, accurate, inexpensive, and reproducible means for assessing the functional

*In speaking with a patient, the word "gangrene" should generally be avoided, since it is often regarded as indicating the need for major amputation.

significance of arterial occlusive disease, the non-invasive vascular laboratory has added greatly to the clinical appraisal of arterial sufficiency in the extremities.[19] It has been used to predict the primary healing of foot lesions with conservative management alone and, when amputation is necessary, noninvasive testing has been used to help determine the appropriate level of amputation.

Two of the most widely used noninvasive tests are segmental systolic pressure measurements taken at the thigh, calf, and ankle levels[21] and pulse volume recordings (PVR)[22] taken at the thigh, calf, ankle, and transmetatarsal (forefoot) levels. Diabetic patients frequently have artificially elevated systolic pressures at all levels thought to be secondary to medial calcification of the peripheral vessels. Previous reports noted that in 5 to 10% of diabetic patients, systolic pressures could not be measured at all because of stiff, non-compressible vessels.[23] Furthermore, because of the predilection for more distal small vessel disease in the diabetic, foot lesions may develop or progress at higher ankle pressures than in the nondiabetic.

The authors[24,25] reported a study of 100 patients undergoing forefoot amputations (toe, toe plus single metatarsal head, transmetatarsal) and 50 patients requiring below-knee amputation. The decision for and level of amputation were based solely on clinical judgment. Of the 100 forefoot amputations, falsely high (> 200 mm Hg) segmental systolic pressures were present in 50% of the evaluations. Of the 82 patients who healed, segmental systolic pressures predicted correctly in only 33% of cases. Of the 18 failures, the segmental systolic pressures predicted correctly in 44%. Ankle systolic pressures predicted failure in 38% of patients who healed and predicted success in 61% of the patients who failed to heal. Segmental pulse volume recordings gave correct predictions in only half of the total group. Flat or slightly positive PVRs were present in 94% of the failed amputations and in 53% of those that healed. In other words, if the noninvasive testing results were the sole determinant of amputation level, a significant number of these patients would have been denied a more distal forefoot amputation. All patients with a strongly positive forefoot PVR trace healed, making this the only noninvasive test result correctly predicting successful outcome.

Of the 50 patients undergoing below knee amputation, segmental systolic pressures were falsely high (> 200 mm Hg) or nonpredictive in 49% of the 48 successful amputations. Individual thigh, calf, and ankle systolic pressures were either falsely high or nonpredictive in over one-half of the cases. There was no correlation between seg-mental and ankle pulse volume recordings and primary healing in this series of amputations.

It is our opinion that no diabetic patient should be denied a more conservative amputation solely on the basis of the unfavorable results of noninvasive laboratory testing. This is especially true when there has already been a major amputation of the other extremity. In the diabetic patient, clinical judgment is still more valuable than noninvasive techniques in determining amputation level and the likelihood of success. As important as predicting the successful level of amputation are the technique and precision used to carry it out. These principles are detailed elsewhere in this chapter.

Treatment of Arterial Insufficiency

Symptomatic arterial insufficiency warrants careful evaluation both because of the presenting problem and also because more serious complications may lie ahead unless some action is taken. The major symptom categories noted previously are claudication, rest pain, and development of areas of gangrene. The treatment of each presents its own set of problems and considerations.

Conservative Treatment. ''Conservative'' here indicates nonoperative, which may not be an entirely accurate definition. Such treatment may include careful control of diabetes, rest, weight reduction, diet, and omission of tobacco. Therapy for minor degrees of claudication may consist only in limitation of walking to distances that do not produce pain. Ischemic pain at rest may be controlled by elevation of the head of the patient's bed on 6-inch blocks. Buerger exercises may help: a cycle of 1 minute of elevation on a simple inclined plane, 3 minutes of sitting with legs dependent, and 6 minutes of rest while lying flat, performed for several half-hour periods per day.

Small areas of gangrene at the tip of a toe or heel may be protected by light dressings using non-allergic tape, a podiatric appliance, and limited walking. Exercise is contraindicated if these areas are on weight-bearing surfaces or are infected.

We have been dissatisfied with the results of treatment with any of the currently available vasodilator drugs. This is not surprising since vasomotor activity is commonly absent in diabetic patients with arterial insufficiency. Medications such as calcium channel blockers, prostaglandins, and pentoxifylline are not recommended for routine use in diabetics but may hold promise for the future.

Arterial Reconstruction. *Indications.* Since 1954 there has been increasing interest in arterial reconstructive procedures in the treatment of patients having localized areas of occlusive arterial disease. Fortunately atherosclerosis in both diabetic and nondiabetic patients is often segmental, and repair may be possible if the areas involved are in the larger arteries, such as the aorta, iliac, femoral or popliteal. Arterial surgery should be considered if a patient with arterial insufficiency has (1) claudication which significantly interferes with work or worthwhile recreational activities, (2) rest pain, or (3) an area of gangrene which does not heal or cannot be removed surgically with success by a local foot operation. Operation is *not* indicated in mild claudication to prevent more serious trouble.

If examination shows a weak or absent femoral pulse, occlusions of the aorta or iliac system are presumed to be present. The extent can be determined preoperatively by aortography and at operation, where if necessary, distal arteriograms can be performed to evaluate the peripheral arteries. If femoral pulses are adequate but the popliteal and pedal pulses are absent, the block is localized to the leg and can be adequately delineated by femoral arteriography. The arteriography is best carried out under local anesthesia by means of a #19 needle in the common femoral artery, through which approximately 25 ml of 50% diatrizoate (Hypaque) or similar dye are injected. The primary purpose is to determine whether, below the block, there is any open artery of sufficient size to use in a reconstruction, and also to evaluate runoff into the distal tibial arteries which must serve in distributing the increased flow of blood brought to the area by a graft. No matter what type of arteriography is performed, one should use as little contrast dye as possible and be sure the patient is adequately hydrated, hoping to minimize the complication of renal shutdown, especially in patients with diminished renal function.

The arteriograms shown in Figures 34–3, 34–4 and 34–5 demonstrate the extremes of situations in which grafts are possible. Figure 34–3 shows an open popliteal artery below the block with patent tibial arteries. Figure 34–4 shows a narrow popliteal artery and further occlusions of the lower leg vessels. Grafts were carried out successfully in both of these patients. In the unfavorable situations in which the graft went to an "isolated segment," enough improvement was secured to rid the patient of rest pain in spite of the persistent distal arterial disease. Figure 34–5 shows a popliteal block with an open tibial artery to which the graft was anastomosed.

A study of the findings of arteriography in diabetic patients has been made by Hoar and colleagues[26] who evaluated 294 arteriograms with regard to the extent of the block, condition of the popliteal artery below the block, and runoff into the three major terminal branches of the popliteal

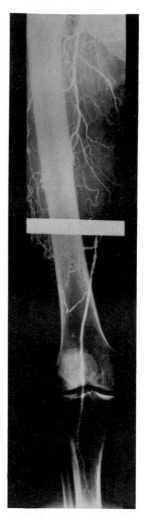

Fig. 34–3. X-ray showing a localized artery block with an excellent popliteal and good distal run-off.

artery. Ninety-eight arterial reconstructions of one type or another were subsequently performed. Since then, techniques for using the calf vessels have been developed, thereby enlarging the number of patients who can benefit from arterial surgery.

Technique. If a block of the aorta and/or iliac arteries is present, and if the symptoms and general condition of the patient permit major surgery, aorto-iliac or aorto-femoral reconstruction is indicated. There are essentially two surgical approaches: artery grafting or thromboendarterectomy. The choice depends on the judgment and experience of the surgeon.

We recently reviewed one hundred patients receiving aortic bifurcation grafts.[26a] Fifty-seven diabetics were compared to forty-three nondiabetics. All patients survived the operation and left the hospital with open grafts. Two-thirds of the operations in diabetics were done for limb salvage as opposed

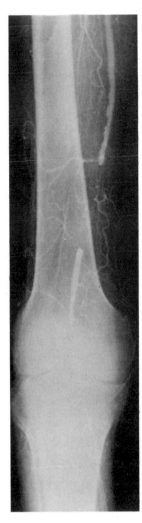

Fig. 34–4. X-ray showing a block in the adductor canal area with a narrow popliteal artery and with further occlusions of the tibial vessels.

obliquely to the side of the artery above and below. Thus, little of the patient's already functioning collateral circulation is disturbed.

If the ipsilateral saphenous vein is too small (less than 4 mm in diameter at the small end), we use the saphenous vein from the opposite leg, and, if necessary, join portions of the right and left saphenous veins (composite or abutting graft) to obtain adequate length. At other times, the cephalic or basilic vein from one or both arms may be used. Hoar and associates[32] have reported good success with these in diabetic patients.

We are hesitant to use plastic grafts in the lower leg since the long-term results are generally so poor. The umbilical vein grafts recently on the market may prove better than plastic, but their use in a large series of diabetic patients has not been reported and long-term patency is still uncertain.

The results of saphenous vein bypass grafts have been reported by Wheelock and Filtzer.[27] Of 104 consecutive operations, 102 patients left the hospital with an open graft (1 patient died of a myocardial infarction and 1 graft failed). Subsequently 27 successful toe or transmetatarsal amputations were carried out to remove areas of gangrene. The long-term patency of these grafts is shown in Table 34–3. Of the 16 grafts which occluded during follow-up, only 8 patients required a major amputation. This experience has now been expanded to include elderly diabetic patients with similar results, especially in terms of limb salvage.[28]

In recent years, encouraged by the reports of Reichle and colleagues,[29] we have been more aggressive in placing grafts to the tibial or peroneal arteries. Using magnifying lenses, vein grafts to arteries 1 to 2 mm in internal diameter can be placed with gratifying results. The majority of these more distal grafts are performed for limb salvage or to relieve severe pain at rest; this procedure is not recommended for claudication alone.

We recently reviewed sixty consecutive femoral to distal tibial/peroneal bypass cases. All patients were diabetic and all operations were performed for limb salvage. There were four early graft failures, all necessitating a major amputation. Four late graft occlusions occurred, none of which resulted in limb loss. This high cumulative patency and limb salvage rate supports an aggressive approach to the ischemic diabetic extremity.

A new development which may increase the patency rate of distal bypass grafts is the "in-situ" method repopularized by Leather and associates.[29a] The technique preserves the vasa vasorum of the vein resulting in minimal endothelial injury. It better matches the sizes of the vein bypass to the arteries it connects and has also allowed for greater utilization of smaller vein segments which might

to one-half in the nondiabetics. Four years later, one-third of the diabetics were dead. Cumulative patency was 94% at five years and was equal for both groups. In the diabetic patients, there was more and progressive distal arterial disease, but we conclude that aortic reconstruction can be safely carried out in diabetics with high graft patency and limb salvage rates.

Femoral artery reconstruction is carried out by means of a graft. A saphenous vein graft is usually preferred if the vein is sufficiently large (4 to 5 mm at the smaller end). This vein makes an almost ideal graft as it has a natural smooth intima, bends without buckling, is easy to suture, is of ample strength, and its use avoids the employment of foreign material. The graft is used as a bypass, usually from the common femoral to the popliteal artery; the opened ends of the vein are sutured

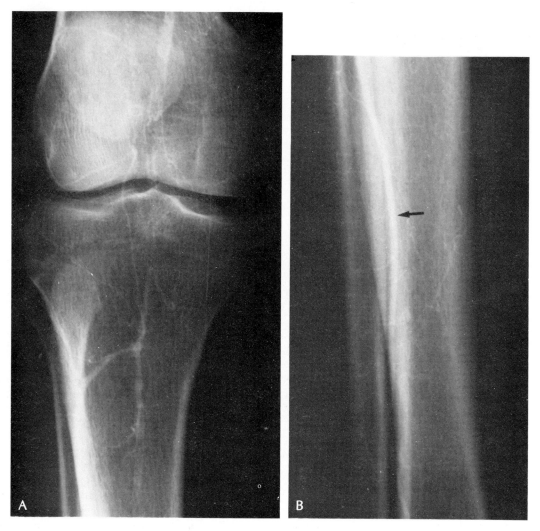

Fig. 34–5. Arteriogram showing popliteal artery occlusion and extensive disease of trifurcation vessels to lower leg. Arrow points to open anterior tibial artery in the lower leg.

Table 34–3. Patency Data of Reconstructed Femoropopliteal Arteries

| Interval in Months | Reconstructed Arteries at Risk (No.) | Reconstructed Arteries Failing (No.) | Reconstructed Arteries not Observed Throughout Interval due to | | Accumulated Patency Rate (%) |
			Death (No.)	Duration of Follow-up (No.)	
0–12	104	4	8	12	96
13–24	80	3	10	20	91
25–36	47	4	4	6	83
37–48	33	1	5	4	80
49–60	23	2	0	5	72
61–72	16	2	2	2	62
73–88	10	0	1	6	62
89–104	3	0	0	3	62

Adapted from Wheelock and Filtzer.[27]

have otherwise been unsatisfactory for a reversed vein graft. Early reports support its superiority for distal tibial bypasses, and it is now our procedure of choice. For this operation, as with all distal bypass grafting, expertise is essential, and the procedure is not recommended for the occasional vascular surgeon.

Transluminal Balloon Dilatation or Angioplasty. Recent advances in angiography and catheter development have made possible non-operative correction of selected arterial blockages and stenoses.[30,31] By means of a small balloon catheter, which is carefully maneuvered into place and distended under fluoroscopy, diseased areas are thought to be crushed into the arterial wall, thereby relieving the obstruction. Pre- and post-dilatation pressures can be used to measure the degree of flow reduction and success.

This procedure requires a great deal of expertise and should not be attempted by those inexperienced or unfamiliar with all aspects of the procedure. Proper surgical back-up is mandatory.

Patient selection is most important. While small, localized arterial stenoses (especially those in the common iliac artery) respond most favorably, as the procedure has become more common and the technique more advanced, so have the indications broadened. Again, caution in the diabetic extremity is needed, especially in those with multisegmental artery disease or disease below the popliteal artery. Careful studies showing long-term patency are still needed in a large series of patients before one can support the use of this procedure routinely. This is especially true when results of by-pass grafting in our experience have been rewarding with quite satisfactory long-term patency.

Sympathectomy. Sympathectomy deserves brief and unenthusiastic comment. It is seldom used since patients with diabetes of longer than 10 years' duration show little evidence of sympathetic activity and in general are not helped by this procedure. Rarely it may be useful in a relatively young diabetic with peripheral vascular disease whose foot can be demonstrated to have the ability to sweat.

AMPUTATIONS

Selection of Site

As mentioned previously, there are two major causes of serious foot problems in diabetic patients—neuropathy and arterial insufficiency. When there has been irreversible destruction associated with neuropathy, the site of amputation of the foot is determined by the area involved. Thus the decisions are relatively easy to make as long as infection has been properly drained and con-

trolled. If arterial insufficiency of some degree is present, more care and thought are required.[33] Our comments will be directed toward the choice of operation in patients with arterial insufficiency. The frequency of the different operations is indicated in Table 34–4 which lists the amputations by site in a typical year.

Transphalangeal Amputation of a Toe. This procedure remains the amputation most commonly performed. If there is evidence of arterial insufficiency, adequate collateral circulation as shown by a venous filling time of 20 seconds or less is necessary. The lesion must be in the distal one-third of the toe, leaving reasonably healthy skin at the point of incision. There should be no dependent rubor of the proximal part of the toe, and all cellulitis and lymphangitis should have cleared prior to operation. Pain, except in the ulcer itself, should have disappeared. To accomplish these ends, up to 3 weeks of in-hospital care may be required. With few exceptions, the aim is to be able to do a closed procedure since open amputations in the presence of diminished circulation do not do well. The skin edges are always approximated with wire or other minimally reactive sutures, and the sutures are left in place for up to 4 weeks. Delicate handling of the skin flaps with avoidance of forceps is mandatory for a successful result.

Amputation of Single Toe and Metatarsal Head. This operation, which removes one toe and its metatarsal head through a racquet shaped incision, leaves a rather large residual space which cannot be surgically closed, particularly when the second, third, or fourth toe is involved. This space must heal by secondary intention with scar formation which eventually pulls the adjacent metatarsals together. The adjacent joint capsules are avascular structures which further delay healing. As one might surmise, the operation is therefore reserved for those patients with quite good collateral circulation. The procedure is actually more useful in the neuropathic rather than the ischemic foot. The lesion most commonly treated by this means is an ulcer under the first or fifth metatarsal head or beneath one of the other metatarsal heads. Usually the incision is closed over its distal 80% and the proximal "racquet handle" is left open for

Table 34–4. Amputations in Diabetic Patients—1979

Guillotine	2
Single toe	105
Transmetatarsal	44
Below-knee	34
Above-knee	22
Total	207

dependent drainage (dependent as the patient lies supine in bed). For the first and fifth toes, the proximal incision is carried along the lateral or medial edge of the foot, off the weight-bearing area. For the others, the incision must extend down the sole.

Sizer[34] reported the results of our digital amputations (692 operations) (Table 34–5). An overall success rate of 94% was achieved. This study substantiates the admonition that in ischemic feet, amputation sites must be closed for maximal success. An analysis by presence or absence of a pedal pulse and by the size of the toe is presented in Table 34–5. Healing of first toe amputation is more difficult because of its size, which means longer flaps to permit closure and thus more chance of flap necrosis.

Transmetatarsal Amputation. In a transmetatarsal amputation one removes all of the toes and metatarsal heads, using a plantar flap, resembling a Turkish slipper, for closure. This results in a short foot, but one that permits walking comfortably without a limp.[35] The lesions for which this amputation may be performed include: (1) one or more distal toe lesions with inadequate circulation at the base of the toes precluding simple toe amputation; (2) one or more proximal toe lesions when ischemia contraindicates a simpler operation; (3) ulcers involving the web space; and (4) ulcers under one or more of the metatarsal heads. Infection must be controlled and the skin of the dorsum and sole of the foot must be healthy. Persistent ischemic pain despite bed rest indicates that circulation is inadequate to permit healing following this type of amputation. In many cases, arterial reconstruction is indicated prior to amputation.

Considerable preparation for the operation may be in order. Small abscesses may need to be drained and necrotic tissue debrided; antibiotics specific for the bacteria involved are administered intravenously for control of active infection. If there has been recent arterial occlusion, enough time must be allowed to permit collateral circulation to build up. If these measures are successful, rest pain will

subside. It may take up to 3 weeks of care in the hospital to prepare the patient for the operation. Many of the failures brought to our attention have been due to haste in operating before a stable and favorable state was achieved.

Pulses need not be present in the foot, but the collateral circulation must meet certain requirements, which include a venous filling time of less than 25 seconds and the absence of dependent rubor at the incision level.

With the patient under spinal or general anesthesia, a fairly straight dorsal incision is made just proximal to the metatarsal heads. A thick plantar flap is fashioned and the metatarsals are divided proximal to their heads. After rongeuring the bone ends to give a smooth contour to the foot, closure is made with one layer of fine wire or other non-reactive sutures.

The results obtained are outlined in Tables 34–6 and 34–7 taken from a report by Wheelock.[36] Table 34–7 demonstrates that peripheral pulses including a popliteal pulse must be present in order to secure successful results. With time, a number of these feet deteriorate further and major amputation may be required. However, the figures indicate a worthwhile limb salvage.

Below-Knee Amputations. When the criteria for a conservative operation on the foot cannot be met or extensive destruction attended with pain or spreading infection demands that the foot be removed, a below-knee amputation should be considered. There is a reasonable and justifiable increase in the selection of this site rather than the supracondylar amputation, since walking with a prosthesis is infinitely more satisfactory following this procedure than after the higher amputation.[37] We select the below-knee level if the patient is expected to use a prosthesis, if the area of gangrene is below the ankle, and if the line of temperature demarcation (between the cold ischemic foot and more nearly normal skin higher up) is at or below the ankle level. A report of our experience by Hoar and Torres[38] in 1962 indicated a low failure rate of 4%, and over the years this has been maintained.

Table 34–5.   Results of 692 Toe Amputations

	Total Number	Initial Success No.	Initial Failure No.	Later Salvage No.
Pedal pulse present—first toe	121	120	1	1
Pedal pulse absent—first toe	85	71	14	10
Pedal pulse present—fifth toe	244	237	7	5
Pedal pulse absent—fifth toe	192	175	17	12
Emergency operation for drainage only:				
First toe	20			10
Fifth toe	30			17

Table 34–6. Results of Transmetatarsal Amputation

Interval Since Amputation	Living Patients	Healed Incisions	
		Number	Percentage
yr.			
2	336	213	63
3	304	173	57
4	281	144	51
5	265	123	46

Table 34–7. Results of Transmetatarsal Amputation According to Level of Pulse Present

Lowest Pulse	Patients No.	Percentage of all Patients	Percentage of Successful Results After 2 yrs
Aorta	11	3	44
Femoral artery	166	39	57
Popliteal artery	190	44	69
Pedal artery	19	4	100
Not recorded	42	10	48
Total	428		

Technically, the amputation is usually accomplished slightly below the mid-lower leg level, using short and equal anterior and posterior flaps, dividing the fibula 1 inch higher than the tibia, and the tibia at a suitable level to permit easy closure. Great care is taken in beveling and contouring the end of the tibia lest a sharp edge cause subsequent ulceration. Occasionally, when there is scarring of the skin over the tibia or the leg is thin, medial and lateral flaps are used. The use of a long posterior muscle flap has seldom been necessary.

Postoperatively a splint is worn for 1 week to reduce the danger of knee contracture. If all goes well, the patient is measured for a prosthesis after 1 week, and ambulation is started near the 14th postoperative day. With an active and well-trained Physical Therapy Department, ambulatory discharge from the hospital is often possible by the 21st day.

Supracondylar Amputations. The mid-thigh amputation is still performed in some hospitals, but should be abandoned in favor of one at the supracondylar level with the incision located at the top of the patella. At this latter site there is less soft tissue to transect, making the procedure especially the closure, easier and faster, important considerations in poor risk or debilitated patients.[33]

The indications for supracondylar amputation include any pathologic condition arising distally that cannot be successfully treated by a more conservative operation on the foot and that do not meet the criteria for a below-knee amputation. In general, the patients undergoing above-knee amputation are in the poor risk groups; many have serious cardiac or renal problems as well as extensive peripheral disease.

CAROTID ARTERY SURGERY

The incidence of stroke in diabetic patients is high. Since many of these can be prevented by carotid surgery,[39] it is imperative to try to identify those at risk. It is well established that a transient ischemic attack (TIA) is often a prelude to a major stroke. Consequently, any patient on our service who has such an event undergoes arteriography and operation if indicated. If an asymptomatic patient is found to have a neck bruit not originating from the chest, noninvasive testing is done.[40,41] If a hemodynamically significant stenosis is detected, an arteriogram is performed. It is recognized that all currently employed noninvasive tests do not identify an ulcerated plaque which may embolize to cause TIA's, but the first event of this origin is usually minor and can be used as an indication for arteriography. If a significant stenosis or an ulcerated plaque is found, carotid endarterectomy is carried out.

Campbell[42] reviewed the results of carotid endarterectomy at the New England Deaconess Hospital and Joslin Clinic. The preoperative stroke rate, the effect of surgery on symptoms, and the long-term follow-up compare well with the results of other large published series (Cf. ref. 39)

NECROBIOSIS LIPOIDICA DIABETICORUM

An occasional diabetic or pre-diabetic patient may develop peculiar flat violaceous skin areas over the shin or around the ankle. The margins may be elevated. Ulceration may develop in these areas, at times becoming quite extensive (see Fig. 34–6, A). Fortunately, the circulation is usually good so skin grafting can be accomplished. Figures 34–6B and C show an extreme case of such necrobiosis pre- and post-grafting. It is important to recognize the nature of this condition and to avoid amputation. This patient had been advised to have bilateral below-knee amputations.

CONCLUSIONS

The diabetic patient may develop certain surgical problems which may be difficult to recognize and which may require specialized surgical treatment. Neuropathy may confuse the diagnosis of acute abdominal problem or create unique foot lesions. Sepsis may be difficult to manage; measures favoring success are more aggressive drainage if appropriate and the energetic use of intravenous antibiotics.

Arterial insufficiency is common but often can

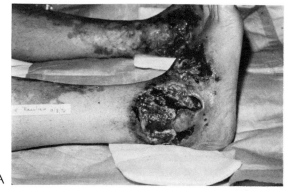

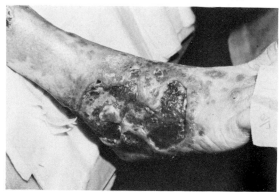

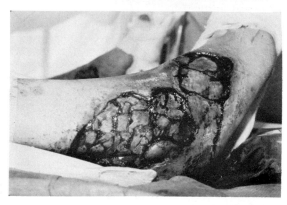

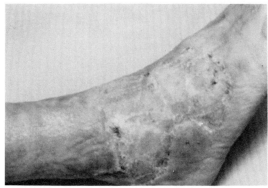

Fig. 34–6. *A.* Necrobiosis lipoidica diabeticorum of lower leg with extensive ulceration and tissue loss. *B.* The same leg immediately before operation. *C.* The same leg following skin grafting. *D.* The same leg six months later.

be helped by appropriate arterial surgery, seldom by sympathectomy. If amputation is indicated, success at all levels can be achieved if certain fundamental principles are followed.

REFERENCES

1. Blackburn, G.L., Gibbons, G.W., Bothe, A., Jr. et al.: Nutritional support in cardiac cachexia. J. Thor. Cardiovasc. Surg. *73*:489, 1977.
2. Dudrick, S.J., Copeland, E.M., Daly, J.M. et al.: A clinical review of nutritional support of the patient. J.P.E.N. *3*:444, 1979.
3. Orr, G., Wade, J., Bothe, A., Jr., Blackburn, G.L.: Alternatives to total parenteral nutrition in the critically ill patient. Crit. Care Med. *8*:29, 1980.
4. Benotti, P., Blackburn, G.L.: Protein and caloric or macronutrient metabolic management of the critically ill patient. Crit. Care Med. *7*:520, 1979.
5. Rosenthal, S., Lerner, B., Dibiase, F., Enquist, I.F.: Relation of strength to composition of diabetic wounds. Surg. Gynecol. Obstet. *115*:437, 1962.
6. Nolan, C.M., Beaty, H.N., Bagdade, J.D.: Further characterization of the impaired bactericidal function of granulocytes in patients with poorly controlled diabetes. Diabetes *27*:889, 1978.
7. Wheat, L.J.: Infection and diabetes mellitus. Diabetes Care *3*:187, 1980.
8. Mundth, E.D.: Cholecystitis and diabetes mellitus. N. Engl. J. Med. *267*:642, 1962.
9. Blumenthal, H.T., Probstein, J.G., Berns, A.W.: Interrelationship of diabetes mellitus and pancreatitis. Arch. Surg. *87*:844, 1963.
10. Bell, E.T.: Carcinoma of the pancreas. I. A clinical and pathologic study of 609 necropsied cases. II. The relation of carcinoma of the pancreas to diabetes mellitus. Am. J. Pathol. *33*:499, 1957.
11. Gramm, H.F., Reuter, K., Costello, P.: The radiologic manifestations of diabetic gastric neuropathy and its differential diagnosis. Gastrointest. Radiol. *3*:151, 1978.
12. Zitomer, B.R., Gramm, H.F., Kozak, G.P.: Gastric neuropathy in diabetes mellitus: clinical and radiologic observations. Metabolism *17*:199, 1968.
13. Louie, T.J., Bartlett, J.G., Tally, F.P., Gorbach, S.L.: Aerobic and anaerobic bacteria in diabetic foot ulcers. Ann. Intern. Med. *85*:461, 1976.
14. Fierer, J., Daniel, D., Davis, C.: The fetid foot: lower extremity infections in patients with diabetes mellitus. Rev. Infect. Dis. *1*:210, 1979.
15. Gibbons, G.W., Eliopoulos, G.M.: Infection of the diabetic foot. In: G.P. Kozak, C.S. Hoar, Jr., F.W. Wheelock, Jr., et al. (Eds.): Management of Diabetic Foot Problems. Philadelphia, W.B. Saunders Co., 1984, pp. 97–103.
16. M.E. Levin, L.W. O'Neal (Eds.): The Diabetic Foot, 2nd ed. St. Louis, C.V. Mosby Co., 1977.
17. Frykberg, R.G., Kozak, G.P.: Neuropathic arthropathy in the diabetic foot. Am. Fam. Physician *17*:105, 1978.
18. LeCompte, P.M.: Vascular lesions in diabetes mellitus. J. Chronic Dis. *2*:178, 1955.
19. Strandness, D.E., Jr.: Evaluation of the patient with peripheral vascular insufficiency. In: J.S. Najarian, J.P. Delaney (Eds.): Vascular Surgery. Miami, Symposia Specialists, 1978, pp. 53–62.
20. Bernstein, E.F.: The noninvasive vascular diagnostic laboratory. In: J.S. Najarian, J.P. Delaney (Eds.): Vascular Surgery. Miami, Symposia Specialists, 1978, pp. 33–46.
21. Yao, J.S., Bergan, J.J.: Application of ultrasound to arterial and venous diagnosis. Surg. Clin. N. Am. *54*:23, 1974.

22. Darling, R.C., Raines, J.K., Brener, B.J. et al.: Quantitative segmental pulse volume recorder: a clinical tool. Surgery 72:873, 1972.

23. Raines, J.K., Darling, R.C., Buth, J., et al.: Vascular laboratory criteria for the management of peripheral vascular disease of the lower extremities. Surgery 79:21, 1976.

24. Gibbons, G.W., Wheelock, F.C., Jr., Hoar, C.S., Jr. et al.: Predicting success of forefoot amputations in diabetic patients by noninvasive testing. Arch. Surg. 114:1034, 1979.

25. Gibbons, G.W., Wheelock, F.C., Jr., Siembieda, C. et al.: Noninvasive prediction of amputation level in diabetic patients. Arch. Surg. 114:1253, 1979.

26. Hoar, C.S., Jr., Wheelock, F.C., Jr., Kellett, M. et al.: Experience with femoral arteriography in diabetic peripheral vascular disease. Surg. Gynecol. Obstet. 123:826, 1966.

26a. Bartlett, F.F., Gibbons, G.W., Wheelock, F.C., Jr.: Aortic reconstruction for occlusive disease: comparable results in diabetics. Submitted for publication, May 1984.

27. Wheelock, F.C., Jr., Filtzer, H.S.: Femoral grafts in diabetics. Resulting conservative amputations. Arch. Surg. 99:776, 1969.

28. Reinhold, R.B., Gibbons, G.W., Wheelock, F.C., Jr., Hoar, C.S., Jr.: Femoro-popliteal bypass in elderly diabetic patients. Am. J. Surg. 137:549, 1979.

29. Reichle, F.A., Rankin, K.P., Tyson, R.R.: Long term results of femoro-infrapopliteal bypass in diabetic patients with severe ischemia of the lower extremity. Am. J. Surg. 137:653, 1979.

29a. Leather, R.P., Shah, D.M., Karmody, A.M.: Infrapopliteal bypass for limb salvage: increased patency and utilization of the saphenous vein used "in situ." Surgery 90:1000, 1981.

30. Abbott, W.M.: Percutaneous transluminal angioplasty: surgeon's view. A.J.R. 135:917, 1980.

31. Greenfield, A.J.: Femoral, popliteal, and tibial arteries: percutaneous transluminal angioplasty. A.J.R. 135:927, 1980.

32. Campbell, D.R., Hoar, C.S., Jr., Gibbons, G.W.: The use of arm veins in femoral-popliteal bypass grafts. Ann. Surg. 190:740, 1979.

33. Wheelock, F.C., Jr.: Amputations: technique and selection of levels. In: J.S. Najarian, J.P. Delaney (Eds.): Vascular Surgery. Miami, Symposia Specialists, 1978, pp. 267–283.

34. Sizer, J.S., Wheelock, F.C., Jr.: Digital amputations in diabetic patients. Surgery 72:980, 1972.

35. Wheelock, F.C., Jr., McKittrick, J.B., Root, H.F.: Evaluation of the transmetatarsal amputation in patients with diabetes mellitus. Surgery 41:184, 1957.

36. Wheelock, F.C., Jr.: Transmetatarsal amputations and arterial surgery in diabetic patients. N. Engl. J. Med. 264:316, 1961.

37. Waters, R.L., Perry, J., Antonelli, D., et al.: Energy cost of walking of amputees: the influence of level of amputation. J. Bone Joint Surg. 58:42, 1976.

38. Hoar, C.S., Jr., Torres, J.: Evaluation of below-the-knee amputation in the treatment of diabetic gangrene. N. Engl. J. Med. 266:440, 1962.

39. Thompson, J.E., Talkington, C.M.: Carotid surgery for cerebral ischemia. Surg. Clin. N. Am. 59:539, 1979.

40. O'Leary, D., Persson, A.V., Clouse, M.E.: Non-invasive testing for carotid artery stenosis. 1. Prospective analysis of 3 methods. A.J.N.R. 2:437, 1981.

41. O'Leary, D.H., Clouse, M.E., Persson, A.V., Edwards, S.: Non-invasive testing for carotid artery stenosis. 2. Clinical application of accuracy assessments. A.J.N.R. 2:565, 1981.

42. Campbell, D.R.: Unpublished data.

35 Foot Lesions in Diabetic Patients: Cause, Prevention, and Treatment

John C. Donovan and John L. Rowbotham

It has long been recognized that persons with diabetes are prone to foot problems. It is likewise well documented that there is increased frequency of both macro- and microvascular disease leading to the ischemia of tissue and poor healing. Diminution of sensation due to peripheral neuropathy is also common in a population of diabetic patients. This leads to lack of protection for both intact and injured tissue.

It is the obligation, therefore, of those dealing with diabetic patients to emphasize the concept of good foot care in the hope of preventing difficulties in the future. This is basically the responsibility of the primary physician who, at each visit, should examine the feet to discover abnormalities and initiate any necessary treatment and instruction. In a hospital setting it is effective to develop a team approach using the services of an internist, surgeon, and podiatrist, as well as those of a nutritionist, physiotherapist, and other specialists as indicated. The role of the team is to treat and to protect vulnerable feet, especially those exposed to increased risk from vascular disease and neuropathy. Treatment provides an excellent opportunity for continuing education of the patient and family in preventive medicine.

RISK FACTORS

Ischemia. This is caused by progressively diminishing circulation in a lower extremity, leading to poor tissue nutrition with the ultimate development of dry, scaly, hairless skin and atrophy of subcutaneous tissue. This predisposes to fissuring, easy blistering, susceptibility to growth of fungi, and a tendency to infection at common sites of injury. Ingrowing toenails, ill-fitting shoes, wrinkled socks or foreign bodies in shoes are also common causes of injury to vulnerable skin. With ischemia of tissues, gangrene can develop quickly and possibly lead to arterial reconstruction and/or amputation.

Neuropathy. Absence of sensation, partial or complete, may cause the patient with neuropathy to ignore development of calluses at various pressure points of the toes and metatarsal heads. Thick calluses often lead to subcallus hematomas with resulting abscesses and osteomyelitis of a metatarsal head or of bones about small joints. Lack of awareness and consequent neglect of these lesions may lead ultimately to surgical intervention.

Ischemia and Neuropathy. In some patients, both neuropathy and ischemia adversely affect healing. It is wise to delineate which is the overriding factor in these situations, realizing that ischemia poses a greater deterrent to healing than neuropathy.

BREAKS IN THE SKIN

In neuropathic and ischemic feet a break in the continuity of the skin may lead to infection. Common sources of such breaks are: fissures, blisters, toenails, trauma, and corns and calluses.

Fissures. Fissures are most frequently caused by dry skin, especially in the area of the heel, around calluses or in the presence of chronic fungal infection. These must be treated with regular application of moisturizing or antifungal creams, some of which are listed below.

Moisturizing	Antifungal	
Eucerin	Haloprogin	(Halofex)
Hydrated lanolin	Tolnaftate	(Tinactin)
Polysorb hydrate	Clotrimazole	(Lotrimin)
	Undecylinic acid	(Desenex)

Maceration of skin between toes due to perspiration also leads to fissures. Following bathing, moisture can be controlled interdigitally by careful blotting with a soft towel. Placing small pledgets of fluffed lamb's wool between the toes or carefully wrapping lamb's wool about the proximal phalanx of the second and fourth toes will promote dryness of all the interspaces. If tinea is present, antifungal solutions are appropriate in this location. It is important to wear clean socks each day. Colored socks contain no poisonous dye, but dirt or stains are more noticeable on white. Shoes should not be worn on 2 consecutive days, but should be allowed to dry out for at least 1 day before being worn again.

Blisters. These are caused most commonly by friction from shoes, sudden increase in walking, wrinkles in socks, and foreign bodies in shoes, as well as exposure to heat, intense cold or chemical irritants. Blisters must be opened or unroofed to relieve the pressure on the underlying tissue, and to permit culture of the exudate. These lesions should then be treated with an antibiotic ointment such as Neosporin (polymixin B-bacitracin-neomycin) or a few drops of one-quarter strength Betadine (10% povidone-iodine).

Hot soaks must never be used. Water macerates and the heat can burn ischemic tissues or be undetected in neuropathic feet. For the same reasons, heating pads, electric blankets and hot water bottles should never be used. All sources of excessive heat and cold should be avoided, and diabetic patients should be taught not to walk barefoot either indoors or outdoors.

All blisters should be considered potential abscesses or gangrene. One must not walk on a blister, but instead should protect the site by using crutches or by complete bed rest. Appropriate antibiotics must be considered if there is any secondary infection.

Toenails. Toenails, even though normal, may be portals of entry of infection due to incorrect cutting. Ingrown toenails, congenital or acquired, result in injury to the nail groove. The inward curling of the nail plate occurs most often in the great toes.

Elderly patients with decreased vision, neuropathy or ischemia are at increased risk, and should have their toenails trimmed and inspected periodically by a podiatrist or responsible family member. Filing with an emery board may be done safely at home. Toenails are better left too long than cut too

short in order to prevent potential irritation of the nail groove and development of a paronychia. If ingrown nails do appear, pressure at the nail plate must be relieved by periodic trimming or by surgery to prevent recurrence of pain and infection.

Trauma. Injury to a sensitive foot is commonly the result of incompatibility of shoes and feet. Improper matching of the shape of the shoe to that of the foot may result in the prompt appearance of abrasions and blisters. Proper fitting may be particularly difficult for feet which lack a protective layer of subcutaneous fat.

Accidental injuries such as lacerations and punctures may provide sources of infection. These episodes, easily overlooked by a patient with sensory neuropathy, emphasize the importance of careful inspection of the feet daily. Sharp objects such as nails and staples may penetrate the sole of a shoe and cause serious infection. This is a common injury to the neuropathic foot and illustrates the need to inspect regularly the shoes as well as the feet. Foreign objects such as stones or other small objects can be "lost" in a shoe and cause irreparable damage to the toes before being suspected or detected.

Corns and Calluses. These arise in predictable patterns over bony prominences where the feet come in contact with shoes or floor. These lesions represent a physiologic response of the skin to irritation, and deserve special evaluation and care, as they are the most common sources of ulcerations in neuropathic skin. They are found most commonly in feet with very low or very high arches, because such feet have more high-pressure areas than the well-balanced foot. If ignored, a hematoma may form under the callus and develop into an abscess with associated osteomyelitis.

TREATMENT OF ULCERS

When ulceration occurs, all necrotic tissue should be gently but completely debrided by the surgeon. A blunt probe is valuable in delineating sinus tracts. Aerobic and, if indicated, anaerobic cultures must be taken. Exposed tissue surfaces are then covered with gauze dressing moistened with antibacterial solutions such as one-quarter strength Betadine (10% povidone-iodine), colistin 75 mg/50 ml saline, or Dakin's solution, one-quarter strength (one-half tablet of Chlorazine [chloramine T] in 30 ml of water). Bed rest or use of crutches to take weight off the foot have proven invaluable by assuring complete relief of pressure and by helping to control edema caused by dependence. Determinations of sensitivity to bacteria allow proper antibiotic selection, but while awaiting results, a broad spectrum antibiotic should be started. With deep sepsis, cellulitis, or lymphangitis, triple antibiotic solutions should be started intravenously at once because in all likelihood there are multiple types of aerobic and anaerobic organisms present. Daily changes of dressing with meticulous debridement of the wound allows granulations to form and prevents pooling of any exudate. Once the ulcer is healed, the patient must return slowly to weight-bearing and attention given to relief of pressure on the healing wound. To prevent recurrence, all factors contributing to formation of ulcers should be eliminated or minimized.

Neuropathic Ulcers. Those ulcers which are small and superficial may be treated successfully on an outpatient basis. However, an ulcer extending to bone and/or joint capsule or tendons usually requires surgical intervention in the hospital to remove or redistribute pressure points. Osteotomy to relocate a protruding metatarsal or resection of a metatarsal head where total pressure relief is needed works well when the circulation is sufficient to heal the surgical wound.

Ischemic Ulcers. Ischemic ulcers or spots of necrosis are less easily treated at home or in the clinic. These are tender infected areas on the toes around the nails or at the base of painful fissures which frequently disable patients. Antibiotics taken orally and frequent visits to the doctor or clinic can provide only limited benefit in such instances. Eventually, especially if the necrosis is spreading, these patients must be hospitalized for vigorous antibiotic therapy, arterial reconstruction and/or some form of ablation, ranging from that of a toe to a major leg amputation.

Superficial Ulcers Caused by Weight-Bearing. These ulcers or digital deformities usually heal once infection is controlled and pressure relieved. Bed rest and crutch walking, although effective, will likely not be continued over a protracted period by an active individual. As weight-bearing is resumed, an "instant healing sandal" (Fig. 35–1) is an effective temporary aid. It consists of a wooden-soled shoe (STAT surgical shoe) lined with materials to cushion points of pressure. The inflexibility of the wooden sole protects by slowing the gait and reducing the length of stride. As a liner, Plastazote (a synthetic, polyethylene foam material) can be heat-molded to the contours of the foot, allowing an even transfer of pressure to the sole. If heat-molding is unnecessary, resilient materials such as Spenco and Poron may be helpful.

Once healing has been achieved, more conventional shoeing is prescribed. Usually, "extra depth" shoes with one-half inch, heat-molded Plastazote inserts provide the depth needed for deformed digits while cushioning metatarsal heads (Fig. 35–2). This combination offers many benefits

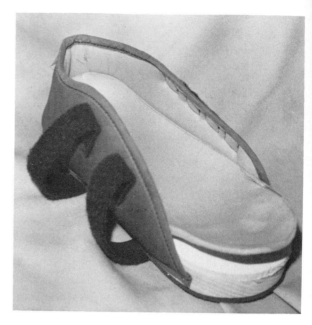

Fig. 35–1. "Instant Healing Sandal." A postoperative wooden-soled shoe that is fitted with a custom heat-molded Plastazote orthotic for the patient who is well on the way to healing a plantar ulceration, but not yet ready for permanent shoeing. The Plastazote is fastened to the shoe with rubber or other cement. Note the Velcro straps. (Courtesy of Geoffrey M. Habershaw, D.P.M.)

including better appearance, reasonable cost, and reduced need for molded shoes.

An additional aid in the treatment of intractable calluses is a rigid sole attained by the use of a full-length shank with a rocker sole below. This arrangement propels the body weight forward and greatly reduces peak loading of pressure on the metatarsal head as weight is thrust forward during walking.

THE FUNCTIONALLY IMPAIRED FOOT

The normal foot is designed to support the body weight easily under a variety of conditions. It is durable, enhances balance, and imparts speed and grace to the human function of walking. However, when support or function is disturbed by vagaries of shape, imbalance of muscles, paralysis, or injuries which alter structure, problems arise. Patients may complain of foot and leg fatigue. Physical examination may disclose deformities of toes and metatarsals, pressure keratoses, and the loss of the smooth rhythm of gait. An unusual form of arthritis, not rare in diabetic patients, is the Charcot joint (neuro-osteoarthropathy) which causes a loss of support of the foot by dissolution of bone with subsequent collapse of the arch and disordered formation of new bone (See Chapter 42). One type

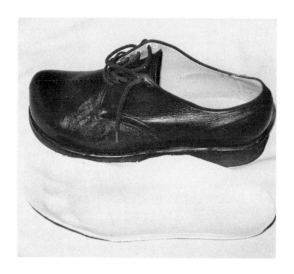

Fig. 35–2. Extra depth shoe with a removable Plastazote orthotic. The Plastazote is heat-molded to conform to the patient's foot. It allows for maximum total contact across the sole of the foot. It is especially useful after healing of a neuropathic ulceration. (Courtesy of Geoffrey M. Habershaw, D.P.M.)

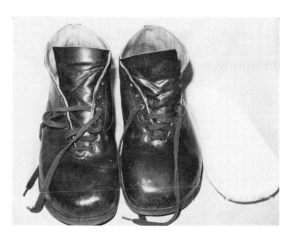

Fig. 35–3. Custom-molded shoe, Chukka style. This shoe is commonly used for deformity too great to be accommodated in a conventional shoe, e.g., Charcot joint, marked hallux valgus with overlapping hammer toe deformity, etc. It extends above the level of the malleoli and gives ankle support, especially desirable for midtarsal, subtalar, or ankle joint Charcot deformity. (Courtesy of Geoffrey M. Habershaw, D.P.M.)

of special shoe to accommodate such deformities is shown in Figure 35–3.

Examination of the patient's shoes may reveal a pattern of irregular wear on the sole, which can make evident destructive forces on that foot. Differences of limb length, presence of joint fusions, and contractures of muscles increase manyfold the

strain to be borne by the foot—strain which some feet cannot bear without breakdown of tissue.

In the foot which has lost toes, metatarsals, or the entire forefoot, the weight-bearing surface area is reduced and the balance of the foot is compromised. Generally, the longer the remaining portion of the foot, the more service it is to the patient. However, if the length of the foot is retained by leaving one or two toes or metatarsal heads, ulcers may develop later. The very fact that an amputation has occurred indicates a high probability that new problems may arise later.

REHABILITATION FOLLOWING PROLONGED BED REST

Bed rest imposed for any length of time leads to muscle wasting. It begins immediately but may not be appreciated for several weeks. Diabetic patients with peripheral vascular or other foot problems may spend many weeks in bed before being allowed up. The average hospital stay for any diabetic person with a foot problem is 6 weeks. It is not uncommon to allow 3 weeks for preparation before doing a transmetatarsal or leg amputation. Following such operations, at least 3 or more weeks in bed or getting ready to ambulate may be necessary.

If one is to avoid serious muscle wasting, a program of rehabilitation must be instituted immediately upon entering the hospital and not delayed until after an operation has been performed.

Rehabilitation is a team affair involving a physiotherapist, a nurse for special dressings and a primary care nurse, as well as the attending physician, surgeon and podiatrist. As soon as expedient, one must begin active bed exercises if possible and passive exercises whenever necessary. Physiotherapy is necessary for every patient hospitalized and bed-ridden because of a foot problem. For those who have surgery, exercises are done up to the time of operation and are resumed as soon as is feasible after surgery. The physiotherapist prepares the patient for walking when the infection or operative wound has healed sufficiently to permit activity.

A program of Buerger exercises is one simple way to accustom the patient to slight activity after a long period at bed rest. The Buerger exercise is a timed program in which the patient lies with legs elevated at 30 to 60 degrees, then sits to dangle them over the side, and finally returns to lying flat in bed. A cycle takes 10 minutes made up, for example, of 1 to 2 minutes elevation, 3 to 4 minutes dependent, and 5 minutes lying. It may be done for 3 to 6 cycles at a time and usually 3 or 4 times a day, depending upon the individual's needs. While Buerger exercises are commonly thought to improve the vasculature of the extremities, they serve primarily to improve muscle tone and strength. They help relieve the monotony of prolonged bed rest and make it much easier to progress from bed to walker to independent walking.

Physiotherapists are indispensable for finding and treating specific weakened muscle groups. Painful feet or legs or amputation stumps are often held flexed and hugged to the body by suffering patients. Great effort must be made to avoid flexion contractures in the limbs of such patients. Splints must be used, either immediately after surgery, or at night when it is so easy to curl the legs up for comfort. These patients require special attention when prosthetics or prostheses are being designed.

The podiatrist plays a special role in the rehabilitation of diabetic patients, serving both as an educator and as a specialist in treating many foot problems. By anticipating that following surgery a foot will swell, muscles will be weaker, bones more fragile, and scars will not have maximum strength, the podiatrist can plan the active phase of rehabilitation after surgery. Dependent edema is common for one or more months after foot surgery or arterial reconstruction. Shoes that formerly would fit will not now do so and can be a source of irritation and blisters. This should be taken into account in considering postoperative shoeing.

In patients with osteoporosis who have been at bed rest for a period of time, a moderately to markedly stiff sole is needed to reduce metatarsal pressure, the risk of stress fractures and possibly Charcot joint disease. A newly healed scar on the plantar surface of the foot cannot tolerate normal weight-bearing for several months after surgical procedure.

A foot that has undergone a transmetatarsal amputation is best fitted with a Clark-Wallabee shoe having a flexible crepe (rather than leather) sole which folds up as the patient walks with a shortened foot (Fig. 35–4). If a toe on one foot is lost because of hallux valgus or bunion with a hammer toe or if one or more toes have been removed with or without the associated metatarsal head, a molded Plastazote insert can help distribute the weight-bearing pressure evenly across the remaining metatarsals. An extra depth shoe with an insert or a molded shoe could accommodate deformities and possibly prevent future contralateral foot problems (Fig. 35–3). Thus, the foot which has had surgery and the opposite intact foot can be protected by mechanical changes in foot gear.

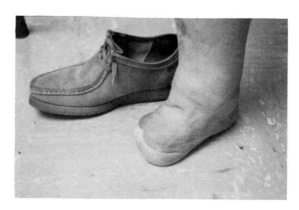

Fig. 35–4. Shoe with a flexible crepe sole (Clark Wallabee) which allows the forward end to fold up. This may be useful for the patient with a transmetatarsal amputation who walks with a shortened foot.

PATIENT EDUCATION REGARDING CARE OF THE FEET

Prevention of foot disease is often a matter of education of the patient and members of the family. The patient, if of suitable age and intelligence, should be impressed with the need for assuming responsibility for care of the feet. Basic rules for foot care include:

1. Careful washing of the feet with a mild soap during regular bathing, followed by thorough drying. At this time the feet (dorsum, sole, and between the toes) should be inspected for lesions.

2. The application of a non-medicated moisturizing cream to prevent dryness and cracking.

3. Clean, non-constrictive stockings or socks of an absorbent material to provide a dry, soft covering.

4. Wearing soft shoes, fitted properly, insulated as well as free from constriction and internal irregularities.

Good support for the structures of the foot is important. Shoes with laces or Velcro closures are preferable to allow for readjustment at mid-day to accommodate any swelling.

If the patient is not well enough physically or emotionally to handle these responsibilities, a family member or Visiting Nurse should be called upon to inspect the feet at frequent intervals, ensure adequate foot care, treat any early indication of disease, and secure podiatric and/or medical care promptly when needed. Continuing attention to the care of the feet is an essential element of long-term success. *Episodic crisis-oriented attention is often incompatible with preservation of a limb.*

36 Infection and Diabetes

Ramachandiran Cooppan

Prior to the advent of modern antimicrobial therapy, infection accounted for much of the mortality of diabetes. In the pre-insulin era from 1914 to 1922, 17.6% of deaths among diabetic patients of Dr. Elliott P. Joslin were reported due to infection (see Table 13–16). Indeed, as late as the period from 1937 to 1943 in the insulin era, 12.6% of the total deaths were ascribed to infection. With the advent of chemotherapeutic and antibiotic agents, fewer and fewer deaths were considered to be due to infection, and in the final period for which statistics are available, 1969 to 1979, only 1.5% were so reported.

If one considers diabetic patients (chiefly those of the Joslin Clinic) who died at the New England Deaconess Hospital, one finds a similar trend in those patients given a post-mortem examination (see Table 14–2). Of 105 deaths up to 1924, 20 (19%) were considered by the pathologist to be due to infection. With the advent of insulin and, later, antimicrobial agents, 88 of 1036 fatalities (8.5%) between 1948 and 1964 and 123 of 1043 deaths

(11.8%) between 1964 and 1980 were ascribed to infection on the basis of autopsy findings. In the last group, the specific causes and number of patients affected were as follows: bronchopneumonia, 58; lobar pneumonia, 1; septicemia, 11; rheumatic fever (including old valvular lesions), 9; pyelonephritis (including necrotizing renal papillitis), 8; peritonitis, 4; endocarditis, 3; meningitis, 2; tuberculosis, 2; gas gangrene, 1; and other infections, 24.

As far as morbidity is concerned, diabetic patients are particularly susceptible to infections of the urinary tract, respiratory tract and skin.

Robbins and Tucker[1] compared the causes of death as determined by autopsy in 307 diabetic patients over the age of 12 years dying between 1932 and 1942 with those in 2800 consecutive nondiabetic patients. They found that the relative incidence of pulmonary and other infections was approximately the same except for acute pyelonephritis and infections of the extremities, which were more frequent in the diabetic patients. Despite the great improvement brought about by insulin and antimicrobial agents, infection still accounts for much of the morbidity and mortality of diabetics. Of 261 adult diabetic patients who died between 1956 and 1960 at the Royal Adelaide Hospital,[2] infection was the direct cause of death in 72 (27.6%), including 3 with pulmonary tuberculosis. Overall infection, whether or not lethal, was found in 152 (58.2%) of the 261 patients; in 51, it was located in the urinary tract.

Cooper and Platt studied the records of all patients with *Staphylococcus aureus* bacteremia who were treated at the New England Deaconess Hospital between 1977 and 1980. The presentation and course of 27 diabetic patients (18 insulin-dependent), largely of the Joslin Clinic, and 34 nondiabetic patients were compared. A primary focus was present in the two groups to a similar degree, 67% and 65%, respectively. They found no difference in mortality between those with and without endocarditis. However, diabetics with staphylococcal bacteremia were more likely than nondiabetics to have endocarditis in the presence of a primary focus.[3]

Infection may be a precipitating or contributing factor in death from diabetic ketoacidosis; this was true especially in the pre-insulin and early antibiotic eras. Tateishi reported from Japan that of 154 patients with diabetes examined at autopsy between 1954 and 1963, in 61 or 40% of the patients, death was due to diabetic coma and in many instances, this was associated with infection.[4] A later study in Japan revealed that of 493 diabetic patients in 384 hospitals examined postmortem in 1968–1970 death was considered to be due to tuberculosis in 1.8%, to pneumonia in 4.2%, and to infection other than these two causes, 5.3% for a total of 11.3%. Incidentally, in 37 (7.5%) death was ascribed to diabetic coma.[4a]

Despite the improvement in mortality regarding infection associated with diabetes, clinical experience indicates that the morbidity due to infection is still a great problem. This is particularly true of the feet, where vascular disease and neuropathy result in a background conducive to soft tissue infection and osteomyelitis (Chapters 34 and 35).

FACTORS INFLUENCING RESISTANCE TO INFECTION

General Considerations

With good control of diabetes, resistance to infection, judged clinically, appears to approach normal. On the other hand, if diabetes is poorly controlled and particularly in the presence of diabetic ketoacidosis, resistance is lowered due in part to impaired leukocyte function. Apart from ketoacidosis, it is the complications of diabetes, especially those of neuropathic and vascular nature, that predispose to infections and lead to a chronic course. Of historical value is the 1960 report of Priscilla White[5] regarding 478 patients who had lived 30 years or more with juvenile onset diabetes. Vascular lesions were associated with a high incidence of infection in this group. There were skin infections in 55% of these patients, urinary tract infections in 28%, pulmonary tuberculosis in 6%, and osteomyelitis in 5% (see Table 36–1).

Table 36–1. Factors Exacerbating Infection in the Diabetic Patient

Likely	Unlikely
1. Dehydration	1. Humoral factors
2. Malnutrition	Defective or inadequate
3. Impaired polymorphonuclear leukocyte function	quate
	Gamma globulin
	Complement
4. Vascular insufficiency	Antibody formation
5. Neuropathy	2. Hormonal factors

Effect of Blood Glucose Level

For years there was no good evidence that the level of blood glucose had any direct effect on infection. However, in an article published in 1978, Nolan and his associates[6] reported that granulocytes from ambulatory, non-hospitalized diabetics with fasting blood glucose values of 200 mg/dl or higher had an impaired ability to engulf and kill opsonized staphylococci. The defects were modest and granulocyte function improved after more intensive management of the diabetes with a reduction in the fasting blood level. The patients in this study were free of infection and, apart from diabetes, were healthy.

More recently, Rayfield and colleagues[6a] reviewed the extensive literature and presented their own data concerning whether diabetic patients are more susceptible to infection than matched nondiabetic controls. They concluded that there is a definite correlation between the prevalence of infection and the mean level of plasma glucose. They found a significant decrease in the intracellular bactericidal activity of leukocytes with *Staphylococcus aureus* and *Escherichia coli* for which serum opsonic activity was lower than in control subjects. They concluded that overall results suggest that good control of blood glucose is a desirable goal.

The effects on infection of dehydration and malnutrition from uncontrolled diabetes are not definitely known. Dubos[7] reported that the bactericidal effect of lactic acid, normally produced by leukocytes in areas of inflammation, is partially reduced for staphylococci in the presence of ketone bodies. The cellular response to infection has received considerable attention. In early studies Marble, White and Fernald[8] found that fresh defibrinated blood and heparinized whole blood of diabetic patients possessed essentially the same phagocytic, bacteriostatic, and bactericidal power against selected strains of streptococci as blood from normal controls. However, the patients in this study were not malnourished, dehydrated, or acidotic, factors that singly or together may play a role.

Defect in Host Defense Mechanisms

A number of studies have now been done to attempt to identify the defect in host defense mechanisms in the diabetic patient. The primary abnormalities appear to be in polymorphonuclear leukocyte (PMN) function, and are most prominent in the poorly controlled patient. Three different aspects of PMN function have been examined: chemotaxis, phagocytosis, and bactericidal activity.

In analyzing the chemotactic aspect with the Rebuck glass cover slip technique, Perillie et al.[9] studied the local exudative cellular response to inflammation in 16 diabetics (10 in good control and 6 in diabetic ketoacidosis) and in 14 nondiabetics, 10 of whom were normal and 4 with uremia and acidosis. The results showed that the early (1 to 3 hours) response of neutrophil granulocytes was impaired in poorly controlled diabetics as compared with findings in normal subjects and well-controlled diabetics. A similar defect was noted in the 4 uremic subjects, suggesting that acidosis played a role since normal cellular responses returned with correction of the acidosis.

The question, however, still remained as to whether the PMN's from diabetic patients had an intrinsic chemotactic defect. In 1970, Brayton et al.[10] reported the effect of alcohol and various diseases, including diabetes on leukocyte mobilization. There was a statistically significant decrease in mobilization in the first 4 hours in 23 diabetic patients as compared with 52 normal controls. Five of these who were in ketoacidosis showed a rate of mobilization which was slower than in the other 18 but the difference was not significant. This defect in migration was not seen in patients with uremia, cirrhosis of the liver, coma as in stroke, or prolonged general anesthesia.

Later, Mowat and Baum,[11] using an in vitro method, measured chemotaxis in 31 diabetic patients. They found the "chemotactic index" to be significantly less than in 31 matched nondiabetic controls. The results were unrelated to therapy (insulin or oral agents), levels of glucose, insulin, and urea nitrogen in blood. However, the defect in chemotaxis of the diabetic leukocyte was corrected by incubation of the cells with insulin and glucose. The amount of immunoglobulin on the surface of the leukocytes did not influence the defect.

On the other hand, Fikrig et al.[12] found no defect in the chemotactic ability of PMN's from adult and juvenile type diabetics in comparison to controls. The authors suggest that differences in technique may explain their results when compared to others.

The cause and the clinical significance of the defect in chemotaxis (reported by some workers) in diabetes have not been determined. The combination of impaired chemotaxis and thickened vascular basement membranes in the diabetic may impair host resistance.

The *phagocytic* function of PMN's in diabetic individuals has been evaluated in a number of studies. Bybee and Rogers[13] compared the phagocytic activity of PMN's obtained from 31 well-controlled diabetics with that from 7 patients with diabetic ketoacidosis and 12 healthy controls. The phagocytic activity of cells from non-acidotic diabetics and controls did not differ significantly but it was suppressed in patients with diabetic ketoacidosis, and this was reversed when the condition was corrected. There were no serum inhibitors of phagocytosis in these tests. A similar defect in phagocytosis was found by Bagdade and co-workers[14] in the blood of poorly controlled diabetics not in ketoacidosis. In a later study by these authors,[15] the phagocytic and *bactericidal* ability of the PMN's for Type 25 pneumococci was studied. Again, a defect, reversible with insulin treatment, was found in both functions. It is believed[16] that insulin is essential for the normal metabolism of glucose to provide energy for phagocytosis and killing of microorganisms.

Cell-Mediated Immune Function

Depressed delayed-type hypersensitivity, abnormal lymphocyte transformation, and granuloma formation have been reported in diabetes;[17] they were more evident when diabetes was poorly controlled. More recently studies in chronically diabetic mice have better defined the changes in the cell-mediated immune system. Roth et al.[18] found that it was not the primary sensitization but the secondary response involving the T lymphocyte or monocyte activity that was severely attenuated. One likely factor for this was insulin deficiency since a significant improvement occurred in the delayed hypersensitivity response with insulin treatment. However, the authors suggest that hyperglycemia and other catabolic factors may also play a role. It also appears with skin testing that the diabetic patient has diminished response to staphylococcal antigen in the lymphocyte transformation assay as well as to Candida antigen.[19,20]

Katz et al.[20a] examined in diabetic patients the phagocytic activity of monocytes which play an important role in the defense against fungi and bacteria and in modulating the immune response. They found a significant reduction in the number of phagocytizing cells when compared with that in controls, although the number phagocytized per cell was similar. The phagocytic capacity of diabetic monocytes was not altered by the addition of insulin. Furthermore, the number of monocytes of control subjects capable of phagocytosis was not affected by the addition of glucose. Their results are in accord with those of Hill et al.[20b]

Influence of Endocrine Systems

The relationship of diabetes to endocrine glands other than the pancreas and the role of other hormones apart from insulin in host resistance to infection are extremely important but still poorly characterized. The anti-inflammatory effect of adrenal steroids is attributed to decreased permeability of the microvasculature, diminished antibody response, and altered function of the reticuloendo-thelial system. The precise role of the thyroid hormones is not fully worked out.

Kass[21] summarized perspectives in these areas and concluded that it is difficult to determine whether the clinical expression of infection in diabetes represents an impaired resistance to invasion or a disturbance of the physiology of host response, increasing the rate of bacterial multiplication once invasion has occurred.

Vascular Insufficiency

Impaired circulation plays a major role in foot infections. In a series of autopsies on persons over 40 years of age performed between 1911 and 1955, Bell,[22] in a now classic paper, reported that infection was an important factor in the development of arteriosclerotic gangrene in 1875 diabetics and only of minor significance in its development in over 50,000 nondiabetics. Gangrene was 53 times as frequent in diabetic as in nondiabetic men and 71 times as frequent in diabetic as in nondiabetic women. The normal response to infection is increased local circulation. The response in the presence of vascular insufficiency is thrombosis and necrosis. An unusual instance of this occurring in the upper extremities was that of a 64-year-old woman with known diabetes for 21 years who developed necrosis of the tips of the left second and the right second and fourth fingers following superficial infections around the nails. There was no evidence of Raynaud's phenomenon. This ultimately led to amputation of the right second finger and subsequent development of osteomyelitis requiring excision of the right first metacarpal head. This patient had gross clinical evidence of diffuse vascular disease as well as chronic uremia secondary to diabetic nephropathy. Her death, approximately a year later at another hospital, was attributed to diabetic nephropathy. Correlation between diabetic vascular disease and urinary tract infections has also been suggested.[23]

Neuropathy

The role of diabetic neuropathy is apparently a local one associated with sensory deficits leading to trauma that is ordinarily avoided by reflex responses, and to delayed treatment once the trauma has occurred. Autonomic neuropathy, by causing paresis of the urinary bladder and stasis of urine in the bladder, predisposes to urinary tract infection, which is common in diabetic patients and may stubbornly resist cure.

INFECTION IN THE PATHOGENESIS OF DIABETES

The question of the role of infection in the pathogenesis of diabetes can be addressed now with greater confidence than in times past. Especially in Type I diabetes, a more definite role for virus infection has been suggested although not proved. Since the suggestion by Harris more than 80 years ago,[24] that a virus might be one of the causes of diabetes in man, there have been many case reports showing a temporal relationship between the onset of certain viral infections and the subsequent development of diabetes.[25] The virus most often thought of clinically has been that of mumps. Indeed, many years ago Gundersen[26] recorded an increased incidence of diabetes during the years immediately following an epidemic of mumps in Norway. It is believed that certain viruses may affect the beta cell and cause an "insulitis"[27] resulting in damage to the cell and subsequent diabetes. In addition, it is believed that certain HLA types may render the host more susceptible to virus damage. For further discussions of viruses as a possible cause of diabetes, see Chapter 2.

For consideration of the relation of chronic pancreatitis to diabetes, see Chapter 40.

SPECIFIC INFECTIONS AND LOCALIZATION OF INFECTIONS IN DIABETES

Urinary Tract Infections. The urinary tract is the site of probably the most common infection in the diabetic. Diabetics have been found at autopsy to have a 5-fold greater frequency of acute pyelonephritis than nondiabetics.[3] However, in the Joslin Clinic series, pyelonephritis has been an infrequent primary—although more frequently a contributory—cause of death (see Chapter 14). Bacteriuria is 2 to 4 times as frequent in diabetic women as in control groups. The incidence in diabetic men is stated to be similar to that in nondiabetic males.[28,29] Although most urinary tract infections in diabetics are relatively asymptomatic, the presence of diabetes predisposes to much more severe infections. Changes in host defense mechanisms, the presence of autonomic neuropathy involving the bladder, and the presence of microvascular disease in the kidneys, may all play a role in this.

Once established, upper urinary tract infections are frequently complicated in diabetic patients as noted by Wheat[30] in his excellent review of the subject of infection and diabetes.

Among 22 patients with emphysematous pyelonephritis, 72% were diabetic.[31] Similarly, of 19 patients with emphysematous cystitis, 80% were diabetic;[32] of 250 with papillary necrosis, 57% were diabetic;[33] of 52 with perinephric abscess, 36% were diabetic;[34] and of 130 patients with metastatic infections, 10% had diabetes.[35]

Emphysematous Pyelonephritis. This is a necrotizing infection with characteristic gas production in and around the kidneys. Most patients have fever and flank pain, and in about 50%, a mass may be felt. In 1978, Spagnola[36] reported 2 cases and found 29 other "true" cases in the literature. In about half of the patients *E. coli* was the causative organism with other gram-negative bacilli isolated in the rest. This is a serious infection associated with bacteremia for which treatment requires the use of parenteral antibiotics and surgery.

Perinephric Abscess. More than a third of patients with this condition have diabetes. The infection occurs insidiously with features of acute pyelonephritis, generally over 4 to 5 days. Most patients have leukocytosis and pyuria. An intravenous pyelogram (IVP) may show non-specific abnormalities but the diagnosis can be more accurately established with ultrasound examination and computerized tomography. The condition does not respond to antibiotic therapy alone; effective treatment requires surgical drainage of the abscess as well.

Papillary Necrosis. This is also an important complication of urinary tract infections in patients with diabetes. Autopsy data indicate that it occurs 5 times more frequently in diabetic persons than in controls.[37] The presentation is of flank pain, fever, chills, and abdominal pain. If a patient with diabetes responds poorly to treatment or if renal insufficiency occurs, this condition must be considered. The diagnosis may be made either by finding fragments of necrotic medullary tissue in strained urine or by retrograde pyelography demonstrating demarcation and separation of the papillae with "ring" shadows due to disappearance of the papillary tip and consequent cavity formation. Intravenous pyelography must be avoided because it may result in acute renal failure from the contrast material, a problem which has become more frequent, especially in diabetics with pre-existing mild renal disease.

Fungal Infections. These infections of the urinary tract are also important. In patients with *Torulopsis glabrata* urinary tract infection, diabetes may be present in 20 to 90%. The majority of fungal infections in the diabetic are clinically insignificant. Candida and *T. glabrata* can cause cystitis, pyelonephritis, renal or perirenal abscesses, fungus balls, and a picture of gram-negative sepsis. A significant infection is present when Candida are found in counts of more than 10,000/ml. However, patients with indwelling catheters may have higher counts with no significant signs of infection. Treatment depends on the site of the infection. Localized bladder infections are treated by irrigation with amphotericin B. The same drug may be used for systemic infections. Another drug that may be used either alone or with amphotericin B is 5-fluoro-cytosine, which is active against Candida and *T. glabrata*.[30]

The long-term effect of urinary infections on the course of diabetes is largely unknown. Because of the increasing likelihood of some microvascular complications with increasing duration of diabetes, all infections of the urinary tract must be properly evaluated and treated. This will reduce the further damage to the kidney that might otherwise result.

Tuberculosis. Root, in reviewing the history of diabetes and tuberculosis, noted that "in the latter half of the 19th century, the diabetic patient appeared doomed to die of pulmonary tuberculosis if he succeeded in escaping coma."[38] In the 1920s and 1930s, tuberculosis continued to be a serious problem for the diabetic. The disease was more extensive and occurred 3 to 16 times more commonly than in nondiabetics. Cheung noted that tuberculosis was far advanced at presentation in more than 50% of cases.[39] Despite the frequent occurrence of tuberculosis in diabetics, patients with tuberculosis did not have an increased incidence of diabetes.

Luntz[40] reviewed results published from 1930 to 1953 and found that within 5 years, 53% of 2010 patients with both diseases had died. Munkner[41] reported in 1953 that 9 of 15 diabetics in a Danish county died within 2 years after the detection of tuberculosis and only 2 remained alive for 4 to 5 years.

In the Philadelphia survey[42] conducted in 1946, the incidence of pulmonary tuberculosis, as determined by x-ray in a series of 3,106 diabetics, was 8.4% compared with 4.3% in a group of 71,767 presumably healthy industrial workers. The proportion of tuberculous patients with active disease was also greater among the diabetics than among the nondiabetics. Age of the patient, duration and severity of diabetes, and underweight were significant factors favoring tuberculosis. Under the age of 40, only 5% of patients with diabetes of less than 10 years' duration had active tuberculosis in contrast to 17% of those with diabetes of more than 10 years' duration. The prevalence rate of active tuberculosis for all diabetics under 40, regardless of duration of the diabetes, was 3 times that for those over 40. A correlation between severity of diabetes and the presence of active tuberculosis was suggested by the finding that 5.3% of those whose diabetes required more than 40 units of insulin daily had the disease in active form. The prevalence of tuberculosis in diabetics, as in nondiabetics, was twice as high among those below standard weight compared with those above standard weight. However, this could in general be accounted for by the fact that the diabetics had a higher percentage of *active* tuberculosis, 31%, as contrasted with 11% in the control group.

Blum and Atagun[43] found that diabetics constituted 3.84% of the 2342 patients admitted to the Tuberculosis Division of Baltimore City Hospitals from January, 1953 to December, 1960. Of the 90 diabetics, 45 were previously known and 30 were newly diagnosed at the time of admission. Fifteen patients later developed symptoms and were then diagnosed as having diabetes. Phillips[44] noted in the 1960s that about half the active new cases of tuberculosis were occurring in those who were at least 45 years old and the relative incidence was highest in those who had passed 65 years. This tendency has apparently continued.[44a] Thus, new cases of tuberculosis are now found most frequently in the age group that has the highest prevalence of diabetes.

Prior to the introduction of specific drugs in the late 1940s, the treatment of tuberculosis presented great problems and the overall mortality was high. Although many patients benefitted from such diverse measures as prolonged bed rest, pneumothorax, pneumonectomy and lobectomy, treatment was tedious, time-consuming, and far from ideal. With widespread usage of antimicrobial agents, treatment has been greatly simplified and the outlook for the patient has improved tremendously. In a paper published as early as 1962, Holden and Hiltz[45] concluded from their 1931 to 1961 series that intensive treatment of both conditions as soon as possible had altered the dread prognosis of the 1930s until it has become equivalent to that of other tuberculous individuals. In the 20 years since, this has been a common experience. Thus, among patients of the Joslin Clinic, tuberculosis was responsible for 4.9% of total deaths in the period of 1914 to 1922. This had fallen to 1.7% by 1944 to 1949, and in the 10-year period of 1969 to 1979, no deaths were ascribed to this infection (See Table 13–16). Nevertheless, at autopsy 2 cases of tuberculosis were found among 1043 diabetic patients examined between 1964 and 1980.

Although drug treatment for tuberculosis has greatly improved the overall prognosis, diabetes, particularly if poorly controlled, may still predispose to reactivation of tuberculosis. In one study,[46] diabetes was found concurrently in 8% of 145 patients with reactivation of tuberculosis. This was second only to the association with severe alcoholism that occurred in 26%. Tuberculosis should be considered in patients with diabetes who have weight loss, fever, and general debility that cannot be fully explained by poor diabetes control alone.

Even though tuberculosis of the lungs is now infrequent, extra-pulmonary sites, especially the urinary tract, must be kept in mind. It may still be advisable to recommend periodic tuberculin testing in diabetic patients who are tuberculin negative. Those with positive reactions or recent conversions who have never been treated, should receive, under close medical supervision, prophylactic treatment with isoniazid and pyridoxine for a year, regardless of age or the radiographic findings, because of the greater severity of tuberculosis in diabetic individuals.

Bacterial Pneumonia. Pneumonia remains an important infection in diabetic patients. It is frequently caused by staphylococci or gram-negative bacilli. In the study of Khurana and associates[47] at the Joslin Clinic it was found that *Klebsiella pneumoniae* and *Staphylococcus aureus* were the most frequent causes of pneumonia in 112 diabetic patients. Nearly 40% of these patients died. Tillotson and Lerner found that diabetes was present in 69% of patients with *E. coli* pneumonia.[48]

In 1969, Winterbauer and co-workers[49] described 158 patients with recurrent pneumonia. Twenty of these had diabetes, which made it the fifth most common association. Mufson et al.[50] described their experience with 264 patients with pneumococcal pneumonia in Cook County Hospital, Chicago. There were 62 deaths with a mortality of 24%. There were 12 diabetics among the 62; 5 of the 12 died.

In a survey by Miller quoted by Moss,[51] pneumonia was diagnosed in 393 patients (5.8%) of 6,765 admissions to the diabetic ward of the Los Angeles County-USC Medical Center. There were 75 deaths, a mortality of 19%. The pneumococcus was identified in 56 patients, 0.8% of the admissions, and in 14% of the pneumonias. Of the 56 in the pneumococcus group, 6 or 11% died. Other pathogenic organisms were identified in the remaining patients with pneumonia; of these, 45 or 13%, died. It would appear therefore from this experience that in the diabetic patient, pneumococcal pneumonia may not be more lethal than other types.

In two studies of bacteremic pneumococcal pneumonia, the diabetic patient fared less well than those who were otherwise in good health and had no underlying chronic disease. Austrian and Gold[52] found a mortality of 17% among 18 diabetics not in ketoacidosis and 7% for those without diabetes. In Mufson's study,[50] there was a mortality of 42% among the 12 diabetics with bacteremic pneumococcal infections.

The question as to whether all diabetic patients should receive pneumococcal vaccine has not been settled. Although some data suggest no benefit with the vaccine, the current recommendation is that elderly patients, those with long duration diabetes with complications of renal disease, coronary artery disease and heart failure, and patients with chronic lung disease should be vaccinated with the hope of preventing pneumococcal pneumonia. Lederman et al.[50a] demonstrated the safety and efficacy of the vaccine in inducing an antibody response. They found no difference between controls and diabetic patients in the magnitude of antibody response (834 ng protein N/ml [controls] versus 1009 ng protein N/ml [diabetics]). Further, there was no correlation with age, sex, duration of diabetes, insulin dose, or glycosylated hemoglobin levels. Results of the study by Feery et al.[50b] substantiated still further the safety and efficacy of the vaccine. Furthermore, Austrian and co-workers[50c] reported a 79% reduction in pneumococcal bacteremia in a field trial involving 4500 normal subjects.

OTHER SPECIAL INFECTIONS IN THE DIABETIC

Emphysematous Cholecystitis.[30] This is an infection with mixed organisms (aerobic and anaerobic) with a characteristic radiologic picture of gas in or around the gallbladder. Over one-third of reported patients with this problem have been diabetic.[53,54]

Clinically, the condition differs from acute cholecystitis in that most patients are male, gangrene of the gallbladder is 30 times more frequent, and perforation occurs 4 times oftener. The overall mortality is 15% (3 times greater) and in patients over the age of 60 years, the mortality is 10 times greater. The presentation clinically is similar with pain in the right upper quadrant, nausea, and vomiting. Gas may be seen in the gallbladder within the first 48 hours of infection and may extend to the surrounding tissues within the next 48 hours. Sequential abdominal x-rays should be done in diabetic patients with findings of acute cholecystitis for at least 4 days.

Bile cultures are positive in more than half the cases and clostridia accounts for 25 to 50% of these. Other organisms isolated have included Pseudomonas aeruginosa, streptococci, staphylococci, and E. coli. Treatment requires early cholecystectomy along with broad spectrum antibiotic therapy. The exact mode of development of the condition is still unclear. Many patients show narrowing of the lumens of the gallbladder arterioles, suggesting a role for arterial insufficiency. Previous attacks of cholecystitis have occurred in a third of patients and about half have gallstones.

Malignant External Otitis. This is an infection unique in diabetics; only rarely has it occurred in other persons. The patients, often elderly, present with persistent ear pain and drainage. Typically, fever and leukocytosis are not present and inspection of the ear shows a polypoid mass of granulation tissue in the canal. About half the patients have a facial palsy, and spread into the bones can lead to other cranial nerve palsies. Rare complications are meningitis and sigmoid sinus thrombosis. Radiographs of the area are not helpful. The commonest organism is Pseudomonas aeruginosa and this can sometimes be recovered from surgically removed tissue.

Most patients require surgical treatment together with a prolonged course of antibiotic therapy. The recommended antibiotics are an aminoglycoside with carbenicillin or ticarcillin.[30] The presence of facial palsy is a bad prognostic sign and at least half of such patients die. The predisposition of the diabetic patient to this infection is not fully understood. It may occur in patients in whom diabetes has been under good control. It is thought that perhaps diabetic microangiopathy in this area may lead to vascular insufficiency and predispose to infection.[55,56] In an article reporting 21 cases of their own and reviewing 130 cases in the literature, Doroghazi et al.[56a] re-emphasized the predominance of diabetes in this infection. Nineteen of 21 patients were diabetic and, most important, they noted that those with central nervous system deficits had a very poor prognosis: six of nine patients died, whereas all patients without neurological deficits survived.

Rhinocerebral Mucormycosis. This rare infection occurs usually in diabetic patients with ketoacidosis. It can occur in other acidotic states, but diabetes has been present in two-thirds of the reported cases of mucormycosis. The fungi belong to the Mucor, Rhizopus, and Absidia genera.

The presentation is with sudden onset of periorbital or perinasal pain, with induration and discoloration associated with a bloody nasal discharge. There may be unilateral headache, lacrimation, and eyelid swelling. The ischemic nasal turbinates are characteristically black and necrotic. Complications of cranial palsies (nerves 2 to 5), hemiparesis, seizures, coma and findings of meningoencephalitis may appear as a result of vascular thrombosis and extension of the infection through the orbital bones into the meninges and brain.[35,57,58]

The presence of unilateral proptosis and chemosis with retinal vein engorgement indicates a possible cavernous sinus thrombosis. Untreated patients die within 1 week. However, about 50 to 85% of patients survive by adequate treatment with amphotericin B along with debridement of necrotic tissue and measures to control diabetes. Regrettably, residual sequelae are common.[35]

Hamill et al.[58a] emphasize that with aggressive treatment of both the infection and the diabetes, rhinocerebral mucormycosis with bilateral brain abscesses can be cured. Their patient, a 31-year-old man with insulin-dependent diabetes, entered the hospital with moderate ketoacidosis and with classic signs of rhinocerebral infection—purulent nasal discharge, induration of the right side of the face, periorbital edema, proptosis of the right eye, total loss of vision, and marked infection and necrosis of the right inner-nasal vestibule. Computerized tomography (CT) scans revealed signs of cerebral involvement. The patient was treated with amphotericin B, penicillin, and nafcillin. Serial CT scans were used to guide the amphotericin B (continued for 4 months) and surgical treatment. The latter consisted of initial debridement followed later by resection of frontal lobe abscesses. The patient was able eventually to return to full-time employment; there were no neurologic sequelae.

Again the cause of the predisposition of diabetic patients to this infection is not fully understood. Acidosis and hyperglycemia play a role in increasing the growth of these fungi. However, cases have been reported in nonketotic diabetes, in which the major problems were dehydration and hyperglycemia.[58] Artis and colleagues[58b] suggest a possible explanation for the growth of the fungus, *Rhizopus oryzae*, in ketotic patients. With acidosis, the iron binding of transferrin is disrupted and, with increased free iron in the serum, the growth of the fungus is promoted.

Soft Tissue and Skin Infections. A general clinical belief is that diabetic patients are predisposed to staphylococcal skin infections. This was certainly true in the pre-insulin era and the results of a study in recent years indicated that staphylococcal colonization correlates with poor glycemic control.[59] It is common clinical experience that, other things being equal, in patients with good diabetes control, resistance to skin infections approaches that in the nondiabetic. In a controlled study by Williams,[60] there was no increase in carbuncles and boils in diabetics when compared to nondiabetics.

The question of postoperative wound infection is unresolved. Results of the study by Cruse and Foord[61] suggested a 5 times greater frequency in diabetes, but Lidgren found no such increase in clean orthopedic wounds.[62]

Necrotizing soft tissue infections with extensive necrosis of skin and subcutaneous tissues or the underlying muscles are uncommon but extremely serious. Necrotizing cellulitis is a life-threatening infection occurring usually in adult Type II diabetics.[63] Usually there is a subcutaneous infection that does not respond to treatment. These patients are very ill and often in diabetic acidosis when admitted; the infection occurs mainly in the lower extremities and perineum. Subcutaneous emphysema is found in about 25% of cases. Anaerobic organisms (bacterioids and anaerobic streptococci)

and other gram-negative bacilli (Pseudomonas and enterococci) may be cultured from the wounds. A bacteremia occurs in half the patients with the above organisms.

Necrotizing fasciitis is less severe and often follows minor trauma and cutaneous infections.[64] Again the perineum and lower extremities are most commonly affected. The skin is often gangrenous. Gram-negative bacilli, streptococci, and staphylococci may be found on culture. Treatment of these infections requires surgery to provide thoroughly adequate drainage and parenteral antibiotics. Repeated debridement may be needed in this condition in which the mortality is still high.

Bone Infections. Foot infections and their treatment are discussed in Chapters 34, 35, and 38. Osteomyelitis has been a frequent complication of these infections. As for infections of the spine, the lumbar and thoracic vertebrae are most often involved. Among 8 patients seen at the Joslin Clinic with vertebral osteomyelitis, all were insulin-dependent and the striking clinical presentation was a long history of low back pain. Six of the patients had peripheral neuropathy and 2 had bladder neuropathy. At the time of admission, a neurologic deficit was present in 4. The erythrocyte sedimentation rate was elevated in all patients and the alkaline phosphatase in 5. Radiographs of the spine showed bony erosion of the body of the affected vertebra. Three patients had disc space abscesses that required drainage. Of the 8 patients, 5 recovered fully with surgery and parenteral antibiotic therapy.[65] Even though there is no definite evidence to show that osteomyelitis is more prevalent in diabetes, it is important to be aware of this possibility because of the morbidity associated with it.

THE MANAGEMENT OF INFECTION IN DIABETES

In the diabetic, for those infections which are amenable to specific medical or surgical therapy, such measures should be applied promptly and the subsequent course should be followed more closely than might be considered necessary for comparable conditions in the nondiabetic. It has been the clinical impression that the diabetic's response to infection differs from that of the nondiabetic in that the diabetic shows fewer diagnostic clues until the condition is far advanced. In acute appendicitis, for instance, the fever and pain may be less in a diabetic patient, especially in the elderly person, than would otherwise be expected. The possibility of acute cholecystitis must always be kept in mind, especially as the complication of gangrene of the gallbladder can occur with minimal physical signs. An unexpected, significant rise in the insulin requirement should lead the clinician to consider an occult infection somewhere.

Choosing an antimicrobial agent for a diabetic patient does not differ from choosing one for a nondiabetic. However, one should be aware that in diabetic gangrene, multiple organisms can be cultured. In the study by Sharp et al.[65a] an average of 2.3 organisms per specimen were found. These were in patients with diabetic gangrene (mainly of the foot) and the predominant organisms were *Proteus* species, enterococcus, and *Staphylococcus aureus*.

Because of the susceptibility to candidiasis, one might consider using nystatin in conjunction with broad-spectrum antibiotics, but routine inclusion of nystatin is not warranted. The possibility of diabetic nephropathy with impaired renal function should be considered in using antibiotics that are excreted by the kidneys.

In the diabetic patient with an infection, the methods for controlling the diabetes do not differ from those employed when no infection is present, but they do need to be applied with more meticulous surveillance than is ordinarily required. Pyogenic infections with fever and/or leukocytosis usually require prompt and large increases in the total daily insulin dosage. The requirement in an individual case can be learned only empirically, and therefore supplementary doses of regular insulin are often necessary to keep the diabetes under reasonable control and prevent persistent acetonuria. Complete euglycemia and aglycosuria are not desirable because the onset of recovery may be associated with prompt abatement of the insulin requirements often to approximately pre-infection levels. The insulin requirement is a sensitive prognostic index.

When it is necessary to prescribe supplementary doses of regular insulin, these may be given at intervals of 4 hours in amounts related to a fraction, such as 10 to 20%, of the patient's usual daily insulin requirement. Twenty percent of the total daily requirement would be an average initial dose of regular insulin for supplementary use when there is considerable glycosuria but no significant acetonuria. If there is moderate to marked acetonuria in the presence of marked hyperglycemia and glycosuria, this dose should be doubled and, as the reports of subsequent urine tests are obtained, even larger amounts may be given if necessary. If supplementation requirements reach these proportions, hospitalization for impending ketoacidosis is usually necessary.

In a patient who has not been taking insulin, the same type of program can be followed, starting with appropriate doses of regular and intermediate-acting (lente or NPH) insulins.

In patients with prominent gastrointestinal symptoms, the anorexia may require slight reduction in the usual morning dose of insulin, particularly the regular insulin. On the other hand, the development of ketoacidosis must be kept in mind and appropriate treatment applied. As in other infections, it is important that the patient take intermediate- or long-acting insulin. If vomiting ensues, insulin requirements usually increase and at times greatly, so that supplementation with regular insulin may be necessary. In non-hospitalized patients in whom vomiting is not intense, salt-containing broth given in tablespoon quantities may help forestall sodium and water depletion until recovery reverses the trend.

The diet must be adjusted to the patient's ability to take food. Low-calorie vegetables are usually omitted and carbohydrate in 'more concentrated form, such as crackers, bread, fruit juices, and ginger ale, is substituted. Ginger ale that has been allowed to decarbonate is often a well-tolerated fluid when taken at room temperature in small amounts, even when nothing else given orally can be retained. Cola syrup (about 50% sugar) may be given in small amounts ranging from sips to a tablespoonful. If oral feeding cannot be tolerated, hospitalization for intravenous fluid therapy is usually required. For further discussion, see ''sick day rules'' in Chapters 17 and 19.

While there is no doubt that angiopathies are the complications most limiting and most threatening to the life of the diabetic patient today, infection still causes a significant morbidity and mortality. In some instances, it tips the scale from a precarious balance between well-being and chronic disability to acute and possible lethal illness. In an overall situation that may be fatal without early diagnosis and prompt and adequate treatment, infection remains an eminent challenge both to clinical acumen and research ingenuity.

REFERENCES

1. Robbins, S.L., Tucker, A.W., Jr.: The cause of death in diabetes: a report of 307 autopsied cases. N. Engl. J. Med. *231*:865, 1944.
2. Seymour, A., Phear, D.: The causes of death in diabetes mellitus. A study of diabetic mortality in the Royal Adelaide Hospital from 1956 to 1960. Med. J. Aust. *50*:890, 1963.
3. Cooper, G., Platt, R.: Staphylococcus aureus bacteremia in diabetic patients. Endocarditis and mortality. Am. J. Med. *73*:658, 1982.
4. Tateishi, R.: The cause of death in diabetes in Japan. A report of 154 autopsied cases. Acta Path. Jap. *15*:133, 1965.
4a. Hirata, Y., Mihara, T.: Principal causes of death among diabetic patients in Japan from 1968 to 1970. In: S. Baba, Y. Goto, I. Fukui (Eds.): Diabetes Mellitus in Asia. Amsterdam-Oxford, Excerpta Medica, 1976, pp. 91–97.
5. White, P.: Childhood diabetes. Its course, and influence

on the second and third generations. Banting Memorial Lecture. Diabetes 9:345, 1960.

6. Nolan, C.M., Beaty, H.N., Bagdade, J.D.: Further characterization of the impaired bactericidal function of granulocytes in patients with poorly controlled diabetes. Diabetes 27:889, 1978.

6a. Rayfield, E.J., Ault, M.J., Keusch, G.T., et al.: Infection and diabetes: The case for glucose control. Am. J. Med. 72:439, 1982.

7. Dubos, R.J.: Effect of ketone bodies and other metabolites on the survival and multiplication of staphylococci and tubercle bacilli. J. Exp. Med. 98:145, 1953.

8. Marble, A., White, H.J., Fernald, A.T.: The nature of the lowered resistance to infection in diabetes mellitus. J. Clin. Invest. 17:423, 1938.

9. Perillie, P.E., Nolan, J.P., Finch, S.C.: Studies of the resistance to infection in diabetes mellitus: local exudative cellular response. J. Lab. Clin. Med. 59:1008, 1962.

10. Brayton, R.G., Stokes, P.E., Schwartz, M.S., Louria, D.B.: Effect of alcohol and various diseases on leukocyte mobilization, phagocytosis, and intracellular bacterial killing. N. Engl. J. Med. 282:123, 1970.

11. Mowat, A.G., Baum, J.: Chemotaxis of polymorphonuclear leukocytes from patients with diabetes mellitus. N. Engl. J. Med. 284:621, 1971.

12. Fikrig, S.M., Reddy, C.M., Orti, E., et al.: Diabetes and neutrophil chemotaxis. Diabetes 26:466, 1977.

13. Bybee, J.D., Rogers, D.E.: The phagocytic activity of polymorphonuclear leukocytes obtained from patients with diabetes mellitus. J. Lab. Clin. Med. 64:1, 1964.

14. Bagdade, J.D., Nielson, K.L., Bulger, R.J.: Reversible abnormalities in phagocytic function in poorly controlled diabetic patients. Am. J. Med. Sci. 263:451, 1972.

15. Bagdade, J.D., Root, R.K., Bulger, R.J.: Impaired leukocyte function in patients with poorly controlled diabetes. Diabetes 23:9, 1974.

16. Bagdade, J.D.: Infection in diabetes: predisposing factors. Postgrad. Med. 59:160, 1976.

17. Wing, E.J., Remington, J.S.: Cell mediated immunity and its role in resistance to infection. West. J. Med. 126:14, 1977.

18. Roth, M.D., Barg, M., Michalski, R., Arquilla, E.R.: Cell-mediated immunity in chronically diabetic mice. Diabetes 29:825, 1980.

19. Casey, J.I., Heeter, B.J., Klyshevich, K.A.: Impaired response of lymphocytes of diabetic subjects to antigen of Staphylococcus aureus. J. Infect. Dis. 136:495, 1977.

20. Plouffe, J.T., Silva, J., Jr., Fekety, R., Allen, J.L.: Cell-mediated immunity in diabetes mellitus. Infect. Immun. 21:425, 1978.

20a. Katz, S., Klein, B., Elian, I., et al.: Phagocytic activity of monocyte chemotactic responses in diabetes mellitus. Diabetes Care 6:479, 1983.

20b. Hill, H.R., Augustine, N.H., Rallison, M.L., Santos, J.I.: Defective monocyte chemotactic responses in diabetes mellitus. J. Clin. Immunol. 3:70, 1983.

21. Kass, E.H.: Hormones and host resistance to infection. Bacteriol. Rev. 24:177, 1960.

22. Bell, E.T.: Atherosclerotic gangrene of the lower extremities in diabetic and nondiabetic persons. Am. J. Clin. Path. 28:27, 1957.

23. Vejlsgaard, R.: Significant bacteriuria in relation to vascular disease of diabetes of long duration. In: E.H. Kass (Ed.): Progress in Pyelonephritis. Philadelphia, F.A. Davis Co., 1964, pp. 492–500.

24. Harris, H.F.: A case of diabetes mellitus quickly following mumps. Boston Med. and Surg. J. 140:465, 1899.

25. Levy, N.L., Notkins, A.L.: Viral infections and diseases of the endocrine system. J. Inf. Dis. 124:94, 1971.

26. Gundersen, E.: Is diabetes of infectious origin? J. Infect. Dis. 41:197, 1927.

27. LeCompte, P.M.: "Insulitis" in early juvenile diabetes. Arch. Path. 66:450, 1950.

28. Kass, E.H.: Bacteriuria and the diagnosis of infections of the urinary tract. Arch. Intern. Med. 100:709, 1957.

29. Pometta, D., Rees, S.B., Younger, D., Kass, E.H.: Asymptomatic bacteriuria in diabetes mellitus. N. Engl. J. Med. 276:1118, 1967.

30. Wheat, L.J.: Infection and diabetes mellitus. Diabetes Care 3:187, 1980.

31. Schainuck, L.I., Fouty, R., Cutler, R.E.: Emphysematous pyelonephritis. A new case and review of previous observations. Am. J. Med. 44:134, 1968.

32. Bailey, H.: Cystitis emphysematosa; 19 cases with intraluminal and interstitial collections of gas. Am. J. Roentgenol. 86:850, 1961.

33. Lauler, D.P., Schreiner, G.E., David, A.: Renal medullary necrosis. Am. J. Med. 29:132, 1960.

34. Thorley, J.D., Jones, S.R., Sanford, J.P.: Perinephric abscess. Medicine (Baltimore) 53:441, 1974.

35. Meyer, R.D., Armstrong, D.: Mucormycosis—changing status. CRC Critic. Rev. Clin. Lab. Sci. 421:51, 1973.

36. Spagnola, A.M.: Emphysematous pyelonephritis. A report of two cases. Am. J. Med. 64:840, 1978.

37. Mandel, E.E.: Renal medullary necrosis. Am. J. Med. 13:322, 1952.

38. Root, H.F.: The association of diabetes and tuberculosis: epidemiology, pathology, treatment and prognosis. N. Engl. J. Med. 210:1, 1934.

39. Cheung, O.T.: Treatment of pulmonary tuberculosis in diabetic patients. Med. Serv. J. Canada, 18:665, 1962.

40. Luntz, G.R.W.N.: Management of the tuberculous diabetic. Follow-up of 84 cases for one year. Brit. Med. J. 1:1082, 1957.

41. Munkner, T.: Incidence of pulmonary tuberculosis among diabetics in the County of Vejle in 1944–51. Acta Tuberc. Scand. 28:355, 1953.

42. Boucot, K.R., Cooper, D.A., Dillon, E.S., et al.: Tuberculosis among diabetics. The Philadelphia Survey. Am. Rev. Tuberc. 65 (Suppl.):1, 1952.

43. Blum, L.V., Atagun, M.: Diabetes mellitus at the Tuberculosis Division of Baltimore City Hospitals. Maryland Med. J. 12:10, 1963.

44. Phillips, S.: A view of the overall problem. In: S. Phillips (Ed.): Current Problems in Tuberculosis. Springfield, Charles C Thomas, 1966, pp. 109–115.

44a. Des Prez, R.: Tuberculosis. In: J.B. Wyngaarden, L.H. Smith (Eds.): Cecil Textbook of Medicine. Philadelphia, W.B. Saunders Co., 1982, p. 1539.

45. Holden, H.M., Hiltz, J.E.: The tuberculous diabetic. Canad. Med. Assoc. J. 87:797, 1962.

46. Edsall, J., Collins, J.G., Gray, J.A.C.: The reactivation of tuberculosis in New York City in 1967. Am. Rev. Respir. Dis. 102:825, 1970.

47. Khurana, R.C., Younger, D., Ryan, J.R.: Characteristics of pneumonia in diabetics. Clin. Res. 21:629, 1973. Abstract.

48. Tillotson, J.R., Lerner, A.M.: Characteristics of pneumonias caused by Escherichia coli. N. Engl. J. Med. 277:115, 1967.

49. Winterbauer, R.H., Bedon, G.A., Ball, W.C., Jr.: Recurrent pneumonia: predisposing illness and clinical patterns in 158 patients. Ann. Intern. Med. 70:689, 1969.

50. Mufson, M.A., Kruss, D.M., Wasil, R.F., Metzger, W.I.: Capsular types and outcome of bacteremic pneumococcal disease in the antibiotic era. Arch. Intern. Med. 134:505, 1974.

50a. Lederman, M.M., Schiffman, G., Rodman, H.M.: Pneumococcal immunization in adult diabetics. Diabetes *30*:119, 1981.

50b. Feery, B.J., Hartman, L.J., Hampson, A.W., Proietto, J.: Influenza immunization in adults with diabetes mellitus. Diabetes Care *6*:475, 1983.

50c. Austrian, R., Douglas, R.M., Schiffman, G., et al.: Prevention of pneumococcal pneumonia by vaccination. Trans. Assoc. Am. Physicians *89*:184, 1976.

51. Moss, J.M.: Pneumococcus infection in diabetes mellitus. Is this a justification for immunization? J.A.M.A. *243*:2301, 1980.

52. Austrian, R., Gold, J.: Pneumococcal bacteremia with especial reference to bacteremic pneumococcal pneumonia. Ann. Intern. Med. *60*:759, 1964.

53. Mentzer, R.M., Jr., Golden, G.T., Chandler, J.G., Horsley, J.S. III: A comparative appraisal of emphysematous cholecystitis. Am. J. Surg. *129*:10, 1975.

54. Abengowe, C.U., McManamon, P.J.M.: Acute emphysematous cholecystitis. Can. Med. Assoc. J. *111*:1112, 1974.

55. Chandler, J.R.: Malignant external otitis: further considerations. Ann. Otol. Rhinol. Laryngol. *86*:417, 1977.

56. Zaky, D.A., Bentley, D.W., Lowry, K., et al.: Malignant external otitis: a severe form of otitis in diabetic patients. Am. J. Med. *61*:298, 1976.

56a. Doroghazi, R.M., Nadol, R.B., Hyslop, N.E., Jr., et al.: Invasive external otitis. Report of 21 cases and review of the literature. Am. J. Med. *71*:603, 1981.

57. Abramson, E., Wilson, D., Arky, R.A.: Rhinocerebral phycomycosis in association with diabetic ketoacidosis. Report of two cases and a review of clinical and experimental experience with amphotericin B therapy. Ann. Intern. Med. *66*:735, 1967.

58. Bauer, H., Ajello, L., Adams, E., Hernandez, D.U.: Cerebral mucormycosis: pathogenesis of the disease. Description of the fungus, Rhizopus Oryzae, isolated from a fatal case. Am. J. Med. *18*:822, 1955.

58a. Hamill, R., Oney, L.A., Crane, L.R.: Successful therapy for rhinocerebral mucormycosis with associated bilateral brain abscesses. Arch. Intern. Med. *143*:580, 1983.

58b. Artis, W.M., Fountain, J.A., Delcher, H.K., Jones, H.E.: A mechanism of susceptibility to mucormycosis in diabetic ketoacidosis: transferrin and iron availability. Diabetes *31*:1109, 1982.

59. Chandler, P.T., Chandler, S.D.: Pathogenic carrier rate in diabetes mellitus. Am. J. Med. Sci. *273*:259, 1977.

60. Williams, J.R.: Does diabetes mellitus predispose the patient to pyogenic skin infections? Study of etiologic relationship of furunculosis and carbuncle. J.A.M.A. *118*:1357, 1942.

61. Cruse, P.J.E., Foord, R.: A five-year prospective study of 23,649 surgical wounds. Arch. Surg. *107*:206, 1973.

62. Lidgren, L.: Post-operative orthopedic infections in patients with diabetes mellitus. Acta Orthop. Scand. *44*:149, 1973.

63. Stone, H.H., Martin, J.D., Jr.: Synergistic necrotizing cellulitis. Ann. Surg. *175*:702, 1972.

64. Rea, W.J., Wyrick, W.J., Jr.: Necrotizing fasciitis. Ann. Surg. *172*:957, 1970.

65. Cooppan, R., Schoenbaum, S., Younger, M.D., et al.: Vertebral osteomyelitis in insulin-dependent diabetics. S. Afr. Med. J. *50*:1993, 1976.

65a. Sharp, C.S., Bessman, A.N., Wagner, W.F., Jr., Garland, D.: Microbiology of deep tissue in diabetic gangrene. Diabetes Care *1*:289, 1978.

37 Disorders of the Blood and Diabetes

Murray M. Bern and Edward J. Busick

The hematologic states pertinent to diabetes, including red blood cell, white blood cell, and coagulation disorders, will be discussed in this chapter. While certain of these are direct complications of diabetes, most are coincidental to the disease. Another review is available which may offer other perspectives.[1]

THE ANEMIAS

Anemias frequently noted in patients with long-duration diabetes are often related to its complications or to intercurrent illnesses. However, there is some evidence that there may be a specific type of anemia associated with long-term diabetes. For example, Burney et al. reported delayed uptake and utilization of iron in diabetic patients with normal renal function and without iron deficiency.[2] Rosen and Tullis noted reduced mobilization of iron in diabetics.[3] Other reports provide some evidence that diabetes is a primary cause of anemia, especially if the glucose is elevated. Red cell survival is abbreviated by 13% when the patient is hyperglycemic and it returns to normal when the diabetes is brought under control.[4]

Diabetic Nephropathy. In the current generation of patients, diabetic nephropathy is found more often than in the past. This is due, at least in part, to the larger number of patients at risk because of longevity consequent to better ways of treatment of diabetes and infections. The anemia associated with diabetic kidney disease is proportional to the severity of the renal failure, unless there has been an intercurrent hemorrhagic episode. The anemia of chronic renal disease is usually normocytic and normochromic. The bone marrow frequently shows depressed activity. Burr cells and occasional fragments of red cells may be seen on the smear. Hematinics, including iron and vitamin B_{12}, are generally ineffective. Injectable androgens may have greater benefit.[5] When symptoms of anemia are present, transfusions may be indicated. Peritoneal dialysis or hemodialysis can correct the dilutional effect of excess volume of the circulating extracellular fluid and, thereby improve the hematocrit reading.

The development of anemia with diabetic nephropathy probably involves several mechanisms, including (a) azotemia, which is often accompanied by anorexia, nausea, and vomiting, resulting in nutritional deficiency; (b) malabsorption of dietary substances necessary for blood formation, such as iron, protein, folic acid, and vitamin B_{12}; (c) decreased iron utilization, despite normal iron stores;

(d) alteration of ferritin metabolism;[6] (e) hemorrhage, especially in the bowel, which occurs in uremia and lowers the number of circulating red cells; (f) shortened survival time of circulating red cells, which often occurs; and (g) bone marrow depression due to the detrimental metabolic effects of uremia as well as the decreased erythropoietin levels in the plasma of uremic patients.[7,8]

Gastrointestinal Neuropathy with Malabsorption. A small percentage of diabetic patients develop a form of visceral neuropathy affecting the gastrointestinal tract, characterized by rapid transit time, episodic diarrhea, and steatorrhea. When severe, it can be accompanied by malnutrition and anemia, because of malabsorption of protein, iron, folic acid, and vitamin B_{12}. The anemia may be macrocytic or microcytic, depending on the level of reticulocytosis and the relative degree of the various deficiencies. It may respond to correction of the transit time and replacement of these nutrients.

Anemia after Hypophysectomy. Patients with diabetic retinopathy, who in the past were treated by surgical pituitary ablation, often developed anemia following operation, with hemoglobin values in the range of 10 to 11 g/dl. This anemia is normochromic, normocytic in type, and resembles that associated with other forms of panhypopituitarism. Its cause is not definitely known. One possibility is a loss of erythropoietin, since some animals have shown decreased erythropoietin after hypophysectomy.[8] The pallor caused by this anemia is similar to the sallow, lemon-yellow color seen in patients with pernicious anemia and hypothyroidism. This characteristic develops promptly after hypophysectomy, independent of the rate of decrease in thyroid function. Hormonal replacement can be useful in correcting the anemia.

Anemias Associated with Hemochromatosis. Primary hemochromatosis is an uncommon cause of diabetes. However, at the Joslin Clinic it has been noted more frequently than has chronic pancreatitis. Anemia is generally not a feature except when hypersplenism or bleeding esophageal varices appear. Sideroblastic anemia, associated with secondary hemochromatosis, has been described.[9] There is evidence of decreased utilization of glycine and succinate in the formation of delta-aminolevulinic acid in heme synthesis in this state. Some consider that excess iron blocks glycine activation and that pyridoxine can overcome that block.[10] When hemochromatosis is complicated further by hepatoma, leukocytosis and erythrocytosis may appear. Contrariwise, anemia may appear as a result of bleeding from esophageal varices as noted above.

Glucose intolerance may be found in states of secondary iron overload.[11] This may occur with transfusion therapy for thalassemia or other chronic anemias; these are characterized by a hypochromic blood picture in the presence of high serum iron and normoblastic hyperplasia of the bone marrow. Treatment with pyridoxine and androgens has been tried for these anemias.

Anemia can become a problem in the phlebotomy therapy of hemochromatosis. Desferrioxamine, an iron-chelating agent, has been of assistance in these cases.[12] Its daily administration promotes renal excretion of iron by forming a complex with circulating iron. This method of removing iron is less efficient than phlebotomy but safer in the presence of anemia. Normal persons excrete iron in the urine at the rate of about 0.5 mg/24 hr; when given desferrioxamine, they excrete 1 to 3 mg/24 hr. When patients with hemochromatosis are given 800 to 1200 mg of desferrioxamine parenterally, the usual response is an output of iron of 15 to 25 mg/24 hr,[13] while weekly venesection removes 200 to 250 mg of iron per 500 ml of whole blood. Increases in urinary iron excretion induced by desferrioxamine are significantly less in diabetics with normal renal function than in nondiabetics.[14]

Pernicious Anemia. The coexistence of diabetes mellitis and pernicious anemia was first reported by Parkinson in 1910.[15] The frequency with which these two diseases are found together was recorded by Root and others.[16] Arapakis and associates[17] reported the incidence of pernicious anemia in nondiabetics as 1 to 1.25 per 1000, whereas in diabetics it was found in various series to range from 2 to 10 per 1000.[18–21]

Munichoodappa and Kozak[21a] found that in a 10-year period (1959–68) 36 verified cases of pernicious anemia were diagnosed among 11,144 Joslin Clinic diabetic patients hospitalized at the New England Deaconess Hospital (3.2 per 1000 patients). In a survey of the literature, they found that the frequency of such association varied widely but averaged 4.2 per 1000 (75 cases in 17,877 diabetic patients). Wintrobe et al.[22] cited the following data from Chanarin:[22a] occurrence of pernicious anemia in a control population, 1.3 to 1.7% and in diabetic patients, 0.4% (4 per 1000). The frequency of diabetes in patients with pernicious anemia is given as 2.4%. They conclude that since diabetes is so prevalent in the general population, a relationship between the two disorders appears not to be significant.

As just observed, in the past there was considerable speculation as to whether or not pernicious anemia occurred more frequently in diabetics than in the general population. Furthermore, in former editions of this book attention was directed to the similarity of symptoms and signs in these two diseases and the possibility of overlooking the diagnosis of one in the presence of the other. Now, however, since evidence is lacking that pernicious anemia occurs in diabetic patients with greater frequency than in persons in the general population, extended discussion is not warranted, especially in view of the current easier access to laboratory tests and treatment. Interested readers are referred to pages 639 to 641 in the 11th edition of this text.

THE HEMOLYTIC ANEMIAS

In addition to the classic causes for congenital hemolytic states, there may be a slightly shortened red cell survival for patients with poorly controlled diabetes.[33,34] Generalized microvascular disease also may cause mild hemolysis. To explain this, it has been postulated that normal red cells are physically damaged by passage through arteries roughened by atherosclerosis, thus causing microangiopathic hemolysis. The part that this mechanism may play in diabetes requires further definition.

Enzyme Defects. Many of the inherited hemolytic anemias have enzyme deficiencies which affect intracellular energy metabolism in the Embden-Meyerhof or hexose-monophosphate shunt pathways. Red cells from diabetics consume normal amounts of glucose via these pathways.[35] A deficiency of glucose-6-phosphate dehydrogenase (G_6PD) causes intravascular hemolysis in the presence of certain drugs and infections. Acute hemolysis, however, can occur also without the participation of such influences[36-39] as in ketoacidotic diabetic patients who are G_6PD-deficient. The mechanisms involved with hemolysis in ketoacidosis are unknown.

In 1964 Chanmugam and Frumin reported finding abnormal glucose tolerance test results in 13 consecutive G_6PD-deficient adults.[40] At that time it was suggested that G_6PD deficiency could in some way influence total body glucose metabolism. This idea remains unproven and requires further study. Another anemia seen with increased incidence in diabetes is the Fanconi's anemia.[41] The reason for this association is unknown.

Hemoglobinopathies. Patients with sickle cell disease may die during ketoacidosis because of diffuse intravascular sickling[42] which may result in brain edema. Sickle cell trait is obviously less dangerous. Thalassemia major has not been noted in Joslin Clinic patients, but many patients with thalassemia minor have been seen. These patients, ranging in age from 7 to 74 years when studied, are chiefly of Italian and Greek ancestry. Patients with sickle cell or thalassemia may have impaired renal concentrating capacity and may become dehydrated more rapidly than normal, thus contributing to hyperosmolar coma in a few cases.[43]

Immune Hemolytic Anemias. These anemias seem to occur following certain viral infections and in association with a variety of primary disorders, including cold hemagglutinin disease, paroxysmal cold hemoglobinuria, collagen diseases, and malignant disease, chiefly of the lymphatic tissues. The red cells are lysed by autoantibodies. Serologic reactions such as the Coomb's test or sugar water test are generally positive. A full discussion of these anemias is beyond the scope of this text as they do not often relate directly to diabetes.

Hemolytic Anemia with Infections. The mechanism for the development of anemia when infections are present is complex. There is evidence of decreased erythropoiesis because of effects on the bone marrow. There is also increased red cell destruction, which is partly related to altered immune mechanisms and splenic hyperplasia. Certain bacteria (e.g., *Clostridium welchii*) produce toxins that damage red cells by direct chemical effect. Other bacteria such as *Bartonella bacilliformis*, *Diplococcus pneumoniae*, *Escherichia coli*, *Haemophilus influenzae*, meningococcus, staphylococcus, salmonella, streptococcus, *Vibrio cholera*, as well as *Plasmodium malariae* and babesia, may also cause hemolysis.

Persons with diabetes, especially if poorly controlled, are prone to infections, particularly of the feet and urinary tract. It would be difficult to assess the frequency of hemolytic anemia in this group since the hemolysis is generally mild, self-limited, and often goes unrecognized. "Dry gangrene" is sometimes associated with hemolytic anemia of varying degree. This association may be due in part to passage of red cells through partially occluded, inflamed, or infected small blood vessels, and in part to the systemic "toxic" effects of gangrene itself and the direct hemotoxic bacteria involved, such as *E. coli* and staphylococci. Many patients with gangrenous limbs have schizocytes in the peripheral blood. Low-grade hemolysis insufficient to cause significant anemia might be found more often in these patients if appropriate tests were done routinely.

Hemolysis Secondary to Drugs. Hemolysis secondary to drugs occurs with a large variety of agents and mechanisms. A few cases of severe hemolytic anemia have occurred in diabetic patients with the administration of sulfonylurea drugs such as chlorpropamide (Diabinese).[44] Many diabetics who have chronic renal failure also have hypertension for which methyldopa (Aldomet) may be prescribed. Since this drug may cause a positive Coombs' reaction, the differentiation of Coombs' positive hemolytic disease from the various other anemias associated with diabetic renal failure, becomes important.

Bone Marrow Failure. Marrow failure does not occur at higher rates because of diabetes per se. However, there may be an overall increased frequency among diabetics related to their higher rates of exposure to potential marrow damaging agents such as chloramphenicol (Chloromycetin) or phenylbutazone (Butazolidine). Chloramphenicol is known for its marrow suppressive effects, causing delayed idiopathic panhypoplasia of the marrow. This drug can also cause cytopenia of varying degrees. If there are specific indications for such drugs, they should be used with caution.

Diabetics have been found to have a relative deficiency of pyroxidine which may be important in searching for causes of sideroblastic anemias in diabetic patients.[45]

IRON DEFICIENCY ANEMIA

Among Joslin Clinic patients, iron deficiency represents one of the most frequent causes of anemia. Inadequate intake of iron, inefficient intestinal absorption, and blood loss are the most frequently noted reasons for deficiency.

Dietary Deficiency. In recent years, inadequate intake has become less common since many foods (e.g., prepared infant formulas, breads, and cereals) are now fortified with additional iron. Dietary deficiency is found most often among food fad dists, young children, and elderly patients who cannot chew, digest or afford meat. Most diabetic patients have a good food iron intake, since the diet is made up of those staple items which, although sugar-poor, are adequate in iron. Joslin Clinic diets call for no special "dietetic foods," but consist of ordinary foods such as meat, vegetables, fruit, milk, and bread, given in measured amounts. If the diet instructions are followed, deficiencies of nutritional factors are not seen on a dietary basis. Many patients use self-prescribed "over-the-counter" vitamin-mineral preparations which contain iron.

Poor Absorption. Failure to absorb iron occurs in association with a wide variety of maladies, including poor dentition and malabsorption syndromes, as well as after gastrectomy and duodenectomy. Ferric iron in food must be converted to ferrous iron for efficient absorption. This is normally accomplished by gastric acid. Even with significant hypo- or achlorhydria, iron absorption usually remains sufficient to maintain normal hemoglobin levels until the achlorhydria has existed for a long time. Atrophic gastritis is often an anatomic cause of achlorhydria, from which occult bleeding can occur and can contribute to this anemia. Since the major portion of iron absorption

occurs in the duodenum, this becomes inefficient when the duodenum is either surgically by-passed or medically diseased. If sufficient dietary iron is provided, such a situation can remain in borderline compensation. However, anemia may develop if the balance is upset by decreased intake, vomiting or stress, creating a greater need for iron. Diabetic gastroenteropathy may be such a stress. The addition of supplemental iron with ascorbic acid or dilute hydrochloric acid can be of some benefit in increasing iron absorption, especially in the elderly.

Chronic Blood Loss. This represents the most frequent cause of iron deficiency in diabetic patients at the Joslin Clinic. This is commonly due to menorrhagia and a large variety of gastrointestinal problems. Primary coagulation defects are usually not encountered and are seldom the causes of chronic blood loss. However, several patients have been seen with anemia caused by occult bleeding while using anticoagulant drugs for various reasons. If bleeding is brisk, the clinical picture can be similar to that of ketoacidosis; both can produce hypotension, tachycardia, labored breathing, pallor, and extreme restlessness. However, in hemorrhage, the eyeballs are firm and the skin moist, whereas in ketoacidosis, dry skin and sunken globes are typical. The laboratory values for hemoglobin, blood glucose, and plasma acetone are obviously differentiating, especially since hemoconcentration in ketoacidosis usually produces an increase in the hematocrit reading. In most cases of advanced diabetic coma, "coffee grounds" material can be aspirated from the stomach, representing superficial bleeding from gastritis. This material gives a positive guaiac reaction. The quantity of blood lost is rarely enough to produce shock or anemia. In such emergencies, careful laboratory evaluation is clearly indicated. Every effort should be made to determine whether ketoacidosis, hemorrhage, or both exist in any given patient.

Chronic bleeding from the genitourinary tract is sometimes associated with iron deficiency anemia. Anemia caused by chronic blood loss occurs in women with menstrual abnormalities and in men with prostatic disease. This type of anemia frequently responds to iron therapy. Bleeding from the upper urinary tract can cause iron deficiency and may be a clue to other important disease. In patients with diabetic nephropathy, small to moderate numbers of red cells may be seen in the urinary sediment.

Pregnancy. Iron deficiency anemia is sometimes noted in women who are pregnant, particularly when the patient has had uterine bleeding in multiple previous pregnancies. Iron, given routinely during pregnancy, is increased in dosage if iron deficiency becomes manifest. The possibility of the so-called "physiologic anemia" of late pregnancy, which may be caused by fluid retention and hemodilution, must be considered. Nutritional causes for anemia, such as iron, folate or vitamin B_{12} deficiency, should be ruled out or corrected, since these states can adversely affect the fetus. However, anemias such as thalassemia minor are not known to affect the fetus unless it carries the same genetic trait. For this latter group, the mother should be treated for symptoms but need not be treated to "help the fetus" unless clear indication exists.

BLOOD GROUPS

Efforts have been made to study the genetic aspects of diabetes by means of statistical studies of the ABO, Rh, and MN blood groups. Conflicting results have been reported. Young diabetics and male diabetics have been found with an increased frequency of blood group A.[46] Overweight diabetics have been reported to belong with decreased frequency to blood group O. However, these findings could not be confirmed.[47,48] It has been suggested that individuals who do not secrete ABO substances are more susceptible to diabetes than are other persons. Buckwalter,[49] on the basis of his own statistical studies and the critical analysis of the work of others, suggested that the results are the reflection of a random distribution of ABO blood groups in diabetics, and that no other specific relationship exists. Macafee,[50] and Berg and co-workers[51] agree with this latter theory.

RED BLOOD CELL FUNCTION

Oxygen transport to the tissues is a multifactorial process which can be altered in diabetes mellitus by changing the oxygen uptake and release from red blood cells. The interactions are complicated and involve 2,3-diphosphoglycerate, pH, and salt concentrations, all of which can be affected by events seen in diabetes.

2,3-Diphosphoglycerate. The accumulation of 2,3-diphosphoglycerate (2,3,-DPG) in red cells occurs in concentrations many times higher than those in any other tissue. It is equimolar to hemoglobin in red cells and affects oxygen hemoglobin dissociation by facilitating oxygen release from hemoglobin.[52–54] The actual level of 2,3-DPG in red blood cells is determined by red cell glycolysis, pH, phosphate levels, blood pyruvate and inosine levels, as well as hypoxia and anemia.[55] As an example, elevation of blood phosphate levels can lead to increased red cell concentrations of 2,3-DPG. The pH also affects 2,3-DPG level and function; alkalosis increases its synthesis by stimulating phosphofructokinase, and simultaneously inhibits its breakdown by suppressing phosphatase.[52] Aci-

dosis, on the other hand, causes 2,3-DPG levels to fall, potentially decreasing oxygen delivery to the tissues. Another minor effect caused by acidosis is to increase 2,3-DPG binding to deoxyhemoglobin. In diabetes this phase of oxygen hemoglobin dissociation can be affected by at least three clinical situations: diabetic ketoacidosis (DKA), chronic hyperglycemia and hyperlipidemia. Overall, the concentrations of 2,3-DPG have been reported to be normal, increased, or decreased in diabetes. This variability must, therefore, be interpreted in view of the patients' vascular disease and their metabolic status.[1,56–59] In ambulatory patients, there is a good correlation between the 2,3-DPG and their vascular status.[56]

Diabetic Ketoacidosis (DKA). During DKA, organic phosphates are liberated into the plasma; renal excretion of phosphate then increases and the total body stores of phosphate fall. Plasma phosphate levels remain compensated until insulin causes a shift of phosphate back into the intracellular compartment. These shifts cause red blood cell 2,3-DPG levels to be lowered by DKA.[53,60–62] There is further lowering as a result of the inhibition of glycolysis by the acidosis.[62]

There is, however, a counterbalancing force on this system. Acidosis increases oxygen delivery by the Bohr effect[62–64] and yet oxygen delivery shows a reduction of about 20%.[65] Therapy of the acidosis has a mixed effect. Correction of acidosis reduces the Bohr effect and simultaneously ends the inhibition of glycolysis. However, the 2,3-DPG levels may take from 1 to 7 days to be restored, leading to a dramatic shift in the oxygen dissociation to the right and a fall in oxygen delivery to the tissues which may be up to 33% of normal.[62,65] During therapy for DKA, serum phosphate may fall dramatically. Thus, replacement of phosphate early in the treatment of DKA may have a role,[66–68] especially if the phosphorus level is low.

Hyperglycemia and Oxygen Delivery. Hyperglycemia can alter oxygen affinity. Ditzel reported in 1972 that diabetics have altered oxygen-hemoglobin dissociation curves with increased oxygen affinity in the hemoglobin and decreased oxygen delivery to tissues.[69] Acute changes in the blood glucose level may produce changes in 2,3-DPG levels[69–71] by shifting phosphates from extracellular to intracellular locations,[67,72–74] thus elevating the levels of 2,3-DPG.[75,76] This effect is balanced by the changes due to increased amounts of hemoglobin A_{1c} in diabetes. This form of hemoglobin causes an increased affinity for oxygen which is unresponsive to changes in 2,3-DPG levels.[77] Glycosylation of hemoglobin at the terminal beta chain affects the area of the hemoglobin molecule involved with 2,3-DPG binding,[77] thus altering somewhat the ability of hemoglobin A_{1c} to respond to changes of 2,3-DPG. To maintain near-normal oxygen hemoglobin dissociation, the 2,3-DPG levels must increase in the remaining normal hemoglobin.[39] This does occur in patients with vascular disease[56] and can be boosted by giving dietary supplements of dicalcium phosphate or by giving etidronate disodium (Didronel).[56,72–75,78,79] Whether increasing phosphate levels will safely benefit patients and reduce long-term complications awaits further investigation. For additional discussion regarding oxygen delivery to tissues, see Chapter 10.

Hyperlipidemia. Hyperlipidemia is a third situation in which diabetic patients develop abnormal oxygen-hemoglobin dissociation. Patients with hypertriglyceridemia and hyperlipoproteinemia (HLP) have increased oxygen affinity and decreased oxygen release.[80] Measurements done on blood from patients with Type I and Type V patterns have P_{50} values that can cause a 30% decrease in oxygen release when tissue pO_2 falls from 60 to 40 mm Hg. Similar changes are found in nondiabetics with familial Types I and V hyperlipidemia. These abnormalities in oxygen-hemoglobin dissociation can be induced by simply incubating red cells in lipemic serum of diabetic patients. It has been theorized that the hypertriglyceridemia decreases the red cell membrane lipids and that this causes increased permeability of red cells for salt which can in turn affect oxygen hemoglobin dissociation.

Red Cells in Diabetes. Red blood cells, granulocytes and monocytes like many other cells have insulin receptors on their surfaces. These receptors can increase following exercise, as indicated by amount of insulin bound.[81] The receptors change concentrations if there is a shift of red cell survival[82] in an inverse exponential fashion[81] and with Types I and II insulin resistance.[83] The red cells also accumulate sorbitol[84] which may be another marker of glucose metabolism, along with hemoglobin A_1.

BLOOD DYSCRASIAS

Malignant disease of the blood-forming organs, as with cancer in general (except of the pancreas),[85] occurs with similar frequency among diabetics and nondiabetics. A number of different blood dyscrasias have been observed in patients of the Joslin Clinic. As of 1974, myeloid metaplasia had been diagnosed in 7, and polycythemia vera in 27, patients.

Leukemias

Leukemias of various types have been noted among diabetic patients of the Joslin Clinic. A total of 60 cases had been recorded until 1974. These were about evenly divided between the lymphatic and myelogenous forms. Thirty-four of the patients were males and 26, females; all were adults. Occasionally insulin resistance has been noted with the development of leukemia.

Levi and Friedman[86] were among the first to report a case of insulin resistance in a diabetic with chronic lymphatic leukemia. There may be multiple reasons why some of these patients develop insulin resistance. Shohl and Field[87] found that leukocytes from diabetic patients bind insulin in vitro, whereas no such effect was observed with leukocytes of nondiabetics. Abnormal proteins that bind insulin also have been found in the serum of diabetic patients with leukemia. Although great progress has been made in recent years in the understanding of insulin resistance, much remains to be learned regarding the mechanism in such special situations as the leukemias.

Lymphomas

Lymphomatous diseases have been diagnosed in many Joslin Clinic patients. These have included Hodgkin's disease, non-Hodgkin's lymphomas of various types, and lymphocytomas. Two of the patients with lymphocytoma have developed lymphatic leukemia. In 1958, Kaufman[88] reported the coexistence of leukemia and diabetes in a patient whose diabetes underwent definite amelioration during x-ray therapy of the abdomen. At the Joslin Clinic several patients have been seen whose diabetes was exacerbated because of the malignancy and improved after its management. One patient's diabetes became more severe as a result of lymphomatous destruction of the pancreas. Insulin resistance coincidental with lymphomatous monoclonal gammopathy has been seen, but that improved when the gammopathy cleared. Finally, bulk effects of the tumor on glucose clearance may enhance the hypoglycemic tendency and reduce the need for insulin.

Multiple Myeloma

As a disease of the hematopoietic system, multiple myeloma warrants attention in a discussion of diabetes because, in some cases, the two diseases share certain features which can create confusion in diagnosis. The hallmarks of multiple myeloma may loosely mimic complications of diabetes.

Myeloma usually begins after the subject is 40 years of age (males: females = 2:1). This brings it into the age group during which diabetes is most frequent, making the coexistence of the two disorders statistically more likely. Also, many diabetics in this age group begin to develop complications. Anemia, urea retention, hyperuricemia, and proteinuria are found in patients with diabetic nephropathy as well as in those with multiple myeloma. Severe, debilitating, peculiar neuralgic pain syndromes occur frequently in association with diabetic neuropathy and can occur with myeloma. The muscle wasting in amyotrophy resembles that seen in some myeloma patients. Both groups are subject to frequent infections. On clinical grounds alone, it is sometimes difficult to separate the symptoms and signs of these disorders in any given case. Statistically, these complications are more common in diabetes than in multiple myeloma, but in the individual difficult case, a high index of suspicion is a useful tool. Appropriate x-ray and laboratory studies should be carried out when a correct diagnosis is not obvious. X-ray study of the bones, bone marrow examination, and electrophoretic studies of serum and urine protein are the most helpful laboratory aids in the diagnosis of multiple myeloma. This disease is not common, but it does occur in diabetics, and no diabetic patient with unusual complaints should be considered with certainty to be suffering from diabetic complications alone until the possibility of multiple myeloma has been ruled out.

Of the 8 cases of myeloma diagnosed in diabetic patients seen at the Joslin Clinic from 1958 to 1974, the range of ages was from 49 to 71 years at time of diagnosis, with an average of 59.5 years. The average duration of diabetes was 11.5 years. All of the patients were under treatment with insulin. The ratio of males to females was about equal. Among the patients were 4 insulin-requiring males with isolated plasma cell tumors. Bence-Jones protein was present in the urine of most of the patients with disseminated multiple myeloma. Abnormalities of serum proteins and anemia were present in all of these patients. Postmortem examination performed on 3 of the patients revealed no evidence of amyloidosis. Renal failure caused by diabetic nephropathy occurred in 2 of the subjects. Pain was present in the spine or rib cage in many of the patients. One patient (Case #20745) had hypercalcemia, the blood calcium level reaching as high as 16.7 mg/dl.

Waldenström's Macroglobulinemia

This condition, with acquired insulin resistance, has been seen in two Joslin Clinic patients. The insulin resistance may respond to plasma exchange or to chemotherapeutic control of the macroglobulinemia. In one case, the M-spike was shown to bind insulin in vitro. The peripheral polyneuropathy was disproportionately severe compared to the expected polyneuropathy of diabetes.[89]

Leukopenia and Aplastic Anemia

Oral hypoglycemic agents have produced adverse hematologic reactions in some few individuals. These responses represent an idiosyncrasy to the drug which is not dose-related and usually appears in the first 6 to 8 weeks of therapy. A few individuals may exhibit hypersensitivity to the sulfonylureas. Leukopenia, hemolysis, and thrombocytopenia have been reported following the use of tolbutamide. Anemia, leukopenia, thrombocytopenia, and eosinophilia have been observed in patients taking chlorpropamide (Diabinese). The use of acetohexamide (Dymelor) has been associated with leukopenia. It must be stressed, however, that adverse hematologic reactions to these drugs are rare.

Agranulocytosis has occurred in 11 patients at the Joslin Clinic; 6 of these were during severe infections. One patient (Case #17292) had a white count of 700 after using phenacetin (acetophenetidin) for 3 days. Two patients (Cases #5672 and #30440) developed low white counts while using sulfadiazine for the treatment of infections. A woman (Case #65228) had a mild depression of the white blood count while being treated with tolbutamide; a leukotoxin test of this drug gave a positive reaction. Symptoms disappeared on discontinuance of the medication. Review of her past history revealed that the patient had had anemia which complicated the use of sulfonamides.

Aplastic anemia has been noted in 2 diabetic patients at the Joslin Clinic. Several hypoplastic marrow syndromes have been seen. In such cases, the etiology is not definitely established since the patients often take a number of medicines.

WHITE BLOOD CELL FUNCTION

It is generally felt that bacterial and fungal infections are more common in diabetic than in nondiabetic populations, though this has not been definitely proven, especially as regards the well-controlled diabetic. Much of the accumulating evidence argues against a difference in the incidence of infections in the two populations. However, problems produced by infection are potentially more threatening in diabetic patients because with infection, the diabetes becomes more difficult to control. Also, complications of diabetes such as impaired circulation and neurogenic bladder, may make an infection of those systems harder to manage. Interest continues high concerning abnormalities of leukocyte function in diabetes. The role of the leukocytes, monocytes, and lymphocytes in combating infections involves a complex series of steps including cell migration, phagocytosis, intracellular bactericidal activities, and responses to mitogenic stimuli.

Leukocytes

Leukocytosis. The movement of leukocytes from the bone marrow and from tissue storage sites is complicated. The kinetics of this process seem altered in diabetes. Diabetic patients have been reported to have a slower but longer neutrophil response to endotoxemia than do control subjects.[90]

Cell Migration. This includes adherence of the leukocyte to the endothelium near the site of inflammation, diapedesis of the leukocyte through the vessel wall, and chemotactic movement of the leukocytes to the actual site of infection. Attempts have been made to study each step separately.

Diapedesis. Ainsworth and Allison[91] achieved blood glucose levels ranging from 495 to 2500 mg/dl in rabbits. They found normal white blood cell adherence to areas of thermal injury, but the number of leukocytes passing into the tissue was reduced in the hyperglycemic animals. Perillie et al.[92] placed a "skin window" over abraded skin and found fewer leukocytes accumulated in patients with diabetic ketoacidosis compared to controls. This defect was reversed when the blood glucose was brought under control. A similar defect has been seen in diabetics with renal failure and acidosis.

Adherence. Van Oss[82] and Peterson et al.[4] found decreased adherence of human leukocytes after the cells had been exposed to increased glucose,[93] in a fashion unrelated to osmolarity. Adherence was corrected when the glucose level improved.[4] MacGregor et al.[94] and Bagdade and co-workers[95] found that leukocytes adhered to nylon fibers either normally or poorly after being exposed to high blood glucose.

Chemotaxis. Chemotaxis describes the movement of leukocytes in a guided fashion along concentrated gradients of leukotactic factors at sites of inflammation. These leukotactic factors include complement factors C3a, C5, 6, and 7. Defects in the ability of the leukocyte to respond could lead to impaired control of bacterial invasion. Mowat and Baum found decreased chemotaxis in the leukocytes of diabetics compared with those of controls, unrelated to the levels of glucose.[96] The defect is worsened when the patient has ketoacidosis.[97,98] The results improved when insulin was added to the test solutions.[96,99] Furthermore, Miller and Baker reported that diabetic sera generated fewer chemotactic factors when tested against normal leukocytes,[99] demonstrating no correlation with cholesterol, triglycerides, or creatinine levels.[100] Molenaar et al. in 1974 reported similar impairment of chemotaxis in the parents

and siblings of juvenile-onset diabetics, suggesting a genetic predisposition for this abnormality.[101]

In spite of these reports, it has not been definitely established that chemotaxis is really impaired in diabetics. Humbert et al. found no difference in the number of leukocytes reaching the attractant.[102] Fikrig et al. (1977), using a Boyden chamber and zymosan, reported no differences in the chemotactic responses between patients with juvenile-onset or adult-onset diabetes and controls.[103] Whether these newer reports mean that chemotaxis really is unimpaired in diabetics, or that we simply need to know more about how the phenomenon takes place, remains to be determined.

Phagocytosis, a major link in the defense against bacteria, includes both entrapment and ingestion of bacteria by leukocytes. The question as to whether phagocytosis is impaired in diabetes has also been controversial.[104,105] Considering that different organisms and different test animals have been used in these studies, it is not surprising that different results have been obtained. Drachman, Root and Wood (1966) reported an interesting in vivo experiment using alloxan-treated rats, infected intrabronchially with pneumococcus bacteria.[106] They showed clear differences in mortality between diabetic and nondiabetic animals at various inoculum sizes. After 36 hours of infection, nearly 10 times as many bacteria were found in the lungs of diabetic animals compared to the non-diabetic control animals. While there was decreased phagocytosis in the diabetics, the number of leukocytes was normal.

Work done in humans has likewise remained controversial. Early work found that white blood cells from diabetic patients were either less effective or unchanged in decreasing viable bacterial counts when bacteria were incubated with blood samples.[107,108] In 1963, Balch and Walters reported impaired phagocytosis in diabetic patients when tested against certain, but not against all, bacteria chosen for testing.[109] Thus, the results of studies may be biased by the bacteria chosen. Miller and Baker, studying ingestion of yeast particles, were unable to detect any difference between controls and diabetics with blood glucose levels ranging from 152 to 472 mg/dl.[99] Bybee and Rogers in 1964 and Crosby and Allison in 1966 detected differences in phagocytosis efficiency when diabetics were in acidosis, leading one to postulate that acidosis may alter the results.[97,110] In 1972, Bagdade et al. reported significant abnormalities in phagocytic capacity in patients whose diabetes was poorly controlled but who were not acidotic.[111,112] They were able to correlate this abnormality with blood glucose values before and after treatment, something that had not been done before.

In 1975, Tan et al., and Nolan et al. in 1978, attempted to differentiate engulfment from intracellular killing. They demonstrated that some leukocytes from patients may engulf bacteria poorly, may have impaired intracellular killing of the bacteria, or may have defects in both functions.[113,114] These results may explain some of the controversies previously reported. Nolan et al. also showed that engulfment of bacteria by leukocytes from diabetics was comparable to controls after 60 minutes' incubation, but was defective if tested after 20 minutes' incubation.[114] Differences could also be demonstrated when the ratio of leukocyte to bacteria was altered. When the bacteria to leukocyte ratios were 10 to 1, there was no difference in entrapment, but when the ratio was 1 to 1 or 2 to 1, there was a significant diminution in the leukocyte function of the diabetics.

In summary, controversy surrounding the ability of the diabetic patient to control infection, still exists. Overall the leukocyte function of the diabetic must be considered to be less than ideal, though it is not clear if it is the cell itself or its milieu that is at fault. The intrinsic metabolic activity of the cell can further affect these outcomes. The neutrophils of diabetes have metabolic changes of glycolysis, phosphofructokinase, and myeloperoxidase. Sulfonylureas inhibit the myeloperoxidase system.[115,116] How these affect the final outcome is not yet defined fully. (See also Chapter 36.)

Lymphocytes

The lymphocytes are another key to control infection. The analysis of subsets of diabetic lymphocytes is discussed elsewhere. Incubation of lymphocytes from diabetic patients with a variety of mutagens causes less blastogenic response than is seen in lymphocytes from normal controls.[117,118] There are differences between the blast transformation seen in well controlled and poorly controlled diabetics, as well as between insulin-dependent and insulin-independent diabetics.[119,120] Insulin added to in vitro test systems improved the response but never enough to equal normal. These defects create delayed hypersensitivity and delayed graft rejection, plus possibly more infections.[120,121]

There is conflicting evidence regarding the metabolic effect of diabetes upon the lymphocytes. There appears to be increased periodic acid-Schiff-positive material in the lymphocytes of diabetic patients.[122] There is also an insulin-responsive synthetic defect for citrate.[123] Insulin does stimulate adenosine triphosphate (ATP) activity and glucose uptake in the lymphocytes.[124]

The clinical relevance of these findings needs further study. How they may relate to the immune attack upon the beta cell of the pancreas, how immunoglobulin synthesis is altered, how response to insulin is affected, plus many other questions require clarification.

COAGULATION DISORDERS

Primary disorders leading to hypocoagulability seem to occur no more frequently among diabetic patients at the Joslin Clinic than would be expected in the general nondiabetic patient population. However, a variety of specific coagulation disorders have been encountered, reflecting the spectrum described in most hematologic texts.[128] There is a tendency toward acceleration of the coagulation scheme which may contribute to the vascular complications of diabetes. This section will deal with both hypo- and, more extensively, hyper-coagulation. In 1962 Fitzhugh,[126] reported the occurrence of diabetes in a patient with hemophilia, in whom the required insulin injections were well tolerated. Other studies[127,128] have reported that hemophilia is not more common in diabetics. Diabetic patients with von Willebrand's disease and with Factor IX deficiency, also have been treated. These patients tolerate insulin injections when appropriate care is given to the injection site.

(Case #55584). A 20-year-old man with newly diagnosed diabetes had had asthma and ulcerative colitis. He developed petechial and subcutaneous bleeding. The platelet adhesion was decreased and the Factor VIII (functional) level was very low. He required insulin for control of the hyperglycemia. By applying pressure over the sites of the injections, they were well tolerated.

Thrombocytopenia

There are unique situations which can be diabetes-specific. Patients with multiple autoantibodies which conceivably might cause diabetes, may also have pernicious anemia due to their cell-specific antibodies. In these cases thrombocytopenia may develop from vitamin B_{12} deficiency. Thrombocytopenia may also develop from haptene-linked thromboagglutinins, wherein an oral hypoglycemic agent serves as the haptene.

(Case #095571). A 68-year-old woman was found to have an acquired thrombocytopenia 3 months after the initiation of treatment with an oral hypoglycemic agent. The platelet count was 36,000 per mm^3. The bleeding time was 19 minutes (control: less than 10 minutes). There was no splenomegaly. The bone marrow contained increased numbers of megakaryocytes. All other coagulation parameters were normal. Oral sulfonylurea-specific platelet agglutinins were discovered in the patient's plasma. Two weeks after the drug was discontinued, the platelet count returned to normal.

Another cause of thrombocytopenia which is

combined with other coagulopathies is the consumptive coagulopathy. Patients with severe diabetic ketoacidosis have been found to have an acute consumptive coagulopathy. Heparin therapy may have a role during the phases of acute management of the metabolic derangements. However, heparin need not be given to all such patients since management of the acidosis will usually bring autocorrection of the coagulopathy.

Hypercoagulation

The potential for thrombosis associated with diabetes is of far greater epidemiologic importance than are the hemorrhagic diseases. Patients with diabetes have many difficulties with occlusive diseases of the large and small vessels. It is useful to understand the cause or causes of these complications since certain preventive or corrective therapy may be offered now, and may become available on a wider scale in the future. Changes of the plasma lipids, the basement membranes, the endothelial cells, platelet functions, the coagulation system, fibrinolytic capacity, and blood viscosity are contributory. Results recorded at a particular moment, such as a "fasting morning sample" may not give a complete picture of the changes which take place during other parts of the day. Similarly, acidosis, hyper- and hypoglycemia may dramatically shift the results of coagulation studies,[129] with a greater tendency toward accelerated thrombosis during hyperglycemia.[130] Thus, patient management should be individualized with attention to all of these components.

Platelets

In studying the acceleration of platelet function in diabetics, it has been suggested that the cause for such changes may be the platelet itself and/or the plasma in which platelets are suspended.[131,132] An example of the former is that the platelet content of phospholipids may be greater in diabetics than in nondiabetic patients. When elevated they return toward normal with improved diabetic control.[133,134] Interest in these changes relates to the role they play in the evolution of the vascular disease of diabetes. At the present time, it remains unknown as to whether pharmacologic control of platelet functions can be used safely and have long-term prophylactic importance, or whether potential adverse effects of the medications may negate their value.

Aggregation. Aggregometry is an informative but artificial system used to measure platelet function. Typically, platelets are tested for their response to adenosine diphosphate, epinephrine, collagen, and arachidonic acid. Changes recorded on the aggregometer should be used carefully because although these may occur as a result of in vivo alteration, they may be induced during in vitro preparation of the platelet-rich plasma. It has been reported that prediabetics (those with two diabetic parents, but who themselves have normal glucose tolerance) have aggregation characteristics equal to those of controls, while latent diabetics (those in whom diabetes is manifest only during a glucose tolerance test) and overt diabetics have increased aggregation after the addition of adenosine diphosphate.[131,132] Others have reported that aggregation is normal in persons with overt diabetes.[135]

Overt diabetics who require insulin or oral hypoglycemic agents have been reported to have delayed disaggregation.[136,137] Diabetics with vascular complications including retinopathy have increased response to adenosine diphosphate (ADP) in aggregation studies and can occasionally form spontaneous aggregates after simple recalcification of the plasma.[138,139] Platelet factors 3 and 4, and B thromboglobulin, which are released during platelet aggregation, were found to be increased in some but not all diabetics.[137,140-143] Platelets from diabetics bind greater amounts of fibrinogen in response to ADP-induced aggregation.[139] It should be remembered that atherosclerosis alone may also affect platelet physiology and that patients with advanced atherosclerosis may have all of the changes of platelet aggregation seen with advanced diabetes alone.[144-146]

Platelet aggregation is dependent upon the prostaglandin pathway. Arachidonic acid, an unsaturated 20-carbon fatty acid, is first released into the platelet. The arachidonate is converted first into the prostaglandins and then into thromboxane A_2, by cyclooxygenase and prostaglandin synthetase enzymes. Some agents, including aspirin, suppress production of the prostaglandins in platelets. They also suppress platelet aggregation production of the natural inhibitor of aggregation, the prostacyclin, PGI_2, in the endothelial cells. Since it is known that diabetics have subnormal production of PGI_2, at least in their vein walls,[147] further suppression may have adverse effects on balance. The platelets then aggregate. Platelets from diabetics make greater amounts of thromboxane A_2,[134,148] especially in those with clinical complications. However, the amount of plasma thromboxane B_2, a stable measure of thromboxane A_2 and of the stable metabolite of PGI_2 may diverge from that found when direct *cell* measurements are made.[149] The plasma levels are probably less important in understanding these phenomena. Therefore, it is not surprising that the results vary when the effect of aspirin on platelet aggregation is tested among diabetics. Agents are being developed that can selectively inhibit the prostaglandin system. Such drugs may be used selectively to affect the patient's clinical course. Dextrans, propranolol, sulfinpyrazone, dipyridamole, and other agents have specific influences. Each of these agents has a different effect on patient physiology and should be used judiciously. The following case history describes the use of dextran and aspirin in a patient at risk.

Case #122889. A 60-year-old man with long-term insulin-dependent, adult-onset diabetes developed peripheral vascular disease with claudication. Angiograms demonstrated diffuse atherosclerosis. Surgical repair with a femoral-to-popliteal graft was planned. Platelet aggregation curves showed a fast onset and maximal second wave development after addition of low concentrations of ADP, epinephrine, and thrombin. In addition, there was spontaneous aggregation when using the stirring bar alone. Platelet adhesion was 87%. The patient was given intravenous dextran during and after operations and was continued thereafter on aspirin to suppress the platelets. He tolerated surgery well and the graft has remained patent. There were no distal emboli from the graft.

Similarly, patients with myocardial ischemia or retinal ischemia may be helped by "anti-platelet" therapy. However, at this moment, this approach should be individualized on the basis of in vitro evidence of accelerated platelet function. The degree of retinopathy has had little or no influence upon the aggregation in some studies.[150] However, in other studies a plasma cofactor which accelerates platelet aggregation to ADP was found to be increased even in juvenile patients with minimal evidence of retinopathy.[151] This substance has a molecular weight of about 21,000 daltons.[152] Trials with large patient populations are now being conducted. Thus, while there is appeal for use of drugs to inhibit the possible harmful "hyperfunctional" platelets, there are still gaps in our knowledge concerning their efficacy and the accompanying suppression of prostacyclin, PGI_2.

There are reports dealing with the effect of insulin or oral hypoglycemic agents on platelet aggregation. Insulin given intravenously accelerated the onset of platelet aggregation and of disaggregation, and when added in vitro caused platelet agglutination.[135,153] Contrariwise, there was no additive effect for insulin or oral agents on the already accelerated platelet aggregation seen in some diabetics.[136,140] To add further to this complex issue, glucose given orally caused the platelets of some patients to have stronger aggregation, but tolbutamide, given intravenously, reversed the accelerated aggregation in diabetics.[132] (It should be appreciated that tolbutamide has a complicated pharmacologic course and that these results should not be analyzed relative to the glucose level alone.) Somatostatin when infused in a cyclic schedule may

create platelet aggregates in vivo without changing platelet aggregation.[154,155] An extremely interesting and important series of experiments were reported by vanZile et al.[156] Their studies demonstrated that soluble immune complexes isolated from diabetic patients enhanced ADP-induced platelet aggregation and release of ATP. Some of these complexes were composed of insulin-anti-insulin complex. The presence of such mechanisms may greatly aid our understanding of accelerated platelet functions in diabetes mellitus.

All of the studies on platelet aggregation have focused on narrow issues during special phases of the patient's day. The effects of exercise, sleep, and hyperglycemic and hypoglycemic swings on platelet function in such studies are not taken into account. Therefore, more investigation is needed to clarify and evaluate the currently available information.

Adhesion. Platelets adhere to foreign surfaces such as glass beads, and this can be used as another measure of platelet function. Adhesion tests are difficult to standardize despite rigorous efforts. Thus the range of "normal" tends to be large. There are shifts of the mean results of the adhesion tests among diabetics compared to normals,[123,136,157] as well as variation in results among diabetics. As an example, diabetic patients without vascular disease, who were receiving oral hypoglycemic agents, had normal or increased adhesion.[158,159] Patients without vascular disease who received dietary therapy alone or with insulin treatment, had increased adhesion using nonanticoagulated blood[157] but decreased adhesion[160] when using anticoagulated blood. Another heterogeneous population of diabetics receiving oral agents or insulin, with or without retinopathy, had normal adhesion by one technique[136] and increased adhesion by another.[161] Glucose added in vitro may increase the adhesiveness.[159,162] Diabetics with coronary artery disease had increased platelet adhesion, which was unrelated to insulin or oral agents.[159,161] Of great importance by comparison, nondiabetics with coronary artery disease had the same increased adhesion. Thus, the adhesion test may be used as an adjunct to understanding the patient's platelet function, but should not be used as a sole determinant.

Platelet Utilization. There are other means of dealing with the complex issue of platelets in diabetes. High rates of platelet turnover in vivo support the idea that excessive utilization of platelets may exist in patients with diabetes mellitus. The platelet-specific β-thromboglobulin is released during platelet aggregation and if found to be elevated in the plasma, would indicate increased release in vivo, or decreased clearance. In fact, elevated plasma levels of β-thromboglobulin may be found in several groups of patients, including those with myocardial infarction, deep vein thrombosis, pre-eclampsia, and diabetes.[163,164] Among the diabetics, some levels of β-thromboglobulin overlap normals. Those that were abnormally elevated did correlate with the degree of vascular disease in some studies, but did not correlate with the duration of diabetes, the treatment provided for the diabetes, or the blood glucose level at the time of plasma sampling in other studies.[143,165,166] The plasma level of β-thromboglobulin did fall toward normal after several weeks of improved control of the blood-glucose levels in the diabetic patients and following 2 weeks of therapy with dipyridamole.[143]

Abbreviated platelet survival times can be found, using radiolabeled platelets in patients with at least two of the following complications: retinopathy, nephropathy, coronary artery disease, or peripheral vascular disease.[167] Estimates of platelet survival also can be made using an analysis of platelet size distribution, since young platelets are larger. Using aspirin-treated platelets as markers of platelet survival, it was found that diabetics have shorter platelet survival curves.[168] Patients without diabetes but with atherosclerotic vascular diseases, as well as diabetics with retinopathy, have larger platelets.[131,169–172] It is not clear, therefore, if the change is due to the diabetes per se, or if it is more a reflection of the atherosclerotic vascular disease.

In regard to this latter point, platelets may contribute to the evolution of the atherosclerotic process in both diabetics and nondiabetics by releasing a low molecular weight, basic, heat-stable glycoprotein which is a mitogenic stimulus for smooth muscle cells and endothelial cells. There can be a piling up of the smooth muscle and endothelial cells in areas of damage in arteries where platelets adhere. Insulin potentiates this effect. Serum factors from patients with poorly controlled non-ketotic non-insulin-dependent diabetes stimulated smooth muscle cells more than did sera from well controlled patients.[173,174] If confirmed, these findings may offer a holistic understanding of one phase of atherosclerosis.

Ristocetin Cofactor. The ristocetin cofactor, or as it is more commonly known, the von Willebrand factor, is a macromolecule which contains immunoreactive antihemophilic globulin and an antihemophilia A-factor VIII (AHF) procoagulant. Part of this molecule is necessary for platelet adhesion. An elevation may cause increased platelet adhesion to areas where endothelial damage has occurred. Insulin-dependent diabetics with atherosclerosis or proliferative retinopathy are known to have elevated levels of the ristocetin cofactor.[131,175–177] Simultaneously, measured factor VIII levels were either normal or elevated.[178] In our studies,[175] those

patients, both diabetic and nondiabetic, with atherosclerosis had greater elevations of the ristocetin cofactor than did diabetics with proliferative retinopathy. Thus, these changes are not simply diabetes-specific, and may be a part of, or in themselves contribute to, the development of atherosclerosis (Table 37–1).

There are only a few reports correlating the level of the ristocetin cofactor and the pharmacologic management of the diabetes.[179] Normal subjects had depressed levels of the cofactor 1 hour after the beginning of a glucose tolerance test (GTT) or after a standard meal. Diabetic patients differed significantly since the cofactor remained depressed for 4 hours of the GTT in accordance with their intolerance to the glucose.

Lamberton, Goodman, and collaborators verified the findings of others that plasma levels of VWF were significantly higher in diabetic than in nondiabetic subjects. However, there was no significant difference in levels of VWF between the diabetics with and without retinopathy or proteinuria. They interpreted their results as suggesting that plasma VWF does not play a primary role in the genesis of microangiopathy. They drew the same conclusion regarding plasma fibronectin, IGF I, and IGF II.[179a]

Plasma Lipids. Changes in the plasma concentration of lipids[142,180,181] and fatty acids[182,183] may affect platelet function. Diets enriched with linoleic acid cause abnormal platelet aggregation to return to normal in diabetics and controls. Diabetic acidosis can change fatty acid production within the platelet.[180] Glucose, added in vitro to platelets of diabetic patients, stimulates incorporation of acetate into fatty acid.[184] We need additional information on the significance of these observations in the daily cycle of insulin-dependent diabetic patients.

Coagulation

In coagulation, a series of molecules possessing stored capacities to convert to enzymes or cofactors, lead finally to fibrin deposition. Each step has physical or chemical breakers to modify its activities. Many reports are available describing normal, accelerated and decreased dynamics of coagulation in diabetic patients.[185–187] Changes toward accelerated coagulation would indicate a distinct risk factor for diabetics since many diabetics suffer from micro- and macrovascular occlusive disease. If consistent changes could be identified, then therapeutic interventions could be designed.

Factors I, V, and VIII are increased while factors VII, IX, XI, and XII have been found to be normal in diabetics.[185] Increased concentration of procoagulants are not necessarily indicative of acceler-

Table 37–1.   Levels of Factor VIII in Three Categories of Diabetic Patients: With No Retinopathy, with Proliferative Retinopathy, and with Atherosclerosis, as Compared with Findings in Normal Controls and Nondiabetic Subjects with Atherosclerosis

Factor VIII Components	Normal Controls	Diabetics			Non-Diabetics
		No Retinopathy	Proliferative Retinopathy	Atherosclerosis	With Atherosclerosis*
Factor VIII Coagulant (% ± SEM) (% of normal)	89 ± 10	158 ± 19	169 ± 25	216 ± 24	184 ± 16
Factor VIII Antigen (% ± SEM) (% of normal)	89 ± 9	265 ± 42	206 ± 65	370 ± 117	273 ± 52
Factor VIII Ristocetin Cofactor (% ± SEM) (% of normal)	79 ± 6	102 ± 16	87 ± 14	139 ± 14	127 ± 7
Hemoglobin A_{1c}	5 ± .25	10 ± .68	10 ± .59	9 ± .47	6 ± .16

*Patients with angiogram-proven atherosclerosis were included in the study if they had no family or personal history of diabetes, no glucose intolerance, were non-smokers, and were not receiving drugs known to be capable of altering platelet physiology.

Study conducted by M.E. Pumphery, J. Horton, and G.L. Davis of Northeastern University and M.M. Bern, New England Deaconess Hospital, Boston, Mass.[175]

ated kinetics of coagulation. Thus kinetic assays are needed to enhance our understanding of each patient. Again, results of studies vary. Thromboplastin conversion times were accelerated among diabetics, but cephalin conversion times were slower than controls.[185] The thrombi produced from plasma of diabetics were larger than those produced from plasma of controls. This difference was most marked when diabetics with vascular disease were studied, possibly reflecting the higher fibrinogen concentrations available for the clot.[170] This is especially true when the patients are hyperglycemic,[187a,187b] a condition correctable with heparin infusion. The transition from normal to accelerated fibrinogen is very fast, if not immediate.[187c] This shift correlated with changes of intravascular volume and increased excretion of the label during fibrinogen clearance studies.[187c] The shift was reversible. Diabetic platelets have increased fibrinogen receptors.[187d] Diabetics also had shortened fibrinogen survival times. Some actually had a small increase of soluble fibrin complexes in their plasma, suggesting minor ongoing intravascular coagulations.[188] There was reduction of recalcification time among the diabetics which, to some degree, was directly related to the duration of diabetes and was independent of vascular disease.[189] Diabetics had increased resistance to heparin but had sensitivity to warfarin therapy.[190] Thus, there appears to be a slight disadvantage for diabetic patients according to these tests. Again, it should be noted that such findings may reflect associated vascular disease and not diabetes per se.

Among the important buffers of the final stages of coagulation are antithrombin III (AT III), alpha-1-antitrypsin and alpha-2-macroglobulin. These molecules inhibit thrombin and other esterales. In the process of binding to thrombin, the AT III is removed from the plasma. Diabetics with and without vascular disease may have low or normal or elevated concentrations of plasma AT III,[191–193] while the alpha-2-macroglobulin and alpha-1-antitrypsin are elevated.[188,194] This latter finding can be used to mark the presence of hypercoagulability. The AT III may fall with stress.[193]

Case #020893. A 48-year-old female diabetic with juvenile-onset atherosclerosis was admitted for evaluation of bilateral carotid bruits. Noninvasive studies and angiography demonstrated significant narrowing of both vessels, and surgical repair was scheduled. Pre-operative evaluation for hypercoagulability demonstrated a partial thromboplastin time (PTT) of 24 seconds (control: 33 seconds); prothrombin time (PT) of 10.0 seconds (control: 11.5 seconds); fibrinogen of 425 mg per 100 ml; and an antithrombin III of 8.9 seconds (control: 18.5 seconds). Surgery was postponed while the patient was given 3 weeks of coumadin at doses designed to allow the antithrombin III to return to normal but not designed to fully anticoagulate the patient. After 3 weeks, the antithrombin III was 38.5 seconds. Surgery was successfully performed.

Fibrinolysis

The fibrinolysis system is necessary for dissolving clots once they are formed, an important corrective therapy for patients with vascular disease. The overall capacity of the fibrinolysis of the plasma can be measured by using the euglobulin lysis time, either with or without exercise stimulation. This measures the time needed for a clot to dissolve in the absence of the inhibitors of fibrinolysis. With this test, the fibrinolysis has been found to be normal in poorly controlled, well controlled, and long-term diabetics.[195,196]

Difficulties exist in deciding how to use the available reports on fibrinolysis.[197–202] In one study, the fibrinolytic response after short exercise was diminished among diabetic men[203] and, if confirmed, would be important to diabetics participating in strenuous exercise programs. Patients recovering from ketoacidosis have increased spontaneous fibrinolysis.[204,205] Patients with diabetic retinopathy have deficiency of the fibrinolysis, which parallels the duration of their retinopathy.[206] Interestingly, patients with no retinopathy had an increase of fibrinolysis in response to stimulation with venous occlusion. Diabetics with quiescent coronary heart disease have been reported to have less fibrinolysis than nondiabetics with the same type of coronary heart disease.[207] It is not yet known how consistent these results are among different investigators or among different patient populations. It is also unknown how the fibrinolysis varies from hour to hour or day to day in diabetics.[208]

An important assay of the release of plasminogen activator from endothelial cells is available in research laboratories using everted segments of veins taken from the dorsum of the hand. Such assays are useful for indicating whether specific patients can be stimulated to create more fibrinolytic capacity. In such studies, diabetics with retinopathy have diminished activation compared to diabetics without retinopathy;[201] but in another study, patients with mild retinopathy had more vein wall activity than those with no retinopathy.[208] Maturity-onset diabetics tended to have poorer plasminogen activator release than the juvenile-onset diabetic patients,[199] and the results were unrelated to the duration of the diabetes.[208] Again results vary. Another study found *no* abnormality of vein wall plasminogen activator for the diabetics.[208] These complex studies need to be repeated with stratification for obesity, age and plasma lipid levels, since these parameters can affect the results.

There have been only a few studies dealing with the systems that inhibit fibrinolysis. In those studies, increases of the concentrations of plasmin and plasminogen inhibitors,[208] elevation of the urokinase inhibitors and elevation of α_2-macroglobulin level[201] were found in the diabetics. These studies also need to be refined with appropriate stratification and attention to the characteristics associated with diabetes.

There is no clinically available drug which consistently increases fibrinolysis in ambulatory patients. Insulin therapy has been reported to reduce,[209] increase[196,210,211] or leave unchanged[206] the levels of spontaneous fibrinolysis. Phenformin and phenformin plus ethylestrenol therapy have improved the fibrinolytic activity in maturity-onset diabetics.[208] Biguanides either enhanced[212] or reduced[213] spontaneous fibrinolysis. Sulfonylureas have consistently and notably reduced the fibrinolytic activity in all studies to date.[196,209,212] These latter reports have importance when considering the controversial statistical observation that sulfonylureas may be associated with an increased incidence of mortality due to heart disease (see Chapter 21). Dietary control alone causes no change in the level of spontaneous fibrinolysis[206] although exercise may improve fibrinolytic capacity. Thus, there are many possibilities to be explored. Can agents with hypoglycemic activity be created which also stimulate fibrinolysis? Can the sulfonylureas be altered so as to have no effect on the lysis system? Otherwise, there are no simple-to-take oral hypoglycemic agents available which stimulate fibrinolysis. (Urokinase and streptokinase are useful only for occlusive events.)

VISCOSITY

Finally, blood viscosity is another complicated consideration in this already multifaceted problem. Blood viscosity measures flow kinetics in vitro and involves all of the cellular and fluid elements contained in the circulating blood. The flow characteristics may contribute to the final occlusive event, assuming there is an antecedent drive toward clotting. The evidence that viscosity contributes to the macrovascular or microvascular disease in diabetes, rests upon clinical correlates. Whole blood viscosity was reported to be increased[212–216] or normal in diabetic patients.[217] Diabetics with proliferative retinopathy had higher viscosities,[218,219] especially at low shear rates. By multiple regression analyses, the viscosity changes correlated best with the plasma fibrinogen concentration. Viscosity did improve with improved levels of HbA_{1c}.[219–222]

Red blood cell deformability has been reported to be decreased among diabetics and worsened in the presence of hyperglycemia, and improved by insulin therapy.[222–224] The loss of deformability seems to relate to ATP concentrations which improve following insulin replacement.[223,224] Red cell aggregates are reported to have greater mechanical integrity[214,214a,217,225–227] in diabetes, due in part to changes of sialic acid content and to changed rates of red cell glycosylation reactions.[225,226] Further change occurs with uremia. The viscosity of white thrombi was also reported to be increased.[214,215] Direct skin window observations made by Branemark found no changes of red blood cell deformability, red cell plasticity, red cell adherence, or aggregation of flowing platelets.[228] Generally, elevated glucose appears to be associated with increased viscosity.[229] Interestingly, red blood cells from diabetics have greater adhesions to endothelial cells than do the red blood cells from normal controls. This unique change was directly related to the degree of vascular disease.[230]

It is difficult to determine how these observations on viscosity should alter our understanding of the vascular occlusive diseases of diabetes. Many pharmacologic research questions have yet to be answered in this field. What is the value of altering the viscosity by reducing fibrinogen concentration? How would changing the intravascular solute load affect the patients? How do the complications of diabetes affect the response? How do drugs, diet, and activity affect the viscosity? These questions may be answered with further basic investigations.

ENDOTHELIAL CELLS AND COAGULATION

The functional interface between the endothelial cell and the fluid plasma has much to do with thrombosis and atherosclerosis.[231] The endothelial cells provide PGI_2, plasminogen-activating substance, and factor-VIII-related antigen, and bind thrombin plus protein C, among other functions. Early evidence points to defective endothelial cell function in the presence of diabetic serum and diabetic substrate. The endothelial cells from human great arteries proliferate less well in diabetic sera as compared to normal sera.[232] Serum from diabetic patients suppresses production/release of prostacyclin PGI_2.[233] Glucose in increasing concentration in the growth media suppresses the growth of human umbilical vein endothelium[234] and is associated with increased factor VIII intracellularly.[235] Insulin elevations also appear to have an effect on endothelial cell function and growth.[236,237] These events need further clinical clarification.

MANAGEMENT OPTIONS

The final process which leads to tissue ischemia generally is a product of two or more of the described variables, with differences existing among different patient groups. While it is possible to pharmacologically attack some of the diabetes-associated problems as described above, there are additional treatable factors which lead to increased propensity to clot. Trigger factors that can move a well-balanced coagulation system toward a hyperfunctional state include, among others, adrenergic stress, acidosis, increased ionized serum calcium, smoking, obesity, hyperlipidemia, elevated free fatty acids, venous occlusion by constricting garments, carcinomas (especially those making mucin), pregnancy, estrogen therapy, hemolysis,

some radiographic contrast materials, surgery, bed rest, dehydration, polycythemia, thrombocytosis, and certain blood groups. When considered individually, some of these can be altered and, thus, the propensity for thrombosis can be reduced.

On an individual basis it appears reasonable to determine with in vitro coagulation tests which individual patients are at unusual risk for thrombosis and to offer specific therapies. This applies particularly to those with transient ischemic attacks of the central nervous system, angina pectoris, peripheral vascular disease, retinopathy and the like. They may have accelerated platelet aggregability and release, or increased platelet adhesion which are reasonable to treat with antiplatelet agents, such as aspirin, low molecular weight dextran, sulfinpyrazone, dipyridamole, or other drugs. Some patients have significant acceleration of coagulation reflected in the kinetic assays. Others may have low concentrations of antithrombin III. Oral anticoagulants may play a role for these patients. In preparation of the patient for vascular surgery, it may be useful to slow coagulation and allow reconstitution of the antithrombin III by giving a course of warfarin-type anticoagulants while at the same time making efforts to reduce the impact of the other trigger factors listed above. The true efficacy of these approaches is under study.

While there are limited data to indicate whether or not diabetic patients are at greater risk than nondiabetics for venous thrombosis, the same approaches may apply. The changes in the procoagulant and fibrinolytic systems described in this chapter are assumed to have impact on the propensity of the diabetic toward venous clots. However, the exact roles are at this moment only speculative. Prophylactic administration of low-dose heparin is advocated for prevention of postoperative thrombophlebitis but there are no comparative studies involving diabetic and nondiabetic patients. The benefits and risks are assumed to be comparable, while clinical proof is pending.

Case #117383. A 64-year-old insulin-dependent diabetic was discovered to have erythrocytosis due to polycythemia vera. He was treated with therapeutic phlebotomies, during the course of which thrombophlebitis developed in the arms and subsequently in the legs. Thereafter, he suffered pulmonary emboli while receiving appropriate anticoagulants. The coagulation parameters were very accelerated and the antithrombin III was depleted. He was heparin-resistant and therefore required unusually large doses. Evaluation to find the source of his unique hypercoagulability turned up an elevated serum acid phosphatase at a time when the prostate examination was benign and bone x-rays were normal. A bone scan did indicate metastatic disease. Later, an orchiectomy was performed for progressive disease. At that time, the carcinoma regressed as did the hypercoagulability. The polycythemia vera remained unchanged.

Finally, a word of caution should be offered. Many of the proposed methods of reducing "hypercoagulability" have not proved to be effective even though they are intuitively logical. Therefore, until the necessary experiments establish the parameters of efficacy and safety, thoughtful exercise of clinical judgment is needed in this complex field.

REFERENCES

1. Jones, R.L., Peterson, C.M.: Hematologic alterations in diabetes mellitus. Am. J. Med. 70:339, 1981.
2. Burney, S.W., Friedell, G.H., Barnett, D.M.: Erythrokinetics in diabetes mellitus. Abstract, Program of the 49th Annual Session of the American College of Physicians, Boston, Ma., April 1–5, 1968, p. 95.
3. Rosen, B.J., Tullis, J.L.: Simplified deferoxamine test in normal, diabetic, and iron over-load patients. J.A.M.A. 195:261, 1966.
4. Peterson, C.M., Jones, R.L., Koenig, R.J., et al.: Reversible hematologic sequelae of diabetes mellitus. Ann. Intern. Med. 86:425, 1977.
5. Neff, M.S., Goldberg, J., Slifkin, R.F., et al.: A comparison of androgens for anemia in patients on hemodialysis. N. Engl. J. Med. 304:871, 1981.
6. Samarel, A., Bern, M.M.: Distribution of iron in splenic ferritin. Lab. Invest. 39:10, 1978.
7. Gallagher, N.I., McCarthy, J.M., Lange, R.D.: Observations on erythropoietic-stimulating factor (ESF) in the plasma of uremic and nonuremic anemic patients. Ann. Intern. Med. 52:1201, 1960.
8. Gurney, C.W., Jacobson, L.O., Goldwasser, E.: The physiologic and clinical significance of erythropoietin. Ann. Intern. Med. 49:363, 1958.
9. Altschule, M.D.: Comment on clinical concepts. Regulation of erythrocyte production. Med. Sci. (Phila.) 7:328, 1960.
10. Gardner, F.H., Nathan, D.G.: Hypochromic anemia and hemochromatosis. Response to combined testosterone, pyridoxine, and liver extract therapy. Am. J. Med. Sci. 243:447, 1962.
11. Zuppinger, K., Molinari, B., Hirt, A., et al.: Increased risk of diabetes mellitus in beta-thalassemia major due to iron overload. Helv. paediatr. Acta 34:197, 1979.
12. Jandl, J.H., Davidson, C.S., Abelmann, W.H., MacDonald, R.A.: Hemochromatosis terminating in polycythemia and hepatoma, with observations on the natural history of hemochromatosis. N. Engl. J. Med. 269:1054, 1963.
13. Moeschlin, S., Schnider, U.: Treatment of primary and secondary hemochromatosis and acute iron poisoning with a new, potent iron-eliminating agent (Desferrioxamine-B). N. Engl. J. Med. 269:57, 1963.
14. Walsh, J.R., Mass, R.E., Smith, F.W., Lange, V.: Desferrioxamine effect on iron excretion in hemochromatosis. Arch. Intern. Med. 113:435, 1964.
15. Parkinson, J.: A case of pernicious anemia terminating in acute diabetes. Lancet 2:543, 1910.
16. Root, H.F.: Diabetes and pernicious anemia. J.A.M.A. 96:928, 1931.
17. Arapakis, G., Bock, O.A., Williams, D.L., Witts, L.J.: Diabetes mellitus and pernicious anemia. Br. Med. J. 1:159, 1963.
18. Wilkinson, J.F.: Diabetes mellitus and pernicious anemia. Br. Med. J. 1:676, 1963.
19. Angervall, L., Dotevall, G., Lehmann, K.E.: The gastric mucosa in diabetes mellitus. A functional and histopathological study. Acta Med. Scand. 169:339, 1961.
20. Beckett, A.G., Matthews, D.M.: Diabetes mellitus and pernicious anemia. Br. Med. J. 1:534, 1963.
21. Moore, J.M., Neilson, J.M.: Antibodies to gastric mucosa and thyroid in diabetes mellitus. Lancet 2:645, 1963.
21a. Munichoodappa, C., Kozak, G.P.: Diabetes mellitus and pernicious anemia. Diabetes 19:719, 1970.
22. Wintrobe, M.M., Lee, G.R., Boggs, D.R., et al.: Clinical Hematology, 8th ed. Philadelphia, Lea & Febiger, 1981, p. 568.
22a. Chanarin, I.: The Megaloblastic Anemias. Philadelphia, F.A. Davis Co., 1969.
23. Aylett, P.: Gastric emptying and secretion in patients with diabetes mellitus. Gut 6:262, 1965.
24. Berger, W., Lauffenburger, T., Denes, A.: The effect of phenformin on the absorption of vitamin B_{12}. Horm. Metab. Res. 4:311, 1972.
25. Jounela, A.J., Pirttiaho, H., Palva, I.P.: Drug-induced malabsorption of vitamin B_{12}. VI. Malabsorption of vitamin B_{12} during treatment with phenformin. Acta Med. Scand. 196:267, 1974.
26. Fixa, B., Komarkova, O., Herout, V., Kos, J.: Morphology of the gastric mucosa in diabetics. Acta Med. Scand. 175:161, 1964.
27. Fixa, B., Komarkova, O., Herout, V., Kos, J.: Gastric secretory disturbances in diabetics. Am. J. Dig. Dis. 9:494, 1964.
28. Dotevall, G.: Gastric secretion of acid in diabetes mellitus during basal conditions and after maximal histamine stimulation. Acta Med. Scand. 170:59, 1961.
29. Dotevall, G.: Gastric function in diabetes mellitus. A clinical and experimental study with special reference to gastric secretion of acid. Acta Med. Scand. 368 (Suppl.):1, 1961.
30. Ungar, B., Stocks, A.E., Martin, F.I.R., et al.: Intrinsic factor antibody in diabetes mellitus. Lancet 2:77, 1967.
31. Ungar, B., Stocks, A.E., Martin, F.I.R., et al.: Intrinsic-factor antibody, parietal-cell antibody, and latent pernicious anemia in diabetes mellitus. Lancet 2:415, 1968.
32. Beckett, A.G., Matthews, D.M.: Vitamin B_{12} in diabetes mellitus. Clin. Sci. 23:361, 1962.
33. Dacie, J.V.: Haemolytic mechanisms in health and disease. Br. Med. J. 429, 1962.
34. Ditzel, J.: Changes in red cell oxygen release capacity in diabetes mellitus. Fed. Proc. 38.2404, 1979
35. Phillips, G.B., Mendershausen, B.: Glucose consumption by red cells of diabetic patients and normal subjects. Effects of ethanol. Clin. Chem. Acta 61:175, 1975.
36. Burka, E.R., Weaver, Z., III, Marks, P.A.: Clinical spectrum of hemolytic anemia associated with glucose-6-phosphate dehydrogenase deficiency. Ann. Intern. Med. 64:817, 1966.
37. Gellady, A.M., Greenwood, R.D.: G-6-PD hemolytic anemia complicating diabetic ketoacidosis. J. Pediat. 80:1037, 1972.
38. Gant, F.L., Winks, G.F., Jr.: Primaquine sensitive hemolytic anemia complicating diabetic acidosis. Clin. Res. 9:27, 1961. (Abstract)
39. Tarlov, A.R., Brewer, G.J., Carson, P.E., Alving, A.S.: Primaquine sensitivity; glucose-6-phosphate dehydrogenase deficiency: an inborn error of metabolism of medical and biological significance. Arch. Intern. Med. 109:209, 1962.
40. Chanmugam, D., Frumin, A.M.: Abnormal oral glucose tolerance response in erythrocyte glucose-6-phosphate dehydrogenase deficiency. N. Engl. J. Med. 271:1202, 1964.

41. Swift, M., Sholman, L., Gilmour, D.: Diabetes mellitus and the gene for Fanconi's anemia. Science *178*:308, 1972.

42. Jurgensen, J.C., Whitehouse, F.W., Oxley, M.J., Saeed, S.M.: Intravascular sickling associated with diabetic ketoacidosis. Diabetes *20*:771, 1971.

43. Simon, G.: Hyperosmolar diabetic state with sickle thalassemia. N.Y. State J. Med. *72*:496, 1972.

44. Logue, G.L., Boyd, A.E., III, Rosse, W.F.: Chlorpropamide-induced immune hemolytic anemia. N. Engl. J. Med. *283*:900, 1970.

45. Davis, R.E., Calder, J.S., Curnow, D.H.: Serum pyridoxal and folate concentrations in diabetics. Pathology *8*:151, 1976.

46. McConnell, R.B., Pyke, D.A., Roberts, J.A.F.: Blood groups in diabetes mellitus. Br. Med. J. *1*:772, 1956.

47. Andersen, J., Lauritzen, E.: Blood groups and diabetes mellitus. Diabetes *9*:20, 1960.

48. Scholz, W., Knussman, R., Daweke, H.: Distribution of blood and serum protein group characteristics in patients with diabetes. Diabetologia *11*:77, 1975.

49. Buckwalter, J.A.: Diabetes mellitus and the blood groups. Diabetes *13*:164, 1964.

50. Macafee, A.L.: Blood groups and diabetes. J. Clin. Pathol. *17*:39, 1964.

51. Berg, K., Aarseth, S., Lundevall, J., Reinskou, T.: Blood groups and genetic serum types in diabetes mellitus. Diabetologia *3*:30, 1967.

52. Harken, A.H.: The surgical significance of the oxyhemoglobin dissociation curve. Surg. Gynecol. Obstet. *144*:935, 1977.

53. Chanutin, A., Curnish, R.: Effect of organic and inorganic phosphates on the oxygen equilibrium of human erythrocytes. Arch. Biochem. *121*:96, 1967.

54. Benesch, R., Benesch, R.E.: The effects of organic phosphates from the human erythrocyte on the allosteric properties of hemoglobin. Biochem. Biophys. Res. Comm. *26*:162, 1967.

55. Alberti, K.G.M.M., Emerson, P.M., Darley, J.H., Hockaday, T.D.R.: 2,3-diphosphoglycerate and tissue oxygenation in uncontrolled diabetes mellitus. Lancet *2*:391, 1972.

56. Kanter, Y., Bessman, S.P., Bessman, H.: Red cell 2,3-diphosphoglycerate levels among diabetics with and without vascular complications. Diabetes *24*:724, 1975.

57. Ditzel, J., Standl, E.: The problem of tissue oxygenation in diabetes mellitus. I. Its relation to the early functional changes in the microcirculation of diabetic subjects. Acta Med. Scand. *578* (Suppl.):49, 1975.

58. Standl, E., Janka, H.U., Dexel, T., Kolb, H.J.: Muscle metabolism during rest and exercise: influence on the oxygen transport system of blood in normal and diabetic subjects. Diabetes *25*:914, 1976.

59. Arturson, G., Garby, L., Robert, M., Zaar, B.: Oxygen affinity of whole blood *in vivo* and under standard conditions in subjects with diabetes mellitus. Scand. J. Clin. Lab. Invest. *34*:19, 1974.

60. Guest, G.M., Rapoport, S.: Electrolytes of blood plasma and cells in diabetic acidosis and during recovery. Proc. Am. Diabetes Assoc. *7*:97, 1947.

61. Guest, G.M., Rapoport, S.: Role of acid soluble phosphorus compounds in red blood cells in experimental rickets, renal insufficiency, pyloric obstruction, gastroenteritis, ammonium chloride acidosis and diabetic acidosis. Am. J. Dis. Child. *58*:1072, 1939.

62. Bellingham, A.J., Detter, J.C., Lenfant, C.: The role of hemoglobin affinity for oxygen and red-cell 2,3-diphosphoglycerate in the management of diabetic ketoacidosis. Trans. Assoc. Amer. Physicians *83*:113, 1970.

63. Ditzel, J.: Changes in rheology and oxygen transport function of erythrocytes in diabetes. In: J. Ditzel, D.H. Lewis (Eds.): Microcirculatory Approaches to Current Therapeutic Problems. Basel, S. Karger, 1971, pp. 123–131.

64. Finch, C.A., Lenfant, C.: Oxygen transport in man. N. Engl. J. Med. *286*:407, 1972.

65. Ditzel, J., Standl, E.: The oxygen transport system of red blood cells during diabetic ketoacidosis and recovery. Diabetologia *11*:255, 1975.

66. Ditzel, J.: Importance of plasma inorganic phosphate on tissue oxygenation during recovery from diabetic ketoacidosis. Horm. Metab. Res. *5*:471, 1973.

67. Ditzel, J.: Oxygen transport impairment in diabetes. Diabetes *25* (Suppl. 2):832, 1976.

68. Andersen, H., Ditzel, J.: Importance of plasma inorganic phosphate in the treatment of diabetic ketoacidosis. (Abstr.). Diabetes *22* (Suppl. 1):293, 1973.

69. Ditzel, J.: Impaired oxygen release caused by alterations of the metabolism in the erythrocytes in diabetes. Lancet *1*:721, 1972.

70. Standl, E., Kolb, H., Standl, A., Mehnert, H.: The effect of diabetes on erythrocyte 2,3-diphosphoglycerate. Diabetologia *9*:91, 1973 (Abstr.).

71. Standl, E., Kolb, H.J.: 2,3-diphosphoglycerate fluctuations in erythrocytes reflecting pronounced blood glucose variation. *In vivo* and *in vitro* studies in normal, diabetic and hypoglycaemic subjects. Diabetologia *9*:461, 1973.

72. Lichtman, M.A., Miller, D.R., Cohen, J., Waterhouse, C.: Reduced red cell glycolysis, 2,3-diphosphoglycerate and adenosine triphosphate concentration and increased hemoglobin-oxygen affinity caused by hypophosphatemia. Ann. Intern. Med. *74*:562, 1971.

73. Travis, S.E., Sugarman, H.J., Ruberg, R.L., et al.: Alterations of red cell glycolytic intermediates and oxygen transport as a consequence of hypophosphatemia in patients receiving intravenous hyperalimentation. N. Engl. J. Med. *285*:763, 1971.

74. Riley, M.S., Schade, D.S., Eaton, E.P.: Effects of insulin infusion on plasma phosphate in diabetic patients. Metabolism *28*:191, 1979.

75. Ditzel, J.: Adaptive changes to tissue hypoxia in ambulatory juvenile diabetics. Diabetes *22* (Suppl.):317, 1973.

76. Ditzel, J., Andersen, H., Peters, N.D.: Increased hemoglobin A_{1c} and 2,3-diphosphoglycerate in diabetes and their effects on red-cell oxygen-releasing capacity. Lancet *2*:1034, 1973.

77. Bunn, H.F., Briehl, R.W.: The interaction of 2,3-diphosphoglycerate with various human hemoglobins. J. Clin. Invest. *49*:1088, 1970.

78. Ditzel, J.: Improved erythrocytic oxygen release following a dietary supplement of calcium diphosphate to diabetic and healthy children. Diabetologia *10*:363, 1974 (Abstr.)

79. Ditzel, J., Hau, C., Dauguaard, N.: Effect of the diphosphonate ethane-1-hydroxy-1, 1-diphosphonate (EHDP) on hemoglobin oxygen affinity of diabetic and healthy subjects. Microvasc. Res. *13*:355, 1977.

80. Ditzel, J., Dyerberg, J.: Hyperlipoproteinemia, diabetes and oxygen affinity of hemoglobin. Metabolism *26*:141, 1977.

81. Pedersen, O., Beck-Nielsen, H., Sørensen, N.S., Heding, L.: Effects of exercise on insulin receptors on erythrocytes and monocytes from insulin-dependent diabetics. Acta Paediatr. Scand. (Supp 283):79, 1980.

82. Eng, J., Lee. L., Yalow, R.S.: Influence of the age of erythrocytes on their insulin receptors. Diabetes *29*:164, 1980.

83. Dons, R.F., Ryan, J., Gorden, P., Wachslicht-Rodbard, H.: Erythrocyte and monocyte insulin binding in man. A

comparative analysis in normal and disease states. Diabetes *30*:896, 1981.

84. Malone, J.I., Knox, G., Benford, S., Tedesco, T.A.: Red cell sorbitol: an indicator of diabetic control. Diabetes *29*:861, 1980.

85. Kessler, I.I.: Mortality experience of diabetic patients: a twenty-six year follow-up study. Am. J. Med. *51*:715, 1971.

86. Levi, J.E., Friedman, H.T.: Insulin resistance in a case of diabetes mellitus and chronic lymphatic leukemia. Report of a case. N. Engl. J. Med. *225*:975, 1941.

87. Shohl, J., Field, J.B.: Insulin binding *in vitro* by leukocytes from normal and diabetic subjects. J. Lab. Clin. Med. *51*:288, 1958.

88. Kaufman, R.E.: Coexistent leukemia and diabetes mellitus. Am. Practit. Dig. Treat. *9*:413, 1958.

89. Rhie, F.H., Ganda, O.P., Bern, M.M., et al.: Insulin resistance and monoclonal gammopathy. Metabolism *30*:41, 1981.

90. Gilbert, H.S., Rayfield, E.J., Smith, H., Jr., Keusch, G.T.: Effects of acute endotoxemia and glucose administration on circulating leukocyte populations in normal and diabetic subjects. Metabolism *27*:899, 1978.

91. Ainsworth, S.K., Allison, F., Jr.: Studies on the pathogenesis of acute inflammation. IX. The influence of hyperosmolality secondary to hyperglycemia upon the acute inflammatory response induced by thermal injury to ear chambers of rabbits. J. Clin. Invest. *49*:433, 1970.

92. Perillie, R.E., Nolan, J.P., Finch, S.C.: Studies of the resistance to infection in diabetes mellitus: local exudative cellular response. J. Lab. Clin. Med. *59*:1008, 1962.

93. Van Oss, C.J.: Influence of glucose levels in the *in vitro* phagocytosis of bacteria by human neutrophils. Infect. Immun *4*:54, 1971.

94. MacGregor, R.R., Spagnuolo, P.J., Lentnek, A.L.: Inhibition of granulocyte adherence by ethanol, prednisone, and aspirin measured with an assay system. N. Engl. J. Med. *291*:642, 1974.

95. Bagdade, J.D., Stewart, M., Waters, E.: Impaired granulocyte adherence: a reversible defect in host defense in patients with poorly-controlled diabetes. Diabetes *27*:677, 1978.

96. Mowat, A.G., Baum, J.: Chemotaxis of polymorphonuclear leukocytes from patients with diabetes mellitus. N. Engl. J. Med. *284*:621, 1971.

97. Bybee, J.D., Rogers, D.E.: The phagocytic activity of polymorphonuclear leukocytes obtained from patients with diabetes mellitus. J. Lab. Clin. Med. *64*:1, 1964.

98. Miller, M.E.: Pathology of chemotaxis and random mobility. Seminars Hematol. *12*:59, 1975.

99. Miller, M.E., Baker, L.: Leukocyte functions in juvenile diabetes mellitus: humoral and cellular aspects. J. Pediatr. *81*:979, 1972.

100. Hill, H.R., Sauls, H.J., Dettloff, J.L., Quie, P.G.: Impaired leukotactic responsiveness in patients with juvenile diabetes mellitus. Clin. Immunol. Immunopathol. *2*:395, 1974.

101. Molenaar, D.M., Palumbo, P.J., Wilson, W.R., Pitts, R.E., Jr.: Impaired leukocyte chemotaxis in non-diabetic relatives of patients with juvenile-onset diabetes. Diabetes *24*:401, 1974. (Abstr.)

102. Humbert, J.R., Hambidge, K.M., Moore, L.L., et al.: Absence of neutrophil chemotactic defect in diabetes. Clin. Res. *24*:180A, 1976. (Abstr.)

103. Fikrig, S.M., Reddy, C.M., Orti, E., et al.: Diabetes and neutrophil chemotaxis. Diabetes *26*:466, 1977.

104. Cruickshank, A.H., Payne, T.P.B.: Anti-pneumococcal powers of the blood in alloxan diabetes in the rabbit. Bull. Johns Hopkins Hosp. *84*:334, 1949.

105. Briscoe, H.F., Allison, F., Jr.: Diabetes and host resistance. I. Effect of alloxan diabetes upon the phagocytic and bactericidal efficiency of rat leukocytes for pneumococcus. J. Bact. *90*:1537, 1965.

106. Drachman, R.H., Root, R.K., Wood, W.B., Jr.: Studies on the effect of experimental nonketotic diabetes mellitus on antibacterial defense. I. Demonstration of a defect in phagocytosis. J. Exp. Med. *124*:227, 1966.

107. Richardson, R.: Immunity in diabetes: influence of diabetes on the development of antibacterial properties in the blood. J. Clin. Invest. *12*:1143, 1933.

108. Marble, A., White, H.J., Fernald, A.T.: The nature of the lowered resistance in diabetes mellitus. J. Clin. Invest. *17*:423, 1938.

109. Balch, H.H., Watters, M.: Blood bactericidal studies and serum complement in diabetic patients. J. Surg. Res. *3*:199, 1963.

110. Crosby, B., Allison, F., Jr.: Phagocytic and bactericidal capacity of polymorphonuclear leukocytes recovered from venous blood of human beings. Proc. Soc. Exp. Bio. Med. *123*:660, 1966.

111. Bagdade, J.D., Nielson, K.L., Bulger, R.J.: Reversible abnormalities in phagocytic function in poorly-controlled diabetic patients. Am. J. Med. Sci. *263*:451, 1972.

112. Bagdade, J.D., Root, R.K., Bulger, R.J.: Impaired leukocyte function in patients with poorly-controlled diabetes. Diabetes *23*:9, 1974.

113. Tan, J.S., Anderson, L., Watanakunakorn, C., Phair, J.P.: Neutrophil dysfunction in diabetes mellitus. J. Lab. Clin. Med. *85*:26, 1975.

114. Nolan, C.M., Beaty, H.N., Bagdade, J.D.: Further characterization of the impaired bactericidal function of granulocytes in patients with poorly-controlled diabetes. Diabetes *27*:889, 1978.

115. Esman, V.: The Diabetic Leukocyte Enzyme *13*:32, 1972.

116. Cech, P., Stadler, H., Widmann, J.J., et al.: Leukocyte myeloperoxidase deficiency and diabetes mellitus associated with Candida albicans liver abscess. Am. J. Med., *66*:149, 1979.

117. Bordy, J.I., Merlie, K.: Metabolic and biosynthetic features of lymphocytes from patients with diabetes mellitus: Similarities to lymphocytes in chronic lymphocytic leukemia. Br. J. Haematol. *19*:193, 1970.

118. Delespesse, G., Duchateau, J., Bastenie, P.A., et al.: Cell-mediated immunity in diabetes mellitus. Clin. Exp. Immunol. *18*:461, 1974.

119. Kaplan, J.H., Vugiris, E.E.: The detection of phytomitogen-induced changes in human lymphocyte surfaces by laser Dappler spectroscopy. J. Immunological Methods. *7*:337–346, 1973.

120. MacCuish, A.C., Urbaniak, S.J., Campbell, C.J., et al.: Phytohemagglutinin transformation and circulating lymphocyte subpopulations in insulin-dependent diabetic patients. Diabetes *23*:708, 1974.

121. Glassman, A.B., Lindsay, J.H., Bennett, C.E., Hodges, E.R., Jr.: Effects of insulin on phytohemagglutinin-P, concanavalin-A, and pokeweed mitogen in diabetic and non-diabetic lymphocytes. Ann. Clin. Lab. Sci. *11*:9, 1981.

122. Ser, I., Czitron, B.: Diagnostic value of the PAS-positive lymphocyte index in diabetes. Isr. J. Med. Sci. *10*:846, 1974.

123. Stern, M.M., Dixit, P.K.: Decreased citrate synthesis by lymphocytes from alloxan-diabetic rat. Proc. Soc. Exp. Biol. Med. *156*:417, 1977.

124. Fabris, N.: Hormones and aging. In: T. Makinodon, E. Yunis (Eds.): Comprehensive Immunology, Vol. I. Immunity and Aging. New York, Plenum Press, 1976, pp. 73–89.

125. Goldstein, H.H.: Disorders of the blood. In: A. Marble, P. White, R.F. Bradley, L.P. Krall (Eds.): Joslin's Diabetes Mellitus, 11th Ed. Philadelphia, Lea & Febiger, 1971. pp. 646–647.
126. Fitzhugh, J.: Diabetes in a hemophiliac. J. Nat. Med. Assoc. 54:479, 1962.
127. Kwzuya, N., Kasaka, K.: Diabetes in Japan. In: S. Lsufi, M. Woda (Eds.): Diabetes Mellitus in Asia. Amsterdam, Excerpta Medica, 1971, pp. 11–21.
128. Pursel, S.E., Sherman, A.K.: Pulmonary resection in hemophilia. Chest 62:342, 1972.
129. Dalsgaard-Nielsen, J., Madsbad, S., Hilsted, J.: Changes in platelet function, blood coagulation, and fibrinolysis during insulin-induced hypoglycaemia in juvenile diabetics and normal subjects. Thromb. Haemost. 47:254, 1982.
130. Porta, M., Maneschi, F., White, M.C., Kohner, E.M.: Twenty-four hour variations of von Willebrand Factor and Factor VIII-related antigen in diabetic retinopathy. Metabolism 30:695, 1981.
131. Colwell, J., Sagel, J., Pennington, R., et al.: Effect of therapy on platelet aggregation in diabetes. Clin. Res. 21:884, 1973.
132. Sagel, J., Colwell, J.A., Crook, L., Laimins, M.: Increased platelet aggregation in early diabetes mellitus. Ann. Intern. Med. 82:733, 1975.
133. Kalofoutis, A., Lekakis, J.: Changes of platelet phospholipids in diabetes mellitus. Diabetologia 21:540, 1981.
134. Butkus, A., Shrinska, V.A., Schumacher, O.P.: Thromboxane production and platelet aggregation in diabetic subjects with clinical complications. Thromb. Res. 19:211, 1980.
135. Hassenein, A.A., el-Garf, T.A., el-Baz, A.: Platelet aggregation in diabetes mellitus and the effect of insulin in vivo on aggregation. Thromb. Diath. Haemorrh. 27:114, 1972.
136. Heath, H., Brigden, W.D., Canever, J.V., et al.: Platelet adhesiveness and aggregation in relation to diabetic retinopathy. Diabetologia 7:308, 1971.
137. Chymielewski, J., Farbiszewski, R.: Platelet factor 4 (PF 4) release during human platelet aggregation in diabetic patients. Thromb. Diath. Haemorrh. 24:203, 1979.
138. Rathbone, R.L., Ardlie, N.G., Schwartz, C.J.: Platelet aggregation and thrombus formation in diabetes mellitus: an in vitro study. Pathol. 2:307, 1970.
139. Lee, H., Paton, R.C., Passa, P., Caen, J.P.: Fibrinogen binding and ADP-induced aggregation in platelets from diabetic subjects. Thromb. Res. 24:143, 1981.
140. Kwaan, H.C., Colwell, J.A., Cruz, S., et al.: Increased platelet aggregation in diabetes mellitus. J. Lab. Clin. Med. 80:236, 1972.
141. Gandolfo, G.M., Afeltra, A., Amoroso, A., Ferri, G.M.: Platelet factor 3 availability in patients affected by pancreatic diabetes. Haematologica 59:316, 1974.
142. Nordöy, A., Rödset, J.M.: Platelet phospholipids and their function in patients with juvenile diabetes and maturity onset diabetes. Diabetes 19:698, 1970.
143. Mühlhauser, I., Schernthaner, G., Silberbauer, K., et al.: Platelet proteins (β-TG and PF 4) in atherosclerosis and related diseases. Artery 8:73, 1980.
144. McDonald, L.: Thrombosis in coronary heart disease. Br. Heart J. 30:151, 1968.
145. Hellem, A.J.: The adhesiveness of human blood platelets in vitro. Scand. J. Clin. Lab. Invest. 12 (Suppl. 51):1, 1960.
146. McDonald, L., Edgill, M.: Changes in coagulability of blood during various phases of ischemic heart disease. Lancet 1:1115, 1959.
147. Silberbauer, K., Schernthaner, G., Sinzinger, H., et al.: Decreased vascular prostocyclin in juvenile onset diabetes. N. Engl. J. Med. 300:366, 1979.
148. Halushka, P.R., Rogers, R.C., Loadholt, C.B., et al.: Increased platelet, prostaglandin and thromboxane synthesis in diabetes mellitus. Horm. Metabolism Res. II (Suppl.) 7, 1981.
149. Ylikorkala, O., Kaila, J.,Viinikka, L.: Prostacyclin and thromboxane in diabetes. Br. Med. J. 283:1148, 1981.
150. Silberbauer, K., Schernthaner, G., Sinzinger, H., Freyler, H.: Platelet aggregation and reversible platelet aggregates in Type I diabetes staged by retinal fluorescein angiography. Atherosclerosis 40:81, 1981.
151. Levin, R.D., Kwaan, H.C., Dobbie, J.G., et al.: Studies of retinopathy and plasma co-factor of platelet hyperaggregation in Type I (insulin-dependent) diabetic children. Diabetologia 22:445, 1982.
152. Levin, R.D., Kwaan, H.C., Dobbie, J.G., et al.: Partial purification and studies of the plasma co-factor that potentiates platelet aggregation in diabetes mellitus. J. Lab. Clin. Med. 98:519, 1981.
153. Kühnau, J., Martin, W., Reutner, H., Tilsner, V.: Effect of insulin on thrombocyte functions in normals and in diabetics. Diabetologia 12:404, 1976 (Abstr. #156).
154. Mielke, C.H., Gerich, J.E., Lorenzi, M., et al.: The effect of somatostatin on coagulation and platelet function in man. N. Engl. J. Med. 293:480, 1975.
155. Coppola, L., Giugliano, D., Tirelli, A., et al.: Circulating platelet aggregates induced by somatostatin in insulin-dependent diabetic subjects. Diabete Metab. 6:245, 1980.
156. vanZile, J., Kilpatrick, M., Laimins, M., et al.: Platelet aggregation and release of ATP after incubation with soluble immune complexes purified from serum of diabetic patients. Diabetes 30:575, 1981.
157. Shaw, S., Pegrum, G.D., Wolff, S., Ashton, W.L.: Platelet adhesiveness in diabetes mellitus. J. Clin. Pathol. 20:845, 1967.
158. Seth, H.N.: Fibrinolytic response to moderate exercise and platelet adhesiveness in diabetes mellitus. Acta Diabetol. Lat. 10:306, 1973.
159. Bridges, J.M., Dalby, A.M., Millar, J.H.D., Weaver, J.A.: An effect of D-glucose on platelet stickiness. Lancet 1:75, 1965.
160. Odegaard, A.E., Skalhegg, B.A., Hellem, A.J.: Increased activity of "anti-Willebrand factor" in diabetic plasma. Thromb. Diath. Haemorrh. 11:27, 1964.
161. Mayne, E.E., Bridges, J.M., Weaver, J.A.: Platelet adhesiveness, plasma fibrinogen and factor VIII levels in diabetes mellitus. Diabetologia 6:436, 1970.
162. Bagchi, A.L., Ghosh, B.P., Sen Gupta, A.N.: Studies on platelet adhesiveness in diabetes mellitus and atherosclerotic heart disease after glucose load. J. Indian Med. Assoc. 54:495, 1970.
163. Preston, F.E., Marcola, B.H., Ward, J.D., et al.: Elevated β-thromboglobulin levels and circulating platelet aggregates in diabetic microangiopathy. Lancet 1:238, 1978.
164. Chesebro, J.H., Fuster, V., Bardsley, W.T., Kazmier, F.J.: Platelet survival half-life in patients with coronary diseases under and over age 50. Council on Arteriosclerosis of American Heart Association (Abstr.). Nov. 12–14, 1979, Anaheim, California, p. 6.
165. Burrows, A.W., Chavin, S.I., Hockaday, T.D.R.: Plasma-thromboglobulin concentrations in diabetes mellitus. Lancet 1:235, 1978.
166. Elving, L.D., Gasparie, A.F., Miedema, K., Russchen, C.J.: Plasma B-thromboglobulin in diabetics with and without microangiopathic complications. (Letter). Diabetologia 21:160, 1981.

167. Abrahamsen, A.F.: Platelet survival studies in man. With special reference to thrombosis and atherosclerosis. Scand. J. Haematol. Suppl. 3:1, 1968.

168. Tindall, H., Paton, R.C., Zuzel, M., McNicol, G.P.: Platelet life-span in diabetics with and without retinopathy. Thromb. Res. 21:641, 1981.

169. Garg, S.K., Lackner, H., Karpatkin, S.: The increased percentage of megathrombocytes in various clinical disorders. Ann. Intern. Med. 77:361, 1972.

170. Ferguson, J.C., Mackay, N., Philip, J.A., Sumner, D.L.J.L.: Determination of platelet and fibrinogen half-life with (75Se) selenomethionine: studies in normal and in diabetic subjects. Clin. Sci. Mol. Med. 49:115, 1975.

171. Nilsson, I.M., Olow, B.: Determination of fibrinogen and fibrinolytic activity. Thromb. Diath. Haemorrh. 8:297, 1962.

172. Steele, P.P., Weily, H.S., Davies, H., et al.: Platelet function studies in coronary artery disease. Circulation 48:1194, 1972.

173. Koschinsky, T., Bünting, C.E., Schwippert, B., Gries, F.A.: Regulation of diabetic serum growth factors for human vascular cells by the metabolic control of diabetes mellitus. Atherosclerosis 39:313, 1981.

174. Koschinsky, T., Bünting, C.E., Schwippert, B., Gries, F.A.: Increased growth stimulation of fibroblasts from rabbits by diabetic serum factors of low molecular weight. Atherosclerosis 37:311, 1980.

175. Bern, M.M., Pumphery, M.E., Horton, J., Davis, G.L.: Factor VIII and von Willebrand's factor in diabetes mellitus. Diabetes 28 (Suppl.):412, 1979. (Abstr.)

176. Weiss, H.J., Hoyer, L.W., Rickles, F.R., et al.: Quantitative assay of a plasma factor deficient in von Willebrand's disease that is necessary for platelet aggregation. J. Clin. Invest. 52:2708, 1973.

177. Bensoussan, D., Levy-Toledano, S., Passa, P., et al.: Platelet hyperaggregation and increased plasma level of von Willebrand factor in diabetics with retinopathy. Diabetologia 11:307, 1975.

178. Coller, B.S., Frank, R.N., Milton, R.C., Gralnick, H.R.: Plasma cofactors of platelet function: correlation with diabetic retinopathy and hemoglobins A_{1a-c}. Studies in diabetic patients and normal persons. Ann. Intern. Med. 88:311, 1978.

179. Lufkin, E.G., Fass, D.N., D'Fallon, W.M., Bowie, E.J.W.: Increased von Willebrand factor in diabetes mellitus. Metabolism 28:63, 1979.

179a.Lamberton, R.P., Goodman, A.D., Kassoff, A., et al.: Von Willebrand factor (VIII R:Ag), fibronectin, and insulin-like growth factors I and II in diabetic retinopathy and nephropathy. Diabetes 33:125, 1984.

180. Hennes, A.R., Awai, K.: Studies of incorporation of radioactivity into lipids by human blood. IV. Abnormal incorporation of acetate 1-C-14 into fatty acids by whole blood and platelets from insulin-dependent diabetics. Diabetes 14:709, 1965.

181. Hennes, A.R., Awai, K., Hammarstrand, K., Duboff, G.S.: Carbon-14 in carboxyl carbon of fatty acids formed by platelets from normal and diabetic subjects. Nature 210:839, 1966.

182. Awai, K., Hammarstrand, K., Hennes, A.R.: Studies of incorporation of radioactivity into lipids by human blood. I. Pattern of incorporation of radioactivity into fatty acids by blood from normal subjects and patients in diabetic acidosis. Metabolism 13:328, 1964.

183. Schmukler, M., Zieve, P.D.: The effect of glucose feeding on fatty acid synthesis in human platelets. J. Lab. Clin. Med. 80:231, 1972.

184. Paterson, R.A., Heath, H., Cranfield, T.: The effect of O-(beta-hydroxyethyl) rutoside on platelet intermediary metabolism in normal and streptozotocin diabetic rats. Biochem. Pharmacol. 23:1591, 1974.

185. Egeberg, O.: The blood coagulability in diabetic retinopathy. Scand. J. Clin. Lab. Invest. 15:533, 1963.

186. Ottaviani, P., Redi, R.: Hemostasis in diabetic retinopathy. Clin. Med. 39:290, 1958.

187. Alberini, B., Tedeschi, G., Lasagna, G.C., Schiavi, L.: Thromboelastographic research in diabetes mellitus. Riforma Med. 75:957, 1961.

187a.Jones, R.L., Peterson, C.M.: Reduced fibrinogen survival in diabetes mellitus: a reversible phenomenon. J. Clin. Invest. 63:485, 1979.

187b.Banerjee, R.N., Sahni, A.L., Kumar, V.: Fibrin coagulopathy in maturity onset diabetes mellitus and atherosclerosis. Thromb. Diath. Haemorrh. 30:123, 1973.

187c.Jones, R.L., Jouvanovic, L., Forman, S., Peterson, C.M.: Time course of reversibility of accelerated fibrinogen disappearance in diabetes mellitus: association with intravascular volume shifts. Blood 63:22, 1984.

187d.Leet, H., Paton, R.C., Passa, P., Caen, J.P.: Fibrinogen binding and ADP-induced aggregation in platelets from diabetic subjects. Thromb. Res. 24:143, 1981.

188. Tsianos, E.B., Stathakis, N.E.: Soluble fibrin complexes and fibrinogen heterogeneity in diabetes mellitus. Thromb. Haemost. 44:130, 1980.

189. Valdorf-Hansen, F.: Coagulability in diabetics. Acta Med. Scand. 467 (Suppl.):147, 1967.

190. Self, T.H., Hood, J., Miller, S.T.: Diabetes mellitus and the hypoprothrombinemic response to warfarin. J.A.M.A. 239:2239, 1978.

191. Banerjee, R.N., Sahni, A.L., Kumar, V., Orya, M.: Antithrombin III deficiency in maturity-onset diabetes mellitus and atherosclerosis. Throm. Diath. Haemorrh. 31:339, 1974.

192. Sowers, J.R., Tuck, M.L., Sowers, D.K.: Plasma antithrombin III and thrombin generation time: correlation with hemoglobin A, and fasting serum glucose in young diabetic women. Diabetes Care 3:655, 1980.

193. Grignani, G., Gamba, G., Geroldi, D., et al.: Enhanced antithrombotic mechanisms in patients with maturity-onset diabetes mellitus without thrombotic complications. Thromb. Haemost. 46:648, 1981.

194. Pozilli, P., DiMario, U., Javicoli, M., et al.: Alpha 2 macroglobulin: its variability in diabetes. Horm. Metab. Res. 12:409, 1980.

195. Tanser, A.R.: Fibrinolytic response of diabetics and non-diabetics to adrenaline. J. Clin. Pathol. 20:231, 1967.

196. MacKay, N., Hume, R.: Fibrinolytic activity in diabetes mellitus. Scot. Med. J. 9:359, 1964.

197. Farid, N.R., Anderson, J., Martin, A., Weightman, D.: Fibrinolytic activity and treatment of diabetes. Lancet 1:631, 1974.

198. Hajjar, G.C., Whissen, N.C., Moser, K.M.: Diurnal variation in plasma euglobulin activity and fibrinogen levels. Preliminary report. Angiology 12:160, 1961.

199. Almer, L.O., Nilsson, I.M.: On fibrinolysis in diabetes mellitus. Acta Med. Scand. 198:101, 1975.

200. Fearnley, G.R., Chakrabarti, R., Avis, P.R.: Blood fibrinolytic activity in diabetes mellitus and its bearing on ischemic heart disease and obesity. Br. Med. J. 1:921, 1963.

201. Almer, L.O., Pandolfi, M., Nilsson, I.M.: Diabetic retinopathy and the fibrinolytic system. Diabetes 24:529, 1975.

202. Fiaschi, E., Barbui, T., Previato, G., et al.: The effects of phenphormin on blood fibrinolysis in diabetes mellitus. Arzneim. Forsch. 19:638, 1969.

203. Cash, J.D., McGill, R.C.: Fibrinolytic response to mod-

erate exercise in young male diabetics and non-diabetics. J. Clin. Pathol. 22:32, 1969.

204. Bogie, W., George, J., Crane, C.W.: Fibrinolytic activity in treatment of diabetes. Lancet 2:312, 1976.

205. Bellet, S., Sandberg, H., Tsitouris, G., et al.: Alterations in fibrinolytic parameters in the human during recovery from diabetic acidosis. Metabolism 10:429, 1961.

206. Almer, L.O., Pandolfi, M.: Fibrinolysis and diabetic retinopathy. Diabetes 25 (Suppl. 2):807, 1976.

207. Badawi, H., el-Sawy, M., Mikhail, M., et al.: Platelets, coagulation, and fibrinolysis in diabetic and non-diabetic patients with quiescent coronary heart disease. Angiology 21:511, 1970.

208. Almer, L.O., Nilsson, I.M.: Fibrinolytic activity and treatment of diabetes. Lancet 1:1342, 1974.

209. Fearnley, G.R., Chakrabarti, R., Vincent, C.T.: Effect of sulphonylureas on fibrinolysis. Lancet 2:622, 1960.

210. Fearnley, G.R., Vincent, C.T., Chakrabarti, R.: Reduction of blood fibrinolytic activity in diabetes mellitus by insulin. Lancet 2:1067, 1959.

211. Farid, N.R., Martin, A., Anderson, J.: Insulin and fibrinolytic activity. Lancet 2:1270, 1973.

212. Fearnley, G.R., Chakrabarti, R.: Pharmacologic enhancement of fibrinolytic activity of blood. J. Clin. Pathol. 17:328, 1964.

213. Ditzel, J.: Whole-blood viscosity and related components in diabetes mellitus. Danish Med. Bull. 15:49, 1968.

214. Barnes, A., Locke, P., Dormandy, J., Dormandy, T.: Abnormal hemorrheology in diabetes mellitus. Bibl. Anat. 16:428, 1977.

214a.Dintenfass, L.: Blood viscosity factors in non-diabetic and diabetic retinopathy. Bibl. Anat. 16:422, 1977.

215. Barnes, A.J., Locke, P., Scudder, P.R., et al.: Is hyperviscosity a treatable component of diabetic microcirculatory disease? Lancet 2:789, 1977.

216. McMillan, D.E., Utterback, N.G., Stocki, J.: Low shear rate blood viscosity in diabetes. Biorheology 17:355, 1980.

217. Volger, E., Schmid-Schönbein, H., Mehnert, H.: Microrheological changes of blood in diabetes mellitus. Bibl. Anat. 13:97, 1975.

218. Dintenfass, L., Sharp, A.: Dynamic blood coagulation, thrombus formation, and degradation in patients with peripheral vascular disease (arteriosclerosis, including diabetic): an in vitro study. Ann. Surg. 170:984, 1969.

219. Poon, P.Y.W., Dornan, T.L., Orde-Peckar, C., et al.: Blood viscosity, glycaemic control and retinopathy in insulin-dependent diabetes. Clin. Sci. 63:211, 1982.

220. Paisey, R.B., Harkness, J., Hartog, M., Chadwick, T.: The effect of improvement in diabetic control on plasma and whole blood viscosity. Diabetologia 19:345, 1980.

221. Juhan, I., Vague, P., Buonocore, M., et al.: Abnormalities of erythrocyte deformability and platelet aggregation

in insulin-dependent diabetics corrected by insulin in vivo and in vitro. Lancet 1:535, 1982.

222. Otsuji, S., Baba, Y., Kamada, T.: Erythrocyte membrane microviscosity in diabetes. Horm. Metab. Res. 11 (Suppl.):97, 1981.

223. Juhan, I., Vague, P., Buonocore, M., et al.: Effects of insulin on erythrocyte deformability in diabetics; relationship between erythrocyte deformability and platelet aggregation. Scand. J. Clin. Lab. Invest. 156 (Suppl.) 159, 1981.

224. LeDevehat, C., Lemoine, A., Cirette, B., Ramet, M.: Red cell filterability and metabolic state in diabetic subjects with macroangiopathy. Scand. J. Lab. Clin. Invest. 41 (Suppl. 156):155, 1981.

225. Gandhi, C.R., Chowdhury, D.R.: Effect of diabetes mellitus on sialic acid and glutathione content of human erythrocytes of different ages. Indian J. Exp. Biol. 17:585, 1979.

226. Fitzgibbons, J.F., Koler, R.D., Jones, R.T.: Red cell age-related changes of hemoglobins A_{1a-b} and A_{1c} in normal and diabetic subjects. J. Clin. Invest. 58:820, 1976.

227. Isogai, Y., Iida, A., Michezaki, K., Abe, K.: Hemorrheological studies on the pathogenesis of diabetic microangiopathy. Throm. Res. 8 (Suppl. II):17, 1976.

228. Branemark, P-I., Langer, L., Fagerverg, S-E, Breine, U.: Studies in rheology of human diabetes mellitus. Diabetologia 7:107, 1971.

229. McMillan, D.E.: Further observations on serum viscosity changes in diabetes mellitus. Metabolism 31:274, 1982.

230. Wautier, J.L., Paton, R.C., Wautier, M.P., et al.: Increased adhesion of erythrocytes to endothelial cells in diabetes mellitus and its relation to vascular complications. N. Engl. J. Med. 305:237, 1981.

231. Ross, R., Glomset, J.A.: The pathogenesis of atherosclerosis. N. Engl. J. Med. 295:369, 1976.

232. Bern, M.M., Zitter, B.A.: Response of human iliac artery endothelial cells to serum from diabetic patients (Submitted for publication).

233. Paton, R.C., Guillot, R., Passa, P., Canivet, J.: Prostacyclin production by human endothelial cells cultured in diabetic serum. Diabete Metab. 8:323, 1982.

234. Stout, R.W.: Glucose inhibits replication of cultured human endothelial cells. Diabetologia 23:436, 1982.

235. Mordes, D.B., Lazarchick, J., Colwell, J.A., Sens, D.A.: Elevated glucose concentrations increase Factor VIII R:Ag levels in human umbilical vein endothelial cells. Diabetes 32:876, 1983.

236. Stout, R.W.: The role of insulin in atherosclerosis in diabetics and nondiabetics: a review. Diabetes 30 (Suppl. 2):54, 1981.

237. King, G.L., Buzney, S.M., Kahn, C.R., et al.: Differential responsiveness to insulin of endothelial and support cells from micro- and macrovessels. J. Clin. Invest. 71:974, 1983.

38 Disorders of the Skin in Diabetes

George P. Kozak and Leo P. Krall

Patients with diabetes, especially if the condition is poorly controlled, are more subject to infections of the skin than are nondiabetics. This was particularly true prior to the availability of insulin and the antimicrobial agents when furunculosis, boils and carbuncles (frequently fatal) were relatively common. Fortunately, with better control of the disease which is possible in the present day, the susceptibility to infection has been largely overcome and approaches that of the nondiabetic.

Nevertheless, unless meticulous glycemic control is achieved, certain abnormalities can be demonstrated. These are concerned chiefly with impairment of granulocyte function,[1] including adherence, chemotaxis, phagocytosis, and bactericidal effect. For comprehensive discussions of infection in diabetes, see Chapter 36 and the review article by Wheat.[2]

Other skin disorders are so much more common in diabetic than in nondiabetic persons that their presence suggests this condition. Such disorders include necrobiosis lipoidica diabeticorum, shin spots, bullosis diabeticorum, and xanthosis.

PATHOPHYSIOLOGY

The entry of glucose into the epidermal cells does not appear to be limited by its passage through the cell membrane, and insulin has no effect on glucose transport in the epidermis. Free glucose is exposed in the intracellular medium to hexokinase and the activity of this enzyme determines the rate of glucose utilization. This hexokinase activity is enhanced by high concentrations of ATP (adenosine-triphosphate) produced in glycolysis and is decreased by high concentrations of ADP (adenosine diphosphate). Hexokinase phosphorylates glucose to form glucose-6-phosphate. About 70 to 75% of this is oxidized through the Embden-Meyerhof pathway to lactic acid; 5% is diverted through the phosphogluconate shunt, 5% is channeled into glycogen, and only 2% is metabolized through the Krebs cycle, while 15% is theoretically available to be broken down to free glucose.[2,3] The identification of phosphoglucomutase and phosphorylase in the skin is evidence of cutaneous synthesis of glycogen and other polysaccharides.[4] Glycogen, however, is not found in the normal adult epidermis and is not present in fetal epidermis until the 6th month of intrauterine life. Inflammation, minor epidermal trauma, and exposure to ultraviolet light cause transitory reappearance of epidermal glycogen.[5]

The ability of human skin to synthesize lipids is well documented. When ^{14}C-acetate is incubated with pieces of human skin, it is incorporated into squalene, sterols and fatty acids. The epidermis is the site of sterol synthesis while the sebaceous glands are responsible for the synthesis of squalene.[6,7] Incorporation of ^{14}C-acetate into skin lipids is higher in the postprandial state than during fasting, and it has been shown in vitro that glucose and insulin stimulate skin lipogenesis. During diabetic acidosis, skin lipogenesis is markedly reduced.[8]

In normal persons, the administration of glucose orally or intravenously is followed by an increase in the content of glucose in the skin. The maximal level attained in the skin occurs later than does the peak level in the blood. The early investigations of Urbach[9,10] showed the skin glucose of diabetics with dermatoses to be higher than that of diabetics without such disorders in spite of comparable blood glucose levels. Urbach called this "skin diabetes" and felt that chemical and clinical improvement followed the use of a low carbohydrate diet with or without insulin. Peterka and Fusaro[11,12] reviewed Urbach's studies and found that the fasting glucose level of the skin reflects the blood glucose level which, in turn, depends on diabetic control. In their studies it was noted that the concentration of glucose in the skin of fasting diabetics was approximately two-thirds that of the blood, whereas in nondiabetic persons it was about one-half that of the blood. However, in the diabetics there was no correlation between high skin/blood glucose ratios and the presence of skin infections.

SKIN AS AN INSTRUMENT OF DIABETES DETECTION

The condition of the skin has long provided clues pointing to the presence of diabetes. These include frequent infections, dryness, and non-specific pruritus. Attempts at correlation of the skin (sweat) and blood glucose have met with only modest success. In one study,[13] the results of simultaneous determinations of blood and urine glucose and detection of skin glucose by means of glucose-oxidase test paper in 86 diabetics, suggested some correlation between elevated levels of glucose in the blood and urine and positive skin reactions. However, West, Rockwell and Wulff[14] found that the skin glucose test was not sufficiently sensitive or specific for the diagnosis of diabetes.

Compared with that of nondiabetics, the skin of the diabetic is said to have structural differences including an increased number of mast cells in the dermis, especially in the superficial layers and around the blood vessels and skin appendages.[15] This has been associated with an increased erythematous reaction to histamine given intradermally. Among other characteristics attributed to the surface capillaries of the skin of diabetic patients have been increased capillary fragility, decreased

temperature changes under the influence of tolazoline (Priscoline), and abnormal plethysmographic and calorigenic responses to nitroglycerin and tetraethylammonium bromide. It has been suggested that blood vessels of the skin in diabetics show decreased circulation, but this has not been conclusively determined. However, newer techniques of light and electron microscopy of the capillaries of the skin have disclosed in diabetics the presence of abnormalities characterized by thickening of the capillary walls due to periendothelial deposits of PAS (periodic acid Schiff)—positive material which appears to have the same density as does the basement membrane.[17] These abnormalities seem to be particularly pronounced in patients with juvenile-onset diabetes, long-term diabetes, and those whose diabetes is associated with retinopathy and nephropathy.[18] However, they have also been noted in prediabetics[19] and in persons with recently diagnosed diabetes.[20] Capillary thickening was also found in nondiabetics with both acute and healed dermatologic lesions.[16]

Binkley[21] noted in diabetics the presence of dermal capillaries with large endothelial cells, endothelial proliferation, PAS-positive material in the cell walls, and sometimes a marked increase in the number of vessels in the upper and lower vascular plexuses.

While none of these changes or the dermatoses to be described later are pathognomonic, they are so frequently found with diabetes in any of its various stages that this association alone may lead to the suspicion of and possible diagnosis of diabetes. The dermatologic conditions found in diabetes may be classified as shown in Table 38–1. Not included in the table is a common complication of diabetes, namely injury to skin in a patient with neuropathy and/or reduced circulation (see Plate V A).

SKIN CONDITIONS USUALLY ASSOCIATED WITH DIABETES

Necrobiosis Lipoidica Diabeticorum

This is the most dramatic skin condition usually associated with diabetes. It is considered to be a rare complication, with a reported frequency of 0.3% in diabetic patients.[22] However, this figure varies with the type of patient seen in any one clinical group. Oppenheim[23] described this lesion in a diabetic patient in 1929 and Urbach[24] reported a case in 1932, coining the name "necrobiosis lipoidica diabeticorum" (NLD). This was descriptive if not acccurate since a small percentage of these lesions occur in nondiabetics and the tendency now is to omit the term "diabeticorum." Cannon[25] has also pointed out that this condition can be found considerably prior to the onset of

Table 38–1. Disorders of the Skin in Diabetes

A. Skin Conditions usually Associated with Diabetes
- Necrobiosis lipoidica diabeticorum
- Diabetic dermopathy (shin spots, brown spots)
- Lipodystrophy
  - Hypertrophy
  - Atrophy
- Insulin allergy
- Skin reactions to oral hypoglycemic agents
- Idiopathic bullae in diabetics (bullosis diabeticorum)

B. Skin Conditions Found Frequently in Patients with Diabetes
- Skin infections
  - Bacterial infections
  - Dermatophytosis
  - Moniliasis
- Xanthomas
  - Tuberous xanthoma
  - Eruptive xanthoma
  - Xanthochromia (carotenemia)

C. Skin Conditions Found Coincidentally with Diabetes
- Pruritus
- Dupuytren's contracture
- Kaposi's sarcoma
- Psoriasis
- Acanthosis nigricans
- Werner's syndrome
- Hemochromatosis
- Lipid proteinosis
- Porphyria
- Glucagonoma syndrome

D. Other Possible Involvements of the Skin in Diabetes
- Reactive perforating collagenosis (RPC)
- Limited joint mobility

overt diabetes. Others[26] have reported that in nearly 1 of 5 cases in the literature, the cutaneous lesions appeared 1 to 5 years before the symptoms of diabetes became obvious.

As described by most authors, the lesion of necrobiosis lipoidica (Plate V B, C, and D) is so distinct clinically that when fully developed, it is difficult either to ignore it or to mistake it for another condition.[27,28] In spite of this, it is frequently missed because (a) it may appear atypical or (b) it may be in one of several stages of development. In general, the earliest lesions are slightly elevated shiny papules 1 to 3 mm in diameter, with fairly sharply outlined borders. They may show a slight scaling or may be moderately erythematous. They do not disappear under pressure. Later they become round, oval, or irregularly shaped plaques with well-defined borders, a firm consistency, and a glistening surface which appears like tightly stretched cellophane. Sometimes wrinkling gives the lesion an atrophic appearance. Still later there may be a circular area of depression with further atrophy and ulceration. The surface may appear as if varnished, may be mottled yellow and traversed by fine blood vessels. At other times it is red to a deep purple and may be so dark-colored that it resembles an area of gangrene. Telangiectasia may be fairly prominent and sometimes there are two zones; a central portion which appears to be healing gradually, and a peripheral one having an "angrier" color.

Necrobiosis is found 3 or 4 times more frequently in the female than in the male,[28] although in one Joslin Clinic series of 37 patients with onset of diabetes at the age of 15 or under, the distribution between the sexes was approximately equal. A more recent study showed 56 females and 24 males in a series of 80. The lesions may be single or multiple and while they may be found on the thighs, arms, hands, abdomen, or back, they appear most frequently on the anterior part of the lower legs, shins, and dorsal part of the foot. Although NLD confined to the face and scalp is rare, this has been reported, and the difficulties of diagnosis are apparent.[29,30] It has also been reported in surgical scars.[31] Since NLD seems to be more prevalent in females, modern dress with significant limb exposure frequently adds up to a situation of cosmetic disaster. While asymptomatic, it is often traumatic to the psyche of the victim. The condition may gradually fade and improve or remain stationary for many years. The greatest danger is that of secondary infection which is aggravated by lack of good surface circulation. The ultimate result can be shallow ulcerations with thin layers of scar tissue that are difficult to conceal. Frequently lesions appear symmetrically on the two legs.

Histologically[32] the lesions show necrobiotic rather than true necrotic changes in the collagen fibers of the connective tissue. Noticeable are foam cells and lipid and vascular changes with perivascular inflammatory infiltrates. Obliterative lesions in the small blood vessels surrounding this infiltrate account for the necrobiotic changes. Lipids are present chiefly in the center of the lesions. Quantitative studies show phospholipids and free cholesterol in these lesions.

Muller and Winkelmann[33] used the cortisone-primed glucose tolerance test to appraise insulin reserves and evaluate the relationship of NLD to diabetes. They reexamined 19 patients who had NLD but who did not have diabetes during previous examinations. Standard glucose tolerance tests gave abnormal results in three of these patients including one who was taking hydrochlorothiazide. Cortisone-primed glucose tolerance tests gave abnormal results in 5 of the remaining 16 patients, and 6 of the 11 without evidence of carbohydrate intolerance had family histories of diabetes. These results confirm the close relationship between the skin and systemic conditions and suggest a relationship to the prediabetic state as well. It is thought that diabetes will eventually develop in the remainder of the patients if they are observed long enough. There is a good deal of debate about the relationship between severity of diabetes and this skin lesion. Halprin[34] believed that diabetes in persons with NLD is usually earlier in onset and more severe than in the general population. Others feel that this lesion bears no relationship to an abnormality of carbohydrate metabolism.[35]

This type of debate indicates progress and increased interest as well as knowledge. Once it was believed that diabetes occurred only with the onset of overt polyuria, polydipsia, and polyphagia. On this basis, arguments that NLD may exist with apparently normal carbohydrate tolerance might have been untenable.[36] If indeed necrobiosis lipoidica is a cutaneous manifestation of microangiopathy,[37] then the conclusion is not necessarily valid that there is no relationship between microangiopathic lesions and carbohydrate abnormality, but rather that, in our present state of knowledge, we are unable to provide sufficiently sensitive indices of intermediate carbohydrate metabolism and its relationship to early vascular disease.

In a fairly large series[38] studied over 4 years, it was found that of 20 patients with NLD, two-thirds had a disturbance of carbohydrate metabolism, and 75% had lipoproteinemia. In another series,[33] the average duration of skin lesions in previously unrecognized diabetes was 10.4 years. There is disagreement as to whether necrobiosis lipoidica is truly a microangiopathic condition, although Sodemann et al.[39] believe that this may be a prerequisite for NLD. The presence of PAS-positive material in the damaged vessels is frequently cited[40] as evidence of such microangiopathy. Although the etiologic basis of diabetic microangiopathy is not clear, the theory has been advanced that the condition is due to increased production of glycoproteins which are deposited within and about the basement membrane of the vessels. Some diabetic patients with NLD have shown this finding.[40,41] Engel and Smith[42] identified by immunologic methods the presence of a protein common to the serum of diabetic patients with vascular lesions and non-

diabetics with necrobiosis lipoidica. Marckwort and Schydlo[43] reported NLD in a 16-year-old diabetic but they could find no involvement of blood vessels.

Apparently the skin lesion of NLD has not been identified in black persons until recently. Whether its predominance in the white population is a valid finding or whether identification of early lesions is difficult in darker-skinned subjects, is a matter of conjecture.[44]

Treatment. There is no specific treatment for NLD and no adequate data to suggest that treatment of diabetes per se will ameliorate this condition. However, uncontrolled diabetes may present hazards of secondary infection or ulceration, even in those who do not have limited circulation.[27] Intradermal steroid injections have been used for treatment of early lesions. Savitt[45] reported a favorable response to cortisone ointment and to injections of hydrocortisone into the lesions. Madison[46] observed ketonuria without glycosuria in 4 diabetics receiving this type of treatment. Apparently ulceration may follow the injection of the lesions. Injection of depo-steroids has been suggested.[28]

Surgical removal of the areas followed by skin grafts has been used from time to time, although necrobiosis lipoidica has recurred in the graft or at its borders.[47] Dubin and Kaplan[48] reported 7 cases of NLD treated surgically at Stanford University Medical Center. No recurrences were noted following surgical excision of the lesions down to the deep fascia, ligation of the associated perforating blood vessels and use of split-skin grafts to cover the defects. Another report[49] documented excellent results from excision and skin grafting which were normal after 24 months. Thus, the varieties of treatment offered intimate that there is nothing specific for this condition except diagnosis (which, by its definiteness, may give some measure of reassurance to the patient), covering the obvious lesions as much as possible for cosmetic reasons, and above all, prevention of trauma with its subsequent problems of infection and ulceration. For active lesions and those which are secondarily infected, bed rest, antibiotics and meticulous wound hygiene are indicated. The chronicity and occasional spontaneous remission of NLD create difficulty in evaluation of various treatment modalities. In isolated cases, favorable response has been observed after treatment with fibrinolytic agents and antiplatelet aggregating drugs.[50,51] Publication of this was followed by a spate of reports from others,[52] claiming success with the same treatment. The theory was that dipyridamole (Persantine) is a potent vasodilator and has an effect on blood platelets. It was thought that the effect of proliferation of blood vessels was an important factor. However, as with all those who have treated NLD, the authors refused to call these results specific for NLD because permanent cure is hard to ascertain with this disorder. In a single case report, the combination of aspirin and dipyridamole produced marked improvement in skin lesions.

Diabetic Dermopathy (Brown Spots, Shin Spots)

Melin[53] called attention to small, round, brownish, atrophic and circumscribed lesions on the skin of the lower extremities of diabetics. These appear isolated or in groups and sometimes show a linear pattern. They vary in number and usually are bilateral, although there is no symmetry in their distribution. They are not painful and do not ulcerate. Patients often assume them to be the result of trauma comparable to the small scars seen on the anterior tibial area of sailors who frequently bruise their shins, going up and down metal ladders. However, in many instances, a history of trauma cannot be obtained. Melin studied 277 diabetics over the age of 15 years and found these lesions in 65% of the males and 29% of the females. In 104 nondiabetic patients, only 7 had this lesion, and in 6 of these, glucose tolerance tests gave abnormal findings. Microscopically there was atrophy of the epidermis and sometimes fibrosis of the dermis. PAS-positive vascular changes in the capillaries of the superficial skin were found. In this series there was increased frequency of the lesions with increased duration of diabetes and the lesions were more prevalent in patients with retinopathy and peripheral vascular disease.

Murphy[54] examined 200 consecutive patients in a diabetic service at the Lahey Clinic, all of whom were over 50 years old. Among the 148 proven diabetics, these atrophic spots were found in 20 patients. No lesions were detected in the nondiabetic group. All patients with skin lesions also had retinopathy or neuropathy. There was no correlation between the atrophic spots and known duration of diabetes. Binkley[21] called these lesions "dermopathy" and suggested that the small blood vessel lesions are the same as those in NLD, but at a much earlier stage and with much less severity of the collagen changes. However, on inspection, there seems to be no surface relationship between the two conditions.

These primary skin lesions as described by Binkley are usually 5 to 12 mm in diameter, round or oval, discrete, flat, dull-red papules, often arranged in linear fashion on the arms and legs. They may have central crusting with inflammation, infiltration, and sometimes vesiculation. Later, atrophy, fibrosis, and small shallow scars appear. Some of the older lesions develop brownish hyperpigmentation near the central involved areas. In the series of Binkley and associates,[55] 16 of 27 males had dermopathy, although only one of 10 diabetic females was found to have these skin lesions. Because of the pretibial site of the lesion, trauma to vulnerable skin seems a logical cause and has often been suspected. However, patients usually deny injuries and Binkley reported that no such lesions occurred in a group of diabetics who were struck repeatedly with a hard rubber mallet.

Danowski and co-workers[56] referred to these lesions as "shin spots" and confirmed the impression that they were found predominantly in diabetics, the likelihood increasing with duration of the diabetes, and the incidence in males higher than in females. Murphy[54] referred to the "spotted leg syndrome," but warned that the diagnosis is not always easy to make clinically because of the atypical forms that may appear. Tornblom[57] expressed concern about the possible relationship to purpura and further results of circulatory deficiency. No specific treatment is indicated.

Lipodystrophy

Since it is nearly always related to the administration of insulin, lipodystrophy must be regarded as a skin condition typically found in diabetes. It can assume either of two forms: (1) hypertrophy of subcutaneous fatty tissue leading to the appearance of muscular hyperdevelopment, or (2) atrophy in which the subcutaneous fatty tissue disappears, leaving areas that seem to be gouged out. Generally patients are more disturbed by atrophies than by hypertrophies. While hypertrophy may sometimes be mistaken for excellent muscular development, atrophy is usually disfiguring and unflattering. Patients often worry needlessly that the atrophy involves loss of muscle tissue, and that it will continue indefinitely (For additional information, see Chapters 19 and 24).

Hypertrophies appear as soft swellings, usually in areas of insulin administration, as in the upper arms, thighs, abdomen, and buttocks. Atrophies, although usually at or near sites of insulin injection, have occasionally been reported to be found remote from the usual sites, i.e., on the face, neck, and breast. The combination of atrophy and hypertrophy may become evident in the same individual, either concurrently or in succession. Sometimes an area of atrophy is surrounded by one of hypertrophy.

The term "lipodystrophy" as used here should not be confused with the classical lipoatrophic diabetes described by Lawrence[58] in 1946. The latter is a generalized condition, in which there is complete absence of subcutaneous, intra-abdominal and perinephric fat, in an insulin-resistant diabetic who has little if any ability to develop ketosis even when insulin administration is omitted. See Chapter 41 and Plate V, E and F).

As an indication of the importance of insulin lipodystrophy in the past, one may cite a 1957 survey[59] of 1096 consecutive diabetic patients of all ages who had taken insulin for 1 year or longer. It was found that 24% had atrophies of some degree. However, among the 342 patients in the series who were under the age of 20 years, atrophies occurred in 44% as contrasted with only 15% in the patients 20 years of age or older. In patients under 20, atrophies were slightly more common in females than in males, while in those 20 years of age and over, the incidence among females was about 7 times as great as that in males. This sex difference may be due to the larger layer of subcutaneous fat in adult females than in adult males. Atrophy gives the appearance of subcutaneous fat having actually melted away, and has been described as a "sharply defined disappearance of the subcutaneous fat without exudative reaction and appreciable fibrosis."[60] Hypertrophy, on the other hand, consists of a mass of scar and fatty tissue beneath the skin. The skin over the mass frequently has considerable loss of sensation, and lipodystrophy has been considered as one possible cause of instability in diabetics. This type of tissue may influence the absorption of insulin after its injection.[61]

Etiologic Factors. Early studies[60] demonstrated that adipose tissue changes were not related to any of the following: preservatives (such as tricresol) in insulin; the presence of a lipase in exogenous insulin; inflammatory processes; the mechanical trauma of injection; or traces of alcohol which might have been left in the syringe before it was loaded with insulin. Studies at the Joslin Clinic[60,62] have shown that: (1) in insulin atrophies, the type of tissue which disappears is neutral fat; (2) the abnormal process consists almost exclusively of fat disappearance with little if any evidence of inflammatory reaction; (3) insulin atrophies or hypertrophies, despite purer insulins, may occur in a small percentage of individuals; (4) insulin pH is not an important factor since atrophies may follow the use of insulin regardless of its neutrality or acidity. (5) It was thought formerly that the change in subcutaneous fat was due to a local metabolic effect of insulin; the studies of Renold, Marble, and Fawcett[63] indicated that hypertrophy of fat was the only adipose tissue change following daily injections of insulin into the groin fat pads of female rats.

Atrophy of fat has been reported after injection of substances other than insulin, such as narcot-

ics.[64] This would suggest that atrophy might be due to mechanical trauma, but histologic studies of tissues in the narcotics cases show inflammatory changes which are not present in insulin atrophy. It has been suggested that patients treated with protamine zinc insulin have a higher incidence of these conditions than those treated with other insulins because of the substances added to slow down the rate of insulin absorption[65] but this impression has not been confirmed.

At the present time a commonly held view is that lipoatrophy is due to a local response, probably of allergic nature, to the impurities present in commercial insulin up until the advent of "single peak" and "single component" insulin. The type of insulin, whether bovine or porcine, may also play a role in such allergies. Now that biosynthetic and semisynthetic human insulins are available, it will be of great interest over the next few years to learn how their use will compare with purified pork insulin in the prevention and treatment of lipodystrophies.

Treatment. There are certain measures which can and should be taken both in prevention and treatment of lipodystrophy.

1. If lipodystrophy is already present, the patient or parents of young patients should be reassured. No one has ever run out of sites for insulin injections. It can be safely said that the course of the lipodystrophies is benign, especially in children, and that in many patients, there will be slow restoration of subcutaneous fat in atrophies if the involved sites are avoided completely in future injections. However, the time required may be very long, perhaps 2 years or more.

2. Insulin injections may be made in the lower layers of subcutaneous fat or even intramuscularly, but not in the superficial layers of subcutaneous fat.

3. The site of injection should be shifted regularly so that no one area 3 cm in diameter receives insulin oftener than once every 3 or 4 weeks. This is receiving less emphasis than formerly because the widespread availability of purer insulins lessens the likelihood of lipodystrophy. However, it is still good practice to shift injection sites until definitive evidence proves it unnecessary.

4. Patients who develop atrophies despite using purified porcine or human insulin, may wish, for cosmetic reasons, to avoid injecting the arms and legs, but rather use parts of the body which are not as frequently exposed to public view. The skin over the abdominal wall, flanks, and buttocks affords excellent sites for injections. Furthermore, loss of fat from these areas often may be welcome.

5. Because of the unconfirmed impression that insulin atrophy may be produced if cold insulin is

injected directly from a refrigerated vial,[66] in the past patients have been told that they may keep the vial of insulin currently in use at room temperature while storing in a refrigerator any reserve supply. This is still reasonable because it is more comfortable to inject insulin kept at the warmer temperature.

6. As early as 1949, Collens and associates[67] suggested that repeated injections of insulin directly into areas of atrophy may result in gradual restoration of lost fat. However, patients or responsible parents are understandably loath to use these sites. In 1971, Watson and Calder[68] repopularized the concept of filling in the atrophic sites when insulin was injected directly into the affected areas in 7 patients. Neutral insulin (Actrapid) and biphasic (Rapitard) insulin were used, and marked improvement of the atrophy occurred. Later, Watson and Vines[69] reported that insulin lipodystrophy prevalence varied with the types of insulin used, with less atrophy occurring in patients using biphasic rather than zinc insulin. Wentworth and associates[70] reported improvement in 88% of 166 patients treated by direct intralesional injection with purified insulins. The authors have also noted improvement with insulin injection at the margins of the atrophic area. The administration of insulin directly into the gouged-out area presumably takes advantage of the hypertrophic effect of insulin. Through 1974, Teuscher[71] noted no lipoatrophy had yet been reported using monocomponent insulins. Asherov et al.[72] reported widespread lipoatrophy in a 19-year-old who had been using bovine insulin. Deep intramuscular injection into the atrophic site with pork insulin caused the atrophy to disappear. Wright et al.[73] observed 511 patients and found cutaneous or subcutaneous abnormalities in 49 of these who had been treated with bovine insulin but no lesions in the group treated during that period with porcine insulin. Maaz[74] reported essentially the same results and concluded that the atrophy was probably due to an antigen-antibody reaction to less purified insulins.

As this complication of insulin treatment is most common in girls and boys under 20 years of age, it may be advisable to treat young diabetics with monocomponent porcine insulin of high purity or with human insulin. Hulst[75] concluded that both the highly purified monocomponent and less purified insulins were suitable for treating insulin-induced lipoatrophy when insulin is injected into the lipoatrophic area.

Whitley et al.[76] reported a remarkable return of fatty tissue by means of subcutaneous injection of dexamethasone-insulin mixture into the atrophic areas in 1 patient. Similar results were noted by Kumar and associates[77] in 6 of 9 patients so treated.

Insulin Allergy

Since insulin is essentially a complex group of 51 diverse amino acids, there are occasions when it may produce a generalized allergic response with not only systemic, but also cutaneous manifestations, usually urticaria. More frequently, there may be localized burning in an area of induration or in an area of erythema and swelling. This is common during the first few weeks of insulin administration in a new patient.

In addition to treatment with antihistamines, changing to an insulin of different animal origin often is helpful, and shifting to human insulin should be the most valuable technique, although instances have been reported of allergy to both semisynthetic[77a] and biosynthetic human insulin.[77b] On rare occasions, it may be necessary to desensitize the patient to insulin (see Chapter 19).

Skin Reactions to Oral Hypoglycemic Agents

Skin manifestations as side effects of oral hypoglycemic agents are discussed in Chapter 21. However, they are mentioned here since the maculopapular eruptions on the arms and legs or even a generalized urticaria might be misinterpreted.

Idiopathic Bullae in Diabetics (Bullosis Diabeticorum)

This lesion is found predominantly on the feet and hands. Some years ago Rocca and Pereyra[78] reported fourteen diabetic patients with rapidly developing bullous lesions of the feet. Most of the patients had long-standing diabetes with neuropathy, and the lesions apparently had developed without trauma. The asymptomatic blisters develop rapidly on the fingers and toes and can be recurrent over a period of years. The multiple tense bullae grossly resemble burns, although erythema is absent at the periphery of the lesions. The lesions heal slowly without scarring unless secondarily infected.

Histologic findings are described in the report of Cantwell and Martz.[79] Microscopic sections showed variably sized intra-epidermal vesicles and mild inflammation of the dermis. The roofs of large vesicles were composed of loose hyperkeratotic cells of stratum corneum. No parakeratosis was noted. The vesicles were filled with amorphous, pale eosinophilic material which contained an occasional degenerated leukocyte. The dermal infiltrate was mild and contained a rare neutrophil and lymphocyte. In the upper dermis, some thickening of blood vessel walls was noted. Gram stain of vesicular fluid was negative.

To speed healing, the larger bullae can be incised and drained and topical antibiotic creams applied.

Healing occurs within several weeks without scarring. The pathophysiology for development of the bullae is not known. Possibly a biochemical substance (chemical vesicant) related to the diabetes is responsible.

SKIN CONDITIONS FOUND FREQUENTLY IN PATIENTS WITH DIABETES

Infections

It is possible that while the onset of infections takes place in diabetics under the same circumstances as in nondiabetics, once established, the infections may advance more rapidly in diabetics. On the other hand, the diabetic has more opportunities for infection because of daily insulin injections, although considering the number of diabetics treated with insulin, the episodes of infection are relatively rare. Once an infection occurs, the question of cause and effect is of only academic interest. A vicious cycle begins with infections interfering with the control of diabetes while the loss of control contributes to persistence of infection and delayed healing. There is no question that patients with poorly controlled diabetes have always had a higher incidence of furuncles than nondiabetics. Prior to insulin therapy and before the advent of antibiotics, carbuncles were a common cause of death among diabetics. Indeed, in the absence of appropriate therapy, it could be a short step from a facial infection, for example, to a furuncle, cellulitis or carbuncle (see Chapter 36).

Bacterial Infections. Bacterial infections of the skin, while still a threat, are now much less common in diabetic patients than when antibiotic therapy was not available. Branom and colleagues[80] reported the occurrence of a severe and uncommon type of skin infection, chancriform pyoderma, in a diabetic. Tuazon et al.[81] reported that in patients with Type I diabetes, the frequency of staphylococcal carriers was more than three times that in normal persons and in those with Type II diabetes.

Although common acne is not limited to diabetics, infections stemming from it may blossom into larger infections and cellulitis even more rapidly than for nondiabetics. A description is scarcely necessary, but warning against spreading infection *is* necessary. Obviously hygienic measures are needed, and the warning not to squeeze or pick these maculopapules is particularly pertinent for those with diabetes. There are four general types: comedones, papules, pustules, and cysts. In addition to the need for cleanliness, there are recent medications that seem helpful, although controlled studies are rare and there is a high incidence of spontaneous remission. Topical treatments include preparations such as Pernox and Fostex, but these entail the hazard of contact sensitization. Some dermatologists recommend ultra-violet light; others recommend vitamin A (retinoic acid preparations). Tetracyclines are useless as lotions but have sometimes been used orally with some success. The number of treatment regimens means that no one is ideal and many dermatologists believe that frequent cleansing of the skin is the most beneficial.

Furuncles and carbuncles should always be regarded as grave infections and in the supposedly nondiabetic, should be a reason for performance of a postprandial blood glucose test to rule out the possibility of diabetes. In diabetics, these infections are dangerous, especially since they may alter the insulin requirement and may be a precipitating factor in acidosis. Muller[35] has pointed out that the severity of infections in diabetics may be worsened by reduction of circulation by arteriosclerosis and degeneration of the nerves to the skin. Hence, an infection in an extremity in the presence of poor circulation or in a site affected by neuropathy can become hazardous. (See Plate VI A.) Prevention of infection by good hygiene and control of diabetes is obviously "worth a pound of cure." Simple measures such as bathing with germicidal soap and regular cleansing are essential. However, once infection has been identified, early treatment with an appropriate antibiotic is imperative.

Dermatophytosis

The usually innocuous epidermophytosis (athlete's foot), simply an annoyance in most people, can in the diabetic lead to serious infection which may result in foot loss. In diabetics, foot hygiene and general foot care must be meticulous.[82] Behrman and Levin[83] found dermatophytosis of the feet to be the most common skin lesion in diabetic patients, and found this more prevalent in diabetic than in nondiabetic persons. Years ago Greenwood[84] in a study of 500 diabetics, found that 198 (40%) had epidermophytosis of the feet. Of this group, one-half of those over 20 years of age had this infection. In diabetics, the open fissures in the depths of the interdigital spaces or on the plantar surfaces of the toes, areas which are usually warm, moist, and well hidden, are sites for severe lesions which may require surgical intervention. In epidermophytosis, cultures from the interdigital spaces will usually yield staphylococci that are secondary to the original infection; these organisms aid in breaking the defensive integument, and the simple "athlete's foot" sometimes becomes cellulitis and then osteomyelitis. (See Chapters 34 and 35.) (See Plate VI B.)

The earlier stages are marked simply by pruritus, erythema, scaling, and maceration between the toes. In the acute form, vesicles and pustules are present. Although the feet are the most common site of infection (tinea pedis), other regions such as the hands and the groin may also be infected.

Below are given measures for prevention and treatment of dermatophytosis. All of them may not be necessary in any individual case, but one or more may be useful.

1. Frequent washing and drying of the feet; not walking with bare feet, particularly on floors where the fungus is readily found, such as gymnasiums, showers, swimming pools, etc.

2. Some of the measures outlined by Muller[35] to prevent undue sweating. These should include, when possible, well-ventilated shoes or sandals rather than rubber-soled shoes, cotton rather than nylon or silk hose, a wisp of lamb's wool between the toes, and the use of talcum powder.

3. Meticulous care of corns, calluses, and nails with pedicure or care by a capable podiatrist.

4. Use of some of the excellent proprietary and prescription medications now available. These include undecylenic acid (Desenex) and tolnaftate (Tinactin). Newer excellent fungicides include clotrimazole (Lotrimin), haloprigin (Halotex), and miconazole (Micatin), which are available either in cream or liquid form.

5. In acute infections of the feet, soaking the feet in a dilute solution of aluminum diacetate or potassium permanganate at room temperature as directed by a physician.

For more severe fungal infections of the skin, hair and nails, griseofulvin (Grisactin or Fulvicin) has proved of value. The use of this drug is not justified in minor infections which will respond to topical agents alone because of the prolonged treatment period required for successful use and also the occasional hypersensitivity to these preparations. When this medication is employed, its use should be continued for 4 to 6 weeks, and if fingernails or toenails are involved, the medication must be given for at least six months. The recommended daily dose is between 0.5 and 1.0 g. Concomitant use of topical agents is usually required, particularly in treatment of tinea pedis. Griseofulvin will not eradicate monilial or bacterial infection. During treatment with griseofulvin the white blood count should be monitored; if granulocytopenia occurs, the drug should be discontinued.

Moniliasis

While normally an inhabitant of the skin and mucous membranes and ordinarily of low pathogenicity, *Candida albicans* is a common yeast skin infection in persons with diabetes mellitus. It is usually manifested by marked erythema and edema affecting the genitalia, perianal region, or medial portions of the thighs as well as the intertriginous areas below the breasts, in the axillae, and between the fingers. Vulvovaginitis due to Candida occurs in about half of diabetic women and is a frequent cause of pruritus.[81] Often small superficial pustules are present at the margins of the involved area, and the area itself is frequently excoriated. The presence of a vaginal "cottage cheese" type of discharge or of a small, white, curd-like series of yeast colonies on the labia minora is of diagnostic value. In rarer instances, thrush may also be present. Candida may also be responsible for balanitis in the male as well as for secondarily infected paronychia.

Mehnert and Mehnert[85] examined urine specimens from 200 diabetic and 100 nondiabetic patients to determine the incidence of yeasts potentially pathogenic for man. They found that the urine of 34.7% of the 150 diabetics with glycosuria contained yeasts as contrasted with only 8% of the 50 diabetics who were aglycosuric. Yeasts were present in the urine of about 10% of the nondiabetics. It would therefore appear that sugar in the urine rather than diabetes per se made the difference. The yeasts isolated were all species of Candida and chiefly of the albicans type. In both diabetics and nondiabetics, the yeasts were found more commonly in female than in male patients. Sonck and Somersalo[86] studied the yeast flora of the anogenital region in 160 diabetic girls, in 92 of whom studies were carried out periodically for several months. C. albicans was found in 69 of 70 patients with clinical signs of vulvitis and there was good correlation between the presence of yeast and clinical symptoms. In 11 patients, C. albicans was found without vulvitis. In 27, other yeasts were present simultaneously or alternating with C. albicans.

The spread of C. albicans may be due to antibiotic or corticosteroid therapy, the glycosuria of diabetes, obesity, alcoholism, the use of oral contraceptives, vascular stasis with poor circulation, hyperhydrosis, and vitamin B deficiency. While moniliasis may be the initial sign of previously undetected diabetes mellitus, it is common in persons with known but poorly-controlled diabetes.

It is more accurate to identify C. albicans by culture than by direct examination of smears. If smears are used, they should be made with scrapings of the floor of pustules or of sloughing areas rather than from swabs alone.[47] If discharge is present, microscopic examination of the exudate is helpful and a fragment of the curd-like material mixed with a few drops of 10% sodium hydroxide solution and stained with ink will show branching pseudomycelia with tiny buds of conidia attached.[87] (See Plate VI C.)

Strict control of diabetes is a necessity both in

the prevention and treatment of moniliasis. Nystatin (Mycostatin) is a specific and effective drug for local therapy. Vaginal tablets with 100,000 units of the substance inserted twice daily, are indicated for vaginal infections, while nystatin ointment or cream may be applied topically to infected surface areas. Another cream, Mycolog, containing nystatin, neomycin, gramicidin, and triamcinolone, has been used with success. In acute, edematous, painful, local inflammations, compresses of aluminum subacetate or diluted vinegar (1 quart of tap water for ½ tablespoonful of white vinegar) applied locally, can relieve the discomfort and clear the skin. For local treatment of vulvovaginal moniliasis (candidiasis), preparations such as miconazole (Monistat) vaginal cream, clotrimazole (Gyne-Lotrimin) vaginal tablets and candicidin (Vanobid) vaginal ointment and tablets have been helpful. Topical forms of amphotericin B (Fungizone) are effective in treatment of cutaneous and mucocutaneous mycotic infections caused by monilial species.

While C. albicans is chiefly a cutaneous and mucous membrane infection, it can involve the gastrointestinal tract, bronchopulmonary system, and other viscera as well. Swartz[88] reiterates the importance of correct diagnosis before treatment is undertaken, and observes that the dermatologist has frequently been called upon to undo the damage caused by the use of strong, irritating local applications prescribed for a nonexistent infection.

The Xanthomas

The xanthomas are a manifestation of tissue lipid deposition in the skin and sometimes in tendons. Histologically they contain giant cells and "foam cells" which are phagocytes loaded with lipid droplets. Generally a connective tissue reaction with fibroblastic proliferation is found surrounding the foam cells. There are four clinical varieties of xanthomas: planus, tuberous, eruptive, and tendinous. The lesions can occur in normolipemic individuals with proliferative disorders of the histiocytes (juvenile xanthogranuloma, xanthoma disseminatum); in patients with hereditary hyperlipoproteinemia (five types according to Fredrickson et al.[89]), and in association with conditions causing secondary hyperlipoproteinemia (biliary cirrhosis, hypothyroidism, nephrosis, von Gierke's disease, pancreatitis, dysglobulinemia, and diabetes mellitus). In diabetics, the development of xanthomas usually indicates poor control of the diabetic state. Patients with poorly-controlled diabetes may exhibit several degrees of secondary hyperlipoproteinemia, usually of the endogenous type, manifested by increases in pre-beta-lipoproteins which cause moderate elevations of choles-

terol and marked triglyceridemia. Occasionally chylomicra are elevated together with the increase in pre-beta-lipoproteins.[90]

Tuberous xanthomas are mildly annoying, but occasionally massive disfiguring lesions are seen, such as those reported by Thomas,[91] which occurred on the knees, elbows, shoulders, buttocks, chest, and face of an untreated diabetic patient with a serum cholesterol of 1000 mg/dl. Eventually the xanthomas disappeared but left keloid scars on this dark-skinned patient.

More commonly, diabetic patients with severe hyperlipoproteinemia develop eruptive xanthomas. These were formerly known as xanthoma diabeticorum, but they may appear in patients having any condition associated with severe hypertriglyceridemia. Characteristically, they are firm, bright red papules, mottled with a deep rose tint, usually appearing on the buttocks and the extremities, particularly on the lateral and dorsal parts of the forearms and about the elbows and knees. An inflammatory halo around the papules is an important diagnostic sign. The lesions may range in size from tiny to as large as 5 mm in diameter. In diabetics they usually disappear when the diabetes is brought under control, although sometimes atrophy and pigmentation remain. Since eruptive xanthomas are a manifestation of severe hypertriglyceridemia, which causes a turbid to milky plasma, concomitant lipemia retinalis may be seen. These lesions may be found in acute states as described by Choutet et al.[92] who described them as a possible manifestation of the ketoacidotic state. It has also been reported that the Köbner phenomenon can be manifested with eruptive xanthoma.[91] This describes the spontaneous eruption in a new location of a rash present elsewhere on the body. This may be brought about by non-specific trauma. While more common in other conditions, it is apparently a rare possibility with the eruptive form of xanthoma. (See Plate VI D, E.)

Xanthelasma. When involving the eyelids, xanthoma planum is called xanthelasma palpebrarum. This is the most common type of xanthoma and begins as one or more pinhead-sized yellow-orange spots covered by normal epidermis. After many months, these spots coalesce and become thicker, eventually forming irregular plaques that may cover almost the entire skin of the lids. The plaques begin near the inner canthus and, as they progress, assume a horseshoe shape. They are usually permanent, progressive, and multiple. The lesions are benign, occurring in nondiabetic as well as diabetic persons. Hypercholesterolemia or hypertriglyceridemia may be found, but there is no relationship between the degree of elevation of serum lipids or the quality of diabetic control and the evolution of these xanthomas. Surgical removal of the lesions is advised only for cosmetic purposes when they become disfiguring.

Xanthochromia. This is a yellowish discoloration of the skin sometimes seen in diabetic patients; it is usually accompanied by an increase in the carotene and cholesterol in the blood. The pigment tends to accumulate in the stratum corneum and becomes particularly noticeable on the palms, soles, and nasolabial folds. It is caused by impairment of the patient's ability to convert carotene to vitamin A in the liver. The carotene is a lipochrome found in large amounts in green and yellow vegetables, egg yolk, and butter. This condition is not confined to diabetics and in one series of cases[93] was found in 9% of 22 patients with renal disease and in 3% of 23 other hospital patients selected at random who did not have diabetes. Treatment consists in restriction of the carotene-rich foods and control of the diabetic condition. Treatment of this disorder has been attempted with clofibrate[94] but the results were not considered satisfactory. Reassurance again is important because, except for the cosmetic effect, xanthochromia is not harmful and causes no symptoms.

SKIN CONDITIONS FOUND COINCIDENTALLY WITH DIABETES

Pruritus

Pruritus occurs so commonly in many diabetics, particularly at the onset of the disease, that it is considered to be one of the cardinal symptoms. However, pruritus of the skin in general is such a non-specific symptom caused by so many conditions, including lymphoma, malignant disease, and other states, that in the truest sense it cannot be considered to be pathognomonic of diabetes. Pruritus pudendi, especially in women, is by far the commonest type in the uncontrolled diabetic and usually subsides after the disappearance of glycosuria unless there is an associated monilial infection. The occurrence of genital pruritus is not easily explained since local application of glucose to the mucous membranes or the skin per se does not lead to itching.[95] Treatment for pruritus is that of the diabetes and the associated dermatosis, when present. Non-specific measures such as strict hygiene, steroid creams, and hydrophilic creams and lotions can be useful. In severe pruritus, cyproheptadine hydrochloride in dosage of 4 mg 3 or 4 times daily, may have a beneficial effect and provide relief.

Dupuytren's Contracture

Dupuytren's contracture (a contraction of the palmar fascia) is included here only because, in its initial stages, it may appear to be a skin condition. It does not seem to be related to diabetes, but its frequency has been variously estimated as from 12 to 32% in diabetics and as only 6% in nondiabetics. The Joslin Clinic experience seems to substantiate this impression. Schneider[96] found that 120 of 381 diabetic patients, whose average age was 61 years, had Dupuytren's contracture. He regards the condition as reversible. Although surgical treatment can be employed when annoying or handicapping contractures of the fingers occur, this is usually not necessary. Spring and Cohen[97] examined 233 consecutive diabetics for changes in the palmar fascia. The group ranged from 30 to 90 years of age, and the overall incidence was 20.6% (49 cases). No correlation was found with any of the facets of the diabetic state, but it was noted that the incidence of this disorder increased progressively with age. Spring and Cohen felt that the condition should suggest the possibility of diabetes (see also Chapter 42).

Kaposi's Sarcoma

The increased association of Kaposi's sarcoma and diabetes has been reported by Hurlbut and Lincoln.[98] Six of their 13 patients had diabetes. Other isolated instances of this association have been reported.[81]

Psoriasis

There has been much controversy as to whether psoriasis and diabetes are really related. Some studies[99] show no relationship; others[100] indicate that the prevalence of diabetes among individuals with psoriasis is 5 times higher than the estimated prevalence in the general population in the United States. Reeds and colleagues[101] found diabetes in 25% of 103 consecutive patients with psoriasis, and family histories in this group showed frequent occurrence of diabetes and psoriasis in relatives. Even more significant was a report from Umbira, Italy,[102] where a group of 200 patients with psoriasis were found to have a statistically significant occurrence of diabetes. Other observations were made in a series of 600 patients in whom the correlation between the two conditions was noted. Here the predominating prevalence was in males under the age of 50.

Acanthosis Nigricans

This is a symmetrical, pigmented, verrucous lesion occurring in the skin folds. In the adult, it is often associated with internal malignant disease. The benign types have been noted in association with endocrine diseases, including pituitary adenoma, Stein-Leventhal syndrome, Addison's disease, Cushing's disease, acromegaly, and lipo-atrophic diabetes as well as diabetes mellitus. Two families with congenital acanthosis nigricans and diabetes have been reported. Patients with this cutaneous disorder should be checked for diabetes.[103]

Kahn and associates[104] have reported two types of insulin-resistant diabetes associated with acanthosis nigricans. In 6 patients with acanthosis nigricans, variable degrees of glucose intolerance, elevated insulin levels and marked resistance to exogenous insulin were found. The insulin resistance was thought to be due to a marked decrease in insulin binding to its membrane receptors. Two unique clinical syndromes were noted: Type A, a syndrome in younger females with signs of accelerated growth or virilization, in whom the receptor defect may be primary, and Type B, seen in older females with signs of an immunologic disease, in whom circulating antibodies to the insulin receptor were found.

Werner's Syndrome

This is a rare disease which appears in adult life and is characterized by features resembling premature aging. Patients exhibit short stature, premature graying of the hair, alopecia, cataracts, skin atrophy, hyperkeratosis, and a sharpening of the nose giving the individual a birdlike appearance. Its description is included here only because it is said that two-thirds of its subjects have a peculiarly mild diabetes characterized by a relative insensitivity to insulin and an absence of ketosis. In the classic review of Epstein and associates,[105] it was stated that diabetes was recognized in 55 of 125 persons with Werner's syndrome reported in the literature. Glucose tolerance and tolbutamide response tests with simultaneous determinations of immunoassayable insulin showed responses characteristic of adult-type stable diabetes, and it was suggested that in persons with Werner's syndrome, a predisposition to develop the adult type of diabetes may be inherited in an autosomal recessive manner (for additional details, see Chapter 24).

Hemochromatosis

While hemochromatosis is discussed in Chapter 37, it is mentioned here because of the slate-gray pigmentation of the skin, associated with it, particularly in areas that are exposed to light. Microscopic examination shows the deposition of hemosiderin around blood vessels and hair follicles.

Lipid Proteinosis

Lipid proteinosis is an extremely rare, hereditary metabolic disturbance characterized by a deposition of lipid proteinous substance in the skin and mucous membranes. It is clinically manifested by white or yellow plaques and nodules in the skin and mucous membranes. Its association with diabetes has frequently been reported.[95]

Porphyria

Although there is no increased incidence of porphyria in diabetes compared with that in the general population, diabetes has been found in as many as 25% of male patients with porphyria cutanea tarda. The reason for this association is not clear. It has been suggested[106] that this particular abnormality results from excessive accumulation of iron, which leads to hemochromatosis with damage to the parenchymatous cells of the pancreas. The rare occurrence of diabetes in females with porphyria has been explained by the fact that females are much less prone to hemochromatosis than males.

Glucagonoma Syndrome

In 1966, McGavran et al.[107] reported the first well-documented case of glucagon-secreting alpha cell glucagonoma of the pancreas. This paper kindled interest in this subject so that Stacpoole[108] in a review published in 1981, listed 84 cases, 52 well-documented and 32 probable. Symptoms include necrolytic migratory erythema, mild diabetes or glucose intolerance, weight loss, anemia, and stomatitis or glossitis. The "glucagonoma syndrome" affects women (chiefly postmenopausal) more than men in a ratio of 4:1. Skin rash may involve any area of the body, more commonly the groin, perineum, buttocks, and thighs. The rash usually appears as erythematous macules, followed by bullous, exudative lesions which desquamate and then heal, leaving hyperpigmented areas. Other lesions appear so that without treatment, it is usually a chronic intermittent process. Plasma glucagon levels (normal, about 100 pg/ml) range from 800 to 6750 pg/ml, and are usually more than 1500 pg/ml.[109] The tumors are often large (5 cm/d); complete removal—usually not feasible—results in cure and remission of signs and symptoms. Medical treatment has been only partly successful; streptozotocin, 5-fluorouracil and dimethyltriazenoimidazole carboxamide (DTIC) have been used.

OTHER POSSIBLE INVOLVEMENTS OF THE SKIN IN DIABETES

Various cases of the skin reflecting problems of diabetes have been illustrated in recent literature. Poliak et al.[110] cited a small series of cases of reactive perforating collagenosis (RPC), in which collagen fibers extrude through the epidermis. Although this rare condition has been reported earlier in the literature, the 6 patients who had multiple umbilicated cutaneous papules in this series all had diabetes mellitus with retinopathy.

Case reports by Rosenbloom et al.[111] and Brink[112] link limited joint mobility to microvascular disease in childhood diabetes. This was commented on in the editorial by Knowles[113] which suggested that the skin condition may be related to hyperglycemia.[114] Although he believes that other factors such as heredity may play a part, Knowles closes with the admonition that "efforts should be continued to control the diabetes as well as possible. . . ."

REFERENCES

1. Bagdade, J.D., Stewart, M., Walters, E.: Impaired granulocyte adherence. A reversible defect in host defense in patients with poorly controlled diabetes. Diabetes 27:677, 1978.
2. Wheat, L.J.: Infection and diabetes mellitus. Diabetes Care 3:187, 1980.
3. Freinkel, R.K.: Metabolism of glucose C-14 by human skin in vitro. J. Invest. Dermatol. 34:37, 1960.
4. Wells, G.C., Sanderson, K.V., McCabe, I.M.: The histochemical localization of the phosphorylases of the skin. Bull. Soc. Franc. Dermatol. Syph. 68:409, 1961.
5. Halprin, K.M., Ohkawara, A.: Glucose and glycogen metabolism in the human epidermis. J. Invest. Dermatol. 46:43, 1966.
6. Nicolaides, N., Reiss, O.K., Langdon, R.G.: Studies of the in vitro lipid metabolism of the human skin. I. Biosynthesis in scalp skin. J. Am. Chem. Soc.77:1535, 1955.
7. Nicolaides, N., Rothman, S.: The site of sterol and squalene synthesis in the human skin. J. Invest. Dermatol. 24:125, 1955.
8. Hsia, S.L., Dreize, M.A., Marquez, M.C.: Lipid metabolism in human skin. II. A study of lipogenesis in skin of diabetic patients. J. Invest. Dermatol. 47:443, 1966.
9. Urbach, E., Lentz, J.W.: Carbohydrate metabolism and skin. Arch. Dermatol. Syph. 52:301, 1945.
10. Urbach, E.: Skin diabetes; hyperglycodermia without hyperglycemia. J.A.M.A. 129:438, 1945.
11. Peterka, E.S., Fusaro, R.M.: Cutaneous carbohydrate studies. I. The glucose content of the skin of the back of normal persons. J. Invest. Dermatol. 44:385, 1965.
12. Peterka, E.S., Fusaro, R.M.: Cutaneous carbohydrate studies. IV. The skin glucose content of fasting diabetics with and without infection. J. Invest. Dermatol. 46:459, 1956.
13. Miller, D.I., Ridolfo, A.S.: The skin-surface glucose test. An aid in the diagnosis of diabetes mellitus. Diabetes 9:48, 1960.
14. West, K.M., Rockwell, D.A., Wulff, J.A.: Value of the skin-surface glucose test as a screening procedure for diabetes. Diabetes 12:50, 1963.
15. Pastras, T., Beerman, H.: Some aspects of dermatology in diabetes mellitus. A review of some recent literature. Am. J. Med. Sci. 247:363, 1964.
16. Bercovici, E., Solomon, L.M., Beerman, H.: Microangiopathy in diabetes mellitus and nondiabetic dermatoses. Am. J. Med. Sci. 248:20, 1964.
17. Aagenaes, O., Moe, H.: Light- and electron-microscopic study of skin capillaries of diabetics. Diabetes 10:253, 1961.
18. McMillan, D.E., Breithaupt, D.L., Rosenau, W., et al.: Forearm skin capillaries of diabetic, potential diabetic and nondiabetic subjects. Changes seen by light microscope. Diabetes 15:251, 1966.
19. Handelsman, M.B., Morrione, T.G., Ghitman, B.: Skin vascular alterations in diabetes mellitus. Arch. Intern. Med. 110:70, 1962.
20. Rees, S.B., Camerini-Davalos, R.A., Caulfield, J.B., et al.: Pathophysiology of microangiopathy in diabetes mellitus. In: M.P. Cameron, M. O'Connor (Eds.): Ciba Foundation Colloquia on Endocrinology, Vol. 15 (Diabetes Mellitus). London, J. & A. Churchill Ltd., 1964, pp. 315–329.
21. Binkley, G.W.: Dermopathy in the diabetic syndrome. Arch. Dermatol. 92:625, 1965.
22. Muller, S.A., Winkelmann, R.K.: Necrobiosis lipoidica diabeticorum. A clinical and pathological investigation of 171 cases. Arch. Dermatol. 93:272, 1966.
23. Oppenheim, M.: Eigentumliche disseminierte Degeneration des Bindesgewebes der Haut bei einem Diabetiker. Zbl. Haut. Beschlechtskr. 32:179, 1929–1930.
24. Urbach, E.: Beiträge zu einer physiologischen und pathologischen Chemie der Haut; ein neue diabetische Stoffwechseldermatose: Nekrobiosis lipoidica diabeticorum. Arch. Dermatol. Syph. 166:273, 1932.
25. Cannon, A.B.: Skin manifestations of some common internal disorders. Southern Med. J. 38:105, 1945.
26. Hildebrand, A.G., Montgomery, H., Rynearson, E.H.: Necrobiosis lipoidica diabeticorum. Arch. Intern. Med. 66:851, 1940.
27. Krall, L.P., Zorrilla, E.: Disorders of the skin in diabetes. In: A. Marble, P. White, R.F. Bradley, L.P. Krall (Eds.): Joslin's Diabetes Mellitus, 11th ed., Philadelphia, Lea & Febiger, 1971, p. 655.
28. Gilgor, R.S., Lazarus, G.S.: Skin manifestations of diabetes mellitus. In: M. Ellenberg, H. Rifkin (Eds.): Diabetes Mellitus Theory and Practice, 3rd ed. New York, Medical Examination Publishing Co., Inc., 1983, pp. 881–883.
29. Metz, G., Metz, J.: Extrakrural Manifestation der Necrobiosis lipoidica. Isolierter Befall des Kopfes. Hautartz 28:359, 1977.
30. Mackey, J.P.: Necrobiosis lipoidica diabeticorum involving scalp and face. Br. J. Dermatol. 93:729, 1975.
31. Sahl, W.J., Jr.: Necrobiosis lipoidica diabeticorum. Localization in surgical scars. J. Cutan. Pathol. 5:249, 1978.
32. Ormsby, O.S., Montgomery, H.: Diseases of the Skin. 8th Ed., Philadelphia, Lea & Febiger, 1954.
33. Muller, S.A., Winkelmann, R.K.: Necrobiosis lipoidica diabeticorum. Results of glucose tolerance tests in nondiabetic patients. J.A.M.A. 195:433, 1966.
34. Halprin, K.M.: Diabetes calling card. Necrobiosis lipoidica diabeticorum. J.A.M.A. 198:175, 1966.
35. Muller, S.A.: Dermatologic disorders associated with diabetes mellitus. Mayo Clin. Proc. 41:689, 1966.
36. Narva, W.M., Benoit, F.L., Ringrose, E.J.: Necrobiosis lipoidica diabeticorum with apparently normal carbohydrate tolerance. Arch. Intern. Med. 115:718, 1965.
37. Bauer, M.F., Hirsch, P., Bullock, W.K., Abdul-Haj, S.K.: Necrobiosis lipoidica diabeticorum. A cutaneous manifestation of diabetic microangiopathy. Arch. Dermatol. 90:558, 1964.
38. Wiemers, U., Hackel, F., Voigt, H.: Studies on the relationship between diabetes mellitus and necrobiosis lipoidica. Z. Gesamte Inn. Med. 30:62, 1975.
39. Sodemann, K., Bruns, W., Linss, G., Rjasanowski, I.: Necrobiosis lipoidica diabeticorum und Serumlipide. Z. Gesamte Inn. Med. 31:270, 1976.
40. Engel, M.F., Hammack, W.J.: Necrobiosis lipoidica diabeticorum; a biochemical, histochemical and plethysmographic study. Arch. Dermatol. 78:73, 1958.

41. Gilliland, I.C., Hanno, M.G., Strudwick, J.I.: Protein-bound polysaccharides in diabetes with and without complications. Biochem. J. *56*:xxxii, 1954.
42. Engel, M.F., Smith, J.G., Jr.: The pathogenesis of necrobiosis lipoidica. Necrobiosis lipoidica, a form fruste of diabetes mellitus. Arch. Dermatol. *82*:791, 1960.
43. Marckwort, H.J., Schydlo, R.: Early onset of necrobiosis lipoidica diabeticorum in juvenile diabetes mellitus. (Author's translation). Monatsschr. Kinderheilkd. *122*:88, 1974.
44. Lunas, J.P., Smith, J.G., Jr.: Necrobiosis lipoidica in a Negro. Arch. Dermatol. *85*:532, 1962.
45. Savitt, L.E.: Favorable response of necrobiosis lipoidica diabeticorum to hydrocortisone suspension. Arch. Dermatol. *71*:506, 1955.
46. Madison, J.F.: Ketonuria after local steroids in necrobiosis lipoidica. Arch. Dermatol. *90*:477, 1964.
47. Andrews, G.G., Domonkos, A.N.: Diseases of the Skin. Philadelphia, W.B. Saunders Co., 1963, p. 473.
48. Dubin, B.J., Kaplan, E.N.: The surgical treatment of necrobiosis lipoidica diabeticorum. Plast. Reconstr. Surg. *60*:421, 1977.
49. Marr, T.J., Traisman, H.S. Griffith, B.H., Schafer, M.A.: Necrobiosis lipoidica diabeticorum in a juvenile diabetic: treatment by excision and skin grafting. Cutis *19*:348, 1977.
50. Tornling, G.: Unge, G., Ljungqvist, A., et al.: Dipyridamole and capillary proliferation. A preliminary report. Acta Pathol. Microbiol. Scand. (A) *86*:82, 1978.
51. Eldor, A., Diaz, E.G., Naparstek, E.: Treatment of diabetic necrobiosis with aspirin and dipyridamole. (Letter). N. Engl. J. Med. *298*:1033, 1978.
52. Fjellner, B.: Treatment of diabetic necrobiosis with aspirin or dipyridamole. (Letter). N. Engl. J. Med. *299*:1366, 1978. (See also Unge, G., and Tornling, G.: (Letter). Ibid., p. 1366).
53. Melin, H.: An atrophic circumscribed skin lesion in the lower extremities of diabetics. Acta Med. Scand. *176* (Suppl. 423): 1, 1964.
54. Murphy, R.A.: Skin lesions in diabetic patients: the "spotted leg" syndrome. Lahey Clin. Found. Bull. *14*:10, 1965.
55. Binkley, G.W., Giraldo, B., Stoughton, R.B.: Diabetic dermopathy. A clinical study. Cutis *3*:955, 1967.
56. Danowski, T.S., Sabeh, G., Sarver, M.E., et al.: Shin spots and diabetes mellitus. Am. J. Med. Sci. *25*:570, 1966.
57. Tornblom, N.: "Shin spots," purpura och gangrän hos diabetespatienter. Lakartidningen *75*:2629, 1978.
58. Lawrence, R.D.: Lipodystrophy and hepatomegaly with diabetes, lipaemia and other metabolic disturbances; case throwing new light on action of insulin. Lancet *1*:724, 1946.
59. Renold, A.E., Winegrad, A.I., Martin, D.B.: Diabète sucré et tissu adipeux. Helv. Med. Acta *24*:322, 1957.
60. Marble, A., Smith, R.M.: Atrophy of subcutaneous fat following injections of insulin. Proc. Am. Diabetes Assoc. *2*:173, 1942.
61. Paley, R.G., Scott, M.H.: Severe insulin lipodystrophy as a possible cause of instability in diabetics. Br. Med. J. *2*:1331, 1958.
62. Marble, A., Renold, A.E.: Atrophy and hypertrophy of subcutaneous fat due to insulin. Trans. Assoc. Am. Physicians *62*:219, 1949.
63. Renold, A.E., Marble, A., Fawcett, D.W.: Action of insulin on deposition of glycogen and storage of fat in adipose tissue. Endocrinology *46*:55, 1950.
64. Mentzer, S.H., DuBray, E.S.: Fatty atrophy from injections of insulin. Calif. West. Med. *26*:212, 1927.
65. Schmidt, V.: Local lipodystrophy after insulin injections. Ugesk. laeger. *111*:1031, 1949.
66. Duncan, G.G.: Diseases of Metabolism, 5th ed. Philadelphia, W.B. Saunders Co., 1964, p. 1019.
67. Collens, W.S., Boas, L.C., Zilinsky, J.D., Greenwald, J.J.: Lipoatrophy following injections of insulin; method of control. N. Engl. J. Med. *241*:610, 1949.
68. Watson, B.M., Calder, J.S.: A treatment for insulin-induced fat atrophy. Diabetes *20*:628, 1971.
69. Watson, D., Vines, R.: Variations in the incidence of lipodystrophy using different insulins. Med. J. Aust. *1*:248, 1973.
70. Wentworth, S.M., Galloway, J.A., Haunz, E.A., et al.: The use of purified insulins in the treatment of patients with insulin lipoatrophy (Abstr.). Diabetes *22*:290A, 1973.
71. Teuscher, A.: Treatment of insulin lipoatrophy with monocomponent insulin. Diabetologia *10*:211, 1974.
72. Asherov, J., Mimouni, M., Laron, Z.: Successful treatment of insulin lipoatrophy. A case report. Diabet. Metab. *5*:1, 1979.
73. Wright, A.D., Walsh, C.H., Fitzgerald, M.G., Malins, J.M.: Very pure porcine insulin in clinical practice. Br. Med. J. *1*:25, 1979.
74. Maaz, E.: Insulin lipoatrophy and its elimination through the use of monocomponent insulin. Z. Gesamte Inn. Med. *31*:941, 1976.
75. Hulst, S.G.Th.: Treatment of insulin-induced lipoatrophy. Diabetes *25*:1052, 1976.
76. Whitley, T.H., Lawrence, P.A., Smith, C.L.: Amelioration of insulin atrophy by dexamethasone injection. J.A.M.A. *235*:839, 1976.
77. Kumar, D., Miller, L.V., Mehtalia, S.D.: Use of dexamethasone in treatment of insulin lipoatrophy. Diabetes *26*:296, 1977.
77a.Altman, J.J., Pehuet, M., Slama, G., Tchobroutsky, C.: Three cases of allergic reaction to human insulin (Letter). Lancet *2*:524, 1983.
77b.Carveth-Johnson, A.O., Mylvaganam, K., Child, D.F.: Generalised allergic reaction with synthetic human insulin. Lancet *2*:1287, 1982.
78. Rocca, F.F., Pereyra, E.: Phlyctenar lesions in the feet of diabetic patients. Diabetes *12*:220, 1963.
79. Cantwell, A.R., Martz, W.: Idiopathic bullae in diabetic. Bullosis diabeticorum. Arch. Dermatol. *96*:42, 1967.
80. Branom, W.T., Jr., Hyman, A.B., Rubin, Z: Chancriform pyoderma. Arch. Dermatol. *87*:736, 1963.
81. Tuazon, C.U., Perez, A., Kishaba, T., Sheagren, J.N.: Staphylococcus aureas among insulin-injecting diabetic patients. J.A.M.A. *231*:1272, 1972.
82. Younger, D.: Infections and diabetes. Med. Clin. N. Am. *49*:1005, 1965.
83. Behrman, H.T., Levin, O.L.: Cutaneous manifestations of systemic disease. J. Mt. Sinai Hosp., N.Y. *13*:257, 1947.
84. Greenwood, A.M.: A study of skin in 500 cases of diabetes. J.A.M.A. *89*:774, 1927.
85. Mehnert, B., Mehnert, H.: Yeasts in urine and saliva of diabetic and nondiabetic patients. Diabetes *7*:293, 1958.
86. Sonck, C.E., Somersalo, O.: The yeast flora of the anogenital region in diabetic girls. Arch. Dermatol. *88*:846, 1963.
87. Rubin, A.: Leukorrhea and vaginitis. Med. Clin. N. Am. *45*:1553, 1961.
88. Swartz, J.H.: Infections caused by dermatophytes. N. Engl. J. Med. *267*:1246, 1962.
89. Fredrickson, D.S., Levy, R.I., Lees, R.S.: Fat transport in lipoproteins—an integrated approach to mechanisms and disorders. N. Engl. J. Med. *276*:273, 1967.

90. Bagdade, J.D., Porte, D., Jr., Bierman, E.L.: Diabetic lipemia. A form of acquired fat-induced lipemia. N. Engl. J. Med. *276*:427, 1967.

91. Thomas, J.E.: Diabetic xanthomatosis in an African. Br. Med. J. 2:999, 1961.

92. Choutet, P., Lamisse, F., Ginies, G., et al.: Xanthomatose eruptive revelant une acidocetose diabètique. Nouv. Presse Med. *8*:782, 1979.

93. Boeck, W.C., Yater, W.M.: Xanthemia and xanthosis (carotinemia); clinical study. J. Lab. Clin. Med. *14*:1129, 1929.

94. Mazovetskii, A.G., Alekseev, I.P., Kliachko, V.R.: Treatment of diabetic xanthomatosis with Atromid. Ter. Arkh. *44*:102, 1972.

95. Eisert, J.: Diabetes and diseases of the skin. Med. Clin. N. Am. *49*:621, 1965.

96. Schneider, T.: Dupuytren's contracture in diabetes mellitus. Med. So. Africa 96, 1957.

97. Spring, M., Cohen, B.D.: Dupuytren's contracture: a warning of diabetes? (Abstr.). Diabetes *15*:547, 1966.

98. Hurlbut, W.B., Lincoln, C.S., Jr.: Multiple hemorrhagic sarcoma and diabetes mellitus; review of series, with report of 2 cases. Arch. Intern. Med. *84*:738, 1949.

99. Gibson, S.H., Perry, H.O.: Diabetes and psoriasis. Arch. Dermatol.*74*:487, 1956.

100. Aschner, B., Curth, H.O., Gross, P.: Genetic aspects of psoriasis. Acta Genet. Statist. Med. (Basel) *7*:197, 1957.

101. Reeds, R.E., Jr., Fusaro, R.M., Fisher, I.: Psoriasis vulgaris. I. A clinical survey of the association with diabetes mellitus. Arch. Dermatol. *89*:205, 1964.

102. Binazzi, M., Calandra, P., Lisi, P.: Statistical association between psoriasis and diabetes: further results. Arch. Dermatol. Res. *254*:43 (Nov.) 1975.

103. Winkelmann, R.K., Sheen, S.R., Jr., Underdahl, L.O.: Acanthosis nigricans and endocrine disease. J.A.M.A. *174*:1145, 1960.

104. Kahn, C.R., Flier, J.S., Bar, R.S., et al.: The syndromes of insulin resistance and acanthosis nigricans. Insulin-receptor disorders in man. N. Engl. J. Med. *294*:739, 1976.

105. Epstein, C.J., Martini, G.:M., Schultz, A.L., Motulsky, A.G.: Werner's syndrome: A review of its symptomatology, natural history, pathologic features, genetics and relationship to the natural aging process. Medicine *45*:177, 1966.

106. Burnham, T.K., Fosnaugh, R.P.: Porphyria, diabetes and their relationship. Arch. Dermatol. *83*:717, 1961.

107. McGavran, M.H., Unger, R.H., Recant, L., et al.: A glucagon-secreting alpha-cell carcinoma of the pancreas. N. Engl. J. Med.*274*:1408, 1966.

108. Stacpoole, P.W.: The glucagonoma syndrome: Clinical features, diagnosis, and treatment. Endocrinol. Rev.*2*:347 (Summer), 1981.

109. Leichter, S.B.: Clinical and metabolic aspects of glucagonoma. Medicine (Baltimore). *59*:100, 1980.

110. Poliak, S.C., Lebwohl, M.G., Parris, A., Prioleau, P.G.: Reactive perforating collagenosis associated with diabetes mellitus. N. Engl. J. Med. *306*:81, 1982.

111. Rosenbloom, A.L., Silverstein, J.H., Lezotte, D.C., et al.: Limited joint mobility in childhood diabetes indicates increased risk for microvascular disease. N. Engl. J. Med. *305*:191, 1981.

112. Brink, S.: Limited joint mobility (LJM) as a risk factor for complications in youngsters with IDDM. Diabetes *32* (Suppl. 1):16A, 1983. (Abstract)

113. Knowles, H.B., Jr.: Joint contractures, waxy skin, and control of diabetes. (Editorial). N. Engl. J. Med. *305*:217, 1981.

114. Buckingham, B.A., Uitto, J., Sandborg, C., et al.: Scleroderma-like syndrome and the non-enzymatic glycosylation of collagen in children with poorly controlled insulin dependent diabetes (IDDM). Pediatr. Res. *15*:(Part 2) 626, 1981.

39 Diabetes and Other Endocrinologic Disorders

George P. Kozak and Ramachandiran Cooppan

Reference has been made repeatedly throughout this text to the close interrelationship between the various glands of internal secretion, particularly the pituitary, thyroid, and adrenal, and their influence upon diabetes. The outstanding feature is the homeostatic or regulating effect of both the anterior pituitary and the adrenal cortical hormones. Certain hormones of the anterior pituitary and of the adrenal cortex have a diabetogenic effect when administered in excess. A number of clinical states may produce a disturbance in the dynamic balance between the rate of insulin production by the pancreas and the insulin requirement of the tissues. The results may be insulin resistance on the one hand, or insulin sensitivity and frequent hypoglycemic episodes on the other.

THE ANTERIOR PITUITARY AND DIABETES

Various clinical observations suggest that abnormalities in pituitary function may play a part in the development and course of diabetes. These include the tendency of diabetic children to be above height for their age at the onset of diabetes and to have bone development a year in advance of their age, the increased incidence of onset of diabetes at puberty, the glycosuria of pregnancy, and the frequent onset of diabetes at or near the menopause.

Acromegaly (Hyperpituitarism)

Acromegaly, a chronic disease with insidious onset, is characterized by progressive overgrowth of body tissues associated with a pituitary tumor or, in rare instances, with hyperplasia of the eosinophilic cells of the anterior lobe of the pituitary gland. Histologically, the tumor may be eosinophilic, poorly granulated, or agranular (chromophobe). Its major effects result primarily from increased production of growth hormone (somatotropin), from the mechanical effects of the expansile growth of a pituitary neoplasm, or from the interference with other normal pituitary functions by pressure of the tumor upon the uninvolved portion of the gland. While the so-called acral changes with overgrowth of the hands, feet and face are the outstanding characteristics, almost all tissues and organs of the body are altered by the excessive production of growth hormone. Increased production of this hormone prior to normal ossification of epiphyseal cartilage may result in gigantism.

The metabolic effects of growth hormone are mediated by the polypeptide somatomedin C. This is a single chain polypeptide that can stimulate incorporation of sulfate into cartilage, DNA synthesis, and multiplication of cells in tissue culture. Measurement of somatomedin C can be used as an index of GH activity and is useful in following treatment.

Assessment of Acromegalic Activity. While full-blown active acromegaly may be obvious, it is difficult at times to decide whether acromegaly in a given case is mildly active or quiescent. The presence of one or more of the following is consistent with excessive growth hormone (GH) activity.

1. Progressive or persistent headaches.
2. Mood changes (increased irritability or depression).
3. Progressive enlargement of the sella turcica.
4. Progressive loss of visual fields.
5. Progressive acral bone enlargement.
6. Active endochondral bone formation (as judged by costochondral junction rib biopsy).
7. Skin and subcutaneous tissue changes.
8. Diabetes mellitus or impaired glucose tolerance.
9. Elevation of plasma GH level.
10. Elevation of plasma insulin level.
11. Elevation of serum phosphorus.
12. Increased urinary hydroxyproline.
13. Increased urinary calcium.

The last three findings, usually accompanied by increased secretion of GH, suggest that the tumor is increasing in size.

The plasma GH level does not always show the the expected elevation, and its interpretation is complicated by the normal diurnal variations and responses to carbohydrate intake and by the effects of age, exercise, anesthesia, and surgery.[1,2] The disturbances in plasma GH and insulin levels in acromegaly have been well documented. They include high GH levels during fasting, associated with an inadequate or absent response to the usual stimuli for the hormone's release or suppression.[1–4] Thus, hypoglycemia in the acromegalic patient seldom results in a further increase of GH level, nor does glucose loading lead to effective suppression.[3,4] Chronic endogenous hypersecretion of GH is associated, in the early phase at least, with an increased plasma insulin response to tolbutamide, and to glucose given orally or intravenously.[4,5] An elevation of serum phosphorus is not a consistent finding, but is helpful diagnostically when present, especially in the adult patient and in the absence of renal insufficiency.

The detection of glucose intolerance or the onset of overt diabetes suggests continuing excessive GH secretion in patients with other features of acromegaly. Personality changes, including "explosive irritability" are noted in a high proportion of patients with active acromegaly and appear to reflect the physiologic effect of excess GH as well as the pathologic effect of an expanding intracranial mass. Increased amounts of hydroxyproline peptides in the urine are associated with excess secretion of GH, thyroid hormone, and pituitary gonadotropins. Increased hydroxyproline excretion has been noted in diabetes, acromegaly, hyperthyroidism, hypergonadotropic conditions, Paget's disease, Marfan's syndrome, and in one patient with the Fanconi syndrome.[6–8] Since rib biopsy reveals chondrogenesis in patients with active acromegaly,[9] and GH promotes collagen formation in vitro,[10] GH influences hydroxyproline excretion by increasing overall collagen synthesis.

Incidence of Diabetes in Acromegaly. A series of 823 cases of acromegaly collected up to the early 1960s, revealed an overall frequency of "diabetes" in 19% of patients.[10a] However, by inclusion of additional patients with lesser degrees of impaired glucose tolerance, the total frequency in acromegaly may be much higher. In 100 patients with proved acromegaly, Davidoff and Cushing[11,12] reported glycosuria in 25% and diabetes in 12%. Coggeshall and Root,[13] in a follow-up of these 100 patients, and 53 others with acromegaly, found that 36% had glycosuria and 17% developed diabetes. In the study of Gordon and associates,[14] diabetes was detected in 18 of 100 acromegalics; in the 82 without frank diabetes, 20 had decreased glucose tolerance. Thus, a diabetic tendency was observed in almost half of the patients in this series. In the 44 acromegalics studied by Ballintine et al.[14a] 6 (14%) had elevated fasting blood glucose levels and an additional 20 (45%) had impaired glucose tolerance. Among the 50 patients of Emmer, Gordon and Roth,[15] 60% had glucose intolerance and of these, 10 had fasting hyperglycemia; 3 of the 50 required insulin in treatment.

It is evident from the above that in reported cases, the frequency of carbohydrate abnormality in acromegaly has varied greatly. This has been due, at least in part, to differing methods and standards as well as the duration of acromegaly and degree of its activity. The more recent reports indicate a frequency of "diabetes" (fasting hyperglycemia) of about 15 to 30% included in a total of 50 to 60% with glucose intolerance.

In the 29 cases of acromegaly and diabetes reported by Coggeshall and Root,[13] the average interval between the onset of acromegaly and that of diabetes was 9.5 years, but there were intervals of from 1 to 22 years, with a majority of cases of diabetes occurring within 15 years. In this series, 10 patients had either irradiation or surgical treatment directed toward the pituitary, but no characteristic difference in the time of appearance of diabetes was evident in these patients. The evaluation of treatment, however, was difficult, since in patients in whom increased intracranial pressure was the initial symptom, a high mortality rate shortened the period of observation. Ten of the patients were males and 19 females. In both sexes, the average age at onset of diabetes was 38.3 years, an average quite different from that found in the general population of diabetics for whom it was approximately 46 years for males and 49 years for females. A family history of diabetes was obtained in 6 of the 29 subjects, whereas in acromegalics without diabetes, a family history of diabetes was found in only 3 of 124 patients. The clinical course of the diabetes varied greatly; but as a whole, showed no greater variations than those noted in any large diabetes clinic.[16]

Jadresic et al.[16a] of the Hammersmith Hospital, London, studied 155 patients with acromegaly of whom 76 were males and 79 females. The series included 41 (27%) with decreased glucose tolerance; 16 of these had clinical and 25 "chemical" diabetes. Among the total of 41 with diabetes, the serum GH level was 189 ng/ml, whereas in 113 without this condition, the corresponding value was 116 ng/ml.

The diabetes of acromegaly is of the stable, maturity-onset type, usually requiring a small amount of insulin. Insulin resistance with a requirement of 200 units or more daily may occur but is not common. In the series of Coggeshall and Root,[13] in 3 of the 16 patients who died, death occurred in diabetic coma, but 2 of these were treated in the pre-insulin era. The common complications of diabetes were found frequently. Arteriosclerosis and pyogenic infections occurred in 7 of the patients. Dietary management was difficult because of the excessive appetite of some of the patients. In general, mere restriction of carbohydrate seemed to have little effect on the fasting blood glucose level.

In the acromegalic series of Gordon et al.,[14] the diagnosis of diabetes and acromegaly was sometimes made at the same time (5 cases), but more often the diabetes appeared some years after acromegaly was manifest (12 cases). In one woman, diabetes seemed to precede the onset of acromegaly. Most patients did not present special problems in management. Ketoacidosis and death did occur in two who showed resistance to insulin, and another diabetic died from overwhelming infec-

tion. Multiple complications related to diabetes were noted in two patients, one of whom had incapacitating peripheral neuropathy.

With improved treatment of acromegaly and its secondary complications, life expectancy has increased with time to permit the development of some of the chronic complications of diabetes. Of 21 acromegalic diabetic patients, McCullagh[17] reported 3 cases of typical nonproliferating retinopathy in patients whose duration of diabetes was only 8, 7, and 2 years respectively. In these three no mention was made of renal involvement characteristic of long-term diabetes.

Pathogenesis of Diabetes in Acromegaly. The unique study of Sönksen and associates[18] investigated the pathogenesis of diabetes in acromegaly. Standard intravenous glucose tolerance tests and measurements of blood glucose, plasma insulin, growth hormone, and free fatty acids were done in 16 acromegalic patients. Seven had impaired carbohydrate tolerance, including 2 with symptomatic diabetes. In 6 patients, serial tests showed the changes that may occur as carbohydrate tolerance deteriorates. Fasting hyperinsulinism was present in 6, and insulin response to intravenous glucose was increased in 10. The pattern of this response varied. In 10, there was a peak in the first 15 minutes, and in 4 the pattern resembled that of maturity-onset diabetes with a gradual rise of plasma insulin concentration toward a peak at 60 minutes. In the 2 patients with overt diabetes, there was no response to glucose given intravenously although the fasting plasma insulin was increased. The data of Sönksen et al. suggest two possible intermediary stages in the development of diabetes associated with acromegaly. The first is the stage of "hyperinsulinism" with a normal or borderline glucose tolerance. At this stage, the peak insulin response occurs promptly but is higher than normal. In the second stage, the peak insulin response is delayed and glucose tolerance may be within normal limits or impaired. This stage would appear potentially reversible following adequate treatment. In the third stage, seen only with established diabetes, the pancreatic response appeared to be maximal in the fasting state and no further rise in insulin concentration occurred after glucose injection.

On the basis of published reports and their own experience, Harrison and Flier[18a] have classified the glucose-insulin abnormalities in acromegaly as shown in Figure 39–1.

In most patients with acromegaly, glucose tolerance improves and plasma insulin levels fall to normal after successful treatment resulting in decreases in GH levels.[18,18b] In a more recent study, Wass et al.[18c] determined the effect of the treatment

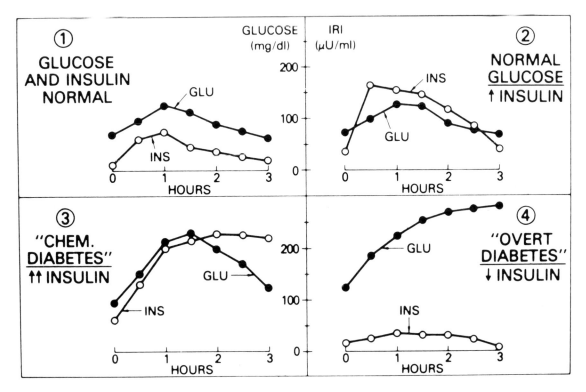

Fig. 39–1. Stages of carbohydrate disturbance in acromegaly as seen in oral glucose tolerance tests. (1) Insulin sensitivity and plasma glucose normal (15 to 20% of patients). (2) Insulin sensitivity mildly decreased; glucose normal (± 20%). (3) Insulin sensitivity decreased; mildly impaired glucose tolerance (± 50%). (4) Insulin secretion markedly impaired; overt diabetes (± 5–10% of patients). (Taken from reference 18a with permission of authors and publisher.)

of acromegaly on the glucose intolerance. They used bromocryptine and found that after 3 months of therapy, there was a highly significant improvement in glucose tolerance in both the diabetic and nondiabetic acromegalics. It was concluded that this was directly due to the reduction in GH by bromocryptine since no improvement was noted when GH levels were not reduced by the drug.

Weight of Viscera in Acromegaly and Diabetes. Davidoff[11] divided the clinical course of acromegaly into three periods: (1) the early period with general overgrowth, gain in weight, and menstrual disturbances in women; (2) the middle period with symptoms caused by pressure in the area of the tumor; visual disturbances, and increases in the size of the sella turcica; and (3) the final period with polyphagia, polydipsia, and the like, because of visceral splanchnomegaly and secondary effects upon the endocrine organs. The splanchnomegaly of acromegaly is a true overgrowth of all tissues and not merely a result of the laying down of excess fat or of increased water in the tissues. It is assumed that the enlargement of the extremities as well as the splanchnomegaly are caused by excessive production of growth hormone or hormones secreted by an anterior pituitary tumor. One might suppose

that development of diabetes in such patients is also due to this same agent acting either directly or indirectly, thereby interfering with the function of the islands of Langerhans. In either case, under the influence of such a substance, one might expect to find some relation between the weight of the pancreas and the weight of other organs of diabetic acromegalic patients.

To test this hypothesis, Coggeshall and Root[13] tabulated the weights of organs in acromegalics with and without diabetes and in non-acromegalic diabetics. The diabetics without acromegaly were divided into three groups, based on the weight of the pancreas: more than 120 g, 100 to 120 g, and less than 40 g. The average weight of the pancreas in 14 patients in group I was 152 g; in 23 patients in group II, 106 g; and in 13 patients in group III, 32 g. The weights of the pancreas in three acromegalics without diabetes were 225, 83, and 140 (av. 149) g, and in three acromegalics with diabetes 150, 118, and 117 (av. 128) g. In this small series, there is no suggestion that the weight of the pancreas in acromegalics with diabetes is influenced by any substance such as that responsible for the enlargement of the skeleton and visceral organs in acromegaly.

At autopsy of 15 acromegalic patients, Gordon and associates[14] observed a general increase in organ weights. However, there was much individual variation. In 1 of the 5 diabetics examined postmortem, insulin assay of the pancreas showed a moderately decreased amount of insulin similar to that usually found in non-acromegalic adult diabetics.[19] Similar assays on 2 other nondiabetic acromegalics showed normal values. The weights of the pancreas of the 2 diabetic acromegalics who died in diabetic coma were 110 and 125 respectively (normal, 100g).

Insulin Resistance in Acromegalics with Diabetes. Fraser and associates[20] noted that the blood glucose response of the nondiabetic acromegalic to exogenous insulin is much less than normal. Galbraith and co-workers[21] demonstrated insulin resistance in acromegalic muscle directly by forearm technique. The degree of insulin resistance did not differ between diabetic and nondiabetic acromegalic patients. In evaluating the pathogenesis of diabetes in acromegaly, Sönksen and associates[18] noted that the alterations of insulin resistance and insulin secretions due to acromegaly are completely reversed by removal of excess growth hormone in the normoglycemic acromegalic. With intravenous glucose loading in normoglycemic acromegalic patients, Cerasi and Luft[5] noted a prompt, vigorous insulin output as measured by radioimmunoassay. Perley and Kipnis[22] showed that acromegalic patients exhibited increases in insulin secretion of 5 to 70 times the normal amount when stimulated with tolbutamide after dexamethasone had been administered. The insulin levels attained by acromegalic subjects far exceeded those of normal or diabetic subjects under similar conditions. The impaired peripheral action of insulin is suggested by the high insulin-resistance index[20] and the absence of reactive hypoglycemia following excessive endogenous insulin release. The triad of compensatory increase in endogenous insulin secretion, resistance to exogenous insulin, and reversal of insulin resistance on removal of the offending factor is seen also in pregnancy, obesity, and Cushing's syndrome, as well as in acromegaly.

Although insulin resistance has not been a common problem in the Joslin series of acromegalics with diabetes, several instructive cases have been noted.

One man (J.C. #17969), aged 44 years at onset of diabetes, was first seen at the Joslin Clinic 3 years later in diabetic coma. His maximum weight had been 245 pounds; his height was 70 inches. After recovery, his weight was 187 pounds. Acromegaly was diagnosed and he subsequently required approximately 250 units of insulin daily. He was rehospitalized a year after first visit because of a large carbuncle, and again was in ketoac-

idosis with blood CO_2 content of 9 mEq/L and blood glucose value of 380 mg/dl. After drainage of the carbuncle, the patient did well for several days until he suddenly developed hemiplegia and died.

Autopsy disclosed a pituitary tumor (25 g; 4 cm in greatest diameter) of the chromaffin type which compressed the hypothalamus and the anterior pituitary. The heart, liver, and kidneys showed overgrowth. In the left cerebral peduncle there was an area of cystic softening which was visible grossly.

Another man (J.C. #58546), has shown a marked, though intermittent, resistance to insulin due presumably to varying degrees of activity of the pituitary tumor. In October, 1960, diabetes was first noted at the age of 37 years. In December, 1961, the patient came to the Joslin Clinic for the first time with classical features of acromegaly. The sella turcica was enlarged with erosion of the sphenoid sinuses, but a pneumoencephalogram did not show suprasellar extension of pituitary tumor. In February, 1962, pituitary irradiation given in total dose of 4000r, was followed by only transient improvement in alleviation of headaches and lowering of elevated serum phosphorus levels. In July, 1962, a sudden change was noted in the character of the diabetes. Whereas it had previously been well regulated on 1.0 g of tolbutamide daily, the patient suddenly began to show a marked increase of the glucose content of urine and blood. Insulin treatment was instituted; the initial requirements were about 150 units daily. In addition to insulin resistance and elevated serum phosphorus levels, costochondral junction biopsy demonstrated excessive growth hormone activity. Surgical hypophysectomy was recommended but was refused by the patient.

A second course of pituitary irradiation (3100r) was given in September, 1962. The diabetes remained difficult to control because of wide swings in blood glucose values, and the insulin requirement was on occasion as high as 500 units daily. During hospitalization in April, 1963, it appeared that the patient's insulin resistance had been broken after 200 units of U-500 regular insulin produced symptoms of hypoglycemia with a blood glucose value of 54 mg/dl. Subsequently, over a 6-day period without insulin, the blood glucose ranged between 160 and 220 mg/dl. Phenformin, 100 mg twice daily, was ineffective, and insulin was resumed in dosage varying between 0 to 500 units daily in a rather cyclic fashion.

During hospitalization in May, 1965, 900 units of U-500 regular insulin were required to bring the blood glucose to a satisfactory range. Subsequently, pork lente insulin in small doses of 6 to 10 units daily, surprisingly resulted in satisfactory control. Serial eye examinations showed moderate generalized constriction of both peripheral fields, but surgery was refused. Reasonable control of the diabetes was obtained by use of pork lente insulin, 12 to 15 units daily, until insulin resistance appeared again after a respiratory infection in January, 1966, requiring 1100 units of insulin. However, in September, 1979, tolazamide, 250 mg daily, gave good diabetes control, but the need for insulin returned so that in 1981 he was receiving 30 units of the NPH type daily.

Hypopituitarism

In adults, hypopituitarism may be caused by tumor, necrosis, vascular disease, infiltrations, and granulomas (noninfectious and infectious) affecting the adenohypophysis. Tumors of the pituitary gland which produce hypopituitarism are most commonly chromophobe adenomas and sometimes craniopharyngiomas. A space-occupying lesion in proximity to the pituitary, including aneurysm, meningioma, or osteoma, may, through local pressure, result in hypopituitarism. Postpartum uterine hemorrhage with hypotension is the most common cause of pituitary infarction (Sheehan's syndrome),[23] but with improvement in obstetric practice, pituitary necrosis resulting in hypopituitarism has become increasingly rare. Other rare vascular causes include extensive diabetic degenerative vascular disease, cavernous sinus thrombosis, and temporal arteritis. Infiltration of the adenohypophysis with hemosiderin-laden macrophages (hemochromatosis) or with sarcoid granulomas has produced hypopituitarism in adults. The triad of diabetes mellitus, skin pigmentation, and hepatomegaly, especially in the presence of heart disease and hypogonadism, should suggest hemochromatosis with pituitary involvement. Cholesterol histiocytosis (Hand-Schüller-Christian disease) may occasionally cause hypopituitarism as well as diabetes insipidus. Infectious causes are now rare but include tuberculosis, syphilis, histoplasmosis, and brucellosis.

Antepartum pituitary necrosis is infrequently diagnosed but perhaps is often overlooked. Characteristic is a severe, deep midline headache lasting 2 to 3 days and requiring hospitalization. The headache secondary to pituitary infarction occurs usually in the third trimester of pregnancy. Amelioration of the diabetes, development of insulin sensitivity, severe hypoglycemic reactions and a marked decrease in insulin requirement, are striking features. The diagnosis of pan- or partial hypopituitarism can be made many years after the acute episode.

In 1971 Schalch and Burday[24] reported their experience with 3 young diabetic women who noted antepartum pituitary insufficiency. All 3 survived the pituitary infarction and delivered viable infants. At that time 4 additional cases were found on literature review. Through the kindness of Dr. Priscilla White, we have studied 6 patients with history of severe "pregnancy headache" for possible hypopituitarism. Pituitary insufficiency was noted in 4 patients; 2 had panhypopituitarism and 2, partial defects. The time span from the presumed acute event to the diagnosis of pituitary insufficiency was 32 years in Joslin Clinic patient #8882. Early recognition during the latter part of pregnancy and appropriate replacement therapy are vital to the health of the mother and fetus in this unusual syndrome. The possibility of a delayed appearance of hypopituitarism should be considered in diabetic patients who had severe headaches of 2 to 3 days' duration during pregnancy.

The functional reserve of the anterior lobe is such that, according to currently available tests, 85% must be destroyed before hypopituitarism causes definite signs and symptoms. In most patients having functional impairment, there is a predictable sequence of hormones showing deficiencies: (1) gonadotropins; (2) somatotropin (children only); (3) thyrotropin, and (4) corticotropin. In mild hypopituitarism, gonadal failure and signs of genital atrophy are the outstanding features. Although pituitary myxedema may occasionally exist out of proportion to other signs, pituitary damage must usually be severe before myxedema or clinically important adrenal insufficiency is seen. The functional impairment in spontaneous hypopituitarism rarely approaches that which results from surgical hypophysectomy.

Cases of selective hormonal pituitary failure of one of the tropic hormones are well documented, although panhypopituitarism is still by far the most common disorder.[26,27] Of the isolated deficiencies, inadequate gonadotropin secretion is most common.[27a] In adults, usually the first indication of failure of pituitary hormones is hypogonadotropic hypogonadism; later thyrotropic and adrenocorticotropic hormone (ACTH) deficiency may develop. Cases of isolated ACTH deficiency are indeed rare; by 1966 only 10 had been reported[28] and by 1982 a total of only 39 cases could be found in the world literature by Stacpoole and co-workers[28a] to which they added 4 new ones.

At least 10 cases of apparent isolated deficiencies of thyroid-stimulating hormone (TSH) had been reported by 1966.[28] Selective or monotropic pituitary failure is seen in some patients with postpartum pituitary necrosis.[25] As yet, diabetes mellitus has not been noted in patients with isolated ACTH deficiency. The case reported years ago by Shuman[29] provided at the time the only example of diabetes mellitus and pituitary myxedema not associated with evidence of other pituitary failure or tumor. By 1971, Miyai et al.[29a] noted that although isolated thyrotropin deficiency is rare, at least 17 cases had been reported. These workers considered that some of the cases were doubtful and that only a few had been confirmed by direct determination of TSH. Their own two patients were sisters with nongoitrous cretinism and the offspring of a consanguineous marriage.

Goldman and colleagues[30] observed a unique

case of fractional hypopituitarism with gigantism in a patient who had diabetic responses to intravenous glucose tolerance tests given before and after cortisone replacement therapy. Hypogonadism, hypothyroidism, and hypoadrenocorticism were present in addition to gigantism stemming from increased quantities or effects of growth hormone. In three patients with similar findings, except for absence of hypothyroidism, reported by Sarver and associates,[31] diabetes was not noted.

Houssay and Biasotti[32] demonstrated that the diabetes which followed pancreatectomy in dogs could be alleviated by hypophysectomy. This Houssay phenomenon has been studied extensively in experimental animals but has been observed only infrequently in man. Martin et al.[33] reported in tabular form 24 cases of coexisting diabetes mellitus and pituitary insufficiency, in which the latter was adequately documented by clinical or pathologic studies, or both. Frey[34] reviewed 30 well-documented cases of coexistent diabetes and pituitary insufficiency, and reported one of his own. These patients could be divided into two groups. The first comprised 25 diabetic patients who subsequently developed pituitary insufficiency; the second was made up of 6 patients including his own, in whom the pituitary disease antedated the onset of diabetes. Not included were the large number of patients who were subjected to either surgical or radiation-induced hypophysectomy in the 1960s for the palliation of degenerative complications of diabetes. The case described by Martin and coworkers[33] was somewhat unique in that it was the third one reported in which the pituitary insufficiency preceded the onset of diabetes. The patient experienced the successive development of renal glycosuria, pituitary insufficiency due to postpartum necrosis (Sheehan's syndrome), and finally, diabetes mellitus.

It is not surprising that diabetes mellitus rarely manifests itself in patients who already have pituitary insufficiency with its characteristic features of spontaneous tendency to hypoglycemia, a pronounced sensitivity to insulin, and diminished gluconeogenesis. In a patient with pre-existing hypopituitarism, the diabetes may be so mild that it is recognized only by testing for glucose tolerance.

Successful hypophysectomy performed in the 1960s for proliferative diabetic retinopathy produced marked and easily recognized changes in carbohydrate metabolism. In addition to increased insulin sensitivity, the amount of insulin required usually falls to less than one-third of that needed prior to the operation. Sensitivity to regular insulin can be extreme: as little as 2 to 4 units of regular insulin can produce profound hypoglycemia. The commonly used sliding scale coverage with regular insulin (20 units for 4 + sugar in the urine, 15 units for 3 +, etc.) should never be employed; severe and sometimes fatal hypoglycemia has been a tragic outcome and a major problem in diabetic patients who have undergone hypophysectomy. The insulin sensitivity and amelioration of diabetes are present despite full replacement doses of glucocorticoids, cortisone, etc.

Aside from patients who were subjected to therapeutic hypophysectomy (either by surgery or proton beam), in the Joslin Clinic series only 8 patients with coexistent diabetes mellitus and pituitary insufficiency have been seen.

THE THYROID GLAND

The thyroid gland is related to diabetes by virtue of variations in the levels of the circulating thyroid hormones, thyroxine, (T4) and triiodothyronine (T3). These levels are influenced by the hypothalamic tripeptide releasing factor (TRH),[35] the thyroid stimulating hormone (TSH)[36] from the anterior pituitary gland, the rate of utilization of the hormones by the body tissues,[37] and the amount of iodine available.[38] The pituitary-thyroid axis normally presents a self-regulating hormonal balance comparable to that between the pituitary on the one hand and the gonads or adrenal cortex on the other.

It is well known that serum growth hormone (GH) during normal life, and in response to different stimuli, is increased in juvenile diabetics, and this hypersecretion of GH has been proposed as a factor in diabetic angiopathy. An increased secretion of GH may represent a generalized hypothalamic dysfunction and, in keeping with this, Raptis et al.[35] in 1971 reported increased levels of TSH in juvenile diabetics both under basal conditions and in response to TRH. However, in a later study by Weeke and Hansen,[36] no difference was noted in the basal TSH levels or following TRH, between 49 patients, 24 women and 25 men, with juvenile-onset diabetes and comparable controls. To date there is no convincing evidence that hypothalamic dysfunction, especially in reference to TSH, has any direct effect on diabetes apart from the thyroidal influence.

In addition to TRH and TSH, other thyroid stimulators have been found in Graves' disease. Apart from the long-acting thyroid stimulator (LATS), a variety of other immunoglobulins have been found, all of which ultimately increase the thyroidal production of hormones. The thyroid gland secretes T4 as well as T3, and most of the metabolically active T3 is derived from peripheral monodeiodination of T4. In fasting, acute illness, with use of glucocorticoids and drugs such as propylthiouracil, and in the fetus, the production of T3 may fall and reverse T3 (rT3) may increase.[37] The serum

T4 is normal or slightly decreased, and normal basal and stimulated levels of TSH are found.

In general, these hormones aid in regulating the rate of metabolism, growth, and development of tissues. The effects on carbohydrate metabolism are not always in direct proportion to the extent of alteration of metabolic rate, whether it be elevated (thyrotoxicosis) or depressed (myxedema).

Theories and Experimental Studies in "Thyrodiabetes"

Experimental evidence indicates that hyperthyroidism exacerbates and hypothyroidism may ameliorate certain defects in carbohydrate metabolism (Table 39–1). Although experimental results have often been contradictory, various theories have been proposed to explain the occurrence of diabetes in thyroid overactivity, as listed below.

(1) Increased absorption of hexoses from intestines.
(2) Increased rate of glucose oxidation and utilization
(3) Insulin sensitivity.
(4) Permanent pancreatic damage—"metathyroid diabetes."
(5) Insulin degradation.
(6) Liver damage and glycogen depletion—decreased hepatic glycogenesis and increased glycogenolysis.
(7) Increased availabilty of fatty acids.
(8) Genetic association.

The *absorption of hexoses* from the intestinal tract is increased by thyroid hormone. Althausen and Stockholm[38] noted this alteration in the intestinal absorption of carbohydrates in persons with hyperthyroidism. Further data from Holdsworth and Besser[39] confirmed this observation. The diabetic type of oral glucose curve associated with hyperthyroidism and the flat curve associated with myxedema, may be due to alterations in the absorption of carbohydrate, as normal curves have been observed when patients are given glucose intravenously.[40] However, the data of Spergel et al.[41] suggest that the abnormal values found in glucose tolerance tests in these patients result from factors other than abnormal intestinal glucose absorption.

Glucose Oxidation and Utilization. Thyroid administration presumably causes an increase and acceleration in total energy expenditure of all body metabolites, including carbohydrate. Mirsky and Broh-Kahn[42] demonstrated this in the thyroid-treated eviscerated rabbit. Other investigators have shown that thyroid overactivity produces a variable response in regard to glucose oxidation and utilization. Normal,[43–46] increased,[40,42,47,48] or decreased[49–55] glucose tolerance or utilization has been described in patients and animals with hyperthyroidism. After administration of glucose, the respiratory quotient in the patient with uncomplicated hyperthyroidism rises as much as in the normal subject and possibly more rapidly.[56,57] The response to a test dose of insulin may be enhanced or diminished in animals treated with thyroid.[45,58,59]

Insulin Sensitivity. Patients with hyperthyroidism or hypothyroidism have been found to be equally and markedly sensitive to a test dose of insulin.[60] Other studies have shown insulin sensitivity or tolerance to be normal,[50,61] decreased,[53,62,63] or increased[43,45,64] in thyrotoxic patients or in animal experiments. Results of investigations have also shown increased,[45,53,65,66] decreased,[54,55] or normal[46,64,67] insulin secretion in hyperthyroidism. Wajchenberg et al.[63] found that during continuous glucose infusion, the mean plasma insulin level and the plasma insulin:glucose ratio were significantly higher for the hyperthyroid state during a control period and during the initial 10 minutes of glucose infusion. Afterward, the ratios were similar for both hyper- and eu- thyroid states. Since basal insulin secretion in man can be modulated by the adrenergic nervous system,[68] the increased adrenergic tonus of hyperthyroidism[69] may play an important role in such primary alterations.

Using the euglycemic clamp technique which

Table 39–1. The Thyroid Gland and Diabetes

	Thyrotoxicosis	Control of Thyrotoxicosis
Diabetes	Aggravated	Ameliorated
Blood glucose	Readily elevated	More stable
Glycosuria	Aggravated	Tends to be corrected
Absorption of hexoses from bowel	Rapid	Depressed
Glycogen		
Hepatic	Reduced	Normal or slightly decreased
Muscle	Reduced	Normal or slightly decreased
Protein catabolism	Increased	Normal
Gluconeogenesis	Stimulated	Normal
Need for insulin	Increased	Reduced
Duration of insulin action	Reduced	Prolonged

allows assessment of insulin sensitivity in the absence of stimulated counterregulatory hormone secretion, McCulloch et al.[69a] studied the basal values for glucose, lactate, pyruvate, alanine, serum insulin, and C peptide in hyperthyroid and control subjects. They found elevated levels of glycerol and 3-hydroxybutyrate in the hyperthyroid patients which remained significantly higher despite euglycemia. They suggested that insulin-stimulated glucose metabolism and inhibition of ketogenesis are normal in hyperthyroidism. In the diabetic, the above changes can be markedly altered in the presence of relative insulin lack. Furthermore, the data suggest that insulin sensitivity is normal in the hyperthyroid state.

A study by Olefsky[70] showed that increased insulin secretion would reduce the number of peripheral receptors and might also reduce the hypoglycemic effect of the secreted insulin.

Permanent Pancreatic Damage. Present data regarding insulin secretion and carbohydrate tolerance in the hyperthyroid state are variable. One possible explanation is that thyroid overactivity produces permanent pancreatic damage. In 1921, Holst[71] proposed that there was islet cell injury in hyperthyroidsm. Houssay[72] was able to produce "metathyroid diabetes" in dogs only if the animals had been subjected to subtotal pancreatectomy. Diabetic animals show relative insulin insufficiency with exacerbation of diabetic symptoms as a result of the feeding of thyroid hormone. In normal animals, the administration of thyroid hormone does not produce diabetes. This seems to be the case in man, since Danowski and collaborators[73] failed to produce glucose intolerance in apparently normal human subjects given large amounts, up to 25 grains (1.5 g) of dessicated thyroid daily.

After partial pancreatectomy or the administration of alloxan or anterior pituitary extract, Houssay noted that in animals, thyroid administration either intensified a pre-exising diabetic state or induced diabetes. Under these conditions, beta cell lesions appeared, but might disappear with cessation of thyroid feeding. Houssay termed this reversible stage "thyroid diabetes." However, if the thyroid hormone is administered for many weeks, irreversible degeneration of the beta cells may produce permanent diabetes. This state, as noted above, has been labeled "metathyroid diabetes."[74-76] Thyroidectomy or thiouracil feeding may delay the onset of diabetes in pancreatectomized rats.[77]

Studies of plasma immunoreactive insulin levels in patients with hyperthyroidism and hyperglycemia have revealed levels lower than expected with the degree of blood glucose elevation.[78,79] A late response of insulin secretion was noted, resembling that of early diabetes. In the series of 51 hyperthyroid patients reported by Kreines et al.,[80] glucose tolerance tests continued to show diabetic responses in 30% of the group after hyperthyroidism had been corrected.

Insulin Degradation. Experimental evidence suggests that thyroid hormone accelerates the degradation of insulin in rats[81,82] and man.[45] Elgee and co-workers,[81] using rats, noted that injection of thyroxine or triiodothyronine increased the degradation of insulin-I[131]. Although such degradation seemed to take place in a number of body tissues, the most active sites appeared to be liver and kidney. In the thyrotoxic patient an increased rate of insulin degradation, without a comparable increase in the rate of insulin production, would result in subnormal amounts of available insulin and a decreased rate of glucose utilization. This effect could possibly explain the diabetogenic action of thyroxine in the partially pancreatectomized dog[74] and the increased insulin requirement in the diabetic patient developing thyrotoxicosis. After hypophysectomy and thyroidectomy, insulin degradation is reduced and hypoglycemic reactions may occur with only a fraction of the insulin dose previously required.

Liver Damage. In 1930, Weller[83] reported that among 44 patients with hyperthyroidism, at autopsy 22 showed well-marked, and 16 slight, hepatitis. Much earlier, Farrant[84] noted that thyroid-fed cats and rabbits demonstrated fatty degeneration of the liver, particularly marked around the center of the lobules. In 1930, hepatic lesions associated with exophthalmic goiter in man were discussed in an editorial.[85] In histologic studies of the livers of rats killed after receiving crystalline thyroxine in nonlethal doses, McIver and Winter[86] found that the cells were similar to those of a starved animal. They attributed this to the fact that hepatic glycogen was markedly diminished. John[87] suggested that the factors influencing the glycogen depletion might be due to toxic substances affecting liver cell parenchyma, or to the high metabolic rate which caused increased consumption of carbohydrate and depleted the insulin stores with a resultant depletion of glycogen. Bodansky and Bodansky[88] questioned whether protein stores as well as glycogen, might be hypermetabolized and depleted.

Increased Availability of Fatty Acids. The metabolism of glucose and nonesterified fatty acid (NEFA) has been shown to be related in such a way that either may reduce the oxidation of the other. Randle and associates[89,90] have described this relationship as the glucose-fatty acid cycle and have suggested that an increased availability of fatty acids for oxidation may be responsible for abnormalities in the results of oral glucose tolerance tests in patients with diabetes mellitus and in normal people on a low carbohydrate dict. Elevation of the fasting plasma NEFA concentration has been noted in association with thyrotoxicosis.[91,92] Abnormal oral glucose tolerance in persons with thyrotoxicosis has been ascribed by Hales and Hyams[78] to insulin resistance resulting from a high plasma concentration of free fatty acids. By reversing the abnormal oral glucose tolerance in thyrotoxicosis with guanethidine, Woeber et al.[93] demonstrated that the abnormality was not due to high plasma free fatty acid levels but rather to an inhibition of insulin release associated with increased sympathetic tone or responsiveness.

Genetic Association. Althausen[94] proposed a possible genetic association between diabetes and hyperthyroidism. A high prevalence of diabetes in close relatives of patients with hyperthyroidism was found by Perlman (36%)[95] and by Kreines et al.[80] These prevalences are greater than those observed by Wilkerson and associates[96] in the general population of the study conducted at Oxford, Massachusetts (18.6%), and compare instead with the 38.6% prevalence of positive family histories for diabetes in diabetic patients of the Oxford community. Other evidence for a possible inherited relationship between diabetes and hyperthyroidism includes: (a) the finding of diabetes and hyperthyroidism in identical twins,[97] (b) the increased prevalence of antithyroid antibodies in patients with diabetes,[98,99] and (c) increased prevalence of large babies born to women subsequently developing hyperthyroidism.[80] The hereditary background of diabetes may be a prerequisite in man if hyperthyroidism is to induce diabetes.

Hyperthyroidism

In uncomplicated hyperthyroidism, disorders of carbohydrate metabolism occur frequently but are relatively mild in most cases. The increased incidence of glycosuria accompanying diseases of the thyroid is due fundamentally to hyperthyroidism. Clinical manifestations of diabetes can also be simulated by features of hyperthyroidism—weight loss, alimentary hyperglycemia, glycosuria, impaired glucose tolerance as shown by the oral test, and tendency to ketosis during relatively short periods of fasting. In 500 patients with thyroid disease reported by Joslin and Lahey,[100] the frequency of glycosuria associated with primary hyperthyroidism was 38.6%; with adenomatous goiter (toxic nodular) with hyperthyroidism, 27.7%; and with nontoxic goiter, 14.8%. In a large control sample the incidence of glycosuria was 13.6%. Clinical diabetes was present in 2.5% of those with primary hyperthyroidism and in 4.3% of those having adenomatous goiter with hyperthyroidism.

Frequency of Diabetes in Hyperthyroid Patients. In patients with potential diabetes, thyrotoxicosis was reported by Wilder to produce an earlier appearance of diabetes than would normally be anticipated. On the other hand, Wilder's reported incidence of 3.3% of diabetes in 1882 patients with hyperthyroidism at the Mayo Clinic (1935–1938),[101,102] was far less than the incidence of diabetes noted among patients with acromegaly or Cushing's syndrome. Reports from large clinics regarding diabetes occurring with hyperthyroidism have ranged from 2 to 3.3%. These figures are actually little different from those expected for genetic overt diabetes in the general population. However, the report of Kreines and colleagues[80] indicates a much higher prevalence of diabetes in clinical hyperthyroidism. Glucose intolerance consistent with diabetes was found in 29 of 51 patients (57%) before, and 13 of 44 patients (30%) after, antithyroid treatment. As noted in other series, diabetes was more common in older patients with toxic nodular goiter than in younger ones with Graves' disease. The occurrence of abnormal glucose tolerance could not be related to the degree of thyrotoxicity. A long-term (11.6 years) follow-up study[103] of the same group of patients showed a 32% incidence of glucose intolerance. Of these patients, 72% (5 of 7) had significant glucose intolerance and in 43% of patients, there were histories suggestive of a diabetic diathesis.

The Diagnosis of Diabetes in Hyperthyroidism. Approximately $1\frac{1}{2}$ to 2 times as many people without known diabetes develop glycosuria and/or hyperglycemia in association with hyperthyroidism, as would be expected in the absence of that condition. Variable degrees of restoration of glucose tolerance toward normal levels have been noted after successful treatment of hyperthyroidism in this group. Interpretation of results in this regard depends on the standards used for the degrees of intolerance.

As previously noted, postprandial hyperglycemia and glycosuria may result from increased glucose absorption associated with hyperthyroidism. Hence, one should be less rigid in using the normal standards for glucose tolerance testing in patients with hyperthyroidism. The phenomenon of increased absorption should not, however, affect the fasting levels or the results of tests made on specimens secured 2 to 3 hours after a glucose load if endogenous insulin is adequate. Since slight abnormalities of carbohydrate metabolism may disappear when treatment for hyperthyroidism is given, one must avoid a diagnosis of diabetes and an assumption that a cure has been achieved. New evaluation by means of postprandial blood sugar determinations or glucose tolerance tests with standard criteria is desirable when the patient has recovered from hyperthyroidism.

We accept the concept that hyperthyroidism alone rarely produces diabetes. Any abnormality of carbohydrate metabolism appearing in a patient with hyperthyroidism means that diabetes is present except (a) when glycosuria is present without hyperglycemia, or (b) when transient alimentary hyperglycemia occurs within 1 hour postprandially or following a glucose load. The persistence of hyperglycemia and glycosuria after a patient has become euthyroid always means that the patient has diabetes, unless some other condition is present that could profoundly interfere with utilization of glucose.

Diabetes Complicated by Hyperthyroidism. Before the days of insulin, antithyroid drugs, radioisotope therapy, and modern surgery, the simultaneous presence of diabetes and hyperthyroidism was a catastrophe. One disease accentuated and accelerated the downward course of the other. Disaster is imminent when ketoacidosis and hyperthyroidism occur together. Ketoacidotic coma may develop with unusual rapidity so that early diagnosis and appropriate therapy are imperative from both the thyroid and diabetic standpoints.

Diagnosis of Hyperthyroidism. The presence of hyperthyroidism should be suspected in diabetic patients with or without thyroid enlargement in the presence of unexplained weight loss, supraventricular tachycardia, increased body warmth, heat intolerance, tremor, unexplained increase in insulin requirement, ketoacidosis, instability of the diabetes, prior symptoms of hyperthyroidsm, or thyroid enlargement. In several instances in the Joslin Clinic experience, inadequately explained atrial fibrillation with or without congestive heart failure, or congestive failure alone in the presence of a demonstrable goiter, led to the diagnosis of hyperthyroidism. One man was seen first in diabetic coma with atrial fibrillation. Although he had no palpable goiter, abrupt increase in the severity of his diabetes and unexplained arrhythmia led to the diagnosis of hyperthyroidism after the patient had recovered from coma.

In 5 Joslin-Lahey Clinic cases, Lakin, et al.[104] noted clinical features which aided in the diagnosis of coexisting diabetic ketoacidosis and acute hyperthyroidism. (a) The temperature in patients with diabetic ketoacidosis is usually normal or subnormal, and remains normal with correction of metabolic abnormalities unless underlying infection is present. However, 3 of the 5 patients of Lakin et al. entered the hospital with an elevated temperature and the remaining two developed fever following correction of the ketoacidosis. (b) Whereas the pulse is usually rapid during ketoacidosis and

becomes normal following its treatment, all 5 of these patients had tachycardia on admission and this persisted despite overcoming of the ketoacidosis. (c) Failure of the tachycardia to respond to adequate digitalization in 2 of the patients prompted thyroid studies. Examination revealed diffusely enlarged thyroid glands in 4 of the patients and a multinodular gland in the 5th. Three patients exhibited exophthalmos, and all gave adequate histories suggestive of hyperthyroidism.

In a review of our more recent experience[105] in 70 patients with diabetes and hyperthyroidism, 9 presented with the disease in masked form. They had experienced severe weight loss and in 5, atrial fibrillation was present. In the group as a whole, the main symptoms were weight loss, palpitation, "nervousness," sweating, and heat intolerance. Deterioration in control of diabetes occurred in 28 of 48 patients on insulin and in 4 of 22 patients on oral hypoglycemic agents. The insulin requirement was increased in 11 patients with a mean increase of 50%. There was no relationship between the severity of the hyperthyroidism and the degree of change in diabetic control. With treatment of the hyperthyroid state, the insulin requirement decreased in 13 patients by a mean of 35%. The diabetic control improved on the average within 10 to 14 days (range 7 to 30 days).

The standard measurements of thyroid function are still useful in the diagnosis of the hyperthyroid state. However, recent data suggest that the turnover of thyroid hormones may be depressed in the poorly-controlled diabetic. Postellon and Foley[106] described a clear correlation of T3 levels to serum pH and the bicarbonate ion level in patients with untreated insulin-dependent diabetes mellitus. The T3 values before and after treatment with insulin rose from 80 ± 118 ng/dL (mean $\pm$ SEM) to 119 ± 5.7 ng/dL. Pittman et al.[107] reported T3 levels of 91 ± 18 ng/dL (mean $\pm$ SD) in 5 patients with poorly-controlled diabetes compared to 126 ± 23 ng/dL in the normal control group. Pittman[108] also showed a rise in the T3 values from 44 ± 26 ng/dL to 113 ± 34 ng/dL in diabetics before and after insulin therapy. Control value in nondiabetics was 173 ± 37 ng/dL.

Furthermore, there are reports now of altered thyroid hormone metabolism in diabetic ketoacidosis. Low serum T3 and elevated reverse T3 (rT3) have been found. Serum T3 levels have been correlated directly with the metabolic clearance rate of glucose and inversely with plasma ketone concentration. This alteration of peripheral thyroid hormone metabolism could decrease the level of serum T3 and result in normal or low T3 levels, thus masking thyrotoxicosis during diabetic ketoacidosis. A case report by Mayfield et al.[109] illustrates this well. Until larger series are reviewed and reported, the currently available tests are still the best way of making the diagnosis, aided by good clinical judgment.

Treatment. Once the diagnosis of hyperthyroidism has been established, treatment is started to improve the patient's general condition and to achieve the euthyroid state. In addition to increased insulin need, the most important factor from the standpoint of diabetic management is liberalization of the diet to correct the weight loss and debilitation that frequently occurs with hyperthyroidism. For all such patients, the diabetic diet should contain at least 2,000 to 2,500 calories per day with ample protein content, i.e., 90 to 100 g or more daily.

Sudden variations in carbohydrate metabolism may take place in association with changing output of thyroid hormone. Treatment with long-acting insulin should be continued and the dose increased by 10 to 20% every 2 days if tests consistently show glycosuria. Supplementary regular insulin should be used in amounts of 10 to 20% of the usual morning dosage and should be administered before the noon and evening meals in accordance with the results of blood glucose tests or of urine test on second morning voidings. Except in patients with stable diabetes, strict control with insistence upon sugar-free specimens, is unwise. With improvement under antithyroid treatment and reduction in the rate of metabolism, the daily insulin requirement may fall abruptly as the euthyroid state is approached. This abrupt fall increases the chance of severe hypoglycemic reactions and should be anticipated and avoided.

At the Joslin Clinic, all diabetic patients with hyperthyroidism are currently being treated with propylthiouracil unless evidence of toxic response to this drug is noted in which case the second agent of choice, methimazole (Tapazole), is employed. Propylthiouracil has been given orally in doses of 100 to 250 mg every 8 hours with good response. Reactions to the drug are idiosyncratic in nature and not dose-related. No increased incidence of toxicity has been noted with increased dosage.

Euthyroid status is usually achieved in 8 weeks on this program. In order to diminish the vascularity of the hyperplastic thyroid gland induced by propylthiouracil therapy, the daily administration of 10 drops of Lugol's solution is begun 10 to 14 days before the time scheduled for thyroidectomy if such is planned. The purpose of iodine therapy is to give the surgeon at operation as firm and avascular a gland as possible. Lugol's solution is unnecessary for the patient with a toxic nodular goiter with hyperthyroidism. In fact, the use of iodine in these patients will exacerbate the hyperthyroid state.

Beta blockade can be useful to control symptoms in the initial treatment phase in severe cases.

If radioactive iodine (I^{131}) treatment seems indicated, it can be instituted at this time when the patient is euthyroid. In the latest series of patients,[105] 30 received therapeutic doses of I^{131}, and 16 underwent surgery. In 12 patients, hypothyroidism developed within 2 to 12 months after I^{131} was used and the possibility of increased sensitivity was raised to I^{131} of glands in these patients. The higher incidence of thyroid microsomal and colloid antibody has been recently reported in a group of insulin-dependent diabetics.[99] It may be that some of the patients with hyperthyroidism had Hashimoto's thyroiditis with hyperthyroidism and thus were more likely to develop hypothyroidism.

Antithyroid medication alone on a long-term basis has had limited use in the Joslin Clinic. Recently it has been reported that short-term oral antithyroid treatment can be successful. However, further long-term follow-up is needed to assess this.

As noted earlier, the use of I^{131} is becoming more popular and is now the treatment of choice in patients over 40 years of age and in those with recurrence of hyperthyroidism following surgery.

Results of I^{131} therapy for toxic nodular goiter with secondary hyperthyroidism are highly variable and are less predictable than with Graves' disease. Multiple doses of I^{131} are frequently required to achieve the euthyroid state.

Frequency of Hyperthyroidism in Diabetic Patients. In a series of diabetics seen at the Joslin Clinic between 1928 and 1965, 604 cases of hyperthyroidism occurred, representing an incidence of about 1.1%. In evaluating this figure, allowance must be made for errors in diagnosis, for readmissions, and for the fact that hyperthyroidism may have developed subsequent to observations.

If the time of onset of either diabetes or hyperthyroidism could be definitely determined, significant conclusions might be drawn as to the part played by one in producing the other. At one time, it appeared that the exact onset of diabetes was fairly easily determined, but its insidious appearance, especially in adults, with long intervals when symptoms may be absent or minimal, has made definite timing difficult. The earlier series of diabetics from predominantly surgical clinics indicated the prior appearance of primary hyperthyroidism in 75 to 85% of patients and of toxic nodular goiter with secondary hyperthyroidism, in 47 to 62%. In diabetics, Regan and Wilder[110] reported the prior appearance of primary hyperthyroidism in 52% and of toxic nodular goiter in 62%. In the Lahey Clinic series of diabetics,[111] the appearance of primary hyperthyroidism before diabetes was noted in 54%; toxic nodular goiter preceded the onset of diabetes in 68%.

In the 1951–1957 Joslin series, only 6 of 86 diabetics developed hyperthyroidism prior to the onset of diabetes. Diabetes preceded primary hyperthyroidism in 66% of the patients and toxic nodular goiter in 67%. Simultaneous onset was noted in 23 patients. In the more recent series of 70 patients (1965–1973),[105] the diabetes preceded the hyperthyroidism in all but 7, who had a simultaneous onset. Diabetic heredity was noted in only 10% of this group, whereas earlier series had a 42% positivity. Bowen and Lenzner[112] found diabetic heredity in 55% of diabetics with primary hyperthyroidism and in 40% of diabetics having toxic nodular goiter.

Age of Diabetics with Hyperthyroidism. In general, in the diabetic, primary hyperthyroidism occurs and is treated 15 to 20 years earlier than is toxic nodular goiter with hyperthyroidism. In studies of diabetics with primary hyperthyroidism, the age range was 16 to 65 years; in those with toxic nodular goiter with hyperthyroidism, it was 21 to 71 years.

Sex Incidence in Diabetics with Hyperthyroidism. Many more female than male diabetics are found to have hyperthyroidism. In the 1951–1957 Joslin series, of the 55 patients with primary hyperthyroidism, 41 (75%) were women. Among 31 patients with adenomatous goiter and hyperthyroidism, 27 (87%) were women.

Hypothyroidism and Diabetes Mellitus

Data supporting a possible autoimmune basis for diabetes mellitus and various endocrine diseases[113] have led to the clinician's active search for hypothyroidism in diabetic patients and to treatment of such when found. In the past, the association of diabetes with primary hypothyroidism was noted rarely at the Joslin Clinic. From 1897 through October, 1957, among approximately 50,000 patients, only 15 cases of spontaneous myxedema were recognized (others may well have been overlooked). The patients were mainly those in whom the diagnosis of myxedema was based on clinical signs, basal metabolic rate, and cholesterol determinations. Twelve were females and 3 males. Five of the females were juveniles, 3 of whom showed features of juvenile myxedema. These 3 had diabetic coma prior to treatment with thyroid extract. The onset of myxedema was manifested in only 4 of the 15 prior to discovery of diabetes. In 1 patient, the possibility of much earlier onset of myxedema was considered but never confirmed. From October, 1957 through September, 1965, an additional 52 cases of primary hypothyroidism (0.24%) were diagnosed among 21,500 "new" diabetic patients.

The possibility that some of the cases were instances of pituitary myxedema cannot be evaluated since responses to thyrotropic hormone, adrenal function tests, and gonadotropin assays were not determined except in the patients seen during the latter part of this period. Known hypothyroidism antedated the diabetes in 10 of the 52 patients.

From a review of the literature, Rupp and associates collected 33 cases and added 2 of their own patients.[114] Baron published 4 cases.[115] Lawrence stated that he had seen both diseases in combination in only "some 50 cases."[116] Hecht and Gershberg found 9 hypothyroid patients among 530 diabetics, a prevalence of 1.7%.[117] In a more recent assessment of the Joslin Clinic experience[118] from 1957 to 1972, 114 cases of primary hypothyroidism were found in 60,073 patients (incidence of 0.19%) (see Table 39–2). This suggests that the two diseases occur together more often than their individual frequencies would indicate. The incidence of spontaneous primary myxedema among total hospital admissions in various large hospitals has been reported to be 0.01% to 0.08%.[119] However, hypothyroidism of varying degrees short of myxedema occurs more frequently. This is more likely to be the by-product of the treatment of Graves' disease or the result of Hashimoto's thyroiditis.

It has been postulated that patients treated with sulfonylureas have a higher frequency of hypothyroidism than those treated with insulin or diet alone.[120] These results have been questioned by other workers.[121] Burdick's studies have shown that treatment with sulfonylureas lowers the protein-bound iodine (PBI) significantly as compared to a matched group treated with diet and insulin or diet alone. This effect is most pronounced with carbutamide (not used clinically in the U.S.A.), but is not seen with tolbutamide in which the amino group is replaced by a methyl group. Furthermore, the doses of sulfonylureas used in the treatment of diabetes are too low to have significant anti-thyroid effects. In the study by Portioli and Rocchi,[122] in 200 patients treated with tolbutamide and followed from 1 to 7 years, thyroid function tests suggested hypothyroidism in 3%, although clinically none of the patients was hypothyroid. At the Joslin Clinic a survey revealed that among approximately 9000 diabetic patients who had ever received "first generation" sulfonylureas, very few—only 14 (0.15%)—had developed hypothyroidism.

As mentioned earlier, both hypothyroidism and diabetes have autoimmune features. Primary hypothyroidism in most instances is due to thyroid atrophy secondary to chronic lymphocyte thyroiditis, a disease that has an autoimmune basis. The presence of thyroid antibodies has been reported in from 8 to 22% of juvenile diabetic patients.[99,123,124]

In a group of 400 diabetic patients, the highest incidence of thyroid autoantibodies was found in young persons with long-term insulin-dependent diabetes.[125] In the Joslin study,[118] 36% of the 99 diabetic patients who later become hypothyroid had had the onset of diabetes before the age of 30 years (Table 39–2b).

The higher frequency of thyroid antibodies in diabetics as well as other evidence suggests an autoimmune basis for diabetes. "Insulitis" or lymphocytic infiltration has been found in the pancreatic islets of juvenile[126] and adult[127] diabetics and has also been found in animals with experimental diabetes. Autoantibodies to endogenous insulin have been noted[128] and the association of diabetes with Addison's disease[129] and pernicious anemia[130] further suggests an underlying autoimmune problem.

Diabetes mellitus in association with congenital cretinism has been reported only rarely.[114,131] Glick's patient,[131] a 34-year-old woman with cretinism since infancy and diabetes since age 7½, was found to be free of degenerative complications after 27 years of marked hyperglycemia, hypercholesterolemia, and frequent insulin reactions. One Joslin Clinic patient with mongolism and cretinism since birth, had had diabetes for 13 years without evidence of degenerative complications when lost to follow-up at age 26. The Joslin Clinic series includes 2 patients with long-term diabetes and juvenile myxedema. One woman, with onset of diabetes at age 9 and of myxedema at an undetermined time before that, developed moderate proliferating retinopathy, renal insufficiency, hypertension, and cardiac decompensation 25 years after the onset of diabetes. Another patient whose diabetes preceded the myxedema by 2 years, had minimal retinopathy 21 years after the onset of diabetes at age 10 years.

Although untreated myxedema may reduce the severity of diabetes and insulin requirements, it does not preclude the occurrence of severe uncontrolled diabetes, ketoacidosis, and coma. Adequate treatment of myxedema will lead to the reappearance of the same severity of the metabolic state that was present prior to the onset of myxedema.

From a clinical standpoint, the presentation of hypothyroidism does not appear to be different in diabetic, as compared to nondiabetic, persons. Since the advent of serum thyroid stimulating hormone (TSH) measurements, many patients are being diagnosed before they develop symptoms or signs.

A difficult problem in differential diagnosis is that of distinguishing the myxedematous patient

Table 39–2. Characteristics of 114 Patients with Associated Diabetes and Hypothyroidism (Joslin Clinic experience, 1957–72)*

Table 2a. Sex Distribution and Presenting Diagnosis

First Diagnosis	Female	Male	Total
Diabetes mellitus	72	22	94
Hypothyroidism	15	0	15
Concurrent	4	1	5
	91	23	114

Table 2b. Age of Patients at Diagnosis of First Disease

Age, yr.	Diabetes Female	Male	Hypothyroidism (All Female)
1–9	5	4	0
10–19	7	3	3
20–29	12	5	2
30–39	10	3	6
40–49	14	3	2
50–59	13	4	2
60–69	8	0	0
70–79	3	0	0

Table 2c. Decrease in Insulin Requirement in 59 of 78 Insulin-Taking Patients Following Development of Hypothyroidism

Decrease in Total Insulin, %	No. of Patients
10	30
10–24	9
25–49	15
50–74	4
75–100	1
	59

*Adapted from Ganz and Kozak.[118]

from the diabetic patient with nephropathy. In addition to becoming more sensitive to insulin and requiring smaller doses, the diabetic who develops nephropathy may have physical findings similar to those of myxedema, i.e., a "slowed-down" manner with facial puffiness and pallor. In addition, failing kidney function tends to distort the results of some thyroid function tests. A combination of tests is again most informative, namely, serum thyroxine (T4), determination of protein-binding capacity of thyroid hormones by resin uptake of triiodothyronine (T3 uptake), and determination of 24-hour radioactive iodine (RAI) uptake. The serum thyroxine is low in both myxedema and nephropathy. Proteinuria results in loss of serum proteins, including thyroxine-binding globulin. In myxedema, the T3 uptake is low, whereas in patients with diabetic nephropathy, it is usually high. In the patients with chronic renal disease, RAI uptake tends to fall to low normal and borderline levels rather than remain in a definitely normal range.

As noted above, the serum TSH assay and T4 level are now used in making the diagnosis. The serum TSH is elevated before any change appears in the serum thyroxine levels. In patients with renal disease, the TSH and free T4 levels are still reliable indices of the thyroid state.

Diabetic patients who develop hypothyroidism are subject to hypoglycemic reactions but not to the same extent as those with primary or secondary adrenal insufficiency. In the Joslin Clinic experience referred to above, only 6 of 78 patients with hypothyroidism (see Table 39–2C) had severe hypoglycemic reactions, and in these, the low blood glucose levels may have been due to delay in the absorption of carbohydrate or a slower rate of insulin degradation or both. After replacement with thyroid medication, no significant increase in insulin requirement was noted.

Miscellaneous Thyroid Disorders

It is of historical interest that in the Joslin Clinic 1951–1957 series of diabetic patients, those with nontoxic goiter numbered at least 327 (Table 39–3), of whom 23 eventually had thyroidectomies. The total number of diabetics with goiter,

Table 39–3. Thyroid Conditions (Excluding Myxedema) in 18,439 Diabetic Patients Admitted to New England Deaconess Hospital Joslin Clinic Experience, 1951–57 series

	No. Cases	Patients Operated Upon
Primary hyperthyroidism	55	38*
Adenomatous goiter with hyperthyroidism	31	18†
Adenomatous goiter without hyperthyroidism	327	23
Chronic thyroiditis	4	4
Hürthle cell adenoma (one with subacute thyroiditis)	3	3
Fibrosarcoma	1	1
Carcinoma	2	2
Total	423	89

*Bilateral subtotal thyroidectomy
†Bilateral subtotal thyroidectomy, 13; hemi-subtotal thyroidectomy, 4; excision of adenoma, 1.

Note: Of the 55 patients with primary hyperthyroidism, 14 were male and 41 female. The average age at onset of diabetes was 30 yr. and at surgery, 36 yr.

Of the 31 patients with adenomatous goiter with hyperthyroidism, 4 were male and 27 female. The average age at onset of diabetes was 49 yr., and at surgery, 60 yr.

exclusive of those having malignant thyroid disease, was 420, or 2.3% of the diabetics admitted to the Deaconess Hospital in this period. Correcting for readmissions, an approximate figure of goiter frequency would be 3.4%. Women again predominated. The prevalence of goiter in diabetics varied considerably according to the region from which the patient came, but undoubtedly goiter was present much more frequently than the above figure indicates. Often the diagnosis is not recorded when thyroid enlargement is clearly not associated with hyperthyroidism or malignant disease and the patient's treatment revolves about diabetes or another condition. Skouby[132] in Denmark, found goiter in 10% of women and 1% of men with diabetes. In diabetics followed for a number of years, Ralli and associates[133] discovered enlarged thyroid glands in 17%, indicating the increasing incidence of goiter in diabetics under observation for many years.

THE ADRENALS AND DIABETES

Clinical disorders involving either the adrenal cortex or the adrenal medulla have important relationships with diabetes. The role of the adrenal cortex in homeostasis is attested to by the inability of the adrenalectomized animal or patient with Addison's disease to cope with the stresses of the environment. In the absence of the pituitary gland, the adrenal cortex becomes inert, at least from the standpoint of glucocorticoid production.

Adrenal Cortex

The most important product of the human adrenal cortex is hydrocortisone (cortisol) which is secreted only in response to stimulation by corticotropin (ACTH). The secretion of ACTH is reciprocally controlled by increases and decreases in cortisol. Most of the other adrenocortical hormones may be regarded as by-products of cortisol since the quantities normally secreted are only weakly active in suppressing pituitary ACTH secretion and in correcting the effects of adrenalectomy. Valuable information concerning the integrity of the pituitary-adrenal axis can be obtained simply by determining plasma cortisol levels and interpreting the results with respect to normal diurnal variations or by determining the quantity of cortisol metabolites (17-hydroxycorticoids) excreted in the urine. Even more useful and informative data can be obtained by studying the effects which certain manipulations of pituitary or adrenal activity have upon plasma or urinary corticoids. The most instructive tests are: (a) adrenocortical reserve (exogenous ACTH stimulation)—capacity to secrete cortisol in response to a standardized infusion of ACTH; (b) pituitary reserve (endogenous ACTH stimulation by metyrapone)—capacity to secrete endogenous corticotropin in response to a reduction in cortisol secretion and lysine vasopressin, probably acting directly on either hypothalamus or anterior pituitary gland to release corticotropin, and (c) pituitary adrenal suppressibility (dexamethasone suppression)—evaluated by decreased endogenous cortisol secretion in response to cortisol-like agents. Aldosterone, the principal electrolyte-regulating hormone of the adrenal cortex, is not significantly regulated by the ACTH governing cortisol secretion.

Adrenocortical Hypofunction (Addison's Disease). Bilateral destruction of adrenocortical secretory tissue results in diminished circulating cortisol. A compensatory increase in corticotropin secretion occurs, and, if there is any remnant of adrenocortical tissue, it is stimulated to maximal secretory activity so that attempts to increase cortisol secretion further by means of corticotropin are futile. Before attaining the final stage of chronic adrenal cortical insufficiency, the patient with Addison's disease may live through periods of less apparent hormonal deficiency. Although the typical brownish pigmentation rarely may be absent, manifestations such as asthenia, weight loss, hypotension, gastrointestinal symptoms, and hypoglycemic episodes may lead to the diagnosis of Addison's disease at an early and treatable stage.

Helpful diagnostic aids and clues include fasting hypoglycemia, microcardia, active or inactive pulmonary tuberculosis, adrenal calcification, increased circulating eosinophils, neutropenia with relative lymphocytosis, a tendency for mild azotemia, hyponatremia, hyperkalemia, and a reduced baseline urinary excretion of 17-ketosteroids and 17-hydroxycorticoids. Complete adrenal insufficiency implies that both the basal production of adrenal hormone and the adrenal reserve function are insufficient. In the partial form of adrenal insufficiency, the basal urinary steroid excretion may be in the low normal range, but there are inadequate adrenal reserves as judged by standard ACTH stimulation tests. Normal subjects show an increase in the 17-hydroxycorticoid urinary excretion by 5 to 25 mg on the first day of ACTH infusion and by 15 to 40 mg on the second day of infusion. The test may be repeated on several successive days if there is a question of adrenal insufficiency secondary to a lack of pituitary endogenous ACTH. The oral glucose tolerance test may show a flat curve because of delayed absorption of glucose. The intravenous glucose tolerance test is hazardous since in nondiabetics, it may be followed by severe hypoglycemia or precipitate acute adrenal insufficiency with hyperpyrexia.

A striking clinical feature in diabetic patients who develop Addison's disease is the increased sensitivity to insulin. This leads to decreased insulin requirement and frequent hypoglycemic reactions. It is well known that in bilaterally adrenalectomized animals, the rate of protein breakdown is decreased and amino acids are diverted to protein synthesis rather than to gluconeogenesis. In the absence of glucocorticoids, the decreased rate of gluconeogenesis is accompanied by a decreased hepatic store of carbohydrate which may be responsible for the increased insulin sensitivity and tendency to hypoglycemia. The diagnosis of adrenal insufficiency, primary or secondary (pituitary), should be suspected when a diabetic patient experiences a decreased insulin requirement or frequent unexplained insulin-induced hypoglycemic reactions. When adrenocortical insufficiency is superimposed on diabetes, the latter is, in a sense, ameliorated with improvement in carbohydrate tolerance. Although the insulin requirement is decreased, the diabetes frequently is more unstable and difficult to manage, particularly from the standpoint of hypoglycemia.

Coexisting Addison's Disease and Diabetes. Addison's disease occurs with a number of other endocrine abnormalities, including hypothyroidism, but the most common association is with diabetes mellitus. This has been the subject of extensive reviews by Stanton and co-workers;[134] Gittler et al.;[135] Beaven and associates;[136] Wehrmacher;[137] Carpenter and co-workers;[129] and by Solomon and colleagues.[138] The last-named review (published in 1965) listed 40 references in a report of 113 cases of coexisting Addison's disease and diabetes.

Joslin Clinic Experience. Yoo and Kazak[139] reported that during the 25-year period from 1949 to 1973, Addison's disease was diagnosed in 19 cases (0.032%) among 59,179 diabetic patients of the Joslin Clinic. By 1982, 12 more instances of coexisting diabetes and Addison's disease were diagnosed, bringing the total to 31 (0.034%) among approximately 90,000 diabetic patients. As may be seen in Table 39–4, 27 of these 31 had developed insulin-dependent diabetes prior to the diagnosis of Addison's disease. In 4 patients, Addison's disease antedated the diagnosis of diabetes. There were 21 females and 10 males. A family history of diabetes was noted in 16 of the 31 (52%). The age at onset of diabetes was between 3 and 63 years and of Addison's disease, between 10 and 64 years. The time between the development of diabetes mellitus and of Addison's disease ranged from 1 to 38 years. The time between onset of symptoms and date of established diagnosis of Addison's was, in the majority of patients, less than 1 year. Two patients had previously undergone subtotal thyroidectomy for hyperthyroidism. In 5 patients, Schmidt's syndrome (Addison's disease and primary hypothy-

Table 39–4. Patients with Diabetes and Addison's Disease Experience of the Joslin Clinic, 1949–79

Patient No.	Sex	Age at Onset of:		Family History of Diabetes	Insulin Dose before Addison's Disease (Units/day)	Insulin dose after Addison's Disease (Units/day)
		Diabetes (years)	Addison's Disease (years)			
1	F	27	41	−	40	18
2	F	7	27	−	40	30
3	M	30	54	−	50	18
4	M	3	10	+	44	12
5	M	16	32	−	50	30
6	M	53	61	+	16	0
7	M	14	17	+	28	28
8	F	22	49	+	40	30
9	M	10	21	+	70	30
10	F	63	64	+	35	0
11	F	30	39	−	26	8
12	F	6	16*	+	75	28
13	F	47	40	+	†	†
14	M	18	19	−	28	22
15	F	26	43	−	28	18
16	F	30	46	+	14	3
17	F	5	9	−	16	6
18	F	21	31	+	55	11
19	F	4	13	+	30	22
20	F	25	38*	+	32	10
21	F	22	43	−	55	19
22	F	38	48	−	40	30
23	M	43	40	−	†	†
24	F	10	48	−	16	3
25	M	18	16	−	†	†
26	F	38	63*	+	35	15
27	F	28	36	−	56	50
28	F	20	52	+	40	16
29	F	11	30*	+	40	6
30	M	11	16*	+	36	26
31	F	38	34	−	†	†

*Schmidt's syndrome (primary thyroid and adrenocortical insufficiency).
†Addison's disease was diagnosed *before* diabetes (see respective ages at onset in columns 3 and 4 of table).
From Yoo and Kozak[139] with permission of publisher.

roidism) was noted. Of the 31 patients, marked insulin sensitivity and severe reactions occurred in 28.

Weakness and weight loss were found in all patients. Thirty of 31 showed pigmentation of the skin and mucosa. In 1 female, pigment changes of the labia had been first noted on pelvic examination 3 years before the diagnosis of Addison's disease. Hypotension (systolic pressure below 90 mm Hg) was found in 28 of the patients. Patients frequently complained of gastrointestinal symptoms with nausea and vomiting, and amenorrhea was common in females.

The association of the two diseases has been noted to occur in childhood.[134,140] In fact, 3 of our 31 diabetic patients developed Addison's at ages 9, 10, and 13 years, respectively, as well as 3 others at 16, 17, and 19 years of age. No definite genetic relationship was noted in hereditary Addison's disease and diabetes by Sunder and associates.[141]

Clinical Studies. The onset of diabetes in a patient with Addison's disease was intensively studied by Thorn and Clinton,[141a] who emphasized the modifying effect of each disease on the other. In their patient, the administration of a single 33-mg dose of cortisone was followed by a loss of glucose tolerance. An increase in urinary sodium and chloride excretion was noted when 33 mg of cortisone and 8 units of regular insulin were given daily. No increase in potassium excretion was observed on this program, whereas a striking increase in potassium excretion accompanied insulin withdrawal. Elevated fasting blood glucose values were noted when cortisone was administered, and the patient's subsequent hypoglycemic states were checked by use of cortisone.[142] From the study of this patient, it appeared that the inability of patients with uncomplicated Addison's disease to maintain an adequate fasting blood glucose level is not dependent solely upon deficiency of adrenal cortical hormone. Increased gluconeogenesis was observed without any increase in adrenal cortical hormone when diabetes supervened.

Gittler and associates[135] noted that in 2 patients, the intensification of adrenal insufficiency produced when diabetes was present as a second complication, could be corrected only partly by administering larger doses of glycocorticoids and mineralocorticoids. In contrast to the improvement in carbohydrate metabolism that occurs when adrenal insufficiency develops in a diabetic, the development of diabetes in a patient with previously well-controlled Addison's disease is characterized by an apparent exacerbation of the adrenal insufficiency. Increasing the glucocorticoid steroid does not correct the abnormality and may actually magnify it by augmenting the glycosuria. Large doses of mineralocorticoids are likewise relatively ineffective in preventing further losses of salt and water. After appropriate treatment with diet and insulin for diabetes has been initiated, the steroid requirement returns to its former level.

The relative time of development of diabetes and Addison's disease is quite variable, judging from reported series. In 2 of the 3 patients studied by Gittler et al.[135] Addison's disease preceded the development of the diabetic state by 15 and 9 years, respectively. Beaven and associates[136] collected data on 63 cases of Addison's disease coexisting with diabetes, including 8 of their own. In 37 of these patients, diabetes preceded Addison's disease; in 21, Addison's disease preceded diabetes; and in 5, the disorders seemed to appear simultaneously. In those patients in whom Addison's disease developed first, the average interval was 3 years before the onset of diabetes, but this was variable and may have been provoked by cortisone replacement therapy. Of the 37 patients in whom diabetes had developed first, 4 also had thyrotoxicosis and 1 had hypothyroidism.

In the 1965 review of Solomon et al.[128] referred to earlier, among 113 patients with coexisting Addison's disease and diabetes, diabetes preceded Addison's disease in 63%, Addison's disease preceded diabetes in 23%, simultaneous onset was noted in 10%, and sequence was not specified in the remaining 4% of the patients. The interval between the apparent onset of the two diseases was less than a year in 20% of the patients. In those in whom the onset of the two diseases was more than one year apart, the average interval was six years. The etiologic basis of Addison's disease in this concurrent diabetic group was idiopathic atrophy of the adrenals in 74%, tuberculosis in 22%, neoplasm in 2%, and other conditions in 2%. Patients with idiopathic Addison's disease showed a higher coincidence of diabetes and/or thyroid dysfunction than did those with the tuberculous type of the disease.

In 1926, Schmidt[142a] described 2 patients with nontuberculous Addison's disease and chronic lymphocytic thyroiditis. Although neither of these patients had clinical signs of thyroid insufficiency, Schmidt postulated that such would have occurred had not the adrenal insufficiency ended their lives. In a review of Schmidt's syndrome by Carpenter and co-workers,[179] 15 new cases were reported, including 10 instances of co-existent diabetes. Thirteen of the 15 patients had circulating antibodies against thyroid tissue and 9 had antibodies against adrenal tissue. It was suggested that Schmidt's syndrome co-existing with diabetes may represent a polyendocrinopathy occurring on an immunologic basis and thus may fit into the galaxy of "autoimmune disorders." In 1978, Nelson et al.[143] reported a case of Schmidt's syndrome in an 11-year-old girl who died 2 years after diagnosis in fulminant diabetic ketoacidosis.

Irvine and colleagues[144] state that diabetes occurs in about 12% of patients with idiopathic Addison's disease, a frequency which considerably exceeds that in the general population. In their experience, more than 80% have insulin-requiring diabetes (Type I) and the age at diagnosis of the two disorders correlates closely. They note that the mean age at diagnosis is approximately 30 years and the sex distribution is about equal. The similar age at onset and the increased prevalence of islet cell antibodies in these patients again suggests a common pathogenesis.

Prognosis. In the past, as recorded in the older literature, the prognosis in patients with both diabetes mellitus and Addison's disease was poor. In Wehrmacher's follow-up[137] of 31 cases through 1961, 19 patients were dead in 1 year (61%), and after 5 years, 30 patients were dead (93.6%). A slightly improved life expectancy was noted in the 1965 study by Solomon and associates[138] in which 50% of the patients died within 1 year. Still greater improvement in outcome was reported in 1969 from the Mayo Clinic.[145] Among 24 patients, 14 (58%) were alive at 1 year and of patients for whom sufficient information was available, 38% (9) were alive at 4 years after the dual diagnosis. In the Joslin Clinic series of 19 patients diagnosed in the period from 1949 to 1973,[139] 13 were still alive and in good health. The longest period of survival after dual diagnosis was 25 years. There were 6 deaths of which 4 occurred in Addisonian crisis due to (1) a short course of nausea and vomiting with no parenteral steroid used; (2) patient with psychologic instability who omitted medication; (3) one who had metastatic pulmonary carcinoma; and (4) one who developed meningo-encephalitis, generalized septicemia, and abscesses with Candida involvement of brain, lungs, and kidneys. A fifth patient developed acute appendicitis and adrenal insufficiency; the sixth died apparently in an Addisonian crisis while being transported to a hospital.

Adrenocortical Hyperfunction. Secretion of excessive quantities of ACTH by an inappropriately overactive pituitary gland induces adrenocortical hyperplasia and excessive secretion of cortisol. Secretion of supraphysiologic amounts of cortisol by adrenocortical tumor suppresses ACTH secretion, in addition to inducing features of Cushing's syndrome. The non-tumorous adrenocortical tissue ceases to secrete cortisol and becomes hypoplastic and unresponsive to ACTH. The most favorable lesion is the unilateral adenoma, in that its removal permits gradual recovery of normal pituitary adrenal function. Removal of pituitary adenoma (microadenectomy) has been reported to be curative.[146,147] This exciting approach negates the need for removal of adrenal tissue. It remains to be seen whether long-term follow-up will confirm the permanency of these favorable results or whether pituitary adenomas might recur because of possible "hypothalamic overdrive."

The ability of adrenocortical secretion to initiate or augment diabetes mellitus in man is noted in patients with Cushing's syndrome and allied disorders (Table 39–5).[148,153]

Lukens and co-workers[148] reported that, among 55 patients with proven tumor or hyperplasia of the adrenal cortex, carbohydrate tolerance was impaired in 49% and well-marked glycosuria was present in 35%. Even more striking are the patients with tumor or hyperplasia associated with chronic hyperglycemia and glycosuria in which the hyperglycemia and glycosuria disappeared completely following subtotal or total resection of adrenocortical tissue. While hyperglycemia can be initiated

by extracts of the anterior pituitary gland, adrenal cortex, and thyroid gland, it is probable that the resulting damage to the pancreas, or underlying genetic predisposition, is responsible for any permanent diabetic conditon. Furthermore, the clinical use of ACTH or cortisone does not result in significant, permanent impairment of carbohydrate tolerance. According to Bookman and associates,[154] diabetes develops in less than 1% of patients given ACTH or cortisone continuously for therapeutic reasons.

Cushing's Syndrome. Cushing's syndrome refers to the constellation of clinical and biochemical signs and symptoms resulting from prolonged exposure to increased amounts of cortisol (glucocorticoids). Characteristic features include truncal obesity, "buffalo hump," "moon" and plethoric facies, purple striae, easy bruisability, poor wound healing, hypertension, impaired glucose tolerance, osteoporosis, asthenia, mental aberrations, hirsutism, and acne. The excess glucocorticoids promote gluconeogenesis from protein sources. In Cushing's syndrome, the protein of lymphatic tissue, skin, bone, and muscle is mobilized and transported to the liver where it is converted to glucose. This process explains the classical skin striae, ecchymoses, muscular weakness, and wasting characteristic of the syndrome. This high gluconeogenetic rate results also in impaired exogenous glucose intolerance and may lead to overt, clinical diabetes, particularly in patients with a diabetogenetic predisposition.

The syndrome may be classified clinically as shown in Table 39–6.

The availability of oral steroid replacement therapy beginning in the early 1950s elevated total bilateral adrenalectomy to the treatment of choice for patients with Cushing's syndrome associated with bilateral adrenal hyperplasia. In favorable cases, pituitary microadenectomy is now perhaps

Table 39–5.　Frequency of Diabetes Mellitus in Cushing's Syndrome

Author	Cushing's Syndrome (No.)	Normal Response in Glucose Tolerance Test (No.)	Abnormal Response in Glucose Tolerance Test (No.)	Clinical Diabetes (No.)	Cushing's Syndrome with Diabetes (%)
Lukens, Flippin, & Thigpen[148]	55	28	27	19	35
Plotz, Knowlton & Ragan[149]	33	2	31	5	15
Cope & Raker[150]	35	6	29	4	11
Sprague & Mayo Associates[151]	67	10	57	22	33
Skillern & McCullagh[152]	34	13	21	7	21
Soffer, Iannaccone, & Gabrilove[153]	50	8	42	10	20
Total	274	67	207*	67	24

*Abnormal response in glucose tolerance test, 76%.

Table 39–6. Clinical Classification of Cushing's Syndrome

A. Endogenous (Spontaneous)	Incidence Percent
1. ACTH dependent	
a. Cushing's disease	
without pituitary tumor	~50
with pituitary tumor	~20
b. Ectopic ACTH secreting tumor	~10
2. ACTH independent	
a. Adenoma	~5
b. Carcinoma	~5
c. Nodular adrenal hyperplasia	~9
d. Adrenocortical rest tumor	<1
B. Exogenous (Iatrogenic)	
1. Prolonged glucocorticoid administration	
2. Prolonged ACTH administration	

the treatment of choice with reservations as mentioned earlier. The development of ACTH-producing pituitary tumors following total adrenalectomy for Cushing's syndrome, despite normal steroid replacement therapy, has constituted a complication in approximately 4 to 5% of the patients undergoing this surgery.[155–157] Another uncommon, perplexing and frustrating problem is the persistence of continued steroidogenesis, despite the removal of both adrenal glands and pituitary irradiation.[158]

The overnight dexamethasone suppression test is still the best test in the initial work-up of suspected adrenal hyperfunction. If abnormal, full work-ups are indicated including a 24-hour urine for free cortisol, low and high dexamethasone suppression and ACTH levels. The 24-hour 17-hydroxycorticoids and 17-ketosteroids still have a role in the diagnosis and approach the accuracy of plasma cortisol levels, especially when related to urinary creatinine.[158a] Details and interpretations of diagnostic tests used in evaluating altered adrenocortical function may be found in the articles cited in references 158a through 166 of this chapter.

Detailed evaluation of carbohydrate metabolism was carried out by Soffer and co-workers[153] in their series of 50 patients with Cushing's syndrome. In 42 of these, laboratory evidence of disturbance in carbohydrate metabolism was present; 2 of the remaining 8 had a flat glucose tolerance curve, and 6 had normal curves. The fasting blood glucose was determined in all patients and in 15 was found to vary from 135 to 200 mg/dl. Of these, 10 had overt diabetes which required suitable dietary regimens and insulin in amounts varying from 10 to 60 units daily. Although significant glycosuria was often present, no ketosis was demonstrated in any of these patients. Glucose tolerance tests were performed in all 50 patients and a diabetic curve was obtained not only in the 15 patients with fasting hyperglycemia, but also in 27 of the 35 patients

who had normal fasting blood glucose levels. In only 2 patients were hyperglycemia and glycosuria requiring insulin therapy, the first manifestations of Cushing's syndrome. In these, diabetes had been present for several months before other clinical manifestations of adrenal cortical hyperfunction became evident. Successful treatment for the Cushing's syndrome in both patients resulted in cure of the diabetes. In a third patient, mild diabetes had been present for 12 years and had never previously required insulin, but with the onset of Cushing's syndrome due to an adrenal carcinoma, 40 units of insulin daily were required for adequate control of the diabetes. In 11 patients who had had some evidence of disturbance in carbohydrate metabolism prior to treatment for Cushing's syndrome, post-treatment fasting blood glucose levels returned to normal limits and glucose tolerance tests gave normal values. Four additional patients with adrenal cortical carcinoma showed an improvement in carbohydrate metabolism following removal of the tumor but reactivation of diabetes occurred with the development of functioning metastatic lesions.

Since 1953, 2 diabetic patients of the Joslin Clinic (cases #32078 and #43693) with Cushing's syndrome secondary to adrenal hyperplasia have undergone bilateral adrenalectomy. Both of the patients were females. An additional case (#64589) was a rare instance of Cushing's syndrome due to an adenoma in a male patient.

While undergoing bilateral adrenalectomy for Cushing's syndrome, Case #78254 was also found to have a pheochromocytoma. In another patient, the findings, although biochemically consistent with adrenal hyperplasia, showed only minimal changes on histologic examination of adrenal tissue. The most recent case was that of a female patient with adrenal carcinoma.

Primary Aldosteronism. Since Conn's original description of primary aldosteronism as a new clinical syndrome,[167–170] a progressive increase in the diagnosis of aldosterone-producing adrenal tumors has occurred. Aldosterone is 20 to 30 times as effective as desoxycorticosterone in maintaining electrolyte balance in Addison's disease, and one-third as effective as cortisone in causing deposition of glycogen in the liver of adrenalectomized animals.

On reviewing reports of the first 145 cases of primary aldosteronism to appear in the literature, Conn and associates[171] noted impaired tolerance for carbohydrate in 21 of 39 patients (54%) who had glucose tolerance tests performed, often without adequate dietary preparation. Since all had normal values for urinary 17-hydroxycorticoids, this remarkably high incidence of carbohydrate intolerance was possibly explained by the effects of potassium depletion on carbohydrate metabolism and/or the known glucocorticoid effects of large amounts of aldosterone. In a subsequent glucose tolerance study of 27 ambulatory patients with primary aldosteronism proven at operation, under controlled conditions (300 g carbohydrate diet and no benzothiadiazine compounds for at least 2 weeks) 14 (52%) exhibited diminished carbohydrate tolerance.[172] On the basis of indirect[173] as well as direct[174] evidence, Conn offered some intriguing speculations regarding hypertension and maturity-onset diabetes seen in middle life. If 15 to 25% of cases of essential hypertension are secondary to primary aldosteronism, this condition could account for the hypertension in 2 to 3 million patients in the U.S.A. alone. If 50% of these are classified as having latent or chemical diabetes on the basis of glucose tolerance tests, a diabetic population of 1 to 1½ million is accounted for. These are indeed astounding figures when one realizes that only a relatively few cases of primary aldosteronism have been reported to date. They would also suggest that a large proportion of the subjects would fall into the normokalemic rather than the hypokalemic category since the measurement of serum potassium is commonly carried out in the evaluation of hypertension.

Strong disagreement against this point of view has been expressed. In a study of 75 patients with thiazide-induced hypokalemia and hypertension, Kaplan[175] found that none of them had primary aldosteronism. Assays of aldosterone content in the small adenomas that occur in association with essential hypertension have shown amounts similar to those in normal adrenal tissue and much less than those in adenomas from patients with primary aldosteronoma.[176] It was Kaplan's conclusion that only a small percentage of patients with essential hypertension have primary aldosteronism.

The impaired carbohydrate tolerance in patients with primary aldosteronism appears to be reversible. In 4 cases reported by Slaton and Biglieri,[177] glucose tolerance returned to normal after surgical removal of the adrenocortical adenomas. Conn[172] demonstrated that the plasma insulin curve which accompanies impaired carbohydrate tolerance in persons with primary aldosteronism is similar to that in patients with "maturity-onset" diabetes. In addition, Conn noted that the carbohydrate defect and defect in plasma insulin response can be shifted to or toward normal by potassium loading preoperatively while the patient still harbors an aldosterone-secreting tumor. Since potassium loading increases aldosterone production in individuals with primary aldosteronism while at the same time it improves carbohydrate tolerance, Conn believes that the hypothesis of impaired carbohydrate tolerance secondary to glucocorticoid effect of large amounts of aldosterone is no longer tenable. Potassium depletion appears to be the key factor, and Conn[172] hypothesized that the impaired carbohydrate tolerance in persons having primary aldosteronism is due to an inability of the beta cells to release insulin quickly in response to a rising blood glucose value, and that this defect is reparable by potassium repletion.

Although diagnostic tests are now readily available (aldosterone excretion studies, aldosterone secretory rates, and plasma renin), primary aldosteronism is not a frequent cause of overt diabetes mellitus. Since Conn's Joslin lecture in 1965,[172] no case of primary aldosteronism has been seen in the Joslin Clinic diabetic population through 1980.

Adrenogenital Syndrome. Cortical hyperfunction with an overproduction of adrenal androgenic hormones has as its chief feature in postnatal development hirsutism and virilization in the female and sexual precocity in the male. Early classifications were intended to apply to cases secondary to adrenal hyperplasia but inadvertently included cases of Cushing's syndrome. Modern classifications have evolved through the suggestions of Broster who divided the adrenogenital syndrome in females into adrenal pseudohermaphroditism, developing in fetal life; adrenal virilism developing later, particularly after puberty; and the Achard-Thiers syndrome, i.e., the diabetes of bearded women.[178–182] In virilizing congenital adrenal hyperplasia, the adrenocortical mechanism for synthesizing cortisol (hydrocortisone) is markedly inefficient, and hence a compensatory increase in ACTH secretion follows. Under this influence of excessive ACTH, the adrenal cortex becomes hyperplastic and secretes large quantities of androgenic by-products of cortisol. In therapy, administration of hydrocortisone, cortisone or synthetic steroid in physiologic doses prevents the compensatory hypersecretion of ACTH, thus promoting the involution of the adrenal cortex and decreasing the secretion of androgenic hormones to normal.

A constellation of signs and symptoms is noted in the adrenogenital syndrome in the adult female. Characteristic features include beard growth, hypertrichosis with masculine distribution, angular baldness with temporal recession, deepening voice, breast atrophy, clitoris enlargement, increased muscle mass with masculine habitus, thickened skin, and tendency for amenorrhea and cessation of ovulation. A paradoxical increase in heterosexual sex drive is noted in some patients. Development of diabetes and a marked beard in postmenopausal women (Archard-Thiers syndrome) is an extreme rarity and is associated with either adrenocortical hyperplasia or an adenoma.

Adrenal Medulla

Pheochromocytoma. Pheochromocytomas are tumors of chromaffin cells which usually arise within the adrenal medulla. Other diverse extra-adrenal sites, such as organs of Zuckerkandl, the bladder, testes, ovaries, kidney parenchyma, and mediastinum, have been noted.[183–185] Familial occurrence with dominant inheritance has been increasingly recognized in addition to association with neurofibromatosis. Early recognition and treatment are essential to prevent irreversibility of this rare but often dramatic cause of secondary, severe hypertension which is potentially curable. Surgical removal is important not only because removal of the tumor or tumors is usually followed by amelioration or permanent cure of the hypertension, but also because approximately 15% of the tumors are malignant.[186] Both benign and malignant tumors produce excess catecholamines (norepinephrine and epinephrine). Predominance of symptomatology depends on relative tumor secretion of epinephrine, which induces metabolic alterations and vasodilation, or of norepinephrine, which produces peripheral vasoconstriction.

Hypertension is so prevalent that it is not feasible to screen every hypertensive patient for pheochromoctyoma. Clinical symptomatology is the most important clue and indication for obtaining special tests. Kvale et al. of the Mayo Clinic[186,187] proposed the following 8 helpful indications: (a) paroxysms, including one or more of the following: headache, palpitation, nervousness, chest or abdominal pain, tremor, hypertension, and excessive sweating (paroxysmal or continuous); (b) thin patients (calories consumed by hypermetabolism; (c) age 35 years or less; (d) basal metabolic rate of +20% or higher without hyperthyroidism; (e) short history of hypertension (2 years); (f) retinopathy, group 3, 4, or severe group 2 (diastolic blood pressure 140 mm); (g) paradoxic response ot blood pressure to ganglion-blocking drugs; (h) severe pressor response during induction of anesthesia. Anxiety-tension states can readily be appreciated as the most difficult and perplexing problem in the differential diagnosis.

The validity of any test for pheochromocytoma may vary from patient to patient and hence the employment of a broad battery of diagnostic procedures would appear reasonable.[188] The specific tests for pheochromocytoma are of two types—chemical and pharmacologic. Pharmacologic tests are now only of historic importance. Chemical assay of plasma or urinary catecholamines or metabolites may establish the diagnosis without need for potentially hazardous and misleading provocative sympatholytic tests. Catecholamine assays may reveal elevated levels of norepinephrine and epinephrine if these are present in plasma and urine, but require a difficult fluorometric laboratory technique. Currently, estimation of the urinary catecholamine metabolite, vanilmandelic acid (VMA), is perhaps the most popular.[189] Food and drugs that give misleading and elevated values include certain fruits such as bananas, vanilla-containing foods, coffee, and salicylates. In the experience of Sjoerdsma and associates[190] and Pisano,[191] the assays for the metanephrines and VMA have proved efficient, specific, and practical for the diagnosis of pheochromocytoma. Urinary metanephrine excretion of greater than 2.0 mg a day is considered diagnostic except during treatment with monoamine oxidase inhibitors. In the presence of monoamine oxidase inhibitors, there may be a considerable increase in metanephrine levels with a decrease in VMA. Probably 90% of patients show elevations of norepinephrine and ephinephrine, VMA, normetanephrine, and metanephrine, so that a reliable assay of any of these will usually suffice.[192]

The formerly popular pharmacologic tests are of two types—provocative and vasodepressor (sympatholytic). The former is exemplified by histamine which produces a reflex sympathetic discharge of catecholamines and thereby provokes a pressor response, and the latter by phentolamine (Regitine) which neutralizes the vasopressor effects of circulating catecholamines and reduces blood pressure. By current concepts, pheochromocytoma tissue is not innervated and hence histamine would not be expected to have a direct effect on the tumor itself. Newer provocative tests include the administration of tyramine intravenously, introduced by Engelman and Sjoerdsma,[193] and the intravenous infusion of glucagon, introduced by Lawrence.[194]

Other than increased catecholamine or metabolite excretion, hyperglycemia and hypermetabolism without hyperthyroidism are the most frequent and striking laboratory findings.

In the review of Gifford and associates[186] of clinical data of 76 patients with pheochromocytoma seen at the Mayo Clinic, hypermetabolism was present in three-fourths and hyperglycemia in two-thirds of those with persistent hypertension. Among other patients with paroxysmal hypertension, these findings were less frequently encountered. In 89 of the patients with sustained hypertension and in 4 with paroxysmal hypertension, the diagnosis of diabetes mellitus had been made before they were seen in the Mayo Clinic. Twenty-one of the 76 patients had the "triad of H's"—hypertension, hyperglycemia, and hypermetabolism—but not hyperthyroidism. It is fortunate that blood thyroxine and triiodothyronine levels and thyroid radioactive iodine uptake are normal in this hypermetabolic state due to pheochromocytoma, in view of its similarity to hyperthyroidism.

In Evans'[195] series of 13 patients with pheochromocytoma, a much higher incidence of diabetes was noted. Eight patients had diabetes when first seen, and in 1 with metastatic pheochromocytoma, diabetes developed after the original tumor was removed. Seven had diabetes with sustained hypertension and only 2 had diabetes with paroxysmal hypertension. Four of the 13 patients with proved pheochromocytoma had hypertension but no diabetes. The incidence of impaired glucose tolerance with pheochromocytoma may be as high as 75% but the hyperglycemia develops after paroxysmal hypertension and is usually mild.[195a,195b] In a series of 72 patients with pheochromocytoma, glucose tolerance was impaired in 19; only 2 required oral hypoglycemic agents and 1 required insulin therapy.[195c]

Cure or marked amelioration of diabetes by removal of a pheochromocytoma has been reported, but no large series is available. The Joslin Clinic experience has been variable in this regard. In 1 patient, removal of a large pheochromocytoma in 1938 had not been followed by a change in severity of diabetes up to the time of death in 1948. From 1954 to 1979, 9 patients with pheochromocytoma have been seen at the Joslin Clinic (Table 39–7). Dramatic amelioration of hyperglycemia and hypertension occurred in 6 of the patients with onset of diabetes shortly before diagnosis of pheochromocytoma was made. Case #17480 with juvenile-onset diabetes was not affected by removal of the pheochromocytoma. He had developed retinopathy and proteinuria 3 years before hypertension was noted. In 2 patients (Cases #74698 and #93904) prior to surgery, treatment had been with small doses of tolbutamide. Others have reported partial or complete remission of the diabetic state following surgical removal of the tumor.[196,197]

Abnormal carbohydrate metabolism associated with pheochromocytoma has been ascribed to the known glycogenolytic effect of excess catecholamines released by these tumors.[198] Spergel et al.[199] have revealed two additional factors: suppression of insulin release and resistance to the hypoglycemic action of endogenous or exogenous insulin. In 2 patients, immediately after removal of the tumor, the response of plasma insulin levels to glucose and tolbutamide was exaggerated, but resistance to the hypoglycemic effects of insulin continued. These findings were attributed to concomitantly elevated plasma cortisol levels. The carbohydrate metabolism reverted to normal with time. Inhibition of insulin secretion by pheochromocytoma has also been reported by Wilber and colleagues.[200] In a later case report, Isles and Johnson[200a] described a patient with new onset diabetes who was started on insulin therapy. During the same admission, a pheochromocytoma was diagnosed. Treatment with beta blockers did not affect the insulin dose but with phenoxybenzamine there was a reduction. This suggests that alpha-2 adrenergic receptors block insulin release in man.

GLUCAGONOMA SYNDROME

The glucagonoma syndrome has striking clinical features characterized by the tetrad of skin rash, anemia, diabetes, and glossitis. Appreciation of this entity was stimulated by the report of 9 cases by Mallinson and co-workers in 1974.[201–203] Eight of the 9 patients were females ranging in age from 48 to 65 years at the time of skin eruption. All initially had the skin problem and were followed at the dermatology clinic. Despite markedly elevated glucagon levels (1500 to 2000 pg/ml), diabetes was noted in only 7 of the 9 patients and was mild in type. All of these patients had pancreatic tumors of which 2 were malignant. The diabetes and skin rash tended to disappear after removal of the tumor. Hypoaminoacidemia was thought to account for the anemia and rash.

The skin rash has been given the impressive name of necrolytic migratory erythema. The initial erythema is followed by superficial blisters which tend to rupture. Gradual spread is noted with central clearing and active margins persisting. Variable degrees of crusting and superficial ulceration can be noted. Major sites of involvement are the perineum, groin, and extremities. In addition, stomatitis and glossitis have been seen frequently (see Chapter 38 for additional comments).

The *sine qua non* of this syndrome remains the presence of elevated glucagon levels (normally less than 100 pg/ml). Another helpful finding in patients with glucagonoma syndrome is the presence of an abnormal glucagon fragment associated with the tumor. However, the assay for such fragments is not widely available. Glucagon determinations are not performed routinely in most laboratories, but extremely low circulating plasma amino acid levels can provide good inferential evidence for the presence of glucagonoma.

Glucagonoma is suspected when a large tumor is observed, with metastases to the liver. Ultrasound and computerized tomography (CT scan) are helpful diagnostic aids. Determination of the size of the tumor and extent of metastases should be made prior to treatment. Cures can be achieved by surgical resection only if the tumor is confined to a single area in the pancreas. Rapid clearing of the skin lesions can be seen following removal of the primary tumor. Chemotherapy has had some suc-

Table 39–7. Diabetes and Pheochromocytoma Experience of Joslin Clinic, 1954–1979

Patient No.	Sex	Onset of Diabetes Age (Years)	Onset of Diabetes Date (Year)	Family History of Diabetes	Date Removal Pheochromocytoma	Insulin Dose Before Surgery (Units/day)	Insulin Dose After Surgery (Units/day)
#40968	F	40	1951	+	Feb 1954	30	0
#46428	M	63	1955	−	Sept. 1955	24	0
#17480	M	14	1934	+	Apr. 1955	80	80
#24607	M	25	1944	+	June 1964	16	0
#74698	M	37	1963	−	July 1968	Tolbutamide, 0.5 g qd	0
#78250	F	54	1969	+	June 1970*	48	Tolbutamide, 0.5 g qd
#93904	F	61	1968	+	May 1974	Tolbutamide, 0.5 g bid	0
#102277	M	61	1975	−	May 1975	50	0
#103053	F	71	1970	+	Aug. 1975	14	0

*Surgery for Cushing's syndrome.

cess in the treatment of metastatic glucagonoma. Streptozotocin (SZ), dimethyltriazenoimidazole carboxamide (DTIC), and 5-fluorouracil (5 FU) are three of the agents used.[204–207]

SOMATOSTATIN

Somatostatin-producing cells (the D cells of pancreatic islets) may occur in the form of tumors both within the pancreas and at times outside that organ in the adjacent area. In general, patients with pancreatic somatostatinomas have diabetes of mild to moderate severity whereas those with extrapancreatic growths do not. The somatostatinoma syndrome effects consist of gallbladder disease, diarrhea, decreased or absent gastric acidity, weight loss, and anemia. The tumors metastasize so that the syndrome may lead to death. Attempts at treatment have been made largely with chemotherapy, although if the tumor is discovered prior to its spread, it may be excised, causing complete disappearance of the diabetes, so that one may speak of a cure.

Studies have usually revealed typical D cells as the chief hormone-producing tissue of the tumors. However, there is evidence from some patients of concomitant production of other hormones, including ACTH, gastrin-producing cells, and probable glucocorticoid excess as well as overproduction of calcitonin.

Radioimmunoassays show marked elevation of plasma somatostatin levels (100–1000 times greater than normal).[207a,207b]

PARATHYROID GLAND

To date no definite relationship has been demonstrated between diabetes and parathyroid disease. In a 1978 report, Akgun and Ertel[208] described a patient with long-duration diabetes who developed hypercalcemia. Following removal of a parathyroid adenoma, repeated hypoglycemic attacks occurred, leading to a 50% decrease in the insulin requirement. Walsh et al.[209] also described 8 patients with co-existing hyperparathyroidism and diabetes; in 1 patient a similar decrease in insulin requirement was noted following tumor removal.

The role of calcium in the dynamics of insulin release is now well documented. The presence of extracellular calcium is an absolute requirement for the secretion of insulin in response to an insulinotropic agent,[210,210a] and glucose has been shown to stimulate the accumulation of Ca^{45} in isolated islets, apparently by inhibiting the efflux of Ca^{++} from the beta cell.[211]

In primary hyperparathyroidism, Kim et al.[212] studied plasma insulin dynamics in 10 patients before and after surgery. Before the operation, fasting plasma insulin concentration and insulin responses to administered glucose, tolbutamide and glucagon were significantly greater than were post-operative values. The hyperinsulinemia was not associated with altered glucose curves during glucose or glucagon tolerance tests, but there was a relatively greater insulin response to tolbutamide that enhanced its hypoglycemic effect. The glucose-lowering effect of insulin given intravenously was slightly impaired before treatment. The authors were able to reproduce the augmented insulin response with parathyroid hormone injections followed by the administration of glucose orally and tolbutamide intravenously. The findings of Kim et al.[212] suggest that chronic hypercalcemia results in a form of endogenous insulin resistance that requires augmented insulin secretion to maintain plasma glucose homeostasis. The exact role of parathyroid hormone in these events has not yet been determined.

The study of Ginsberg et al.[213] indicated that the quantitative effects of primary hyperparathyroidism on glucose and insulin metabolism are modest. This is in keeping with other clinical surveys that have failed to show significant carbohydrate intolerance in patients with hyperparathyroidism.[214] In the study by Yasuda et al.[215] of 5 patients with hypoparathyroidism, a decreased insulin response during an oral glucose tolerance test was found without any abnormality of the glucose response. These results are in keeping with the in vitro studies of Curry et al.[216] who found that the amount of insulin released by glucose was proportionate to the calcium concentration in the perfusate over the range of 0.5 to 4 mEq/L.

Diabetic Osteopenia

In 1949 Albright and Reifenstein[217] reported the occurrence of osteoporosis in patients with long-standing and poorly-controlled diabetes. This was also documented by Berney in 1952[218] and Menczel[219] in 1972. In Menczel's study, the diabetic patients had a 22% incidence of proximal hip fractures. Levin et al.[220] studied skeletal mass in 35 patients with insulin-dependent juvenile-onset diabetes and in 101 patients with maturity-onset diabetes. Using the photon absorption method, they found a significant loss of bone mass in the mineral content of the forearm in both groups. The decrease was already present in patients with diabetes of less than 5 years' duration. Bone loss and duration of diabetes did not correlate. The greatest degree of bone loss occurred in patients receiving oral agents. Others have confirmed this reduction in bone mass,[221,222] and still others have not.[223–225]

Heath et al.[226] could detect no changes in a number of elements of calcium homeostasis to account for the osteopenia. The earlier work of Schneider and associates in the diabetic rat model[227,228] had suggested a possible pathogenetic mechanism for osteopenia in diabetes. It was thought that the diabetic state could somehow impair hydroxylation of 25-hydroxy-vitamin D and so decrease the 1,25, dihydroxy-vitamin D (1,25 (OH)$_2$D) level which is most active in the gut in calcium absorption. Taken together with the evidence in clinical or experimental conditions[229,230] showing that oral glucose loading produces significant changes in urinary calcium excretion, these events could lead to calcium loss and secondary hyperparathyroidism, preserving plasma calcium at the expense of bone.

The results of studies in a group of young insulin-dependent diabetics and age-matched controls were reported recently by Witt and colleagues.[230a] They found that there was a continuous spectrum of calcium excretion from normal values to those seen in the recovery phase of hypercalcemia in renal failure. The authors suggest that there is a component of intestinal calcium hyperabsorption in

these patients which together with resulting decreased parathyroid hormone and vitamin D level may lead to defective remodelling and decreased cortical thickness of bone.

In a study of 45 insulin-dependent diabetics aged 7 to 18 years, Frazer et al.[230b] found a reduction in 1,25(OH)$_2$D, elevated circulating 24,25(OH)$_2$D and low normal levels of immunoreactive parathyroid hormone (PTH) levels in these patients. The authors suggest that these alterations could relate to the decrease in the cortical bone mass observed in these patients. These results and interpretations demonstrate the difficulty in extrapolating results in animals such as those obtained by Heath[226] to patients with diabetes. It may well be that diabetic osteopenia is an acquired defect of bone formation which may be partially or completely correctible with insulin treatment as proposed by Levin et al.[220]

In summary, there is a great deal of evidence for the presence of significant osteopenia in patients with diabetes mellitus. The exact etiology has not yet been established and, for the present, no definite preventive measures are available. McNair et al.[231] assessed the significance of different risk factors for the development of bone loss in diabetes. They found that residual insulin and quality of metabolic control are major factors in determining mineral content in insulin-treated patients. Therefore, striving for the best possible control of diabetes remains the only way for the present.

Pancreatitis

The association between hyperparathyroidism and acute pancreatitis has been emphasized in recent years. In 1957, Cope and associates[232] postulated that pancreatitis is another diagnostic clue to hyperparathyroidism on the basis of experience with 2 patients who had both conditions concomitantly. In 1962, Mixter et al.[233] reviewed 62 reported cases of hyperparathyroidism associated with pancreatitis or pancreatic calcification, or both. Cope and associates emphasized the point that a normal serum calcium value during an attack of acute pancreatitis does not rule out the possibility of hyperparathyroidism since pancreatitis is known to be associated with a depressed serum calcium level. An elevated serum calcium value in pancreatitis (initially thought to be a laboratory error because a lowered calcium level had been anticipated) has occasionally been a key diagnostic clue.[234,235] The association of the two diseases needs further emphasis, as surgical cure of the hyperparathyroidism may be followed by relief of the pancreatitis.

At the Massachusetts General Hospital between 1950 and 1959, pancreatitis occurred at least 11 times in 155 patients (7%)[235] with proven hyperparathyroidism. In the Mayo Clinic series of 380 cases of primary hyperparathyroidism[236] only 10 patients (2.6%) appeared to have had some form of pancreatitis whereas "serendipity" was the diagnostic clue in 45 patients. Of the 45 patients in whom the diagnosis was made by chance calcium determinations, 18 had no signs or symptoms which could be ascribed to hyperparathyroidism, even on careful review. The incidence of peptic ulcer appears more significant and more than coincidental in hyperparathyroidism. Reported estimates of the frequency with which these conditions co-exist have varied from 10 to 30%. In the Mayo Clinic series,[236] an incidence of peptic ulcer of 15.5% (59 of 380 patients) was noted. The therapeutic disaster of parathyroid storm may be precipitated by treatment of peptic ulcer with the Sippy regimen (calcium carbonate) in a patient with co-existing severe, but unrecognized, hyperparathyroidism.

In a patient in Gross' series,[237] recurrent renal calculi were noted, followed by relapsing pancreatitis with subsequent diabetes, and finally hyperparathyroidism. The father of this patient, a 40-year-old man, did have diabetes. The association of recurrent pancreatitis with hereditary hyperparathyroidism has been noted. In Jackson's remarkable family,[238] 6 and possibly 7 cases of hyperparathyroidism occurred in members of two generations; this was associated with recurring pancreatitis in at least 2 of these patients. Without doubt, two members of this extraordinary family had diabetes.

DIABETES INSIPIDUS AND DIABETES MELLITUS

Diabetes insipidus may result from injury to the hypothalamus, the posterior lobe of the pituitary gland, or the bilateral pathways connecting the hypothalamus with the posterior lobe. It is a syndrome due to deficiency of antidiuretic hormone (ADH) and is characterized by extreme thirst leading to the drinking of large amounts of fluid and excretion of dilute urine in quantities varying from 3 to 15 liters daily. It occurs when there is a failure either to produce or release ADH or, rarely, failure of renal response to ADH (nephrogenic diabetes insipidus).

Current concepts postulate that ADH is produced in the supraoptic and paraventricular nuclei of the hypothalamus and migrates down the nerve tracts to the posterior lobe of the pituitary for storage prior to release into the blood stream. Some of the nerve tracts end in the median eminence and pituitary stalk which can take over the storage function of the posterior lobe if the latter is destroyed.

Lesions which involve the hypothalamus may destroy the nuclei which produce ADH, whereas lesions involving the pituitary stalk may interrupt the nerve tracts which transport ADH to structures lower in the hypothalamico-neurohypophyseal system.

Since polydipsia and polyuria are cardinal manifestations of both diabetes insipidus and diabetes mellitus, the differential diagnoses of the two diseases and their simultaneous presence in the same patient are of interest. The association of the two conditions appears to be fortuitous. An exception is the rare instance in which a hyperfunctioning eosinophilic adenoma of the pituitary may be the causal factor of both conditions, as in the case report of Natelson.[239] His patient, a 46-year-old Mexican woman who entered the hospital in diabetic acidosis (blood glucose 720 mg/dl and serum CO_2 11 mEq/L), had coexistent diabetes insipidus, acromegaly, and diabetes mellitus. A photograph taken 3 years prior to her hospital admission showed obvious acromegalic prognathism, coarsening of the features, macroglossia, and spade-like hands. Autopsy revealed a large, eosinophilic adenoma of the pituitary with extensive degeneration and hemorrhage. The extrasellar portion invaginated the adjacent portion of the hypothalamus.

The association of diabetes mellitus and diabetes insipidus had been reported in 46 patients in the world's literature from 1897 thorugh 1964.[240–243] Only 7 of the patients were children. The familial presence of the two diseases had not been recorded until Raiti and associates[242] reported finding their occurrence in two sisters. Joslin Clinic records show only 8 patients, with the coexistence or the occurrence at different times, of diabetes mellitus and diabetes insipidus.

DIABETES MELLITUS, DIABETES INSIPIDUS AND OPTIC ATROPHY (DIDMOAD)

A unique association is that of diabetes mellitus, diabetes insipidus, and primary optic atrophy.[244–247] Familial occurrence has been noted and it is thought to be probably of genetic origin. Diagnoses have usually been established during childhood. In addition to visual difficulties, generalized episodic seizures and hearing problems are frequent. It has not been determined whether the seizures are provoked by acute metabolic derangements such as hypoglycemia and water intoxication or whether they are related to a primary convulsive disorder. From a therapeutic standpoint, some favorable results have been noted with the use of chlorpropamide (Diabinese) and lysine vasopressin nasal spray. Subsequent refractoriness to chlorpropamide has been noted in the pediatric age group of patients with co-existing diabetes mellitus, diabetes insipidus, and optic atrophy. Three such patients have been seen at the Joslin Clinic.

THE GONADS AND DIABETES

Men and women with adequately controlled diabetes have reproductive capacities comparable to those of healthy nondiabetic individuals.[248-250] Diabetic women may indeed have somewhat increased fertility. When reproductive histories of 198 men were compared with those of a matched nondiabetic population, no significant differences were noted in the number of pregnancies among the wives of the men in the two groups.[249]

However, premature impotence is frequently seen in diabetic men and is especially common after many years of poorly-controlled diabetes in those with the juvenile-onset type of disease. Diabetic autonomic neuropathy presumably is responsible. Impotence is occasionally the first symptom for which medical aid is sought and the diabetes is then discovered. Impotence that arises while the diabetes is poorly controlled, often disappears when good control is established. If impotence develops when the diabetes is under adequate control, it is much more likely to be permanent. The study of 198 diabetic men by Rubin and Babbott showed an incidence of permanent impotence from 2 to 5 times greater than that of the general population.[250,251] Of the diabetic men in their 30s, 25% were impotent. An incidence of 38% was noted for men in their 40s and 54% for those 50 to 54 years of age. Libido tended to persist for some time after these patients had lost their coital abilities. Among impotent diabetic men over 55 years old, libido was often diminished or completely lost. All diabetic men should be questioned about their potency and all impotent men should be investigated for diabetes. For a detailed discussion of sexual disorders in diabetes, see Chapter 32.

Calcification of the vas deferens can be seen occasionally on x-ray of the scrotal contents. Wilson and Marks[252] found such calcifications to be 6 times more frequent in diabetics than in the normal population. In view of the much higher frequency of impotency, the calcifications apparently have little or no causal relationship.

At the present time, there is no known alteration of primary nature in the function of the gonads, either ovaries or testes, that is causally associated with diabetes mellitus.

Forbes and Engel[253] called attention to the high incidence of diabetes mellitus in a series of 41 patients with gonadal dysgenesis who were examined at an average age of 38 years. Six (15%) manifested diabetes after the age of 30 years. In 20 patients there was a family history of diabetes and in 14 the diabetes occurred in paternal members

only. Since more than half the patients had either diabetes or a family history of it, an association of diabetes mellitus and gonadal dysgenesis is suggested. The unproven possibility exists that the metabolic consequence of congenital hypogonadism or genetic consequence of damage to an X chromosome may have contributed to the occurrence of diabetes in the patients.

Diabetes also appears to be prevalent in patients with Klinefelter's syndrome. In 24 patients with this syndrome seen at the Massachusetts General Hospital, overt diabetes was present in 2, 5 others had an abnormal reaction to glucose tolerance tests, and 11 gave a family history of diabetes.[254]

REFERENCES

1. Daughaday, W.H., Parker, M.L.: Human pituitary growth hormone. Ann. Rev. Med. *16*:47, 1965.
2. Glick, S.M., Roth, J., Yalow, R.S., Berson, S.A.: The regulation of growth hormone secretion. Rec. Prog. Horm. Res. *21*:241, 1965.
3. Hartog, M., Gaafar, M.A., Meisser, B., Fraser, R.: Immunoassay of serum growth hormone in acromegalic patients. Br. Med. J. *2*:1229, 1964.
4. Beck, P., Schalch, D.S., Parker, M.L., et al.: Correlative studies of growth hormone and insulin plasma concentrations with metabolic abnormalities in acromegaly. J. Lab. Clin. Med. *66*:366, 1965.
5. Cerasi, E., Luft, R.: Insulin response to glucose loading in acromegaly. Lancet *2*:769, 1964.
6. Prockop, D.J., Sjoerdsma, A.: Significance of urinary hydroxyproline in man. J. Clin. Invest. *40*:843, 1961.
7. Benoit, F.L., Theil, G.B., Watten, R.H.: Hydroxyproline excretion in endocrine disease. Metabolism *12*:1072, 1963.
8. Sjoerdsma, A., Udenfriend, S., Keiser, H., LeRoy, E.C.: Hydroxyproline and collagen metabolism: clinical implications. Combined Clinical Staff Conference at the National Institutes of Health. Ann. Intern. Med. *63*:672, 1965.
9. Jones, D.R., Bahn, R.C., Randall, R.V., Sullivan, C.R.: The human costochondral junction. II. Patients with acromegaly. Mayo Clin. Proc. *44*:330, 1969.
10. Daughaday, W.H., Mariz, I.K.: Conversion of proline-U-C14 to labeled hydroxyproline by rat cartilage in vitro: effects of hypophysectomy, growth hormone, and cortisol. J. Lab. Clin. Med. *59*:741, 1962.
10a.Kozak, G.P.: Diabetes and other endocrinologic disorders. In: A. Marble, P. White, R.F. Bradley, L.P. Krall (Eds.): Joslin's Diabetes Mellitus, 11th Ed., Philadelphia, Lea & Febiger, 1971, Table 24–1, p. 667.
11. Davidoff, L.M.: Studies in acromegaly. II. Historical note. III. The anamnesis and symptomatology in one hundred cases. Endocrinology *10*:453, 461, 1926.
12. Davidoff, L.M., Cushing, H.: Studies in acromegaly: the disturbances of carbohydrate metabolism. Arch. Intern. Med. *39*:751, 1927.
13. Coggeshall, C., Root, H.F.: Acromegaly and diabetes mellitus. Endocrinology *26*:1, 1940.
14. Gordon, D.A., Hill, F.M., Ezrin, C.: Acromegaly: a review of 100 cases. Canad. Med. Assoc. J. *87*:1106, 1962.
14a.Ballintine, J., Foxman, S., Gorden, P., Roth, J.: Rarity of diabetic retinopathy in patients with acromegaly. Arch. Intern. Med. *141*:1625, 1981.
15. Emmer, M., Gorden, P., Roth, J.: Diabetes in association

with other endocrine disorders. Med. Clin. N. Am. 55:1057, 1971.

16. Wilder, R.M.: Clinical Diabetes Mellitus and Hyperinsulinism. Philadelphia, W.B. Saunders Co., 1940, p. 71.

16a.Jadresic, A., Banks, L.M., Child, D.F., et al.: The acromegaly syndrome. Relation between clinical features, growth hormone values and radiologic characteristics of the pituitary tumours. Quart. J. Med. NS LI, No. 202, 189, 1982.

17. McCullagh, E.P.: Diabetogenic action of the pituitary; clinical observations. Diabetes 5:223, 1956.

18. Sönksen, P.H., Greenwood, F.C., Ellis, J.P., et al.: Changes of carbohydrate tolerance in acromegaly with progress of the disease and in response to treatment. J. Clin. Endocrinol. 27:1418, 1967.

18a.Harrison, L.C., Flier, J.S.: Diabetes associated with other endocrine diseases. In: S. Podolsky, M. Viswanathan (Eds.): Secondary Diabetes. The Spectrum of the Diabetic Syndromes. New York, Raven Press. 1980, pp. 269–286.

18b.Eastman, R.C., Gorden, Ph., Roth, J.: Conventional supervoltage irradiation is an effective treatment for acromegaly. J. Clin. Endocrinol. Metab. 48:931, 1979.

18c.Wass, J.A.H., Cudworth, A.G., Bottazzo, G.F., et al.: An assessment of glucose intolerance in acromegaly and its response to medical treatment. Clin. Endocrinol. 12:53, 1980.

19. Wrenshall, G.A., Bogoch, A., Ritchie, R.C.: Extractable insulin of pancreas: correlation with pathological and clinical findings in diabetic and nondiabetic cases. Diabetes 1:87, 1952.

20. Fraser, R., Joplin, G.F., Opie, L.H., Rabinowitz, D.: The augmented insulin tolerance test for detecting insulin resistance. J. Endocrinol. 25:299, 1962.

21. Galbraith, H.J.B., Ginsburg, J., Paton, A.: Decreased response to intra-arterial insulin in acromegaly. Diabetes 9:459, 1960.

22. Perley, M., Kipnis, D.M.: Effect of glucocorticoids on plasma insulin. N. Engl. J. Med. 274:1237, 1966.

23. Sheehan, H.L.: Simmonds' disease due to postpartum necrosis of the anterior pituitary. Quart. J. Med. 8:277, 1939.

24. Schalch, D.S., Burday, S.Z.: Antepartum pituitary insufficiency in diabetes mellitus. Ann. Intern. Med. 74:357, 1971.

25. Smith, C.W., Jr., Howard, R.P.: Variations in endocrine gland function in postpartum pituitary necrosis. J. Clin. Endocrinol. 19:1420, 1959.

26. Ganong, W.F., Hume, D.M.: Effect of graded hypophysectomy on thyroid, gonadal and adrenocortical function in the dog. Endocrinology 59:293, 1956.

27. Peters, J.P., German, W.J., Mann, E.B., Welt, L.G.: Functions of gonads, thyroid and adrenals in hypopituitarism. Metabolism 3:118, 1954.

27a.Marshall, J.C., Harsoulis, P., Anderson, D.C., et al.: Isolated pituitary gonadotrophin deficiency: gonadotrophin secretion after synthetic luteinizing hormone and follicle stimulating hormone-release hormone. Br. Med. J. 4:643, 1972.

28. Odell, W.D.: Isolated deficiencies of anterior pituitary hormones. Symptoms and diagnosis. J.A.M.A. 197:1006, 1966.

28a.Stacpoole, P.W., Interlandi, J.W., Nicholson, W.E., Rabin, D.: Isolated ACTH deficiency: a heterogenous disorder. Critical review and report of four new cases. Medicine 61:13, 1982.

29. Shuman, C.R.: Hypothyroidism due to thyrotropin deficiency without other manifestations of hypopituitarism. J. Clin. Endocrinol. 13:795, 1953.

29a.Miyai, K., Azukizawa, M., Kumahara, Y.: Familial isolated thyrotropin deficiency with cretinism. N. Engl. J. Med. 285:1043, 1971.

30. Goldman, J.K., Cahill, G.F., Jr., Thorn, G.W.: Gigantism with hypopituitarism. Am. J. Med. 34:407, 1963.

31. Sarver, M.E., Sabeh, G., Fetterman, G.H., et al.: Fractional hypopituitarism with gigantism and normal sella turcica. N. Engl. J. Med. 271:1286, 1964.

32. Houssay, B.A., Biasotti, A.: La diabetes pancreatica de los perros hipofisoprivos. Rev. Soc. Argent. de Biol. 6:251, 1930.

33. Martin, M.H., Salassa, R.M., Sprague, R.G.: Clinics on endocrine and metabolic diseases. 3. The development of diabetes mellitus in a patient with pituitary insufficiency and renal glycosuria. Mayo Clin. Proc. 35:414, 1960.

34. Frey, H.M.: The development of diabetes mellitus during pituitary insufficiency. Acta Med. Scand. 175:523, 1964.

35. Raptis, S., Rothenbuchner, G., Birk, J., et al.: Insulin dependent diabetes mellitus and HGH, TSH in serum following thyrotrophin releasing factor (TRF). Abstract 182). Acta Endocrinol. (Suppl. 155) (Kbh):182, 1971.

36. Weeke, J., Hansen, Aa.P.: Serum thyrotropin during daily life and in response to thyrotropin releasing hormone in normal subjects and juvenile diabetics. Diabetologia 10:101, 1974.

37. Schimmel, M., Utiger, R.D.: Thyroidal and peripheral production of thyroid hormones. Review of recent findings and their clinical implications. Ann. Intern. Med. 87:760, 1977.

38. Althausen, T.L., Stockholm, M.: Influence of thyroid gland on absorption in digestive tract. Am. J. Physiol. 123:577, 1938.

39. Holdsworth, C.D., Besser, G.M.: Influence of gastric emptying rate and of insulin response on oral glucose tolerance in thyroid disease. Lancet 2:700, 1968.

40. Amatuzio, D.S., Schultz, A.L., Vanderbilt, M.J., et al.: The effect of epinephrine, insulin and hyperthyroidism on the rapid intravenous glucose tolerance test. J. Clin. Invest. 33:97, 1954.

41. Spergel, G., Levy, L., Goldner, M.: The impaired carbohydrate metabolism of thyroid disease. Diabetes 17 (Suppl. 1):345, 1968.

42. Mirsky, I.A., Broh-Kahn, R.H.: Effect of experimental hyperthyroidism on carbohydrate metabolism. Am. J. Physiol. 117:6, 1936.

43. Macho, L.: The influence of endocrine glands on carbohydrate metabolism. II. The glucose tolerance and clearance of glucose in healthy subjects and in patients with hypo- and hyper thyroidism. Acta Med. Scand. 160:485, 1958.

44. Gorowski, T., Wolanska, A.: Statistical analysis of clinical value of blood sugar tolerance curve in case of hyperthyroidism and in neutral goiter. Pol. Arch. Med. Wewnet. 27:909, 1957.

45. Elrick, H., Hlad, C.J., Jr., Arai, Y.: Influence of thyroid function on carbohydrate metabolism and a new method for assessing response to insulin. J. Clin. Endocrinol. 21:387, 1961.

46. Andreani, D., Menzinger, G., Fallucca, F., et al.: Insulin levels in thyrotoxicosis and primary myxedema: response to intravenous glucose and glucagon. Diabetologia 6:1, 1970.

47. Holman, E.F.: Hypoglycemia in exophthalmic goiter. A preliminary report. Bull. Johns Hopkins Hosp. 34:69, 1923.

48. Sanger, B.J., Hun, E.G.: The glucose mobilization rate in hyperthyroidism. Arch. Intern. Med. 30:397, 1922.

49. Baumgarten, F.: Die Kombination von physiologischer Belastung und Entlastung als diagnostisches Prinzip, (Ein Beitrag zur Einfuhrung der Prazisions-Dauerinfusion und

eines hochempfindlichen Insulintests in die funktionelle Diagnostik). Z. Klin. Med. *152*:174, 1953.

50. Kellen, J.: Über Strörungen des Kohlenhydratstoffwechsels bei erhöhter Tätigkeit der Schilddrüse. Z. Ges. Inn. Med. *11*:368, 1956.

51. Kellen, J.: Stoffwechselstörungen im Kohlehydrathaushalt bein Thyreotoxikose Zur Frage der Insulinresistenz. Z. Ges. Inn. Med. *11*:368, 1956.

52. Crawford, T.: Carbohydrate tolerance in hypothyroidism and hyperthyroidism. Arch. Dis. Child. *15*:184, 1940.

53. Doar, J.W.H., Stamp, T.C.B., Wynn, V., Audhya, T.K.: Effects of oral and intravenous glucose loading in thyrotoxicosis: Studies of plasma glucose, free fatty acid, plasma insulin and blood pyruvate levels. Diabetes *18*:633, 1969.

54. Renauld, A., Andrade, L.L., Sverdlik, R.C., Rodriguez, R.R.: Serum insulin response to glucose infusion in hyperthyroid dogs. Horm. Metabl. Res. *6*:400, 1974.

55. Cavagnini, F., Peracchi, M., Raggi, U., et al.: Impairment of growth hormone and insulin secretion in hyperthyroidism. Eur. J. Clin. Invest. *4*:71, 1974.

56. Dubois, E.F.: Basal Metabolism in Health and Disease, 3rd ed. Philadelphia, Lea & Febiger, 1936, p. 333.

57. Wilder, R.M.: Clinical Diabetes Mellitus and Hyperinsulinism. Philadelphia, W.B. Saunders Co., 1940, pp. 244–261.

58. DeBodo, R.C., Altszuler, N.: Insulin hypersensitivity and physiological insulin antagonists. Physiol. Rev. *38*:389, 1958.

59. Hagen, J.H.: Effect of insulin on the metabolism of adipose tissue from hyperthyroid rats. J. Biol. Chem. *235*:2600, 1960.

60. Meythaler, F., Mann, H.: Über den Einfluss der Schilddrüse auf den Kohlehydratstoffwechsel; die Wirkungsintensität des Insulins bei Basedow und Myxödem. Klin. Wschr. *16*:983, 1937.

61. Lazarus, S.S., Volk, B.W.: The estimation of insulin sensitivity by the modified glucose insulin tolerance test. J. Lab. Clin. Med. *39*:404, 1952.

62. Cramer, W.: On the glycogenic function of the liver and its endocrine control. Br. J. Exp. Path. *5*:128, 1924.

63. Burn, J.H., Marks, H.P.: The relation of the thyroid gland to the action of insulin. J. Physiol. (London) *60*:131, 1925.

64. Marecek, R.L., Feldman, J.M.: Effect of hyperthyroidism on insulin and glucose dynamics in rabbits. Endocrinol. *92*:1604, 1973.

65. Wajchenberg, B.L., Cesar, F.P., Leme, C.E., et al.: Carbohydrate metabolism in thyrotoxicosis: studies on insulin secretion before and after remission from the hyperthyroid state. Horm. Metab. Res. *10*:294, 1978.

66. Federspil, G., Zaccaria, M., Casara, D., et al.: Plasma insulin response to glibornuride in thyrotoxicosis. Diabete Metab. (Paris) *2*:27, 1976.

67. Levy, L.J., Adesman, J.J., Spergel, G.: Studies on the carbohydrate and lipid metabolism in thyroid disease: effects of glucagon. J. Clin. Endocrinol. Metab. *30*:372, 1970.

68. Robertson, R.P., Porte, D., Jr.: Adrenergic modulation of basal insulin secretion in man. Diabetes *22*:1, 1973.

69. Wiener, L., Stout, B.D., Cox, J.W.: Influence of beta sympathetic blockade (propranolol) on the haemodynamics of hyperthyroidism. Am. J. Med. *46*:227, 1969.

69a. McCulloch, A.J., Home, P.D., Heine, R., et al.: Insulin sensitivity in hyperthyroidism: measurement by the glucose clamp technique. Clin. Endocrinol. *18*:327, 1983.

70. Olefsky, J.M.: The insulin receptor: its role in insulin resistance of obesity and diabetes. Diabetes *25*:1154, 1976.

71. Holst, J.: Glycosuria and diabetes in exophthalmic goiter. Acta Med. Scand. *55*:302, 1921.

72. Houssay, B.A.: Thyroid and metathyroid diabetes. Endocrinology *35*:158, 1944.

73. Danowski, T.S., Bonessi, J.V., Saraver, M.E., Moses, C.: Hydrocortisone and/or dessicated thyroid in physiologic dosage. XIII. Carbohydrate metabolism during large dose thyroid (proloid) therapy. Metabolism *13*:739, 1964.

74. Houssay, B.A.: Thyroid and diabetes. Vitamins and Hormones *4*:187, 1946.

75. Houssay, B.A., Foglia, V.G., Martinez, C.: The influence of the thyroid on alloxan and pancreatic diabetes in the rat. Endocrinology *39*:361, 1946.

76. Kinash, B., Haist, R.E.: The influence of the thyroid gland on the islets of Langerhans and the pancreas. Can. J. Biochem. Physiol. *33*:380, 1955.

77. Houssay, B.A.: The action of the thyroid on diabetes. Rec. Progr. Horm. Res. *2*:277, 1948.

78. Hales, C.N., Hyams, D.E.: Plasma concentrations of glucose, non-esterified fatty acid, and insulin during oral glucose tolerance tests in thyrotoxicosis. Lancet *2*:69, 1964.

79. Klink, D., Estrich, D.: Plasma insulin concentration in Cushing's syndrome and thyrotoxicosis. Clin. Res. *12*:354, 1964. (Abstr.)

80. Kreines, K., Jett, M., Knowles, H.C., Jr.: Observations in hyperthyroidism of abnormal glucose tolerance and other traits related to diabetes mellitus. Diabetes *14*:740, 1965.

81. Elgee, N.J., Williams, R.H., Lee, N.D.: Distribution and degradation studies with insulin I[131]. J. Clin. Invest. *33*:1252, 1954.

82. Cohen, A.M.: Interrelation of insulin activity and thyroid function. Am. J. Physiol. *188*:287, 1957.

83. Weller, C.V.: Hepatic lesions associated with exophthalmic goiter. Trans. Assoc. Am. Physicians *45*:71, 1930.

84. Farrant, R.: Hyperthyroidism: its experimental production in animals. Br. Med. J. *2*:1363, 1913.

85. Editorial: Hepatic lesions associated with exophthalmic goiter. Ann. Intern. Med. *4*:501, 1930.

86. McIver, M.A., Winter, E.A.: Deleterious effects of anoxia on the liver of the hyperthyroid animal. Arch. Surg. *46*:171, 1943.

87. John, H.J.: Carbohydrate metabolism in hyperthyroidism. In: G. Crile (Ed.): Diagnosis and Treatment of Diseases of the Thyroid Gland. Philadelphia, W.B. Saunders Co., 1932, p. 209.

88. Bodansky, M., Bodansky, O.: Diseases of the thyroid. In: Bodansky, M.: Biochemistry of Diseases, 2nd Ed. New York, Macmillan, 1942, p. 634.

89. Randle, P.J., Garland, P.B., Hales, C.N., Newsholme, E.A.: The glucose fatty-acid cycle. Its role in insulin sensitivity and the metabolic disturbances of diabetes mellitus. Lancet *1*:785, 1963.

90. Hales, C.N., Randle, P.J.: Effects of low-carbohydrate diet and diabetes mellitus on plasma concentrations of glucose, non-esterified fatty acid, and insulin during oral glucose tolerance tests. Lancet *1*:790, 1963.

91. Rich, C., Bierman, E.L., Schwartz, I.L.: Plasma nonesterified fatty acids in hyperthyroid states. J. Clin. Invest. *38*:275, 1959.

92. Marks, B.H., Kiem, I., Hills, A.G.: Endocrine influences on fat and carbohydrate metabolism in man. I. Effect of hyperthyroidism on fasting serum non-esterified fatty acid concentration and on its response to glucose ingestion. Metabolism *9*:1133, 1960.

93. Woeber, K.A., Arky, R., Braverman, L.E.: Reversal by guanethidine of abnormal oral glucose tolerance in thyrotoxicosis. Lancet *1*:895, 1966.

94. Althausen, T.L.: The disturbance of carbohydrate metabolism in hyperthyroidism; nature and management. J.A.M.A. *115*:101, 1940.
95. Perlman, L.V.: Familial incidence of diabetes in hyperthyroidism. Ann. Intern. Med. *55*:796, 1961.
96. Wilkerson, H.L.C., Krall, L.P., Butler, F.K.: Diabetes in a New England town. IV. 12-year progress report on the 70 diabetics found in the original Oxford, Mass., study. J.A.M.A. *179*:652, 1962.
97. Berkle, T.K.: Diabetes mellitus and hyperthyroidism in identical twins. Z. Menschl. Vererb. Konstitutionsl. *32*:68, 1953.
98. Landing, B.H., Pettit, M.D., Wiens, R.L., et al.: Antithyroid antibody and chronic thyroiditis in diabetes. (Letter to the Editor). J. Clin. Endocrinol. *23*:119, 1963.
99. Brink, S.J.: Thyroiditis and juvenile diabetes mellitus. Pediatr. Res. *13*:376, 1979.
100. Joslin, E.P., Lahey, F.H.: Diabetes and hyperthyroidism. Am. J. Med. Sci. *176*:1, 1928.
101. Wilder, R.M. Ref. 57, p. 46.
102. Wilder, R.M., Browne, H.C., Butt, H.R.: Diseases of metabolism and nutrition; review of certain recent contributions. Arch. Intern. Med. *65*:390, 1940.
103. Maxon, H.R., Kreines, K.W., Goldsmith, R.E., Knowles, H.C., Jr.: Long term observations of glucose tolerance in thyrotoxic patients. Arch. Intern. Med. *135*:1477, 1975.
104. Lakin, M., Bradley, R.F., Bell, G.D.: Acute hyperthyroidism in severe diabetic ketoacidosis. Am. J. Med. Sci. *241*:344, 1961.
105. Cooppan, R., Kozak, G.P.: Hyperthyroidism and diabetes mellitus. An analysis of 70 patients. Arch. Intern. Med. *140*:370, 1980.
106. Postellon, D.C., Becker, D.J., Foley, T.P., Jr.: Alterations in triiodothyronine (T3) and reverse triiodothyronine (rT3) concentrations in newly diagnosed patients with juvenile diabetes mellitus. (Abstract). Diabetes *27*:498, 1978.
107. Pittman, C.S., Suda, A.K., Chambers, J.B., Jr., et al.: Impaired 3,5,3'-triiodothyronine (T3) production in diabetic patients. Metabolism *28*:333, 1979.
108. Pittman, C.S., Suda, A.K., Chambers, J.B., Jr., et al.: Abnormalities of thyroid hormone turnover in patients with diabetes mellitus before and after insulin therapy. J. Clin. Endocrinol. Metab. *48*:854, 1979.
109. Mayfield, R.K., Sagel, J., Colwell, J.A.: Thyrotoxicosis without elevated serum triiodothyronine levels during diabetic ketoacidosis. Arch. Intern. Med. *140*:408, 1980.
110. Regan, J.F., Wilder, R.M.: Hyperthyroidism and diabetes. Arch. Intern. Med. *65*:1116, 1940.
111. Allan, F.N., Lahey, F.H., Murphy, R.: Hyperthyroidism and diabetes. An evaluation of anti-thyroid drugs. Trans. Am. Assoc. Study Goiter, 1940, p. 248.
112. Bowen, B.D., Lenzner, A.R.: The use of propylthiouracil in hyperthyroidism and diabetes. A study of forty-one cases. N. Engl. J. Med. *245*:629, 1951.
113. Volpe, R.: The role of autoimmunity in hypoendocrine and hyperendocrine function with special emphasis on autoimmune thyroid disease. Ann. Intern. Med. *87*:86, 1977.
114. Rupp, J.J., DiGeorge, A.M., Paschkis, K.E.: Hypothyroidism and diabetes mellitus. Diabetes *4*:393, 1955.
115. Baron, D.N.: Hypothyroidism and diabetes mellitus. Lancet *2*:796, 1955.
116. Lawrence, R.D.: The Diabetic Life, 17th Edn. London, J. & A. Churchill, 1965, p. 155.
117. Hecht, A., Gershberg, H.: Diabetes mellitus and primary hypothyroidism. Metabolism *17*:108, 1968.
118. Ganz, K., Kozak, G.P.: Diabetes mellitus and primary hypothyroidism. Arch. Intern. Med. *134*:430, 1974.
119. DeGroot, L.J., Stanbury, J.: The Thyroid and Its Diseases. New York, McGraw-Hill Book Co., 1975.
120. Hunton, R.B., Wells, M.V., Skipper, E.W.: Hypothyroidism in diabetics treated with sulphonylurea. Lancet *2*:449, 1965.
121. Burdick, R.E., Brice, L.T.: Hypothyroidism after sulphonylurea. Lancet *1*:97, 1968.
122. Portioli, I., Rocchi, F.: Sulphonylureas and hypothyroidism. Lancet *1*:681, 1969.
123. Goldstein, D.E., Drash, A., Gibbs, J., et al.: Diabetes mellitus: the incidence of circulating antibodies against thyroid, gastric and adrenal tissue. J. Pediatr. *77*:304, 1970.
124. Pettit, M.D., Landing, B.H., Guest, G.M.: Antithyroid antibody in juvenile diabetics. (Letter to the Editor). J. Clin. Endocrinol. Metab. *21*:209, 1961.
125. Whittingham, S., Matthews, J.D., Mackay, I.R., et al.: Diabetes mellitus, autoimmunity and aging. Lancet *1*:763, 1971.
126. LeCompte, P.M.: "Insulitis" in early juvenile diabetes. Arch. Pathol. *66*:450, 1958.
127. LeCompte, P.M., Legg, M.A.: Insulitis (lymphocytic infiltration of pancreatic islets) in late onset diabetes. Diabetes *21*:762, 1972.
128. Renold, A.E., Gonet, A.E., Vecchio, D.: Immunopathology of the endocrine pancreas. In: P.A. Miescher, H.J. Müller-Eberhard (Eds.): Textbook of Immunopathology. New York, Grune & Stratton, 1968, Vol. 2, pp. 595–601.
129. Carpenter, C.C., Solomon, N., Silverberg, S.G., et al.: Schmidt's syndrome (thyroid and adrenal insufficiency). A review of the literature and a report of fifteen new cases including ten instances of coexistent diabetes mellitus. Medicine *43*:153, 1964.
130. Munichoodappa, C., Kozak, G.P.: Diabetes mellitus and pernicious anemia. Diabetes *19*:719, 1970.
131. Glick, S.M.: Diabetes mellitus and cretinism: report of a case free of complications after 27 years. Metabolism *10*:788, 1961.
132. Skouby, A.P.: Clinical endocrine disturbances in diabetics; their relation to late diabetic lesions. Acta Med. Scand. *155*:401, 1956.
133. Ralli, E.P., Street, E., Pell, S.: The course and complications of diabetes mellitus. Data in 331 cases observed regularly in a diabetic clinic. Diabetes *4*:456, 1955.
134. Stanton, E.R., Jones, H.W., Jr., Marble, A.: Coexisting diabetes mellitus and Addison's disease: observations and report of a case in a 10-year-old boy. Arch. Intern. Med. *93*:911, 1954.
135. Gittler, R.D., Fajans, S.S., Conn, J.W.: Coexistence of Addison's disease and diabetes mellitus: report of three cases with a discussion of metabolic interrelationships. J. Clin. Endocrinol. *19*:797, 1959.
136. Beaven, D.W., Nelson, D.H., Renold, A.E., Thorn, G.W.: Diabetes mellitus and Addison's disease: a report on eight patients and a review of 55 cases in the literature. N. Engl. J. Med. *261*:443, 1959.
137. Wehrmacher, W.H.: Addison's disease with diabetes mellitus. Treatment with tolbutamide. Arch. Intern. Med. *108*:114, 1961.
138. Solomon, N., Carpenter, C.C.J., Bennett, I.L., Jr., Harvey, A.M.: Schmidt's syndrome (thyroid and adrenal insufficiency) and coexistent diabetes mellitus. Diabetes *14*:300, 1965.
139. Yoo, J., Kozak, G.P.: Diabetes and Addison's disease. Postgrad. Med. *55*:62, 1974.
140. Gould, K.S., Shlevin, E.L.: Addison's disease compli-

cating diabetes mellitus in adolescence. Ann. Intern. Med. *43*:1092, 1955.

141. Sunder, J.H., Bonessi, J.V., Balash, W.R., Danowski, T.S.: Hereditary Addison's disease in relation to diabetes mellitus. N. Engl. J. Med. *272*:818, 1965.

141a.Thorn, G.W., Clinton, M., Jr.: Metabolic changes in a patient with Addison's disease following the onset of diabetes mellitus. J. Clin. Endocrinol. *3*:355, 1943.

142. Thorn, G.W., Forsham, P.H., Frawley, T.F., et al.: Advances in the diagnosis and treatment of adrenal insufficiency. Am. J. Med. *10*:595, 1951.

142a.Schmidt, M.B.: Eine biglandulare Erkrankung (Nebennieren und Schilddruse) bei Morbus Addisonii. Verh. Dtsch. Ges. Pathol. *21*:212, 1926.

143. Nelson, R.P., Traisman, H.S., Deddish, R.B., Green, O.C.: Schmidt's syndrome in a child with diabetes mellitus. Diabetes Care *1*:37, 1978.

144. Irvine, W.J., Taft, A.D., Feek, C.M.: Addison's disease. In: V.H.T. James (Ed.): The Adrenal Gland. New York, Raven Press, 1979, pp. 131–164.

145. Gharib, H., Gastineau, C.F.: Coexisting Addison's disease and diabetes mellitus; report of 24 cases with review of literature. Mayo Clin. Proc. *44*:217, 1969.

146. Hardy, J.: Transsphenoidal surgery of hypersecreting pituitary tumors. In: P.O. Kohler, T.G. Ross: Diagnosis and Treatment of Pituitary Tumors. New York, American Elsevier, 1973, pp. 179–194.

147. Tyrrell, J.B., Brooks, R.M., Fitzgerald, P.A. et al.: Cushing's disease. Selective transsphenoidal resection of pituitary microadenomas. N. Engl. J. Med. *298*:753, 1978.

148. Lukens, F.D.W., Flippin, H.F., Thigpen, F.M.: Adrenal cortical adenoma with absence of the opposite adrenal. Report of a case with operation and autopsy. Am. J. Med. Sci. *193*:812, 1937.

149. Plotz, C.M., Knowlton, A.I., Regan, C.: The natural history of Cushing's syndrome. Am. J. Med. *13*:597, 1952.

150. Cope, O., Raker, J.W.: Cushing's disease: the surgical experience in the care of 46 cases. N. Engl. J. Med. *253*:119, 165, 1955.

151. Sprague, R.G., Randall, R.V., Salassa, R.M., et al.: Cushing's syndrome: a progressive and often fatal disease; a review of 100 cases seen between July 1945 and July 1954. Scientific exhibit. Arch. Intern. Med. *98*:389, 1956.

152. Skillern, P.G., McCullagh, E.P.: Hyperfunction and hypofunction of endocrine glands and diabetes mellitus. J. Indiana Med. Assoc. *50*:701, 1957.

153. Soffer, L.J., Iannaccone, A., Gabrilove, J.L.: Cushing's syndrome: a study of fifty patients. Am. J. Med. *30*:129, 1961.

154. Bookman, J.J., Drachman, S.R., Schaefer, L.E., Adlersberg, D.: Steroid diabetes in man; the development of diabetes during treatment with cortisone and corticotropin. Diabetes *2*:100, 1953.

155. Nelson, D.H., Meakin, J.W., Dealy, J.B., Jr., et al.: ACTH-producing tumor of the pituitary gland. N. Engl. J. Med. *259*:161, 1958.

156. Salassa, R.M., Kearns, T.P., Kernohan, J.W., et al.: Pituitary tumors in patients with Cushing's syndrome. J. Clin. Endocrinol. *19*:1523, 1959.

157. Nelson, D.H., Meakin, J.W., Thorn, G.W.: ACTH-producing pituitary tumors following adrenalectomy for Cushing's syndrome. Ann. Intern. Med. *52*:560, 1960.

158. Kozak, G.P., Paul, G.L., Vagnucci, A.I., et al.: Adrenal secretion after bilateral adrenalectomy for Cushing's syndrome. Ann. Intern. Med. *64*:778, 1966.

158a.Gold, E.M.: The Cushing syndrome: changing views of diagnosis and treatment. Ann. Intern. Med. *90*:829, 1979.

159. Laidlaw, J.C., Reddy, W.J., Jenkins, D., et al.: Advances in the diagnosis of altered states of adrenocortical function. N. Engl. J. Med. *253*:747, 1955.

160. Liddle, G.W.: Tests of pituitary-adrenal suppressibility in the diagnosis of Cushing's syndrome. J. Clin. Endocrinol. *20*:1539, 1960.

161. Forsham, P.H.: Abnormalities of the adrenal cortex. Clin. Sympos. *15*:35, 1963.

162. Lipsett, M.B., Hertz, R., Ross, G.T.: Clinical and pathophysiologic aspects of adrenocortical carcinoma. Am. J. Med. *35*:374, 1963.

163. Paris, J.: On the diagnosis of Addison's disease and Cushing's syndrome.

164. Herrera, M.G., Cahill, G.F., Jr., Thorn, G.W.: Cushing's syndrome: diagnosis and treatment. Am. J. Surg. *107*:144, 1964.

165. Pavlatos, F.C., Smilo, R.P., Forsham, P.H.: A rapid screening tests for Cushing's syndrome. *193*:720, 1965.

166. Nugent, C.A., Nichols, T., Tyler, F.H.: Diagnosis of Cushing's syndrome: single dose dexamethasone suppression test. Arch. Intern. Med. *116*:172, 1965.

167. Conn, J.W.: Potassium-losing nephritis. (Corresp.) Br. Med. J. *2*:1415, 1954.

168. Conn, J.W.: Presidential address: Pt. I Painting background. Pt. II. Primary aldosteronism, a new clinical syndrome. J. Lab. Clin. Med. *45*:3, 1955.

169. Conn, J.W.: Primary aldosteronism: progress report. J. Lab. Clin. Med. *45*:661, 980, 1955.

170. Conn, J.W., Louis, L.H.: Primary aldosteronism: a new clinical entity. Trans. Assoc. Am. Physicians *68*:215,1955.

171. Conn, J.W., Knopf, R.F., Nesbit, R.M.: Clinical characteristics of primary aldosteronism from analysis of 145 cases. Am. J. Surg. *107*:159, 1964.

172. Conn, J.W.: Hypertension, the potassium ion and impaired carbohydrate tolerance. N. Engl. J. Med. *273*:1135, 1965.

173. Conn, J.W.: Plasma renin activity in primary aldosteronism. Importance in differential diagnosis and in research of essential hypertension. J.A.M.A. *190*:222, 1964.

174. Conn, J.W., Cohen, E.L., Rovner, D.R., Nesbit, R.M.: Normokalemic primary aldosteronism: a detectable cause of curable"essential" hypertension. J.A.M.A. *193*:200, 1965.

175. Kaplan, N.M.: Hypokalemia in the hypertensive patients, with observations on the incidence of primary aldosteronism. Ann. Intern. Med. *66*:1079, 1967.

176. Kaplan, N.M.: The steroid content of adrenal adenomas and measurements of aldosterone production in patients with essential hypertension and primary aldosteronism. J. Clin. Invest. *46*:728, 1967.

177. Slaton, P.E., Biglieri, E.G.: Hypertension and hyperaldosteronism of renal and adrenal origin. Am. J. Med. *38*:324, 1965.

178. Broster, L.R., Vines, H.W.C.: The Adrenal Cortex. London, H.K. Lewis & Co., 1933.

179. Broster, L.R., Patterson, J., Camber, B.: Adrenal pseudohermaphroditism. Br. Med. J. *2*:1288, 1953.

180. Archard, C., Thiers, J.: Le virilisme pilaire et son association à l'insuffisance glycolitique (diabète des femmes à barbe). Bull. Acad. Méd. (Paris) 3e sér. *86*:51, 192.

181. Bongiovanni, A.M., Root, A.W.: The adrenogenital syndrome. N. Engl. J. Med. *268*:1283, 1342, 1391, 1963.

182. New, M.I., Dupont, B., Grumbach, K., Levine, L.S.: Congenital adrenal hyperplasia and related conditions. In: J.B. Stanbury, J.B. Wyngaarden, D.S. Fredrickson, et

al. (Eds.): The Metabolic Basis of Inherited Disease. 5th Edn. New York, McGraw-Hill Book Co., 1983, pp. 973–1000.

183. Soffer, L.J., Dorfman, R.I., Gabrilove, J.L.: The Human Adrenal Gland. Philadelphia, Lea & Febiger, 1961, p. 12.

184. Flint, L.D., Bartels, C.C.: Ten years' experience with 125 operated cases of pheochromocytoma. Surg. Clin. North Am. *42*:721, 1962.

185. Carman, C.T., Brashear, R.E.: Pheochromocytoma as an inherited abnormality: report of the tenth affected kindred and review of the literature. N. Engl. J. Med. *263*:419, 1960.

186. Gifford, R.W., Jr., Kvale, W.F., Maher, F.T., et al.: Clinical features, diagnosis and treatment of pheochromocytoma: a review of 76 cases. Mayo Clin. Proc. *39*:281, 1964.

187. Kvale, W.F., Roth, G.M., Manger, W.M., Priestley, J.T.: Present-day diagnosis and treatment of pheochromocytoma: a review of fifty-one cases. J.A.M.A. *164*:854, 1957.

188. Crout, J.R., Pisano, J.J., Sjoerdsma, A.: Urinary excretion of catecholamines and their metabolites in pheochromocytoma. Am. Heart J. *61*:375, 1961.

189. Gitlow, S.E.: The vanilmandelic acid test for pheochromocytoma. Heart Bull. *11*:21, 1962.

190. Sjoerdsma, A., Engelman, K., Waldmann, T.A., et al.: Pheochromocytoma: current concepts of diagnosis and treatment. Combined Clinical Staff Conference at the National Institutes of Health. Ann. Intern. Med. *65*:1302, 1966.

191. Pisano, J.J.: A simple analysis for normetanephrine and metanephrine in urine. Clin. Chim. Acta *5*:406, 1960.

192. von Studnitz, W., Käser, H., Sjoerdsma, A.: Spectrum of catecholamine biochemistry in patients with neuroblastoma. N. Engl. J. Med. *269*:232, 1963.

193. Engelman, K., Sjoerdsma, A.: A new test for pheochromocytoma. Pressor responsiveness to tyramine. J.A.M.A. *189*:81, 1964.

194. Lawrence, A.M.: Glucagon provocative test for pheochromocytoma. Ann. Intern. Med. *66*:1091, 1967.

195. Evans, J.A.: Difficulties in the diagnosis of pheochromocytoma. Med. Clin. N. Am. *44*:411, 1960.

195a.Sudre, Y., Becq-Giraudon, B., Pouget-Abadie, J.F., et al.: Le diabète du phéochromocytome. Sem. Hop. Paris *52*:1893, 1976.

195b.Emmer, M., Gorden, Ph., Roth, J.: Symposium of diabetes mellitus: diabetes in association with other endocrine disorders. Med. Clin. N. Am. *55*:1057, 1971.

195c.Modlin, I.M., Farndon, J.R., Shepherd, A., et al.: Phaeochromocytoma in 72 patients: clinical and diagnostic features, treatment and long-term results. Br. J. Surg. *66*:456, 1979.

196. Duncan, L.E., Jr., Semans, J.H., Howard, J.E.: Adrenal medullary tumor (pheochromocytoma) and diabetes mellitus: disappearance of diabetes after removal of tumor. Ann. Intern. Med. *20*:815, 1944.

197. Goldner, M.G.: Pheochromocytoma with diabetes: case report and discussion. J. Clin. Endocrinol. *7*:716, 1947.

198. Cori, D.F.: Mammalian carbohydrate metabolism. Physiol. Rev. *11*:143, 1931.

199. Spergel, G., Bleicher, S.J., Ertel, N.H.: Carbohydrate and fat metabolism in patients with pheochromocytoma. N. Engl. J. Med. *278*:803, 1968.

200. Wilber, J.F., Turtle, J.R., Crane, N.A.: Inhibition of insulin secretion by phaeochromocytoma. Lancet *2*:733, 1966.

200a.Isles, C.G., Johnson, J.K.: Phaeochromocytoma and diabetes mellitus: further evidence that alpha-2 receptors in-

hibit insulin release in man. Clin. Endocrinol. *18*:37, 1983.

200b.Metz, S.A., Hulter, J.B., Robertson, R.P.: Induction of defective insulin secretion and impaired glucose tolerance by clonidine: selective stimulation of metabolic alpha adrenergic pathways. Diabetes *27*:554, 1978.

201. Mallinson, C.N., Bloom, S.R., Warin, A.P., et al.: A glucagonoma syndrome. Lancet *2*:1, 1974.

202. Weir, G.C., Novelline, R.A.: The glucagonoma syndrome. Am. Fam. Physician *16*:83, 1977.

203. Kessinger, A., Lemon, H.M., Foley, J.F.: The glucagonoma syndrome and its management. J. Surg. Oncol. *9*:419, 1977.

204. R.E. Scully (Ed.): Case records of the Massachusetts General Hospital. Case 20–1975. N. Engl. J. Med. *292*:1117, 1975.

205. Kessinger, A., Foley, J.F., Lemon, H.M.: Use of DTIC in the malignant carcinoid syndrome. Cancer Treat. Rep. *61*:101, 1977.

206. Strauss, G.M., Weitzman, S.A., Aoki, T.T.: Dimethyltriazenoimidazole carboxamide therapy of malignant glucagonoma. Ann. Intern. Med. *90*:57, 1979.

207. Moertel, C.G., Hanley, J.A., Johnson, L.A.: Streptozotocin alone compared with streptozotocin plus fluorouracil in the treatment of advanced islet-cell carcinoma. N. Engl. J. Med. *303*:1189, 1980.

207a.Krejs, G.J., Orci, L., Conlon, J.M., et al.: Somatostatinoma syndrome. N. Engl. J. Med. *301*:285, 1979.

207b.Ganda, O.P., Weir, G.C., Soeldner, J.S., et al.: "Somatostatinoma": a somatostatin-containing tumor of the endocrine pancreas. N. Engl. J. Med. *296*:963, 1977.

208. Akgun, S., Ertel, N.H.: Hyperparathyroidism and coexisting diabetes mellitus. Altered carbohydrate metabolism. Arch. Intern. Med. *138*:1500, 1978.

209. Walsh, C.H., Soler, N.J., Malins, J.M.: Diabetes mellitus and primary hyperparathyroidism. Postgrad. Med. J. *51*:446, 1975.

210. Grodsky, G.M., Bennett, L.L.: Cation requirement for insulin secretion in the isolated perfused pancreas. Diabetes *15*:910, 1966.

210a.Milner, R.D.G., Hales, C.N.: The role of calcium and magnesium in insulin secretion from rabbit pancreas studied *in vitro*. Diabetologia *3*:47, 1967.

211. Malaisse, W.J., Brisson, G.R., Baird, L.E.: Stimulus secretion coupling of glucose induced insulin release. X. Effect of glucose on Ca^{++} efflux from perfused islets. Am. J. Physiol. *224*:389, 1973.

212. Kim, H., Kalkhoff, R.K., Costrini, N.Y., et al.: Plasma insulin disturbances in primary hyperparathyroidism. J. Clin. Invest *50*:2596, 1971.

213. Ginsberg, H., Olefsky, J.M., Reaven, G.M.: Evaluation of insulin resistance in patients with primary hyperparathyroidism. (38665). Proc. Soc. Exp. Biol. Med. *148*:942, 1975.

214. Purnell, D.C., Smith, L.H., Scholz, D.A., et al.: Primary hyperparathyroidism: a prospective clinical study. Am. J. Med. *50*:670, 1971.

215. Yasuda, K., Hurukawa, Y., Okuyama, M., et al.: Glucose tolerance and insulin secretion in patients with parathyroid disorders. Effect of serum calcium on insulin release. N. Engl. J. Med. *292*:501, 1975.

216. Curry, D.L., Bennett, L.L., Grodsky, G.M.: Requirement for calcium ion in insulin secretion by the perfused rat pancreas. Am. J. Physiol. *214*:174, 1968.

217. Albright, F., Reifenstein, E.C., Jr.: The Parathyroid Glands and Metabolic Bone Disease. Selected Studies. Baltimore. Williams & Wilkins, 1948, p. 150.

218. Berney, P.W.: Osteoporosis and diabetes mellitus. Report of a case. J. Iowa Med. Soc. *42*:10, 1952.

219. Menczel, J., Makin, M., Robin, G., et al.: Prevalence of diabetes mellitus in Jerusalem: its association with presenile osteoporosis. Isr. J. Med. Sci. 8:918, 1972.

220. Levin, M.E., Boisseau, V.C., Avioli, L.V.: Effects of diabetes mellitus on bone mass in juvenile and adult onset diabetes. N. Engl. J. Med. 294:241, 1976.

221. Santiago, J.V.,: McAlister, W.H., Ratzan, S.K., et al.: Decreased cortical thickness and osteopenia in children with diabetes mellitus. J. Clin. Endocrinol. Metab. 45:845, 1977.

222. Rosenbloom, A.L., Lezotte, D.C., Weber, F.T., et al.: Diminution of bone mass in childhood diabetes. Diabetes 26:1052, 1977.

223. Meema, H.E., Reid, D.B.W.: The relationship between skin and cortical bone thickness in old age with special reference to osteoporosis and diabetes mellitus: a roentgenographic study. J. Gerontol. 24:28, 1969.

224. Meema, H.E., Meema, S.: The relationship of diabetes mellitus and body weight to osteoporosis in elderly females. Can. Med. Assoc. J. 96:132, 1967.

225. DeLeeuw, I., Abs, R.: Bone mass and bone density in maturity-type diabetics measured by the ¹²⁵I photon-absorption technique. Diabetes 26:1130, 1977.

226. Heath III, H., Lambert, P.W., Service, F.J., Arnaud, S.B.: Calcium homeostasis in diabetes mellitus. J. Clin. Endocrinol. Metab. 49:462, 1979.

227. Schneider, L.E., Wilson, H.D., Schedl, H.P.: Effects of diabetes and Vitamin D depletion on duodenal and ileal calcium transport in the rat. Acta Diabetol. Lat. 14:18, 1977.

228. Schneider, L.E., Schedl, H.P., McCain, T., Haussler, M.R.: Experimental diabetes reduces circulating 1.25 dihydroxyvitamin D in the rat. Science 196:1452, 1977.

229. DeFronzo, R.A., Goldberg, M., Agus, Z.S.: The effects of glucose and insulin on renal electrolyte transport. J. Clin. Invest. 58:83, 1976.

230. Fleming, L.W., Stewart, W.K.: Effect of carbohydrate intake on the urinary excretion of magnesium, calcium and sodium in fasting obese patients. Nephron. 16:64, 1976.

230a. Witt, M.F., White, N.H., Santiago, J.V., et al.: Use of oral calcium loading to characterize the hypercalcemia of young insulin-dependent diabetics. J. Clin. Endocrinol. Metab. 57:94, 1983.

230b. Frazer, T.E., White, N.H., Hough, S., et al.: Alteration in circulating vitamin D metabolites in the young insulin–dependent diabetic. J. Clin. Endocrinol. Metab. 53:1154, 1981.

231. McNair, P., Madsbad, S., Christiansen, C., et al.: Bone loss in diabetes. Effects of metabolic state. Diabetologia 17:283, 1979.

232. Cope, O., Culver, P.J., Mixter, C.G., Jr., Nardi, G.L.: Pancreatitis, a diagnostic clue to hyperparathyroidism. Ann. Surg. 145:857, 1957.

233. Mixter, C.G., Jr., Keynes, W.M., Cope, O.: Further experience with pancreatitis as a diagnostic clue to hyperparathyroidism. N. Engl. J. Med. 258:265, 1962.

234. Hoar, C.S., Jr., Gorlin, R.: Hyperparathyroidism and acute pancreatitis. N. Engl. J. Med. 258:1052, 1958.

235. Lacher, M.J., Goldberg, J.A., Thomas, D.F., Calvy, G.L.: Hyperparathyroidism and pancreatitis: report of a case. N. Engl. J. Med. 261:239, 1959.

236. Keating, F.R., Jr.: Diagnosis of primary hyperparathyroidism. Clinical and laboratory aspects. J.A.M.A. 178:547, 1961.

237. Gross, J.B.: Some recent developments pertaining to pancreatitis. Ann. Intern. Med. 49:796, 1958.

238. Jackson, C.E.: Hereditary hyperparathyroidism associated with recurrent pancreatitis. Ann. Intern. Med. 49:829, 1958.

239. Natelson, R.P.: Co-existent acromegaly, diabetes mellitus and diabetes insipidus. Ann. Intern. Med. 40:788, 1954.

240. Randall, R.V., Clark, E.C., Bahn, R.C.: Classification of the causes of diabetes insipidus. Mayo Clin. Proc. 34:299, 1959.

241. Riggs, B.L.J., Randall, R.V.: Clinics on endocrine and metabolic diseases. 2. Diabetes insipidus and diabetes mellitus: report of a case. Mayo Clin. Proc. 35:30, 1960.

242. Raiti, S., Plotkin, S., Newns, G.H.: Diabetes mellitus and insipidus in two sisters. Br. Med. J. 2:1625, 1963.

243. Zatuchni, J., Armento, D.F., Mensel, P.H.: Pitressin-resistant diabetes insipidus and diabetes mellitus with bilateral hydronephrosis. Am. J. Med. Sci. 247:445, 1964.

244. Bretz, G.W., Baghdassarian, A., Graber, J.D., et al.: Co-existence of diabetes mellitus and insipidus and optic atrophy in two male siblings. Am. J. Med. 48:398, 1970.

245. Page, M.McB., Asmal, A.C., Edwards, C.R.W.: Recessive inheritance of diabetes: the syndrome of diabetes insipidus, diabetes mellitus, optic atrophy and deafness. Quart. J. Med. (New Series 45):505, 1976.

246. Cremers, C.W., Wijdeveld, P.G., Pinckers, A.J.: Juvenile diabetes mellitus, optic atrophy, hearing loss, diabetes insipidus, atonia of the urinary tract and bladder, and other abnormalities (Wolfram syndrome). A review of 88 cases from the literature with personal observations on 3 new patients. Acta Paediatr. Scand. 264 (Suppl.) 1–16, 1977.

247. Gossain, V.V., Sugawara, M., Hagen, G.A.: Co-existent diabetes mellitus and diabetes insipidus, a familial disease. J. Clin. Endocrinol. Metab. 41:1020, 1975.

248. Babbott, D., Rubin, A., Ginsburg, S.J.: The reproductive characteristics of diabetic men. Diabetes 7:33, 1958.

249. Rubin, A.: Studies in human reproduction. II. The influence of diabetes mellitus in men upon reproduction. Am. J. Obstet. Gynecol. 76:25, 1958.

250. Rubin, A.: Sexual behavior in diabetes mellitus. Medical Aspects of Human Sexuality 1:23, 1967.

251. Rubin, A., Babbott, D.: Impotence and diabetes mellitus. J.A.M.A. 168:498, 1958.

252. Wilson, J.L., Marks, J.H.: Calcification of vas deferens: its relation to diabetes mellitus and arteriosclerosis. N. Engl. J. Med. 245:321, 1951.

253. Forbes, A.P., Engel, E.: The high incidence of diabetes mellitus in 414 patients with gonadal dysgenesis, and their close relatives. Metabolism 12:428, 1963.

254. Federman, D.D.: Abnormal Sexual Development. Philadelphia, W.B. Saunders Co., 1967, p. 30.

40 The Digestive System and Diabetes

Kenneth R. Falchuk, Charles Trey, John F. Sullivan, and B. Dan Ferguson

Disturbances of the digestive tract are common in diabetic patients. Most of these are not directly related to diabetes whereas others, such as those due to diabetic neuropathy, may be regarded as specific complications. Among the latter, hypotonia and altered motility of hollow viscera are the most frequently encountered abnormalities.

ORAL CAVITY

Many changes may be observed in the oral cavity of diabetic patients, some of which are related to the current and/or long-term degree of control of diabetes. These include dry mouth, burning sensations in the buccal mucosa and tongue, painful fissures, and coating of the tongue. Of long-term importance is an increased prevalence of periodontal disease, with hyperemic and swollen gingival tissues, polypoid gingival proliferation, and finally alveolar bone destruction and loosened teeth. Indeed, symptoms related to such findings may first bring the patient with undiagnosed diabetes to the physician or dentist. However, despite numerous experimental and clinical investigations, opinions vary regarding the relationship of diabetes to disease of the mouth. Definite mechanisms by which diabetes may affect the periodontium remain a matter for discussion, but it is reasonable to assume that lowered resistance to infection, sub-optimal healing of wounds, and microangiopathy which are found in patients with chronically poor control of diabetes, play significant roles. Unfortunately, often in studies along this line, subjects have been chosen without due regard to age, type of diabetes (insulin-dependent or noninsulin-dependent), degree of control of hyperglycemia, duration of diabetes, and accompanying vascular and neurologic disease.

In a longitudinal study of 21 female diabetic patients, aged 19 to 35 years, Cohen et al. found highly significant differences in the gingival and periodontal scores as compared with nondiabetic control subjects. These differences remained over 3 successive years of study.[1] Golub and co-workers outlined some of the basic pathophysiologic considerations of diabetes, stating that disease accelerates periodontal breakdown and impairs healing of wounds.[2]

Glavind and associates[3] found that diabetics aged 30 to 40 years had significantly greater loss of periodontal support compared to controls in the same age group. Greater periodontal damage was present in those who had had diabetes for more than 10 years and in whom retinal vascular changes had taken place. These findings were in keeping with the results of earlier work such as that of Finestone and Boorujy who noted that the prevalence and severity of periodontal disease increased with the duration of diabetes, variance of blood glucose levels, and the presence of systemic complications.[4] As a result of their studies on albino rats with alloxan diabetes, Glickman, Smulow and Moreau concluded that healing following surgical resection of marginal gingival tissue was retarded by inhibition of fibroplasia and bone formation.[5] Sznajder et al., in a study of diabetic and nondiabetic patients with periodontal disease, found that loss of periodontal support was significantly more severe in the diabetics who were over 30 years of age than in the nondiabetic controls.[6]

Gingival capillary basement membranes in healthy patients, nondiabetic patients with periodontal disease, and diabetics with periodontal disease were examined by Frantzis and co-workers.[7] They found that in the diabetics with periodontal disease the basement membrane was 4 times thicker than in subjects in the other two groups. Histologic studies with light and electron microscopy suggested a higher prevalence of gingival vascular changes in diabetics than in nondiabetics.[8,9] Biopsies of human gingiva with periodontitis showed significantly lower concentrations of cyclic adenosine monophosphate (cAMP) when compared with biopsies of healthy gingiva.[10] This nucleotide is believed to play a role in the regulation of normal cell growth and to act as an inhibitor to excessive cell growth. A comparison by Grower and associates of gingival fluids in diabetics and nondiabetics, showed a decreased level of cAMP in the diabetics.[11]

Bernick et al. studied 50 diabetic children and an age-matched control group of 36 nondiabetic children. He reported that with the same measures of oral hygiene, there was a greater frequency of gingival inflammation and radiographic bone loss in the diabetic group.[12]

In contrast to the above studies that show that diabetes may have a deleterious effect on gingival and periodontal tissues, other investigators have reported that in persons with well-controlled diabetes, the response of gingival tissues is comparable to that in nondiabetic persons. In an early study by Benveniste, Bixler and Conneally which included both diabetics and nondiabetics aged 5 to 72 years, the results indicated that although the frequency of gingivitis and calculus formation was higher in the diabetic patients, the differences were not statistically significant.[13] The conclusions of Hove and Stallard[14] and of Mackenzie and Millard[15] supported those of Benveniste and co-workers.

Dental Care in the Patient with Diabetes

The examination and treatment of the patient with diabetes is similar to that in the nondiabetic person. However, prior to treating a diabetic patient, the dentist should take a detailed history including such items as the usual degree of control of diabetes achieved by the patient, and the absence or presence of complications, particularly those related to microangiopathy, i.e, retinopathy and nephropathy. Despite controversy, particularly in the past, as to the relationship of diabetes to periodontal disease, evidence in the last decade or two has mounted to indicate that if diabetes can be controlled to the extent that the blood glucose oscillates within a normal or near-normal range, other metabolic indices tend to return toward normal. It is reasonable to predict, other things being equal, that resistance to infection and wound-healing likewise become normal or approach such unless the abnormality is too far advanced.

Dental plaque or gingival debris (composed almost entirely of bacteria), deposited on the tooth surface close to the gingival tissue, is the principal cause of gingival and periodontal disease. This inflames and infects the gingival tissue and as it becomes more pronounced, spreads into the deeper periodontal structures with loss of alveolar bone and eventually loss of teeth. Obviously, attempts at prevention should include consistently good control of diabetes as well as daily cleansing of the teeth by brushing and flossing.

Using a multiple imprint culture technique, Tapper-Jones and colleagues[15a] found that the oral carrier rate and density of *Candida albicans* were higher in a group of 50 diabetic patients (mean age, 52.5 years) than in 50 comparable control subjects. Surprisingly, the patient's age, duration of diabetes, type of treatment, or degree of control were not correlated with the presence or absence of *C. albicans*. Local influences such as the wearing of dentures and smoking did appear to be predisposing factors, especially in the diabetic group.

Treatment of Gingivitis. When gingivitis and/or periodontitis are present, a treatment plan of scaling and plaque control with oral hygiene instruction may suffice if the inflammatory processes are located within the gingival tissue and if the gingival defects are small. When deeper defects show radiographic evidence of alveolar bone loss, resection of infected gingival tissue, mucoperiosteal flaps of the facial and lingual gingival tissues, osseous correction of alveolar bone defects, suturing of the tissues, and placement of a periodontal pack are required. When healing has taken place, usually in about 2 weeks, the tooth root surfaces are scaled and curetted and the patient is educated to an exacting level of oral hygiene and plaque removal, using an electric tooth brush, dental floss, rubber-tipped interdental stimulation, and waterpick. Careful instructions are also given for gingival massage with the electric tooth brush. After the active phase of periodontal treatment is completed, the patient should return every 2 or 3 months for care designed to maintain a healthy periodontium.

Any dental procedure requiring general anesthesia should be carried out in a hospital operating room, where there are appropriate personnel and equipment to deal with both anesthetic and medical emergencies. Those procedures requiring local anesthesia may be handled in the office.

Patients whose diabetes is well treated on a daily basis may not require specific antibiotic coverage for these procedures. However, appropriate antibiotic prophylaxis should be used in the same instances as in the patient without diabetes

DISORDERS OF THE ESOPHAGUS

Esophageal motor dysfunction, characterized by absence or marked decrease in the primary peristaltic wave, delays esophageal emptying and the presence of frequent spontaneous contractions, and has been demonstrated by both cineradiographic and manometric studies in certain diabetic patients.[16-20] Such motor abnormalities have been found to have a strong association with peripheral neuropathy; moreover, there is a correlation between the severity of the motor dysfunction and that of peripheral neuropathy.[21] Some workers have reported a decrease of pressure in the lower esophageal sphincter and the development of gastroesophageal reflux,[19,22] whereas other investigators have been unable to find any differences in this regard between diabetic and normal individuals.[21]

Studies on the neuropathology of the esophagus have demonstrated degenerative changes in the nerve trunks of the esophageal plexus and about the celiac ganglia.[22] In the diabetic, the myenteric plexus is functionally intact and there is no hypersensitivity to cholinergic agents as seen in achalasia, in which there is degeneration of the myenteric plexus.[23]

When a diabetic complains of significant symptoms referable to the esophagus, a complete evaluation should be made with radiographic as well as endoscopic studies to exclude disorders such as reflux esophagitis, moniliasis, or even carcinoma of the esophagus. Diabetes predisposes to the development of gastrointestinal moniliasis. Although a barium swallow can demonstrate esophageal involvement by candida, demonstration of the yeast forms from material recovered during endoscopy remains the best method of diagnosis. Most patients with candidiasis respond to nystatin given orally. If such treatment fails, flucytosine (Ancobon), low-dose amphotericin B given intravenously, or oral ketoconazole (Nizoral) may be used successfully.[24-26]

DISORDERS OF THE STOMACH

Motor Abnormalities

Gastric motor abnormalities occur in 20 to 30% of diabetic patients,[27] often without noteworthy clinical manifestations. Rundles[16] in 1945 was the first to describe a marked decrease in gastric motility in diabetes. In 1958, Kassander[28] introduced the term "gastroparesis diabeticorum" to describe atony and delayed gastric emptying.

Gastroparesis. In the majority of patients, gastroparesis is associated with generalized diabetic neuropathy. Symptomatically the effects of gastric stasis are quite variable: many patients are asymptomatic, while others describe vague abdominal symptoms. Nausea, postprandial fullness, early satiety, and epigastric pain are the most frequent complaints. In advanced cases, there may be protracted vomiting severe enough to suggest gastric outlet obstruction.[29] Glycemic control may be difficult to maintain, especially in insulin-dependent diabetics; frequent hypoglycemic episodes may occur.[30]

Diabetic gastric neuropathy occurs most frequently in the presence of other diabetic complications such as peripheral neuropathy, retinopathy, and nephropathy. Radiographically, the stomach can be large, distended, and with diminished peristalis. Marked gastric retention of barium and food particles can be demonstrated for hours or even days in extreme cases. Duodenal bulb atony and dilatation without evidence of organic obstruction has been reported in 34% of diabetics with gastroparesis.[31] Because a conventional upper gastrointestinal barium study is an insensitive approach to the detection of gastric stasis, we recommend the use of a "barium-burger" (barium-bread meal) radiologic study, or preferably an isotopic scintiscanning (radio-labeled egg white) technique[32] to evaluate those patients with abnormality of gastric emptying.

Diabetic patients with gastroparesis have either markedly depressed antral motor function or ineffectual peristalsis. The antral circular muscle appears to be normal as assessed by the pharmacologic response to bethanechol.[33] The etiology of gastric stasis has not been fully elucidated. The delay in gastric emptying has been attributed to vagal damage as part of a more generalized autonomic neuropathy,[34,35] but other mechanisms may contribute to the etiology of this disorder. Although hyperglycemia and also glucagon may have a role by inhibiting gastric motility,[36] the concentrations of glucagon required to effect emptying are greater than the physiologic range.[37] Furthermore, a similar effect of hyperglycemia has not been demonstrated in diabetics.[38]

The treatment of the symptomatic patient with gastroparesis has been generally disappointing. Antibiotics may provide some temporary relief, and small feedings should be encouraged. At times, brief periods of intravenous alimentation are required. Various anticholinesterase preparations have been tried without much success.[29,31] Drugs such as bethanechol (Urecholine) and metoclopramide (Reglan) which increase gastric motility, have been somewhat helpful clinically.[39,40] Metoclopramide increases the strength of gastric contractions and accelerates gastric emptying. It is thought to act as a dopamine antagonist, enhancing the local effect of acetylchloline on gastric smooth muscle.[39] In recent studies, metoclopramide was found to be significantly superior to placebo in reducing the symptoms associated with delayed gastric emptying.[41,42] Various surgical procedures have been performed, mostly with little benefit except for an occasional report of good results after a pyloroplasty.[43]

Secretory Abnormalities

The results of studies of gastric secretion in diabetes are conflicting. Dotevall[44] found that both basal and histamine-stimulated gastric secretions were less in diabetic patients than in a control group. Others have not found significant differences in acid secretion between diabetics and nondiabetics.[45] The gastric mucosa in diabetics becomes atrophic more commonly and at an earlier age than in nondiabetics. As many as 65% of diabetics may have partial or complete atrophy of the gastric mucosa, possibly explaining the reported diminished gastric secretion. Parietal cell and intrinsic factor antibodies are increased in diabetics.[46] The frequency of diabetes in patients with pernicious anemia is about 2%,[47] while that of pernicious anemia in insulin-dependent diabetics has been reported to be 4%.[48] In addition to hyperglycemia and increased glucagon secretion,[49] which have been found to inhibit gastric secretion, the diminished acid secretion in diabetics can also result from vagal neuropathy.[50]

Gastric and Duodenal Ulcer

Dotevall[44] in a study of 1218 diabetics reported a lower incidence of duodenal ulcer in these patients than in nondiabetics. This finding may be related to the decrease in gastric secretion found by the same investigator. However, a more recent report raises some questions about the incidence of peptic ulcer in patients with diabetes.[51] Gastric ulcers occur with the same frequency as in nondiabetics. The complication of ulcer disease tend to be more severe in diabetics. Bleeding from an ulcer may be more profuse and difficult to control because of the vascular changes associated with diabetes. In addition, symptoms of gastric outlet obstruction are often accentuated because of decreased gastric motility in those patients with autonomic neuropathy.[52]

DISORDERS OF THE INTESTINE

Absorption

The absorption of glucose in diabetics has been reported as normal by some[53] and increased by others.[54] The enzymatic activity of brush border hydrolases, including disaccharidases and peptidases, have been found to be normal in both juvenile and maturity onset types of diabetes.[55] Experimentally in diabetic rats, the increased enzymatic activity of a representative disaccharidase (such as sucrase) is the consequence of an increase in sucrase-isomaltase protein which develops because of a decrease in its rate of degradation.[56] In most studies, the jejunal absorption of water and electrolytes in patients with diabetic diarrhea has been found similar to that of nondiabetic controls.[57]

Diabetic Diarrhea and Steatorrhea

The term "diarrhea of diabetes" was first used by Bargen and associates of the Mayo Clinic[58] to describe the intractable diarrhea in patients with severe diabetes, usually in association with peripheral or autonomic neuropathy.[59] Other causes of prolonged diarrhea must always be excluded. Enteric infections, gluten enteropathy, and chronic pancreatitis should be considered among the many etiologic possibilities of diarrhea and steatorrhea in diabetics. Commonly, no obvious cause other than the diabetic state is detected. In these patients, the term "diabetic diarrhea" is applied.

Patients with diabetic diarrhea commonly have insulin-dependent, poorly-controlled diabetes complicated by neuropathy. Characteristically, young male diabetics (aged 20 to 40 years) are most affected. The diarrhea tends to be intermittent, watery, profuse, and to occur more frequently at night.[60] These patients often experience other manifestations of autonomic neuropathy such as impotence, defective sweating, postural hypotension, and bladder dysfunction. Diabetic diarrhea undergoes unexplained periods of remission and exacerbation. While the pathogenesis of the diarrhea, with or without steatorrhea, has not been clearly established, several mechanisms have been postulated, including not only autonomic neuropathy, but also bacterial overgrowth, exocrine pancreatic insufficiency, and intestinal mucosal alterations. Diabetic diarrhea is frequently characterized by motor abnormalities of the small bowel such as a progressive decrease in upper small intestinal tone and an increase in the frequency and amplitude of large waves.[61]

Radiographic features of diabetic diarrhea often relate to the autonomic neuropathy, and include delayed gastric emptying and a prolonged, disorderly transit of intestinal contents through the small bowel.[27,61] The caliber of the gut lumen may show considerable variation; localized segments of dilated intestine with segmentation and coarsening of the mucosal folds may be present. Because these radiologic findings lack specificity, primary mucosal abnormalities such as gluten enteropathy must be excluded. In the majority of patients with diabetic diarrhea, the intestinal mucosa is normal despite significant steatorrhea.[62,63] The absorption of d-xylose and vitamin B_{12} as well as sodium and water transport, is usually normal.[57] It has been suggested that afferent sympathetic innervation is impaired, whereas the efferent pathways are uninterrupted in patients with autonomic neuropathy.[57] Although lesions of the dendritic processes of the para- and pre-vertebral sympathetic ganglia have been reported,[62,64] there is no conclusive evidence of histologic abnormalities affecting the intestinal sympathetic or parasympathetic nerves or the submucosal or myenteric plexus.[59,62]

It has been stated that steatorrhea represents a more intense manifestation of diabetic diarrhea.[63] The mechanism of steatorrhea in diabetes is usually not clear, but in some patients it may be due to (1) exocrine pancreatic insufficiency; (2) bacterial overgrowth, or (3) concomitant celiac disease. Abnormalities of pancreatic exocrine function have been reported in 20 to 70% of diabetics,[65] but clinically significant exocrine insufficiency is uncommon,[59] and pancreatic enzyme replacement therapy usually does not ameliorate the steatorrhea.

In a small number of diabetics, intestinal bacterial overgrowth may result in deconjugation of bile salts with defective micellar formation and fat malabsorption. Whenever bacterial overgrowth is suspected, a 2-week trial of broad spectrum antibiotics (e.g., tetracycline) is indicated. Although various reports have documented clinical improvement after antibiotic therapy,[66,67] there has been no controlled trial of antibiotics in diabetic diarrhea, and direct evidence for intestinal bacterial overgrowth has been obtained in very few patients.[57,67,68] In some diabetics, bile acid malabsorption has been implicated in the etiology of diarrhea and in certain of these patients, the use of cholestyramine (Questran) has resulted in symptomatic improvement[69] while, in others, therapy with this bile acid binding resin was unsuccessful.

Primary Malabsorption and Diabetes

Steatorrhea in the diabetic should lead to a careful search for celiac disease, since these two bowel disorders may co-exist. Thompson[70] concluded that the incidence of diabetes in children with celiac disease is 4 times that expected. Other studies[71,72] also seem to indicate that celiac disease may occur more frequently in insulin-dependent diabetics than would be expected by chance alone. However, Boyer and Andersen[73] stated that there was no significant relationship between diabetes and celiac disease in the families of patients with and without celiac disease, and Carter, Sheldon, and Walker[74] found no cases of diabetes in 88 patients with glutein-induced enteropathy. Thus, the status of this possible association remains unclear.

In recent years, the histocompatability antigen $HLA-B_8$ has been shown to be associated with both celiac disease[75] and juvenile-onset diabetes.[76] In view of this association, it is possible that a gene (or genes) linked to, and in disequilibrium with, certain loci (B and D) of the HLA complex, is important in the pathogenesis of celiac disease and diabetes. To establish the diagnosis of celiac disease, an intestinal biopsy showing the typical celiac sprue lesion is needed in addition to a clinical response to treatment with a gluten-free diet. Some suggest that re-challenge with gluten after an apparent response to gluten withdrawal is needed to establish the diagnosis unequivocally. At the New England Deaconess Hospital, we have been able to confirm an association between gluten-sensitive enteropathy, insulin-dependent diabetes, and the HLA-B8 antigen in 80% of cases. In our patients, prompt clinical improvement followed the withdrawal of gluten from the diet.

The management of patients with diabetic diarrhea without a specific etiology, represents a challenge to the physician and to the patient. In some diabetics, cholinergic drugs such as metacholine[35] may be helpful. In others, the use of diphenoxylate with atropine (Lomotil) or loperamide (Imodium) may result in clinical improvement. At times certain opiate derivatives such as codeine phosphate may benefit a small number of patients in whom other modalities of therapy have failed. At present, empirical therapy is all that one can offer those diabetics in whom a specific cause for diarrhea has not been found.

Constipation

Constipation is a common gastrointestinal complaint of diabetic patients as indeed it is with non-diabetics. As many as 20% of diabetics may be constipated.[16] This symptom reflects the end result of the visceral neuropathy which impairs colonic motility leading to atony and dilatation of the colon. This may occasionally cause fecal impaction simulating intestinal obstruction. It is important to emphasize that constipation is also common in diabetics with autonomic neuropathy. Treatment consists of a bowel training program as well as the use of a high-fiber diet supplemented by psyllium hydrophilic mucilloid (Metamucil).

PANCREAS

Since the endocrine pancreas is central to any discussion of diabetes, it is reasonable to wonder as to any functional relationship to the exocrine portion of the organ of which it comprises fully 95% of the weight. One keeps in mind the common embryologic origin of the apparently distinct two portions of the organ.

In the section which follows, two main topics—pancreatic tumors and pancreatitis—will be discussed from the standpoint of the gastroenterologist.

Pancreatic Tumors

Pancreatic carcinoma is now the second most frequent gastrointestinal malignancy and the fourth most frequent cause of all deaths from cancer in the Unites States. The results of recent studies show an increase in the incidence of carcinoma of the pancreas in diabetics[77-79] as well as in nondiabetics. This tumor appears to be about twice as common in diabetics as in the general population and in the Joslin Clinic experience, it comprises 12 to 13% of all malignancies in diabetics.[80] However, the reported incidence varies considerably depending on the population under study. This frequency is strongly correlated with age, being rare in individuals less than 25 years old, while the occurrence in males over 75 years of age is 8 to 10 times that in the general population.[81]

The diagnosis of pancreatic carcinoma should be considered when diabetes develops de novo in an elderly non-obese subject without a family history of diabetes, or if instability of diabetic control develops in a previously well-controlled diabetic, particularly if weight loss or vague abdominal symptoms are also present.

Abdominal ultrasound and computerized tomography are noninvasive techniques which may facilitate the diagnosis of pancreatic tumors when grounds for suspicion exist.[82] Endoscopic retro-grade pancreatography and cytologic study of pure pancreatic juice are sensitive and specific tests for the detection of pancreatic carcinoma, providing a positive diagnosis in 88 to 93% of patients with cancer of the pancreas.[83,84] In recent years, with the development of percutaneous aspiration biopsy of the pancreas under ultrasound guidance, the diagnosis of pancreatic carcinoma can be made without resorting to more expensive and uncomfortable diagnostic procedures or laparotomy.[85] Selective angiography is proving to be increasingly helpful, especially in localizing small tumors.[86]

To date, the therapy for this neoplasm is usually palliative by the creation of a biliary bypass for relief of obstructive jaundice. Pancreatoduodenectomy should be limited to those patients with small tumors. This procedure is associated with an operative mortality of 20% and with a 5-year survival of less than 5%.[87] In addition, nonoperative techniques, such as the percutaneous insertion of a transhepatic catheter with external or internal drainage,[88] have been developed for the relief of obstructive jaundice in patients with carcinoma of the head of the pancreas.

In chapters 14, 42 and 43 tumors of the endocrine pancreas are discussed. A summary of the various reported tumors is shown in Table 40-1.

Pancreatitis

Blumenthal et al.[65] studied the relationship between diabetes and pancreatic disease by reviewing the findings in 3821 autopsies carried out over a period of 35 years; of these 281 were on diabetic patients, 277 of whom were over the age of 20 years at time of death. Pancreatitis was found to occur twice as frequently in the diabetics as in the nondiabetics. This increased frequency was similar to that of vascular related diseases such as myocardial, cerebrovascular, or renal vessel infarction. However, arterial occlusion usually results in pancreatic infarction but not pancreatitis.

The relationship of diabetes to pancreatitis, acute and chronic, is discussed at length in the monograph edited by Podolsky and Viswanathan[89] on secondary diabetes. Diminished exocrine pancreatic function is characteristic of insulin-dependent diabetes. In 80% of 20 juvenile-onset diabetics, endocrine function tests, such as output of bicarbonate, trypsin, and amylase enzyme in response to intravenous secretin and cholecystokinin pancreozymin, were reduced in direct relationship to the duration of diabetes.[90] The cause is not known, but repeated vascular infarcts must be considered. Viral or autoimmune causes have also been postulated. Islet cell antibodies (ICA) are significantly increased in the blood of newly diagnosed insulin-dependent diabetics in contrast to the nondiabetic

Table 40–1. Clinical Syndromes Associated with Endocrine Tumors of the Pancreas

Clinical Syndrome	Type of Lesion	Predominant Hormonal Product	Clinical Features
Zollinger-Ellison	Tumor (gastrinoma) Hyperplasia	Gastrin	Gastric hypersecretion Peptic ulceration Diarrhea
Verner-Morrison	Tumor (vipoma)	Vasoactive intestinal polypeptide	Refractory watery diarrhea Hypokalemia Achlorhydria
Glucagonoma	Tumor	Glucagon	Migratory necrolytic erythema Diabetes Stomatitis Anemia Diarrhea
Somatostatinoma	Tumor Hyperplasia	Somatostatin	Diabetes Steatorrhea Hypochlorhydria Cholelithiasis
Insulinoma	Tumor Hyperplasia	Insulin	Hypoglycemia
Carcinoid	Tumor (mid-gut variety)	ACTH Gastrin	Clinical syndrome when associated with hepatic metastases
Nesidioblastosis	β-cell hyperplasia Microadenomatous transformation	Insulin	Hypoglycemia in infants and children

population (29.2% in 1848 insulin-dependent diabetics vs. 6.3% in 851 noninsulin-dependent diabetics and 1.3% in 1716 nondiabetics.[91] The ICA titers gradually decrease over months of time.

Acute pancreatitis from many causes is associated with transient glucose intolerance in about 30% of patients. The glucose intolerance usually disappears when the attack subsides. In a large multicenter prospective epidemiologic project, the Copenhagen Pancreatitis Study,[92] 5% of patients with acute pancreatitis were noted to be under treatment for diabetes while 20% of patients with chronic pancreatitis were receiving such treatment. In the patient with chronic pancreatitis, the development of diabetes is usually due directly to the destruction of the pancreas.

Etiology. The etiology of pancreatitis varies in different areas. The commonest cause of acute and chronic pancreatitis in the United States, France, and South Africa is alcoholism, which is noted in 75% of patients with this disease. The quantity of alcohol necessary to induce pancreatic damage has not been established, but it would appear that a period of 6 to 12 years of steady or "binge" consumption is necessary before symptoms become manifest. The mechanism for the production of pancreatic damage has not been determined. Chronic consumption of alcohol may produce irreversible damage to the pancreas. It is not known,

however, whether in diabetic patients, the pancreas is more affected by alcohol than in nondiabetics.[93]

Other causes for pancreatitis include gallbladder disease, which appears to be the most frequent cause of this disorder in Great Britain, and the second most frequent in the United States. In a large study in England by Trapnell[94] concerning the etiology in 590 patients, biliary tract disease was present in 316, 203 were idiopathic, 26 were thought due to alcoholism, and other causes such as mumps, carcinoma, hyperparathyroidism, and steroids accounted for the rest.

Prevalence. Chronic pancreatitis is found predominantly in two regions of the world.[95] The first includes those nations (United States, France, and South Africa) mentioned above in which alcohol usage is high. In these countries as well as in Italy, Portugal, and Switzerland, inhabitants consume a diet rich in proteins and lipids, which may also give rise to pancreatitis of gallbladder origin. In these countries, males are most affected in ages ranging from 35 to 40 years.

In the second region, Asia and Africa, the onset of chronic calcifying pancreatitis begins in childhood, and is usually due to childhood malnutrition. An example of this variety is observed in Kerala, South India, where chronic calcifying pancreatitis is frequently noted with an incidence of 5.47% of the autopsied population, more than 10 times the rate in Marseilles. In Kerala, the age at onset of calcific pancreatitis is about 12.5 years, and 40% of the patients are females. Alcoholism is rare and diabetes is a frequent complication. The diet here is low in protein and the staple food is cassava (tapioca). It is considered possible that the cassava consumption leads to the disease since cassava metabolites include cyanogenic glycosides which undergo acid hydrolysis with release of hydrocyanic acid. Protein malnutrition interferes with the detoxification of cyanide, leading to pancreatitis with secondary calculus formation. In Kerala, radiologic examination of patients with "pancreatic diabetes" demonstrates calculi in about 85% of them. In Madras, calcification of the pancreas in the same age group is evident radiologically in only 13% of cases.[96]

Chronic relapsing pancreatitis is rare in Great Britain. However, there are reports of increasing incidence of this disorder due to an increase in alcoholism.[97] Trapnell[94] noted that transient hyperglycemia occurred in 9% of acute pancreatic attacks, but found no instances of patients progressing later to full-blown diabetes. Pancreatitis is therefore considered a rare cause of diabetes in that country.

Calcific pancreatitis formerly was a rare disease in Japan, occurring in only 0.1% of all Japanese diabetics. This incidence has increased recently due presumably to increase in alcohol consumption.[98]

Clinical Picture of Pancreatitis in Diabetic Patients.[99,99a] Acute pancreatitis rarely precipitates diabetic ketoacidosis. The first cases were reported by Root,[100] but since then few additional cases have been published. Hyperparathyroid crisis and acute necrotizing pancreatitis can present as diabetic ketoacidosis.[101] In a ketoacidotic patient with abdominal pain and shock, underlying pancreatitis should be considered. Abdominal pain, also a common symptom of ketoacidosis, is more severe in acute pancreatitis. The patient is usually more obtunded and frequently in shock. Serum amylase is elevated (but may also be in diabetic ketoacidosis) and hypercalcemia is present in severely affected patients. Treatment for shock in acute pancreatitis should include colloid or fresh frozen plasma and intramuscular volume expanders such as human albumin. The effect of acute pancreatitis is similar to that of severe burns with much loss of fluid and plasma at the site of pancreatic necrosis, making fluid replacement critical.

Chronic Pancreatitis and Diabetes. About two-thirds of patients with chronic pancreatitis have abnormal glucose tolerance tests. Approximately 20% have clinical diabetes and the majority of these may need treatment with insulin. Insulin regimens vary, but usually the requirements are less than in primary diabetes and the hyperglycemia is easier to control.

It is important to consider the possibility of disturbances of exocrine pancreatic function when diabetes is present. If there seems to be a possibility of malabsorption, the patient should be studied for fat soluble vitamin deficiency, B_{12} deficiency, and fat malabsorption. If these are present, vitamin supplements, including injections of B_{12}, should be prescribed. Pancreatic enzymes should be administered orally if the patient has steatorrhea. These measures will facilitate control of diabetes and promote adequate nutrition.

Patients with chronic pancreatitis who have peripheral neuropathy should be investigated for diabetic and alcoholic etiologies. Each attack of relapsing acute or chronic pancreatitis should be carefully treated and followed. Gall stones require investigation with ultrasound procedures. If present, their role in precipitating attacks should be reviewed, and if indicated, cholecystectomy should be performed after recovery from attacks, unless there is associated biliary obstruction.

The complication of pseudocyst should be considered, and ultrasound of the pancreas should be repeated, especially if acute pancreatitis continues for longer than 3 weeks.

Treatment. Treatment and follow-up care of pancreatitis in diabetic patients is the same as in nondiabetics. However, the special nutritional requirements of the diabetic and susceptibility to infection must be considered. If the patient is unable to consume an adequate diet, parenteral hyperalimentation should be instituted, keeping in mind that this may require more energetic treatment of the diabetes.

As there is a higher incidence of pancreatic malignancy in diabetic patients, a patient with recent onset of diabetes and pancreatitis who does not respond well to treatment should be investigated for the possibility of pancreatic carcinoma.

Diabetes following traumatic pancreatitis is rare, but has been reported. This can occur later and is usually due to an automobile accident. The interval between acute and chronic relapsing pancreatitis and onset of established diabetes varies from 14 months to 12 years, with an average of 3.7 years.

Trauma sustained during automobile accidents in which the steering wheel compresses the abdomen, has become an important cause of pancreatitis. There are only rare reports of the appearance of diabetes later.[102] The longer the interval between the accident and the development of diabetes, the more difficult it is to establish a relationship since the diabetes may well be of the usual primary type.

LIVER DISEASE AND DIABETES

Liver disease and diabetes can be considered in three categories: (a) the effect of diabetes on the liver; (b) conditions in which liver disease and diabetes are both present as part of a clinical syndrome (of which the best illustration is idiopathic familial hemochromatosis); and (c) the effect of liver disease and its treatment on the diabetic patient.

Effect of Diabetes on the Liver

An effect of diabetes on the liver is often seen in patients with uncontrolled or poorly-controlled diabetes. In the acute, uncontrolled state, the patient may complain of right upper quadrant pain and examination may reveal an enlarged and tender liver. Diffuse abdominal pain may be the initial presentation of ketoacidosis. In one series, hepatic enlargement was noted in all patients with ketoacidosis, in about 60% of those with uncontrolled diabetes, and in only 9% of those with well-controlled diabetes.[103] In a review of 1759 liver biopsies, fatty changes were found in 25 to 78% of patients and were more common in those with maturity-onset diabetes.[104] The pathologic condition noted in these studies included fatty infiltration of the hepatocytes with eccentric nuclei but no inflammatory response. The pathophysiology of this event is complex but seems related to an increased influx of fatty acids, which may lead to increased formation of triglycerides and lipoproteins. In severe ketoacidosis there is also impaired excretion of lipoproteins and fatty acids from the liver.

It is unclear whether fatty liver in the diabetic progresses to cirrhosis. The results of some studies suggest that cirrhosis may occur, but the data are inconclusive.[104] Autopsy studies reveal an increased prevalence of cirrhosis in the diabetic with frequencies ranging from 5.7 to 21.4%. In one such study, cirrhosis was present in 16.4% of the diabetics as compared to 8.4% in nondiabetic subjects;[105] other studies, however, have failed to document significant differences.[106]

Adler and Schaffner[107] studied 29 overweight patients by liver biopsy and divided the pathologic findings into four groups: fatty liver; fatty liver with hepatitis; fatty liver with hepatitis and fibrosis; and fatty liver with cirrhosis. The numbers of patients were about equal in each of these groups; females predominated. Ten patients had a history of diabetes in relatives. Diabetes was stated to have been present in 61% of the 29 patients with equal frequency in each of the 4 groups named above. Lipoprotein abnormalities, especially Type IV, was found in the two less affected pathologic groups. The biochemical derangement included mild elevation of the alkaline phosphatase and serum glutamic oxaloacetic transaminase (SGOT) in about 50% of the patients. Data regarding sedimentation rate were not reported. The emphasis of this study is on the contribution of obesity to fibrosis.

The authors (K.R.F. and C.T.) studied 5 female patients with maturity-onset diabetes (only 2 required insulin) and hepatomegaly. All were moderately obese with body weights not more than 50% over the calculated ideal. None had experienced episodes of ketoacidosis. None gave a history of alcohol intake nor had a jejuno-ileal bypass procedure. Biopsies showed fatty liver, pericentral fibrosis, and intracellular hyaline with collagen surrounding the hepatocytes.[108] In 3 of the patients fibrotic bridging between central veins and portal tracts was present. These findings were unlike those in alcoholic hepatitis in that polymorphonuclear neutrophils and regenerative nodules were not seen.

In the patients described above, the biochemical abnormalities included elevated alkaline phosphatase levels in the range of 120 to 216 mU/ml in 4 of the 5 patients. There was concomitant elevation of the 5^1 nucleotides and gamma glutamyl transferase. The SGOT and serum glutamic pyruvic transaminase (SGPT) were modestly elevated at levels about 110 mU/ml. The striking feature in all patients was a persistent elevation of the erythrocyte sedimentation rate to between 55 and 75 mm per hour. It was the alkaline phosphatase and the sedimentation rate which necessitated the study of a liver biopsy which yielded findings different from those described by Adler and Schaffner,[107] and could be compared to those in patients with ileojejunal bypasses. Pericentral sclerosis has been well documented in our patients, and studies in other patients with these features have shown that this pathologic lesion can progress to cirrhosis.[109] Perhaps our patients are in a pre-cirrhotic stage but will need to be followed to determine this possibility.

Oral Hypoglycemic Agents and Their Effects on the Liver

The effects of oral hypoglycemic agents on the liver have been well documented.[110] Sulfonylureas can in some instances, especially with excessive dosage, lead to significant liver injury. In most patients, however, the effect is slight and may be masked by the fatty liver and the mild elevation of liver enzymes often noted in diabetics. Granulomatous reactions have been observed.[110a] Two of the early sulfonylureas, carbutamide and metahexamide (never marketed), produced serious and even fatal liver injury in 0.5 to 1.5% of cases, leading to their withdrawal from clinical trial in the United States. Chlorpropamide (Diabinese) when given in dosage larger than recommended may cause cholestatic changes in about 5% of patients. Current use of lower dosages (not more than 500 mg per day) of chlorpropamide have resulted in a greatly reduced incidence of this. A skin rash and hypersensitivity reaction should alert the physician to the possibility of hepatotoxicity in patients receiving sulfonylureas, and the need for discontinuance of the drug. Acetohexamide (Dymelor) rarely causes hepatic injury; tolbutamide (Orinase) has even less tendency to do so with only 6 such patients reported to date. Tolazamide (Tolinase) and azepenamide (not marketed in U.S.A.: see Table 21–2) have rarely been associated with hepatotoxicity. Cholestasis should be considered as part of a generalized hypersensitivity in patients receiving sulfonylureas and need not lead to any permanent hepatic damage.

While biguanides interfere with hepatic metabolism, thereby leading to lactic acidosis, hepatic injury has been reported in only 2 instances in which jaundice was noted.

Hemochromatosis

Hemochromatosis is an example of the clinical association of diabetes and liver disease because of a pathologic defect in iron storage, especially in the liver and pancreas. Overt diabetes occurs in 60 to 80% of hemochromatosis patients of whom about 70% ultimately require insulin.[111,112] Diabetes is frequently noted before frank cirrhosis is manifest. The complications commonly associated with diabetes such as neuropathy, nephropathy, and retinopathy may be present. Thus the establishment of the diagnosis of hemochromatosis in an individual is important, as the specific treatment of venesection can improve the diabetes and other manifestations of iron overload. Early detection in family members can allow initiation of phlebotomies in them at an early stage of the disease.[113]

Iron storage diseases may be classified into three large groups according to their effects on the body.[114] (a) Hemosiderosis, the commonest, is seen in patients who have had multiple transfusions or in patients with hemolysis in whom there is an increase in total body iron without tissue damage. The iron is stored largely in the reticuloendothelial system. However, after transfusions of about 100 units of blood, iron may accumulate to an extent approaching tissue levels seen in hemochromatosis. Tissue damage is unusual except in excessive hemolysis when deposits may occur in the liver and heart. (b) Hemochromatosis, a rare condition seen in the familial form of iron storage disease, is caused by an increase in total body iron with concomitant tissue damage. Excessive iron is found diffusely in the parenchyma of various organs. This definition includes patients who have sustained organ damage secondary to iron excess but have failed to mobilize the iron by therapeutic phlebotomy; such patients are those with alcoholic cirrhosis and iron overload. (c) The third group is comprised of persons with asymptomatic pre-cirrhotic familial hemochromatosis who have excessive iron but no tissue damage. It is presumed that they will ultimately develop clinical hemochromatosis unless appropriate treatment is instituted. They usually are relatives of patients with overt hemochromatosis.

Iron Absorption. Iron absorption from the gastrointestinal tract is a finely regulated system because there is no physiologic mechanism for removal of excess body iron. Iron loss via kidney or skin is negligible. Patients with hemochromatosis absorb more iron from the gastrointestinal tract than is normal, leading to accumulation of excess stores of body iron. Thus, while the normal adult male absorbs approximately 1 mg of iron per day to maintain a total body store of 600 to 1000 mg, patients with hemochromatosis absorb several times that amount and eventually may develop iron stores in excess of 20 g. Normally, patients who are iron-depleted have an alteration in their intestinal absorption of iron to a higher threshold, and perhaps this normal mechanism is increased in patients with hemochromatosis. However, the iron distribution in the intestinal villi of patients with idiopathic hemochromatosis seems to differ from that in patients with hemosiderosis, and this may be the result of different routes of iron accumulation. The macrophages isolated from patients with hemochromatosis are more numerous and have an intercellular pattern of iron distribution which differs from cells isolated from patients with other storage disorders.[113]

Hereditary Pattern. The hereditary pattern of hemochromatosis seems variable. Initially it was considered to follow autosomal dominance;[115] however, family studies in France and in Utah[116,117] by HLA typing showed a higher frequency in HLA-A3 and HLA-B14 antigens than in control populations, and have shown the disease in overt form to be recessive but not completely so since the heterozygote has some of the symptoms. There may be a spectrum of hemochromatosis with different modes of inheritance. Thus there have been family reports of autosomal recessives with expression in heterozygotes as well as reports of autosomal dominance with incomplete expressivity.

The pathologic changes seen in hemochromatosis are best shown in the liver. There is deposition of iron in the hepatocyte with variably associated cirrhosis which progressively can result in portal hypertension with splenomegaly. Progression of the disease can lead to ascites and esophageal varices with a propensity to bleeding.

Iron deposition less marked than that seen in the liver is found also in various organs already mentioned. The iron deposition in the pancreas leads to endocrine deficiencies resulting eventually in both diabetes and less commonly in exocrine insufficiency. The cardiac involvement will depend on the sites of iron deposition. If these are near the conducting bundles, arrhythmias may occur or if iron is deposited in the myocardial cells, myocardopathies leading to congestive cardiac failure may follow and prove to be resistant to treatment.

There is one report of idiopathic hemochromatosis in monozygotic twins, showing identical patterns of organ involvement. There has been considerable controversy as to whether true hemochromatosis represents simply an increase in hemosiderosis, but because of reports in families, there appears to be conclusive evidence for an hereditary basis.[118]

Clinical Presentation. The clinical manifestations are variable and depend on the extent and predominant sites of iron deposits. The disease is manifest usually in the 4th to 5th decade of life in the male and about 10 years later in the female, presumably because of blood loss from menses and childbirth. Formerly, it had been considered to occur almost entirely in males. Excessive alcohol intake with the associated increase in iron stores and recurrent hepatic damage may hasten the clinical presentation of the liver disease.

The commonest finding in hemochromatosis is hepatomegaly which is seen in 93% of patients on initial diagnosis.[113] Despite a palpable liver, less than 50% of patients exhibit abnormal liver function tests. The hepatomegaly may precede diabetes by many years, but the occurrence of both diabetes and hepatomegaly should alert the clinician to this syndrome and appropriate studies should be initiated.[7]

Hemochromatosis in Younger Patients. There is a syndrome of idiopathic hemochromatosis in the younger age group.[119] Fifty-three such patients have been reported as having heart failure, insulin-dependent diabetes, hepatomegaly, and in the female, secondary amenorrhea. The symptoms improve with phlebotomy. In these younger patients, there is an equal sex ratio and the symptoms are usually those of cardiomyopathy and congestive cardiac failure. The case presented by Lamon et al. was associated with an autosomal recessive mode of inheritance.[119] The patient responded well to repeated phlebotomies. Diabetes is less frequent than in older patients: only 34% of those under the age of 30 years had diabetes. Hepatomegaly was frequently observed in both the young and old

groups and liver biopsy showed in all patients heavy iron deposition in the hepatocytes, but the extent of portal fibrosis varied. Hypogonadism as manifested by secondary amenorrhea, diminished libido, and loss of sexual hair, was observed in 64% of patients under 30 as compared to 30% in the older group. Autopsy studies have demonstrated iron deposits in the pituitary, adrenals, and gonads as well as in the thyroid and parathyroids. The cardiac disorder in the younger age group is predominantly that of constrictive cardiomyopathy; this occurred initially in 58.5% of the young patients as opposed to 35% of the older age group. Cardiac manifestations because of deposition of iron in the myocardium are usually progressive unless appropriate treatment is instituted. The cardiomyopathy may mimic constrictive pericarditis.

Skin manifestations, occurring in 98% of patients, are initially due to an increase in melanin deposits in the melanocytes and only later when the slate gray color is more obvious, are there excessive iron deposits which can be diagnosed on biopsy of the skin. Additional cutaneous manifestations include hair thinning, icthyosis, and nail abnormalities. Koilonychia is seen in about 50% of patients; it is an especially distressing symptom which is difficult to treat if the diabetes is poorly controlled. Deposits of iron in the exocrine sweat glands are a finding unique to hemochromatosis and should alert one to this diagnosis.

Arthropathy commonly occurs in about 35% of patients with hemochromatosis, but the symptoms are variable and are more manifest in older patients. Radiologic findings in the joints are fairly characteristic and should alert one to the diagnosis. There is alteration of the bony cortex with subarticular cysts in the smaller bones and chondrocalcinosis in the larger joints.[120] Hypogonadism is frequently seen; iron deposits in the testes as well as in the pituitary have been noted with some decrease in the plasma luteinizing hormone.[121]

The diagnosis of hemochromatosis is thus suspected by the clinical presentations and the presence of a family history. Laboratory tests give variable results. Fifty percent of the patients with hepatomegaly have normal liver function tests. There is an increase in the serum iron with a reduced total iron binding capacity; the percentage of transferrin saturation is increased in 90% of patients with the overt disease. Serum ferritin is increased[122] to a greater degree than that seen in other diseases, such as rheumatoid arthritis or Hodgkin's disease. However, the correlation between serum ferritin levels and hemochromatosis is not a constant one, and values vary greatly, especially in the pre-cirrhotic form of the disease.

The detection of pre-cirrhotic hemochromatosis

by study of asymptomatic relatives is most important in the prevention of the full-blown syndrome. Measurements of iron-binding saturation or of ferritin have not always correlated well with total body iron stores in some families. However, if serum ferritin is elevated, this information is useful in detecting patients at risk of developing idiopathic hemochromatosis. The only way to determine the presence of iron overload in persons at risk is by percutaneous liver biopsy. It this is positive, phlebotomies three or four times a year as well as close follow-up of the patient, are available. The effectiveness of the prophylactic treatment in precirrhotic hemochromatosis needs to be established by prospective studies.

Treatment. Deferoxamine (Desferal) has been useful in documenting iron overload. This drug chelates iron, forming a stable complex which is readily soluble in water and passes easily through the kidneys. In a normal person, one gram of deferoxamine given intramuscularly will result in the urinary excretion of less than 2 mg of iron per 24 hours. Patients with idiopathic hemochromatosis similarly treated, may excrete over 10 mg in 24 hours, although this may vary from 2 to 10 mg.

Ultimately, the diagnosis of hemochromatosis resides in demonstrating the excessive iron stores in the liver. The normal liver contains less than 0.25% iron expressed as dry weight, whereas patients with idiopathic hemochromatosis have values in excess of 2%.[123]

The prognosis in patients with idiopathic hemochromatosis is influenced by treatment and is also dependent on the extent of iron storage and the effectiveness of its removal. Venesection is the most efficient form of therapy since with this method 250 mg of iron may be removed in 500 ml of whole blood, whereas an intramuscular injection of 1 g of deferoxamine will remove at most only 10 to 20 mg of iron in the urine per 24 hours. Since phlebotomies are contraindicated in patients with conditions of hemolysis and associated iron overload, here the use of deferoxamine either by injection or by continuous infusion, is the treatment of choice.

There are now many studies showing improvement of survival by use of repeated venesections. In 85 patients with idiopathic hemochromatosis treated with phlebotomies, the 5- and 10-year survival from the time of clinical diagnosis was 66% and 32% respectively as opposed to 18% and 6% in the control group.[124] In another report,[113] 20 of 49 patients showed a decrease in insulin requirement and 4 discontinued taking insulin during the course of treatment. Reversibility is thus not completely predictable, but improvement is the usual result. Although it has been considered that ar-

thropathy with iron deposition in the synovial joints, is the form of hemochromatosis most resistant to treatment, we have seen relief of pain in 2 patients who have been phlebotomized over a period of 2 years.

Cardiomyopathy and congestive cardiac failure are frequently improved by repeated phlebotomies.[125] We phlebotomize our patients at weekly or biweekly intervals, depending on the severity of the disease, until the excess iron stores are depleted as measured by hematocrit and serum iron estimations. Patients given folic acid and vitamin supplements are frequently tested for blood in the feces because of the association of cirrhosis with bleeding varices and the increased frequency of peptic ulcers. Concomitant treatment is necessary for other common manifestations of cirrhosis such as portal hypertension, peptic ulcer and, in about 12% of cases, ascites.

Hepatoma. Hepatomas develop in 6 to 12% of older patients with idiopathic hemochromatosis. Since venesection does not influence the development of liver cell carcinoma, it is important that continual observation and examination of the patient be carried out to watch for this possibility. Development of pain over the liver, sudden rise of serum enzymes reflecting disturbed liver function, and rise in the serum α-fetoprotein are warning signs of the possible development of hepatoma and deserve investigation. We usually perform an α-fetoprotein estimation annually on our patients, and on many occasions a sudden rise of this value is associated with either the multifocal development of hepatomas or extension of the hepatomas beyond easily resectable boundaries. The development of sudden ascites in the patient also deserves investigation for hepatoma.

The initial tests to perform are a liver scan and ultrasound. If one is more suspicious of a possible hepatoma, computerized axial tomography (CAT scan) of the liver and pancreas is performed. When considered necessary because of a small hepatoma (under 1.2 cm) which might be missed by a liver scan, a laparoscopy may be carried out in the hope of being able to detect an easily resectable hepatoma. If suspicions are high but the above measures are not diagnostic, one resorts to angiography and laparotomy. The difference in survival following resection of a hepatoma versus other forms of treatment, is highly significant. Palliative treatment of hepatomas by radiotherapy may give relief of pain arising from a stretched capsule.

For a brief discussion of hemochromatosis from the viewpoint of the pathologist, see Chapter 14.

Effect of Liver Disease and its Treatment on the Diabetic Patient

Defective carbohydrate metabolism has been observed in patients with cirrhosis or other liver diseases.[126,127] Hypoglycemia is rare and if severe, is associated usually with fulminant hepatic failure and a grave prognosis. The cause of hypoglycemia can be impaired gluconeogenesis or glycogen synthesis and in some instances decrease in the metabolism of insulin.[128] Mild hypoglycemia has been noted in acute viral hepatitis. Hypoglycemia has also been reported in toxic damage secondary to acetaminophen usage although in the early stage, hyperglycemia has been noted. Early consideration and detection of acetaminophen toxicity is important, as specific treatment with N-acetylcysteine or cysteamine may lead to prompt improvement. Hepatoma can cause hypoglycemia. The hypoglycemia associated with excessive alcohol ingestion is caused by inhibition of hepatic gluconeogenesis as a consequence of increased $NADH_2/NAD$ ratio and decreased reserves of hepatic glycogen. Recognition and treatment of this entity are mandatory as there is a reported 11% mortality in adults and 25% in children in untreated cases.[129] Hyperglycemia during an oral or intravenous glucose tolerance test is frequently noted in patients with cirrhosis. They also show abnormal intravenous tolbutamide tests. Cirrhotic patients usually do not show evidence of the complications encountered in diabetes such as retinopathy, nephropathy, and neuropathy. The mechanism of impaired glucose tolerance includes decreased parenchymal mass, portal systemic shunting of glucose, impaired insulin action on the liver, decreased degradation of insulin, or poor nutrition. Perhaps the contributions of most of the above are concomitant.[176,127] Studies of C-peptide which is not degraded by the liver, have shown that hyperinsulinism is frequently present in liver disease because of slowed degradation of insulin itself.[130] Hyperinsulinism in the cirrhotic patient is commonly associated with impaired glucose tolerance.

Occasionally hyperglycemia is also associated with severe pancreatic damage. Impaired glucose tolerance is common both in acute and chronic liver disease but is not of clinical importance. Alberti and Johnson[127] appeal for discontinuance of glucose tolerance testing in patients with alcoholic cirrhosis as this would save much time and work, would not cause significant loss of knowledge, and might stimulate workers to have new ideas and enlightened approaches.

Treatment of chronic active hepatitis in the diabetic patient could lead to worsening of diabetes and even ketoacidosis. However, in most, after the reduction of the initial high dose of steroids or the addition of azathioprine (Imuran), diabetes can be better controlled. The treatment of liver disease and portal hypertension with associated hepatitis is similar in patients with or without diabetes and is well discussed in monographs on liver disease.[127] However, in patients with both diabetes and liver disease, the sudden exacerbation of the liver disease or the aggravation of hepatic encephalopathy should alert the clinician to possible underlying sepsis or poorly controlled diabetes with concomitant fluid and electrolyte abnormalities. Early treatment should be instituted and if the patient has ascites, diagnostic paracentesis should be performed to consider spontaneous peritonitis.

Covert alcoholism with liver disease, poses a diagnostic and therapeutic problem in the diabetic. These patients may develop lactic acidosis as well as ketoacidosis, and the hepatic disease and jaundice become more obvious during the course of the illness. About 10 to 20% may also present with a cholestatic phase of alcoholic hepatitis and associated polymorphonuclear leukocyte response and fever, and must be distinguished quickly from patients with mechanical obstruction and infection. In these patients, liver biopsies can help in diagnosing the typical pathologic condition of alcoholic hepatitis from that of other forms of liver disease. Liver biopsy should be considered in the patient with diabetes if the findings do not conform to those in the usual syndromes of liver disease. Biopsy results can serve to identify liver diseases which have specific pathologic problems such as alcoholic or granulomatous liver disease, primary biliary cirrhosis, or hemochromatosis, and if bile infarcts are present, mechanical obstruction of the biliary tree.

For a more detailed discussion of the investigation of patients with liver disease, see standard texts on the subject. With due regard to diabetes, the type and extent of studies are the same in the diabetic as in the nondiabetic patient.

GALLBLADDER DISEASE

Acute cholecystitis and cholelithiasis are more frequently seen in the diabetic, possibly because of the delayed emptying of the gallbladder and associated stagnant bile. Most of this increased frequency has been noted at autopsy. Cholecystitis in diabetic patients has a higher morbidity and mortality rate than in nondiabetic persons. In the acute phase when emergency surgery was indicated, mortality in the 1950s ranged from 15 to 20% in the diabetic, about 5 times that seen in the control group. In elective surgery the operative morbidity and mortality have been similar to that in nondiabetics, although the degree of control of the diabetes at the time of surgery influences the prognosis.[131]

In view of the above, the diabetic patient with symptomatic gallstones and a history of gallbladder colic or cholecystitis in the past, should be advised to have surgery as soon as possible. Cholecystitis should be treated with an appropriate antibiotic at once and considered for early surgery. It is important, too, that during surgery, cultures of the bile duct be taken and that antibiotic treatment be continued in the postoperative period. This has been a standard practice by most surgeons at the New England Deaconess Hospital because studies have shown that it provides a significant decrease in morbidity and mortality. The antibiotic of choice should be one which has adequate bactericidal action on the suspected bacteria; the fact that certain antibiotics are more easily dispersed in the bile should not influence one's choice in this respect.

Patients should be watched for complications in the postoperative period, and it is advisable to provide antibiotic coverage if T-tube cholecystography is necessary. The T-tube should be cultured to identify any organisms present. Also in the pre- or postoperative phase, if percutaneous transhepatic cholangiography is needed, the patient should be protected with appropriate antibiotics. There have been catastrophic instances in the pre- and immediate postoperative phases, of patients developing fulminant *Clostridium welchii* infection. Sudden bilirubinemia rising from a near normal to about 12 mg/dl or more in one day, is commonly seen, and appropriate therapy should be initiated immediately.

Postoperative cholecystitis can occur as a complication of certain surgical procedures, especially hip joint replacement or cardiac surgery. However, in reported cases, there has been no higher incidence of post-operative cholecystitis in the diabetic than in the nondiabetic patient. There is a higher incidence related to age and susceptibility to infection; in a group of 20 patients, half had this complication without concomitant gallstones.[132] The entity of cholecystitis without gallstones does, indeed, exist with a frequency of between 1 to 10% of patients. It is important to consider this disorder in the diabetic patient who has all the signs and symptoms of acute cholecystitis but in whom investigations including ultrasound and cholecystography are negative.

If a diabetic patient is found to have asymptomatic gallstones, the gallbladder function may be assessed by means of an oral cholecystogram. Since a significant number, about 30%, yield a false positive result on one administration of iopanoic acid (Telepaque), we administer the preparation on 2 consecutive days before performing the x-rays. This test provides a correct diagnosis in about 95% of patients, if the bilirubin is normal and if the patient does not have diarrhea due to an idiosyncrasy to the drug.

Echography also has an overall accuracy of about 96% in gallstone determination, even in the presence of jaundice. Therefore it is especially useful in patients who are allergic to iopanoic acid and in pregnant patients in whom exposure to radiation is undesirable.

Treatment of Gallstones. In the presence of gallstones in a non-functioning gallbladder, the patient should be advised to have the gallbladder removed because of the real danger of the development of cholecystitis. Gallstones in asymptomatic patients with normally functioning gallbladders have remained asymptomatic in follow-up studies in 50% of cases over a 20-year period. In the rare patient, a single gallstone followed over a period of 10 years can disappear. Statistics indicate that there is a 50% likelihood of an asymptomatic patient with gallstones developing symptoms. Seventy-five percent of patients who do develop these symptoms will experience biliary colic, but in the diabetic there is a greater risk of infection. Thus, in the elderly diabetic, fever and shock may be the initial signs of acute cholecystitis. Consequently, it seems appropriate to advise cholecystectomy in patients under 50 years of age, as there is a 50% chance of their developing cholecystitis over the next 20 years. In elderly asymptomatic patients with gallstones and a normally functioning gallbladder, the decision for surgery is more difficult. Cholecystectomy is thus advised in all diabetic patients with symptomatic gallstones and in all patients with a demonstrable non-functioning gallbladder and the presence of stones. Patients who refuse the suggestion of operation or whom one would clinically prefer to watch, should be followed carefully.

Medical dissolution of gallstones with the oral administration of either chenodeoxycholic acid or ursodeoxycholic acid is rarely effective in patients with pigment and radiopaque stones. The prerequisites of a normally functioning gallbladder and long term maintenance therapy exclude most of our patients from nonsurgical intervention. The administration of bile salt also incurs the risk of diarrhea in 50% of patients, abdominal discomfort in a similar percentage, and the recurrence of stones once treatment is neglected. Another advantage of cholecystectomy is that following this procedure, there is a change in the bile salt composition with an increase in the bile salt pool. This may explain the infrequency of recurrent stone formation after cholecystectomy.

REFERENCES

1. Cohen, D.W., Friedman, L.A., Shapiro, J., et al.: Diabetes mellitus and periodontal disease: two-year longitudinal observations. (Part I). J. Periodontol. *41*:709, 1970.
2. Golub, L.M., Schneir, M., Ramamurthy, N.S.: Enhanced

collagenase activity in diabetic rat gingiva: in vitro and in vivo evidence. J. Dent. Res. *57*:520, 1978.

3. Glavind, L., Lund, B., Loe, H.: The relationship between periodontal state and diabetes duration, insulin dosage and retinal changes. J. Periodontol. *39*:341, 1968.
4. Finestone, A.J., Boorujy, S.R.: Diabetes mellitus and periodontal disease. Diabetes *16*:336, 1967.
5. Glickman, I., Smulow, J.B., Moreau, J.: Post-surgical periodontal healing in alloxan diabetes. J. Periodontol. *38*:93, 1967.
6. Sznajder, N., Carraro, J.J., Kugna, S., Sereday, M.: Periodontal findings in diabetic and nondiabetic patients. J. Periodontol. *49*:445, 1978.
7. Frantzis, T.G., Reeve, C.M., Brown, A.L., Jr.: The ultrastructure of capillary basement membranes in the attached gingiva of diabetic and nondiabetic patients with periodontal disease. J. Periodontol. *42*:406, 1971.
8. Ray, H.G., Organ, B.: Gingival structures in diabetes mellitus. J. Periodontol. *21*:85, 1950.
9. Listgarten, M.A, Ricker, F.H., Jr., Laster, L., et al.: Vascular basement lamina thickness in the normal and inflamed gingiva of diabetics and nondiabetics. J. Periodontol. *45*:676, 1974.
10. Schieffer, L.D., Alster-Krakowski, A., Slambaugh, R.: Cyclic AMP content in normal and diseased gingival biopsies. J. Dent. Res. *53*:221, 1974.
11. Grower, M.F., Ficara, A.J., Chandler, D.W., Kramer, G.D.: Differences in cAMP levels in the gingival fluid of diabetics and nondiabetics. J. Periodontol. *46*:669, 1975.
12. Bernick, S.M., Cohen, D.W., Baker, L., Laster, L.: Dental disease in children with diabetes mellitus. J. Periodontol. *46*:241, 1975.
13. Benveniste, R., Bixler, D., Conneally, P.M.: Periodontal disease in diabetics. J. Periodontol. *38*:271, 1967.
14. Hove, K.A., Stallard, R.E.: Diabetes and the periodontal patient. J. Periodontol. *41*:713, 1970.
15. Mackenzie, R.S., Millard, D.H.: Interrelated effects of diabetes, arteriosclerosis and calculus on alveolar bone loss. J. Am. Dent. Assoc. *66*:191, 1963.
15a.Tapper-Jones, I. M., Aldred, M.J., Walker, D.M., Hayes, T.M.: Candidal infections and populations of *Candida albicans* in mouths of diabetics. J. Clin. Pathol. *34*:706, 1981.
16. Rundles, R.W.: Diabetic neuropathy; general review with report of 125 cases. Medicine *24*:111, 1945.
17. Horgan, J.H., Doyle, J.S.: A comparative study of esophageal motility in diabetics with neuropathy. Chest *60*:170, 1971.
18. Mandelstam, P., Lieber, A.: Esophageal dysfunction in diabetic neuropathy-gastroenteropathy. J.A.M.A. *201*:88, 1967.
19. Mandelstam, P., Siegel, C.I., Lieber, A., Siegel, M.: The swallowing disorder in patients with diabetic neuropathy-gastroenteropathy. Gastroenterol. *56*:1, 1969.
20. Vix, V.A.: Esophageal motility in diabetes mellitus. Radiology *92*:363, 1969.
21. Hollis, J.B., Castell, D.O., Braddom, R.L.: Esophageal function in diabetes mellitus and its relation to peripheral neuropathy. Gastroenterol. *73*:1098, 1977.
22. Stewart, I.M., Hosking, D.J., Preston, B.J., Atkinson, M.: Esophageal motor changes in diabetes mellitus. Thorax *31*:278, 1976.
23. Kramer, P., Ingelfinger, F.J.: Esophageal sensitivity to Mecholyl in cardiospasm. Gastroenterol. *54*:771, 1968.
24. Medoff, G, Dismukes, W.E., Mead, R.H., Moses, J.M.: A new therapeutic approach to Candida infection. Arch. Intern. Med. *130*:241, 1972.
25. Rutgerts, L., Verhaegen, H.: Intravenous miconazole in

the treatment of chronic esophageal candidiasis. Gastroenterol. *72*:316, 1977.
26. Graybill, J.R., Drutz, D.J.: Ketoconazole: a major innovation for treatment of fungal infections. Ann. Intern. Med. *93*:921, 1930.
27. Goyal, R.K., Spiro, H.M.: Gastrointestinal manifestations of diabetes mellitus. Med. Clin. N. Am. *55*:1031, 1971.
28. Kassander, P.: Asymptomatic gastric retention in diabetics (gastroparesis diabeticorum). Ann. Intern. Med. *48*:797, 1958.
29. Marshak, R.H., Maklansky, D.: Diabetic gastropathy. Am. J. Dig. Dis. *9*:366, 1964.
30. Campbell, A., Conway, H.: Gastric retention and hypoglycemia in diabetes. Scottish Med. J. *5*:167, 1960.
31. Zitomer, B.R., Gramm, H.F., Kozak, G.P.: Gastric neuropathy in diabetes mellitus. Clinical and radiologic observations. Metabolism *17*:199, 1968.
32. Campbell, I.W., Heading, R., Tothill, P., et al.: Gastric emptying in diabetic autonomic neuropathy. Gut. *18*:462, 1977.
33. Fox, S., Behar, J.: Pathogenesis of diabetic gastroparesis: a pharmacologic study. Gastroenterol. *78*:757, 1980.
34. Wooten, R.L., Meriwether, T.W.: Diabetic gastric atony: a clinical study. J.A.M.A. *176*:1082, 1961.
35. Vinnik, L.E., Kern, F., Jr., Struther, J.E., Jr.: Malabsorption and the diarrhea of diabetes mellitus. Gastroenterol. *43*:507, 1962.
36. Aylett, P.: Gastric emptying and change in the blood sugar level as affected by glucagon and insulin. Clin. Sci. *22*:171, 1962.
37. Bloom, S.R.: Gastrointestinal hormones. Internat. Rev. Physiol. *12*:71, 1977.
38. Aylett, P.: Gastric emptying and secretion in patients with diabetes mellitus. Gut *6*:262, 1965.
39. Malagelada, J.R., Rees, W.D.W., Mazzotta, L.J., Go, V.L.W.: Gastric motor abnormalities in diabetic and postvagotomy gastroparesis: Effect of metoclopramide and bethanechol. Gastroenterol. *78*:286, 1980.
40. Brady, P.G., Richardson, R.: Gastric bezoar formation secondary to gastroparesis diabeticorum. Arch. Intern. Med. *137*:1729, 1977.
41. Snape, W.J., Jr., Battle, W.M., Schwartz, S.S., et al.: Metoclopramide to treat gastroparesis due to diabetes mellitus. A double-blind, controlled trial. Ann. Intern. Med. *96*:444, 1982.
42. McCallum, R.W., Ricci, D.A., Rakatansky, H., et al.: A multicenter placebo-controlled clinical trial of oral metoclopramide in diabetic gastroparesis. Diabetes Care *6*:463, 1983.
43. Roon, A.J., Mason, G.R.: Surgical management of gastroparesis diabeticorum. Calif. Med. *116*:58, 1972.
44. Dotevall, G.: Gastric secretion of acid in diabetes mellitus during basal conditions and after maximal stimulation. Acta Med. Scand. *170*:59, 1961.
45. Marks, I.N., Shuman, C.R., Shay, H.: Gastric acid secretion in diabetes mellitus. Ann. Intern. Med. *51*:227, 1959.
46. Irvine, W.J., Clarke, B.F., Scarth, L., et al.: Thyroid and gastric autoimmunity in patients with diabetes mellitus. Lancet *2*:163, 1970.
47. Ungar, B., Stocks, A.E., Martin, F.I.R., et al.: Intrinsic factor antibody, parietal cell antibody and latent pernicious anemia in diabetes mellitus. Lancet *2*:415, 1968.
48. Wilkinson, J.F.: Diabetes mellitus and pernicious anemia. Br. Med. J. *1*:676, 1963.
49. Solomon, S.P., Spiro, H.M.: The effects of glucagon and glucose on the human stomach. Am. J. Dig. Dis. *4*:775, 1959.

50. Hosking, D.J., Moody, F., Stewart, I.M., Atkinson, M.: Vagal impairment of gastric secretion in diabetic autonomic neuropathy. Br. Med. J. 2:588, 1975.

51. Manson, R.R.: Duodenal ulcer as a second disease. Gastroenterol. 59:712, 1970.

52. Wood, M.N.: Chronic peptic ulcer disease in 94 diabetics. Am. J. Dig. Dis. 14:1, 1947.

53. Genel, M.D., London, D., Holtzapple, P.G., Segal, S.: Uptake of alpha-methylglucoside by normal and diabetic human jejunal mucosa. J. Lab. Clin. Med. 77:743, 1971.

54. Vinnik, I.E., Kern, F., Jr., Sussman, K.E.: The effect of diabetes mellitus and insulin on glucose absorption by the small intestine in man. J. Lab. Clin. Med. 66:131, 1965.

55. Caspary, W.F., Winckler, K., Creutzfeldt, W.: Intestinal brush border enzyme activity in juvenile and maturity onset diabetes mellitus. Diabetologia 10:353, 1974.

56. Olsen, W.A., Korsmo, H.: The intestinal brush border membrane in diabetes. Studies of sucrase-isomaltase metabolism in rats with streptozotocin diabetes. J. Clin. Invest. 60:181, 1977.

57. Whalen, G.E., Soergel, K.H., Geens, J.E.: Diabetic diarrhea: a clinical and pathophysiological study. Gastroenterol. 56:1021, 1969.

58. Bargen, J.A., Bollman, J.L., Kepler, E.J.: The "diarrhea of diabetes" and steatorrhea of pancreatic insufficiency. Mayo Clinic Proc. 11:737, 1936.

59. Malins, J.M., French, J.M.: Diabetic diarrhea. Quart. J. Med. 26:467, 1957.

60. Katz, L.A., Spiro, H.M.: Gastrointestinal manifestations of diabetes. N. Engl. J. Med. 275:1350, 1966.

61. McNally, E.F., Reinhard, A.E., Schwartz, P.E.: Small bowel motility in diabetics. Am. J. Dig. Dis. 14:163, 1969.

62. Berge, K.G., Sprague, R.G., Bennett, W.A.: The intestinal tract in diabetic diarrhea. A pathologic study. Diabetes 5:289, 1956.

63. Wruble, L.D., Kalser, M.H.: Diabetic steatorrhea: a distinct entity. Am. J. Med. 37:587, 1968.

64. Hensley, G.T., Soergel, K.H.: New pathologic findings in diabetic diarrhea. Arch. Path. 85:587, 1968.

65. Blumenthal, H.T., Probstein, J.G., Berns, A.W.: Interrelationship of diabetes mellitus and pancreatitis. Arch. Surg. 87:844, 1963.

66. Green, P.A., Berge, K.G., Sprague, R.G.: Control of diabetic diarrhea with antibiotic therapy. Diabetes 17:385, 1968.

67. Goldstein, F., Wirts, C.W., Kowlessar, O.D.: Diabetic diarrhea and steatorrhea. Microbiologic and clinical observations. Ann. Intern. Med. 72:215, 1970.

68. Sumi, S.M., Finlay, J.M.: On the pathogenesis of diabetic steatorrhea. Ann. Intern. Med. 55:994, 1961.

69. Condon, R., Suleman, M.I., Fan, Y.S., McKeown, M.D.: Cholestyramine and diabetic and post-vagotomy diarrhea. Br. Med. J. 4:423, 1973.

70. Thompson, M.W.: Hereditary, maternal age and birth order in etiology of celiac disease. Am. J. Human Gen. 3:159, 1951.

71. Green, P.A., Wollaeger, E.E., Sprague, R.G., Brown, A.L., Jr.: Diabetes mellitus associated with nontropical sprue. Report of 4 cases. Diabetes 11:388, 1962.

72. Mann, J.G., Brown, W.R., Kern, F., Jr.: The subtle and variable clinical expressions of gluten induced enteropathy. Am. J. Med. 48:357, 1970.

73. Boyer, P.H., Andersen, D.H.: Genetic study of celiac disease: incidence of celiac disease, gastrointestinal disorders, and diabetes in pedigrees of children with celiac disease. J. Dis. Child. 91:131, 1956.

74. Carter, C., Sheldon, W., Walker, C.: Inheritance of celiac disease. Ann. Human Genet. 23:266, 1959.

75. Falchuk, Z.M., Rogentine, G.N., Strober, W.: Predominance of histocompatibility antigen HL-A8 in patients with gluten-sensitive enteropathy. J. Clin. Invest. 51:1602, 1972.

76. Cudworth, A.G., Woodrow, J.C.: Evidence for HLA-linked genes in "juvenile diabetes mellitus." Br. Med. J. 3:133, 1975.

77. Bell, E.T.: Carcinoma of the pancreas. I. Clinical and pathologic study of 609 necropsied cases. II. Relation of carcinoma of pancreas to diabetes mellitus. Am. J. Pathol. 33:499, 1957.

78. Clark, C.G., Mitchell, P.E.G.: Diabetes and primary carcinoma of the pancreas. Br. Med. J. 2:1259, 1961.

79. Cohen, G.F.: Early diagnosis of pancreatic neoplasm in diabetics. Lancet 2:267, 1965.

80. Joslin, E.P., Lombard, H.L., Burrows, R.E., Manning, M.D.: Diabetes and cancer. N. Engl. J. Med. 260:486, 1959.

81. Morgan, R.G.H., Wormsley, K.G.: Cancer of the pancreas. Progress report. Gut 18:581, 1977.

82. Barkin, J., Vining, D., Miale, A., et al.: Computerized tomography, diagnostic ultrasound and radionucleide scanning. Comparison of efficiency in diagnosis of pancreatic carcinoma. J.A.M.A. 238:20, 1977.

83. Hatfield, A.R.W., Smithies, A., Wilkins, R., Levi, A.J.: Assessment of endoscopic retrograde cholangiopancreatography in patients with pancreatic disease. Gut 17:14, 1976.

84. Di Magno, E.P., Malagelada, J.R., Taylor, W.F., Go, V.L.W.: A prospective comparison of current diagnostic tests for pancreatic cancer. N. Engl. J. Med. 297:737, 1977.

85. Smith, E.H., Bartrum, R.J., Chang, Y.C., et al.: Percutaneous aspiration biopsy of the pancreas under ultrasonic guidance. N. Engl. J. Med. 292:825, 1975.

86. Boijsen, E.: Pancreatic angiography. In: H.L. Abrams (Ed.): Angiography, 2nd ed. Vol. 2. Boston, Little, Brown & Co., 1971. p. 953.

87. Silverberg, B.S., Grant, R.N.: Cancer statistics, 1970. CA 20:11, 1970

88. Pereiras, R.V., Owen, J.R., Hutson, D., et al.: Relief of malignant obstructive jaundice by percutaneous insertion of a permanent prosthesis in the biliary tree. Ann. Intern. Med. 89:589, 1978.

89. Podolsky, S., Viswanathan, M. (Eds.): Secondary Diabetes. The Spectrum of the Diabetic Syndromes. New York, Raven Press, 1980.

90. Frier, B.M., Saunders, J.H.B., Wormsley, K.G., Bouchier, I.A.D.: Exocrine pancreatic function in juvenile-onset diabetes mellitus. Gut 17:685, 1976.

91. Kaldany, A.: Autoantibodies to islet cells in diabetes mellitus. Diabetes 28:102, 1979.

92. The Copenhagen Pancreatitis Study Group: An interim report from a prospective epidemiological multicentre study. Scand. J. Gastroenterol. 16:305, 1981.

93. Singer, M.V., Sarles, H.: Chronic pancreatitis in Western Europe. In: Ref. 89, pp. 89–103.

94. Trapnell, J.E.: Patterns of pancreatitis in Great Britain—with special reference to diabetes. In: Ref. 89, pp. 77–88.

95. Viswanathan, M.: Pancreatic diabetes in India. An overview. In: Ref. 89, pp. 105–116.

96. McMillan, D.E., Geevarghese, P.J.: Dietary cyanide and tropical malnutrition. Diabetes Care 2:202, 1979. See also ref. 89, pp. 239–247.

97. James, D., Agnew, J.E., Bouchier, I.A.D.: Chronic pancreatitis in England: a changing picture. Br. Med. J. 2:34, 1974.

98. Ikeda, Y., Saito, H., Tajima, N., Abe, M.: Pancreatic

diabetes with pancreatolithiasis in Japan. In: Ref. 93, pp. 159–164.

99. Dreiling, D.A., Greenstein, A.: Diagnosis of pancreatic disease. In: L.C. Carey (Ed.): The Pancreas. St. Louis, C.V. Mosby Co., 1973, pp. 61–95.

99a. Bank, S.: Acute and chronic pancreatitis. In: T.L. Dent, F.E. Eckhauser, A.I. Vinik, and J.G. Turcotte (Eds.): Pancreatic Disease. Diagnosis and Therapy. New York, Grune & Stratton, 1981, pp. 167–188.

100. Root, H.F., Diabetic coma and acute pancreatitis with fatty liver. J.A.M.A. 108:777, 1937.

101. Payne, J.E., Jr., Tanenberg, R.J.: Hyperparathyroid crisis and acute necrotizing pancreatitis presenting as diabetic ketoacidosis. Am. J. Surg. 140:698, 1980.

102. Sinha, S.K.: Pancreatic diabetes in man. Clinical features and management. In: Ref. 89, pp. 197–214.

103. Goodman, G.I.: Hepatomegaly and diabetes mellitus. Ann. Intern. Med. 39:1077, 1953.

104. Creutzfeldt, W., Fredricks, H., Sickniger, K.: Liver disease and diabetes mellitus. In: H. Popper, F. Scheffner (Eds.): Progress in Liver Disease, Vol. 3. New York, Grune & Stratton, 1973, pp. 380–407.

105. Jacques, W.E.: The incidence of portal cirrhosis and fatty metamorphosis in patients dying with diabetes mellitus. N. Engl. J. Med. 249:442, 1953.

106. Macdonald, R.A., Mallory, C.K.: The natural history of post-necrotic cirrhosis. Am. J. Med. 241:334, 1958.

107. Adler, M., Schaffner, F.: Fatty liver hepatitis and cirrhosis in obese patients. Am. J. Med. 67:811, 1979.

108. Falchuk, K.R., Fiske, S.C., Haggitt, R.C., et al.: Pericentral hepatic fibrosis and intracellular hyalin in diabetes. Gastroenterol. 78:535, 1980.

109. Edmondson, H.A., Peters, R.L., Frankel, H.H.: The early stage of liver injury in the alcoholic. Medicine (Baltimore) 46:119, 1967.

110. Zimmerman, H.J.: Hepatotoxicity. New York, Appleton-Century-Croft, 1978. pp. 455–459.

110a. Bloodworth, J.M.B., Jr., Hamwi, G.J.: Histopathologic lesions associated with sulfonylurea administration. Diabetes 10:90, 1961.

111. Stokes, A.E., Powell, L.W.: Carbohydrate intolerance in idiopathic hemochromatosis and cirrhosis of the liver. Quart. J. Med. 42:733, 1973.

112. Dymock, I.W., Cassar, J., et al.: Observations on pathogenesis, complications and treatment of diabetes in 115 cases of hemochromatosis. Am. J. Med. 52:203, 1972.

113. Finch, S.C., Finch, C.A.: Idiopathic hemochromatosis in iron storage disease. A. Iron metabolism in hemochromatosis Medicine 34:301, 1955.

114. Popp, J.W., Jr., Wands, M.D.: Recent views on the recognition of hemochromatosis. In: C.S. Davidson (Ed.): Problems in Liver Disease. New York, Stratton Intercontinental Medical Book Corporation, 1979, pp. 187–201.

115. Walters, G.O., Jacobs, A., Worwood, M., et al.: Iron absorption in normal subjects and patients with idiopathic hemochromatosis; relationship with serum ferritin concentration. Gut 16:188, 1975.

116. Beaumont, C., Simon, M., Fauchet, R.: Serum ferritin as a possible marker of the hemochromatosis allele. N. Engl. J. Med. 301:169, 1979.

117. Cartwright, G.E., Edwards, C.Q., Kravitz, K., et al.: Hereditary hemochromatosis. Phenotypic expressions of the disease. N. Engl. J. Med. 301:175, 1979.

118. Kidd, K.K.: Genetic linkage and hemochromatosis. N. Engl. J. Med. 301:209, 1979.

119. Lamon, J.M., Marynick, S.P., Roseblatt, R., Donnelly, S.: Idiopathic hemochromatosis in a young female. A case study and review of the syndrome in young people. Gastroenterol. 76:178, 1979.

120. Jensen, P.S.: Hemochromatosis: a disease often silent but not invisible. Am. J. Roentgenol. 126:343, 1976.

121. Stokes, A.E., Powell, L.W.: Pituitary function in hemochromatosis. Am. J. Med. 45:839, 1968.

122. Lipschitz, D.A., Cook, J.D., Finch, C.A.: A clinical evaluation of serum ferritin as an index of iron stores. N. Engl. J. Med. 290:1213, 1974.

123. Barry, M.: Progress report. Iron and liver. Gut 15:324, 1974.

124. Bomford, A., Williams, R.: Long term results in venesection therapy in idiopathic hemochromatosis. Quart. J. Med. 19:611, 1976.

125. Easley, R.M., Schreiner, B.F., Yu, P.N.: Reversible cardiomyopathy associated with hemochromatosis. N. Engl. J. Med. 287:866, 1972.

126. Johnson, D.G., Alberti, K.G.M.M.: Carbohydrate metabolism in liver disease. Clin. Endocrinol. Metab. 5:675, 1976.

127. Alberti, K.G.M.M., Johnson, D.G.: Carbohydrate. In: R. Wright, K.G.M.M. Alberti, S Karran, M. Ward-Sadler (Eds.): Biliary and Liver Disease. Philadelphia, W.B. Saunders Co., 1979, pp. 44–62.

128. Samson, R.I., Trey, C., et al.: Fulminant hepatitis with recurrent hypoglycemia and hemorrhage. Gastroenterol. 53:291, 1967.

129. Madison, L.L., Lochner, A., Wolff, J.: Ethanol induced hypoglycemia. II. Mechanism of suppression of hepatic glyconeogenesis. Diabetes 16:252, 1967.

130. Johnson, D.G., Alberti, K.G.M.M., Wright, R., et al.: C-Peptide and insulin in the liver. Diabetes 27 (Suppl. 1):201, 1978.

131. Mundth, E.D.: Cholecystitis and diabetes mellitus. N. Engl. J. Med. 267:642, 1962.

132. Howard, R.J., Delaney, J.P.: Post-operative cholecystitis. Am. J. Dig. Dis. 17:213, 1972.

41 Lipoatrophic Diabetes

Aldo A. Rossini

Lipoatrophic diabetes and generalized lipodystrophy are synonymous terms for a syndrome characterized by overall absence of adipose tissue in association with insulin-resistant diabetes mellitus. Although the description may appear straightforward, the diagnosis is often not readily evident; by no means does every thin patient with uncontrolled diabetes have lipoatrophic diabetes. Indeed, overdiagnosis has led to considerable confusion. It is the intent of this chapter to clarify terminology and highlight the criteria which must be used to make the diagnosis. The task is not a simple one because this disease may represent but one extreme of a wide spectrum of unusual clinical conditions, all of which may prove to be different expressions of the same pathogenic mechanism. In addition to true lipoatrophic diabetes, this spectrum includes such diverse disease states as leprechaunism,[1] diencephalic syndrome of emaciation,[2] cerebral gigan-

tism,[3] congenital muscular hypertrophy with mental defect,[4] and the syndrome of macroglossia, gigantism, and exomphalos.[5] There are also individuals with partial lipodystrophy in which only part of the body lacks fat. This review will attempt to provide a uniform and relatively precise categorization of lipoatrophic diabetic states.

DEFINITIONS

Zeigler[6] has been credited with the first report of generalized lipoatrophy. Hansen and McQuarrie[7] then described the association of generalized lipoatrophy and diabetes mellitus. However, it remained for Lawrence[8] to present in 1946 the first comprehensive case report from which could be derived strict criteria on which to base a diagnosis of lipoatrophic diabetes. His five major criteria were: (1) generalized absence of fat; (2) insulin-resistant diabetes mellitus; (3) absence of ketosis; (4) elevated basal metabolic rate; and (5) severe hyperlipidemia with consequent hepatomegaly. Adhering closely to these criteria, in 1974 the writer (A.R.) was able to identify approximately 80 well-documented cases which had been described in the world literature.

After careful study of reported cases, in 1971 Seip[9,10] was able to define two subcategories of lipoatrophic diabetes, acquired and congenital. The distinction between these subcategories is of considerable interest.

Acquired Lipoatrophic Diabetes (The Lawrence Syndrome)

The acquired type of lipoatrophic diabetes accounts for approximately 40% of all cases. Its occurrence is entirely sporadic, and in no instance has familial transmission been observed. Affected patients usually have the onset of generalized lipoatrophy in childhood or young adulthood, followed an average of 4 years later by diabetes. Rarely, diabetes may precede the lipoatrophy. Sex distribution is stated to be equal in the congenital type with a female preponderance (2:1) in the acquired type. Often an antecedent viral illness is documented prior to the onset of lipoatrophy. Pertussis, varicella, rubella, infectious mononucleosis, and an undefined febrile illness with diarrhea have all preceded the acquired syndrome. This association has engendered speculation that a virus may initiate the disorder, but proof of any sort is lacking. Other features of the acquired type of lipoatrophic diabetes include a high incidence of severe acanthosis nigricans, and marked cirrhosis, the complications of which may prove fatal.

Congenital Lipoatrophic Diabetes (The Berardinelli-Seip Syndrome)

The more common type of lipoatrophic diabetes is congenital[11] which accounts for some 60% of cases. Transmission of this syndrome seems to be autosomal recessive. Onset of lipoatrophy occurs in infancy; the diabetes appears later in childhood with mean onset at 12 years of age. A high incidence of parental consanguinity has been noted, as has an equal sex distribution.[12] Various forms of intracerebral disorders, most commonly in the area of the third ventricle, are common findings and may be important in the pathogenesis.[11] Other congenital defects associated with the congenital lipodystrophic syndrome include abnormalities of the heart, kidneys, and ovaries.[13–16] Mental retardation and the development of psychiatric disturbances have also been reported.[17] Growth and maturation of bone are frequently accelerated.[10] Patients with congenital lipoatrophic diabetes usually have a milder form of acanthosis nigricans and less severe cirrhosis than do those with the acquired disease.

CLINICAL MANIFESTATIONS

Many of the physical characteristics and clinical signs present in patients with lipoatrophic diabetes are seen in both forms of the disorder. While no findings are pathognomonic, the presentation of patients with lipoatrophic diabetes is rather stereotyped, and suspicion should be high when the findings listed below are encountered.

Generalized Lipodystrophy

The most striking finding in patients with lipoatrophic diabetes is the absence of fat. Not only is there an obvious paucity of subcutaneous fat, but also an occult absence of fat in areas where it usually remains present despite severe nutritional emaciation. The perirenal, buccal, retroperitoneal, and epicardial fat pads may all be absent.[9] Interestingly, mammary fat tissue alone may be preserved.[12,18] The loss of adipose tissue makes certain anatomic structures prominent. The thyroid gland and peripheral veins often appear enlarged. Thyromegaly and phlebomegaly appear to represent genuine increases in the size of the affected tissue;[8,9] loss of

surrounding fatty tissue then further accentuates the increase in size (Fig. 41–1).

Acanthosis Nigricans

Acanthosis nigricans is a dermatosis characterized by brown-black hyperpigmented areas of confluent papillomata which produce a sandpaper-like sensation on palpation. The lesions usually affect the axilla, groin, neck, umbilicus, and nipple, but occasionally have been described on the dorsum of hands and feet. These lesions are more prominent in the acquired than in the congenital type of lipoatrophic diabetes.[9,19,20] Acanthosis nigricans is known to occur in association with malignancy,[21] particularly intestinal neoplasia. In addition, this skin disorder is now known to be associated with insulin resistance and diabetes mellitus.[22] The basis for the peculiar association of insulin resistance with acanthosis nigricans remains an unsolved riddle. What information is available will be discussed more fully below.

Acromegaloid and Herculean Features

Patients with generalized lipodystrophy exhibit a striking accentuation of the muscular features of their anatomy. Not only are muscles prominent, but they may be hypertrophied as well.[23,24] Elevated urinary creatinine, increased muscle glycogen, and body composition studies using radioisotopes confirm this clinical impression.[25] Acromegaloid facial features along with thick skin and large hands, feet and ears are also classic. Growth velocity in the first 4 to 5 years of life is increased in congenital lipoatrophy, an observation documented both by growth grids and by demonstration of accelerated skeletal maturation.[9] Genitalomegaly has also been mentioned as a feature of congenital type lipoatrophic diabetes. However, onset of puberty does not reflect the skeletal age but rather the chronologic age of the patient.[9]

Thick Curly Hair. An interesting observation in patients with lipoatrophic diabetes is the presence of thick curly hair. In one striking case studied at the Joslin Research Laboratory, an American Indian with lipoatrophic diabetes developed this typical hair pattern. Family members, all of whom had straight black hair, ostracized the patient.[26] Hypertrichosis and low neck hair lines have also been described.[27]

Hyperhidrosis. Although not often a prominent feature of this syndrome, profuse sweating may be present,[9,26] especially post-prandially. It is believed that increased oxidation of calories occurs following a meal in patients with lipoatrophic diabetes. Profuse sweating is then an important physiologic mechanism by which heat is dissipated and severe body core hyperthermia avoided.

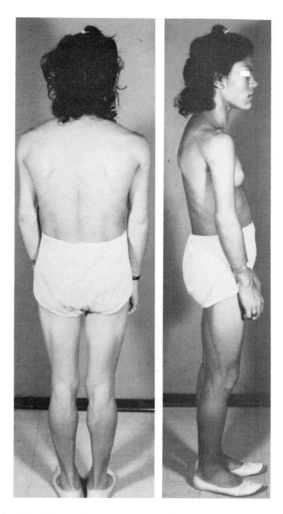

Fig. 41–1. Patient (M. O'F.) showing characteristic appearance of lipoatrophic diabetes.

Abdominal Signs. Because of concurrent hepatomegaly and absence of subcutaneous fat, the patient with lipoatrophic diabetes often presents with marked abdominal protuberance. Although the degree of liver enlargement varies from case to case, it is not uncommon to find the liver edge below the iliac crest.[26] In at least 1 case, the liver was observed to decrease markedly in size (by approximately 50%) following a fast. This conspicuous improvement was probably due to mobilization of lipids and/or glycogen from the liver. Conversely, a diet high in fat and carbohydrate increases liver size. An unfortunate consequence of the hepatomegaly is progression to cirrhosis and, eventually, to portal hypertension with splenomegaly.[7,8] In a few reported cases of acquired lipoatrophic diabetes, death has been attributed to the sequelae of portal hypertension and cirrhosis.[28–30]

Splenomegaly may occur in the absence of cirrhosis, and lymph node enlargement in the neck and groin, along with enlargement of tonsils and adenoids, are frequently encountered.[31] These findings are probably due to hyperlipemia and secondarily increased fat content in the lymph glands. Fat globules in the cytoplasm of reticulum cells of lymph glands have been reported.[8]

Hyperlipidemia. Hyperlipidemia in the patient with lipoatrophic diabetes may be signaled clinically by the presence of eruptive xanthomas and lipemia retinalis.[26,32] Not infrequently patients will have serum triglyceride levels greater than 5000 mg/dl.[26,32]

Other. There is one report of a case of lipoatrophic diabetes which occurred in association with the sicca syndrome—the triad of keratoconjunctivitis sicca, xerostomia, and other connective tissue disorders.[33] Irregular menses and polycystic ovaries are also common findings.[8,26,34–37]

LABORATORY OBSERVATIONS

Elevated Metabolic Rate

Lawrence was the first to observe an elevation of oxygen consumption (basal metabolic rate or

BMR) in a patient with acquired lipoatrophic diabetes.[8] On several occasions, the BMR was recorded above $+150\%$ (N $= -5\%$ to $+15\%$). He initially attributed this observation to hyperthyroidism. Although the patient was clinically euthyroid, a thyroidectomy was performed which resulted in a fall in BMR. However, the patient soon became clinically hypothyroid, and when thyroid replacement therapy was instituted, the BMR returned to an elevated level. Since this first report, marked hypermetabolism has been considered a characteristic of lipoatrophic diabetes. Recent studies have shown that oxygen consumption in these patients is increased following meals, and is decreased during brief starvation. In 1 case, the BMR index value was $+75\%$ to $+100\%$ (65 to 75 kcal hr/sqm) and fell after 3 days of fast to -17% to $+12\%$ (31 to 35 kcal/hr/sqm).[26] Other studies have suggested that protein more than fat or carbohydrate, results in this increase in metabolic rate.[38] The exact mechanism by which dietary intake induces excessive thermogenesis in lipoatrophic diabetes is unknown, but one line of speculation relates it to fluctuations in T_3 (triiodothyronine) concentration.

Insulin-Resistant Diabetes Mellitus

Another hallmark of lipoatrophic diabetes is marked insulin resistance.[8,24] Elevated basal insulin levels in the postabsorptive state as well as normal increases in circulating insulin levels following various beta cell stimuli suggest that beta cell function is normal.[16,39] Proinsulin to insulin ratios are also normal.[40] Biologic assay of circulating insulin as well as the half-life of the insulin are normal.[24,26,39] There is no evidence of insulin antibodies, circulating inhibitors, or anti-receptor antibodies.[26,32] However, some patients reportedly have normal receptor binding or affinity, while others have either decreased or increased binding.[41,42] The data suggest that the pathogenesis of insulin resistance in lipoatrophic diabetes is heterogeneous and may involve both receptor and postreceptor abnormalities.[42] There is some suggestion that insulin resistance may derive from reversible loss of coupling of a normal insulin receptor to metabolic pathways. This antagonist may be diet-dependent.[43]

In some cases of lipoatrophic diabetes, large quantities of insulin have been used in an attempt to achieve glucose homeostasis; up to 9,000 units have been administered in 1 day.[26] The insulin resistance appears not to be related solely to caloric intake since it persists even during fasting.

Interestingly, both insulin resistance and acanthosis nigricans can occur without lipoatrophy. Kahn, Flier, et al.[22,44] have classified this syndrome into three groups. Type A patients are young females with virilization, increased growth, and decreased insulin receptor concentrations without circulating insulin receptor inhibitors. Type B patients appear to have a disturbance of the immune mechanism with circulating antibodies to insulin receptors. Type C patients have no receptor defect, and the pathologic process is therefore believed to be a postreceptor abnormality. The relationship of insulin resistance, insulin receptors, and acanthosis nigricans in all of these syndromes is unknown, but the data suggest a complicated pathogenic process that must be much better understood before a definitive classification can be made. The possibility of a genetic deficiency of insulin receptors has been supported by the results of a number of studies.[44a,44b]

Lipid Status

Severe hyperlipemia has been a consistent and extensively studied abnormality in cases of lipoatrophic diabetes. In the postabsorptive state, a Type V hyperlipemia is present with its characteristic lactescent serum. The deposition of the circulating lipid into lymphoreticular tissue, particularly liver, spleen, and lymph nodes has been discussed above.[6] Following a carbohydrate meal, triglyceride levels increase significantly in most cases; following a fast, the levels fall.[26,39] Lipoprotein lipase levels are variable, and both decreased clearance and increased synthesis may be involved in the pathogenesis of the hyperlipidemia.[32,39,45] In one report of a patient with partial lipodystrophy, kinetic studies performed after injection of autologous radioiodinated VLDL indicated that VLDL was over-produced, and the authors suggest that insulin was responsible for the overproduction.[46]

The most intriguing aspect of lipid metabolism in patients with lipoatrophic diabetes is resistance to ketone production.[8,32] In the absence of insulin (as occurs in the insulin-dependent diabetic) lipolysis occurs with resultant production of ketones. In contrast, the patient with lipoatrophic diabetes has both a paucity of stored fat and elevated circulating insulin levels. These two factors account for the resistance to ketone production despite the concomitant resistance to insulin. It should be noted, however, that resistance to, not absence of, ketogenesis is implied. During a 48-hour fast, circulating levels of insulin decrease and evidence of slight ketone production may be observed.[26] Accordingly, Lawrence's original criterion of absence of ketosis for the diagnosis of lipoatrophic diabetes must be modified to resistance to ketosis. No patients with lipoatrophic diabetes, however, have yet been reported to develop ketoacidosis.

Other Hormone Studies

Thyroid hormone levels are normal in lipo-atrophic diabetes.[26,47] Occasionally, intercurrent thyroid disorder does occur, but its relationship to lipoatrophic diabetes is unclear and may be coincidental.[26] Glucagon levels are reported to range from normal to marked elevation.[26,45,48] Gonadotropin levels are normal,[24] although in some cases of congenital lipoatrophic diabetes, polycystic ovaries compatible with the Stein-Leventhal syndrome have been reported.[6,12,34,37] One possible explanation for the overproduction of testosterone is that it is due to a direct effect of hyperinsulinemia on the ovary.[48a] Adrenal function is generally described as normal.[19,23] In 2 of 3 cases of lipoatrophic diabetes in one study, there were no increases in norepinephrine and epinephrine concentrations following hypoglycemia induced by high doses of insulin. In the third case, only epinephrine rose.[48]

Probably the greatest discrepancies among case reports pertain to the results of growth hormone studies. The acromegaloid appearance of patients with lipoatrophic diabetes leads one to suspect hypersecretion of growth hormone, but measurements are inconsistent. Some investigators report a hypersecretion,[49] while others report normal levels and lack of response following administration of common perturbants of growth hormone.[26,50] These discrepancies most likely reflect the great heterogeneity of patients with lipoatrophic diabetes. Just as there appear to be subtypes of lipoatrophic patients with insulin resistance and acanthosis nigricans, there may be as yet unclassified subtypes with respect to growth hormone secretion. It is also conceivable that in some cases there may be secretion of an abnormal peptide which is measured by some growth hormone immunoassays and not by others.

Radiographic Findings

The most striking radiologic feature of the patient with lipoatrophic diabetes is absence of fat.[47,51,52] Loss of fat beneath the skin, between muscle bundles, in the retroperitoneum, and around such organs as the heart and kidneys causes an abnormal image of these structures. Complete absence of perinephric fat can cause disappearance of renal outlines. Another characteristic radiographic feature of this syndrome is osteosclerosis of long bones with thickened cortex extending into the shafts and replacing part of the marrow cavity. Occasionally, elongation of unfused epiphysis is also demonstrated.[47,51] The sclerotic changes are believed due in some way to replacement of hematopoietic marrow by fat, this fatty deposition being in turn secondary to the persistent hyperlipemia. It has been proposed that marrow fat may be transformed into osteogenic cells (liposkeletogenic modulation).[53]

Although skeletal changes are more often seen in the congenital syndrome, they can also occur in acquired lipoatrophic diabetes. Not uncommonly, multiple, discrete, well-defined areas of sclerosis are seen; these have been termed cystic angiomata.[12] In congenital lipoatrophic diabetes, associated congenital defects of the heart and other organs may produce their characteristic roentgen picture. Enlargement of the heart is not uncommonly seen radiographically; it is believed to reflect increased cardiac output secondary to the chronic hypermetabolic state. Enlarged kidneys may be seen on urographic examination, and there may be bilateral ureteroceles with dilatation of the ureters. The latter finding is thought to be the result of chronic polyuria secondary to hyperglycemia,[29,52] since similar changes are observed in patients with diabetes insipidus.

Morbidity and Mortality

As in other patients with chronic diabetes mellitus, long-term complications are observed in patients with lipoatrophic diabetes. Classic Kimmelstiel-Wilson renal disease with proteinuria and hypertension is commonly encountered.[16,39,47] Diabetic retinopathy and peripheral neuropathy have also been described in lipoatrophic diabetics. In a patient with lipodystrophy for 19 years and diabetes for 6 years, quantitative examination of muscle capillaries revealed severely thickened basement membrane.[54] Curiously, although these patients have both diabetes mellitus and chronic hyperlipidemia, atherosclerotic changes are not a constant finding.[9] One 29-year-old female with congenital lipoatrophic diabetes did, however, show generalized atherosclerosis at autopsy.[28] In other cases, calcification of the vas deferens has been described. Reportedly the most common cause of death is liver disease. Cirrhosis may lead to portal hypertension, esophageal varices, liver failure, and hepatic coma.[9,28] A patient with congenital lipoatrophic diabetes of 11 years' duration developed the nephrotic syndrome with progressive glomerulosclerosis. Renal transplantation was successfully performed but within 1 month renal failure developed. Biopsy revealed massive lipid deposition in renal tubular cells with necrosis and hemorrhage, but with minimal evidence of graft rejection. The authors conclude that serum lipids must be lowered prior to renal transplantation in patients with lipoatrophic diabetes.[55]

ETIOLOGY

Although both congenital and acquired lipoatrophic diabetes have similar clinical appearances, there is no reason to assume that they have similar etiologies. The autosomal recessive inheritance of the congenital form suggests a missing gene or enzyme. On the other hand, the frequent history of infectious disease prior to the onset of acquired lipodystrophy tempts one to suspect a virus as the initiating factor in the acquired syndrome. Other hypothesized etiologies are those listed below.

Lipid Mobilizing Factor

A polypeptide substance capable of mobilizing fat has been isolated from the urine of patients with lipoatrophic diabetes.[56,57] This material also appears to cause insulin resistance and has diabetogenic as well as adipokinetic properties.[58] This substance is thought to cause rapid turnover of stored fat through the continuous hydrolysis of triglycerides to free fatty acids and glycerol. However, this polypeptide has also been found in proteinuric diabetes without evidence of lipoatrophic diabetes,[57] and in the pituitary glands of normal cows, hogs, and sheep.[59–61] The role of a lipid-mobilizing factor in lipoatrophic diabetes remains purely speculative. The concept of an abnormal circulating factor remains an enticing one, however. Some abnormal peptide might, for example, directly stimulate the secretion of growth hormone, thus accounting for the clinical finding of acromegaloid features and organomegaly. The variable growth hormone levels reported in lipoatrophic diabetes could then be attributed to variation in circulating peptide.

Insulin Receptor and Other Hormonal Receptor Abnormalities

As noted earlier, there appear to be abnormalities of insulin receptors in some patients with lipoatrophic diabetes.[41,42,62] Absence of either cell membrane receptors or receptors at the nuclear level is possible. It may be hypothesized that other hormone receptors are similarly defective in some way, causing such associated disorders as acanthosis nigricans, polycystic ovaries, and abnormal growth hormone physiology. Another alternative hypothesis holds that there could be alterations in intracellular signals elicited by insulin and other hormones. Such erroneous signals theoretically could account for the fall in circulating amino acids after exogenous insulin administration, as well as hypertrophied muscles and increased organ size.

Hypothalamic Etiology

Certain studies have found an increase in hypothalamic releasing factors (corticotropin releasing factor, melanocyte stimulating hormone, follicle-stimulating hormone) in the circulation of patients with lipoatrophic diabetes.[63–66] Some investigators hypothesize that the increase in these releasing factors is secondary to an accumulation of dopamine within the hypothalamus. Dopamine hydroxylase, which catalyzes the conversion of dopamine to norepinephrine, is theorized to be absent in patients with lipoatrophic diabetes. Thus, normal inhibition of releasing factors does not occur, and the stimulatory effects of dopamine proceed unimpeded. In support of these ideas, it has been reported that pimozide, a narcoleptic which decreases hypothalamic dopamine levels, is capable of reversing various metabolic and clinical features of lipoatrophic diabetes.[67,68] However, other studies using this drug have proven unsuccessful.[26,69,70] Another drug said to be beneficial in treating subjects with lipoatrophic diabetes is fenfluramine. This drug, a blocker of dopamine, also lowers brain serotonin levels and was found to increase sensitivity to exogenous insulin in patients with lipoatrophic diabetes.[69,70] Further studies clearly are necessary to establish the efficacy of these drugs.

The possibility that a hypothalamic lesion may be important has also been suggested by other lines of evidence. One is the frequent finding of tumors in the third ventricle of patients with congenital lipoatrophic diabetes. Another is the clinical picture in the diencephalic syndrome of infancy. In this syndrome there is absence of fat, elevation of basal metabolic rate, and acceleration of growth associated with anterior hypothalamic tumors but not with diabetes. Other syndromes such as leprechaunism, cerebral gigantism, and congenital muscular hypertrophy with mental deficiency may all be different expressions of lipoatrophic diabetes, but at the present time, the diagnosis of true lipoatrophic diabetes should be reserved for those patients fulfilling all five accepted criteria. Recently, a boy with lipoatrophic diabetes and stenosis of the aqueduct of Sylvius, underwent a ventriculo-cisternal shunt operation to relieve intracranial pressure. Following surgery, a dramatic improvement in his diabetic state ensued. The authors concluded that abnormal hypothalamic function may be responsible for the disturbed carbohydrate and lipid metabolism.[71]

PARTIAL LIPODYSTROPHIES

Partial lipodystrophy is somewhat more common than generalized lipodystrophy, although it must be remembered that both are rare. The most common variety of partial lipodystrophy is characterized by loss of fat above the waist, while below it, adiposity is normal or even increased.[72,73] This type of lipodystrophy is also known as cephalothoracic lipodystrophy, lipodystrophia progressiva, Barroquer-Simons disease, or "Florid Venus of the

Ultra Rubens Style.''[9,74] Many investigators believe that partial lipodystrophy represents a less severe variant of the generalized type.[75] Indeed, glucose intolerance, insulin resistance, and, in at least 40% of cases, hypermetabolism have been observed.[76,77] In both acquired generalized lipoatrophic diabetes and partial lipodystrophy, the syndrome usually develops in childhood and may be preceded by an infectious process. Familial occurrence has been described, however.[9] At least 1 case of partial lipodystrophy appears to have evolved into the complete or generalized type of lipodystrophy.[75] The partial lipodystrophies are associated with a high incidence of brain tumors.[78]

Another interesting association in patients with partial lipodystrophy is the presence of renal disease. Mesangiocapillary (membrano-proliferative) glomerulonephritis has been confirmed by biopsy, and not infrequently has resulted in the nephrotic syndrome.[79,80] In this regard, as in patients with mesangiocapillary nephritis without lipoatrophy, there frequently is hypocomplementemia.[77,81] A possible mechanism has been postulated in which complement deficiency may predispose subjects to infections which may then lead to lipodystrophy and/or mesangiocapillary nephritis.[81] In 1 case, a patient with partial lipodystrophy had increased susceptibility to infection. Interestingly, she was also found to have a clinical picture compatible with systemic lupus erythematosus. The patient's serum contained low C_3 levels and abnormal C_3-cleaving activity resulting in the presence of circulating C_3 breakdown products.[82] In total lipodystrophy, however, no abnormalities of the complement system have been found.

The line of demarcation of lipoatrophy in partial syndromes often follows a dermatomal distribution. A defect associated with a certain neuroanatomic level would favor a local environmental factor or hormone which renders limited regions of tissue different from similar distant regions. Perhaps the susceptibility of an area is mediated through the autonomic nervous system. Indeed, one study found abnormal fat cells associated with autonomic dysfunction.[83,84] More perspiration was observed in the atrophic region, and some investigators believe that there is hypersecretion of norepinephrine in such areas.[84,85] However, in another study, autonomic dysfunction with normal fat cells was observed.[86]

Probably the most interesting studies, suggesting that a local environmental factor is important in the pathogenesis of lipodystrophy, were experiments involving autotransplantation of adipose tissue.[86,87] When normal adipose tissue was transplanted to an area of lipodystrophy, the transplant lost fat. Conversely, if lipoatrophic tissue was brought to an area of normal adiposity, the previously lipoatrophic tissue tended to gain fat.

Although no inflammatory responses have been reported in the skin or adipose tissue, swelling of the fat cells has occasionally been described prior to atrophy. Thus, there does exist the possibility that lipoatrophy is the result of an immunologic mechanism in which the fat cell is the target tissue. However, this hypothesis does not account well for the partial lipodystrophies, particularly those affecting, for example, half the body or only the ankles.[88]

Final Comments

It should be clear that speculation and hypotheses regarding lipoatrophic diabetes are abundant, but facts are few. What can be said in summary is that there appear to be two major types of lipoatrophic diabetes, one acquired and one congenital. Certain clinical and laboratory characteristics of lipoatrophic diabetes confirm the diagnosis. The partial lipodystrophies, diencephalic hypothalamic syndrome, leprechaunism, and the syndrome of acanthosis nigricans and insulin resistance probably represent variations in the expression of the same disease state. The etiologic factor or factors remain unknown and are the subject of numerous reviews.[9,79,89] To make the diagnosis of lipoatrophic diabetes per se, 5 criteria must be met: (1) insulin resistant diabetes; (2) ketosis resistance; (3) markedly elevated metabolic rate; (4) severe hyperlipidemia and hepatomegaly; and (5) generalized absence of fat.

REFERENCES

1. Donohue, W.L., Uchida, I.: Leprechaunism: a euphemism for a rare familial disorder. J. Pediatr. 45:505, 1954.
2. Russell, A.: A diencephalic syndrome of emaciation in infancy and childhood. Arch. Dis. Child. 26:274, 1951.
3. Sotos, J.F., Dodge, P.R., Muirhead, D., et al.: Cerebral gigantism in childhood. A syndrome of excessively rapid growth with acromegalic features and a nonprogressive neurologic disorder. N. Engl. J. Med. 271:109, 1964.
4. Bruck, F.: Über ein Fall von congenitaler Makroglossie, combiniert mit allgemeiner wahrer Muskelhypertrophie und Idiotie. Dtsch. Med. Wschr. 15:229, 1889.
5. Wiedemann, H.R.: Complexe malformatif familial avec hernie ombilicale et macroglossie—un ''syndrome nouveau?'' J. Genet. Hum. 13:223, 1964.
6. Ziegler, L.H.: Lipodystrophies: report of seven cases. Brain 51:147, 1928.
7. Hansen, A.E., McQuarrie, I.: Serum and tissue lipids in a peculiar type of generalized lipodystrophy (lipohistiodiaresis). Am. J. Dis. Child. 60:754, 1940.
8. Lawrence, R.D.: Lipodystrophy and hepatomegaly with diabetes, lipaemia, and other metabolic disturbances. A case throwing new light on the action of insulin. Lancet 1:724, 1946.
9. Seip, M.: Generalized lipodystrophy. Ergeb. Inn. Med. Kinderheilkd. 31:59, 1971.
10. Seip M., Trygstad, O.: Generalized lipodystrophy. Arch. Dis. Child. 38:447, 1963.

11. Berardinelli, W.: An undiagnosed endocrinometabolic syndrome: report of two cases. J. Clin. Endocrinol. *14*:193, 1954.

12. Brunzell, J.D., Shankle, S.W., Bethune, J.E.: Congenital generalized lipodystrophy accompanied by cystic angiomatosis. Ann. Intern. Med. *69*:501, 1968.

13. Witzgall, H.: Hyperlipämiche Lipoatrophie, ein klinischer Beitrag zur Regulation des Fettstoffwechsels. Aerztl. Wschr. *12*:1093, 1957.

14. Senior, B., Gellis, S.S.: The syndromes of total lipodystrophy and of partial lipodystrophy. Pediatr. *33*:593, 1964.

15. Senior, B.: Lipodystrophic muscular hypertrophy. Arch. Dis. Child. *36*:426, 1961.

16. Tourniaire, J., Guinet, P., Mornex, R., et al.: Diabète lipoatrophique. Étude clinique et biologique d'un cas atypique. Sem. Hôp. Paris *44*:3289, 1968.

17. Jolliff, J.W., Craig, J.W.: Lipoatrophic diabetes and mental illness in three siblings. Diabetes *16*:708, 1967.

18. Miller, M., Shipley, R.A., Shreeve, W.W., et al.: The metabolism of C-14 glucose in normal and diabetic subjects. Trans. Assoc. Am. Physicians *68*:199, 1955.

19. Reed, W.B., Dexter, R., Corley, C., Fish, C.: Congenital lipodystrophic diabetes with acanthosis nigricans. Arch. Dematol. *91*:326, 1965.

20. Janaki, V.R., Premalatha, S., Rao, N.R., Thambiah, A.S.: Lawrence-Seip syndrome. Br. J. Dermatol. *103*:693, 1980.

21. Newbold, P.C.H.: Skin markers of malignancy. Arch. Dermatol. *102*:680, 1970.

22. Kahn, C.R., Flier, J.S., Bar, R.S., et al.: The syndromes of insulin resistance and acanthosis nigricans. Insulin-receptor disorders in man. N. Engl. J. Med. *294*:739, 1976.

23. Ruvalcaba, R.H., Samols, E., Kelley, V.C.: Lipoatrophic diabetes. I. Studies concerning endocrine function and carbohydrate metabolism. Am. J. Dis. Child. *109*:279, 1965.

24. Seip, M.: Lipodystrophy and gigantism with associated endocrine manifestations: a new diencephalic syndrome? Acta Paediatr. *48*:555, 1959.

25. Meguid, M.M., Rossini, A.A., Boyden, C.M., Moore, F.D.: Body composition in lipoatrophic diabetes. Endocrine Society Program and Abstracts, 57th Ann. Meeting. Abstr. *478*:290, 1975.

26. Rossini, A.A., Self, J., Aoki, T.T., et al.: Metabolic and endocrine studies in a case of lipoatrophic diabetes. Metabolism *26*:637, 1977.

27. Dorasamy, D.S.: Congenital lipodystrophy: a case report. S. Afr. Med. J. *58*:417, 1980.

28. M.G.H. weekly clincopathological exercises. Case 1-1975. N. Engl. J. Med. *292*:33, 1975.

29. Wesenberg, R.L., Gwinn, J.L., Barnes, G.R., Jr.: The roentgenographic findings in total lipodystrophy. Am. J. Roentgen. *103*:154, 1968.

30. Fontan, A., Verger, P., Couteau, J.M., Pery, M.: Hypertrophie musculaire généralisée à début précoce, avec lipodystrophie faciale, hépatomégalie et clitoridienne chez une fille de 11 ans. Arch. Fr. Pediatr. *13*:276, 1956.

31. Brubaker, M.M., Levan, N.E., Collipp, P.M.: Acanthosis nigricans and congenital total lipodystrophy. Associated anomalies observed in two siblings. Arch. Dermatol. *91*:320, 1965.

32. Schwartz, R., Schafer, I.A., Renold, A.E.: Generalized lipoatrophy, hepatic cirrhosis, disturbed carbohydrate metabolism and accelerated growth (lipoatrophic diabetes): longitudinal observation and metabolic studies. Am. J. Med. *28*:973, 1960.

33. Ipp, M.M., Howard, N.J., Tervo, R.C., Gelfand, E.W.: Sicca syndrome and total lipodystrophy. A case in a fifteen-year-old female patient. Ann. Intern. Med. *85*:443, 1976.

34. De Gennes, J.L., Salticl, H., Tremolieres, J., et al.: Révision de l'exploration métabolique et endocrinienne d'un cas de diabète lipoatrophique. Presse. Med. *75*:2605, 1967.

35. Jimenez-Diaz, C., Rodriguez-Minon, J.L., Arrieta, F.: El syndrome de lipodystrofia, esteatosis hepatica y diabetes resistente. Rev. Clin. Esp. *86*:9, 1962.

36. Pavel, I., Cimpeanu, S., Niculescu, M., et al.: Le diabète lipoatrophique est-il un diabète lipidique? Presse. Med. *71*:1279, 1963.

37. Huseman, C.A., Johanson, A.J., Varma, M.M., Blizzard, R.M.: Congenital lipodystrophy. II. Association with polycystic ovarian disease. J. Pediatr. *95*:72, 1979.

38. Robbins, D.C., Danforth, E., Jr., Burse, R.L., et al.: Hypermetabolism of total lipoatrophic diabetes. Clin. Res. *26*:311A, 1978.

39. Hamwi, G.J., Kruger, F.A., Eymontt, M.J., et al.: Lipoatrophic diabetes. Diabetes *15*:262, 1966.

40. Sovik, O., Oseid, S., Oyassaeter, S.: Studies in congenital generalized lipodystrophy. V. Circulating insulin and proinsulin. Acta Endocrinologica *73*:731, 1973.

41. Oseid, S., Beck-Nielsen, H., Pedersen, O., Sovik, O.: Decreased binding of insulin to its receptor in patients with congenital generalized lipodystrophy. N. Engl. J. Med. *296*:245, 1977.

42. Wachslicht-Rodbard, H., Muggeo, M., Saviolakis, G.A., et al.: Evidence for heterogeneity in the pathogenesis of lipoatrophic diabetes as demonstrated by ^{125}I-insulin binding to circulating cells. Clin. Res. *27*:379A, 1979.

43. Keenan, B.S., Kirland, R.T., Garber, A.J., et al.: The effect of diet upon carbohydrate metabolism, insulin resistance, and blood pressure in congenital total lipoatrophic diabetes. Metabolism *29*:1214, 1980.

44. Flier, J.S., Kahn, C.R., Roth, J., Bar, R.S.: Antibodies that impair insulin receptor binding in an unusual diabetic syndrome with severe insulin resistance. Science *190*:63, 1975.

44a. Scarlett, J.A., Kolterman, O.G., Moore, P., et al.: Insulin resistance and diabetes due to a genetic defect in insulin receptors. J. Clin. Endocrinol. Metab. *55*:123, 1982.

44b. Podskalny, J.M., Kahn, C.R.: Cell culture studies on patients with extreme insulin resistance. I. Receptor defects on cultured fibroblasts. J. Clin. Endocrinol. Metab. *54*:261, 1982.

45. Kem, D., Collins, D., Martin, C.: Immunoreactive glucagon in total lipodystrophy. Clin. Res. *18*:122, 1970.

46. Chait, A., Janus, E., Mason, A.S., Lewis, B.: Lipodystrophy with hyperlipidaemia: the role of insulin in very low density lipoprotein over-synthesis. Clin. Endocrinol. *10*:173, 1979.

47. Marcus, R.: Retinopathy, nephropathy and neuropathy in lipoatrophic diabetes. Case report and discussion. Diabetes *15*:351, 1966.

48. Huseman, C., Johanson, A., Varma, M., Blizzard, R.M.: Congenital lipodystrophy: an endocrine study of three siblings. I. Disorders of carbohydrate metabolism. J. Pediatr. *93*:221, 1978.

48a. Taylor, S.I., Dons, R.F., Hernandez, E., et al.: Insulin resistance associated with androgen excess in women with autoantibodies to the insulin receptor. Ann. Intern. Med. *97*:851, 1982.

49. Tzagournis, M., George, J., Herrold, J.: Increased growth hormone in partial and total lipoatrophy. Diabetes *22*:388, 1973.

50. Oseid, S.: Studies in congenital generalized lipodystrophy. III. Growth hormone levels. Acta Endocrinologica *73*:427, 1973.

51. Gold, R.H., Steinbach, H.L.: Lipoatrophic diabetes mellitus (generalized lipodystrophy): roentgen findings in two brothers with congenital disease. Am. J. Roentgen. *101*:884, 1967.

52. Griffiths, H.J., Rossini, A.A.: A case of lipoatrophic diabetes. Radiology *114*:329, 1975.

53. Johnson, L.C.: Morphologic analysis in pathology; the kinetics of disease and general biology of bone. In: H.M. Frost (Ed.): Bone Biodynamics. Boston, Little, Brown & Co., 1964, pp. 644–647.

54. Goebel, F.D., Dörfler, H., Goebel, H.H., Zöllner, N.: Muscle capillary basement membrane thickness in lipoatrophic diabetes. Res. Exp. Med. *171*:271, 1977.

55. Casali, R.E., Resnick, J., Goetz, F., et al.: Renal transplantation in a patient with lipoatrophic diabetes. A case report. Transplantation *26*:174, 1978.

56. Louis, L.H., Conn, J.W., Minick, M.C.: Lipoatrophic diabetes: isolation and characterization of an insulin antagonist from urine. Metabolism *12*:867, 1963.

57. Louis, L.H., Conn, J.W.: A diabetogenic polypeptide from hog and sheep adenohypophysis similar to that found in lipoatrophic diabetes. Metabolism *17*:475, 1968.

58. Louis, L.H., Conn, J.W.: A urinary diabetogenic peptide in proteinuric diabetic patients. Metabolism *18*:556, 1969.

59. Trygstad, O., Foss, I.: Inhibition by human serum of the adipokinetic effect of a human pituitary lipid-mobilizing factor (LMF) in rabbits. Acta Endocrin. (Kbh) *56*:649, 1967.

60. Trygstad, O.: The lipid-mobilizing effect of some pituitary gland preparations. Preparation of a human pituitary lipid-mobilizing factor (LMF) with hypocalcaemic and hyperglycaemic effects in rabbits. Acta Endocrin. (Kbh) *57*:81, 1968.

61. Bray, G.A., Trygstad, O.: Lipolysis in human adipose tissue: comparison of human pituitary hormones with other lipolytic agents. Acta Endocrin. *70*:1, 1972.

62. Dörfler, H., Wieczorek, A., Wolfram, G., Zöllner, N.: Binding of insulin to fibroblasts in lipoatrophic diabetes. Res. Exp. Med. *170*:161, 1977.

63. Mabry, C.C., Hollingsworth, D.R., Upton, G., Corbin, A.: Pituitary-hypothalamic dysfunction in generalized lipodystrophy. J. Pediatr. *82*:625, 1973.

64. Upton, G.V., Corbin, A.: Albright's syndrome and lipoatrophic diabetes. Lancet *2*:544, 1972.

65. Upton, G.V., Corbin, A.: Hypothesis: Hypothalamic dysfunction and lipoatrophic diabetes. Yale J. Biol. Med. *46*:314, 1973.

66. Mabry, C.C., Hollingsworth, R.: Failure of hypophysectomy in generalized lipodystrophy. J. Pediatr. *81*:990, 1972.

67. Upton, G.V., Corbin, A., Mabry, C.C.: Management of lipoatrophic diabetes. N. Engl. J. Med. *292*:592, 1975.

68. Corbin, A., Upton, G.V., Mabry, C.C., et al.: Diencephalic involvement in generalized lipodystrophy: rationale and treatment with the neuroleptic agent, pimozide. Acta Endocrinol. *77*:209, 1974.

69. Trygstad, O., Foss, I.: Congenital generalized lipodystrophy and experimental lipoatrophic diabetes in rabbits treated successfully with fenfluramine. Acta Endocrinol. *85*:436, 1977.

70. Trygstad, O., Seip, M., Oseid, S.: Lipodystrophic diabetes treated with fenfluramine. Int. J. Obes. *1*:287, 1977.

71. Hager, A., Heding, L.G., Larsson, Y., et al.: Pancreatic B cell function and abnormal urinary peptides in a boy with lipoatrophic diabetes and stenosis of the aqueduct of Sylvius. Acta Paediatr. Scand. *69*:537, 1980.

72. Mitchell, S.W.: Singular case of absence of adipose matter in the upper half of the body. Am. J. Med. Sci. *90*:105, 1885.

73. Weber, F.P.: Lipodystrophia progressiva. Proc. Roy. Soc. Med., Part 2, Neurol. Sect. *6*:127, 1912–1913.

74. Taylor, W.B., Honeycutt, W.M.: Progressive lipodystrophy and lipoatrophic diabetes. Review of the literature and case reports. Arch. Derm. *84*:31, 1961.

75. Murray, I.: Lipodystrophy. Br. Med. J. *2*:1236, 1952.

76. Piscatelli, R.L., Vieweg, W.V.R., Havel, R.J.: Partial lipodystrophy. Metabolic studies in three patients. Ann. Intern. Med. *73*:963, 1970.

77. Steinberg, T., Gwinup, G.: Lipodystrophy, a variant of lipoatrophic diabetes. Diabetes *16*:715, 1967.

78. Gellis, S.S., Green, S., Walker, D.: Chronic renal disease in children with lipodystrophy. Am. J. Dis. Child. *96*:605, 1958.

79. Podolsky, S.: Lipoatrophic diabetes and miscellaneous conditions related to diabetes mellitus. In: A. Marble, P. White, R.F. Bradley, L.P. Krall (Eds.): Joslin's Diabetes Mellitus, 11th Ed. Philadelphia, Lea & Febiger, 1971, pp. 722–766.

80. Sissons, J.G.P., West, R.J., Fallows, J., et al.: The complement abnormalities of lipodystrophy. N. Engl. J. Med. *294*:461, 1976.

81. Jasin, H.E.: Systemic lupus erythematosus, partial lipodystrophy and hypocomplementemia. J. Rheumatol. *6*:43, 1979.

82. Clarkson, P.: Lipodystrophies. Plast. Reconstr. Surg. *37*:499, 1966.

83. West, R.J., Fosbrooke, A.S., Lloyd, J.K.: Metabolic studies and autonomic function in children with partial lipodystrophy. Arch. Dis. Child. *49*:627, 1974.

84. Davidson, M.B., Young, R.T.: Metabolic studies in familial partial lipodystrophy of the lower trunk and extremities. Diabetologia *11*:561, 1975.

85. Bernstein, R.S., Pierson, R.N., III, Ryan, S.F., Crespin, S.B.: Adipose cell morphology and control of lipolysis in a patient with partial lipodystrophy. Metabolism *28*:519, 1979.

86. Langhof, H., Zabel, R.: Über lipodystrophia progressiva. Arch. Klin. Exp. Dermat. *210*:313, 1960.

87. Shelley, W.B., Izumi, A.K.: Annular atrophy of the ankles. A case of partial lipodystrophy. Arch. Dermatol. *102*:326, 1970.

88. Rossini, A.A., Cahill, G.F., Jr.: Lipoatrophic diabetes. In: L.J. DeGroot, G.F. Cahill, Jr., W.D. Odell, et al. (Eds.): Endocrinology, Vol. 2. New York, Grune & Stratton, 1979, pp. 1093–1097.

42 Diverse Abnormalities Associated with Diabetes

Stephen Podolsky and Alexander Marble

This chapter deals with a variety of conditions associated with diabetes. Clinicians and investigators have, over many years, created an extensive literature regarding these subjects. The topics discussed may have a definite, probable, and possible association with diabetes and include musculoskeletal and neuromuscular disorders, gout, certain trace elements and cations, and malignant disease. The information available is summarized and evaluated insofar as possible.

MUSCULOSKELETAL DISORDERS

Definite Associations

Neuroarthropathy (Charcot Joint). Although neuropathic joint disease is definitely associated with diabetes, and may be considered a complication, this abnormality occurs in a variety of diseases.[1-3] Diabetes is the most common cause of neuroarthropathy (Charcot joint) which in one study was estimated to occur in 1 of 680 diabetics[4] (Fig. 42–1).

Neuroarthropathy most often occurs in patients with long-standing poorly-controlled diabetes already complicated by diabetic peripheral neuropathy. Vascular insufficiency is usually not present. The tarsometatarsal joints are most commonly involved, presenting with painless soft tissue, with or without bony deformity. Various authorities

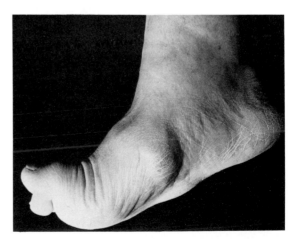

Fig. 42–1. Bony deformity on the medial aspect of the foot, resulting from tarsal neuroarthropathy (Charcot joint). (With permission of Shailendra K. Sinha, from unpublished material.)

have classified diabetic neuroarthropathy as a type of either peripheral (somatic) or autonomic (visceral) diabetic neuropathy.[5] The foot is most often involved, particularly the metatarsal, metatarsophalangeal, and ankle joints. Occasionally the knee,[6] upper extremities,[6,7] or spine[8] may be involved. The highest prevalence of Charcot joints is said to be in patients who have had diabetes for 12 to 18 years.[9] The onset of joint symptoms occurs typically in the sixth decade, but occasionally earlier.[10] There were 90 patients with Charcot joints observed over a 13-year period (1959–1972) at the New England Deaconess Hospital.[11] The sex ratio appears equal.[4]

Characteristically a recent minor trauma or sprain is followed by a markedly swollen, often painless, foot. When there is some pain or discomfort, it is far less than would be expected considering the deformity of the foot. Often there is subluxation of the midtarsal region or of the metatarsophalangeal joints which results in the typical "rocker sole" appearance of the foot. The foot in appearance is anything but ischemic, it is warm to the touch, and may be anhydrotic or hyperhydrotic (if other signs of autonomic diabetic neuropathy are present). Pedal pulses are usually palpable. Further examination of the joint shows some degree of hypermobility (Fig. 42–2).

X-ray findings in diabetic neuroarthropathy are no different from those of Charcot joints due to any etiology. There is joint destruction and disorganization with irregular narrowing, fragmentation and juxta-articular sclerosis. Sometimes there is new bone formation and remodeling.

Management of diabetic neuroarthropathy has not been satisfactory, although one group stated that the disease process could be halted in most cases.[12] Conservative measures such as joint rest and avoidance of weight-bearing are especially important (see Chapters 34 and 35). These, together with patient education regarding proper foot care will often arrest or ameliorate the process, although premature resumption of weight-bearing may result in further joint destruction. Redistribution of weight with special shoes is helpful. Partial non-weight-bearing has been induced by patellar tendon-bearing arthrodesis.[13] Lumbar sympathectomy has been used as therapy,[14] but has been abandoned because of lack of effectiveness. Surgical procedures such as arthrodesis require further evaluation, and in the diabetic patients with vascular disease, may be complicated by wound infection, poor healing, and non-union of bone.[15,16]

The pathogenesis of Charcot joint is not entirely clear. Hypermobility of the joint may be related to loss of proprioception sense that normally inhibits hypermobility.[17] Charcot joint probably occurs as

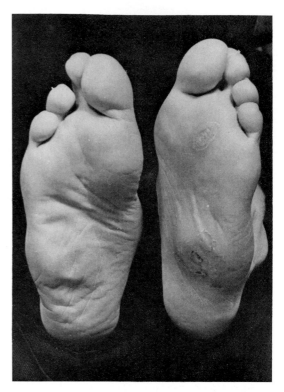

Fig. 42–2. Bilateral neuropathy. Downward collapse of tarsal or tarso-metatarsal areas results in one or two "rocker soles." Blistering and callus formation may occur and, if a break in the skin appears, infection may take place, as seen on the left foot above. (With permission of Shailendra K. Sinha, from unpublished material.)

a result of a combination of this proprioceptive defect, plus impairment of pain perception, which lead to joint injury from repeated mechanical trauma. It has also been suggested that autonomic diabetic neuropathy leads to defective temperature regulation and hypotonic vessels, which may play a role in pathogenesis. It cannot be over-emphasized, however, that repeated trauma is at least one prerequisite for progression of joint destruction.[4] Even in experimental animal models of Charcot joint, it has been found that repetitive trauma is harmful and reduction of the trauma leads to improvement.[16]

Diabetic neuropathic arthropathy should be differentiated from diabetic osteopathy or osteolysis (see below), which does not affect the interarticular space, is generally accompanied by plantar ulcer, and often is reversible. As for osteomyelitis, the destructive joint changes seen in that condition are more severe and are accompanied by signs of inflammation such as erythema, heat, and tenderness.

Diabetic Osteopathy (Osteolysis). Osteolysis detected on x-ray, occurring in the absence of symptoms and without evidence of infection, is definitely associated with diabetes. It has been referred to as diabetic osteopathy.[18] This complication most commonly involves the distal foot, usually the distal metatarsals and proximal phalanges. It usually starts at the metaphysis as an ill-defined loss of bone cortex, extends through the subarticular bone, and eventually destroys the entire bone end but spares the central part of the diaphysis. The articular surface may remain intact even though completely dissociated from the destroyed head of a metatarsal bone or base of a phalanx. The most striking thing about osteolysis in the diabetic is that it may be reversible, at least in part.

Clinical examination may reveal good arterial pulses, a warm foot, and absence of diabetic neuropathy, despite severe destructive osteolysis and demineralization. Infection is often absent. The absence of diabetic peripheral neuropathy differentiates diabetic osteopathy from diabetic neuroarthropathy. The end result of this destructive process is complete absence of the tips of phalanges. The bone becomes fragmented and soft tissue infection may occur. The x-ray appearance resembles that of osteomyelitis, but the osteolysis of diabetes is far more destructive. It is important to recognize that almost complete reconstruction of previously demineralized bone may occur. Pogonowska and co-workers[19] reported 2 patients who had had cellulitis of a foot for several months and in whom the distal and middle phalanges of a toe appeared to be completely destroyed. However, examination a year later showed that the phalanges were almost normal in shape and structure, joint spaces were preserved, and ankylosis had not occurred. Similar changes have been described by other observers[7,21–26] (Fig. 42–3).

An important lesson to be learned from the reversibility of diabetic osteopathy is that x-ray evidence of bone destruction in a diabetic must not be the sole basis for amputation of the toe or lower extremity. However, this reversion of destroyed bone to normal is not seen in osteomyelitis.

The pathogenesis of diabetic osteopathy is unknown, and the complete clinical picture cannot be explained on the basis of neuropathy alone. Increased blood flow is required for osteolysis to occur, and it is likely that hyperemia, diminished pain sensation, and trauma are all involved.[7] An interesting point is that osteolysis of the end bone closely resembles that seen in the anesthetic form of leprosy.[26]

Having outlined the case for diabetic osteopathy (osteolysis) as a condition set apart from bone infection, it is only fair to state that some workers such as Whitehouse and Weckstein[27] have challenged this view and concluded that the presence of diabetic osteopathy implies previous osteomyelitis.

Osteopenia. Although a number of reports indicate that patients with either insulin-dependent (IDDM) or noninsulin-dependent diabetes (NIDDM) have moderately reduced bone mass (osteopenia),[28–31] the controlled studies of Heath et al.[32] indicated that diabetes is not a risk factor for skeletal fracture. These authors concluded that "any reduction of bone mass in diabetics that is revealed by sophisticated analysis, is of no medical or economic importance to the patients or their physicians."

Diabetic Hand Syndrome (Joint Contractures and Waxy Skin). In an editorial in the New England Journal of Medicine in 1981, Knowles[33] summarized reports of contractures of the finger joints in patients with IDDM. A variety of terms have been used for this condition, including "joint stiffness," "diabetic hand syndrome," "juvenile diabetic cheiroarthropathy," and "limited joint mobility."

In 1971 Jung and co-workers[34] described 23 patients with diabetes who had contractures of the finger joints. The mean age of the patients was 43 years and the mean duration of diabetes was 17 years. Most of the adult patients had evidence of diabetic peripheral neuropathy. In 1974 Rosenbloom and Frias[35] described three adolescents with long-term IDDM who had restricted mobility of small and large joints, thick, tight, waxy skin, impaired growth, and maturational delay. These multiple joint contractures developed 8 to 14 years after the onset of diabetes. Rosenbloom's group[36] then reported in 1976 that 65 of 229 (28.4%) campers with diabetes had contractures, and that the frequency of this finding increased with the duration of diabetes. Only 2 of 210 nondiabetic controls matched for age and sex had this finding. Subsequently Traisman and co-workers[37] reported that 8.4% of 310 diabetic children aged 1 to 18 years were affected. Traisman et al. found joint contractures in 9.4% of 106 nondiabetic siblings of the patients and a 2% frequency in 19.9 nonsibling control children. Glucose tolerance was impaired in 4 of 9 siblings and 2 of 3 nonsiblings with joint contractures (Fig. 42–4).

In 1981, Rosenbloom et al.[38] reported further observations, finding that 92 of 309 patients (30%) with diabetes (ages 1 to 28 years) had limited mobility of small and large joints. To demonstrate joint mobility, the patients were asked to approximate the palmar surfaces of the interphalangeal joints of both hands tightly, with fingers fanned. To confirm any observed limitation, the examiner passively extended the patient's finger. (Extension should be to 180° or more at the proximal interphalangeal

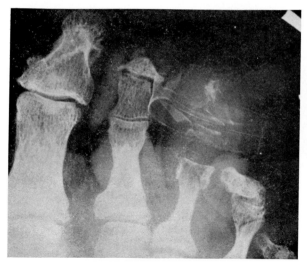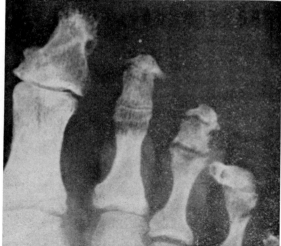

Fig. 42–3. *Left.* Severe osteolysis (diabetic osteopathy) in third toe. *Right.* Remarkable reversal of osteolysis 1 year later, with disappearance of all inflammatory signs.

joints, and the metacarpal phalangeal joints should extend to 60°). The presence of joint contractures could not be related to race, sex, dose of insulin, or estimated control of diabetes. Studies carried out at Joslin Clinic confirmed these observations.[38a,38b]

One-third of Rosenbloom's patients with contractures had thick, tight, waxy skin, particularly over the dorsum of the hands. There is evidence that the waxy skin is associated with an abnormality of collagen metabolism. Hamlin et al.[39] found a stiffening of tendon collagen at autopsy in three juvenile diabetics, which they suggested was due to an increase in cross-linking by metabolites in diabetes. Other studies in diabetic patients have also suggested they have decreased elasticity of skin collagen[40] or lung collagen.[41] Increased cross-link formation with accumulation of inflexible collagen and decrease in response to collagenase has been demonstrated in experimentally diabetic rats.[42]

Improvement of control of hyperglycemia following the use of an insulin pump for 3 months resulted in decrease in skin thickness in several patients with IDDM and waxy skin.[43]

Rosenbloom and associates[38] also found an extraordinary association of joint contractures with diabetic microangiopathy. Knowles[33] states: "The data appear to show a definitive positive relation." Joint lesions preceded the findings of microangiopathy. After 16 years of diabetes, patients with joint contractures had an 83% probability of microvascular complications, whereas those without contractures had only a 2 to 5% risk for such. The overall risk for microangiopathy by the 16th year of diabetes for all of Rosenbloom's[38] patients was 42%, which is comparable to data on retinopathy reported by others.[44,45] Rosenbloom makes the point that the finding of joint contractures may be of clinical value because it indicates a high risk for subsequent microangiopathy as was the case with the Joslin Clinic patients (see Chapter 38).

Probable Associations

Periarthritis. The common clinical impression that bursitis and periarthritis, particularly involving the shoulder, seem to occur more frequently in diabetics than in nondiabetics, has been confirmed by several controlled studies as described below.

Bridgman[46] reviewed the medical records of 800 diabetics and found evidence of periarthritis in 10.8%, compared with 2.3% in a control group of 600 nondiabetics. The difference in incidence was highly significant (p = .005). Periarthritis was more common in those with IDDM but did not seem to be unduly increased in those with peripheral or autonomic diabetic neuropathy. Bilateral involvement of the shoulders was much more common in the diabetics (42%) than in a control group (5%).

Kaklamanis et al.[47] "blindly" reviewed the x-rays of 200 diabetic and 100 nondiabetic outpatients and found the frequency of periarthritis of the shoulders with calcification to be 22 and 8% respectively (p = .01). They confirmed Bridgman's[46] observations on the increased frequency of symptoms and signs in diabetics, the preponderance of insulin-dependent patients, and

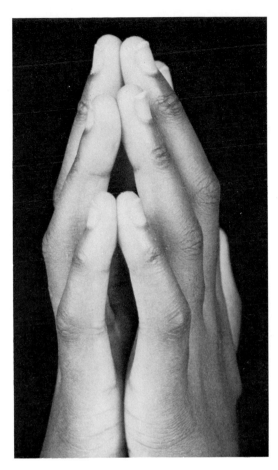

Fig. 42–4. Attempted approximation of the palmar surfaces of the proximal and distal interphalangeal joints. Inability to approximate the palmar surfaces demonstrates the limited mobility of all the joints. (From Rosenbloom et al.,[38] with permission of authors and publisher.)

the fact that almost half of the diabetics had bilateral shoulder involvement.

Earlier, Laul[48] had reported that 36 to 40 patients with "frozen shoulder" syndrome (severe periarthritis) had elevated fasting blood glucose levels in the range of 134 to 150 mg/dl.

Shoulder-hand syndrome (glenohumeral periarthritis accompanied by vasomotor changes in one or both hands) is also said to be associated with diabetes, particularly when there is bilateral involvement.[49] However, to our knowledge, no controlled studies of this association have been carried out.

Ankylosing Hyperostosis. Ankylosing hyperostosis (hyperostotic spondylosis) is a common disease of the spine in which thick, calcific bony bridges form between the anterior and lateral surfaces of the vertebral bodies. It usually involves the thoracic vertebrae and has a predilection for the right side.[50] While pain and limitation of motion

occasionally occur, the condition is often asymptomatic and is discovered as an incidental abnormality on x-rays.[51] Males are affected more often than females, and the disease has a predilection for obese individuals.

Diabetes has been found in a high proportion of patients with ankylosing hyperostosis.[52,53] Two controlled studies by Julkunen and co-workers[54,55] confirm this relationship. They found that 13% of 510 diabetics had ankylosing spondylosis on a lateral chest x-ray.[55] They then took a subgroup of 122 older diabetics (60 to 69 years) and compared them to 148 nondiabetic controls matched for age and weight. Radiographic characteristics of ankylosing hyperostosis were present in 21% of the diabetics and 4% of the nondiabetics (p = .001). They found no correlation between the severity of hyperglycemia and the extent of hyperostosis. In one study Julkunen and co-workers[55] found abnormal glucose tolerance to be present in 23% of 164 patients with ankylosing hyperostosis, and in 9% of 164 matched control subjects.

Ankylosing hyperostosis was found in 6 of 21 patients with acromegaly.[54] The frequency of this condition in diabetics and acromegalics led to the suggestion that increased production of growth hormone promoted the development both of bone proliferation and hyperglycemia.[52] Although circulating growth hormone levels have not been found to be abnormally elevated in patients with ankylosing spondylosis without acromegaly, an increased sensitivity of bone to normal concentrations of growth hormone has not been excluded.

Dupuytren's Contracture. Contraction of the palmar fascia has been known for centuries. Larsen[56] commented that the apostolic blessing may have been originated by some long forgotten cleric who was unable to extend his ring and little fingers because of this condition. In 1834, Dupuytren[57] classically described fibrous palmar nodules causing finger contractures in a coachman, and the deformity has subsequently borne his name. Since then, contraction of the palmar fascia frequently has been reported to occur more often among older diabetics than among nondiabetics, especially in the European literature.

In most or all of these studies and others, a higher frequency of abnormal glucose tolerance was found in patients with Dupuytren's contracture than in controls. One group even reported that diabetes was "definitely present" in 179 of 185 patients with Dupuytren's contracture (96.7%)![58]

Possible Associations

Gout. More than 200 years ago Whytt[59] suggested an association between diabetes mellitus and gout. In 1881 Charcot,[60] in his book entitled *Dis-*

ease of Old Age, wrote that inheritance of a common underlying character could lead to the development of either diabetes mellitus or gouty arthritis.

According to Joslin et al.,[61] however, writing in 1952, the presence of gout in patients with diabetes is an unusual occurrence, being "1 in 1500." Joslin et al.[62] later wrote that "the number of cases of gout occurring in our clientele is trifling." Other studies of diabetics also revealed a low frequency of gout.[63,64] The Tecumseh, Michigan survey of 6000 people failed to discover both gouty arthritis and diabetes in a single subject.[65] The Framingham, Massachusetts study of 5000 people aged 30 to 59 years also was unable to confirm a relationship between gouty arthritis and diabetes mellitus,[66] finding not a single case of clinical diabetes in persons with gout. More recently, Herzberg[67] found only one patient with gout in a group of 314 diabetics. Studies of serum uric acid levels in patients with diabetes have shown either no difference from controls[66,68] or even lower mean serum uric acid levels than in nondiabetics.[62,64,69,70]

There is, therefore, a long-standing controversy over whether the incidence of either clinical diabetes or abnormal glucose tolerance is increased in patients with gouty arthritis.[50,71-73] Some studies have not defined abnormal carbohydrate tolerance precisely, and most were not controlled for advanced age, obesity, amount of physical exercise, etc.

In one study of oral glucose tolerance tests performed in 30 patients with gout, the frequency of abnormal carbohydrate tolerance varied from 7 to 55%, depending upon which criteria were used to interpret the glucose tolerance test.[74] Of two controlled studies, in one no difference was found in the results of oral or intravenous glucose tolerance tests.[75] In the other, an increased frequency of abnormal glucose tolerance in gouty subjects was noted, as compared to controls of normal weight, but no difference was found when compared with weight-matched control subjects.[76] Gray and Gotlieb,[49] however, believe that the weight of present evidence favors the thought that the frequency of glucose intolerance is greater in patients with gout than would be anticipated.

Glucose loading in both normal and diabetic persons has been found to cause increased urinary clearance of uric acid.[77] This may account for the lower mean serum uric acid levels in diabetics, and also explain the finding that gout may improve with the onset of diabetes.

Obesity and disturbances of lipid metabolism are common in both diabetes and gout. Elevated levels of triglyceride and pre-beta lipoprotein occur in patients with gout.[78,79] Most patients with gout who have abnormal glucose tolerance are obese, and have increased insulin secretion as well.[80] Similar to diabetics, patients with gout or asymptomatic hyperuricemia have higher systolic blood pressures, higher cholesterol levels,[81] more platelet abnormalities and more vascular disease than do control populations.[82]

Results of a study of 1605 Polynesians and 432 Europeans living in the South Pacific area suggested a genetic correlation between hyperuricemia, gout, and diabetes.[83]

Among the Europeans, 1.5% of males and 3.9% of females had diabetes. However, 9.2% of New Zealand Maori males and 7.0% of the females had diabetes. In a group of town-dwelling Rarotongans in the Southern Cook Islands, diabetes was present in 4.5% of males and 3.9% of females. The prevalence of diabetes was less (males 9.5% and females 2.1%) among inhabitants of Pukapuka, an isolated coral atoll in the Northern Cook Islands. More than 40% of both males and females in all three Polynesian groups were hyperuricemic by accepted standards.[84] Among males, the attack rate for clinical gout in New Zealand Maoris was 10.2%; in Rarotongans, 2.5%; and in Pupapukans, 5.3%.

Ten of 34 diabetic male New Zealand Maoris had clinical gout, as did 2 of 27 diabetic females.[83] Gout was present in only 1 of 11 males in Rarotonga. Ten of the 38 gouty Maoris also had diabetes, which developed after the onset of gout in all but 1 of 10. The difference between Polynesians and Europeans points to important genetic factors contributing to hyperuricemia, gout, and diabetes. Obesity and hypertension were also common in the gouty New Zealand Maoris, but not in the Cook Islanders.

It is apparent that all three Polynesian groups have a strong genetic predisposition to hyperuricemia. However, gout, diabetes, hypertriglyceridemia, and hypertension were far greater in those exposed to a Western life style than in those who were isolated and maintained their primitive life style in Pukapuka. The largest amount of alcohol consumed was by "Westernized" New Zealand Maoris. Those exposed to a Western life style also consumed higher fat, higher caloric diets and had more obesity, which probably contributes to their greater prevalence of diabetes.[84-86]

Heyden[87] has emphasized the importance of weight reduction and proper nutrition for "health maintenance despite health risks," in hypertension, diabetes, gout, and hyperlipidemia.

In summary, despite 2 centuries of discussion regarding the possible association of diabetes and gout, the subject remains controversial due partly to a paucity of controlled studies. However, the weight of evidence indicates that clinical gout is uncommon in patients with overt diabetes. As for the frequency of clinical diabetes in persons with gout, this also seems not greater than in non-gouty subjects. Exceptions to these general statements rest on a number of variables including criteria used for the designation of "diabetes" and whether clinical gout or simply hyperuricemia are used for the designation of "gout." Other important items include age, sex, dietary habits, body weight, genetic factors, and differing ethnic (e.g., certain Polynesians) and racial groups and their life styles.

Pseudogout. The diagnosis of pseudogout is suggested by typical clinical signs and symptoms plus the radiologic finding of chondrocalcinosis, and confirmed by identifying weakly positive birefringent rhomboid-shaped crystals in the synovial fluid, using a polarizing microscope.[88] Four of the first 7 patients with the pseudogout syndrome reported by McCarty and colleagues[89] were diabetic. Although some reports have indicated an association between diabetes and pseudogout, McCarty et al.[90] were unable to confirm this in a matched study among elderly patients. In 15 to 27 subjects with, and 10 of 22 without, chondrocalcinosis, their results were more statistically similar, using blood glucose levels greater than 100 mg/dl fasting and greater than 140 mg/dl 2 hours postprandially, as criteria for the presence of diabetes.

Osteoarthritis. Although osteoarthritis is the most common rheumatic disease, there have been few studies of the possible association between it and diabetes. However, there is some evidence that such a relationship may exist.[91–93]

In a postmortem study of 200 sternoclavicular joints, Silberberg and co-workers[91] found a positive correlation between degenerative changes and diabetes. Waine et al.[92] in a controlled clinical study carried out some years ago, evaluated radiologic evidence of osteoarthritis in 30 diabetics, aged 19 to 55 years, and in 30 age- and sex-matched nondiabetic controls. The patients with diabetes had a higher frequency, greater severity, and earlier age of onset of osteoarthritis.

Since phosphorylated glucose intermediates are precursors of both the galactosamine and glucuronic acid moieties of glycosaminoglycans, impaired glucose utilization might lead to diminished formation of polysaccharides, in keeping with the biochemical abnormalities of osteoarthritis.[94]

Hyperostosis Frontalis Interna. There have been two reports that hyperostosis frontalis interna occurs more frequently in diabetics than in the general population.

Messerer and Frank[95] compared skull films in 100 randomized diabetics to a group of 100 carefully matched healthy controls. While there was no difference in the diffuse pattern of hyperostosis

frontalis interna, the tuberose pattern type was much more frequent in the diabetics. Forgacs[96] reported that hyperostosis frontalis interna was more common in diabetics.

Flexor Tenosynovitis. Flexor tenosynovitis (trigger finger, stenosing tenosynovits) is a common disorder in which the patient complains of painful snapping of the finger on motion, and sometimes locking of the finger in a flexed position. It is due to inflammation of flexor tendons or tendon sheaths. There is a marked female preponderance, and the right hand (thumb, middle, or ring finger) is more often involved.[58]

Many of the patients with trigger finger are said to be diabetic.[97] In a preliminary report it was stated that diabetes was present in 11 of 63 patients presenting with multiple palmar flexor tenosynovitis.[98]

Carpal Tunnel Syndrome. Compression of the median nerve within the carpal tunnel at the wrist is the most common entrapment neuropathy, and occurs 3 times as frequently in women as in men. Phalen[99] reported that diabetes was present in 63 of 379 patients with carpal tunnel syndrome (16.6%), and that a family history of diabetes was elicited in 40 additional patients.

Other workers have reported a 5 to 6% frequency of diabetes in patients with carpal tunnel syndrome,[100,101] but to our knowledge, no controlled studies have been reported. It is possible that underlying diabetic neuropathy renders the median nerve of the diabetic more susceptible to compression.

Severe diabetic neuropathy involving the upper extremities may result in atrophy of the interosseous muscles of the hands, as well as other symptoms and signs that are indistinguishable from carpal tunnel syndrome. The ulnar nerve is also frequently affected, and its decreased nerve conduction velocity will help differentiate this from carpal tunnel syndrome. It is thus important that diabetics with hand muscle atrophy or contractures be studied thoroughly by electrodiagnostic techniques when considering surgery to correct a presumed nerve entrapment.

Sudeck's Atrophy. In 1900, Sudeck[102] described painful bone atrophy due to injury. This "reflex sympathetic dystrophy" may occur after a relatively minor injury. Its mechanism is unknown. The process appears to be more acute and diffuse than can be explained on the basis of atrophy due to disuse. There is usually severe atrophy of bone and soft tissues with accompanying sympathetic hyperactivity in the ankle, wrist, or shoulder, somewhat similar to that seen in the "shoulder-hand syndrome."

Although some diabetologists have the impression that Sudeck's atrophy is seen more frquently in diabetics than in nondiabetics, it is difficult to find confirmation of this in the literature. It has been noted that Sudeck's atrophy of the hand may be associated with Dupuytren's contracture.[103]

Fibrous Dysplasia of Bone. This rare disorder, associated with precocious puberty when it occurs in females, is also known as Albright's syndrome.[104,105] Diabetes has occurred as part of the polyendocrinopathy of this condition,[106] but hyperthyroidism is much more frequently seen. Oral glucose tolerance testing of one young girl with classic fibrous dysplasia of bone accompanied by sexual precocity and thyrotoxicosis, demonstrated an excessively elevated plasma insulin response to stimulation by glucose.[106] Abnormalities of growth hormone were also found.[107]

NEUROMUSCULAR DISORDERS ASSOCIATED WITH DIABETES

Muscle Atrophy of Polyneuropathy

Muscle atrophy due to impairment of neuronal motor function is not as common as sensory involvement in peripheral diabetic neuropathy (diabetic polyneuropathy). Paralysis with subsequent atrophy of the interosseus muscles of the feet is the most common motor nerve alteration of polyneuropathy. Next most common is atrophy of the interosseus muscles of the hands, also due to diabetic neuropathy. These abnormalities are usually bilateral and symmetrical (See Chapter 31).

Diabetic Amyotrophy

A syndrome of pain and asymmetric muscle weakness and atrophy, usually limited to the quadriceps femoris and psoas, is another type of muscle disorder seen in diabetics. These muscles often exhibit marked wasting. Sensory impairment occurs but is not striking. This syndrome, called diabetic amyotrophy, typically occurs in elderly males although it affects females as well. There is variable but often marked elevation of the protein content of the cerebrospinal fluid.[108] The diagnosis of diabetic amyotrophy is confirmed by biopsy of the affected muscle[109] which reveals a characteristic pattern of single fiber atrophy, unrelated to vascular changes. The disease is self-limited but recovery is usually slow over a period of 1 to 2 years. Characteristically unilateral, the process often later involves the other extremity (See a detailed discussion in Chapter 31).

Inherited Muscular Dystrophies and Neuromuscular Degenerative Disorders

In recent years it has been recognized that glucose intolerance is an integral feature of a large number of distinct genetic syndromes, including the muscular dystrophies and some of the neuro-muscular degenerative disorders. In certain of these such as the muscular dystrophies and at least some of the neurodegenerative diseases (e.g., Friedreich's ataxia), the glucose intolerance may be due to factors such as delay in disposal of glucose because of the reduced muscle mass, relative inactivity, and perhaps poor nutrition. Nevertheless, when diabetes is associated with Friedreich's ataxia, it is usually in a form that it is insulin-dependent, ketosis-prone, and predisposed to vascular complications.[110,111] Sibling pairs have been reported in which both members are afflicted with Friedreich's ataxia and diabetes mellitus. Friedreich's ataxia is transmitted as an autosomal recessive trait.

Two other genetic syndromes with an autosomal recessive mode of transmission, Werner's and ataxia telangiectasia, are typically associated with an insulin-resistant, nonketosis-prone form of diabetes.[112,113] However, these two conditions differ in that individuals with Werner's syndrome usually die from severe atherosclerotic complications, while those with ataxia telangiectasia often succumb to lymphomatous malignancy.

In some neuromuscular disorders, e.g. hereditary chorea (Huntington's disease) and myotonic dystrophy, impaired glucose tolerance may be associated with hyperinsulinemia.[113-117] Since carbohydrate intolerance usually has not been demonstrated prior to the diagnosis of the neuro-muscular degeneration, one cannot exclude the possibility that the metabolic disorder is somehow caused by the muscular abnormality. Huntington's disease is an autosomal dominant disease with late onset (4th decade of life), characterized by uncontrollable movements and progressive dementia. Patients usually do not live long enough after diagnosis for any potential vascular complications of the associated diabetes to develop.

The diabetes associated with myotonic dystrophy is similar to that present in many patients with Huntington's disease, being of an insulin-resistant, maturity-onset type. Patients with myotonic dystrophy who develop diabetes frequently survive long enough to develop typical vascular complications. It appears that the incidence of diabetic microangiopathy in patients with myotonic dystrophy is no different than in the usual noninsulin-dependent diabetic patient.

Glycogen Storage Disease

The various forms of glycogen storage disease include other examples of myopathies associated with disordered carbohydrate metabolism.[118] These metabolic myopathies are characterized by abnormal accumulations of glycogen resulting from a defect in certain specific enzymes. Four of the glycogen storage diseases affect skeletal muscle: (a) Type II (acid maltase deficiency; Pompe's disease); (b) Type III (deficient debrancher system; Cori's disease); (c) Type V (phosphorylase deficiency); and (d) Type VII (phosphofructokinase deficiency).

GENITOURINARY DISORDERS

Cystitis Emphysematosa

Emphysematous pyelonephritis and cystitis have already been mentioned in Chapter 36. Emphysematous cystitis is characterized by collections of gas in the urinary bladder and in small vesicles in its wall.[118a] The gas (carbon dioxide) is due to infection with *Escherichia coli* and *Aerobacter aerogenes,* usually plus some impaired emptying of the bladder, presumably on a neuropathic basis. Because of the active infection, tests of the urine may indicate little or no sugar despite hyperglycemia.

Treatment involves (1) institution and maintenance of as good control of blood glucose as possible; (2) energetic and prolonged antimicrobial therapy; and (3) attempts to correct the bladder paresis if such exists. The last-named basic problem is a difficult one which will require the cooperation of a urologist.

Calcification of the Vas Deferens

This relatively specific and rather common complication may be noted by x-ray in men with diabetes, usually of 10 to 20 years' duration. A landmark article was that by Marks and Ham[118b] from the New England Deaconess Hospital and published in 1942. Reports differ considerably, but it appears that at least 70% of patients noted to have this condition have diabetes.[118c] In fact, of 215 patients with this lesion seen at the Deaconess Hospital, over 98% had diabetes,[118d] a figure probably biased due to the high percentage of diabetic patients in this hospital.

The calcification is found in the muscular wall of the vas deferens and may extend through the inguinal canal into the scrotum. In one series of 60 patients, calcification was bilaterally symmetrical. It is of note that in this particular series, no woman became pregnant after calcification of the vasa deferentia was noted in her husband.[118e]

This condition must, of course, be differentiated from arterial calcification, but this usually causes no difficulty if the possibility of vas calcification is kept in mind. However, calcification of the vasa deferentia is not uncommonly associated with generalized arterial calcification. There are no symptoms and no specific treatment is known.

TRACE METALS, CATIONS, AND DIABETES

Zinc

Insulin is stored as zinc crystals in the beta cells of the pancreas in most mammalian species. Zinc has been found regularly within the pancreas of humans, rabbits, dogs, cats, rats, pigs, mice, and fish, but is almost absent in the islets of the guinea pig. Zinc may be concerned with the binding or storage of insulin in an inactive form, pending release in response to appropriate stimuli. While it readily complexes with insulin, causing structural changes in the insulin crystal,[119] zinc is not required for biologic activity as zinc-free insulin is fully potent.[120]

Zinc concentration in the beta cells decreases following acute stimulation of insulin secretion.[121,122] Administration of zinc does not affect insulin release,[121] although in-vitro studies indicate that it may increase the binding of insulin to mouse liver and decrease the degradation of insulin.[119]

Quarterman and co-workers[123] found that zinc-deficient rats had a reduced secretion of insulin and a reduced sensitivity to the hormone. Hendricks and Mahoney[124] confirmed that zinc-deficient rats had abnormal parenteral glucose tolerance, but found that oral glucose tolerance was not impaired. Huber and Gershoff[125] documented the presence of significantly reduced circulating insulin levels in zinc-deficient rats which were not affected by high zinc diets. Insulin levels are also reduced in zinc-deficient hamsters.[126]

Prout et al.[127] found serum zinc levels in patients with diabetes to be the same as in nondiabetic persons. Numerous later reports also indicated no significant difference between serum zinc levels in diabetics and normals, as well as no correlation between serum zinc and glucose concentrations.[128–132] The zinc content of white and red blood cells and blood plasma appears to be normal in diabetic individuals.[133] Alcoholic pancreatitis is one disorder in which patients are at high risk for acute zinc deficiency.[134]

Thus, except for reduced serum or plasma zinc concentration in patients with uncontrolled diabetes given intensive fluid therapy intravenously, no correlation has been found between the serum zinc level, duration of diabetes, severity of the disease, blood glucose level, presence of acetonuria, vascular complications of diabetes, etc.

Although serum zinc concentrations are seldom abnormal in diabetics, urinary excretion of zinc may be increased.[135–137] Pidduck and co-workers[137] did a controlled study in which diabetics were found to have significant hyperzincuria as compared to healthy subjects. The presence of proteinuria in long-standing diabetes could account for increased zincuria because of the great affinity of this metal for protein.[136]

While there is no substantial evidence that zinc deficiency in man is related to diabetes, other endocrine abnormalities occur, including failure of growth and retarded bone development, hypogonadism, apparent depression of endogenous ACTH production, and increased sensitivity to insulin. Oral glucose tolerance tests demonstrate delayed absorption, but response to intravenous glucose tolerance tests is normal to accelerated. Treatment with zinc reverses the clinical features.

In Iran and Egypt, children with zinc deficiency develop a syndrome including dwarfism and hypogonadism, which resembles idiopathic hypopituitarism.[138] Zinc deficiency in these individuals apparently is caused by a paucity of this mineral in diets made up mostly of cereal, and possibly worsened by zinc loss due to excessive sweating and/or blood loss due to hookworm infestation.

Magnesium

Several enzymes involved in carbohydrate metabolism require magnesium as a co-factor (Embden-Myerhoff pathway, glycogen storage, and pentose monophosphate shunt). One-half of the total body magnesium is present in bone, and all but 1% of the remainder is inside body cells, being second only to potassium as an active intracellular cation. Rats with experimental diabetes have decreased intestinal transport of magnesium and calcium, although that of magnesium is depressed later albeit to a lesser degree than calcium.[139–141]

Although marked hypomagnesemia may occur during therapy of diabetic ketoacidosis, particularly with protocols which include the use of the phosphate salt of potassium,[142] there are conflicting reports of serum or plasma magnesium concentrations in diabetic outpatients. Low,[143] normal,[133] and elevated[134] mean magnesium levels have been reported in the past. In a controlled study of 582 unselected ambulatory diabetics, Mather and colleagues[145] found the mean plasma magnesium to be significantly lower than in 140 control subjects. Atomic absorption spectrophotometry was used to make the measurements. Plasma magnesium levels correlated best with blood glucose concentrations.

There has been speculation that hypomagnesemia might predispose to ischemic heart disease in diabetics.[146,147] Persons with diabetes are certainly at increased risk for this vascular complication.

McNair and co-workers[148] investigated possible risk factors in two groups of patients who had had diabetes for 10 to 20 years (26 with and 45 without advanced diabetic retinopathy) and in 194 normal controls. The mean serum magnesium level was significantly lower (0.74 ± 0.012 mmol/L) in the diabetics than in the normal controls (0.83 ± 0.007 mmol/L). In addition, the group of diabetics with severe retinopathy had a significantly lower serum magnesium (0.72 ± 0.018 mmol/L) than those with normal fundi or only minor changes, (0.75 ± 0.014 mmol/L. The two groups of diabetics did not differ significantly from controls with respect to serum concentrations of potassium calcium, glucose, lipids, parathyroid hormone and C-peptide. Furthermore, the patients with more diabetic retinopathy included a higher proportion of smokers than those without retinopathy. This reinforces earlier observations that there is an association between smoking and diabetic retinopathy.[149] There was no evidence that serum magnesium concentrations were related to smoking habits.

This work was singled out in an editorial in Lancet[150] in which it was stated that "low concentrations of magnesium may be an additional risk factor in the development of diabetic retinopathy." As with potassium, serum magnesium levels are not necessarily a good indication of the intracellular concentration; thus, the intracellular magnesium content in diabetic patients may well be decreased even more than the serum level. Since magnesium salts have a low level of toxicity, the editorial writer suggested that the cautious administration of magnesium salts might have a beneficial effect in both diabetic retinopathy and in ischemic heart disease.

Isolated cases of hypomagnesemia have been reported in infants of mothers with insulin-dependent diabetes.[151] In a prospective study, Tsang et al.[152] found that 21 of 56 infants of diabetic mothers had serum magnesium levels below normal on at least one occasion during the first 3 days of life. Serum magnesium concentration in these hypomagnesemic infants did not demonstrate the normal increase with postnatal age that was present in normomagnesemic infants. There was no correlation with neuromuscular irritability in the infants. It was speculated that this fairly common transitory neonatal hypomagnesemia which occurs in infants of diabetic mothers, may be caused by maternal hypomagnesemia or neonatal hyperphosphatemia, and that it in turn is related to neonatal hypocalcemia and functional hypoparathyroidism.[152]

Of somewhat related interest is the finding of one investigator that during oral glucose tolerance tests, serum calcium and magnesium levels decline less in diabetic children and adolescents than in normals.[153]

Chromium

The amount of chromium in human tissue declines from birth to old age, but some is always present.[154] Chromium is the only element in which such a decline has been detected, in marked contrast to the known accumulation of other elements (particularly certain heavy metals from the environment).[155] Deficiency of chromium in the diet has been suggested as the cause of this aging-related decline in chromium content, which is unique among the trace metals.[156]

In 1959 Schwartz and Mertz,[157] working with rats, demonstrated for the first time the occurrence of chromium deficiency. They found that the trivalent form of chromium improved the impaired intravenous glucose tolerance of animals fed a diet containing Torula yeast. The replacement of Torula yeast by an equivalent amount of brewers' yeast maintained glucose utilization at the initial level.[154] (Both yeasts are similar in their nutrient content, except that Torula yeast contains low amounts of chromium in a poorly available form). Trivalent chromium was subsequently shown to be the active ingredient in a hypothetical dietary agent termed "glucose tolerance factor." The gross chemical composition of glucose tolerance factor appears to be that of a nicotinic acid-chromium complex.[154]

Restriction of chromium intake in rats results in progressive impairment of carbohydrate tolerance.[157-159] Similar effects of chromium deficiency and/or dietary chromium or "glucose tolerance factor" supplementation, have been observed in the squirrel monkey[160] and in the genetically obese diabetic mouse.[161] However, Woolliscroft and Barbosa,[162] in more recent studies, were able to find only a mild degree of carbohydrate intolerance in chromium-deficient rats.

In humans, fasting plasma chromium levels have no correlation with glucose tolerance, but absence of a rise in plasma chromium following a glucose load has been thought to suggest a deficiency of available chromium stores in tissues.[163] Glinsmann and Mertz[164] reported that oral supplementation with 150 to 1000 mcg of chromium III (trivalent chromium) for 15 to 120 days, was associated with improvement in glucose tolerance in 3 of 6 diabetics as shown by oral and intravenous tests. Chromium administration had no effect on persons with normal glucose tolerance. Studies of children with protein-calorie malnutrition in Jordan, Nigeria, and Turkey, have demonstrated that their impaired carbohydrate tolerance can be normalized by increased chromium intake.[165,166] However, a similar study of malnourished children in Egypt failed to show a significant effect of chromium on glucose tolerance, possibly because of the previously high chromium intake of these subjects and the lack of a true chromium deficiency.[167]

There have been variable results with chromium supplementation of the diets of diabetics in the United States. Levine et al.[168] gave 150 mcg of chromium daily to 10 elderly people who had abnormal glucose tolerance; this became normal in 4, but remained abnormal in 6. While serum chromium levels were normal in all patients, those who did not respond to chromium supplementation by improvement in glucose tolerance had a smaller rise in serum chromium than did the others. The conclusion drawn was that chromium deficiency may lead to impairment of glucose tolerance in some elderly subjects.

The beneficial effect of chromium supplementation on glucose tolerance in humans with diabetes is by no means universal. Sherman and co-workers[169] in a double-blind cross-over study lasting 16 weeks, demonstrated that dietary supplementation with chromium did not improve hyperglycemia in any of their 10 diabetic subjects.

For supplementation of diets with biologically active forms of chromium to be beneficial in the treatment of diabetes, there must be evidence of a clinical chromium deficiency state. It is not yet established that chromium deficiency is present in human diabetes and if so, in what subgroup of diabetic patients it occurs. Chromium is rapidly cleared from the blood stream and therefore the plasma concentration is a poor indicator of nutritional deficiency of chromium.[159]

Using atomic absorption spectrophotometry, Hambidge et al.[170] found the chromium content of hair to be significantly lower in 19 male children with insulin-dependent diabetes than in 33 age-matched nondiabetic males. Chromium concentration in the hair of Thai females with adult-onset diabetes was also found to be significantly lower than in matched normal controls.[171] Morgan[172] found in postmortem studies that the chromium content of the liver was significantly lower in 31 diabetics than in 61 nondiabetic controls (18 with ischemic heart disease, 19 with hypertensive cardiovascular disease, and 24 without either). Patients with malignancies were excluded from this study because of the widely variable hepatic trace metal content in neoplasia.

The most recent and extensive investigations of the chromium status in diabetes were carried out by Rabinowitz, Levin, and Gonick[173] who studied 46 male outpatients with diabetes and 20 nondiabetic age-matched male controls. They measured fasting and postprandial total chromium in plasma, red blood cells and urine, total chromium in hair, and volatile and ultrafiltrable chromium in plasma and urine from all subjects. The range of chromium values extended over a factor of 10, and both the diabetics and the normals displayed this wide individual variation in chromium concentration in each body fluid or tissue which was sampled. Nevertheless, the plasma chromium range was similar to that found in another recent study[174] in which ketosis-prone, insulin-dependent diabetics were found to have significantly higher plasma chromium levels than either the other diabetics or the controls. Of interest is the new finding that non-ketosis-prone, nonobese diabetics had elevated urinary chromium output when compared to the other groups. A significant inverse relationship was seen between erythrocyte chromium and fasting plasma glucose in the patients with diabetes. However, men with low hair chromium were not identical with those having low erythrocyte chromium. Although the authors could not confirm the presence of chromium deficiency in this male diabetic population, their findings provide suggestive evidence for a relationship between certain body pools of chromium and carbohydrate metabolism in diabetes.

The most direct evidence of chromium deficiency in humans resulting in impaired carbohydrate tolerance comes from studies of patients sustained on total parenteral nutrition, with inadequate chromium intake.[175,176] This type of secondary diabetes appears to be clearly responsive to chromium administration. The patient of Jeejeebhoy et al.[175] who had received total parenteral nutrition for 5 years, had a negative chromium balance, and developed glucose intolerance and neuropathy. These changes were corrected by the addition of chromium to her infusate.

It is apparent that additional observations and studies are required before one can recommend supplementation of conventional diabetic diets with chromium, "glucose tolerance factor," or the recently synthesized substance with glucose tolerance factor activity.[177] In 1976 Mertz[155] wrote: "Chromium supplementation can have practical importance only if chromium deficiency can be expected to exist in the population, or at least in individual subjects."

Manganese

Manganese is an essential cofactor for several enzymatic processes. Cotzias[178] reviewed the absorption, distribution, transport, fate, and physiologic role of manganese in the body. Manganese deficiency in young chicks leads to a defect in bone growth and leg deformities,[179] but such deficiency is not known to occur in humans.

Hassanein et al.[180] studied carbohydrate metabolism in 11 patients with chronic manganism. In all instances, there was an exaggerated, prolonged hypoglycemia in response to an acute intravenous glucose load. The cause of this reactive hypoglycemia was not clear. Rubenstein and co-workers[181] administered 5 mg of a manganese salt daily to try to control the hyperglycemia in a patient

with diabetes, who then became hypoglycemic. They suggested that the manganese salt might act peripherally or directly upon the pancreas to increase insulin release or inhibit glucagon secretion.

Potassium

The potassium ion is an essential activator in many enzymatic processes, including those associated with the transfer of high energy phosphate in carbohydrate metabolism. Potassium is quantitatively the most prominent intracellular cation with a normal concentration of approximately 150 to 155 mEq/L of cell water. Almost all of the body's potassium content is located inside cells, with 70% inside muscle tissue.

More than 30 years ago Gardner et al.[182] and Fuhrman[183] reported that severe potassium depletion in animals results in abnormal glucose tolerance. Shortly thereafter, Hastings and co-workers,[184] studying liver slices, demonstrated alterations in carbohydrate metabolism in potassium-deficient rats which were similar to those seen with insulin deficiency. Sagild et al.[185] induced potassium depletion of 200 to 500 mEq in human volunteers by the oral administration of a cation exchange resin for 5 days. The potassium depletion was accompanied by considerable impairment of glucose tolerance, even with normal serum potassium levels. They suggested that decreased endogenous insulin production might be responsible for the changes observed. Mild diabetes and a reduced insulin response to glucose are found in hypokalemic rats treated with desoxycorticosterone acetate.[186] Potassium has been shown to stimulate insulin release from the isolated perfused rat pancreas.[187] These observations may be relevant to patient care because potassium depletion and carbohydrate intolerance not infrequently occur together.

Hypokalemia and potassium depletion due to excessive loss of potassium in the urine frequently occur in primary aldosteronism, and the impaired carbohydrate tolerance and subnormal insulin response in these patients may be reversed by repleting deficient potassium stores.[187,188]

Potassium depletion may occur in hepatic cirrhosis for a variety of reasons (including inadequate dietary intake, vomiting, diarrhea, secondary hyperaldosteronism, and the use of diuretic drugs) and is associated with impaired glucose tolerance.[189] Whereas most patients with hepatic cirrhosis and noninsulin-dependent diabetes have paradoxically excessive insulin response to glucose stimulation, the subgroup of potassium-depleted diabetic cirrhotics have a decreased insulin (and growth hormone) response to stimulation.[190-193]

Podolsky and co-workers[190] found that 7 of 17

patients with cirrhosis and impaired carbohydrate tolerance had potassium depletion despite the fact that their serum potassium levels were within the normal range. Using a whole body counter to measure total body potassium, they observed rises of from 12.7 to 35.8% of the initial value during potassium chloride supplementation. Cautious administration of 180 mEq of potassium chloride daily for a period of 2 or more weeks resulted in increased body potassium, improved glucose tolerance, and marked increases in the previously subnormal insulin and growth hormone responses in the 7 potassium-depleted cirrhotic patients (Fig. 42–5). On the other hand, there was no significant change in any of these measurements in any of the 10 patients without potassium depletion (who were otherwise clinically and biochemically similar).[191]

In keeping with these findings, cirrhotics who spontaneously develop severe potassium depletion suffer deterioration in glucose tolerance and impairment of insulin and growth hormone response to stimulation.[194]

One of the most urgent considerations of any discussion of potassium metabolism in relation to diabetes is the recognition and prevention of iatrogenic hypokalemia following administration of insulin in the treatment of diabetic ketoacidosis or hyperosmolar nonketotic coma. This problem is discussed in detail in Chapter 26.

It is not sufficiently recognized that despite a normal level of serum potassium, depletion may occur in severely uncontrolled diabetes, due to potassium loss with osmotic diuresis. This is especially apparent in both diabetic ketoacidosis and in hyperosmolar nonketotic coma.[195–198] Reduction of body potassium stores is probably even greater in hyperosmolar nonketotic coma because of the generally longer period of illness. A vicious cycle may develop in the noninsulin-dependent diabetic with hyperosomolar coma in whom this decrease in tissue potassium stores may further reduce the already limited insulin reserves, which in turn worsens the hyperglycemia.

Diurëtic therapy may result in hypokalemia and hyperglycemia in nondiabetics and worsening of hyperglycemia in noninsulin-dependent diabetics. The presence of at least partially functioning beta cells seems to be required in order for blood glucose levels to increase to clinically significant levels in association with diuretic-induced hypokalemia, since this effect is not seen in insulin-dependent diabetics.[199]

After poor dietary compliance as the most common problem, the second most frequent cause of poor control of hyperglycemia in noninsulin-dependent diabetics may be potassium depletion due to thiazide or other diuretic therapy given for concomitant hypertension. This effect can be reversed by administration of potassium chloride to treat the hypokalemia or replete the depleted potassium stores. It is not yet clear whether long-term diuretic therapy can also lead to normokalemic body potassium depletion,[200] as occurs in potassium wasting disorders.

Hyperkalemia stimulates the release of both insulin[201] and aldosterone,[202] resulting in increased renal potassium excretion and movement of potassium into cells. Recent findings indicate that some patients with diabetes have an impairment of potassium homeostasis that is probably related to combined insulin and aldosterone deficiency.[203] It appears that diabetics may be particularly at risk for developing hyperkalemia because of an apparent propensity toward development of a hyporeninemic hypoaldosteronism syndrome.[204,205] Indeed, marked hyperkalemia has been reported in diabetics with hypoaldosteronism and mild to moderate renal insufficiency,[204,205] and during the use of potassium-sparing diuretics even when normal or near normal renal function exists.[206,207] Furthermore, although administration of glucose to normal subjects lowers potassium levels because increased insulin release facilitates the intracellular movement of both glucose and insulin,[208] the intravenous administration of glucose to diabetics with hypoaldosteronism may result in paradoxical increases in serum potassium levels.[209] Similar par-

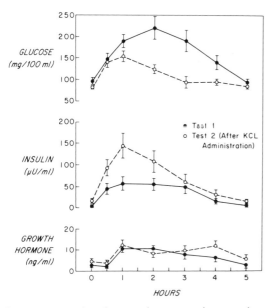

Fig. 42–5. Results of assays for serum glucose, plasma insulin, and growth hormone during an oral glucose tolerance test in seven K-depleted patients, before and after administration of potassium. Circles represent means, and bars, standard error. (From Podolsky, et al.,[192] with permission of authors and publisher.)

adoxical hyperkalemia has developed during intravenous glucose tolerance testing of diabetics receiving the potassium-sparing diuretics triamterene (Dyrenium)[210] or amiloride (Midamor).[206]

These observations indicate that the use of oral potassium supplementation or potassium-retaining diuretics may be particularly hazardous to diabetic patients with hyporeninemic hypoaldosteronism. These abnormalities may predispose to unexpected and occasionally life-threatening hyperkalemia, particularly in the setting of diminished renal function, severe hyperglycemia or acidosis.

Calcium

Grodsky and Bennett[187] in studies with the isolated perfused rat pancreas found calcium to be an absolute requirement for insulin release. Glucose had no stimulating effect on insulin release when serum calcium concentration was greatly lowered. Numerous experimental studies have demonstrated the critical importance of the calcium ion for production and release of insulin from the beta cell.[211-214] In addition, the convulsive action of insulin in mice has been noted to be potentiated by calcium and also by magnesium.[215] Rats made diabetic experimentally have decreased intestinal transport of calcium and to a lesser degree, of magnesium.[139-141]

Most dairy cows go through a period of hypocalcemia and hyperglycemia during or shortly after parturition.[216-218] Postpartum cows with the most severe hypocalcemia had diabetic glucose tolerance tests with low levels of endogenous insulin. Infusion of calcium borogluconate caused an abrupt and marked rise in plasma insulin levels, accompanied by a decrease in blood glucose levels. Even cows with only slightly decreased plasma calcium and normal glucose tolerance were found to have decreased insulin response.[216]

Patients with hypocalcemia due to idiopathic hypoparathyroidism have a subnormal insulin response to a glucose load, although glucose tolerance itself was generally normal.[219] Only 2 of Yasuda's[216] 8 patients with idiopathic hypoparathyroidism had slightly abnormal glucose tolerance curves. Normalization of the serum calcium level with treatment did not result in improvement of glucose tolerance in these 2 hyperglycemic patients. Normal glucose tolerance tests have also been found in patients with postoperative hypoparathyroidism,[220] although abnormal results have been reported in pseudohypoparathyroidism.[221,222] Although the serum calcium levels in all these patients did not fall to the severely low levels (3.7 mg/dl) seen in hyperglycemic postpartum cows, there was a clear relation between the serum calcium level and insulin response to an oral glucose load in the patients with hypocalcemia.[216] Conversely, patients with hypercalcemia due to primary hyperparathyroidism have an increased insulin response to an oral glucose load, with normal glucose tolerance.[216,223]

The use of newer treatment protocols for the management of diabetic ketoacidosis which call for administration of the phosphate salt of potassium (rather than chloride salt) have led to profound hypocalcemia and hyperphosphatemia.[142,224] Hypomagnesemia has also sometimes been induced during therapy of diabetic ketoacidosis with potassium phosphate. Such hypomagnesemia may impair the release of parathyroid hormone,[225] leading to worsening of the hypocalcemia induced by phosphate loading.

Hypocalcemia has also been reported in about 1 in 4 infants of diabetic mothers.[152,226-228] Neuromuscular irritability manifested by twitching, as well as respiratory difficulty, cyanosis and congestive heart failure, may occur in the infant. The cause of the hypocalcemia may be a temporary hypoparathyroid state in the newborn related to elevated serum calcium in the diabetic mother and elevated serum phosphate in the infant,[226] or to neonatal hypomagnesemia, when it is present.[152]

CANCER AND DIABETES

Cancer is reported to have been responsible for more than 400,000 deaths in the United States in 1980.[228a] It is a leading cause of death, second only to heart disease. Diabetes mellitus is 7th in rank, with over 34,000 deaths in 1980. It is generally recognized, however, that this number is deceptively low since diabetic angiopathy contributes heavily to the mortality from cardiovascular-renal disease, and yet diabetes may not even be mentioned on the death certificate.[229,230]

Particularly in the past, questions have been raised as to the possible relationship of cancer and diabetes. Is cancer more common in individuals with diabetes than in those without it? Also, is diabetes more common in persons with cancer? It is now possible to give more definitive answers to these questions than formerly.

It is difficult indeed to plan and execute a study along these lines because of the many factors which may influence the results. Among these are the following: (1) The diagnosis of diabetes is subject to standards which vary from worker to worker. Throughout the world there are many millions of persons with varying degrees of intolerance to glucose ranging all the way from slight deviations from normal (with much difference of opinion as to what is normal) up to that of overt, insulin-dependent diabetes. In the classification of diabetes and diabetes-like states proposed in 1979 (see Table

1 in Chapter 15), a definitive category of impaired glucose tolerance (IGT) was set up as a designation for asymptomatic and lesser degrees of abnormality.[231] It was suggested that in such instances, the diagnosis should be IGT rather than diabetes. Obviously, this is at variance with the custom of many physicians, both past and present, and lends confusion to the type of study under discussion. (2) Both cancer and diabetes are more common in older persons who, it has become increasingly apparent, have a tendency to IGT, the interpretation of which varies widely. (3) For diverse reasons, various chronic diseases including arthritis and neurologic disorders, are associated with IGT as are other states such as physical inactivity or low carbohydrate diet prior to glucose testing (see Chapter 15). (4) As noted above, the use of death certificates as a means of identifying causes of death is fraught with great error due to the lack of care often taken in the completion of such certificates.

Frequency of Cancer in Diabetic Patients

Reports during the first 2 or 3 decades of the insulin era suggested that cancer occurs more commonly in diabetics than in nondiabetics.[232-234] More recent data do not bear this out. In a study of 6317 autopsy records (1212 with malignancy), Herdan[235] found that malignant tumors occurred in 10.1% of diabetics, whereas the frequency in nondiabetics was 19.5%. Similarly, in postmortem studies, Aronson and co-workers[236] found a smaller percentage of intracranial neoplasms in 1011 patients with clinically verified diabetes than among 1943 nondiabetics (2.9 versus 11.4%).

Ragozzino et al.[237] of the Mayo Clinic studied those persons who had been residents of Rochester, Minnesota for at least 1 year prior to diagnosis of diabetes. These 1135 diabetic patients, about equally divided between males and females, were then followed for over 9800 person-years. During the 25 years of observation (1945–1969), 120 malignancies were detected, of which cancer of the cervix and non-melanomatous skin cancer were excluded because of the lack of reliable incidence rates for the general population. In a 1982 report, the authors concluded that the overall risk of the diabetics for the development of malignant disease (1.2 for men and 1.1 for women) was not significantly different from that in persons in the general population. However, among individual types of malignancy, the relative risk for cancer of the pancreas was 3.8 in men and 4.4 in women, which was significant (p < 0.05). When this risk was calculated to exclude development of cancer in the first year of follow-up, it fell to 2.7 for men and 2.5 for women which was just below the level of significance.

Table 42–1. Frequency of Cancer Among 34,499 Deceased Diabetics, 1897–1979* (Experience of the Joslin Clinic)

Period	Total Deaths	Cancer Deaths	Percent Cancer Deaths of All Deaths
1897–1914	326	5	1.5
1914–1922	843	32	3.8
1922–1936	4160	362	8.7
1937–1943	3641	327	9.0
1944–1949	4154	403	9.7
1950–1959	9925	1042	10.5
1960–1968	7160	752	10.5
1969–1979	4290	515	12.0

*Based on deaths reported through July, 1979. Data prior to 1969 were obtained and analyzed with the cooperation of the Statistical Bureau, Metropolitan Life Insurance Company.

Table 42–2. Ratio of Cancer Deaths to Total Deaths in Massachusetts*

	Percentage of Deaths Due to Cancer			
Year	All Ages	40–49 Years	50–59 Years	60–69 Years
1895	3.5	7.5	10.3	8.9
1900	4.1	8.7	11.1	9.4
1910	5.8	10.4	13.2	11.3
1920	7.8	12.0	17.1	15.0
1930	11.7	14.5	19.1	17.3
1940	14.3	17.7	20.0	18.4
1950	17.6	22.5	24.3	21.8
1960	17.0	23.1	25.9	22.5
1970	18.9	26.4	27.9	25.7
1980	22.7	31.9	36.0	32.6

*Figures for 1895 to 1930 were compiled from Table 102 in Bigelow and Lombard: Cancer and Other Chronic Diseases in Massachusetts, Boston, Houghton Mifflin Company, 1933. Data for 1930–50 were kindly supplied by Dr. Herbert L. Lombard; for 1960 by Dr. Leslie Lipworth; and for 1970 and 1980 by Dr. Sharon L. Rosen, all of the Masschusetts Department of Public Health.

Experience of the Joslin Clinic. In the series of Warren, LeCompte, and Legg[238] comprising 1854 diabetic patients (largely from the Joslin Clinic service at the New England Deaconess Hospital) on whom postmortem examinations were performed, 224 (12.1%) were found to have malignant disease. This figure may be somewhat misleading because the Deaconess Hospital is a center for the treatment of cancer as well as diabetes. Additional data regarding the frequency of cancer among Joslin Clinic patients are shown in Table 42–1. It will be noted that with the advent of insulin in 1922, there began a rise in the percentage of deaths from cancer compared with the total number of deaths, reflecting the increasing longevity of diabetic individuals. During 1969–79 cancer deaths amounted to 12.0% of 4290 total deaths tabulated (see also Table 16 in Chapter 13). As is evident from Table 42–2, deaths from cancer for all ages comprised 22.7% of all deaths in the general population of Massachusetts in 1980. This was much greater than that in diabetic individuals (12.0% in 1969–79 as shown in Table 42–1). The Massachusetts figures for deaths from cancer at all ages are in the same general range as those for the United States as a whole (20.6% in 1978). The lower ratio for deaths from cancer associated with diabetes may reflect the facts that, at comparable ages, the life expectancy of diabetic persons is still less than that of persons in the general population and death from some type of vascular disease takes a greater toll than in the nondiabetic.

Beginning in 1933 and continuing over some years,[239] studies were carried out at the Joslin Clinic to determine the frequency of malignant disease among diabetic patients. The results suggested that the frequency of cancer (other than pancreatic and questionably endometrial cancer) was no greater than that in persons of the same age and sex in the general population.

Warren, LeCompte, and Legg[238] in 1966 reported that of 214 diabetic women who died of cancer and were examined at autopsy at the New England Deaconess Hospital, 23 or 10.7% had cancer of the endometrium in contrast to a frequency of about 5% in nondiabetic females who died of cancer. However, this difference has not been borne out in subsequent experience at the Deaconess.[239a]

These analyses were expanded later by Kessler[239b] who studied the frequency of death from cancer among 21,447 diabetic patients (Massachusetts residents) of the Joslin Clinic who had been seen first at the Clinic during the 26 years ending in 1956 and who had survived for at least a year beyond the date of the first visit. Observations were made through 1959 and the report was published in 1971. Only 0.7% of the patients were untraced. The observed numbers of deaths from cancer were compared with the numbers expected according to the age- and sex-specific rates in the general Massachusetts population over the same period of time. A total of 902 deaths from cancer was recorded.

Kessler found that among males in the group studied, there were fewer deaths from cancer than expected (358 versus 421). Total cancer deaths among the diabetic females were at about the expected frequency (544 versus 530). Kessler attributed the decreased cancer risk in males to excessive risk of death from other causes, especially coronary heart disease.

Kessler's results confirmed the usual finding of a significantly increased risk of death from cancer of the pancreas; among males, 30 deaths were observed when 20 were expected, and among females, 48 were observed when 23 were expected. Mortality from lung cancer was reduced significantly among the male diabetics but not among the females. In contrast to the findings of certain other workers, the study suggested that diabetic women do not have an increased risk of death from cancer of the body of the uterus.

Among 267 males and 463 female cancer decedents for whom adequate information was available, the onset of diabetes had preceded the onset of cancer in 98% of the males and 94% of the females. Prior onset of diabetes was true also for patients who died from cancer of the pancreas; among those for whom adequate data were available, the onset of diabetes preceded that of cancer of the pancreas in 22 of 30 males and in 33 of 48 females.

Frequency of Diabetes in Persons with Cancer

The development and frequency of diabetes among persons who have cancer is a different matter. Interest in this question has waxed and waned since 1885, when Freund[240] reported finding hyperglycemia in 62 of 70 patients with cancer. In a study of this long-debated subject, Marks and Bishop[241] found that the rate of disappearance of glucose given intravenously was significantly slower in individuals with cancer than in control subjects. Their patients were stated to have been well-nourished and non-cachectic. Not surprisingly, Edmonson[242] noted impaired glucose tolerance and increased fatty acid utilization in 20 cachectic patients with advanced cancer as compared to findings in 17 normal control subjects. Lisker, Brody and Beitzer[243] reported that the results of oral glucose tolerance tests were abnormal in 52% of 66 patients with malignant disease (myelo- and lympho-proliferative disorders, Hodgkin's sarcoma, and reticulum cell sarcoma). In matched controls the frequency of abnormal results was only 8.5%.

Glicksman and Rawson[244] and Glicksman, Myers and Rawson[245] performed oral glucose tolerance tests in 950 patients admitted consecutively to the Memorial Center for Cancer and Allied Diseases in New York City. Findings rated as abnormal were obtained in 36.7% of 628 patients in whom the diagnosis of cancer was made by tissue examination, as contrasted with abnormal findings in only 9.3% of the control group of 322 patients with lesions proven to be benign. Known diabetics made up 4.4% of the control group and 13% of the cancer group. Considering only those sites in which cancer was found in 10 or more of the patients concerned, a high frequency (up to 70%) of a diabetic response was found.

Noteworthy is the finding of Glicksman et al.[245] that 64% of patients with endometrial carcinoma showed abnormal responses of glucose tolerance tests, while in only 16% of those with epidermoid carcinoma of the cervix were the results abnormal. Similar findings were obtained by Lynch and co-workers[246] who noted a 42% frequency of abnormal response to tests in 154 patients with endometrial carcinoma. In the same way, Benjamin and Romney,[247] in a study of 50 patients with uterine cervical carcinoma and 75 patients with endometrial carcinoma, found a high and statistically greater frequency of diabetes and disturbed glucose tolerance in the endometrial carcinoma group than in control subjects (22%) without malignant disease. Their results were the same for the two populations studied, one in New York City and the other in Capetown, South Africa.

As noted earlier, the interpretation of results of glucose tolerance tests obtained from patients with cancer must take into account the age group concerned, since most workers have found that the frequency of abnormal results is surprisingly high in supposedly healthy, elderly persons in the general population. Furthermore, the results are known to be influenced greatly by such factors as previous diet, state of nutrition (obese or lean), and physical activity. With this in mind, Weisenfeld, Hecht, and Goldner[248] performed oral and intravenous glucose tolerance, glucose-insulin sensitivity, tolbutamide response, and glucagon response tests in a group of hospitalized patients, 47 of whom had cancer and 48 of whom had no known cancer. All showed a decreased tolerance to glucose given orally despite a normal fasting level of blood glucose. Except in a few instances, the other tests mentioned, particularly the intravenous glucose tolerance test, failed to corroborate derangement of carbohydrate metabolism in either group. They concluded that the decreased tolerance to glucose given orally in patients with cancer is not a specific response to this disease but a nonspecific phenomenon accompanying chronic illness.

Tumors of the Pancreas

Exocrine Pancreas. Cancer of the pancreas has surpassed stomach cancer as the second most common gastrointestinal cancer (after colo-rectal cancer) in the general population of the United States.[249] The number of deaths yearly from pancreatic cancer approaches closely its incidence (approximately 22,600 versus 25,000), reflecting the short survival after diagnosis. The current death rate of this disease places it sixth among all cancer deaths, and its incidence appears to be rising.

Conceivably, glucose intolerance may develop in patients with cancer of the pancreas because of encroachment of tumor tissue leading to impairment of insulin secretion. However, destruction of 90 to 95% of the pancreas is said to be necessary to produce diabetes in experimental animals, so extensive replacement of the gland by tumor would be required.

Relevant to the above was the study of Murphy and Smith[250] who found that of 251 Lahey Clinic patients with primary carcinoma of the pancreas, the glucose tolerance test gave frankly diabetic results in 37.4% The frequency of positive results was no greater when the tumor was located in the body or tail than in the head of the pancreas. Levison noted that occasionally overt diabetes is not present even when the pancreas is almost replaced by cancer.[251]

Certain ethnic groups appear to have a higher risk of cancer of the pancreas, particularly black men and women. Hawaiian men have almost twice the risk for pancreatic cancer as do Caucasian males in mainland United States, but Hawaiian women have rates that are at or below those of Caucasian women. Rates for cancer of the pancreas are higher than average in chemists, metal workers, coke and gas plant workers, and several other occupational groups.[252] Cohen[253] suggested that difficulty in control of diabetes may be an early clue to the diagnosis of cancer of the pancreas in diabetics. Measurement of serial blood carcinoembryonic antigen (CEA) levels following therapy of pancreatic carcinoma, may be clinically useful.

Green and co-workers[254] analyzed the clinical and autopsy records of 209 consecutive patients with primary carcinoma of the pancreas, and found that 9 (4.3%) were known to be diabetic prior to the onset of symptoms of cancer, and 32 (15.3%) developed diabetes after the onset of the cancer. In at least two-thirds of the 32 patients in whom diabetes was found after the symptoms of cancer appeared, there did not seem to be enough postmortem evidence of damage to islet tissue by fibrosis, tumor invasion, or inflammation to account for the development of diabetes.

Dashiell and Palmer[255] earlier found a diabetic type of glucose tolerance test result in 18 of 21 patients with carcinoma of the pancreas. Glicksman and Rawson[244] noted some intolerance in 4 of their 5 patients with cancer of the pancreas. Clark and Mitchell[256] reported that of 65 patients with confirmed primary carcinoma of the pancreas, 10 (15.4%) also had diabetes. In all 10, symptoms of diabetes preceded those of cancer by only a few weeks, or asymptomatic diabetes was discovered incidentally in the hospital.

Summary. Interpretation of the varying results

of studies regarding the relationship of diabetes and carcinoma of the exocrine pancreas is difficult. This is true because of influences which include differing diagnostic standards of diabetes and glucose intolerance, the older age, lowered state of nutrition, reduced food intake, and decreased physical activity. However, one may reasonably conclude that cancer of the pancreas occurs more commonly in diabetic than in nondiabetic individuals.

Endocrine Pancreas. These tumors include insulinoma, glucagonoma, somatostatinoma, gastrinoma, vipoma, and carcinoid tumor. Glucagonomas (see Chapters 38 and 39) and somatostatinomas are associated with a diabetes-like state.

Cancer and Hypoglycemia. Insulin-secreting tumors of the islet cells of the pancreas may be malignant or benign, and lead to fasting hypoglycemia. These insulinomas, discussed also in Chapter 43, are the most common of the several hormone-producing tumors of the pancreas.

In 1971 Laurent and co-workers[257] reviewed 850 cases of insulinomas and speculated as to the possible relationship between hyperglycemia or diabetes and the natural history of insulinoma. Assan et al.[258] reported a diabetic woman who developed an insulinoma, and reviewed 22 cases of insulinoma in patients with documented diabetes. Marks and Samols[259] also commented on the strong association between insulinoma and family incidence of diabetes. However, Ganda and Soeldner[260] more recently reviewed the numerous reports of insulinomas in patients with known diabetes, and concluded that in some of them, the tumors may have been of the glucagon-secreting type rather than the insulin-secreting variety.

Tragl and Mayr[261] reported a family with multiple islet-cell adenomatosis and diabetes in various members. The diabetes was of the noninsulin-dependent type. It was speculated that the genetic transmission, probably autosomal dominant, produced hypertrophy of the beta cell in certain members, while inducing "hypofunction" in others, perhaps depending on certain environmental influences.

Surprisingly little long-term follow-up information is available on the development of diabetes in patients after resection of insulinomas. If pancreatic excision is extensive, as in the removal of a malignant insulinoma, one would expect diabetes to occur secondarily as a natural outcome. Dunn[262] reported that diabetes occurred in 2 of 7 patients as a late complication of resection of insulinoma (14 to 16 years after surgery). In 4 other patients there was some impairment of insulin secretion in response to oral glucose following surgical treatment of insulinoma.

Two of 8 patients with successfully removed

insulinomas who were studied at the Joslin Research Laboratory were found to have diabetes-like glucose tolerance test results several years following surgery.[260] Two other patients had glucose tolerance findings which were in the "borderline" range. Abnormalities of insulin response were also found. It was thought that these relatively common abnormalities noted in oral glucose tolerance tests following removal of insulinomas, were usually *not* primarily due to the extensiveness of the removal of pancreatic tissue.

Large extrapancreatic tumors are also sometimes associated with fasting hypoglycemia.[263–265] These malignancies seldom, if ever, produce insulin, but may produce "insulin-like growth factor" (ILGF) formerly called "nonsupressible insulin-like activity" (NSILA).[266] Extrapancreatic cancers may produce a compound that inhibits gluconeogenesis.[267] Cachectic patients with massive mesenchymal cancers and fasting hypoglycemia may have a diabetic type of glucose tolerance test.[263]

REFERENCES

1. Calabro, J.J., Garg, S.L.: Neuropathic joint disease. Am. Fam. Phys. 7:90, 1973.
2. Peitzman, S.J., Miller, J.L., Ortega, L., et al.: Charcot arthropathy secondary to amyloid neuropathy. J.A.M.A. 235:1345, 1976.
3. Harrison, R.B.: Charcot's joint: two new observations. Am. J. Roentgenol. 128:807, 1977.
4. Sinha, S., Munichoodappa, C.S., Kozak, G.P.: Neuroarthropathy (Charcot joints) in diabetes mellitus: clinical study of 101 cases. Medicine 51:191, 1972.
5. Faerman, I., Jadzinsky, M., Podolsky, S.: Diabetic neuropathy and sexual dysfunction. In: S. Podolsky (Ed.): Clinical Diabetes: Modern Management. New York, Appleton-Century-Crofts. 1980, pp. 294, 330.
6. Feldman, M.J., Becker, K.L., Reefe, W.E., et al.: Multiple neuropathic joints, including the wrist, in a patient with diabetes mellitus. J.A.M.A. 209:1690, 1969.
7. Schwartz, G.S., Berenyi, M.R., Siegel, M.W.: Atrophic arthropathy and diabetic neuritis. Am. J. Roentgenol. 106:523, 1969.
8. Feldman, F., Johnson, A.M., Walter, J.F.: Acute axial neuroarthropathy. Radiology 111:1, 1974.
9. Frykberg, R.G., Kozak, G.P.: Neuropathic arthropathy in the diabetic foot. Am. Fam. Phys. 17:105, 1978.
10. Robillard, R., Gagnon, P.A., Alarie, R.: Diabetic neuroarthropathy: report of four cases. Can. Med. Assoc. J. 91:795, 1964.
11. Clouse, M.E., Gramm, H.F., Legg, M., et al.: Diabetic osteoarthropathy. Clinical and roentgenographic observations in 90 cases. Am. J. Roentgenol. 121:22, 1974.
12. Lippmann, H.I., Perotto, A., Farrar, R.: The neuropathic foot of the diabetic. Bull. N.Y. Acad. Med. 52:1159, 1976.
13. Gristina, A.G., Nicastro, J.F., Clippinger, F., et al.: Neuropathic foot and ankle patellar-tendon-bearing orthosis as an adjunct to patient management. Orthop. Rev. 6:53, 1977.
14. Parsons, H., Norton, W.S.: Management of diabetic neuropathic joints. N. Engl. J. Med. 224:935, 1951.
15. Johnson, E.W.: Surgical management of diabetic complications. W. Va. Med. J. 54:157, 1958.

16. Johnson, J.T.: Neuropathic fractures and joint injuries. Pathogenesis and rationale of prevention and treatment. J. Bone Joint Surg. (Am.) 49:1, 1967.

17. Finby, N., Kraft, E., Spyropoulos, E., et al.: Diabetic osteopathy of the foot and ankle. Am. Fam. Phys. 14:90, 1976.

18. Morgano, G.: Osteopatie diabetiche ed osteopatie senili. G. Gerontol. 18:379, 1979.

19. Pogonowska, M.J., Collins, L.C., Dobson, H.L.: Diabetic osteopathy. Radiology 89:265, 1967.

20. Azérad, E., Lubetzki, J., Stuhl, L., Slotime, M.: Les osteopathies du diabetes sucre. Ouest Med. May, 1964, 529.

21. Pomeranze, J., King, E.J.: Neuropathic ulcers in diabetes mellitus. Geriatrics 20:353, 1965.

22. Mirouze, J., Jaffiol, C., Schmouker, Y., et al.: Faux panaris de Morvan récidivant avec osteolyse curable au cours d'une neuropathie diabétique. Diabete 14:39, 1966.

23. Gondos, B.: Roentgen observations in diabetic osteopathy. Radiology 91:6, 1968.

24. Steinberg, G.: Trophoneuropathic bone changes versus osteomyelitis in diabetes mellitus. Geriatrics 26:111, 1971.

25. Campbell, W.L., Feldman, F.: Bone and soft tissue abnormalities of the upper extremity in diabetes mellitus. Am. J. Roentgenol. 124:7, 1975.

26. Harris, J.R., Brand, P.W.: Patterns of disintegration of the tarsus in the anesthetic foot. J. Bone Joint Surg. (Br.) 48:4, 1966.

27. Whitehouse, F.W., Weckstein, M.: On diabetic osteopathy: a radiologic study of 21 patients. Diabetes Care 1:303, 1978.

28. Forgacs, S., Halmos, T., Salamon, F.: Bone changes in diabetes mellitus. Isr. J. Med. Sci. 8:782, 1972.

29. Levin, M.E., Boisseau, V.C., Avioli, L.V.: Effects of diabetes mellitus on bone mass in juvenile and adult-onset diabetes. N. Engl. J. Med. 294:241, 1976.

30. Santiago, J.V., McAlister, W.H., Ratzan, S.K., et al.: Decreased cortical thickness and osteopenia in children with diabetes mellitus. J. Clin. Endocrinol. Metab. 45:845, 1977.

31. Rosenbloom, A.L., Lezotte, D.C., Weber, F.T., et al.: Diminution of bone mass in childhood diabetes. Diabetes 26:1052, 1977.

32. Heath, H., III, Melton, L.J., III, Chu, C-P: Diabetes mellitus and risk of skeletal fracture. N. Engl. J. Med. 303:567, 1980.

33. Knowles, H.B., Jr.: Joint contractures, waxy skin, and control of diabetes. (Editorial) N. Engl. J. Med. 305:217, 1981.

34. Jung, Y., Hohmann, T.C., Gerneth, J.A., et al.: Diabetic hand syndrome. Metabolism 20:1008, 1971.

35. Rosenbloom, A.L., Frias, J.L.: Diabetes mellitus, short stature and joint stiffness—a new syndrome. Clin. Res. 22:92A, 1974.

36. Grgic, A., Rosenbloom, A.L., Weber, F.T., et al.: Joint contracture—common manifestation of childhood diabetes mellitus. J. Pediatr. 88:584, 1976.

37. Traisman, H.S., Traisman, E.S., Marr, T.J., et al.: Joint contractures in patients with juvenile diabetes and their siblings. Diabetes Care 1:360, 1978.

38. Rosenbloom, A.L., Silverstein, J.H., Lezotte, D.C., et al.: Limited joint mobility in childhood diabetes indicates increased risk for microvascular disease. N. Engl. J. Med. 305:191, 1981.

38a. Starkman, H., Brink, S.: Limited joint mobility of the hand in Type I diabetes mellitus. Diabetes Care 5:534, 1982.

38b. Brink, S.: Limited joint mobility (LJM) as a risk factor for complications in youngsters with IDDM. Diabetes 32 (Suppl. 1):16A, 1983.

39. Hamlin, C.R., Kohn, R.R., Luschin, J.H.: Apparent accelerated aging of human collagen in diabetes mellitus. Diabetes 24:902, 1975.

40. Francis, M.J., Ellis, J.P., Hockaday, T.D.: Skin collagen in diabetes mellitus in relation to treatment. Proc. R. Soc. Med. 67:35, 1974.

41. Schuyler, M.R., Niewoehner, D.E., Inkley, S.R., et al.: Abnormal lung elasticity in juvenile diabetes mellitus. Am. Rev. Respir. Dis. 113:37, 1976.

42. Chang, K., Uitto, J., Rowold, E.A., et al.: Increased collagen cross-linkages in experimental diabetes: reversal by B-aminopropionitrile and D-penicillamine. Diabetes 29:778, 1980.

43. Lieberman, L.S., Rosenbloom, A.L., Riley, W.J., et al.: Reduced skin thickness with pump administration of insulin. N. Engl. J. Med. 303:940, 1980.

44. Knowles, H.C., Jr.: Long-term juvenile diabetes treated with unmeasured diet. Trans. Assoc. Am. Phys. 14:95, 1971.

45. Pirart, J.: Diabetes mellitus and its degenerative complications: a prospective study of 4,400 patients observed between 1947 and 1973. Diabetes Care 1:168, 1978.

46. Bridgman, J.F.: Periarthritis of the shoulder and diabetes mellitus. Ann. Rheum. Dis. 31:69, 1972.

47. Kaklamanis, P., Rigas, A., Giannatos, J., et al.: Calcification of the shoulders and diabetes mellitus. N. Engl. J. Med. 293:1266, 1975.

48. Laul, V.S.: Frozen shoulder syndrome. Indian Practnr. 20:787, 1967.

49. Gray, R.G., Gottlieb, N.L.: Rheumatic disorders associated with diabetes mellitus: literature review. Semin. Arthritis Rheum. 6:19, 1976.

50. Pastan, R.S., Cohen, A.S.: The rheumatologic manifestations of diabetes mellitus. Med. Clin. N. Am. 62:829, 1978.

51. Forestier, J., Lagier, R.: Ankylosing hyperostosis of the spine. Clin. Orthop. 74:65, 1971.

52. Hájková, Z., Středa, A., Škrha, F.: Hyperostotic spondylosis and diabetes mellitus. Ann. Rheum. Dis. 24:536, 1965.

53. Harris, J., Carter, A.R., Glick, E.N., et al.: Ankylosing hyperostosis. I. Clinical and radiological features. Ann. Rheum. Dis. 33:210, 1974.

54. Julkunen, H., Kärävä, R., Viljanen, V.: Hyperostosis of the spine in diabetes mellitus and acromegaly. Diabetologia 2:123, 1966.

55. Julkunen, H., Heinone, O.P., Pyörälä, K.: Hyperostosis of the spine in an adult population. Ann. Rheum. Dis. 30:605, 1971.

56. Larsen, R.D.: Dupuytren's contracture. In: J.E. Flynn (Ed.): Hand Surgery. Baltimore, Williams & Wilkins, 1966, p. 992.

57. Dupuytren, B.: Permanent retraction of the fingers, produced by an affection of the palmar fascia. Lancet 2:222, 1834.

58. Davis, J.S., Finesilver, E.M.: Dupuytren's contraction, with a note on the incidence of the contraction in diabetes. Arch. Surg. 24:933, 1932.

59. Whytt, R.: The Works of Robert Whytt. Edinburgh, Beckett, 1978, p. 707.

60. Charcot, J.M.: Disease of Old Age. Baltimore, William Wood & Co., 1881, pp. 75–78.

61. Joslin, E.P., Root, H.F., White, P., Marble, A.: The Treatment of Diabetes Mellitus, 9th Ed. Philadelphia, Lea & Febiger, 1952, p. 93.

62. Joslin, E.P., Root, H.F., White, P., Marble, A.: The

Treatment of Diabetes Mellitus, 10th Ed., Philadelphia, Lea & Febiger, 1959, pp. 92, 93.

63. Beckett, A.G., Lewis, J.G.: Gout and the serum uric acid in diabetes mellitus. Quart. J. Med. 29:443, 1960.

64. Whitehouse, F.W., Cleary, W.J., Jr.: Diabetes mellitus in patients with gout. J.A.M.A. 197:73, 1966.

65. Mikkelsen, W.M.: The possible association of hyperuricemia and/or gout with diabetes mellitus. Arthritis Rheum. 8:853, 1965.

66. Hall, A.P., Barry, P.E., Dawber, T.R., et al.: Epidemiology of gout and hyperuricemia. A long-term population study. Am. J. Med. 42:27, 1967.

67. Herzberg, L.: Diabetes mellitus, serum urate and gout. A study in 314 patients. Acta Diabetol. Lat. 10:1202, 1973.

68. Crepaldi, G., Salandin, F., Tiengo, A., et al.: Serum levels of uric acid in diabetes mellitus. (Abstr.) Diabetologia 2:146, 1966.

69. Herman, J.B., Mount, F.W., Medalie, J.H., et al.: Diabetes prevalence and serum uric acid. Observations among 10,000 men in a survey of ischemic heart disease in Israel. Diabetes 16:858, 1967.

70. De Coek, N.M.: Serum urate and urate clearance in diabetes mellitus. Aust. Ann. Med. 14:205, 1965.

71. Buchanan, K.D.: Diabetes mellitus and gout. Semin. Arthritis Rheum. 2:157, 1972.

72. Newcombe, D.S.: Endocrinopathies and uric acid metabolism. Semin. Arthritis Rheum. 2:281, 1973.

73. Kmoch, J.: Relationship between diabetes mellitus and gout. Knitr. Lek 24:1060, 1978.

74. Varney, J.M., Sato, M.M.: Diabetes in Hawaii: arthritis, rheumatism and gout in Hawaii: some statistical analyses. Hawaii Med. J. 38:197, 1979.

75. Denis, G., Launay, M.P.: Carbohydrate intolerance in gout. Metabolism 18:770, 1969.

76. Boyle, J.A., McKiddie, M., Buchanan, K.D., et al.: Diabetes mellitus and gout. Blood sugar and plasma insulin responses to oral glucose in normal weight, overweight and gouty patients. Ann. Rheum. Dis. 28:374, 1969.

77. Padova, J., Patchefsky, A., Onesty, G., et al.: The effect of glucose loads in renal uric acid excretion in diabetic patients. Metabolism 13:507, 1964.

78. Bluestone, R., Lewis, B.,., Mervert, I.: Hyperlipoproteinaemia in gout. Ann. Rheum. Dis. 30:134, 1971.

79. Mielants, H., Veys, E.M., De Weerdt, A.: Gout and its relation to lipid metabolism. I. Serum uric acid, lipid, and lipoprotein levels in gout. Ann. Rheum. Dis. 32:506, 1973.

80. Diamond, H.S., Carter, A.C., Feldman, E.B.: Abnormal regulation of carbohydrate metabolism in primary gout. Ann. Rheum. Dis. 33:554, 1974.

81. Fessel, W.J., Siegelaub, A.B., Johnson, E.S.: Correlates and consequences of asymptomatic hyperuricemia. Arch. Intern. Med. 132:44, 1973.

82. Bluhm, G.B., Riddle, J.M.: Platelets and vascular disease in gout. Semin. Arthritis Rheum. 2:355, 1973.

83. Prior, I.A., Davidson, F.: The epidemiology of diabetes in Polynesians and Europeans in New Zealand and the Pacific. New Zeal. Med. J. 65:375, 1966.

84. Prior, I.A., Rose, B.S., Harvey, H.P.: Hyperuricaemia, gout and diabetic abnormality in Polynesian people. Lancet 1:333, 1966.

85. Zimmet, P.: Epidemiology of diabetes and its macrovascular manifestations in Pacific populations: the medical effects of social progress. Diabetes Care 2:144, 1979.

86. Zimmet, P.: Type 2 (noninsulin-dependent) diabetes—an epidemiological overview. Diabetologia 22:399, 1982.

87. Heyden, S.L. The working man's diet. II. Effect of weight reduction in obese patients with hypertension, diabetes, hyperuricemia and hyperlipidemia. Nutr. Metab. 22:141, 1978.

88. Bjelle, A., Sunden, G.: Pyrophosphate arthropathy: a clinical study of fifty cases. J. Bone Joint Surg. 56B:246, 1974.

89. McCarty, D.J., Jr., Kohn, N.N., Faires, J.S.: The significance of calcium phosphate crystals in the synovial fluid of arthritic patients: the "pseudogout syndrome." I. Clinical aspects. Ann. Intern. Med. 56:711, 1962.

90. McCarty, D.J., Silcox, D.C., Coe, F., et al.: Diseases associated with calcium pyrophosphate dihydrate crystal deposition. A controlled study. Am. J. Med. 56:704, 1974.

91. Silberberg, M., Frank, E.L., Jarrett, B.S., et al.: Aging and osteoarthritis of the human sternoclavicular joint. Am. J. Pathol. 35:851, 1959.

92. Waine, H., Nevinny, D., Rosenthal, J., Jaffe, J.B.: Association of osteoarthritis and diabetes mellitus. Tufts Folia Med. 7:13, 1961.

93. Ghanem, M.H., Said, M.: Diabetes mellitus and osteoarthritis. Egypt. Rheum. 4:1, 1967.

94. Lee, P., Rooney, P.J., Sturrock, R.D., et al.: The etiology and pathogenesis of osteoarthritis: a review. Semin. Arthritis Rheum. 3:189, 1974.

95. Messerer, U., Franke, E.: Hyperostosis frontalis interna beim Diabetes mellitus. Z. Gesamte Inn. Med. 28:562, 1973.

96. Forgacs, S.: Hyperostotische Knochenveränderung bei Diabetikern. Radiologe 13:167, 1973.

97. Weilby, A.: Trigger finger. Incidence in children and adults and the possibility of a predisposition in certain age groups. Acta Orthop. Scand. 41:419, 1970.

98. Mackenzie, A.H.: Final diagnosis in 63 patients presenting with multiple palmar flexor tenosynovitis. Arthritis Rheum. 18:415, 1975.

99. Phalen, G.S.: Reflections on 21 years' experience with the carpal tunnel syndrome. J.A.M.A. 212:1365, 1970.

100. Yamaguchi, D.M., Lipscomb, P.R., Soule, E.H.: Carpal tunnel syndrome. Minnesota Med. 48:22, 1965.

101. Frymoyer, J.W., Bland, J.: Carpal tunnel syndrome in patients with myxedematous arthropathy. J. Bone Joint Surg. (Am.) 55A:78, 1973.

102. Sudeck, P.: Über die acute enzuendliche Knochenatrophie. Arch. Klin. Chir. 62:147, 1900.

103. Dickson, J.W.: Association of Sudeck's atrophy with Dupuytren's contracture. Lancet 2:1150, 1964.

104. Albright, F., Butler, A.M., Hampton, A.O., et al.: Syndrome characterized by osteitis fibrosa disseminata, areas of pigmentation and endocrine dysfunction with precocious puberty in females. Report of five cases. N. Engl. J. Med. 216:727, 1937.

105. McCune, D.J., Bruch, H.: Osteodystrophia fibrosa: Report of a case in which the condition was combined with precocious puberty in females, pathologic pigmentation of skin and hyperthyroidism, with a review of the literature. Am. J. Dis. Child. 54:806, 1937.

106. Peck, F.B., Sage, C.V.: Diabetes mellitus associated with Albright's syndrome (osteitis, fibrosa disseminata, areas of skin pigmentation, and endocrine dysfunction with precocious puberty in females); report of a case. Am. J. Med. Sci. 208:35, 1944.

107. Podolsky, S., Bryan, R.S.: Albright's syndrome (polyostotic fibrous dysplasia of bone) with sexual precocity, dermoid cyst of ovary, hyperthyroidism, and insulin and growth hormone abnormalities. In: B. Frame, A.M. Parfitt, H. Duncan (Eds.): Clinical Aspects of Metabolic Bone Disease. Amsterdam, Excerpta Medica, 1973, pp. 484–486.

108. Locke, S., Lawrence, D.G., Legg, M.A.: Diabetic amyotrophy. Am. J. Med. 34:775, 1963.

109. Goldstein, S., Poldolsky, S.: The genetics of diabetes mellitus. Med. Clin. N. Am. 62:639, 1978.

110. Podolsky, S., Sheremata, W.A.: Insulin-dependent diabetes mellitus and Friedreich's ataxia in siblings. Metabolism 19:555, 1970.

111. Podolsky, S., Pothier, A., Jr., Krall, L.P.: Association of diabetes mellitus and Friedreich's ataxia. A study of two siblings. Arch. Intern. Med. 114:533, 1964.

112. Epstein, C.J., Martin, G.M., Schultz, A.L.: Werner's syndrome. A review of the symptomatology, natural history, pathologic features, genetics and relationship to the natural aging process. Medicine (Baltimore) 45:177, 1965.

113. Schalch, D.S., McFarlin, D.E., Barlow, M.H.: An unusual form of diabetes mellitus in ataxia telangiectasia. N. Engl. J. Med. 282:1396, 1970.

114. Kobayashi, M., Meek, J.C., Streib, E.: The insulin receptor in myotonic dystrophy. J. Clin. Endocrinol. Metab. 45:821, 1977.

115. Podolsky, S., Sax, D.S., Leopold, N.A.: Increased frequency of diabetes mellitus in patients with Huntington's chorea. Lancet 1:1356, 1972.

116. Podolsky, S., Leopold, N.A.: Growth hormone abnormalities in Huntington's chorea: effect of L-dopa administration. J. Clin. Endocrinol. Metab. 39:36, 1974.

117. Podolsky, S.: Hormone studies in patients with Huntington's disease. Age 2:17, 1979.

118. Zacks, S.I.: Myopathies related to diabetes mellitus and other metabolic diseases. Ann. Clin. Lab. Sci. 5:248, 1975.

118a. Bailey, H.: Cystitis emphysematosa. 19 cases with intraluminal and interstitial collections of gas. Am. J. Roentgenol. 86:850, 1961.

118b. Marks, J.H., Ham, D.P.: Calcification of the vas deferens. Am. J. Roentgenol. 47:859, 1942.

118c. Culver, G.J., Tannenhaus, J.: Calcification of the vas deferens in diabetes. J.A.M.A. 173:648, 1960.

118d. Kellett, M.A.: The radiologic features of diabetes mellitus. Radiol. Clin. N. Am. 5:239, 1967.

118e. Wilson, J.L., Marks, J.H.: Calcification of the vas deferens. Its relation to diabetes mellitus and atherosclerosis. N. Engl. J. Med. 245:321, 1951.

119. Arquilla, E.R., Packer, S., Tarmas, W., et al.: The effect of zinc on insulin metabolism. Endocrinology 103:1440, 1978.

120. Grodsky, G.M., Forsham, P.II.: Insulin and the pancreas. Ann. Rev. Physiol. 28:347, 1966.

121. Logothetopoulos, J., Kaneko, M., Wrenshall, G.A., et al.: Zinc, granulation and extractable insulin of islet cells following hyperglycemia or prolonged treatment with insulin. In: S.E. Brolin, B. Hellman, H. Knutson (Eds.): The Structure and Metabolism of the Pancreatic Islets. New York, Macmillan Co., 1964, pp. 333–347.

122. Engelhart, K., Kief, H.: Über das funktionelle Verhalten von Zink und Insulin in den B-Zellen des Rattenpankreas. Virchows Arch. Abt. B. Zellpathol. 4:294, 1970.

123. Quarterman, J., Mills, C.F., Humphries, W.R.: The reduced secretion of, and sensitivity to, insulin in zinc deficient rats. Biochem. Biophys. Res. Commun. 25:354, 1966.

124. Hendricks, D.G., Mahoney, A.W.: Glucose tolerance in zinc-deficient rats. J. Nutr. 102:1079, 1972.

125. Huber, A.M., Gershoff, S.N.: Effect of zinc deficiency in rats on insulin release from the pancreas. J. Nutr. 103:1739, 1973.

126. Boquist, L., Lernmark, A.: Effects on the endocrine pancreas in Chinese hamsters fed zinc-deficient diets. Acta Pathol. Microbiol. Scand. 76:215, 1969.

127. Prout, T.D., Asper, S.P., Jr., Lee, T., et al.: Zinc metabolism in patients with diabetes mellitus. Metabolism 9:109, 1969.

128. Reusch, C.S., Bunch, L.D.: Serum zinc level in diabetes. J.A.M.A. 210:2285, 1969.

129. Pidduck, H.G., Wren, P.J.J., Price Evans, D.A.: Plasma zinc and copper in diabetes mellitus. Diabetes 19:234, 1970.

130. Kumar, S., Rao, K.S.: Blood and urinary zinc levels in diabetes mellitus. Nutr. Metab. 17:231, 1974.

131. Mateo, M.C., Bustamante, J.B., Cantalapiedra, M.A.: Serum zinc, copper and insulin in diabetes mellitus. Biomedicine (Express) 29:56, 1978.

132. Alexander, F.W.: The role of zinc in childhood diabetes mellitus. Proc. Nutr. Soc. 38:106A, 1979.

133. Rosner, F., Gorfien, P.C.: Zinc and magnesium levels in diabetes. Letter to the Editor. J.A.M.A. 211:2156, 1970.

134. Williams, R.B., Russel, R.M., Dutta, S.K.: Alcoholic pancreatitis: patients at high risk of acute zinc deficiency. Am. J. Med. 66:889, 1979.

135. Meltzer, L.E., Rutman, J., George, P., et al.: The urinary excretion pattern of trace metals in diabetes mellitus. Am. J. Med. Sci. 244:282, 1962.

136. Dettwyler, W.: Quelques aspects du métabolisme du zinc chez le diabétique. Diabetologia 2:75, 1966.

137. Pidduck, H.G., Wren, P.J.J., Price Evans, D.A.: Hyperzincuria of diabetes mellitus and possible genetical implications of this observation. Diabetes 19:240, 1970.

138. Sandstead, H.J., Prasad, A.S., Schulert, A.R., et al.: Human zinc deficiency, endocrine manifestations and response to treatment. Am. J. Clin. Nutr. 20:422, 1967.

139. Schneider, L.E., Schedl, H.P.: Effects of alloxan diabetes on magnesium metabolism in the rat. Proc. Soc. Exp. Biol. Med. 147:494, 1974.

140. Miller, D.L., Schedl, H.P.: Effects of diabetes on intestinal magnesium absorption in the rat. Am. J. Physiol. 231:1039, 1976.

141. Fort, P., Lifshitz, F., Wapnir, I.L.: Magnesium metabolism in experimental diabetes mellitus. Diabetes 26:882, 1977.

142. Winter, R.J., Harris, C.J., Phillips, L.S., et al.: Diabetic ketoacidosis. Induction of hypocalcemia and hypomagnesemia by phosphate therapy. Am. J. Med. 67:897, 1979.

143. Stutzman, F.L., Amatuzio, D.S.: Blood serum magnesium in portal cirrhosis and diabetes mellitus. J. Lab. Clin. Med. 41:215, 1953.

144. Becket, A.G., Lewis, J.G.: Serum magnesium in diabetes mellitus. Clin. Sci. 18:597, 1959.

145. Mather, H.M., Nisbet, J.A., Burton, G.H., et al.: Hypomagnesemia in diabetes. Clin. Chim. Acta 95:235, 1979.

146. Seeling, M.S., Heggvelt, H.A.: Magnesium interrelationships in ischemic heart disease: a review. Am. J. Clin. Nutr. 27:59, 1974.

147. Chipperfield, B., Chipperfield, J.R.: Magnesium and the heart. Editorial. Am. Heart J. 93:679, 1977.

148. McNair, P., Christiansen, C., Madsbad, S., et al.: Hypomagnesemia, a risk factor in diabetic retinopathy. Diabetes 27:1075, 1978.

149. Paetkau, M.E., Boyd, T.A.S., Winship, B., et al.: Cigarette smoking and diabetic retinopathy. Diabetes 26:46, 1977.

150. Editorial: Hypomagnesaemia and diabetic retinopathy. Lancet 1:762, 1979.

151. Green, J., Sweet, R.: Diabetes in pregnancy. In: S. Podolsky (Ed.): Clinical Diabetes: Modern Management.

New York, Appleton-Century-Crofts, 1980, pp. 481–508.

152. Tsang, R.C., Strub, R., Brown, D.R., et al: Hypomagnesemia in infants of diabetic mothers: perinatal studies. J. Pediatr. 89:115, 1976.

153. Rosenbloom, A.L.: Serum calcium and magnesium decline during oral glucose tolerance testing in children and adolescents with preclinical diabetes mellitus less than in normals. Metabolism 26:1033, 1977.

154. Schroeder, H.A., Balassa, J.J., Tipton, I.H.: Abnormal trace metals in man—chromium. J. Chronic Dis. 15:941, 1962.

155. Mertz, W.: Chromium and its relation to carbohydrate metabolism. Med. Clin. N. Am. 60:739, 1976.

156. Boyle, E., Jr., Mondschein, B., Dash, H.J.: Chromium depletion in the pathogenesis of diabetes and atherosclerosis. South Med. J. 70:1449, 1977.

157. Schwartz, K., Mertz, W.: Chromium (III) and the glucose tolerance factor. Arch. Biochem. 85:292, 1959.

158. Schroeder, H.A.: Chromium deficiency in rats: a syndrome simulating diabetes mellitus with retarded growth. J. Nutr. 88:439, 1966.

159. Mertz, W.: Chromium occurrence and function in biological systems. Physiol. Rev. 49:163, 1969.

160. Davidson, I.W.K., Blackwell, W.L.: Changes in carbohydrate metabolism of squirrel monkeys with chromium dietary supplementation. Proc. Soc. Exp. Biol. Med. 127:66, 1968.

161. Tuman, R.W., Doisy, R.J.: Studies in the genetically diabetic mouse: effect of glucose tolerance factor (GTF) and clofibrate (CPIB) on the diabetic syndrome. In: proceedings of the Second International Symposium on Trace Element Metabolism in Animals. Baltimore, University Park Press, 1974, pp. 678–681.

162. Woolliscroft, J., Barbosa, J.: Analysis of chromium induced carbohydrate intolerance in the rat. J. Nutr. 107:1702, 1977.

163. Glinsmann, W.H., Feldman, F.J., Mertz, W.: Plasma chromium after glucose administration. Science 152:1243, 1966.

164. Glinsmann, W.H., Mertz, W.: Effect of trivalent chromium on glucose tolerance. Metabolism 15:510, 1966.

165. Hopkins, L.L., Jr., Ransome-Kuti, O., Majaj, A.S.: Improvement of impaired carbohydrate metabolism by chromium (III) in malnourished infants. Am. J. Clin. Nutr. 21:203, 1968.

166. Gürson, C.T.: Sauer, G.: Effect of chromium on glucose utilization in marasmic protein-calorie malnutrition. Am. J. Clin. Nutr. 24:1313, 1971.

167. Mertz, W., Toepfer, E.W., Roginski, E.E., et al.: Present knowledge of the role of chromium. Fed. Proc. 33:2275, 1974.

168. Levine, R.A., Streeten, D.H.P., Doisy, R.J.: Effects of oral chromium supplementation on the glucose tolerance of elderly human subjects. Metabolism 17:114, 1968.

169. Sherman, L., Glennon, J.A., Brech, W.J., et al.: Failure of trivalent chromium to improve hyperglycemia in diabetes mellitus. Metabolism 17:439, 1968.

170. Hambidge, K.M., Rodgerson, D.O., O'Brien, D.: Concentration of chromium in the hair of normal children and children with juvenile diabetes mellitus. Diabetes 17:517, 1968.

171. Benjanuvatra, N.K., Bennion, M.: Hair chromium concentration of Thai subjects with and without diabetes mellitus. Nutr. Report Int. 12:325, 1975.

172. Morgan, J.M.: Hepatic chromium content in diabetic subjects. Metabolism 21:313, 1972.

173. Rabinowitz, M.B., Levin, S.R., Gonick, H.C.: Comparisons of chromium status in diabetic and normal men. Metabolism 29:355, 1980.

174. Vir, S, Love, A.H.: Chromium status of the aged. Int. J. Vit. Nutr. Res. 48:402, 1978.

175. Jeejeebhoy, K.N., Chu, R.C., Marliss, E.B., et al.: Chromium deficiency, glucose tolerance and neuropathy reversed by chromium supplementation in a patient receiving long-term total parenteral nutrition. Am. J. Clin. Nutr. 30:531, 1977.

176. Freund, H., Atamian, S., Fischer, J.E.: Chromium deficiency during total parenteral nutrition. J.A.M.A. 241:496, 1979.

177. Tuman, R.W., Bilbo, J.T., Doisy, R.J.: Comparison and effects of natural and synthetic glucose tolerance factor in normal and genetically diabetic mice. Diabetes 27:49, 1978.

178. Cotzias, G.C.: Manganese in health and disease. Physiol. Rev. 38:503, 1958.

179. Wilgus, H.S., Jr., Norris, L.C., Heuser, G.F.: The role of certain inorganic elements in the cause and prevention of perosis. Science 84:252, 1936.

180. Hassanein, M., Ghaleg, H.A., Haroun, E.A., et al.: Chronic manganism: preliminary observations on glucose tolerance and serum proteins. Br. J. Indust. Med. 23:67, 1966.

181. Rubenstein, A.H., Levin, N.W., Elliott, G.A.: Manganese-induced hypoglycaemia. Lancet 2:1348, 1962.

182. Gardner, L.I., Talbot, N.B., Cook, C.D., et al.: The effect of potassium deficiency on carbohydrate metabolism. J. Lab. Clin. Med. 35:592, 1950.

183. Fuhrman, F.A.: Glycogen, glucose tolerance and tissue metabolism in potassium-depleted rats. Am. J. Physiol. 167:314, 1951.

184. Hastings, A.B., Renold, A.E., Teng, C.T.: Cationic and hormonal influences on carbohydrate metabolism of rat liver in vitro. Trans. Assoc. Am. Physicians 66:129, 1953.

185. Sagild, U., Andersen, V., Andreasen, P.B.: Glucose tolerance and insulin responsiveness in experimental potassium depletion. Acta Med. Scand. 169:243, 1961.

186. Spergel, G., Schmidt, P., Stern, A., et al.: Effects of hypokalemia on carbohydrate and lipid metabolism in the rat. Diabetes 16:312, 1967.

187. Grodsky, G.M., Bennett, L.L.: Cation requirements for insulin secretion in the isolated perfused pancreas. Diabetes 15:910, 1966.

188. Conn, J.W.: Hypertension, the potassium ion and impaired carbohydrate tolerance. N. Engl. J. Med. 273:1135, 1965.

189. Podolsky, S., Melby, J.C.: Improvement of growth hormone response to stimulation in primary aldosteronism with correction of potassium deficiency. Metabolism 25:1027, 1976.

190. Podolsky, S., Zimmerman, H.J., Burrows, B.A.: Relationship between total body potassium and growth hormone and insulin response in cirrhosis. (Abstr.) J. Clin. Invest. 49:75A, 1970.

191. Podolsky, S., Gutman, R.A., Zimmerman, H.J., Burrows, B.A.: Effects of potassium on insulin, proinsulin and growth hormone release in cirrhotics with abnormal carbohydrate tolerance. (Abstr.) Diabetes 20:372, 1971.

192. Podolsky, S., Zimmerman, H.J., Burrows, B.A., et al.: Potassium depletion in hepatic cirrhosis: a reversible cause of impaired growth hormone and insulin response to stimulation. N. Engl. J. Med. 288:644, 1973.

193. Conn, H.O.: Cirrhosis and diabetes. IV. Effect of potassium chloride administration on glucose and insulin metabolism. Am. J. Med. Sci. 259:394, 1970.

194. Samaan, N.A., Stone, D.B., Eckhardt, R.D.: Serum glu-

cose, insulin and growth hormone in chronic hepatic cirrhosis. Arch. Intern. Med. *124*:149, 1969.

195. Podolsky, S., Melissinos, C., Burrows, G.A.: Potassium depletion in fatal diabetic ketoacidosis. High serum potassium with low body potassium and similar skeletal muscle and myocardial potassium values. (Abstr.) Diabetes *23*:381, 1974.

196. Podolsky, S.: Hyperosmolar nonketotic coma in the elderly diabetic. Med. Clin. N. Am. *62*:815, 1978.

197. Podolsky, S.: Hyperosmolar nonketotic coma. Underdiagnosed and undertreated. In: S. Podolsky (Ed.): Clinical Diabetes: Modern Management. New York, Appleton-Century-Crofts, 1980, pp. 209–235.

198. Podolsky, S., Emerson, K., Jr.: Potassium depletion in diabetic ketoacidosis (KA) and in hyperosmolar nonketotic coma (NHC). Diabetes *22*:299, 1973.

199. Graybiel, A.L., Sode, J.: Diuretics, potassium depletion, and carbohydrate intolerance. Lancet *2*:265, 1971.

200. Podolsky, S., Burrows, B.A.: Does long-term diuretic therapy of hypertension cause potassium depletion? Effects of "K-losing" and "K-sparing" diuretic regimens on serum and body potassium in essential hypertension. Prevent. Med. *7*:123, 1978.

201. Santeusanio, F., Faloona, G.R., Knochel, J.P., et al.: Evidence for a role of endogenous insulin and glucagon in the regulation of potassium homeostasis. J. Lab. Clin. Med. *81*:809, 1973.

202. Dluhy, R.G., Axelrod, L., Underwood, R.H., et al.: Studies of the control of plasma aldosterone concentration in normal man. II. Effect of dietary potassium and acute potassium infusion. J. Clin. Invest. *51*:1950, 1972.

203. Perez, G.O., Lespier, L., Knowles, R., et al.: Potassium homeostasis in chronic diabetes mellitus. Arch. Intern. Med. *137*:1018, 1977.

204. Oh, M.S., Carroll, H.J., Clemmons, J.E., et al.: A mechanism for hyporeninemic hypoaldosteronism in chronic renal disease. Metabolism *23*:1157, 1974.

205. Schambelan, M., Stockigt, J.R., Biglieri, E.G.: Isolated hypoaldosteronism in adults. A renin-deficiency syndrome. N. Engl. J. Med. *287*:573, 1972.

206. McNay, J.L., Oran, E.: Possible predisposition of diabetic patients to hyperkalemia following administration of potassium-retaining diuretic, amiloride (MK870). Metabolism *19*:58, 1970.

207. Cohen, A.B.: Hyperkalemic effects of triamterene. Ann. Intern. Med. *65*:521, 1966.

208. Knochel, J.P., White, M.G.: The role of aldosterone in renal physiology. Arch. Intern. Med. *131*:876, 1973.

209. Goldfarb, S., Cox, M., Singer, I., et al.: Acute hyperkalemia induced by hyperglycemia: Hormonal mechanisms. Ann. Intern. Med. *84*:426, 1976.

210. Walker, B.R., Capuzzi, D.M., Alexander, F., et al.: Hyperkalemia after triamterene in diabetic patients. Clin. Pharmacol. Ther. *13*:643, 1972.

211. Milner, R.D.G., Hales, C.N.: The role of calcium and magnesium in insulin secretion from rabbit pancreas studied *in vitro*. Diabetologia *3*:47, 1967.

212. Malaisse, W.J., Brisson, G., Malaisse-Lagae, F.: The stimulus-secretion coupling of glucose-induced insulin release. I. Interaction of epinephrine and alkaline earth cations. J. Lab. Clin. Med. *76*:895, 1970.

213. Harter, H.R., Santiago, J.W., Rutherford, W.E., et al.: The relative roles of calcium, phosphorus, and parathyroid hormone in glucose- and tolbutamide-mediated insulin release. J. Clin. Invest. *58*:359, 1976.

214. Malaisse, W.J., Herchuelz, A., Davis, G., et al.: Regulation of calcium fluxes and their regulatory roles in pancreatic islets. Ann. N.Y. Acad. Sci. *307*:562, 1978.

215. Planchart, A.: Potentiation of insulin action by calcium and magnesium. Diabetes *14*:430, 1965.

216. Yasuda, K.: Hyperglycemia caused by hypocalcemia or calcium depletion. In: S. Podolsky, M. Viswanathan (Eds.): Secondary Diabetes: The Spectrum of the Diabetic Syndromes. New York, Raven Press, 1980, pp. 449–454.

217. Blum, J.W., Wilson, R.B., Kronfeld, D.S.: Präpartuale Hyperinsulinämie und kalziumabhängige Insulinsekretion bei der Kuh. Schweiz Med. Wochenschr. *103*:849, 1973.

218. Littledike, E.T., Witzel, D.A., Whipp, S.C.: Insulin: evidence for inhibition of release in spontaneous hypocalcemia. Proc. Soc. Exp. Biol. Med. *129*:135, 1968.

219. Yasuda, K., Hurukawa, Y., Okuyama, M., et al.: Glucose tolerance and insulin secretion in patients with parathyroid disorders. Effect of serum calcium on insulin release. N. Engl. J. Med. *292*:501, 1975.

220. Halver, B.: Glucose metabolism in parathyroid disease. Acta Med. Scand. *182*:737, 1967.

221. Potts, J.T., Jr., Deftos, L.J.: Parathyroid hormone, calcitonin, Vitamin D, bone and bone metabolism. In: P.K. Bondy, L.E. Rosenberg (Eds.): Duncan's Diseases of Metabolism, 7th Ed. Philadelphia, W.B. Saunders Co., 1974.

222. Laron, Z., Rosenberg, Th.: Inhibition of insulin release and stimulation of growth hormone release by hypocalcemia in a boy. Horm. Metab. Res. *2*:121, 1970.

223. Kim, H., Kalkhoff, R.K., Costrini, N.V., et al.: Plasma insulin disturbances in primary hyperparathyroidism. J. Clin. Invest. *50*:2596, 1971.

224. Zipf, W.B., Bacon, G.E., Spencer, M.L., et al.: Hypocalcemia, hypomagnesemia, and transient hypoparathyroidism during therapy with potassium phosphate in diabetic ketoacidosis. Diabetes Care *2*:265, 1979.

225. Anast, C.S., Winnacker, J.L., Forte, L.R., et al.: Impaired release of parathyroid hormone in magnesium deficiency. J. Clin. Endocrinol. Metab. *42*:707, 1976.

226. Warner, R.A., Cornblath, M.: Infants of gestational diabetic mothers. Am. J. Dis. Child. *117*:678, 1969.

227. Tsang, R.C., Kleinman, L.I., Sutherland, J.M., et al.: Hypocalcemia in infants of diabetic mothers. Studies in calcium, phosphorus, and magnesium metabolism and parathormone responsiveness. J. Pediatr. *80*:384, 1972.

228. Raker, R.K., Gartner, L.M.: The infant of the diabetic mother. In: H. Rifkin, P. Raskin (Eds.): Diabetes Mellitus, Volume V. Bowie, Maryland. Robert J. Brady Co., 1981, pp. 179–184.

228a. Reports of the Division of Vital Statistics: Mortality from ten leading causes of death. Unites States, 1980, 1979, and 1978. National Center for Health Statistics.

229. Tokuhata, G.K., Miller, W., Digon, E., et al.: Diabetes mellitus: An underestimated health problem. J. Chron. Dis. *28*:23, 1975.

230. West, K.M.: Epidemiology of Diabetes and its Vascular Lesions. New York, Elsevier, 1978, pp. 177–178.

231. National Diabetes Data Group: Classification and diagnosis of diabetes mellitus and other categories of glucose intolerance. Diabetes. *28*:1039, 1979.

232. Wilson, E.B., Maher, H.C.: Cancer and tuberculosis with some comments on cancer and other diseases. Amer. J. Cancer *16*:227, 1932.

233. Ellinger, F., Landsman, H.: Frequency and course of cancer in diabetics. New York J. Med. *44*:259, 1944.

234. Jacobson, P.H.: A statistical study of cancer among diabetics. Milbank Mem. Fund. Quart. *26*:90, 1948.

235. Herdan, G.: The frequency of cancer in diabetes mellitus. Br. J. Cancer *14*:449, 1960.

236. Aronson, S.M., Aronson, B.E., Okazaki, H., Browder, E.J.: Intracranial neoplasms and diabetes mellitus: data indicating an inverse syntropy. Trans. Amer. Neurol. Assoc. *84*:155, 1959.

237. Ragozzino, M., Melton, L.J., III, Chu, C-P., Palumbo, P.J.: Subsequent cancer risk in the incidence cohort of Rochester, Minnesota residents with diabetes mellitus. J. Chron. Dis. 35:13, 1982.
238. Joslin, E.P., Lombard, H.L., Burrows, R.E., Manning, M.D.: Diabetes and cancer. N. Engl. J. Med. 260:486, 1959.
239. Warren, S., LeCompte, P.M., Legg, M.A.: The Pathology of Diabetes Mellitus, 4th ed. Philadelphia, Lea & Febiger, 1966, p. 514.
239a. Legg, M.A.: Personal communication.
239b. Kessler, I.I.: Mortality experience of diabetic patients: a twenty-six-year follow-up study. Am. J. Med. 51:715, 1971.
240. Freund, E.: Zur Diagnose des Carcinoms. Wien. Med. Bl. 8:268, 1885.
241. Marks, P.A., Bishop, J.: Alteration in carbohydrate metabolism associated with neoplasia in man. Proc. Am. Assoc. Cancer Res. 2:131, 1956 (Abstr.)
242. Edmonson, J.H.: Fatty acid mobilization and glucose metabolism in patients with cancer. Cancer 19:277, 1966.
243. Lisker, S.A., Brody, J.I., Beizer, L.H.: Abnormal carbohydrate metabolism in patients with malignant blood dyscrasias. Am. J. Med. Sci. 252:282, 1966.
244. Glicksman, A.S., Rawsom, R.W.: Diabetes and altered carbohydrate metabolism in patients with cancer. Cancer 9:1127, 1956.
245. Glicksman, A.S., Myers, W.P.L., Rawson, R.W.: Diabetes mellitus and carbohydrate metabolism in patients with cancer. Med. Clin. N. Am. 40:887, 1956.
246. Lynch, H.T., Krush, A.J., Larsen, A.L., Magnuson, C.W.: Endometrial carcinoma: multiple primary malignancies, constitutional factors, and heredity. Am. J. Med. Sci. 252:381, 1966.
247. Benjamin, F., Romney, S.: Disturbed carbohydrate metabolism in endometrial carcinoma. Cancer 17:386, 1964.
248. Weisenfeld, S., Hecht, A., Goldner, M.G.: Tests of carbohydrate metabolism in carcinomatosis. Cancer 15:18, 1962.
249. Cancer Facts and Figures, 1980. New York, American Cancer Society, Inc., 1981.
250. Murphy, R., Smith, F.H.: Abnormal carbohydrate metabolism in pancreatic carcinoma. Med. Clin. N. Am. 47:397, 1963.
251. Levison, D.A.: Carcinoma of the pancreas. J. Pathol. 129:203, 1979.

252. Kessler, I.I.: Cancer and diabetes mellitus. A review of the literature. J. Chron. Dis. 23:579, 1971.
253. Cohen, G.F.: Early diagnosis of pancreatic neoplasms in diabetics. Lancet 2:267, 1965.
254. Green, R.C., Jr., Baggenstoss, A.H., Sprague, R.G.: Diabetes mellitus in association with primary carcinoma of the pancreas. Diabetes 7:308, 1958.
255. Dashiell, G.F., Palmer, W.L.: Carcinoma of the pancreas: diagnostic criteria. Arch. Intern. Med. 81:173, 1948.
256. Clark, C.G., Mitchell, P.E.G.: Diabetes mellitus and primary carcinoma of the pancreas. Br. Med. J. 2:1259, 1961.
257. Laurent, J., Debry, G., Floquet, J.: Hypoglycaemic Tumours. Amsterdam, Excerpta Medica, 1971.
258. Assan, R., Hanania, G., Lambert, P., et al.: Tumeur bêta-langerhansienne insulino-sécrétante chez une femme atteinte de diabete sucré. Une observation et revue de la littérature. Ann. Med. Interne. (Paris) 120:173, 1969.
259. Marks, V., Samols, E.: Insulinoma: natural history and diagnosis. Clin. Gastroenterol. 3:559, 1974.
260. Ganda, O.P., Soeldner, J.S.: Relationship between insulin-secreting islet-cell tumors and diabetes mellitus. In: S. Podolsky, M. Viswanathan (Eds.): Secondary Diabetes: The Spectrum of the Diabetic Syndromes. New York, Raven Press, 1980, pp. 297–306.
261. Tragl, K-H, Mayr, W.R.: Familial islet-cell adenomatosis. Lancet 2:426, 1977.
262. Dunn, D.C.: Diabetes after removal of insulin tumors of pancreas: A long-term follow-up survey of 11 patients. Br. Med. J. 2:84, 1971.
263. Marks, L., Steinke, J., Podolsky, S., Egdahl, R.: Hypoglycemia associated with neoplasia. Ann. N.Y. Acad. Sci. 230:147, 1974.
264. Wanebo, H.J., Schlessinger, I., Tashima, C.K.: Severe hypoglycemia associated with terminal lymphomas. Cancer 19:1451, 1966.
265. Papaioannou, A.: Tumors other than insulinomas associated with hypoglycemia, a collective review. Surg. Gynecol. Obstet. 123:1093, 1966.
266. Subauste, C., Calderón, R., Llerena, L.A., Carrion, E.: Insulin and insulin-like activity in tumor tissue and plasma of a patient with a fibrosarcoma associated with hypoglycemia. Metabolism 14:881, 1965.
267. Ensinck, J., Menahan, L., Stoll, R., et al.: Hypoglycemia and mesothelioma: Isolation of an antigluconeogenic substance from the tumor. Diabetes 19:354, 1970 (Abstr.)

43 Hypoglycemia

Robert J. Smith

CHARACTERISTICS AND CLASSIFICATION

Definition

Glucose is an important metabolic fuel for essentially all mammalian tissues. As food intake and energy requirements vary, the circulating glucose concentration is maintained within a relatively narrow range by a complex homeostatic mechanism. The normal lower limit for blood glucose is difficult to define because of wide variation between individuals that results in part from differences in sex and diet.[1] As shown in Table 43–1, glucose concentration declines progressively during fasting and reaches lower levels in women than in men.[1a] After an overnight fast, whole blood glucose concentrations less than 50 mg/dl in males or 40 mg/dl in females are unlikely to occur in normal persons.

(Note that plasma glucose concentration is approximately 15% higher than whole blood glucose.) Before making the diagnosis of hypoglycemia, especially in patients with borderline glucose levels, it is important to consider the clinical setting and the presence or absence of associated symptoms.

Signs and Symptoms

The clinical manifestations of hypoglycemia result either directly as a consequence of tissue glucose deficiency, or indirectly as effects of hormones released in response to the low glucose (Table 43–2). As blood glucose concentrations decline, a complex hormonal response develops that includes the release of epinephrine, glucagon, glucocorticoids, and growth hormone. In addition to the effects of these hormones on glucose turnover and insulin release, epinephrine causes a number of symptoms, such as tachycardia, diaphoresis, and tremulousness. These "adrenergic" symptoms are especially prominent when blood glucose falls rapidly. Signs of central nervous system glucose deficiency or "neuroglycopenia" are more closely correlated with the actual level of glucose. These symptoms, whose biochemical basis is still not completely understood,[2] are highly varied, including headache, visual changes, mental status changes, focal neurologic signs, and ultimately coma and death. Prompt restoration of glucose to normal usually leads to complete reversal of symptoms, but prolonged hypoglycemia can cause irreversible neurologic damage.

Physiology of Glucose Regulation

Before considering the pathophysiology and therapy of disorders causing hypoglycemia, it is important to understand the mechanisms that normally maintain circulating glucose levels. These regulatory processes assure glucose homeostasis both in the immediate postprandial state when glucose absorption exceeds tissue requirements, and during fasting when endogenous glucose production is required. The normal North American diet contains 200 to 400 g of carbohydrate, accounting for approximately 45% of total calories.[3] This mixture of simple sugars and complex polysaccharides

Table 43–1.   Standards of Normality for Plasma Glucose Concentration at 24-Hour Intervals during 3 Days of Fasting

Subjects	Plasma Glucose* mg/100 ml	−1 SD†	−2 SD‡
24 hr:			
Women (44)§	57.7±11.6	46.1	34.5
Men (12)	79.1±12.9	67.0	55.3
48 hr:			
Women (35)	49.6± 6.4	43.2	36.8
Men (12)	74.6±12.3	62.3	50.0
72 hr:			
Women (45)	41.3±13.4	27.9	14.5
Men (12)	67.5± 8.6	58.9	50.3

*Mean ± SD.
†Obtained by subtraction of the SD given under plasma glucose.
‡2.5 percentile value chosen arbitrarily as lower limit of normal.
§Figures in parentheses denote no. of subjects.
   With permission of authors and publisher.[1a]

Table 43–2.   Symptoms and Signs of Hypoglycemia

Sympathetic		Neuroglycopenic	
Faintness	Irritability	Blurred Vision	Inappropriate Affect
Weakness	Hunger	Diplopia	Bizarre Behavior
Pallor	Palpitations	Lethargy	Motor Incoordination
Tremulousness	Tachycardia	Headache	Sensory Dysfunction
Nervousness	Diaphoresis	Inability to Concentrate	Paralysis
Anxiety		Loss of Memory	Seizures
		Confusion	Coma

is efficiently hydrolyzed and absorbed in the small intestine as monosaccharides (80% glucose, 15% fructose, 5% galactose).[4] About half of the resulting portal vein glucose load is removed by the liver and converted to glycogen,[5] thereby never reaching the peripheral circulation. The remainder of the absorbed glucose is taken up by both insulin-dependent and insulin-independent tissues. The actual rate and amount of insulin secreted is governed by a number of factors, including circulating glucose and enteric hormones (e.g., gastric inhibitory polypeptide).[6] Typically, the blood glucose concentration may rise as much as 2-fold following a meal and then return to normal over the next few hours. The levels of glucose and insulin that result from ingestion of a standardized oral glucose load are depicted in Figure 43–1.

As glucose absorption declines following a meal, free fatty acids and ketone bodies gradually replace glucose as a fuel in most peripheral tissues. Glucose adequate for tissues that cannot utilize these alternate fuels is derived from breakdown of glycogen and from gluconeogenesis. Hepatic glycogenolysis begins at about 2 to 3 hours after a meal, triggered by a complex regulatory system that includes substrate and hormone effects on phosphorylase and glycogen synthase activities.[7] The hepatic glycogen pool can be rapidly mobilized, but it is small in size and therefore is entirely depleted after 24 hours of fasting.[8] Gluconeogenesis, which is the de novo formation of glucose from glycerol, lactic acid and amino acids, also begins several hours after a meal. The rate of gluconeogenesis depends upon the supply of precursors and the influence of insulin, glucagon, and other hormones.[9] After an overnight fast, gluconeogenesis accounts for about 75% of endogenous glucose production[10] and in longer term fasting it is the only important endogenous source of glucose.

The processes that reduce glucose utilization and generate glucose endogenously following caloric restriction or the acute lowering of blood glucose are largely under hormonal control (glucocorticoids, catecholamines, glucagon, and growth hormone). Each hormone promotes increased blood glucose levels through several different mechanisms (Table 43–3), and deficiency of any one counterregulatory hormone theoretically could lead to hypoglycemia.

Classification

The differential diagnosis of hypoglycemia in adults is outlined in Table 43–4. Although the list may appear to be long at first glance, the appropriate diagnostic possibilities in a given patient can usually be reduced significantly on the basis of the

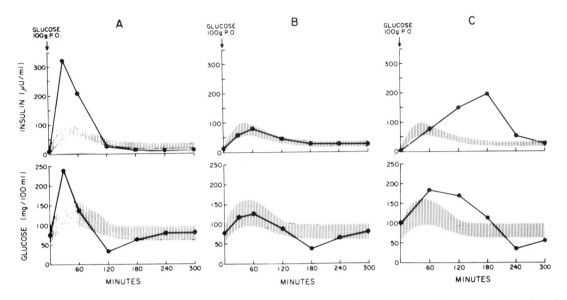

Fig. 43–1. Typical results of oral glucose tolerance testing in patients with: A. alimentary hypoglycemia, B. idiopathic hypoglycemia, and C. hypoglycemia associated with early diabetes mellitus. Shaded areas represent the normal ranges of plasma insulin and glucose.

Table 43–3. Effects of the Counterregulatory Hormones on Glucose Homeostasis

	Increased Hepatic Gluconeogenesis	Increased Hepatic Glycogenolysis	Decreased Peripheral Glucose Utilization	Increased Lipolysis	Increased Muscle Amino Acid Release	Decreased Insulin Release
Glucocorticoids	+	−	+	+	+	−
Epinephrine	−	+	+	+	−	+
Glucagon	+	+	−	+	−	−
Growth Hormone	−	−	+	+	−	+

The + sign indicates that the hormone has an effect; the − sign indicates the absence of a hormonal effect.

clinical history. In the following sections, the pathophysiology, diagnosis, and treatment of each cause of hypoglycemia will be reviewed in detail. This chapter is limited to a discussion of hypoglycemia in adults. Insulin-induced hypoglycemia in diabetics is reviewed in Chapters 19 and 24.

REACTIVE HYPOGLYCEMIA

The various causes of reactive or postprandial hypoglycemia account for approximately 75% of all cases of spontaneous hypoglycemia. In general, patients with these disorders have normal blood glucose levels in the fasting state with the onset of symptomatic hypoglycemia occurring within 5 hours after the ingestion of a meal. The symptoms are predominantly adrenergic and usually are transient. Although the clinical history is extremely useful, it is important to point out that it may be difficult to establish with certainty whether hypoglycemic symptoms occur in the postprandial or in the fasted state. In addition, some diseases associated with fasting hypoglycemia, e.g., insulinomas, can occasionally cause both reactive and fasting hypoglycemia.

Alimentary Hypoglycemia

A form of reactive hypoglycemia designated "alimentary hypoglycemia" or "early phase reactive hypoglycemia" develops in 5 to 10% of patients who have undergone gastrectomy, gastrojejunostomy, or pyloroplasty with or without vagotomy.[11] Rarely, a similar syndrome occurs in patients who have not had gastric surgery.[12] Hypoglycemia associated with adrenergic symptoms usually develops between 90 and 180 minutes after food ingestion. Although neuroglycopenic symptoms generally are thought to be unusual in disorders causing reactive hypoglycemia, recent work suggests that they commonly occur in alimentary hypoglycemia with associated risks of neuropsychiatric sequelae.[13]

It is clear that alimentary hypoglycemia is pre-

Table 43–4. Differential Diagnosis of Hypoglycemia in Adults

I. Reactive Hypoglycemia
   1. Alimentary
   2. Idiopathic, functional
   3. Early diabetes mellitus
II. Fasting Hypoglycemia
   1. Insulinoma
   2. Islet cell hyperplasia
   3. Extrapancreatic neoplasms
   4. Adrenocortical deficiency
   5. Growth hormone deficiency
   6. Hepatic failure
   7. Renal failure
   8. Autoimmune hypoglycemia
III. Pharmacologic Hypoglycemia
   1. Insulin reactions
   2. Factitious insulin injections
   3. Sulfonylureas
   4. Ethanol
   5. Beta blocking agents
   6. Other medications (rare)
IV. Artifactual Hypoglycemia
   1. Leukocytosis
   2. Hyperlipidemia

cipitated by loss of the reservoir function of the stomach. Dumping of food into the small intestine leads to rapid digestion and absorption of carbohydrate. Blood glucose rises above normal postprandial levels, followed by excessive insulin secretion that drives glucose into the hypoglycemic range.[14] Although excess insulin release was originally thought to occur in response to the early hyperglycemia, more recent work has suggested a role for intestinal factors in stimulating insulin release. In particular, gastric inhibitory polypeptide, enteroglucagon, and possibly cholecystokinin are hypersecreted in patients following gastric surgery and can stimulate insulin release.[15,16]

Alimentary hypoglycemia has also been designated the "late dumping syndrome" to distinguish it from the "early dumping syndrome," a separate disorder that is caused by the rapid entry of gastric contents into the small bowel. Early dumping results from the introduction of a large solute load into the jejunum leading to osmotic swelling and presumably the release of as yet unidentified vasoactive factors, either directly from the intestinal wall or as a result of transient hypovolemia.[11] Characteristic symptoms of weakness, flushing, palpitation, fatigue, nausea, and somnolence develop within 60 minutes of food ingestion. Early dumping is described only to make clear that it is predominantly a vasomotive phenomenon and is not primarily associated with hypoglycemia.

The diagnosis of alimentary hypoglycemia is suggested by a past history of gastric surgery and the temporal relationship between symptoms and

food intake. The characteristic early glucose rise followed by symptomatic hypoglycemia can be documented with an oral glucose tolerance test (Fig. 43–1A). Intravenous glucose tolerance tests are generally normal and thus rule out diabetes.

In the past, patients have been treated by reducing dietary carbohydrate and by dividing food intake into multiple small meals. Anticholinergics given prior to meals have also been used to delay gastric emptying. More recently, several other pharmacologic agents have been suggested. In small groups of patients, propranolol (10 mg) before meals has been shown to decrease the early glucose peak, reduce the severity of hypoglycemia, and alleviate symptoms.[17] In other studies, dietary fiber (e.g., pectin) has been equally effective.[18] Ultimately, a series of glycoside-hydrolase inhibitors that delay carbohydrate digestion may offer the most effective treatment.[19] As a last resort, in patients with debilitating symptoms, surgical correction can be attempted with the insertion of an antiperistaltic loop of small intestine.[20]

Idiopathic (Functional) Hypoglycemia

Approximately 70% of adults with spontaneous hypoglycemia fit into a poorly defined syndrome that is variably designated as idiopathic, functional, or vagotonic hypoglycemia.[21] Following its initial clinical description, it was suggested that idiopathic hypoglycemia occurs in patients with increased vagal tone that leads secondarily to accelerated gastric emptying and excessive insulin secretion. Subsequent work has failed to document any consistent gastrointestinal or pancreatic defect.[22] The oral glucose tolerance test typically shows a normal rate of rise and peak of blood glucose, with a transient dip into the hypoglycemic range usually after 2 to 4 hours (Fig. 43–1B). Insulin secretory patterns are generally normal, with a tendency toward a slight delay in the insulin peak.[23] There are no other documented abnormalities in glucose regulation. Since the etiology of the symptomatic hypoglycemia remains unknown, it is possible that the syndrome represents a heterogeneous group of disorders.

Interest in idiopathic hypoglycemia has increased tremendously in recent years because of the suggestion that many people with chronic lethargy, fatigue, and depression actually are experiencing symptomatic hypoglycemia. The weight of scientific evidence now indicates that most of these patients do not in fact have demonstrable hypoglycemia,[24] but instead often suffer from primary psychiatric disturbances.[25] Idiopathic hypoglycemia, on the other hand, refers to a disorder of glucose homeostasis with symptoms that correlate with low glucose levels and resolve with appropriate therapy.

The clinical history and the response to oral glucose are the criteria currently used to establish the diagnosis of idiopathic hypoglycemia. Interpretation of the results of glucose tolerance testing is difficult, however, since more than 20% of normal individuals develop blood glucose levels less than 50 mg/dl between 2 and 5 hours after an oral glucose load, differing only in their lack of symptoms.[26] It has recently been suggested that the "hypoglycemic index" (the decline in blood glucose during a 90-minute period before reaching the nadir, divided by the glucose concentration at the nadir) allows the identification of patients with true idiopathic hypoglycemia solely on the basis of a glucose tolerance test.[27] Until the usefulness of the "hypoglycemic index" has been confirmed in larger groups of patients, however, the diagnosis must still depend upon the careful correlation of blood glucose levels and symptoms. Once symptomatic hypoglycemia has been documented, it still may be necessary to rule out other causes, such as alimentary hypoglycemia, mild diabetes mellitus, and insulinoma. For practical considerations, it may be appropriate to treat some patients conservatively for presumed idiopathic hypoglycemia with close follow-up, rather than immediately to attempt to rule out other causes.

The usual treatment consists of dietary manipulation, with reduction in carbohydrate and division of food intake into smaller meals, especially with mid-morning and mid-afternoon snacks. Elimination of caffeine and cigarettes, plus the use of minor tranquilizers such as diazepam, may aid some patients but has not been clearly shown to be beneficial. The symptoms in patients who do not respond to changes in diet may be alleviated by using anticholinergics (7.5 mg propantheline 45 minutes before meals)[28] or propranolol (10 mg before meals).[29] Most patients with demonstrable symptomatic hypoglycemia will respond to a combination of these relatively benign therapies.

Early-Onset Diabetes Mellitus

If oral glucose tolerance tests are performed early in the course of maturity-onset diabetes mellitus, blood glucose levels not infrequently fall below 50 mg/dl between 3 and 5 hours after ingesting glucose. Associated symptoms are rare, but a small percentage of patients experience typical adrenergic symptoms of hypoglycemia.[30] Therefore, the possibility of early diabetes must be considered when patients are evaluated for reactive hypoglycemia. Similar reactive hypoglycemia in juvenile-onset diabetes is rare, perhaps because juvenile diabetics progress relatively rapidly to marked insulin deficiency. Occasionally, hypoglycemic seizures can be the first sign of diabetes in infants.[31] In adults it is important to distinguish early-onset diabetes from idiopathic hypoglycemia, because the pathogenesis, treatment, and prognosis are quite different. It can be predicted that diabetes-related hypoglycemia will resolve in time as glucose intolerance worsens.

The pathogenesis of hypoglycemia in early diabetes is believed to relate to a defect in β cell release of insulin. During an oral glucose tolerance test (Fig. 43–1C), fasting glucose is frequently noted to be elevated or high in the normal range. Following glucose ingestion, blood glucose levels rise normally at first but reach a delayed, elevated peak before declining to hypoglycemic levels. Simultaneous measurements of insulin show a marked lag in insulin secretion that eventually becomes excessive after 2 to 4 hours.[32] The reason for occurrence of symptoms in only a small percentage of patients with low blood glucose levels is not known.

In persons being evaluated for reactive hypoglycemia, the possibility of diabetes may be suggested by obesity and/or a family history of diabetes. Ultimately, the diagnosis depends upon the demonstration of glucose intolerance followed by the development of low blood glucose and symptoms. In a few patients, the glucose tolerance test may be indistinguishable from the pattern seen in idiopathic hypoglycemia (Fig. 43–1B) and the diagnosis will become clear only with the passage of time.

The most effective form of treatment of early-onset diabetes at least in obese patients, is weight reduction.[33] All patients should eventually be placed on diabetic diets with total caloric intake adjusted to ideal body weight. Planned morning, afternoon, or evening snacks can be used to prevent hypoglycemic episodes that occur repeatedly at particular times of day. It is important to remember that the patients have early diabetes and thus require close follow-up.

FASTING HYPOGLYCEMIA

As glucose absorption tapers off after a meal, a number of interrelated mechanisms prevent blood glucose from declining below normal levels. As discussed above, peripheral glucose utilization falls and hepatic glucose production rises as a result of decreased secretion of insulin and increased secretion of several "counterregulatory" hormones. The failure of one or more of these responses can lead to fasting hypoglycemia, usually occurring more than 5 hours after a meal. Fasting hypoglycemia is often more prolonged and more severe than reactive hypoglycemia, frequently resulting in neuroglycopenic symptoms.

Functioning Pancreatic β-Cell Tumors (Insulinomas)

Both benign and malignant insulin-producing tumors can arise from the pancreatic β cells. These uncommon tumors occur at any age, but most often are diagnosed in the fourth to the sixth decade with an equal sex distribution. Patients usually present with symptoms of hypoglycemia that are most marked in the fasting state and often are exacerbated by exercise. The decline in blood glucose is gradual, and for this reason, symptoms of neuroglycopenia predominate. Aberrant behavior and loss of consciousness are common, but almost any pattern of neurologic dysfunction can develop, ranging from chronic lethargy and fatigue to focal paralysis. Occasionally the timing and pattern of symptoms can be more characteristic of reactive than of fasting hypoglycemia.[34] Although patients may learn to treat or prevent episodes of hypoglycemia by eating,[35] excessive hunger and obesity are uncommon. Especially with benign adenomas, the progression of symptoms can be very gradual and extend over many years before the diagnosis is made.[36]

Approximately 75% of insulinomas are autonomously functioning, benign, single adenomas. They are small in size; 75% are less than 3 cm in diameter.[21] Therefore, symptoms usually are related to excess insulin secretion rather than to local tumor mass effects. About 10% of insulinomas occur as multiple, benign adenomas scattered throughout the pancreas. Another 10% occur as malignant β cell carcinomas, which are usually larger in size than adenomas with lower insulin content per gram of tumor. In addition to insulin, carcinomas can secrete other hormones including glucagon, gastrin, adrenocorticotropic hormone (ACTH), melanocyte stimulating hormone (MSH), secretin, parathyroid hormone (PTH), and vasopressin.[37–40] Carcinomas metastasize to reional nodes and the liver, typically resulting in death in 2 to 3 years.[21]

In infants and young children, a well-described form of hypoglycemia results from excess insulin production by diffusely hyperplastic islets of Langerhans.[41] The syndrome, termed nesidioblastosis, is thought to be caused by a failure in islet cell differentiation that leads to continued replication.[42] Although similar diffuse hyperplasia was originally thought to be extremely rare in adults, more recent studies have suggested that hyperplasia may account for up to 5 to 10% of cases of hypoglycemia caused by excess endogenous insulin production in adults.[43,44] The relationship between pediatric and adult β cell hyperplasia is not clear.

The diagnosis of insulinoma requires the demonstration of (1) symptomatic hypoglycemia associated with inappropriately high insulin levels and (2) a pancreatic tumor. Whipple's triad,[45] which consists of symptoms of hypoglycemia, documented low blood glucose at the time of symptoms, and immediate relief of symptoms by glucose ingestion or infusion, occurs with hypoglycemia from many different causes and does not prove the existence of an insulinoma. In many patients, excessive secretion of insulin is almost continuous and the diagnosis is evident on the basis of one or two random blood samples. In most cases, however, insulin secretion by the tumors is intermittent or only mildly abnormal, so that multiple overnight fasting blood specimens, prolonged fasting, or the infusion of insulin secretagogues are required to confirm the diagnosis. After an overnight fast, approximately 50% of patients with proven insulinomas exhibit whole blood glucose values less than 60 mg/dl.[46] The percentage is markedly increased by analyzing two or three blood samples after overnight fasts. In patients who do not become hypoglycemic after fasting overnight, an extended 72-hour fast probably is the most definitive test. Only rare patients with functioning islet cell tumors can tolerate 72 hours of fasting without developing hypoglycemia. The measurement of insulin as well as glucose levels is useful in identifying patients with insulinomas during a fast. The normal ratio of immunoreactive insulin (μU/ml) to glucose (mg/dl) is less than 0.30.

$$\frac{\text{Insulin } (\mu U/ml)}{\text{Glucose } (mg/dl)} \leq 0.30$$

Suppression of insulin secretion during fasting in normal persons results in a decline in the ratio. In contrast, the insulin/glucose ratio is frequently greater than 0.30 in patients with insulinomas and, more importantly, it rises during fasting.[47] It obviously is important that patients with suspected insulinomas be closely observed during fasting, since profound hypoglycemia can develop rapidly at any time.

In addition to fasting, a number of diagnostic tests have been designed that take advantage of altered responsiveness of islet cell tumors to insulin secretagogues, e.g., tolbutamide, glucagon, leucine, and calcium. In the intravenous tolbutamide test, two baseline blood samples for glucose and insulin are drawn after an overnight fast. One gram of sodium tolbutamide is then given as an intravenous infusion over 3 minutes, and blood samples are drawn at frequent intervals over the next 3 hours. In patients with insulinomas, the blood glucose should decrease by 50% or more in the first

30 minutes after infusion of tolbutamide and will often remain depressed for the entire 3 hours.[48] Extending the fast for several more hours reportedly will identify even a higher percentage of patients with insulinomas,[49] although this may increase the risk of severe hypoglycemia.

The usefulness of the test is based on the marked stimulation by tolbutamide of insulin secretion from most islet cell tumors. Therefore, care must be taken to avoid precipitating severe, prolonged hypoglycemia. Patients with starting blood glucose values less than 45 mg/dl should not be given tolbutamide and all other patients should be monitored closely for symptoms of hypoglycemia and given 50% dextrose as soon as hypoglycemia develops. The use of a bedside glucose analyzer, in addition to clinical parameters, can greatly help in deciding whether or not to terminate the test. As a further precaution, the test can be stopped after 30 minutes in all patients, and the insulin levels can be used to identify insulinomas even if hypoglycemia never develops.[50]

Glucagon (1.0 mg given intravenously over 3 minutes) also stimulates excessive insulin secretion from neoplastic β cells.[46] By following plasma insulin levels for 60 minutes following glucagon injection, a high percentage of insulinomas can be identified. Severe hypoglycemia is less likely to occur than with tolbutamide, since glucagon stimulates hepatic glucose production as well as insulin secretion. Nevertheless, the same precautions with close monitoring of the patient for hypoglycemia are advisable. The responses to leucine given orally[46] and calcium administered intravenously[51] also are exaggerated in patients with insulinomas, although these agents do not discriminate as clearly between normal persons and patients with tumors.

Besides the risk of precipitating severe hypoglycemia, the usefulness of all of the stimulation tests is limited by the occurrence of false negatives and false positives (e.g., in the presence of obesity, acromegaly, and certain drugs). Outside of the research laboratory, they are most useful in patients with equivocal responses to 72-hour fasting or in monitoring the response of patients to therapy.

A further diagnostic tool for identifying insulinomas is the measurement of proinsulin. In normal β cells, insulin is synthesized as a single proinsulin chain and then cleaved to insulin and the fragment designated "C-peptide" prior to release (See Fig. 2 in Chapter 5). The efficiency of conversion is altered in many insulinomas, leading to excess secretion and high circulating levels of proinsulin. The secretion of proinsulin appears to be especially high in patients with carcinomas, such that up to 90% of total insulin immunoreactivity can exist as proinsulin.[52] Although proinsulin levels greater than 20% of total insulin are suggestive of an insulinoma, proinsulin alone cannot be used to make a diagnosis.

When the diagnosis has been established through the above biochemical tests, successful treatment almost always requires surgical excision of the tumor. Approximately 65% of lesions can be localized by subselective angiography prior to surgery. Ultrasound and computerized axial tomography are usually not useful, since the tumors are too small. Transhepatic venography with sampling of pancreatic venous radicles entering the splenic vein is still an experimental tool.

If a tumor cannot be localized angiographically or by palpation of the pancreas at surgery, subtotal resection of the pancreas should be undertaken with careful intraoperative pathologic examination. Almost all insulinomas can be visualized grossly if the pancreas is cut into approximately 2 mm sections. Since total pancreatectomy has considerable morbidity, the problem is one of deciding how much pancreas to resect if a tumor cannot be located. On the chance that hypoglycemia may result from diffuse hyperplasia or from an islet cell tumor arising in pancreatic rests elsewhere along the gastrointestinal tract, 10 to 20% of the pancreas should generally be left if a tumor cannot be identified.[53] It should be remembered also that removal of a single adenoma does not assure a cure, since about 10% of benign tumors are multiple. The use of continuous, intraoperative glucose monitoring has been advocated as a means of documenting effective tumor removal,[54] since blood glucose should begin to rise shortly after excision of the tumor. In my experience, however, intraoperative manipulation of an insulinoma without its actual removal can result in a transient decrease in insulin secretion and a rise in blood glucose that lasts for several hours.

Hypoglycemia caused by unresectable or recurrent malignant insulinomas is generally difficult to treat. If frequent high-carbohydrate feedings and oral diazoxide[55] fail to maintain blood glucose, palliation with streptozotocin is currently the treatment of choice.[56] Other drugs that may be useful in selected cases include propranolol,[57] mithramycin,[58] and L-asparaginase.[59] Embolization of hepatic metastases has been attempted with transient success.[60] In one patient with a recurring benign insulinoma, local embolization with microfibrillar collagen resulted in elimination of hypoglycemia for several months.[61]

The relationship between diabetes mellitus and insulin-producing tumors of the pancreas is not clear. In a series of patients with insulinomas seen at the Mayo Clinic, 24% of the patients had a family history of diabetes.[62] There have also been a number of anecdotal reports of insulinomas occurring in patients with maturity-onset diabetes.[63] Abnormal glucose tolerance is common several years after successful removal of insulinomas,[64] but the role of postoperative pancreatitis with islet destruction is difficult to evaluate. Careful prospective studies will be required to establish whether common genetic or etiologic factors link diabetes mellitus with islet cell tumors. In addition to the possible associations with diabetes, the occurrence of other forms of endocrine tumors in patients with insulinomas should always be considered. In the syndrome termed multiple endocrine neoplasia Type I, multiple, benign functioning islet cell adenomas are accompanied by tumors or hyperplasia of the parathyroid, pituitary, and gastrin-secreting cells.[65]

Extrapancreatic Neoplasms Associated with Hypoglycemia

Non-islet cell tumors occasionally cause fasting hypoglycemia. The clinical picture may be identical to that produced by β cell tumors, except that symptoms and signs of a space-occupying lesion frequently are present. Many tumor types have been associated with the syndrome, and they probably cause hypoglycemia through a number of different mechanisms. A total of approximately 250 cases have been reported;[66] the specific tumor types are summarized in Table 43–5. As would be expected with such diverse tumor types, the syndrome can occur at any age, although the incidence is highest between the 5th and 7th decades.[67] The tumors are generally large; the smallest ones reported have weighed approximately 400 g. Hypoglycemia can be the presenting symptom, but usually occurs as a terminal or preterminal event.

The mechanisms of tumor-associated hypoglycemia are still poorly understood. In spite of early reports to the contrary, there are no well-documented cases of ectopic insulin production by extrapancreatic neoplasms.[68] Since the tumors typically are large, it was at one time thought that the hypoglycemia resulted from accelerated glucose consumption by the tumor tissue. Studies of glucose utilization, however, have not generally indicated accelerated glucose turnover.[69] Instead, the neoplasms in most cases appear to produce a yet unidentified substance that results in decreased hepatic gluconeogenesis and decreased glycogenolysis. It is possible that the substance is an insulin-like growth factor (IGF), or somatomedin, produced and secreted by the tumors. The insulin-like growth factors are a family of polypeptides of 5 to 10 thousand molecular weight that are believed to mediate cell growth. They have many structural homologies with insulin and are capable of pro-

ducing the full spectrum of insulin activities at very high concentrations.[70] It is not yet clear what percentage of cases of hypoglycemia associated with extrapancreatic neoplasms can be attributed to IGF over-production. Confusion may relate in part to the heterogeneous nature of the growth factors. Using a radioreceptor assay, increased IGF levels in one study were found to be associated with hypoglycemia in 19 of 52 patients with non-islet cell tumors.[71] Other investigators, however, have not found elevated circulating levels of IGF,[72] perhaps because they have used other types of assays. While further work is required to resolve the controversy, it seems likely that the insulin-like growth factors will be found to be one of several mechanisms responsible for hypoglycemia in patients with extrapancreatic neoplasms.

At present, the diagnosis usually depends upon the demonstration of a large tumor in a patient with fasting hypoglycemia and appropriately low insulin levels. Unlike insulinomas, the tumors do not usually respond to tolbutamide or other insulin secretagogues. Treatment is directed toward control of the neoplasm. Frequent high carbohydrate feedings or parenteral glucose may be useful temporary measures, but long-term control of the hypoglycemia is generally not possible unless the tumor is removed.[66]

Endocrinopathies Associated with Hypoglycemia

The normal counterregulatory response to hypoglycemia results from the secretion of glucagon, glucocorticoids, growth hormone and catecholamines (Table 43–3). Theoretically, a deficiency of any one of these hormones might be expected to lead to symptomatic hypoglycemia. This clearly can occur in cases of isolated glucocorticoid insufficiency or growth hormone insufficiency. Based upon a limited number of case descriptions, it is possible but not proven that hypoglycemia occurs

Table 43–5. Origin of Extrapancreatic Tumors Associated with Hypoglycemia

Tumor Origin	Percent
Mesenchymal	
Fibrosarcomas and other fibroblastic tumors	38
Muscle tumors	6
Lymphosarcomas and lymphomas	3
Hepatic	
Hepatomas	21
Other hepatic	5
Adrenal Cortex	11
Epithelial (GI, GU, pulmonary)	7
Miscellaneous	9

Adapted with modifications from Laurent et al.[67]

as a rare complication of isolated glucagon deficiency.[73] Catecholamine insufficiency, arising spontaneously or resulting from bilateral adrenalectomy, does not appear to be associated with hypoglycemia.[21]

Adrenocortical Insufficiency

Mild fasting hypoglycemia is relatively common in patients with glucocorticoid insufficiency. Their sensitivity to exogenous insulin is markedly increased, as exemplified by diabetics in whom the onset of adrenocortical insufficiency may be heralded by an increased frequency of insulin reactions. In most nondiabetic patients, signs and symptoms of glucocorticoid deficiency are obvious before hypoglycemia develops.

Any form of glucocorticoid insufficiency can be associated with hypoglycemia, including primary adrenal insufficiency, hypopituitarism,[74] and the adrenogenital syndrome.[75] Hepatic gluconeogenesis decreases through changes in glucocorticoid-dependent pathways. The activity of pyruvate carboxylase, a rate-limiting enzyme for gluconeogenesis, is diminished in the absence of glucocorticoids.[76] In addition, the release of amino acid precursors for gluconeogenesis from skeletal muscle requires glucocorticoids.[77] There also appears to be an increased tendency to develop symptoms of hypoglycemia, since glucocorticoid replacement sometimes results in elimination of symptoms without significantly elevating blood glucose.[78]

The diagnosis of glucocorticoid insufficiency is usually suggested by other signs and symptoms by the time that overt symptomatic hypoglycemia develops. It can be documented in suspected cases by measuring morning cortisol levels or by the use of appropriate adrenocortical stimulation tests. The hypoglycemia is successfully treated with normal replacement doses of glucocorticoids.

Growth Hormone Deficiency

Symptomatic fasting hypoglycemia develops in children with a number of types of inherited, isolated growth hormone deficiency.[79] Any form of pituitary disease in other age groups can similarly lead to growth hormone deficiency and hypoglycemia. In one series, approximately 10% of patients with panhypopituitarism experienced episodes of symptomatic fasting hypoglycemia in spite of adequate glucocorticoid levels.[80] The diagnosis is not difficult, since patients usually have signs and symptoms of panhypopituitarism and may have a radiologically abnormal sella turcica. Since human growth hormone is not generally available for treatment of hypoglycemia, treatment usually consists of increasing the carbohydrate content of the diet and the frequency of feedings. If necessary,

glucocorticoids can be given at slightly higher than normal replacement levels.

Hepatic Failure

Since the liver plays such an essential role in glucose homeostasis both in the postprandial and fasting states, it is not surprising that liver disease can result in hypoglycemia. Studies in experimental animals, however, have shown that more than 80% of the liver must be removed surgically before hypoglycemia ensues.[81] Therefore, it is not surprising that hypoglycemia is a rare complication of acquired human liver disease, because such extensive hepatocellular destruction is usually rapidly fatal. Almost any type of diffuse, severe liver disease is occasionally associated with hypoglycemia, including infectious,[82] toxic[83] and infiltrative disorders. The only requirement appears to be massive hepatocellular dysfunction that develops rapidly. For this reason, the most common causes are infectious hepatitis with acute yellow atrophy and severe toxic hepatitis. Hypoglycemia is much less common in hepatic cirrhosis and metastatic disease.[84] Hepatic disease severe enough to cause hypoglycemia, e.g., in severe right heart failure, is not necessarily irreversible.[85]

Typically, patients with hepatic failure have abnormally high levels of glucose postprandially that gradually decline to hypoglycemic levels after 4 to 5 hours. Hepatic uptake of glucose for glycogen synthesis is diminished in the immediate postprandial period, and both glycogenolysis and gluconeogenesis are reduced in the fasting state. Decreased clearance of insulin by the liver and diminished food intake may also contribute to hypoglycemia.

The diagnosis is usually obvious because of the severity of the underlying liver disease. It is important to note that occurrence of hypoglycemia does not correlate with the degree of abnormality of conventional liver function tests, such as serum transaminase and alkaline phosphatase activities.[21] Thus, the likelihood of hypoglycemia cannot be predicted by liver function tests. Glucose levels can usually be restored to normal by frequent high carbohydrate meals or by infusions of glucose parenterally. Although the long-term prognosis depends on the course and nature of the underlying liver disease, restoration and maintenance of blood glucose are equally critical for the patient's survival.

Renal Failure

It is well known that patients with chronic renal failure frequently develop glucose intolerance[86]; on the other hand, the insulin requirements of diabetics often decline when renal failure develops.[87]

In the past 10 years, there also have been approximately 20 reported cases of fasting hypoglycemia developing in both diabetics and nondiabetics with severe chronic renal failure.[88,89] The pathophysiology of the hypoglycemia is unknown, but it is suspected to be multifactorial. Hepatic glucose production from glycogenolysis may be decreased in the fasting state because of chronic cachexia and associated glycogen depletion. In addition, gluconeogenesis may be decreased because of a deficiency of alanine substrate.[90] The sensitivity of peripheral tissues to insulin appears to be normal[89] and the counterregulatory hormones appear to be secreted in adequate amounts. There is no temporal correlation between episodes of hypoglycemia and dialysis. Although the severity of renal failure does not correlate closely with the occurrence of hypoglycemia, patients with both chronic renal failure and hypoglycemia generally have a poor prognosis.

Autoimmune Hypoglycemia

Since the first description in 1970,[91] there have been approximately 20 reported cases of hypoglycemia occurring secondary to high levels of insulin-binding antibody in patients who have never received exogenous insulin. The symptoms can be either of the adrenergic type or related to central nervous system glucopenia, and the hypoglycemia can occur in the fasting or postprandial state.[92] The patients appear to have unusually high levels of circulating insulin, often greater than 1000 μUnits/ml, in double-antibody radioimmunoassays. In actuality, endogenous anti-insulin antibodies compete with the antibody and result in falsely high insulin levels. Such endogenous antibodies apparently can arise in patients who have not had previous immunization with insulin, although it is not possible to distinguish them from antibodies that arise as a result of exogenous insulin injection.[92] The syndrome is not associated with other autoimmune diseases with the exception of a few patients who have also had Graves' disease.[93] It has been suggested that insulin antibodies may arise in some patients as part of an idiosyncratic response to methimazole or α-mercaptoproprionyl glycine.[94]

The mechanism of autoimmune hypoglycemia is unknown but suspected to result from the gradual, unregulated release of insulin from a large circulating antibody-bound pool. Clinical experience has not been extensive enough to establish treatment strategies other than non-specific maneuvers directed toward correction of the hypoglycemia. In some patients, the disorder has been noted to resolve spontaneously.[94]

PHARMACOLOGIC AND TOXIC CAUSES OF HYPOGLYCEMIA

There are many examples of drugs and toxic agents that have on very rare occasions been associated with symptomatic hypoglycemia either by acting directly or by potentiating the action of sulfonylureas or other durgs. This discussion will be limited to a few of the most common pharmacologic causes of hypoglycemia. The single most common cause, unintentional insulin reactions in diabetic patients, is discussed in detail in Chapters 19 and 24.

Factitious Insulin Administration

There have been many reported cases of intentional insulin-induced hypoglycemia in psychiatrically disturbed individuals. Most patients are medical and paramedical personnel, diabetics, or their relatives. The clinical picture is quite variable, depending on when a patient decides to inject insulin. Since insulin levels are elevated, suspicion of islet cell tumors has led to unnecessary laparotomies and partial pancreatectomies.[95,96] Factitious insulin administration should thus be considered in all patients with hypoglycemia and documented hyperinsulinemia, especially before undertaking invasive procedures.

The diagnosis of factitious hypoglycemia can be quite difficult, depending for the most part upon the discovery of hidden insulin vials through careful detective work. The presence of insulin antibodies in non-diabetic patients strongly suggests exogenous insulin administration, although recent reports have documented that insulin antibodies can arise spontaneously.[92] In centers where reliable radioimmunoassays for C-peptide are available, the diagnosis is somewhat simplified since C-peptide levels in the blood correlate well with insulin levels in both the basal and stimulated states.[97] The administration of exogenous insulin suppresses secretion of both endogenous insulin and C-peptide.[98] Since commercially available insulins do not contain significant amounts of C-peptide, factitious insulin administration results in a pathognomonic triad of hypoglycemia, hyperinsulinemia, and low circulating C-peptide. Although insulin antibodies do not interfere with the C-peptide radioimmunoassay, it is important to note that high levels of proinsulin arising from an insulinoma can cross-react with some C-peptide assays. Therefore, antibody-bound proinsulin must be removed with polyethylene glycol prior to C-peptide determination.[99] In a recent report,[100] the problems of cross-reactivity in the C-peptide assay were avoided by measuring insulin levels with a human specific insulin antibody. This method may never be of practical use, however, since anti-human insulin antibody is not generally available, and human insulin is now commercially available.

Sulfonylureas

In a recent review of all known cases of drug-induced hypoglycemia occurring over the past 40 years, sulfonylureas were found to be responsible in 504 of 778 cases.[101] It is estimated that 5% of all patients on sulfonylureas have hypoglycemic reactions.[21] Acute or chronic malnutrition almost always accompanies the hypoglycemia. Other predisposing factors include advanced age, hepatic or renal insufficiency, and adrenocortical insufficiency. In addition, the action of sulfonylureas can be potentiated by ethanol, salicylates, sulfonamides, and other drugs.[101] Hypoglycemia is assumed to result both from excess insulin release and from direct inhibition of hepatic glucose output.

The diagnosis depends strongly upon the history as well as on clinical suspicion. Elevated blood levels of sulfonylureas can be confirmed by direct measurements. All patients suspected of having sulfonylurea-induced hypoglycemia should be hospitalized, since the drug effects can last for many hours or even for days. Chlorpropamide deserves special mention because of its slow excretion and long-lasting effects. Suicidal or accidental overdoses can be especially difficult to manage. It may be impossible to maintain normal glucose levels with routine glucose infusions, in which case slow intravenous infusions of diazoxide may be beneficial.[102,103] Sulfonylureas are not removed effectively by dialysis, since the drugs are tightly bound to plasma proteins.[103]

Ethanol-Induced Hypoglycemia

Excessive alcohol consumption can lead to severe hypoglycemia with blood glucose levels as low as 10 mg/dl.[104] Although most persons who develop this condition are chronic alcoholics, hypoglycemia can occur in nonalcoholics following the ingestion of large amounts of ethanol. The syndrome appears to occur most often in persons who have depleted hepatic glycogen stores as a result of a binge or as a result of fasting prior to alcohol ingestion. In addition to the severe hypoglycemia caused by high doses of alcohol, recent evidence suggests that the ingestion of small amounts may commonly lead to milder reactive hypoglycemia.[105] Ingestion of as little as 1 ounce of ethanol appears to promote glucose-induced insulin release, leading to hypoglycemia.

Alcohol-induced hypoglycemia develops in patients with totally normal liver function. It is believed that the conversion of ethanol to acetaldehyde and acetate results in marked elevation of the NADH/NAD$^+$ ratio.[106] This in turn shifts key intracellular equilibrium reactions and blocks tricarboxylic acid cycle functions such that precursors for gluconeogenesis (e.g., pyruvate and α-ketoglutarate) are unavailable. Starvation further promotes the hypoglycemia by depleting hepatic glycogen stores.

The diagnosis usually is based upon the clinical setting of hypoglycemia in an intoxicated patient. It is important to note, however, that there is not always a good correlation between blood ethanol levels or symptoms of intoxication and hypoglycemia, since ethanol levels can be declining at the time that hypoglycemia develops.[107] Patients generally respond rapidly to the intravenous infusion of glucose and do not require long-term glucose replacement. Recognition and treatment of alcohol-induced hypoglycemia is extremely important; the mortality rate in adults was estimated some years ago to be approximately 10%.[107]

Beta-Blocking Agents

In the past 15 years, it has been noted that propranolol and other β-blocking agents can occasionally cause symptomatic hypoglycemia. The initial observations were in insulin-dependent diabetics,[108] but β-blockade has subsequently been noted to cause hypoglycemia in non-diabetic patients. In the latter, hypoglycemia secondary to β-blockers most often develops in association with acute or chronic malnutrition, ethanol ingestion, or extreme exercise.[109] The mechanisms of the β-blocker effects are unclear, but most probably involve the inhibition of hepatic gluconeogenesis. It has been suggested that selective β_1-blockers may have less marked effects on glucose homeostasis,[110] but further studies are required.[111]

ARTIFACTUAL HYPOGLYCEMIA

In leukemia or leukemoid reactions, excessive glycolysis by blood leukocytes between the time of blood drawing and the time of glucose determination can result in artifactually low glucose levels.[112] Although fluoride is supposed to inhibit glycolysis, it has been shown that normally adequate amounts of fluoride may not entirely inhibit glucose consumption in the presence of high levels of leukocytes.

Marked hyperlipidemia also can lead to a mild artifactual lowering of blood glucose through a different mechanism. Since glucose distributes throughout the aqueous phase of blood, the concentration may be underestimated if the space occupied by the non-aqueous lipid phase is not taken into account. In most cases of marked hypertriglyceridemia, the blood can be centrifuged at high speed and glucose can be determined in the aqueous infranatant layer. Even without correction for the space occupied by lipids, however, triglyceride levels are seldom high enough to account for more than approximately a 15% underestimation of actual glucose levels.

APPROACH TO THE DIAGNOSIS OF HYPOGLYCEMIA

On first considering the rather lengthy list of possible etiologies, it may seem that it is inevitably a difficult and expensive task to establish the cause of hypoglycemia. In most patients, however, the process can be greatly simplified by considering the history and clinical setting. For example, if hypoglycemic symptoms occur in response to meals (reactive), there may be a history of gastrointestinal surgery suggesting alimentary hypoglycemia or a family history of diabetes indicating possible early diabetes in the patient. In hypoglycemia occurring in the fasting state, there may be a history or obvious physical evidence of hepatic failure, renal failure, or adrenocortical or pituitary insufficiency. Hypoglycemia caused by pharmacologic or toxic agents often presents as an emergency, usually with a positive history of the ingestion of sulfonylureas, ethanol, propranolol, or other drugs. Thus, the exact approach to any patient is greatly influenced by the history, the clinical setting, any previous documentation of hypoglycemia, and the severity of the hypoglycemic episodes. For patients in whom symptoms occur in response to food ingestion, the 5-hour oral glucose tolerance test is the most useful initial study. Since the response to oral glucose and other insulin stimulatory agents is affected by nutritional status, patients should receive if possible a diet containing 250 to 300 g of carbohydrate per day for at least 3 days prior to testing.

When an islet cell tumor or other cause of fasting hypoglycemia is suspected, the most definitive single test probably is the carefully monitored 72-hour fast. Its usefulness can be even further increased by measuring both glucose and insulin and by calculating the insulin/glucose ratio. It may be elected to precede the fast with several glucose and insulin determinations after overnight fasts. In patients with equivocal responses to a 72-hour fast, stimulatory tests with tolbutamide and glucagon may be helpful. When indicated, other appropriate information can be gathered, including insulin antibody levels, proinsulin levels, C-peptide levels, sella turcica x-rays, other x-rays, serum cortisol levels, etc.

It is important to recognize that a definitive diagnosis need not be established at the time of initial evaluation in patients with reactive hypoglycemia with mild, non-progressive symptoms. For some patients, it may be reasonable to follow the response to therapy before undertaking expensive diagnostic studies.

REFERENCES

1. Soeldner, J.S., Park, B.N.: Implications from oral glucose tolerance testing. In: L.I. Rose, R.L. Lavine (Eds.): New Concepts in Endocrinology and Metabolism. New York, Grune & Stratton, 1977, pp. 107–124.
1a. Merimee, T.J., Tyson, J.E.: Stabilization of plasma glucose during fasting. Normal variations in two separate studies. N. Engl. J. Med. *291*:1275, 1974.
2. Ferrendelli, J.A.: Hypoglycemia and the central nervous system. *In:* D.H. Ingvar, N.A. Lassen (Eds.): Brain Work. The Coupling of Function, Metabolism and Blood Flow in the Brain. Proceedings of the Alfred Benzon Symposium VIII. Copenhagen, Munksgaard, 1975, pp. 298–311.
3. Committee on Dietary Allowances, National Research Council: Recommended Dietary Allowances. Washington, D.C., Natl. Acad. Sci., 1980.
4. Gray, G.M.: Intestinal digestion and maldigestion of dietary carbohydrates. Ann. Rev. Med. *22*:391, 1971.
5. Felig, P., Wahren, J., Hendler, R.: Influence of oral glucose ingestion on splanchnic glucose and gluconeogenic substrate metabolism in man. Diabetes *24*:468, 1975.
6. Brown, J.C., Dryburgh, J.R., Ross, S.A., Dupré, J.: Identification and actions of gastric inhibitory polypeptide. Recent Prog. Horm. Res. *31*:487, 1975.
7. Hers, H.G., De Wulf, H., Stalmans, W., Van Den Berghe, G.: The control of glycogen synthesis in the liver. Adv. Enzyme Regul. *8*:171, 1970.
8. Hultman, E., Nilsson, L.H.: Liver glycogen in man. Effect of different diets and muscular exercise. *In:* B. Pernow, B. Saltin (Eds.): Muscle Metabolism during Exercise. New York, Plenum Press, 1971, pp. 146–151.
9. Exton, J.H.: Gluconeogenesis. Metabolism *21*:945, 1972.
10. Felig, P.: The glucose-alanine cycle. Metabolism *22*:179, 1973.
11. Meyer, J.H.: Chronic morbidity after ulcer surgery. *In:* M.H. Sleisenger, J.S. Fordtran (Eds.): Gastrointestinal Disease. Philadelphia, W.B. Saunders Co., 1978, pp. 947–969.
12. Permutt, M.A., Kelly, J., Bernstein, R., et al.: Alimentary hypoglycemia in the absence of gastrointestinal surgery. N. Engl. J. Med. *288*:1206, 1973.
13. Leichter, S.B.: Alimentary hypoglycemia: a new appraisal. Am. J. Clin. Nutr. *32*:2104, 1979.
14. Schultz, K.T., Neelon, F.A., Nilsen, L.B., Lebovitz, H.E.: Mechanism of postgastrectomy hypoglycemia. Arch. Intern. Med. *128*:240, 1971.
15. Thomford, N.R., Sirinek, K.R., Crockett, S.E., et al.: Gastric inhibitory polypeptide: Response to oral glucose after vagotomy and pyloroplasty. Arch. Surg. *109*:177, 1974.
16. Marco, J., Baroja, I.M., Diaz-Fierros, M., et al.: Relationship between insulin and gut glucagon-like immunoreactivity (GLI) secretion in normal and gastrectomized subjects. J. Clin. Endocrinol. Metabol. *34*:188, 1972.
17. Leichter, S.B., Permutt, M.A.: Effect of adrenergic agents on postgastrectomy hypoglycemia. Diabetes *24*:1005, 1975.
18. Jenkins, D.J.A., Bloom, S.R., Albuquerque, R.H., et al.: Pectin and complications after gastric surgery: normalization of postprandial glucose and endocrine responses. Gut *21*:574, 1980.
19. McLoughlin, J.C., Buchanan, K.D., Alam, M.J.: A gly-

coside-hydrolase inhibitor in treatment of dumping syndrome. Lancet 2:603, 1979.

20. McGuigan, J.E.: Peptic ulcer. *In* R.G. Petersdorf, R.D. Adams, E. Braunwald, et al.: Harrison's Principles of Internal Medicine, 10th Ed. New York, McGraw-Hill Book Co., 1983, p. 1708.

21. Ensinck, J.W., Williams, R.H.: Disorders causing hypoglycemia. *In:* R.H. Williams (Ed.): Textbook of Endocrinology, 6th ed. Philadelphia, W.B. Saunders Co., 1981, pp. 844–875.

22. Permutt, M.A.: Postprandial hypoglycemia. Diabetes 25:719, 1976.

23. Hofeldt, F.D., Lufkin, E.G., Hagler, L., et al.: Are abnormalities in insulin secretion responsible for reactive hypoglycemia? Diabetes 23:589, 1974.

24. Yager, J., Young, R.T.: Non-hypoglycemia is an epidemic condition. N. Engl. J. Med. 291:907, 1974.

25. Ford, C.V., Bray, G.A., Swerdloff, R.S.: A psychiatric study of patients referred with a diagnosis of hypoglycemia. Am. J. Psych. 133:290, 1976.

26. Cahill, G.F., Jr., Soeldner, J.S.: A non-editorial on non-hypoglycemia. N. Engl. J. Med. 291:905, 1974.

27. Hadji-Georgopoulos, A., Schmidt, M.I., Margolis, S., Kowarski, A.A.: Elevated hypoglycemic index and late hyperinsulinism in symptomatic postprandial hypoglycemia. J. Clin. Endocrinol. Metab. 50:371, 1980.

28. Permutt, M.A., Keller, D., Santiago, J.: Cholinergic blockade in reactive hypoglycemia. Diabetes 26:121, 1977.

29. Arky, R.A.: Hypoglycemia. *In:* L.J. DeGroot, G.F. Cahill, Jr., L. Martini, et al. (Eds.): Endocrinology. Vol. 2. New York, Grune & Stratton, 1979, pp. 1099–1123.

30. Seltzer, H.S., Fajans, S.S., Conn, J.W.: Spontaneous hypoglycemia as an early manifestation of diabetes mellitus. Diabetes 5:437, 1956.

31. Rosenbloom, A.L., Sherman, L.: The natural history of idiopathic hypoglycemia of infancy and its relation to diabetes mellitus. N. Engl. J. Med. 274:815, 1966.

32. Seltzer, H.S., Allen, E.W.: Evidence that the primary lesion in diabetes mellitus is biochemical inertia of the beta cell. J. Lab. Clin. Med. 108:1014, 1963. (Abstr.)

33. Permutt, M.A.: Is it really hypoglycemia? If so, what should you do? Med. Times 108:35, 1980.

34. Connor, H., Scarpello, J.H.B.: An insulinoma presenting with reactive hypoglycaemia. Postgrad. Med. J. 55:735, 1979.

35. Scholtz, D.A., ReMine, W.H., Priestley, J.T.: Clinics on endocrine and metabolic diseases. 3. Hyperinsulinism: Review of 95 cases of functioning pancreatic islet cell tumors. Proc. Staff Meeting Mayo Clinic 35:545, 1960.

36. Crain, E.L., Jr., Thorn, G.W.: Functioning pancreatic islet cell adenomas: A review of the literature and presentation of two new differential tests. Medicine 28:427, 1949.

37. Broder, L.E., Carter, S.K.: Pancreatic islet cell carcinoma. I. Clinical features of 52 patients. Ann. Intern. Med. 79:101, 1973.

38. Hammar, S., Sale, G.: Multiple hormone producing islet cell carcinomas of the pancreas. Human Pathol. 6:349, 1975.

39. Tiengo, A., Fedele, D., Marchiori, E., et al.: Suppression and stimulation mechanisms controlling glucagon secretion in a case of islet-cell tumor producing glucagon, insulin, and gastrin. Diabetes 25:408, 1976.

40. Murray, F.T., Nakhooda, A.F., Roe, P., et al.: Remission of hypoglycemia after partial resection of a metastatic islet cell tumor. Am. J. Surg. 135:846, 1978.

41. Heitz, P.U., Klöppel, G., Häcki, W.H., et al.: Nesidio-

blastosis: the pathologic basis of persistent hyperinsulinemic hypoglycemia in infants. Diabetes 26:632, 1977.

42. Shermeta, D.W., Mendelsohn, G., Haller, J.A.: Hyperinsulinemic hypoglycemia of the neonate associated with persistent fetal histology and function of the pancreas. Ann. Surg. 191:182, 1980.

43. Woodtli, W., Hedinger, C.: Inselzelltumoren des pankreas und ihre syndrome. I. Insulinome, organische hyperinsulinismus. Schweiz. Med. Wochenschr. 107:685, 1977.

44. Stefanini, P., Carboni, M., Patrassi, N., Basoli, A.: Beta-islet cell tumors of the pancreas: Results of a study on 1067 cases. Surgery 75:597, 1974.

45. Whipple, A.O., Frantz, V.K.: Adenoma of islet cells with hyperinsulinism: a review. Ann. Surg. 101:1299, 1935.

46. Khurana, R.C., Klayton, R., Jung, Y., et al.: Insulin and glucose patterns in control subjects and in proved insulinoma. Am. J. Med. Sci. 262:115, 1971.

47. Fajans, S.S., Floyd, J.C.: Fasting hypoglycemia in adults. N. Engl. J. Med. 294:766, 1976.

48. Fajans, S.S., Schneider, J.M., Schteingart, D.E., Conn, J.W.: The diagnostic value of sodium tolbutamide in hypoglycemic states. J. Clin. Endocrinol. Metab. 21:371, 1961.

49. Steinke, J.: Hypoglycemia. *In:* A. Marble, P. White, R.F. Bradley, L.P. Krall (Eds.): Joslin's Diabetes Mellitus. 11th ed., Philadelphia, Lea & Febiger, 1971, pp. 797–817.

50. Roth, J., Gorden, P.: Clinical applications of the insulin assay. *In:* S. Berson, R.S. Yalow (Eds.): Peptide Hormones. Methods in Investigative and Diagnostic Endocrinology, Vol. 2B. New York, Elsevier, 1973, pp. 876–883.

51. Roy, B.K., Abuid, J., Wendorff, H., et al.: Insulin release in response to calcium in the diagnosis of insulinoma. Metabolism 28:246, 1979.

52. Gutman, R.A., Lazarus, N.R., Penhos, J.C., et al.: Circulating proinsulin-like material in patients with functioning insulinomas. N. Engl. J. Med. 284:1003, 1971.

53. Kavlie, H., White, T.T.: Pancreatic islet beta cell tumors and hyperplasia: Experience in 14 Seattle hospitals. Ann. Surg. 175:326, 1972.

54. Karam, J.H., Lorenzi, M., Young, C.W., et al.: Feedback-controlled dextrose infusion during surgical management of insulinomas. Am. J. Med. 88:675, 1979.

55. Marks, V., Samols, E.: Diazoxide therapy of intractable hypoglycemia. Ann. N. Y. Acad. Sci. 150:442, 1968.

56. Broder, L.E., Carter, S.K.: Pancreatic islet cell carcinoma. II. Results of therapy with streptozotocin in 52 patients. Ann. Intern. Med. 79:108, 1973.

57. Shaklai, M., Aderka, D., Blum, I., et al.: Suppression of hypoglycemic attacks and insulin release by propranolol in a patient with metastatic malignant insulinoma. Diabete Metab. 3:155, 1977.

58. Kiang, D.T., Frenning, D.H., Bauer, G.E.: Mithramycin for hypoglycemia in malignant insulinoma. N. Engl. J. Med. 299:134, 1978.

59. Sadoff, L.: Control of hypoglycemia with L-asparaginase in a patient with islet cell cancer. J. Clin. Endocrinol. Metab. 36:334, 1973.

60. Doppman, J.L., Girton, M., Kahn, C.R.: Proximal versus peripheral hepatic artery embolization: Experimental study in monkeys. Radiology, 128:577, 1978.

61. Moore, T.J., Peterson, L.M., Harrington, D.P., Smith, R.J.: Successful arterial embolization of an insulinoma. J.A.M.A. 248:1353, 1982.

62. Breidahl, H.D., Priestley, J.T., Rynearson, E.H.: Clinical aspects of hyperinsulinism. J.A.M.A. 160:198, 1956.

63. Ganda, O.P., Soeldner, J.S.: Relationship between in-

sulin-secreting islet-cell tumors and diabetes mellitus. *In:* S. Podolsky, M. Viswanathan (Eds.): Secondary Diabetes: The Spectrum of the Diabetic Syndromes. New York, Raven Press, 1980, pp. 297–306.

64. Dunn, D.C.: Diabetes after removal of insulin tumours of pancreas: A long-term follow-up survey of 11 patients. Br. Med. J. *2*:84, 1971.

65. Levin, M.E.: Endocrine syndromes associated with pancreatic islet cell tumors. Med. Clin. N. Am. *52*:295, 1968.

66. Kahn, C.R.: The riddle of tumour hypoglycaemia revisited. Clin. Endocrinol. Metab. *9*:335, 1980.

67. Laurent, J., Debry, G., Floquet, J.: Hypoglycaemic tumours. Amsterdam, Excerpta Medica, 1971.

68. Skrabanek, P., Powell, D.: Ectopic insulin and Occam's razor: Reappraisal of the riddle of tumour hypoglycaemia. Clin. Endocrinol. *9*:141, 1978.

69. Unger, R.H.: The riddle of tumor hypoglycemia. Am. J. Med. *40*:325, 1966.

70. Zapf, J., Schoenle, E., Froesch, E.R.: Insulin-like growth factors I and II: Some biological actions and receptor binding characteristics of two purified constituents of nonsuppressible insulin-like activity of human serum. Eur. J. Biochem. *87*:285, 1978.

71. Gorden, P., Hendricks, C.M., Kahn, C.R., et al.: Hypoglycemia associated with non-islet cell tumor hypoglycemia and insulin-like growth factors: A study of the tumor types. N. Engl. J. Med. *305*:1452, 1981.

72. Zapf, J., Rinderknecht, E., Humbel, R.E., Froesch, E.R.: Nonsuppressible insulin-like activity (NSILA) from human serum: Recent accomplishments and their physiologic implications. Metabolism *27*:1803, 1978.

73. Bleicher, S.J., Levy, L.J., Zarowitz, H., Spergel, G.: Glucagon-deficiency hypoglycemia: A new syndrome. Clin. Res. *18*:355, 1970. (Abstr.)

74. Woeber, K.A., Arky, R.: Hypoglycaemia as the result of isolated corticotrophin-deficiency. Br. Med. J. *2*:857, 1965.

75. White, F.P., Sutton, L.E.: Adrenogenital syndrome with associated episodes of hypoglycemia. J. Clin. Endocrinol. *11*:1395, 1951.

76. Baxter, J.D., Forsham, P.H.: Tissue effects of glucocorticoids. Am. J. Med. *53*:573, 1972.

77. Bondy, P.K., Ingle, D.J., Meeks, R.C.: Influence of adrenal cortical hormones upon the level of plasma amino acids in eviscerate rats. Endocrinology *55*:354, 1954.

78. Frawley, T.F.: The role of the adrenal cortex in glucose and pyruvic acid metabolism in man including the use of intravenous hydrocortisone in acute hypoglycemia. Ann. N. Y. Acad. Sci. *61*:464, 1955.

79. Rimoin, D.L., Schimke, R.N.: Genetic Disorders of the Endocrine Glands. St. Louis, C.V. Mosby Co., 1971.

80. Brasel, J.A., Wright, J.C., Wilkins, L., Blizzard, R.M.: An evaluation of seventy-five patients with hypopituitarism beginning in childhood. Am. J. Med. *38*:484, 1965.

81. Mann, F.C.: The effects of complete and of partial removal of the liver. Medicine (Baltimore) *6*:419, 1927.

82. Samson, R.I., Trey, C., Timme, A.H., Saunders, S.J.: Fulminating hepatitis with recurrent hypoglycemia and hemorrhage. Gastroenterology *53*:291, 1967.

83. Marks, V., Rose, F.C.: Hepatogenous hypoglycaemia. *In:* V. Marks, F.C. Rose (Eds.): Hypoglycaemia. Philadelphia, F.A. Davis Co., 1965, pp. 166–172.

84. Zimmerman, H.J., Thomas, L.J., Scherr, E.H.: Fasting blood sugar in hepatic disease with reference to infrequency of hypoglycemia. Arch. Intern. Med. *91*:577, 1953.

85. Hedayati, H.A., Beheshti, M.: Profound spontaneous hypoglycaemia in congestive heart failure. Curr. Med. Res. Opin. *4*:501, 1977.

86. DeFronzo, R.A., Andres, R., Edgar, P., Walker, W.G.: Carbohydrate metabolism in uremia: a review. Medicine (Baltimore) *52*:469, 1973.

87. Hatch, F.E., Watt, M.F., Kramer, N.C., et al.: Diabetic glomerulosclerosis. A long-term follow-up study based on renal biopsies. Am. J. Med. *31*:216, 1961.

88. Peitzman, S.J., Agarwal, B.N.: Spontaneous hypoglycemia in endstage renal failure. Nephron. *19*:131, 1977.

89. Langlois, M., Robert, G., Nawar, T., Caron, C.: Hypoglycémie spontanée et insuffisance rénale chronique. Can. Med. Assoc. J. *118*:1083, 1978.

90. Garber, A.J., Bier, D.M., Cryer, P.E., Pagliara, A.S.: Hypoglycemia in compensated chronic renal insufficiency. Substrate limitation of gluconeogenesis. Diabetes *23*:982, 1974.

91. Hirata, Y., Ishizu, H., Ouchi, N., et al.: Insulin autoimmunity in a case with spontaneous hypoglycemia. J. Jap. Diabetes Assoc. *13*:312, 1970.

92. Goldman, J., Baldwin, D., Rubenstein, A.H., et al.: Characterization of circulating insulin and proinsulin-binding antibodies in autoimmune hypoglycemia. J. Clin. Invest. *63*:1050, 1979.

93. Hirata, Y., Tominaga, M., Ito, J.I., Noguchi, A.: Spontaneous hypoglycemia with insulin autoimmunity in Graves' disease. Ann. Intern. Med. *81*:214, 1974.

94. Ichihara, K., Shima, K., Saito, Y., et al.: Mechanism of hypoglycemia observed in a patient with insulin autoimmune syndrome. Diabetes *26*:500, 1977.

95. Safrit, H.F., Young, C.W.: Factitious hypoglycemia. N. Engl. J. Med. *298*:515, 1978 (Letter).

96. Stellon, A., Townell, N.H.: C-peptide assay for factitious hyperinsulinism. Lancet *2*:148, 1979 (Letter).

97. Horwitz, D.L., Starr, J.I., Mako, M.E., et al.: Proinsulin, insulin, and C-peptide concentrations in human portal and peripheral blood. J. Clin. Invest. *55*:1278, 1975.

98. Horwitz, D.L., Rubenstein, A.H., Reynolds, C., et al.: Prolonged suppression of insulin release by insulin induced hypoglycemia: Demonstration by C-peptide assay. Horm. Metab. Res. *7*:449, 1975.

99. Kuzuya, H., Blix, P.M., Horwitz, D.L., et al.: Determination of free and total insulin and C-peptide in insulin-treated diabetics. Diabetes *26*:22, 1977.

100. Bauman, W.A., Yalow, R.S.: Differential diagnosis between endogenous and exogenous insulin-induced refractory hypoglycemia in a nondiabetic patient. N. Engl. J. Med. *303*:198, 1980.

101. Seltzer, H.S.: Severe drug-induced hypoglycemia: A review. Compr. Therapy *5*(4):21, 1979.

102. Johnson, S.F., Schade, D.S., Peake, G.T.: Chlorpropamide-induced hypoglycemia. Successful treatment with diazoxide. Am. J. Med. *63*:799, 1977.

103. Pfeifer, M.A., Wolter, C.F., Samols, E.: Management of chlorpropamide-induced hypoglycemia with diazoxide. S. Med. J. *71*:606, 1978.

104. Marks, V., Medd, W.E.: Alcohol-induced hypoglycaemia. Br. J. Psychiat. *110*:228, 1964.

105. O'Keefe, S.J.D., Marks, V.: Lunchtime gin and tonic a cause of reactive hypoglycemia. Lancet *1*:1286, 1977.

106. Krebs, H.A., Freedland, R.A., Hems, R., Stubbs, M.: Inhibition of hepatic gluconeogenesis by ethanol. Biochem. J. *112*:117, 1969.

107. Madison, L.L.: Ethanol-induced hypoglycemia. Adv. Metab. Dis. *3*:85, 1968.

108. Deacon, S.P., Karunanayake, A., Barnett, D.: Acebutolol, atenolol and propranolol and metabolic responses to acute hypoglycaemia in diabetics. Br. Med. J. *2*:1255, 1977.

109. Uusitupa, M., Aro, A., Pietikäinen, M.: Severe hypo-

glycemia caused by physical strain and pindolol therapy. A case report. Ann. Clin. Res. *12*:25, 1980.

110. Lager, I., Blohmé, G., Smith, U.: Effect of cardio-selective and nonselective β-blockade on the hypoglycaemic response in insulin-dependent diabetics. Lancet *1*:458, 1979.

111. Viberti, G.C., Keen, H., Bloom, S.R.: Beta blockade and diabetes mellitus: Effect of oxprenolol and metoprolol on the metabolic, cardiovascular, and hormonal response to insulin-induced hypoglycemia in normal subjects. Metabolism *29*:866, 1980.

112. Goodenow, T.J., Malarkey, W.B.: Leukocytosis and artifactual hypoglycemia. J.A.M.A. *237*:1961, 1977.

113. Oyer, P.E., Cho, S., Peterson, J.D., Steiner, D.F.: Studies on human proinsulin. Isolation and amino acid sequence of the human pancreatic C-peptide. J. Biol. Chem. *246*:1375, 1971.

44 Diabetes in its Psychosocial Context

David M. Holmes

INTRODUCTION

This chapter describes confluent biologic, social and psychologic influences on the quality, and even length of life of the person who has diabetes. It also provides suggestions for the treating physician and those developing treatment programs. While studies based on the biomedical model have enormously increased the physician's knowledge and effectiveness, the more complex biopsychosocial model[1-1c] used in this chapter permits a deeper understanding of the person with a chronic medical condition. This in turn increases the effectiveness of almost everything the physician does.[1d] Up to half of this country's burden of illness and mortality from medical conditions such as diabetes, costing about 8% of our gross national product, can be traced to behavioral-lifestyle risk factors such as nonadherence to effective medication regimens and unhealthy responses to social pressures.[2] This fact underscores the research and therapeutic potential of this approach.

Most of the generalizations and case reports presented here are drawn from my assessments of 400 patients referred for psychiatric consultation by internists at the Joslin Diabetes Center. Although there are limits to the general applicability of inferences drawn from data in a group of people seeing a psychiatrist, over three-quarters of these patients came for consultation about common challenges related to diabetes. Half the cases described here simply illustrate clinical phenomena. The other half illustrate treatment. Readers should not dismiss the dreams and other psychologic phenomena described in this chapter as unpleasant symptoms limited to an unfortunate few who required psychiatric consultation.

I acknowledge a profound debt to Dr. Priscilla White for her guidance and counsel over more than three and one-half decades.

Diversity. People with diabetes make up the most diverse group imaginable, including members of both sexes, with all degrees of health, and from different walks of life. Pre-school children, television stars, retired teachers, professional athletes, physicians, welfare recipients and working mothers—all can have diabetes. This diversity, along with the facts that diabetes can occur at any time in the lifespan, from infancy to old age, and does not go away, accounts for the wide range of associated biopsychosocial issues.

Multiple stresses which range from insulin reactions to permanent physical complications occur in three phases of health and function.[3] The first phase is the year after onset of diabetes, with emotional upheaval attendant on diagnosis; the midphase of relative well-being and full function usually lasts several years, and occasionally several decades; the third phase begins if and when the person needs to make allowances for one or more permanent physical complications.

Similarity. All people with diabetes, from the 3-year-old girl with insulin-dependent diabetes to the 65-year-old obese man with noninsulin-dependent diabetes, usually find it upsetting to learn and to be reminded daily that they have a serious, even life-threatening condition that will not go away. They tend to view the prospect of complications as bleak. The disorder may impede their development or maintenance of autonomy, increase their vulnerability to pessimism and disability, and shorten their expected life spans.

COPING WITH DIABETES AT ONSET

The stress in the first phase is the impact of the presenting symptoms, the diagnosis, and its implications for the individual and the family. Several authors have examined the psychologic challenge posed by the onset of a chronic medical condition, such as diabetes.[3-12] Some emotional upheaval seems to be universal. Transient reactions range from mild to major adjustment disorders, with increased anxiety, depression, anger, withdrawal from others, diminished ability to feel intimate and playful, and impaired ability to learn and work. The sense of helplessness, anger, and anxiety felt by those confronted by newly diagnosed diabetes is usually far less intense than the feelings experienced by children who have been kidnapped, women who have been raped, or soldiers who have seen companions die in combat. However, unlike these types of trauma, the real threat of diabetes persists. Both clinical experience and the literature on coping in crisis suggest that psychologic intervention in the first year after onset may be especially helpful to individuals and families in establishing relatively healthy ways of living with diabetes in later years.[9,13,14] There are many possible places to intervene, for the first response and early adaptation to diabetes are influenced by a number of psychologic and circumstantial factors[15-19] such as:

(a) the ability of the adult patient or the parents of a newly diagnosed child to grasp available knowledge and apply it to increase well-being;

(b) self-esteem, equanimity about depending on oneself and others, and confidence, based on having overcome previous difficulties;

(c) the events surrounding onset;

(d) availability of information about alternative outcomes and steps to increase well-being at a time when this information can be grasped and used;

(e) economic, interpersonal, and medical circumstances which determine availability of help with concrete tasks, help in thinking logically; and

(f) state-of-the-art treatment, including timely psychiatric intervention, such as treatment of depression in a spouse or parent and eliciting worst fears of the patient and family.

Shock of Diagnosis

In the United States 5000 to 10,000 children develop insulin-dependent diabetes each year.[20] There is reason to hope that, with future advances in understanding and management, the life expectancy of the child with diabetes will continue to increase and will eventually approach closely that of nondiabetic peers. In addition, retrospective studies of children with diabetes followed into adulthood indicate that, in cognitive and psychosocial development, some will surpass their nondiabetic peers. However, parents who are informed that their child has diabetes often react with disbelief or shock. This is followed by bewilderment, anxiety, a sense of helplessness, and a deepening grief for the child whom they recently knew to be healthy. A number of authors have noted the extensive turmoil occurring in most families when informed that a child is diabetic.[4,5,7,8,21-25] The parents' distress and sense of vulnerability of their child to catastrophe without warning is intensified by the often dramatic onset in children: unquenchable thirst, bed-wetting, vulvitis, extreme tiredness and weakness, rapid emaciation, and sometimes a lapse into a stuporous or comatose state. With its implication that a child may become disabled or die early, diabetes tends to increase any feeling that parents may have already that they did something wrong. Parents try not to take out their fears and frustrations on the child with diabetes or on their other children, and try not to abuse each other emotionally.[23] Ideally parents should be supported in ways that prevent such problems and help the whole family. The section on treatment will describe some preventive therapeutic interventions.

Some of the reactions of the parents to the diagnosis of diabetes in their child are inevitably picked up by the child and manifested in a manner reflecting age and family style. For example, while some families have a quiet style, others such as these parents and their newly diagnosed child, express their fear and resentment dramatically:

A 7-year-old boy's mother and father told the doctor they were "shocked" and "shattered," respectively, by the onset of his diabetes, 6 months earlier. The mother openly acknowledged resenting the responsibility for managing his diabetes and of feeling panicky lest he die when he had an insulin reaction. She was concerned that he might interpret her refusing to give him certain foods that he wanted as lack of love on her part. In the previous 6 months, he had had temper tantrums and once had hit a nurse in the Diabetes Treatment Unit of a hospital. After one insulin reaction, he threw himself weeping into his mother's arms and confided that he did not think he would live to age 8.

The manner in which parents and children express the feelings of fear that are stirred up in them by the diagnosis, varies widely. Although these feelings often remain unacknowledged, extrapolating from what they say, they do appear to be more similar than different. For example, the parents of a girl with diabetes, diagnosed at age 7, had not told her exactly what could happen if she ate more than prescribed on her meal plan. However, within a year of diagnosis, she "knew" that she would die if she ate even a bite of ice cream or pretzel that was not part of her meal plan. Her apprehension gave way to relief at camp at age 12 when she saw apparently healthy children with diabetes, who had occasionally eaten more food than their meal plans specified, and yet survived.

Younger children master some of the more disturbing aspects of the first year with diabetes through their play. Socially competent children have been known to invite friends to see their syringes and needles and urine sugar kits, and some, reminiscent of Tom Sawyer, have even allowed their nondiabetic friends the "privilege" of measuring sugar in urine.[26]

In the older child or youth, the onset of diabetes often seems to invite upsetting comments, bits of folklore, and reminiscences from others, perhaps those trying to come to terms with their own mortality. Many children and adolescents with recently diagnosed diabetes can recount such disturbing encounters:

In an attempt to console a grammar school girl who had recently returned home following hospitalization with ketoacidosis and diagnosis of insulin-dependent diabetes, the postman told her that at least mosquitoes would not bite her since they do not like diabetic blood.

On his first day of school following hospitalization with ketoacidosis and diagnosis of insulin-dependent diabetes, the teacher of a 13-year-old youth told him that the treatment of diabetes had advanced since twins known to her had died of diabetes in infancy and were buried in identical tiny white coffins.

The first seven adolescents referred to me for psychiatric consultation within months of diagnosis made their way through a series of phases similar to those traversed by young adults. With or without initial transient disbelief of the diagnosis, there was the first shock of having a life-long potentially life-threatening condition. Occasionally this was briefly ameliorated by the relief of knowing that the condition is compatible with many years of life, rather than a disease associated with more imminent death. After the initial shock following diagnosis, came a deepening sense of helplessness and anger or anxiety, colored by past experience, as in the following patient:

A 15-year-old youth had wondered if his grandfather had died, not from brain tumor, but because a stranger had hit him in the head. Within a year his other grandfather had died of cancer, his father had left home, and he had developed diabetes. Now fearful of becoming blind from diabetes, he reported the following nightmare:

"A man in a black shirt chased me. I ran and hid in the closet. He found me and shot me in the face with a shotgun."

Bereft of both grandfathers and father, he perceived the onset of diabetes as a catastrophe. He wondered what could warrant such a shocking attack. Children often wonder how they "caused" a parent to leave home. This boy wondered if he would be "let off" with blindness.

There are always attempts to account for the onset of diabetes, and often patients and parents of newly diagnosed youths blame themselves or others. Occasionally, a patient will try to bargain a way back to good health, as illustrated here:

An emaciated newly diagnosed 13-year-old youth wondered if the onset of his diabetes was punishment for masturbation. He made a deal with God to forego masturbation for return to good health.

For the adolescent, like the adult, the sense of helplessness and anxiety that follows the diagnosis of diabetes is ameliorated by minimizing mentally, on the one hand, the distressing implications of the condition and, on the other hand, seeking new information about diabetes and its management to feel as well as possible and doing what can be done to prevent physical complications.

Even for some adults, the impact of the diagnosis seems unbearable, particularly in families beset by troubles or in those lacking successful experience in coping with chronic medical conditions. In such families, the empathy, warmth, realism and tact exhibited by staff professionals seem to help swing the outcome from the development or accentuation of tenacious personality problems (often with less than ideal management of diabetes) toward a relatively serene mid-phase. The following case is an illustration, drawn from the sixth of the diabetic population with onset between ages 18 and 44:

A 30-year-old mother of two had developed insulin-dependent diabetes 8 months earlier. She was referred by her home physician to the Diabetes Treatment Unit because she was omitting insulin on Saturdays and had begun drinking milkshakes, which she said she had previously abhorred. She was inclined to believe that her doctors had misdiagnosed her as a diabetic. In monthly meetings with a psychiatrist over the next 7 months, she explained that she came from a family with Christian Science ties that had little tolerance for helplessness. The prevailing attitude toward medical problems was: "Never mind, they'll go away." She awakened from a dream in panic:

"I was walking at night from one closed store to another, trying to buy the insulin I needed to keep myself alive."

During the "third of the time" that she acknowledged herself to be diabetic, she felt insulted and angry, with "knots in the stomach," and she feared becoming blind. She was afraid that others would see that she was "weak and sick." With follow-up by her physician at home and working with the Joslin Clinic physician and her psychiatrist, she came to feel that they understood. Her growing sense that she was not alone was reflected in another dream:

"I was injured, helpless, and furious in a strange emergency ward. When my own doctor arrived, I fell asleep, because I had come to trust him."

Within 7 months, she began taking insulin every day, tolerated her daughter's asking her about her diabetes, and began to arrange educational meetings to help others with diabetes in her community.

To many whose diabetes is newly diagnosed, it seems that the world is fairly crammed with aunts, uncles, and acquaintances with amputations of their feet or legs as a result of diabetes. Such reminders of special vulnerability and mortality are not easily avoided. However, some unnecessary trauma is prevented by design of large clinical programs, such as those at the Joslin Diabetes Center, which encourage natural groupings of diabetics of all ages. Staff members encourage each group to attend only relevant training exercises. In the inpatient treatment program, for example, while the white-haired patient with impaired peripheral circulation is attending a session about foot care, the adolescent has the benefit of much-needed ordinary youth activities, such as playing a game of volleyball or learning how to substitute certain foods on social occasions.

CHILD'S TRANSITION FROM MATERNAL TO SELF-CARE

Heightened awareness of a child's physiologic homeostasis is generally characteristic of able mothers of both nondiabetic infants and older diabetic children. When these children with diabetes have grown up and have children of their own, they often say that their mothers are still able to tell what their blood glucose level is by looking at them or even by talking with them on the telephone. While such maternal vigilance is helpful in childhood, some diabetic children tend to incorporate their mothers' fear that death will overtake them if they are left alone, and this becomes a clear developmental liability after about age 11. These children find it somewhat harder to separate themselves from their parents as they develop peer relationships outside the home.

Experimentation

While the majority with onset of diabetes before age 11 gradually assume responsibility for managing their diabetes, the transition from maternal to self-care, usually accelerating sharply at age 11 or 12, poses an extra developmental hurdle. At about this age, when most children appropriately begin to give themselves insulin injections, they often carry out experiments to test the hypothesis that they do *not* have diabetes. These are conducted to see what will happen if parental instructions about insulin and diet are not followed. Such experiments usually indicate a child's preparation for increasing separation from parents. Although these activities are usually carried out secretly, in one instance, a child took her mother into her confidence:

A 12-year-old girl with onset of diabetes at age 4 asked her mother for permission to omit her insulin until she was sure she had diabetes. With trepidation her mother gave her permission and kept herself awake to monitor her daughter's condition while insulin was omitted for 2 days. On the first day the girl felt proud. Then she became so thirsty and tired that she concluded she had diabetes, ended her experiment, and resumed its management.

The transition from parental management of diabetes to self-management can be premature. In the following case a serious problem arose when too much responsibility was given prematurely; this problem was quickly resolved once the physician understood the girl's primary concern:

An 11-year-old girl, with onset of diabetes at age 9, had had 50 (sic) episodes of ketoacidosis since age 10, when she had begun self-injection of insulin. She publicly attributed the ketoacidosis to eating over her diet. The fact that she had become distressed by lumps on her legs at the sites of insulin injections a year earlier had probably led her to omit insulin many days in the past year. Members of the medical staff helped her to take measures to minimize or prevent development of unsightly lumps in the future while taking her insulin.

Mismanagement of diabetes during the transition

from parental care to self-care may also reflect other mechanisms, such as attempts to attract attention from distant, disinterested, or overwhelmed parents[27] or may show the child's mixed feelings about overprotection by an intrusive mother, as in this case:

This 19-year-old woman extended the transition to self-care throughout adolescence. The mother gave meticulous attention to the diabetes. Under her mother's threat of complications, she took her insulin, followed the diet, and gave her mother a urine sample for testing 4 times daily. After she had been out with friends who did not know she had diabetes, she began diluting the urine which she gave her mother, then tinted the water she gave her mother with yellow dye, and finally started omitting insulin now and then to lose weight. At age 19, after an elderly neighbor developed gangrene of the toes, she moved out of her parents' home and dreamed on the eve of her 20th birthday:

> She had hidden her legs in black bandages for too long, despite her mother's warning. When she removed the bandages, she found little gangrenous bumps inside tiny clam shells opening on each big toe.

She felt angry at herself for acting as if the diabetes was her mother's instead of her own and for not taking better care of herself. With her mother's help, she made an appointment with a psychiatrist. She accepted his referral to a diabetes specialist. She moved back home on her own, where she felt "like a baby" at times. She took her insulin regularly. With difficulty, she started measuring the glucose in the urine and began to follow the meal plan. She no longer had bad dreams.

Occasionally females are motivated to take care of their diabetes only with the appearance of a symptom or sign which they believe may be a complication. Males who make an easy transition to self-care as far as metabolic control goes, sometimes continue into mid-life to show evidence of difficulty freeing themselves from overdependence on their mothers or maternal substitutes.

Prolonged Parental Protection and Autonomy

The dramatic onset of diabetes in a child before age 11 has usually made the mother aware of her child's vulnerability to medical emergencies. Also, within the first 2 years of onset she is the parent most likely to find her child clammy and unresponsive during inevitable insulin reactions, and to believe for a moment that her child has died. Such traumatic experiences increase her fear that the child will die if left alone, and increase the intensity and rapidity with which an able mother responds to minor fluctuations in the well-being of her child. The vigilantly protective attitude of such mothers is reminiscent of the experiment in which the muscle tonus of several nondiabetic mothers exactly

paralleled that of their nondiabetic infants whom they held while the muscle tension of each was being recorded by electromyograph.[28] The child with diabetes picks up the mother's tension about "going it alone." The sense that something awful will happen tends to reach a peak when the child is both hypoglycemic and alone. This shared tension, when the two are separated, can become a clear problem in adolescence, when the youth should be striking out independently; meanwhile the parents stand on the sidelines, ready to help when asked. Some pre-teenagers and adolescents, mostly girls, anxiously test the dangers of autonomous function by covertly mismanaging insulin, meal plans, exercise, and the stress-related lability of diabetes in a way which invites the mother to remain over-involved with even minor fluctuations in the well-being of the child. Experience with the family described below illustrates the genesis of prolonged parental protectiveness and impaired autonomy, and how to nip them in the bud:

In the year following onset of a girl's diabetes at age 8, her mother rapidly mastered the basic skills needed to maintain her daughter's life, although she had found her daughter in bed cool, perspiring and unresponsive during more than one insulin reaction, and had thought each time that her daughter had died. A year and a half after diagnosis and after going to a camp for children with diabetes where she learned to give her own insulin injections, the daughter became contrary about several issues, including management of diabetes. Her father said he was inclined to deal with her as a contrary child who happened to have diabetes. Her mother still feared her daughter would die in an insulin reaction while she (the mother) slept. Her sense of her daughter's vulnerability to death rendered her helpless to deal with her daughter's obstinacy. After her mother voiced and explored her worst fear, and digested more facts about hypoglycemia, she felt relieved and became more able to absorb information which helped her believe that it would be better for her to be firm with her daughter and then turn her attention elsewhere.

Most pre-teenagers and parents know that moving out into the world with friends promises the most for the future, and that ultimately the patient will become the person in the best position to manage the diabetes, but the simultaneous occurrence of two of several conditions can temporarily delay autonomous development[29] (Table 44–1).

Beyond such normal transient setbacks, especially when children become diabetic before age 5, over-dependency can become a significant problem in adolescence or adulthood. Depending on the strictness of the criteria used, I have identified between 19 and 26 adolescents or adults (15 to 20% of the 130 with onset of diabetes before age 11) in whom anxiety had slowed age-appropriate separation from their mothers and hindered the devel-

Table 44–1.   Biopsychosocial Conditions Determining Health and Function

Feeling, Functioning Relatively Well: Biopsychosocial Homeostasis	versus	Discomfort, Compromised Function: Biopsychosocial Regression
1. Sense of continuity, connection, safety		Threat of separation, injury
2. Sense of mastery		Uncertainty, helplessness demoralization, despondency, hopelessness
3. Vigor		Fatigue
4. Optimism about life span		Pessimism about life span
5. Autonomy		Dependence
6. Equanimity		Anxiety
7. Reasonable assertiveness		Timidity or recklessness
8. Regularity of pattern of meals, exercise, medicines, sleep		Disruption of regular pattern
9. Mutually beneficial relationships		Sense of being isolated, different, using symptoms to obtain care of others
10. Resistance to infection		Vulnerability to infection, fever
11. Self-esteem		Falling self-esteem, depressive disorder
12. Well-being and function relatively unimpaired by bodily symptoms		Feeling ill with symptoms to which patient is predisposed, such as hyper- and hypoglycemia, nausea, aches, pains, dyspnea

opment of realistic independence. Prolonged over-protectiveness before age 11 could only be inferred by the time these adolescents or adults were seen in psychiatric consultation. Such over-protection was inferred half as often in males as in females, perhaps because gender roles make it even harder for most males to acknowledge difficulty in breaking away from their mothers. In 1971, a Joslin Clinic physician referred a "mother and daughter combination" for psychiatric consultation. Both the wording of the referral and the psychiatrist's report described prolonged parental over-protection resulting in dependency inappropriate to age:

Probably before, and off and on since this 13-year-old girl, seen at a time of hospitalization, first left home for public school at age 6, she and her mother had felt tense about being separated. Despite excellent advice and probably excellent management of most aspects of her diabetes since the age of 20 months, when called upon to function separately from her mother, the daughter's tension tended to disrupt her smooth social and academic development. Since age 12, the daughter felt able to stay in school only 3 hours before calling her mother to pick her up and take her home because of headaches and nausea. The daughter's development of competence in managing her diabetes had apparently been a bit retarded, too, as reflected in the fact that until this hospitalization the mother had been giving her daughter insulin injections. The ambivalence which children in our culture normally have about relinquishing dependent roles with parents for independent roles with peers had been heightened in this daughter by the combination of diabetes and her mother's anxieties about her. Neither mother nor daughter directly acknowledged the latter (although at age 8 after a bout with the "flu," her mother had her child repeat a grade despite marks good enough to warrant promotion).

The patient reported a dream in which the boundaries

between the malefactors and the innocent, and who was responsible for what, were ill-defined:

She escaped from a pursuing giant foot, and met two reformed bank robbers. She discovered that she had a six-shooter strapped to each hip, and someone robbed a bank. Accused, she tried to extricate herself.

This mother had managed her daughter's life and the details of her health care for so long, it was hard for her to stand back and wait for her daughter to function on her own. At one point during the interview, the mother answered the psychiatrist's questions to her daughter about what she would like to do later in life, before the daughter could respond for herself. Past medical emergencies such as an episode of ketoacidosis at age 5 had reinforced the mother's tendency to perceive emergencies when there were none, so that she overreacted and reacted too quickly to normal developmental tensions in her daughter. Uncurbed, the mother's tendency would have handicapped the daughter in feeling basically optimistic, in savoring life, and in keeping pace with her peers. With continued counsel and support, the mother was capable of delaying her manifest response to what she perceived as emergencies. She needed help to delay reacting to tension in her daughter, giving her time to reflect on the alternatives, and allowing the mother to gain experience standing on the sidelines, ready to help sometimes when asked.

The patient's usual route to autonomy is to supplement age-inappropriate dependency on the mother with a heterosexual relationship with a peer. A new age-inappropriate dependency may develop with that person, often with over-dependence on a partner who minimizes risks. This new over-dependence usually passes as normal, helping the patient to develop additional, more autonomous relationships. A majority in our series of 19 to 26 overprotected, over-dependent adolescents and adults achieved at least a slight increase in equanimity while accumulating experience with more autonomous functioning.

SPECIAL CHALLENGES FOR THE ADOLESCENT AND YOUNG ADULT

The impact of the onset of diabetes and its management is even greater for the adolescent than the adult, and poses some special challenges. The male adolescent in good health typically feels himself in the position of the youngest son about to set out to slay the metaphorical dragon and win princess and kingdom against all odds; he feels he needs stout heart and a little magic if he is to achieve his challenging goal.[30] At this critical juncture, when he needs to feel confident, lucky, and indestructible, the onset of diabetes confronts the adolescent with bad luck and his vulnerability to early disability and death. He is advised to measure the glucose in his urine or blood, eat carefully and differently from his friends, and inject himself with insulin one, two, or even more times daily before crossing the threshold of his parents' home to meet the world.

Using inner resources and help from others, the child entering adolescence then tackles these tasks (Table 44–2) and in mastering them gradually acquires the competence, confidence, and bearing that maintain acceptance by peers and then as an adult by other adults.

Sense of Vulnerability and Feeling "Different"

Adolescents with diabetes at the Clara Barton Birthplace Camp recounted experiences that had reinforced their sense of being different:

A nondiabetic acquaintance who was unaware that the girl to whom she was speaking had diabetes, learned that a third girl had diabetes. She said that she could tell that the third girl had diabetes because her home "smelled different."

Table 44–2.   Major Tasks Facing the Child Entering Adolescence

1. Modifying concepts of parents so that, failing to find others to play the role of all-wise, omnipotent counsellor, whatever knowledge and competence the youth achieves comes to be seen as residing within and as part of self.
2. Building two-way relationships with valued peers.
3. Forging moral standards which are acceptable to self and others.
4. Creating an adult sexual role.
5. Refining goals and making educational and vocational decisions that will tend to shape the future.

On learning that another camper had diabetes, a nondiabetic acquaintance said, "But you don't *look* diabetic!"

The adolescent's sense of personal vulnerability to catastrophe may be increased by severe hypoglycemic episodes. Swift et al.[31] and Krosnick[5] found the tendency toward anxiety 3 to 4 times more prevalent and more manifest in adolescents with diabetes. This awareness of vulnerability along with feeling different, separates diabetic adolescents from their nondiabetic peers, and frequently makes it harder for them to feel attractive and confident, and to form friendships. It also undercuts willingness to be more aware of diabetes.[32] This process is described in the literature on alienation[33] and by Covelli in his autobiography,[34] as exemplified in the following case history:

An 18-year-old student nurse with onset of diabetes at age 6 had grown up in a middle-class suburban home. Her mother, with help from the Joslin Clinic, had managed her diabetes until she took charge in adolescence. The patient expected a lot of herself in handling her diabetes, in her performance in school, and in other ways. Sometimes she ate over her diet, but usually she did not. Until age 15, her mother thought she was developing well except for the fact that she had no particular friend. At age 15 her usual outer poise began to give way to tearful bouts of castigating herself or being unable to joke and get along comfortably with peers. She left home at age 18 to attend nursing school. She was disappointed when a young man stopped visiting her. She began getting lower marks. She ate over her meal plan more often, and finally began turning to her mother for reassurance and advice. Her diabetes specialist referred her for psychiatric consultation. In the second interview, she reported this dream:

"I was walking in a group of student nurses. Without warning, my teeth started falling out. I hoped that the girls wouldn't notice. I felt awful, but told myself, 'Oh, well, I can't be perfect.'"

Her dream suggests that she felt that she was alone and unlike her acquaintances, was vulnerable to sudden, unexpected physical catastrophe which, in this case, was the loss of her teeth, which were part of a lovely smile, but implicated in eating. Her diabetes increased her awareness of her differentness from those around her. In her dream, as in her life, surrounded by those who, if she had been more open, might have proven friends, she kept herself very much alone and hoped others would not notice her defect. She told the psychiatrist of hating "feeling wobbly-kneed and drunk" during insulin reactions and spoke of guilt about eating over her diet. Within 2 months of reporting this dream, by minimizing and denying problems, she was once again her usual cheerful self. Over the next 3 years her dissatisfaction with herself periodically broke through her surface poise. She maintained pleasant, superficial relationships with acquaintances, completed nursing school, and started college. By age 21 she was suspended between her considerable fear of exposing herself to others and her growing wish to look more directly at her problems, to take a chance, and to become more open with others.

Perhaps 1% of those with insulin-dependent diabetes now use insulin pumps, but distress about appearing different keeps at least as many young people from starting.[35,36]

Subjective Life Expectancy

Many adolescents and others with diabetes fluctuate in their expectations of the future, from an unexamined sense that they will live happily ever after, to the equally unrealistic notion that they will drop dead in a moment. A typical daydream during a pessimistic phase is that the person will become blind, develop gangrene leading to amputation of both legs, and become totally dependent once again on now aging parents, before dying at a very young age.

Interpreting reports[37,38] of subjective life expectancy among nondiabetic adolescents, one finds that most adolescents think little about death, but when they do, they tend to feel deeply afraid. At least in one group of nondiabetic adults, men were slightly more apt to put off thinking realistically about death than were women.[39] However, having diabetes gives credence to extreme pessimism. Two of the four circumstances cited in Table 44–1 as delaying autonomous development, may also lead the adolescent or young adult to give up temporarily normal optimism about the future, and to dwell instead on the prospect of an early death. The comfort or discomfort a person feels at the moment tends to determine which notion of the future is in ascendancy at that time.[40]

An 18-year-old woman with onset of diabetes at age 9 left home for college, where her notion of herself was shaken by the realization that she was neither brighter nor more gifted than some other bright people. Going to see the dentist for an extraction, she became preoccupied with her personal finiteness and the inevitability of her death. She revised her estimate of how long she would live from age 49 to age 39. In the context of a relationship with a psychiatrist for another problem, she formed a solid friendship with another woman and became less anxious about her diabetes. Her pessimism decreased somewhat, and she began to think of herself as living to age 50 rather than age 39.

A sense of well-being, self-esteem, and equanimity about depending on oneself and others, and a measure of success in the face of difficulties, enhances the ability of a person with diabetes to maintain an optimistic faith about length and quality of life.

Personal Development in Adolescence

The person under acute stress tends to have a blurred self-concept.[41] The modified self-concept and defenses emerging in the child or youth following the diagnosis of diabetes tend to persist. These may be observed years later, in the setting of impending separation from important people. This young woman illustrates how the prospect of separation from family led to reemergence of turmoil after years of relative equanimity, buttressed by denial, suppression, reaction formation, and counterphobic defenses:

Within the past year, the last sibling of this 16-year-old had left home. As the imminence of her own separation from home loomed larger, she began having headaches. Referred to a psychiatrist, she reported that within a year of the onset of her diabetes at age 7, she had dreamt:

"I was alone in a boat. A big boa constrictor tipped over the boat. I thought something might reach up from the silt of the river bottom and grab my feet."

Although this adolescent thought of herself as "open," she could remember no dream since that one at age 7 or 8, and her only thought about it was that she loved snakes. She was referred to a psychiatrist in her home state for help in recognizing some of her currently unacknowledged fears and fantasies about her diabetes, and to help her find more adaptive ways of dealing with them, leaving her less vulnerable to unexplained bodily symptoms.

Although earlier attempts to link diabetes with a particular personality type have been discredited, a person with diabetes, especially when diagnosed before age 17, readily becomes cautious, anxious or pessimistic about the future. These traits can impede evolvement or maintenance of autonomy and slow the development of peer relationships. People with onset of diabetes in childhood, adolescence or young adulthood are actively deciding how they will stand on their own and work with others, what they value and who they are, sexually and vocationally. Since diabetes in youth is temporally associated with evolution of adult identity, and such patients even later as adults tend to remain fascinated by the influence of diabetes on their lives. Separations, symptoms, failures or ambiguities in later life will tend to bring the influence and implication of the onset of diabetes back into focus.

We need to understand the mechanisms by which diabetes affects the development of the person's self-image, self-esteem, and ability to play and enjoy life, empathize and otherwise share with others, set limits, renounce, identify, make commitments, and give free rein to imagination and creative self-expression. This is especially true for the 8% of the diabetic population who develop diabetes before age 17. Hauser and Jacobson[41,42] are carrying out a prospective longitudinal study of early adolescents with diabetes and their families, comparing their development with that of adolescents without diabetes. Early results suggest that diabetes may slow psychologic development of adolescents, the boys lagging characteristically behind the girls. The adolescent patients studied were not likely to be as impulsive, dependent, exploitive or given to fear or stereotyping as were psychiatric patients. However, they were more likely to be concerned with acceptance and status and less likely to be as complex, self-aware, or to place as much value on mutuality or individuality as non-patient volunteers of the same age. In the future we should like to better understand the mechanisms by which diabetes may foster the development of both compensatory strengths and coping skills, and maladaptive traits and life patterns such as inhibition, avoidance, clinging, or acting on a sense of entitlement.

Despite the need of adolescents to pull away from the direct supervision of their parents, they usually observe closely but furtively the parents' feelings and concerns. They are likely to assert that their parents' misconceptions are a handicap as they try to complete their physical and psychosocial development. They are less likely to admit how much their parents' example, realism, practicality, tolerant appreciation of their individualities and encouragement, help them to measure themselves realistically against their peers, bolster their sense of well-being and optimism, and aid them in finding the strength to complete the five major tasks of adolescence (Table 44–2). They need parents to learn from, shove off from, and check in with as they try to make a place for themselves in the world of peers.

Family circumstances and attitudes shape both health and psychosocial development in those with growth-onset diabetes far more than does specific age at onset. The onset of diabetes creates a family crisis; it poses two new responsibilities—managing the diabetes itself and coming to terms with its existence within the family—which somewhat complicates the course of the adolescent's psychosocial development. Most early adolescents pass through transitory periods of devaluating parents, rebelliousness, and intergenerational conflict in their attempts to achieve autonomy. The outcome is benign perhaps 9 times out of 10 but this struggle for autonomy is more difficult in youths with diabetes, because the need to manage their diabetes increases their dependence on the guidance and good will of their parents.

Age 17: A Turning Point. By age 17 to 20, young people without diabetes have usually become disenchanted with parents who can no longer protect them from the threatening world which they regard with great interest, and into which they are now moving with their peers.[43] White noted that as early as age 17, the inconsistent management

of diabetes often seen in the adolescent, may begin to give way to resignation and a settling for the benefits of managing the diabetes in feeling as well as possible.[44] By this time, the fortunate adolescent feels comfortable enough to explore and reveal inner aspects of self which have been relatively veiled since about age 8.[45] This is also the age at which, if the earlier relationships with parents were basically sound, the adolescent with diabetes tends to begin to open up more with the physician, and then with parents. In the years that follow, fortunate children and parents gradually reshape their relationships on a more nearly equal footing.

The usual movement from a shifting combination of minimizing and denial mechanisms and hypervigilant tensing, toward a self-respecting acceptance of oneself with diabetes and its implications, seems to begin as early as age 17. This process may be completed as early as age 35, at which time most people, without long-standing chronic conditions, are just starting to come to terms with their limitations and mortality.[46] This process gives rise to the only two benefits which can accrue to those with onset of diabetes in youth. The first is reinforcement of the ability to empathize with disadvantaged people, including mentally retarded children and people with health problems. This, together with the need for active mastery of the diabetes and identification with the physician, contributes to the fact that a relatively high proportion of youths with diabetes (7% in my group) later enter the medical professions, where some have made significant contributions to medical knowledge. This process also gives rise to a second, bittersweet benefit: a head start in coming to terms with one's limitations and mortality.[46a]

Presenting Psychiatric Problems. Although only about 5% of people with diabetes have had the onset before age 11, there is a striking overrepresentation of this early onset group among those referred for psychiatric consultation. This reflects multiple factors, including the high degree of physician interest in promoting the well-being of each member of this group, with whom a physician has worked or will work for years. In addition to significant slowing of the development of autonomy in about a fifth of these patients, as discussed earlier, these patients, half of them now in their late teens, tend to come with one of seven presenting problems, shown in Table 44–3. All seven of these problems and the timing of turning to consultation were usually linked with at least two of the circumstances mentioned earlier which transiently undercut well-being, including autonomy (Table 44–1).

Without addressing diabetes specifically, Akiskal stated that with onset of certain chronic medical

Table 44–3. Presenting Psychiatric Problems in Patients with Insulin-Dependent Diabetes Onset under age 11; present age 4–48 (midphase)

	Patients	
	Number	Percent
Fearful, pessimistic attitudes evident in context of separation in adolescence or adult life.	35	33
Mismanagement of diabetes by a school or college age youth, usually female, as a means of asserting pseudo-independence from mother while simultaneously stimulating the mother's fear of the danger of separation.	13	12
Persistent anxiety, bad dreams or nightmares, often associated with school age child's conflict with the parent of the same sex.	9	8
Mismanagement of diabetes by a child or adolescent to try to hold parents together, to justify staying home from school, or force other family behavior.	9	8
Guilty, anxious, upset parent of a child with diabetes under age 10.	8	7
Depressive disorder occurring at any age in connection with a recent important loss	7	7
Adolescent girl or young woman becoming pregnant in context of conflict-ridden relationship with mother	6	6
Other problems	20	19
Total	107	100%

conditions in childhood, such as neurologic and rheumatologic disorders, mild protracted depression is woven into personality, and parallels vicissitudes of the underlying medical condition.[47] The prevalence of gross pessimism (33%) and depressive disorder (7%) in our group was at least as high as the 32 to 40% prevalence of depressed mood in patients in the general population referred for psychiatric consultation and higher than the 20 to 24% prevalence of depressed mood reported in the general population.[48–53] This finding has implications for development of personal relationships and even for avoiding recklessness by people with onset of diabetes before age 11[54–59] (Table 44–1). The following case illustrates the interplay between the implications and complications of diabetes, relationships in the family while growing up, and present relationships and self-concept.

This 28-year-old unemployed college graduate had grown up in a middle-class family. He had a father who was understanding but remote and an easily enraged mother whom he tried to avoid. He developed diabetes at age 5. Growing up, he often felt himself to be a burden to his parents. Lacking confidence that he could develop and sustain a relationship with a woman who might come to depend on him, he substituted romantic-erotic encounters and cocaine for open-ended relationships. At times he felt he would live only a day or a week, and usually did not plan beyond that day. At other times he imagined he would live almost as long as his nondiabetic sister. His pessimism was increased by the appearance of a single small retinal hemorrhage.

In the context of helpful relationships with his doctors and a job as a legal secretary, he gave up first cocaine and then tobacco, and fine-tuned his diabetes control. He felt that without moving from a pessimistic stance,

he would be unable to sustain and then build a relationship with a woman. After meeting a man his age in the Diabetes Treatment Unit who had diabetes but who also had a family and a "future," he came to see that his pessimism was rooted not only in his diabetes, but also in his experience in his particular family. In the context of his 3-year relationship with a woman whom he saw as dependable and kind, he gained experience talking out differences of opinion. At age 32, he described his evolving image of himself and his life.

"I walk through my house, closing doors as I move from room to room and floor to floor, farther and farther from the crazy tunnels in the basement."

The next year, with a new job as a legal assistant, he trusted himself and the future looked bright enough for him to take the plunge into marriage.

DIABETES WITH ONSET AFTER THE MID-FORTIES

The person with diabetes diagnosed after age 45 is provided an abrupt and concrete reminder of mortality. These mid-life and older patients who make up two-thirds of the population with diabetes must now live with a disease which makes them more imminently vulnerable to sickness, loss of function, loss of body parts, and disability, than their spouses, contemporaries, and most younger people with diabetes. Those over age 45 may react to stressful life events with fewer symptoms than younger people, but they tend to feel the impact deeply and their symptoms tend to persist longer. If they have suffered more recent losses than positive life events, they become vulnerable to falling self-esteem and the reemergence of unresolved conflicts.[60] The positive aspects of self-concept should be shored up, conflict resolved and morale restored. Furthermore, since heredity plays a stronger role in noninsulin-dependent diabetes than in insulin-dependent diabetes, many of the over-45 patients have known relatives who suffered physical complications of diabetes—neuropathy, cataracts, heart disease, amputations, and strokes. The stresses which accompany diabetes and which make it somewhat harder for children and youths to achieve their full potential, also make it harder for people after their mid-forties to grow older with relative equanimity.

The onset of diabetes at any age is an unsettling event that increases uncertainty about the future. Working people over age 45 wonder if they will be able to keep their jobs or find new ones, and if they can maintain life, health and hospital insurance. Menopausal women with diabetes wonder if they will be able to hold up their side of the marriage, take care of themselves and still be energetic, attractive, and have interests to share with their partners. Men wonder if they will become impotent. People of both sexes tend to worry about becoming blind, losing one or both legs, and becoming "basket cases," dependent on others who may then become indifferent, contemptuous or even revolted.

The person over 45 with diabetes shares certain health and preventive issues with a nondiabetic person of the same age. Both should eat well-balanced, nutritious diets, exercise, achieve and maintain ideal body weight, accept more personal responsibility for their health, and maintain and even increase their independence.[61] However, the lifestyle of an adult who has had many years to form prediabetic living patterns and practice ways of finding comfort, may become maladaptive with the onset of diabetes. These patterns may need to be changed at a time in life when they are firmly rooted. Before diabetes, patients may have sought comfort in ways that involved social eating and drinking with others. After diagnosis, however, lack of information and experience in selecting the proper type and amount of food increases the strain of these activities and diminishes the comfort they can afford. Food can be a dependable, available comfort in itself, and treatment of diabetes plus overweight, involves specifying and limiting food, thereby decreasing the effectiveness of this form of comfort. Those who previously talked about commonly shared fears and other feelings with a close friend or family member, may now feel constrained by lack of information and by the sense of being different and placing a potential burden on the confidant.

A patient's misperception of the physician as threatening physical complications unless the patient complies with the doctor's recommendations, may undercut their relationship, increase pessimism and thereby undermine the patient's management of the diabetes. Fortunately, more relaxed assimilation of the risks of complications and how to minimize those risks—a process which may extend over years—usually helps the patient manage the diabetes more effectively.

For the older diabetic patient in fair health, learning how to manage diabetes in order to feel as well as possible and to retain as much of the structure of the previous lifestyle as possible, may be all that is needed to maintain a sense of wholeness necessary to attend to work, relationships, and diversions more interesting than diabetes.[62] Concerns of partners, spouses and other family members can also be alleviated by specific information presented with the intention of preserving as many of the former living patterns as possible.

Only 34 (9%) of the first 400 people with diabetes referred for psychiatric consultation had the onset of diabetes at age 45 or later. Books about living with diabetes, with a light touch, may be helpful for these patients.[63,64] Such patients provide a contrast with people with onset of diabetes in youth, who tend to take their disorder quite seriously. In the absence of illness, those who become diabetic in mid-life more easily succeed in diverting themselves from their diabetes and other unpleasantnesses. Most of the 34 patients with onset after age 45 were referred for psychiatric consultation only because of a substantial crisis unrelated to diabetes, and they usually saw the psychiatrist only once or twice.

Four months earlier this 55-year-old woman, with onset of diabetes at age 49, had participated with her husband in the decision for an elective operation to bring his dangerous obesity under control. She felt very guilty when he died of a heart attack after the operation, and the fact that her husband had appeared in the dreams of their two sons, while she could recall no dreams, seemed to confirm her guilt. She started working three jobs to save enough money to carry out her promise to her husband to put their youngest son through medical school. Whenever she stopped working, she thought about taking an overdose of sleeping medicine, but knew she would not do so. She did not follow the psychiatrist's advice to return for a second interview, but did drop one of her three jobs. Nine months later, the psychiatrist saw her dancing with a new husband.

A few of the 34 people with maturity-onset diabetes coming for consultation in their late 40s and 50s did come for extended, but not intensive psychiatric treatment. They were intelligent, down-to-earth, articulate, open, and proficient in work involving other people. Unlike younger patients, they did not seek help in dealing with themselves as people with diabetes. They wanted help in coming to terms with the loss of a person important to them or help in dealing with some other painful problem that was not usually connected with diabetes.

A 53-year-old man rarely drank hard liquor until his late 40s, when a series of changes began to occur: he became diabetic; his diabetic mother died; he slept less; he married for the first time and to a woman who reminded him of his mother; marital sex declined; his senile father-in-law moved in; he took on more church and Masonic activities; he ate less; and he was promoted over a life-long friend at work. With his new position came greater corporate responsibilities, including supervising two long-term acquaintances whose job performances had declined over the years. With these changes, totalling over 400 points on the Holmes-Rahe stress scale,[65] he began drinking more to sleep, became addicted, and finally consumed up to a pint of vodka a day. Two months after his promotion he allowed himself to be seen taking a drink in a parking lot at work. His supervisors warned him, and he sought psychiatric consultation. He started reviewing the stresses in his life in his first interview, and subsequently limited his drinking to two light beers after dinner. He related no dreams but talked of seeing a Mexican mother feed her shriveled infant tea because she had no milk. He returned to talk with the psychiatrist three times a year, enjoyed these sessions, and believed they protected him from returning to heavy drinking.

The Depressed Patient. A patient who meets four or five of the following Washington University research criteria for depression[66] usually benefits from anti-depressant medication: poor appetite or weight loss; sleep disturbance, including sleeping more or less than usual; fatigue, loss of energy; agitation or being slowed; loss of interest in usually stimulating activities such as job, hobbies, social activities or sex; less ability to concentrate; self-reproach or guilt; or recurrent thoughts of death or suicide, including the wish to be dead.

All tricyclic and tetracyclic antidepressants pose risks of postural hypotensive, cardiotoxic, and anticholinergic side effects, which increase the risks of treatment of people with diabetes over the age of 45.[67] This is especially true when a patient has known vascular disease, a family history of glaucoma, or an enlarged prostate. In these patients, and in those showing a pre-treatment fall in blood pressure of at least 15 mm Hg after standing quietly for 3 minutes, certain of these drugs, such as desipramine (Norpramin, Pertofrane), pose a relatively low risk of either postural hypotensive or anticholinergic side effects. In elderly patients in whom dose requirements are usually 15 to 50% of the usual adult prescription, side effects should be monitored and may be minimized by dividing daily quantities into two or three doses and increasing the dose relatively slowly.

Trazodone (Desyrel), chemically unrelated to the drugs discussed above, has little anticholinergic activity or cardiovascular toxicity. However, a tendency to cause postural hypotension, usually evident in the first 4 days of treatment, can increase the risk of falling.

DIABETES AND OBESITY

Both physiologic and psychosocial factors are known to increase the tendency to obesity. Damage to the hypothalamic satiety center, reduced activity of the sodium "pump," endogenous opioid peptide production,[68] and certain endocrine diseases such as hyperadrenocorticism and hypothyroidism are some physical reasons. Family and cultural patterns of eating, persistent high caloric intake in persons whose level of activity has dropped, and certain overeating behaviors triggered by separation and loneliness[69] are some psychosocial factors. In addition, an overeating-dieting pattern, to which women may be especially vulnerable in our culture, may undermine efficient natural appetite and eating control mechanisms.[70]

Eating over the meal plan frequently threatens the well-being of patients with both insulin-dependent and non-insulin-dependent diabetes, at all ages.[71] The psychologic goal is to identify the particular, widely varying problems that contribute to a patient's compulsion to overeat, and to help each person come to grips with them in order to regain control of eating habits and move toward more normal blood glucose levels and desired weight.

Behavior Modification, Peer Pressure, Diet Counseling, and Psychotherapy

Although behavior modification programs and peer pressure often lead to weight loss, the results of one study suggest that psychotherapy is likely to be a helpful supplement for patients who become obese by age 11, while diet counseling is likely to be an effective adjunct for patients who become obese after age 19.[72] Having settled on a tentative treatment plan, the doctor may continue as the primary therapist for obesity, often with a supplemental referral to a weight reduction support group, a nutritionist, therapeutic dietitian or teaching nurse with appropriate training in behavior modification. Since women with a pattern of upper body obesity are 8 times more likely to develop diabetes than other women, and since this pattern is associated with fat cells capable of shrinking, many obese women with diabetes can lose weight relatively easily by sticking to a prescribed meal plan. The woman with lower body obesity will find it relatively difficult to lose weight, even when she sticks to her meal plan faithfully. Even if she succeeds, her upper body may become thin while she remains obese from the hips down.[73]

Weight loss can usually be achieved by a program of diet, exercise, psychologic support, education, cognitive and behavioral reinforcement, and sometimes spouse and peer pressure. Although intermittent administration of sympathicomimetic appetite suppressant such as fenfluramine, diethylproprion, or phentermine, may be a useful short-term adjunct,[74–76] prolonged use of such drugs should be avoided.

Those who lose weight during the initial program and then regain it may need a maintenance program, based on the concept that until we learn more, theirs is a problem that will require lifetime effort. Patients who actively adhere to their maintenance programs are rewarded by their growing sense of active mastery and the knowledge that they are treating themselves well. For further discussion of obesity and diabetes, see Chapter 18.

WORST FEARS

Adult onset patients tend to imagine the same worst fears as those with onset in youth.

> "After I become blind, my gangrenous limbs will be amputated and I shall be totally dependent on others. Ultimately, people will withdraw. At the end, I shall be helpless and friendless, in strange surroundings."

Relative dependence on family and one or more daily injections of insulin make it difficult for an adolescent to divert attention from the implications of having diabetes for more than a few hours at a time. Because the onset of diabetes in youth is profoundly upsetting, these patients are often driven, like trauma victims, alternately to avoid the subject and not to talk about it. In those with onset of diabetes as adults, this worst fear is further from awareness and less of a backdrop for the rest of their lives. As long as they feel well, they turn their attention to other matters with relative ease.

A key step in helping people to relax is to ask them their worst fear.[77] Sometimes the physician can lead the patient and the partner, when both are rested and feeling fairly well, to share and exchange their worst fears, so that both will feel less tense and closer to each other. This exchange tends to undercut the tendency for inhibition in talking freely together to spread to other areas. Ideally the internist inquires about worst fears or delegates this task to the psychiatrist or someone supervised by a psychiatrist.

HYPOGLYCEMIA

Under certain circumstances both insulin and oral hypoglycemic agents can cause the blood glucose to fall below 40 mg/dl. This stimulates counter-regulatory hormones, giving rise to a protean range of signs and symptoms, and functional impairment. The epinephrine response to rapidly falling blood glucose, with tremor and sweating, often accompanied by weakness, hunger, unsteady movements and blurred vision, is relatively easy for a patient to identify, except that in middle-aged women, occasionally it may be mistaken for a menopausal hot flash. With the passage of years, some people with diabetes develop neuropathy of the autonomic nervous system, dampening the helpful glucagon and epinephrine responses to rapid fall in blood glucose,[79–82] and resulting in "insulin reactions without warning."

Patients with panic attacks may believe they are hypoglycemic; home glucose monitoring settles such questions. If panic attacks occur frequently without hypoglycemia, patients should be referred for psychiatric evaluation and treatment.

In contrast to acute hypoglycemia, gradual fall in blood glucose to low levels, especially likely to occur at night, shows up in slow, confused thinking, passivity, drowsiness, and impaired initiative, sometimes with transiently impaired memory and lessened ability to judge the passage of time. In the latter type of hypoglycemia, ideally the patient makes the self-diagnosis of hypoglycemia when the blood glucose is low enough to notice, yet still high enough to permit the judgment that thinking is slowed. The decision at this "window" must be made without the aid of dramatic neuromuscular signs or outpouring of epinephrine. At a blood glucose of about 60 mg/dl, patients recall mathematical facts more slowly, and in order to add correctly they do so more slowly.[82a] If the patient fails to make the self-diagnosis at that point, either because of preoccupation or sleep, judgment will become too impaired to do so. At this stage, mental incompetence becomes grossly and painfully apparent to others.

If hypoglycemia goes undetected and untreated with carbohydrate or glucagon for many hours and the patient's blood glucose falls to extremely low levels despite rise in counterregulatory hormones, the patient may lose consciousness. Ultimately, after some hours, the blood glucose begins to rise, the patient regains consciousness and, after a period of daze, almost invariably recovers full neurologic function. However, with much circulating insulin, hours of profound hypoglycemia can cause central nervous system damage similar to that caused by hypoxia.[82b,82c]

In addition to any transient or permanent impairment of brain function, repeated hypoglycemic episodes have the cumulative deleterious effect of undercutting the patient's and partner's sense that the patient is dependable. Hypoglycemia may harm the marital relationship, academic achievement, and performance on the job.

Patients should be taught that the pessimism or plummeting self-esteem which accompanies a flagging sense of competence is usually a useful subjective clue that they are hypoglycemic and should signal them to ingest glucose immediately. Other emotional and cognitive signs of hypoglycemia include slowing to maintain accuracy, slowed grasp of spoken or written information, difficulty in recalling people's names, place names or titles, loss of emotional delicacy, a euphoric conviction of being extraordinarily self-sufficient despite appearances to the contrary,[82d] or, conversely, the impression that others possess extraordinary mental acuity (See also Chapters 19 and 24).

STRESS AND DIABETES

Ideally, to minimize fluctuations in blood glucose, a patient should balance not only medication, meal plans, and exercise, but also stress. Stressful changes in the life circumstances and psychophysiologic state of a person with diabetes may conceivably lead to changes in levels of circulating hormones and to deviations from normal blood glucose levels—even though insulin or oral hypoglycemic agents, meal plans, and exercise—are held relatively constant. Such hormones include cortisol, catecholamines, glucagon, growth hormone, and beta-endorphin.[83] Common stressful changes include not only menstruation, infection, febrile illness, injury, or hypoglycemia itself, which can cause uncomfortable rebound to high blood glucose levels, but also overload of responsibility and other adversely stressful challenges from relationships and circumstances. In those with insulin-dependent diabetes, stress of sufficient intensity can lead to rise of blood glucose and ketones, and may even lead to ketoacidosis if insulin is not increased. Fluctuations in blood glucose from such stresses can often be anticipated and prevented.

One busy mother learned to take two extra units of insulin with the onset of premenstrual tension and to drop this extra insulin on the second day of her period.

A law student noticed a week of steadily rising blood glucose while studying for his final examinations. He appropriately and gradually raised his insulin dose until he was taking an extra six units, 110% of his usual dose each day. Within 5 minutes of handing in his final examination, he became quite confused and uncoordinated from rapidly falling blood glucose. He avoided a repetition when he took his law board examination by eating candy as he neared the end of the examination.

The emotional sustenance, information and material aid provided by a partner, family, friends and others help to maintain well-being and prevent illness in times of stress.[54-58] Healthy young people can usually name about two dozen people important to them. However, one confidant, physician or friend can have great effect.

Jacobson and colleagues provide a review of some of the observations made and experiments carried out on effects of stress on the homeostasis of the person with diabetes.[84] Groups in Boston, Wichita, Durham, Albuquerque, and Jacksonville have begun developing programs to help patients reduce the fluctuations in blood glucose which result from adverse psychosocial stress. Methods range from teaching progressive muscular relaxation to exercising regularly and joining a mutual support group.[85]

Early Complications Related to Stress

A majority of those with onset of diabetes before age 11 referred for psychiatric consultation, felt physically well and were free from late physical complications of diabetes. However, within this group of 155 predominantly healthy patients, there were 43 (28%) with early physical complications (see Table 44–4). Twelve of the 15 patients who had developed permanent physical complications within 2 to 19 years after onset of diabetes had stressful parental influences as shown in Table 44–5.

Viewed retrospectively, these family-related stresses seemed to have caused fluctuations in blood glucose and to have diverted attention or mischanneled efforts needed to manage insulin, meal plan, exercise and stress to feel as well as possible. By history, these children had inadequate metabolic control, as did children in the chaotic families that Koski described as having internal cliques and showing severe conflicts, helplessness, and poor cooperation.[86] In predisposed families, these parental characteristics and events apparently contribute to metabolic mismanagement and probably to early appearance of complications. Evaluation of families with a member whose glyco-

Table 44–4. Permanent Physical Complications in 155 Patients Referred for Psychiatric Consultation with Onset of Diabetes Before Age 11

Ages of Patients Referred	Number of Patients	Patients with Permanent Physical Complications	
		Number	(%)
0–10	15	0	0
11–12	8	2	25
13–19	54	9	17
20–45	71	28	39
46+	7	4	57
All ages	155	43	28%

Table 44–5.   Parental Characteristics or Events Affecting 12 (80%) of 15 Patients with Insulin-Dependent Diabetes Mellitus (IDDM) with Onset Before Age 11, and with Permanent Physical Complications Within 2–19 Years

Male Patients	Female Patients
Father could not accept son with IDDM.	Father was grossly depressed.
Father was grossly depressed.	Father left family in difficult straits when daughter was age 4.
Mother with IDDM disliked son with IDDM.	Mother was grossly depressed.
Mother was ineffective caretaker.	Mother with IDDM mismanaged her own IDDM.
	Mother died in accident when daughter was age 21, followed by daughter's gross mismanagement of diabetes.

sylated hemoglobin remains markedly elevated before age 11, may identify points at which modest psychosocial efforts may increase and extend well-being and may possibly even extend life for some at high risk for early complications (Table 44–5).

Achievement and Stress

Selye showed the severe damaging effects of stress on animal and human organisms.[87] He also emphasized the beneficial effects of light and moderate stress. Immigrant achievement in America may be an example of beneficial response to stress. The most that could be achieved under the severe and constant life threat of a prisoner in a Nazi concentration camp was to add a deeper meaning to one's life and to remain brave, dignified and unselfish, an extraordinary feat.[88]

Patients with both juvenile and adult-onset diabetes have made promising original contributions in writing, medical science, and the arts, and have achieved or maintained preeminence in sports, entertainment, writing, painting, and medical science. For example, George R. Minot, whose life was prolonged by insulin after onset of Type I diabetes in his twenties, discovered the treatment for pernicious anemia working with Murphy and Whipple.

COMPLICATIONS

In a country where advances in treatment of infectious diseases have greatly reduced morbidity and mortality, diabetes has become the leading cause of disability over the age of 45 and the lead-

ing cause of new blindness. The incidence of terminal kidney failure is increased 17 times, that of amputation 15 times, and that of coronary infarct and stroke doubled, when diabetes is present. Impairments are manifested by angina, claudication, myocardial or central nervous system infarction, visual impairment at times progressing to blindness, hypertension and proteinuria progressing to renal insufficiency, and persistent troublesome muscular weakness, numbness, erectile impotence, or diarrhea. Persistent hyperglycemia in children can lead to short stature in adults. Profound, prolonged hypoglycemia can lead to a permanent encephalopathy. Cosmetically embarrassing skin complications include lipodystrophy and necrobiosis lipoidica. Stillbirths and the births of children with distressing congenital anomalies have profound lasting impact on the would-be mother with diabetes.

Adaptation. The way in which a patient experiences each phase of diabetes is determined by what a person's present circumstances evoke from past experiences. The third and last phase of living with diabetes is characterized by permanent physical complications and the need to adapt to them. These tend to threaten self-esteem, stir up anxiety about losing hard-won skills and competence, bodily functions and parts, and produce guilt, shame, fear of retaliation for shortcomings, and anxiety about losing the approval, affection and respect of family, friends, and people at work. These stresses are greatly magnified by any physical distress and increasing disability. The literature on chronic illness suggests that those who adapt most readily to complications have a vital interest in life and the affection and respect of others; membership in a group that will come to one's aid, flexibility to manage under changing circumstances; freedom from oversensitivity; congeniality; willingness to shoulder responsibility; and adequate income and housing.[89]

Patients with the least tolerance for distress, those with labile diabetes, those with angina, and those with fluctuating mental acuity may be most inclined to minimize, forget, and compartmentalize distressing problems, fears, and feelings of helplessness. These patients may believe that to face feelings and to deal with interpersonal conflict may cause deterioration of health. At the same time, a patient's fear of alienating those who give access to medical care may curb open expression of anger or resentment, thereby increasing passive-aggressive or passive-dependent behavior. To continue to rigidly avoid emotional distress delays resolution of conflict and increases the family's burden and the patient's frustration, anger, and despair. In this way the patient's prolonged avoidance impedes rehabilitation and ultimately increases morbidity and mortality. If the patient's behavior suggests that serious psychologic problems are present, the primary physician should arrange further evaluation. Ideally, this will be done by a psychiatrist experienced in work with patients with diabetes, or by a psychiatrist-supervised nurse, social worker, psychologist, or other professional counselor. As Strain[12] has noted for chronic illness in general, the nature and quality of the patient's adaptation in this phase of the diabetes is determined by (a) the degree of regression to earlier patterns of behavior under stress; (b) the conflict in the patient and between the patient and others stirred up by that regression; and (c) the nature and quality of the patient's relationships with others.

With onset of serious complications of diabetes, the patient comes to draw on the reserves of family members. When a nuclear family has only two adult members, is isolated from the extended family, and both parents are working, it is less likely to be equipped to carry on with this extra burden. Such a nuclear family, like many single parent families and single adults under stress, may be unable to sustain both its healthy and chronically sick members, for the demands are heavy, physically and emotionally, as illustrated here.

A 70-year-old widow with many years of poorly controlled, noninsulin-dependent diabetes had a myocardial infarction. This was followed by 3 months of despondency during which she wanted to fight off this feeling with activities, such as helping others, which were previously appropriate but now physically unwise. After the heart attack and death of a neighbor, she developed more chest pain, relieved some by nitroglycerine, and became frankly depressed. She wanted to help others instead of being a burden, but her agitation was so great that her married daughters felt the need to telephone her 10 to 12 times daily.

A person refusing to enter into new and more onerous living arrangements required by lower levels of function may reject his situation by suicide, divorce, or abandonment. While a patient with renal insufficiency may talk of suicide, further exploration usually reveals that person wants to live on as long and as well as possible.[90] The chronically ill, as well as many of their partners, family members and close friends, are remarkably able to accommodate to simpler levels of interaction and style. Because of what the relationship means to them, they strive artfully and tenaciously to keep their interactions, their relationships and their lives as much the same as possible. They learn to help each other regard the changes and differences between them as unimportant.[91]

Visual Impairment. Blank has described the profound difference between being born without sight and losing one's sight.[92] Fitzgerald concisely described the phenomonology of new blindness, including recurrent denial of aspects of blindness, visual illusions during the day and frequently, heightened vividness of colors in dreams. He noted that initial reactions to visual impairment included depression and anxiety, withdrawal, bodily complaints, anger, thoughts of suicide, sleeplessness, guilt, shame, and self-blame, usually limited in duration. Use of the white cane ususally signals accepting oneself as blind and ready for rehabilitation as a blind person. In three-fourths of the recently blind, one or two particular experiences continue to trigger pangs of sadness, regret, anger, or low self-esteem.[93] The author confirmed these findings and noted that all confrontations with blindness tend to stir up other past losses, and some confrontations, like this one, precipitate depression:

A 62-year-old widowed grandmother with onset of insulin-dependent diabetes at age 10 had adapted well to 20 years of progressive visual loss. Recently she started wearing dark-tinted glasses to make the most of her remaining 30% vision in one eye. When her favorite grandson, age 7, kept distance between them and said, "Don't wear those dark glasses," she became depressed and decided she did not want to "live blind."

The following case illustrates the difficulty of coming to terms with fluctuating visual impairment.

An 18-year-old college freshman with onset of insulin-dependent diabetes at age 6 had 2 months of fluctuating vision, followed by light-shadow vision alternating with blindness, before becoming totally blind. The patient made a suicidal gesture, and her fiance left her. Her imaginings of the life she would have had with this man were filled with light and colors, showing how hard it was for her to separate her longings for life with him from longings to see. While taking atropine eye drops, she had a recurrent vision:

> "A line of 4- or 5-year-old boys, dressed in brightly colored plaid shirts, are jumping up and down on very green grass, waving their fists all around."

At first this intense vision of the children frightened her because she could not stop it, but as the atropine was reduced, it stopped, and she "wished they'd come back." After 8 months of blindness, she learned to use a white cane. She returned to college and began dating a young man whom she liked. Twice her vision returned to the point that she could read and just as quickly deteriorated. She made a second suicidal gesture. She wished she would either go permanently blind or get better. It was impossible to plan; she felt anguished and "in limbo."

Oehler has written a series of papers which describe the psychologic phases through which she and other blind people with diabetes have passed, and their special problems of rehabilitation.[94–96] Others have noted that the discovery that loss of sight does not entail loss of sexual potency becomes a part of recovery, and, furthermore, that multiple aids and agencies exist to improve the quality of life for the visually handicapped person—resources which all too often have been unknown to the doctor.[97–100]

Peripheral Vascular Disease and Amputation. Levin wrote that approximately 30% of people with diabetes eventually develop peripheral vascular disease.[101] There are indirect preventive steps such as stopping smoking, following antihypertensive and foot care regimens, and attention to insulin, meal plans, and exercise. For some patients with larger arterial blockage, endarterectomy, bypass surgery and transcutaneous angioplasty are helpful, but others eventually require amputation. Both a patient with amputation of a limb and those closest to the patient feel the amputation personally and deeply. Some relatives may have just as much trouble accepting the patient with the amputation as does the patient, further impeding the amputee's self-acceptance,[102] as illustrated here:

A 25-year-old single man with onset of insulin-dependent diabetes at age 2 had had a below-knee amputation. After learning that he would be going home without a permanent prosthesis, he lay for a week curled up in his hospital bed, refusing to get up to be weighed or to allow blood to be drawn. He said that he had given up and added, apparently without sarcasm:

"I need to give myself a boot to get going."

He reported two dreams:

"I was on the police force, running after this guy who'd broken into a store. I cornered him, caught him, booked him, and locked him up."
"The Babe Ruth Baseball League didn't want me any more."

His mother refused to talk with the psychiatrist until his father insisted. She felt unable to subject herself to the anguish of investing herself in his rehabilitation. She felt it was hopeless, since he would not live long, and had given up. After listening to the psychiatrist discuss how his parents could help their son through his despondency, she asked his father with tearful irritation, "Why did you do this to me?" Both the patient and his mother told the psychiatrist separately that the patient was "a failure," as if the amputation had set his value and set it low. This put up a wall between them, limited them to "small talk," and delayed his self-acceptance and rehabilitation.

The patient's post-amputation adjustment depends on pre-surgery physical and psychologic characteristics of patient and family, and their preparation. If both are properly prepared for the am-

putation, the patient is more likely to regard the artificial limb as part of himself.[103–105]

Neuropathy and Erectile Impotence. As a complication of diabetes, neuropathy can cause such disparate symptoms as numbness, foot drop, diarrhea, pain, and total erectile impotence. The last-named condition is especially distressing. While some men with diabetes do not have to cope with long-term impotence, in a significant proportion of those who do, neuropathy is present. Levine provides a sound overview of erectile dysfunction.[106] Schiavi and Hogan reviewed the literature on impotence as a complication of diabetes and the effect of diabetes on female sexual response.[107]

The causes of erectile impotence are many, both physiologic and psychologic, transient and permanent. With so many possible causes, it is small wonder that sometimes a case cannot be classified as either psychologic, situational or organic; it is a combination. In the absence of regular use of narcotic or certain antihypertensive medications, a history of diabetes and more than a year of gradually increasing penile flaccidity despite sexual desire, even with genital stimulation is presumptive evidence of diabetic erectile impotence.

For 3 years, this 58-year-old man with onset of insulin-dependent diabetes at age 6, had had increasing difficulty sustaining a full erection long enough to have intercourse. The 55-year-old wife of 7 years had been upset, wondering if she was fulfilling her role as a wife if he was not sexually satisfied. He had felt waves of sexual excitement and frustration holding his wife, and felt his erectile impotence might make the relationship mean less for her. Two weeks earlier he had dreamt:

"My wife and I were trying to paddle up the river in a canoe. We'd make a little progress, lose it, wind up in the water. We were struggling, trying to make it, not succeeding."

Absent or incomplete sleep-related erections are confirmatory. As a manifestation of an autonomic neuropathy, erectile impotence usually accompanies incomplete emptying of the bladder, postural hypotension, relatively small dark-adapted pupils, slow initial iris response to light or retrograde ejaculation into the bladder.[108–112] More rarely, it stems from aortic or iliac artery atherosclerosis.[112]

Once diabetic impotency is diagnosed, one of three types of stiffening penile implants may be warranted.[112] A penile implant may be especially good when a personal relationship exists between the patient and his sexual partner. In view of the complexities and subtleties of sexuality and relationships, it is well to suggest that the patient bring in his partner so that the physician may talk with them both singly and together to discuss (a) their past sexual histories, (b) their expectations of the implant, (c) the objective advantages and disadvantages of each of these courses of action, and (d) any issues which have arisen between them. Ideally, before the patient makes his decision, he should be offered the opportunity to talk by telephone with someone who faced a similar situation and elected to try the procedure. About 25,000 men with diabetes now have such implants, which allow them to engage in coitus, experience orgasm and ejaculate. In one study, 81% of men were satisfied with the implant; outside of the few complications, only 1% were displeased.[113] Usually wives can accept their husbands' ability to have intercourse with the presence of the implant.

See Chapters 31 and 32 of this book for additional comments regarding erectile impotence.

Heart and Kidney Complications. Angina, myocardial infarction, and heart or kidney insufficiency are especially distressing to patients who become symptomatic and limited in function in their 20s and 30s. Having known an active life, they see themselves as having reached only the threshold of adult life. While the psychopathologic tradition emphasizes the undependable and unsatisfactory nature of gross denial as a way of dealing with the unpleasant, everyone uses denial at moments throughout life. Work with patients in the acute recovery phase of myocardial infarction and patients on renal dialysis suggests that while marked denial of the illness and its dangers produces problems, the recall of reassuring facts and the minimizing of other facts with frightening implications helps many patients achieve equanimity and survive.[114] For patients with coronary insufficiency, fury at the dinner table may be all that is needed to precipitate severe anginal episode. Such patients can learn to manage their rising rage and other emotional states in order to minimize the chance of overtaxing compromised circulation. Cassem and Hackett have noted the usefulness of defining, by means of metabolic equivalents, safe activity levels for patients recovering from myocardial infarctions. Depression calls for treatment, for there is evidence that following myocardial infarction, patients who are clinically depressed have a more complicated hospital course of recovery[115] and are less likely to survive 5 years.[116] Post-infarction patients and patients with angina, heart or kidney insufficiency often become despondent without meeting the criteria for treatment with antidepressants. Cassem described how the physician may, by personal exchanges, improve and maintain such a patient's self-esteem and sense of well-being.[117–119]

Crises in Treatment of the Patient with Kidney Problems. The beginning of either dialysis or a kidney transplant is a crisis for the patient and the family. The combination of the patient's and family members' fears and strongly held attitudes, the force of the rapidly changing medical needs of the patient, plus the medical organization's forceful way of moving to meet those needs, frustrates the patient in his desire to be his own prime mover.[120] Especially in the patient with a high creatinine level, neuropsychiatric symptoms and signs include malaise, fatigue, diminished appetite, diminished ability to cooperate, restlessness, irritability with angry outbursts, erratic short and intermediate memory, and fluctuating ability to concentrate.[121,122] One engineer, for example, could work only 15 minutes on a good day to complete a difficult mathematical problem. With the large shifts in water and other blood components from the patient to the dialysis machine and back again, the patient may experience drowsiness, headache, thirst and weight gain. These problems may be minimized by sophisticated application of available technical knowledge.[123,124]

Also, the patient is likely to hate intensely the machine which sustains life only if he is obedient to a rigid schedule. At the same time, he is likely to become intensely afraid of being separated from it. Reichman and Levy have described three successive phases of adaptation to maintenance hemodialysis and the complicating intensity of relationships developing between the patient and the nurses who spend 15 hours a week with him in administering this life-sustaining treatment.[125] It may be that continuous ambulatory peritoneal dialysis (CAPD) will prove not only less expensive than hemodialysis, but also a practical means of freeing the patient from much of the tyranny of the hemodialysis program.[126,127]

Piening[128] has described how behavior of patients with renal insufficiency may regress to resemble behavior at the time of initial diagnosis of diabetes. Expectations are shattered, family roles change, and marriages are severely stressed. Whether or not the marriage survives, both spouses need help in dealing with their feelings and worries and those of their children.[120]

Campbell and Campbell describe the demeaning process of finding money for the expensive treatments of dialysis and transplant, and the heavy personal toll extracted from a couple engaged in home dialysis.[129] Not surprisingly, the patients who do best on chronic hemodialysis have high frustration tolerance and families with a strong parental partnership, respect for individuality in a context of closeness and warm, affectionate, optimistic behavior with other family members.[130,131]

In one study, only 23% of patients with diabetes on dialysis were able to carry out productive physical activities.[132] Patients receiving kidney transplants from a living relative may feel guilt, overwhelming obligation, some sense of being mixed up with the donor, or the sense that more than a kidney has been donated. They need to be concerned enough to take practical precautions without being disabled by fear of losing the transplant.[133] Patients with kidney transplants, like other patients who are continually confronted with the uncertainty of life, feel it is dangerous to remain quiet and passive, and echo Satchel Paige, the pitcher who said, "Don't look back, something may be gaining on you," as illustrated in this case:

A 35-year-old divorced man with insulin-dependent diabetes since age 20 noticed deteriorating vision after his father died, when the patient was 31 years old. Now he was blind, with kidney insufficiency. His body had rejected the kidney transplanted from his mother. His mother said, "We're a corporation," and added, "He can have both my kidneys and both of my eyes if I get a guarantee." When the patient was introduced to the psychiatrist in a small group, he joked about the "Kaffee Klatsch" and said he had survived so far because of a good sense of humor. In the interview which followed, the psychiatrist remained relatively quiet in the hope of helping this blind, dying man to deal with his fears of helplessness. The patient said he had become panicky while shaving, fearing he was bleeding in some way "too horrible" to describe. He also joked that he had asked for a "meat-eating kidney" but had received a "milk-drinking kidney" instead.

The following illustration of a patient whom I followed from the time of her transplant until her death, reveals both the ambivalence such a patient feels about family and physicians, and its ultimate resolution. She also illustrates how young adults under adverse circumstances of transplant and steroid complications may choose to look inward, attending to their dreams, coming to terms with their worst fears instead of running, and regaining appreciation of emotional nuances. Some develop themselves and their relationships, learn, and achieve a great deal:

A high school graduate and secretary, with onset of insulin-dependent diabetes at age 11, had kidney insufficiency followed by a kidney transplant from her mother at age 24. Avoiding introspection for some months, she finally related this dream:

"I was dressed in black, pedaling a black and white bicycle as fast as I could on a road with white exit signs and no trees. I was being chased by three men in a black limousine who wore white shirts and black suits. It was getting dark and there were no street lights."

She awoke terrified. She thought that the men in the dream might be malevolent undertakers or members of the underworld. Her psychiatrist encouraged her to find out more about these men by "meeting" them as she finished her dream on another night. The patient's bad dreams did not disappear, but they became less frequent and the content of the dreams became less frightening as more details emerged from them. For example, one of the men in the limousine turned out to behave kindly and to wear a brightly colored sports shirt.

The patient wanted to compress a lifetime into whatever time she had and wanted to make some contribution. In the 9 years following her transplant, she reaffirmed life by cultivating 150 house plants, learned to play the flute proficiently, and worked for the Kidney Foundation as a speaker and volunteer visitor to other patients facing transplants. She participated in educational programs of the American Diabetes Association, fought her way into and graduated with highest honors from college and nursing school, helped write a manual used to interpret intelligence test results, and wrote articles published in nursing journals and Diabetes Forecast. She was named one of Ten Outstanding American Women of the year and received the Distinguished Graduate Award and an appointment to the Adjunct Faculty of the school of nursing which had refused at first to admit her. Even as she was finishing school, publishing, and receiving these honors, she was having many stress fractures, infections, and operations, including amputation of a toe. She developed cataracts, retinopathy, muscle weakness, and severe ischemic pain of both hands. As these complications accumulated, she had a recurrent dream which she first experienced as dismal, frightening and hopeless:

"I'm in the middle of a circle of people who continue to wrap a huge rope around me and then to wrap others in the group wearing brightly colored clothing with the same rope until I'm crunched in the center of a sea of people. They all look at me, without pushing or shoving, but I am unable to get loose."

In later dreams which repeated this theme as her complications progressed, the slack in the rope decreased and the people were wrapped ever more closely around her. The patient had lived 9 years between the discomfort of feeling suffocated by the reasonable care of her family and doctors and the fear of being torn from people and life. She focused on trying to become "more tolerant" of the feelings her constricting circumstances evoked. She wrote her friends, most of them doctors and nurses by now, on stationary decorated with a tree pushing up a rainbow. She died during an operation a few hours after having telephoned her mother to say she loved her, having lived over 9 years with her mother's transplanted kidney, far longer than any person with diabetes and a kidney transplant had yet lived. Her mother sent her doctors notes of thanks on stationary decorated with a colored butterfly flying through dusk. To use the patient's image, like Dante's traveler, she seemed to become reconciled to being part of a huge circle of care and concern without need to run.

TREATMENT

Most visits to a primary care physician, most hospitalizations, and most referrals for psychiatric consultation follow alterations in the balance within two or more of the pairs of conditions listed in Table 44–1. Occasionally a patient will develop very troublesome bodily symptoms while continuing to enjoy most or all of the other conditions usually associated with feeling and functioning well. More commonly, a change in the balance within only two of these pairs tends to influence the associated conditions and alters the patient's comfort, well-being, and level of function accordingly.

At least a third of patients who visit a primary care physician have no physical or biomedical ailment,[1a] and the timing of most hospitalizations of patients with diabetes appear to hinge at least partly on nonmedical events such as the loss of a boy friend. Helping a patient change one or more psychosocial conditions (which the patient may not have mentioned initially) often helps that patient to feel and function rather more effectively, without expensive hospitalization, tests, procedures, or loss of time from work or other responsibilities. Although patients tend to detest what they see as manipulation, the likelihood of mutual respect and good feeling all around is high when the doctor conveys respect and interest, clarifies choices, and works out an agreement with the patient on treatment goals.

Patient-Physician Relationship

Much of the therapeutic task of the primary care physician is educational.[134] The doctor must help the patient and family to learn specific steps which support maintenance of relative euglycemia and well-being, even in the context of stressful circumstances, which range from infection to feeling alone in the face of an extreme challenge. Physicians attribute therapeutic value to the patient-doctor relationship, especially in chronic medical conditions. This is reflected in the presumption that the best treatment includes continuity of care. A growing literature confirms that an empathic relationship can cushion the adverse impact of stresses which would otherwise disrupt homeostasis and well-being. The physician supports development or maintenance of both the patient's independence and interdependence with peers. Directly or working through others, the primary care physician can often help the patient and family to feel and function better and manage the diabetes as well as possible by taking some of the following steps:

Demonstrate acceptance of the just-diagnosed pre-school child by affectionately holding or touching the child while informing the parents of the diagnosis.

Encourage patient and spouse, or parents of a child when the child is not present, to describe and exchange upsetting experiences and worst fears (i.e., unduly pessimistic fears of failing in care or of the patient dying). Explore similarities and dissimilarities between current and past, even remote, situations. The patient and family may explain the roots and sources of the worst fears to the primary physician or psychiatrist, social worker or nurse. This helps re-establish the perspective needed to become relaxed enough in the care of the person with diabetes.[23,77]

Treat or refer for psychiatric evaluation and treatment any patient, spouse, parent or other member of the family with a depressive disorder.

Encourage all in the family to collaborate actively from the outset (e.g., in partnership with the mother, the father can become more actively involved in their children's care in ways that will strengthen the parents' partnership.[23,135,137]

Encourage the patient's active exploration, understanding, organizing, and taking responsibility. Make it plain that ultimately, the person with diabetes will probably become the person best able to manage it.

Explain treatment positively, in terms of feeling well, a full life, and lengthened life expectancy, rather than in terms of consequences and non-adherence[138] (e.g., warmly and respectfully acknowledge the primary importance of the patient's having taken the appropriate dose of insulin regularly and add that by following the meal plan, the patient may feel and function even better). Join patient and family in ingeniously preserving pleasant, healthful living patterns; pass along other patients' creative solutions to problems of living with diabetes.[91] In discussing diabetes and its management with patient and family, use clear, neutral language. Terms such as "eating over the meal plan" sound better than "cheating on the diet," even if the latter is said with a smile. "Managing the meal plan, insulin and exercise to feel well" is clearer and more neutral than "achieving good control." "Measuring blood or urine glucose" has a more pleasant sound than "testing." "Renal insufficiency" sounds better than "renal failure." Patients prefer being described as "people who happen to have diabetes" and not "diabetics."

Provide follow-up, weekly or quarterly, depending on needs.

Encourage members of the family to talk with corresponding members of a family of a similar patient. When a patient discusses experiences with a similar patient, when the patient's spouse discusses experiences with another spouse, or when parents discuss with other parents of diabetic children their experiences with their child, all feel more understood, less alone, and more confident.[21,22]

Encourage a hesitant patient and family to take a chance when a new independent effort by the patient is quite likely to succeed. By simultaneously expressing realistic concerns about another family member, the physician may direct the limelight away from the patient. The respite may help the patient take the autonomous step, while family attention is diverted to the other family member.[137]

Benefits of the Peer Group

Certain activities with peers are likely to provide a youth with models for self-respecting identification, increase self-acceptance with diabetes, and enhance development of interdependence with friends. Examples of such activities include participation in camp activities with other campers and counselors with insulin-dependent diabetes; working in committees of diabetic youths in carrying out executive and social functions; and taking part in mutual support groups. The finding in two studies, that self-esteem in adolescents at a diabetes camp was usually as high or higher than in nondiabetic campers, probably reflects the beneficial effect of being with diabetic peers who are in relatively good health.[139,140] When peers with diabetes are counselors, running the camp with obvious proficiency and flair, the effect is greatly magnified; one new arrival at camp in the 1970s described this experience as "Diabetic Power." Confidants and peer support help to modify developmental arrests in adolescents exposed to war trauma,[141–143] and may go far in preventing problems and enhancing development in adolescents with diabetes.

The powerful influence of peer groups has not been fully used in Western medicine up to now, perhaps as Marmor suggests, because of the strong individualistic theme in our culture.[144] In the future, physicians will probably make more effective use of the group as a therapeutic influence, especially in chronic medical conditions such as diabetes.

Rehabilitation After Permanent Loss of Function

In addition to some of the therapeutic steps mentioned in the previous list, including treating depressive disorders in any member of the family, the personal physician[89] attempts to:

Maintain open communication with the patient who should feel that the physician is someone in whom to confide and who improves the patient's quality of life.

Elicit the worst fears of the patient and key family member, and explore their perceptions of similarities and differences between the present family situation and past circumstances.

Help the family understand that part of a patient's regression after a medical event may be temporary.

Help the family grasp that partial disability of a parent or spouse with diabetes, even though significant, is not total. With support, the patient can sometimes carry out responsible activities which help the family, such as supervising the children, bringing in income, and with help, running the household.

Help the family tolerate the patient's expression of fears

and feelings that recovery may never take place or that death may occur.

Help dispel the patient's dread of abandonment by the family, yet help the patient to function as autonomously as possible.

Help mobilize any needed support from outside the family.

Help the family abstain from explicit or implicit criticism when the patient is unable to carry on as before.

Tailor rehabilitation goals so that, rather than seeming to be discouragingly impossible, some progress toward those goals is definitely possible.

Convey the attitude that the patient is worth the effort of medical personnel and that learning to live despite complications is possible and worth the patient's effort.

Recurring Themes in Treatment

The patient's sense of medical availability and constancy encourages persistence in managing medication, meal plans, and exercise, especially in the face of stress, thereby smoothing out perturbations in that patient's psychophysiologic well-being. I have the impression that most outpatients with chronic medical conditions thrive on follow-up at least 4 times a year, with frequency increasing after concurrence of two of several conditions implicated before in undercutting well-being, including autonomy or subjective life expectancy, and leading to psychiatric referral (see Table 44–1). This follow-up may include the patient's use of a "hotline" for advice, delegation by the physician of clinical responsibilities to another member of the treatment team, or referral to a psychiatrist for consultation. Partly by example, the physician encourages the patient to take interest in both the external aspects of life including meal plan, medication and exercise, and the inner, subjective aspects of experience. Both are important and both are valid.[85] There are a variety of ways to do the latter, ranging from asking how the patient sees things to asking the patient to recount a recent dream. Clinical experience[144a] and a bit of experimental evidence[144b] suggest that such a personal approach engages the patient and enhance collaboration with the physician.

Ideally, the physician keeps aware of his or her own responses to the patient's clinical problems and crises. For example, the physician's understandable concern about being overwhelmed by a patient's dependency needs could lead the doctor to discourage a feeling of closeness from the patient. Recognizing the source of the concern allows the doctor to remember how effectively the physician can reduce the patient's isolation and anxiety, and thus reduce the intensity of the patient's demands. If the doctor notes a pattern of setting aside too little time for the patient to ask questions and discuss fears, perhaps partly because of uncertainty about the appropriateness or effectiveness of the biopsychosocial approach, an experiment is in order. In one such experiment,[145] the physician asks all patients three questions: (1) what sort of worries or tensions the patient experiences; (2) whether the patient has been depressed recently, especially in conjunction with an illness; and (3) whether the patient is having any problems in close personal relationships, especially with those persons with whom the patient lives. There is no substitute for a full history, empathic listening and warmth. The resulting deepened understanding strengthens the patient-doctor relationship and increases the therapeutic effectiveness of almost everything the physician does.

REFERENCES

1. Engle, G.L.: Sounding board—the biopsychosocial model and medical education. N. Engl. J. Med. 306:802, 1982.
1a. Cohen-Cole, S.A.: On teaching the new (and old) psychobiology. In: C.P. Friedman, E.F. Purcell (Eds.): New Biology and Medical Education. New York, Josiah Macy Jr. Foundation, 1983, pp. 133–134.
1b. Cohen-Cole, S.A.: On teaching the new (and old) psychobiology. In: C.P. Friedman, E.F. Purcell (Eds.): New Biology and Medical Education. New York, Josiah Macy Jr. Foundation, 1983, pp. 133–134.
1c. American Hospital Association and Centers for Disease Control: Strategies to promote self-management of chronic disease. Chicago, U.S. Dept. of Health and Human Services and American Hospital Association, 1982.
1d. Tarlov, A.R.: Shattuck Lecture: The increasing supply of physicians, the changing structure of the health-service system, and the future practice of medicine. N. Engl. J. Med. 308:1235, 1983.
2. D.A. Hamburg, G.R., Elliott, D.L. Parron (Eds.): Health and Behavior: Frontiers of Research in the Biobehavioral Sciences. Washington, D.C., National Academy Press, 1982.
3. Isenberg, P.L., Barnett, D.M.: Psychological problems in diabetes mellitus. Med. Clin. N. Am. 49:1125, 1965.
4. Kimball, C.P.: Emotions and psychosocial aspects of diabetes mellitus. Med. Clin. N. Am. 55:1007, 1971.
5. Krosnick, A.: Psychiatric aspects of diabetes: In: M. Ellenberg, H. Rifkin (Eds.): Diabetes Mellitus: Theory and Practice. New York, McGraw-Hill Book Co., 1970, pp. 920–933.
5a. Jacobson, A.M., Hauser, S.T.: Behavior and psychological aspects of diabetes. In: M. Ellenberg, H. Rifkin (Eds.): Diabetes Mellitus. Theory and Practice, 3rd Ed. New Hyde Park, N.Y. Medical Examination Publishing Co., 1983, pp. 1037–1052.
6. Guthrie, D.W., Guthrie, R.A.: Diabetes in adolescence. Am. J. Nurs. 75:1740, 1975.
7. Kravitz, A.R., Isenberg, P.L., Shore, M.F., Barnett, D.M.: Emotional factors in diabetes mellitus. In: A. Marble, P. White, R. Bradley, L. Krall (Eds.): Joslin's Diabetes Mellitus, 11th Ed. Philadelphia, Lea & Febiger, 1971, pp. 767–782.
8. White, P.: Life cycle of diabetes in youth. 50th anniversary of the discovery of insulin (1921–1971). J. Am. Med. Wom. Assoc. 27:293, 1972.
9. Tietz, W., Vidmar, J.T.: The impact of coping styles on the control of juvenile diabetes. Psychiatry in Med. 3:67, 1972.
10. Vandenberg, R.L.: Emotional aspects. In: K. Sussman (Ed.): Juvenile-Type Diabetes and its Complications: Theoretical and Practical Considerations. Springfield, Charles C Thomas, 1971, pp. 411–438.
11. Tarnow, J.D., Tomlinson, N.: Juvenile diabetes: impact on the child and family. Psychosomatics 19:487, 1978.
12. Strain, J.J.: Psychological Interventions in Medical Practice. New York, Appleton-Century-Crofts, 1978.
13. Galatzer, A., Amir, S., Gil, R., et al.: Crisis intervention program in newly-diagnosed diabetic children. Diabetes Care 5:414, 1982.
14. Caplan, G.: Principles of Preventive Psychiatry. New York, Basic Books, 1964.
15. Moos, R.H., Tsu, V.D.: The crisis of physical illness: an overview. In: R.H. Moos (Ed.): Coping with Physical Illness. New York, Plenum Press, 1977, pp. 3–22.
16. Caplan, G.: Mastery of stress: psychosocial aspects. Am. J. Psychiatry 138:413, 1981.
17. G.V. Coelho, D.A. Hamburg, J.E. Adams (Eds.): Coping and Adaptation. New York, Basic Books, 1974.
18. Haan, N.: Coping and Defending: Process of Self-Environment Organization. New York, Academic Press, 1977.
19. Cohen, F., Lazarus, R.S.: Coping with the stresses of illness. In: G.C. Stone, F. Cohen, N.E. Adler et al. (Eds.): Health Psychology. A Handbook: Theories, Applications, and Challenges of a Psychological Approach to the Health Care System. San Francisco, Jossey-Bass, 1979, pp. 217–254.
20. Cahill, G.F., Jr., McDevitt, H.O.: Insulin-dependent diabetes mellitus: the initial lesion. N. Engl. J. Med. 304:1454, 1981.
21. Leibovich, J.B.: Parents of diabetic youngsters look at themselves. Part I. Diabetes Forecast 30:10, 1977.
22. Mattsson, A.: Long-term physical illness in childhood: a challenge to psychosocial adaptation. In: R.H. Moos (Ed.): Coping with Physical Illness. New York, Plenum Press, 1977, pp. 183–200.
23. Hoover, J.: The emotional impact of diabetes on the patient and his family. Diabetes Conquest (Australia Diabetes Society) March, 1978, pp. 9–12.
24. Benedek, T.: An approach to the study of the diabetic. Psychosom. Med. 10:284, 1948.
25. Koski, M-L.: The coping processes in childhood diabetes. Acta Paediatr. Scand. Suppl. 198:1, 1969.
26. Kovacs, M.: Depression and "adaptation" in juvenile diabetics. In: B.A. Hamburg, L.F. Lipsett, G.E. Inoff, A.L. Drash (Eds.): Behavioral and Psychosocial Issues in Diabetes. Washington, D.C.: U.S. Department of Health and Human Services, 1980, NIH Publ. No. 80–1993.
27. Belmonte, M.M., Bunn, T., Gonthier, M.: The problem of "cheating" in the diabetic child and adolescent. Diabetes Care 4:116, 1981.
28. Wolf, P.: Personal communication.
29. Young, S., Holmes, D.: Living with growth onset diabetes from age 8 to 30. (videotape). Boston Veterans Administration Medical Center, 1981.
30. Bettelheim, B.: The Uses of Enchantment. The Meaning and Importance of Fairy Tales. New York, Alfred A. Knopf, 1976.
31. Swift, C.R., Seidman, F., Stein, H.: Adjustment problems in juvenile diabetes. Psychosom. Med. 29:555, 1967.
32. Myers, G., Marrero, D., Golden, M., et al.: Diabetes

and adolescence: the patient's view. Diabetes *30* (Suppl. 1):49A, 1981 (Abstr.)

33. Manderschied, R.W., Silbergeld, S., Dager, E.Z.: Alienation: a response to stress. J. Cybernet *5*:91, 1975.
34. Covelli, P.: Borrowing Time: Growing Up With Juvenile Diabetes, New York, T.Y. Crowell, 1979.
35. Bolic, T., Walker, M.: Psychological correlates of insulin pump therapy. Diabetes *30* (Suppl 1):49A, 1981 (Abstr.)
36. Bonheim, R.: The 'pump.' Diabetes Forecast *13*:22, 1982.
37. Alexander, I.E., Colley, R.S., Adlerstein, A.M.: Is death a matter of indifference? J. Psychol. *43*:277, 1957.
38. Kastenbaum, R.: Time and death in adolescence. In: H. Feifel (Ed.): The Meaning of Death. New York, McGraw-Hill, 1959, pp. 99–113.
39. Handal, P.J. The relationship between subjective life expectancy, death anxiety and general anxiety. In: H.W. Montefiore, J.R. Cautela, R.N. Butler (Eds.): Death Anxiety: Normal and Pathological Aspects. New York, MSS Corp. 1973, pp. 119–122.
40. Wohlford, P.: Extension of personal time, affective states and expectation of personal death. J. Personality Soc. Psychol. *3*:559, 1966.
41. Hauser, S.T., Jacobson, A.M., Noam, G., Powers, S.: Ego development and self-image complexity in early adolescence: longitudinal studies of psychiatric and diabetic patients. Arch. Gen. Psychiatry *40*:325, 1983.
42. Jacobson, A.M., Hauser, S.T., Powers, S., Noam, G.: Ego development in diabetics: a longitudinal study. In: Z. Laron, A. Galatzer (Eds.): Psychosocial Aspects of Diabetes in Children and Adolescents. Basel, Karger, 1983, p. 1–8.
43. Sarwer-Finer, G.J.: Denial of death and the unconscious longing for indestructability and immortality in the terminal phase of adolescence. Can. Psychiatr. Assoc. J. *17* (Suppl. 2):SS51, 1972.
44. White, P.: The child with diabetes. Med. Clin. N. Am. *49*:1049, 1965.
45. Bornstein, B.: On latency. In: R.S. Eissler, A. Freud, H. Hartmann, E. Kris (Eds.): The Psychoanalytic Study of the Child. Vol. 6. New York, International University, 1952. pp. 69–81.
46. Jacques, E.: Death and the mid-life crisis. Int. J. Psychiatry *46*:502, 1965.
46a.Pray, L.M.: Journey of a Diabetic. New York, Simon and Schuster, 1983.
47. Akiskal, H.S.: Dysthymic disorders: psychopathology of proposed depressive subtypes. Am. J. Psychiatry *140*:11, 1983.
48. Boyd, J.H., Weissman, M.: Epidemiology of affective disorders. Arch. Gen. Psychiatry *38*:1039, 1981.
49. Nielsen, A.C., Williams, T.A.: Depression in ambulatory medical patients: prevalence by self-report questionnaire and recognition by nonpsychiatric physicians. Arch. Gen. Psychiatry *37*:999, 1980.
50. Lipowsky, Z.J.: Psychiatric illness among medical patients. Lancet *1*:478, 1979.
51. Moffic, H.S., Paykel, E.S.: Depression in medical inpatients. Br. J. Psychiatry *126*:346, 1975.
52. Weissman, M.M., Myers, J.K., Thompson, W.D.: Depression and its treatment in a U.S. urban community—1975–1976. Arch. Gen. Psychiatry *38*:417, 1981.
53. Murphy, J.M.: Continuities in community-based psychiatric epidemiology. Arch. Gen. Psychiatry *37*:1215, 1980.
54. Parker, G.B., Brown, L.B.: Coping behaviors that mediate between events and depression. Arch. Gen. Psychiatry *39*:1386, 1982.
55. House, J.S., Robbins, C., Metzner, H.L.: The association of social relationships and activities with mortality: pro-

spective evidence from the Tecumseh Community Health Study. Am. J. Epidemiol. *161*:123, 1982.
56. Berkman, L.F., Syme, S.L.: Social networks, host resistance and mortality: a nine-year follow-up study of Alameda County residents. Am. J. Epidemiol. *109*:186, 1979.
57. Cobb, S.: Social support as a moderator of life stress. Psychosom. Med. *38*:300, 1976.
58. Greenblatt, M., Becerra, R.M., Serafetinides, E.A.: Social networks and mental health: an overview. Am. J. Psychiatry *139*:977, 1982.
59. Pattison, E.M., Liamas, R., Hurd, G.: Social network mediation of anxiety. Psychiatric Ann. *9*:56, 1979.
60. Horowitz, M.J.: Unpublished paper, 1983.
61. Fries, J.F.: Aging, natural death, and the compression of morbidity. N. Engl. J. Med. *303*:130, 1980.
62. Felton, B.J., Hinrichsen, G.A., Revenson, T., Ellenberg, M.: Coping strategies and emotional adjustment among middle-aged and elderly diabetics. Diabetes *28*:370, 1979. (Abstr.)
63. Sims, P.F. (Ed.): Diabetes: Reach for Health and Freedom. St. Louis, C.V. Mosby Co., 1984.
64. Bierman, J., Toohey, B.: The Diabetic's Total Health Book. Los Angeles, J.P. Tancker, Inc., 1980.
65. Holmes, T.H., Rahe, R.H.: The social readjustment rating scale. J. Psychosom. Res. *11*:213, 1967.
66. Feighner, J.P., Robins, E., Guze, S.B.: Diagnostic criteria for use in psychiatric research. arch. Gen. Psychiatry *26*:57, 1972.
67. Thompson, T.L., II, Moran, M.G., Nies, A.S.: Medical intelligence: psychotropic drug use in the elderly. N. Engl. J. Med. *308*:194, 1983.
68. Mandenoff, A., Fumeron, F., Apfelbaum, M., Margules, D.L.: Endogenous opiates and energy balance. Science *215*:1536, 1982.
69. Hillard, J.R., Lobo, M.C., Keeling, R.P.: Bulimia and diabetes: a potentially life-threatening combination. Psychosomatics *24*:292, 1983.
70. Harmatz, M.G.: Eating-dieting syndrome may alter normal control. Psych. News *15* (20):7, 1980.
71. Rusting, R.: Just one more bite. Diabetes Forecast *13*:(6) 14, 1982.
72. Grinker, J.: Behavioral and metabolic consequences of weight reduction. J. Am. Diet Assoc. *62*:30, 1973.
73. Maugh, T.H., II: A new marker for diabetes. Science *215*:651, 1982.
74. Salmela, P.I., Sotaniemi, E.A., Viikari, J., et al.: Fenfluramine therapy in non-insulin-dependent diabetic patients: effects on body weight, glucose homeostasis, serum lipoproteins, and antipyrine metabolism. Diabetes care *4*:535, 1981.
75. Bigelow, G.E., Griffiths, R.R., Liebson, I., Kaliszak, J.E.: Double-blind evaluation of reinforcing and anorectic actions of weight control medications. Arch. Gen. Psychiatry *37*:1118, 1980.
76. Silverstone, T.S.: Obesity: Pathogenesis and Management. Acton, Mass., Public Sciences Group, 1975.
77. Holmes, D.M.: Issues in psychiatric referrals. In: B.A. Hamburg, L.F. Lipsett, G.E. Inoff, A.L. Drash (Eds.): Behavioral and Psychosocial Issues in Diabetes. Washington, D.C. U.S. Department of Health and Human Services, 1980, NIH Publ. No. 80–1993.
78. Hoover, J.: What the patient expects from the doctor. Practical Diabetology *1*:1, 1982.
79. Polonsky, K., Bergenstal, R., Pons, G., et al.: Relation of counterregulatory responses to hypoglycemia in Type I diabetes. N. Engl. J. Med. *307*:1106, 1982.
80. White, N.H., Skow, D.A., Cryer, P.E., et al.: Identification of Type I diabetic patients at increased risk for

hypoglycemia during intensive therapy. N. Engl. J. Med. *308*:485, 1983.

81. Cryer, P.E., Gerich, J.E.: Relevance of glucose counterregulatory systems to patients with diabetes: critical roles of glucagon and epinephrine. Diabetes Care *6*:95, 1983.

82. Barbosa, J., Johnson, S.: Severe hypoglycemia during maximized insulin treatment of diabetes in a randomized clinical trial. Diabetes Care *6*:62, 1983.

82a. Bolli, G.B., Dimitriadis, G.D., Pehling, G.B., et al.: Abnormal glucose counterregulation after subcutaneous insulin in insulin-dependent diabetes mellitus. N. Engl. J. Med. *310*:1706, 1984.

82b. Holmes, C.S., Hayford, J.T., Gonzalez, J.L., Weydert, J.A.: A survey of cognitive functioning at different glucose levels in diabetic persons. Diabetes Care *6*:180, 1983.

82c. Stewart, T.: Growing up. Diabetes Forecast, *36*:July–Aug., 1980.

82d. Franceschi, M., Cecchetto, R., Minicucci, F., et al.: Cognitive processes in insulin-dependent diabetes. Diabetes Care *7*:228, 1984.

83. Feldman, M., Kiser, R.S., Unger, R.H., Li, C.H.: Beta-endorphin and the endocrine pancreas: studies in heatlhy and diabetic human beings. N. Engl. J. Med. *308*:349, 1983.

84. Jacobson, A.M., Daffner, K., Hauser, S.T., Younger, D.: Psychological aspects of diabetes mellitus. In: T.C. Manschreck (Ed.): Psychiatric Medicine Update: Massachusetts General Hospital Reviews for Physicians. New York, Elsevier, 1981, pp. 119–128.

85. Schade, D.S.: The stress factor. Diabetes Forecast *13* (2):18, 1982.

86. Koski, M-L., et al.: A psychosomatic follow-up. Acta Paedopsychiatr *42*:(Basel) 12, 1976.

87. Selye, H.: Stress Without Distress, 1st Ed. Philadelphia, J.B. Lippincott Co., 1974.

88. Ehrentheil, O.F.: The effect of various degrees of social pressure. Mental Health Soc. *5*:14, 1979.

89. Dudley, D.L., Glaser, E.M., Jorgenson, B.N., Logal, D.L.: Psychosocial concomitants to rehabilitation in COPD. Chest *77*:413, 1980.

90. Piening, S.: Personal communication. 1982.

91. Strauss, A.L., Glaser, B.G.: Chronic Illness and the Quality of Life. St. Louis, The C.V. Mosby Co., 1975.

92. Blank, H.R.: Psychoanalysis and blindness. Psychoanal. Quart. *26*:1, 1957.

93. Fitzgerald, R.G.: Visual phenomenology in recently blind adults. Am. J. Psychiatry *127*:1533, 1971.

94. Oehler-Giarratana, J., Fitzgerald, R.G.: Group therapy with blind diabetics. Arch. Gen. Psychiatry *37*:463, 1980.

95. Oehler-Giarratana, J.: Personal and professional reactions to blindness from diabetic retinopathy. New Outlook for the Blind *70*:237, 1976.

96. Oehler-Giarratana, J.: Meeting the psychosocial and rehabilitative needs of the visually impaired diabetic. J. Visual Impair. Blind: *72*:358, 1978.

97. Carroll, T.: Blindness. Boston, Little, Brown & Co., 1961.

98. Vanderkolk, C.J.: Counseling and psychotherapy with the visually impaired: an annotated bibliography. New Outlook for the Blind *70*:109, 1976.

99. Chevigny, H., Braverman, S.: The Adjustment of the Blind. New Haven, Yale University Press, 1950, pp. 158–172.

100. Stetten, D., Jr.: Sounding board: Coping with blindness. N. Engl. J. Med. *305*:458, 1981.

101. Levin, M.E.: Peripheral vascular disease. Diabetes Forecast *13*(1):40, 1982.

102. Dembo, T., Leviton, G.L., Wright, D.A.: Adjustment to misfortune—a problem of social-psychological rehabilitation. Artif. Limbs *3*:4, 1956.

103. Fishman, S.: Amputation. In: J.F. Garrett, E.S. Levine (Eds.): Psychological Practices with the Physically Disabled. New York, Columbia University Press, 1961.

104. Mital, M.A., Pierce, D.S.: Amputees and Their Prostheses. Boston, Little, Brown & Co., 1971, pp. 25–39.

105. Thomas, K.R., David, R.M., Hochman, M.E.: Correlates of disability acceptance in amputees. Rehab. Counseling Bulletin (March) 508, 1976.

106. Levine, S.B.: Marital sexual dysfunction: erectile dysfunction. Ann. Intern. Med. *85*:342, 1976.

107. Schiavi, R.C., Hogan, B.: Sexual problems in diabetes mellitus: psychological aspects. Diabetes Care *2*:9, 1979.

108. Podolsky, S.: Sexual function in diabetic men. Practical Diabetology *1* (1):1, 1982.

109. Karacan, I.: Nocturnal penile tumescence as a biologic marker in assessing erectile dysfunction. Psychosomatics *23*(4)349, 1982.

110. Beylot, M., Marion, D., Noel, G.: Ultrasonographic determination of residual urine in diabetic subjects: relationship to neuropathy and urinary tract infection. Diabetes Care *5* (5):501, 1982.

111. Pfeifer, M., Cook, D., Brodsky, J., et al.: Quantitative evaluation of sympathetic and parasympathetic control of iris function. Diabetes Care *5*:518, 1982.

112. Krosnick, A., Podolsky, S.: Diabetes and sexual dysfunction: restoring normal ability. Geriatrics *36*:92, 1981.

113. Beaser, R.S., van der Hoek, C., Jacobson, A.M., et al.: Experience with penile prostheses in the treatment of impotence in diabetic men. J.A.M.A. *248*:943, 1982.

114. Cassem, N.H., Hackett, T.P.: Psychological aspects of myocardial infarction. Med. Clin. N. Am. *61*:711, 1977.

115. Pancheri, P., Bellaterra, M., Matteoli, S., et al.: Infarct as a stress agent: life history and personality characteristics in improved versus not-improved patients after severe heart attack. J. Human Stress *4*:16, 1978.

116. Bruhn, J.G., Chandler, B., Wolf, S.: A psychological study of survivors and nonsurvivors of myocardial infarction. Psychosom. Med. *31*:8, 1969.

117. Cassem, N.H.: Depression. In: T.P. Hackett, N.H. Cassem (Eds.): Massachusetts General Hospital Handbook of General Hospital Psychiatry. St. Louis, The C.V. Mosby Co., 1978, pp. 210–216.

118. Cassem, N.H.: The dying patient. In: Ibid. pp. 303–314.

119. Cassem, N.H.: Treatment decisions in irreversible illness. In: Ibid. pp. 573–574.

120. D'Elia, J.A., Piening, S., Kaldany, A., et al.: Psychosocial crisis in diabetic renal failure. Diabetes Care *4*:99, 1981.

121. Marshall, J.R.: Neuropsychiatric aspects of renal failure. J. Clin. Psychiatry *40*:81, 1979.

122. Patterson, M., Miller, F.: Neuropsychiatric complications in a patient on hemodialysis. Psychomatics *22*:61, 1981.

123. Friedman, E.A., Lundin, A.P., III: Environmental and iatrogenic obstacles to long life on hemodialysis. N. Engl. J. Med. *306*:167, 1982.

124. Wirth, J.B., Folstein, M.F.: Thirst and weight gain during maintenance hemodialysis. Psychosomatics *23*:1125, 1982.

125. Reichsman, F., Levy, N.B.: Problems in adaptation to maintenance hemodialysis. A four-year study of 25 patients. Arch. Intern. Med. *130*:859, 1972.

126. Amair, P., Khanna, R., Leibel, B., et al.: Continuous ambulatory peritoneal dialysis in diabetics with end-stage renal disease. N. Engl. J. Med. *306*:625, 1982.

127. Harrington, J.T.: Chronic ambulatory peritoneal dialysis. N. Engl. J. Med. *306*:670, 1982.

127a.Luke, R.G.: Renal replacement therapy. N. Engl. J. Med. *308*:1593, 1983.

128. Piening, S.: Family stress in diabetic renal failure. Health Soc. Work *9*:134, 1984.

129. Campbell, J.D., Campbell, A.R.: The social and economic costs of end-stage renal disease. A patient's perspective. N. Engl. J. Med. *299*:386, 1978.

130. Steidl, J.H., Finkelstein, F.O., Wexler, J.P., et al.: Medical condition, adherence to treatment regimens, and family functioning: their interactions in patients receiving long-term dialysis treatment. Arch. Gen. Psychiatry *37*:1025, 1980.

131. N.B. Levy (Ed.): Psychonephrology One: Psychological Factors in Hemodialysis and Transplantation. New York, Plenum Press, 1981.

132. Gutman, R.A., Stead, W.W., Robinson, R.R.: Physical activity and employment status of patients on maintenance dialysis. N. Engl. J. Med. *304*:309, 1981.

133. Milne, J.E.: Psychosocial aspects of renal transplantation. Urology *9*: (Supp.) 82, 1977.

134. Watts, F.N.: Behavioral aspects of the managemnent of diabetes mellitus: education, self-care and metabolic control. Behav. Res. Ther. *18*:171, 1980.

135. Anderson, B.J., Auslander, W.F.: Research on diabetes management and the family: a critique. Diabetes Care *3*:696, 1980.

136. Rusting, R.: The year in research. Diabetes Forecast *13* (5):34, 1982.

137. Minuchin, S.: Families and Family Therapy. Cambridge, Harvard University Press, 1974.

138. McNeil, B.J., Pauker, S.G., Sox, H.C., Tversky, A.: On the elicitation of preferences for alternative therapies. N. Engl. J. Med. *306*:1259, 1982.

139. Hauser, S.T., Pollets, D.: Psychological aspects of diabetes mellitus: a critical review. Diabetes Care *2*:227, 1979.

140. Sullivan, B-J.: Self-esteem and depression in adolescent diabetic girls. Diabetes Care *1*:18, 1978.

141. Egendorf, A.: The postwar healing of Vietnam Veterans: recent research. Hosp. Community Psychiatry *33*:901, 1982.

142. Berman, S., Price, S., Gusman, F.: An inpatient program for Vietnam combat veterans in a Veterans Administration Hospital. Hosp. Community Psychiatry. *33*:919, 1982.

143. Killilea, M.: Social support systems and their relation to health and illness. In: B.A. Hamburg, L.F. Lipsett, G.E. Inoff, A.L. Drash (Eds.): Behavioral and Psychosocial Issues in Diabetes. Washington, D.C.: U.S. Department of Health and Human Services. 1980, NIH Publ. No. 80–1993.

144. Marmor, J.: Recent trends in psychotherapy. Am. J. Psychiatry *137*:409, 1980.

144a.LaCroix, A.M., Assal, J.Ph.: Active listening: how to make sure that we heard was what the patient really meant. In: J.Ph. Assal, M. Berger, N. Gay, J. Canivet (Eds.): Diabetes Education: How to Improve Patient Education. Amsterdam, Excerpta Medica, 1983, pp. 236–248.

144b.Cartwright, R.D., Tipton, L.W., Wicklund, J.: Focusing on dreams: a preparation program for psychotherapy. Arch. Gen. Psychiatr. *37*:275, 1980.

145. Waring, E.M.: An interpersonal model for teaching psychiatry to medical students. Psychosomatics *21*:998, 1980.

45 Life Cycle in Diabetes: Socioeconomic Aspects

Leo P. Krall, Paul S. Entmacher, and Thomas F. Drury

INTRODUCTION

Here, near the end of this 12th edition, it is evident that diabetes mellitus as we know it today is not the same in everyone labeled as diabetic. Diabetes is almost capricious in its deviousness: there are patients with occasional postprandial hyperglycemia at one end of the spectrum and long-term patients with almost constantly elevated blood glucose levels and dire complications at the other. Most of us would like to look at a medical condition as clearly definitive and readily understandable. This was the thinking about diabetes until the last several decades when it was discovered that in pathologic states, change begets change. Roger North in *Examen* in 1940 mentioned that men like to think that changes take place in a static situation and then said ''. . . Many changes are dynamic and set in motion many other changes.'' How better to describe diabetes than to understand its differences with each change in the life cycle? In the young, the onset is often like a forest fire with a conflagration starting in dry leaves. In later years, the onset may be insidious. In the very old, at onset the apparently symptomless state of diabetes may linger for years before being discovered, but there are exceptions to each phase of the life cycle. The ''majority diabetic,'' and possibly the most neglected one, is the older person who is, in the opinion of many, likely to have other physical problems, and has so many minor complaints that more serious conditions may inadvertently be buried among these. More detailed information concerning diabetes in the elderly may be found in Chapter 25.

The stage of the diabetes cycle also affects the patient's involvement with the economic factors of life which can have an effect on diabetes. Diabetes is simpler to treat among the affluent and those educated to expect superior medical care. But what about those in approximately half of the world who do not have optimal nutrition or potable water to drink and with little or no medical care? So economic considerations do play an important role in the life cycle of the diabetic and indeed the life style caused by diabetes in the patient may often influence the socioeconomic style as well.

This chapter describes the following. Who are the diabetics? What are their problems? What resources do they have and what help can they get? Finally, what is in store for them?

As in earlier chapters, the experience of the Joslin Clinic staff and patients in dealing with the many issues which arise throughout the lifespan of a person with diabetes are discussed in the context of national and international developments related to these issues. Where possible, summaries of extant literature have been supplemented with findings and tabulations from the National Health Interview Survey (NHIS) carried out by the National Center for Health Statistics (NCHS) of the Department of Health and Human Services.[1] The NHIS is one of the major sources of national statistics on the health of the civilian, noninstitutionalized population of the United States. In specific years, scientifically-selected subsamples of persons who have been told by their physicians that they have diabetes are included in the NHIS. At appropriate places in the discussion, information from the NHIS on the health and health-related characteristics of adults with known diabetes is introduced. References containing detailed descriptions of the procedures used in the NHIS are available elsewhere.[1]

DIABETES IN THE YOUNG

In reading Chapter 23, it becomes apparent that although diabetes is often at its most virulent in the young, in the developed part of the world these young people may be least affected by socioeconomic influences. Certainly the diabetic young have problems which are not only pathophysiologic but emotional as well, and these have been adequately described. Also, the young may be in a sheltered state. Parents are likely to take care of them and most of them are in an orderly system of schools, camps, and social groups. Many of these organized programs have been valuable in implementing independence in preparation for life. Indeed, a relatively large portion of funding for care and treatment is focused on this group. Except for school problems and the ever-present one of acceptance by both the patient and his peers, it is in the approach to adulthood that life problems become magnified. There are certain avenues that may help, however. One of these involves the summer camp program,[2,2a] which has been valuable both in implementing the independence of the young diabetic and in giving the parents of these children a hiatus in the constant responsibilities of diabetes care. For a full discussion of camps, see Chapter 24.

Almost all children, including those with diabetes, attend school. While it is important for the growing child to have as good diabetes regulation as possible, it is also important to maintain blood glucose levels high enough to prevent insulin reactions, particularly during active periods such as when traveling to school and when exercising during recess and in the gymnasium. It must also be remembered that many youngsters have a lowered renal threshold for sugar and indeed glucose may be found in "first void" or any urine specimen even though the blood glucose level at the time may be normal. Thus, for active children, it is sometimes better not to have urine glucose tests completely negative. This potential problem is now mitigated by the availability of home blood glucose monitoring, in that more meticulous attention to metabolic control can be obtained with greater safety.

Obviously the teacher, while aware of the diabetes, must not shelter or overprotect the child. Teachers must not make obvious special allowances for diabetes since youngsters do not want to appear different from their classmates. What is told to the schoolteacher is most important for the child and the diabetes. There should be enough information but not too much. Of primary importance are the fact of diabetes, the possibility of insulin reactions, and their treatment. It is likewise important that the teacher permit snack times as unobtrusively as possible and without fanfare. The needed information can be printed on cards to be distributed to schoolteachers (see also Chapter 24 and Fig. 24–4).

By the time young persons with diabetes go to college, many have mastered control of their condition and are self-sufficient, so that they will do well when they leave home. The personal physician to be consulted depends a good deal on the assessment of the young person's ability to care for him- or her-self. Virtually no admission restrictions are placed on diabetics who apply for college entrance. However, the school medical authorities should also be aware of the diabetes and the particular needs of the student. With recent stress on computer technology and other so-called white collar occupations, the diabetic of the future may be in a more favorable environment than ever and those who learn professions or specialized skills will be on an equal footing with nondiabetics.

Into Adulthood. How does one define adulthood? Is it completely age-related? States have different definitions in permitting driving, drinking, and until quite recently, voting. Completing education, choosing careers, and possibly marriage and parenthood are fairly specific parameters of adulthood. However, in any case, the proper approach to diabetes in the earlier stage will have considerable bearing on entrance into adulthood. Those who have not accepted diabetes have a limited knowledge of it, and already are involved with complications, have a definite handicap that is sometimes difficult to overcome. At this point in life, there is a tremendous yearning for "a normal life," usually as measured by the lifestyle of peers. It is wrong for a physician to insist that the diabetic can "live a perfectly normal life" although with the use of improving generations of insulin pumps, this goal may appear closer. The person with diabetes, however, can lead a useful, productive, and satisfactorily happy life. However, "normal" as defined by most persons would indicate that one would have to think about nothing concerning his state of health. The alleged joys of skipping meals, overindulging in food, and not being concerned with work habits, hours of the day, etc., are not possible for most Type I diabetics. When one must test blood or urine for glucose frequently, adjust insulin doses, eat regularly, and avoid insulin reactions as well as scrupulously avoid infections, and plan the logistics of a vacation trip like a military campaign, this is no longer a normal lifestyle. John Philpot Curran (1790) pointed out that eternal vigilance was the price of liberty. This also applies to successful care of diabetes. While patients should, as much as possible, adjust the diabetes to their lifestyle rather than be subdued because of it, those who have been aware of their diabetes and conquered life's problems in spite of it, have fared much better than those who ignored it.

PROBLEMS OF LIVING

Marriage and the Diabetic Patient

A physician faces a delicate diplomatic problem when giving advice to a diabetic contemplating marriage to a nondiabetic, and an even more delicate one when discussing this with the parents of the nondiabetic member of the potential marriage. Many decades ago, Dr. Elliott P. Joslin wrote that "It is a great advantage for a diabetic to be married because of the intimate protection and care thereby attained." However, as Dr. Joslin pointed out, there are certain matters to be faced by the diabetic and by the nondiabetic partner. Since diabetics, like anyone else, will probably marry regardless of what anyone else thinks, it is useful for those considering marriage to have genetic counseling, and certainly nondiabetic partners must be aware of the problems and possible complications. They must also be aware of the everyday emergencies that can occur. The stigma of marriage to diabetics has disappeared in recent years, since those with diabetes live reasonably close to normal life spans in many cases. The possibility of inheritance as a major factor in diabetes, while still present, is much less definite than previously thought. Increasing numbers of diabetics live 50 years or longer, many without any major complications. The outlook for those with diabetes as a class is much more optimistic than it was 20 or even 10 years ago. It must be recognized that the techniques of helping to prevent or to ameliorate complications are much better and are still improving. However, the prospective bride and groom should know that complications of the disease may occur after a period of years despite the best possible control, and may possibly result in disability or even premature death. With diabetic females, the fact must be faced that while the chances of having a stillborn infant have decreased tremendously, they are still greater for her than for the person without diabetes. Likewise, the possibility of congenital anomalies, sometimes of a major nature, is greater in children born to a diabetic mother than to mothers without diabetes (see Chapter 33). For males, the problems of sexual dysfunction may arise (Chapter 32). Decreased potency, possibly due to neuropathy, is a factor in the minds of many people. There will be special problems involved in obtaining insurance and employment although this situation is improving, as discussed later in this chapter.

However, in advising those who are considering marriage, apart from any other benefits that generally result from a good marriage such as increased support and care, the happiness of the patient should be the main concern of the physician. Magoun's advice[3] written 3 decades ago, "In our culture, mature happiness depends more upon finding the right choice of a mate and subsequent good interpersonal relationships in marriage than any other single factor," is still true.

Operating Motor Vehicles

One of the most cherished and measurable tribal rites of adulthood is the insatiable desire of almost every young person to drive and own an automobile. With the complications of modern life and the distances necessary for travel to or as part of employment, the ability to obtain a driver's license becomes increasingly important. While the laws regulating drivers' licenses vary greatly from state to state, the trend appears to be toward more strict requirements for drivers with chronic medical conditions. All 50 states allow adults with diabetes to drive provided they demonstrate road sense and safety knowledge, although some states require that the diabetic obtain a physician's report, certifying that the diabetes is in good control and that the diabetic has no complications and has never suffered periods of unconsciousness. Some states require periodic examinations for all drivers. One problem is that the states do not set definite standards to guide the physician, who must therefore base his certification of a patient's ability to drive safely on one state's regulation which appeared some time ago, i.e., that the applicant not be subject to "fits and fainting spells." The Federal government insists on minimal standards for drivers before states may qualify for federal funds to be used for highway construction.[4]

Among the most common potential problems described by Krosnick[5] are hypoglycemia, temporarily blurred vision which is possible during periods of hyperglycemia, and defective reflexes or sensation in the feet due to diabetic neuropathy as well as possibly impaired circulation. Motor vehicle authorities in New Jersey require a diabetic driver who is cited for a motor violation or who had an accident to complete a diabetes history form. In addition, the driver's physician must submit an exhaustive report concerning the patient's history, complications, etc., and express an opinion concerning whether or not diabetes would interfere with highway safety. This document is then reviewed by a medical advisory panel who make recommendations to the Director of the Division of Motor Vehicles as to the final decision. Moreover, present federal regulations prohibit insulin-dependent diabetics from driving trucks and other large commercial vehicles interstate, although intrastate driving is permitted by most states.

Unquestionably, motor vehicle accidents are a leading cause of death in the United States after heart, cardiovascular diseases, and cancer.[6] In one study,[7] drivers with diabetes, along with those who had epilepsy and other chronic conditions, all averaged about twice as many accidents per million miles of driving as did drivers in the control group. Another problem is that many persons with diabetes do not declare this fact on their applications for a license. For example, a recent study[8] showed that of 250 patients with insulin-dependent diabetes in England, 42.8% had not declared this fact on their applications for a driver's license. The problem here is that failure to declare medical facts is of major importance, since under these circumstances, a license is not valid, and this may affect the validity of insurance coverage. The American Medical Association[9] has published a guide to assist physicians in determining drivers' limitations.

It must be clearly recognized that to drive a vehicle is not a right but a privilege which can be revoked at any time. While regulations covering the use of high-powered boats, snowmobiles and other powered vehicles have not yet been defined, insulin reactions are no less dangerous when these vehicles are used. Drivers must never skip a meal or be late for needed nourishment and they must carry concentrated carbohydrate in their cars within easy reach for emergencies. Increasing numbers of accidents among diabetics, whether caused by insulin or oral hypoglycemic agents, will only threaten the privilege of driving for all diabetics.

Other "Lifestyle" Problems

There are a number of miscellaneous "vices" which must be mentioned. They are included here not because physicians have any doubts about the proper answers to the questions but because patients are becoming increasingly ingenious in their reading habits and, having more time than most physicians, manage to choose those bits of evidence which apparently condone their lifestyle choices, while ignoring others.

Alcohol. In a true physiologic sense, almost no physician would state that large-scale drinking of alcoholic beverages is beneficial for anyone, diabetic or nondiabetic. Drinking, however, has become a social and business custom worldwide, and in recent years, the drinking of alcohol by diabetics has become a fact of life. This is so widely accepted that a list of wines allegedly suitable for diabetics was approved some years ago by the British Diabetic Association.[10] Included was the delightful admonition that "two ordinary glasses of a wine containing 0.4% sugar will contribute 1 g of sugar to the diet. The calories are contributed by the alcohol as well as by the sugar, and those diabetics who are on a reducing diet must count the calories as part of their daily diet." Basically the problem of drinking for persons with diabetes breaks down into three areas: (1) the effect of alcohol itself; (2) its effect as a cause of hypoglycemia, and (3) its effect on other aspects of the life of the diabetic such as driving, etc. In spite of its caloric production, alcohol is not a food; it furnishes no carbohydrate, protein, fat, vitamins, or minerals, and is not useful for nutrition. One g of alcohol yields 7 calories which can be metabolized and stored for future use. The amount of alcohol is determined by the proof. One-half of the proof is the percentage of alcohol in the drink. For example, 80 proof whiskey has 40% alcohol. One ounce (30 g) of straight whiskey contains about 85 calories. Adding sweetened liquids such as ginger ale or cocktail mixes and freely available hors d'oeuvres results in still more calories. Beer averages about 4 to 5% alcohol in the United States and as high as 12 to 14% in other parts of the world. Overall, beer provides about 14 calories an ounce or 150 calories per 12-ounce can or bottle. Wines vary from highly fortified sherries and ports to dry white table wines which may be lower in both sugar and alcoholic content. Since wine is often consumed with meals, there is less risk of decreased glucose levels.

Although the results of certain studies suggest that the slight or moderate use of ethanol may be of value in the prevention and treatment of coronary artery disease,[10a,10b] its benefit to health is controversial. In fact, in some persons even a modest intake may have detrimental effects on various parts of the body and over-use may do serious damage. Recently, alcohol has been linked to increasing plasma triglyceride levels,[11] increasing symptomatic peripheral neuropathy,[12] and impaired platelet function,[134] among a whole litany of unfavorable effects. Obviously, it is best for diabetics not to drink, but if they do, it should be done thoughtfully and intelligently. A drink containing $1\frac{1}{2}$ ounces (45 g) of whiskey should be consumed preferably with water or soda (unsweetened), or "on the rocks." Occasionally ingestion of dry white wine with a meal poses no great problem. The physician is not nearly as concerned about the patient who drinks rarely or occasionally, or perhaps has a glass of champagne at his daughter's wedding, as he is about the person who habitually drinks "socially." In the United States, this could be a frequent occurrence.

Another danger posed by alcohol for diabetics is the depressing effect of alcohol on the capacity of the liver for gluconeogenesis, thereby favoring hypoglycemia.[14] Sugar is not freely available when needed and the hypoglycemic reaction that ensues can be profound and prolonged. In addition, there is the fact that drinking can mask the signals of low blood glucose. Adding the problems of symptom-masked hypoglycemia to the considerable dangers of driving on modern highways makes alcohol, when used injudiciously, an increased risk for diabetics, who are already often high on the risk list.

Smoking. At this time in the United States, it is easy to be adamant against smoking by anyone, and especially diabetics. While patients may differ in their personal beliefs about drinking, the feeling against cigarette use is increasingly negative. It is now appreciated that the time and effort spent by physicians in convincing patients not to smoke cigarettes will produce more useful years of life than almost all of the surgical miracles put together. The increased risks of cancer and emphysema for the smoker in the general population are well documented. For diabetics, the fact that the risk of cardiovascular complications is enormously greater than in nondiabetics should be an added deterrent to smoking. There is also evidence that tobacco increases constriction of smaller blood vessels, further impeding an already diminishing circulation. Fortunately, in many segments of the population,

the use of tobacco is decreasing and in those with diabetes, it should be absolutely banned.

Travel. As the world gets smaller and travel becomes easier, it is apparent that about one-third of the American population make a trip each year. Travel has become so highly organized that a visit to major centers, particularly in Europe, the Caribbean, most parts of South America and some parts of Asia, should cause little or no concern. Obviously, patients with unstable diabetes who are prone to insulin reactions without warning should get their condition into as stable a situation as possible before leaving. It is also best for them to travel with a companion who is knowledgeable about diabetes.

Since patients will ask their physicians for advice pertaining to health and other matters, it is best rapidly to review some of the important areas.

(a) Before Leaving. It is almost impossible to start preparations too early for a trip. It is useful to make certain that the traveler's health insurance applies to the areas that will be visited or, if not, temporary health and accident insurance may be purchased to cover the trip. Inoculations should be brought up to date as needed. Although smallpox vaccinations are no longer required, there are certain areas of the world where diseases such as cholera, plague, and yellow fever are endemic and preventive inoculations should be in force. These change from time to time. Information concerning which immunizations are proper may be obtained from the local Health Department, the U.S. Public Health Service, or the Communicable Disease Center in Atlanta, Georgia. The pamphlet, *Immunization Information for International Travel,* can be obtained from the Superintendent of Documents, U.S. Government Printing Office, Washington, D.C. 20402.

Prevention against malaria is important in much of the world, and recently a new strain of P. falciparum has been described which is not affected by the usual malaria medications. Newer, stronger medications, unavailable several years ago, may be obtained to cope with this.

(b) Anyone with a chronic condition (including diabetes) should carry a note stating the current medical condition and listing required medications by their generic rather than trade names. Diabetes identification is important at home and even more vital abroad. Although customs officers have become quite sophisticated about the need for syringes and needles by diabetics, a huge supply of these can raise eyebrows in some parts of the world, and it is best to have a note from the physician, stating that this person is diabetic.

(c) Personal medications should be carried with the traveler. Generally the diabetic patient can carry enough insulin for most trips. This need not be refrigerated but may be carried with the traveler. A supply of medications for the next several days should be in the person's handbag or carry-on luggage since checked luggage generally arrives with the passenger, but not always.

(d) Those with diabetes should fly in the United States during daylight hours when possible. However, going east across the Atlantic or west across the Pacific, this is usually not possible. Most people need a day after a major trip to return to normal circadian rhythms. While the speed of the jet plane shortens trips, it also shortens the day going east, or lengthens the day going west. Most flights to Europe start at an hour when the diabetic has already had an evening meal. About an hour or two after take-off, another meal is generally served. After a too short or non-existent sleep, the traveler arrives in Europe at 9 A.M., when his body tells him that it is still about 4 A.M. The daily insulin injection should be given before the breakfast meal, wherever it is, and preferably at the hotel. The first day's dose should be cut by about 25%. This applies particularly to intermediate insulins. If the patient uses regular insulin as well, this might be eliminated for the first day if the tests are negative. Persons taking oral agents are less likely to have problems. Returning westward, there is not much difficulty because the day is longer and the person is awake and generally eating. However, a small supplemental dose of insulin may be required on arrival at home.

(e) The chance of hypoglycemia while flying is minimal, because there is little activity but plenty of food. In this jet age, relatively few people get airsick, but for these susceptible persons, the physician should prescribe meclizine (Antivert; Bonine), cyclizine (Marezine), or dimenhydrinate (Dramamine) before the departure. Passengers should also walk up and down the aisle at intervals to avoid possible clotting in the legs or increasing the chance of phlebitis.

(f) Diarrhea, the Curse of Travel. A number of articles have been written, recommending one or another of numerous medications for travelers' diarrhea. In one study,[15] doxycycline, 100 mg/day, apparently helped prevent episodes of travelers' diarrhea. It should be noted that any compound, even this, may cause annoying adverse effects. Furthermore, some strains of enterotoxigenic agents such as E. coli are resistant to tetracyclines. Another recent study[16] has suggested that 1 tablet daily of double strength trimethoprim/sulfamethoxazole (Bactrim DS, Septra DS) may also be helpful—again with awareness of the possibility of adverse reactions to drugs. Symptomatic treatment for mild cases of travelers' diarrhea, which is usu-

ally fairly self-limiting, might consist of Lomotil (diphenoxylate with atropine). Kaolin-pectin preparations such as Kaopectate have been helpful with some people. When there is severe diarrhea with large losses of water and electrolytes, oral rehydration is necessary. Where medical attention is not readily available, most pharmacists can mix some replacement solution with table salt, sodium bicarbonate, and table sugar, and a person with severe diarrhea should sip about a quart (liter) every 6 hours. However, at this stage, medical care is imperative. Most hotels abroad have access to English-speaking physicians, as do the United States embassy or consulates in each country. An organization called Intermedic, 777 Third Avenue, New York, NY 10017, has lists of English-speaking physicians who treat patients for a set fee. There are few places in the world without adequate medical service, and into those remote places, only the best-trained and most self-reliant diabetics should venture.

Discrimination against Diabetics. Unquestionably there has been and is discrimination against people with diabetes, just as there often is against anyone who is different. Having some of the stigmata of diabetes is bad enough, and when these include impairments of appearance such as obvious necrobiosis lipoidica. lipoatrophy, or lipohypertrophy, the situation becomes more distressing, causing the patient to feel a difference that is often interpreted as a feeling of discrimination. This becomes worse when there are diminished physical or mental performance, frequent absences from school or work, or any other factors which make the condition more obvious. However, this bias goes much further according to Petrides[17] who cited the results of a pair of studies in the British Medical Journal.[18,19] In one of these surveys, a group of schools of nursing in England were asked if they were willing to accept as students young women with diabetes. Although 111 were if the applicants had completely controlled diabetes, 34 had strong reservations, and suggested that other careers might be preferable. Twelve others stated that they would automatically reject all persons with diabetes without even an explanation. There are many examples of this type of discrimination. This prejudice also carries over into types of employment such as airline flight attendants. In this regard, while a case is cited later in this chapter, there is no consistent policy among all airlines.[20] Needless to say, increasingly efforts are being made to provide equality and full participation for anyone capable of employment. In 1981, the World Health Organization proclaimed that year to be the International Year of Disabled Persons (IYDP).[21] While this attempt to step up worldwide cooperation includes assistance for persons with conditions much more debilitating than diabetes, nevertheless the fight against discrimination is a real one. Many states now have statutes prohibiting discrimination in employment, but generally they are so broad and cover so many other facets and areas that the person with diabetes finds it much easier to go underground and not reveal the condition. Uruguay recently enacted the first and a most comprehensive law for the employment of diabetics in all of Latin America. This may indeed be a landmark for much of the rest of the world. The law states: "Diabetes will not cause, by itself, inability for the commencement or execution of work either in public or private organizations except in those areas where severe complications may interfere with the working ability" (Article 70, Law 14032, 1971, Uruguay).[22] Nancy Eriksson[23] has stated that a real equality among diabetic and nondiabetic people does not exist anywhere. It is obvious that the physician as well as other members of the medical profession can be influential in reducing this discrimination against persons who are willing and able to function as relatively normal members of society.

SOCIOECONOMIC PROBLEMS

The socioeconomic aspects of diabetes have with few exceptions been the province of the foreign literature. Most American texts do not cover these, considering that diagnosis, treatment, and care of complications are the physician's only involvement with the disease. In fact, many years ago diabetes was considered to be a disease of the rich, and the 19th century physicians of Europe recognized the association between affluence and diabetes at that time. In fact, some considered diabetes to be a sign of Heaven's disapproval of the prosperous who allegedly made their profits from the backs of the laboring poor. Dr. E. P. Joslin and associates recognized in the earliest edition of this book that the way persons with diabetes live and their ability to make a living have much to do with the success of treatment. The mere fact that they are diabetic makes them somewhat strange in the eyes of colleagues. As a result, diabetics tend to fit this picture and have been described as less aggressive, less impulsive, and less spontaneous with a greater need for social contact.[24] The fact is that economics in all its aspects plays a major role in the lives of most of us and even more so with diabetics. The choice of employment and the ability to get insurance and to make an adequate living are important to everyone. However, the person with a lifelong condition such as diabetes has the burden of extra expenses with fewer means of earning enough to cover them.[25]

Central Europeans, of course, with their centrally planned economies, have done an extraordinary job in the socioeconomic field.[26] In addition to medical care provided by the Ministry of Health of the German Democratic Republic (GDR), for example, a central institute coordinates the work of all outpatient stations for diabetes. Starting with the newborn and for as long as necessary, all patients are advised about their individual social problems, especially regarding choice of jobs, parenthood, and all other aspects of life. The patients receive medical instruction and remain under systematic observation and treatment in almost all phases of their lives. Obviously the sociomedical problems of diabetes must vary from nation to nation, but since the economic systems of the world are such that part of the world suffers from a lack of any medical attention while other areas have an over-abundance, it is hard to find an average. However, unquestionably the structures of education and the economic facts of life have a marked influence on the diabetes of persons so afflicted. The goal of medicine has been to keep the patient living as long and as healthy as possible. This is no longer enough. Increasingly it is being understood that the quality of life is as important as the quantity, and in this respect, socioeconomic factors play an important part.

OCCUPATIONAL PROBLEMS: EMPLOYMENT POSSIBILITIES AND CHOICES

For obvious reasons, the occupation and employment of persons with diabetes probably have been emphasized more than any other problem relating to the diabetic life. A person who cannot qualify for proper employment or who is suboptimally employed will suffer drastic changes in lifestyle. The young diabetic entering the labor market today continues to have problems. Because of federal and state legislation enacted in the last decade, the situation has eased somewhat. Admittedly the enthusiastic support of various diabetes associations and societies has also added pressure against employment discrimination. The older person developing diabetes is more likely to be employed, because generally members of this group are already working when their diabetes becomes apparent. Either they have established adequate work records or they keep their condition secret. At any rate, the onset of diabetes does not jeopardize their employment status to the extent that it does with the younger person. Since about 600,000 new cases are said to be diagnosed annually in the United States and with the condition increasing by 6% each year, opportunities must be available for diabetics to be employed according to their abilities. Diabetes is a registrable disability in Great Britain, although the great majority of diabetics are not in any sense disabled. Since employers of more than 30 persons are compelled by law to employ a certain proportion of "disabled" persons, it is to the diabetic's advantage to be registered through the local office of the Department of Employment and Productivity.[27] A major problem in this respect is whether or not a person is truly disabled or whether others, including present or future employers, consider the individual disabled. For example, there are many persons without diabetes who find it difficult to perform certain occupation-related functions. In this regard, the recent literature has described an increased number of hand difficulties among musicians. The majority of these musicians were at the peak of their careers. These difficulties led to loss of control, diminished facility, or loss of speed and ability to perform fast finger movements.[28] Since most of these persons were self-employed or kept their problems secret, in most cases they were able to survive. However, if they had been known to have diabetes, it might have been more difficult, even among those who lived the disciplined but relatively independent lives of musicians.

Participation in the Work Force

Regardless of how participation in the work force is assessed, it would appear that in the United States, about a third of all adult diabetics are actively involved on a regular basis in the work force. Based on information collected through the National Health Interview Survey (NHIS), one of the major general population surveys carried out annually by the National Center for Health Statistics, it has been estimated that in 1976 slightly less than two-fifths (36.9%) of all diabetics 20 years of age and older were in the labor force (Table 45–1). Since the vast majority (93.8%) of all labor force

participants in the general population actually had a job or business in which they were engaged, it follows that about a third (34.6%) of all adult diabetics were employed in 1976 during an average 2-week period. Other indicators of work participation, taking into account a person's experience over a 12-month period, show comparable estimates of work-force participation levels. Based on 1977 NHIS measurements, it is estimated that about 3 of 10 (31.2%) adult diabetics 20 years of age and older had year-round work experience (i.e., worked at a job or business during all 12 months of the previous year). This same 1977 NHIS survey[29] also provided information indicating that as many as two-fifths of adult diabetics had worked at a job or business during at least one of the past 12 months. These data are not significantly different from the National Health Survey Interview material for the period 1959 to 1961.

Variations in the Participation of Diabetics in the World of Work. In the general population, participation in the world of work varies with age, sex, race, education, health status, and many other factors. Comparable variations in the work force occur among adult diabetics (data not shown). Work force participation is inversely associated with age. Within age categories, diabetic men are almost twice as likely as diabetic women to participate in the work force. Black diabetics have lower rates of participation than do white diabetics. Those with fewer years of educational attainment have lower rates of work force participation than do those with more years. Diabetics with activity limitations due to their diabetes or some other chronic condition or impairment are less likely to participate in the work force than those without such limitations. These variations occur irrespective of whether workforce participation is measured by labor force participation rates, work experience, or usual activity during the past 12 months.

Employability Guidelines. Actually, few restrictions must be placed on well-controlled diabetics. Employment standards for persons with diabetes were first recommended by the American Diabetes Association (ADA) in 1972[30] and have been updated since. The introduction to the 1980 standards states: "Guidelines for employment and the placement of the diabetic in industry have been updated. These guidelines are intended to help the physician in his recommendations to management for hiring and job placement so that a safe work environment is insured for both the diabetic and the nondiabetic." Still later, however, in 1982,[31] the ADA Board of Directors decided to abandon specific employment standards and instead stated: "Any diabetic, whether insulin-dependent or non-insulin-dependent, should be able to accept any

Table 45–1. Percent of Persons 20 Years of Age and Over with Known Diabetes in Labor Force by Age and Sex, United States, 1976*

	Total 20 years and over	20–44 years	45–64 years	65 years and over
	Percent in Labor Force			
Both sexes	36.9%	67.4%	48.7%	9.9%
Men	54.0	91.1	68.9	18.6
Women	23.9	53.7	30.0	4.1

*Computed by the Division of Epidemiology and Health Promotion, National Center for Health Statistics, from 1976 National Health Interview Survey data provided by the Division of Health Interview Statistics.

employment for which he or she is individually qualified.''

Since the passage of the Rehabilitation Act of 1973 by the Federal government, most employers cannot deny employment to handicapped persons because of their medical history. In effect, this shifted the focus to job placement rather than employability. The key question is whether or not an individual can perform a specific job. If so, he must be hired. The recent ADA recommendation is consistent with this aspect of the law since it urges that individual consideration be given to determine if a diabetic job applicant is qualified to perform the specific available job. The prior ADA standards were intended to inform personal physicians of diabetics and employers about what jobs were suitable. The ADA recognized that warnings about insulin-dependent diabetics not being placed in jobs where insulin reactions might cause harm to themselves or other employees might unnecessarily limit the employability of diabetics. Petrides and co-workers[32] give in detail comprehensive standards and tests applicable to various job abilities and limitations.

However, in spite of this, insulin-dependent diabetics still do not qualify for commercial pilots' licenses; nor, as mentioned previously, are they permitted to drive buses or trucks in interstate commerce. On the other hand, diabetics who are controlled with oral hypoglycemic agents, while unable to qualify as commercial pilots, are permitted to drive commercial vehicles.

In 1980, the United States Department of Transportation guidelines[33] stated that persons with uncontrolled diabetes should not drive any motor vehicle. However, they divided persons with diabetes and other metabolic conditions into three groups: Group A—Individuals with no episode of altered consciousness for the previous 3 years, who are not taking any medication, can drive any vehicle. Group B—Individuals without any such episode within a year, whether or not on medication, can drive large single vehicles, but are not to haul passengers for hire or hazardous cargo, or drive emergency vehicles. Group C—Individuals who have had an episode of altered consciousness in the previous year, whether or not on medication, are limited to driving passenger vehicles and trucks weighing less than 24,000 pounds, and also cannot have passengers for hire or hazardous cargo or drive emergency vehicles.

Even though airline pilots as a group are extremely responsible people, the medicolegal implications of piloting a jet at barely subsonic speeds with a cargo of several hundred people aboard, are so great that even the suspicion of hypoglycemia-induced poor judgment could be catastrophic. In 1979, 317 million persons were transported by the nation's scheduled airlines compared to 170 million passengers at the start of the decade. So it can be clearly understood that no risk can be taken and the Federal Aviation Administration (FAA) regulations are quite explicit in stating that diabetes requiring any medication for control, oral or otherwise, is disqualifying.[34] However, in the *Guide for Aviation Medical Examiners* dated October, 1981, paragraph 21k states that the finding of glycosuria or proteinuria at the time of examination is cause for deferral by the examiner. Although diabetes mellitus requiring hypoglycemic drugs for control is disqualifying, a past history of need for such medication may not be disqualifying. While a history of diabetes of itself is not disqualifying, a period of control of at least 90 days by diet alone is required.

This strict regulation against the potential dangers of flying while under treatment with anti-diabetic agents has led to some extraordinarily successful regulation of diabetes by diet alone in this most motivated and technically educated work population. In a Joslin Clinic series cited in the previous edition,[35] reference was made to a number of pilots whose diabetes was found early and whose glucose intolerance was unquestionably diabetes but who, with early diagnosis and vigorous dietary treatment, were able to continue flying, sometimes for a number of years. In this age group in a relatively sedentary and generally well-nourished population, diabetes ranks third in frequency for medical groundings. At present, educational efforts are reaching the aviation industry and pilots, either voluntarily or at the request of their medical departments, are being checked for earlier evidences of diabetes before it becomes an obvious clinical entity. Weight reduction programs and diet regulation have salvaged many pilots from what otherwise would have aborted their careers, sometimes many years before their retirement age. However, these are exceptionally motivated persons and one wonders what would happen in the general population with the same desire to diet.

There is a gray area, however, with non-operating personnel such as flight attendants. Apparently each company determines its own rules in this matter. Some have without exception prohibited cabin attendants from flying while under treatment with antidiabetic agents. The justification for this appears to be that in case of an accident of any proportion, the cabin attendant who is responsible for many functions including emergency evacuation, might be suffering from a hypoglycemic reaction and be unable to perform. On the other hand, in a selected group like these attendants and at their ages, the risk of having any significant number of diabetics among them is extremely remote. More-over, most flights now have anywhere from four to a dozen or more flight attendants. Thus, the risk of having a flight attendant in a severe hypogly-cemic reaction at the time of a non-total cata-strophic accident is so remote as to be statistically minuscule. Recently a landmark decision was reached in an out-of-court settlement between a flight attendants' union and a major airline. This decision, taking into consideration that the attend-ant with diabetes had for several years maintained exceptional control, had suffered no hypoglycemic reactions, had an Hb$_{A1c}$ within normal limits, and had been extremely responsible, restored her to her former employment. It agreed in principle that em-ployees in this category should be judged as in-dividuals rather than as a class, and that poor dia-betes regulation with evidence of hypoglycemic reactions would be a subject for disciplinary action as would poor handling of any other medical con-dition. This places the burden where it should be in this particular group of employed individuals, although in this case, the person involved had an exceptional employment record to begin with. The same rules probably would not apply to someone with diabetes attempting to find employment in this type of position. It is, however, an important step forward in understanding the rights of employees who develop diabetes.

To demonstrate the significant changes in atti-tude in several recent decisions,[36] the National Transportation Safety Board has issued orders to the Federal Aviation Administration for medical certification of pilots with surgically treated coro-nary artery disease, thus returning them to active flight status, although with some qualifications. In view of the rapid advance and progress in the use of insulin pumps and the future possibility of pan-creas transplantation, it is apparent that even this area will undergo constant revision. For example, with the new definitions of diabetes as agreed to by the American Diabetes Association, the World Health Organization and the International Diabetes Federation, it may be necessary for the FAA to re-evaluate its standards for diagnosis of diabetes as well.

The Characteristics of Employment

Data from the 1976 NHIS show that with regard to occupation (Table 45–2), about one-half (48.9%) of all employed diabetics were in "white-collar" occupations, another third (32.8%) were in "blue collar" jobs, 14.5% were in service jobs, and another 3.2% were farm workers. Women with diabetes were more likely to be in white-collar and service jobs while a greater proportion of men were in blue-collar and farm jobs.

Since most cases of diabetes are diagnosed after people have settled into an occupation, the forces shaping the occupational distribution of diabetic men and women are probably similar to those af-fecting the nondiabetic population. It is often sug-gested that the expanding array of white-collar oc-cupations may offer diabetics, particularly if diabetes is diagnosed early, a more satisfactory person-job match. It is useful to see if there are differences among time-of-diagnosis categories of employed diabetics with respect to their occupa-tional composition. Table 45–3 shows such data. Men and women diagnosed before their 20th birth-day differ from those diagnosed at later ages with respect to occupational groups. However, while men diagnosed before their 20th birthday were more likely to be in blue-collar jobs than men di-agnosed in later years, the early diagnosed women were more likely to be in white-collar jobs than were women diagnosed later in life. Findings such as these raise a variety of questions. Does diabetes in one's youth affect the capacity to stay in school? Does it reduce the chances of getting sufficient education to compete for a better-paying job? Or, since among entry-level jobs, many blue-collar jobs pay better than white-collar ones, does the tendency for men diagnosed early to be in blue-collar work reflect accommodation to the tempo-rary betterment of economic circumstances, espe-cially if a man is the chief source of family income at the time he enters the labor market?

As far as work setting is concerned, in 1976 currently employed diabetics were primarily found in service industries (27.7%), manufacturing (24.2%), and wholesale and retail settings (20.2%). The remainder were spread among public administration (7.7%), transportation and public utilities (5.8%), insurance and real estate (4.6%), agriculture (4.2%) and construction industries (4.0%). The vast majority of employed diabetics were in privately paid jobs (68.6%) although this percentage declined with age. Almost 1 of 5 (18.3%) worked for government at the local, state, or federal level, and about 1 of 10 (11.8%) were self-employed. The lower proportions in private or public employment differ somewhat from the class-of-worker profile in the general population. These data would lead one to ask: (1) Is it possible that age-related differences in self-employment reflect cohort differences in types of employment which will disappear as younger cohorts of diabetics re-place older cohorts? Self-employment has been de-clining steadily for several decades as a proportion of total employment. (2) Also, one could wonder if the greater proportion of self-employed diabetics reflects either an attempt at security or the avoid-ance of revealing diabetes to a possibly unsym-

Table 45–2. Percent Distribution of Currently Employed Adult Diabetics 20 Years of Age and Over by Occupational Group According to Age and Sex, United States, 1976*

Sex and Age Years	Total	Occupational Group‡				
		White Collar	Blue Collar	Service	Farm	Unknown
		Percent Distribution				
Both sexes						
≥20	100.0%	48.9%	32.8%	14.5%	3.2%	0.6%
20–44	100.0	51.4	31.6	14.9	1.1	1.1
45–64	100.0	47.9	35.2	12.9	3.5	0.4
≥65	100.0	47.3	22.9	22.3	7.5†	—
Male						
≥20	100.0	46.0	40.4	8.9	4.3	0.4†
20–44	100.0	49.2	43.1	5.4†	1.4†	0.9†
45–64	100.0	45.2	42.0	8.1	4.4†	0.3†
≥65	100.0	44.8	27.8	18.8†	8.6†	—
Female						
≥20	100.0	53.8	19.6	24.4	1.5†	0.8†
20–44	100.0	53.4	20.7	23.8	0.8†	1.3†
45–64	100.0	53.9	20.3	23.6	1.7†	0.5†
≥65	100.0	55.0	8.0†	32.7†	4.2†	—

*Computed by the Division of Epidemiology and Health Promotion, National Center for Health Statistics, from 1976 National Health Interview Survey data provided by the Division of Health Interview Statistics.
†Relative standard error greater than 30%.
‡Employed persons are classified by occupation to code categories in the Classified Index of Occupations and Industries of the U.S. Bureau of the Census used for the 1970 Decennial Census. Detailed occupational categories have been condensed into four categories as follows:
"White collar" includes professional, technical, and kindred workers, managers and administrators (except farm), sales workers, and clerical and kindred workers.
"Blue collar" includes craftsmen and kindred workers, operatives (except transport), transport equipment operatives, and laborers (except farm).
"Service" includes service workers (except private household) and private household workers.
"Farm" includes farmers and farm managers, farm laborers, and farm foremen.

Table 45–3. Percent Distribution of Employed Diabetics 20 Years of Age and Over by Occupational Group, According to Age at Diagnosis of Diabetes and Sex, United States, 1976*

Sex and Age at Diagnosis Years	Total	Occupational Group‡				
		White Collar	Blue Collar	Service	Farm	Unknown
		Percent Distribution				
Male						
All ages at diagnosis	100.0	45.4	40.9	9.1	4.1	0.5
<20	100.0	33.2	60.6	3.2	2.9	—
20–39	100.0	48.1	44.9	5.2	1.7	—
40–49	100.0	45.0	40.0	11.4	2.8	0.8
50–59	100.0	46.3	37.7	10.3	4.9	0.9
≥60	100.0	43.4	34.8	11.5	10.3	—
Female						
All ages at diagnosis	100.0	52.3	20.2	25.0	1.7	0.9
<20	100.0	65.9†	13.4†	16.5†	—	4.2†
20–39	100.0	49.0	23.7	26.5	—	0.8
40–49	100.0	56.0	18.2	21.4	4.5	—
50–59	100.0	50.7	22.6	23.4	3.3	—
≥60	100.0	49.1	8.1†	42.7†	—	—

*Computed by the Division of Epidemiology and Health Promotion, National Center for Health Statistics, from 1976 National Health Interview Survey data provided by the Division of Health Interview Statistics.
†Relative standard error greater than 30%.
‡See footnote to Table 45–2.

pathetic employer. Or (3) since stress is thought to be one of the factors in the onset of diabetes in persons genetically predisposed, does the stress associated with a private business or self-employment increase the vulnerability to the condition of those who are borderline or might become diabetic? Probably not, but it is interesting to contemplate.

Employment Experience

Employed Population. The overall impression gained from studies of work experience is that most diabetics have the same experience as their fellow employees without diabetes. For example, studies at the Du Pont Company as well as the Ford Motor Company[37–39] showed that over 70% of the diabetics had completely satisfactory records of absenteeism due to sickness.[39] However, as a result of a less favorable experience in the remainder of the diabetics, the entire group of employed diabetics in both companies had a less satisfactory record of absenteeism for sickness than matched control groups.

The Du Pont Company also did a 10-year follow-up survey of diabetics identified in a 1957 survey and found that about 44% of the diabetics and 60% of matched controls were still active employees at the end of that period. Mortality was 2.6 times greater among the diabetics than the controls, and disability pensions were much more common among the diabetics. The authors commented, however, that "first, the question of what policy to adopt regarding the hiring of diabetics is to a large extent academic because the onset of the disease in most cases occurs after the age of 40 when people are less likely than younger ones to look for new jobs. The second point is that although morbidity and mortality were increased in the diabetic group, the majority of diabetics are still active employees after 10 years of follow-up or have worked to the mandatory retirement age of 65. Thus, a substantial portion of diabetics present no problem with regard to early retirement."

In 1974, Moore and Buschbom[40] reported their findings in a review of studies relating to the employment experience of diabetics. They concluded that one of the major reasons that investigators in 13 studies commencing in 1943 reported higher absentee rates for diabetics, was the fact that the age distributions for the diabetic samples were different from control groups. They analyzed the work records of the diabetics employed at the Hanford Operations in Richland, Washington, for observation periods ranging from 1 year to 5.7 years for an average of 4.3 years. In every category, the absentee rate of diabetics was lower than that of a matched group of nondiabetic employees. The work experience of the Hanford diabetics also com-

pared favorably to Department of Labor absentee rate estimates for heavy industry employees and to estimates from the National Interview Survey from 1965 through 1970.

General Population. General population data show that, compared to nondiabetics of similar age, persons with diabetes tend to have less favorable work-loss profiles (Table 45–4). During 1976, for example, currently employed diabetics averaged 10.8 work-loss days per person compared to 5.4 for nondiabetics. Among diabetics, work-loss days were higher for persons 20 to 44 years of age (14.2 days per person), somewhat lower among persons 45 to 65 years (10.4 days per person), and lowest among the elderly employed (3.8 days per person). Diabetic men in each of these age groups had lower rates than did diabetic women. In the nondiabetic population there was little variation by age.

Unfortunately, however, these overall aggregate comparisons do not reveal the vast individual variation among diabetics with respect to health-related absences from work. Nor do these aggregate statistics highlight the fact that a minority of all currently employed diabetics account for the majority of work-loss days among diabetics. In 1976, about 33.5% of all currently employed diabetics were limited in their activities due to their diabetes or to some other chronic condition or impairment. Nonetheless, this minority of all employed dia-

Table 45–4. Work-loss Days per Year Associated with Acute and Chronic Conditions per Currently Employed Person 20 Years of Age and Over by Diabetic Status, Age, and Sex, United States, 1976*

Sex and Age Years	Total	Diabetic	Non-Diabetic
	Number of Work-loss Days per Person per Year		
Both sexes			
Total, ≥20	5.5	10.8	5.4
20–44	5.2	14.2	5.1
45–64	6.1	10.4	6.0
≥65	4.0	3.8	4.1
Male			
Total, ≥20	5.2	8.4	5.2
20–44	4.8	10.1	4.8
45–64	6.3	9.6	6.1
≥65	3.2	—	3.4
Female			
Total ≥20	5.8	14.9	5.6
20–44	5.7	18.0	5.6
45–64	5.9	12.3	5.8
≥65	5.7	15.3	5.3

*Computed by the Division of Epidemiology and Health Promotion, National Center for Health Statistics, from 1976 National Health Interview Survey data provided by the Division of Health Interview Statistics.

betics accounted for the majority (56.4%) of the work-loss days. These national survey findings are consistent with findings from studies of individual companies which have demonstrated the fallacy of making inferences about the work-loss profile of a particular diabetic person based only on an aggregate level of statistics for all employed diabetics.

Rehabilitation Act of 1973

The Rehabilitation Act of 1973, Public Law 93–112, has been previously summarized. In brief, the intent was (1) to prevent discrimination in the employment of handicapped persons; (2) to insure that after handicapped persons are employed, there are no unfair barriers against advancement and (3) to require affirmative action programs for the hiring of the handicapped. How has this law functioned? Data from the Office of Federal Contract Compliance Programs show that from the time the Rehabilitation Act of 1973 went into effect until May 1, 1979,[41] there were about 7,500 cases of alleged discrimination against handicapped persons, and of these, 224 or 3% were identified as diabetics. During the period from May 1, 1979 to December 31, 1980, there were 3,199 complaints of which 94 or 2.9% were identified as diabetic. This seems to indicate an increasing rate of complaints in the more recent period although the percentage of complaints involving diabetics has remained constant. There is no evidence available on the resolution of the complaints.

Second Injury Laws. Over the years, employers have been reluctant to hire handicapped persons because of a belief that such persons were prone to accidents, resulting in payment of higher premiums for workers' compensation insurance. This type of insurance is compulsory in 48 of the 50 states, being elective only in New Jersey and Texas. It provides monetary benefits to workers who sustain job-related injuries whether or not the injured employee was at fault. The passage of second injury laws has helped to relieve some of the financial burden imposed on a company by the prolonged disability, not only of diabetics, but of any person with known impairment when hired.

The main provision of these laws is to provide a fund to help defray the expenses of an impaired person who sustains a subsequent injury on the job. These laws limit significantly the employer's liability when such an injury occurs. This serves to encourage employers to hire handicapped people. In addition, second injury laws increase the chances that the injured person will be fully compensated for the period of disability. The laws vary a great deal, being more generous in some states than in others, but they are of direct benefit to diabetics and to employers who knowingly hire them.

Labor Market Problems as Determined by the 1976 NHIS. Despite the Rehabilitation Act of 1973 and the second-injury laws, many diabetics have difficulty in obtaining employment. There has been improvement since the survey done in 1957,[42] which indicated that among companies polled, 60% of the small and 71% of the large organizations hired no known diabetics, which figures, incidentally, were not much greater than those reported in a survey almost 25 years previously. However, there has been increasing pressure upon employers to regard persons with diabetes as functionally useful employees. The International Diabetes Federation acknowledged the existence of the problem on a world-wide scale as far back as 1963. In 1965, the World Health Organization Expert Committee on Diabetes took a strong stand on this problem and has continued to emphasize the need for diabetics to have an equal opportunity to obtain and perform work for which they are medically and vocationally suitable.[43]

Unemployment was also found in the 1976 NHIS to be a major problem for some diabetics, particularly males aged 20 to 44 years and females 45 to 64 years (Table 45–5). Elderly diabetics of both sexes appeared to have fewer problems finding employment, but the fact that virtually all the elderly labor-force diabetics in the 1976 NHIS sample were currently employed may simply be due to the fact that traditional unemployment statistics do not adequately reflect worker discouragement in even looking for a job when economic times are bad.

Labor Market Needs of Diabetics with Some Chronic Limitation of Activity. About half of all adult diabetics have some limitation of activity due to their diabetes or some other chronic condition or impairment. These limitations severely restrict the extent of their participation in the work force. Among diabetic adults, those with a limitation, as compared with those with no limitation, are less likely to be in the labor force and, if working, are less likely to have worked year-round or to be currently employed. (Table 45–6). The labor market situation of diabetics between the ages of 20 and 44 with only a high school or less education is especially severe. While most other age-education categories of diabetics in the labor force had an employment rate in 1976 of approximately 90%, young diabetics with a high school or less education had an employment rate of 74% or lower during that period. This means that the unemployment rate in the lower education categories of young diabetics with some restricted activity is about 25%. Despite the apparently severe labor market difficulties which these less-educated, relatively young

Table 45–5. Percent Distribution of Persons 20 Years of Age and Over in the Labor Force by Current Employment Status, According to Diabetic Status, Age and Sex, United States, 1976*

Sex and Current Employment Status	Total ≥ 20 years		20–44 years		45–64 years		65 years and over	
	Diabetic	Non-Diabetic	Diabetic	Non-Diabetic	Diabetic	Non-Diabetic	Diabetic	Non-Diabetic
Men								
Total in labor force	100.0	100.0	100.0	100.0	100.0	100.0	100.0	100.0
				Percent Distribution				
Employed	94.7	94.3	88.8	93.6	95.9	95.6	100.0	95.0
Unemployed	5.3	5.7	11.2†	6.4	4.1†	4.4	—	5.0
Women								
Total in labor force	100.0	100.0	100.0	100.0	100.0	100.0	100.0	100.0
				Percent Distribution				
Employed	92.5	92.1	91.5	90.9	92.2	94.1	100.0	95.8
Unemployed	7.5	7.9	8.5†	9.1	7.8†	5.9	—	4.2

*Computed by the Division of Epidemiology and Health Promotion, National Center for Health Statistics from 1976 National Health Interview Survey data provided by the Division of Health Interview Statistics.
†Relative standard error greater than 30%.

diabetics experience, only 11% of them were estimated in 1977 to have received any job training, counseling or placement assistance in the previous 12 months.

HEALTH CHARACTERISTICS OF ADULT DIABETICS

Since we have been discussing the influence of health on employability and the general lifestyle of diabetics, it is time to discuss the health status of adults to determine more precisely the extent of their limitations and disabilities. Adult diabetics are 2 to 3 times more likely than nondiabetics to perceive their health as only "fair" or "poor" and these assessments are more prevalent among older persons and those with fewer years of formal schooling.

In 1976, only 15.3% of nondiabetics considered their health as fair or poor, while close to half (48.1%) of all adult diabetics did so. Moreover, although this 3-fold difference in perceived fair or poor health is diminished somewhat for some age-education categories, there is still at least a 2-fold difference in each age-education comparison shown in Table 45–7. Among persons 20 to 44 years of age with 13 or more years of schooling, there is a 7-fold difference, with 3.9% of the nondiabetics and 27.8% of the diabetics reporting that they were in only fair or poor health.

Disability Days and Limitation of Activity. There are many specific ways to measure the health status of a person or a group. One general approach is to think of health as the capacity to perform daily familial and social obligations. Within this frame-

work, illness can be thought of as the incapacity to perform these duties. This social dysfunction approach can be used (1) to estimate the magnitude of illness events associated with acute and chronic conditions among various categories of the population or (2) to estimate the percentage of persons with long-term limitation of activity due to chronic conditions or impairments.

Table 45–8 presents data on each of these types of health indicators for diabetics and nondiabetics based on the 1976 NHIS. Even when age differences are taken into account, the levels of restricted-activity days and bed-disability days, as well as the prevalence of chronic activity limitation, are at least double for diabetics as compared to nondiabetics.

However, among diabetics as among the general population, persons limited in activity due to a chronic condition or impairment account for a disproportionate share of restricted-activity and bed-disability days. Moreover, what is true in this regard for all types of chronic activity limitation is also true specifically for diabetes as a cause of chronic activity limitation. Data collected through the 1975 NHIS make it possible to estimate the percent of persons with diabetes for whom diabetes was reported as causing their limitation of activity (Table 45–9). It is also possible from this same data source to estimate the volume and rate of restricted-activity and bed-disability days reported by diabetics as due to their diabetes. Overall, diabetes was reported as a *cause* of activity limitation in 30.9% of those for whom diabetes was estimated to cause chronic activity limitation. In 15.3% of

Table 45–6. Selected Indicators of Workforce Participation among Diabetics 20 Years of Age and Over by Education, Chronic Activity Limitation, and Age, United States, 1976*

Limitation of Activity and Education	Labor Force Participation				Currently Employed				Year-round Employment‡			
	≥20	Years of Age			≥20	Years of Age			≥20	Years of Age		
		20–44	45–64	≥65		20–44	45–64	≥65		20–44	45–64	≥65
	Percent in labor force				Percent currently employed§				Percent with year-round employment			
Limited in Activity Years of Schooling												
All levels	23.7	52.8	33.1	7.2	91.9	79.3	94.8	100.0	16.3	36.8	22.2	6.5
<12	16.2	32.2	24.9	7.0	90.9	68.5†	92.1	100.0	9.6	16.2	14.0	5.7
12	36.0	61.9	42.5	7.1	91.4	74.2	98.7	100.0	23.5	43.9	26.7	6.6†
≥13	42.9	75.9	49.1	11.8†	94.2	93.2	93.8	100.0†	36.4	62.0	46.1	11.3†
Not limited in Activity Years of Schooling												
All levels	52.9	74.7	68.8	14.3	94.9	94.0	94.7	100.0	46.6	57.8	60.0	16.8
<12	42.3	71.7	60.1	12.8	91.4	86.4	91.8	100.0	33.9	39.2	53.2	10.8
12	62.1	71.7	78.3	12.7†	97.1	96.4	97.3	100.0†	55.4	63.3	63.4	20.9†
≥13	66.8	81.7	74.6	26.5†	97.5	100.0	100.0	100.0†	61.3	68.6	69.4	34.9

*Computed by the Division of Epidemiology and Health Promotion, National Center for Health Statistics, from 1976 and 1977 National Health Interview Survey data provided by the Division of Health Interview Statistics.
†Relative standard error greater than 30%.
‡Data from 1977.
§Percent of labor force.

Table 45–7. Percent of Persons 20 Years of Age and Over Who Perceived Themselves as Only in Fair or Poor Health, by Education, Diabetic Status, and Age, United States, 1976*

Education	≥20 Years of Age			20–44 Years of Age			45–64 Years of Age			≥65 Years of Age		
	Total	Non-Diabetic	Diabetic	Sub-Total	Non-Diabetic	Diabetic	Sub-Total	Non-Diabetic	Diabetic	Sub-Total	Non-Diabetic	Diabetic
All levels	16.4	15.3	48.1	8.7	8.4	36.3	22.2	20.6	51.2	31.2	29.5	49.6
<12 years	30.0	28.3	56.8	18.9	18.3	49.0	34.1	32.2	61.3	36.9	35.1	54.5
12 years	12.0	11.3	39.1	7.9	7.7	31.4	16.7	15.7	42.0	23.8	22.5	40.6
≥13 years	6.6	6.1	31.4	4.1	3.9	27.8	9.9	9.0	33.9	17.5	16.7	31.4

*Computed by the Division of Epidemiology and Health Promotion, National Center for Health Statistics from 1976 National Health Interview Survey data provided by the Division of Health Interview Statistics.

Table 45–8.   Days of Disability and Limitation of Activity Among Persons 20 Years of Age and Over by Diabetic Status, United States, 1976*

Type of Disability Day and Extent of Limitation	Number of Disability Days per Person per Year			
	Unadjusted for Age		Age-Adjusted	
	Nondiabetic	Diabetic	Nondiabetic	Diabetic
Type of Disability Day				
Restricted-Activity Days	20.9	55.0	21.2	46.9
Bed-Disability Days	7.7	21.6	7.3	19.3

Limitation of Activity due to Chronic Conditions	Percent of Persons with Limitation of Activity			
	Unadjusted for Age		Age-Adjusted	
	Nondiabetic	Diabetic	Nondiabetic	Diabetic
Limited	18.6	55.9	18.9	46.4
Limited in major activity	14.3	48.6	14.6	37.7
Unable to perform usual activity	4.8	19.9	4.9	12.7
Limited, but not in major activity	4.3	7.3	4.3	8.9

*Computed by the Division of Epidemiology and Health Promotion, National Center for Health Statistics, from 1976 National Health Interview Survey data provided by the Division of Health Interview Statistics.

Table 45–9.   Percent Distribution and Rate per Person per Year of Restricted Activity Days Associated with Known Diabetes, by Diabetes as a Cause of Chronic Activity Limitation, and Age in Persons 20 Years of Age and Over, United States, 1975*

Diabetes as a Cause of Chronic Activity Limitation	Persons 20 Years and Over with Known Diabetes			
	Total	20–44 years	45–64 years	65 years and over
Total: Number (in thousands)	4,668	735	2,166	1,767
Percent	100.0	100.0	100.0	100.0
Diabetes reported as cause of chronic activity limitation	Percent Distribution			
Yes	30.9	24.2	30.3	34.5
Main Cause	15.3	17.8	14.7	14.9
Secondary Cause	15.7	6.5	15.7	19.5
No	69.1	75.6	69.7	65.6
	Restricted Activity Days Associated with Known Diabetes			
Total: Number (in thousands)	88,156	12,296	35,310	40,549
Percent	100.0	100.0	100.0	100.0
Diabetes reported as cause of chronic activity limitation	Percent Distribution			
Yes	63.2	61.7	56.9	69.2
Main Cause	37.3	43.1	27.7	43.8
Secondary Cause	26.0	18.6	29.1	25.5
No	37.0	38.3	43.1	30.8
	Number of Restricted Activity Days Associated with Known Diabetes per Person per Year			
Total	18.9	16.7	16.3	22.9
Diabetes reported as cause of chronic activity limitation				
Yes	38.6	42.6	30.6	46.1
Main Cause	46.1	40.5	30.8	67.2
Secondary Cause	31.2	47.6	30.4	30.0
No	10.1	8.5	10.1	10.8

*Computed by the Division of Epidemiology and Health Promotion, National Center for Health Statistics, from 1975 National Health Interview Survey data provided by the Division of Health Interview Statistics.

the cases it was reported as the *main cause* (See top panel of Table 45–9).

There are some important age variations in the distribution of diabetes as a cause of activity limitation. However, two general points are important and require comment. (1) Some 30% of diabetics (See top panel of Table 45–9) account for about 63% of all the restricted-activity days associated with diabetes (See middle panel of Table 45–9); (2) Among diabetics for whom their diabetes is not a cause of chronic activity limitation, the number of restricted-activity days per person per year associated with diabetes is only 10.1 days, contrasted with 38.6 days for diabetics for whom their diabetes is a cause of activity limitation (See bottom panel of Table 45–9). Findings presented earlier in this chapter on absence from work due to illness or injury (Table 45–4) show a similar pattern and argue the need for looking closely at individual differences if one is not to make false inferences about diabetics from statistics on diabetics as a group.

Prevalence of Selected Chronic Conditions. One reason why diabetics have higher rates of disability days than nondiabetics is that diabetics are more likely to have additional complicating chronic conditions. In 1976, as shown in Table 45–10 diabetics and nondiabetics were asked in the NHIS if they had ever had cataracts, glaucoma, arteriosclerosis, hypertension, a heart attack, other cardiac problems, a "stroke," or kidney trouble. Even with age taken into account, diabetics were at least twice as likely as nondiabetics to report ever having had any of these conditons.

Utilization of Health Services. Given the levels of activity limitation and complicating chronic illnesses among diabetics, one would expect them to make greater use of physicians and hospitals than persons without such problems, and they do. Even

after the older age of diabetics is taken into account, diabetics are about twice as likely to visit physicians and to use short-stay hospitals as are nondiabetics. In 1976 (Table 45–11) the age-adjusted number of physician visits per person per year was 11.6 for diabetics and only 5.3 for nondiabetics. The age-adjusted annual number of discharges (not counting discharges for deliveries) from short-stay hospitals per 1000 persons was 38.8 for diabetics and only 15.0 for nondiabetics. The average length of stay for these discharges was about 2 days longer for diabetics than it was for nondiabetics—11.0 days and 8.9 days respectively. In the course of the 12-month period prior to their 1976 NHIS interview, 25.8% of diabetics, but only 12.6% of nondiabetics, had been in a short-stay hospital overnight at least once.

In contrast to their greater use of physicians and hospitals, diabetics make less use of dentists than do nondiabetics. In 1976, the age-adjusted percent of persons contacting a dentist one or more times in the preceding 12 months was 39.4% for diabetics and 47.6% for nondiabetics. The fact that the number of dental visits per person per year is similar for nondiabetics and diabetics (1.7 vs 1.8 respectively) might indicate a greater number of dental visits among diabetics who use dentists than among nondiabetics. However, actually the relative frequency of visiting a dentist among adults who use dentists at all, is about the same; in 1976, the annual rate of dental visits per person among such individuals was 3.4 in nondiabetics and 4.2 in diabetics. Perhaps there is a small proportion of diabetics who use dentists with an unusually high number of visits. (Data regarding dental care are not shown in a table; however, see Table 45–14.)

LIFE INSURANCE

The demonstration of improved life expectancy as well as the better understanding of different

Table 45–10.   Prevalence of Selected Chronic Conditions Reported in Household Interviews Among Persons 20 Years of Age and Over by Diabetic Status, United States, 1976*

| Chronic Condition | Persons 20 Years of Age and Over | | | |
| | Nondiabetic | Diabetic | Nondiabetic | Diabetic |
	Unadjusted Rate Per 1,000 Persons		Age-Adjusted Rate Per 1,000 Persons†	
Cataracts	34.0	121.4	35.4	68.5
Glaucoma	9.5	39.4	9.8	26.4
Arteriosclerosis	24.5	115.4	25.4	67.5
Hypertension	159.8	464.4	162.6	382.8
Heart Attack	29.3	131.6	30.3	76.8
Other Heart Trouble	47.1	172.9	48.1	123.2
Stroke	12.2	65.2	12.7	35.6
Kidney Trouble	65.7	144.0	66.1	139.8

*Computed by the Division of Epidemiology and Health Promotion, National Center for Health Statistics, from 1976 National Health Interview Survey data provided by the Division of Health Interview Statistics.
†Age adjusted by the direct method to the 1976 civilian noninstitutionalized population, using 3 age intervals.

Table 45–11. Selected Measures of Health Care Utilization Among Persons 20 Years of Age and Over by Diabetic Status, United States, 1976*

Measures of Utilization	Persons 20 Years of Age and Over			
	Nondiabetic	Diabetic	Nondiabetic	Diabetic
	Unadjusted Rate or Percent		Age-Adjusted Rate or Percent†	
Physician Visits				
Number per Person per Year	5.3	11.0	5.3	11.6
Percent of Persons with Visits in Past Year	76.0	91.8	75.8	91.5
Dental Visits				
Number per Person per Year	1.6	1.4	1.7	1.8
Percent of Persons with Visits in Past Year	40.1	34.1	47.6	39.4
Hospitalization				
Number of Discharges per 1000 Persons per Year	16.7	39.4	16.8	41.9
Number of Discharges (Excluding Deliveries) per 1000 Persons per Year	14.9	38.4	15.0	38.8
Average Length of Stay in Days	8.3	11.8	8.4	10.5
Average Length of Stay (Excluding Deliveries) in Days	8.8	12.0	8.9	11.0
Percent of Persons with one Hospital Episode or More in Past Year	12.6	25.6	12.6	25.8

*Computed by the Division of Epidemiology and Health Promotion. National Center for Health Statistics, from 1976 National Health Interview Survey data provided by the Division of Health Interview Statistics.
†Age-adjusted by the direct method to the 1976 civilian noninstitutionalized population using 3 age intervals.

types of diabetes has led, in some instances, to a more liberal approach to life insurance for diabetics. Most diabetics today qualify for individual life insurance policies and many are issued policies at standard rates.[44] Nevertheless, in spite of improvement in this regard, many persons with diabetes have difficulty obtaining insurance without paying a higher premium. Because of many early evidences of possible future complications, and because the longevity of diabetic persons, although vastly improved, is not as great as in persons without diabetes, many diabetics are classified as substandard risks.

The experience of insurance companies has tended to corroborate the rationale behind the revised classification of diabetes mellitus and other categories of glucose intolerance proposed by the National Diabetes Data Group.[45] Type I, or insulin-dependent, diabetes mellitus is associated with the highest mortality rates. Major studies of insured diabetics carried out by the Equitable Life Assurance Society of the United States,[46] Lincoln National Life Insurance Company,[47] New York Life Insurance Company,[48] and Metropolitan Life Insurance Company[49] have all shown that excess mortality, as measured by the mortality ratios, was highest among those diabetics whose onset of disease was at the very young ages and who presumably had insulin-dependent diabetes. The lowest mortality ratios were found in the older age groups, comprised mostly of persons with noninsulin-de-

pendent diabetes. The mortality tended to increase with duration following the issuance of insurance, with a leveling off or decrease at the longest durations. In all categories, there was an extremely unfavorable impact on mortality if proteinuria was found at the time of examination for insurance, with mortality ratios of over 10-fold. This undoubtedly resulted from the presence of diabetic nephropathy as well as generalized small vessel disease. The presence of minor cardiovascular abnormalities, demonstrated primarily by hypertension or by electrocardiographic changes with no history of myocardial infarction, had an adverse effect on mortality but not as severe as that associated with proteinuria. Overweight caused only a modest increase in mortality.

An analysis of mortality among insured diabetics by Metropolitan Life[50] showed that there was an improvement in mortality among diabetics issued insurance during the period 1961 to 1973 and traced to January 1, 1979, as compared to those diabetics issued insurance in 1961 to 1965 and traced to January 1, 1968. In all likelihood, this reflects the generally decreased mortality ratios among diabetics in recent years.

An important contribution of the new classification of diabetes mellitus is that impaired glucose tolerance and gestational diabetes are in separate categories and are not considered to be stages of diabetes. This is also true of previous and potential abnormalities of glucose tolerance. The prognosis of all of these categories is considered to be favorable, and, from an insurance viewpoint, standard insurance can be issued.

Most insurance companies, when evaluating diabetic insurance applicants, consider the following factors to be important:

1. Type of diabetes (insulin-dependent or non-insulin-dependent).
2. Duration of the disease.
3. Adequacy of control.
4. Severity of the disease as indicated by size of insulin dose.
5. Presence or absence of complications of the disease.

Noninsulin-dependent diabetics without complications of the disease may be issued standard insurance, and those using effective oral hypoglycemic drug therapy are considered as favorably as patients able to control their condition by diet alone. Insulin-dependent diabetics are generally issued substandard insurance; if complications are present, they are evaluated on an individual basis and may be rejected or issued coverage, but in a substandard classification.

Many persons with diabetes are covered by group life and/or health insurance at their places of employment. When a group insurance contract is issued to a company, all of the employees actively at work at the time or within a specified period prior to the time the contract goes into effect are automatically covered by the insurance if they indicate their desire to be covered. This is true regardless of what medical conditions they may have at the time. If a person develops diabetes after being employed for a period of time and while covered by the policy, he cannot have the insurance canceled while he remains in the employ of the company.

Diabetes associations are becoming increasingly aggressive in seeking insurance coverage for their members and are sometimes able to participate in group plans at more reasonable rates than an individual can obtain.

PROBLEMS OBTAINING AND PAYING FOR HEALTH CARE

Access to Health Care

With the possible exception of dental care, it would appear that most diabetics have fairly good access to adequate health care. Access, however, has many facets which are not always evident in utilization statistics. Some minimal aspects of access to health care which should be assessed include: (1) having a well-defined point of entry into the health care system, (2) having a personal phy-

sician in whatever health care setting is utilized, (3) freedom from problems getting health care when needed and (4) actually getting the needed health care.

Concerning a well-defined entry point, it would appear from 1978 NHIS data that diabetics are well positioned vis-a-vis the health care system. When asked whether they had a particular place or doctor they could turn to for help or advice about their health, more than 90% of diabetics reported affirmatively. Moreover, among the 6% of diabetics who reported no one particular source of medical care, about half stated that they generally saw different physicians depending on their particular problem at the time. Among those with a regular source of care, the majority reported that they routinely went to a private physician's office or clinic. One of 10 diabetics with a regular source of care made routine use of hospital outpatient departments. As for access to a physician, about 4 of 5 diabetics with a regular source of care indicated that they had a particular doctor at their usual place for health care.

There are still, however, some important problem areas. Among diabetics with a regular source of care, as many as 39% of economically deprived blacks reported a hospital outpatient department as their place of care, whereas an average of only about 5% of other poor/non-poor categories of diabetics reported regular use of outpatient facilities. In the same vein, while at least 9 of 10 diabetics in most poor/non-poor categories had a particular doctor to whom they usually went, only about 7 of 10 poorer black diabetics reported having their own physician at their usual source of care.

The process of getting medical care also presents problems for some diabetics. In 1977, diabetics and nondiabetics alike were asked by NHIS interviewers whether they had had any problems getting medical care in the past 12 months because of one or more of the following problems: (1) no care was available when needed; (2) the cost of care; (3) they did not know where to go; (4) they had transportation problems; or (5) hours were not convenient. While about 9.2% of all nondiabetics reported having had one or more of these problems, some 15.3% of diabetics had at least one of them. Among young diabetics, 20 to 44 years of age, as many as 24% reported having one or more problems getting health care in contrast to about 11% of their nondiabetic counterparts. The specific problem identified most frequently by both diabetics (9.3%) and nondiabetics (5.1%), was the cost of health care. Young persons with diabetes were twice as likely (18%) to identify costs as a problem as were diabetics generally, and about three times as likely as young nondiabetics.

All persons who reported having a problem getting medical care were asked in the 1977 NHIS whether the problem had prevented them from securing medical care. Based on their responses, it is estimated that overall, about 8.3% of adult diabetics were unable to get health care that they thought they needed, compared to about 5% of all nondiabetics. Young diabetics were twice as likely as diabetics in general to be unable to get needed care, and more than twice as likely as young nondiabetics to be prevented from receiving needed health care.

That health care costs are particularly burdensome for young diabetics is evidenced from information obtained during the 1974 NHIS on perceptions and reasons for unmet heath care needs. In that earlier survey, respondents were asked whether or not they believed they were getting all the health care they needed. About 9% of diabetics generally and about 11% of young diabetics felt that they were not. However, while about 60% of all diabetics with unmet needs cited the cost of health care as a reason for this, as many as 73% of young diabetics with unmet health care needs reported cost to be the reason.

In addition to these problems of health care accessibility with which small but substantial minorities of diabetics are burdened, there are problems of accessibility in the area of preventive health services. These other problems are less visible, however, because in many areas of preventive health services, diabetics are either slightly more likely or as likely as their nondiabetic counterparts to have recently received the service. In comparing diabetics and nondiabetics with respect to recent use of selected preventive health services such as eye examinations including glaucoma tests, chest x-rays, and electrocardiograms (Table 45–12), it appears that diabetics are just as likely if not more likely than nondiabetics to have obtained these services in the recent past. However, given the greater relative risk of eye and cardiovascular complications among diabetics, it might be argued that the differences between diabetics and nondiabetics should be greater in the use of certain of the services than the data in Table 45–12 indicate to be the case.

Health Care Coverage

Everyone firmly believes that diabetics require a good deal of medical care and hospitalization since this is a chronic, multi-system condition. Given the rising costs of health care, it has been speculated that a major reason that some diabetics experience problems with the costs of their diabetes, is that they lack adequate health care coverage. Until quite recently, information on the per-

Table 45–12. Use of Selected Preventive Health Services, According to Diabetes Status and Age, United States, 1973*

Preventive Health Service and Age	Total	Diabetes Status	
		Diabetic	Nondi-abetic
		Percent of Persons	
Eye Examination†			
Total	50.3	57.0‡	50.1‡
20–44 years	48.1	58.6	48.0
45–64 years	54.5	56.8	54.4
65 years and over	48.4	52.4	48.1
Glaucoma Test†			
Total	33.3	40.5‡	33.0‡
40–44 years	26.4	42.7	26.1
45–64 years	34.8	39.5	34.6
65 years and over	34.0	41.3	33.3
Chest x-ray†			
Total	44.6	59.3‡	44.1‡
20–44 years	43.9	59.2	43.7
45–64 years	47.2	63.3	46.4
65 years and over	41.5	51.2	40.7
Electrocardiogram†			
Total	33.0	51.8‡	32.0‡
40–44 years	26.1	41.2	25.8
45–64 years	32.7	54.3	31.7
65 years and over	37.3	52.4	36.0

*Drury, T.F., Harris, M., Lipsett, L.F.: Prevalence and Management of Diabetes. Health-United States, 1981. U.S. Department of Health and Human Services, December, 1981, p. 27.
†During past 2 years.
‡Age-adjusted by the direct method to the 1973 civilian noninstitutionalized population, using 3 age intervals.

centages of diabetics with private health insurance and other types of health care coverage has been unavailable. In 1978, however, the NHIS obtained such information for diabetics in a one-third subsample of households. With these data (Table 45–13), it is now possible for the first time to estimate the percentage of diabetics in various age categories of the population with private health insurance coverage, Medicare coverage, Supplemental Security Income coverage, Medicaid coverage, military (CHAMPUS) or Veterans Administration health benefits coverage, as well as the percentage with any of these types of coverage.[51]

In 1978, about 7 of 10 diabetics were estimated to have some form of private health insurance, compared to about 8 of 10 nondiabetics. This difference in private health insurance coverage between diabetics and nondiabetics primarily reflects the situation of diabetics 20 to 64 years of age. Among the elderly, there appears to be little or no difference in private health insurance coverage. Because Medicare charges are handled locally by intermediary insurance companies, such as Blue

Cross/Blue Shield, it is suspected that some Medicare recipients who receive copies of paid invoices for their personal medical records from intermediary insurance companies misinterpret this to mean that they have private health insurance when they actually do not. This source of response bias is adjusted for, however, in the estimate of the elderly who have either private health insurance or Medicare, and from these latter data it would appear that virtually all elderly persons have at least one of these types of health care coverage irrespective of whether they are diabetic (98.1%) or nondiabetic (97.3%).

Persons under age 65 may receive health services under Medicare if they are disabled. Presumably, the higher rates of Medicare coverage for diabetics 20 to 64, particularly among diabetics 45 to 64, as compared to similarly aged nondiabetics, reflect the higher rate of disabling illnesses among these younger and especially middle-aged diabetics.

A small minority of diabetics also have some health services paid for by the Supplemental Security Income (SSI) (6.9%) and Medicaid (11%) programs. Participation in these two programs is relatively higher for diabetics than it is for nondiabetics, but these differences in SSI and Medicaid participation rates primarily reflect differences in both groups from 20 to 64 years of age. In the case of Medicaid participation, young diabetics are about 4 times more likely than similarly aged nondiabetics to participate in the program, with 15.5% of young diabetics and 4.4% of young nondiabetics participating in the program in some fashion in 1978.

In 1978, 11.3% of adult diabetics were identified by NHIS as having either military or Veterans Administration (V.A.) health benefits coverage, compared to 6.6% of nondiabetics with one of these coverages. Most of this difference reflects the greater percentage of diabetics 45 to 64 years of age having military or V.A. health care coverage in comparison with nondiabetics in the same age

Table 45–13. Percent of Persons 20 Years of Age and Over with Selected Types of Health Care Coverage by Diabetic Status and Age, United States, 1978*

Type of Health Care Coverage and Diabetic Status	Persons 20 Years of Age and Over				
	20 Yrs. and Over	20–64 Years	20–44 Years	45–64 Years	65 Yrs. and Over
	Percent of Persons with Coverage				
Private Health Insurance Coverage					
Total	79.4	81.7	80.6	83.7	67.3
Nondiabetic	79.7	82.0	80.7	84.3	67.1
Diabetic	70.8	71.7	68.2	72.9	69.4
Medicare					
Total	16.6	2.0	1.0	4.3	93.5
Nondiabetic	15.7	1.8	1.0	3.9	93.3
Diabetic	41.3	8.7	4.5†	10.2	95.9
Private Health Insurance Coverage or Medicare					
Total	85.1	82.8	81.0	85.8	97.3
Nondiabetic	85.1	82.9	81.1	86.2	97.3
Diabetic	84.6	76.6	72.0	78.2	98.1
Supplemental Security Income					
Total	2.1	1.1	1.0	1.6	7.3
Nondiabetic	1.9	1.0	1.0	1.4	7.2
Diabetic	6.9	5.4	5.1†	5.6	9.4
Medicaid					
Total	4.8	4.1	4.5	3.3	8.8
Nondiabetic	4.6	3.9	4.4	3.0	8.6
Diabetic	11.0	10.6	15.5	8.9	11.6
Military or V.A.					
Total	6.8	5.6	3.6	9.1	13.0
Nondiabetic	6.6	5.5	3.6	8.9	13.1
Diabetic	11.3	10.9	3.5	13.6	11.8
Any of Above Types of Coverage					
Total	90.0	88.5	87.0	91.2	98.9
Nondiabetic	89.9	88.3	86.8	91.2	98.8
Diabetic	91.7	87.1	84.5	88.0	99.4

*Computed by the Division of Epidemiology and Health Promotion, National Center for Health Statistics, from 1978 National Health Interview Survey data provided by the Division of Health Interview Statistics.
†Relative standard error greater than 30%.

group—13.6% compared to 8.9%. Since diabetes with onset early in life is usually disqualifying for military service, this suggests that the disease started during or after military service, and many such patients continue their diabetes care through the Veterans Administration.

Further analysis of the above data reveals that the vast majority of diabetics have at least one or more of the above types of health care coverage. Of all diabetics 20 years of age and over, 91.7% were identified in 1978 as having either private health insurance, Medicare, SSI, Medicaid or military or V.A. health benefits coverage. Young diabetics were least likely (84.5%) to have any of these types of health care coverage while virtually all (99.4%) elderly diabetics had some form of coverage.

Out-of-Pocket Health Care Costs

Cost is the major reason which diabetics, particularly younger diabetics, give for not getting all the health care they feel they need. The basis for this is not difficult to discern when the average out-of-pocket health expenditures of diabetics are examined. Table 45–14 compares the per capita out-of-pocket costs for various types of expenses borne by diabetics and nondiabetics during the calendar year 1975. Table 45–15 shows related information on the average expenses of diabetics and nondiabetics with expenses during the same time period. These data were obtained from households interviewed in the NHIS during the first quarter of 1976.

Differentials in the use of physicians and short-stay hospitals (already noted) translate into far greater out-of-pocket expenditures for diabetics both on a per capita basis and in terms of average expenses for persons with any expense. The per capita information on dental expenses is consistent with data discussed previously which showed the average annual number of dental visits per person to be about the same for diabetics and nondiabetics. The average dental expenses, however, show a higher expenditure for diabetics, suggesting that diabetics either have more complicated dental work done or a small number of diabetics have an unusually large number of dental visits. In view of the fact that most adult diabetics use insulin or oral hypoglycemic agents and that others often are on medication for hypertension or other complications, it is not surprising that diabetics average higher out-of-pocket costs for prescribed medicines. Optical expenses, however, are quite similar for diabetics and nondiabetics. The per capita costs of health insurance premiums are also about the same for diabetics and nondiabetics, possibly because the vast majority of diabetics already have health insurance before they are diagnosed as having diabetes.

The higher average expense for health insurance premiums among diabetics who have such coverage may reflect the higher costs of substandard health insurance coverage for many diabetics. It is possible, however, that the slight difference in average expenses for health insurance simply reflects the manner in which these family health expenditures have been allocated to individuals in this survey.

With this in mind, the total age-adjusted out-of-pocket health expenses, including the allocated costs for insurance premiums, for diabetics who

Table 45–14. Per Capita Out-of-Pocket Health Expenses Among Persons 20 Years of Age and Over, by Type of Expense and Diabetic Status, United States, 1975*

Type of Expense	Persons 20 Years of Age and Over			
	Nondiabetic	Diabetic	Nondiabetic	Diabetic
	Unadjusted per capita expense in dollars		Age-adjusted‡ per capita expense in dollars	
All Types†				
Including Insurance Premiums	$296	$537	$299	$473
Excluding Insurance Premiums	220	442	222	405
Hospital	37	84	37	68
Physician	76	145	77	139
Dental	47	42	47	49
Prescription medicine	38	139	38	131
Optical	18	22	18	16
Health Insurance Premium	75	91	76	78
Other	8	19	8	11

*Division of Health Interview Statistics, National Center for Health Statistics: Unpublished data from the 1976 First Quarter National Health Interview Survey.
†Since estimates for specific expenses are based on slightly different item response rates, per capita expenses for specific types of expense do not add to total per capita expenses.
‡Age adjusted by the direct method to the first quarter 1976 civilian noninstitutionalized population, using three age intervals.

Table 45–15. Average Out-of-Pocket Health Expenses for Persons 20 Years of Age and Over with Such Expense by Type of Expense and Diabetic Status, United States, 1975*

Type of Expense	Persons 20 Years of Age and Over			
	Nondiabetic	Diabetic	Nondiabetic	Diabetic
	Unadjusted average expenses in dollars		Age-adjusted† average expenses in dollars	
All Types				
Including Insurance				
Premiums	$332	$594	$335	$536
Excluding Insurance				
Premiums	275	524	277	477
Hospital	294	400	289	320
Physician	125	211	125	196
Dental	108	145	109	147
Prescription Medicine	67	181	66	172
Optical	69	69	68	62
Health Insurance Premiums	122	135	119	131
Other	119	159	105	112

*Division of Health Interview Statistics, National Center for Health Statistics. Unpublished data from the 1976 First Quarter National Health Interview Survey.
†Age-adjusted by the direct method to the first quarter 1976 civilian noninstitutionalized population, using 3 age intervals.

had any expenses, were approximately $536 in 1975; for their nondiabetic counterparts, the comparable costs in 1975 were about $335 (Table 45–15). If the allocated costs of family health insurance premiums are excluded, the total age-adjusted average out-of-pocket health bill for individual diabetics in 1975 was about $477; for individuals without diabetes it was around $277. Comparable figures for 1983 or 1984, if they were available, would be much higher.

Although it is evident that modern trends have made it possible for diabetics to obtain some form of health insurance, there are those who feel there is considerable room for improvement. As Rifkin and Mazze[52] have pointed out, many who want to improve their diabetes control in order to attempt to prevent complications, are kept from many of the modern benefits such as home blood glucose testing, use of insulin pumps, and diabetes education classes because the costs are too high. Indeed, many who turn to health insurers find that their system is basically set up to cover only standard hospital costs. There is some hope for the future, however, because the Centers for Disease Control (CDC), which oversee diabetes control programs, are developing figures on the money saved on hospitalization after preventive efforts are carried out. In some states, Blue Cross/Blue Shield and Medicare/Medicaid programs are participating in a 3-year trial of reimbursement for preventive medicine and education. If as anticipated, cost savings are demonstrated, insurance for these types of services may become more readily available.

During the period 1950–1977, the Consumer Price Index rose 150% while health care costs increased 280%.[53] The situation is, of course, much worse for older persons, including those with diabetes, because although the average American had a 16% likelihood of being hospitalized in 1975, this probability increased to 29% for those over age 55, 36% for those over 65, and 54% at age 85.[54] The British, through the efforts of the British Diabetic Association, have made notable strides in this area. They have arranged for diabetic persons to get insurance at favorable premiums if they are in good health and under age 65. However, some companies in Great Britain for undetermined reasons, reject diabetics who take more than 70 units of insulin a day.[55] Personal accident insurance is also available with an extra premium, depending on the nature of the applicant's occupation, as is short-term medical expense insurance for travel abroad. It is apparent, therefore, that although medical services have become much more available to diabetics, there are still gaps which should and must be filled.

ECONOMIC IMPACT OF DIABETES

It is estimated that in 1980 the overall cost to the United States resulting from diabetes was $9.7 billion. This cost has been increasing steadily since 1969.

The total cost is divided into indirect costs which result from loss of productivity due to morbidity and mortality, and direct costs which reflect expenditures for medical and related services. Table 45–16 shows that the total cost associated with morbidity from diabetes in 1980 was approximately $8.240 billion, with the direct cost for medical and related services being $4.80 billion, and the indirect cost due to loss of productivity and earning losses among employed diabetics, diabetic women keeping house, and totally disabled diabetics, being $3.44 billion. The indirect economic cost of mortality in 1980 was $1.46 billion. This was measured in terms of the discounted present value of lifetime earnings of diabetics who died in 1980. The estimated earnings loss of employed diabetics who died in 1980 was $100 million. This compares to about $80 million in 1975. The cost associated with earnings loss due to mortality has been increasing since 1975 despite the fact that deaths have decreased from approximately 37,000 in 1975 to 34,000 in 1980. It is also of interest that the total number of person-years of work lost due to diabetes has been increasing steadily. In 1980, it was 212,000 days.

The direct costs of morbidity due to diabetes (Table 45–17) amounted to $4.8 billion, with the largest expenditure of $2.2 billion resulting from hospital care. The second largest expenditure of $1.24 billion was due to nursing home care, and the cost of physicians' services was $840 million.

While methodology has been developed to estimate the cost of illness, these estimates must be considered significantly under the true costs of diabetes. There is no satisfactory way yet to allocate costs when multiple diagnoses are present. For example, when diabetes and coronary artery disease present together, should the costs of medical care and disability be ascribed to diabetes or to coronary artery disease or to both? If the last, what proportions should be used? All too frequently, even though diabetes is the underlying disease, the economic costs are considered to be due to complications of the disease such as coronary artery disease or blindness.

Unquestionably, the matter of economics and funding for health care are closely related. Around the world and even in socialistic countries, as the costs for health care increase, there is pressure to cut back the price paid for this care first, and secondly, as far as is politically possible, to try to trim back the available care. Great Britain is a case in point. Although the economic base from which health and social programs are financed has been heavily eroded, the advantage of a health service continues, at a cost which is remarkably low compared to that of other nations. According to recent figures, the National Health Service costs about 6% of the gross national product (GNP) as compared to Germany, the Netherlands, and Sweden where health care spending is close to 10% of the GNP.[56] The problems of health care provided by nations facing economic pressures are increasing worldwide. Yet there is another side to the coin. As Ibrahim[57] states, "The gross national product is the result of material and human input." However, the contribution of this human input depends on health and technical competence of people and their ability to work. This work capacity can be effective only with good health. In a remarkable study, quoted by Ibrahim,[57] with regard to the social cost of diabetes medical care in 1981, it was shown that after deducting costs of treatment and maintenance, society got benefits several times greater than the costs involved. In trying to solve this problem, some ingenious methods are being developed. Breslow and Somers[58] have proposed that a lifetime health monitoring program would combine cost-effective and health-effective preventive measures that would avert many long-term complications, and have suggested a series of health goals and professional services for every stage of life from birth to 75 years of age and over. Health screening techniques have been known for approximately 40 years, but have never really been accepted on a large scale. At this point, everyone recognizes that economic and social forces are intimately tied to the health of any nation. However,

Table 45–16. Trends in Cost of Diabetes, 1969–80 As Estimated by the Statistical Bureau of the Metropolitan Life Insurance Company (dollars expressed in millions)

	1969	1973	1975	1977	1980
Total	$ 2,589	$ 4,015	$ 5,270	$ 6,780	$ 9,700
Morbidity*	1,460	2,630	4,200	5,740	8,240
Direct	996	1,650	2,520	3,400	4,800
Indirect	464	980	1,680	2,340	3,440
Mortality†	1,129	1,385	1,070	1,040	1,460
No. Deaths	38,530	38,208	37,000	33,570	34,000
Man-Years Lost	73,000	112,000	164,000	194,000	212,000

*Morbidity = Illness during year named. Direct = costs due to loss of productivity including earnings. Indirect = costs of medical and related services.
†Mortality = death during year named.
Figures include both direct and indirect costs. Direct costs include estimated $100 million attributed to earnings loss of employed diabetics in 1980.

Table 45–17. Estimated Direct Costs of Morbidity Due to Diabetes by Type of Expenditure, United States, 1980*

Type of Expenditure	Amount (in millions)
Total	$4,800
Hospital Care	2,200†
Physicians' Services	840‡
Drugs	380
Nursing Home Care	1,240
Other Medical Professional Services	140

*Excludes expenditures for dentists' services, eyeglasses and appliances, prepayment and administration, government and other health services, research and medical facilities construction.

†Based on days of care in short-stay hospitals.

‡Cost of patient visits to physicians.

Source: Estimated by the Statistical Bureau of the Metropolitan Life Insurance Company.

although many view the situation with alarm, a satisfactory and definitive answer has not yet been developed.

PROBLEMS OF AGING

In considering the life cycle, it is not possible to escape discussion of the penultimate stage of aging. Whether one regards aging as a good or bad process, it is inevitable. The poet Browning wrote:

"Grow old along with me!
The best is yet to be,
The last of life, for which the first was made. . ."

Seneca described it thus: "Old age is an incurable disease." In any case, many nations with western culture and developed societies are facing the problems of aging. For a discussion of the treatment of diabetes in the elderly, see Chapter 25.

ORGANIZATIONS TO AID DIABETICS

Fortunately throughout the world there is an increasing role for diabetes societies and organizations to help in the detection of diabetes and improvement of education and medical care. These local and national diabetes societies, most often non-profit organizations, are in their infancy, although some countries have more sophisticated services than others.

In general, there are two types of organizations that can be extremely useful for all diabetics. These, of course, will vary with the country.

Governmental Agencies

The World Health Organization (WHO) is a prime example of governmental approaches to the amelioration of diseases and their complications. The WHO, a part of the United Nations, does not deal directly with private institutions, voluntary organizations, or individuals. The constitution of this organization and numerous World Health Assembly resolutions have reaffirmed that health is a basic human right and a worldwide social goal.[59] In 1977, the 30th World Health Assembly resolved that the main social target of governments and WHO would be "the attainment by all citizens of the world by the year 2000 of a level of health that will permit them to lead a socially and economically productive life" and the principal goal, "Health for All," was further adopted by the 34th World Health Assembly. This was brought about by the fact that more than half and possibly as much as two-thirds of the world do not have adequate health care, with a tremendous gap between the developed and developing countries. It must also be remembered that in much, if not most, of the world, health activities are organized or initiated by governmental structures. The World Health Organization has many problems besides diabetes and, indeed, in many parts of the world, diabetes is not the main objective. However, it is being found increasingly that as nations "develop," with greater prosperity, diabetes burgeons. Whereas formerly other pressing problems took precedence, in many cases now diabetes is a subject of real concern for the first time.

Since WHO deals with governments, it is convenient and often mandatory for governments to reach practicing physicians and patients by means of voluntary organizations. Governments can set policies but frequently require a good deal of reinforcement to make certain that these are carried out. Accordingly, a joint executive committee on diabetes was established in 1980 by WHO and the International Diabetes Federation (IDF). This working relationship with the IDF gives WHO connections with the national associations and institutions. A network of WHO-collaborating centers is being established to deal with specific problems. International teaching seminars on the epidemiology and public health aspects of diabetes were held in July of 1981 and 1983, and seminars on laboratory technology have been organized. WHO always considers that diabetes services must be an integral part of existing national health services as well as a part of primary health care, rather than a vertically structured "diabetes empire."

Voluntary Associations

International Diabetes Federation. The focal point of the world attack on diabetes is the IDF with headquarters in London. It consists of some 80 national diabetes organizations and societies of which the American Diabetes Association is one. Its Board of Management and Executive Board are responsible to the General Council with representation from all the nations of the world. Rolf Luft,[60] past President, has aptly pointed out that a good working relationship between IDF and WHO is vital so that diabetes may be included in the improvement of the general health care systems. On the other hand, WHO has many other responsibilities and challenges, and the IDF must be involved with encouragement and coordination of research, education and patient care activities. While physicians have traditionally placed the welfare of individual patients above all else, increasingly they are discovering that they also have an obligation to the health and welfare of others in society. Through its national organizations, the IDF can better reach into local areas and community programs, encouraging improved health technology in both prevention and treatment.[61]

National Associations. These associations are, as mentioned previously, private, non-profit groups which were generally started by interested physicians, enthusiastic diabetics, or relatives of those with diabetes. Yet after many years, they are involved with at most only 5 to 10% of the diabetics in their countries. One of the problems concerns the limited or non-existent relationships with communities and governments. The American Diabetes Association (ADA), 2 Park Avenue, New York, NY 10016, has made remarkable progress and, along with other cooperating organizations such as the Juvenile Diabetes Foundation and numerous other groups and individuals, helped enact a law in 1976, authorizing the creation of the National Diabetes Advisory Board, which advises the Government about the needs of the nations's diabetics. The ADA consists of numerous local chapters and affiliates. This group gives diabetics a direct voice in the future of their own health. Much of this positive effect is due to the increasing visibility of the person with diabetes. There was a time when those with diabetes were considered pariahs because of their condition, which few understood. In fact, some of the early publications of the ADA were mailed in brown paper wrappers. Later, this practice was discarded on the grounds that no one would give money to a secret society. At present the Centers for Disease Control have established community-based diabetes control demonstration projects in cooperation with state health departments in 20 states. The ADA affiliates in all of them work closely with state personnel to improve the quality, accessibility and effectiveness of diabetes care according to the needs of the community.[62]

Local organizations can do a great deal to improve the lot of the diabetic. For example, the Massachusetts ADA affiliate, after 2 years of struggle, helped enact a law climinating a sales tax on syringes and needles. Still more recently, Wisconsin mandated insurance coverage for insulin infusion pumps and equipment used in the treatment of diabetes.[63] There is a chain which ensures the finest type of self-help and the proper influence of diabetes organizations. This begins when individuals form a group. (There are now 67 ADA affiliates). ADA then becomes one of the 80 national organizations that comprise the IDF which, in turn, cooperates with WHO. Thus, in a sense, the individual diabetic has a direct, positive voice in world affairs toward success in the struggle for Health for All by the Year 2000.

Throughout the world, diabetes organizations perform services that are vital to diabetes care. In Great Britain and New Zealand, for example, where social programs provide much of the medical care, there is a vast educational effort. In Colombia, donors "adopt" young diabetics who would not be able to afford insulin, and underwrite this life-saving medication for them. Each organization performs according to its needs. What is crucial, however, is for diabetes organizations somehow to locate the 90% of the world's diabetics whom they do not know, and bring them into the fold. There should be one umbrella representing all diabetes organizations, and accommodations must be made so that no one is left out. In unity there is strength and even as brooks become streams that flow into rivers and into bays and oceans, if the diabetics of the world could somehow unite and work together, the impetus they would create could not be stopped.

LOOKING AHEAD

After this discussion of the disease or syndrome known as diabetes in all its ramifications, and description of the lot of the diabetic, both good and bad, the "bottom" line really is, as diabetics often ask: "What about me?" One cannot blame persons with a lifetime disorder for being concerned about themselves and their families. The plethora of research and improvement in clinical treatment over the past 20 years give hope for the future. Advances in basic research include such information as the fact that insulin-dependent diabetes is associated with certain genetically determined histocompatibility antigens;[64] the influence of genetic factors on other forms of diabetes; and the possibility that viral infection may induce the onset of insulin-dependent diabetes in susceptible persons. There are exciting data that define the problem in the obese diabetic who may be insulin-resistant, possibly because of a decrease in the number or diminished sensitivity of insulin receptors. Of tremendous importance is the demonstration in a nationwide multicenter study[65] that laser beam photocoagulation not only slows the progression of diabetic retinopathy, but may prevent blindness in a large percentage of afflicted persons. Other exciting advances include the finding that careful monitoring of diabetes control during pregnancy has a profound effect on perinatal morbidity and mortality in infants of diabetic mothers as well as in the prevention of congenital anomalies. The development of new techniques for the treatment of kidney complications has added to the life span of numerous diabetics so affected.

However, even more exciting are those advances which are on the threshold of being perfected. For example, there is an increasing body of data in experimental diabetes highly suggestive that hyperglycemia and microvascular disease may be related. However, there is as yet no complete clinical evidence that rigid control of diabetes can prevent all vascular complications. Nor, on the other hand, is there evidence that microvascular complications are independent of hyperglycemia.[66] Now that vastly improved varieties of insulins have become available, first as highly purified all pork and recently as biosynthetic insulins, the main problem remaining is the delivery of insulin. Pancreatic transplants have not been generally satisfactory except in isolated cases. The transplanting of islet cell tissue has had some success in animals but not in humans. Great progress has been made with the open-loop system pumps, which are helpful to many patients. The closed-loop system, whereby the device could measure current blood glucose levels and determine how much insulin to give, has not yet become practical. However, research and increased knowledge in many areas of diabetes and its treatment provide considerable hope for the future of the person with diabetes.

At the first annual meeting of the American Diabetes Association in 1941, the minutes noted that "the associate members pay the same dues as the active members, namely, Two Dollars per year," and in his address, the President went on to say: "The diabetic mortality is rising at an alarming rate. This may indicate a deficiency on the part of the lay public to realize the value of modern medical procedures, or to appreciate the significance of their early symptoms."[67] It is evident that enormous strides have been made since that time, because in this and many other countries, mortality due to diabetes is actually dropping. Tremendous numbers of diabetics are living longer and better than ever before, and many without significant complications. Since 1970, more than 700 persons have received the bronze medal of the Joslin Diabetes Center, which is given to recognize the courage and endurance of those who have had well-documented, insulin-dependent diabetes for 50 years or more.

Possibly the best way to summarize the practical advances in diabetes care is to compare the lot of the diabetic patient today with that of the patient of only 25 years ago. It is possible to measure this progress at the Joslin Clinic where since 1897 an attempt has been made to follow patients throughout life. This program has been handicapped in recent years by the increasing high cost of such a follow-up but currently special studies of selected segments of this large diabetic population are yielding valuable information.

Twenty-five years ago there was little to offer patients with retinopathy; indeed, it was just beginning to be recognized as a problem. Now with the laser beam properly used, the threat of blindness has greatly diminished. The morbidity and mortality rates of infants of diabetic mothers have been reduced tremendously. Although at that time there were approximately three floors in the New England Deaconess Hospital where patients were given the best possible care for that period, there were a tremendous number of limb amputations. There still are occasional major amputations, but there are many fewer, and although much surgery is done, often it is either corrective or uses vascular bypasses to improve circulation. Little could be accomplished for the patient with diabetic nephropathy. Now active measures are being taken to prolong the life span, which is improving and will continue to do so. Research efforts which were confined to a few rooms in the Baker Building of the Deaconess Hospital, have now expanded to fill two complete floors at the Joslin Diabetes Center, with various auxiliary projects in other areas. Probably most dramatic of all is the simple fact that 25 years ago, when patients had survived for 20 years with insulin-dependent diabetes, they would be personally congratulated by Dr. Elliott P. Joslin, and treated as survival heroes. At this time, on any Clinic day, there are patients who have lived 30, 40, or even 50 or more years with diabetes without exciting any particular attention.

It is easy to become discouraged if one has diabetes. However, patients should be assured that if they do indeed have diabetes, this is absolutely the best time in history to have it!

REFERENCES

1. Data Systems of the National Center for Health Statistics. Programs and Collection Procedures, Series 1, No. 16, Vital and Health Statistics. U.S. Department of Health and Human Services, Public Health Service, National Center for Health Statistics.
2. Lebovitz, F.L., Ellis, G.J., III, Skyler, J.S.: Performance of technical skills of diabetes management: increased in-

dependence after a camp experience. Diabetes Care *1*:23, 1978.

2a. Fernandez, F., McCamman, S., Ling, L., et al.: Combined summer camp for non-diabetic and diabetic children. The Diabetes Educator, Spring, 1977, p. 22.

3. Magoun, F.A.: Love and Marriage. New York, Harper & Brothers, 1956, p. xi.

4. U.S. Department of Transportation. Federal Highway Administration: Motor carrier safety regulations. Revised Part 391, Qualification of Drivers. MCSR Amendment No. 10. Federal Register *35*:6458, April 22, 1970.

5. Krosnick, A.: Yes, you can get a driver's license. Diabetes Forecast *35*:(Jan.–Feb.) 16, 1982.

6. Wetzler, H.P.: Loss of working years in accidents. (Letter to the Editor). N. Engl. J. Med. *294*:1348, 1976.

7. Waller, J.A.: Chronic medical conditions and traffic safety. Review of the California experience. N. Engl. J. Med. *273*:1413, 1965.

8. Frier, B.M., Matthews, D.M., Steel, J.M., Duncan, L.J.P.: Driving and insulin-dependent diabetes. Lancet *1*:1232, 1980.

9. American Medical Association: Physician's Guide for Determining Driver Limitation. Chicago, Americal Medical Association, 1973.

10. Wines and the diabetic. Harveys of Bristol. 1964–1965.

10a. Hennekens, C.H., Willett, W., Rosner, B., et al.: Effects of beer, wine, and liquor in coronary deaths. J.A.M.A. *242*:1973, 1979.

10b. Marmot, M.G., Shipley, M.J., Rose, G., Thomas, B.J.: Alcohol and mortality: a U-shaped curve. Lancet *1*:580, 1981.

11. Ginsberg, H., Olefsky, J., Farquhar, J.W., Reaven, G.M.: Moderate ethanol ingestion and plasma triglyceride levels. Ann. Intern. Med. *80*:143, 1974.

12. McCulloch, D.K., Campbell, I.W., Prescott, R.J., Clarke, B.F.: Effect of alcohol intake on symptomatic peripheral neuropathy in diabetic men. Diabetes Care *3*:245, 1980.

13. Haut, M.J., Cowan, D.H.: The effect of ethanol on hemostatic properties of human blood platelets. Am. J. Med. *56*:22, 1974.

14. O'Keefe, S.J.D., Marks, V.: Lunchtime gin and tonic a cause of reactive hypoglycaemia. Lancet *1*:1286, 1977.

15. Sack, D.A., Kaminsky, D.C., Sack, R.B., et al.: Prophylactic doxycycline for travelers' diarrhea. N. Engl. J. Med. *298*:758, 1978.

16. Immunizations and chemoprophylaxis for travelers. The Medical Letter *23*:December 11, 1981.

17. Petrides, P.: Discrimination of juvenile diabetics in various professions. Pediatr. Adolesc. Endocrinol. *11*:50, 1983.

18. Bagshaw, E.: Careers for diabetic girls in nursing. (Letter to the Editor). Br. Med. J. *280*:1227, 1980.

19. Hardwick, D., Bloom, A.: Careers for diabetic girls in nursing. (Letter to the Editor). Br. Med. J. *280*:1616, 1980.

20. Mott, D.R.: Personal communication from Director of Safety, Association of Flight Attendants. Sept. 19, 1979.

21. N'Kanza, Z.: International year of disabled persons. Full participation and equality. IDF Bulletin. Delivery of Health Care for Diabetics in Developing Countries *2*:Sept. 1, 1981, pp. 2–5.

22. Ley de Lucha Antidiabetic., Art. 70, Ley no. 14032. 8 de Octobre de 1971, Uruguay.

23. Eriksson, N.: Liberty, equality and solidarity for diabetics. IDF Bulletin *26*:114, 1971.

24. Meuter, F., Thomas, W., Gries, F.A., et al.: Persönlichkeitspsychologische Untersuchungen an Patienten mit Diabetes mellitus. Diagnostik *15*:912, 1982.

25. Petrides, P.: Socio-medical problems of diabetes and their possible solutions. IDF Bulletin *26*:8 (Feb.), 1981.

26. Bibergeil, H.: Education and other social performances in the "Zentralinstitut fur Diabetes Gerhardt Katsch," Karlsburg, GDR. Diab. Croat. *1*:299, 1972.

27. Oakley, W.G., Pyke, D.A., Taylor, K.W.: Diabetes and Its Management. 2nd Edn. Oxford, Blackwell Scientific Publications, 1975, pp. 176–181.

28. Hochberg, F.H., Leffert, R.D., Heller, M.D.: Hand difficulties among musicians. J.A.M.A. *249*:1859, 1983.

29. Drury, T.F., Lipsett, L.F.: Complications of diabetes. Selected data on known diabetes and disability among persons 20 years and over in the United States. Presentation at American Diabetes Association meeting. Washington, D.C., June 17, 1980.

30. American Diabetes Association: Employment of diabetics. A statement of the Committee on Employment and Insurance. Diabetes *21*:834, 1972.

31. Zagoria, R.B.: Your right to work. Diabetes Forecast *35*:20 (May/June), 1982.

32. Petrides, P., Weiss, L., Loffler, G., Wieland, O.H.: Diabetes Mellitus: Theory and Management. Baltimore—Munich, Urban and Schwarzenberg, 1978, pp. 114–115.

33. Guidelines for Motor Vehicle Administrators: Functional Aspects of Driver Impairment, A guide for State Medical Advisory Boards. Superintendent of Documents, U.S. Government Printing Office, Washington, D.C., 1980.

34. U.S. Department of Transportation. Federal Aviation Administration. 14 CFR Part 67. Special Issuance of Airman Medical Certificates. Federal Register *47*:No. 73. April 15, 1982. Rules and Regulations.

35. Entmacher, P.S., Marks, H.E.: Socioeconomic considerations in the life of the diabetic. In: A. Marble, P. White, R.F. Bradley, L.P. Krall (Eds.): Joslin's Diabetes Mellitus, 11th Ed. Philadelphia, Lea & Febiger, 1971, p. 793.

36. Sands, M.J., Jr.: Aviator medical certification after coronary artery surgery. N. Engl. J. Med. *307*:52, 1982.

37. Pell, S., D'Alonzo, C.A.: Diabetes mellitus in an employed population. J.A.M.A. *12*:1000, 1960.

38. Pell, S., D'Alonzo, C.A.: Sickness absenteeism in employed diabetics. Am. J. Public Health *57*:253, 1967.

39. Nasr, A.N.M., Block D.L., Magnuson, M.J.: Absenteeism experience in a group of employed diabetics. J. Occup. Med. *8*:621, 1966.

40. Moore, R.H., Buschbom, R.L.: Work absenteeism in diabetes. Diabetes *23*:957, 1974.

41. Unpublished correspondence with J.W. Cisco (Jan. 1980) and K.G. Patton (June, 1980), Acting Directors, Division of Program Policy, U.S. Department of Labor, Employment Standards Administration. Washington, D.C.

42. Committee on Employment, American Diabetes Association: Analysis of a survey concerning employment of diabetics in some major industries. Diabetes *6*:551, 1957.

43. World Health Organization: Employment and placement of diabetics. In: Diabetes Mellitus. Report of a WHO Expert Committee. Technical Report Series NO. 310, Geneva, WHO, 1965, pp. 31–34.

44. Entmacher, P.S., Bale, G.S.: Insurability and life expectancy of diabetics. In: H. Rifkin and P. Raskin (Eds.): Diabetes Mellitus, Vol. 5, Bowie, Md. Robert J. Brady Company, 1981, pp. 341–345.

45. National Diabetes Data Group: Classification and diagnosis of diabetes mellitus and other categories of glucose intolerance. Diabetes *28*:1039, 1979.

46. Goodkin, G., Wolloch, L., Gottcent, R.A., Reich, F.: Diabetes: A twenty-year mortality study. Trans. Assoc. Life Insurance Med. Directors of America *58*:217, 1974.

47. Barch, J.W.: Diabetes—a continuing mortality study. Proc. Home Office Life Underwriters Assoc. *52*:66, 1971.

48. Levinson, L., Singer, R.B.: Methodology. Chapter 2. In: Medical Risks. Lexington Books. Lexington, Mass., D.C. Heath & Co., 1976, pp. 9–19.

49. Entmacher, P.S.: An insurance-clinical dialogue on diabetes. Trans. Assoc. Life Insurance Medical Directors of America 55:205, 1971.

50. Metropolitan Life Insurance Co.: Unpublished data.

51. National Center for Health Statistics: Health care coverage under private health insurance, Medicare, Medicaid, and military or Veterans Administration health benefits: United States, 1978. Advance Data from Vital and Health Statistics. No. 71. DHHS Pub. No. (PHS) 81-1250. Public Health Service. Hyattsville, Maryland, June 29, 1981.

52. Rifkin, H., Mazze, R.: Health insurance policies: a plea for change (Editorial). Diabetes Forecast 35 (Nov–Dec.):4, 1982.

53. Tucker, F.A.: Insurance. In: T.G. Duncan (Ed.): Over 55. A Handbook on Health. Philadelphia. Franklin Institute Press, 1982, pp. 549–559.

54. Aden, G.T.: The hospital. In: Ibid., pp. 511–528.

55. Oakley, W.G., Pyke, D.A., Taylor, K.W.: Diabetes and Its Management. 2nd Edn. Oxford, Blackwell Scientific Publications, 1975, p. 180.

56. Abel-Smith, B.: Health care in a cold economic climate. Lancet 1:373, 1981.

57. Ibrahim, M.: The economics of diabetes health care. In.: L.P. Krall, K.G.M.M. Alberti (Eds.): World Book of Diabetes in Practice, 1982. Amsterdam, Excerpta Medica, 1982, pp. 186–189.

58. Breslow, L., Somers, A.R.: The lifetime health-monitoring program. N. Engl. J. Med. 296:601, 1977.

59. WHO Expert Committee on Diabetes Mellitus. Second Report. Geneva, World Health Organization, TRS No. 646, 1980.

60. Luft, R.: The status of diabetes mellitus today. In: L.P. Krall, K.G.M.M. Alberti (Eds.): World Book of Diabetes in Practice, 1982, Amsterdam, Excerpta Medica, 1982, pp. 1–3.

61. Renold, A.E.: Global opportunities in diabetes. In: Ibid., pp. 209–212.

62. Clark, C.M., Jr.: States on the move. Diabetes Forecast 34:18–21 (May/June), 1981.

63. Behnke, R.E.: Well done, Wisconsin. (Letter). Diabetes Forecast 36:9, (Jan./Feb.), 1983.

64. Salans, L.B.: Diabetes mellitus. A disease that is coming into focus. J.A.M.A. 247:590, 1982.

65. DRS Research Group (U.S.A.): Clinical application of Diabetic Retinopathy Study (DRS) results. In: L.P. Krall, K.G.M.M. Alberti (Eds.): World Book of Diabetes in Practice, 1982. Amsterdam, Excerpta Medica, 1982, pp. 117–119.

66. Raskin, P.: Transplants, artificial pancreas, and new pharmacologic advances. In: H. Rifkin, P. Raskin (Eds.): Diabetes Mellitus, Vol. V. Bowie, Md., Robert J. Brady Company, 1981, pp. 367–373.

67. Striker, C.: The President's Address, First Annual Meeting, Cleveland, Ohio, June 1, 1941. Proc. Am. Diabetes Assn. 1:23, 1941.

Appendices

A. Food composition source books.
B. Joslin Clinic Form for the dietary prescription and meal plan.
C. Food lists.
    1. Milk.
    2. Vegetables.
    3. Fruit.
    4. Bread.
    5. Meat.
    6. Fat.
    7. Miscellaneous foods.
    8. Snack list.
    9. "Free" food group.
    10. Glycemic index.
D. "No added salt" diet (3 to 4 gm sodium per day).
E. Additional guidelines for patients.
F. Height and weight tables.
    1. Comparison of 1959 and 1983 Metropolitan height and weight tables.
        a. Men.   b. Women.
    2. Changes in average weights for men and women between 1959 and 1979. Weight in pounds (without clothing) according to height and age.
    3. 1983 Metropolitan height and weight tables for men and women on metric basis. According to frame, ages 25 to 59.
    4. Heights and weights (without clothing) of young persons ages 2 to 18 years (at 5th, 50th and 95th percentiles).
G. Traditional Joslin Clinic lists of food values.
    1. Carbohydrate, protein, fat and calories in basic foods.
    2. Approximate utilizable carbohydrate content of certain vegetables and other common foods.
    3. Approximate amounts (grams) of fruits, fresh or canned (water-packed), which yield respectively, 10 and 15 g of carbohydrate.
    4. Approximate substitutes for foods on diet sheet.

APPENDIX A
FOOD COMPOSITION SOURCE BOOKS

Watt, B.K., Merrill, A.L.: Composition of Foods—Raw, Processed, Prepared. Agriculture Handbook No. 8, Washington, D.C., U.S.D.A., 1963. Revised and reprinted, Dec. 1975. Some 2,500 foods are included. Values are presented for 100 grams, edible portion of food and edible portion of 1 pound of food "as purchased". Does not include household portions.

Agriculture Handbook No. 8, Composition of Foods—Raw, Processed, Prepared. Revised Sections.

    8–1   Dairy and Egg Products (revised 1976)
    8–2   Spices and Herbs (revised 1977)
    8–3   Baby Foods (revised 1978)
    8–4   Fats and Oils (revised 1979)
    8–5   Poultry Products (revised 1979)
    8–6   Soups, Sauces, and Gravies (revised 1980)
    8–7   Sausages and Luncheon Meats (revised 1980)
    8–8   Breakfast Cereals (revised 1982)
    8–9   Fruits and Fruit Juices (revised 1982)

Data are presented on the basis of 100 grams in two common measures, and in the edible portion of 1 pound as purchased. Values are provided for refuse, energy, water, protein, lipids, carbohydrate and ash, seven mineral elements, nine vitamins, individual fatty acids, cholesterol, total phytosterols and 18 amino acids.

Agriculture Handbook No. 456, Nutritive Value of American Foods in Common Units. December 1975. This publication contains basically the same material as was published in the 1963 edition of Agriculture Handbook No. 8 except that data have been converted to various household measures and market units of food.

Home and Garden Bulletin No. 72, Nutritive Value of Foods. Provides nutrient data for over 700 commonly consumed food items in household units, such as cups, ounces, quarts, etc. It is easy to use.

All of the publications cited above are available from the Superintendent of Documents, U.S. Government Printing Office, Washington, D.C. 20402.

Pennington, J.A.T., Church, H.N.: Bowes & Church's Food Values of Portions Commonly Used, 13th ed., Philadelphia, J.B. Lippincott Co., 1980. Data are presented for portions in household units and grams whenever possible. Sources used for food values include Ohio State Data Bank; USDA Handbook No. 456; USDA Handbook No. 8; food industry and journal articles. This includes many brand name foods. It is easily used.

Paul, A.A., Southgate, D.A.T.: McCance and Widdowson's Composition of Foods, 4th rev. ed. of Special Report No. 297, London, Her Majesty's Stationery Office, Elsevier/North-Holland Biomedical Press, 1978. The content of dietary fiber is given for a wide variety of foods.

GUIDE BOOKS FOR TEACHING OF DIETS

Kozak, G.P., Holleroth, H.J., Gordon, C., et al.: Diabetes Teaching Guide. Boston, Joslin Diabetes Center, 1983.

American Diabetes Association, American Dietetic Association: Lists for Meal Planning. New York and Chicago, 1976. Copies are available from each of these organizations.

APPENDIX B

FORM USED AT JOSLIN CLINIC FOR THE DIETARY PRESCRIPTION AND MEAL PLAN

Meal Plan

Name: _____ Dietitian: _____

Date: _____ Phone: _____

CHO _____ PRO _____ FAT _____ Calories _____

MEAL	SPECIAL INSTRUCTIONS	EXAMPLES
BREAKFAST No. of Time _____ Choices		
_____ MILK		
_____ FRUIT		
_____ BREAD		
_____ MEAT		
_____ FAT		
MORNING SNACK Group Time		
LUNCH No. of Time _____ Choices		
_____ MILK		
_____ VEGETABLE		
_____ FRUIT		
_____ BREAD		
_____ MEAT		
_____ FAT		
AFTERNOON SNACK Group Time		
DINNER No. of Time _____ Choices		
_____ MILK		
_____ VEGETABLE		
_____ FRUIT		
_____ BREAD		
_____ MEAT		
_____ FAT		
EVENING SNACK Group Time		

APPENDIX C

FOOD LISTS

In the teaching of patients regarding food types and amounts, a liberal investment of skill, time and patience often yields large dividends in terms of health and longevity. At the outset, food should be measured or weighed to promote familiarity with the amount of a given item called for on the diet plan. Cooperative patients soon learn to estimate such with reasonable accuracy so that on occasion they may feel free to eat in restaurants, in the homes of friends and relatives, etc.

The food lists which follow represent a blending of material used by the Joslin Clinic and that contained in "Exchange Lists for Meal Planning" of the American Dietetic and American Diabetes Associations. Foods are grouped about 1 of 6 key items: milk, vegetables, fruit, bread, meat, and fat.

In each list, the carbohydrate, protein, fat, and kilocalorie content of one portion appears just above the columns of foods. Measures and equivalents used are: one cup = 8 oz (240 g or ml); one teaspoonful = 5 ml or g; one tablespoonful = 15 ml or g. Obviously, for a variety of reasons, measurements and calculations are rough and approximate, but they do furnish helpful guides to patients.

In the lists and accompanying material, statements are presented in the second person as in the instruction of patients.

LIST 1.

MILK (Includes whole, low fat (1%), skim milk and milk substitutes)

Each of the following food items in the portion size indicated, is considered 1 whole milk choice, 1 low-fat milk choice, or 1 skim milk choice.

Select one of the items listed for each milk choice indicated on your plan for each meal. Use whole, low-fat or skim milk choices depending on which one is indicated on your meal plan.

Per portion of milk: Whole   C 12   P 8   F 8   kcal 152
                      Low fat C 12   P 8   F 4   kcal 116
                      Skim   C 12   P 8   F 0   kcal 80

ITEM	Portion
Whole milk:	
Fresh whole milk	1 cup
Evaporated milk	½ cup
Reconstituted powdered milk	1 cup plus 2 fat choices
Yogurt (plain) made from	
partially skimmed milk	1 cup
Low-fat milk	1 cup
Skim milk:	
Fresh skim milk	1 cup
Powdered milk	⅓ cup
Reconstituted powdered milk	1 cup
Buttermilk made from skim milk	1 cup
Evaporated skim milk	½ cup

C = carbohydrate; P = protein; F = fat; kcal = kilocalories.

LIST 2

VEGETABLES (Includes fresh, frozen and canned vegetables)

Each of the following food items, in the portion size indicated, is considered 1 vegetable choice. Unless otherwise indicated, the portion sizes are for both raw and cooked vegetables. Select one of the items listed for each vegetable choice indicated on your meal plan.

Some vegetables such as *corn, lima beans, parsnip, peas, squash, potatoes, tomato paste,* and *tomato puree* provide more carbohydrate. Because of their high carbohydrate content, they must be used as a bread choice. These items, and the appropriate portions to use, appear on the bread list. (see List 4).

Most leafy green vegetables may, within reason, be eaten freely. However, anything added, as salad dressing, must be taken into account.

Per portion: C 5   P 2   F 0   kcal 28

ITEM	PORTION	ITEM	PORTION
Artichoke	½	Mushrooms (raw)	1 cup
Asparagus	1 cup	Mustard greens (cooked)	1 cup
Bamboo shoots	½ cup	Okra	½ cup
Bean sprouts	½ cup	Onions	½ cup
Beets	½ cup	Pimento	Free list
Beet greens	1 cup	Pumpkin	¼ cup
Broccoli	½ cup	Radishes	1 cup
Brussel sprouts	½ cup	Red pepper	1 cup
Cabbage	1 cup	Rutabagas	½ cup
Cabbage (Chinese)	2 cups	Sauerkraut	½ cup
Carrots	½ cup	Spinach	
Cauliflower	1 cup	raw	2 cups
Celery	1 cup	cooked	½ cup
Chicory	2 cups	Squash	
Collard greens	1 cup	summer	1 cup
Cucumber	1½ cup	zucchini	1 cup
Eggplant	½ cup	Swiss chard	1 cup
Endive	2 cups	Tomato (ripe)	1 medium
Green beans	1 cup	Tomato sauce	⅓ cup
Green pepper	1 cup	Turnips	½ cup
Kale	½ cup	Vegetables, mixed	¼ cup
Kohlrabi	½ cup	Wax beans	1 cup
Leeks	½ cup	Water chestnuts	5
Lettuce	2 cups	Watercress	4 cups

LIST 3

FRUIT (includes fresh fruit, pure fruit juices, and canned, dried, cooked or frozen fruit without added sugar). Canned fruit should be water-packed.

Each of the following food items, in the portion size indicated, is considered 1 fruit choice. Select one of the items listed for each fruit choice indicated on your meal plan.

Per portion: C 10   P 0   F 0   kcal 40

ITEM	PORTION	ITEM	PORTION
Apricots:		Honeydew melon	⅛ melon
raw	2 small	Mango	¼ cup diced
canned	3 halves	Nectarine (2½ inch	
*dried	4 halves	diameter)	½
Apple	1 small	Orange (3 inch diameter)	1
Apple juice	⅓ cup	Orange juice	½ cup
Applesauce	½ cup	Papaya (3½ inch diameter)	⅓
Banana (8 inch length)	½	cubed	¾ cup
Blackberries (raw or		Peach (2½ inch diameter)	1
frozen)	½ cup	Pear	
Blueberries	½ cup	fresh	1 small
Canteloupe (5 inch		canned, drained	2 halves
diameter)	¼ melon	Pineapple	
Casaba (7 inch diameter)	¹⁄₁₀ melon	canned, drained	⅓
Cherries (sweet)		raw, diced	½ cup
raw	10	Plums (2 inch diameter)	2
canned	⅓ cup	*Prunes (dried, medium	
Cherries (sour)		size)	2
canned	⅓ cup	Prune juice	¼ cup
Cranapple juice (diet)	1 cup	*Raisins	2 tablespoons
Cranberry juice (low			(10)
calorie)	5½ ounces	Raspberries	¾ cup
Cranberry sauce (diet)	¼ cup	Rhubarb (raw, diced)	2 cups
Figs	1 large	Strawberries	¾ cup
Fruit cocktail	½ cup	Tangerine (2½ inch	
Grapefruit (4 inch		diameter)	1
diameter)	½	**Tomato juice, V-8	1 cup
Grapefruit juice	½ cup	Watermelon (diced)	1 cup
Grapes	12		

*Avoid dried fruits to which sodium benzoate has been added.
**Avoid tomato juice if you are on a moderate salt (sodium) diet.

LIST 4

BREAD (Includes bread, cereal, pasta, starchy vegetables, and other selected items).

Each of the following food items, in the portion size indicated, is considered 1 bread choice. Select one of the items listed for each bread choice indicated on your meal plan for each meal.

Per portion: C 15 P 2 F 0 kcal 68

ITEM	PORTION	ITEM	PORTION
BREADS:		**PASTA:**	
White, whole wheat, rye, etc.	1 slice	Macaroni	½ cup (cooked)
Syrian (pocket—4 inch diameter)	½ pocket	Noodles	½ cup (cooked)
Italian and French bread	1 slice (1 oz.)	Shells	½ cup (cooked)
Thin sliced	1½ slices	Spaghetti	½ cup (cooked)
Bagel	½ medium	**OTHER:**	
Muffins: English, bran, corn, or plain	½ medium	Bread crumbs	3 tablespoons
Rolls:		Cornstarch	2 tablespoons
Hamburger	½ medium	Flour	2 tablespoons
Frankfurter	1 whole	Rice (plain brown or white)	⅓ cup (cooked)
Dinner	1 small plain	Stuffing mix	⅓ cup = 1 bread + 1 fat
Bulkie	½ small		
Crackers (see snack list)		**CRACKERS EQUAL TO 1 BREAD CHOICE**	
Matzoh	1 (6″ square)	Animal Crackers	9
Melba Toast	5 thin slices	Arrowroot Biscuits™	5
Tortilla (6 inch diameter)	1 each	†Bacon Thins™	12
*STARCHY VEGETABLES:		†Bugles™	1 ounce
Corn	⅓ cup	Butter Thins™	5
Dried beans, limas, peas and lentils	½ cup	†Cheese Tidbits™	30
Parsnips	⅔ cup	Fortune Cookies	3
Peas	½ cup	Ginger Snaps	5
Squash, winter	½ cup	†Goldfish™	38
Potato (white)		Graham Crackers	2 squares
Mashed or boiled	½ cup	Lorna Doones™	3
Baked	½ medium	Onion Toasts™	8
Sweet potato:		**Oyster Crackers	30
Baked	½ medium	**Norwegian Flat Bread™ (thin)	3 wafers
Mashed	¼ cup	Popcorn	3 cups
Tomato paste	⅓ cup	†Pretzels	2
Tomato puree	¾ cup	Rice Cakes	2
CEREALS:		†Ritz Crackers™	8
Cooked (oatmeal, farina, etc.)	½ cup	†Rye Krisp™	3
Grits	½ cup	Rye Thins™	9
Bran cereals	½ cup	†**Saltines	6
Puffed wheat or rice	1 cup	†Triscuits™	5
Other dry cereals	¾ cup	Uneedas™	3
Wheat germ	2 tablespoons	Vanilla Wafers	6
		†Waverly Thins™	6
		†Wheat Thins™	12

*While these items are vegetables, they must be used as a bread choice because of their carbohydrate content.
**These crackers are low in fat but high in sodium.
†These products are high in sodium. Limit your use of these products if you are on a salt (sodium) restricted diet.

LIST 5

MEAT (Includes meat, fish, poultry, eggs, cheese, and meat substitutes)

Each of the following food items, in the portion size indicated, is considered 1 meat choice. Select one of the items listed for each meat choice indicated on your meal plan for each meal. Leaner selections of meat are recommended. Trim all visible fat before cooking. Bake or broil your selections when possible. Weigh your portions *after* cooking. Do not include bones.

Per portion: C 0   P 7   F 5   kcal 73

ITEM	PORTION
Beef: chipped beef, chuck, flank steak, hamburger with 15% fat, rib eye, rump, sirloin, tenderloin, top and bottom round	1 ounce
Lamb: except breast	1 ounce
Pork: except deviled ham, ground pork and spare ribs	1 ounce
Veal: except breast	1 ounce
Poultry without skin: chicken, turkey or Cornish hen	1 ounce
Fish and other seafood:	
Fresh or frozen (except shrimp)	1 ounce
Canned:	
Water-packed salmon, tuna, crab, lobster	¼ cup
Water-packed oysters, clams	5 or 1 ounce
Sardines, drained	3
Cheese:	
Cottage, pot	¼ cup
Part-skim mozzarella, part-skim ricotta, farmer, Neufchatel, Monterey Jack	1 ounce
Parmesan	3 tablespoons
Egg substitutes	½ cup

RECOMMENDED SUBSTITUTES FOR MEAT PORTION

Tofu	3 ounces
Peanut butter	1 tablespoon
Dried beans, peas and lentils, cooked	½ cup = 1 meat + 1 bread

DUE TO HIGH FAT OR CHOLESTEROL CONTENT, THE FOLLOWING MEAT CHOICES SHOULD BE USED SPARINGLY:

Beef: brisket, club or rib steaks, corned beef, regular hamburg with 20% fat, rib roast, short ribs	1 ounce
Lamb: breast	1 ounce
Pork: deviled ham, ground pork, spare ribs, sausage	1 ounce
Veal: breast	1 ounce
Poultry: capon, duck, goose	1 ounce
Cheese: blue, brie, cheddar, Colby, feta, muenster, provolone, Swiss, pasteurized processed	1 ounce
Luncheon meats: bologna, bratwurst, braunschweiger, frankfurter, knockwurst, liverwurst, pastrami, Polish sausage, salami	1 ounce
Shrimp	5 shrimp or 1 ounce
Organ meats: liver, heart, kidney	1 ounce
Egg, medium size	1

LIST 6

FAT (Includes butter, margarine, cream, mayonnaise, nuts, salad dressings, vegetable oils, and other selected items.)

Each of the following food items, in the portion size indicated, is considered 1 fat choice. Select one of the items listed for each fat choice indicated on your meal plan for each meal. Items which are high in saturated fat are identified with an asterisk. These should be used sparingly. Polyunsaturated fats such as corn, cottonseed, safflower, and sunflower oils, as well as margarines made from these oils, should be used whenever possible.

Per portion: C 0   P 0   F 5   kcal 45

ITEM	PORTION	ITEM	PORTION
Avocado (4 inch diameter)	⅛ whole	Peanuts	10 single nuts
*Bacon	1 strip	Pecans	4 halves
‡Butter	1 teaspoon	Walnuts	4 halves
*Cream		Oil: corn, olive, peanut,	
Half and Half	2 tablespoons	safflower	1 teaspoon
Heavy	2 teaspoons	Olives:	
Light	1 tablespoon	black	2 large
Sour	4 teaspoons	green	6 medium
Whipped	2 teaspoons	Salad dressings: Italian,	
*Cream cheese	1 teaspoon	French, Thousand Island[1]	1 tablespoon
‡Margarine[1]	1 teaspoon	Seeds:	
Mayonnaise[1]	1 teaspoon	Pumpkin	1 tablespoon
†Nuts		Squash	1 tablespoon
Almonds	1 tablespoon	Sunflower	1 tablespoon
Cashews	1 tablespoon	Sesame	1 tablespoon

*These items are high in saturated fat and should be used sparingly.

†Nuts contain some carbohydrate and protein as well as fat. If used in quantities larger than those listed above, they should be considered as part of your daily requirement for carbohydrate, protein and fat.

‡Equal portions of butter and margarine have the same number of calories and may be substituted for each other. Butter, however, is made of animal fat while margarine is made of vegetable fat. Your physician or nutritionist will advise you about which to use.

[1]When using low calorie versions of margarine, mayonnaise or salad dressing, use amounts equal to 50 calories.

LIST 7

MISCELLANEOUS LIST

Because of their ingredients, some foods are considered a combination of choices from several food groups. A plain doughnut, for instance, is considered not only two bread choices, but also 2 fat choices because of its high fat content. Some "mixed" foods such as doughnuts can be incorporated into a meal plan by substituting them for choices from more than one food group. A sample list of such foods appears below.

ITEM	PORTION	EQUALS
SOUP		
Rice or noodle with broth	10 ounces (½ can)	1 bread
Vegetable	10 ounces (½ can)	1 bread
Cream soup prepared with skim milk	10 ounces (½ can)	1 bread, 1 fat, 1 cup skim milk
Chicken soup	10 ounces (½ can)	1 bread
OTHER FOODS		
Plain cheese pizza	1 slice	2 bread, 1 meat, 1 fat
Potato chips	15	1 bread, 2 fat
Plain doughnut	1	2 bread, 2 fat
Pancake	2 (4 inch diameter)	1 bread, 1 fat
Waffle (made with egg and milk)	1 (5½ inch diameter)	2 bread, 1 fat
Whipped topping	5 tablespoons	½ fruit, 1 fat
Frozen iced milk	½ cup	1 bread, 1 fat
Ice cream (vanilla)	½ cup	1 bread, 2 fat
Pudding (D'Zerta) made with non-fat milk)	½ cup	½ milk, ½ bread
Beefstew (homemade)	1 cup	3 meat, 1 bread
Taco (tortilla with meat or cheese filling)	1	2 meat, 1 vegetable, 1 bread

LIST 8

SNACK LIST

For each snack listed on your meal plan, choose a snack from the appropriate snack group below. Be sure to choose snacks from the group or groups indicated on your meal plan form. The snacks include various combinations of bread, regular and low fat meat, and whole and skimmed milk choices. You can create your own snacks as long as they include the correct number of choices from each food group.

Many snacks can include crackers as the bread choice. To provide you with variety, a list of many of the crackers you will find in your grocery store appears in List 4 (Bread). The list tells you how many crackers of each variety is equal to one (1) bread choice.

Group 1	Group 3

One meat choice,
Plus one bread choice.
15 grams carbohydrate, 9 grams protein and 5 or more grams of fat.
Examples:
  1 ounce of roast beef plus ½ English muffin;
  1 ounce of cheese plus 4 melba toast;
  1 tablespoon peanut butter plus 6 saltines;
  1 ounce ham plus 1 slice whole wheat bread;
  4 crackers plus 1 tablespoon peanut butter
	One-half whole milk choice,
	Plus one-half bread choice.
	14 grams carbohydrate, 6 grams protein and 4 grams fat.
	Examples:
	  ½ cup whole milk plus 4 animal crackers;
	  ½ cup whole milk plus 6 Wheat Thins™;
	  ½ cup whole milk plus ⅓ cup dry cereal;
	  ½ cup plain low-fat yogurt plus 4 Rye Thins™;
	  1½ fruit plus 1 ounce low fat cheese.

Group 2	**Group 4**

One low fat meat choice,
Plus one bread choice
15 grams carbohydrate, 9 grams protein and 3 or less grams fat.
Examples:
  ¼ cup low fat cottage cheese plus 6 saltines;
  1 ounce chicken plus 1 slice whole wheat bread;
  ¼ cup tuna packed in water plus 1 slice bread
  1 ounce low fat cheese plus ½ pocket Syrian bread.
	One-half skim milk choice,
	Plus one bread choice.
	21 grams carbohydrate and 6 grams protein.
	Examples:
	  ½ cup skim milk plus 3 Rye Krisps™;
	  ½ cup skim milk plus 2 graham cracker squares;
	  ½ cup skim milk plus ¾ cup dry cereal.

LIST 9

"FREE" FOOD GROUP

The following foods contain few calories and may be used freely in your meal plan. Items marked with an asterisk* should not be used, however, if you are on a salt (sodium) restricted diet.

GENERAL

*Bouillon cubes

*Broth (clear)

"Calorie free" soft drinks (be careful—some of these contain carbohydrate)

*Catsup (1 tablespoon daily—unless calculated as part of the total daily calories)

Coffee

*Consomme

Cranberries

Decaffeinated coffee

Extracts (See list below)

Gelatin (unsweetened)

Herbs (See list below)

Horseradish

Lemon and lime juice

Lemon rind/lime rind

*Mustard (prepared)

Orange rind

*Pickles (unsweetened)

Postum (limited to 3 cups daily unless calculated as part of the total daily calories)

Rennet tablets

Saccharin

Seasonings and condiments (see list below)

*Soy sauce

Spices

*Steak sauce

Sugarless chewing gum

Tabasco sauce

Taco sauce

Tea

Unprocessed bran (1 tablespoon)

Vinegar (cider, white, apple, wine)

Yeast (dry or cake)

SPICES, HERBS AND EXTRACTS

Allspice

Almond extract

Anise extract

Anise seed

Baking powder

*Baking soda

Basil

Bay leaf

Black cherry extract

*Bouillon cube

Butter flavoring

*Butter salt

Caraway seeds

Cardamon

*Celery salt (seeds, leaves)

Chives

Chocolate extract

Cilantro (Mexican coriander)

Cinnamon

Cloves

Cream of tartar

Cumin

Curry

Dill

Fennel

Garlic

Ginger

Lemon extract

Mace

Maple extract

Mint

Mustard (dry)

Nutmeg

Onion (1 tablespoon)

Orange extract

Oregano

Paprika

Parsley

Pepper

Peppermint extract

Pimiento

Poppy seed

Poultry seed

Poultry seasonings

Saccharin

Saffron

Sage

*Salt

Savory

LIST 10

GLYCEMIC INDEX

The area under the blood glucose response curve for each food expressed as a percentage of the area after taking the same amount of carbohydrate as glucose* (data from normal persons).

100%	60%–69%	40%–49%	20%–29%
Glucose	Bread (white)	Spaghetti (whole meal)	Kidney beans
80%–90%	Rice (brown)	Porridge oats	Lentils
Corn flakes	Muesli	Potato (sweet)	Fructose
Carrots‡	Shredded Wheat	Beans (canned navy)	**10%–19%**
Parsnips‡	"Ryvita"	Peas (dried)	Soya beans
Potatoes (instant mashed)	Water biscuits	Oranges	Soya beans (canned)
Maltose	Beetroot‡	Orange juice	Peanuts
Honey	Bananas	**30%–39%**	
70%–79%	Raisins	Butter beans	
Bread (whole meal)	Mars bar	Haricot beans	
Millet	**50%–59%**	Blackeye peas	
Rice (white)	Buckwheat	Chick peas	
Weetabix	Spaghetti (white)	Apples (Golden Delicious)	
Broad beans (fresh)‡	Sweet corn	Ice cream	
Potato (new)	All-Bran	Milk (skim)	
Swede‡	Digestive biscuits	Milk (whole)	
	Oatmeal biscuits	Yogurt	
	"Rich Tea" biscuits	Tomato soup	
	Peas (frozen)		
	Yam		
	Sucrose		
	Potato chips		

*From Jenkins, D.J.A.: Lente carbohydrate: a newer approach to the dietary management of diabetes. Diabetes Care 5:634, 1982. Used by permission of the author and publisher.

‡25-gm carbohydrate portions tested.

APPENDIX D

"NO ADDED SALT" DIET FOR DIABETIC PATIENTS
3 to 4 g Sodium per Day

DIRECTIONS TO PATIENTS

1. Use no salt at the table.
2. Use only a VERY SMALL amount of salt in cooking, at most about ½ teaspoon per day.
3. Do not use sodium bicarbonate ("baking soda").
4. Avoid foods that contain much salt; these are listed below.
5. This diet will not change your diabetes meal plan. Your substitutions will simply be limited to those items low in salt.
6. If your medical condition is such that the "no added salt" diet furnishes too much sodium, your physician will prescribe a meal plan which provides an even lower intake.

SUBSTITUTION LIST	ALLOWED WITHIN MEAL PLAN AMOUNTS	AVOID
Bread	All regular bread, pasta, rice, rolls, cereals, muffins, potato, corn, lima beans, shell beans, and salt-free canned or homemade soups	Salted crackers, popcorn, canned soups and tomato sauce
Fruit	All fresh or water-packed fruit	Canned tomato juice
Vegetables	All fresh, frozen or canned vegetables except those in the "avoid" column	Sauerkraut, tomato sauce, and the juice from canned vegetables
Milk	All whole and skim milk	Limit buttermilk to 1 cup per day
Meat	All fresh chicken, fish, meat, shellfish, poultry, organ meat, cottage cheese, peanut butter, tuna canned in water, eggs, and salt-free hard cheese	Tuna canned in oil, dried or corned beef, cold cuts, frankfurters, pastrami, cheese, ham, sausage, cured or smoked meat and fish, anchovies, sardines, and meat made kosher by salting
Butter	Regular butter, margarine, all oils, salad dressings, sour cream, cream cheese, mayonnaise, unsalted nuts, and avocado	Bacon fat, salt pork, lard, bacon, salted nuts, and olives
Items with little food value, seasonings, and condiments	Sugar substitutes, sugar-free tonic, powdered coffee additives, sugar-free gelatin, salt-free catsup and mustard, or other substances not containing significant amounts of sodium	Salt, monosodium glutamate, garlic salt, and other seasoning salts, bouillon, pickles, relish, catsup, mustard, steak sauce, Worcestershire sauce, soy sauce, horseradish, meat tenderizers, combination seasonings, chili sauce, and meat sauce

APPENDIX E

ADDITIONAL GUIDELINES FOR PATIENTS

SODIUM

While a moderate as opposed to an excessive use of sodium is generally considered desirable, discuss the issue with your physician before making a change in your eating patterns. If your physician recommends a reduction of sodium, you can still eat a wide selection of foods while consuming only a moderate amount. Suggestions on how much to limit the amount of sodium appear below.

HOW TO DECREASE SODIUM IN YOUR MEAL PLAN

1. Taste your food before adding salt. If you must salt your food during cooking or at the table, do it lightly.
2. Rely less on convenience, canned and packaged foods. In general, the more a food is processed, the more sodium it contains.
3. Switch to lower sodium snacks. Potato chips, salted nuts and most crackers are loaded with salt. Use lower sodium snacks such as raw vegetables, yogurt, unsalted nuts and fruits.
4. Discover new flavor enhancers. Instead of salt, mustard, catsup, sauces, and other salt-filled flavoring, use herbs and spices, onion, green pepper, lemon juice, and vinegar.
5. Eat sparingly of smoked or cured meats such as bacon, frankfurters, and cold cuts to name a few. Use, instead, sliced turkey, lean roast beef, peanut butter, and hamburger.
6. Read "between the lines" on food labels. When sodium is listed among the first four or five items in the ingredient list, there is a good chance the food is high in sodium.

CHOLESTEROL AND SATURATED FAT

Reducing the amount of cholesterol and saturated fat you eat is another way to care for your health. Cholesterol is a fat-like substance found in animal and dairy fats and egg yolks. Some cholesterol is also made by your body. Saturated fats also come from animal products. Palm oil and coconut oil are saturated fats even though they come from plants.

Research links excess cholesterol and fat levels in the blood with coronary heart disease. Because people with diabetes have a tendency toward heart disease, many physicians recommend that they limit the amount of cholesterol and saturated fat in their meal plans.

Suggestions on how to reduce the amount of cholesterol and saturated fat you eat appear below. For more detailed and specific advice, consult your physician or dietitian.

HOW TO DECREASE CHOLESTEROL AND SATURATED FAT IN YOUR MEAL PLAN

1. Trim all visible fat from meats. Decrease use of red meats, including luncheon meats, frankfurters, and sausage. Use fish, chicken, and turkey.
2. Limit eggs to 2 per week. Use low cholesterol egg substitutes.
3. Use skim or low-fat milk and milk products.
4. Instead of butter, use a soft margarine made from corn or safflower oil.
5. Instead of lard, bacon fat, or hardened vegetable shortenings, use polyunsaturated oil or margarine.
6. Bake, broil, roast, boil, or steam foods instead of frying them.

APPENDIX F

HEIGHT AND WEIGHT TABLES

For many years, physicians and other health professionals have used the height and weight tables prepared by the Metropolitan Life Insurance Company. Most widely and most recently used were those prepared in 1959 from pooled data of 26 insurance companies in the United States and Canada.[1] In 1983, the Metropolitan published new tables (based on a 1979 survey) which indicated that those persons experiencing the greatest longevity now weigh more than shown in the 1959 tables.[2] In both studies, those with major diseases such as heart disease, cancer or diabetes, were screened out to isolate the effect of weight on longevity. The new tables have led to much discussion among individuals and agencies who have long recommended avoidance of being overweight and now prefer to continue to follow the 1959 guidelines. At any rate, the figures shown in both the 1959 and 1983 tables are below the averages for those of the general population. Paul S. Entmacher, M.D., Vice-President and Chief Medical Director of the Metropolitan, is quoted as saying "It does not mean that people have a license to gain. It simply indicates that many people may have fewer pounds to lose." Furthermore, since the earlier height and weight tables have been called "ideal" or "desirable," causing misinterpretation, the Metropolitan stresses that both the 1959 and 1983 tables simply indicate the weights at which people have had the greatest longevity. They stress that "the new height and weight tables are a health education tool—a guideline."[3]

In Tables 1A and 1B, weights associated with the greatest longevity for men and women are listed for the two surveys together with columns for the change in the 20-year period. In Table 2, the data for *average* weights are arranged according to sex, height, and age groups. It will be noted that increases in weight for tall men and women are not as great as those for short persons or for those of medium height. On a percentage basis, the increase was 10% for short men, 5% for those of medium height, and 1% for tall men. Corresponding increases for women were 9%, 6%, and 2%, respectively. In Table 3 are listed the 1983 height and weight data in metric equivalents. Finally, in Table 4 data are given for young persons 2 to 18 years of age as prepared by the National Center for Health Statistics.

[1]Metropolitan Life Insurance Col: New weight standards for men and women. Statistical Bulletin *40*:1, 1959.
[2]Idem: 1983 Metropolitan Height and Weight tables. Statistical Bulletin *64*:2, 1983.
[3]For one viewpoint of the problem see the paper by Knapp, T.R.: A methodological critique of the "ideal weight" concept. J.A.M.A. *250*:506, 1983.

Table 1. Comparison of 1959 and 1983 Metropolitan Height and Weight Tables

A. MEN

Weight in Pounds (Without Clothing)

Height (Without Shoes) Feet Inches	SMALL FRAME 1959	1983	Change Since 1959	Percent Change	MEDIUM FRAME 1959	1983	Change Since 1959	Percent Change	LARGE FRAME 1959	1983	Change Since 1959	Percent Change
5 1	105–113	123–129	18 16	17 14	111–122	126–136	15 14	14 11	119–134	133–145	14 11	12 8
5 2	108–116	125–131	17 15	16 13	114–126	128–138	14 12	12 10	122–137	135–148	13 11	11 8
5 3	111–119	127–133	16 14	14 12	117–129	130–140	13 11	11 9	125–141	137–151	12 10	10 7
5 4	114–122	129–135	15 13	13 11	120–132	132–143	12 11	10 8	128–145	139–155	11 10	9 7
5 5	117–126	131–137	14 11	12 9	123–136	134–146	11 10	9 7	131–149	141–159	10 10	8 7
5 6	121–130	133–140	12 10	10 8	127–140	137–149	10 9	8 6	135–154	144–163	9 9	7 6
5 7	125–134	135–143	10 9	8 7	131–145	140–152	9 7	7 5	140–159	147–167	7 8	5 5
5 8	129–138	137–146	8 8	6 6	135–149	143–155	8 6	6 4	144–163	150–171	6 8	4 5
5 9	133–143	139–149	6 6	5 4	139–153	146–158	7 5	5 3	148–167	153–175	5 8	3 5
5 10	137–147	141–152	4 5	3 3	143–158	149–161	6 3	4 2	152–172	156–179	4 7	3 4
5 11	141–151	144–155	3 4	2 3	147–163	152–165	5 2	3 1	157–177	159–183	2 6	1 3
6 0	145–155	147–159	2 4	1 3	151–168	155–169	4 1	3 1	161–182	163–187	2 5	1 3
6 1	149–160	150–163	1 3	1 2	155–173	159–173	4 0	3 0	166–187	167–192	1 5	1 3
6 2	153–164	153–167	0 3	0 2	160–178	162–177	2 –1	1 –1	171–192	171–197	0 5	0 3
6 3	157–168	157–171	0 3	0 2	165–183	166–182	1 –1	1 –1	175–197	176–202	1 5	1 3

B. WOMEN

Weight in Pounds (Without Clothing)

Height (Without Shoes) Feet Inches	SMALL FRAME 1959	1983	Change Since 1959	Percent Change	MEDIUM FRAME 1959	1983	Change Since 1959	Percent Change	LARGE FRAME 1959	1983	Change Since 1959	Percent Change
4 9	90–97	99–108	9 11	10 11	94–106	106–118	12 12	13 11	102–118	115–128	13 10	13 8
4 10	92–100	100–110	8 10	9 10	97–109	108–120	11 11	11 10	105–121	117–131	12 10	11 8
4 11	95–103	101–112	6 9	6 9	100–112	110–123	10 11	10 10	108–124	119–134	11 10	10 8
5 0	98–106	103–115	5 9	5 8	103–115	112–126	9 11	9 10	111–127	122–137	11 10	10 8
5 1	101–109	105–118	4 9	4 8	106–118	115–129	9 11	8 9	114–130	125–140	11 10	10 8
5 2	104–112	108–121	4 9	4 8	109–122	118–132	9 10	8 8	117–134	128–144	11 10	9 7
5 3	107–115	111–124	4 9	4 8	112–126	121–135	9 9	8 7	121–138	131–148	10 10	8 7
5 4	110–119	114–127	4 8	4 7	116–131	124–138	8 7	7 5	125–142	134–152	9 10	7 7
5 5	114–123	117–130	3 7	3 6	120–135	127–141	7 6	6 4	129–146	137–156	8 10	6 7
5 6	118–127	120–133	2 6	2 5	124–139	130–144	6 5	5 4	133–150	140–160	7 10	5 7
5 7	122–131	123–136	1 5	1 4	128–143	133–147	5 4	4 3	137–154	143–164	6 10	4 6
5 8	126–136	126–139	0 3	0 2	132–147	136–150	4 3	3 2	141–159	146–167	5 8	4 5
5 9	130–140	129–142	–1 2	–1 2	136–151	139–153	3 2	2 1	145–164	149–170	4 6	3 4
5 10	134–144	132–145	–2 1	–1 1	140–155	142–156	2 1	1 1	149–169	152–173	3 4	2 2

Note: Prepared by Metropolitan Life Insurance Company.
Source of basic data: Build Study, 1979, and Build and Blood Pressure Study, 1959, Society of Actuaries and Association of Life Insurance Medical Directors of America. These are not average weights but are weights associated with the greatest longevity.

Table 2. Changes in Average Weights for Men and Women Between 1959 and 1979

Weight in Pounds (Without Clothing) According to Height and Age

Height (Without Shoes)		Ages 20–24		Ages 25–29		Ages 30–39		Ages 40–49		Ages 50–59		Ages 60–69	
Feet	Inches	Average Weight 1979	Change Since 1959	Average Weight 1979	Change Since 1959	Average Weight 1979	Change Weight 1979	Average Weight 1979	Change Since 1959	Average Weight 1979	Change Since 1959	Average Weight 1979	Change Since 1959
MEN													
5	1	125	4	129	2	133	3	135	2	136	1	135	3
5	2	131	6	135	4	138	4	139	2	140	2	139	4
5	3	134	5	138	4	142	4	144	3	145	3	144	5
5	4	138	6	142	5	146	4	149	4	150	4	148	5
5	5	143	8	147	6	151	5	153	4	154	4	153	6
5	6	148	10	151	7	155	5	158	4	159	4	158	6
5	7	152	10	156	8	160	6	162	4	163	4	162	6
5	8	158	12	161	9	165	7	167	5	168	5	167	6
5	9	162	12	166	10	169	6	171	4	172	4	171	5
5	10	166	12	170	10	174	7	176	5	177	4	176	5
5	11	171	12	176	11	179	7	181	5	182	4	181	5
6	0	177	14	181	11	185	9	187	7	188	6	186	5
6	1	182	15	186	11	190	9	192	7	193	6	191	5
6	2	188	17	192	13	196	10	198	8	199	7	195	4
6	3	193	19	197	14	201	9	203	7	204	6	202	5
WOMEN													
4	8	98	0	103	0	107	−4	111	−7	115	−6	117	−6
4	9	102	1	107	1	110	−3	115	−5	118	−5	120	−5
4	10	107	3	109	0	112	−4	118	−5	122	−4	124	−3
4	11	109	1	111	−1	115	−4	120	−6	124	−5	127	−3
5	0	113	2	116	−1	118	−4	124	−5	128	−4	130	−3
5	1	117	3	118	0	121	−4	126	−6	130	−6	133	−4
5	2	121	4	122	1	125	−3	130	−6	134	−6	137	−4
5	3	124	3	125	0	128	−3	133	−6	138	−6	140	−5
5	4	127	2	129	0	131	−4	136	−7	141	−7	144	−5
5	5	130	2	131	−1	134	−4	140	−7	144	−7	147	−6
5	6	134	2	135	−1	138	−4	144	−7	149	−7	152	−5
5	7	138	2	139	−1	142	−4	147	−8	153	−7	155	−5
5	8	143	3	145	1	147	−3	152	−8	156	−9	158	*
5	9	146	1	147	−2	150	−5	155	−10	159	−11	160	*
5	10	152	2	153	−1	156	−4	159	−11	163	−13	164	*

*Not calculated because of insufficient data in 1959.
Note: Prepared by Metropolitan Life Insurance Company.
Source of basic data: *Build Study, 1979*, and *Build and Blood Pressure Study, 1959*, Society of Actuaries and Association of Life Insurance Medical Directors of America

Table 3. 1983 Metropolitan Height and Weight Tables for Men and Women on Metric Basis

According to Frame, Ages 25–59

MEN

Height (In Shoes)† Centimeters	Weight in Kilograms (In Indoor Clothing)*		
	Small Frame	Medium Frame	Large Frame
158	58.3–61.0	59.6–64.2	62.8–68.3
159	58.6–61.3	59.9–64.5	63.1–68.8
160	59.0–61.7	60.3–64.9	63.5–69.4
161	59.3–62.0	60.6–65.2	63.8–69.9
162	59.7–62.4	61.0–65.6	64.2–70.5
163	60.0–62.7	61.3–66.0	64.5–71.1
164	60.4–63.1	61.7–66.5	64.9–71.8
165	60.8–63.5	62.1–67.0	65.3–72.5
166	61.1–63.8	62.4–67.6	65.6–73.2
167	61.5–64.2	62.8–68.2	66.0–74.0
168	61.8–64.6	63.2–68.7	66.4–74.7
169	62.2–65.2	63.8–69.3	67.0–75.4
170	62.5–65.7	64.3–69.8	67.5–76.1
171	62.9–66.2	64.8–70.3	68.0–76.8
172	63.2–66.7	65.4–70.8	68.5–77.5
173	63.6–67.3	65.9–71.4	69.1–78.2
174	63.9–67.8	66.4–71.9	69.6–78.9
175	64.3–68.3	66.9–72.4	70.1–79.6
176	64.7–68.9	67.5–73.0	70.7–80.3
177	65.0–69.5	68.1–73.5	71.3–81.0
178	65.4–70.0	68.6–74.0	71.8–81.8
179	65.7–70.5	69.2–74.6	72.3–82.5
180	66.1–71.0	69.7–75.1	72.8–83.3
181	66.6–71.6	70.2–75.8	73.4–84.0
182	67.1–72.1	70.7–76.5	73.9–84.7
183	67.7–72.7	71.3–77.2	74.5–85.4
184	68.2–73.4	71.8–77.9	75.2–86.1
185	68.7–74.1	72.4–78.6	75.9–86.8
186	69.2–74.8	73.0–79.3	76.6–87.6
187	69.8–75.5	73.7–80.0	77.3–88.5
188	70.3–76.2	74.4–80.7	78.0–89.4
189	70.9–76.9	74.9–81.5	78.7–90.3
190	71.4–77.6	75.4–82.2	79.4–91.2
191	72.1–78.4	76.1–83.0	80.3–92.1
192	72.8–79.1	76.8–83.9	81.2–93.0
193	73.5–79.8	77.6–84.8	82.1–93.9

WOMEN

Height (In Shoes)† Centimeters	Weight in Kilograms (In Indoor Clothing)*		
	Small Frame	Medium Frame	Large Frame
148	46.4–50.6	49.6–55.1	53.7–59.8
149	46.6–51.0	50.0–55.5	54.1–60.3
150	46.7–51.3	50.3–55.9	54.4–60.9
151	46.9–51.7	50.7–56.4	54.8–61.4
152	47.1–52.1	51.1–57.0	55.2–61.9
153	47.4–52.5	51.5–57.5	55.6–62.4
154	47.8–53.0	51.9–58.0	56.2–63.0
155	48.1–53.6	52.2–58.6	56.8–63.6
156	48.5–54.1	52.7–59.1	57.3–64.1
157	48.8–54.6	53.2–59.6	57.8–64.6
158	49.3–55.2	53.8–60.2	58.4–65.3
159	49.8–55.7	54.3–60.7	58.9–66.0
160	50.3–56.2	54.9–61.2	59.4–66.7
161	50.8–56.7	55.4–61.7	59.9–67.4
162	51.4–57.3	55.9–62.3	60.5–68.1
163	51.9–57.8	56.4–62.8	61.0–68.8
164	52.5–58.4	57.0–63.4	61.5–69.5
165	53.0–58.9	57.5–63.9	62.0–70.2
166	53.6–59.5	58.1–64.5	62.6–70.9
167	54.1–60.0	58.7–65.0	63.2–71.7
168	54.6–60.5	59.2–65.5	63.7–72.4
169	55.2–61.1	59.7–66.1	64.3–73.1
170	55.7–61.6	60.2–66.6	64.8–73.8
171	56.2–62.1	60.7–67.1	65.3–74.5
172	56.8–62.6	61.3–67.6	65.8–75.2
173	57.3–63.2	61.8–68.2	66.4–75.9
174	57.8–63.7	62.3–68.7	66.9–76.4
175	58.3–64.2	62.8–69.2	67.4–76.9
176	58.9–64.8	63.4–69.8	68.0–77.5
177	59.5–65.4	64.0–70.4	68.5–78.1
178	60.0–65.9	64.5–70.9	69.0–78.6
179	60.5–66.4	65.1–71.4	69.6–79.1
180	61.0–66.9	65.6–71.9	70.1–79.8
181	61.6–67.5	66.1–72.5	70.7–80.2
182	62.1–68.0	66.6–73.0	71.2–80.7
183	62.6–68.5	67.1–73.5	71.7–81.2

*Indoor clothing weighing 2.3 kilograms for men and 1.4 kilograms for women.
†Shoes with 2.5 cm. heels
Source of basic data Build Study, 1979, Society of Actuaries and Association of Life Insurance Medical Directors of America.
Copyright 1983 Metropolitan Life Insurance Company.

Table 4.   Heights and Weights (without Clothing) of Young Persons Ages 2 to 18 Years (at 5th, 50th, and 95 Percentiles*)

Age Years	Net Height: inches (centimeters)			Net Weight: pounds (kilograms)		
	5th P	50th P	95th P	5th P	50th P	95th P
Males						
2	32.5 (82.5)	34.3 (86.8)	37.3 (94.4)	23.3 (10.49)	27.3 (12.34)	34.3 (15.5)
3	35.0 (89.0)	37.3 (94.9)	40.3 (102.0)	26.5 (12.05)	32.3 (14.62)	39.3 (17.77)
4	37.8 (95.8)	40.5 (102.9)	43.3 (109.9)	30.0 (13.64)	36.8 (16.69)	44.8 (20.27)
5	40.3 (102.0)	43.3 (109.9)	46.0 (117.0)	33.8 (15.27)	41.3 (18.67)	51.0 (23.09)
6	42.5 (107.7)	45.8 (116.1)	48.5 (123.5)	37.3 (16.93)	45.5 (20.69)	58.0 (26.34)
7	44.5 (113.0)	48.0 (121.7)	51.0 (129.7)	41.0 (18.64)	50.3 (22.85)	66.5 (30.12)
8	46.5 (118.1)	50.0 (127.0)	53.5 (135.7)	45.0 (20.40)	55.8 (25.30)	76.0 (34.51)
9	48.5 (122.9)	52.0 (132.2)	55.8 (141.8)	49.0 (22.25)	62.0 (28.13)	87.3 (39.58)
10	50.3 (127.7)	54.3 (137.5)	58.3 (148.1)	53.8 (24.33)	69.3 (31.44)	99.8 (45.27)
11	52.3 (132.6)	56.5 (143.3)	61.0 (154.9)	59.0 (26.80)	77.8 (35.30)	113.5 (51.47)
12	54.3 (137.6)	59.0 (149.7)	64.0 (162.3)	65.8 (29.85)	87.8 (39.78)	128.0 (58.09)
13	56.3 (142.9)	61.5 (156.5)	66.8 (169.8)	74.3 (33.64)	99.0 (44.95)	143.3 (65.02)
14	58.5 (148.8)	64.1 (163.1)	69.5 (176.7)	84.3 (38.22)	112.0 (50.77)	159.0 (72.13)
15	61.0 (155.2)	66.5 (169.0)	71.5 (181.9)	95.0 (43.11)	125.0 (56.71)	174.5 (79.12)
16	63.5 (161.1)	68.3 (173.5)	73.0 (185.4)	105.3 (47.74)	137.0 (62.10)	188.8 (85.62)
17	65.0 (164.9)	69.3 (176.2)	73.8 (187.3)	113.5 (51.50)	146.3 (66.31)	201.3 (91.31)
18	65.3 (165.7)	69.5 (176.8)	73.8 (187.6)	119.0 (53.97)	151.8 (68.88)	211.0 (95.76)
Females						
2	32.3 (81.6)	34.3 (86.8)	36.8 (93.6)	22.0 (9.95)	26.0 (11.80)	31.3 (14.15)
3	34.8 (88.3)	37.0 (94.1)	39.5 (100.6)	25.5 (11.61)	31.0 (14.10)	38.0 (17.22)
4	37.5 (95.0)	40.0 (101.6)	42.8 (108.3)	29.0 (13.11)	35.3 (15.96)	44.0 (19.91)
5	39.8 (101.1)	42.8 (108.4)	45.5 (115.6)	32.0 (14.55)	39.0 (17.66)	49.8 (22.62)
6	42.0 (106.6)	45.0 (114.6)	48.3 (122.7)	35.5 (16.05)	43.0 (19.52)	56.8 (25.75)
7	44.0 (111.8)	47.5 (120.6)	51.0 (129.5)	39.0 (17.71)	48.3 (21.84)	65.5 (29.68)
8	46.0 (116.9)	49.8 (126.4)	53.5 (136.2)	43.3 (19.62)	54.8 (24.84)	76.5 (34.71)
9	48.0 (122.1)	52.0 (132.2)	56.3 (142.9)	48.0 (21.82)	62.8 (28.46)	89.5 (40.64)
10	50.3 (127.5)	54.5 (138.3)	58.8 (149.5)	53.8 (24.36)	71.8 (32.55)	104.0 (47.17)
11	52.5 (133.5)	57.0 (144.8)	61.5 (156.2)	60.0 (27.24)	81.5 (36.95)	119.0 (54.00)
12	55.0 (139.8)	59.8 (151.5)	64.0 (162.7)	67.3 (30.52)	91.5 (41.53)	134.0 (60.81)
13	57.3 (145.2)	61.8 (157.1)	66.3 (168.1)	75.3 (34.14)	101.8 (46.10)	148.3 (67.30)
14	58.5 (148.7)	63.3 (160.4)	67.5 (171.3)	83.3 (37.76)	110.8 (50.28)	161.0 (73.08)
15	59.3 (150.5)	63.8 (161.8)	68.0 (172.8)	90.3 (40.99)	118.3 (53.68)	171.5 (77.78)
16	59.8 (151.6)	64.0 (162.4)	68.3 (173.3)	95.8 (43.41)	123.3 (55.89)	178.5 (80.99)
17	60.0 (152.7)	64.3 (163.1)	68.3 (173.5)	98.8 (44.74)	125.0 (56.60)	181.8 (82.46)
18	60.5 (153.6)	64.5 (163.7)	68.3 (173.6)	99.8 (45.26)	124.8 (56.62)	181.8 (82.47)

*Adapted from: National Center for Health Statistics: NCHS Growth Charts, 1976. Monthly Vital Statistics Report, Vol. 25, No. 3, Supp. (HRA) 76-1120. Rockville, Md., Health Resources Administration, June 22, 1976.

APPENDIX G

TRADITIONAL JOSLIN CLINIC LISTS OF FOOD VALUES

For the use of physicians, dietitians, and other diabetes educators who may wish to follow the method of instruction used at the Joslin Clinic for many years, the tables below and on the following pages are provided (See also the relevant text in Chapter 17).

Table 1. Carbohydrate, Protein, Fat and Calories in Basic Foods

30 Grams (1 oz) Contain Approximately	Carb. (g)	Prot. (g)	Fat (g)	Calories
Bread, 1 large slice	15	2.5	0	70
Crackers, 2½ × 2½ inches, 4	20	3	2	110
Cereal (dry, 12 gm; cooked, 120 gm)	10	2.5	1	59
Vegetables, 3%†	1	0.5	0	6
6%	2	0.5	0	10
20%	6	1	0	28
Milk, whole	1.5	1	1	19
skimmed or buttermilk	1.5	1	0	10
Egg, 1 medium (50 gm)	0	6	6	78
Meat, lean, and fish‡	0	7	5	73
Chicken (all poultry and fowl)	0	8	3	59
Oysters, clams (raw)	1	3	0.5	21
Lobster	0	5	0.5	25
Cheese, cheddar	0	8	10	122
cottage	0	6	0	24
cream	0	3	12	120
Bacon, 4 long strips	0	5	15	155
Cream, 20% (light)	1	1	6	62
40% (heavy)	1	1	12	116
Butter or margarine	0	0	25	225

†Unlimited amounts of 3% vegetables may be eaten.
‡Certain fish contain less fat and calories.

Table 2. Approximate Utilizable Carbohydrate Content of Certain Vegetables and other Common Foods

3% Vegetables		
Asparagus	Cucumber	Peppers, green
Bean sprouts	Dill pickle	Radishes
Beans, string,	Egg plant	Rhubarb
very young	Endive	Sauerkraut
Broccoli	Greens	Spinach
Cabbage	Kohlrabi	Swiss chard
Cauliflower	Lettuce	Water cress
Celery	Mushrooms	

6% Vegetables		20% Carbohydrate Foods
Beans, string,	Okra	Beans (shell,
green and wax	Onions	lima, baked)
Beets	Parsley	Corn
Brussels sprouts	Peas	Macaroni
Carrots	Pumpkin	Potato
Chives	Rutabagas	Rice
Collards	Squash	Spaghetti
Kale	Turnips	Sweet potatoes
		Yams

Table 3. Approximate Amounts (Grams) of Fruits, Fresh or Canned (Water-Packed), Which Yield Respectively, 10 and 15 Grams of Carbohydrate

	Carbohydrate	
	10 g	15 g
Grapefruit pulp	150	225
Strawberries	150	225
Watermelon	150	225
Cantaloupe	150	225
Blackberries	120	180
Orange pulp	100	150
Pears	90	135
Peaches	90	135
Apricots	80	120
Raspberries	80	120
Plums	80	120
Pineapple	70	105
Apple	70	105
Honeydew melon	70	105
Blueberries	70	105
Cherries	60	90
Banana	50	75
Prunes (cooked)	50	75

Commercial ice cream, allowed for occasional use as a substitute for fruit, contains approximately 20% carbohydrate.

Table 4. Approximate Substitutes for Foods on Diet Sheet

Substitutes for 1 ounce (30 g) of lean meat (any kind)
  1 egg
  2 full-sized strips bacon (15 g)
  1 ounce fish or fowl (30 g)
  5 oysters, clams, shrimps, scallops (all small) plus 1 teaspoon butter
  1 ounce or 1 slice American cheese (30 g) omit 1 teaspoon butter
  1 ounce creamed cottage cheese (30 g)
  1 tablespoon peanut butter (15 g)
  2 ounces meat = 1 pound live chicken lobster plus 2 teaspoons butter

Substitutes for two Uneedas (food value of following = 10 grams carbohydrate)
  2 graham crackers   15 oyster crackers
  2 double squares Ry-Krisp (13 grams)   ⅔ slice bread (20 g)
  3 arrow root biscuits   ½ cup cooked cereal (oatmeal) (120 g)
  4 saltines   12 grams dry prepared cereal (cornflakes, etc.) (¾ cup)
  5 Ritz (also Cheese Ritz)   100 grams orange (small)
  3 Ginger snaps   5 small vanilla wafers
  3 Butter thins   1 cup popped corn (15 g)
  8 Wheat thins   3 Chocolate snaps (8.1 g)

Substitutes for 1 slice bread (30 g) (following foods = 15 g carbohydrate)
        Always use regular bread, dark or white. *Do not use* protein or gluten breads ("diet breads").

  2½ ounces (medium) potato (75 g)—½ cup whipped
    Add 20 g to baked potato to allow for skin
  ⅓ cup corn, lima beans, shell beans (75 g)
  ¾ cup parsnips
  ⅓ cup cooked rice (75 g)
  ½ cup cooked macaroni, spaghetti, noodles (75 g)
  1 medium bran muffin without raisins (30 g)
  1 slice pumpernickel (30 g)
  1 Pilot cracker
  1 Matzoth (20 g)
  Medium orange (150 g)
  1 small corn muffin (30 g)
  ½ English muffin (30 g)

Substitutes for 1 teaspoon butter (5 g = 4 g fat)
  1 teaspoon margarine   1 tablespoon French dressing
  1 teaspoon mayonnaise   1 tablespoon light cream (15 g)
  1 teaspoon salad oil   2 teaspoons cream cheese
  1 teaspoon peanut butter   1 slice bacon
  For 2 teaspoons butter: 1 tablespoon sour cream
                          1 tablespoon heavy cream
                          1 heaping tablespoon whipped
                             cream

Table 4. *Continued*

Substitutes for fruits and other foods
   All fruits fresh or dietetic water-packed. All fruit juices unsweetened. All fruits cooked without sugar. Weight of fruit equal to the weight of the fruit juice.

Substitutes for 100 g of Orange (small)*

½ medium grapefruit (150 g)   1 small apple (70 g)
1 cup strawberries (150 g)   ¼ cup pineapple (70 g)
¾ cup watermelon (150 g)   ¼ cup applesauce (80 g)
½ cantaloupe (150 g)   ⅓ honeydew melon (70 g)
½ cup blackberries (120 g)   ½ small mango (55 g)
1 small pear (90 grams)   9 cherries (60 g)
½ cup fruit cocktail (90 g)   ½ small banana (50 g)
1 medium peach (90 g)   3 prunes without sugar (50 g)
½ cup raspberries (80 g)   ¾ serving Jello (50 g) (regular)
2 medium plums (80 g)   Ice cream (50 g), plain, once or twice a week
¼ cup stewed apricots (80 g)   1 cup tomato juice (240 g)
⅓ medium papaya (100 g)   1 large tangerine (100 g)
½ cup blueberries (70 g)

ADDITIONAL SUBSTITUTIONS

1. Canned soups. *Avoid bean and bacon soups*
   ⅓ can soup plus water (100 grams soup plus water) = 150 g 3% plus 75 g 6% vegetable at one meal. Or 20 g (⅔ slice) bread.
   Exchange remaining ⅓ slice bread for 1 Uneeda if desired.
2. Creamed soups or chowders
   ⅓ can concentrated soup plus ½ cup milk = 1 slice bread plus 1 ounce meat
3. Baked custard 120 g = 100 g orange plus 1 ounce meat
4. Sponge cake (plain) 30 g = 1 slice bread—use occasionally—or 150 g orange
5. Beans and pork (canned) ½ cup (130 g) = 1 slice bread plus 2 vegetables at one meal plus 2 teaspoons butter
6. Doughnut (plain, small, 30 g) = 1 slice bread plus 2 teaspoons butter
7. Potato chips (30 g) = 1 slice bread plus 2 teaspoons butter

Substitutes for usual afternoon snack of 2 Uneeda Biscuits (or equivalent) and ½ cup of milk.
1. ¾ cup dry prepared cereal plus ½ cup milk
2. 3 crackers plus 1 tablespoon peanut butter (no milk)
3. 3 crackers plus ½ ounce (15 grams) American cheese (no milk)
4. 2 crackers plus 1 teaspoon butter plus ½ cup skim milk
5. 1 package peanut butter 'NABS' (4 sandwiches) (no milk)

*If called for on the meal plan, servings 50% larger may be used by appropriate calculation.

Index

Page numbers in italics refer to illustrations. Page numbers followed by t indicate tables.

Borderline diabetes, 336
Brain
   abnormalities due to hypoglycemia, 402
   edema. *See* Cerebral edema
   glucose metabolism by, 402
   in hypoglycemia, 324
   pathology in diabetes, 314
Bread, in meal plan, 943
Breast, mammary duct pathology in diabetes, 321
Broad-beta disease, 221
Brown spots, 773
Buerger exercises, 723, 735-736
Buformin. *See also* Biguanides
   trade names, 414t
Bulbocavernosus reflex, 690
Bullosis diabeticorum, 775-776
Bursitis, 846-847

Calcification, of vas deferens, 851
Calcium, 856
   in insulin release, 807-808, 856
   in insulin secretion, 71
   metabolism in renal osteodystrophy, 638
   mobilization in beta cells, 71
   postpartum levels, 856
   role in insulin action, 94
Calcium channel blockers, 566
Callus(es), foot, 718-719, 733
Camps, diabetic, 514-516
   benefit of peer group in, 902
Cancer. *See also* Neoplasms
   cholesterol lowering and, 228
   diabetes mellitus associated with, 856-860
   difficulty in studying relationship to diabetes, 856-857
   frequency in diabetic patients, 323, 857-858
   frequency of diabetes in patients with, 858-859
   hypoglycemia related to, 860
   impaired glucose tolerance in, 858-859
   pancreatic. *See* Pancreatic carcinoma
Candida infections. *See* Moniliasis
Capillaries. *See also* Microangiopathy
   damage in renal-retinal syndrome, 645-646
Captopril
   complications, 591t
   dosage, 594t
   in hypertension, 593
Carbohydrates. *See also* Glucose; Glycogen
   amount present in body, 138
   in diet of diabetic, 367-368
   energy storage capability of, 138
   metabolism. *See also* Glucose tolerance
      in aldosteronism, 803-804
      chromium role, 853
      in Cushing's syndrome, 803
      glucagon effects on, 161
      in hyperthyroidism, 791, 793-794
      insulin effect compared with glucagon, 161t
      magnesium role, 852
      manganese role, 854
      in pheochromocytoma, 806
      potassium role, 854-855
Carbonic anhydrase inhibitors, in glaucoma, 604, 605
Carboxyhemoglobin, and atherogenesis of smoking, 231
Carbuncle, 776
Carbutamide, 413, 416
   liver damage due to, 427
   trade names, 414t
Carcinoid syndrome, 823t
Cardiac catheterization, in renal insufficiency, 642-643, 643t, 644t
Cardiac output
   in hypertension, 584
   increase in nephropathy, 587

Cardiomyopathy, 571-574
   in hemochromatosis, 828
   in infant of diabetic mother, 575
   microangiopathy related to, 572, 574
   pathology, 571, *572, 573*
   in renal insufficiency, 643-644
Cardiovascular disease risk factors. *See* Risk factors
Carnitine acyl-transferase, in diabetic ketoacidosis, 530
Carotenemia, in xanthochromia, 779
Carotid artery, surgery in arterial disease, 729
Carp, Japanese, toxin-induced diabetes in, 126
Carpal tunnel syndrome, 669-670, 849
Case control study, 251-252
   patient selection in, 252
Cataracts, 193, 606-607
   cortical spokes, 606
   diabetic, 606
   disulfide bonds related to, 193
   floccular, 606
   nuclear sclerotic, 606
   pathology in diabetes, 312
   posterior subcapsular, 606
   prevalence in diabetes, 606
   after renal transplantation, 657
   sorbitol pathway in, 201
   surgery effect on neovascularization, 607, 608t
   totally opaque lens, 606
   treatment, 606-607
   after vitrectomy, 627
Catecholamines, 173-174. *See also* Epinephrine;
      Norepinephrine
   actions, 173-174
   assays in pheochromocytoma, 805
   in atherosclerosis pathogenesis, 237-238
   in autonomic neuropathy of heart, 570
   beta blockers inhibition of release, 592
   in diabetic ketoacidosis, 530
   in exercise, 455-456
   in hypoglycemia symptoms, 592
   and insulin, 173
   in myocardial infarction, 561
   in type A personality, 233
Cavernous sinus thrombosis, in mucormycosis, 743
Celebese ape
   atherosclerosis in, 126
   diabetic model in, 121
Celiac disease, diabetes association with, 821
Cell surface abnormalities, 188
Cell-mediated immunity, 739
   in diabetes, 56
Cellulitis
   necrotizing, 744
   orbital, 631
Central nervous system. *See also* Neuropathy
   arteriosclerosis in diabetes, 676
Cerebellar dysfunction, diabetes with, 493
Cerebral edema
   in diabetic ketoacidosis, 506-507, 538-539, 542
      causes, 538-539
      diagnosis, 539
      incidence, 538
      prevention during fluid therapy, 533
      treatment, 539, 542, 675
   in hyperglycemic hyperosmolar nonketotic coma, 545
Cerebral infarction, 676
Cerebrospinal fluid
   in neurologic disorders, 677
   pH in coma, 675
Cerebrovascular disease. *See also* Atherosclerosis
   in diabetes, 314, 676
   obesity associated with, 374
   treatment, 677
Cesarean section, management in diabetes, 708
Chalones, and atherosclerosis, 219